Taylor and Kelly's Dermatology for Skin of Color

Taylor and Kelly's Dermatology for Skin of Color

Second Edition

Editors

A. Paul Kelly, MD
Professor of Medicine, Division of Dermatology
Charles Drew University of Medicine and Science
Chief Emeritus, Division of Dermatology
Martin Luther King Jr. Medical Center
Los Angeles, California
Clinical Professor of Medicine: Dermatology
The David Geffen School of Medicine at UCLA
FAMCO: Dermatology Unit
Sultan Qaboos University/Hospital
Muscat, Sultanate of Oman

Susan C. Taylor, MD
Founding Director
Skin of Color Center
Division of Dermatology
St. Luke's-Roosevelt Hospital Center
New York, New York
Assistant Clinical Professor of Dermatology
College of Physicians and Surgeons
Columbia University Medical Center
New York, New York

Co-Editors

Henry W. Lim, MD
Dermatologist
Chairman and C.S. Livingood Chair
Department of Dermatology
Senior Vice President for Academic Affairs
Henry Ford Health System
Incoming President Elect, 2015
American Academy of Dermatology
Detroit, Michigan

Ana Maria Anido Serrano, MD
Consultant Dermatologist
FAMCO Family Medicine & Public Health
Dermatology Unit
Sultan Qaboos University Hospital
Sultan Qaboos University
OMSB, Faculty
Dermatology Residency Program
Muscat, Oman

Mc
Graw
Hill
Education

New York   Chicago   San Francisco   Athens   London   Madrid   Mexico City
Milan   New Delhi   Singapore   Sydney   Toronto

10   LKV   23 22

ISBN 978-0-07-180552-0

MHID 0-07-180552-4

This book was set in Minion by Cenveo® Publisher Services.
The editors were Karen G. Edmonson and Regina Y. Brown.
The production supervisor was Richard Ruzycka.
The illustration manager was Armen Ovsepyan.
The illustration manager Muscat, Oman was Nassir Masoud.
Project management was provided by Kritika Kaushik, Cenveo Publisher Services.
The designer was Alan Barnett; the cover designer was Dreamit, Inc.
LSC Communications was printer and binder.
This book is printed on acid-free paper.

Library of Congress Cataloging-in-Publication Data

Taylor and Kelly's Dermatology for Skin of Color, Second Edition / [edited by] Susan Taylor, A. Paul Kelly, Henry W. Lim,
   Ana Maria Anido Serrano.—2e.
         p. ; cm.
      Includes bibliographical references and index.
      ISBN 978-0-07-180552-0 (hardcover :alk. paper)—ISBN 0-07-180552-4 (hardcover : alk. paper)
   I. Taylor, Susan C., editor.   II. Kelly, A. Paul, editor.   III. Lim, Henry W., editor.   IV. Anido Serrano, Ana Maria, editor.
      [DNLM: 1. Skin Diseases.   2. Ethnic Groups—psychology.   3. Skin Diseases—ethnology.   4. Skin Pigmentation—physiology.
   WR 140]
      RL73.4.B63
      616.50089—dc23
                                                                                                                      2015001230

McGraw-Hill books are available at special quantity discounts to use as premiums and sales promotions, or for use in corporate training programs. To contact a representative, please visit the Contact Us pages at www.mhprofessional.com.

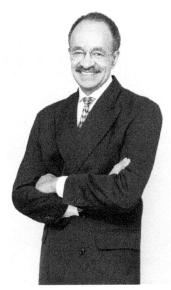

Courtesy of Jim Dennis Photography, Oakland, California.

DEDICATION/IN MEMORIAM FOR DR. A. PAUL KELLY

The second edition of *Taylor and Kelly's Dermatology for Skin of Color* is dedicated to co-editor A. Paul Kelly, who died in May of 2014 in Muscat, the Sultanate of Oman, from complications of Parkinson disease. Dr. Kelly was a pioneer in dermatology, an institution builder, scholar, researcher, educator, lecturer, and author. His lifelong dream of publishing a textbook specifically about skin diseases affecting people of color was realized with the first edition of *Dermatology for Skin of Color*.

Born in 1938, in Asheville, North Carolina, he was the son and grandson of physicians and graduated from Brown University and Howard University's College of Medicine. He was Chief of Dermatology for 35 years at King/Drew Medical Center in Los Angeles, where he developed a world-class residency program that trained more than a hundred dermatology residents and medical students.

Dr. Kelly was editor-in-chief of the *Journal of the National Medical Association* from 1997 to 2004. He was the second African American member of the American Dermatological Association and later its president. He was the first African American president of the Association of Professors of Dermatology, and of the Pacific Dermatologic Association. He was also elected to the Alpha Omega Alpha Honor Medical Society and received the Outstanding Professor Award from the Charles R. Drew University of Medicine and Science's academic senate.

Throughout his career, Dr. Kelly researched skin diseases in people of color, particularly keloidal scarring. After retirement, he became a Fulbright Regional Research Scholar and brought his keloid research project to Sultan Qaboos University in Oman. There he assembled an extraordinary team of dermatologists and geneticists from many countries to carry out an ongoing epidemiologic and genetic study on familial keloids.

Paul is survived by his wife of 48 years, Beverly Baker-Kelly, PhD, EdD, Esq, who was also a Fulbright Scholar in Oman, thus making them the first African American couple in history to both be Fulbright Scholars. They have two daughters, Traci and Kara, two son-in-laws, Brian and Rahsaan, and two granddaughters, Keiley and Hayden Kelly-Thompson.

It was through Dr. Kelly's extraordinary efforts and dedication to excellence that the second edition of *Taylor and Kelly's Dermatology for Skin of Color* was completed while he lived in Muscat, Oman. This is a part of his enduring legacy.

Susan C. Taylor
Henry W. Lim
Ana A. Serrano

Contents

Contributors

Naurin E. Ahmad, MD

Dermatologist
Medical Arts and Associates
Moline, Illinois

Andrew F. Alexis, MD, MPH

Chairman
Department of Dermatology
Mount Sinai St. Luke's and Mount Sinai Roosevelt
Director
Skin of Color Center
Mount Sinai Health System
New York, New York

Frances O. A. Ajose, MRCP (UK), FRCP (London)

Consultant Physician Dermatologist/Senior Lecturer
Department of Medicine
Faculty of Clinical Sciences
Lagos State University College of Medicine
Lagos, Nigeria

Faiza Mohamed Al Ali, MD

Consultant Dermatologist & Dermatopathologist
Dermatology Centre
Dubai Health Authority
Dubai, United Arab Emirates

Salam Al-Kindi, MD

Associate Professor
Department of Hematology
Sultan Qaboos University Hospital
Sultan Qaboos University
Muscat, Sultanate of Oman

Ahmed Al Waily, MD

Senior Consultant
FAMCO Family Medicine & Public Health
Dermatology Unit
Sultan Qaboos University Hospital
Sultan Qaboos University
Muscat, Sultanate of Oman

Chia-Chun Ang, MBBS, MMed (in Med), MRCP (UK)

Associate Consultant
Department of Dermatology
Changi General Hospital
Singapore

Chere Lucas Anthony, MD

Dermatologist
Boca Raton, Florida
Voluntary Faculty
Department of Dermatology
University of Miami, Miller School of Medicine
Miami, Florida

Collette Ara-Honore, MD

Dermatologist
Howard University Medical Center
Department of Dermatology
Washington, DC

María-Ivonne Arellano-Mendoza, MD

Dermatologist and Cutaneous Oncologist
Hospital General de México, "Dr. Eduardo Liceaga"
Professor Universidad Autónoma de México
Universidad La Salle and Universidad Anáhuac,
Mexico City, Mexico

Saundrett G. Arrindell, MD

Dermatological Consultant
Brentwood, Tennessee

Nasir Aziz, MD

Department of Dermatology
Veterans Affairs Medical Center
Assistant Professor of Dermatology
Howard University College of Medicine
Department of Dermatology
Washington, DC

Sonia Badreshia-Bansal, MD

Clinical Instructor
Department of Dermatology
University of California, San Francisco
San Francisco, California
Elite MD Advanced Dermatology, Laser, and Plastic Surgery
Institute
Danville, California

Degambar D. Banodkar, MBBS, MCPS, DDV, DVD, MD(DERM), FRCP(I)

Senior Consultant Dermatologist
Emirates Medical Center
Muscat, Sultanate of Oman

Kruti Pravin Banodkar, DNB (India), DD (Glasgow, UK)

Consultant Dermatologist
Hithwardhar Trust Hospital
Mumbai, India

Pravin Degambar Banodkar, DNB (India), DD (Glasgow, UK)
Consultant Dermatologist
Cumballa Hill Hospital
Mumbai, India

Priyanka G. K. Banodkar MBBS, MRCGP (UK), DPD (Cardiff)
General Practioner-Dermatology
Knoll Medical Practice
Orpinton, Kent, London

Diane Baras
L'Oreal Recherche
Typology Manager for Instrumental Make Up Evaluation
Chevilly-Larue, France

Victoria Holloway Barbosa, MD, MPH, MBA
Millennium Park Dermatology
Assistant Professor
Department of Dermatology
Rush University
Chicago, Illinois

Elma D. Baron, MD
Associate Professor, Dermatology
Director of Photomedicine
Director of Skin Studies Center
Department of Dermatology
University Hospitals of Cleveland Case Medical Center
Cleveland, Ohio

Ardeshir Bayat, BSc (Hons), MBBS, MRCS, PhD
Principal Investigator/Group Leader
Bayat Laboratory
Plastic and Reconstructive Surgery Research
Manchester Institute of Biotechnology
University of Manchester
Manchester, United Kingdom

Carol A. Bibb, PhD, DDS
Associate Dean for Student Affairs
Division of Oral Biology and Medicine
University of California at Los Angeles, School of Dentistry
Los Angeles, California

Michael Bigby, MD
Associate Professor
Department of Dermatology
Harvard Medical School and Beth Israel Deaconess Medical Center
Boston, Massachusetts

Curley L. Bonds, MD
Associate Professor and Chair
Department of Psychiatry and Human Behavior
Charles R. Drew University of Medicine and Science
Health Sciences Clinical Professor
Department of Psychiatry
David Geffen School of Medicine at the University of California Los Angeles
Medical Director
Didi Hirsch Mental Health Services
Los Angeles, California

Khari H. Bridges, MD, MBA
Dermatologist Miami Dermatology and Cosmetics
Miami, Florida

Karen Chen Broussard, MD
Division of Dermatology
Department of Medicine
Vanderbilt University School of Medicine
Nashville, Tennessee

Stella M. Bulengo, MD
Athens-Oconee Skin Cancer & Dermatology, LLC
Watkinsville, Georgia
Adjunct Clinical Professor
Department of Pathology
Medical College of Georgia
Augusta, Georgia

Daniel Butler, MD
Harvard Medical School
Beth Israel Deaconess Medical Center
Department of Dermatology
Boston, Massachusetts

Laurence Caisey
Worldwide Director for Makeup Evaluation
L'Oreal Recherche
Chevilly-Larue, France

Daniel Callaghan, MD
Georgetown University School of Medicine
Medstar Washington Hospital Center
Washington, DC

Jeffrey P. Callen, MD
Professor of Medicine (Dermatology)
Chief, Division of Dermatology
University of Louisville
Louisville, Kentucky

Valerie D. Callender, MD
Associate Professor of Dermatology
Howard University College of Medicine
Washington, DC
Medical Director
Callender Dermatology and Cosmetic Center
Glenn Dale, Maryland

Henry H.L. Chan, MBBS (London), MD (London), PhD (HK), FRCP (London, Edinburgh, Glasgow), FHKCP, FHKAM (Medicine)
Specialist in Dermatology
Hon. Clinical Professor
Division of Dermatology, Department of Medicine,
University of Hong Kong
Hong Kong Dermatology and Laser Center
Central, Hong Kong

Siew Eng Choon, MD, FRCP
Senior Consultant Dermatologist
Head, Department of Dermatology
Hospital Sultanah Aminah Johor Bahru
Clinical Associate Professor
Monash University Sunway Campus
Clinical School Johor Bahru
Johor Bahru, Malaysia

Richard A.F. Clark, MD
Vice-Chair for Research and Professor of Dermatology
Professor of Biomedical Engineering
Founding Chair of Dermatology
Director, Burn and Nonscar Healing Program
RCCC, Armed Forces Institute of Regenerative Medicine
Health Sciences Center
State University of New York, Stony Brook
New York, New York

Raechele Cochran Gathers, MD
Senior Staff Physician
Multicultural Dermatology Center
Henry Ford Health System
Department of Dermatology
Detroit, Michigan

Sharif Currimbhoy, MD
Department of Dermatology
University of Texas Southwestern Medical Center
Dallas, Texas

Maria Suzanne L. Datuin, MD, FPDS
Consultant Dermatologist
St. Luke's Medical Center Global City
Taguig City, Philippines

Jennifer David, DO, MBA
Research Fellow
Society Hill Dermatology
Philadelphia, Pennsylvania

Vincent DeLeo, MD
Chairman
Department of Dermatology
St. Luke's Roosevelt Hospital Center
New York, New York

Nicole DeYampert, MD
Staff Dermatologist
Department of the Army
Andrew Rader U.S. Army Health Clinic
Fort Myer, Virginia

Angela D. Dillard, PhD
Director, The Residential College
Professor of Afro-American & African Studies
University of Michigan
Ann Arbor, Michigan

Ncosa C. Dlova, MBChB, FCDerm
Dermatology Department
Nelson R Mandela School of Medicine
University of Kwa-Zulu Natal
Durban, South Africa

Christy B. Doherty, MD
Kaiser Permanente Medical Group
Department of Dermatology
Roseville, California

Sean D. Doherty, MD
Kaiser Permanente Medical Group
Department of Dermatology
Roseville, California

Sridhar Dronavalli, MD
Assistant Professor
Department of Dermatology
University of Maryland School of Medicine
Baltimore, Maryland

Nada Elbuluk, MD, MSc
Assistant Professor
Ronald O. Perelman Department of Dermatology
NYU Langone Medical Center
New York, New York

Boni E. Elewski, MD
Professor of Dermatology
University of Alabama
Department of Dermatology
Birmingham Alabama

Nasim Fazel, MD, DDS
Department of Dermatology
University of California Davis School of Medicine
Sacramento, California

Seth B. Forman, MD
Principal Investigator
Forward Clinical Trials
Florida Dermatology and Skin Cancer Specialists
Forman Dermatology Division
Tampa, Florida

Algin B. Garrett, MD
Professor and Chairman
Department of Dermatology
Medical College of Virginia/Virginia Commonwealth University
Health System
Richmond, Virginia

Jewell Gaulding, MD
Department of Dermatology
Henry Ford Health System
Detroit, Michigan

Jorge Gaviria, MD
General Surgeon
Chief Medical Officer
Gaviria Medical Hair and Research
Miami Beach, Florida

Amy Geng, MD
Dermatologist
Los Altos Hills, California

Aanand Geria, MD
Clinical Instructor
Icahn School of Medicine at Mount Sinai
New York, New York

Lisa R. Ginn, MD
Dermatologist & Cosmetic Laser Surgeon
Skin@LRG, LLC
Chevy Chase, Maryland

Marcia J. Glenn, MD
Dermatologist
Director, Odyssey MediSpa
Marina Del Rey, California

Chee Leok Goh, MD, MMed, MRCP (UK), FRCPE
Clinical Professor
Faculty of Medicine
National University of Singapore
National Skin Centre (NSC)
Department of Dermatology
Singapore

Narendra Gokhale, MMBS, MD
Dr. Narendra Gokhale's SKLINIC
Consultant Dermatologist
CHL Apollo Hospital
Indore, Madhya Pradesh, India

Pearl E. Grimes, MD
Director
Vitiligo & Pigmentation Institute of Southern California
Clinical Professor
Division of Dermatology
David Geffen School of Medicine, UCLA
Los Angeles, California

Aditya K. Gupta, MD, PhD, MBA, FRCPC
Professor
Division of Dermatology
Department of Medicine
Sunnybrook and Women's College
Health Sciences Center
University of Toronto
Toronto, Ontario
Mediprobe Research Inc.
London, Ontario

Nawal A. Habiballah Joma, MD, PhD
Consultant Dermatologist
Med Art Clinics
Dhahran, Saudi Arabia

Rebat M. Halder, MD
Chief, Department of Dermatology
Howard University College of Medicine
Washington, DC

Jennifer Haley, MD
Department of Dermatology
Southern California Permanente Medical Group
Associate Clinical Professor
Division of Dermatology
Department of Internal Medicine
David Geffen School of Medicine at UCLA
Los Angeles, California

Iltefat H. Hamzavi, MD
Senior Staff Physician
Multicultural Dermatology Center
Henry Ford Health System
Department of Dermatology
Detroit, Michigan

Evangeline B. Handog, MD, FPDS
Chair
Department of Dermatology
Asian Hospital and Medical Center
Muntinlupa, Philippines

Candrice R. Heath, MD
Department of Dermatology
Mount Sinai St. Luke's and Mount Sinai Roosevelt
Medical Center
New York, New York

Karen A. Heidelberg, MD
Heidelberg Dermatology
Faculty, Dermatology Residency Program
St. Joseph Mercy Livingston Hospital
Detroit, Michigan

Claudia Hernandez, MD
Associate Professor
Department of Dermatology
University of Illinois at Chicago,
Chicago, Illinois

Dóris Hexsel, MD
Dermatologist and Dermatologic Surgeon
Preceptor of Cosmetic Dermatology
Department of Dermatology
Main Investigator of the Brazilian Center for Studies in Dermatology
Pontifícia Universidade Catolica do Rio Grande do Sul (PUC-RS)
Porto Alegre, Brazil

Lori M. Hobbs, MD
Dermatologist & Cosmetic Laser Surgeon
Martin Luther King, Jr. Multi-Service Ambulatory Care Center
Los Angeles, California

Thomas J. Hornyak, MD, PhD
Associate Professor of Dermatology and Biochemistry and
Molecular Biology
University of Maryland School of Medicine
Chief, Dermatology Service
VA Maryland Health Care System
Baltimore, Maryland

Richard H. Huggins, MD
Senior Staff Physician
Department of Dermatology
Henry Ford Health System
Detroit, Michigan

Sotonye Imadojemu, MD
Departments of Dermatology and Medicine
University of Pennsylvania
Philadelphia, Pennsylvania

Marvi Iqbal, MD, MPH
Dermatologist
La Palma, California

Norihisa Ishii, MD, PhD
Director, Leprosy Research Center (LRC)
National Institute of Infectious Diseases (NIID)
Tokyo, Japan

Mouhiba Jamoussi, MA, MA, PhD
Head of the Department
Associate Professor
Humanities and Social Sciences/General Education
Modern College of Business and Science
Muscat, Sultanate of Oman
Associate Professor
Faculty of Language Studies
Arab Open University, Kuwait Branch
Kuwait

Julie Jefferson, MD
Department of Dermatology
Johns Hopkins School of Medicine
Baltimore, Maryland

A. Paul Kelly, MD
Professor of Medicine, Division of Dermatology
Charles R. Drew University of Medicine and Science
Chief Emeritus, Division of Dermatology
Martin Luther King Jr. Medical Center
Los Angeles, California
Clinical Professor of Medicine
Division of Dermatology
The David Geffen School of Medicine at UCLA
Los Angeles, California
Scholar in Residence 2009–2014
Fulbright Regional Research Scholar
FAMCO Family Medicine & Public Health
Dermatology Unit
Sultan Qaboos University Hospital
Sultan Qaboos University
Muscat, Sultanate of Oman

Farhan Khan, MD, MBA
Center for Clinical Studies
Houston, Texas

Lawrence S.W. Khoo, MD, MBBS (Singapore), MRCP (London), FAMS (Dermatology)
Consultant Dermatologist
Skin and Laser Specialist
Dermatology Associates
Singapore

Chesahna Kindred-Weaver, MD
Dermatologist
MedStar Medical Group
Department of Dermatology
Baltimore, Maryland

Sheila M. Krishna, MD
Department of Dermatology
Medical College of Virginia/Virginia Commonwealth University
Health System
Richmond, Virginia

Roopal V. Kundu, MD
Associate Professor
Director, Center for Ethnic Skin
Department of Dermatology
Northwestern University Feinberg School of Medicine
Chicago, Illinois

Angela Kyei, MD, MPH
Director
Multicultural Skin & Hair Center
Dermatology & Plastic Surgery Institute
Cleveland Clinic
Cleveland Ohio
Cosmopolitan Dermatology Inc
Cleveland, Ohio

Anh D. Le, DDS, PhD
Department of Oral & Maxillofacial Surgery
Robert Schattner Center
School of Dental Medicine
University of Pennsylvania
Department of Oral & Maxillofacial Surgery and Oral
Rehabilitation
Hospital of the University of Pennsylvania
Penn Medicine
University of Pennsylvania
Philadelphia, Pennsylvania

Johnathan J. Ledet, MD
Dermatologist
NEA Baptist Clinic
Jonesboro, Arkansas

Jennifer Lee, MD
Medical Director
REN Dermatology
Franklin, Tennessee

Sylvia Li, MD
Department of Dermatology
University of Illinois at Chicago
Chicago, Illinois

Henry W. Lim, MD
Chairman and C.S. Livingood Chair
Department of Dermatology
Senior Vice President for Academic Affairs
Henry Ford Health System
Incoming President Elect, 2015
American Academy of Dermatology
Detroit, Michigan

Joyce Teng Ee Lim, MBBS, FRCPI, FAMS
Consultant Dermatologist
Joyce Lim Skin and Laser Clinic
Singapore

Yi-Ling Lin, DDS, DMSc
Assistant Professor
University of California at Los Angeles
School of Dentistry UCLA School of Dentistry Los Angeles,
California

Zhong Lu, MD, PhD
Professor, Director of Laser Center
Dermatology Department
Huashan Hospital
Fudan University
Shanghai, China

Maria Juliet E. Macarayo, MD, FPDS
Consultant Dermatologist
Angeles University Foundation Medical Center
Angeles City, Pampanga, Philippines

Shoshana Marmon, MD, PhD, MScEPB
Senior Research Associate
Hong Kong Dermatology and Laser Centre
Central, Hong Kong

Claudio Cayetano Martinez, MD
Dermatologist
Mexico City, Mexico

Joni M. Mazza, MD
Assistant Professor
Hofstra North Shore-LIJ School of Medicine
Department of Dermatology
Manhasset, New York

Charles McDonald, MD
Chair Emeritus
Department of Dermatology
The Warren Alpert Medical School of Brown University
Department of Dermatology
Providence, Rhode Island

Lynn McKinley-Grant, MD
Associate Professor of Medicine/Dermatology
Georgetown University School of Medicine
Medstar Washington Hospital Center
Washington, DC

Amy McMichael, MD
Chair and Professor of Dermatology
Department of Dermatology
Wake Forest University School of Medicine
Winston-Salem, North Carolina

Lauren S. Meshkov, MD
Department of Dermatology
Mount Sinai St. Luke's and Mount Sinai Roosevelt
New York, New York

Diana V. Messadi, DDS, MMSc, DMSc
Professor and Chair
Section of Oral Medicine and Orofacial Pain
Division of Oral Biology and Medicine
University of California Los Angeles, School of Dentistry
Los Angeles, California

Allison Nicholas Metz, MD
Consultant Dermatologist
San Francisco, California

Ginat W. Mirowski, DMD, MD
Associate Professor
Department of Oral Pathology, Medicine, and Radiology
Indiana University School of Dentistry
Indianapolis, Indiana

Vineet Mishra, MD
Director of Mohs Surgery and Procedural Dermatology
Assistant Professor of Dermatology
University of Texas Health Science Center - San Antonio
San Antonio, Texas

Richard S. Mizuguchi, MD
Assistant Clinical Professor
Department of Dermatology
Mount Sinai St. Luke's and Mount Sinai Roosevelt
New York, New York

Pamela A. Morganroth, MD
Dermatologist
Portland, Oregon

Anisa Mosam, FCDerm, MMed, PhD (SA)
Dermatology Department
Nelson R. Mandela School of Medicine
University of Kwa-Zulu Natal
Durban, South Africa

Gabriela Munhoz-da-Fontoura, MD
Dermatologist
Rio de Janeiro, Brazil

Jenny Murase, MD
Assistant Clinical Professor
Department of Dermatology
University of California, San Francisco
San Francisco, California
Director of Phototherapy
Palo Alto Foundation Medical Group
Mountain View, California

Harrison P. Nguyen, MD, MBA, MPH
Department of Dermatology
Baylor College of Medicine
Houston, Texas

Kim Nichols, MD
Dermatologist
Director, Nichols MD of Greenwich
Greenwich, Connecticut

Rajiv I. Nijhawan, MD
Department of Dermatology
St. Luke's-Roosevelt Hospital Center and Beth Israel Medical Center
Fellow
Procedural Dermatology/Mohs Micrographic Surgery
Memorial Sloan-Kettering Cancer Center & Weill Cornell Medical College
New York, New York

Temitayo A. Ogunleye, MD
Clinical Instructor
Hospital of the University of Pennsylvania
Department of Dermatology
Philadelphia, Pennsylvania

Ashley E. Ojeaga, MPH
Center for Clinical Studies
Houston, Texas

Emmanuel Olaniyi Onayemi, MBBS, FMCP
Professor/Consultant Dermatologist & Venereologist
Department of Dermatology & Venereology
Obafemi Awolowo University Teaching Hospital
Ile-Ife, Nigeria

Chinwe Laura Onyekonwu, MBBS, FMCP, MPH (Liverpool)
Senior Lecturer/Consultant Physician/Dermatologist
College of Medicine, University of Nigeria, Enugu Campus
Department of Dermatology
University of Nigeria Teaching Hospital, Ituku-Ozalla
Enugu, Nigeria

Mobolaji Opeola, MD
Dermatologist
Dermatology Associates of San Antonio
San Antonio, Texas

Cindy E. Owen, MD
Assistant Professor
Division of Dermatology
University of Louisville
Louisville, Kentucky

Patricia Oyetakin-White, MD
Department of Dermatology
University Hospitals of Cleveland Case Medical Center
Cleveland, Ohio

David Ozog, MD
Director of Cosmetic Dermatology
Division of Mohs and Dermatological Surgery
Vice-Chair Department of Dermatology
Henry Ford Health System
Detroit, Michigan

Gladys Angela Ozoh, BM, BCH, FWACP
Senior Lecturer, Dermatologist
College of Medicine, University of Nigeria, Enugu Campus
Department of Dermatology
University of Nigeria Teaching Hospital, Ituku-Ozalla
Enugu, Nigeria

So Yeon Paek, MD
Assistant Professor of Dermatology
The Warren Alpert Medical School of Brown University
Department of Dermatology
Providence, Rhode Island

Amit G. Pandya, MD
Professor
Department of Dermatology
University of Texas Southwestern Medical Center
Dallas, Texas

Justine Park, MD
Assistant Professor of Dermatology
University of Southern California
Keck School of Medicine
Director of Pediatric Dermatology
Children's Hospital Los Angeles
Los Angeles, California

Kelly K. Park, MD, MSL
Dermatologist
Loyola University
Stritch School of Medicine
Division of Dermatology
Maywood, Illinois

Anabella Pascucci, MD
Department of Dermatology
University of California Davis School of Medicine
Sacramento, California

Mayha Patel, DO
Western University of Health Sciences
Oak Park, California

Jon Klint Peebles, MD
Department of Dermatology
University of Wisconsin Hospital and Clinics
Madison, Wisconsin

Maritza I. Perez, MD
Dermatologist
Director, Advanced DermCare
Danbury, Connecticut

Francisco Pérez-Atamoros, MD
Dermatologist
Director
Centros Dermatologicos Tennyson
México DF, México

Manoela Porto, MD
Dermatologist
Member of Brazilian Society of Dermatology
Researcher at Brazilian Center for Studies in Dermatology
Porto Alegre, Brazil

Frederick N. Quarles, MD
Dermatologist
Virginia Beach and Hampton, Virginia

Chemene R. Quinn, MD
Dermatology Consultant, PLLC
Jackson, Mississippi

Shobita Rajagopalan, MD, MPH
Professor of Medicine
Internal Medicine/Infectious Disease
Charles R. Drew University of Medicine and Science
Los Angeles, California
Associate Medical Director
Office of the Medical Director
Los Angeles County Department of Public Health Office of AIDS
Programs and Policy
Los Angeles, California

Marigdalia K. Ramirez-Fort, MD
Department of Radiation Oncology
SUNY Downstate Medical Center
Postdoctoral Research Associate Weill Cornell Medical College
New York, New York

Marcia Ramos-e-Silva, MD, PhD
Associate Professor and Chair
Sector Dermatology
School of Medicine and University Hospital
Federal University of Rio de Janeiro
Rio de Janeiro, Brazil

Ashraf M. Reda, MD
Consultant Dermatologist
Mediclinic Welcare Hospital
Dubai, United Arab Emirates

Virginia J. Reeder, MD
Department of Dermatology
Tulane University School of Medicine
New Orleans, Louisiana

Nianda Reid, MD, MBA
Department of Dermatology
The Warren Alpert Medical School of Brown University
Providence, Rhode Island

Marta I. Rendon, MD
Medical Director
Rendon Center for Dermatology & Aesthetic Medicine
Boca Raton, Florida
Voluntary Clinical Associate Professor
Department of Dermatology
University of Miami, Miller School of Medicine
Miami, Florida

Phoebe Rich, MD
Adjunct Professor Dermatology
Director of the Nail Disorder Clinic
Oregon Health & Sciences University
Portland, Oregon

Shelly Rivas, MD
Department of Dermatology
North Shore-LIJ Health System
Manhasset, New York

Wendy E. Roberts, MD
Dermatologist
Director, Desert Dermatology Skin Institute
Rancho Mirage, California

Leslie Robinson-Bostom, MD
Director of Dermatopathology/Professor of Dermatology
The Warren Alpert Medical School of Brown University
Providence, Rhode Island

Ife J. Rodney, MD
Assistant Professor of Dermatology and Pathology
Department of Dermatology
Howard University
Washington, DC

Sanna Ronkainen, MD
Associate Professor of Medicine/Dermatology
Georgetown University School of Medicine
Medstar Washington Hospital Center
Washington, DC

Theodore Rosen, MD
Professor of Dermatology
Baylor Department of Dermatology
Houston, Texas

Uche Rowland Ojinmah, MBBS, FMCP
Lecturer
College of Medicine, University of Nigeria, Enugu Campus
Department of Dermatology
University of Nigeria Teaching Hospital, Ituku-Ozalla
Enugu, Nigeria

Dakara Rucker Wright, MD
Physician Lead, Pediatric and Adult Dermatologist
Mid-Atlantic Kaiser Permanente
Halethorpe, Maryland

Shirley Russell, PhD
Center for Human Genetics Research
Division of Dermatology
Department of Medicine
Vanderbilt University School of Medicine
Nashville, Tennessee

Miguel Sanchez, MD
Associate Professor
Ronald O. Perelman Department of Dermatology
NYU School of Medicine
NYU Langone Medical Center
New York, New York

Rashmi Sarkar, MD
Department of Dermatology
Maulana Azad Medical College
Bahadur Shah Zafar Marg
New Delhi, India

Amado Saúl-Cano, MD
Professor of Dermatology
Universidad Nacional Autonoma de México
Mexico City, Mexico

Richard K. Scher, MD, FACP
Professor of Clinical Dermatology and Head, Nail Section
Weill Cornell Medical College
New York, New York

Heddie Sedano, DDS, DrOd
Lecturer
Division of Clinical Specialties and Craniofacial Clinic
University of California Los Angeles, Schools of Dentistry and Medicine
Los Angeles, California

Ana Maria Anido Serrano, MD
Consultant Dermatologist
FAMCO Family Medicine & Public Health
Dermatology Unit
Sultan Qaboos University Hospital
Sultan Qaboos University
OMSB, Faculty
Dermatology Residency Program
Muscat, Oman

John Seykora, MD, PhD
Associate Professor
Departments of Dermatology and Pathology
Perelman School of Medicine at the University of Pennsylvania
Philadelphia, Pennsylvania

Dwana Shabazz, MD, MPH
Dermatologist
Director, Renascance Dermatology
Fairfax, Virginia

Sudhanshu Sharma, MD
Department of Dermatology
Maulana Azad Medical College
Bahadur Shah Zafar Marg
New Delhi, India

Nanette B. Silverberg, MD
Pediatric Dermatologist
Department of Dermatology
St. Luke's-Roosevelt Hospital Center and Beth Israel Medical Center
New York, New York

Chandra Smart, MD
Associate Clinical Professor
Department of Pathology and Laboratory Medicine
University of California Los Angeles
Los Angeles, California

Titilola Sode, MD
Georgetown University School of Medicine
Washington, DC

Seaver L. Soon, MD
Staff Physician
Division of Dermatology & Dermatologic Surgery
Scripps Clinic & The Scripps Research Institute
La Jolla, California

Allen G. Strickler, MD, PhD, MPH
Dermatopathology Fellow
Geisinger Medical Center
Danville, Pennsylvania

George P. Stricklin, MD, PhD
Professor of Medicine (Dermatology)
Director, Division of Dermatology
Vanderbilt University School of Medicine
Department of Medicine
Nashville, Tennessee

Flora N. Taylor, PhD
Psychologist and Organizational Development Consultant
Adjunct Professor
Columbia University
New York, New York
Group and Organizational Dynamics
Instructor
University of Pennsylvania
Philadelphia, Pennsylvania

Susan C. Taylor, MD
Founding Director
Skin of Color Center
Division of Dermatology
St. Luke's-Roosevelt Hospital Center
New York, New York
Assistant Clinical Professor of Dermatology
College of Physicians and Surgeons
Columbia University Medical Center
New York, New York

Andrew J. Thompson
Baylor College of Medicine
Houston, Texas

Gisela Torres Bonilla, MD
Suncoast Medical Clinic
St. Petersburg, Florida
Volunteer Clinical Instructor
University of Central Florida College of Medicine
Orlando, Florida

Patricia A. Treadwell, MD
Professor of Pediatrics
Indiana University School of Medicine
Indianapolis, Indiana

Stephen K. Tyring, MD, PhD, MBA
Clinical Professor
The University of Texas Medical School at Houston
Houston, Texas

Sabrina Uddin, MD
Department of Dermatology
University of Illinois at Chicago
Chicago, Illinois

Neelam A. Vashi, MD
Assistant Professor of Dermatology
Director of Research in Cosmetic and Laser Medicine
Director, Boston University Center for Ethnic Skin
Cosmetic and Laser Center
Boston University School of Medicine
Boston Medical Center
Boston, Massachusetts

Carl V. Washington, Jr., MD
Dermatology Associates of Georgia
Clinical Associate Professor of Dermatology
Emory University School of Medicine
Atlanta, Georgia

Mari Wataya-Kaneda, MD, PhD
Associate Professor
Department of Dermatology
Graduate School of Medicine, Osaka University
Osaka, Japan

Jeffrey M. Weinberg, MD
Associate Clinical Professor of Dermatology
Department of Dermatology
St. Luke's-Roosevelt Hospital Center and Beth Israel Medical Center
New York, New York

Victoria Werth, MD
Chief
Division of Dermatology
Philadelphia Veteran's Affairs Medical Center
Professor
Department of Dermatology
Perelman School of Medicine
University of Pennsylvania
Philadelphia, Pennsylvania

Adam Whittington, MD
Northwestern University Feinberg School of Medicine
Chicago, Illinois

Sharona Yashar, MD
Staff Dermatopathologist
UCLA Departments of Dermatology and Dermatopathology
David Geffen School of Medicine at UCLA
Los Angeles, California

Angeline Anning Yong, MBBS (Singapore), MRCP (UK), MRCS (Edinburgh), FRCP (Edinburgh), FAMS
National Skin Centre
Singapore

Yuichi Yoshida, MD
Division of Dermatology
Department of Medicine of Sensory and Motor Organs
Faculty of Medicine
Tottori University
Yonago, Japan

Rie Roselyne Yotsu, MD, MIPH, PhD
Department of Dermatology
National Center for Global Health and Medicine
Tokyo, Japan

Cherie M. Young, MD
Director of Research
Callender Skin and Laser Center
Mitchellville, Maryland

Jasmine Yun, MD, MBA
Assistant Clinical Professor of Dermatology
University of Southern California
Keck School of Medicine
Los Angeles, California

Preface

Historically, mainstream dermatologic research, literature, and training had little focus on skin of color. In addition to the paucity of reliable information regarding the pathology, physiology, and reactivity of more darkly hued skin, there were misconceptions based on myth, folklore, and prejudice. Fortunately, by the end of the twentieth century, new interest and attention had turned to the burgeoning field of skin of color. This is most relevant as the demographics of patient populations are changing worldwide. For example, in the United States, it is estimated that black, Hispanic, and Asian Americans will comprise approximately 50% of the population by the year 2050.

Textbooks first by Johnson and then by Halder and Grimes served to create a foundation upon which an understanding of ethnic skin, pigmented skins, and darker skin types has been built. Efforts by the Skin of Color Society, the Dermatology section of the National Medical Association, and the American Academy of Dermatology have also aided in advancing understanding of skin of color.

The first edition of *Dermatology for Skin of Color* was published in 2009. It was a comprehensive textbook and photographic atlas written by dozens of nationally and internationally recognized experts in the field. The two editors involved in the edition, A. Paul Kelly and Susan C. Taylor, were extremely gratified by the favorable reception of the textbook. With the evolving knowledge of the field, this second edition is intended as both a textbook and as an up-to-date reference for all physicians, especially dermatologists, medical students, dermatology residents, and physician extenders. It contains chapters on structure, function, biology, and the myriad of diseases occurring in patients of color as well as cosmetic issues. In addition, *Dermatology for Skin of Color* provides a rich understanding of the cultural habits, practices, beliefs, and use of alternative medicine by patients of diverse backgrounds. It concludes with a section on comparative dermatology from Africa, Asia, and Latin America and a spectacular atlas of skin of color dermatology.

As our population grows increasingly multiracial, multicultural, and multiethnic, dermatologists will be challenged with the task of recognizing how darker skin differs from lighter skin, what is normal versus pathologic, which treatments have the highest efficacy and lowest morbidity, and how to interact with patients in a culturally competent manner. It is our hope that this book will serve as an invaluable tool to help dermatologists and the larger medical community meet those challenges.

A. Paul Kelly
Susan C. Taylor
Henry W. Lim
Ana A. Serrano

Acknowledgments

Emotional sustenance became very important to me as I undertook and progressed with my editorial tasks on the second edition of *Dermatology for Skin of Color* while my body was being progressively ravaged by Parkinson disease. My wife of 48 years, Beverly Baker-Kelly, was my indispensible partner throughout each phase of the production of this second edition. She did double duty as a Scholar-in-Residence in business law at the Modern College of Business and Science in Muscat, Oman, all the while acting as my *sous chef* in editing this book.

Our daughters, Traci and Kara Kelly; their spouses, Brian Crump and Rahsaan Thompson; our granddaughters, Keiley and Hayden Kelly-Thompson, ages 10 and 13, respectively; and my 95-year-old mother-in-law, Connie Baker, all of California, endured our absences from family holidays and special occasions. They understood that my dual missions were to finish this textbook and to make significant headway on my keloid research project while I was residing in Muscat. Keiley, my oldest granddaughter, took the first edition of the textbook to her school to show it around. I was glad to hear from her teachers how proud my granddaughter was about the book and the adventurous lives of her grandparents in the Arabian Gulf.

Collaboration has always been invigorating and intellectually stimulating for me. I count myself lucky to have assembled an expert, supportive, and energetic editorial staff in Muscat and in the United States. I owe a debt of gratitude to my editorial assistants, Natasha Savoy Smith, Rachel Schiera, Charlotte Woon, Ayshe Ismail, and Louise Morgan in Muscat, and to Patricia Elmore, their counterpart in California. Each editorial assistant delivered expertly finished products.

The skills displayed by Nassir Masoud and Nivu Hussain of Muscat and Gabriel Silva and Tijani Mohammed of Oakland, California, to research, format, organize, and creatively position figures in each of our assigned chapters helped to develop the uniqueness of our book.

Words cannot express the depth of my gratitude to Dr. Muneer Al Maskery, Dean Ahmed Al Naamany, and Mr. Saleh Al Kindi of the Modern College of Business and Science in Muscat for providing spacious office accommodations where our editorial team could meet 24/7, if necessary, to swim through the "molasses" of editorial tasks.

Dr. Art Papier, CEO, and Heidi Halton, Image Collection Manager, at Logical Images supplied wonderfully illustrative images to augment my comprehensive collection of slides featuring skin of color disorders.

A big round of applause goes to Sarah M. Granlund, our developmental editor with McGraw-Hill Medical Publishing, who paid expert attention to the gestalt and minutiae of each chapter in order to produce a textbook of the finest quality. Karen Edmonson and Regina Brown are also to be praised for their commitment to having this book published after taking up the cudgels from Anne M. Sydor.

Thanks are in order to many of my dermatology colleagues, particularly Drs. Pearl Grimes, Fred Quarles, and Howard Maibach, for their input. Many members of the Section on Dermatology of the National Medical Association donated photos for both versions of the textbook and shared their therapeutic pearls of wisdom.

My appreciation also goes to my co-editors, Drs. Susan C. Taylor, Henry Lim, and Ana Maria Anido Serrano. I can remember when Anne Sydor, our magnificently supportive McGraw-Hill publisher, floated the idea to us of the possibility of publishing a second edition of this book. Susan, Henry, and Ana all stepped up to the plate and said, "Count me in," notwithstanding their fixed commitments and academic responsibilities. It is my deepest hope that generations of dermatologists, medical practitioners, and the general public will benefit from our joint efforts and commitment to excellence.

A. Paul Kelly

It is with great pride and joy that we present the second edition of *Dermatology for Skin of Color,* which is more comprehensive and expansive than the first edition. This occurred through the dedication of two new editors, whom I thank, Drs. Henry Lim and Ana Maria Anido Serrano, who took up the gauntlet and helped produce a text with global reach. I marvel at the singular determination and dedication of my co-editor, Prof. A. Paul Kelly, who completed this edition despite so many challenges. I thank you, Paul, for being an exemplary friend and colleague. This project would not have come to fruition without the vision and support of Anne M. Sydor, our extraordinary McGraw-Hill Editor, as well as our developmental editor, Sarah M. Granlund. Finally, I acknowledge the love and support of my wonderful family: my husband, Kemel Dawkins, and my daughters, Morgan Elizabeth and Madison Lauren, with whom all things are possible.

Susan C. Taylor

It has been a privilege and pleasure for me to join A. Paul Kelly and Susan Taylor—both longstanding colleagues and friends, and Ana Anido Serrano as co-editor of *Dermatology for Skin of Color.* The first edition, with Paul and Susan as co-editor, has become a standard textbook on this subject. This expanded second edition is the result of the excellent contribution of the authors, all recognized experts on the topics. My special recognition goes to Paul who motivated all of us to move forward with the project, and to Beverly Baker-Kelly, who assisted us in completing it. The team from McGraw-Hill, Anne M. Sydor, Sarah M. Granlund, and Kritika Kaushik, has been superb in bringing this book to fruition.

My deep gratitude goes to my wife of 39 years, Mamie Wong Lim, MD, who is a loving wife, mother to our children Christopher and Kevin, and grandmother to Julian, Madelaine, and Dylan. Her patience and support have made this and many other projects possible.

Henry W. Lim

In both the Sultanate of Oman, where I have lived and practiced dermatology for the past 21 years, and Cuba, where I was born and studied medicine, the people are known to cultivate and exhibit intense feelings of loyalty and deference toward those they respect and cherish. In this instance, I am proud to fit this mold. Loyalty and deference perfectly describe my feelings regarding Prof. Kelly, as we called him from the first day he came to our dermatology department in 2009 at the Sultan Qaboos University Hospital in Muscat, Oman, with his epidemiology and genetics keloid research project.

Our professional relationship soon morphed into a fruitful and productive partnership, culminating in my being invited to become a co-editor for this textbook along with my highly esteemed colleagues, Drs. Susan C. Taylor and Henry W. Lim, both internationally recognized giants in the field of dermatology.

Prof. Kelly, our co-editors, and I worked tirelessly to identify eminent dermatologists from all over the world, including the Arabian Peninsula, India, Malaysia, China, Japan, Europe, Canada, Africa, Latin

America, Mexico, and the United States, who could be invited to contribute their expertise to this second edition of our textbook. To these distinguished contributors, I would like to extend my sincere gratitude. Your expertise, commitment, and diligence will have a huge impact on patient care for countless dermatologists and medical practitioners the world over for many years to come.

But I would be remiss if I did not give equal praise to our team here in Muscat, Oman, who joined hands with us and made this book their own. Our expert editorial staff was headed by Natasha Savoy Smith, an extremely skilled editor—secretly called "barracuda" by the rest of us—who was able to make corrections and discern errors that escaped our trained eyes. Likewise, our other equally dedicated and expert editors, Rachel Schiera, Charlotte Woon, Aisha Ismail, and Louise Morgan, are to be commended.

My thanks to our digitally minded computer experts, Nassir Masoud and Nivu Hussain, who literally worked with us night and day, consistently going the extra mile to help consolidate, arrange, match up and ultimately transform our images and texts into the beautifully expressive finished product you hold in your hands today.

Also, my highly detail-oriented friend and colleague, Dr. Beverly Baker-Kelly, cannot be thanked enough for her unfailing dedication to the organization and execution of this incredible project. She was our 'go-to person' on every aspect of the textbook as she diligently planned and ensured that every task was executed to make our book a *magnum opus*.

Finally, I would like to take this opportunity to express my profound gratitude from the depth of my heart to my beloved parents, Aramis and Xiomara, to my sister, Laura, to Salim, and to Loay, our son, for their love and continuously unwavering spiritual support.

Ana Maria Anido Serrano

Foreword

FOREWORD TO TAYLOR AND KELLY'S DERMATOLOGY FOR SKIN OF COLOR, 2ND EDITION

Acclaimed by *The Journal of the American Medical Association* as the first comprehensive reference on the subject, the first edition of *Dermatology for Skin of Color* won two PROSE Awards from the Association of Academic Publishers for excellence in Clinical Medicine and for excellence in Biology and Life Sciences. The book was recognized not only for the importance of the topic, but for the quality of the text, photographs, organization, and features.

This second edition is significantly expanded, with 21 new chapters written by experts in the field of dermatology, many more clinical pictures, and improved organization. New chapters cover dermatology for geriatric, adolescent, and pregnant patients, as well as topics on depigmenting agents, viral infections, cutaneous manifestations of internal malignancy, neurofibromatosis, tuberous sclerosis, photoaging, photosensity, laser treatment for skin tightening, toxins and fillers, cosmetic practices in Mexico, effects of tattooing and piercing, sickle cell disease, drug eruptions, and the biology of oral mucosa.

Most importantly, this edition takes a more global approach, covering not only Africa, Asia, and Latin America, but also Arab countries. New or augmented chapters address common skin diseases prevalent in each. Other chapters address cultural beliefs and traditions that dermatologists should respect.

The concluding history section now includes Asian American, Hispanic, and African American pioneers in dermatology in the United States.

As the opening chapter states, while race is merely a socially constructed concept, there is a need to focus medically on skin of color to understand and treat various cutaneous diseases. DNA analysis looks promising for helping dermatologists unlock the mysteries of skin.

Pearl E. Grimes, MD
Director, The Vitiligo & Pigmentation Institute of Southern California
Clinical Professor of Dermatology, University of California, Los Angeles

Taylor and Kelly's Dermatology for Skin of Color

CHAPTER 1

Skin of Color: A Historical Perspective

A. Paul Kelly

Mouhiba Jamoussi

KEY POINTS

- Myth and religion provided the earliest explanations of skin color.
- Most early rational explanations ascribed skin color to climate.
- Nineteenth-century pseudoscientific theories often supported the polygenist school, which stated that there were separate origins of the "races."
- Pseudoscientific misinformation, based on faulty or undocumented evidence, justified early twentieth-century sociopolitical prejudices.
- The theory of evolution ended the polygenist argument and subsequently led to theories of skin color based on evolution.
- Modern research led to the vitamin D/sunlight theory and an understanding of the evolutionary process behind skin color.
- The Fitzpatrick skin type scheme classifies skin types by the response of the skin to sun exposure. A few dermatologists use this scheme to classify skin types, although sometimes without fully understanding its correlation to sun exposure.
- Understanding of the biology of the melanin pigmentary system is based on research using light and electron microscopy.
- The Human Genome Project, along with advances in DNA and the mapping of the genes, should help dermatologists to further understand skin diseases and their treatment.

Throughout history, the subject of skin of color has been shrouded in mystery, misconception, mystique, and misunderstanding. Since antiquity, people have sought answers to various questions, such as where skin color comes from, the skin color of the first humans, and why humans developed different skin colors [**Table 1-1**].[1]

Naturally, ancient people sought to answer these questions through mythology. One of the earliest explanations for skin color was proposed by the ancient Greeks. According to their mythology, Phaeton, the son of Helios, the sun god, persuaded his father to let him drive the sun chariot for a day. Because of his inexperience and inability to control the fiery steeds, Phaeton drove the chariot too near the earth over certain lands, burning the people black, and too far from the earth over other regions, causing the people to turn pale and cold [**Figure 1-1**].[2] The early Greeks probably had brown skin tones that were midway between fairer and darker pigmented skin.

According to an early African myth, early humans quarreled over the first ox slaughtered for food. The color of their descendants thus was determined by the distribution of the meat; those who ate the liver had black children, those who took the lungs and blood had red children, and those who ate the intestines had white children.[3]

One North American Indian legend claims that both black and white people were created before the "Earth-maker" had mastered his baking technique. In baking the first human, the creator cooked him too long, and he emerged black. The white person was also a culinary failure because he was not baked long enough and consequently turned out pale-skinned. It was only with the third attempt that the creator was able to produce the properly baked, golden-brown North American Indian.[4]

A different North American Indian legend attributes differences in skin color to the order in which three men went swimming in a body of water. The first man to dive in left the water dirty but came out clean, and from him there descended white people. The second man jumped into the now somewhat muddied water and exited slightly dirtier than the previous man. Indians were said to have descended from this man. The last man came out of the water black and went on to father all black people.[5]

RELIGIOUS EXPLANATIONS FOR SKIN OF COLOR

Every religion seems to have its own doctrine on the origin of skin of color, especially on the source of black versus white skin. In the Abrahamic religions, one of the most widely cited religious explanations is that the biblical Ham and his descendants became black because he was cursed by Noah. In actuality, there is no mention in the chapter of Genesis regarding the descendants of Ham or of his son Canaan being black; this belief seems to originate in the *Talmud, Midrash Rabbah*, and other rabbinical writings from the second to the fifth centuries AD as different interpretations of the chapter of Genesis (9:20–27).[6]

There are several versions of this story, with the most popular version being that Noah forbade all the people and animals on the ark to have sexual intercourse. His son, Ham, disobeyed this order and was cursed by being turned black, and subsequently became the ancestor of all black people.[7]

Another version is that Ham laughed at his father while Noah was drunk and lying naked on the ground, spilling his semen. Noah's other sons, walking backward so as not to see their father's nakedness, covered Noah with a garment. Noah punished Ham by having the curse fall on his son, Canaan. The descendants of Ham, through Canaan, therefore had dark skin as a result of Ham observing his father's nakedness; they also had "misshapen" lips because Ham spoke to his brothers about Noah's condition and curly hair because Ham twisted his head around to observe his father's nakedness [**Figure 1-2**].[8]

Yet another version of the story asserts that Ham was cursed with black skin because he resented the fact that his father desired a fourth son. To prevent the birth of a rival heir, Ham is said to have castrated his father.[7]

The *Genesis Rabbah*, Chapter 37, gives yet a different version. It states that in the quarrel between Ham and Noah, Noah said, "You have prevented me from doing something in the dark, ie, sexual intercourse; therefore, your seed will be ugly and dark-skinned,"[6] thus giving rise to another commonly held rationale behind the origin of black skin.

The "curse of Ham" has been used by some members of Abrahamic religions to justify racism and the historical enslavement of people of African ancestry, who were believed to be descendants of Ham. They were often called Hamites. This racist theory was widely held during the eighteenth to twentieth centuries but has been largely abandoned since the mid-twentieth century by even the most conservative theologians.[9]

In another biblical story, Cain slew his brother Abel because of jealousy over God's favor. Cain became an outcast, but a protecting mark was placed on him by God in order to shield him from vengeful hands. The brand he bore associated Cain and his kind with evil. Many who wanted to prove that black people were inferior claimed that Cain's protecting mark was black skin [**Figure 1-3**].[9]

TABLE 1-1   **Summary of historical perspectives on skin of color**

Originator of theory	Date of theory	Theory on skin of color
Native American Indians	Exact date unknown	The creator had not yet perfected his cooking technique while creating humans, burning or undercooking the first humans and thereby causing differences in skin color.
		Early men jumped into a body of water, progressively dirtying the water and coloring men's skin darker and darker.
African tribes	Exact date unknown	Distribution of the meat of an ox resulted in differing skin colors in those who ate different parts.
Ancient Greeks	c. 1500–400 BC	Phaeton flew the sun chariot too close to or too far from the earth, burning black those to whom he flew too close, and turning others pale when he flew too far away.
Abrahamic religions	c. 1400 BC	Cain slew Abel in jealousy over God's favor, and God put a dark mark on Cain and all of his descendants as punishment.
		Ham was cursed with blackness because he disobeyed the prohibition against sexual intercourse aboard the ark.
		Noah cursed Ham when he looked upon his father's nakedness, resulting in a black mark of shame on all of Ham's descendants.
		Gehazi, servant of Elisha, was cursed with leprosy and the resulting white skin for having solicited money from Naaman.
Leonardo da Vinci	c. 1470 AD	Humans' different skin colors could be explained by the differences in environment.
Paracelsus	1520	Black and white people (termed the children of Adam) had entirely separate origins.
Isaac de La Peyrère	1655	Man descended from either an Adamite or a pre-Adamite race, with natives of Africa, Asia, and the New World being descended from pre-Adamites.
Johann F. Blumenbach	1795	Differences in human skin color were produced by a combination of climate and other factors. Black colored skin was thought to result from embedded carbon due to the heat of tropical climates.
Samuel Stanhope Smith	1810	Skin color was attributable mainly to climate, but skin color could eventually become hereditary.
Benjamin Rush	1812	Black skin was a hereditary illness.
Johann Meckel	1816	Skin color emanated from the cortical part of the brain.
Julien-Joseph Virey	1837	Based on observations of changes in newborns' skin color, it was determined that external factors had little or no effect on skin color.
Joseph Smith Jr.	1840	The Lamanites had once been white but were cursed by God and turned black.
Robert Chambers	1844	Nonwhite people were in the process of developing to the highest race as Caucasians.
Samuel G. Morton	1847	Black and white people were not varieties of a single race but entirely different species; this was based on the conviction that "half-breeds" cannot propagate themselves indefinitely.
Charles Darwin	1871	The theory of evolution left no doubt that all humans belong to the same species.
Rudolph Matas	1896	The chemical composition of pigment in black skin was identical to white skin.
MODERN SCIENTIFIC THEORIES OF SKIN OF COLOR		
Vitamin D/sunlight theory		
Charles Loring Brace IV	1987	The need for protection from ultraviolet radiation leads to darker skin color.
Thomas B. Fitzpatrick	1988	The Fitzpatrick skin type scheme classifies skin types I to VI by the response of the skin to sun exposure, in terms of the degree of burning and tanning of the skin. However, many dermatologists have adopted Fitzpatrick's skin type classifications without correlating the amount of sun exposure to the skin type category.
Nina Jablonski and George Chaplin	2010	Skin pigmentation is the result of natural evolutionary processes trying to balance between protecting the skin from harmful ultraviolet rays and the absorption of vitamin D.
Biology of the melanin pigmentary system		
George Szabó	1959	The use of light and electron microscopes led to the understanding that melanocytes are symmetrically distributed and do not differ significantly in size, shape, or population density between the various races.
Walter Quevedo Jr.	1971	Pigmentation of the skin is related to the formation and melanization of melanosomes in melanocytes. The amount of melanin present in keratinocytes is the essential factor in determining skin color.
Genetics and the DNA of skin of color		
Human Genome Project (HGP)	1990–2003 and ongoing	The HGP is helping redefine who humans are and how we have evolved. This project may help us answer questions about the evolution of the color of skin. The mapping of DNA has proven that human beings are genetically the same and that skin color is simply a variation.

Source: Used with permission from Dr. Beverly Baker-Kelly, Dr. Mouhiba Jamoussi, Ms. Natasha Savoy Smith, and Ms. Rachel Schiera.

Joal Augustus Rogers (1883–1966), better known as J. A. Rogers, a respected Jamaican American self-trained historian and author, noted that some black ministers have viewed the story of Cain and Abel in a different light. According to their interpretations, Cain was originally black when he killed Abel; when God shouted at him in the Garden of Eden, he turned white from fright and his features shrank up.[10]

Another biblical story is that white skin is the result of leprosy. The ancestor of white people is said to have been Gehazi, the servant of Elisha,

who was cursed with leprosy for having solicited money from Naaman (II Kings 5:21–27) [**Figure 1-4**].[11] As in the previous case, white skin is portrayed negatively, as the result of a disease. However, this interpretation is a deviation from the usual positive connotations associated with white skin color.

The Mormon prophet, Joseph Smith Jr. claimed that the Lamanites, a white people, were changed to black by God for their sins. The *Book of Mormon*, II Nephi, verse 21, reads:

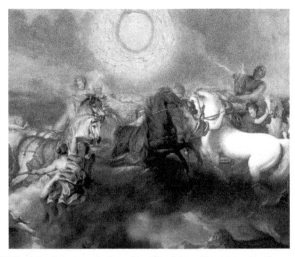

FIGURE 1-1. An early myth about the origin of skin color explains that Phaeton burnt some people black by driving too close to the earth and turned others white by driving too far from it. (Used with permission from Marisol LLC, Muscat, Sultanate of Oman.)

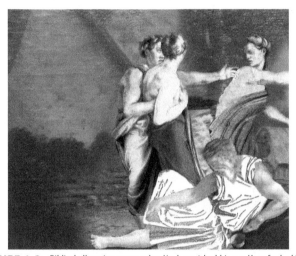

FIGURE 1-2. Biblical allegories suggest that Noah punished his son Ham for looking at his nakedness, ensuring that the descendants of Ham would have dark skin and curly hair. (Used with permission from Marisol LLC, Muscat, Sultanate of Oman.)

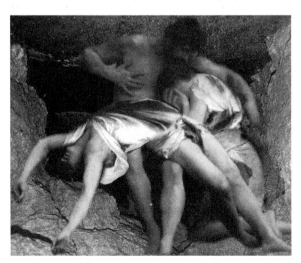

FIGURE 1-3. The allegorical protective mark of black skin that God put upon Cain has been associated with evil and inferiority. (Used with permission from Marisol LLC, Muscat, Sultanate of Oman.)

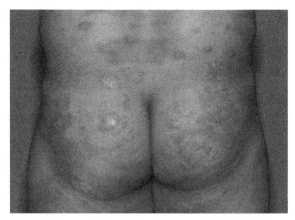

FIGURE 1-4. Some biblical writings refer to white skin as a curse resulting from leprosy, as seen in this patient.

And he caused the cursing to come upon them, yet, even a sore cursing, because of their iniquity. For behold they had hardened their hearts against him, that they had become like unto a flint; wherefore, as they were white, and exceedingly fair and delightsome, that they might not be enticing unto my people the Lord God did cause a skin of blackness to come upon them.[12]

EUROPEAN THOUGHT ON SKIN OF COLOR

In 1520, Paracelsus (1493–1541), a Swiss physician, declared that the children of Adam occupied only a small part of the Earth, and that black people and other non-white people had a wholly separate origin: "God could not endure to have the rest of the world empty so by his admirable wisdom filled the world with other men."[13] Likewise, Isaac de La Peyrère (1596–1676), a French Protestant theologian, argues in a book published in 1655 that there had been two separate creations of humans.[14] In the first chapter of Genesis, a man and a woman are given domain over every living thing, but not until the second chapter is anything said of the creation of Adam and Eve. Furthermore, Cain chose his wife from the earlier race when he was cast off by his own people for the murder of Abel. De La Peyrère believed that it was from this pre-Adamite race that the natives of Africa, Asia, and the New World were descended.[15]

Leonardo da Vinci (1452–1519) had already taken a different perspective from those interpretations that relied on mythologies or religion to explain differences in skin color. He was convinced that humankind was really unified and that the physical differences among races could be explained by environment. He thought that people born in hot countries were black because they found the cool, dark nights refreshing and did much of their work at that time, thus becoming dark. Likewise, the people of northern climates were white because they worked during the day.[16]

Johann Friedrich Blumenbach (1752–1840), Professor of Medicine at the University of Göttingen in Germany, made a lifelong study of racial differences. It was he who coined the term *Caucasian* to describe the white race. The term *Caucasian* is based on the study of a single skull in Blumenbach's collection that came from the Caucasus Mountain region of Russia [**Figure 1-5**]. Blumenbach thought that the differences in human color were produced by a combination of climate and other factors. Although he had no solution to the question of race and color, he speculated that the black color of darker-skinned people might be caused by a tendency in the tropics for carbon to be imbedded in the skin, reasoning that carbon on contact with oxygen darkens over a period of time. He also postulated that there might be some connection between the black coloration that white women sometimes develop during pregnancy and the permanent skin color of darker-skinned people.[17]

In 1837, Julien-Joseph Virey (1775–1846) disagreed with the idea that climate and external factors had an effect on skin color. He observed that newborn darker-skinned children developed areas of reddish or yellowish color with a brownish hue on some parts of their bodies, such

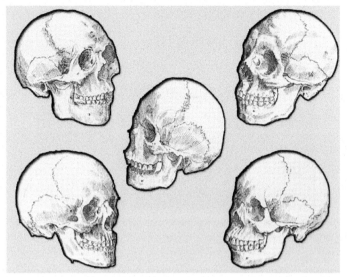

FIGURE 1-5. John F. Blumenbach, a comparative anatomy professor, categorized people by physical appearance instead of geography. The term *Caucasian* is based on his study of a single skull that came from Georgia in the Caucasus Mountain region of Russia around 1779. He did craniological research and divided the human species into five races. (Used with permission from Marisol LLC, Muscat, Sultanate of Oman.)

as around their fingernails, toes, and genital organs. Soon after birth, their skin darkened permanently, whether they were in a cold or warm climate or whether they were exposed to the sunlight or kept in a dark place. Therefore, Virey concluded that because black skin seemed to be hereditary in all countries and in all generations, external causes probably had little, if any, effect on the determination of skin color.[18]

Johann Meckel (1781–1833) and other eighteenth- and nineteenth-century anatomists thought that the complexion of black people was caused by skin color being determined in the cortical part of the brain. It was Meckel's opinion that nerves emerging from the brain's *medulla oblongata* convey a black color to all of the body, including the skin.[19]

AMERICAN TREATISES ON RACE AND SKIN OF COLOR

One of the first American treatises on race and skin color was proposed by Samuel Stanhope Smith (1751–1819), a Presbyterian minister and Professor of Moral Philosophy at the College of New Jersey (now Princeton) and later its president. In *An Essay on the Causes of the Variety of Complexion and Figure*, Smith attributed color mainly to climate, stating that as "one moved towards the tropics one would find successively darker shades of skin."[20] He maintained that dark skin might well be considered one universal freckle, and in time, the dark color would become hereditary.[20]

The case of Henry Moss seemed to be a dramatic confirmation of Smith's theory on the influence of climate on human skin color. Born a slave in Virginia, Moss fought in the Revolutionary War and then moved to the North. After many years there, he developed white spots on his body, which could have been vitiligo, and in 3 years, he became almost completely white [**Figure 1-6, A and B**]. In 1796, he was exhibited in Philadelphia, Pennsylvania as a scientific curiosity. Smith, of course, claimed Moss was living proof that the different races were a single human species and that black people would, in time, become white in a northern climate. Smith noted that, "wherever there were vents in the thin clothes that covered Moss there were generally seen the largest spots of black," proving that the sun was the determinant of dark skin color.[20] He thought that if black people were perfectly free, could own property, and were allowed to liberally participate in the society, rank, and privileges of their former masters, their African "peculiarities" of skin and large lips and noses would change much faster.[20] Nevertheless, no matter how great a curiosity Moss was to the white

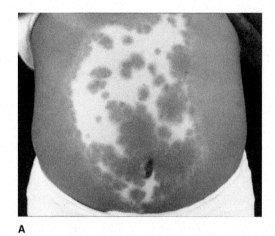

A

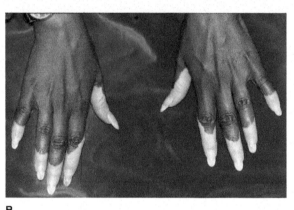

B

FIGURE 1-6. After moving from the Southern state of Virginia to the North, Henry Moss, an African slave, may have exhibited cutaneous manifestations of vitiligo similar to these patients with vitiligo (**A and B**). At the time, this change in skin color of a formerly dark-skinned man seemed to confirm Samuel Stanhope Smith's theory that climate influenced skin color.

community of Philadelphia, there was denial that white people could turn black even though a black man could, apparently, "turn white."[21]

Benjamin Rush (1745–1813), a Founding Father of the United States and an eminent physician of the late eighteenth century, was another scientist fascinated by Moss's case. He based his argument on "scientific findings" that being black was a hereditary illness, which he referred to as "negroidism." In an address to the American Philosophical Society, Rush said that the only evidence of a "cure" occurred when the skin color turned white. Rush drew the conclusion that, "blackness was a mild form of a non-contagious disease."[22] He postulated that Black skin color, as it is called in Negroes, was derived from leprosy (or perhaps vitiligo) but that Moss was, for some reason, undergoing a cure induced by nature itself and was thus reverting to his natural white color [**Figure 1-7, A and B**].[23]

PSEUDOSCIENTIFIC THEORIES ON SKIN OF COLOR

Pseudoscientific theories of race and skin color abounded in the nineteenth century. Various arguments seemed to support either one or the other of the two main camps: the monogenist or polygenist school of thought. The monogenist theory of human origins proposed a common ancestry for all human races. The polygenist theory, on the other hand, held that human races were descendants of more than two ancestral racial types. The leader of the polygenist school was Samuel Morton (1799–1851), a famous physician and researcher in natural history. According to Morton, the key to the separate origin of races was found in hybrids, or "mulattoes." It was his opinion that mulatto women bore children only with great difficulty, and if these women mated only with other mulattoes, their children were less fertile, and so the progeny would eventually die out. Since the middle of the eighteenth century,

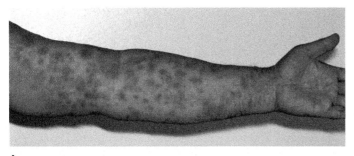

A

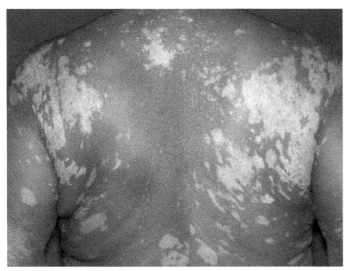

B

FIGURE 1-7. Benjamin Rush, a Founding Father of the United States and eminent physician of the late eighteenth century, proposed that **(A)** black skin color was derived from leprosy, as seen in this patient, or **(B)** that a change in skin color could have resulted from vitiligo, as seen in this patient.

when Carl Linnaeus (1707–1778) founded the science of taxonomy and classified organisms, the test of species in natural history has been the ability of two organisms to produce fertile offspring. From his conviction that "half-breeds" could not propagate themselves indefinitely, Morton concluded that black and white people were not varieties of a single race but entirely separate species.[24,25]

In the nineteenth century, the theory of maternal impression resurfaced, revitalizing an earlier explanation for why some white women had black babies and some black women had white ones. The theory is attributed to Hippocrates, the ancient Greek physician, who saved the honor of a princess accused of adultery because she bore a black baby by saying that the princess, while having intercourse with her husband, had accidentally seen a picture of a black person cohabitating with a white woman.[26]

The *Midrash Rabbah* also supports this theory of maternal impression, with the story of an Ethiopian wife who presented her dark-skinned husband with a light-colored child. The husband told the rabbi that the child was not his. The rabbi then asked whether there had been a picture of a man in the room at the moment of intercourse. When he was told that there was in fact such a picture, the rabbi asked whether the man in the picture was white or black. When told that the man in the picture was white, the rabbi answered that this picture was the cause of the light color of the child.[27]

Aleš Hrdlička (1869–1943), an anthropologist, believed that the "pure strains" of people of color would not show a red mark on the skin when fingernails were drawn over the chest with pressure. However, if there was any intermixture with white people, the lines would show as fairly broad, red marks, and the flush would be of some duration. Both of these features would be more prevalent depending on the percentage of "white blood" present in the individual examined.[28]

THEORIES OF EVOLUTION

The theories of evolution formulated by Charles Darwin (1809–1882) ended the monogenist/polygenist controversy over race. Darwin left no doubt that all human races belong to the same species. He wrote:

Although the existing races of man differ in many respects, as in color, hair, shape of skull, proportions of the body, yet if their whole organization be taken into consideration they are found to resemble each other closely in a multitude of points. Many of these points are of so unimportant or of so singular a nature that it is extremely improbable that they should have been independently acquired by aboriginally distinct species or races.[29]

An earlier evolutionary concept of race and color had been advanced by Robert Chambers (1802–1871), an Edinburgh publisher and amateur scientist. In 1844, he anonymously published *Vestiges of the Natural History of Creation*, in which he argued that humans began as Africans, passed through Malay, Indian, and Mongolian phases, and finally emerged as Caucasian. Non-white people were thus simply a representation of phases of development to the highest evolutionary stage–Caucasian.[30]

An oft-quoted twentieth-century opinion on the origin of skin of color was that of Charles Loring Brace IV (b. 1930). He wrote that early humans lived in the tropics and exchanged their anthropoidean fur coats for an improved sweat gland system that allowed them to run down game in the heat of the day. The loss of body hair thus exposed the early hominoids to the dangers of skin cancer; the need for protection from ultraviolet (UV) radiation damage led to the development of black skin. Successful and extensive human occupation of the northern temperate zones as a permanent habitat did not occur until the last glaciation period, approximately 70,000 years ago. While the previous glaciation periods had forced people to areas closer to the equator, by the end of the third interglacial movement, they had developed technologies to resist the cold further north, where large game abounded. There, the adaptive significance of melanin was substantially reduced, with the inevitable result that mutations detrimental to melanin production allowed people without black skin to survive and multiply.[31]

PSEUDOSCIENTIFIC DATA ON SKIN OF COLOR

Controversy regarding skin of color continued to abound throughout the late nineteenth and early twentieth centuries when scientists discussed the data concerning the anatomic and/or physiologic differences between black skin and white skin. One of the main reasons for this controversy was the undocumented evidence published by "experts" on the subject.

Pseudoscientific information was propagated by leading authorities, such as Edward A. Balloch (1857–1948). Although honored for his deanship at the historically black college, Howard University College of Medicine, Balloch stated that "the Negro differs from the Caucasian anatomically, physiologically and pathologically."[32] He carried his erroneous clinical observations further by asserting that "the dominant physiologic peculiarity of the Negro is the lessened sensibility of the nervous system. The Negro bears surgical operations remarkably well: he seldom suffers from shock, and wounds of all kind heal with quickness, and that is certainly delightful to the surgeon."[32]

An approach closer to modern theories was put forth by the surgeon Rudolph Matas (1860–1957). Although he did not have the luxury of modern investigative tools, he was still able to determine that the chemical composition of pigment in black skin was identical to white skin [**Figure 1-8**]. In a monumental publication in 1896, Matas made the following groundbreaking pseudoscientific statement: "this melanin of the Negro differs from that of whites in quantity and general distribution rather than in quality."[33]

An early-twentieth-century publication by H. Fox, which was probably influenced by Matas' findings, is a classic example of the contemporary beliefs regarding the difference between black and white skin. Fox made such pseudoscientific statements as, "the skin of the Negro,

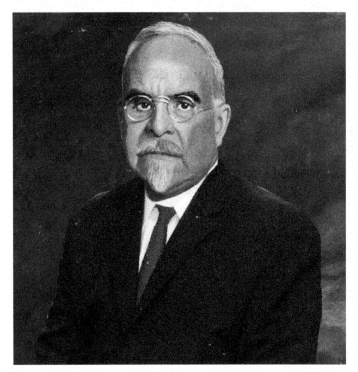

FIGURE 1-8. In the late nineteenth century, Rudolph Matas and colleagues stated that the composition of pigment in black and white individuals was identical and that the "melanin of the Negro differs from that of the white in quantity and general distribution rather than in quality."[33] (Used with permission from Marisol LLC, Muscat, Sultanate of Oman.)

especially the dermis, is thicker than that of the white. This is also true of the subcutaneous tissues, as exemplified by the characteristic thick lips of the Negro."[34,35]

These types of findings persisted well into the twentieth century. In the introductory paragraph of his article *Abnormalities of Pigmentation in the Negro,* Meyer L. Niedelman states that "the skin of persons of the Negro race differs from that of members of the white race not only in structure and physiology but in its reaction to trauma and infection."[36]

Many eminent scientists have used pseudoscientific data to advance, justify, and defend some of the prejudicial sociopolitical doctrines of their day. Examples of how erroneous cutaneous data were used in a direct or indirect fashion to propagate some of these beliefs abound: "It is well known that the blacker the Negro the healthier and stronger he is," and "any diminution in color of the pure race, outside of albinism, is a mark of feebleness or ill health."[37,38] Unfortunately, much of this misinformation was disseminated throughout the scientific literature, and some pseudoscientific data continued to be regarded as fact rather than fiction up until the early twenty-first century.

MODERN SCIENTIFIC THEORIES ON SKIN OF COLOR

THE VITAMIN D/SUNLIGHT THEORY

A widely accepted modern explanation of skin of color is the vitamin D/sunlight theory. It is known that the first humans lived in a very warm climate, such as the one found in Africa. Only those with dark skin were protected from the damaging effects of UV light; those with lighter skin were less successful and not chosen as mates, and so, after thousands of years, they essentially vanished, according to the theory.[39]

The assumption is that early humans were hunters, and as nearby game was depleted, they followed their prey into cooler areas. There, dark skin, which had protected them from UV rays, now screened out too much of the sun's light, resulting in the lower synthesis of vitamin D. Insufficient amounts of vitamin D in infants could have resulted in

bowed legs, knock knees, scoliosis, and other manifestations of rickets and similar ossification defects in older children. Women deprived of adequate vitamin D during puberty, pregnancy, and lactation may have been predisposed to osteomalacia. However, away from the equator, people with lighter skin would have thrived, whereas for those with darker skin, excessive amounts of vitamin D could often lead to kidney stones and other metastatic calcifications in infants.[40]

When humans moved north of the Mediterranean Sea and the latitude of 40°N, where the winter sun is less than 20° above the horizon and most of the needed UV light is removed by the powerful filtering action of the atmosphere, the more deeply pigmented infants could have developed the grossly bent legs and twisted spines characteristic of rickets, crippling their ability to hunt game as adults and making them undesirable as mates.[41] The realization that infants born in the spring and summer had fewer growth defects may have led to the popularity of June weddings.

Another argument for the vitamin D/sunlight theory is that most infants of all races have lighter skin at birth, which may gradually develop into darker skin of color as they mature, paralleling the declining need for vitamin D.[42] A notable exception to the correlation between latitude and skin color is the Inuit. Although they have medium brown skin and endure long, dark Arctic winters, they remain completely free of rickets.[41] A plausible explanation is that they receive large quantities of vitamin D in other forms (eg, in their diet, which is heavy in fish oil and meat), making it unnecessary to have light skin to prevent rickets.

The vitamin D/sunlight theory seems to offer a better explanation for the evolution of skin of color than the initial early sunlight and heat theories, especially since studies by J. S. Weiner and colleagues show that black Yoruba skin reflects only 24% of the incident light, whereas untanned European skin reflects as much as 64%.[42] Therefore, one would expect that individuals with heat-absorbing black skin would be found in the cold northern climates and those with reflective white skin near the equator. Also, according to William F. Loomis of the University California, San Diego, UV regulation, rather than heat regulation, explains why Caucasians are white in the winter and pigmented in the summer.[39,43] The contemporary work of Nina Jablonski (b. 1954) and George Chaplin (b. 1953), of the California Academy of Sciences, relates the differences of skin color to evolution and reproduction. They conclude that modern humans probably originated in the tropics, where there are high levels of UV light, which breaks down the essential vitamin B_9 that is needed for cell division and the production of new DNA. This led to the evolution of melanin-rich skin, which protects against UV light. However, when humans moved into regions with less UV light, their skin became paler to compensate for the reduction in vitamin D production. Therefore, according to Jablonski and Chaplin, skin color "basically becomes a balancing act between the evolutionary demands of photo-protection and the need to create vitamin D in the skin."[44]

Until 1988, people's skin color was classified according to their hair and eye color phenotypes, but since then, the scale developed by Thomas B. Fitzpatrick (1919–2003) of Harvard University has proven to be widely accepted.[45] Fitzpatrick's scale includes factors such as the natural color of unexposed skin, the individual's ability to tan, and the reaction of the individual's skin to staying out in the sun too long.[45,46] Fitzpatrick's skin type scheme can be seen below and in [**Figure 1-9**][46]:

- Skin type I: Always burns, never tans (pale white skin)
- Skin type II: Burns easily, tans minimally (white skin)
- Skin type III: Burns moderately, tans uniformly (light brown skin)
- Skin type IV: Burns minimally, always tans (moderate brown skin)
- Skin type V: Rarely burns, tans profusely (dark brown skin)
- Skin type VI: Never burns (deeply pigmented dark brown to black skin)

At present, this is the most commonly used system to classify skin type. However, a few dermatologists seem to use this scheme without correlating skin color categories to the skin's response to the sun, in terms of burning or tanning. The skin type categories, however, are still very useful for dermatologists because individuals of different skin types

Type I	Type II	Type III	Type IV	Type V	Type VI

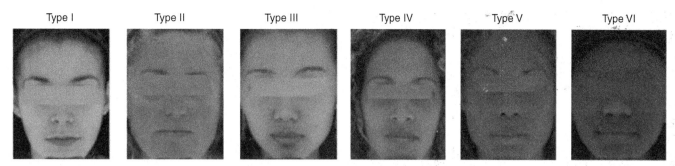

FIGURE 1-9. Thomas B. Fitzpatrick (1919–2003) developed his eponymous skin type classification system in 1988. This commonly used system classifies a person's skin type by their response to sun exposure in terms of the degree of burning and tanning.[45-47] (Used with permission from Marisol LLC, Muscat, Sultanate of Oman.)

will react differently to various procedures and medications, as well as suffer from type-specific skin complaints.[47]

BIOLOGY OF THE MELANIN PIGMENTARY SYSTEM

Although there has been much philosophical, religious, and scientific speculation on the causes of skin of color, light and electron microscopes have provided us with the biological answer to our clinical observations [**Figure 1-10**]. George Szabó of Harvard University demonstrated that melanocytes are symmetrically distributed and do not differ significantly in size, shape, or population density in the various races.[48,49] The skin of the forehead, cheek, and genital areas contains over 2000 melanocytes/mm^2, whereas the skin of the trunk has less than 1000 melanocytes/mm^2, variations that impart the clinical differences in skin color. Also, we know that melanin pigmentation results from the melanin produced in melanocytes versus keratinocytes. Because the ratio of melanocytes in the epidermis is 36:1, it must be the amount of melanin present in keratinocytes that is the essential factor in determining the color of skin. Walter Quevedo Jr. (1930–2010), of Brown University [**Figure 1-11**], was also a seminal thinker on the topic of skin of color. According to Quevedo and colleagues, pigmentation of the skin is related to four biological processes[50]:

1. Formation of melanosomes in melanocytes

2. Melanization of melanosomes in melanocytes

3. Secretion of melanosomes into keratinocytes, with and without degradation in lysosomal-like granules

4. Transportation of melanosomes by keratinocytes to the epidermal surface

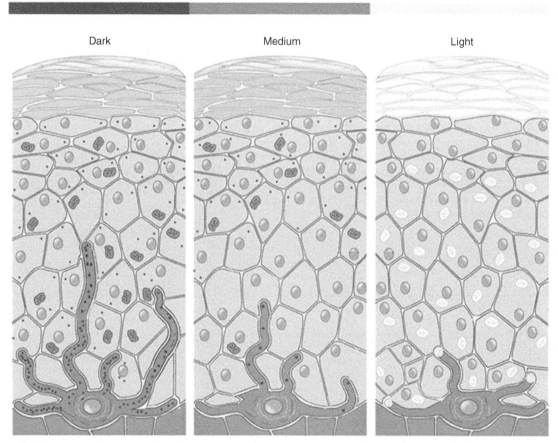

Dark	Medium	Light

FIGURE 1-10. Although darker and lighter skin have the same number of melanocytes, those in darker skin have more dendrites and are biologically more active as compared to the melanocytes in lighter skin. In lighter skin, melanosomes are small and grouped together, overall there is less melanin and little melanin is contained in the keratinocytes in the upper layer of the skin. In darker skin, melanosomes are larger and contain more melanin which is released and dispersed more uniformly throughout the epidermis. (Used with permission from Marisol LLC, Muscat, Sultanate of Oman.)

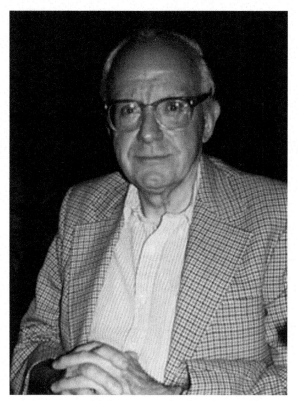

FIGURE 1-11. Walter Quevedo Jr. of Brown University, Division of Biology and Medicine, was a great thinker on the topic of skin of color. Along with his colleagues, Thomas Fitzpatrick and George Szabó, he used light and electron microscopy to research the biology of the melanin pigmentary system. (Used with permission from Mrs. Mercedes Quevedo, wife of Walter Quevedo Jr., PhD)

The first biological process is essentially the same in all races. People with very dark skin of color, with almost all stage IV melanosomes, have more melanization of their melanosomes than people with white skin, who have mostly stage II and III melanosomes. In melanocytes of all races, the melanosomes are discrete particles; but in the keratinocytes of Caucasians, Mongoloids, and American Indians, melanosomes are aggregated into groups of 2 to 8 surrounded by a membrane. The importance of these conclusions on the biology of the melanin pigmentary system is that it essentially proves that there is only one "race" of humans.

◼ GENETICS AND THE DNA OF SKIN OF COLOR

One of the more recent influences on the concept of race and skin color are the findings from the Human Genome Project (HGP), which began in 1990 and sought to understand the genetic makeup of the human species. The HGP has given us "the ability, for the first time, to read nature's complete genetic blueprint for building a human being."[51] The HGP may help us answer questions about the evolution of the color of skin.[52] Importantly, DNA research has also shown that all humans are genetically the same, regardless of the color of their skin and other small "surface" variations.[44] In terms of application to patient care, the mapping of genes and DNA advances should be of help to dermatologists in understanding their patients' skin diseases.

In conclusion, the study of human skin pigmentation remains of the highest importance in understanding the evolution of skin color, despite evidence that races do not exist as separate, invariable, biological entities and that the idea of race is merely a socially constructed concept.[53,54]

Whereas this chapter has traveled through the long historical journey that has brought us to the current point in time, the chapters that follow examine the differences between lighter and darker skin pigmentation in a medical context. We acknowledge that there is a need to focus medically on skin of color to understand various skin diseases and to understand the natural evolution of skin color in a historical context. The use of DNA analysis appears promising for helping dermatologists unlock the mysteries of skin.

Let us hope that our long history of classifying people based solely on skin color is nearing an end and that people of the twenty-first century and beyond accept that we are all members of the same human family. The real differences between darker and lighter skin have too often gone unrecognized, often resulting in incorrect treatment. The following chapters will examine those differences and their implications for dermatologists.

REFERENCES

1. Khaldun I. *The Muqaddimah: An Introduction to History*. Vol I. Rosenthal F, trans. Princeton, NJ: Princeton University Press; 1996:34-36.
2. Watts AE. *The Metamorphoses of Ovid*. Berkeley, CA: University of California Press; 1955:24-35.
3. Ananikian, M, Werner A. Armenian, African. In: Gray LH, ed. *African Mythology on the Mythology of All Races*. Vol VII. New York, NY: Cooper Square Publishers; 1964:150.
4. Brown DM. Indian fireside tales. In: *Wisconsin Folklore Society Booklet*. Madison, WI: Wisconsin Folklore Society; 1947:3-4.
5. Swanton JR. Myths and tales of the southeastern Indians. In: *Bulletin 88*. Washington, DC: Smithsonian Institution Bureau of American Ethnology; 1919:74.
6. Freedman H, Simon M. *Midrash Rabbah, Genesis*. Vol III. London, United Kingdom: Soncino Press; 1929:213, 674.
7. Goldberg DM. *The Curse of Ham, Race and Slavery in Early Judaism, Christianity and Islam: Jews, Christians, and Muslims from the Ancient to the Modern World*. Princeton, NJ: Princeton University Press; 2003:154-160.
8. Schwartz RM. *The Curse of Cain: The Violent Legacy of Monotheism*. Chicago, IL: University of Chicago Press; 1997:226-236.
9. Haynes SR. *Noah's Curse: The Biblical Justification of American Slavery*. New York, NY: Oxford University Press; 2002:56-87.
10. Rogers JA. *Sex and Race*. Vol III. St. Petersburg, FL: Helga M Rogers; 1944:316-317.
11. Blank W: The Church of God daily bible study, a ministry of God's Word. http://www.keyway.ca. Accessed December 30, 2012.
12. Smith J. *The Book of Mormon*. Salt Lake City, UT: The Church of Jesus Christ of Latter-Day Saints; 1921:61.
13. Wiesner-Hanks ME. *Early Modern Europe 1450 to 1789*. 2nd ed. Cambridge, United Kingdom: Cambridge University Press; 2013:374.
14. de La Peyrère I. *Men before Adam, or, a Discourse upon the twelfth, thirteenth, and fourteenth verses of the Fifth Chapter of the Epistle of the Apostle Paul to the Romans*. Private publication, 1656:122.
15. Campbell A. *White Attitudes Toward Black People*. Ann Arbor, MI: Institute for Social Research; 1971:12-14.
16. Vasari G. *The Lives of Artists*. Oxford, United Kingdom: Oxford University Press; 1998:186.
17. Bendyshe MA. *The Anthropological Treaties of Johann Friedrich Blumenbach*. London, United Kingdom: Longman, Green, Longman, Roberts and Green; 1865:210, 221.
18. Virey JJ. *Natural History of the Negro Race*. Guenebault LJ, Beile B, trans. New York, NY: Babcock & Co.; 1837:22-23.
19. Meckel JF. *Deutsches Archiv für die Physiologie*. Vol 2. Berlin, Germany: Nabu; 1816:287-875.
20. Zilversmith A, ed. An essay on the causes of the variety of complexion and the figure. In: Smith SS, ed. *The Human Species*, 1810. *William Mary Q*. 1966;23:506.
21. Yokota KA. Common-place: a cabinet of curiosities. http://www.common-place.org/vol-04/no-02/yokota/. Accessed May 2, 2013.
22. Rush B. *The Autobiography of Benjamin Rush: "Travels Through Life" Together With His Commonplace Book for 1789-1813*. Indianapolis, IN: Bobbs-Merrill; 1812:78.
23. Brodsky A. *Benjamin Rush: Patriot and Physician*. New York, NY: Truman Talley Books/St Martin's Press; 2004:102-105.
24. Smith CH. *The Natural History of the Human Species*. Edinburgh, United Kingdom: Gould and Lincoln; 1848:160.
25. Bondeson J. *A Cabinet of Medical Curiosities*. Ithaca, NY: Cornell University Press; 1897:146.

26. Zonta M. *A Hebrew Translation of Hippocrates' De Superfoetatione: Historical Introduction and Critical Edition.* Bloomington, IN: Indiana University Press; 2003:97-102.

27. Ginzberg L. *The Legend of the Jews.* Vol 5. Philadelphia, PA: Jewish Publication Society of America; 1925:56, 169-170.

28. Hrdlička A. Anthropometry. *Am J Phys Anthropol.* 1919;2:17.

29. Darwin CR. *The Descent of Man, and Selection in Relation to Sex.* Vol I. London, United Kingdom: John Murray; 1871:231-232.

30. Chambers R. *Vestiges of the Natural History of Creation.* London, United Kingdom: George Rutledge and Sons; 1844:226-228.

31. Brace CL. *The Stages of Human Evolution.* 3rd ed. Englewood, NJ: Prentice-Hall; 1987:75, 104-105.

32. Balloch EA. The relative frequency of fibroid processes in dark skinned races. *Med News.* 1894;2:29-35.

33. Matas R. The surgical peculiarities of the Negro. *Transact Am Surg Assoc.* 1896;14:483-606.

34. Fox H. Observations on skin diseases in the Negro. *J Cutan Dis.* 1908;26:67-79.

35. Rogers JA. *Nature Knows No Color-Line: Research Into the Negro Ancestry in the White Race.* New York, NY: Helga M. Rogers; 1952:21.

36. Niedelman ML. Abnormalities of pigmentation in the Negro. *Arch Dermatol.* 1945;51:1-9.

37. Stanton W. Leopard spots. In: *Scientific Attitudes Towards Race in America, 1815-1859.* Chicago, IL: University of Chicago Press; 1960:5-6.

38. De Montellane BRO. Melanin, Afrocentricity, and pseudoscience. *Am J Phys Anthropol.* 1993;36:33-58.

39. Loomis WF. Skin-pigment regulation of vitamin-D biosynthesis in man. *Science.* 1967;157:501-506.

40. Kirchweger G. The biology of skin color: black and white. The evolution of race was as simple as the politics of race is complex. *Discover.* 2001;22:78-80.

41. Thomas WA. Health of a carnivorous race: a study of the Eskimo. *JAMA.* 1927;88:1559-1560.

42. Weiner JS, Harrison GA, Singer R, et al. Skin color in southern Africa. *Hum Biol.* 1964;36:294-307.

43. Quevedo WC Jr, Fitzpatrick TB, Pathak MA, et al. Light and skin colour. In: Pathak MA, Harber LC, Seiji M, et al, eds. *Sunlight and Man: Normal and Abnormal Photobiologic Responses.* Tokyo, Japan: University of Tokyo Press; 1974:165-194.

44. Iqbal S. A new light on skin color. http://ngm.nationalgeographic.com/ngm/0211/feature2/online_extra.html. Accessed July 13, 2013.

45. Fitzpatrick TB. The validity and practicality of sun-reactive skin types I through VI. *Arch Dermatol.* 1988;124:869-871.

46. Australian Radiation Protection and Nuclear Safety Agency. Fitzpatrick skin type. http://www.arpansa.gov.au/pubs/RadiationProtection/FitzpatrickSkinType.pdf. Accessed July 15, 2013.

47. Shah SK, Alexis AF. Defining skin of color. In: Alam M, Bhatia A, Kundu R, et al, eds. *Cosmetic Dermatology for Skin of Color.* New York, NY: McGraw-Hill Professional; 2009:1-4.

48. Szabó G. Quantitative histological investigations on the melanocyte system of the human epidermis. In: Gordon M, ed. *Pigment Cell Biology.* New York, NY: Academic Press; 1959:99-125.

49. Szabó G, Gerald AB, Pathak MA, Fitzpatrick TB. Racial differences in the fate of melanosomes. *Nature.* 1969;222:1081-1082.

50. Fitzpatrick TB, Quevedo WC, Szabó G, et al. Biology of the melanin pigmentary system. In: Fitzpatrick TB, Arndt KA, Clark WH, et al, eds. *Dermatology in General Medicine.* New York, NY: McGraw-Hill; 1971:117-146.

51. National Human Genome Research Institute. http://www.genome.gov/10001772. Accessed March 30, 2013.

52. Callister P, Didham R. Who are we? The Human Genome Project, race and ethnicity. *Soc Pol J N Z.* 2009;36:63-76.

53. Jablonski NG. The evolution of human skin coloration. *J Hum Evol.* 2000;39:57-106.

54. Jablonski N. Lecture from 2010. http://www.youtube.com/watch?v=QOSPNVunyFQ. Accessed March 30, 2013.

CHAPTER 2

Defining Skin of Color

Susan C. Taylor
Angela Kyei

KEY POINTS

- The term *skin of color* identifies individuals of racial groups with skin darker than Caucasians, such as Asians, Africans, Native Americans, and Pacific Islanders.

- Patients with skin of color often have distinctive cutaneous and hair characteristics, disorders, and reaction patterns, as well as diverse cultural practices affecting skin care.

- There is a diversity of skin hues, cutaneous diseases, and responses to cutaneous stimuli within each racial or ethnic group.

- Top dermatologic diagnoses in patients with skin of color include alopecia, keloidal scarring, and seborrheic dermatitis in African Americans; seborrheic dermatitis in Asians; and dyschromias in Hispanics.

- The rapid increase of the population with skin of color in the United States and worldwide requires dermatologists and other physicians to study texts focusing on the distinct cutaneous disorders, reaction patterns, and cultural practices of this population.

HOW DO WE DEFINE *SKIN OF COLOR?*

The term *skin of color* identifies individuals of particular racial and ethnic groups who share similar cutaneous characteristics and disorders, as well as reaction patterns to those disorders. In general, these individuals have darker skin hues and tend to fall into the first four of the five racial categories created by the U.S. Census [**Table 2-1**]. It is important to recognize that using the term *race* as a surrogate for biological or genetic inheritance is not ideal and is controversial. When using the term *race*, it is important to bear in mind that no single gene, trait, or characteristic distinguishes all members of one race from all members of another.[1] Because humans have always mixed freely and widely, the vast majority of the human gene pool is shared. For example, 85% of all human variation can be found in any local population, and 94% can be found on any continent.[2] Thus, regardless of racial classification, the vast majority of humans share a common genetic pool. Moreover, race does not completely represent ancestry because individuals may have mixed racial backgrounds. Thus, someone racially identified as African American may have parents with primarily European ancestry; nevertheless, because of a distant relative of African ancestry, they are still classified as African American, a categorization that ignores any European ancestry and genetic pool. Some genetic studies suggest that "geographic ancestry" may be a better proxy than "race" for a shared genetic pool because geographical isolation of populations over time can result in genetic diversity.[1,3]

Despite the shortcomings of racial classifications, there are cutaneous characteristics and disorders that disproportionately affect members of the same racial group, and to further study these traits, there needs to be an easily understood categorization of these groups. For example, many people of African ancestry have tightly curled hair. Furthermore, there are certain cutaneous disorders, such as acne keloidalis nuchae and pseudofolliculitis barbae, that primarily occur in patients with this hair structure. To study these disorders, these patients need to be classified, and terms such as *race* and *ancestry* attempt to do just that. It is undeniable that the current classification is far from ideal, but this shortcoming should not undermine much needed studies of these diseases in this population.

In addition, genetics is not the only determinant of disease; environment and social factors are also important. To this end, people have

TABLE 2-1	Five categories for race in the United States[a]

1. American Indian or Alaska Native
   - Native American, Eskimo, Aleut
2. Asian
   - Filipino, Chinese, Japanese, Korean, Vietnamese, Thai, Malaysian, Laotian, Hmong, Indian, Pakistani
3. Black
   - African, African Caribbean, African American
4. Native Hawaiian or other Pacific Islander
5. White

[a]Data from the United States Census 2010.

been classified based on ethnicity. Although the terms *race* and *ethnicity* are often used interchangeably, *ethnicity* refers to a group of people who share a common culture, language, religion, history, and other sources of group identification without regard to race or ancestry. Because culture is related to behavior and behavior affects health and disease, it is important to also consider ethnicity when studying skin of color.

In summary, patients with skin of color represent a diverse population with different races and ancestral origins as well as multiple ethnicities. The study of this group involves an understanding of common and unique disorders that disproportionately affect them, in addition to understanding the cultural underpinning of disease development in this population. Thus, the subspecialty of skin of color is used to bring together patients, clinicians, and scientists interested in the treatment and investigation of disorders that occur in these individuals.

WHO ARE INDIVIDUALS WITH SKIN OF COLOR AND FROM WHERE DID THEY ORIGINATE?

Individuals with skin of color encompass multiple racial and ethnic groups who tend to share cutaneous characteristics, the most notable of which is increased pigmentation. These individuals include four races defined by the U.S. Census: American Indian or Alaska Native, Asian, Black, and Native Hawaiian or other Pacific Islander [Table 2-1].

The most widely accepted evolutionary theory explaining human origins and skin pigmentation focuses on two major evolutionary selective pressures: the folic acid theory and the vitamin D theory.[4-6] According to the folic acid theory, early man developed in an ultraviolet (UV)-rich environment of equatorial Africa and thus developed a dark, photoprotective, eumelanin-rich pigmentation as a means to protect himself from the harmful effects of the sun. This darkly pigmented skin

was important for preventing photolysis of folate, a process by which folate is depleted by reactive oxygen species generated by UVA, which is present at high levels year-round near the equator. Because folic acid is important in cell division, DNA repair, and melanogenesis, depletion of this supplement results in multiple deformities, including neural tube defects. This depletion would result in offspring less fit for survival. Thus, those who were darkly pigmented had a survival advantage in the African environment because dark skin prevented the depletion of folic acid. In addition, it is theorized that tightly curled dark hair, which is most adept at deflecting UV radiation and keeping the scalp cool, was also selected for during this time. Thus, early man possessed dark skin and thick, tightly curled hair because this was the best fit for his environment[4,5] [**Figures 2-1 and 2-2**].

As mankind began to migrate out of Africa, around 150,000 to 200,000 years ago, different selection pressures were faced. According to the vitamin D theory of race, as man moved away from equatorial Africa, he encountered colder environments with a lower UV index and thus required less photoprotection. In fact, the lower ultraviolet B (UVB) index in these areas presented the new challenge of producing adequate levels of vitamin D for bone synthesis and other vital functions dependent on vitamin D. It is postulated that lighter skin was selected for these environments because it impacted the survival of progeny. Those who were lighter with straight and light-colored hair were able to absorb more UVB to make vitamin D and thus prevent rickets and other deformities resulting from inadequate vitamin D synthesis. Thus, the different shades of the human skin color spectrum are believed to be a result of the UV index and its impact on two important vitamins, folic acid and vitamin D[6].

The evolution of mankind from a darkly pigmented common ancestor from Africa is also supported by genetic data. Recent genetic data involving mitochondrial DNA analysis and polymorphisms associated with the non-recombining portion of the Y chromosome have provided evidence of a common African heritage for all humankind.[7] Mitochondrial DNA analysis has determined that all women in the world descended from three African women, identified as L1, L2, and L3.[8] Descendants of L1 and L2 populated Africa, whereas descendants of L3 migrated to and populated the remaining continents. Presumably, these African ancestors had darker skin hues, or skin of color.

Underhill et al[7] analyzed DNA from 1062 men from 21 populations and demonstrated 131 unique haplotypes. These haplotypes were used to trace the microevolutionary trajectory of global modern human genetic diversification [**Table 2-2**]. Early humans first populated Africa, then Southeast Asia and Japan, Australia, New Guinea, and Central Asia, and finally, the remainder of the continents.

As early humankind migrated into and populated the six continents, they provided the basis for the modern-day concept of racial groups.

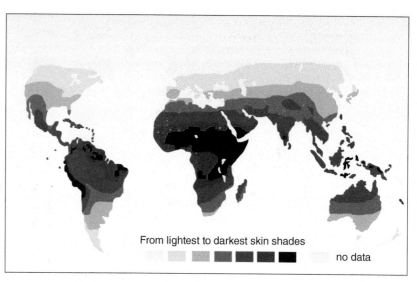

FIGURE 2-1. World population by race, 2007. (Reproduced with permission from Chaplin G. Geographic distribution of Environmental Factors influencing human skin coloration, *Am J Phys Anthropol* 2004 Nov;125(3):292-302.)

From lightest to darkest skin shades   no data

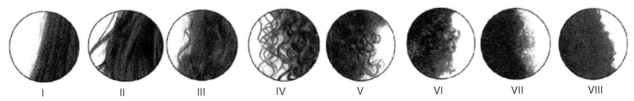

FIGURE 2-2. The eight types of human hair in terms of degree and type of curl, as described by Loussouarn et al. (Reproduced with permisison from Loussouarn G, Garcel AL, Lozano I, et al: Worldwide diversity of hair curliness: a new method of assessment, *Int J Dermatol.* 2007 Oct;46 Suppl 1:2-6).[5a]

Rosenberg[9] demonstrated that it is possible to cluster persons into population groups based on geographic origin (continent) with high statistical accuracy. Likewise, Stephens[10] demonstrated that single-nucleotide polymorphisms or their corresponding haplotypes enable some degree of classification of humans according to continent. Selectively neutral, nonexpressed genes from populations from Africa, Eurasia, East Asia, Oceania, and America, correspond with self-reported population ancestry or the concept of racial classifications (see Chapter 3, Epidemiology of Cutaneous Diseases).[10]

The migration across continents resulted in changes in skin color, craniofacial features, and hair texture and color. The differences displayed in the appearance of various racial groups are felt to be due to environmental, dietary, and adaptive factors. Recently, Lamason[11] identified the *SLC24A5* gene, localized to melanosomes, that determines skin pigmentation. West Africans with the normal form of *SLC24A5* have brown skin, whereas fairer-skinned Europeans have a modified form of the gene. The modified form accounts for fewer and smaller melanosomes and, hence, white skin. This gene, however, does not play a role in determining skin tones among Asian individuals, which are determined by yet another gene.[11]

In summary, individuals with skin of color represent a diverse population of multiple racial and ethnic groups who, in general, have darker skin color compared to Caucasians. Theories explaining the origins of humans indicate that mankind originated from a common African ancestor, whose offsprings migrated to populate the rest of the world and, in the process, underwent adaptation of different skin colors based on the UVB index and multiple selection pressures.

WHY IS IT USEFUL TO IDENTIFY AND HIGHLIGHT INDIVIDUALS WITH SKIN OF COLOR?

Understanding the important differences between skin of color and Caucasian skin is the underpinning of this textbook, with the ultimate goal of educating others so that they may improve the dermatologic health of this group. People with skin of color have increased cutaneous melanogenesis compared to Caucasians. In addition, hair characteristics such as hair follicle shape, density, and moisture content tend to differ in many populations with skin of color compared with Caucasians. Furthermore, skin reactivity to injury, an important factor when administering topical medications and performing common dermatologic procedures, differs by race and thus merits special consideration when evaluating populations with skin of color. These and other differences merit further investigation to maximize and improve care to these populations.

The macroscopic differences highlighted thus far can serve as a basis for further evaluation on the microscopic level. Given the ongoing explosion of knowledge in the field of genetics, studying populations with skin of color may lead to a better understanding of differential

susceptibility to disease and responses to pharmacologic agents. Geneticists are actively discovering polymorphisms that lead to disease susceptibility among different racial groups. For example, there are specific polymorphisms that may make African Americans more prone to diabetes and hypertension. Others confer differential responses to pharmacologic agents and drugs commonly used to treat heart disease that are known to be less effective in individuals of African descent relative to individuals of European descent.[12]

An increased understanding of differential susceptibility to disease based on genetic variation among people with skin of color is also important in the field of dermatology. Certain cutaneous disorders disproportionately affect populations of color such as lupus, dermatomyositis, and keloids in Asians and Africans,[13-16] and cutaneous T-cell lymphoma, sarcoidosis, and hidradenitis in African Americans.[17-19] Thus, a greater understanding of the genetic diversity that exists within these groups will, in the future, lead to more effective, as well as individualized, dermatologic therapy. These advancements occur most efficiently when there is a deliberate focus and study of these populations, which is a goal of this textbook.

Besides the biological and genetic variations that merit study within this group, cultural differences influence skin and hair care practices and, thus, are important components of studying populations with skin of color. Well-documented health disparities and poor outcomes tend to disproportionately affect populations with skin of color.[20] Why is it that despite the low incidence of melanoma in populations with skin of color, morbidity and mortality due to this form of skin cancer tend to be higher in Hispanics and African Americans in the United States?[1] Why do African Americans have a 19-fold increase in keloid formation?[21] Why does central centrifugal cicatricial alopecia primarily affect African Americans?[22] Why do Asians develop nasopharyngeal carcinoma more frequently in association with dermatomyositis?[15] These are examples of the types of questions that remain unanswered in populations with skin of color and warrant further investigation. This book and the study of populations with skin of color aim not only to educate, but also to stimulate interest in this field to foster further research to resolve many questions that currently remain unanswered.

In the next few decades, it will be increasingly important to serve the populations with skin of color given their seismic demographic changes projected in the United States. The total number of individuals in the United States with skin of color was approximately 77 million in the year 2010.[23] The U.S. Census Bureau projections for the year 2050 indicate that this population will approximately equal or surpass the non-Hispanic white population[24] [**Figure 2-3**]. The changing face of America, as well as the remainder of the globe, highlights the importance of understanding this population. Their population growth, coupled with the ease of international travel and immigration into the United States, means that dermatologists will be faced with the challenge of diagnosing and treating skin diseases in racially and ethnically diverse populations.

WHAT ARE SOME OF THE CUTANEOUS DISORDERS THAT OCCUR IN INDIVIDUALS WITH SKIN OF COLOR?

The subspecialty of skin of color is relatively young. As such, epidemiologic data highlighting incidence of skin diseases and outcomes are limited. Insight into diseases in various populations is often based

TABLE 2-2	Global trajectory of modern human populations
Groups I and II: Africans (Khoisan, Bantu, Pygmy, Sudanese, Ethiopian, and Malian)	
Groups III and IV: Africans, Southeast Asians/Japanese	
Group V: Australians, New Guineans, Southeast Asians, Japanese, and Central Asians	
Groups VI–X: Migration across the remainder of the world (except sub-Saharan Africa)	

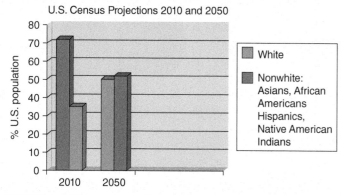

FIGURE 2-3. U.S. census projections for 2050, based on U. S. census data for 2010.

TABLE 2-4	Reasons for visits to dermatologists for Asian American patients	
Rank order	Diagnosis	Percentage
1	Acne	19
2	Dermatitis	18
3	Benign neoplasm	6
4	Psoriasis	5
5	Seborrheic keratosis	5
6	Atopic dermatitis	5
7	Warts	4
8	Urticaria	3
9	Cysts	3
10	Seborrheic dermatitis	3

on healthcare service utilization data such as retrospective private and clinic practice surveys, as well as dermatologists' published reports of their personal experience.[25,26] Although these data are useful, they are limited by several factors, including the location of the practice, patient demographics, patient access to healthcare, patient customs and practices, the genetics of the populations, and the time period of the study. In the United States, the largest surveys have been conducted by the National Center for Health Statistics, including the National Ambulatory Care Survey (NAMCS).[27] In this survey, samples of a nationally representative group of visits to the offices of non–federally employed physicians in the United States are obtained. The NAMCS provides the primary diagnosis for dermatologists by race and ethnicity. A review of the data for the years 1993 to 2009 suggest that about 50% of the most frequent 10 cutaneous diagnoses in the United States are shared regardless of racial origin. For example, acne is first or second diagnosis across all races and cultures. Common dermatoses such as warts, psoriasis, and dermatitis are high on the list for all demographics [**Tables 2-3, 2-4, 2-5, and 2-6**]. There are differences, however. For example, alopecia and seborrheic dermatitis appear in the top 10 diagnoses among African Americans, whereas they do not occur in the top 10 diagnoses among Caucasian Americans. Another striking difference is the lack of malignant skin cancer on the Asian, African American, and Hispanic lists, whereas this diagnosis is in the top five among Caucasian Americans. Keloids also appear on the African American and Asian lists, whereas it is absent on the Caucasian American list.[27]

In addition to these differences, some skin disorders disproportionately affect certain populations with skin of color. What follows is an overview of the various skin conditions and their incidences and mortalities in patients with skin of color compared to Caucasian Americans. Highlighting these disparities empowers the clinician to improve outcomes in these groups.

SKIN CANCER AND RACE

Lymphoma Cutaneous T-cell lymphoma refers to a group of non-Hodgkin lymphomas that primarily involve the skin but can spread to the lymph nodes and internal organs. The two main forms are Sézary syndrome and mycosis fungoides (MF), with MF representing the most common form.[28,29] This skin cancer is derived from T-helper lymphocytes and has the potential to transform into a high-grade T-cell lymphoma.[30] The incidence of MF is 0.29 cases per 100,000 per year, comprising 2.2% of all reported lymphomas. MF is more common in African Americans than Caucasian Americans, with an incidence 1.7 times higher and a mortality rate 2.4 times higher among African Americans compared with Caucasians.[29] Furthermore, many patients with skin of color present with a hypopigmented clinical variant of MF. The reasons for these disparities are unclear, but greater surveillance and early detection and treatment are most likely part of the solution (see Chapter 47, Cutaneous T-Cell Lymphoma).

Melanoma Melanoma represents a small proportion of skin cancers seen in all racial groups but accounts for over 75% of all skin cancer deaths. Melanoma tends to occur in sun-exposed areas in Caucasians, whereas in racial minorities, it tend to develop in non–sun-exposed areas. For example, an acral site is the most common site among African Americans, and the trunk is the most common site for Native Americans. Although the incidence of melanoma is low among skin of color groups, it is increasing among Asian Americans and Hispanic Americans in the United States.[1] Moreover, 5-year survival rates for African Americans and Hispanic Americans are much lower compared to Caucasian Americans. This is partly due to the fact that African Americans and Hispanic Americans present with significantly more advanced stages of the disease compared to Caucasian Americans.[31] The reasons behind the increase in melanoma among Asian Americans and Hispanic Americans

TABLE 2-3	Reasons for visits to dermatologists for African American patients	
Rank order	Diagnosis	Percentage
1	Acne	22
2	Dermatitis	14
3	Seborrheic dermatitis	8
4	Atopic dermatitis	6
5	Dyschromia	5
6	Psoriasis	4
7	Alopecia	4
8	Keloids	3
9	Warts	3
10	Cysts	3

TABLE 2-5	Reasons for visits to dermatologists for Caucasian American patients	
Rank order	Diagnosis	Percentage
1	Actinic keratosis	15
2	Acne	15
3	Benign neoplasm	8
4	Dermatitis	8
5	NMSC	7
6	Seborrheic keratosis	6
7	Warts	6
8	Psoriasis	4
9	Rosacea	4
10	Cysts	4

TABLE 2-6 Reasons for visits to dermatologists for Hispanic American patients

Rank order	Diagnosis	Percentage
1	Acne	22
2	Dermatitis	13
3	Psoriasis	7
4	Benign neoplasm of skin	6
5	Viral warts	5
6	Actinic keratosis	4
7	Seborrheic keratosis	4
8	Sebaceous cyst	4
9	Rosacea	3
10	Dyschromia	3

TABLE 2-7 Common/exclusive cutaneous disorders in Asian populations

Mongolian spots

Nevus of Ota

Nevus of Ito

Hori nevus

Kawasaki disease

Primary cutaneous amyloidosis (lichen, macula, anosacral)

Kikuchi-Fujimoto disease

Lipodystrophia centrifugalis abdominalis infantilis

Conditions as a result of alternative medicine (eg, cupping, coin-rubbing, and moxibustion)

Source: Data from Lee CS, Lim HW. Cutaneous disease in Asians. *Dermatol Clin.* 2003;21(4):669-677.

are not clear, but the study of this trend is important as part of the subspecialty of skin of color (see Chapter 44, Melanomas).

Nonmelanoma Skin Cancers Nonmelanoma skin cancer is the most common cancer in the United States. However, it is less common in darker-skinned patients due to photoprotection resulting from their more melanized skin. Despite the low rates among darker-skinned patients, they suffer disproportionately, having greater morbidity and mortality. Squamous cell carcinoma (SCC) is the most common type of skin cancer among African Americans and the second most common among Japanese and Asians. SCC tends to occur on non–sun-exposed sites in those with skin of color, unlike their fairer-skinned counterparts. African Americans with SCC have a mortality rate as high as 29%, presumably because of delayed diagnosis and potentially more biologically aggressive tumors. Basal cell carcinoma is the most common type of skin cancer in Hispanics and Asians and, again, tends to occur in photoprotected sites.[31,32] Despite the low incidence of nonmelanoma skin cancer among darker-skinned patients, it is clear from the epidemiologic trends that this population needs greater surveillance (see Chapter 45, Squamous Cell Carcinoma, and Chapter 46, Basal Cell Carcinoma).

■ PIGMENTARY DISORDERS AND RACIAL ORIGINS

Pigmentary disorders consistently rank high on the list of common skin complaints among patients with skin of color, including those of African, Arab, and Southeast Asian origins.[33] Certain pigmentary disorders seem to occur frequently in Asian populations. Melasma is one such common pigmentary disorder. The frequency of melasma has been reported to range from 0.25% to 4.0% in several Southeast Asian populations. There are several disorders that either occur almost exclusively in Asian populations or are very common in this group, including Hori nevus, nevus of Ota, nevus of Ito, and Mongolian spots, and all represent dermal melanosis.[34] Alternative medicine is often practiced in Asian cultures, which may result in self-inflicted skin abnormalities.[34] These practices can be misdiagnosed as child abuse when their results are seen in children. It is important for dermatologists to be knowledgeable about these practices and disorders [**Table 2-7**] (see Section 7, Pigmentary Disorders).

■ SYSTEMIC DISEASES WITH SKIN MANIFESTATIONS

Sarcoidosis Sarcoidosis is a multisystem granulomatous disease affecting the skin and multiple internal organs, including the lungs, mediastinal and peripheral lymph nodes, eyes, kidneys, spleen, liver, and central nervous system.[35] Skin involvement occurs in 25% of cases, and often patients have only cutaneous disease. Sarcoidosis affects all races and ethnicities, but in the United States, it is more common in African Americans, with a three- to four-fold higher risk of disease in

darker-skinned individuals compared with their fairer-skinned counterparts [**Table 2-8**]. Moreover, African Americans have an earlier onset and are more likely to have progressive disease resulting in death[36,37] (see Chapter 74, Sarcoidosis).

Systemic Sclerosis Systemic sclerosis occurs disproportionately in African Americans, with an earlier onset, more widespread disease, and more severe lung involvement. Darker-skinned women tend to have a lower survival rate than fairer-skinned women with this disease. It is unclear why these differences exist even after taking into consideration socioeconomic status. Genetics may explain the disparity; however, relatively insulated groups such as the Choctaw Native Americans were also found to have increased prevalence of the disease. Moreover, different racial groups tend to have specific human leukocyte antigen disease associations conferring different disease severity. Thus, variations in genetic polymorphisms and serologic and immunologic data among different racial groups are key to understanding and treating this disorder among patients with skin of color.[38,39]

Systemic Lupus Erythematosus Systemic lupus erythematosus (SLE) is another autoimmune disorder that tends to affect people with skin of color more often than Caucasian Americans. African Americans are three to four times more likely to be affected compared to their Caucasian American counterparts. In addition, Asians, including Chinese, Filipinos, and Japanese, have been found to have significantly higher rates of SLE compared with Caucasians. Both African Americans and Hispanic Americans have a higher mortality from this disease and have an earlier onset of the disease compared to Caucasian Americans.[3,16] It is not clear what factors account for these differences, but there are racial and ethnic differences in the autoimmune profile of this disorder. For example, anti-Ro antibody is more prevalent among Southern Chinese and Northern Africans. In addition, anti-Smith antibodies are increased in African Americans, North Africans, South Africans, Saudis from the Arabian Gulf, and Vietnamese. The reason for these racial and ethnic differences is unclear but warrants further study.[16]

TABLE 2-8 Disorders with increased incidence in African Americans compared to Caucasian Americans

Cutaneous T-cell lymphoma

Sarcoidosis

Keloids

Hidradenitis suppurativa

Pseudofolliculitis barbae

Acne keloidalis nuchae

Central centrifugal cicatricial alopecia

Systemic lupus erythematosus

Dermatomyositis

Systemic sclerosis

Dermatomyositis Dermatomyositis is a multisystem disease that affects all races. In Asians, it is associated with an increase in nasopharyngeal carcinoma; thus greater surveillance of this population is warranted.[15] In addition, there is some evidence to suggest that East Asians with amyopathic dermatomyositis have an increased risk of interstitial lung disease.[40] Dermatomyositis/polymyositis is four-fold more common in African Americans than white Caucasian Americans. Given these differences in the Asian and African populations, further study is warranted.[2]

◾ SKIN DISORDERS WITHOUT SYSTEMIC MANIFESTATIONS

Hidradenitis Suppurativa Hidradenitis suppurativa is a chronic inflammatory skin condition affecting apocrine-bearing sites. It has a predilection for intertriginous areas such as the axillae, inframammary region, groin, and buttocks. This is yet another condition that disproportionately affects African Americans.[19] Treatment of this condition often requires multiple specialists including dermatologists and plastic surgeons. Despite the availability of surgical and medical therapies, complete resolution of this condition often proves difficult (see Chapter 43, Hidradenitis Suppurativa).

Keloids Keloids are benign tumors that represent an overgrowth of dense, fibrous scar tissue that develops as a result of cutaneous injury, spreading beyond the site of injury.[21] Keloids can occur in response to surgery, trauma, burns, or inflammatory conditions and do not regress spontaneously.[13,21] Moreover, keloids can be extremely disfiguring and may limit joint mobility. Studies show significant impairment of quality of life in patients with keloids and hypertrophic scars. Keloids disproportionately affect African Americans and Asian Americans compared with fairer-skinned individuals, with incidence ratios ranging from 2:1 to 16:1. It is unclear why keloids occur in these groups, although a genetic predisposition is theorized[13] (see Chapter 33, Keloids).

◾ HAIR DISORDERS

Racial differences in hair density, structure, and texture are well documented [**Table 2-9 and Figures 2-4 and 2-5**].[41] For example, African Americans and those of African origins with natural, tightly coiled hair tend to have lower hair follicle density and less moisture in the hair compared with their Caucasian American and Asian American counterparts. In addition, the natural hair has an elliptical shape on cross-section, compared with the round shape of Asian American hair and the oval shape of Caucasian American hair. The shape of the hair of African Americans leads to a tightly curled mesh of spirals, which is primarily responsible for the hair pathology seen in this group. In African Americans, sebum tends to be less efficiently transferred from the scalp to tightly curled hair so that this oily substance tends to sit on the scalp, leading to drier hair follicles and possibly more seborrheic dermatitis of the scalp.[42] Tightly curled hair has also been implicated in the pathology of several hair disorders including pseudofolliculitis barbae and acne keloidalis nuchae[43] (see Chapter 39, Pseudofolliculitis Barbae, and Chapter 34, Acne Keloidalis Nuchae).

In addition, there is a robust culture of hair grooming that is unique to African Americans related to the challenges they face because of the unique properties of their hair. Treating hair disorders in this population requires knowledge of these hairstyles, including braids, weaves,

TABLE 2-9	Hair growth rate by race
	growth rate (mm/d)
Caucasians	0.165–0.506
Asian Americans	0.244–0.611
African Americans	0.129–0.436

Source: Data from Loussouarn G, El Rawadi C, Genain G. Diversity of hair growth profiles. *Int J Dermatol.* 2005;44(Suppl 1):6-9.

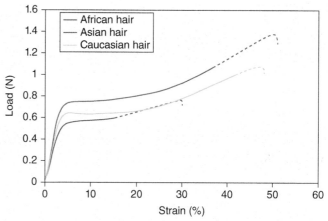

FIGURE 2-4. Differences in hair strength by race. (Reproduced with permission from Franbourg A, Hallegot P, Baltenneck F, et al: Current research on ethnic hair, *J Am Acad Dermatol* 2003 Jun;48(6 Suppl):S115-S119)

chemical relaxers, and locks. The most common scarring hair disorder seen in African Americans, central centrifugal cicatricial alopecia, has been linked to wearing tight braids. Thus, understanding the biological and cultural differences in this group is key to adequately addressing their dermatological needs[22] (see Chapter 37, Hair Care Practices: Complications, Treatments, and Prevention).

◾ COSMETIC DERMATOLOGY

In 2010, people with skin of color made up more than 25% of all patients seeking cosmetic procedures in the United States, and this number is projected to increase by the year 2050.[44,45] Traditionally, cosmetic dermatology has focused on antiaging measures primarily focusing on addressing rhytids. Multiple surveys conducted among populations with skin of color including Americans of Asian, Hispanic, and African origins suggest that pigmentary disorders such as postinflammatory hyperpigmentation and melasma rank higher as a cosmetic concern compared with rhytids. Currently, tools that exist to address pigmentation concerns, such as lasers and chemical peels, are less widely used in patients with skin of color, given the increased risk of scarring and pigmentary alteration in this population. Recently, dermatologists specializing in skin of color cosmetics have demonstrated that most cosmetic procedures including lasers can be safely performed in patients with skin of color and produce satisfactory cosmetic outcomes. As the population with skin of color grows and there is more demand for treatment of pigmentary alteration, dermatologists with experience in performing cosmetic procedures in this population will be in high demand.

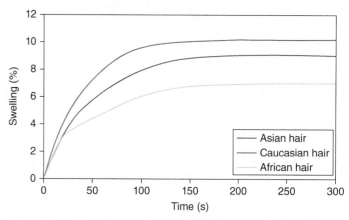

FIGURE 2-5. Water content of hair by race. (Reproduced with permission from Franbourg A, Hallegot P, Baltenneck F, et al: Current research on ethnic hair, *J Am Acad Dermatol* 2003 Jun;48(6 Suppl):S115-S119.)

CONCLUSION

The rapid increase in the populations with skin of color worldwide, coupled with their distinct cutaneous disorders, reaction patterns, and cultural habits and practices, ensures that textbooks highlighting skin of color are important and necessary for dermatology students, residents, physicians, and physician extenders. This textbook will provide both an informative reference guide and an in-depth view of all aspects of skin of color.

REFERENCES

1. Shoo BA, Kashani-Sabet M. Melanoma arising in African-, Asian-, Latino- and Native-American populations. *Semin Cutan Med Surg.* 2009;28:96-102.
2. PBS. *Go Deeper: Human Diversity.* A PBS Documentary on Race: The Power of an Illusion. www.pbs.org/race/000_About/002_04-godeeper.htm. Accessed January 7, 2015.
3. Piram M, Maldini C, Mahr A. Effect of race/ethnicity on risk, presentation and course of connective tissue diseases and primary systemic vasculitides. *Curr Opin Rheumatol.* 2012;24:193-200.
4. Jablonski NG, Chaplin G. Human skin pigmentation as an adaptation to UV radiation. *Proc Natl Acad Sci USA.* 2010;107:8962-8968.
5. Jablonski NG, Chaplin G. The evolution of human skin coloration. *J Hum Evol.* 2000;39:57-106.
5a. Loussouarn G, Garcel AL, Lozano I, et al. Worldwide diversity of hair curliness: a new method of assessment. *Int J Dermatol.* 2007;46(Suppl 1):2-6.
6. Chaplin G, Jablonski NG. Vitamin D and the evolution of human depigmentation. *Am J PhysAnthropol.* 2009;139:451-461.
7. Underhill PA, Passarino G, Lin AA, et al. The phylogeography of Y chromosome binary haplotypes and the origins of modern human population. *Ann Hum Genet.* 2001;65:43-62.
8. Brown MD, Hosseini SH, Torroni A, et al. MtDNA haplogroup X: An ancient link between Europe/western Asia and North America? *Am J Hum Genet.* 1998;63:1852-1861.
9. Rosenberg NA. Genetic structure of human populations. *Science.* 2003;300:1877.
10. Stephens JC. Haplotype variation and linkage disequilibrium in 313 human genes. *Science.* 2001;293:489-493.
11. Lamason RL. SLC24A5, a putative cation exchanger, affects pigmentation in zebrafish and humans. *Science.* 2005;310:1782-1786.
12. Campbell M, Tishkoff SA. African genetic diversity: implications for human demographic history, modern human origins and complex disease mapping. *Annu Rev Genomics Hum Genet.* 2008;9:403-433.
13. Seifert O, Mrowietz U. Keloid scarring: bench and bedside. *Arch Dermatol Res.* 2009;301:259-272.
14. Wolfram D, Tzankov A, Pülzl P, Piza-Katzer H. Hypertrophic scars and keloids: a review of their pathophysiology, risk factors, and therapeutic management. *Dermatol Surg.* 2009;35:171-181.
15. Liu WC. An 11 year review of dermatomyositis in Asians patients. *Ann Acad Med Singapore.* 2010;39:843-847.
16. Lau CS, Mok MY. Ethnic and geographical differences in systemic lupus erythematosus: an overview. *Lupus.* 2006;15:715-719.
17. Westney GE, Judson MA. Racial and ethnic disparities in sarcoidosis: from genetics to socioeconomics. *Clin Chest Med.* 2006;27:453-462.
18. Hinds GA, Heald P. Cutaneous T-cell lymphoma in skin of color. *J Am Acad Dermatol.* 2009;60:359-375.
19. Hicks-Graham S. Hidradenitis suppurativa. In: Kelly PA, Taylor SC, eds. *Dermatology for Skin of Color.* New York, NY: McGraw-Hill; 2009:276-280.
20. Sue S, Dhindsa MK. Ethnic and racial health disparities research: issues and problems. *Health Educ Behav.* 2006;33:459-469.
21. Kelly AP. Update on the management of keloids. *Semin Cutan Med Surg.* 2009;28:72-76.
22. Kyei A, Bergfeld W. Medical and environmental risk factors for the development of central centrifugal cicatricial alopecia. A population study. *Arch Dermatol.* 2011;147:909-914.
23. U.S. Census Bureau. Population Statistics 2010. www.census.gov/population/prod/cen2010/briefs/c2010br.pdf. Accessed January 7, 2015.
24. U.S. Census Bureau. Population Projections. www.census.gov/population/projections/data/national/2012/summarytables.html. Accessed January 7, 2015.
25. Taylor SC. Epidemiology of skin diseases in ethnic population. *Dermatol Clin.* 2002;21:601-607.
26. Taylor SC. Epidemiology of skin diseases in people of color. *Cutis.* 2003;71:271-275.
27. National Center for Health Statistics. Ambulatory healthcare data. www.cdc.gov/nchs/about/major/ahcd/sampnam.htm. Accessed January 7, 2015.
28. Orenstein A, Haik J, Tamir J, et al. Photodynamic therapy of cutaneous lymphoma using 5-aminolevulinic acid topical application. *Dermatol Surg.* 2000;26:765-769.
29. McDonald HC, Pandya AG. Cutaneous T-cell lymphoma. In: Kelly AP, Taylor SC, eds. *Dermatology for Skin of Color.* New York, NY: McGraw-Hill; 2009:300-305.
30. Hinds GA, Heald P. Cutaneous T-cell lymphoma in skin of color. *J Am Acad Dermatol.* 2009;60:359-375.
31. Bradford PT. Skin cancer in skin of color. *Dermatol Nurs.* 2009;21:170-206.
32. Jackson BA. Nonmelanoma skin cancer in persons of color. *Semin Cutan Med Surg.* 2009;28:93-95.
33. Sivayathorn A. Melasma in Orientals. *Clin Drug Invest.* 1995;10:34-63.
34. Lee CS, Lim HW. Cutaneous disease in Asians. *Dermatol Clin.* 2003;21:669-677.
35. Westney GE, Judson MA. Racial and ethnic disparities in sarcoidosis: from genetics to socioeconomics. *Clin Chest Med.* 2006;27:453-462.
36. Cozier YC, Berman JS. Sarcoidosis in black women in the United States. Data from the Black Women's Health Study. *Chest.* 2011;139:144-150.
37. Jacyk WK. Cutaneous sarcoidosis in black South Africans. *Int J Dermatol.* 1999;38:841-845.
38. Mayes MD. Race, scleroderma, and survival: why is there a difference? *J Rheumatol.* 2005;32:1873-1874.
39. Nietert PJ, Mitchell HC. Racial variations in clinical and immunological manifestations of systemic sclerosis. *J Rheumatol.* 2006;33:263-268.
40. Cao H, Pan M, Kang Y, et al. Clinical manifestations of dermatomyositis and clinical amyopathic dermatomyositis patients with positive expression of anti-melanoma differentiation-associated gene 5 antibody. *Arthritis Care Res.* 2012;64:1602-1610.
41. Camacho-Martinez FM. Hypertrichosis and hirsutism. In: Bologna JL, Jorizzo JL, Rapini RP, eds. *Dermatology.* Rio de Janeiro, Brazil: Elsevier Ltd.; 2003:1007-1018.
42. Loussouarn G. Diversity of hair growth profiles. *Int J Dermatol.* 2005;44:6-9.
43. Kelly AP. Pseudofolliculitis barbae and acne keloidalis nuchae. *Dermatol Clin.* 2003;21:645-653.
44. American Society of Plastic Surgeons. Cosmetic procedures up in all ethnic groups except Caucasians. http://www.plasticsurgery.org/News-and-Resources/Press-Release-Archives/2009-Press-Release-Archives/Cosmetic-Procedures-Up-in-All-Ethnic-Groups-Except-Caucasians-in-2008.html. Accessed January 15, 2015.
45. American Society of Plastic Surgeons. Briefing paper: plastic surgery for ethnic patients. http://www.plasticsurgery.org/news/plastic-surgery-for-ethnic-patients.html. Accessed January 15, 2015.

Epidemiology of Cutaneous Diseases

CHAPTER 3

Michael Bigby

KEY POINTS

- The epidemiology of a cutaneous disease can be expressed using the following four standard measurements: mortality, incidence, prevalence, and utilization of healthcare services.

- Commonly used racial classification systems lack biological validity, are inherently racist, and can be misleading.

- The incidence and mortality of melanoma are lower in people with skin of color.

- Data indicate that different racial groups seek treatment for different dermatologic disorders.

- Establishing a rapport and channels of honest communication with patients is more important in healthcare than pigeonholing patients into racial categories.

- Every patient deserves culturally competent care.

THE EPIDEMIOLOGY OF CUTANEOUS DISEASES

Cutaneous diseases—otherwise known as diseases of the skin—are very common. They can cause morbidity and have a significant impact on quality of life. With a few notable exceptions (eg, melanoma, toxic epidermal necrolysis, cutaneous T-cell lymphoma, and autoimmune bullous diseases), deaths from skin diseases are uncommon. This chapter will review the data on the descriptive epidemiology of cutaneous diseases using four commonly used measures: mortality, incidence, prevalence, and utilization of healthcare services.

The term *mortality* is used to indicate the number of deaths from a specific disease occurring in a population over a defined period of time. The *incidence* of a disease is the number of new cases occurring in a population over a defined period of time. Incidence and mortality are commonly expressed as numbers of cases or deaths, respectively, per 100,000 people per year. Accurate incidence and mortality data can be obtained only if cases or deaths are reliably identified and reported. It is mandatory to report a death and the cause of death in the United States. Therefore, fairly accurate estimates of mortality rates for skin diseases are available. In the United States, accurate incidence data for skin diseases are available only for a few diseases, including melanoma, nonmelanoma skin cancer, Kaposi sarcoma, and cutaneous T-cell lymphoma.

The *prevalence* of a disease is the number of cases in a population at a given time. It is a "snapshot" of the frequency at which a disease is present in a given population at a given time. Prevalence is best determined by performing a randomized survey of the population. *Healthcare service utilization* can be measured by determining the number of visits to physicians over a defined period of time for specific reasons (for instance, by looking at diagnoses or complaints). Such information can be obtained from data collected for other purposes (often in billing records or drug dispensations), or it can be obtained specifically to study resource utilization. To understand the data on the epidemiology of skin diseases in people with skin of color, the problems that arise from attempts to racially classify human populations must be addressed.

RACIAL CLASSIFICATION SYSTEMS: INHERENTLY RACIST AND LACKING BIOLOGICAL VALIDITY

The first scientific attempt to classify human populations into races in 1735 was written by Carl Linnaeus (1707–1778).[1] He divided the races into four groups that were described as follows: *white* (Europeans), who were "acute, gentle, and inventive"; *red* (Native Americans), who were "obstinate, merry, and free"; *dark* (Asians), who were "stiff, haughty, and avaricious"; and *black* (Africans), who were "phlegmatic, indolent, and negligent."[1]

The dictionary definition of a Caucasian is "a member of the peoples traditionally classified as the Caucasian race, especially those peoples having light to fair skin: no longer in technical use."[2] It was Johann Blumenbach (1752–1840) who introduced the term *Caucasian* into the medical lexicon in 1795.[3] He divided the races into five groups (ie, Caucasian, Mongolian, Ethiopian, American, and Malayan) and described Caucasians as "a beautiful people who derive their name from Mount Caucasus," referring to the Caucasus Mountain Range in the southwestern Soviet Union between the Black and Caspian seas. In fact, these people were not all "white," and this idea was actually derived from Jean Chardin (1643–1713), a French explorer who had traveled to Mount Caucasus and described the people.[3] As noted by Holubar, "When saying Caucasian, we should be aware of the historical origin of this term, of the fact that it is a misnomer, of the time when it entered scientific literature and what we may understand it to mean (and what not)."[3]

Thus, we come to the question: Who is "black" in America? It is also important to remember that race in America is a pervasive political and social construct. The designation of racial classifications is a product of our nation's history and has often been used to justify prejudice, discrimination, and segregation—for instance in separating those with rights (people with fairer skin) from those who could be sold as property (people with darker skin). It is a pervasive idea that is accepted legally and in the medical community that any person with a discernible feature of black skin of color *is* "black." This practice (known as the "one drop rule," which refers to one drop of "black" blood) makes a mockery of the notion that racial classifications can be of genetic or biological usefulness.[4]

The information collected regarding race has changed significantly over time from the inception of the U.S. Census in 1790, and it makes for fascinating reading.[5,6] Recognizing the inadequacy of the data collection system and the significant change in the demographics of the American population, the Census now classifies people into larger groups (using categories such as black, white, Asian, Pacific Islander, American Indian, Eskimo or Aleut, and many others), with the additional category of Hispanic (any of whom can also choose to classify themselves as one of the aforementioned racial groups).[5,6] The 2010 Census included 5 categories of "Hispanic" origin and 15 racial categories that could be chosen in separate questions.[7] Thus, there were potentially 75 different ethnic/origin groups. This system clearly makes as little sense genetically or biologically as its predecessors. Nonetheless, we are currently forced to deal with this morass of nomenclature; in this chapter, groups of people are referred to using the terms employed in the original references.

Modern genetic analyses have been used to separate people into genetically determined groups. Based on polymorphisms in mitochondrial DNA or in the Y chromosome, it is estimated that modern humans first appeared in East Africa about 44,000 years ago. Using polymorphisms in the Y chromosome, Underhill et al[8] were able to divide human populations into 21 distinct groups that roughly corresponded to the regions in the world where they were located. Similar results were obtained using polymorphisms in mitochondrial DNA.[9] Based on 100 Alu element polymorphisms examined in 565 people, four distinct groups were identified—two sub-Saharan African groups (Mbuti Pygmies and other), Europeans, and East Asians.[10] Alternatively, based on 375 short tandem repeats examined in 1000 people from 52 ethnic groups, five distinct groups were identified (sub-Saharan Africans, Europeans and Asians west of the Himalayas, East Asians, New Guineans, and Melanesians).[10] If a large enough number of polymorphisms are studied (ideally in the thousands), even smaller divisions of populations sharing genetic similarities can be made (for instance, in differentiating Chinese and Japanese groups, or Hispanic, African American, and European American groups).[11]

It is important to remember, however, that even when using modern genetic techniques to attempt to divide populations into distinct groups based on the frequency of genes expressed, the genetic variation within groups is greater than the variation between them. The average nucleotide diversity between two randomly chosen people is about 1 in 1000 to 1 in 500, or 0.2 to 3 million base pairs.[10,11] The nucleotide diversity between a human and a chimpanzee is about 1 in 100. Most human genetic variance is within the population variance (85% to 90%), with only 10% to 15% represented by between-population variance.[10,11]

The implicit assumption made in identifying a person's race in clinical medicine is that this racial group identification imparts useful genetic, and therefore biological, information about the person. Unfortunately, this is often not the case.[11-14] For example, recent attention has been paid to differences in the responsiveness between African Americans and European Americans to angiotensin-converting enzyme (ACE) inhibitors. A meta-analysis revealed that the mean difference in systolic blood pressure (BP) reduction between African Americans and European Americans was 4.6 mm Hg.[11,12] The standard deviation of the change was 12 and 14 mm Hg in African Americans and European Americans, respectively, indicating that the group's responses overlapped considerably and that a large number of African Americans will have significant diastolic BP reduction using ACE inhibitors.

At its worse, identifying a person's race in clinical medicine can be destructive or completely misleading. Thus the diagnosis of rosacea is often not considered in patients with skin of color because of the mistaken (or at least unsubstantiated) belief that rosacea is uncommon in this group.[14,15] A "black" patient with pityriasis rosea is more likely to be thought to have secondary syphilis (and have a rapid plasma reagin

[RPR] test done) than a "white" patient, even though the need for serologic testing in patients with a typical herald patch and rash is doubtful.[16] Therapeutic assumptions based on racial classification also abound. Many physicians are reluctant to use topical retinoids for "black" patients in the fear of provoking postinflammatory hyperpigmentation, despite a randomized, controlled clinical trial indicating that tretinoin is beneficial in reducing hyperpigmentation in patients with dark skin of color suffering from acne.[17,18]

EPIDEMIOLOGY OF CUTANEOUS DISEASES

MORTALITY

Skin diseases were estimated to cause 12,650 deaths in 2013, with melanoma (9480 deaths) and nonepithelial skin cancer (3170 deaths) accounting for this figure.[19] Melanoma mortality data by race and gender are available in the Surveillance, Epidemiology, and End Results (SEER) Program. Mortality from melanoma is significantly lower in people with skin of color [**Table 3-1**].[19]

Other nonepithelial mortality rates by race and gender are available using SEER Program statistics [**Table 3-2**]. Again, rates are highest in people classified as "whites," but only by a factor of two to three.

INCIDENCE

Melanoma incidence by race and gender are available from the SEER Program [**Table 3-3**].[20] The incidence of melanoma is significantly lower in people with skin of color. Fairly accurate estimates of the incidence of some skin cancers (eg, Kaposi sarcoma or cutaneous T-cell lymphoma) are available based on SEER data [**Table 3-4**].[20] Estimates are also available for several reportable diseases that have cutaneous manifestations (eg, syphilis, leprosy, or measles) based on reports to health departments. With these data, underreporting is a potential problem or limitation.

PREVALENCE

The only systematically collected data on the prevalence of skin diseases in the general population in the United States was collected as part of the National Health and Nutrition Examination Survey (NHANES).[21] Whereas 75% of participants were examined as part of this survey, with more than 20,000 Americans aged between 1 and 74 years old examined, the survey has three major weaknesses that limit its usefulness for determining the prevalence of disease in people with skin of color. First, the data were collected more than 20 years ago (1971 to 1974), and

TABLE 3-2	Other nonepithelial skin cancer mortality trends 2006–2010, per 100,000 people per year	
	Mortality	
Race/Ethnicity	Male	Female
All races	1.5	0.4
White	1.6	0.5
Black	0.8	0.2
Asian/Pacific Islander	0.3	0.1
American Indian/Alaska Native	1	^
Hispanic	0.7	0.2

Source: Reproduced with permission from Surveillance, Epidemiology, and End Results. SEER Stat Fact Sheets: other non-epithelial skin. http://seer.cancer.gov/statfacts/html/othskin.html. Accessed September 28, 2012.

therefore, the results do not reflect the demographics of today's population and may not reflect the current disease prevalence. Second, the only "race" categories included were "black," "white," and "other." Third, this racial category was "marked by observation." According to records, the interviewers were instructed to assume that the race of all related persons was the same as the respondent unless otherwise learned. The respondents were only asked about their race if the appropriate category could not be determined by observation. Because there were only three broad categories, interviewers were instructed to record persons who responded with something other than "white" or "black"—such as Japanese, Chinese, American Indian, Korean, Hindu, or Eskimo—as "other." Furthermore, they were told to include Mexicans, Puerto Ricans, and other persons of Latin American descent in the "white" category unless definitely "black," American Indian, or of another "nonwhite" race.[21]

These limitations notwithstanding, nearly a third of those examined had at least one skin lesion warranting a physician visit. The most common skin diseases were diseases of the sebaceous glands (acne), dermatophytosis, tumors, seborrheic dermatitis, atopic dermatitis, contact dermatitis, and ichthyosis/keratoses [**Table 3-5**].

More recently, the NHANES collected data on participants aged 20 to 59 years between 2005 and 2012. This included data regarding the number of moles, hair color, susceptibility to sunburn, personal and family history of melanoma, and presence of eczema or contact dermatitis. Additionally, photographs were taken to assess the presence of psoriasis or hand dermatitis. Race/ethnicity was determined by asking the participants and

TABLE 3-1	Melanoma mortality trends 2005–2009, per 100,000 people per year		
	Mortality		
Race/Ethnicity	All	Male	Female
All races	2.7	4.1	1.7
White[a]	3.1	4.6	2
White Hispanic	0.8	1.1	0.6
White non-Hispanic	3.4	5	2.1
Black	0.4	0.5	0.4
Asian/Pacific Islander	0.4	0.5	0.3
American Indian/Alaska Native	1.1	1.7	0.8
Hispanic[a]	0.8	1	0.6

[a]Hispanic and non-Hispanic are not mutually exclusive from whites, blacks, Asian/Pacific Islanders, and American Indians/Alaska Natives. Incidence data for Hispanics and non-Hispanics are based on the NAACCR Hispanic Identification Algorithm and exclude cases from the Alaska Native Registry. The 2005 to 2009 Hispanic and non-Hispanic death rates exclude deaths from the District of Columbia, North Dakota, and South Carolina. The 2000 to 2009 Hispanic and non-Hispanic mortality trends exclude deaths from Connecticut, the District of Columbia, Maine, Maryland, Minnesota, New Hampshire, New York, North Dakota, Oklahoma, South Carolina, and Vermont.

Source: Reproduced with permission from Surveillance, Epidemiology, and End Results. SEER Stat Fact Sheets: melanoma of the skin. http://seer.cancer.gov/statfacts/html/melan.html#incidence-mortality. Accessed October 22, 2012.

TABLE 3-3	Melanoma incidence trends 2005–2009, per 100,000 people per year		
	Incidence		
Race/Ethnicity	All	Male	Female
All races	21	27.2	16.7
White	24.7	31.6	19.9
White Hispanic[a]	4.5	4.7	4.6
White non-Hispanic[a]	28.8	36.4	23.5
Black	1	1.1	0.9
Asian/Pacific Islander	1.4	1.6	1.2
American Indian/Alaska Native	4.1	4.3	4
Hispanic[a]	4.5	4.7	4.6

[a]Hispanic and non-Hispanic are not mutually exclusive from whites, blacks, Asian/Pacific Islanders, and American Indians/Alaska Natives. Incidence data for Hispanics and non-Hispanics are based on the NAACCR Hispanic Identification Algorithm and exclude cases from the Alaska Native Registry. The 2005 to 2009 Hispanic and non-Hispanic death rates exclude deaths from the District of Columbia, North Dakota, and South Carolina. The 2000 to 2009 Hispanic and non-Hispanic mortality trends exclude deaths from Connecticut, the District of Columbia, Maine, Maryland, Minnesota, New Hampshire, New York, North Dakota, Oklahoma, South Carolina, and Vermont.

Source: Reproduced with permission from Surveillance, Epidemiology, and End Results. SEER Stat Fact Sheets: melanoma of the skin. http://seer.cancer.gov/statfacts/html/melan.html#incidence-mortality. Accessed October 22, 2012.

TABLE 3-4	Other nonepithelial skin cancer incidence trends 2006–2010, per 100,000 people per year	
	Incidence	
Race/Ethnicity	**Male**	**Female**
All races	2.7	1.4
White	2.9	1.4
Black	1.2	1.1
Asian/Pacific Islander	0.9	0.8
American Indian/Alaska Native	^	1.2
Hispanic	1.2	1

Source: Reproduced with permission from Surveillance, Epidemiology, and End Results. SEER Stat Fact Sheets: other non-epithelial skin. http://seer.cancer.gov/statfacts/html/othskin.html. Accessed September 28, 2012.

was first categorized as either Hispanic/Latino or non-Hispanic/Latino. The participants could then choose among one or more of the following: white, black/African American, Native American Indian, Alaskan Native, Native Hawaiian, Guamanian, Samoan, Asian Indian, Chinese, Filipino, Japanese, Korean, Vietnamese, or other Asian. Data from this survey were not readily available for analysis but may soon be.[22]

UTILIZATION OF HEALTHCARE RESOURCES

Several studies have been published that measured the reasons that people with skin of color seek dermatologic care [**Tables 3-6 to 3-9**].[23-28] In several instances, the frequencies of visits for different disorders were compared in different groups in the same locale. Halder et al[23] compared the reasons for visits to a predominantly black practice and a predominantly white practice in the Washington, DC, area. Pigmentary disorders, seborrheic dermatitis, dermatophytosis, alopecia, pityriasis versicolor, and keloids were the most common disorders prompting visits by patients with skin of color.

Alexis et al[24] compared the reasons for visits to the Skin of Color Center at St. Lukes-Roosevelt Hospital Center, New York, from August 2004 to July 2005. The most common disorders for patients with skin of color were acne, dyschromia, contact dermatitis, eczema, and seborrheic dermatitis [Table 3-6].

Davis et al[25] compared the reasons for visits to dermatologists and nondermatologists from 1993 to 2009 in the National Ambulatory Medical Care Survey (NAMCS). Acne, dermatitis, seborrheic dermatitis, atopic dermatitis, and dyschromia were the leading disorders prompting visits by African American patients to a dermatologist. In contrast, Caucasian patients were most commonly diagnosed with acne, dermatitis, actinic keratoses, viral warts, and sebaceous cysts [Table 3-7]. Visits that resulted in a single diagnosis of a dermatologic condition by any

TABLE 3-6	Reasons for visits to a hospital in New York, NY, United States	
	Percentage of visits (rank)	
Diagnosis	**Black**	**White**
Acne	28 (1)	21 (1)
Dyschromia	20 (2)	—
Dermatitis	9 (3)	11 (4)
Alopecia	8 (4)	—
Seborrheic dermatitis	7 (5)	7 (6)
Lesion or unspecified behavior	4 (6)	21 (2)
Hirsutism	4 (7)	—
Folliculitis	4 (8)	4 (10)
Atopic dermatitis	4 (9)	—
Keloid	3 (10)	—
Vitiligo	3 (11)	—
Sebaceous cyst	2 (12)	—
Other diseases of the sebaceous glands	2 (13)	—
Seborrheic keratosis	2 (14)	—
Benign neoplasm of the torso	—	12 (3)
Psoriasis	—	7 (5)
Rosacea	—	6 (7)
Actinic keratosis	—	6 (8)

physician are shown in Table 3-8. An interesting observation in this study was that African American and Hispanic patients were less likely than other groups to see a dermatologist for a sole diagnosis of a dermatologic condition, in terms of number of visits per year per population of 100,000.

Child et al[26] compared the reasons for visits to a single practice in London by individuals in the racial categories of black, white, and Asian patients [Table 3-9].[26] The population in the surrounding community was roughly 50% black, 40% white, and 10% Asian. Therefore, if the prevalence of disease was the same in each group, and each group was motivated to seek dermatologic care for similar reasons, it would be expected that, for each diagnosis, 50%, 40%, and 10% of the patients would be black, white, or Asian, respectively. However, the overwhelming majority of visits for acne keloidalis were by individuals in the black category. A disproportionately high percentage of visits for atopic dermatitis, alopecia areata, and keloids were from Asian patients. Similarly, hyperpigmentation was excessively high in the Asian and black patient groups. Additionally, psoriasis was extremely common in the Caucasian ethnic group compared with other groups.

TABLE 3-5	Prevalence of skin diseases					
		Prevalence by race				
Skin condition	**Number of cases**	**All**	**White (n = 16,351)**	**Black (n = 4163)**	**Other (n = 235)**	
Dermatophytosis	1227	0.059	0.057	0.067	0.094	
Acne vulgaris	1198	0.058	0.059	0.054	0.068	
Seborrheic dermatitis	436	0.021	0.022	0.017	0.009	
Atopic dermatitis	337	0.016	0.015	0.017	0.056	
Psoriasis	145	0.007	0.008	0.002	0.000	
Ichthyosis/keratosis	120	0.006	0.005	0.007	0.000	
Vitiligo	95	0.005	0.004	0.006	0.000	
Verruca vulgaris	91	0.004	0.005	0.002	0.004	
Folliculitis	70	0.003	0.004	0.002	0.000	
Herpes simplex	61	0.003	0.004	0.001	0.000	

Source: Reproduced with permission from National Health and Nutrition Examination Survey (NHANES). Public use data tape documentation: dermatology, ages 1–74, tape number 4151. www.cdc.gov/nchs/data/nhanes/nhanesi/4151.pdf. Accessed September 28, 2012.

TABLE 3-7   Reasons for visits to dermatologists

	Reason for visit (%)		
African American	Asian or Pacific Islander	White	Hispanic
Acne (22)	Acne (19)	Actinic keratosis (15)	Acne (22)
Dermatitis (14)	Dermatitis (18)	Acne (15)	Dermatitis (13)
Seborrheic dermatitis (8)	Benign neoplasm (6)	Benign neoplasm (8)	Psoriasis (7)
Atopic dermatitis (6)	Psoriasis (5)	Dermatitis (8)	Benign neoplasm (6)
Dyschromia (5)	Seborrheic keratosis (5)	NMSC (7)	Warts (5)
Psoriasis (4)	Atopic dermatitis (5)	Seborrheic keratosis (6)	Actinic keratosis (4)
Alopecia (4)	Warts (4)	Warts (6)	Seborrheic keratosis (4)
Keloids (3)	Urticaria (3)	Psoriasis (4)	Cysts (4)
Warts (3)	Cysts (3)	Rosacea (4)	Rosacea (3)
Cysts (3)	Seborrheic dermatitis (3)	Cysts (4)	Dyschromia (3)

Abbreviation: NMSC, nonmelanoma skin cancer.

Source: Data from Davis SA, Narahari S, Feldman SR, et al. Top dermatologic conditions in patients of color: an analysis of nationally representative data. *J Drugs Dermatol.* 2012 Apr;11(4):466-473.

TABLE 3-8   Reasons for visits to physicians for a sole diagnosis of a dermatologic condition

	Reasons by race/ethnicity				
Rank order	African American	Asian/Pacific Islander	White	Hispanic/Latino	Non-Hispanic
1	Dermatitis	Dermatitis	Acne	Dermatitis	Dermatitis
2	Acne	Acne	Dermatitis	Acne	Acne
3	Dermatophytosis	Atopic dermatitis	Actinic keratosis	Cysts	Actinic keratosis
4	Cysts	Urticaria	Viral warts	Viral warts	Viral warts
5	Cellulitis/abscess	Psoriasis	Cysts	Cellulitis/abscess	Cysts
6	Atopic dermatitis	Viral warts	Nonmelanoma skin cancer	Psoriasis	Nonmelanoma skin cancer
7	Candidiasis	Rash/skin eruption	Benign neoplasm	Rash/skin eruption	Benign neoplasm
8	Rash/skin eruption	Cellulitis/abscess	Psoriasis	Scabies	Psoriasis
9	Dermatophytosis	Benign neoplasm	Unspecified skin disorder	Urticaria	Unspecified skin disorder
10	Keloid scar	Cysts	Cellulitis/abscess	Atopic dermatitis	Cellulitis/abscess

Source: Data from Davis SA, Narahari S, Feldman SR, et al. Top dermatologic conditions in patients of color: an analysis of nationally representative data. *J Drugs Dermatol.* 2012 Apr;11(4):466-473.

TABLE 3-9   Comparison of frequency of reasons for visits to a single practice in London, United Kingdom, by racial group

Disorder	African origin (%)	Caucasian origin (%)	Asian origin (%)
Acne	51	41	8
Acne keloidalis	95	5	0
Atopic dermatitis	32	50	18
Psoriasis	7.5	82	11
Keloids	60	8.5	32
Pityriasis versicolor	48	35	17
Hyperpigmentation	73	9	18
Alopecia areata	29	48	24
Dermatofibroma	13	75	13
Urticaria	32	53	15
Sarcoidosis[a]	100	0	0
Lupus[a]	47	41	12
Traction alopecia[a]	100	0	0
Pigmentation of the nail/sole[a]	100	0	0

[a]Few patients seen.

Source: Adapted with permission from Child FJ, Fuller LC, Higgins EM, et al. A study of the spectrum of skin disease occurring in a black population in south-east London. *Br J Dermatol.* 1999 Sep;141(3):512-527.

TABLE 3-10	Recommendations for caring for patients from different cultures
Be courteous.	
Understand missed or late appointments.	
Be self-aware.	
Avoid stereotyping and labeling.	
Understand "maladaptive" behaviors.	
Be aware of potential patient distrust.	
Be aware of your and your patient's energy.	
Discover the patient's experiences.	
Learn the patient's attribution.	

Source: Data from Levy DR. White doctors and black patients: influence of race on the doctor-patient relationship. *Pediatrics.* 1985;75:639-643. Used with permission.

The most common reasons for dermatologic consultations have been studied among adults with dark skin of color in the United Kingdom,[21] as well as in children in Singapore and Kuwait.[27,28] Interestingly, what is most striking about the results is that the reasons for the dermatologic consultations are so similar between the populations.

Nevertheless, it is important to remember that the reasons for dermatologic visits cannot be taken as a proxy for the prevalence of disease in different groups. Many other factors, such as the severity, the impact on quality of life, the availability and cost of care, and other competing concerns, play a role in why and when patients seek medical attention.

CONCLUSION

WHAT DO PATIENTS WANT?

In caring for patients, establishing communication is far more important than pigeonholing them into racial categories. Effective communication between the doctor and patient, a skill not emphasized in medical education programs, is essential for patient satisfaction and optimal patient care. In many teaching hospitals, the doctor is commonly white and middle class, and the patient is "of color" and indigent. Racial and cultural differences, even in the absence of social class differences, may have a negative impact on the quality of the physician–patient relationship. Levy[29] reviewed the impact of racism on healthcare delivery and made recommendations to enhance the relationship between doctors and patients [**Table 3-10**]. His recommendations are even more germane given the increasing diversity of populations of patients and medical care providers in all countries. All patients deserve culturally competent care.[29,30]

REFERENCES

1. Morro J. Race: is it a valid issue? http://www-personal.umich.edu/~jonmorro/race.html. Accessed September 28, 2012.
2. Dictionary.com. Caucasian. http://dictionary.reference.com/browse/caucasian?s=t. Accessed September 28, 2012.
3. Holubar K. What is a Caucasian? *J Invest Dermatol.* 1996;106:800.
4. Davis FJ. *Who Is Black? One Nation's Definition.* University Park, PA: Pennsylvania State University Press; 1991.
5. Wikipedia. Race and ethnicity in the United States Census. http://en.wikipedia.org/wiki/Race_and_ethnicity_in_the_United_States_Census. Accessed September 28, 2012.
6. U.S. Census Bureau. What is race? Updated April 29, 2013. http://www.census.gov/population/race/. Accessed October 21, 2013.
7. Population Reference Bureau. The 2010 census questionnaire: seven questions for everyone. http://www.prb.org/Articles/2009/questionnaire.aspx. Accessed September 28, 2012.
8. Underhill PA, Shen P, Lin AA, et al. Y chromosome sequence variation and the history of human populations. *Nat Genet.* 2000;26:358-361.
9. Jorde LB, Watkins WS, Bamshad MJ, et al. The distribution of human genetic diversity: a comparison of mitochondrial, autosomal, and Y-chromosome data. *Am J Hum Genet.* 2000;66:979-988.
10. Bamshad MJ, Olson SE. Does race exist? *Sci Am.* 2003;289:78-85.
11. Jorde LB, Wooding SP. Genetic variation, classification and "race." *Nat Genet.* 2004;36:S28-S33.
12. Lorusso L. The justification of race in biological explanation. *J Med Ethics.* 2011;37:535-539.
13. Witzig R. The medicalization of race: scientific legitimization of a flawed social construct. *Ann Intern Med.* 1996;125:675-679.
14. Bigby M, Thaler D. Describing patients' "race" in clinical presentations should be abandoned. *J Am Acad Dermatol.* 2006;54:1074-1076.
15. Alexis AF. Rosacea in patients with skin of color: uncommon but not rare. *Cutis.* 2010;86:60-62.
16. Horn T, Kazakis A. Pityriasis rosea and the need for a serologic test for syphilis. *Cutis.* 1987;39:81-82.
17. Bulengo-Ransby SM, Griffiths CE, Kimbrough-Green CK, et al. Topical tretinoin (retinoic acid) therapy for hyperpigmented lesions caused by inflammation of the skin in black patients. *N Engl J Med.* 1993;328:1438-1443.
18. Chan R, Park KC, Lee MH. A randomized controlled trial of the efficacy and safety of a fixed triple combination (fluocinolone acetonide 0.01%, hydroquinone 4%, tretinoin 0.05%) compared with hydroquinone 4% cream in Asian patients with moderate to severe melisma. *Br J Dermatol.* 2008;159:697-703.
19. Surveillance, Epidemiology, and End Results. Previous version: browse the SEER Cancer Statistics Review 1975-2009. http://seer.cancer.gov/csr/1975_2009_pops09/browse_csr.php?section=16&page=sect_16_table.15.html. Accessed September 28, 2012.
20. Surveillance, Epidemiology, and End Results. SEER Stat Fact Sheets: other nonepithelial skin. http://seer.cancer.gov/statfacts/html/othskin.html. Accessed September 28, 2012.
21. Centers for Disease Control and Prevention. National Health and Nutrition Examination Survey. http://www.cdc.gov/nchs/nhanes/nhanesi.htm. Accessed September 28, 2012.
22. Centers for Disease Control and Prevention. National Health and Nutrition Examination Survey: Dermatology Procedures Manual. http://www.cdc.gov/nchs/data/nhanes/nhanes_03_04/dermmanual_03_04.pdf. Accessed September 28, 2012.
23. Halder RM, Grimes PE, McLaurin CI, et al. Incidence of common dermatoses in a predominantly black dermatologic practice. *Cutis.* 1983;32:388-390.
24. Alexis AF, Sergay AB, Taylor SC. Common dermatologic disorders in skin of color: a comparative practice survey. *Cutis.* 2007;80:387-393.
25. Davis SA, Narahari S, Feldman SR, et al. Top dermatologic conditions in patients of color: an analysis of nationally representative data. *J Drugs Dermatol.* 2012;11:466-473.
26. Child FJ, Fuller LC, Higgins EM, et al. A study of the spectrum of skin disease occurring in a black population in south-east London. *Br J Dermatol.* 1999;141:512-517.
27. Chua-Ty G, Goh CL, Koh SL. Pattern of skin diseases at the National Skin Center (Singapore) from 1989-1990. *Int J Dermatol.* 1992;31:555-559.
28. Nanda A, Al-Hasawi F, Alsaleh QA. A prospective survey of pediatric dermatology clinic patients in Kuwait: an analysis of 10,000 cases. *Pediatr Dermatol.* 1999;16:6-11.
29. Levy DR. White doctors and black patients: influence of race on the doctor-patient relationship. *Pediatrics.* 1985;75:639-643.
30. Dy SM, Purnell TS. Key concepts relevant to quality of complex and shared decision-making in healthcare: a literature review. *Soc Sci Med.* 2012;74:582-587.

CHAPTER 4

Multicultural Competence in Dermatologic Practice

Flora N. Taylor
Raechele Cochran Gathers

KEY POINTS

- Limitations on treatment time and lack of cultural understanding often cause culturally competent care to be sidelined.
- To empathize with a patient's cultural issues, the physician should explore his or her own background, using the tools provided in this chapter.
- Intake procedures should incorporate a cultural assessment, and provisions should be made for non–English-speaking patients.
- Multiculturally competent care can improve patient outcomes.

In the current healthcare community, the skills associated with providing culturally competent healthcare are more greatly appreciated than ever before. Unfortunately, many healthcare professionals still fail to provide health services that respect the health beliefs, practices, and cultural and linguistic needs of their patients. For a variety of reasons, including limited treatment time and ignorance, providing culturally competent healthcare may be sidelined in the service of expediting patient visits. A common physician complaint is that there is not enough time to focus on anything beyond the patient's presenting illness. The approach described in this chapter attempts to help practitioners identify the value of putting healthcare in a multicultural context and how this can actually help physicians to provide better medical care to their patients. A very important step toward this is to build a connection with patients by learning to value one's own cultural identity. To this end, this chapter begins with exercises for clinicians aimed at improving their personal understanding of the potential importance of a patient's individual cultural identity.

A LOOK WITHIN

Some might question the necessity of physicians investigating their own cultural identity in order to provide culturally competent care for their patients. However, this process is very significant because a fundamental component of the physician–patient relationship is empathy, which requires the capacity to vicariously identify with the feelings or experiences of others. With respect to identity, we are unfortunately well aware that empowered groups can lose touch with—or perhaps never understand to begin with—the difficulties that are faced by those who are less privileged. Psychologically, it takes more effort to empathize with others than to ignore them; this may be due to a variety of reasons, most pertinently an instinct for self-protection. Hence, it may be easier and less time consuming for physicians to ignore the cultural identities of their patients; however, this does a great disservice to the patient and undermines the doctor–patient relationship.

The current demographics of the United States are changing rapidly, and it is estimated that the majority of American citizens by 2050 will be individuals with skin of color. The Hispanic population, already the nation's largest minority group, will triple in size and will account for most of the nation's population growth through 2050. Additionally, Hispanic Americans will compose 29% of the population of the United States by this time, compared with 14% in 2005. Similarly, the Asian American population is expected to grow to almost 10% of the population. In contrast, the Caucasian American population will increase more slowly than other racial and ethnic groups; it is estimated that this group will be a minority by 2050 (at 47%).[1,2]

The relevance of cultural competence is most evident in the area of healthcare disparities. Health disparities are defined as the "differences in incidence, prevalence, morbidity, mortality, and burden of diseases, [as well as] other adverse health conditions that exist among specific population groups."[3,4] Cultural differences between the patient and provider, if left unaddressed, may contribute to poor health outcomes through misunderstandings, value conflicts, and disparate concepts of what constitutes health and illness.[5] One of the most conspicuous examples of health disparity within the dermatologic field is the rates of diagnosis and survival of skin cancer for Latino and African American patients compared to Caucasian patients. In 2009, a retrospective analysis study in Florida examined the incidence of melanoma and the stage of the tumors at diagnosis among patients with lighter or darker skin of color between 1990 and 2009. The authors reported that both Hispanic and Africa American patients had significantly more advanced melanoma (at the regional or distant stage) upon presentation (18% and 26%, respectively) compared with Caucasian patients (12%).[6] Another study, conducted in California, found that 15% of Hispanic male patients were diagnosed with a melanoma after it had already metastasized, compared with only 6% of non-Hispanic white male patients.[7] These disparities are alarming because a late diagnosis means that the disease has a greater chance of rapid progression, distant metastases, and higher morbidity and mortality. The 5-year melanoma survival rate has been reported as 74.1% for black patients, compared with 92.9% for white patients. Furthermore, although nonmelanoma skin cancer is relatively rare in black individuals, with an incidence of 3.4 per 100,000, there is a greater risk of these individuals presenting with both later stage and more aggressive squamous cell carcinomas.[8]

The explanations for these health disparities are wide-ranging, encompassing possible biological factors that make certain subtypes of aggressive melanoma and nonmelanoma skin cancers more common in non-Caucasian populations; sociocultural factors, including the potentially limited access to quality healthcare among ethnic minorities, lack of transportation, and decreased health literacy; traditional or cultural health beliefs, such as poor insight into skin cancer risk factors[9]; and the lack of public education targeted at non-Caucasian patients on the importance of sun protection and skin cancer screening. Although public health campaigns aimed at educating the public about common risk factors for skin cancer, such as having light eyes, hair, and skin, have been both robust and successful, they may inadvertently suggest to those with differing physical characteristics that they are less at risk for skin cancer and that sun protection and skin cancer screening are less of a concern.[10] Research has shown that the lack of a perceived risk is a barrier to reducing the incidence of skin cancers.[11] It is important that both dermatologists and public health groups carefully tailor their messages of the risk of skin cancer and the importance of sunscreen and dermatologic check-ups to ensure that all at-risk groups are adequately and effectively targeted.

Patients, although they may be reluctant to state it, keenly feel the personal interest, or lack thereof, of their doctor. Sometimes patients will keep such observations private, out of embarrassment or for fear of creating an even greater distance between the doctor and themselves. Alternatively, some patients may simply choose to see another physician instead or continue seeing their current doctor and limit visits to absolute emergencies due to their uncomfortable rapport. In a study evaluating several domains from the Consumer Assessment of Healthcare Providers and Systems Cultural Competence measure, diabetic patients' reports of trust in their primary care physician were associated with better glycemic control. This study provided empirical evidence for an association between the patient–physician relationship and a measurable health outcome.[12] Empathy and a good doctor–patient rapport have been found to be more important to minority patients than to nonminority patients.[13] Similarly, African American, Hispanic, and Asian patients have been found to rate concern, courtesy, and respect as the most important factors in their interactions with healthcare providers.[14-16] Acknowledging and exploring their own identities will allow physicians to appreciate the value of a cultural identity for their patients. This will result in a more holistic standard of care, with patients feeling that they are seen as individuals, and not simply as carriers of a particular disease constellation or lesion. In this scenario, the patient and the physician can form a more effective partnership (or a group if the patient's extended family is involved), and this will result in greater health benefits for the patient. Toward this goal, please take a moment to complete the questions found in **Table 4-1** that are designed to encourage healthcare providers to reflect on their own multicultural heritage and attitudes.

Physicians are encouraged to take a moment to think about what may have surprised them in their answers to this self-quiz. The following questions may occur: Have you thought about these issues before? Are you a person who tends to give a great deal of meaning to cultural or multicultural issues? Are you a person who tends to give little attention to the cultural aspects of identity? Physicians may then wish to consider what might happen if these questions, and the corresponding answers, are discussed with those with whom they work most closely. The self-quiz was designed to help practitioners develop greater cultural empathy by providing a basis for understanding how a physician's own cultural identity and attitudes may interact with and affect their treatment of patients.

TABLE 4-1	Physicians' cultural self-quiz

1. Do you know your maternal and paternal ethnic/racial designation(s)? What are they? Do they affect the way you think about your identity?

2. Have you ever considered how your cultural background might shape the way in which you respond to the healthcare system when seeking medical services?

3. Can you recall stories about how your family has responded to the healthcare system (eg, refusals to seek treatment because of "old-fashioned" fears, a blanket reverence toward all doctors, a blanket distrust of healthcare providers as a group, or an acceptance of healthcare providers due to a certain gender, race, or organizational affiliation only)?

4. With which cultural groups do you associate yourself? In answering this question, do you consider regional affiliation, religion, gender, or sexual orientation? These, too, are considered to be culture-loaded designations.

Exacerbated by the economic pressure that managed healthcare may add to an already heavy workload, many doctors are encouraged to treat their patients as quickly as possible. This means that it is all too easy to lose touch with patients, particularly regarding the cultural components of a person's identity. It is also easy to assume that, if a patient looks or talks like you, he or she will automatically feel understood on a cultural level. Additionally, many doctors may conclude that a patient who looks like them is of the same cultural group. Neither of these assumptions may be true. Similarly, the opposite assumption may apply, with practitioners, rightly or not, assuming alternate cultural backgrounds for patients who have different physical appearances. Although some practitioners may be more careful to ensure that communication is smooth and accurate, they may quite often unintentionally ignore other possible cultural implications of the patient's behavior. Many doctors treat their patient's lesion, ache, or pain, assuming that this will be sufficient—it is, after all, why the patient has come to see them. Are patients well served by physicians and other healthcare providers working from this assumption?

So, what *is* the point? How does culture relate to healthcare provision? We will argue that, although it may sometimes be outside of the provider's awareness, the provision of healthcare is nonetheless deeply affected by the cultural aspects of the interaction. How the individual physician and patient see and understand health and illness is very much tied to their respective cultures. If culture affects the way in which an individual beholds the world, then it will also affect the way this individual sees health and illness. A practitioner who appreciates the influence of culture on a patient's receptivity to treatments is better positioned to connect with the patient, form a strong working alliance with the patient, and subsequently elicit the patient's cooperation in his or her own treatment.

DEFINING OUR TERMS

Perhaps some definitions of the concepts used in this chapter will help the reader with terminology that may initially appear to be amorphous, including terms such as *culture, multicultural, cultural competence,* and *multiculturally competent healthcare. Culture* is a commonly used term, but one that is not so easily defined. This is largely due to the broadness of the term, because it can be used to refer to periods of time (for instance, as in the culture of the 1980s), regional distinctions (as one can refer to *culture shock* after moving to a different country or region), ethnic/racial distinctions, religious distinctions, and even workplace distinctions (as in *corporate culture*). When a group is referred to as being *of the same culture,* this may indicate people who associate themselves with each other according to many possible dimensions. For example, geographical boundaries may suggest some cultural affiliations—on the national level, as well as the subnational level (eg, the differences in culture between southern, eastern, and midwestern states), and maybe even within the same region (eg, the culture of the suburbs compared with the city). Therefore, culture, which is often immediately interpreted as racially or ethnically based and visually identifiable by variations in dress, food, music, language, and the like, can alternatively be charged with regional, religious, political, economic, and other affiliations. Essentially, the crucial factor to remember about culture is that individuals acknowledge the affiliation that groups them into a particular culture and that customs, beliefs, and worldviews are, in part, shaped by this affiliation.[17,18]

Hidalgo[18] parses the term *culture* into three levels: concrete, behavioral, and symbolic. At the concrete level, she refers to the cultural factors *that can be seen,* such as food, dress, and music. These elements might be thought of as the "fun" aspects of a culture. At the behavioral level, she refers to the behaviors and actions *that people do,* such as the language people use and the way in which they speak, as well as how they construct family, gender, and other social roles. Therefore, although less visible than, for instance, the type of food that is eaten, this level of culture could be said to describe who provides for, buys, prepares, eats, and then cleans up the food. At the third level, the symbolic level, which is even less visible than the preceding two levels, Hidalgo isolates how individuals within a group *define themselves,* such as through intellectual or spiritual concepts such as a religion, worldview, spiritual beliefs, traditional customs, and many others. Continuing with food as our example to unify the three levels, the symbolic application would be why an individual does or does not eat certain foods and how the eating (or not) of certain foods helps to define who that individual is.

Differentiating these three levels of culture is helpful to the practitioner. An awareness of the concrete level of culture will help patients to feel that they are *seen* by their doctor. On the other hand, recognition of the behavioral level will enable doctors to understand how their patient fits within their external social system. The social system in which an individual lives is likely to affect or impact his or her health. For example, whose role is it to bring children to seek medical care? Is there a familial or social role that forbids illness or a specific set of illnesses associated with undesired lifestyle choices or habits? Finally, an awareness of the third symbolic level on the part of the healthcare provider will enhance a broader understanding of the world and the way in which this patient and his or her affiliations fit into that context. For example, in the excellent nonfiction film, *Worlds Apart,* a Western doctor comes to understand and accept a Laotian mother's hesitation about allowing crucial heart surgery for her daughter, based on fears that the child will become too scarred to subsequently be accepted into the afterlife.[19] In this way, the opportunity for continued care is sustained by receptivity and acceptance, rather than potentially being destroyed by intolerance, impatience, and misunderstanding.

Multiculturalism is a term that became prominent in the early 1980s and had its initial introduction in the early 1960s within educational disciplines.[20] Some of the pioneers to promote the importance of multicultural classrooms were Canadian. Margai and Frazier[21] posit that the term multiculturalism in the United States came about in the 1960s, during the Civil Rights Movement, as a reaction by African Americans to the "melting pot" theory. This theory promoted the development and advancement of one greater American identity despite the actual diversity of the American populace. However, as the U.S. population grew to include a greater proportion of Asian and Latin immigrants and, following that, other minority groups including the gay and disabled communities, "this required a more inclusive multiculturalism, one seeking social tolerance and a broader representation from a diverse American population in the discussion of global, national and local matters."[21] Concretely, a multicultural classroom is one that has posters and other audiovisual materials that reflect the backgrounds of the children who are learning in that particular classroom. Behaviorally, it means recruiting and admitting students who represent a broad spectrum of cultures and nationalities. Symbolically, it means integrating the students' differences—whether these are religious, racial, or socioeconomic differences—into the fabric of the educational institution (eg, in the school calendar or the teachers' and professors' training) in such a way that the success of a multicultural student body is supported by the entire institution.

The term *multiculturalism* is hard to define. It is a simple term, yet seeks to encompass within its meaning most of the other terms used within this chapter. It is often defined as a doctrine that promotes the idea that "several different cultures (rather than one national culture) can coexist peacefully and equitably in a single country."[22] As a term, it does not refer exclusively to ethnic and racial groupings, although these are often included within its meaning. In an absolute sense, multiculturalism "recognizes the broad scope of [the] dimensions of race, ethnicity, language, sexual orientation, gender, age, disability, class status, education, religious/spiritual orientation, and other cultural dimensions."[19] Multiculturalism may be thought of as a theoretical "container" that allows more space to explore and contain the intricacies of an individual's identity. This includes understanding and respecting the many different ways in which individuals choose to identify themselves. Furthermore, multiculturalism also allows a community to avoid the monopolization or domination of a single culture within a setting. For example, in a multicultural classroom, it is expected that the readings, materials, posters, students, and teachers will represent a combination of cultures—in this way, all cultures will feel valued.

One way to determine the level of awareness regarding an individual's multicultural thumbprint is to complete a sociogram [**Figure 4-1**]. The template seen here can help the reader think about his or her multiculturalism. The circle in the center of the diagram represents the individual, with the spokes of the wheel representing branches of the individual's identity. These may include, for example, level of education, religion, religiosity, regional background, sexual orientation, marital status, parenthood status, race, occupation, ethnicity, socioeconomic status, and gender, among others. It is advised that readers take a few minutes to create their own sociogram. It would be appropriate for individuals to use the aspects of identity that hold the most meaning for them and, if desired, to add spokes to their wheel. Once the sociogram is completed, readers may wish to consider the follow-up questions: (1) What emotions were felt upon completion of the sociogram? Emotion elicited from this exercise may include familiarity/unfamiliarity, comfort/discomfort, and satisfaction/distaste. (2) Were certain aspects of identity more difficult than others? How so? (3) Are there others who would know without being told the aspects identified on the sociogram? (4) Imagine that each patient has a sociogram that describes important aspects of his or her identity. Would recognition of this fact (either with or without knowing the full details of such a sociogram) allow the physician to connect more fully with the patient?

It is important to go one step further with this issue by considering how awareness of multiculturalism in individuals can be helpful to

Guide for Self-Reflection

• Identify the cultural groups to which you belong. Label each circle (add or subtract circles as per your unique experience).

• Note an experience that you associate with each group membership in each circle.

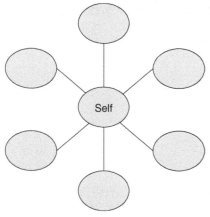

FIGURE 4-1. A sociogram template.

patients in an institutional context. If, for example, the professional and administrative staff of a large practice has an appreciation for and an understanding of the importance of multicultural factors in patient care, it can be understood that this practice is developing its multicultural competence. The definition of *cultural competence* is "a set of congruent behaviors, attitudes, and policies that come together in a system, agency, or among professionals that enables effective work in cross-cultural situations."[22] This includes providing services that are respectful of and responsive to the health beliefs, practices, and cultural and linguistic needs of diverse patient populations.[22]

The significance of cultural competence in dermatologic care cannot be overemphasized. The dermatologic specialty is a largely visual and external one, focusing on maladies of culturally laden entities, such as the hair, skin, and nails. Therefore, issues of diversity of cultures are likely to come up daily in many dermatologic practices. Concerns about acne and dyspigmentation have been cited to be the top two reasons for seeking care among African American patients.[23] It is imperative that the treating dermatologist should have a thorough knowledge of the unique presentation and sequelae of acne in patients with skin of color. Although a practitioner may understandably be more focused on controlling the condition, this may not be the case for the patient. For example, patients with skin of color suffering from acne may be significantly distressed by the scars, dark marks, and dyspigmentation left behind by the acne and not by the acne lesions themselves.[24] With an understanding of cultural competency, the dermatologist will be able to address not just the acne, but also the patient's significant distress due to any subsequent dyspigmentation. In this way, the dermatologist may prescribe acne medication for the primary condition, as well as medications aimed at limiting any dyspigmentation. Additionally, the dermatologist would also address the significance of sunscreen, which is often underused by patients with skin of color, in ameliorating the condition.

Another area in which cultural competence is relevant to dermatologic care is in the management of cosmetic concerns. Patients with skin of color represent the fastest growing group of consumers seeking cosmetic dermatologic care. Between 1999 and 2005, the percentage of African Americans and Latinos seeking skin rejuvenation increased by 49% and 89%, respectively. Even as an increasing numbers of patients with skin of color seek out cosmetic rejuvenation procedures, key areas of difference in skin of color must be respected. The treating physician should be knowledgeable regarding the response of skin of color to certain types of chemical peels, laser treatments, and light and heat modalities, which can often lead to complications such as dyspigmentation or scarring. Similarly, certain surgical procedures may elicit a keloid response more commonly in patients with skin of color, and it is incumbent on the treating physician to recognize this and take both detailed personal and family scar histories, as well as appropriately counsel patients on their individual risk factors before recommending any procedure.

Issues of cultural competence may be especially prevalent in encounters with black patients suffering from hair or scalp issues. Issues regarding the hair or scalp are an exceedingly common reason for black patients to seek dermatologic care. Alopecia has been reported as the fourth most common reason for black patients to visit a dermatologist. In contrast, alopecia does not even rank in the top 10 diagnoses among white patients.[23] With this knowledge, it logically follows that practicing dermatologists should expect to encounter a fair number of hair and scalp complaints among their black patients and should be well versed in both the differential diagnosis of common hair and scalp diseases in these patients and the importance of offering culturally competent treatments. For example, the clinician should be familiar with differences in hair growth and morphology patterns in black patients and should be aware of differences in shampoo frequency and the preference for ointment or oil-based medications versus lotion or solution-based medications. Additionally, the clinician should recognize popular hairstyles and grooming techniques in different patient populations and understand both the dermatologic pitfalls and best practices associated with these techniques. For example, for a black woman who braids her hair, a simple recommendation to take out the braid if it begins to cause pain can significantly reduce the likelihood of this patient developing traction alopecia. Similarly, for a patient suffering from seborrheic dermatitis, the straightforward suggestions of washing hair weekly instead of monthly and the application of a topical corticosteroid oil or ointment can have a positive impact on both the treatment outcome and patient compliance. Likewise, educating a black patient regarding the maladies of tight and frequent hair weaving, the ills associated with irritating weave and wig glues, and the risk of hair breakage and scalp damage that can occur with hair relaxers if applied too frequently or incorrectly will go a long way toward improving the outcome. It is paramount that treating physicians should seek out information on cultural groups, particularly regarding potentially unique disorders with which they may be unfamiliar.

Any discomfort that is felt by the care provider does not go unnoticed by the patient. In an unpublished study from the metropolitan region of Detroit, Michigan, 28% of African American women sought physician care for a hair or scalp concern. However, only 32% of these patients felt that their treating physician understood African American hair. Therefore, it is not surprising that, in a U.S. survey, 47% of dermatologists and dermatology residents reported that their medical training was inadequate in educating them on skin conditions in black patients.[25] In another study, only 52.4% of dermatology chief residents and 65.9% of program directors reported that their programs integrated education on skin of color skin into the curriculum.[26] These statistics support the necessity for greater exposure among dermatology trainees to measures designed to enhance education on skin of color dermatology. These may take the form of lectures, peer-reviewed literature, immersion experiences, texts, guest lecturers, and teaching staff with a focus and expertise in skin of color dermatology. These measures will increase awareness, knowledge, and confidence among dermatologists as they care for an increasingly diverse patient population and will allow them to deliver the highest quality of care to their patients.

Kleinman[27] offers a list of cultural assessment questions [shown in **Table 4-2**] that practitioners may choose to include in their intake procedures to collect more culturally sensitive information.[27] Information like this could be collected from the patient by a medical assistant should the physician feel that there is insufficient time to gather these data within a clinical interview. In this case, the interviewer must be trained in identifying, as well as quickly and reliably communicating, any key information so that the physician can then make use of the information in the initial patient assessment.

Once intake procedures integrate more fully the multicultural identities of patients, dermatologists will have access to additional information concerning their patients. This may enable them to consider the patient as a whole and thereby discover interesting and informative patterns of epidemiologic behavior or incidence. The questions in **Table 4-3** are designed to aid a physician in eliciting their patients' cultural fingerprints.

Physicians may identify patterns that describe the patients they tend to treat. These patterns will have implications for multicultural competence. If, for example, a dermatologist is based in West Philadelphia, Pennsylvania, which has a large community of recent Hmong immigrants and first- and second-generation Hmong children, the dermatologist may require a professional translator. Additionally, the dermatologist may also need to educate himself regarding Hmong medical decision-making practices and hierarchies and to understand the role of traditional healers within the culture. Forms, resource pamphlets, and the like may need to be provided in multiple languages to the patient. For these scenarios, as well as others, the physician may find it useful to consider the practice issues outlined in **Table 4-4**.

CONCLUSION

Humans have a tendency, long-honed during their race for survival, to cling to the familiar. The desire for familiarity can be found in many different aspects of identity, including race, ethnicity, gender, sexual orientation, age, and religion, among others—all aspects of culture, as we have attempted to convey in this chapter. Given this understanding, we

TABLE 4-2	Cultural assessment questions to incorporate in the patient intake procedure

Cultural assessment

1. Where were you born?
2. If you were born outside of the United States, how long have you lived in this country?
3. Who are the people you depend on the most for help (family members, friends, community services, church, etc.)?
4. Are there people who depend on you for care? Who are they? What kind of care do you provide?
5. What languages do you speak?
6. Can you read and write in those languages?
7. What is the first thing you do when you feel ill?
8. Do you ever see a native healer or other type of practitioner when you don't feel well?
9. What does this native healer or other type of practitioner do for you?
10. Do you ever take any herbs or alternative/traditional medicines that are commonly used in your native country or cultural group?
11. What are these herbs or alternative/traditional medicines, and what do you take them for?
12. What foods do you generally eat? How many times a day do you eat?
13. How do you spend your day?
14. How did you get here today?
15. Do you generally have to arrange for transportation when you have appointments?

Health beliefs

1. What do you call your health problem? What name does it have?
2. What do you think caused your health problem?
3. Why do you think your health problem started when it did?
4. What does your sickness do to you? How does it work?
5. How severe is your health problem? Will it have a short or long course?
6. What do you fear most about your disorder?
7. What are the chief problems that your sickness has caused for you?
8. What kind of treatment do you think you should receive? What are the most important results you hope to receive from treatment?

Further questions to consider

1. Do individuals in this culture feel comfortable answering questions?
2. Does the patient or family perceive a provider asking questions as a lack of knowledge?
3. Who should be told about the illness?
4. Does the family need a consensus, or can one person make health-related decisions?
5. Does the patient feel uncomfortable because of the gender of the provider?
6. Is the quantity of medicine associated by the patient with the severity of the illness?
7. Is the absence of medication associated by the patient with health?
8. Does the patient prefer to feel the symptoms or mask them?
9. Does the patient prefer one solution or multiple choices of treatment?
10. Does the patient want to hear about his or her risks?

can anticipate that patients presenting themselves for care may hesitate to let go of their preexisting beliefs, even in the face of seemingly incontrovertible scientific evidence. Here is a final anecdote to illustrate the problem as well as a proposed solution:[28]

A 40-year-old African American female patient approached Dr. Susan Taylor, one of the editors of this textbook, with a scalp condition that requires the application of medication to the wet scalp. At the follow-up visit, the patient complained that she had become sick as a result of leaving her home with wet hair. Attempts to reason with the patient were unsuccessful, with the patient stating that she had heard the information before but that there was nothing that could be said to change her mind on the issue. Dr. Susan Taylor proceeded to consult with Dr Flora Taylor in order

TABLE 4-3	Questions to aid the physician in identifying patient populations

- Who is your patient base? Take a moment to consider your patient base.
- Do you treat more women than men?
- Do you treat more Caucasians than Asians?
- Do you treat more Hispanics than African Americans?
- Do you treat more West Indians than African Americans?
- Do you treat more Caucasians of northern versus southern European decent?
- Is there an enclave of ethnic immigrants that your practice serves?
- Do you serve more first-, second-, or third-generation immigrants?
- Do you serve more high-, middle-, or low-income clients?
- Do you serve more rural, urban, or suburban dwellers?
- Do you treat a large number of patients who speak English as a first language?
- Do you treat a large number of patients who speak English as a second language or perhaps no English at all?
- Do you treat a large number of patients who are extremely religious versus patients who are not at all religious?
- What religions are practiced by the patients you serve?
- Do you treat more older, middle-age, or younger clients?
- Do you serve gay clients who are open regarding their sexual preference?
- Do you serve gay clients who are "closeted" or secretive regarding their sexual preference?
- Which groups of patients do you serve that are not culturally described by the preceding questions?

to find a culturally competent frame through which to understand and resolve the problem.

The real question is this: What is the patient's investment in maintaining the belief that wet hair can lead to a cold, despite considerable scientific evidence to the contrary? The patient must clearly gain something from her beliefs and actions or there would be no reason for her to cling to them so insistently. Dr. Flora Taylor shared with Dr. Susan Taylor some potential explanations for the patient's viewpoint and persistence: (1) that the patient's mother and grandmother may have inculcated this belief; (2) that to go against this belief may seem to be a sign of disrespect to her ancestors; and (3) that her belief had probably been reinforced coincidentally on many occasions, much in the same way that superstitions develop. It is important to remember that familial and cultural beliefs are extremely powerful! We cling to them just as we cling to parts of our identity, and we may even feel gratified by the "folksiness" of

TABLE 4-4	Questions to determine whether a practice is culturally sensitive

- Does the practice provide magazines, posters, signs, and other reading material in languages that all or most of the patients can understand?
- Does the practice provide or have access to a translator, especially a professional one, when clients need one (and not only when they ask for one)?
- Is the receptionist trained to skillfully and sensitively handle patients who can neither read nor write English or perhaps any language?
- Does the practice provide resource information relevant to the life issues of clients who sit in the waiting room?
- Do the practitioners know enough about their patients' culture to be able to ask pertinent questions about how their culture and their perception of their illness may interface?
- If the medical assistant flags a multicultural item on intake, does the practitioner feel sufficiently comfortable to discuss it with their patient?
- Does the practitioner include any multicultural questions in their own face-to-face interview of the patient that elevates the importance of those questions in the patient's perception?
- Would the practice consider having a consultant visit their office anonymously to assess its multicultural competence without informing staff?

a belief. Dr. Flora Taylor recommended that Dr. Susan Taylor try sharing a personal belief of her own as a way of aligning herself with the patient and building trust.

Beyond that, as a physician, it is sometimes necessary to compromise with a patient in order to encourage the patient's compliance with a medical regimen. To this end, Dr. Susan Taylor suggested that the patient wear a hat over her wet hair when leaving the house.

This anecdote offers an example of how the perception of illness can be influenced by culture. This chapter has attempted to provide information about the importance and methods of providing multiculturally competent medical care to patients. This includes, on the medical side, analysis of the results from several dermatologic studies that specifically inform the practitioner of patient concerns. Furthermore, on the psychological side, this chapter has offered several exercises that physicians can perform to help raise their awareness of the cultural aspects of their identities. The premise for this chapter is the notion that, by becoming both culturally and multiculturally aware, clinicians can provide more comprehensive and, therefore, superior care to their patients; in turn, these patients will respond by being more cooperative with their physician. These two factors combined will likely result in better outcomes for patients. To conclude, one small but extremely important improvement toward cultural sensitivity that healthcare providers could implement, which would take relatively little effort but reap a huge benefit, would be to learn to pronounce each patient's name fully and correctly upon their first meeting.[21] At the very least, patients have a right to expect that the very basics of their identity, as represented by their first and last name, will be respected by their doctor. Any potential stumbling and/or repetition that may be required to accomplish this task is small payment for the benefits reaped in the patient–physician relationship. In the end, not only is a multicultural approach a winning one, but it is also increasingly the only viable approach available, as demographic patterns continue to change worldwide.

REFERENCES

1. U.S. Census Bureau. U.S. Census Bureau projections show a slower growing, older, more diverse nation a half century from now. http://www.census.gov/newsroom/releases/archives/population/cb12-243.html. Accessed September 25, 2013.
2. U.S. Census Bureau. Population projections. www.census.gov/population/projections/data/national/2012/summarytables.html. Accessed September 15, 2013.
3. National Institutes of Health. Strategic research plan and budget to reduce and ultimately eliminate health disparities. Volume I: fiscal years 2002-2006. http://www.nimhd.nih.gov/our_programs/strategic/pubs/VolumeI_031003EDrev.pdf. Accessed July 5, 2009.
4. Hernandez C, Mermelstein RJ. A conceptual framework for advancing melanoma health disparities research. *Arch Dermatol.* 2009;145:1442-1446.
5. Lie D, Carter-Pokras O, Braun B, et al. What do health literacy and cultural competence have in common? Calling for a collaborative health professional pedagogy. *J Health Commun.* 2012;17:13-22.
6. Hu S, Parmet Y, Allen G, et al. Disparity in melanoma: a trend analysis of melanoma incidence and stage at diagnosis among whites, Hispanics, and blacks in Florida. *Arch Dermatol.* 2009;145:1369-1374.
7. Cress RD, Holly EA. Incidence of cutaneous melanoma among non-Hispanic whites, Hispanics, Asians, and blacks: an analysis of California Cancer Registry data, 1988-93. *Cancer Causes Control.* 1997;8:246-252.
8. Buster KJ, Stevens EI, Elmets CA. Dermatologic health disparities. *Dermatol Clin.* 2012;30:53-59.
9. Pipitone M, Robinson JK, Camara C, et al. Skin cancer awareness in suburban employees: a Hispanic perspective. *J Am Acad Dermatol.* 2002;47:118-123.
10. Taylor SC, Heath C. Cultural competence and unique concerns in patients with ethnic skin. *J Drugs Dermatol.* 2012;11:460-465.
11. Buster KJ, You Z, Fouad M, et al. Skin cancer risk perceptions: a comparison across ethnicity, age, education, gender, and income. *J Am Acad Dermatol.* 2012;66:771-779.
12. Fernandez A, Seligman H, Quan J, et al. Associations between aspects of culturally competent care and clinical outcomes among patients with diabetes. *Med Care.* 2012;50:S74-S79.

13. Ngo-Metzger Q, Telfair J, Sorkin D, et al. Cultural competency and quality of care: obtaining the patient's perspective. http://www.commonwealthfund.org/Publications/Fund-Reports/2006/Oct/Cultural-Competency-and-Quality-of-Care–Obtaining-the-Patients-Perspective.aspx. Accessed October 20, 2013.

14. Murray-García JL, Selby JV, Schmittdiel J, et al. Racial and ethnic differences in a patient survey: patients' values, ratings, and reports regarding physician primary care performance in a large health maintenance organization. *Med Care*. 2000;38:300-310.

15. Nápoles-Springer AM, Santoyo J, Houston K, et al. Patients' perceptions of cultural factors affecting the quality of their medical encounters. *Health Expect*. 2005;8:4-17.

16. Weech-Maldonado R, Carle A, Weidmer B, et al. The consumer assessment of healthcare providers and systems (CAHPS) cultural competence (CC) item set. *Med Care*. 2012;50:S22-S31.

17. American Psychological Association. Guidelines on multicultural education, training, research, practice, and organizational change for psychologists. www.apa.org/pi/multiculturalguideleines/definitions.html. Accessed March 6, 2004.

18. Hidalgo N. Multicultural teacher introspection. In: Fraser J, Perry T, eds. *Freedom's Plow: Teaching in the Multicultural Classroom*. New York, NY: Routledge; 1993:99-106.

19. Grainger-Monsen M, Haslett J. *Worlds Apart: A Four-Part Series on Cross-Cultural Healthcare*. http://www.fanlight.com/catalog/films/912_wa.php. Accessed October 29, 2013.

20. Gorski PC. The challenge of defining "multicultural education." http://www.edchange.org/multicultural/initial.html. Accessed October 20, 2013.

21. Margai FM, Frazier JW. Multiculturalism and multicultural education in the United States: the contributory role of geography. http://www.sunypress.edu/pdf/62241.pdf. Accessed October 29, 2013.

22. U.S. Department of Health and Human Services, Office of Minority Health. What is cultural competency? http://minorityhealth.hhs.gov/templates/browse.aspx?lvl=2&lvlID=11. Accessed September 5, 2013.

23. Alexis AF, Sergay AB, Taylor SC. Common dermatologic disorders in skin of color: a comparative practice survey. *Cutis*. 2007;80:387-394.

24. Jones E, Downie J. African-American skin remedies and folk healing practices. In: Kelly AP, Taylor SC, eds. *Dermatology for Skin of Color*. Beijing, China: McGraw-Hill Medical; 2009:48-52.

25. Buster KJ, Yang L, Elmets CA. Are dermatologists confident in treating skin disease in African-Americans? *J Invest Dermatol Meeting Abstr*. 2011; abstract 235.

26. Nijhawan RI, Jacob SE, Woolery-Lloyd H. Skin of color education in dermatology residency programs: does residency training reflect the changing demographics of the United States? *J Am Acad Dermatol*. 2008;59:615-618.

27. Kleinman A. *Patients and Healers in the Context of Culture: An Exploration of the Borderland Between Anthropology, Medicine, and Psychiatry*. Oakland, CA: University of California Press; 1980.

28. Taylor S. Dr. Taylor and Dr. Taylor solve a problem. http://www.huffingtonpost.com/dr-susan-taylor/dr-taylor-and-dr-taylor-solve-a-problem_b_3307480.html. Accessed October 29, 2013.

CHAPTER
5

Impact of Traditional Cultures on Healthcare Practices: An Overview

Marta I. Rendon
Jorge I. Gaviria

KEY POINTS

- Physicians need to understand the traditional cultural attitudes, beliefs, and values of their African, Asian, and Hispanic patients, because these may affect healing practices.

- Genetic, environmental, ethnic, and socioeconomic factors may play roles in the etiology and treatment of a disease.

- Minority Americans typically receive poorer healthcare than Caucasian Americans.

- The increased awareness of racial and cultural differences has encouraged more egalitarian healthcare delivery systems in America.

More than 5000 distinct ethnic groups exist in the world today. As people migrate to the United States and other developed countries in search of jobs, they bring along a broad collection of traditional customs and cultural beliefs. In its relatively short existence, the United States has become a melting pot of colors and cultures. In 1998, only 28% of the U.S. population was comprised of ethnic and racial minorities. By 2060, this figure is expected to reach 57%.[1,2] In many metropolitan areas, cultural diversification has become the norm; Miami, for example, has the largest foreign-born population of any city in the world and is home to African Americans, Caucasian Americans, and Americans from Cuba, Central America, South America, and the Caribbean. New York and Los Angeles also have large foreign-born populations.[3] Even historically homogeneous states—like Wisconsin or Iowa in the American Midwest, for example—are seeing a dramatic influx of immigrants, which is changing their demographic profiles.

Little has been published in the dermatologic literature on how cultural influences affect healthcare practices or physician–patient relationships. This chapter will attempt to shed light on this issue. It is clear that, as physicians, our cultural backgrounds influence how we communicate with patients and how patients respond to us. To deliver the best possible care, we must understand culturally driven, health-related behaviors and adapt our practices to accommodate them. Failure to do so may result in noncompliance or potentially harmful interactions between folk remedies and prescription medications, as well as missed opportunities for prevention or intervention.[4,5]

Attitudes toward illness have changed dramatically since the 1970s, to the benefit of physicians and patients alike, when the dominant model of illness was strictly biomedical. No room was left for the cultural, behavioral, psychological, or social dimensions that affect illness. Fortunately, it is generally accepted today that the social sciences can be used to bridge the gap between clinical medicine and specific cultural groups; biopsychosocial models are now being incorporated into medical school curricula, research, and teaching.

THE PROBLEM OF DEFINING RACIAL AND ETHNIC GROUPS

Defining the criteria for a specific ethnic group can be difficult. The term *African American* implies a family origin in Africa. The first Africans with skin of color were brought to the New World by Spanish conquistadors and slave traders in the sixteenth century. The first colonies were located in northern South American countries, such as Colombia and Venezuela, and in the Caribbean countries of Cuba, the Dominican Republic, Jamaica, Haiti, the Antilles, and Puerto Rico. Shortly thereafter, slaves were introduced to the English colonies of the current United States. Contemporary African Americans represent, inter alia, a mixture of Africans, Caucasians, and Native Americans.

Many native English-speaking people with skin of color in the United States consider themselves African Americans, whereas people with skin of color from Spanish- and French-speaking heritages tend to identify with their country of origin rather than Africa and prefer to be known as a descendant of that country—for example, as a Cuban American or Haitian American—rather than as an African American.

The term *Hispanic* is used widely in reference to people born in Central and South America, and the official use of the name in the United States has its origins in the 1970 Census.[6] The terms *Latino* and *Hispanic* are often used interchangeably.

The term *Asian American* refers to those of Asian heritage; Asian Americans are the second fastest growing population after Hispanics and the most ethnically diverse minority group in the United States. In the Census, *Asian* is used to designate individuals with heritages from any countries lying between Europe and the Pacific Ocean. In common practice, however, it describes people from countries in western Asia.

As a note, *Indian* literally means "from India." Originally, Christopher Columbus incorrectly called Native Americans "Indians," because he believed he had arrived in India, and did not realize that he had alighted in the New World. The correct term for the indigenous people of the continental United States is *Native Americans*; in Alaska, it is *Alaska Natives*; in Canada, it is *Canadian Natives* or *Canadian Aboriginals*; in South America, it is *Colombian, Peruvian, Bolivian,* or *Brazilian Natives*.

The conventional practice of clustering individuals into the four broad categories mentioned earlier—those of African, Asian, Caucasian, or Hispanic origin—risks perpetuating outdated stereotypes. Calling all Asians "Chinese" or all those with skin of color "African Americans" results in the bracketing together of people from very different cultures and socioeconomic strata who may have very little in common. A fairer-skinned individual from the Dominican Republic living in the United States may have nothing in common with a Dominican or a Mexican with dark skin of color, even though they may all speak Spanish. In contrast, a Haitian with skin of color may have no common ground with a Jamaican, an Ethiopian, or a Cuban with skin of color.

It behooves every physician to be aware of the differences between various cultures and to treat patients in a manner that reflects an understanding of their unique cultural characteristics.[5] Respect is key, and an open mind is essential in understanding how patients' beliefs can affect their health and their responses to treatment suggestions. Patients bring their cultural and ideological beliefs with them when they seek healthcare. As a dermatologist, these traditional beliefs may challenge or contradict professional opinions on the best medical practice or approach. Cultural insensitivity and/or disrespect may result in patient noncompliance or ineffective physician–patient relationships. Understanding and respecting cultural beliefs are critical to gaining a patient's trust and respect and in establishing a relationship that will ultimately benefit the patient.

COMMUNICATION AND LANGUAGE BARRIERS

Communication presents one of the biggest challenges faced by physicians and other healthcare providers. Language barriers, the real meaning of certain words, the use of telephones, and how much information is given and by whom are all important issues. Interpreters are not always accessible or available, and some groups—for example, South Asians (those from Afghanistan, Bangladesh, Bhutan, India, Nepal, Pakistan, or Sri Lanka) and those from China, Hong Kong, Korea, or Vietnam—may prefer same-sex physicians, nurses, and translators. In certain cultures, some patients are uncomfortable discussing sexual matters, sexually transmitted diseases, or illegal drug use. For instance, Hispanic Americans or those of Arab origin are generally too embarrassed to discuss personal and sexual matters with their physicians. For Hispanics, discussing or admitting to mental illness is taboo, with strong social prohibitions; they may have great difficulty communicating about mental illness issues in close family members. Others can be reluctant to communicate using the telephone, preferring face-to-face discussions. African Americans and Hispanics are less likely than Caucasian Americans to find the prescription of antidepressant medications acceptable.[7,8] A study found that physicians are 1.52 times more likely to prescribe antidepressant medication for Caucasian Americans than for Hispanics or African Americans with the same disorder. Whether this is due to institutionalized racism or because sociologic factors influence prescribing behaviors is unknown.[8]

Although diversities exist among the Hispanic subcultures, a fundamental value is *confianza* (trust and confidence); non-Hispanic healthcare providers may encounter patient resistance if they do not actively seek to establish trust prior to providing care.[9] Furthermore, patients expect their healthcare interactions to be friendly, personal, and respectful. Concepts of *simpatia* (compassion) and *respeto* (respect) are also highly valued in Hispanic/Latino culture. Verbal and nonverbal communications with Hispanic patients usually demonstrate *respeto*; it is extremely important that this is reciprocal, especially when the patients are older.[9]

In patients for whom English is a second language, communicating complex medical information can be a challenge. Some Asian languages—for example, the one spoken by the Hmong population of Laos—lack specific medical terminology, making a direct translation impossible. Language barriers in healthcare present a challenge that

requires culturally competent providers; this can obviously lead to serious misunderstandings.[10,11] To help reduce the impact of miscommunication, multilingual resources and high-quality, carefully verified translations of necessary information should be used by healthcare providers who treat substantial numbers of patients from particular backgrounds.

TRADITIONAL ATTITUDES, BELIEFS, AND PERCEPTIONS

It is important to become familiar with the traditional healing techniques and preferences used by various racial and ethnic groups to integrate these practices into individual healthcare plans. A good place to start is the report on policies and strategies regarding traditional medicine released by the World Health Organization (WHO).[12] In addition, the National Center for Complementary and Alternative Medicine (NCCAM), a division of the National Institutes of Health, offers meetings, workshops, and financial support for clinical trials designed to increase understanding of alternative and complementary medicines used in the United States.[13]

▇ AFRICAN AMERICANS

Four centuries of African American history in the United States have ensured that a large portion of the population has very specific health needs, markedly different cultural beliefs, and socioeconomic disparities—all of which affect their healthcare. Two questions that arise from studies of healthcare in African Americans, which can also be extrapolated to some Asian American and Hispanic groups, are as follows: (1) Why do these groups receive poorer quality healthcare than Caucasian Americans? (2) Why do they suffer from some diseases more often than Caucasian Americans?

African Americans as a whole suffer disproportionally from diseases such as stroke, hypertension, diabetes, obesity, and peripheral vascular disease[14,15]; yet cultural factors may play a role in the lower number of referrals for surgery.[16] Substantial delays exist between the diagnosis and treatment of breast cancer in African American women versus Caucasian American women between the ages of 20 and 54 years, but the exact contribution of cultural beliefs, diet, and genetics is unclear.[17] It is significant that although Caucasian American women have the highest incidence rate for breast cancer, African American women are still most likely to die from the disease.[18] African American men tend to bear a disproportionate burden for disease compared to other ethnic and racial groups[19]; for example, African American men have the highest incidence rate for prostate cancer in the United States and are more than twice as likely to die of this disease as Caucasian men.[18] Due to the differences between the genders, African American men are more likely to hold attitudes and beliefs that negatively affect their well-being, including beliefs related to masculinity.[19]

A recent survey of the health beliefs of African American patients provided evidence that most patients hold unconventional beliefs about the origins of asthma and lung cancer and the risks of smoking. Furthermore, these patients tended to have negative opinions of standard medical and surgical treatments and preferred using complementary or alternative medicines. In fact, it was found that the vast majority of complementary/alternative medicines and health behaviors were considered safe, with very few being thought of as unsafe.[20] Therefore, it is very important for healthcare providers to discuss any unconventional beliefs with the patients, in a respectful way, because there is an increased risk that these patients will resort to potentially dangerous alternative treatments.[20]

Unfortunately, there are still prejudices within the healthcare system in the United States. A survey by Peek et al in 2010 focused on factors that influence the process of shared decision-making, in which the patient and physician work together to agree on a healthcare plan. Participants identified two main issues that could influence the physician's behavior toward the patient: physician bias or discrimination and cultural discordance. This was often evidenced by the healthcare provider being less likely to share information, such as test results, and more likely to be domineering with African American patients.[21] However, mistrust of non–African American physicians and internalized racism were recorded as patient-related issues on the part of African American patients. In these ways, patients were less forthcoming with their health-care provider about health information and were less likely to adhere to treatment regimens.[21] These patient- and physician-related barriers may significantly hinder the relationship and process of shared decision-making between African American patients and their physicians.[21]

ASIAN AMERICANS

Asians tend to treat healthcare providers with respect and view them as authority figures. Asian patients may not ask questions concerning treatment options or other health-related issues because asking questions is often considered disrespectful in their culture. Patient information is usually discussed with the family and not the patient. Most South Asian patients are not accustomed to being informed of every detail of their diagnosis, particularly if the diagnosis is negative. In these circumstances, the family acts as a buffer to determine what the patient should and should not be told.

Unlike Caucasian Americans, higher levels of education, average household income, and insurance are not associated with better access to healthcare among Asian Americans.[22] Nevertheless, Asian Americans with high school or college degrees have 41% to 53% lower odds of having a regular healthcare provider compared with those with graduate degrees, as well as those without insurance.[22]

In terms of religion and spirituality, those who follow Buddhist or Confucian doctrines may view illness as a natural way of life. Symptoms may be seen as simply bad luck, misfortune, the result of poor karma, or potentially as payback for something done in the past. They also may view health as a balance between complementary energies, such as cold and hot, and traditional treatments are often preferred over Western medications.

Bracelets, beads, and other symbolic jewelry are sacred for some Hindus, Muslims, and Sikhs, and cannot be removed without family permission to do so. In addition, observant Sikhs do not cut their hair. When hair must be cut or jewelry removed for surgery, physicians are advised to discuss the dilemma with a family member or a religious leader of the patient's faith.

HISPANICS

Both Hispanics who have recently arrived in the United States and those born and raised there may share similar values, languages, and health-care beliefs. Although they may share Spanish as a common language, marked differences in socioeconomic status among their countries of origin and the presence of very different cultures create strong differences between Hispanics of Caribbean, Central American, and South American origin. A recent study by Erwin et al[23] demonstrated that country of origin and current residential location in the United States significantly impacted the perspectives of Hispanic/Latino women on many issues, including their anatomic knowledge, experiences within the medical system, and access to healthcare services.

In the 1970s and early 1980s, Latino immigrants primarily came from lower socioeconomic classes. A lower socioeconomic class is generally accompanied by a lack of medical insurance and perhaps a tendency toward noncompliance with physicians' recommendations. Starting in the 1990s, the United States began experiencing a wave of educated middle- and upper-class immigrants leaving South America to escape political instability.

For Hispanics, alternative treatment can be seen as a way of life. In one particular survey, 17% of Hispanics initially sought healthcare from a folk healer, 32% used a healthcare professional, and the remainder opted for self-treatment.[12] Some Hispanics tend not to have regular healthcare, and Hispanics are twice as likely to use emergency room services as the general population.[24] Hispanics in lower socioeconomic circumstances are not accustomed to making use of routine medical care. Some of them do not have access to adequate healthcare due to either a lack of insurance or a lack of knowledge regarding the healthcare system.

Therefore, some medical issues are left untreated, and these patients may eventually end up in an emergency room for acute or critical care. A survey of Puerto Rican patients suffering from hypertension revealed that 21% relied solely on herbal preparations or teas to treat their condition. Although Puerto Rico has been a territory of the United States for more than 100 years, a lack of education, the absence of healthcare policies, and different cultural beliefs regarding medical treatments continue to interfere with proper medical treatment.[25] Food plays an important cultural role in every Caribbean, Central American, and South American country, and poor dietary habits and traditional cultural practices may well account for the propensity of these ethnic groups toward diabetes, hypertension, and obesity.[26]

Culturally, family loyalty (which may extend to members of the extended family and not solely the immediate family) is considered to overshadow the needs of the individual. This concept is known as *familismo*.[27] This means that decisions regarding the patient's treatment options or lifestyle changes will need to be discussed with the entire family, lengthening the decision-making process; however, it is also a strong motivational tool and support setting for patients who have diseases that require self-management.[27] Additionally, traditional gender roles tend to apply in Hispanic families, with men as providers and women as the primary caretakers[9]; as a result, women may have more healthcare knowledge. This may mean that male Hispanic or Latino patients will refer to their wives and mothers for healthcare advice, rather than visiting a physician or healthcare practitioner, or that these female family members may accompany male patients on healthcare visits.[27]

The Hispanic *machismo* (attitudes associated with masculinity that mean men are expected to behave in certain ways) may discourage certain patients from scheduling an appointment in the first place—particularly because pain is often seen as a sign of weakness.[27] Furthermore, this cultural attitude may affect the patient's lifestyle, in that the patient may indulge in negative behaviors such as heavy drinking and risk-taking.[27]

Another cultural belief that may influence health behavior is *personalismo*, which is the patient's expectation of developing a personal relationship with his or her healthcare provider. Thus, some Hispanic patients may prefer their physician or healthcare provider to engage in close physical contact and show genuine interest in their life and activities beyond what is considered to be professional. In this case, a perceived lack of *personalismo* may result in patient dissatisfaction and, ultimately, in patients choosing not to return.[27] However, physical or verbal overfamiliarity (eg, in the casual use of first names) is not appreciated early in the patient–physician relationship.[9]

Traditional remedies may include psychotropic compounds, herbs, roots, stones, and seeds. Some of these remedies may have no scientific rationale and may even cause harm. Physicians should be reminded to ask about the use of home remedies and folk medicines to avoid any adverse reactions that may occur when these are combined with prescription drugs.[28,29]

RELIGION AND HEALTH

Among city-dwelling Hispanics, the use of *curanderos* is very common, particularly when the illness or disease is believed to have a supernatural cause. *Curanderos* are traditional healers believed to have received healing powers from God. *Sobadores* (masseuses) and *yerbateros* (herbalists) are also traditional healers.

One example of a traditional superstition in which diseases are caused supernaturally is the *mal de ojo*, or "evil eye," which is essentially a curse: Somebody causes harm to another just by looking at them or saying something about the future. To be cured, one must supposedly place an egg over the body and then keep this egg overnight in a bowl under the pillow. If the egg appears cooked by the morning, this is not only proof of the *mal de ojo*, but also a guarantee that it has now been removed from the victim. It is also believed that placing red and white seeds in a colorful wristband on a child's wrist within the first hours of life affords some protection from the evil eye.

In the Hispanic culture, many believe that God's will ultimately controls every aspect of an individual's life, such as disease. This is termed *fatalismo*, which refers to the belief that the disease process is a part of an individual's destiny and cannot be changed. This may result in patients being less likely to adhere to treatment plans or to actively manage their condition by changing their lifestyles.[27]

Although not a popular practice, *brujeria* (witchcraft) plays an important role in some cultures. A hex (*hechizo* or *maldicion*) can be placed on someone by a black witch (*bruja*) or another person who knows witchcraft. Symptoms often vary, but the cure usually involves Catholic prayers, herbs, massages, chili powder, medicinal enemas, showering with spices and vegetables, and making crosses with water and olive oil.

Santería (also called *Candomble, Quimbanda,* and *Umbanda* in Brazil), is an Afro-Cuban religious tradition derived from the traditional beliefs of people from Nigeria. This religious practice is similar to *Voodoo* and is often common to the people of the Caribbean, Brazil, and other countries in Central and South America. *Santería* comes from the Spanish word *santo,* meaning "saint," and practitioners are called *santeros.* Although slaves brought to the Caribbean Islands and Central and South America from Africa were converted to Catholicism, they preserved some of their traditions, fusing their traditional beliefs and rituals with elements of Catholicism. Today, any city with a large Latino population has many practicing *santeros* as well as Catholics, with many people choosing to practice both.

In cities such as Miami, New York, and Los Angeles, *botanicals* are a fundamental construct of some Latino communities. These are locations where *Santería* paraphernalia can be found. The practice of *Santería* and the use of recommended products from *botanicals* may replace physician advice and treatment or be used concomitantly with physician-prescribed medications.

Voodoo comes from an African word for "spirit." Slaves from Nigeria brought the religion with them to the New World, and although it was suppressed by colonial governments, it survived through the formation of underground societies. More than 60 million people practice *Voodoo;* they are located primarily in Haiti, the Dominican Republic, Ghana, Togo, and the southern United States (particularly Florida and Louisiana).[30-33] Ultimately, *Voodoo* is a fatalistic religion in that the *loa* (spirits) are forces that interact with people; although they can provide protection and luck, they can also bring about negative consequences, such as illness.[34] *Voodoo* priests (*houngan*) and priestesses (*mambo*) treat every conceivable ailment, from acquired immunodeficiency syndrome (AIDS) and cancer to lovesickness. Services include healing, rituals to contact or potentially calm the *loa,* prophecy, dream interpretation, spell casting, the creation of protection charms or potions, and revenge.[34] *Voodoo* practitioners may sometimes recommend working in tandem with Western physicians and sometimes interfere outright with a physician's recommendations. Unfortunately, some diseases are thought to be curable only by a *Voodoo* practitioner; seizure and psychiatric disorders are examples of problems that are traditionally thought to require treatment by a *houngan* or *mambo.*[34]

GENETIC RESPONSE TO DISEASE

Environmental conditions, ethnic and racial differences, genetic factors, and socioeconomic status play a complex role in the presence of disease.[35,36] Although the incidence of cancer has decreased in the African American, Asian American, and Hispanic populations, mortality rates remain higher for these groups than for Caucasian Americans.[18,37] Moreover, African Americans continue to suffer the greatest burden for each of the most common types of cancer.[18] Cigarette smoking and obesity are prevalent in the Latino population and may play a role in the higher incidence of cancer and other diseases related to these lifestyle factors. This being said, the age-adjusted death rates for cancer, heart disease, and stroke are lower for Hispanics than for African Americans or Caucasian Americans.[38,39]

Genetic factors found in different populations can affect the patient's response to certain medications; additionally, polymorphisms can cause differences in drug levels due to the absence or presence of drug-catabolizing enzymes. For example, Asians are known to be rapid metabolizers of codeine and suffer more adverse effects. In particular, Chinese individuals are more sensitive to the emetic effect of morphine and less sensitive to respiratory depression and hypotension. They also require less heparin and warfarin than Caucasian Americans to produce the same effects.

One area where racial differences are already well recognized is in the incidence and management of hypertension. Some research suggests that African Americans may carry a gene that makes them more sensitive to salt, which increases the risk of high blood pressure.[15] Changes in hypertension treatments are necessary to accommodate the different response by the renin-angiotensin system in people of African and Caribbean origin. The Joint National Committee on Prevention, Detection, Evaluation, and Treatment of High Blood Pressure advises low doses of thiazide diuretics as a first-line treatment in patients with skin of color. In contrast, they recommend angiotensin-converting enzyme (ACE) inhibitors or ß-blockers in young Caucasian American patients and ACE inhibitors for Caucasian or white patients over the age of 50 years. Asian Americans metabolize propranolol faster than African Americans, Hispanics, and Caucasian Americans. In general, Asian American patients achieve better hypertension control with calcium antagonists, diuretics, and ß-blockers.[40] Genetics play only a small part in the racial and ethnic differences in the health of a patient. Cultural and environmental factors may play a more influential role on health than genetics.

AN UNEQUAL HEALTHCARE DELIVERY SYSTEM

Minority groups do not fare as well as the Caucasian American majority in the U.S. healthcare system. Even after adjustments for insurance status and income, racial and ethnic minorities tend to have less access to healthcare and receive lower quality healthcare than nonminorities.

In an analysis of 150,391 visits by Medicare patients to 4300 primary care doctors, researchers from the Memorial Sloan-Kettering Cancer Center and the Center for Studying Health System Change verified this inequality. African American and Caucasian American patients were treated by different doctors. Physicians who treated African American patients were less qualified academically. Doctors in the study who cared for African American patients were less likely to be board certified in a specialized area of medicine than those treating Caucasian American patients (77.4% vs 86.1%). These noncertified doctors were less likely to diagnose conditions and more likely to simply treat symptoms.[41]

When asked specifically whether they were able to provide access to high-quality care for all their patients, 27.8% of primary care physicians treating African American patients responded negatively compared with 19.3% of physicians treating Caucasian patients. More physicians treating African American patients, versus physicians treating white patients, also answered that they were unable to always provide access to high-quality specialty services (overall: 24% vs 17.9%; diagnostic imaging: 24.4% vs 16.6%; nonemergency hospital admissions: 48.5% vs 37.0%; and quality ancillary services: 36.6% vs 27.7%).[41]

Another study showed that being foreign-born was negatively related with access to healthcare; this included owning health insurance and having access to either routine or emergency care.[42] Evidence suggests that immigrants often experience barriers to healthcare utilization, particularly when it comes to preventive care and screening services.[42]

Hatzenbuehler et al[43] state that stigma is one of the major social determinants of population health, due to its pervasiveness and disruption of multiple lifestyle factors; this includes resources, social relationships, and coping behaviors.

This type of discrimination is not a consequence of intentional malpractice but the result of a greater proportion of African Americans, Hispanics, and Caribbean Americans living in poorer neighborhoods with fewer high-quality clinics and fewer well-paid physicians.[44] Also, minorities, in general, are less represented in the healthcare professions.[45]

The American College of Physicians has identified specific disparities affecting racial and ethnic minorities in the U.S. healthcare system. These important issues are being addressed through continued research, increasing access to quality healthcare, better patient care, addressing provider issues and societal concern, and improving systems that deliver healthcare.[46] Healthcare professionals, patients, insurance companies, and society as a whole should be made aware of the gap in healthcare quality between minority and nonminority groups.[45] Furthermore, health systems should improve minority patients' access to care, for instance, by ensuring that the financial incentives of the physicians do not bias them against minority patients and increasing the number of minority health professionals.[45]

FOCUS OF RESEARCH

There is a wealth of evidence that ethnic and racial disparities exist in our healthcare system; this remains an inconsistency between the democratic principles and egalitarian commitments of this nation and the realities of its racial/cultural policies and medical practices. These policies and practices need to be quantified to improve the quality of healthcare and reduce racial disparities.[45,47-50] Even when factors such as income and insurance are controlled, minorities tend to receive a lower quality of healthcare; these disparities are due, in part, to health systems and the administrative/bureaucratic process, as well as the healthcare providers and patients themselves.[45]

More ethnographic studies need to be conducted to determine the perspectives and beliefs of specific groups from different cultures and how these can influence the experience of seeking Western medical care. Most published studies are biased and lack a cultural understanding of the issues faced by racial and ethnic minorities. Data should not originate solely from the medical establishment; there is a great need to explore the cultural competence of physicians from the patient's point of view.

In designing a prospective study to evaluate the impact of traditional cultural beliefs on healthcare practices by African Americans, Asian Americans, and Hispanic Americans, core variables must be applied to reflect their economic, geographic, and social diversity. Comparative approaches should be used to focus on the diverse manifestations of disease among different racial and ethnic groups, aiming to incorporate traditional beliefs and cultural aspects of illness into the clinical arena. Studies must go beyond epidemiology to explain the factors that give rise to the data and to help us better understand how traditional cultural beliefs affect the delivery of medical care to African Americans, Asian Americans, and Hispanics.

The reality is that physicians will continue to encounter a higher number of patients with cultural backgrounds that differ from their own. In response, physicians must learn to conduct a comprehensive cultural assessment of their patients. Only by evaluating a patient's traditional, ethnic and racial background will physicians be able to understand the genetic and cultural variables that may impact the patient's response to medications, as well as their compliance with treatment and prevention suggestions.

CONCLUSION

As physicians, we must make a serious effort to understand the beliefs, cultures, expectations, perceptions, and realities of the patients we serve. However, we cannot do this alone; cultural sensitivity training must start in medical school. Fortunately, medical schools are beginning to teach medical students and residents about the presentation of common skin conditions in populations with different backgrounds.

The University of Georgetown founded a National Center for Cultural Competence (NCCC) that helps underserved communities interact with the health system.[51] The University of California, San Francisco, started a cultural competence initiative in 1999 with a collection of resources for physicians and the public. Their goal is to motivate medical professionals and the public to create behavioral and institutional changes that respect the multiple cultures of their patients. The Baylor College of Medicine has an ethnocultural introduction program that promotes communication issues with patients from different ethnic, racial, and religious backgrounds. Similarly, the George Washington University

Medical Center offers interdisciplinary student–community–patient education services in their curricula. Additionally, the Community College of San Francisco has a healthcare interpreter certification program. Even the U.S. government is finally getting into the act. An initiative from the Department of Health and Human Services, termed Healthy People 2020, has made the reduction of racial disparities a national health priority.[47,52]

In some ways, the focus on cultural differences has been beneficial, resulting in the creation of a wide variety of resources designed to better know and understand diverse communities. Yet insufficient resources are available to overcome the provider bias, and insufficient research has been conducted on the impact of race on healthcare.

One of the most challenging factors in raising cultural sensitivity is the origin of medical students. There continues to be a disproportionate representation of Caucasian Americans in medical schools. Few African Americans and Hispanics are represented in the ranks of physicians, regardless of socioeconomic class. The increased presence of African American, Asian American, and Hispanic physicians would play an important role in caring for people of lower socioeconomic status and members of minority groups.[48,53]

The increased awareness of cultural differences has started a trend toward more egalitarian healthcare delivery. For example, articles have been published in the field of dermatology on skin of color in response to a growing interest in the specific skin conditions and reactions of African Americans, Asian Americans, and Hispanics.[49,50,52-57] The increasing importance of minority groups has led to the creation of societies such as the Skin of Color Society, whose primary purpose is the understanding of and further research into skin diseases of people with skin of color. They also hope to educate society about the dermatologic conditions that affect many other population groups, apart from Caucasian Americans.

REFERENCES

1. U.S. Census Bureau. Population Projections. www.census.gov/population/projections/data/national/2012/summarytables.html. Accessed September 15, 2013.
2. U.S. Census Bureau. U.S. Census Bureau projections show a slower growing, older, more diverse nation a half century from now. http://www.census.gov/newsroom/releases/archives/population/cb12-243.html. Accessed September 25, 2013.
3. United Nations Development Program. Human Development Report 2011: sustainability and equity—a better future for all. http://hdr.undp.org/en/reports/global/hdr2011/. Accessed September 15, 2013.
4. Brach C, Fraser I. Can cultural competency reduce racial and ethnic health disparities? A review and conceptual model. *Med Care Res Rev.* 2000;57: 18-217.
5. Brown MT, Bussell JK. Medication adherence: WHO cares? *Mayo Clin Proc.* 2011;86:304-314.
6. Cohn D. Census history: counting Hispanics. http://www.pewsocialtrends.org/2010/03/03/census-history-counting-hispanics-2/. Accessed September 25, 2013.
7. Cooper LA, Gonzales JJ, Gallo JJ, et al. The acceptability of treatment for depression among African-American, Hispanic, and white primary care patients. *Med Care.* 2003;41:479-489.
8. Castillo M. CBS News: whites more likely to get antidepressant prescription than African-Americans, Hispanics. http://www.cbsnews.com/8301-504763_162-57415853-10391704/study-whites-more-likely-to-get-antidepressant-prescription-than-african-americans-hispanics/. Accessed September 24, 2013.
9. Kim-Godwin Y, McMurry MJ. Perspectives of nurse practitioners on healthcare needs among Latino children and families in the rural Southeastern United States: a pilot study. *J Pediatr HealthCare.* 2012;26:409-417.
10. Johnson SK. Hmong health beliefs and experiences in the Western healthcare system. *J Transcult Nurs.* 2002;13:126-132.
11. Singleton K, Krause EMS. Understanding cultural and linguistic barriers to health literacy. *Ky Nurse.* 2010;58:4, 6-9.
12. World Health Organization. *Legal Status of Traditional Medicine and Complementary/Alternative Medicine: A Worldwide Review.* Geneva, Switzerland: World Health Organization; 2002:43-48.

13. National Center for Complementary and Alternative Health. Program announcement: developmental/pilot projects in cancer complementary and alternative medicine (CAM). http://grants.nih.gov/grants/guide/pa-files/PAR-02-040.html. Accessed September 15, 2013.

14. Selvin E, Erlinger TP. Prevalence of and risk factors for peripheral arterial disease in the United States: results from the National Health and Nutrition Examination Survey, 1999-2000. *Circulation.* 2004;110:738-743.

15. American Heart Association. African-Americans and heart disease, stroke. http://www.heart.org/HEARTORG/Conditions/More/MyHeartandStroke-News/African-Americans-and-Heart-Disease_UCM_444863_Article.jsp. Accessed September 24, 2013.

16. Haithcock B, Velanovich V. Comparison of antireflux surgery among ethnicity. *J Natl Med Assoc.* 2004;96:535-541.

17. Gwyn K, Bondy ML, Cohen DS, et al. Racial differences in diagnosis, treatment, and clinical delays in a population-based study of patients with newly diagnosed breast carcinoma. *Cancer.* 2004;100:1595-1604.

18. National Cancer Institute. Fact sheet: cancer health disparities. http://www.cancer.gov/cancertopics/factsheet/disparities/cancer-health-disparities. Accessed September 24, 2013.

19. Harvey IS, Alston RJ. Understanding preventive behaviors among mid-Western African-American men: a pilot qualitative study of prostate screening. *J Mens Health.* 2011;8:140-151.

20. George M. Health beliefs, treatment preferences and complementary and alternative medicine for asthma, smoking and lung cancer self-management in diverse black communities. *Patient Educ Couns.* 2012;89:489-500.

21. Peek ME, Odoms-Young A, Quinn MT, et al. Race and shared decision-making: perspectives of African Americans with diabetes. *Soc Sci Med.* 2010;71:1-9.

22. Chang E. Effect of acculturation on variation in having a usual source of care in Asian American versus non-Hispanic white adults in California. 141st American Public Health Association Annual Meeting, Boston, MA, November 5, 2013. Presentation 282794.

23. Erwin DO, Treviño M, Saad-Harfouche FG, et al. Contextualizing diversity and culture within cancer control interventions for Latinas: changing interventions, not cultures. *Soc Sci Med.* 2010;71:693-701.

24. Diaz VA Jr. Cultural factors in preventive care: Latinos. *Prim Care.* 2002;29:503-517.

25. Vergara C, Martin AM, Wang F, et al. Awareness about factors that affect the management of hypertension in Puerto Rican patients. *Conn Med.* 2004;68:269-276.

26. Sharma S, Cruickshank JK. Cultural differences in assessing dietary intake and providing relevant dietary information to British, African-Caribbean populations. *J Hum Nutr Diet.* 2001;14:449-456.

27. Caballero AE. Understanding the Hispanic/Latino patient. *Am J Med.* 2011;124:S10-S15.

28. Boyd EL, Taylor SD, Shimp LA, et al. An assessment of home remedy use by African Americans. *J Natl Med Assoc.* 2000;92:341-353.

29. Chen XW, Serag ES, Sneed KB, et al. Clinical herbal interactions with conventional drugs: from molecules to maladies. *Curr Med Chem.* 2011;18:4836-4850.

30. Mami Wata West African Diaspora Vodoun. A brief history of Vodoun. http://mamiwata.com/voodoohistory.html. Accessed September 15, 2013.

31. Le Peristyle Haitian Sanctuary: America's First Church of Voodoo. What is Voodoo? http://leperistylehaitiansanctuary.com/voodoo.html. Accessed September 15, 2013.

32. The Guardian. Young Haitian-Americans turn to voodoo for cultural and spiritual connection. http://www.theguardian.com/world/2009/feb/11/voodoo-usa-haiti. Accessed September 25, 2013.

33. BBC News. Is voodoo a force for good or bad? http://news.bbc.co.uk/2/hi/africa/4588262.stm. Accessed September 25, 2013.

34. Etienne MO, Pavlovich-Danis SJ. Cultural considerations for Haitian patients. http://ce.nurse.com/content/ce592/cultural-considerations-for-haitian-patients/. Accessed September 24, 2013.

35. Cooper RS. Race, genes, and health: new wine in old bottles? *Int J Epidemiol.* 2003;32:23-25.

36. Hernandez LM, Blazer DG, eds. Sex/gender, race/ethnicity, and health. In: *Genes, Behavior, and the Social Environment: Moving Beyond the Nature/Nurture Debate.* Washington, DC: National Academies Press; 2006.

37. Glanz K, Croyle RT, Chollette VY, et al. Cancer-related health disparities in women. *Am J Public Health.* 2003;93:292-298.

38. Centers for Disease Control and Prevention National Center for Health Statistics. Table 29: Age-adjusted death rates for selected causes of death, by sex, race, and Hispanic origin: United States, selected years 1950–2004, in: Health, United States, 2006. http://www.cdc.gov/nchs/data/hus/hus06.pdf#029. Accessed September 15, 2013.

39. Centers for Disease Control and Prevention. Minority health. http://www.cdc.gov/minorityhealth/index.html. Accessed September 24, 2013.

40. Pearce N, Foliaki S, Sporle A, et al. Genetics, race, ethnicity, and health. *BMJ.* 2004;328:1070-1072.

41. Bach PB, Pham HH, Schrag D, et al. Primary care physicians who treat blacks and whites. *N Engl J Med.* 2004;351:575-584.

42. Ye J, Mack D, Fry-Johnson Y, et al. Healthcare access and utilization among US-born and foreign-born Asian Americans. *J Immigr Minor Health.* 2012;14:731-737.

43. Hatzenbuehler ML, Phelan JC, Link BG. Stigma as a fundamental cause of population health inequalities. *Am J Public Health.* 2013;103:813-821.

44. Epstein AM. Healthcare in America: still too separate, not yet equal. *N Engl J Med.* 2004;351:603-605.

45. Smedley BD, Stith AY, Nelson AR, eds. *Unequal Treatment: Confronting Racial and Ethnic Disparities in HealthCare.* Washington, DC: National Academies Press; 2009.

46. Groman R, Ginsburg J, American College of Physicians. Racial and ethnic disparities in healthcare: a position paper of the American College of Physicians. *Ann Intern Med.* 2004;141:226-232.

47. van Ryn M, Fu SS. Paved with good intentions: do public health and human service providers contribute to racial/ethnic disparities in health? *Am J Public Health.* 2003;93:248-255.

48. Geiger HJ. Race and healthcare: an American dilemma. *N Engl J Med.* 1996;335:815-816.

49. Rendon MI, Del Rosso JQ. Current assessment of melasma in Hispanic populations—focus on approaches to management and quality of life issues. Poster presented at: American Academy of Dermatology Annual Summer Meeting; July 28-August 1, 2004; New York, NY.

50. Rendon MI, Benitez, AL, Gaviria JI. Telangiectatic melasma: a new entity? *J Cosmet Dermatol.* 2007;20:17-22.

51. National Center for Cultural Competence. Bridging the cultural divide in healthcare settings: the essential role of cultural broker programs. http://www11.georgetown.edu/research/gucchd/nccc/documents/Cultural_Broker_Guide_English.pdf. Accessed October 25, 2012.

52. Healthy People. About Healthy People. http://www.healthypeople.gov/2020/about/default.aspx. Accessed September 25, 2013.

53. Komaromy M, Grumbach K, Drake M, et al. The role of black and Hispanic physicians in providing healthcare for underserved populations. *N Engl J Med.* 1996;334:1305-1310.

54. Halder RM, Nandedkar MA, Neal KW. Pigmentary disorders in ethnic skin. *Dermatol Clin.* 2003;21:617-628.

55. Taylor SC. Skin of color: biology, structure, function, and implications for dermatologic disease. *J Am Acad Dermatol.* 2002;46:41-62.

56. Rendon MI, Ciocca GR, Gaviria J. The challenge of diagnosing melasma in Hispanic populations. Poster presented at: 61st Annual Meeting of the American Academy of Dermatology; March 21-16, 2003; San Francisco, CA; poster 576.

57. Rendon MI. Melasma and postinflammatory hyperpigmentation. *J Cosmet Dermatol.* 2003;16:9-17.

Impact of Traditional African American Cultures on Healthcare Practices

CHAPTER 6

Victoria Holloway Barbosa

KEY POINTS

- Over 15.5% of the world's population is made up of people of African descent, whether based in sub-Saharan Africa or living elsewhere. In the United States, there were more than 42 million residents of African descent in 2010, representing over 13% of the population. Additionally, the number of individuals self-identifying as "multiracial" has grown substantially in the last 10 years.

- Cultural and racial identities have a direct impact on a patient's diagnosis, treatment options, and healthcare practices. Therefore, it is vital that treating physicians recognize the beliefs and cultural context of each patient so as to fully understand the patient's individual health concerns and conditions and subsequently be able to recommend effective treatments.

- Although much of African American culture in the United States originates from African traditions, a distinctly African American experience is now apparent, separate from the "traditional" African culture. As time passes, African American culture will continue to change and evolve with each new generation.

- There are significant disparities in health status and service utilization between African Americans and other ethnic groups. Certain factors have been identified that play a role in this disparity between patient populations, including the accessibility of care, differences in treatment-seeking behaviors between groups, and a lack of trust in physicians and the medical system in general.

- In the African American community, hair care is considered vitally important, and individual hairstyles may have social, political, and esthetic implications. Today, a vast selection of hairstyles is currently in fashion among African American individuals, each of which can have various associated dermatologic concerns, such as pomade acne, irritant contact dermatitis, or relaxer-induced scarring alopecia.

- Many African American patients hold inaccurate beliefs regarding skin and hair care, for instance, regarding the need for sun protection or ways to encourage hair growth. Physicians should take a thorough history from each patient so as to be able to dispel these common misconceptions and perhaps prescribe a more effective treatment for any underlying conditions.

INTRODUCTION

The population of individuals of African descent in the United States is comprised of a dynamic and increasingly complex diaspora. Much of African American culture is rooted in African traditions, with countless similarities found in various aspects of life, such as food, music, dance movements, and hair and skin care practices. However, distance, time, and creativity have shaped a distinctly African American experience that stands on its own, apart from its African heritage. In fact, visiting many cities in Africa can reveal the influence that African American music and fashion have on African popular culture.

One of the fascinations of studying culture is observing the ways in which each culture evolves. Recent trends in immigration show an increase in the number of first-generation Africans and Afro-Caribbeans in the United States, adding a new layer to the existing population.[1] This demographic shift continues to broaden the range of perspectives, beliefs, and healthcare practices of people of African descent in the United States and will undoubtedly continue to shape African American culture in the future.

The physician's office is a microcosm of society. The increasing diversity of people of African descent in the United States will be reflected in the patient population served by physicians. Understanding the disease processes and health risks of individuals of different skin of color groups or ethnicities is only one part of the considerations for successful patient interactions and effective care. To establish meaningful patient–physician relationships, it is important to also understand the belief systems of the individual and their cultural context to recognize the patient's concerns, to communicate effectively, and to make treatment recommendations that will encourage patient compliance and follow-through (see Chapter 4, Multicultural Competence in Dermatologic Practice).

The question arises as to whether skin of color classifications, as well as ethnicity, should be considered at all within the field of healthcare. There has been much discussion throughout history regarding the validity of the concept of "race" and, by extension, the importance of ethnicity, and the significance of each on healthcare practices (see Chapter 1, Skin of Color: A Historical Perspective). Both historically and in modern times, the conversation about skin of color and ethnicity is complicated, particularly because the terms used frequently change and are sometimes confusing to healthcare professionals. Most patients, however, are not involved in these types of historical, anthropologic, or

biological debates—they simply want excellent healthcare. Racial and cultural factors may impact perceptions of disease, the utilization of health services, and disease outcomes. Consequently, an understanding of the cultural context of the patient and his or her disease is paramount.

DEMOGRAPHICS OF AFRICAN AMERICANS AND PEOPLE OF AFRICAN DESCENT WORLDWIDE

The world's population is approaching more than 7 billion people.[1] With almost 936 million Africans in sub-Saharan Africa and a further 186 million individuals of African origin living elsewhere, 15.5% of the world's population is made up of people of African descent.[2,3] Of course, these figures are subject to modification for several reasons. First, the sub-Saharan region of Africa hosts many people of European and Asian descent who would not be counted in the calculation of "people of African descent" when the term is used as a proxy to indicate darker skin of color or "race" rather than the individual's continent of origin. Second, inhabitants of eight countries composing northern Africa, the Western Sahara, Morocco, Algeria, Tunisia, Libya, Egypt, Sudan, and South Sudan, are not usually included in demographic population calculations for people of African descent. These people identify with and are heavily influenced in terms of religion and culture by the Middle East, Europe, and Asia.[4] Finally, the calculation of people of African descent living outside Africa includes both so-called "single-race" and "mixed-race" individuals, with varying calculations in the perceptions and tabulations of race and ethnicity by country. The official distribution of this diaspora includes approximately 22 million people of African descent in the Caribbean, 111 million in South America, 44 million in North America, and almost 8 million in Europe.[3]

At present, the diaspora encompassing the population of individuals of African descent in the United States is growing and becoming more diverse. At the time of the 2010 U.S. Census, there were more than 42 million people of African descent living in the United States.[5] This represented over 13% of the population and was almost a 15% increase in the size of the population compared with the preceding census in 2000.[5] This number includes people who were considered to be, in the terminology used by the census, "Black or African American alone" or "in combination" thereof. Almost 13% of the total population was considered "Black or African American alone"[5]; this option was chosen if they listed one entry, either checking the "Black or African American" box or recording that they were from a sub-Saharan African country or an Afro-Caribbean country like Nigeria or Haiti. Conversely, 1% of the total population was considered "Black or African American in combination," where they listed more than one category, including "Black or African American."[5] Of note, this "multiple race" group has grown substantially by approximately 75% since the 2000 U.S. Census.[5] The rapid emergence of groups that self-identify as "multiracial" or multiethnic has direct implications for patients' diagnoses, treatments, and healthcare practices.

In addition to the increase in diversity that accompanies the increasing numbers of individuals who identify as multiracial, immigration has also played its part in fostering cultural diversity. In 2010, there were more than 1.5 million African immigrants in the United States, 74% of whom were individuals with darker skin of color; this is double the number of African immigrants residing in the United States in 2000.[6] The states with the largest African foreign-born populations in 2010 were California, New York, Texas, Maryland, and Virginia.[6] The African foreign-born population continues to increase, with estimates from the more recent 2012 American Community Survey suggesting that over 3 million people from sub-Saharan Africa now live in the United States [**Figure 6-1**].[7] It was also estimated in the survey that there were approximately 2.8 million non-Hispanic West Indians in the United States in 2012, of whom Jamaicans and Haitians made up over 70%.[7] The complete distribution of countries can be found in **Figure 6-2**. Specific demographic data concerning racial identity for these populations in the United States are not provided; however, these countries comprise many individuals of African descent, although there is a significant amount of racial fusion, as with African Americans.[7]

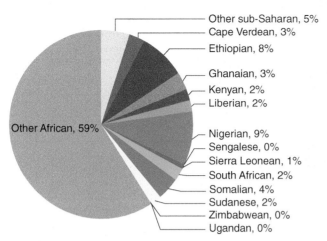

FIGURE 6-1. Chart detailing the ancestry of sub-Saharan Africans living in the United States in 2012. (Data from U.S. Census Bureau. 2012 American Community Survey 1-Year Estimates.[7])

In general, African Americans, Africans, and Afro-Caribbeans recognize their shared ancestry, although most view themselves as distinct ethnic groups. First- and second-generation Africans and Afro-Caribbeans often identify predominantly with their country of origin and continue many of their traditional cultural practices while living in the United States. On the whole, relationships among those of the African diaspora are cordial, and there is an attitude of receptiveness toward other cultures. The impact of newer African and Afro-Caribbean cultures on the "traditional" African American culture can be expected in the years ahead.

Finally, it is important to stress that many people of African descent are of mixed race and that racial and ethnic heritage are not always apparent based on the appearance of the individual, just as not everyone with lighter fair skin is purely of Caucasian or European descent. Patients should be afforded the opportunity to self-identify their racial and ethnic background, alleviating the necessity of having assumptions made by their healthcare providers based on physical attributes. In the future, the use of deoxyribonucleic acid (DNA) genome sequencing may be beneficial in identifying genetically determined diseases. Information regarding a patient's racial and ethnic self-identity should be gathered routinely, and new intake forms should be designed for the purposes of medical history-taking.

DISPARITIES IN HEALTHCARE STATUS AND HEALTH SERVICES UTILIZATION FOR PATIENTS WITH SKIN OF COLOR

Currently, a crisis in healthcare exists for African Americans and other patients with skin of color. Although the causes are complex and often debated, the evidence of this crisis is clear, with significant and well-documented disparities in health status between African Americans and other groups, particularly Caucasians. These disparities take many forms: the infant mortality rate is 2.2 times higher for African American babies than for Caucasian infants[7,8]; the age-adjusted obesity rate in African Americans is 47.6% versus 32.6% in non-Hispanic whites; the risk of stroke is almost twice as high for those with darker skin of color as opposed to fairer-skinned patients[9,10]; African Americans make up 44% of new human immunodeficiency virus (HIV) cases each year, despite comprising only 13.4% of the population[11]; and women with darker skin of color are 40% more likely to die from breast cancer than Caucasian women.[12] These are just a few examples of the readily apparent health disparities faced by the African American patient population.

Unfortunately, there is a paucity of research on health disparities in the field of dermatology, except for an awareness of the disparities in melanoma stage, diagnosis, and resulting outcomes. A total of 26% of African American patients with melanoma have regional or distant metastases upon presentation compared with 12% of fairer-skinned individuals.[13] Additionally, the 10-year survival rate is lower for patients with darker skin of color than for fairer-skinned patients (73% and 88%, respectively).[14] A recent study by Lott and Gross[15] sheds light on the disparities that exist with conditions other than skin cancer. Upon examining mortality from nonneoplastic skin diseases over a 10-year period, Lott and Gross[15] demonstrated that the age-adjusted mortality from these skin diseases was 3.4 times greater for individuals with skin of color. It is hoped that these recent findings will stimulate additional dermatologic research on African Americans and individuals with skin of color in the United States and, indeed, worldwide.

Racial and ethnic differences have also been reported among patients' reasons for visiting a dermatologist, both in the United States and Europe. In a study by Alexis et al,[16] the five most common diagnoses listed for African Americans visiting a dermatology practice were (1) acne, (2) dyschromia, (3) contact dermatitis and other eczema, (4) alopecia, and (5) seborrheic dermatitis [**Figures 6-3 to 6-7**].[16] Interestingly, the conditions of dyschromia and alopecia, common among African American patients, were not among the top diagnoses in Caucasian patients. The top five diagnoses for Caucasians were (1) acne, (2) lesions of uncertain behavior on the trunk, (3) benign neoplasms on the trunk, (4) contact dermatitis and other eczema, and (5) psoriasis.[16] Similar patterns have been noted among individuals of African descent in other parts of the world. For instance, a study of 1000 patients in Jamaica noted that the four most common diagnoses were acne, seborrheic

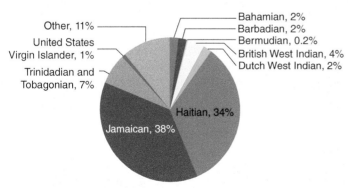

FIGURE 6-2. Chart detailing the ancestry of non-Hispanic Caribbean Americans living in the United States in 2012. (Data from U.S. Census Bureau. 2012 American Community Survey 1-Year Estimates.[7])

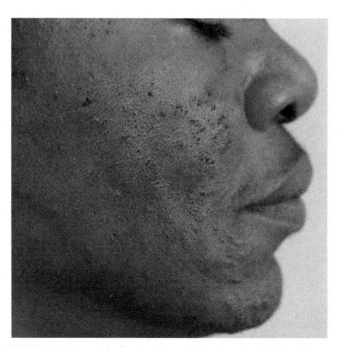

FIGURE 6-3. An example of acne scarring on the face of a patient with skin of color.

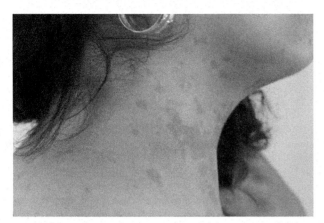

FIGURE 6-4. Photograph showing dyschromia in the form of post inflammatory hyperpigmentation on the neck of a patient.

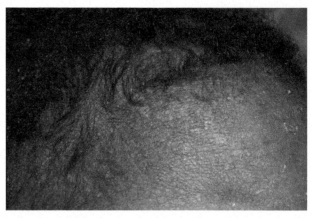

FIGURE 6-7. An African American female with seborrheic dermatitis on the scalp and forehead.

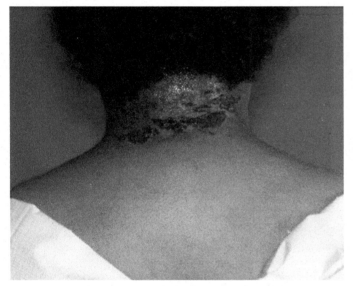

FIGURE 6-5. A patient suffering from allergic contact dermatitis.

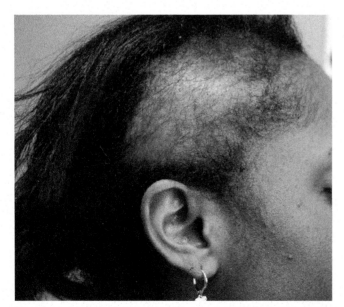

FIGURE 6-6. An African American female with hair miniaturization and thinning on the temporoparietal scalp, with preservation of the marginal hairline. These are symptoms consistent with traction alopecia. (Used with permission from Meena Singh, MD, Shawnee Mission, KS.)

eczema, pigmentary disorders, and atopic eczema.[17] Also, a study performed in Paris, France, on adults of African and Afro-Caribbean decent found that the most common diagnoses were acne, dyschromia, alopecia, and eczema.[18]

In an attempt to understand the cultural considerations needed in treating the dermatologic needs of African American patients and in addressing the current health disparities among racial and ethnic groups, many questions come to mind. Factors such as (1) access to care, (2) barriers to treatment, (3) perceptions of the medical system, (4) treatment-seeking behaviors, (5) trust in physicians, and (6) willingness to participate in clinical research have all been explored in the medical literature in general; however, there is a lack of specific studies pertaining to dermatologic care. This is an extremely important frontier for future research and study.

COMMON MISCONCEPTIONS AMONG AFRICAN AMERICANS ABOUT HAIR AND SKIN

In the African American community, knowledge and beliefs about the care and treatment of hair and skin may come from many sources, and the dermatologist is often not the first source of this information. Patients may come to their medical appointment armed with folk wisdom gathered from a variety of sources, such as information passed down from mother to daughter, heard from other relatives or friends, or gleaned from the Internet. Knowledge is also sought from other resources, such as beauty magazines or salon hairdressers. Unfortunately, not all the information passed on or gathered from these various sources is correct, and there are many beauty and health misconceptions that are often accepted as fact. Dermatologists should be aware of common misconceptions about the care and treatment of skin and hair so that they can dispel them during patient visits.

To explore commonly held health and beauty misconceptions among African Americans, an Internet search was performed using the terms "African American beauty, skin or hair myths." The 10 most popular posts from beauty blogs, magazine, and radio websites, as well as other online resources, were analyzed for common themes. Commercial websites selling cosmetic products or containing press releases were excluded. The five most frequently found misconceptions by African Americans regarding skin and hair are presented below, along with strategies for dispelling them.

◼ MISCONCEPTIONS ABOUT SKIN

Five main misconceptions regarding African American skin were found [**Table 6-1**]. It is not surprising that three of these erroneous beliefs relate directly or indirectly to sun exposure and protection. African Americans in general are aware that darker pigmentation offers some protection from the sun; however, many patients mistakenly believe that the modest protection provided by darker skin of color compared with

TABLE 6-1	The five most frequent African American misconceptions regarding skin or skin care
	Misconceptions
1	African Americans do not get sunburned.
2	African Americans do not contract skin cancer.
3	African Americans do not wrinkle.
4	Cocoa butter can be used to fade or minimize the appearance of dark spots.
5	African American skin is oily and does not need to be moisturized.

TABLE 6-2	The five most frequent African American misconceptions regarding hair or hair care
	Misconceptions
1	Hair of African Americans does not grow.
2	Trimming the ends of the hair will ensure hair growth.
3	Wearing braids will ensure hair growth.
4	Washing hair too often will dry it out.
5	It is necessary to grease the scalp to combat dry skin or a dry scalp.

fairer skin eliminates the possibility of burning, wrinkling, or developing skin cancer. Consequently, sunscreen use is lower among African Americans, with Pichon et al[19] reporting that 63% of the African American adults studied never wore sunscreen. Sunscreen use is also infrequent among adolescents, with Hall et al[20] demonstrating significantly lower sunscreen use for African American high school students than for their Caucasian counterparts (4.8% vs 16.5%, respectively). Additionally, knowledge regarding melanoma is low among individuals with skin of color in the United States. In a recent study by Robinson et al,[21] focus groups of African Americans, Hispanics, and Asians revealed the common theme that skin cancer was considered irrelevant.

This lack of information about skin cancer is particularly concerning given the fact that melanomas in people with darker skin of color and Hispanics are more likely to metastasize and have poorer outcomes than those among Caucasians.[13,22] One recommendation is to raise the topics of sun protection and skin cancer prevention with patients of African descent and all patients with skin of color. Even a few minutes of discussion and education on these topics can be key to the early prevention and detection of skin cancer for at-risk patients and may ultimately prove to be life saving for the patient. Discussing the role of sunscreen in maintaining an even complexion can be an additional motivating factor for these patients, because this is an issue that often resonates among patients with darker skin of color due to the fact that this patient group is more prone to conditions such as melasma and postinflammatory hyperpigmentation.[23]

The high prevalence of dyschromia among individuals of African descent has given rise to a number of folk remedies and is the reason for the fourth most common misconception about skin among African Americans—that the application of cocoa butter will fade areas of skin discoloration. In addition, cocoa butter is also believed to improve the appearance of scars and stretch marks. Hence, cocoa butter is an ingredient that is very popular in African American skin care products. Cocoa butter is an excellent moisturizer and is prized for its rich, creamy texture and pleasant aroma. It is not, however, a skin-lightening agent. Furthermore, several studies demonstrate that the utilization of coca butter does not prevent or improve stretch marks.[24,25]

In many parts of Africa and in cosmetic markets worldwide, high-potency topical corticosteroids, prescription-strength hydroquinone, or mercury-containing bleaching products are sold as treatments to fade dark spots, even out skin complexion, or lighten the skin. Over-the-counter skin products in the United States are marketed as fading, bleaching, or lightening skin creams. It is noteworthy that these same types of skin creams are available from regional manufacturers in Africa, Asia, Latin America, the Middle East, and the Arabian Gulf regions. Lighter skin seems to be valued as a mark of beauty in many societies around the world; however, hopefully this standard of beauty is changing to encompass a broader range of skin color. Consequently, taking a thorough patient history, focusing particularly on the patient's history of product use, might bring misconceptions to the fore and provide an opportunity for the physician to prescribe a more effective treatment. Furthermore, thorough history-taking might reveal the use of potentially dangerous folk treatments.

There are conflicting data regarding the fifth most common skin misconception among African Americans, which is that skin of color is oily and does not need moisturizing. To date, medical opinion remains divided on this issue, and it has yet to be either confirmed or refuted. Again, there is a paucity of information on variations in sebaceous gland size and sebum secretion among differing populations. In fact, although some African Americans do have oily skin, many others suffer from dry skin, often referred to as having "ashy" skin. Additionally, seasonal variations in temperature and humidity, as well as age-related decreases in sebum production, will affect the rate of oil production within the skin of any given individual.

In light of these common misconceptions regarding skin, physicians should habitually inquire about their patients' skin care routines and beliefs. Many African Americans do not realize that their beliefs and attitudes toward skin care are inaccurate and may in fact be worsening or exacerbating an underlying condition. At the very least, informing patients of the reality behind certain skin care misconceptions may save them time, effort, and money in the long term.

MISCONCEPTIONS ABOUT HAIR CARE

There are five common misconceptions by African American regarding hair care [**Table 6-2**]. Three of these five erroneous beliefs are related to the issue of hair growth. They are that (1) the hair of individuals with skin of color does not grow, (2) hair will grow when the ends are trimmed, and (3) hair grows when it is worn in braids. In fact, Afro-textured, or "spiraled," hair does grow, although it does not grow as quickly as the common Caucasian or Asian hair type, and it breaks off more easily than that of other groups, whether it is virgin hair or chemically treated.[26,27] These factors are often interpreted by African Americans to mean that their hair is not growing. Additionally, trimming the ends of hair does not alter the rate of hair growth. It can, however, decrease hair breakage due to damaged ends.

In regard to hair styling, braids and twists are often worn by African Americans and are traditionally left in place for 6 to 8 weeks or longer [**Figures 6-8 and 6-9**]. During that time, the hair is not exposed to heat or chemicals and is not combed or brushed daily. Consequently, there is no "weathering" of the hair that normally leads to breakage of the hair ends; hence, when the braids or twists are removed or "taken down," the hair is noticeably longer. Although the braided style did not change the rate of hair growth, it did perceptibly reduce the amount of breakage. Of note, patients are sometimes concerned due to hair loss during the removal of their braids. They should be reassured that, normally, individuals will lose approximately 100 hair strands per day; these hairs remain trapped in the braids for the duration of the hairstyle and are then removed all at once when the braids are taken down. For instance, if a patient were to wear their braids for a 2-month period, they would notice a hair loss of approximately 6000 strands when the braids were removed. Although this seems like a large amount, this hair loss is normal.

The fourth mistaken belief is that washing the hair too much dries it out. This is related to the fact that shampoo products intend to remove sebum and dirt from the hair and some formulas are more aggressive in achieving this goal than others. However, it is not the cleansing process itself that damages African American hair, but rather that wet hair has a lower tensile strength and is more easily broken than dry hair, so even the act of combing wet hair can lead to breakage. In addition, the use of very hot styling implements, including blow dryers, cap dryers, curling irons, and flat irons, on recently shampooed hair can cause additional

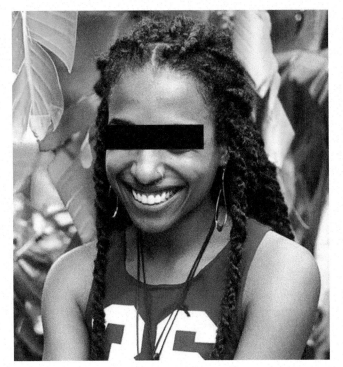

FIGURE 6-8. An example of braided hair on a young African American girl. (Used with permission from Meena Singh, MD, Shawnee Mission, KS.)

breakage. Deep conditioners and leave-in conditioners can be used to decrease the amount of force needed to comb hair, as well as provide protection from heated styling implements.

Lastly, the application of an oily product to the scalp, otherwise known as "greasing," is a common practice among African Americans to combat dry hair and/or a dry scalp. However, older products often use heavy pomades containing mineral oil or petroleum, neither of which penetrates the hair shaft and both of which can contribute to pomade acne. As part of the new movement promoting "natural" hair, many women are embracing the use of pure natural oils obtained at health food or organic grocery stores. Olive, coconut, and argan oils are popular choices. Women with very dry hair often choose to use butters, such as shea, cocoa, or mango butter. The use of these products on the hair can be helpful to moisturize and condition the hair. However, "greasing" the scalp is unnecessary. Additionally, some people who believe that they have a dry scalp actually suffer from seborrheic dermatitis and would receive far greater benefit from using prescription medicine or over-the-counter products.

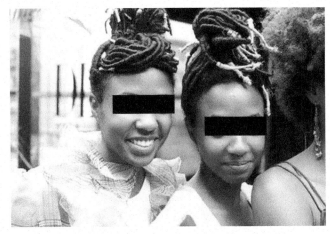

FIGURE 6-9. Other examples of braided hair on young African American girls. (Used with permission from Meena Singh, MD, Shawnee Mission, KS.)

Many African Americans do not realize that dermatologists treat hair and scalp conditions in addition to skin diseases. Therefore, they may not realize when dealing with these conditions that their provider is an excellent resource for them. Physicians should take the time to inquire about their patient's hair grooming practices as part of the medical history-taking and be sure to examine the patient's scalp during a full-body examination.

THE CULTURE OF HAIR CARE AND STYLING

The importance of hair care in the African American community cannot be overstated. For many women of African descent, their hair is considered their "crowning glory." This biblical reference means that, for many women of faith, healthy and aesthetically pleasing hair is more than simply a cosmetic ideal, but truly the word of God. For women of African descent, hairstyle has had political and commercial implications, in addition to being a marker of changing social norms.

No history lesson concerning African American hair care is complete without discussing Madame C. J. Walker (1867–1919), the first female self-made millionaire in the United States, who made her fortune by selling hair products [**Figure 6-10**]. Since her time, countless women have supported their families by earning money as licensed beauty parlor beauticians or "kitchen beauticians," most without a state license. Many families have amassed fortunes by founding hair care companies like Johnson & Johnson, Soft Sheen-Carson, and Dudley Beauty Corp, LLC, continuing in the tradition of Madame C. J. Walker.

The last several decades have seen hairstyles change and revert back to more natural hair styles, as women and men went from wearing "conks"

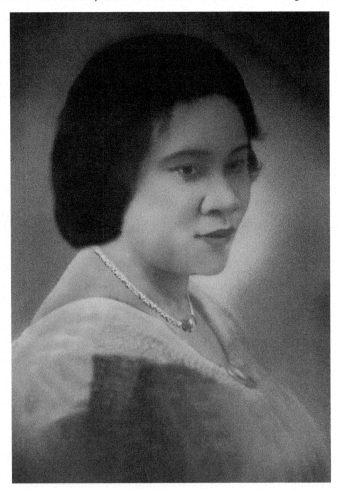

FIGURE 6-10. Madam C. J. Walker (1867–1919) was the first female self-made millionaire of any race in America, making her fortune by developing and marketing a range of beauty and hair products for women with skin of color. (Used with permission from Marisol LLC, Muscat, Sultanate of Oman.)

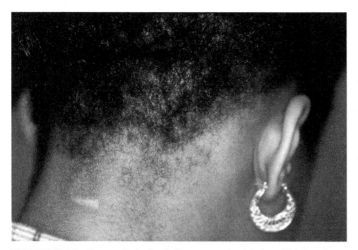

FIGURE 6-11. Photograph of a chemical burn on a patient's neck resulting from the use of a heated styling appliance.

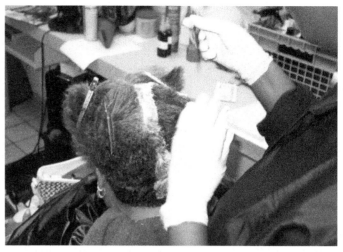

FIGURE 6-13. An African American woman undergoing chemical relaxation to straighten her hair.

(ie, chemically straightened hair) in the 1950s and 1960s to *afros* as a sign of racial pride in the 1970s. In the 1980s and 1990s, the use of relaxers was widespread, but the new millennium saw a return to braided and twisted styles, a huge upsurge in the popularity of hair extensions, and the continued fashion for straightened hair. Today's culture is one of "anything goes," so all of the hairstyles mentioned above are likely to be seen and have various different problems associated with them.

Hair straightening can be accomplished with the use of heat or more permanently with the use of chemicals. Heated styling appliances such as blow dryers, curling irons, hot combs, and flat irons temporarily rearrange the hydrogen bonds to straighten the hair. Professional styling appliances are readily available at most beauty supply stores, and therefore, many patients may have access to styling tools that can reach temperatures of 450°F.

There are two main challenges that result from the use of heated appliances. First, chemical burns are common and result from the direct contact of the heated appliance on the scalp, face, or neck [**Figure 6-11**]. Second, hair breakage (which may sometimes be immediate) may occur due to the application of high temperatures directly onto the hair shaft, leading to hair degradation [**Figure 6-12**]. In addition, heat can cause a condition known as bubble hair syndrome, an acquired deformity of the hair shaft that leads to hair breakage over time. The characteristic "bubbles" that can be seen in the hair shaft under the microscope are actually pockets of gas that occur because of the rapid water vaporization

resulting from the heat. The areas where bubbles occur are subsequently more prone to breakage in the future.

Hair can be permanently straightened with the use of relaxers. Strong alkalis, such as sodium hydroxide and calcium hydroxide, are used to permanently rearrange the disulfide bonds in the hair. Relaxer reapplication every 8 weeks or so is recommended to address the issue of new hair growth. In the short term, people may experience irritant contact dermatitis from the accidental application of the relaxer to the scalp. In addition, breakage may occur from hair that is repeatedly chemically processed. Relaxers have been demonstrated to lower the tensile strength of hair even after one application. Therefore, patients should be counseled to extend relaxer application sessions to at least every 8 weeks, and the product should only be applied to the new hair growth [**Figure 6-13**].

The impact of undergoing long-term straightening with relaxers is still to be determined. There have been reports of relaxer-induced scarring alopecia, irritant dermatitis followed by bacterial infection, and Stevens-Johnson syndrome, all following relaxer application.[28-30] Perhaps the most commonly debated topic is the role of relaxers in the development of central centrifugal cicatricial alopecia among women of African descent.

Twisted and braided hairstyles are one of many African American traditions borrowed directly from African culture. There are many reasons why women choose to wear their hair in these styles, whether making a fashion statement or a political one, enjoying the convenience of not having to style their hair on a weekly basis, or enjoying a protective style that gives the hair a "rest" from heat and chemicals and allows it to grow. These styles may be simple or intricate and may use the patient's own hair or include additional hair extensions. The main problem with these styles is that wearers can develop traction alopecia as a result of the hair being pulled too tightly from the braids or twists. The challenges from straightening hair with heat or chemicals or braiding hair present multiple dermatologic problems that may require close attention by physicians and their patients.

THE CULTURE OF SKIN CARE

For many African Americans, skin care has mainly been focused on achieving an even complexion. Partly due to the natural variation in facial skin tones among individuals and partly due to the frequency among African Americans of postinflammatory hyperpigmentation from conditions like acne, an even complexion can sometimes be elusive. Skin-lightening agents have been in use for decades in the African American community. In earlier times, when certain benefits were afforded to lighter-skinned individuals, fade creams were occasionally used for the purpose of lightening the complexion. Fortunately, it is hoped that society has since

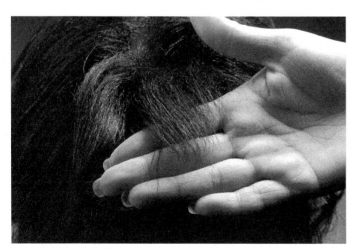

FIGURE 6-12. Photograph demonstrating hair breakage due to the use of styling tools heated to high temperatures. This hair breakage can sometimes be immediate and can lead to hair degradation.

advanced beyond this way of thinking and that most women with skin of color embrace and are proud of their skin's natural shade. Currently, there is a huge demand for products that even or brighten the skin without changing its natural color. Hydroquinone and alternatives like vitamin C serums, licorice, and arbutin are commonly used.

An example of the ways in which African culture can influence African American culture can be observed in the use of skin care products. In many cities in Africa, products such as high-potency topical steroids, high concentrations of hydroquinone, and mercury-containing compounds can easily be purchased from street vendors. Although these products are either available only by prescription or are entirely illegal in the United States, they can sometimes be found in African stores and readily purchased. For obvious safety reasons, it is vital that this practice be discouraged among all patients, including African American patients.

UNDERUTILIZATION OF THE HEALTHCARE SYSTEM

History and culture shape how African Americans view and use the healthcare system. Unfortunately, there are many historical instances of African Americans being used for medical research in ways that were at best unkind or inappropriate, and at worst dangerous and life-threatening. The best known example of this is the Tuskegee Study of Untreated Syphilis in the Negro Male, an infamous clinical study that was conducted from 1932 until 1972 and has been widely documented. In short, the U.S. Public Health Service conducted a 40-year experiment in which 600 males, 399 of whom had syphilis, were told they were being treated for "bad blood." Free medical examinations, meals, and burial insurance were provided. The subjects were not, however, informed of their actual illness and did not give consent, nor were they provided with adequate medical treatment, even after penicillin became the clear treatment of choice in 1947.[31] Although this may now seem like distant history, cases like this had a lasting impact in terms of fostering a lack of trust in physicians, the medical care system, and clinical research in general among African Americans.

As participants within a society and an era, physicians are unfortunately also affected by the stereotypical thinking that occurs within the general population; in fact, "racial folklore" has impacted all of the disciplines and subspecialties of medicine.[32] It is difficult to change the established mind-set of the current U.S. medical system and to encourage acknowledgement of and learning from current and past medical prejudice. For these reasons, as stated by Hoberman, "racial enlightenment will not reach medical schools until the current 'race-aversive' curricula include new historical and sociological perspectives."[32]

The far-reaching implications of medical racism include problems like African American patients being less willing to go to the doctor or less willing to follow medical advice and being reluctant to participate in medical research that could ultimately help physicians to treat the African American population.

CONCLUSION

Ultimately, caring for the African American patient is no different than caring for any other patient. It is incumbent on the physician to respect the culture of their patients, to listen to the patient's needs and concerns, and to be aware that there may be issues that need to be raised due to reluctance on the part of the patient or because the patient may not realize the extent of the physician's knowledge. Key areas for dermatologists to address include sun protection, skin cancer prevention, and hair grooming practices, since these are areas where patients may have incomplete information or hold inaccurate beliefs.

ACKNOWLEDGMENTS

A special thanks to Meena Singh, MD, dermatologist, Shawnee Mission, KS, and Stacey Gambrell Hunt, MD, Department of Dermatology, Kaiser Permanent, Walnut Creek, CA, who both so graciously acted as auxiliary consultants on skin and hair care practices and figures for this chapter.

REFERENCES

1. U.S. Census Bureau. U.S. and world population clock. www.census.gov/popclock/. Accessed July 26, 2014.
2. The World Bank Group. Data: sub-Saharan Africa (developing only). www.data.worldbank.org/region/sub-saharan-africa. Accessed July 26, 2014.
3. Central Intelligence Agency. The World Fact Book. www.cia.gov/library/publications/the-world-factbook/fields/2075.html. Accessed August 9, 2014.
4. Berglee R. North Africa and Southwest Asia. In: *Regional Geography of the World: Globalization, People, and Places.* www.2012books.lardbucket.org/books/regional-geography-of-the-world-globalization-people-and-places/s11-north-africa-and-southwest-asi.html#. Accessed August 9, 2014.
5. U.S. Census Bureau. The black population: 2010. www.census.gov/prod/cen2010/briefs/c2010br-06.pdf. Accessed August 9, 2014.
6. Immigration Policy Center, American Immigration Council. African Immigrants in America: a demographic overview. www.immigrationpolicy.org/just-facts/african-immigrants-america-demographic-overview. Accessed August 9, 2014.
7. U.S. Census Bureau. 2012 American community survey 1-year estimates. www.factfinder2.census.gov/faces/tableservices/jsf/pages/productview.xhtml?pid=ACS_12_1YR_C04003&prodType=table. Accessed August 9, 2014.
8. Centers for Disease Control and Prevention. Morbidity and Mortality Weekly Report. QuickStats: infant mortality rates, by race and Hispanic ethnicity of mother: United States, 2000, 2005, and 2010. www.cdc.gov/mmwr/preview/mmwrhtml/mm6301a9.htm?s_cid=mm6301a9_w%20infant%20mortality. Accessed August 9, 2014.
9. Centers for Disease Control and Prevention. Overweight and obesity: adult obesity facts. www.cdc.gov/obesity/data/adult.html. Accessed August 9, 2014.
10. Centers for Disease Control and Prevention. Stroke facts. www.cdc.gov/stroke/facts.htm. Accessed August 9, 2014.
11. Centers for Disease Control and Prevention. HIV/AIDS: HIV among African Americans. www.cdc.gov/hiv/risk/racialethnic/aa/facts/index.html. Accessed August 9, 2014.
12. Hunt BR, Whitman S, Hurlbert M. Increasing Black:White disparities in breast cancer mortality in the 50 largest cities in the United States. *Cancer Epidemiol.* 2014;38:118-123.
13. Hu S, Parmet Y, Allen G, et al. Disparity in melanoma: a trend analysis of melanoma incidence and stage at diagnosis among whites, Hispanics, and blacks in Florida. *Arch Dermatol.* 2009;145:1369-1374.
14. Collins KK, Fields RC, Baptiste D, et al. Racial differences in survival after surgical treatment for melanoma. *Ann Surg Oncol.* 2011;18:2925-2936.
15. Lott JP, Gross CP. Mortality from nonneoplastic skin disease in the United States. *J Am Acad Dermatol.* 2014;70:47-54.
16. Alexis AF, Sergay AB, Taylor SC. Common dermatologic disorders in skin of color: a comparative practice survey. *Cutis.* 2007;80:387-394.
17. Dunwell P, Rose A. Study of the skin disease spectrum occurring in an Afro-Caribbean population. *Int J Dermatol.* 2003;42:287-289.
18. Arsouze A, Fitoussi C, Cabotin PP, et al. Presenting skin disorders in black Afro-Caribbean patients: a multicentre study conducted in the Paris region. *Ann Dermatol Venereol.* 2008;135:177-182.
19. Pichon LC, Corral I, Landrine H, et al. Sun-protection behaviors among African Americans. *Am J Prev Med.* 2010;38:288-295.
20. Hall HI, Jones SE, Saraiya M. Prevalence and correlates of sunscreen use among US high school students. *J Sch Health.* 2001;71:453-457.
21. Robinson JK, Joshi KM, Ortiz S, et al. Melanoma knowledge, perception, and awareness in ethnic minorities in Chicago: recommendations regarding education. *Psychooncology.* 2011;20:313-320.
22. Rouhani P, Hu S, Kirsner RS. Melanoma in Hispanic and black Americans. *Cancer Control.* 2008;15:248-253.
23. Davis EC, Callender VD. Postinflammatory hyperpigmentation: a review of the epidemiology, clinical features, and treatment options in skin of color. *J Clin Aesthet Dermatol.* 2010;3:20-31.
24. Buchanan K, Fletcher HM, Reid M. Prevention of striae gravidarum with cocoa butter cream. *Int J Gynaecol Obstet.* 2010;108:65-68.
25. Osman H, Usta IM, Rubeiz N, et al. Cocoa butter lotion for prevention of striae gravidarum: a double-blind, randomised and placebo-controlled trial. *BJOG.* 2008;115:1138-1142.
26. Loussouarn G. African hair growth parameters. *Br J Dermatol.* 2001; 145: 294-297.
27. McMichael AJ. Hair breakage in normal and weathered hair: focus on the black patient. *J Invest Dermatol Symp Proc.* 2007;12:6-9.
28. Khumalo NP, Pillay K, Ngwanya RM. Acute 'relaxer'-associated scarring alopecia: a report of five cases. *Br J Dermatol.* 2007;156:1394-1397.

29. Kaur BJ, Singh H, Lin-Greenberg A. Irritant contact dermatitis complicated by deep-seated staphylococcal infection caused by a hair relaxer. *J Natl Med Assoc.* 2002;94:121-123.

30. Booker MJ. Stevens-Johnson syndrome triggered by chemical hair relaxer: a case report. *Cases J.* 2009;2:7748.

31. Centers for Disease Control and Prevention. U.S. Public Health Service Syphilis Study at Tuskegee. www.cdc.gov/tuskegee/timeline.htm. Accessed August 9, 2014.

32. Hoberman J. *Black and Blue: The Origins and Consequences of Medical Racism.* Los Angeles, CA: University of California Press; 2012.

Impact of Traditional Asian American Cultures on Healthcare Practices

CHAPTER 7

Richard S. Mizuguchi

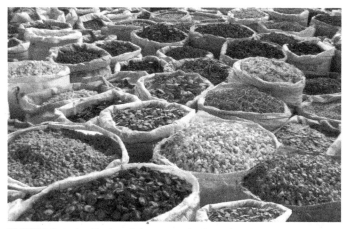

FIGURE 7-1. Dried herbs and plant portions for Chinese herbology in China. (Used with permission from Marisol LLC, Muscat, Sultanate of Oman.)

KEY POINTS

- Traditional Chinese medicine (TCM) involves herbs, dietary therapy, massage, and acupuncture.

- Herbal remedies are often effective but may cause allergic reactions and side effects, including dermatitis.

- Traditional Asian practices of cupping, coining, and moxibustion can cause bruises and lesions that are sometimes mistaken for physical abuse; however, these are distinguishable by their regular circular appearance.

- Physicians should realize that TCM is not quackery; many of the therapies in this chapter are currently used in Western hospitals, and some have shown efficacy in double-blind studies.

It is important for dermatologists to be familiar with the traditional cultural practices of the Asian and Asian American population in the United States. According to the 2010 Census report, the Asian and Pacific Island population currently represents about 5.6% of the U.S. population but is projected to increase to more than five times the current size by the year 2050, reaching 41 million people. The Asian population would then represent 10.3% of the U.S. population.[1] Because Asians represent a fast-growing segment of the population, dermatologists should become familiar with the specifics regarding the treatment of Asian skin of color and also have a basic knowledge of some of the more common cultural practices of Asians.

The history of the Asian population in the United States displays a long tradition of using alternative medicine. Asian immigrants, like many other immigrants and refugees who settle in the United States, tend to visit physicians within their local communities. Therefore, many cultural practices may go unnoticed by healthcare providers outside of the Asian community. A study of a Vietnamese refugee community in San Diego, California, showed that most of the Vietnamese participants preferred both Vietnamese entertainment and health services, even after settling in the United States. These refugees continued to use traditional health practices, such as coining, steam inhalation, and acupuncture.[2] However, sometimes an emergency or moving locations requires patients to seek treatment from dermatologists outside of their habitual communities. Therefore, the dermatologist should be aware of the potential side effects of traditional Asian treatments. In the current milieu of alternative medicine, both Asian and non-Asian patients may present with side effects to certain remedies, including contact allergic and irritant dermatitis. This chapter reviews some of the more common cultural habits and practices within the Asian culture, including traditional Chinese medicine, acupuncture, and the practice of coining. As with most communities, there are also myths and misconceptions which abound. Many patients seek out "natural" remedies, believing that no side effects will occur as a result of their use. However, as this chapter illustrates, this is not always the case; some of the side effects and reactions resulting from certain alternative treatments can be extremely serious.

TRADITIONAL CHINESE MEDICINE

As an alternative method of therapy, traditional Chinese medicine (TCM) is practiced throughout China and East Asia by millions of people. Until the middle of the nineteenth century, alternative medicine provided by botanical healers, midwives, chiropractors, homeopaths, and an assortment of other lay healers was the fundamental method used by humans to treat diseases and to preserve their health.[3] The current prevalence of alternative medicine suggests that patients are looking for more therapeutic options than are widely available in conventional healthcare settings[3] and are searching for a more holistic approach to healthcare. Typically, TCM involves medical practices that use herbs, cannabis, dietary therapy, massage, and acupuncture [**Figures 7-1 to 7-3**]. The use of medicinal herbs that are chosen and combined specifically for each individual patient is stressed. Shen Nung's herbal book, dated 2700 BC, is considered the oldest Chinese medical book and contains details of the medicinal uses of over 300 plants [**Figure 7-4**].[4]

Among the Asian population, TCM is a very popular method of treating systemic and dermatologic diseases. The use of alternative medicine in Western countries ranges between 35% and 69%.[5,6] This popularity,

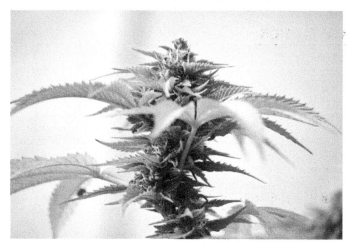

FIGURE 7-2. Cannabis is one of the 50 "fundamental" herbs of traditional Chinese medicine and is prescribed for a broad range of ailments. (Used with permission from Marisol LLC, Muscat, Sultanate of Oman.)

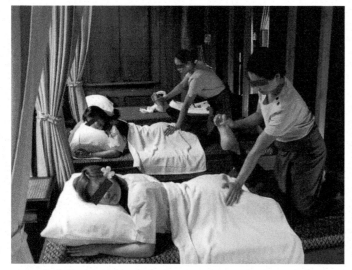

FIGURE 7-3. Thai massage is a system of massage and assisted stretching developed in Thailand and influenced by the traditional medicine systems of India, China, and Southeast Asia. (Used with permission from Marisol LLC, Muscat, Sultanate of Oman.)

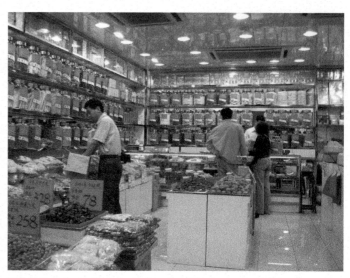

FIGURE 7-5. Medicines for dietary purposes. Patients seek out alternative medicine stores after becoming frustrated with modern medicine. (Used with permission from Marisol LLC, Muscat, Sultanate of Oman.)

which extends beyond the Asian population, is based on the misconception that alternative therapies are always safe and cost less than Western medicine. Additionally, patients who are increasingly frustrated by modern medicine also tend to seek alternative medical therapy [**Figure 7-5**]. In the United States, alternative therapy in 2007 generated expenditures estimated at around $14 billion.[7] Due to the increasing popularity of TCM, it is important to address the safety of some of the more common treatments and practices.

Herbal treatments are becoming increasingly popular and are often used for dermatologic conditions. Despite the common misconception that TCM herbal remedies have no adverse effects due to their "natural" composition, possible adverse effects such as hepatotoxicity have occurred. The most common adverse reactions with topical TCM treatments are contact dermatitis and irritant dermatitis. Topical TCM

treatments are often adulterated with the allergen, balsam of Peru, which is a natural resinous balsam from the trunk of a Central American tree; additionally, the North American standard patch tray now includes allergens such as tea tree oil and ylang-ylang [**Figure 7-6**], which are also commonly found in TCM.

Many dermatologists remain unaware of the existence of placebo-controlled studies involving TCM. Sheehan et al,[8] working in conjunction with the Chinese herbalist Luo in London, England, conducted one of the first placebo-controlled, double-blind studies involving atopic dermatitis. Therapeutic agents—including *Potentilla chinensis, Tribulus terrestris, Rehmannia glutinosa, Lophatherum gracile, Clematis armandii, Ledebouriella seseloides, Dictamnus dasycarpus, Paeonia lactiflora, Schizonepeta tenuifolia,* and *Glycyrrhiza glabra*—were compared with placebo herbs that had had no known efficacy for the treatment of atopic

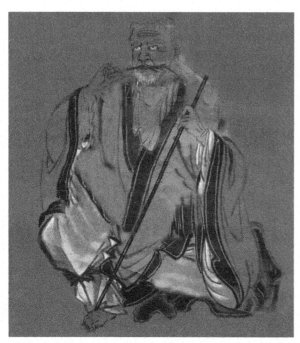

FIGURE 7-4. Shen Nung's herbal book, dated 2700 BC, is considered the oldest Chinese medical book and contains details of more than 300 plants. (Used with permission from Marisol LLC, Muscat, Sultanate of Oman.)

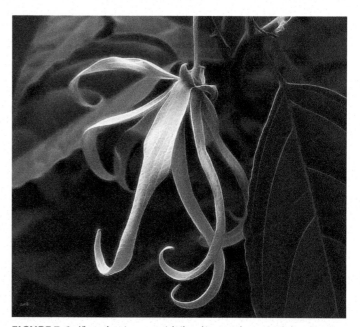

FIGURE 7-6. Ylang-ylang is an essential oil used in aromatherapy. It is believed to relieve high blood pressure, normalize sebum secretion for skin problems, and is considered to be an aphrodisiac. (Used with permission from Marisol LLC, Muscat, Sultanate of Oman.)

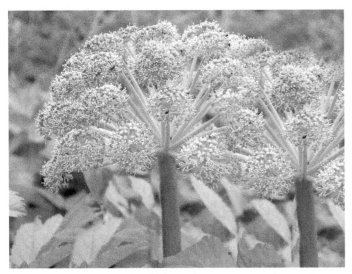

FIGURE 7-7. *Angelica dahurica* is a herb, known by its Latin name, *Radix angelicae dahuricae*, or by its Chinese name, *Bai Zhi*, and is used medicinally in traditional Chinese medicine. (Used with permission from Marisol LLC, Muscat, Sultanate of Oman.)

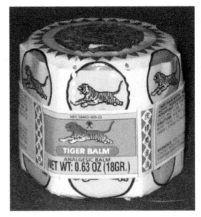

FIGURE 7-8. Tiger Balm can be used to treat muscle aches. It produces a warming effect when applied to the skin.

dermatitis. The results revealed that erythema was decreased by 91.4% with the active herbs compared with only 10.6% with the placebo herbs. The safety of these agents was demonstrated, and liver function tests, renal function tests, and complete blood cell counts were stable during the study period.[8]

Furocoumarins, a class of organic chemical compounds produced by various plants, are found in many Chinese herbal medicines that are used in the treatment of psoriasis. Several studies have been conducted with herbal medicines containing herbs such as Radix angelicae dahuricae (*Angelica dahurica*) [**Figure 7-7**] that have demonstrated efficacy in conjunction with ultraviolet A (UVA) radiation.[9] The difference in the efficacy between psoralen plus ultraviolet A (PUVA) and Radix angelicae dahuricae plus UVA was not statistically significant, and there was an increase in dizziness and nausea in the patients. However, a similar herb, Radix angelicae pubescentis, although equally successful in the treatment of psoriasis, showed increased lens changes.[10] Therefore, the side effects of certain alternative treatments may warrant a more conventional therapy with close medical supervision, even though the active herb may be effective therapeutically.

As the previously mentioned studies demonstrate, there is a very real possibility that certain TCM treatments may have efficacy beyond that of a simple placebo effect. However, associated adverse effects can sometimes occur that may prove fatal. In one case, a 66-year-old female patient developed Stevens-Johnson syndrome, a life-threatening skin condition, after drinking a health drink containing ophiopogonis tuber.[11] She tested positive in a drug lymphocyte stimulation test and on rechallenge with 1/1000 of the original dose.

TOPICAL TRADITIONAL MEDICINE

The use of traditional medicated oils and ointments is increasing in the United States. It is important to note that certain brand names do not indicate the actual ingredients contained within the treatments; for example, the popular brands Tiger Balm and 3-Snake Oil do not actually contain any material from these two animals [**Figure 7-8**]. One of the frequent arguments of using topical TCM by patients is the supposed absence of topical corticosteroids. However, many of the most common and prevalent adulterants in herbal creams are indeed corticosteroids.[12-18] More alarmingly, oral formulations have also been found to contain corticosteroids.[19-21] In a large-scale study from Taiwan, 2609 samples of traditional Chinese remedies were analyzed, and 24% were found to contain corticosteroids, some with significant amounts of clobetasol propionate.[22] In a study from London, 8 of 11 creams analyzed contained dexamethasone at concentrations inappropriate for use on the face or by children.[23] Other investigators reported the presence of triamcinolone acetonide in a phytocosmetic cream marketed in Europe as a skin care cosmetic product.[24,25] Unfortunately, both adults and infants may use products such as these for long periods of time, unaware of the potential adverse effects.

Herbal remedies frequently cause allergic reactions,[26] and the list of reported reactions in the medical literature is too extensive to be reviewed here. Some of the more common ingredients are discussed below, and other rare adverse effects are listed in **Table 7-1**.[27-35] Essential oils used topically for aromatherapy and in herbal creams have been responsible for photosensitization.[36] Bergamot has been implicated in some cases because it contains 5-methyoxyposor alen, and St. John's Wort, a best-selling herbal antidepressant, has photosensitivity as an adverse effect as well.[37] This may be significant in patients who require phototherapy for dermatologic conditions. The contamination of oral herbal preparations has also been reported, resulting in cases of arsenic and mercury poisoning.[38] Therefore, it is prudent to gain a detailed history of TCM use for patients presenting with either arsenical dermatoses or symptoms of mercury poisoning, because this may determine the cause of the poisoning.

As these studies indicate, some herbal medications have been demonstrated to improve dermatologic conditions in placebo-controlled studies. However, dermatologists should be aware that herbal treatments are by no means free of dermatologic adverse effects. It is important to realize that many TCM remedies have the potential to cause allergic contact dermatitis or photosensitization. A patch test or photo-patch test may be necessary to determine the offending herb.

ACUPUNCTURE

Acupuncture is an ancient system of healing developed over thousands of years as part of traditional medicine in China, Japan, and other Eastern countries. The earliest records of acupuncture date back over 4700 years ago, and it was described by Huang Ti Nei Ching Wen in

TABLE 7-1	Rare side effects of traditional Chinese medicine other than allergic reactions or contact dermatitis
Ingredient	**Adverse reactions**
Arnica extracts, paprika	Sweet's syndrome[27,28]
Arsenic	Arsenic dermatoses[29-31]
Garlic	Urticaria, angioedema[32]
Kakkon-to	Fixed drug eruption[33]
Kombucha tea	Pellagra[34]
Mercury	Mercury poisoning[38]
Piperaceae	Contact leukomelanosis[35]

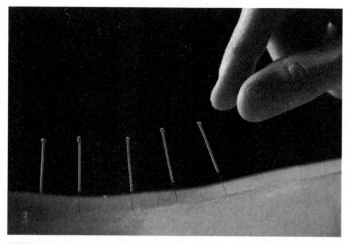

FIGURE 7-9. Acupuncture is an ancient system of healing developed over thousands of years as a part of the traditional medicine.

The Yellow Emperor's Classic of Internal Medicine, which is considered the authoritative text of Ancient Chinese medicine.[39] According to the National Health Interview Survey, an estimated 3.1 million adults and 150,000 children in the United States used acupuncture in 2007.[40]

The practice of acupuncture is thought to have begun with the discovery that the stimulation of specific areas on the skin affects the functioning of certain organs of the body. Acupuncture uses fine needles to stimulate the body's own healing process through lines of energy in the body or the vital energy—otherwise known as *Qi*. The *Qi* is thought to flow through channels know as *meridians* (meaning the elements of wood, water, metal, fire, and earth). When the free flow of this energy is obstructed, a symptom appears. The aim of acupuncture is to remove these obstructions, thus allowing the energy to flow freely and the symptom to disappear. This is done by the insertion of fine needles into acupuncture meridian points just beneath the skin [**Figures 7-9 and 7-10**]. Magnets are also used on acupuncture meridian points and are most commonly secured with tape or a bandage, as shown in **Figure 7-11.**

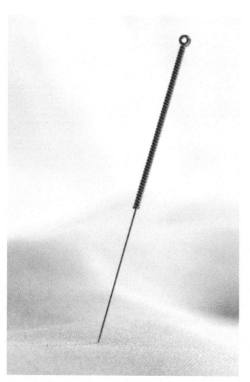

FIGURE 7-10. Needles are commonly used for acupuncture. (Used with permission from Marisol LLC, Muscat, Sultanate of Oman.)

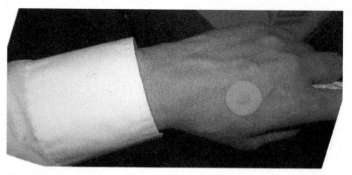

FIGURE 7-11. Magnets are also used on acupuncture meridian points and are most commonly secured with a tape or a bandage.

Acupuncture is used in a number of dermatologic conditions, such as atopic dermatitis, urticaria, and psoriasis.[41]

It is important for physicians to be aware of and understand some cultural practices, including moxibustion, cupping, and coining, because they may mimic symptoms of physical abuse. However, the lesions are usually transient, although there are reported cases of permanent scarring from moxibustion.[42,43]

MOXIBUSTION

Moxibustion is a procedure practiced most commonly in Southeast Asia and almost exclusively by the Mien.[44] *Moxibustion* is a word derived from the words *moxa* and *combustion*. *Moxa* is a herb derived from the plant mugwort, or *Artemisia vulgaris*. It is believed that this herb, when burned on acupuncture points, can restore the flow of *Qi*. The procedure consists of heat application with use of the herb *moxa* on acupuncture points.

Similar to acupuncture, moxibustion can be used either directly or indirectly to treat a variety of ailments, such as anemia, chronic stasis, acute lymphangitis, and immune suppression.[45] In the direct method, *moxa* is simply placed on the skin and lighted with an incense stick. The burning *moxa* is then pinched out or taken away by the therapist before it burns down completely to the skin. In the indirect method, the burning *moxa* is placed at the head of an inserted acupuncture needle. Japanese acupuncturists tend to prefer the direct method, and Chinese acupuncturists prefer the indirect method.[46] Patients often report a rush of warmth throughout their body during the treatment.

A great deal of training is required for a therapist to master moxibustion techniques. The lesions may mimic physical abuse, similar to cupping and coining,[47] because permanent burn scars can occur from an improper technique.[48] Physicians unfamiliar with these practices may suspect abuse, especially if the patient presenting with cutaneous lesions resulting from this traditional health practice is a woman or a child. Misdiagnosis could lead to grave consequences; for example, in one case, a false accusation of child abuse resulted in the suicide of a Vietnamese father.[49]

CUPPING

In cupping, a bottle is placed over a candle and coin with the bottle lip in direct contact with the skin [**Figure 7-12**]. As the candle consumes the oxygen, a vacuum is produced. This vacuum is intended to draw out the "fire wind" (pain). With this procedure, blood is drawn to the surface of the skin by the suction of the glass vessel on the skin. The cups are placed on areas in need of treatment, such as the chest, back, buttocks, chin, and dorsum of the foot. The cups are left on these specific areas of the skin until they adhere to the skin due to the negative pressure. They are then removed, leaving raised red patches that represent superficial skin inflammation. The lesions produced by cupping are round or annular as a consequence of both the suction and the mild burn caused by the heated bottle before the lack of oxygen extinguishes the flame. This

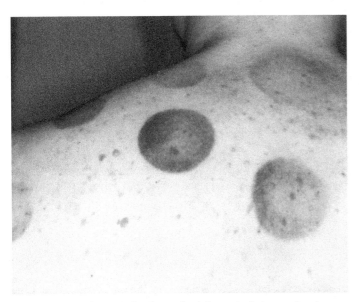

FIGURE 7-12. Cupping is thought to reduce inflammation in deeper adjacent organs. Both pain and infection are thought to be alleviated by the effect of the counterirritation. Shown are bruises on the back of an Asian male as a result of cupping.

is thought to reduce inflammation in adjacent organs deeper under the skin. Both pain and infection are thought to be alleviated through the effect of counterirritation.

COINING

Coining is a Vietnamese practice used commonly to treat a variety of illnesses, including febrile illnesses, headaches, myalgia, and malaise. This folk remedy is also known as *cao gio*. Coining is the process of applying hot mentholated oil or Tiger Balm to the chest and back. The edge of a coin is rubbed over the spine and ribs, producing linear petechiae and ecchymoses [**Figure 7-13**].[50] When found in Vietnamese children, lesions produced by coining have sometimes been misdiagnosed as

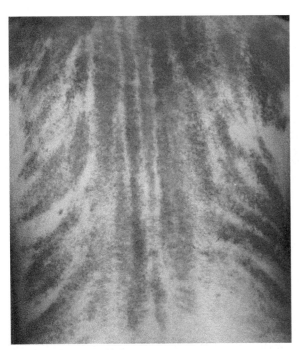

FIGURE 7-13. Coining is a Vietnamese practice used commonly to treat a variety of illnesses, including febrile illnesses, headaches, myalgia, and malaise. (Used with permission from Marisol LLC, Muscat, Sultanate of Oman.)

child abuse, and legal actions have been brought against the parents. Fortunately, in some of the cases, physicians acquainted with this practice testified that coining was not a form of child abuse but a type of alternative therapy.[50]

The most common complications of coining have been minor burns. There is an isolated report of a 45-year-old female patient who caught fire during a coining treatment and sustained full-thickness burns, requiring admission to a burn unit.[51] There was one report of coining, or brainstem compression, secondary to the practice of coining, and this seems to be an idiosyncratic reaction.[52] Because many Vietnamese Americans and other Southeast Asians living in the United States fear criticism from their physicians for practicing coining, the true incidence of the custom is unknown. It is probably much higher than appreciated. In a survey of a clinic in Washington, DC, coining was the most commonly used practice among Cambodian (70%), Chinese (35%), and Laotian (10%) patients.[44]

Another Asian healing practice, pinching, uses the same principle as coining. In this case, pressure is applied by pinching the skin between the thumb and index finger in order to produce a contusion.

CONCLUSION

In conclusion, the fast-growing Asian populations of the United States have a diverse range of cultural customs and practices that affect healthcare. Additionally, some cultural practices and habits are being adapted by many non-Asians for the treatment of certain medical illnesses. It is important for clinicians to be knowledgeable of these cultural practices and habits, and this is especially true for those practicing in urban regions, which generally have higher immigrant populations.

There are many myths regarding the practice of TCM, and it is important to realize that certain TCM treatments and customs should not automatically be designated as unscientific superstition. Many traditional therapies are currently being used in Western hospitals, such as the use of acupuncture for treatment of stress and aches. Some therapies have shown efficacy in double-blind studies. However, like most over-the-counter and prescription medications, both topical and oral herbal medications have been known to cause significant side effects, particularly allergic contact dermatitis and photosensitization.

Finally, it is important to be aware of traditional practices such as coining and moxibustion so as to ensure that their results are not misconstrued as spousal or child abuse. An increased awareness and understanding of various Asian cultural habits and practices will hopefully facilitate communication between patient and physician as well as provide insight into various signs and symptoms during clinical examinations.

REFERENCES

1. U.S. Census Bureau. The Asian population: 2010. http://www.census.gov/prod/cen2010/briefs/c2010br-11.pdf. Accessed October 31, 2013.
2. Ries AL, Picchi MA, Nguyen LH, et al. Asthma in a Vietnamese refugee population. *Am J Respir Crit Care Med.* 1997;155:1895-1901.
3. White House Commission on Complementary and Alternative Medicine Policy. Chapter 2: overview of CAM in the United States: recent history, current status, and prospects for the future. http://www.whccamp.hhs.gov/fr2.html. Accessed November 2, 2013.
4. U.S. National Library of Medicine. Classics of traditional Chinese medicine. http://www.nlm.nih.gov/exhibition/chinesemedicine/emperors.html. Accessed November 2, 2013.
5. Ernst E, Pittler MH, Stevinson C. Complementary/alternative medicine in dermatology: evidence-assessed efficacy of two diseases and two treatments. *Am J Clin Dermatol.* 2002;3:341-348.
6. Smith N, Shin DB, Brauer JA, et al. Use of complementary and alternative medicine among adults with skin disease: results from a national survey. *J Am Acad Dermatol.* 2009;60:419-425.
7. Davis MA, Weeks WB. The concentration of out-of-pocket expenditures on complementary and alternative medicine in the United States. *Altern Ther Health Med.* 2012;18:36-42.
8. Sheehan MP, Rustin MH, Atherton DJ, et al. Efficacy of traditional Chinese herbal therapy in adult atopic dermatitis. *Lancet.* 1992;340:13-17.

9. Zhang GW, Wang HJ, Zhou YH, et al. Treatment of psoriasis by photochemotherapy: a comparison between the photosensitizing capsule of *Angelica dahurica* and 8-MOP. *Zhonghua Yi Xue Za Zhi (Taipei).* 1983;63:16-19.

10. Li FQ, Fang FY, Li SH. A long-term follow-up of 58 cases of psoriasis treated with traditional Chinese medicine *Angelica dahurica* and long wave ultraviolet. *Chin J Phys Ther.* 1984;7:154-155.

11. Mochitomi Y, Inoue A, Kawabata H, et al. Stevens-Johnson syndrome caused by a health drink (Eberu) containing ophiopogonis tuber. *J Dermatol.* 1998;25:662-665.

12. Ahmed S, Riaz M. Quantitation of cortico-steroids as common adulterants in local drugs by HPLC. *Chromatographica.* 1991;31:67-70.

13. Wood B, Wishart J. Potent topical steroid in a Chinese herbal cream. *N Z Med J.* 1997;110:420-421.

14. Ernst E. Adverse effects of herbal drugs in dermatology. *Br J Dermatol.* 2000;143:923-929.

15. Allen BR, Parkinson R, Hollman A, et al. Chinese herbs for eczema. *Lancet.* 1990;336:177.

16. O'Driscoll J, Burden AD, Kingston TP. Potent topical steroid obtained from a Chinese herbalist. *Br J Dermatol.* 1992;127:543-544.

17. Graham-Brown RA, Bourke JF, Bumphrey G. Chinese herbal remedies may contain steroids. *BMJ.* 1994;308:473.

18. Hughes JR, Higgins EM, Pembroke AC. Oral dexamethasone masquerading as a Chinese herbal. *Br J Dermatol.* 1994;130:261.

19. Van Stricht BI, Parvais OE, Vanhaelen-Fastré RJ, et al. Safer use of traditional remedies: remedies may contain cocktail of active drugs. *BMJ.* 1994;308:1162.

20. Morice A. Adulteration of homeopathic remedies. *Lancet.* 1987;1:635.

21. Joseph AM, Biggs T, Garr M, et al. Stealth steroids. *N Engl J Med.* 1991;324:62.

22. Huang WF, Wen KC, Hsiao ML. Adulteration by synthetic therapeutic substances of traditional Chinese medicines in Taiwan. *J Clin Pharmacol.* 1997;37:344-350.

23. Keane FM, Munn SE, Vivier AW, et al. Analysis of Chinese herbal creams prescribed for dermatological conditions. *BMJ.* 1999;318:563.

24. Vena GA, Cassno N, Mastrolonardo M, et al. Management of inflammatory dermatoses with a cosmetic preparation containing antioxidant/anti-inflammatory agents. *J Ital Dermatol Venerol.* 1998;133:373-380.

25. Bircher AJ, Niederer M, Hohl C, et al. Stealth triamcinolone acetonide in a phytocosmetic cream. *Br J Dermatol.* 2002;146:531-532.

26. Mäntyranta T, Haahtela T. Allergic reactions caused by alternative drugs. *Duodecim.* 1993;109:301-308.

27. Greer JM, Rosen T, Tschen JA. Sweet's syndrome with an exogenous cause. *Cutis.* 1993;51:112-114.

28. Delmonte S, Brusati C, Parodi A, et al. Leukemia-related Sweet's syndrome elicited by pathergy to arnica. *Dermatology.* 1998;197:195-196.

29. Kew J, Morris C, Aihie A, et al. Arsenic and mercury intoxication due to Indian ethnic remedies. *BMJ.* 1993;306:506-507.

30. Wong SS, Tan KC, Goh CL. Cutaneous manifestations of chronic arsenicism: review of seventeen cases. *J Am Acad Dermatol.* 1998;38:179-185.

31. Tay CH. Cutaneous manifestations of arsenic poisoning due to certain Chinese herbal medicine. *Australas J Dermatol.* 1974;15:121-131.

32. Asero R, Mistrello G, Roncarolo D, et al. A case of garlic allergy. *J Allergy Clin Immunol.* 1998;101:427-428.

33. Fujimoto N, Tajima S. Extensive fixed drug eruption due to the Japanese herbal drug "kakkon-to." *Br J Dermatol.* 2003;149:1303-1305.

34. Wood B, Rademaker M, Oakley A, et al. Pellagra in a woman using alternative remedies. *Australas J Dermatol.* 1998;39:42-44.

35. Liao YL, Chiang YC, Tsai TF, et al. Contact leukomelanosis induced by the leaves of Piper Betle L. (Pieperaceae): a clinical and histopathologic survey. *J Am Acad Dermatol.* 1999;40:583-589.

36. Cocks H, Wilson D. Dangers of the intake of psoralens and subsequent UV exposure producing significant burns. *Burns.* 1998;24:82.

37. Stevinson C, Ernst E. Safety of hypericum in patients with depression. *CNS Drugs.* 1999;11:125-132.

38. Ernst E, de Smet PAGM. Risks associated with complementary therapies. In: Dukes MNG, ed. *Meyler's Side Effects of Drugs.* 13th ed. Amsterdam, the Netherlands: Elsevier Science; 1996:1427.

39. Veith I. *The Yellow Emperor's Classic of Internal Medicine.* Vol 18. Berkeley, CA: University of California Press; 1984:56-78.

40. National Center for Complementary and Alternative Medicine. Acupuncture: an introduction. http://nccam.nih.gov/health/acupuncture/introduction. htm#ususe. Accessed November 2, 2013.

41. Chen CJ, Yu HS. Acupuncture treatment of urticaria. *Arch Dermatol.* 1998;134:1397-1399.

42. Crutchfield CE III, Bisig TJ. Images in clinical medicine: coining. *N Engl J Med.* 1995;332:1552.

43. Wong HC, Wong JK, Wong NY. Signs of physical abuse or evidence of moxibustion, cupping or coining? *CMAJ.* 1999;160:785-786.

44. Buchwald D, Panwala S, Hooton T. Use of traditional health practices by Southeast Asian refugees in a primary care clinic. *West J Med.* 1992;156:507-511.

45. Zhou W. Acute lymphangitis treated by moxibustion with garlic in 118 cases. *J Tradit Chin Med.* 2003;23:198.

46. Wilcox F. *Moxibustion: The Power of Mugwort Fire.* Boulder, CA: Blue Poppy Press; 2008.

47. Look KM, Look RM. Skin scraping, cupping, and moxibustion that may mimic physical abuse. *J Forens Sci.* 1997;42:103-105.

48. Condé-Salazar L, Gonázlez MA, Guimarens D, et al. Burns due to moxibustion. *Contact Dermatitis.* 1991;25:332-333.

49. Nong TA. "Pseudo-battered child" syndrome. *JAMA.* 1976;236:2288.

50. Yeatman GW, Dang VV. Cao gío (coin rubbing): Vietnamese attitudes toward healthcare. *JAMA.* 1980;244:2748-2749.

51. Amshel CE, Caruso DM. Vietnamese "coining": a burn case report and literature review. *J Burn Care Rehabil.* 2000;21:112-114.

52. Ponder A, Lehman LB. "Coining" and "coning": an unusual complication of unconventional medicine. *Neurology.* 1994;44:774-775.

CHAPTER 8

Impact of Traditional Hispanic American Cultures on Healthcare Practices

Sabrina Uddin

Sylvia Li

Claudia Hernandez

KEY POINTS

- The increased ethnic diversity in the United States is resulting in an increase in different types of traditional medical practices and beliefs.

- The Hispanic population in the United States will triple by 2050, representing 29% of the population; thus, practicing physicians should be aware of the traditional health beliefs and popular folk remedies used widely by this group.

- Traditional medicine, also known as indigenous or folk medicine, is used largely by elderly Mexican Americans for chronic health problems; however, this population will often deny their attachment to these kinds of treatments due to their negative cultural connotations.

- *Curanderos, naturistas,* and *sanadores* are lay healers who may provide healthcare services to the Hispanic community.

- Folk illnesses, such as *mal de aire* and *mal de ojo,* are recognized in certain cultures as legitimate causes of illness.

- Botanical remedies that are intended to cure or alleviate dermatologic conditions are the most common folk-healing products used by Hispanics.

- Folk remedies are most often applied to treat skin conditions like acne, alopecia, and atopic dermatitis.

INTRODUCTION

During the twentieth and twenty-first centuries, medicine in the United States has borne witness to a new and unique challenge—physician practices have become more complex because providers have to care for patients who belong to an ever-increasing range of cultural and racial groups. This growing complexity has risen out of the large-scale transformations that have taken place in the U.S. population. The country's shifting immigration patterns, along with the growth of certain geographical regions and settlements that attract a concentration of immigrant populations, have led to cultural changes in local communities that will naturally have an impact on practicing physicians.

The key minority groups in the United States, according to the U.S. Office of Management and Budget, are *Hispanic* or *Latino*, *African American* or *Black*, *Asian American*, *Native Hawaiian* or other *Pacific Islander*, *American Indian*, and *Alaskan Native*.[1] Apart from the Asian group, the remaining groups are all considered to have disadvantaged status because these minorities are burdened with a disproportionate number of the nation's poor health outcomes, which is also an example of the health disparities among populations.[2,3] These disparities are preventable and the result of multiple factors, including poor access, sociolinguistic barriers, poverty, and differences in healthcare expectations.[4,5] Further contributing to these disparities is a poor understanding of the traditional cultural beliefs and practices of many patients. Traditional medicine remains a commonly sought-out alternative for many patients in part due to its affordability, its correspondence to the patient's ideology, the reduced linguistic barriers, and the patient's dissatisfaction with the perceived results of modern medical therapies.[6] Over 75% of Hispanics use or practice alternative therapies, although few patients will share this with their healthcare provider.[7,8] Improving the quality of healthcare for minority patients will require improvements in the treating physician's recognition and sensitivity to these traditional practices. This chapter explores traditional Hispanic health beliefs and popular folk remedies used for dermatologic conditions.

BACKGROUND

The U.S. government mandated the use of the terms *Hispanic* and *Latino* nearly four decades ago to categorize this diverse population group; these terms are still used interchangeably to describe individuals of various regions of origin and do not indicate a specific ethnic group. Although they are used interchangeably, the two terms nevertheless differ significantly in their meaning. *Hispanic*, derived from the ancient Roman provinces of Hispania, is used to denote individuals from countries that were once under Spanish rule. On the other hand, *Latino* categorizes someone of Latin American origin and is believed to have derived from the shortening of the Spanish term *latinoamericano*.[9,10] The context in which the word is used is important because one term may be more correct than the other; for example, a native of Spain would fall under the category of *Hispanic* but not *Latino*.

The U.S. Census Bureau lists 28 Hispanic or Latino American groups.[11] These groups are not homogenous and have significant cultural differences, although most speak Spanish. Despite the use of these pan-ethnic terms, most Hispanics (51%) still prefer to refer to themselves by their family's country of origin (eg, as Cuban or Dominican), according to the Pew Hispanic Center. However, if forced to use one of these two terms, most prefer the term *Hispanic* over *Latino* by a ratio of 2 to 1.[12] Because this chapter deals with residents of the United States, most of whom are from the Latin American countries, the terms *Hispanic* and *Latino* will be used interchangeably.

Hispanics have replaced African Americans as the most populous minority group in the United States. In 2005, there were 42 million Hispanics living in the United States, and this number is expected to rise to 128 million by 2050. This means that the Hispanic population will have tripled by 2050 and form 29% of the total population. A total of 31% of the adult working-age population and 35% of the child population are predicted to be Hispanic by 2050.[13] Mexicans are the largest Hispanic group by country of origin, followed by Puerto Ricans, Cubans, Central Americans, South Americans, Dominicans, and Spaniards.[11]

TRADITIONAL, ALTERNATIVE, AND FOLK MEDICINE

Traditional medicine, also known as indigenous or folk medicine, can be defined as "the knowledge, skills and practices based on the theories, beliefs and experiences indigenous to different cultures, used in the maintenance of health and in the prevention, diagnosis, improvement or treatment of physical and mental illness."[14] Traditional medicine often reflects the prevailing practices, philosophies, and geographical

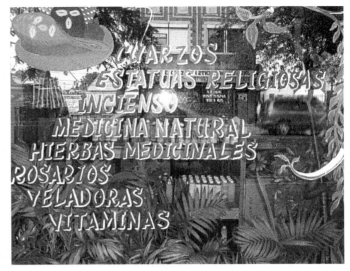

FIGURE 8-1. The storefront of a local natural remedies shop, or *botánica*, in a Hispanic neighborhood. The items available for sale include medicinal herbs, crystals, and religious items.

conditions of a certain area. It often has a holistic approach, focusing on the overall health of a patient and on achieving an equilibrium between the body, mind, and environment.[15] Although traditional medicine is at times referred to as alternative medicine, this may not always be correct. Alternative (or complementary) medicine is a "broad set of healthcare practices that are not part of [the] country's own tradition and not integrated into the dominant healthcare system."[16] Additionally, folk healing is also disparate from the two previous types of medicine because it involves the "use of culturally known herbs and remedies, either self-administered or obtained through a folk healer, for curing sickness and illnesses."[17-19] All cultures practice some form of folk healing, including the Hispanic cultures. Latino immigrants may combine a range of approaches, often including conventional medicine, folk healers who use alternative treatments, and religious beliefs and rituals [**Figure 8-1**].[20]

CURANDERISMO

Although Hispanics tend to seek out modern medicine for major health problems, traditional healing practices remain a commonly sought-out alternative for chronic health problems. This is especially true of elderly Mexican Americans who often approach the use of health resources in a different manner from second- or third-generation individuals born in the United States.[21] *Curanderismo* originates from the term *curar*, meaning "to heal," and is an umbrella term for a wide variety of Mexican folk-healing practices. The central tenements of *curanderismo* espouse achieving a harmony and balance with nature, along with aspects of spirituality. The healing process is conducted by an individual who is believed to have a gift or calling for this type of healing, known as *el don* or *curandero*.[22] The *curandero* incorporates the patients' religious beliefs into the process, provides counseling and spiritual cleansing, and administers or recommends herbal medications.[20,21] The *curandero* remains an important health resource in the border communities but can be found anywhere in the United States. Many Latinos will deny having any communication with them and may even view the word *curandero* with negative connotations. Instead, *naturista* (herbal medication specialist) and *sanador* (healer) appear to be increasingly popular as terms to refer to these folk healers.[20] Although the *curandero* is the best-known term for a folk healer, there are many lay individuals who provide healthcare services within and catering to the Latino community [**Table 8-1**].

SANTERÍA

Santería is a fusion of philosophy and religion originally brought over by West African slaves that has since been combined with Christian cultural elements. It is particularly popular among Cubans, Puerto Ricans, and Dominicans. In the past, slaves were forbidden to pray to *orishas*

TABLE 8-1	Types of Hispanic folk medicine practitioners
Practitioner	**Description**
Curandero/a	This is the best-known type of folk healer. They are known to have clear expertise in the community as a lay healer. They are recognized by the community as being able to treat spiritual, physical, and psychosomatic illnesses. They may also be known as *sanador*.
Espiritualisto/a	Psychic medium.
Huesero	Bone therapist.
Partera	Midwife.
Señor/a	They are usually the first folk healer consulted. They may read tarot cards and may also be an elder (*abuela* or grandmother).
Sobadoro/a	Muscle therapist who primarily gives massage therapy.
Yerbero/a	Herbalist who specializes in herbal remedies.

Source: Data from Trotter and Chavira[21] and Tafur et al.[22]

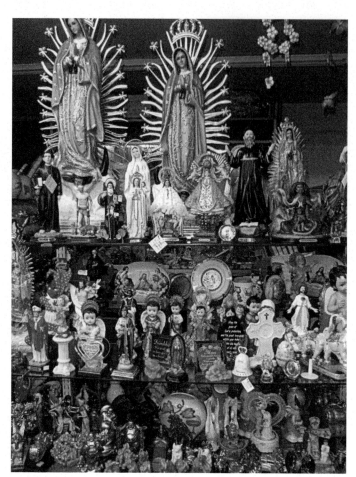

FIGURE 8-3. Religious statues available at a natural remedy store, or *botánica*. Although Christian figures dominate the shelves of this store, other figures such as Buddhas, seen on the bottom shelf, are also for sale.

(deities of *Santería*), so they substituted Catholic saints to symbolize these folk deities to trick their owners.[23,24] *Orishas* are believed to control nature, and the individual gods possess various powers that correspond to specific symbols, objects, and jewelry.[25] By attributing the causes of illness to supernatural forces, *Santería* attempts to explain why some stay well while others get sick. *Santería* helps to maintain or reinstate balance and a sense of control over one's life by dispelling malignant forces, mobilizing beneficial forces, and decreasing an individual's uncertainty and stress regarding their illness.[25,26] *Santeros* are the priests and only official practitioners of *Santería* [**Figure 8-2**].

RELIGION AND HEALING

In Christianity, both in the Old and New Testament, there are many accounts of the faithful seeking and being rewarded with cures through prayers and sacrifice. These cures are ascribed to the power of God and many of the Catholic Church's canonized saints. Many communities in Latin America have canonized their own saints (often termed folk saints), many of whom have a "Robin Hood" outlaw image befitting their image as protectors. The veneration of these folk saints coexists with reverence for the officially canonized Christian saints in many Latino cultures.[27] To symbolize their confidence in and devotion to these saints, many individuals will possess copies of images of the saints and participate in devotional pilgrimages. This spiritualism is felt to have salutogenic effects.[28] For many, prayer is an important coping mechanism used to gain some emotional stability when facing difficult situations such as poor health [**Figure 8-3**].[20]

LATINO FOLK MEDICINE CONSTRUCTS

Folk illnesses are diseases that are recognized only within a specific cultural or societal context; these may be referred to as culture-related, culture-bound, or culture-specific syndromes. Latino patients can experience a variety of these syndromes, including *mal de aire* (bad or malevolent wind), *susto* and *espanto* (sudden fright), *robo de alma* (theft of the soul), and *mal de ojo* (evil eye).[29] These conditions may present

with a wide constellation of possible patient symptoms and are common disorders. They may carry psychological or religious overtones and are deeply rooted in the Latino culture. When Latino patients are treated by physicians unfamiliar with these cultural-specific illnesses, the true nature of their complaint could be lost or mislabeled as fabrications or malingering. Culture-related syndromes may be best compared to psychosomatic disorders; however, within their own specific culture, they are recognized diseases and treated with the folk medicine of that culture.[30] It is recommended for physicians to consult with those familiar with the culture to learn more regarding other common general syndromes seen in Latinos.

However, some diseases are clearly recognized as being the consequence of a biological process and not the result of spiritual or supernatural forces. For example, infections are recognized as a biological process and are not treated using only a spiritual ritual or with folk medicines. Skin complaints are generally classified as a biological process due to their clinically visible nature and are not typically treated with rites or folk medicines.

FOLK-HEALING REMEDIES

Botanical remedies are the most common folk-healing products used by Hispanics. Many treatments involve applying the plants or plant products externally on the skin, even for internal ailments. These products are usually purchased at local stores called *botánicas* or *hierberías*, which are local herbal shops commonly found in Hispanic neighborhoods. These establishments may also sell amulets, statues of saints, candles, and solutions to protect the buyer from misfortune or to restore health [**Figures 8-4 and 8-5**]. No regulation of herbal products currently exists in the United States, except for dietary supplements, so there is little to

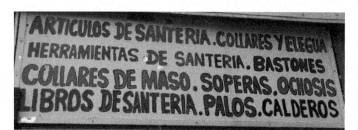

FIGURE 8-2. A natural remedy store named for *Eleguá*, a powerful orisha in *Santería*.

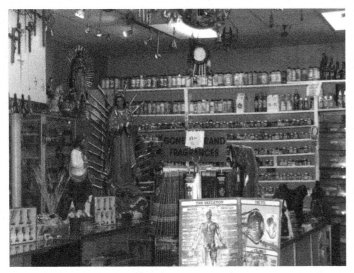

FIGURE 8-4. A *botánica* store in a predominantly Hispanic neighborhood in Chicago, IL. Religious, medicinal, and other "good luck" items are for sale.

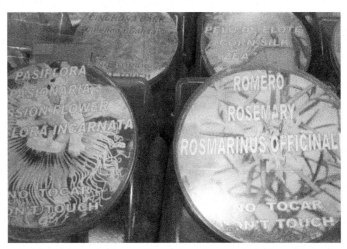

FIGURE 8-6. Local *botánicas* or herb shops generally have a selection of dried herbs. Customers may ask the shopkeepers for advice on the correct combination and preparation of herbs to use for their particular health problems.

no standardization of the respective purity, active ingredients, or concentrations of herbal remedies. It is likely that many herbal remedies are sold or prescribed for conditions for which they may have no significant scientific evidence of effectiveness [**Figure 8-6**].[31]

Teas and herbs are the typical starting point for Latino traditional medicine. Botanical products are also boiled, with the resulting solution being used for compresses, or are mixed with a variety of oils to be compounded into creams, pastes, or poultices.[21] A poultice, also known as a cataplasm, is a soft moist mass containing an adhesive substance that is spread on cloth and applied while warm to an inflamed area of the body or on aching joints.[32] Other preparations include syrups, salves, capsules, and tablets containing the powdered form of a botanical product.

Minerals are inorganic natural compounds formed through geologic processes; unlike botanical products, they are not grown or plant-based in origin. They include trace elements such as calcium, zinc, and various salts.[33] Both minerals and vitamins are widely used as dietary supplements in the Hispanic community for disease treatment or prevention. The most commonly used supplements are one-a-day multivitamin/multimineral supplements. Hispanic women are more likely to use dietary supplements than men; however, overall, Hispanics will use these less frequently than non-Hispanic in the United States.[34,35] Zootherapies are remedies made or resulting from animals, or made from their products. An example of a product made from animals would be lanolin, because it is made by the sebaceous glands of wool-bearing animals. Apitherapy (bee sting/bee venom therapy) is used by many Latinos for arthritic or joint pains. In many cases, live bees are used to deliver the venom. Folk remedies may also include man-made or industrial elements; examples include the use of soot and coal tar.[36]

TREATMENTS FOR DERMATOLOGIC CONDITIONS

After gastrointestinal disorders, skin disorders are the most common ailments for which natural remedies are used in South America.[37] Popular natural remedies can be found under search terms such as *remedios caseros* (home remedies), *remedios naturales* or *medicina natural* (natural remedies), and *remedios de la abuela* (grandmother's cures/therapies). Many of these remedies have been passed down for generations through oral traditions and folk practices. The retention of these practices within the Latino community can be explained by the close proximity of their traditional homelands in Mexico or South America as well as the continuing influx of immigrants who reinforce these practices. The following sections describe remedies used by many Hispanics for some common dermatologic conditions. As previously stated, there may be little scientific evidence supporting the effectiveness of such remedies. These natural medicinal products are summarized in **Table 8-2**.[38-42]

ACNE

The majority of acne home remedies are topical and make use of different fruits, vegetables, and herbs. Acids within the fruit, specifically

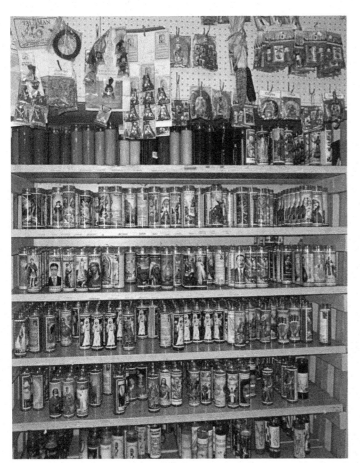

FIGURE 8-5. A large selection of candles with images of religious figures available for sale at a *botánica*. This is one of three shelves displaying hundreds of votive candles.

TABLE 8-2 Botanicals, minerals, nutrients, and other traditional products used by Hispanics for medicinal purposes

Traditional botanical products used medicinally

Botanical product	Spanish name	Dermatologic use	Contraindications
Almonds	*Almendra*	Used topically as a poultice for burns.	• None
Aloe vera	*Zábila*	Used topically for acne, atopic dermatitis, blisters, burns, rosacea, sunburn, tinea pedis, urticaria, and verrucae. Used topically and orally for psoriasis.	• None with topical use
Apple cider vinegar	*Vinagre de sidra de manzana*	Used topically for acne, atopic dermatitis, pediculosis, rosacea, and sunburn.	• Moderate interaction with digoxin, insulin, and potassium-sparing diuretics
Arnica	*Árnica*	Used topically for psoriasis.	• Moderate interaction with anticoagulants (aspirin, clopidogrel, ibuprofen, dalteparin, enoxaparin, heparin, and warfarin)
Avocado	*Aguacate*	Used topically for dermatophytosis, hair loss prevention, and pediculosis.	• Moderate interaction with antidiabetic medications
Basil	*Albahaca*	Used topically for acne.	• Moderate interaction with anticoagulants
Bitter melon	*Cundeamore*	Used topically for anorectal herpes, cutaneous abscesses and wounds, and psoriasis.	• Moderate interaction with antidiabetic medications • Should not be taken orally if pregnant or breastfeeding
Burdock	*Bardana*	Used topically for atopic dermatitis. Used orally by boiling and then ingesting as a tea.	• Moderate interaction with anticoagulants
Cabbage	*Repollo*	Used topically for blisters by boiling in milk and applying to the skin.	• None
Calendula	*Caléndula*	Used topically for acne scars by crushing the fresh petals and applying to the skin. Used topically for atopic dermatitis by applying as a tea.	• Moderate interaction with CNS depressants • Should not be taken if pregnant or breastfeeding
Carrot	*Zanahoria*	Used topically for acne, atopic dermatitis, blisters, furuncles (boils), melasma, and sunburn.	• None
Cat's claw	*Uña de gato*	Used orally for wound healing and alopecia.	• Moderate interaction with drugs changed by the cytochrome P450 system, antihypertensives, and immunosuppressants • Should not be used in individuals with leukemia or autoimmune disorders
Celery	*Apio*	Used topically for urticaria by boiling and then applying the cooled liquid.	• Moderate interaction with levothyroxine, lithium, photosensitizing drugs, and CNS depressants
Chamomile	*Manzanilla*	Used topically for atopic dermatitis, minor injuries, sunburn, and rosacea. Used orally for urticaria as a tea.	• Moderate interaction with oral contraceptive pills, estrogen, benzodiazepine, CNS depressants, tamoxifen, and warfarin • Minor interaction with medications changed by cytochrome P450 system • Should not be used in patients with conditions worsened by exposure to estrogen (eg, breast cancer, uterine cancer, ovarian cancer, endometriosis, and fibroids)
Comfrey leaves	*Consuelda*	Used topically for acne.	• Major interaction with hepatotoxic drugs • Moderate interaction with drugs changed by cytochrome P450 system • Should not be used on broken skin or in those with liver disease
Cornstarch	*Maicena*	Used topically for atopic dermatitis, sunburn, and urticaria.	• None
Cucumber	*Pepino*	Used topically for acne, burns, eczema, rosacea, and sunburn by soaking and applying the liquid.	• Moderate interaction with antidiabetic medications
Dandelion	*Diente de león*	Used topically for lentigines and verrucae. Used orally for acne and seborrheic dermatitis by boiling and ingesting.	• Moderate interaction with quinolone antibiotics, lithium, potassium-sparing diuretics, and medications changed by the cytochrome P450 system
Fig	*Higo*	Used topically for furuncles (boils).	• Moderate interaction with insulin and other antidiabetic drugs
Garlic	*Ajo*	Used topically for acne, arthropod bites, blisters, comedones, furuncles (boils), dermatophytosis, pediculosis, psoriasis, tinea pedis, and verrucae.	• Major interaction with isoniazid and NNRTIs • Moderate interaction with oral contraceptive pills, cyclosporine, medications changed by the cytochrome P450 system, and anticoagulants
Ginger	*Jengibre*	Used topically for analgesia and burns. Used topically for tinea pedis by boiling and applying.	• Moderate interaction with anticoagulants • Minor interaction with antidiabetic agents and calcium channel blockers

(Continued)

TABLE 8-2   Botanicals, minerals, nutrients, and other traditional products used by Hispanics for medicinal purposes (continued)

Traditional botanical products used medicinally

Botanical product	Spanish name	Dermatologic use	Contraindications
Honey	*Miel*	Used topically for burns, dermatophytosis, and seborrheic dermatitis. Used topically for scars by adding sugar and used as an exfoliant.	• None
Horseradish	*Rábano picante*	Used topically for lentigines.	• Large amounts should not be ingested if the patient is pregnant or breastfeeding or has gastric or intestinal ulcers, hypothyroidism, or renal disease • Moderate interaction with levothyroxine
Lavender oil	*Aceite esencial de lavanda*	Used topically for atopic dermatitis, blisters, pediculosis, seborrheic dermatitis, and tinea pedis.	• None
Lemon juice	*Jugo de limón*	Used topically for acne, dermatophytosis, hyperhidrosis, lentigines, and melasma.	• Large amounts should not be ingested by those with renal disease
Lettuce	*Lechuga*	Used topically for furuncles (boils).	• Major interaction with CNS depressants
Lime	*Cal*	Used topically for arthropod bites.	• Moderate interaction with drugs broken down by the cytochrome P450 system • Side effects include increased photosensitivity
Mint	*Menta*	Used topically for burns.	• Moderate interaction with drugs broken down by the cytochrome P450 system • Minor interaction with antacids
Oatmeal	*Avena*	Used topically for acne, atopic dermatitis, psoriasis, and sunburn.	• Should not be used on large open wounds
Olive oil	*Aceite de oliva*	Used topically for pediculosis, psoriasis, and rosacea.	• None topically
Onion	*Cebolla*	Used topically for lentigines by applying the juice. Used topically for burns, and urticaria by applying the skins.	• Moderate interaction with aspirin, lithium, antidiabetic agents, and anticoagulants
Orange skin	*Piel de naranja*	Used topically for acne.	• None
Oregano	*Orégano*	Used topically for acne, arthropod bites (including spider bites), dermatophytosis, psoriasis, rosacea, seborrheic dermatitis, tinea pedis, varicose veins, and verrucae.	• Moderate interaction with lithium
Parsley	*Perejil*	Used topically for skin blemishes and urticaria as a poultice.	• None
Persimmons	*Nísperos*	Used topically for scars by boiling, soaking a cloth with the boiled liquid, and applying.	• Moderate interaction with antihypertensives
Plantain leaves	*Llantén*	Used topically for acne and tinea pedis.	• Unknown
Potatoes	*Patata*	Used topically for burns.	• Moderate interaction with thrombolytic drugs
Rose hips	*Rosa de Castilla*	Used topically for skin infections as an eyewash.	• Moderate interaction with vitamin C
Rosemary	*Romero*	Used topically for alopecia and seborrheic dermatitis.	• Possible exacerbation of seizure disorders
Sage	*Salvia*	Used topically for arthropod bites, atopic dermatitis, sunburn, and as a deodorant. Used orally for hyperhidrosis.	• None
Sarsaparilla	*Zarzaparrilla*	Used topically for furuncles (boils) by boiling and applying the liquid. Used orally for urticaria.	• Moderate interaction with digoxin or lithium • Should not be used by those with renal disease
St. John's wort	*Hierba de San Juan*	Used topically for cuts and wounds.	• May cause photosensitivity in large doses • Should not be taken in conjunction with other antidepressants • May interfere with the action of oral contraceptives • May diminish the effectiveness of protease inhibitors in patients with HIV
Tea tree oil	*Esencias del árbol del té*	Used topically for acne, arthropod bites, blisters, dermatophytosis, pediculosis, seborrheic dermatitis, tinea pedis, and as a deodorant.	• Should not be ingested
Thyme	*Tomillo*	Used topically for alopecia areata, and atopic dermatitis.	• May affect thyroid activity
Tomato	*Tomate*	Used topically for furuncles (boils), rosacea, sunburn, and urticaria.	• None
Turmeric	*Cúrcuma*	Used topically for lentigines by combining with buttermilk and used as a scrub.	• Moderate interaction with anticoagulants
Vinegar	*Vinagre*	Used topically for tinea pedis, and arthropod bites.	• Moderate interaction with digoxin, insulin, and diuretics

(Continued)

TABLE 8-2   Botanicals, minerals, nutrients, and other traditional products used by Hispanics for medicinal purposes (continued)

Traditional botanical products used medicinally

Botanical product	Spanish name	Dermatologic use	Contraindications
Witch hazel	*Agua de hamamelis*	Used topically for atopic dermatitis, sunburn, and urticaria.	• None
Wormwood	*Estafiate*	Used topically for healing wounds, arthropod bites, and as a counterirritant to reduce pain.	• Should not be used if pregnant or breastfeeding or in those with seizure disorders or taking antiepileptics
Yerba mansa	*Yerba manza*	Used topically for skin wounds as a poultice.	• Not recommended if pregnant or breastfeeding • May cause increased drowsiness/sedation

Traditional mineral and nutritional products used medicinally

Mineral/nutritional product	Spanish name	Dermatologic use	Contraindications
Egg	*Huevo*	Used topically for burns, melasma, rosacea, and sunburn. Used topically for furuncles (boils) by applying the egg membrane. Used topically for scars by applying the egg shell and hydrogen peroxide.	• None
Fish oil	*Aceite de pescado*	Used topically for psoriasis.	• Moderate interaction with oral contraceptive pills, antihypertensives, and tetrahydrolipstatin (orlistat) • Minor interaction with anticoagulants
Milk	*Leche*	Used topically for sunburn.	• None
Milk of magnesia	*Leche de magnesia*	Used topically for urticaria.	• None
Vitamin B	*Vitamina B*	Used orally for rosacea.	• None
Vitamin E	*Vitamina E*	Used topically for scars and verrucae.	• Moderate interaction with cyclosporine, medications changed by the cytochrome P450 system, chemotherapy agents, anticoagulants, statins, and niacin
Yogurt	*Yogur*	Used topically for atopic dermatitis, burns, melasma, sunburn, tinea pedis, and urticaria.	• Moderate interaction with tetracyclines, ciprofloxacin, and immunosuppressants
Zinc	*Zinc*	Used topically for psoriasis.	• Moderate interaction with quinolones, tetracycline, cisplatin, and penicillamine • Minor interaction with amiloride

Other traditional products used medicinally

Other traditional products	Spanish name	Dermatologic use	Contraindications
Alcohol	*Alcohol*	Used topically for acne.	• None
Baking soda	*Bicarbonato de sosa*	Used topically for acne, burns, psoriasis, sunburn, tinea pedis, urticaria, verrucae, and as a deodorant.	• None
Sea salt	*Sal marina*	Used topically for burns and psoriasis.	• None

Abbreviations: CNS, central nervous system; HIV, human immunodeficiency virus; NNRTI, nonnucleoside reverse transcriptase inhibitor.

Source: Data from Wellness Library,[38] Howell et al,[39] Dole et al,[40] Rivera et al,[41] and WebMD.[42]

glycolic, malic, tartaric, gluconolactone, and citric acids, have been demonstrated to have some effectiveness on the condition due to their exfoliative properties.[31,43] Lemon juice is one of the most common substances applied to acne-prone skin by Latinos; others include orange peels mixed with yogurt, cooked/puréed carrots, and garlic oil, which is applied specifically to reduce open comedones.[38,44] Certain treatments to reduce acne scarring also involve the use of fruit juices (lemons and oranges), orange peels, and garlic cloves, which are applied directly onto the scar. However, irritation can result with the prolonged exposure of the skin to fruit and fruit juices.[45] Other herbal remedies for acne include the use of garden sorrel (*Rumex acetosa*), often simply called sorrel. The sorrel, a leafy vegetable, is mixed with alcohol and vinegar to dry out acne lesions.

Another plant that may frequently be found in Latino homes is *Aloe vera*. The aloe leaf is renowned in many cultures for its soothing properties. The aloe leaves produce a gel that can be freshly squeezed from the plant onto acne lesions for a calming or soothing effect or for decreasing pruritus. Aloe vera has been found to accelerate the healing process, possibly via reductions in thromboxane A$_2$ and B$_2$ as well as prostaglandin 2α, which increases dermal perfusion and reduces tissue loss by localized ischemia.[46]

ALOPECIA

Alopecia remedies often involve topical treatments made from different oils and plants. In reviewing the literature, it is not always possible to specifically denote what type of hair loss is being treated with which remedy. Instead, many of these recommendations appear to be used for several types of hair loss. One recommended mixture is made from thyme, rosemary, lavender, cedar wood, grape seed, and jojoba, which is then massaged into the scalp.[47,48] Aloe vera is also used to reduce hair loss and promote growth; the aloe vera is rubbed into the scalp, allowed to dry, and then rinsed with water. Fish oils, lemon juice mixed with onion juice, and coconut milk are additionally used as scalp massage lotions. Another lotion is made from boiling nettle leaves (of the *Urticaceae* family), which are then rubbed into the scalp and left on overnight before being rinsed off the next morning.[49] Nettle leaves have stinging hairs that contain serotonin, formic acid, and histamine. Cases of acute urticaria have been reported after handling nettle leaves.[50]

ARTHROPOD BITES AND BURNS

Although wounds, burns, and insect bites often require different treatment approaches, aloe vera is often recommended for all of these conditions due to its soothing effect on the injuries.[15] The salicylic acid present in aloe vera acts as an analgesic and anti-inflammatory agent via the inhibition of prostaglandin production, while the magnesium lactate inhibits histidine decarboxylase to reduce pruritus.[31,51] Another remedy for burns is to cover the affected area with a paste of frozen mashed potatoes, honey, and onions. Honey contains catalase whose debriding properties likely assist in wound healing.[52] Burn wounds dressed with honey have been known to show an early reduction of acute inflammatory changes, reduced infections, and rapid wound healing.[53] Olive oil and sea salt are believed to prevent blister development in burns. Other remedies to treat burns include plain yogurt or milk; a paste made of crushed olives, egg whites, and tomatoes; and sliced tomatoes.[45]

Arthropod bites may be treated with lemon juice, vinegar, garlic cloves, and/or ice to decrease the swelling.[45] Meat tenderizer can be mixed with a few drops of water and applied to bites. Unseasoned meat tenderizer contains an enzyme called papain (bromelain) that is believed to dissolve toxins.[54] Sage leaves (*Salvia officinalis*) are often rubbed onto wasp stings to reduce itching and promote rapid healing, whereas tea tree oil may be applied to prevent the bites from becoming infected.[55]

ATOPIC DERMATITIS AND PRURITUS

One folk remedy for atopic dermatitis (AD) is to create a paste from cornstarch mixed with a quarter cup of apple cider vinegar for application to affected skin. Short-term topical applications of puréed carrots, aloe vera (either in gel or leaf form), honey, and lavender oil have all been used as topical agents to decrease the pruritus associated with AD.[38] Witch hazel, produced from the leaves and bark of the witch hazel shrub, is believed to have a soothing and antipruritic effect on the skin when applied as a cream, ointment, or compress.[56] Witch hazel bark is rich in tannins that assist by coagulating exudates and surface proteins to form a protective layer on the skin, reducing secretions and skin permeability. Tannins are also believed to have antimicrobial properties that may benefit AD patients because superinfections are common in this disease.[57-59]

Arnica, a flowering plant in the *Asteraceae* family, is frequently used for dermatitis because it appears to help reduce inflammation. This effect may be due to the inhibition of the activation of the transcription factor known as nuclear factor κ light-chain enhancer of activated B cells (NF-κB).[60] Particles isolated from this plant have also shown activity against Gram-positive bacteria, including methicillin-resistant *Staphylococcus aureus* (MRSA). However, arnica contains sesquiterpene lactones, and allergic contact dermatitis may occur with use. It is not recommended for use on open wounds or broken skin.[31,61]

Teas ingested as an AD treatment may include burdock tea (also used topically by some Latino folk healers); juniper, sage, and thyme tea (1 tablespoon of each); and chamomile tea. All are used to minimize skin inflammation.[39] Chamomile, another plant from the *Asteraceae* family, is said to have anti-inflammatory properties that are attributed to its essential blue oil. This oil contains flavonoids, chamazulene, α-bisabolol, and sesquiterpene alcohol. These substances inhibit cyclooxygenase and lipoxygenase (in vitro); the flavonoids inhibit histamine release; and α-bisabolol may assist in wound healing. Chamomile is also available in topical formulations that have been reported to cause contact dermatitis.[58,62]

Soaks are also commonly recommended for AD/pruritus, with most mixtures prepared by boiling ingredients, cooling them, and then applying the resulting products to the affected areas during a bath or adding them directly to the bath water. For example, a handful of strawberry leaves and a handful of plum leaves can be boiled, allowed to cool, and then applied to lesions during a bath. Plant horsetail (*Equisetum*) can be used as another soak; again, it is prepared by boiling, cooling, and then adding it to bath water. It appears to be a good source of antioxidants.[63,64] Colloidal oatmeal can also be used as a bath soak. When mixed with liquid, oats can form a coating for the skin that assists in sealing in the moisture. This effect is attributed to the gluten content of the oats.[31] Another popular soak is made from watermelon rinds and vinegar.[38]

BACTERIAL INFECTIONS

Echinacea is a group of popular flowering plants often used as antimicrobial agents. Prior to the introduction of sulfonamide antibiotic drugs, echinacea plants were widely used as a treatment for infections. Their polysaccharides, inulins and alkylamides, are believed to increase T-cell and natural killer cell activity, improving immune system function. Due to these effects, there is concern that the use of echinacea may worsen autoimmune diseases and decrease the effectiveness of immunosuppressants, including systemic corticosteroids.[65] Tea tree oil is obtained from the leaves of the *Melaleuca alternifolia* tree and has demonstrated in vitro activity against a wide variety of microorganisms, including *Propionibacterium acnes*, *S. aureus* (including MRSA), and *Escherichia coli*.[66] Tea tree oil is toxic when ingested and may cause allergic contact dermatitis when applied topically. It has been found to have cytolytic effects on fibroblasts as well as epithelial cells and should not be used on open wounds or burns.[67] The presence of tea tree oil in styling products is one of the suspected causes of gynecomastia in young boys.[68]

FUNGAL INFECTIONS

Tinea pedis, also known as "athlete's foot," is often treated topically with lavender oil (*Lavandula*), which is recognized to have some antiseptic properties possibly related to its tannin content.[38] It is photosensitizing and has also been implicated in cases of gynecomastia in young boys.[31,68] Vinegar and baking soda (sodium bicarbonate) are other popular remedies to treat this infection, because their application will dry the lesions and create an unfavorable growth environment for the fungi.[38] Yogurt is also applied to the affected skin due to the belief that the *Lactobacillus acidophilus* in yogurt can successfully compete with the infecting fungi, thus making the environment less favorable for the continued growth of the fungi.[69]

Tinea corporis can be treated by using lemon juice combined with boiled plantains and the ever popular boiled garlic.[38] Garlic (*Allium sativum*) contains ajoene, a chemical compound that has been shown to have antifungal properties.[70] Contact dermatitis has been reported when garlic is used topically for extended periods of time, whereas prolonged bleeding can occur with the oral ingestion of garlic.[71,72] Crushed, dried burdock plants (*Arctium*) can be made into a poultice and used to try and clear tinea corporis. Burdock extracts have been found to be rich in phytosterols and the essential fatty acids that can kill fungi.[73] Additionally, tea tree oil has recently been found to show activity against *Candida*, *Trichophyton mentagrophytes*, and *Trichophyton rubrum*.[66] Thyme oil (extracted from *Thymus vulgaris*) is also used topically as an antibacterial and anticandidal agent. It contains between 20% and 54% thymol, which likely accounts for its effectiveness against various fungi.[31,71]

Tinea capitis is often treated with avocado oil; a poultice made from crushed watercress (*Nasturtium officinale*) leaves; castor oil and avocado; or a mixture of honey with chopped peach leaves. Most of these remedies are left on overnight under a plastic cap and then rinsed off in the morning.[38]

PSORIASIS

One of the most commonly recommended folk remedies for psoriasis is garlic oil. Its main effect is believed to be the loosening of the scale generated by this disease. Various oils, including olive, fish, and soy, are used primarily for moisturizing and smoothing psoriatic skin.[45] Oil of arnica (as discussed in the AD section) can be prepared by cooking arnica flowers in olive oil and then applying the cooled mixture to the affected skin.[38] Other alternative remedies used by Latinos include aloe vera, extract of licorice (the root of *Glycyrrhiza glabra*), oatmeal (in the form of baths or wraps), sunbathing, and combining sunbathing with the application of seawater (or salt water).[38]

Some herbal teas used for the treatment of psoriasis include using the roots of the dandelion (of the *Taraxacum* genus), burdock, or horsetail plants. These plants can also be directly consumed.[45] Contact dermatitis has been reported when handling dandelions; this is likely due to the latex found in the leaves and stems. Care should be taken when prescribing potassium-sparing diuretics because the use of dandelions can increase potassium levels.[74,75]

Not surprisingly, tars are also recommended folk therapies for psoriasis. Tars are antiproliferative agents that also can reduce pruritus. It can be isolated from juniper (*Juniperus*), birch (*Betula*), or beech (*Fagus*) trees. Although dermatologists are familiar with their use, it is still worth remembering that these tars are photosensitizing compounds.[31] Herbal remedies (both topical and oral) containing furocoumarins reduce the proliferation of epithelial cells when coupled with sunlight exposure (specifically ultraviolet A [UVA]). Parsnips, celery, and parsley have high concentrations of furocoumarins, whereas lower concentrations are found in citrus fruits, sweet fennel, and figs. High levels of consumption of these foods are required to cause photosensitization; a combination of extreme consumption plus UVA exposure results in peeling and the formation of vesicles on exposed skin.[76]

SCARS

The exfoliative properties of lemon juice likely account for any of the benefits seen when using this product with scars. Lemon juice has been combined with water or blended with other ingredients such as milk.[45] Some believe that it also acts as a skin-whitening agent, making the scars less noticeable. Others use aloe vera combined with honey, castor oil, and cocoa butter; boiled persimmons; or vitamin E (the topical application of capsule contents).[38,77] Rosehip seed oil from rose seeds (either *Rosa moschata* or *Rosa rubiginosa*) is also frequently used for lightening scars. The *R. rubiginosa* rose bush grows in the southern Andes mountains, and its seed oil contains vitamin A, vitamin C, and essential fatty acids.[78,79] Some Latinos combine rosehip oil with sage and almond oils for scar treatment.[38]

VERRUCAE

One of the most common recommendations for the treatment of verrucae is to use a crushed clove of garlic and tape it directly onto the verruca.[45] However, failure to protect the surrounding skin during this treatment may lead to blistering.[80] Another folk remedy uses onions that have been cut in half, hollowed out, and filled with salt. As the salt draws the juice out of the onion, the liquid is applied to the wart several times a day.[81] Other topical remedies used to remove warts include the application of vitamin E oil; aloe vera; rubbing the site with a piece of pig skin daily; lemon slices soaked in apple cider; or castor oil either singly or combined into a paste with baking soda.[38]

DRUG INTERACTIONS

Many Hispanics use traditional medicine concurrently with prescription pharmaceuticals, increasing the likelihood of dangerous and adverse effects. The potential interactions of the plants and herbs used in folk remedies with prescription pharmacologic agents remains poorly understood. Some known examples of interactions include arnica with anticoagulants (aspirin, clopidogrel, ibuprofen, dalteparin, enoxaparin, heparin, and warfarin); chamomile with oral contraceptive pills, benzodiazepines, and warfarin; and the substantial interaction of vinegar with digoxin and insulin. Physicians should take thorough medical histories of their patients, including a history of their over-the-counter drug use and use of folk medicines, to detect and prevent potential interactions. Table 8-2 has a more complete list of potential interactions between folk remedies and prescription drugs.

CONCLUSION

Unfortunately, Hispanics often report that their experiences of Western health resources and physicians are not entirely positive; this may in part help to explain the persistence of traditional healthcare beliefs and practices in this cultural group, even among young urban Hispanics.

The prevailing medical education curriculum encourages cultural sensitivity toward and an awareness and recognition of folk belief systems. The goal of a folk healer is ultimately the same as that of the physician: to improve and enhance the patient's health. An improved understanding of the strengths and weaknesses of folk medicine by Western healthcare personnel could ultimately benefit all of the cultural groups living in the United States.

REFERENCES

1. The White House Office of Management and Budget. Revisions to the standards for the classification of federal data on race and ethnicity. www.whitehouse.gov/omb/fedreg_1997standards/. Accessed January 5, 2013.
2. National Institutes of Health Research Portfolio Online Reporting Tools (REPORT). Health disparities. www.report.nih.gov/nihfactsheets/viewfactsheet.aspx?csid=124. Accessed January 1, 2013.
3. Centers for Disease Control and Prevention. Health disparities. www.cdc.gov/healthyyouth/disparities/. Accessed January 6, 2013.
4. Díaz-Duque OF. Communication barriers in medical settings: Hispanics in the United States. *Int J Soc Lang.* 1989;79:93-102.
5. Hernandez C, Mermelstein RJ. A conceptual framework for addressing melanoma health disparities research. *Arch Dermatol.* 2009;145:1442-1446.
6. Lopez RA. Use of alternative folk medicine by Mexican American women. *J Immigr Health.* 2005;7:23-31.
7. Bushy A. Cultural considerations for primary healthcare: where do self-care and folk medicine fit? *Holist Nurse Pract.* 1992;6:10-18.
8. Rivera JO, Ortiz M, Lawson ME, et al. Evaluation of the use of complementary and alternative medicine in the largest United States–Mexico border city. *Pharmacotherapy.* 2002;22:56-264.
9. Wolfe L. Which is politically correct: Latino or Hispanic: what is the difference between Hispanic and Latino? www.womeninbusiness.about.com/od/businessetiquette/a/pc-hispanic.htm. Accessed January 5, 2013.
10. Merriam-Webster. Latino. http://www.merriam-webster.com/dictionary/latino. Accessed November 30, 2013.
11. U.S. Census Bureau. The Hispanic Population 2010: 2010 Census briefs. www.census.gov/prod/cen2010/briefs/c2010br-04.pdf. Accessed November 29, 2013.
12. Taylor P, Lopez MH, Martínez J, Velasco G. When labels don't fit: Hispanics and their views of identity. www.pewhispanic.org/2012/04/04/when-labels-dont-fit-hispanics-and-their-views-of-identity/. Accessed January 3, 2013.
13. Passel JS, D'Vera C. U.S. Population Projections: 2005–2050. Available at: www.pewhispanic.org/files/reports/85.pdf. Accessed December 31, 2012.
14. World Health Organization. Traditional medicine. www.who.int/topics/traditional_medicine/en/. Accessed December 12, 2012.
15. Wachtel-Galor S, Benzie IFF. Herbal medicine: an introduction to its history, usage, regulation, current trends, and research needs. In: Benzie IFF, Wachtel-Galor S, eds. *Herbal Medicine: Biomolecular and Clinical Aspects.* 2nd ed. Boca Raton, FL: CRC Press Group; 2011:1-9.
16. World Health Organization. Traditional medicine: definitions. www.who.int/medicines/areas/traditional/definitions/en/index.html. Accessed December 12, 2012.
17. Applewhite SL. Curanderismo: demystifying the health beliefs and practices of elderly Mexican Americans. *Health Soc Work.* 1995;20:247-253.
18. Hufford DJ. Folk medicine and health culture in contemporary society. *Prim Care.* 1997;24:723-741.
19. Leininger MM. The theory of culture care diversity and universality. In: Leininger MM, McFarland M. *Culture Care Diversity and Universality: A Worldwide Nursing Theory.* 2nd ed. Sudbury, MA: Jones & Barlett Learning; 2005:5-72.
20. Ransford HE, Carrillo FR, Rivera Y. Healthcare-seeking among Latino immigrants: blocked access, uses of traditional medicine, and the role of religion. *J HealthCare Poor Underserved.* 2010;21:862-878.
21. Trotter RT II, Chavira JA. *Curanderismo: Mexican American Folk Healing.* Athens, GA: University of Georgia Press; 1997:1-40.
22. Tafur MM, Crowe TK, Torres E. A review of curanderismo and healing practices among Mexicans and Mexican Americans. *Occup Ther Int.* 2009;16:82-88.
23. Sandoval MS. Santeria. *J Fla Med Assoc.* 1983;70:620-628.
24. Figueroa I. Santería: brief overview. www.elboricua.com/AfroBorinquen_Santeria.html. Accessed January 5, 2013.
25. Alison newby C, Riley DM, Leal-Almeraz TO. Mercury use and exposure among Santeria practitioners: Religious versus folk practice in northern New Jersey, USA. *Ethn Health.* 2006;11:287-306.

26. Pasquali EA. Santería. *J Holist Nurs.* 1994;12:380-390.

27. Ortiz FA, Davis KG. Latina/o folk saints and marian devotions: popular religiosity and healing. In: McNeill B, Cervantes JM, eds. *Latina/o Healing Practices: Mestizo and Indigenous Perspectives.* New York, NY: Taylor & Francis Group; 2008:29-62.

28. Antonovsky A. *Health, Stress and Coping.* San Francisco, CA: Jossey-Bass Inc.; 1979.

29. Lewis-Fernandez R, Guarnaccia PJ, Patel S, et al. Ataque de nervios: anthropological, epidemiological, and clinical dimensions of a cultural syndrome. In: Georgiopoulos AM, Rosenbaum JF, eds. *Perspectives in Cross-Cultural Psychiatry.* Philadelphia, PA: Lippincott Williams & Wilkins; 2005.

30. American Psychiatric Association. *DSM-IV-TR: Diagnostic and Statistical Manual of Mental Disorders, Text Revision.* 4th ed. Washington, DC: American Psychiatric Association; 2000:898-901.

31. Shenefelt PD. Herbal treatment for dermatologic disorders. In: Benzie IFF, Wachtel-Galor S, eds. *Herbal Medicine: Biomolecular and Clinical Aspects.* 2nd ed. Boca Raton, FL: CRC Press Group; 2011:383-403.

32. The Free Dictionary by Farlex. Poultice. www.thefreedictionary.com/poultice. Accessed December 19, 2012.

33. The Free Dictionary by Farlex. Mineral. www.medical-dictionary.thefreedictionary.com/mineral. Accessed November 30, 2013.

34. Rock CL. Multivitamin-multimineral supplements: who uses them? *Am J Clin Nutr.* 2007;85:277S-279S.

35. Murphy SP, Wilkens LR, Monroe KR, et al. Dietary supplement use within a multiethnic population as measured by a unique inventory method. *J Am Diet Assoc.* 2011;111:1065-1072.

36. Quave CL, Pieroni A, Bennett BC. Dermatological remedies in the traditional pharmacopoeia of Vulture-Alto Bradano, inland southern Italy. *J Ethnobiol Ethnomed.* 2008;4:5.

37. Dajas F, Rivera-Megret F. Herbal medicines in the developing world: South America. In: Bagetta GC, Corasanti M, Tiziana M, eds. *Herbal Medicines: Development and Validation of Plant-Derived Medicines for Human Health.* Boca Raton, FL CRC Press; 2011:439-455.

38. Wellness Library. Atopic dermatitis. www.livingnaturally.com/ns/DisplayMonograph.asp?StoreID=3ED1FF6A18BD42979FFF73C8E8CD4512&DocID=allergy-atopicdermatitis. Accessed November 30, 2013.

39. Howell L, Kochhar K, Saywell R Jr, et al. Use of herbal remedies by Hispanic patients: do they inform their physician? *J Am Board Fam Med.* 2006;19: 566-578.

40. Dole EJ, Rhyne RL, Zeilmann CA, et al. The influence of ethnicity on use of herbal remedies in elderly Hispanics and non-Hispanic whites. *J Am Pharm Assoc (Wash).* 2000;40:359-365.

41. Rivera JO, González-Stuart A, Ortiz M, et al. Guide for herbal product use by Mexican Americans in the largest Texas-Mexico border community. *Tex Med.* 2006;102:46-56.

42. WebMD. Vitamins & Supplements Center. www.webmd.com/vitamins-supplements/. Accessed January 3, 2013.

43. Hunt MJ, Barnetson RS. A comparative study of gluconolacone versus benzoyl peroxide in the treatment of acne. *Australas J Dermatol.* 1992;33:131-134.

44. Buzzle. Clearing acne naturally. www.buzzle.com/articles/clearing-acne-naturally.html. Accessed December 28, 2012.

45. Innatia. Remedios naturales. www.remedios.innatia.com/. Accessed January 3, 2013.

46. Klein AD, Penneys NS. Aloe vera. *J Am Acad Dermatol.* 1988;18:714-720.

47. Levin C, Maibach H. Exploration of "alternative" and "natural" drugs in dermatology. *Arch Dermatol.* 2002;138:207-211.

48. Hay IC, Jamieson M, Ormerod A. Randomized trial of aromatherapy: successful treatment for alopecia areata. *Arch Dermatol.* 1998;134:1349-1352.

49. Mariquita Farm. Nettle recipes. www.mariquita.com/recipes/nettles.html. Accessed January 9, 2013.

50. Fu HY, Chen SJ, Chen RF, et al. Identification of oxalic acid and tartaric acid as major persistent pain-inducing toxins in the stinging hair of the nettle, *Urtica thunbergiana. Ann Bot.* 2006;98:57-65.

51. Robinson MC, Heggers JP, Hagstrom WJ Jr. Myth, magic, witchcraft, or fact? Aloe vera revisited. *J Burn Care Rehabil.* 1982;3:157-163.

52. Efem SE. Clinical observations on the wound healing properties of honey. *Br J Surg.* 1988;75:679-681.

53. Maghsoudi H, Salehi F, Khosrowshahi MK, et al. Comparison between topical honey and mafenide acetate in treatment of burn wounds. *Ann Burns Fire Disasters.* 2011;24:132-137.

54. Ross EV Jr, Badame AJ, Dale SE. Meat tenderizer in the acute treatment of imported fire ant stings. *J Am Acad Dermatol.* 1987;16:1189-1192.

55. Carson CF, Hammer KA, Riley TV. Melaleuca alternifolia (tea tree oil): a review of antimicrobial and other medicinal properties. *Clin Microbiol Rev.* 2006;19:50-62.

56. Bedi MK, Shenefelt PD. Herbal therapy in dermatology. *JAMA Dermatol.* 2002;138:232-242.

57. Thring TS, Hili P, Naughton DP. Antioxidant and potential anti-inflammatory activity of extracts and formulations of white tea, rose, and witch hazel on primary human dermal fibroblast cells. *J Inflamm (Lond).* 2011;8:27.

58. Brown DJ, Dattner AM. Phytotherapeutic approaches to common dermatologic conditions. *Arch Dermatol.* 1998;134:1401-1404.

59. Peirce A. *The American Pharmaceutical Association Practical Guide to Natural Medicines.* New York, NY: The Stonesong Press, Inc.; 1999.

60. Gilmore TD. Introduction to NF-kappaB: players, pathways, perspectives. *Oncogene.* 2006;25:6680-6684.

61. Ernst E, Pittler MH. Efficacy of homeopathic arnica: a systematic review of placebo-controlled clinical trials. *Arch Surg.* 1998;133:1187-1190.

62. Science Daily. Chamomile tea: new evidence supports health benefits. www.sciencedaily.com/releases/2005/01/050104112140.htm. Accessed December 30, 2012.

63. Cetojević-Simin DD, Canadanović-Brunet JM, Bogdanović GM, et al. Antioxidative and antiproliferative activities of different horsetail (*Equisetum arvense* L.) extracts. *J Med Food.* 2010;13:452-459.

64. University of Maryland Medical Center. Horsetail. www.umm.edu/health/medical/altmed/herb/horsetail. Accessed January 8, 2013.

65. Graf J, Sanchez, MR. Alternative and complementary medicines in dermatology. In: Freedberg IM, Sanchez MR, eds. *Current Dermatologic Diagnosis and Treatment.* Philadelphia, PA: Lippincott Williams & Wilkins; 2001:222-223.

66. Hammer KA, Carson CF, Riley TV. In-vitro activity of essential oils, in particular *Melaleuca alternifolia* (tea tree) oil and tea tree oil products, against *Candida* spp. *J Antimicrob Chemother.* 1998;42:591-595.

67. Faoagali J, George N, Leditschke JF. Does tea tree oil have a place in the topical treatment of burns? *Burns.* 1997;23:349-351.

68. Henley DV, Lipson N, Korach KS, et al. Prepubertal gynecomastia linked to lavender and tea tree oils. *N Engl J Med.* 2007;365:479-485.

69. Peacefulmind.com. Athlete's foot. www.peacefulmind.com/athletes_foot.htm. Accessed January 10, 2013.

70. Ledezma E, DeSousa L, Jorquera A, et al. Efficacy of ajoene, an organosulphur derived from garlic, in the short-term therapy of tinea pedis. *Mycoses.* 1996;39:393-395.

71. Fleming T. *PDR for Herbal Medicines,* 2nd ed. Montvale, NJ: Medical Economics Company; 2000:1184.

72. McGuffin M, Hobbs C, Upton R, et al, eds. *American Herbal Products Association's Botanical Safety Handbook.* Boca Raton, FL: CRC Press; 1997.

73. Balch PA. Prescription for herbal healing: an easy-to-use A-Z reference to hundreds of common disorders and their herbal remedies. New York, NY: Avery Trade; 2002:38.

74. Church B. *Medicinal Plants, Trees, & Shrubs of Appalachia: A Field Guide.* Raleigh, NC: Lulu.com; 2006:28.

75. Rodriguez-Fragoso L, Reyes-Esparza J, Burchiel SW, et al. Risks and benefits of commonly used herbal medicines in Mexico. *Toxic Appl Pharmacol.* 2008;227:125-135.

76. Lawley R, Curtis L, Davis J. Biological toxins. In: Lawley R, Curtis L, Davis J, eds. *The Food Safety Hazard Guidebook.* Cambridge, United Kingdom: Royal Society of Chemistry; 2008:179-287.

77. University of Hawaii. Persimmon: general crop information. www.extento.hawaii.edu/kbase/crop/crops/i_persim.htm. Accessed January 10, 2013.

78. Livestrong.com. What are the benefits of rose hip oil on the face? http://www.livestrong.com/article/228464-what-are-the-benefits-of-rose-hip-oil-on-the-face/. Accessed November 30, 2013.

79. Fromm M, Bayha S, Kammerer DR, et al. Identification and quantitation of carotenoids and tocopherols in seed oils recovered from different *Rosaceae* species. *J Agric Food Chem.* 2012;60:10733-10742.

80. Drury S. Plants and wart cures in England from the seventeenth to the nineteenth century: some examples. *Folklore* 1991;102:97-100.

81. Alleman G. Herbal remedies for warts. www.health.howstuffworks.com/wellness/natural-medicine/herbal-remedies/herbal-remedies-for-warts.htm. Accessed January 4, 2013.

CHAPTER 9

Impact of Traditional Arabian Gulf Cultures on Healthcare Practices

Ashraf M. Reda

Faiza Mohamed Al Ali

KEY POINTS

- In general, people from the Arabian Gulf countries have similar cultures, habits, beliefs, and practices.

- The medical beliefs and practices of people from these countries are the result of their rich history, tribal traditions, and the involvement and importance of religion in all aspects of life.

- Understanding and respecting these beliefs can facilitate communication with patients from these countries, as well as positively impact health outcomes and treatment.

- Certain cultural traditions may impact the patient–physician relationship, particularly between members of the opposite gender. Physicians should be aware that a refusal by the patient to touch, maintain eye contact, or speak directly to a member of the opposite gender should not be considered insulting. Patients may prefer to be treated by a member of the same gender; if this is impossible, the patient may request that a family member or a nurse/interpreter of the same gender be present during the consultation.

- Consanguinous marriage rates in the Arab Gulf countries are among the highest in the world. This may result in increased incidence of autosomal recessive disorders and atopic diseases.

- Physicians should understand and respect religious practices that may impact healthcare, such as fasting during *Ramadan*, daily praying, and the prohibition of certain *haram* food products.

- Traditional Arabian healthcare treatments include *hijama* (cupping/bloodletting) and *kaiy* (cautery). Many older patients may still use these procedures or may bear scars from past treatments.

INTRODUCTION

The Gulf Cooperation Council (GCC) is a political and economic union of the Arab states of Bahrain, Kuwait, Oman, Qatar, Saudi Arabia, and the United Arab Emirates [**Figure 9-1**]. These states are also sometimes referred to as the Arabian Gulf countries. People from these countries display a great degree of similarity in their cultures, habits, beliefs, and practices. This similarity may be influenced by the shared language of Arabic, the prevailing belief in Islam and its traditions, and the common history and geographical environment of these states. The economic standards of these countries are among the highest in the world. As a result, people from these countries often travel to the United States and Europe; the reasons for travel may include business, tourism, education, or training, as well as a desire for medical treatment.

Although people from these countries are Arabs and Muslims, they may differ from the Arab and Muslim immigrants living in the United States because they may not have adapted to the culture and healthcare system of the United States. The middle-aged and older generations of this cultural group are particularly bound to their local culture, beliefs, and habits. Healthcare providers may face challenges when dealing with patients from these countries because they may have unique cultural and religious beliefs. To provide improved clinical care, healthcare providers must be familiar with the cultural beliefs and practices of this group because these may directly affect their healthcare needs.

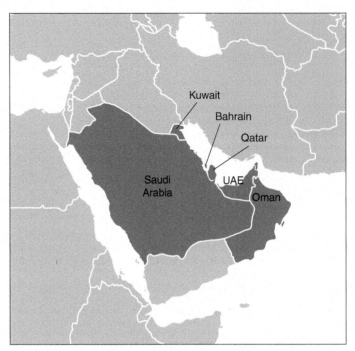

FIGURE 9-1. Arabic states are members of the Gulf Cooperation Council (GCC). The region is also called the Arabian Gulf.

BACKGROUND OF THE ARABIAN GULF CULTURE[1,2]

The GCC area is home to a rich cultural heritage that has been strongly influenced by the geographical cohesiveness of the Arabian Peninsula, which is characterized by a shared desert interior region and bound by the exterior coastline. The harsh environment of the region has dictated the traditional lifestyles that have evolved over the centuries. Furthermore, the tribal structure of the society has created strong ties between its inhabitants. In such a social structure, each family member is traditionally bound by obligations to his immediate relatives, as well as to the tribe as a whole. These obligations are based on the concept of mutual assistance. The vast majority of Gulf Arabians are ethnically Arab, and large numbers of the population are able to trace their ancestry back through the many generations who have lived in the same area. Nearly all of the Gulf Arabians speak Arabic. Since the Islamic expansion of the mid-seventh century, most Arabians have been Muslims. In these countries, Islam is not merely a religion, but a way of life; it is used as a guide for all aspects of life, including religious practices, morality, familial and social relationships, marriage, divorce, and economics.

After discovery of the rich natural reserves of oil in the Middle East, the GCC area evolved and several of the states are now among the richest countries in the world. The standards of living improved dramatically in these countries, and this aided in the emergence of new generations of educated citizens. The economic wealth has attracted many immigrants to move to and work in these countries. Currently, there are considerable expatriate communities in all six of the GCC states; in some of them, expatriate inhabitants constitute the majority of the population.

CULTURAL HABITS

■ DRESS CODE

The Arabian people of the GCC, as with most Arabs and Muslims, are very particular about limiting the exposure of the body. In terms of dress code, the Islamic requirement for women is to dress so as to cover all parts of the body except the face and hands. Additionally, clothes should not be revealing or transparent. Most women in the GCC countries wear a head covering (or veil) called a *hijab* and a long black overgarment called an *abaya*. Some women will choose to cover their face with the *niqab* or *burqaa*. Traditionally, women wear this clothing at all times while in public places or around strangers, removing it only when absolutely necessary, such as during a medical examination. In such situations, Muslim patients—both men and women—should be allowed to wear long gowns (preferably floor length with long sleeves) that can be securely tied in the back or should be offered a robe or sheet to preserve their modesty. Alternatively, a patient may choose to wear a shawl or coat over their gown in order to cover up.[3]

While examining a Gulf Arabian patient, it is advisable to uncover only one part of the body at a time, recovering the other parts of the body as necessary, because patients will usually feel very uncomfortable exposing large areas of their body. In some cases, female patients may only show one part of the body even if the lesion or condition is widespread. Full-body exposure is unacceptable, and any suggestion to expose the whole body will be taken with suspicion. The recognition of these sensitivities by the healthcare provider or technician will help the patient to relax.

TOUCHING AND SHAKING HANDS

Muslim and Arab patients avoid excessive touching between members of the opposite gender; this includes forms of touching such as shaking hands, hugging, or patting on the shoulder.[3] However, touching and holding hands while walking in the street may be acceptable between members of the same gender and with certain close family members. Because of this, the practitioner may extend their hand as a courtesy, remaining aware that a refusal from the other party to do the same should not be considered insulting.

SAME-GENDER PREFERENCE IN HEALTHCARE SETTINGS

Outside of the extended family unit, men and women in traditional GCC communities do not tend to interact socially. In a healthcare setting, the patient may have a strong preference to be treated by a health provider of the same gender; this is especially the case for female patients. Nevertheless, Islam does not ban treatment or care from a doctor, nurse, or technician of the opposite sex if it cannot be avoided; however, if a male provider must examine a female patient, she may feel more comfortable if another family member or a female nurse or interpreter is present.

GENDER ROLES

In the cultural and religious traditions of most Gulf Arabian communities, the male is the head of the household and is the official decision-maker responsible for the financial support of his family and the protection of his family's health and honor. During a medical consultation, men will usually accompany their wife, mother, or daughter. The man may answer medical questions directed at the female patient and may also sign any consent forms on her behalf. It is common for a woman to avoid eye contact with a male healthcare provider, and she may not answer his questions directly, unless her husband or father is unavailable or she has an agreement with her husband or father that she may respond to the healthcare provider's questions. Therefore, for a male healthcare provider, asking permission from an accompanying male to address a female patient is considered a sign of good intentions.

DISCLOSING PRIVATE INFORMATION

The disclosure of personal information is not guaranteed or easily obtained from the patient, even if this personal information is directly related to the patient's illness or healthcare. In particular, questions related to sexual activity or history are very sensitive and may cause embarrassment or be considered offensive. Muslims and Arabs tend to be very private about personal and family matters; therefore, clarifying

the medical reason for a question, or indirectly asking personal questions, may help to ease the tension and aid the patient's disclosure.

CONSANGUINEOUS MARRIAGES

Consanguineous marriage rates in the Arab Gulf countries are among the highest in the world, with rates between 30% and 50% compared with rates of less than 5% in the United States and Europe.[4] For example, in Oman, 52% of all marriages are consanguineous, with marriages between first cousins being most common; these make up 39% of all marriages and 75% of all consanguineous marriages.[5] Similarly high rates of consanguineous marriages exist in Saudi Arabia (58%), Mauritania (60%), and Sudan (65%).[5] Social, religious, cultural, and economic factors play significant roles in maintaining the high rates of consanguineous marriages in these countries. Traditionally, consanguineous marriages promote family ties, reduce dowries, and help keep family property within families. Islam et al[5] also reported a relationship between consanguinity and early marriages; their findings indicated that women who had a consanguineous marriage were 37% more likely to have married early. The main impact of consanguinity is an increase in the rate of homozygotes for autosomal recessive genetic disorders.[6] Bener and Janahi[7] reported a significant association between childhood atopic disease and parental atopic disease in a population with high consanguinity in Qatar.

RELIGIOUS BELIEFS AND PRACTICES

PROPHETIC MEDICINE

Prophetic medicine refers to the actions and words of the Islamic Prophet, Mohammad, that dealt with sicknesses, hygiene, and health in general. Muslims are required by their religion to seek medical advice whenever they are ill, and they believe that every disease has a cause and a cure. Many Muslims, including those of the GCC countries, may use prophetic medicine as part of their system of healthcare, alongside seeking modern medical treatment.

PRAYER

Muslim men and women are obliged to recite prayers five times each day, preferably at a mosque, at various times between dawn and nightfall. Prayer nodules [**Figure 9-2, A and B**] are well-known, asymptomatic, chronic skin changes that consist mainly of thickening, lichenification, and hyperpigmentation. They develop over a long period of time as a consequence of the repeated, extended pressure against hard, rough floors during prayer on the bony prominences, such as the forehead, the dorsum of the feet, and the ankles.[8,9]

Before prayer, Muslims must engage in a cleansing process called ablution or *Wudu*. The steps of ablution include washing the face, hands, arms, legs, and feet, using running water. The increased prevalence of tinea pedis has been reported in Muslim communities due to the prolonged wetness of the feet caused by frequent ablution.[10] Moreover, the common tradition of sitting cross-legged may, over time, induce a macerated pressure-reaction hyperkeratosis in the toe webs of overweight individuals, where the webs become colonized by environmental germs.[11]

PROHIBITIONS IN FOOD AND MEDICATIONS

Alcohol, pork, and narcotics are strongly prohibited in Islam. Most Muslims stringently avoid such products, regardless of their level of religious devotion. Patients may refuse to take medications that contain any of these ingredients. This may pose an ethical issue if the patients are not informed of the contents of such medications. However, Islamic law will allow the use of such medications, but only if the patient's condition is critical and there is no other alternative medicine.

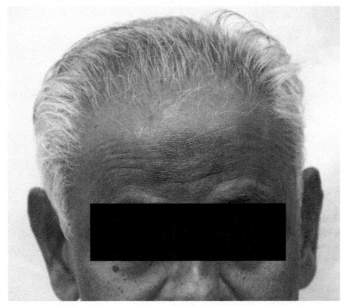

A

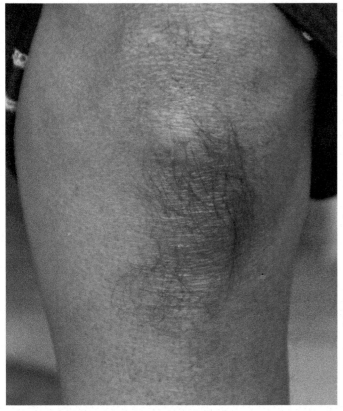

B

FIGURE 9-2. (A) A prayer nodule on the forehead of a Muslim man that is acquired after repeated *sajdah*, which is the practice of bending down to touch the head to the floor during prayer. **(B)** Hyperpigmentation on the knees due to extended and repeated pressure from kneeling during Islamic prayers. (Used with permission from Nivu Hussain.)

Approved foods in Islam are known as *halal* [**Figure 9-3**]. Forbidden products, on the other hand, are known as *haram*. This includes the products previously mentioned (alcohol and pork or pork byproducts), as well as blood and blood byproducts, and the meat from carnivorous animals, animals that were dead prior to slaughtering, and animals that were not slaughtered properly or not slaughtered in the name of *Allah*. The Jewish dietary *kosher* meat is roughly equivalent to *halal* meat for

Muslims. In the GCC countries, as in other Arab and Muslim countries, *halal* food is a very important and fundamental issue.

FASTING DURING *RAMADAN*

The ninth month of the lunar calendar, *Ramadan*, is considered a holy month by most Arabian Gulf communities. As part of their religious practices, Muslims are supposed to refrain from eating or drinking from dawn until dusk. This fasting includes any oral medications. However, patients may also be unwilling to undergo injectable treatments during these hours of fasting. If possible, healthcare providers should discuss safe methods to adapt the medication schedules, or medication doses, of their patients. For example, medications to be taken once or twice per day are preferable because they will not interfere with fasting. It is important to know that acutely or chronically ill patients, people who are traveling, and women who are menstruating, pregnant, or breastfeeding are exempt from fasting. Nevertheless, if a patient chooses to fast under such circumstances, the healthcare provider should discuss with the patient the potential health concerns of doing so. In a life-threatening situation, the healthcare provider should seek a family member or a leader from the Muslim community to help convince the patient that complying with treatment does not breach Islamic teachings.

RUQYAH (SPIRITUAL HEALING)

Many Muslims believe that reading verses from the Quran or reading statements of the Prophet will give the power to heal body, mind, and soul. This is called *Ruqyah*. Many Muslims use this type of spiritual healing as part of their treatment plan. It is very common to see patients or family members uttering religious words during difficult times, such as in the case of severe illness or before a surgery.

USE OF TRADITIONAL PLANT AND FOOD PRODUCTS

The use of plants in traditional therapy is common in the GCC countries. Many plants and foods traditionally used as home remedies in the GCC countries are based on the recommendations of the Prophet. Some products are used widely based on these recommendations.

HONEY

Honey is widely used as a natural remedy for various ailments throughout the Middle East [**Figure 9-4**]. Expensive mixtures of honey and other products are still used and sold in the Arabian Gulf countries, claiming to cure coughs, treat burns, heal stomach ulcers, and relieve allergies. The use of honey and black seed (*Nigella sativa*) products are particularly widespread in the GCC area as preventative medicines and treatments for a variety of gastrointestinal and dermatologic ailments [**Figure 9-5**].[7,12]

SENNA

Another common plant product used traditionally is senna, which is a shrub that grows to about 1 m in height and is found in hot and humid climates. It is used to relieve constipation, relax the muscles, and improve hair; it is also used as an aid against lice, headaches, rashes, and epilepsy.[13] Senna is also used as a hair conditioner to make the hair thick and glossy and to nourish and strengthen the scalp.

SIWAK

Siwak (also known as *miswak*) is a twig used as a natural toothbrush, toothpaste, and dental floss. It comes from the *Arak* tree (*Salvadora persica*), and the twigs are usually a hand span in length and of medium thickness [**Figure 9-6**]. *Siwak* contains tannin, which helps to strengthen the gums. It is believed to help remove the bad smell from the mouth.[14] Modern medicine has confirmed the benefits of *siwak* in improving dental plaque score and gingival health when it is used as an adjunct to modern teeth brushing.[15] In addition, the use of *siwak* was reported to promote gingival health in patients with orthodontic appliances.[16]

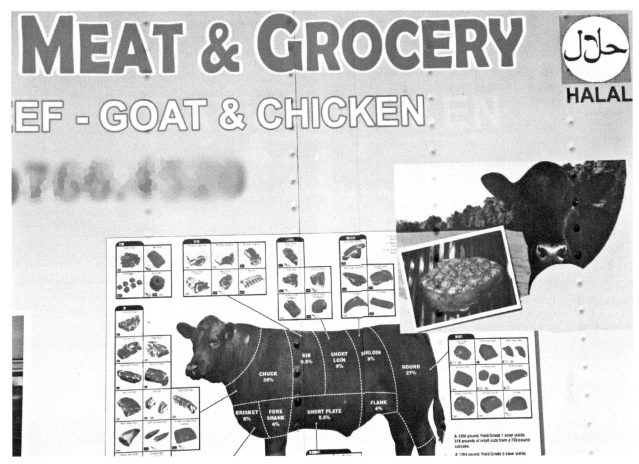

FIGURE 9-3. *Halal* foods are allowed under Islamic dietary guidelines.

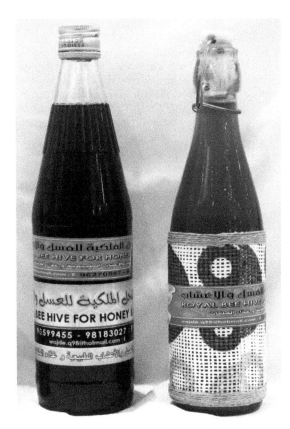

FIGURE 9-4. Honey is widely used as a natural remedy for various ailments throughout the Middle East. (Used with permission from Nivu Hussain.)

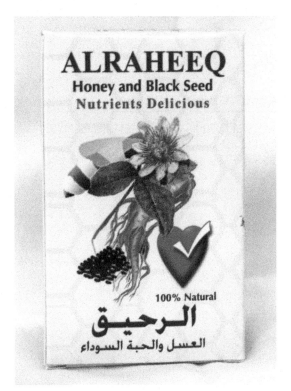

FIGURE 9-5. The use of honey and black seed (*Nigella sativa*) products is particularly widespread in the Arabian Gulf in preventative medicine. (Used with permission from Nivu Hussain.)

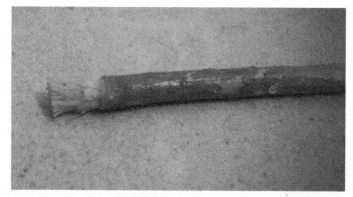

FIGURE 9-6. The trimmed end of the *siwak* stick is often used for tooth cleaning in the Arabian Gulf countries. It is also used by some Muslims for teeth cleansing prior to each of the five daily prayers.

HERBS AND SEEDS

Specialized *Etara* shops are common and sell different mixtures and compounds of herbs [**Figure 9-7**] to cure many diseases. The composition of these products is not standardized and is based on the individual experience and preference of the herbalist.

The following are some of the most widely used plants.[17] The seeds of *Senna italica*, the senna plant previously mentioned, are often used as a laxative, and many Arabs of the Bedouin tribe claim that they will heal any kind of stomach pain. The seeds of the desert squash, *Citrullus colocynthis*, are highly acclaimed as a cure for diabetes. The bitter sap of the milkweed, *Calotropis procera*, is dried and used to fill aching, hollow teeth; the woody parts of this plant are burned to make charcoal, which was an ingredient for gunpowder in the past. Poultices made of the leaves are applied to joints to heal rheumatism. *Salsola imbricata* and several of the *Suaeda* genus of plants are dried and powdered to be used in snuff form to clear the sinuses. In the Arab culture, the best-known cosmetically used plant is henna (*Lawsonia inermis*), which is used to dye hair and to decorate the hands and feet. The poisonous plant *Rhazya stricta* is used in small quantities to settle gastrointestinal problems. An important plant for combating fevers is *Teucrium stocksianum*, a very fragrant herb that is similar to sage. The seeds of the Arab gum tree (*Acacia nilotica*) are grounded to a powder to dry out second-degree burns.

THERAPEUTIC PROCEDURES

HIJAMA (WET CUPPING OR BLOODLETTING CUPPING)[18]

The Arabic word *hijama* means "sucking." It is a therapeutic procedure where blood is drawn from a small skin incision by a vacuum created

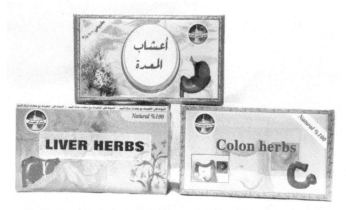

FIGURE 9-7. Different herbal mixtures that are used for treating the liver and colon. (Used with permission from Nivu Hussain.)

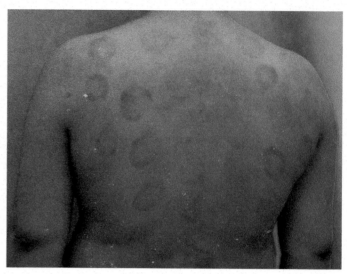

FIGURE 9-8. Circular marks on the back of a man after *hijama* (bloodletting cupping), which is a traditional practice in the Arabian Gulf for treating numerous afflictions, including headaches, stomach problems, poisoning, magic spells, bruising, pain, and skin sores.

with the aid of suction cups [**Figure 9-8**]. *Hijama* can be performed almost anywhere on the body, but it is often done at the site of an ache or pain to ease or alleviate it. Islamic teaching considers cupping to be both a cure and a blessing. Early Muslims used *hijama* to treat numerous afflictions, including headaches, stomach problems, poisoning, magic spells, bruising, pain, skin sores, and more. This procedure continues to be practiced by Muslims today, and it is very popular in the GCC area. Current practitioners claim that dry cupping therapy is beneficial in treating pain, muscular and joint problems, circulatory problems, colds, indigestion, arthritis, congestion in the throat and lungs, headaches, fever, and more. The mechanism of *hijama* is not exactly known. However, there is a marked difference in the composition of blood drawn through the technique of cupping compared with blood drawn intravenously (eg, via a phlebotomy or venesection), suggesting that *hijama* may produce its beneficial effect through a mechanism different than that of drawing blood intravenously.[19] Recent studies have suggested a beneficial effect of wet cupping in the treatment of several diseases, such as rheumatoid arthritis,[20] herpes zoster,[21] and low back pain.[22]

KAIY (CAUTERY)

Kaiy, the Arabic term for cautery, is one of the most ancient forms of therapy used by Arabs over the centuries. In the Arabian Gulf, *kaiy* involves the use of metal sticks or iron nails that are heated over hot charcoal until they glow red and are then placed on a specified area of the skin for a few seconds. The choice of location for the application of the metal depends on the patient's individual complaints.[23] This practice was often used in the past to manage internal pain, clean wounds, and treat psychiatric conditions. Although *kaiy* is rarely seen now, cautery scars can nevertheless still be seen on the skin of elderly people who have come from or been raised in Bedouin areas. The Bedouin are a distinct desert-dwelling Arabian ethnic group within the GCC countries.

ORIGINS OF ILLNESSES

HASSAD (ENVY)

One popular belief in the Arabian Gulf culture is *hassad* (envy). In Islam, *hassad* occurs when a person envies others for something good that they possess; this envy is accompanied by a wish to inflict misfortune on them or for them to be deprived of their good fortune. Muslims believe that a look or a comment by the envious person may initiate an adverse event, such as an ailment, mental illness, or a failure in relationships or in business. It is not uncommon that, once they have established trust in their healthcare provider, some patients may consider *hassad* to be the cause of their suffering. Dismissing this notion may offend the patient, potentially breaking trust and creating a barrier in the patient–provider relationship. The physician should remain respectful of the patient's beliefs. It is believed that the reversal of *hassad* is possible by reading special verses of the Quran.

WILL OF GOD

In general, the Islamic view tends to stress the will of God as the origin of all actions, fates, and events. Accordingly, illnesses are often regarded as divine punishment for having committed a sin or as a gift from God to purify the soul. Those who exert patience and accept their illnesses are believed to be praised and rewarded by God. Many Muslims also believe that the cure for their suffering can only be received from God and that any treatment given by a healthcare provider is merely the execution of God's will. Muslims are required to seek medical treatment, while also praying, reading verses of the Quran, and reciting invocations.

JINN AND EVIL FORCES

Although uncommon, some patients believe in the role of unseen forces, mostly *jinn* or evil spirits, in causing diseases, especially in cases of mental illness and for diseases of unknown cause. Some believe that wearing amulets containing verses from the Quran can protect the individual from the harm of *jinn*.

BEAUTY STANDARDS AND PRACTICES IN THE ARABIAN GULF

SKIN LIGHTENING

In the Arabian Gulf, standards of beauty have changed over time, based on the changing cultural values. Despite the influence of the media, which perpetuates a supposedly "global" standard of ideal beauty, there is a distinction in the perception of beauty that is evident in different parts of the world. In the GCC countries, most Fitzpatrick skin types range between III and V; nevertheless, a fair complexion is considered to be the most beautiful among the majority of women. This has resulted in a dramatic increase in the use of skin-lightening products, even when the safety of such products has not been established, in an attempt to lighten the skin tone [**Figure 9-9**]. However, over the last few years, a noticeable number of the younger generations, including both males and females, have become more interested in skin tanning.

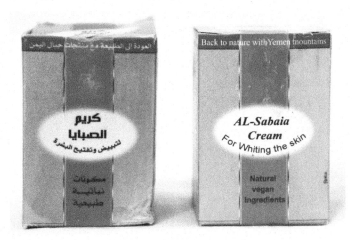

FIGURE 9-9. Skin-lightening creams are often used by many women in an attempt to lighten their skin tone. (Used with permission from Nivu Hussain.)

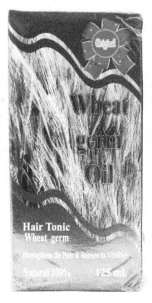 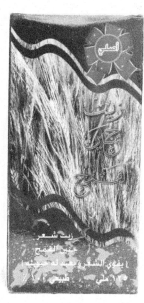

FIGURE 9-10. Wheat germ oil is often used by women as a hair conditioner. (Used with permission from Nivu Hussain.)

HAIR PREFERENCES

Most women in the GCC area strongly believe that long and straight hair is cosmetically pleasing. A lot of locally made oil mixtures are sold for the purposes of strengthening and lengthening the hair [**Figure 9-10**]. Even so, many young women are now experimenting with changing fashions, for instance by having curly, short, or lighter colored hair.

HENNA

Henna (*L. enermis*) is a plant that is widely used in the GCC countries to dye the hair and temporarily tattoo the skin. The name is often misused for other skin and hair dyes, such as black henna or neutral henna, that do not actually contain henna plant products. Black henna may be derived from the indigo plant (*Indigofera tinctoria*) or *S. italica* and may contain unlisted dyes and chemicals such as *p*-phenylenediamine (PPD), which can quickly stain the skin black. However, PPD can also cause severe allergic reactions such as blistering, intense itching, permanent scarring, and permanent chemical sensitivities.[24,25] The U.S. Food and Drug Administration (FDA) specifically forbids PPD to be used for such a purpose.

In several parts of the world, henna is traditionally used in various festivals and celebrations. Decorative henna has been used for over 5000 years and has become a symbol of good luck, health, and sensuality in the Arab world [**Figure 9-11**].[26] Henna decorating is considered an art form and is practiced widely in the GCC countries. The most popular traditional use of henna is in wedding celebrations and during bridal preparations. For dyeing or tattooing the skin, a paste of henna (either prepared from a dried powder or from the freshly ground leaves) is applied to the skin and left for a period of time ranging from a few hours to overnight. Henna stains can last from a few days to a month depending on the quality of the paste, the individual skin type, and the duration of time that the paste has been left in contact with the skin.[25] Various shades of colors can be procured by mixing henna with the leaves and fruit of other plants, such as indigo, tea, coffee, cloves, and lemon. In addition to its decorative use, henna is also applied to the palms and soles during hot weather because it acts as a cooling agent. As a temporary tattoo, henna is acceptable from the religious point of view; this is in contrast to any permanent tattoos, which are strongly forbidden in Islam. Many Muslims who have had a permanent tattoo at some point in their life often later seek tattoo removal by laser or surgery.

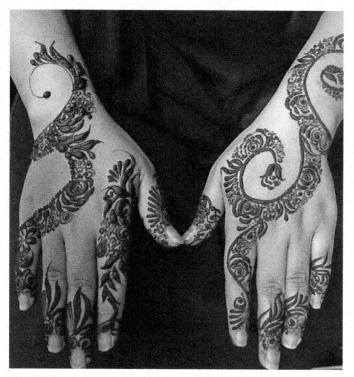

FIGURE 9-11. Decorative *henna* has been used for over 5000 years and has become a symbol of good luck, health, and sensuality in the Arab world.

13. Al-Jawziyya IQ. *Medicine of the Prophet*. 1st ed. Johnstone P, transl. Cambridge, United Kingdom: The Islamic Texts Society; 1998.
14. Prophet Medicine. Siwak. www.prophetmedicines.com/article.php?id=142. Accessed March 8, 2013.
15. Patel PV, Shruthi S, Kumar S. Clinical effect of miswak as an adjunct to tooth brushing on gingivitis. *J Indian Soc Periodontol*. 2012;16:84-88.
16. Al-Teen RM, Said KN, Abu Alhaija ES. Siwak as an oral hygiene aid in patients with fixed orthodontic appliances. *Int J Dent Hyg*. 2006;4:189-197.
17. United Arab Emirates National Media Council. UAE Yearbook 2006: traditional use of plants. www.uaeyearbook.com/Yearbooks/2006/ENG/. Accessed March 10, 2013.
18. Hajar Albinali HA. Chairman's reflections: blood-letting. *Heart Views*. 2004;5:74-85.
19. Bilal M, Alam Khan R, Ahmed A, et al. Partial evaluation of technique used in cupping. *J Basic Appl Sci*. 2011;7:65-68.
20. Ahmed SM, Madbouly NH, Maklad SS, et al. Immunomodulatory effects of blood letting cupping therapy in patients with rheumatoid arthritis. *Egypt J Immunol*. 2005;12:39-51.
21. Cao H, Zhu C, Liu J. Wet cupping therapy for treatment of herpes zoster: a systematic review of randomized controlled trials. *Altern Ther Health Med*. 2010;16:48-54.
22. Farhadi K, Schwebel DC, Saeb M, et al. The effectiveness of wet-cupping for nonspecific low back pain in Iran: a randomized controlled trial. *Complement Ther Med*. 2009;17:9-15.
23. Hajar Albinali HA. Special section. *Heart Views*. 2003;4:5.
24. Singh M, Jindal SK, Kavia ZD, et al. Traditional methods of cultivation and processing of henna. In: *Henna, Cultivation, Improvement and Trade*. Jodhpur, India: Central Arid Zone Research Institute; 2005:21-24.
25. Hema R, Kumaravel, Gomathi S, et al. Gas chromatography–mass spectroscopic analysis of *Lawsonia inermis* leaves. *New York Sci J*. 2010;3:141-143.
26. Cvitanic M. Henna: an enduring tradition. www.habiba.org/culture.html. Accessed December 13, 2013.

CONCLUSION

The deeply rooted cultures, habits, beliefs, and practices of people from the Arabian Gulf countries appear to affect many aspects of healthcare practices. Awareness by healthcare providers of the different cultures and habits of people from this region of the world will help to ensure proper care and management of many illnesses, including skin diseases.

REFERENCES

1. Encyclopaedia Britannica. Arabia. www.britannica.com/EBchecked/topic/31551/Arabia. Accessed March 8, 2013.
2. UAEinteract. Traditional culture. www.uaeinteract.com/culture/. Accessed March 8, 2013.
3. Boston University School of Medicine. Islam and health: general guidelines. www.bu.edu/bhlp/Resources/Islam/health/guidelines.html. Accessed March 8, 2013.
4. Bittles AH, Black M. Global prevalence of consanguinity. www.consang.net/index.php/Global_prevalence. Accessed January 28, 2014.
5. Islam MM, Dorvlo AS, Al-Qasmi AM. The pattern of female nuptiality in Oman. *Sultan Qaboos Univ Med J*. 2013;13:32-42.
6. Tadmouri GO, Nair P, Obeid T, et al. Consanguinity and reproductive health among Arabs. *Reprod Health*. 2009;6:17.
7. Bener A, Janahi I. Association between childhood atopic disease and parental atopic disease in a population with high consanguinity. *Coll Antropol*. 2005;29:677-682.
8. English JSC, Fenton DA, Wilkinson JD. Prayer nodules. *Clin Exp Dermatol*. 1984;9:97-98.
9. Monk BE. Prayer nodules. *Clin Exp Dermatol*. 1982;7:225-226.
10. Ilkit M, Tanir F, Hazar S, et al. Epidemiology of tinea pedis and toenail tinea unguium in worshippers in the mosques in Adana, Turkey. *J Dermatol*. 2005;32:698-704.
11. Lestringant GG, Saarinen KA, Frossard PM, et al. Etiology of toe-web disease in Al-Ain, United Arab Emirates: bacteriological and mycological studies. *East Mediterr Health J*. 2001;7:38-45.
12. Alireza MA. Honey: food and medicine. www.arabnews.com/node/324985. Accessed December 13, 2013.

CHAPTER 10

Psychiatric Aspects of Skin of Color

Curley L. Bonds

KEY POINTS

- Skin color is the major contributor to race consciousness and prejudice, with psychological implications for the individual that are often overlooked.
- Dermatologic conditions are frequently linked to psychiatric disorders such as anxiety, depression, and social phobia.
- Medications for skin imperfections sometimes induce depression or suicidal thoughts.
- Skin abnormalities should be evaluated to determine if they represent an underlying psychiatric disorder.
- Some psychotropic medications are associated with a wide range of skin lesions that can be serious or even life-threatening.
- Skin bleaching, tattooing, and branding are culturally specific forms of self-mutilation in people with skin of color.
- Shared management and close collaboration among clinicians treating individuals with psychocutaneous disorders are important for the best outcome.

Skin color, texture, and tone are among the first things that we notice about a person. In a culture where appearances and first impressions dominate interpersonal interactions, it is appropriate that we consider the role that the skin plays in psychological health. Although race is largely a sociopolitical concept, skin color is perhaps the single largest contributor to race consciousness, whereas other, less prominent physical characteristics play a secondary role.

For centuries, social inequalities have been linked to race and, as a result, to the characteristics of one's skin. The institution of slavery for African Americans was predicated in large part on the ability to distinguish one group of individuals from another based on the color of their skin. However, other examples of bias based on skin tone and color exist throughout the globe and across most cultures. Brazilians identify social classifications along lines of skin color rather than racial ancestry.[1] In fact, Brazilian Portuguese has more than 30 words to describe various skin colorations. In preapartheid South Africa, elaborate social classification schemata were developed based on skin tone and other racial features. For healthcare providers, it is essential to recognize the interrelationships between colored skin and mental health.

Research has demonstrated that cultural stereotypes exist based on skin tone bias. This is true for both Caucasians and minorities. An illustration of this fact comes from a historic rhyme popular among African Americans in the mid-1900s: "If you're white, you're all right; if you're yellow, you're mellow; if you're brown, stick around; if you're black, get back."[2] In *The Future of Race*, Henry Louis Gates Jr. described being subjected to the "paper bag principle" during a social event that he encountered at Yale University in the late 1960s.[3] The party involved a traditional discriminatory practice that illustrates skin tone bias in the southern United States. People darker than a brown paper bag placed on the door of the party were denied entry.[3] Although empirical evidence about the relative advantages of lighter or darker skin is limited, several examples in the literature demonstrate that many people attribute positive personality characteristics to lighter-skinned individuals and negative traits to those with darker skin.[4-9]

The observed preferences for lighter skin extend to members of various ethnic groups. Discrimination based on skin tone within an ethnic group is referred to as *colorism* and can be associated with profoundly negative social and interpersonal consequences, including low self-esteem and discrimination. Keith and Herring[10] studied African Americans and skin tone variance and demonstrated that higher occupational prestige, educational achievement, and family income were linked to lighter skin tones.[10] The long-term psychological implications of coping with the effects of skin tone bias are poorly understood but should be considered when working to provide mental health interventions.

From early embryonic development, the ectoderm and neuroectoderm are connected and remain so throughout life. As a result, a strong association between dermatologic and psychiatric disorders exists. Up to a third of dermatologic conditions coexist with psychiatric disorders. A number of psychiatric, behavioral, and medical presentations have unique presentations in skin of color. A few examples will be presented in this chapter, but the list is by no means exhaustive.

PSYCHIATRIC DISORDERS WITH DERMATOLOGIC SYMPTOMS

BODY DYSMORPHIC DISORDER

Body dysmorphic disorder (BDD) is a somatoform spectrum illness characterized by a preoccupation with an imagined bodily defect. Patients initially may present to primary care physicians or dermatologists with concerns about their skin. The psychopathology is the perception that a flaw or imperfection exists in the skin. The patient may be convinced that the coloring of their skin is abnormal or that his or her skin's elasticity is amiss. The patient also may perceive imagined imperfections such as scars, acne, moles, or cellulite. The focus of attention is frequently the face. Sigmund Freud's "Wolf Man" was excessively concerned about his nose and is the classic example of BDD.

BDD occurs in 10% to 14% of dermatology patients and 1% of the general population. Women are affected more commonly than men. The age of onset is between 15 and 20 years. Up to 60% of patients have concurrent comorbid depression, and the lifetime risk of depression in BDD patients is 80%. About a third of patients suffer from social phobia, usually because they are fearful of others seeing their defects. Treatment

with selective serotonin reuptake inhibitors (SSRIs) helps to reduce the intensity of symptoms in about 50% of patients. In those who fail to respond fully to SSRIs, augmentation with buspirone, clomipramine, lithium, or methylphenidate may be helpful.[11]

Surgical, dermatologic, and other medical interventions should be avoided because they typically worsen the patient's condition. Cognitive behavioral psychotherapy has also been shown to reduce the impairment caused by symptoms.

MOOD AND ANXIETY DISORDERS

Skin lesions and disfigurement resulting from dermatologic conditions may have a profound impact on psychological functioning. Visible scars and depigmented or hyperpigmented patches of skin often become the focus of depressive thoughts in those who are prone to mood disorders. Social anxiety and reclusive behavior may result from severe disfigurement. The stress of living with chronic acne, warts, herpes, or psoriasis may trigger feelings of shame, depression, rage, and hopelessness.

Cultural stigma associated with mental health treatment means that patients of color are much more likely to consult a dermatologist or primary care provider, hoping that treatment of the perceived skin lesion may improve their sense of well-being. Patients who experience permanent visible scarring, such as those with keloids [**Figure 10-1**] or cystic acne, should be questioned about psychosocial functioning and mood symptoms during the clinical interview. Assessing the seriousness of depressive symptoms is important for these patients so that appropriate treatment can be initiated. Depression as a clinical syndrome requires the presence of at least five of nine cardinal symptoms, including:

1. Depressed mood
2. Sleep disturbance (hyposomnia or hypersomnia)
3. Appetite disturbance (increased or anorexia)
4. Decreased interest in usual activities
5. Poor energy (or restless energy)
6. Problems with concentration
7. Guilty thoughts
8. Psychomotor slowing or agitation
9. Suicidal thoughts (or recurrent death-themed fantasies)

Depressed individuals also may report low self-worth and feelings of hopelessness and helplessness. The presence of these symptoms in the absence of clearly precipitating changes in psychosocial circumstances is suggestive of a major depressive episode. Psychosis may complicate severe depression. The psychosis may take the form of delusional thoughts, including somatic delusions focused on skin abnormalities.

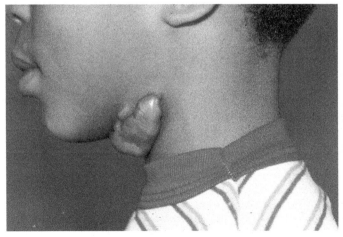

FIGURE 10-1. Large keloids on children, as pictured above, can cause psychological problems.

Although some skin conditions certainly may cause depression and anxiety, there exist psychophysiologic disorders in which the dermatologic condition is precipitated or aggravated by stress.[12] The list includes atopic dermatitis, *acne excoriée des jeune filles*, hyperhidrosis, urticaria, seborrheic dermatitis, rosacea, and pruritus. In most cases, treatment of the comorbid psychological distress helps the skin condition to improve.

It is important to note that several medications used to treat dermatologic conditions may induce depression as a side effect. The most common offenders include isotretinoin, interferon, prednisone, and other steroids. In February 1998, Roche Laboratories issued a letter to all physicians warning of the increased risk of depression with isotretinoin:

> Psychiatric disorders: Accutane may cause depression, psychosis and, rarely, suicidal ideation, suicide attempts and suicide. Discontinuation of Accutane therapy may be insufficient; further evaluation may be necessary. No mechanism of action has been established for these events.[13]

The product labeling now states that discontinuation of therapy in some patients resulted in a reduction in depression but that depression recurred when the drug was reinstituted. Clinicians should be cautious in using this agent, especially in patients who have a history of depression.

In many cases, the medication-induced depression is severe and may lead to suicidal thoughts or plans. This level of depression is considered a psychiatric emergency, and the inciting drug should be stopped or tapered immediately and the patient referred for a full psychiatric assessment.

TRICHOTILLOMANIA

Trichotillomania is an impulse-control disorder characterized by recurrent hair pulling resulting in visible hair loss. Patients often report an increase in anxiety or tension prior to the pulling out of hair that is resolved by the act. Attempts to resist the behavior result in escalating anxiety and tension, making the behavior difficult to resist. Symptoms usually worsen when the individual is under stress. However, some individuals pull or twist their hair in an absent-minded, distracted fashion when they are bored or inactive. The scalp is most commonly affected. However, the hairs of eyebrows, eyelashes, the pubic area, the extremities, and the trunk also may become targets.[14] In about a quarter of patients, the onset is linked to some stressful event. Diagnostic criteria include a sense of pleasure, gratification, or relief when hair pulling occurs. The activity of hair pulling must cause clinically significant distress or impairment in social, occupational, or other important areas of functioning.

Although the condition may be benign, effective treatments usually involve co-management by a psychiatrist and dermatologist. Psychopharmacologic options include clomipramine (a serotonergic tricyclic antidepressant), SSRIs, lithium, and naltrexone. Antipsychotic agents, particularly pimozide or the newer atypical antipsychotics, may be useful to augment the effects of serotonergic drugs. Nonpharmacologic psychiatric interventions that have shown some success include hypnosis, relaxation training, biofeedback, and behavior therapy. Recently, Lee et al[15] described a novel dermatologic approach to trichotillomania in a case report of laser hair removal as a treatment option. The patient's illness involved hairs on the legs only, so the ability to generalize this approach to other patients is limited.

Pathologic skin picking is a distinct illness, but it is related to trichotillomania because both fall into the spectrum of body-focused repetitive behaviors (BFRBs). Skin picking has also been linked to obsessive-compulsive disorder and BDD. Patients with the condition may spend minutes to hours of each day picking. Individuals with BDD may specifically focus their picking behaviors on areas of skin that they feel are abnormal. Eventually, the picking itself leads to scarring, which then can intensify the attention paid to the area, creating a vicious cycle of inspection, picking, and tissue damage. Multiple medications have been studied, but none are approved by the U.S. Food and Drug Administration (FDA) for this disorder. Unfortunately, most trials have been open label and limited in size. Drug interventions showing the greatest effectiveness are similar to those used to treat trichotillomania: SSRIs and tricyclic antidepressants, dual norepinephrine and serotonin

reuptake inhibitors, and lamotrigine. Naltrexone, an opioid antagonist used to treat alcohol dependence and opioid dependence, has shown some promise in individuals who have co-occurring substance abuse and mental illness and may hold promise for those suffering from skin picking.[16,17]

PSYCHOGENIC SKIN DISORDERS

DELUSIONS OF PARASITOSIS

Delusions are firm and fixed beliefs that can occur in a variety of forms. Classic paranoid delusions involve thoughts that someone is following, watching, or monitoring the individual, usually with malicious intent. Other delusional disorders may involve grandiose, jealous, erotic, or somatic themes. Delusions of parasitosis (DOP) are classified as somatic and consist of the belief that parasites are living beneath the skin. Patients with this condition should be differentiated from those experiencing formication (the sensation of bugs crawling and biting beneath the skin). Unlike those with DOP, those with formication do not hold the delusion of something living beneath the skin.[18] Formication is frequently experienced during cocaine withdrawal.

MORGELLONS DISEASE

A condition related to delusions of parasitosis is Morgellons disease. In addition to the sensations of insect-like creatures crawling beneath the skin, patients with Morgellons disease also experience debilitating fatigue, cognitive dysfunction, and fiber-like filaments, granules, or crystals beneath the skin that can be extracted from their lesions. This disorder has gained a strong following of self-proclaimed sufferers who have developed support groups and proposed diagnostic criteria. Patients usually present to dermatologists for care. Individuals may bring in "samples" of the alleged offending organism wrapped in paper tissue or cellophane wrap. They may spend an inordinate amount of time scratching, picking, and surveying their epidermis in efforts to locate parasites or other organisms thought to be responsible for their infestation. Pimozide traditionally has been the gold standard of treatment, but newer atypical antipsychotics also should be considered and may be better tolerated.[19,20]

Published studies about psychiatric interventions for this disorder are sparse because affected individuals often reject psychiatric diagnoses or care. The best approach to the patient is to avoid excessive biopsies and manipulations of the skin to prove or disprove the existence of invaders. The clinician should provide support and reassure the individual that he or she is aware of the distress that the alleged parasites cause despite their origins. Patients sometimes can be convinced to take medications if they learn that they may increase their ability to cope with what appears to be a medically unsolvable situation.

DERMATOLOGIC AND MEDICAL DIAGNOSES

DERMATITIS ARTEFACTA AND OTHER SELF-INFLICTED LESIONS

A great number of dermatologic conditions have unique psychological components when they occur in pigmented skin. Dermatitis artefacta is the deliberate production of skin wounds to resolve an unconscious psychological conflict or emotional need. It is considered to be a factitious disorder because the patient is aware of his or her behavior but denies responsibility for the lesions. Although rare overall, some forms of dermatitis artefacta are worth mentioning here because of cultural factors that may place people of color at increased risk for them. In the clinical assessment, looking for a life-altering event or trauma is important because the onset of self-inflicted skin injury frequently follows an emotional disturbance.[21]

SELF-MUTILATION

The incidence of self-mutilating or cutting behaviors appears to be increasing. This is particularly true among adolescents, who have a 12%

to 14% rate of this behavior and in whom awareness of this behavior is increasing.[22] Self-mutilation may be associated with personality disorders and, in fact, is an essential feature listed in the diagnostic criteria for borderline personality disorder.[23]

Usually the individual cuts, pierces, or picks at his or her skin in efforts to replace psychic pain with physical pain. Patients often report an increase in mental tension or anxiety prior to an episode of self-mutilation. This tension may be released after the act of cutting, resulting in a powerful but temporary sense of well-being and calmness. Patients may go to great lengths to disguise marks or place them only on private skin so that the behavior is not easily detected.

The highest risk group for self-mutilation remains young Caucasian women; however, in jail and prison settings, inmates often engage in self-injury in efforts to gain attention and medical or mental health treatment. In emergency departments, roughly 50% of patients who self-mutilate have a psychiatric diagnosis.[24] When a patient presents for medical care of a self-inflicted wound, the clinician should seize the opportunity to screen for psychiatric illness and to offer a referral for mental health services when appropriate. In some native African and aboriginal tribes, ritual mutilation may be a culturally sanctioned practice and therefore not considered to be psychopathological.

TATTOOING

Over the last two decades, social norms have shifted and moved tattoos (see Chapter 36, Tattoos, Body Piercing, and Scarification) into the mainstream. Earlier literature linked tattooing to antisocial and other unstable personality traits. The popularity of tattooing renders these perspectives dated and obsolete today. An online poll conducted in 2012 by Harris Interactive showed that 21% of American adults had at least one tattoo, with the number increasing to 38% for those between the ages of 30 and 39.[25] Themes and images present in tattoos can give the clinician insight into how the individual views himself or herself and his or her relationship with the world.

Gang affiliations are often memorialized with tattoos. This, of course, creates problems when the individual opts to make a lifestyle change because these semipermanent marks serve as a reminder of past affiliations and behaviors. Self-inflicted tattoos, common among teens and inmates, can have specialized meanings. For instance, in Mexican gangs and prison culture, a teardrop tattoo worn on the face sometimes indicates that the individual has committed murder but can also mean that a relative or friend has been killed.[26] The symbol is intended to indicate one's gang allegiance, memorialize a fallen friend or relative, intimidate viewers, or warn them that the tattooed individual is dangerous and powerful.[26] In Filipino culture, a tattoo of a question mark anywhere on the body indicates membership in the notoriously violent and dangerous *Bahala Na Gang* (BNG, or "Come What May").[27] Understanding the meaning behind tattoos requires knowledge of local and regional codes that may change over time.

In other settings, intoxicated individuals may wake up from a night on the town during which a tattoo was obtained and live to regret their impulsive decision. Only about 14% of Americans in the Harris poll mentioned earlier expressed regret about their tattoos.[25] The risk factors most commonly cited for regret include being a Republican, living in the South, and having a person's name in the tattoo. Fortunately, laser technology has made tattoo removal possible.[28] Unfortunately, the effectiveness of the equipment on darker skin and the cost can be prohibitive for many minority patients. However, the importance of erasing distinctive gang tattoos from visible skin should not be underestimated in the full psychosocial rehabilitation of patients who aspire to move beyond past life choices.[29]

BRANDING

Some African American fraternity brothers use self-inflicted wounds caused by branding to indicate a sense of group identity and belonging. This controversial rite of passage for inductees to African American

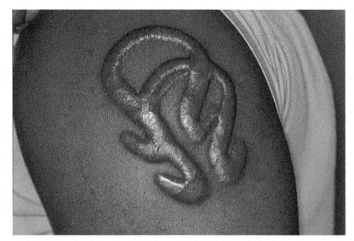

FIGURE 10-2. Bicep showing scarring in the shape of a Greek letter as a result of fraternity branding.

Greek letter organizations creates unpredictable results. Some brand wounds heal with neatly raised scars outlining an emblem or symbol; in other cases, a flat scar occurs [**Figure 10-2**]. Some individuals intentionally pick at scabs that form on the wound in hopes of creating a keloid. In a psychological context, the history of using branding in colonial courts to mark criminals or among plantation owners to mark slaves as property is difficult to overlook.[30,31] One interpretation of an individual's independent decision to undergo branding is that he is advertising his ability to make choices for himself.[32]

Generally, self-inflicted branding does not represent a psychiatric symptom but rather a form of self-expression.[33] Ironically, branding can be viewed by disapproving outsiders as a form of identification with a historical aggressor because pain is inherent to the process of branding. Branding also may be used in some tribal cultures as a form of therapeutic healing.[34] The complications of branding that may require medical attention include infections, transmission of blood-borne pathogens, allergic reactions, and injuries related to a third-degree burn.

SKIN BLEACHING

The desire to have lighter skin leads some individuals with skin of color to extreme measures, sometimes going so far as to bleach their children's skin.[35] Skin bleaching agents are aggressively marketed to Asian and African consumers, who sometimes will go to great lengths to lighten their complexions. The psychological motivation among Asians and Africans as well as others with darker skin is the rationale that lighter skin is associated with greater marriageability, higher status, and a greater competitiveness in the global job market.[35,36] Many of the commercially available products are poorly regulated and may contain ingredients such as hydroquinone in dangerous quantities.[37]

VITILIGO

Vitiligo results in a marked loss of skin pigmentation, which is more easily noticeable in individuals with naturally dark skin color [**Figure 10-3**]. Individuals with this autoimmune depigmenting disorder can experience extreme shame and depression related to the seemingly uncontrollable and unpredictable course of the disease. Retreat from society because of "anticipated rejection" is common, especially in children, who can be subjected to extremely hurtful and humiliating comments. Michael Jackson's public disclosure that he had vitiligo during a 1993 interview with Oprah Winfrey resulted in greater public awareness of the illness.[38] Prior to this, even he was the victim of many unkind comments from critics who saw his progressive depigmentation, along with facial plastic surgery, as an attempt to transform himself into a Caucasian (see Chapter 49, Vitiligo).[39]

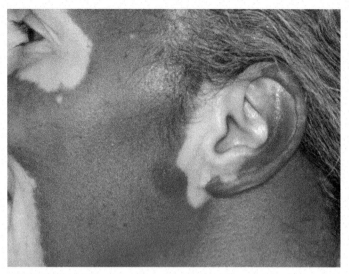

FIGURE 10-3. Vitiligo of the ear, eye, and lips with surrounding patches of hypopigmentation.

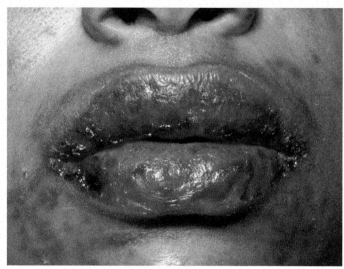

FIGURE 10-5. A patient with Stevens-Johnson syndrome.

PSYCHOTROPIC MEDICATIONS AND DERMATOLOGIC SIDE EFFECTS

▇ MOOD STABILIZERS

Lithium remains a mainstay for treatment of bipolar disorder. It is an excellent mood stabilizer that has the reputation of decreasing the risk of completed suicides in depressed patients. In addition, it may be used in lower doses to augment antidepressants. It also may cause or worsen acne and psoriasis, with an occurrence rate of up to 45%, and should be avoided in patients with these preexisting conditions because compliance may be adversely affected.[40] Male patients are at greater risk than female patients.[41] Gupta et al[42] reported a case of lithium-induced hidradenitis suppurativa [**Figure 10-4**] and also found that other cutaneous side effects of lithium include folliculitis, alopecia, and maculopapular/macular eruption. Hair also may lose its curl or wave. Lithium-related cutaneous lesions are also slower to respond to conventional therapy while the patient continues to receive lithium.[42]

▇ ANTICONVULSANT MOOD STABILIZERS

Lamotrigine is an anticonvulsant mood stabilizer that is also indicated by the FDA for treatment of major depression.[43] The primary

dermatologic concern with this medication is that it may cause Stevens-Johnson syndrome, or toxic epidermal necrolysis [**Figure 10-5**]. The incidence is low, and the syndrome may be prevented when proper dosing guidelines are followed. Serious rashes from lamotrigine are usually confluent and located on the face, neck, soles, and palms. The rash may have a purpuric or hemorrhagic appearance and may be associated with fever, malaise, pharyngitis, anorexia, or lymphadenopathy.[44] The patient should stop the drug immediately and seek emergency medical attention. Critical care in an intensive care unit setting is usually warranted. The risk of rash increases exponentially when valproic acid is coadministered with lamotrigine. Thus, when the two drugs are used simultaneously, the initial dose and rate of dose escalation of lamotrigine should be adjusted accordingly. Calabrese et al[45] published a thorough review of lamotrigine-related rashes, including a detailed discussion of clinical management.

Other anticonvulsant mood stabilizers include valproic acid and carbamazepine. Carbamazepine is much more likely to cause rashes, but most of these are benign. Oxcarbazepine is a newer alternative to carbamazepine and appears to cause fewer rashes. About 75% of patients who develop skin lesions with carbamazepine will tolerate oxcarbazepine.[46] Valproate is known to interfere with liver function and may cause elevated clotting times. Visible bruises may be the first warning that liver function has been adversely affected. Valproate is also known to cause alopecia. This can be addressed by administering a multivitamin containing zinc and selenium.[47]

Other classes of psychotropic medications are also associated with multiple dermatologic diagnoses.

CONCLUSION

The interrelationships between psychological and dermatologic disorders are complex. Treating these conditions in patients with skin of color presents the clinician with added challenges. The best approach to psychocutaneous disorders involves shared management between medical and mental health professionals working toward agreed-on treatment goals. The overall health status of all patients can be improved if psychological factors are considered during the treatment of dermatologic disorders.

REFERENCES

1. Telles EE. *Race in Another America: The Significance of Skin Color in Brazil*. Princeton, NJ: Princeton University Press; 2004:1.
2. Brown KT. Consequences of skin tone bias for African-Americans: resource attainment and psychological/social. *Afr Am Res Perspect*. 1998;4:1-9.

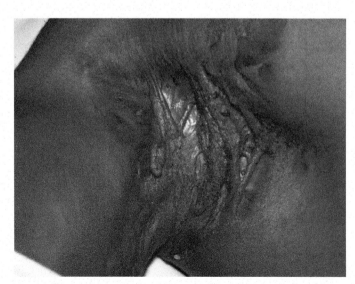

FIGURE 10-4. Hidradenitis suppurativa abscesses in the skin of the underarms due to the involvement of apocrine glands.

3. Gates HL. *The Future of Race*. New York, NY: Vintage Books; 1997:18.

4. Seeman M. Skin color values in three all-Negro school classes. *Am Sociol Rev.* 1946;11:315-321.

5. Porter CP. Social reasons for skin tone preferences of black school-age children. *Am J Orthopsychiatry.* 1991;61:8149-8154.

6. Goering JM. Changing perceptions and evaluations of physical characteristics among blacks. *Phylon.* 1971;33:231-241.

7. Robinson TL, Ward JV. African-American adolescents and skin color. *J Black Psychology.* 1995;21:256-274.

8. Bond S, Cash FT. Black beauty: skin color and body images among African-American college women. *J Negro Ed.* 1992;46:76-88.

9. Hall RE. Bias among African-Americans regarding skin color: implications for social work practice. *Res Social Work Prac.* 1992;2:479-486.

10. Keith VM, Herring C. Skin tone and stratification in the black community. *Am J Sociol.* 1991;97:760-778.

11. Phillips KA, Hollander E. Treating body dysmorphic disorder with medication: Evidence, misconceptions, and a suggested approach. *Body Image.* 2008;5:13-27.

12. Jafferany M. Psychodermatology: a guide to understanding common psychocutaneous disorders. *Prim Care Companion J Clin Psychiatry.* 2007;9:203-211.

13. RxList. Accutane. http://www.rxlist.com/accutane-drug/warnings-precautions.htm. Accessed February 12, 2013.

14. Hautmann G, Hercogova J, Torello L. Trichotillomania. *J Am Acad Dermatol.* 2003;45:807-826.

15. Lee SJ, Park SG, Kang JM, et al. Laser hair removal as an option for treatment of trichotillomania: a case report. *Eur Acad Dermatol Venereal.* 2006;21:1413-1450.

16. Drake RE, Mueser KT, Brunette MF. Management of persons with co-occurring severe mental illness and substance use disorder: program implications. *World Psychiatry.* 2007;6:131-136.

17. Petrakis IL, Nich C, Ralevski E. Psychotic spectrum disorders and alcohol abuse: a review of pharmacotherapeutic strategies and a report on the effectiveness of naltrexone and disulfiram. *Schizophr Bull.* 2006;32:644-654.

18. Wong JW, Koo JYM. Delusions of parasitosis. *Indian J Dermatol.* 2013;58:49-52.

19. Reid EE, Lio PA. Successful treatment of Morgellons disease with pimozide therapy. *Arch Dermatol.* 2010;146:1191-1193.

20. Morgellons Disease. Morgellons disease treatment. http://www.morgellonsdisease.net/tag/atypical-antipsychotics/. Accessed February 12, 2013.

21. Fabish W. Psychiatric aspects of dermatitis artefacta. *Br J Dermatol.* 1980;102:29-34.

22. Lukomski J, Folmer T. Self-mutilation: information and guidance for school personnel. http://www.nasponline.org/resources/principals/nasp_mutil.pdf. Accessed February 12, 2013.

23. Simeon D, Stanley B, Frances AJ, et al. Self-mutilation in personality disorders: psychological and biological correlates. *Am J Psychiatry.* 1992;149:221-226.

24. Olfson M, Gameroff MJ, Marcus SC, et al. Emergency treatment of young people following deliberate self-harm. *Arch Gen Psychiatr.* 2005;62:1122-1128.

25. Harris Interactive. One in five U.S. adults now has a tattoo. http://www.harrisinteractive.com/NewsRoom/HarrisPolls/tabid/447/mid/1508/articleId/970/ctl/ReadCustom%20Default/Default.aspx. Accessed February 12, 2013.

26. Walker R. Street gang and prison gang tattoos. Why are tattoos used by gangs? What do gang tattoos mean? http://www.gangsorus.com/gang_tattoos.html. Accessed February 12, 2013.

27. Kowalski E. Filipino gangs in the Philippines. http://www.zimbio.com/The+Philippines/articles/PR2SNUkbmGf/Filipino+Gangs+Philippines. Accessed February 12, 2013.

28. Bernstein EF. Laser tattoo removal. *Semin Plast Surg.* 2007;21:175-192.

29. Federal Bureau of Investigations. Honoring community leaders. http://www.fbi.gov/about_us/partnerships_and_outreach/community_outreach/dcla/2009/saltlakecity. Accessed February 12, 2013.

30. Colonial Williamsburg Foundation. Colonial punishments. http://www.history.org/Foundation/journal/Spring03/brankslideshow/2.html. Accessed February 12, 2013.

31. Thomas H. The branding (and baptism) of slaves. http://www.ralphmag.org/slave2.html. Accessed February 12, 2013.

32. Posey SM. Burning messages: interpreting African-American fraternity brands and their bearers. *Voices.* 2004;30:3-4.

33. Karamanoukian R, Ukatu C, Lee E, et al. Aesthetic skin branding: a novel form of body art with adverse clinical sequela. *J Burn Care Res.* 2006;27:108-110.

34. Kumar S, Kumar PR. Skin branding. *J Postgrad Med.* 2004;50:204.

35. Fokuo KJ. The lighter side of marriage: skin bleaching in post-colonial Ghana. *African Asian Studies.* 2009;8:125-146.

36. Hunter ML. Buying racial capital: skin-bleaching and cosmetic surgery in a globalized world. http://www.jpanafrican.com/docs/vol4no4/HunterFinal.pdf. Accessed February 13, 2013.

37. Parsand D, Prasand S, Kumarasing W. *Psychosocial Implications of Pigmentary Disorders in Asia.* Singapore: PanAmerican Society for Pigment Cell Research Commentary; 2006.

38. The Oprah Winfrey Show. The Michael Jackson interview: Oprah reflects. http://www.oprah.com/entertainment/Oprah-Reflects-on-Her-Interview-with-Michael-Jackson/3. Accessed February 11, 2013.

39. Anomalies Unlimited. A photographic history of Michael Jackson's face. http://anomalies-unlimited.com/Jackson.html. Accessed February 11, 2013.

40. Yeung CK, Chan HH. Cutaneous adverse effects of lithium: epidemiology and management. *Am J Clin Dermatol.* 2004;5:3-8.

41. Chan H, Wing Y, Su R. A control study of the cutaneous side effects of chronic lithium therapy. *J Affect Disord.* 2000;57:107-113.

42. Gupta AK, Knowles SR, Gupta MA, et al. Lithium therapy associated with hidradenitis suppurativa: case report and a review of the dermatologic side effects of lithium. *J Am Acad Dermatol.* 2004;32:382-386.

43. Lamictal (prescribing information). In: *Physicians' Desk Reference.* 59th ed. Montvale, NJ: Medical Economics Company; 2005.

44. Guberman A, Besag F, Brodie M, et al. Lamotrigine-associated rash: risk/benefit considerations in adults and children. *Epilepsia.* 1999;40:985-991.

45. Calabrese JR, Sullivan JR, Bowden CL, et al. Rash in multicenter trials of lamotrigine in mood disorders: clinical relevance and management. *J Clin Psychiatr.* 2002;63:1012-1019.

46. Ketter TA, Wang PW, Post RM. Carbamazepine and oxcarbazepine. In: Schatzberg AF, Nemeroff CB, eds. *Essentials of Clinical Psychopharmacology.* Washington, DC: American Psychiatric Publishing; 2006.

47. Hurd RW, Van Rinsvelt HA, Wilder BJ, et al. Selenium, zinc, and copper changes with valproic acid: possible relations to drug side effects. *Neurology.* 1984;34:1393-1395.

CHAPTER

11

Structure and Function of Skin

Sonia Badreshia-Bansal
Mayha Patel
Susan C. Taylor

KEY POINTS

- Epidermal differences include stratum corneum structure, lipid content, and melanin dispersion.
- Dermal differences include varied structural organization and concentration of dermal components.
- Although few definitive conclusions can be made with sparse research, biological skin differences do exist.
- These biological differences in skin structure and function account for lower rates of skin cancers and less pronounced photoaging, but also increased incidence of keloids and a variety of pigmentary disorders.

STRATUM CORNEUM

STRUCTURE AND FUNCTION

The stratum corneum forms the interface between the external environment and the body and influences barrier function and subsequently the potential for irritant reactions. The stratum corneum contains approximately 12 to 16 layers of corneocytes, each with a mean thickness of 1 μm. The primary function of the stratum corneum is to prevent evaporative water loss from the aqueous interior cell layers. The stratum corneum also protects against mechanical insults, foreign chemicals, microorganisms, and ultraviolet (UV) light. This layer was initially thought to be biologically inert, offering only a layer of protection for the more active layers underneath. However, in the past 30 years, the stratum corneum has been also found to have important biological properties.

The stratum corneum consists of a two-compartment system, termed *bricks and mortar*, that is composed of polyhedral corneocytes surrounded by a matrix of lipid-enriched membranes. The corneocytes are filled with keratin filaments and osmotically active small molecules, including filaggrin, loricrin, and involucrin, which also play an important role in natural moisturizing and the elastic properties of the skin. Additionally, the mechanical strength and chemical resistance of the skin barrier are due to these extensively cross-linked proteins into the corneocyte cornified envelope. Lipids in the intercellular spaces of the stratum corneum are organized into elaborate multilammelar structures composed of ceramides, cholesterol, and long-chain saturated fatty acids. These lipids maintain an optimal ratio to mediate the permeability barrier against excessive water and electrolyte loss. Corneodesmosomes connect adjacent corneocytes in the stratum corneum and comprise various proteins such as desmosomal cadherins, desmogleins, and desmocollins. The site of corneodesmosome hydrolysis, where proteolytic enzymes are involved in the desquamation and shedding process, is termed the *aqueous pore pathway* for water, drug, and xenobiotic movement in the epidermis.[1] In a variety of pathologic conditions, the structure, composition, and organization of the stratum corneum may be altered, leading to a reduced capacity to hold water and increased transepidermal water loss (TEWL).

STRUCTURAL DIFFERENCES

Attention has been focused on the thickness, density, and compactness of the stratum corneum when comparing skin of color with white skin. The thickness of the stratum corneum in white and black skin is generally thought to be similar.[2] A comparative study investigating the number of tape strips required to completely remove the stratum corneum (a measure of the number of layers of the stratum corneum) demonstrated a greater variability in tape strippings in black subjects compared with white subjects. Black subjects required a higher number of tape strippings than white subjects.[2-6] The degree of pigmentation had no correlation with the number of cell layers observed in a few studies.[2-7] Microscopic differences also included a greater average number of stratum corneum layers in black skin compared with white skin. This led to the conclusion that since thickness was equal in both groups, the stratum corneum in black skin is more cohesive and compact.[2]

This observation was confirmed when comparing skin phototypes V and VI with phototypes II and III.[5] Subjects with darker skin phototypes required more tape strippings to disrupt the epidermal barrier. This led to the conclusion that more cornified compact cell layers in darker skin could display superior epidermal barrier function and faster recovery from barrier damage. No differences in the number of strippings were found between Caucasians and Asians. Hence, in this study, structural differences were demonstrated to be related to skin phototype and not race. The above conclusion was confirmed in another study.[8]

Other investigators reported that the composition of lipids varied between the racial groups, with the lowest ceramide level found in African Americans,[9] followed by Caucasians, Hispanics, and Asians.[10] Ceramide levels were inversely correlated with TEWL and directly related to water content, suggesting that darker skin has poor water retention capacity and the highest evaporative water loss.

In examining corneocyte surface area, the data are inconsistent. A comparative study among African Americans, Caucasian Americans, and Asians of Chinese descent showed no difference in corneocyte surface area, but there was increased spontaneous corneocyte desquamation in African Americans, which was attributed to a difference in the composition of the lipids of the stratum corneum.[11] This contrasts with another study that found a greater desquamation index of corneocytes of the cheeks and foreheads of white subjects compared with black subjects.[12]

A recent study evaluated structural differences in barrier properties in African Americans, Caucasians, and East Asians (Chinese, Japanese, and Koreans).[9] Ceramide levels and cohesion in the uppermost layers of the stratum corneum were found to be similar in Caucasian and East Asian skin. African Americans had low ceramide levels, larger corneocyte size, and greater corneocyte density determined by tape strippings, suggesting a slow desquamation rate and thus accounting for potential xerosis, scaliness, and ashiness.[9] Qualitative and quantitative changes in these lipids, specifically reduced ceramide levels, have resulted in defective barrier function and impaired water retention capacity, and have been shown to be a characteristic of dry skin, particularly in atopic dermatitis patients.[13] The level of ceramides appears to have an impact on cellular cohesion and, therefore, may control the amount of scaliness.

In contrast to these observations, one study reported a trend toward a thicker stratum corneum in darker skin compared with lighter skin.[14]

However, these finding have not been substantiated using standard methodologies.

FUNCTIONAL DIFFERENCES

The barrier properties of the skin depend on an intact stratum corneum, among several other factors.[15] Skin permeability is related to the thickness of the epidermis and density of cutaneous appendages, which affect penetration into the capillary system in the dermis.[16-18] Studies of racial differences in percutaneous absorption have demonstrated conflicting results. Small study numbers do not allow for unequivocal conclusions. Wickrema-Sinha et al[19] and Guy et al[20] investigated skin by several methodologies, including evaluation of vasodilatation or laser Doppler velocimetry (LDV) in response to percutaneous absorption of methyl nicotinate. Guy et al[20] found that there was no difference in absorption between black versus white skin. However, Gean et al[21] demonstrated greater LDV output in both black and Asian skin versus white skin.

Skin irritation is another controversial area where multiple poorly designed studies offer conflicting results. Methodologic flaws include studies relying on investigator observation of erythema induced by various chemicals as a primary end point in pigmented skin.[2,22-25] As a result, this subjective assessment led these researchers to conclude that darker skinned subjects were less susceptible to irritants than lighter skinned subjects. Irritation was inversely proportional to skin color, so lighter skinned subjects were most susceptible to irritation.[26,27] Also, interindividual variability to irritants can be a confounding variable leading to inaccurate conclusions.

Instead of using the subjective measurement of erythema, more recent studies have relied on TEWL and other objective measures of irritancy.[28-35] However, these studies have their own limitations. Topical sodium lauryl sulfate (SLS) was applied with occlusion on normal skin, skin that had been stripped of stratum corneum, and skin that had been preoccluded (hence had increased water content). The irritant effect of SLS was secondary to disruption in stratum corneum integrity that used objective measurements, including TEWL (evaporimetry), capacitance (water content), and LDV (microcirculation). These studies concluded that individuals with skin of color (1) display a stronger skin irritant reaction, (2) have more sensitive skin, and (3) display less erythema, blood vessel reactivity, and cutaneous blood flow than white subjects. They also concluded that Hispanic subjects showed (1) strong irritant reaction similar to individuals with darker skin of color, (2) strong irritant reactions when injured, and (3) similar erythematous reactions when compared with lighter skinned subjects.

It is important to note that these conclusions are based only on an altered preoccluded skin model. A compromised skin barrier undoubtedly will result in increased susceptibility to irritants. However, for the untreated normal skin model, there were no significant differences in stratum corneum integrity. Therefore, the conclusions noted earlier would be better substantiated if these values were observed in an untreated skin model.[36]

A comparative study by Goh and Chia[33] of skin complexion among fair-skinned Chinese, darker-skinned Malaysians, and dark-skinned Indians found no difference in irritation indices measured by TEWL to 2% SLS. A follow-up study in black, Caucasian, and Asian subjects by Kompaore et al,[34] which evaluated only TEWL and LDV without exposure to irritants or chemicals that disrupt the stratum corneum, showed an increase in baseline TEWL in Asian and black subjects. This led to the conclusion that black and Asian subjects have a more compromised barrier function that would likely be more susceptible to irritants.[34] Higher TEWL at higher temperatures in black cadaveric skin was observed by Wilson et al[31] in another study. However, studies by DeLuca et al[35] and Pinnagoda et al[37] have found no apparent difference. A more recent study by Hicks et al[38] evaluating irritant contact dermatitis using confocal microscopy in vivo interestingly demonstrated more severe reactions in white forearm skin, which was characterized by parakeratosis, spongiosis, perivascular inflammatory infiltrate, and microvesicle formation. In addition, when comparing reactions to 2% and 4% SLS, white skin

had a greater mean increase in TEWL after exposure to 4% SLS than did black skin. These results support the theory that those with darker skin of color are more resistant to irritants and have a more intact and robust stratum corneum.

Key functional differences in the stratum corneum were noted among female African Americans, East Asians, and Caucasian volunteers.[9] First, maturation index (a measure for the tranglutaminase-1–dependent cross-linking in the cornified envelope) was found to be highest in African Americans and lowest in East Asians. Hence, this incomplete maturation process and thus weaker barrier observed in the East Asian subjects may partially account for their greater skin sensitivity and supports a stronger barrier function in African Americans. However, African Americans had low proteolytic activity, an important step in corneodesmosome degradation and an integral part of the differentiation process. These results may contribute to slower desquamation and thicker stratum corneum layers, resulting clinically in xerosis in African Americans. Dry, detached corneocytes scatter light strongly, appear bright white,[39] and are often observed as ashiness in darker skin.

More recently, skin pigment–related differences in epidermal barrier function have been attributed to the pH of the stratum corneum. Skin phototypes IV–V has been shown to have a lower pH, which is a key regulator for serine protease activity in the epidermis and for lipid processing,[40] although evidence for this has been conflicting. Limitations in studying skin pH include the presence of other variables such as gender, body site, and skin environment (skin temperature, hydration of the stratum corneum, rate of sebum excretion, TEWL, and sweating).[41]

The architecture of the outer stratum corneum appears different between ages, body sites, and skin color. One study showed that corneocyte detachment observed by dermoscopy was more prevalent with increasing age, on sun-exposed sites, and Caucasian subjects when compared with African American subjects.[42] As African Americans age, intercellular bonds in the stratum corneum appear to maintain their strength better than Caucasians. Minimal changes were noted in water-handling properties, including TEWL and conductivity. However, this study was limited by use of subjective scaling assessments.

Another study in women of various ages demonstrated greater skin hydration capacity in African American facial skin across all age groups when compared with age-matched white and Asian Indian skin.[43] This parallels another study that showed that skin dryness was increased in lighter skin tones, such as those of Asian descent and Caucasians, when compared with sun-exposed or nonexposed sites in African American and darker-skinned Mexican women.[44] The proposed mechanism involves the protective factor of melanin and the ability of the stratum corneum to retain its water content, creating a synergistic defense against harmful UV rays and protecting against dryness. However, with the aging process, skin dryness became greater in African American and Caucasian women than in Chinese and Mexican women, with a higher percent increase in Caucasian women.

Although there are several published studies discussing variations in stratum corneum structure and function with skin color, the data are difficult to compare and have limitations due to several confounding variables when evaluating epidermal barrier, stratum corneum hydration, surface pH, and surface lipids. For example, in healthy individuals, barrier strength is also known to be influenced by external factors, such as temperature, humidity, and seasonal variations, and internal factors, such as age, gender, hormonal status, anatomic site, and stress.[45-48] Conflicting reports warrant further studies to confirm these skin differences.

EPIDERMAL-MELANIN UNIT

STRUCTURE AND FUNCTION

Melanocytes are an important component of the epidermis that display differences in structure among the various racial groups. Derived from neural crest cell precursors, melanocytes migrate through the mesenchyme into the basal layer of the epidermis, the hair matrix and outer root sheath of hair follicles, epithelia of various mucous membranes, leptomeninges, the cochlea in the inner ear, and the uveal tract of the eye. Immunohistochemical staining reveals that primitive melanocytes first appear diffusely throughout the dermis of the head and neck region during the eighth week of fetal life.[49] Melanocytes are identified in the epidermis at as early as day 50 of gestation, and by 120 days, melanosomes are recognizable by electron microscopy.[50] At the end of gestation, active dermal melanocytes disappear, presumably as a result of programmed cell death. The arborization of melanocytes among 30 to 40 neighboring keratinocytes occurs during development with subsequent transfer of melanosomes into the keratinocytes.[51] This relationship of cells is termed the *epidermal-melanin unit*. Melanin functions to provide the skin with natural protection from the effects of daily UV radiation, as well as contributing to the color of the skin.

Recent research into evolutionary genetics demonstrates that skin color variation stems from mutations in the many genes that compose the pigmentation pathway, including differences in tyrosinase activity, the rate-limiting step for melanogenesis.[52] Skin pigmentation is one of the best examples of natural selection acting on a human trait,[53] with more than 25 pigmentation genes showing evidence of natural selection.[52] Whereas one trait supports dark pigmentation and photoprotection against UVA and UVB near the equator, the other trait favors light pigmentation to promote seasonal, UVB-induced photosynthesis of vitamin D_3 near the poles.[54] Intermediate latitudes with their seasonally high loads of UVB favored the evolution of moderate pigmentation capable of tanning. The lifetime course of pigmentation also varies and reflects its importance in reproduction and evolution. Infants are born more lightly pigmented and develop their genetically determined maximum level of pigmentation only in their peak fertility years in their late teens or early 20s.[53] In middle and old age, pigmentation fades and the potential for tanning decreases due to a decline of active melanocytes.[55]

▪ STRUCTURAL DIFFERENCES

Pigment cell biology has determined that the number of melanocytes is constant among races.[56,57] However, the activity of melanocytes does vary among the races, as well as from one individual to another and among different anatomic regions of the body.[58] Pigmentation of the skin depends on an orderly transfer of melanosomes from melanocytes to keratinocytes. The amount, density, and distribution of melanin within the melanosome, as determined by melanocyte activity, are the primary determinants of the variability of human skin color.[49,56-65] Differences in melanosome size, density, and aggregation correlate closely with skin color. **Figure 11-1** illustrates these differences in various skin hues. For example, early stage I or II melanosomes, seen in fair-skinned individuals, are small, clustered in groups or aggregations, and degraded more quickly in the stratum spinosum. This is in contrast to late stage IV melanosomes, seen in darker-skinned individuals, which are larger, individually dispersed, and degraded more slowly and remain in the stratum corneum longer. In general, darker-skinned subjects tend to have larger, nonaggregated, dense, and more oval melanosomes than subjects with lighter skin. Although skin of color contains melanosomes that tend to be larger and nonaggregated, this is not absolute. The size and distribution of melanosomes within individuals vary with skin hues and skin phototypes. For example, African Americans with lighter skin tones have a unique combination of single, large as well as small, aggregated melanosomes.[60] Similar variability also occurs in Caucasian and Asian subjects of darker and lighter hues.

Melanosomal distribution throughout the epidermis has racial variability. In darker skin, melanosomes are distributed throughout the entire epidermis, which is in contrast to unexposed fair skin, in which melanosomes are confined to the stratum basale and absent in the upper epidermal layers.[62,66] Sun exposure can play an important role in melanosomal distribution and groupings. The distribution of melanosomes in sun-exposed, deeply tanned Caucasian skin was noted to be similar to the distribution of melanosomes in darker skin of color.[62,66] A study in deeply tanned Thai patients showed that melanosomes in these subjects tended to have dense clusters in the basal layer with distribution

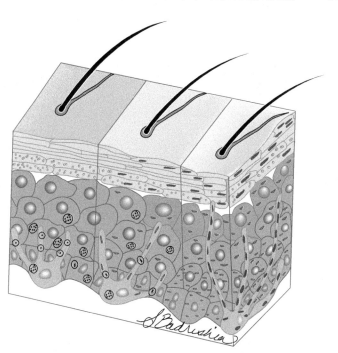

FIGURE 11-1. Schematic representation illustrating differences in melanosome organization in dark skin (right), tan skin (middle), and light skin (left).

throughout the epidermis and heavy pigmentation in the stratum corneum.[67]

A small study confirmed that more melanosomes were transferred into basal keratinocytes in the skin of subjects of African descent compared with Caucasian subjects.[68] Tyrosinase, which was found to be more active in darker skin, was also found to be controlled by melanosomal pH. A lower pH was seen in melanocytes of lighter-skinned individuals than in those of African descent. It has also been demonstrated that protease-activated receptor-2 (PAR-2), a seven-transmembrane G-protein–coupled receptor, regulates phagocytosis in keratinocytes. Darker skin exhibits a higher expression of PAR-2 compared with lighter skin, confirming the finding that inhibition of PAR-2 lightens skin complexion.

There appears to be a size requirement that dictates melanosomal aggregation in a membrane. Melanosomes in fair skin are smaller than 0.35 μm and can group into a membrane-bound unit called a phagosome.[58,63] However, melanosomes in dark skin are larger than 0.35 μm and therefore cannot be complexed and aggregated physically. As expected, total melanin content has been found to be greater in darker skin than in lighter skin, as determined through melanocyte cultures.[60] Darker skin has a higher eumelanin (brown-black) to pheomelanin (yellow-red) ratio compared with light skin.

▪ FUNCTIONAL DIFFERENCES

The amount, density, and distribution of melanin that correlates with human skin color are related to photoprotection and the incidence of skin cancer. It has been established that melanin confers protection from UV radiation.[63,64,69] In skin of color, the higher number of nonaggregated stage IV melanosomes absorb more UV radiation than the aggregated, smaller melanosomes in fair-skinned patients.[69] Skin color, rather than stratum corneum thickness, is responsible for differences in skin color reflectance measurements, as demonstrated by the similarities between albino Africans and European Caucasians.[70] Darkly pigmented skin of color had average minimal erythema doses (MEDs) 15 to 33 times greater than fairer skin, depending on skin tone.[63,69] The melanin pigment in darker skin, with high content of eumelanin, is considered a neutral-density filter, reducing the transmission wavelengths of light equally.[69] A similar trend occurs in other populations with skin of color. In a study of Asian skin, Japanese women demonstrated that greater

TABLE 11-1   Comparison of the epidermis across three racial groups[9,36,78]

Characteristic	Caucasian descent	African descent	Asian descent
Stratum corneum thickness	Equal	Equal	
Stratum corneocyte size	Equal	Equal	Equal
Stratum corneum layers	Less	More	Less
Stratum corneum lipids	Low	High	
Ceramide concentration	High	Low	High
Melanin	Low	High	Intermediate
Melanosomes	Small, aggregated	Large, dispersed	Mixed
Melanocyte number	Same	Same	Same
Melanosome distribution	Stratum basale	Entire epidermis	Mixed
Vitamin D production	High	Low	Intermediate
Minimal erythema dose	Low	High	Intermediate
Photodamage	High	Minimal	Intermediate
Glutathione (reduced state)	High	Low	
Glutathione reductase	High	Low	

melanin content, as evidenced by darker complexion, reacted less severely to the sun.[71] Reflectance spectroscopy in African and Caucasian subjects confirmed changes in melanin concentration due to racial differences and tanning, and also observed that differences in epidermal thickness and blood volume were related to anatomic location.[72]

Although melanin in pigmented skin confers protection from UV radiation, pigmented skin is not immune from damage. Individuals with this skin type have the ability to experience significant photodamage, including atypia, atrophy, collagen and elastin damage, and hyperpigmentation.[66,67] A study of Thai women found that melanin is not an efficient absorber of UV light of longer wavelengths, including UVA and infrared rays.[67] Furthermore, melanin also can be photoreactive, with the production of damaging oxygen free radicals.[73] Another recent study measured differences in oxidative stress in sun-exposed versus sun-protected sites in Japanese and French subjects. The antioxidant capacity, as measured by catalase activity, and parameters relating to skin hydration and barrier function were superior in Japanese subjects. However, the study was limited by confounding data, because there was no consideration of age, sex, lifestyle, stress, diet, and smoking habits, important factors affecting skin conditions.[74] Another study reported lower concentrations of most antioxidants, but also lower oxidative DNA damage levels, in African American than in Caucasian American subjects.[75] Investigations should be repeated in a larger number of volunteers of comparable lifestyle and nutritional habits to detect genuine skin of color differences.

Variability in melanin protection correlates with differences in extrinsic and intrinsic aging among racial groups. In general, there is a marked difference in atrophy and cell cytology between darker and lighter skin, with the former displaying fewer changes.[56] Chronologic aging in black subjects does occur with more pronounced changes, such as epidermal thinning, effaced rete ridges, and dyskeratosis occurring in older individuals.[66] This parallels findings in a study performed on Thai subjects over the age of 50 years with heavy sun exposure, who were noted to have greater disordered epidermal differentiation and atrophy.[67]

However, melanin is not the only skin factor that influences aging or responses to environmental stresses. One study found that skin aging in Korean, Vietnamese, and Singaporean subjects was directly related to TEWL and wrinkle characteristics and inversely related to skin hydration, sebum excretion, melanin index, and skin temperature.[41] The authors concluded that maintaining a low pH through skin hydration and increased sebum may be useful to slow skin aging.

Glutathione may play a role in genetically determined differences in skin color among different races.[76] This sulfhydryl-containing epidermal compound plays a role in melanin formation. The tripeptide glutathione (γ-glutamyl-cysteinyl-glycine) is present in the human epidermis in sufficient concentrations to be the inhibitor of melanin formation from

tyrosine by tyrosinase.[76] Glutathione in its reduced state (GSH) and the enzyme glutathione reductase, which maintains GSH levels, were found in lower concentrations in African skin than in Caucasian skin.

Additionally, there have been recent reports of differences in epidermal methylation patterns in Africans, Caucasians, and Asians. For example, the 5′ gene body of the *VWCE* (von Willebrand factor C and EGF domains) gene, which was predicted to be hypermethylated in African Americans, showed increased methylation in the 454 profiles collected from African samples.[77] It showed 61% methylation in Africans as compared with 37% and 36% in Asians and Caucasians, respectively. The confirmed presence of methylation differences may help elucidate the complex networks of genetic regulation, predict disease risk, and contribute to complex traits, such as drug response.

Tables 11-1 and 11-2 summarize the evidence discussed earlier regarding differences in the epidermal structure and function of the various racial groups.

TABLE 11-2   Possible clinical implications in skin of color based on epidermal differences[9,36,78]

Skin of color	Properties	Possible clinical implications
African descent	More compact cell layers	Superior barrier function, decreased penetration, more resistance to irritants, and faster barrier recovery
	Reduced ceramides	
	Suboptimal ratio of lipids	Xerosis, increased transepidermal water loss
	High maturation index[a]	Superior barrier function, improved recovery from stressors
	Poor degree of differentiation[b]	Increased scaliness
	Increased desquamation	Increased ashiness
Asian descent	Less compact cell layers	Slower barrier recovery, weak barrier function
	Increased ceramides	Less dryness
	Low maturation index (East Asian)[a]	Weak barrier function, increased skin sensitivity
	High degree of differentiation[b]	Less scaliness

[a]Maturation index is a measure of the amount of cross-linking in the cornified envelope.

[b]Differentiation is a measure of the amount of proteolytic activity required for corneodesmosome degradation.

DERMIS

STRUCTURE AND FUNCTION

The dermis is a highly vascular structure made up of several components, including collagen, elastin, and ground substance, as well as various glands. The cells of the dermis are derived from primitive mesenchymal cells, including fibroblasts, which produce collagen, elastin, and the matrix, and several specialized cells, including histiocytes, mastocytes, lymphocytes, plasma cells, and eosinophils.

Eccrine sweat glands, a key part of the body's thermoregulatory system, form in the fourth month of gestation from a downward budding of the epidermis. The coiled secretory portion is located in the reticular dermis, which then spirals upward onto the skin's surface, forming the acrosyringium, the excretory portion of the duct that secretes hypotonic saline. There are an estimated 2 to 5 million eccrine ducts located throughout the skin, with the densest population present in the axillae, palms, soles, and forehead, where they are under sympathetic cholinergic control.[79]

Apocrine glands are phylogenetic remnants of the mammalian sexual scent gland and function very similar to the eccrine ducts.[79] These glands are outgrowths of the pilosebaceous unit, and they deposit their contents into the infundibulum of hair follicles. Apocrine glands are densely populated in the axillae, perineum, areolae, and external auditory canal. They become active just before puberty, generating odorless sweat by decapitation secretion that develops an odor after interacting with the skin's bacteria. Apocrine sweat glands are innervated by sympathetic adrenergic nerve fibers.

Sebaceous glands compose the third gland found in the dermis, and they produce sebum, which consists of various lipids, including squalene, cholesterol, cholesterol esters, wax esters, and triglycerides, that traverse the follicular canal to the skin surface. These lipids function as the skin's natural moisturizer.

STRUCTURAL AND FUNCTIONAL DIFFERENCES

The existence of well-documented racial differences in the quantity, structure, and function of the eccrine sweat glands is not confirmed.[36] Most of the literature suggests no significant differences. Because of the premise that races evolved as a result of environmental selection, it is plausible that differences in sweat glands between races exist due to adaptation to hot, humid climates versus colder climates. It is unclear whether these differences would be based on genetics or strictly environmental adaptations.

The literature does not support difference in the number of eccrine glands between racial groups.[80,81] However, a racial differential in the functional activity of eccrine sweat glands has been noted. Higher sweating rates by white subjects during physical labor[82] or by cholinergic stimulation by pilocarpine tests[83,84] have been seen compared with both dark skin of color Africans and Asian Indians. The sodium content in sweat was lower in Africans, suggesting a more efficient electrolyte conservation system.[85] Electrophysiologic studies showed higher skin resistance and therefore greater eccrine gland activity in black subjects compared with white subjects.[86-89] Interestingly, in Hispanic and Spanish subjects, gland activity was between black and white eccrine gland activity.[86] This would suggest that skin color correlates with eccrine activity and that darker individuals have higher skin resistance than fair-skinned individuals.

There are limited and less than optimal studies in the literature regarding racial differences in apocrine glands.[36] Three early studies with a small study design concluded that black subjects had larger apocrine glands[90] in greater numbers[90,91] and with more turbid secretions.[92] However, the small study design and lack of investigator-blinded assessment preclude definitive conclusions.

An apoeccrine gland, also called a mixed sweat gland, develops at puberty from an eccrine gland that underwent apocrinization in the axilla, perineum, and nasal skin.[93] The secretory rate in an apoeccrine gland is 10 times more than that in an eccrine gland. Although there is great interindividual variation, one study found a greater number of apoeccrine glands in black versus white facial skin.[62,94] The significance of this finding is unclear.

Racial differences in sebaceous gland size and activity have been suggested. However, there are limited studies that seem contradictory due to a lack of well-controlled protocols, methodologic flaws, and small study populations. The literature suggests that black subjects tend to have higher sebum levels and larger glands than white subjects.[95,96] However, another study found a trend toward increased sebum production on the foreheads of black versus white men, although it did not reach statistical significance. The opposite finding was true when comparing black and white females. In a more recent study, there was no statistical difference when measuring sebum excretion among white, black, and Asian patients.[97] Finally, a study of Japanese women demonstrated a positive correlation between the amount of skin surface lipids and darker pigmentation.[71]

Although there are no differences in caliper-assisted skin thickness encompassing both epidermis and dermis, there may be differences at the cellular level between the dermis of black and white individuals.[78] Fibroblasts in black female facial skin were larger, binucleated or multinucleated, and of greater quantity than in white female facial skin.[62] There was greater interindividual variability in white subjects compared with blacks. Collagen fiber bundles in black skin were smaller, were more closely stacked, and ran more parallel with more collagen fibrils and glycoprotein fragments in the interstices versus larger, more sparse fiber fragments in white skin. Under transmission electron microscope (TEM), the ultrastructure of black skin showed some densely stained proteoglycans between the collagenous fibrils.[98] Fibroblast hyperreactivity is the result of the interaction among mast cells, cytokines, and fibroblasts. Number and size of mast cells are constant between the two racial groups.[62] However, there are more and larger macrophages in the papillary dermis, along with a decrease in collagenase, in black skin. This may explain in part the propensity for keloid formation in black individuals.

A small study in young Asians (Koreans) and Caucasians evaluated differences in endothelial function as it related to response of local heat and vascular occlusion to blood flow. Skin blood flow responses were significantly higher for all temperatures and following vascular occlusion in Caucasians than Asians, suggesting that genetic variations exist to account for the lower endothelial function found in Koreans.[99]

Just as hair color and hair structure vary among diverse racial groups,[100] follicle morphology may also vary, but with minor influence on the follicular penetration of applied agents.[101] One study demonstrated that Caucasians have significantly more hair follicles in the forehead area and increased follicular infundibulum than Africans and Asians.[102] Another small study in these three groups confirmed larger follicular infundibulum on the scalp in Caucasians. However, this larger volume is not completely available for incorporation of topically applied substances but, instead, is filled with sebum and desquamated cells.[103] Paradoxically, larger amounts of sodium fluorescein penetration were noted in the follicles and stratum corneum after 24 hours in the Asian group. This was contrary to another study that showed that no differences exist in penetration of different substances into the stratum corneum by tape stripping in Caucasians, Asians, and Africans.[104] The differences observed in penetration in the Asian group were explained by the cultural habits and weather conditions, which may have influenced storage capacity. Interestingly, no statistically significant differences were found in skin physiologic parameters including TEWL, skin moisture, pH, sebum excretion, skin roughness, and β-carotene or lycopene concentrations across all three groups.

This study also found differences in hair diameter and hair density across the three groups. Asians showed a significantly larger mean terminal hair diameter on the scalp, although there were large interindividual differences. In contrast, the African volunteers had significantly larger vellus hair shaft diameters in the calf region than Caucasians.

TABLE 11-3 Comparison of dermal structure between individuals of Caucasian and African descent[9,36,98]

Characteristic	Caucasian descent	African descent
Dermis	Thin and less compact	Thick and compact
Papillary and reticular layer	More distinct	Less distinct
Collagen fiber bundles	Large	Small, close stacking; proteoglycans between collagen fibrils
Fiber fragments	Sparse	Prominent and numerous
Melanophages	Few	Numerous and larger
Lymphatic vessels	Moderate, dilated	Dilated empty channels
Fibroblasts	Few	Numerous, large, binucleated and multinucleated
Elastic fibers	Several, elastosis	Few, elastosis uncommon
	Normal arrangement in papillary dermis	Abnormal arrangement in papillary dermis
	Surround secretory eccrine glands	Surround secretory eccrine glands
Superficial blood vessel	Sparse to moderate	Numerous, mostly dilated
Glycoprotein	Variable	Numerous in the dermis

Higher vellus hair density was noted in Asians in the calf region, contrary to other reports demonstrating higher density of hair follicles on the scalp in Caucasians,[105-107] and in the forehead region in Caucasians.[102,108] More studies are needed with larger numbers of volunteers and varying body sites, taking into consideration cultural habits and seasonal variations, to better understand differences in follicle morphology and follicular penetration.

In summary, several racial differences in the structure, function, and biology of the skin have been documented. The most conclusive data regarding the epidermis support a greater number of stratum corneum layers, lower ceramide concentrations, and higher levels of melanin packaged in larger, singly dispersed melanosomes in blacks. The dermal structure in darker skin of color individuals consists of a thicker and more compact dermis, compared with fair-skinned individuals, with closely stacked collagen bundles and prominent and numerous fiber fragments. **Tables 11-3 and 11-4** summarize these findings and their implications for clinical disease in skin of color.

TABLE 11-4 Therapeutic implications of key biologic differences in skin of color[9,36,78,98]

Biologic factor	Clinical implications
Epidermis	
Increased melanin content	Lower rates of skin cancer
Increased melanosome dispersion	Less pronounced photoaging
	Pigmentation disorders due to both biologic predispositions and cultural practices
Dermis	
Multinucleated and larger fibroblasts	Greater incidence of keloids
Thick and compact dermis	Less wrinkling of the skin

REFERENCES

1. Darlenski R, Sassning S, Tsankov N, et al. Non-invasive in vivo methods for investigation of the skin barrier physical properties. *Eur J Pharm Biopharm.* 2009;72:295-303.
2. Weigand DA, Haygood C, Gaylor JR. Cell layers and density of Negro and Caucasian stratum corneum. *J Invest Dermatol.* 1974;62:563-568.
3. Freeman RG, Cockerell FG, Armstrong J, et al. Sunlight as a factor influencing the thickness of epidermis. *J Invest Dermatol.* 1962;39:295-297.
4. Thomson ML. Relative efficiency of pigment and horny layer thickness in protecting the skin of Europeans and Africans against solar ultraviolet radiation. *J Physiol (Lond).* 1955;127:236-238.
5. Reed JT, Ghadially R, Elias PM. Effect of race, gender, and skin type on epidermal permeability barrier function. *J Invest Dermatol.* 1994; 102:537.
6. McKnight A, Momoh AO, Bullocks JM. Variations of structural components: specific intercultural differences in facial morphology, skin type, and structures. *Semin Plast Surg.* 2009;23:163-167.
7. Berardesca E, Rigol J, Leveque JL. In vivo biophysical differences in races. *Dermatologica.* 1991;182:89-93.
8. La Ruche G, Cesarini JP. Histology and physiology of black skin. *Ann Dermatol Venereol.* 1992;119:567-574.
9. Muizzuddin N, Hellemans L, Van Overloop L, et al. Structural and functional differences in barrier properties of African American, Caucasian and East Asian skin. *J Dermatol Sci.* 2010;59:123-128.
10. Sugino K, Imokawa G, Maibach HI. Ethnic difference of stratum corneum lipid in relation to stratum corneum function. *J Invest Dermatol.* 1993;100:597.
11. Corcuff P, Lotte C, Rougier A, et al. Racial differences in corneocytes. *Acta Derm Venereol.* 1991;71:146-148.
12. Warrier AG, Kligman AM, Harper RA, et al. A comparison of black and white skin using noninvasive methods. *J Soc Cosmet Chem.* 1996;47: 229-240.
13. Imokawa G, Abe A, Jin K, et al. Decreased level of ceramides in stratum corneum of atopic dermatitis: an etiologic factor in atopic dry skin? *J Invest Dermatol.* 1991;96:523-526.
14. Johnson BL Jr. Differences in skin type. In: Johnson BL Jr, Moy RL, White GM, eds. *Ethnic Skin: Medical and Surgical.* St Louis, MO: Mosby; 1998: 3-5.
15. Bereson PA, Burch GE. Studies of diffusion through dead human skin. *Am J Trop Med Hyg.* 1971;31:842.
16. Malkinson FD, Gehlman L. Factors affecting percutaneous absorption. In: Drill VA, Lazar P, eds. *Cutaneous Toxicology.* New York, NY: Academic Press; 1977.
17. Scheuplein RJ, Blank IH. Permeability of the skin. *Physiol Rev.* 1971;51:702.
18. Marzulli FN. Barriers to skin penetration. *J Invest Dermatol.* 1962;39:387.
19. Wickrema-Sinha AJ, Shaw SR, Weber DJ. Percutaneous absorption and excretion of tritium-labeled diflorasone diacetate: a new topical corticosteroid in the rat, monkey and man. *J Invest Dermatol.* 1978;7:372-377.
20. Guy RH, Tur E, Bjerke S, et al. Are there age and racial differences to methyl nicotinate-induced vasodilatation in human skin? *J Am Acad Dermatol.* 1985;12:1001-1006.
21. Gean CJ, Tur E, Maibach HI, et al. Cutaneous responses to topical methyl nicotinate in black, Oriental and Caucasian subjects. *Arch Dermatol Res.* 1989;281:95-98.
22. Marshall EK, Lynch V, Smith HV. Variation in susceptibility of the skin to dichloroethylsulfide. *J Pharmacol Exp Ther.* 1919;12:291-301.
23. Schwartz L, Tulipan L, Birmingham DJ. *Occupational Diseases of the Skin.* Philadelphia, PA: Lea & Febiger; 1939.
24. Shelley WB. Newer understanding of ecology in dermatology. In: Rees RB, ed. *Dermatosis Due to Environmental and Physical Factors.* Springfield, IL: Charles C. Thomas; 1962:12.
25. Frosch RJ, Kligman AM. The chamber scarification test for assessing irritancy of topically applied substances. In: Drill VA, Lazar P, eds. *Cutaneous Toxicology.* New York, NY: Academic Press; 1977:150.
26. Marshall J, Heyl T. Skin diseases in western Cape Province. *S Afr Med J.* 1963;37:1308.
27. Marshall J. New skin diseases in Africa. *Trans St Johns Hosp Dermatol Soc.* 1970;56:3-10.
28. Berardesca E, Maibach HI. Racial differences in sodium lauryl sulfate–induced cutaneous irritation: black and white. *Contact Dermatitis.* 1988;18:65-70.
29. Berardesca E, Maibach HI. Sodium-lauryl-sulphate–induced cutaneous irritation comparison of white and Hispanic subjects. *Contact Dermatitis.* 1988;19:136-140.

30. Berardesca E. Racial differences in skin function. *Acta Derm Venereol.* 1994;185:44-46.

31. Wilson D, Berardesca E, Maibach HI. In vivo transepidermal water loss: differences between black and white skin. *Br J Dermatol.* 1988;119:647-652.

32. Berardesca E, Maibach HI. Sensitive and ethnic skin: a need for special skin care agent? *Dermatol Clin.* 1991;9:89-92.

33. Goh CL, Chia SE. Skin irritability to sodium-lauryl sulphate: as measured by skin water vapor loss—by sex and race. *Clin Exp Dermatol.* 1988;13:16-19.

34. Kompaore F, Marty JP, Dupont C. In vivo evaluation of the stratum corneum barrier function in blacks, Caucasians and Asians with two non-invasive methods. *Skin Pharmacol.* 1993;6:200-207.

35. DeLuca R, Balestrieri A, Dinle Y. Measurement of cutaneous evaporation: 6. Cutaneous water loss in the people of Somalia. *Boll Soc Ital Biol Sper.* 1983;59:1499-1501.

36. Taylor SC. Skin of color: biology, structure, function, and implications for dermatologic disease. *J Am Acad Dermatol.* 2002;46:S41-S62.

37. Pinnagoda J, Tupker RA, Agner T, et al. Guidelines for transepidermal water loss (TEWL) measurement. *Contact Dermatitis.* 1990;22:164-178.

38. Hicks SP, Swindells KJ, Middelkamp-Hup MA, et al. Confocal histopathology of irritant contact dermatitis in vivo and the impact of skin color (black vs white). *J Am Acad Dermatol.* 2003;48:727-734.

39. Kollias N. The physical basis of skin color and its evaluation. *Clin Dermatol.* 1995;13:361-367.

40. Gunathilake R, Schurer NY, Shoo BA, et al. pH-regulated mechanisms account for pigment-type differences in epidermal barrier function. *J Invest Dermatol.* 2009;129:1719-1729.

41. Jung YC, Kim EJ, Cho JC, Suh KD, Nam GW. Effect of skin pH for wrinkle formation on Asian: Korean, Vietnamese and Singaporean. *J Eur Acad Dermatol Venereol.* 2013;27:e328-e332.

42. Chu M, Kollias N. Documentation of normal stratum corneum scaling in an average population: features of differences among age, ethnicity and body site. *Br J Dermatol.* 2011;164:497-507.

43. Fantasia J, Liu JC, Chen T. Comparison of skin hydration levels among three ethnic populations in the United States. *J Am Acad Dermatol.* 2010;62:AB60.

44. Diridollou S, de Rigal J, Querleux B, et al. Comparative study of the hydration of the stratum corneum between four ethnic groups: influence of age. *Int J Dermatol.* 2007;46(Suppl 1):11-14.

45. Akutsu N, Ooguri M, Onodera T, et al. Functional characteristics of the skin surface of children approaching puberty: age and seasonal influences. *Acta Derm Venereol.* 2009;89:21-27.

46. Muizzuddin N, Marenus KD, Schnittger SF, et al. Effect of systemic hormonal cyclicity on skin. *J Cosmet Sci.* 2005;56:311-321.

47. Garg A, Chren MM, Sands LP, et al. Psychological stress perturbs epidermal permeability barrier homeostasis: implications for the pathogenesis of stress-associated skin disorders. *Arch Dermatol.* 2001;137:53-59.

48. Halkier-Sørensen L, Menon GK, Elias PM, et al. Cutaneous barrier function after cold exposure in hairless mice: a model to demonstrate how cold interferes with barrier homeostasis among workers in the fish-processing industry. *Br J Dermatol.* 1995;132:391-401.

49. Bolognia JL, Orlow SJ. Melanocyte biology. In: Bolognia JL, Jorizzo JL, Rapini RP, eds. *Dermatology.* St Louis, MO: Mosby; 2003:935.

50. Holbrook KA, Underwood RA, Vogel AM, et al. The appearance, density, and distribution of melanocytes in human embryonic and fetal skin revealed by the anti-melanoma monoclonal antibody, HMB-45. *Anat Embryol.* 1989;180:443-455.

51. Jimbow K, Quevedo WC Jr, Fitzpatrick TB, et al. Some aspects of melanin biology: 1950–1975. *J Invest Dermatol.* 1976;67:72-89.

52. Quillen E, Shriver M. Unpacking human evolution to find the genetic determinants of human skin pigmentation. *J Invest Dermatol.* 2011;131:E5-E7.

53. Jablonski N, Chaplin G. Human skin pigmentation as an adaptation to UV radiation. *Proc Natl Acad Sci USA.* 2010;107:8962-8968.

54. Chaplin G, Jablonski NG. Vitamin D and the evolution of human depigmentation. *Am J Phys Anthropol.* 2009;139:451-461.

55. Quevedo WC, Szabó G, Virks J. Influence of age and UV on the populations of dopa-positive melanocytes in human skin. *J Invest Dermatol.* 1969;52:287-290.

56. Szabo G. Mitochondria and other cytoplasmic inclusions. In: Gordon M, ed. *Pigment Cell Biology.* New York, NY: Academic Press; 1959.

57. Starkco RS, Pinkus S. Quantitative and qualitative data on the pigment cell of adult human epidermis. *J Invest Dermatol.* 1957;28:33.

58. Toda K, Pathak MA, Parrish JA, et al. Alteration of racial differences in melanosome distribution in human epidermis after exposure to ultraviolet light. *Nat New Biol.* 1972;236:143-144.

59. Johnson BL Jr. Differences in skin type. In: Johnson BL Jr, Moy RL, White GM, eds. *Ethnic Skin: Medical and Surgical.* St Louis, MO: Mosby; 1998:3-5.

60. Masson P. Pigment cells in man. In: Miner RW, Gordon M, eds. *The Biology of Melanosomes.* Vol IV. New York, NY: New York Academy of Sciences; 1948:10-17.

61. Szabo G, Gerald AB, Pathak MA, et al. Racial differences in the fate of melanosomes in human epidermis. *Nature.* 1969;222:1081-1082.

62. Montagna W, Carlisle K. The architecture of black and white facial skin. *J Am Acad Dermatol.* 1991;24:929-937.

63. Olson RL, Gaylor J, Everett MA. Skin color, melanin, and erythema. *Arch Dermatol.* 1973;108:541-544.

64. Mitchell R. The skin of the Australian Aborigines: a light and electron microscopical study. *Australas J Dermatol.* 1968;9:314.

65. Smit NM, Kolb RM, Lentjes EM, et al. Variations in melanin formation by cultured melanocytes from different skin types. *Arch Dermatol Res.* 1998;290:342-349.

66. Herzberg AJ, Dinehart SM. Chronologic aging in black skin. *Am J Dermatopathol.* 1989;11:319-328.

67. Kotrajaras R, Kligman AM. The effect of topical tretinoin on photodamaged facial skin: the Thai experience. *Br J Dermatol.* 1993;129:302-309.

68. Yoshida-Amano Y, Hachiya A, Ohuchi A, et al. Essential role of RAB27A in determining constitutive human skin color. *PLoS One.* 2012;7:e41160.

69. Kaidbey KH, Agin PP, Sayre RM, et al. Photoprotection by melanin: a comparison of black and Caucasian skin. *J Am Acad Dermatol.* 1979;1:249-260.

70. Thomson, ML. Relative efficiency of pigment and horny layer thickness in protecting the skin of Europeans and Africans against solar ultraviolet radiation. *J Physiol.* 1955;127:236-238.

71. Abe T, Arai S, Mimura K, et al. Studies of physiological factors affecting skin susceptibility to ultraviolet light irradiation and irritants. *J Dermatol.* 1983;10:531-537.

72. Yudovsky D, Pilon L. Retrieving skin properties from in vivo spectral reflectance measurements. *J Biophotonics.* 2011;4:305-314.

73. Hill HZ, Li W, Xin P, et al. Melanin: a two-edged sword? *Pigment Cell Res.* 1997;10:158-161.

74. Yamashita Y, Okano Y, Ngo T, et al. Differences in susceptibility to oxidative stress in the skin of Japanese and French subjects and physiological characteristics of their skin. *Skin Pharmacol Physiol.* 2012;25:78-85.

75. Hesterberg K, Lademann J, Patzelt A, et al. Raman spectroscopic analysis of the increase of the carotenoid antioxidant concentration in human skin after a 1-week diet with ecological eggs. *J Biomed Opt.* 2009;14:024039.

76. Halprin K, Ohkawara A. Glutathione and human pigmentation. *Arch Dermatol.* 1966;94:355-357.

77. Winnefeld M, Brueckner B, Grönniger E, et al. Stable ethnic variations in DNA methylation patterns of human skin. *J Invest Dermatol.* 2012;132:466-468.

78. Whitmore SE, Sago NJ. Caliper-measured skin thickness is similar in white and black women. *J Am Acad Dermatol.* 2000;42:76-79.

79. Hurley HJ. Diseases of the eccrine sweat glands. In: Bolognia JL, Jorizzo JL, Rapini RP, eds. *Dermatology.* St Louis, MO: Mosby; 2003:567.

80. Johnson LG, Landon MM. Eccrine sweat gland activity and racial differences in resting skin conductance. *Psychophysiology.* 1965;1:322-329.

81. Montagna W, Parakkal PF. *The Structure and Function of Skin.* 3rd ed. New York, NY: Academic Press; 1974.

82. Robinson S, Dill D, Wilson J, et al. Adaptation of white men and Negroes to prolonged work in humid heat. *Am J Trop Med.* 1941;21:261-287.

83. McCance RA, Purohit G. Ethnic differences in response to the sweat glands to pilocarpine. *Nature.* 1969;221:378-379.

84. McCance RA, Rutishauser IH, Knight HC. Response to sweat glands to pilocarpine in the Bantu of Uganda. *Lancet.* 1968;1:663-665.

85. Calhoun DA, Oparil S. Racial differences in the pathogenesis of hypertension. *Am J Med Sci.* 1995;310:S86-S90.

86. Homma H. On apocrine sweat glands in white and Negro men and women. *Bull Johns Hopkins Hosp.* 1956;38:365.

87. Johnson LC, Corah NL. Racial differences in skin resistance. *Science.* 1960;139:766-767.

88. James CL, Worland J, Stern JA. Skin potential and barometer responsiveness of black and white children. *Psychophysiology.* 1976;13:523-527.

89. Juniper K Jr, Blanton DA, Dykman RA. Skin resistance, sweat-gland counts, salivary flow, and gastric secretion: age, race, and sex differences, and intercorrelations. *Psychophysiology.* 1967;4:216-222.

90. Schiefferdecker P. Dsaabel (vollkomin Mitt). *Zoologica.* 1922;27:1-154.

91. Homma H. On apocrine sweat glands in white and Negro men and women. *Bull Johns Hopkins Hosp.* 1926;38:365.

92. Hurley HJ, Shelley WB. The physiology and pharmacology of the apocrine sweat gland. In: *The Human Apocrine Sweat Gland in Health and Disease.* Springfield, IL: Charles C Thomas; 1960.

93. Ito T. Morphological connections of human apocrine and eccrine sweat glands: occurrence of the so-called "mixed sweat glands"—a review. *Okajimas Folia Anat Jpn.* 1988;65:315-316.

94. Goldsmith LA. Biology of eccrine and apocrine sweat glands. In: Freedberg IM, Eisen AZ, Wolff K, et al, eds. *Fitzpatrick's Dermatology in General Medicine.* Vol 1. New York, NY: McGraw-Hill; 1999.

95. Kligman AM, Shelley WB. An investigation of the biology of the sebaceous gland. *J Invest Dermatol.* 1958;30:99-125.

96. Champion RH, Gillman T, Rook AJ, et al. *An Introduction to the Biology of the Skin.* Philadelphia, PA: FA Davis; 1970:418.

97. Abedeen SK, Gonzales M, Judodihardjo H, et al. Racial variation in sebum excretion rate. Program and Abstracts of the 58th Annual Meeting of the American Academy of Dermatology; March 10-15, 2000; San Francisco, CA; abstract 559.

98. Prota G, Kenney J, Montagna W. *Black Skin: Structure and Function.* New York, NY: Academic Press; 1993.

99. Yim J, Petrofsky J, Berk L, et al. Differences in endothelial function between Korean-Asians and Caucasians. *Med Sci Monit.* 2012;18:CR337-CR343.

100. Franbourg A, Hallegot P, Baltenneck F, et al. Current research on ethnic hair. *J Am Acad Dermatol.* 2003;48(6 Suppl):S115-S119.

101. Luther N, Darvin ME, Sterry W, et al. Ethnic differences in skin physiology, hair follicle morphology and follicular penetration. *Skin Pharmacol Physiol.* 2012;25:182-191.

102. Mangelsdorf S, Otberg N, Maibach HI, et al. Ethnic variation in vellus hair follicle size and distribution. *Skin Pharmacol Physiol.* 2006;19:159-167.

103. Teichmann A, Jacobi U, Ossadnik M, et al. Differential stripping: determination of the amount of topically applied substances penetrated into the hair follicles. *J Invest Dermatol.* 2005;125:264-269.

104. Lotte C, Wester RC, Rougier A, et al. Racial differences in the in vivo percutaneous absorption of some organic compounds: a comparison between black, Caucasian and Asian subjects. *Arch Dermatol Res.* 1993;284:456-459.

105. Lee HJ, Ha SJ, Lee JH, et al. Hair counts from scalp biopsy specimens in Asians. *J Am Acad Dermatol.* 2002;46:218-221.

106. Loussouarn G, El Rawadi C, Genain G. Diversity of hair growth profiles. *Int J Dermatol.* 2005;44(Suppl 1):6-9.

107. Sperling LC. Hair density in African Americans. *Arch Dermatol.* 1999;135:656-658.

108. Mangelsdorf S, Otberg N, Maibach HI, et al. Ethnic variation in vellus hair follicle size and distribution. *Skin Pharmacol Physiol.* 2006;19:159-167.

CHAPTER

12

Histology

Jennifer Haley
Chandra Smart

KEY POINTS

- Racial differences in pigmentation are due to the number, size, and aggregation of melanosomes in the melanocytes and adjacent keratinocytes.

- Individuals of African descent have a more compact stratum corneum when compared to Caucasian skin.

- Racial differences in distribution and secretions of apocrine glands have been observed.

- African Americans have higher lipid content in their hair due to higher amounts of sebum production when compared to Caucasians.

- There are racial differences in hair pattern, elastic fiber and melanosome distribution, total hair density, and ultrastructure of the hair.

- Racial differences in dermal organization and cellularity have been observed.

NORMAL SKIN PHYSIOLOGY

Skin, the largest organ in the body, serves as a protective barrier that is integral in thermal regulation, serves as an important sensory organ, and plays an important role in immunologic function. The skin is divided into three main anatomic layers: epidermis, dermis, and subcutis [**Figure 12-1**]. Epidermal appendages include pilosebaceous units and apocrine and eccrine glands.

■ EPIDERMIS

The epidermis derives from the ectoderm and is the most superficial layer of the skin. It is composed of several layers: stratum corneum, stratum granulosum, stratum spinosum, and stratum basale [**Figure 12-2**]. The stratum spinosum and stratum basale together are sometimes referred to as the *malpighian layer.*

Stratum Basale The stratum basale, or basal cell layer, is composed of proliferating stem cells separated from the dermis by a thin basement membrane composed of type IV collagen.[1] In histologic sections, these cells are seen as a single layer above the basement membrane.[1] The daughter cells differentiate and undergo keratinization as they migrate upward toward the surface of the skin. The process of regeneration takes place every 28 to 40 days.

Stratum Spinosum The stratum spinosum lies above the basal cell layer. This layer is composed of several layers of keratinocytes. These cells differentiate from basal cells and accumulate keratin as they approach the surface of the epidermis. Desmosomes, or cell adhesion molecules, are responsible for the "spiny" appearance of this layer and hence its name.

Stratum Granulosum In the granular layer, cells continue to accumulate keratin and basophilic keratohyaline granules. These granules, coupled with the desmosomes, help to form a waterproof barrier, protecting the body from excessive water loss. They also serve as promoters for aggregation of keratin filaments in the cornified layer via the protein filaggrin.[1]

Stratum Corneum The stratum corneum is the thickest of the epidermal layers. Cells are anucleate, flattened, and filled with keratin. As cells migrate up to this layer, it is thought that rupture of lysosomal membranes releases enzymes that eventually cause cell death. These dead cells then take on the characteristic flattened, eosinophilic morphology and are eventually shed from the surface of the skin.[1]

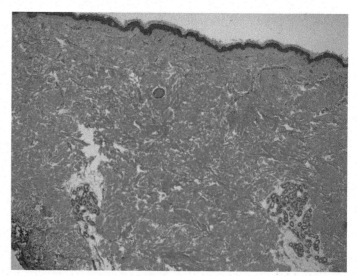

FIGURE 12-1. Normal skin. There are three anatomic layers of the skin: epidermis, dermis, and subcutis. Epidermal appendages include pilosebaceous units and eccrine glands.

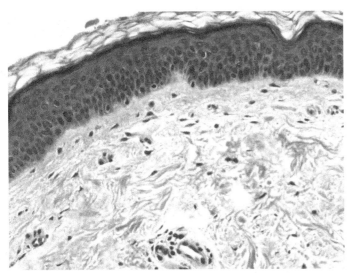

FIGURE 12-2. Normal skin. The subdivisions of the epidermis are the cornified layer, the spinous layer, and the granular cell layer. The dermis is divided into the papillary dermis and the wider, deeper reticular dermis.

EPIDERMAL CELL TYPES

Keratinocytes Keratinocytes constitute the major cell population of the epidermis, accounting for approximately 80% of all cells.[2] They are subclassified by their location in the epidermis.

Melanocytes Melanocytes are derived from neural crest cells and migrate to the epidermis during the first 3 months of development. Melanocytes are located in the basal layer of the skin and contain melanosomes. Melanosomes are the cellular organelles where the synthesis of melanin takes place via the enzyme tyrosinase. This enzyme is responsible for converting tyrosine into dihydroxyphenylalanine, one of the key steps in melanin production.[3] Developing melanosomes containing melanin are transferred to neighboring basal and hair follicular cells via phagocytosis of the dendritic tips of melanocytes by surrounding keratinocytes. Melanin can either be yellow to reddish-brown (pheomelanin) or brown to black (eumelanin).[1] The most important function of melanin is to protect against the effects of ultraviolet (UV) radiation.[1] The number of melanocytes in normal skin is constant in all races, with a ratio of one melanocyte per every 4 to 10 keratinocytes.[1] Melanocytes appear as cuboidal cells with clear cytoplasm along the basal layer [**Figure 12-3**].

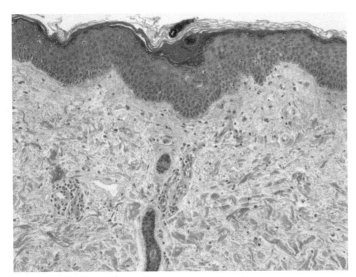

FIGURE 12-3. Pigmented skin. Melanocytes appear as cuboidal cells with clear cytoplasm along the basal layer. Langerhans cells may resemble melanocytes with hematoxylin and eosin stain but are located in the middle to upper dermis.

Langerhans Cells Langerhans cells may resemble melanocytes when stained with hematoxylin and eosin but are located in the middle to upper part of the epidermis.[1] Langerhans cells are derived from precursor cells in the bone marrow and serve as the antigen-presenting cells integral to immune surveillance in the skin. These dendritic cells process and present antigens to helper T-cells and are related in function to tissue macrophages, forming an important immunologic barrier of the skin.

Merkel Cells Merkel cells are thought to be responsible for mediating tactile sensation.[1] They are located predominantly in the basal layer of the epidermis and are found in increased concentration in the glabrous skin of the digits, lips, and oral cavity. Their site of origin is debatable, with some authors postulating a neural crest origin and others favoring differentiation from adjacent keratinocytes.[1]

DERMIS

The dermis is derived from the mesoderm and serves as the connective tissue support structure for the skin. It contains the blood vessels, nerves, and cutaneous appendages. The dermis consists of two layers: papillary dermis and reticular dermis. The papillary dermis is composed of loosely arranged type I and III collagen fibers, elastin fibers, abundant ground substance, capillaries of superficial plexuses, and fibroblasts.[1] It is named after the dermal papillae, or protrusions of dermal connective tissue, that indent the base of the epidermis. The reticular dermis is composed of predominantly type I collagen, forming layers that are thick, densely packed, and arranged parallel to the epidermis. The cellular makeup of the reticular dermis includes fibroblasts, dendritic cells, macrophages, and mast cells.[1] Dermal elastic fibers give the skin elasticity and resilience. The elastic fibers in the papillary dermis are arranged vertically, and are arranged horizontally in the reticular dermis.

DERMAL-EPIDERMAL JUNCTION

The dermal-epidermal junction represents the interface between the lower part of the epidermis and the underlying dermis. This complex structure is composed of the lamina lucida, the lamina densa, and adhesion proteins including hemidesmosomes, anchoring filaments, and anchoring fibrils. The relevance of these proteins in skin adhesion is apparent in both genetic and autoimmune disorders in which components of the basement membrane zone are defective, absent, or damaged.

SUBCUTIS

The subcutis is arranged into lobules of mature adipocytes separated by fibrous connective tissue septa. There are two types of fat: brown fat and white fat. Deposits of brown fat may be seen in infants and young children, and are characterized by a pink granular cytoplasm and a more centrally placed nucleus. Mature subcutaneous fat is composed of adipocytes with an expanded cytoplasm, displacing the nucleus to an eccentric location. The lipid dissolves in routinely processed specimens. The thickness of the subcutis varies with gender, nutritional status of the individual, and anatomic location.[2]

SKIN APPENDAGES

Eccrine Glands These glands are the true sweat glands, important in regulating temperature. The eccrine gland is composed of a secretory coil (pictured) that leads into a coiled proximal duct and then a straight duct which eventually passes through the epidermis [**Figure 12-4**]. The intraepidermal portion of the eccrine duct is also known as the acrosyringium and follows a spiral course through the epidermis. The acrosyringium is composed of one layer of inner cells and two or three layers of outer cells. The intradermal eccrine duct is composed of two layers of basophilic cuboidal or columnar cells. The secretory portion of the duct is composed of two cell types, pale staining cells and dark basophilic cells. Eccrine glands are found predominantly in the palms, soles, forehead, and axillae. Eccrine glands produce an isotonic to hypertonic secretion that is modified by the ducts to emerge on the skin surface as sweat.[2]

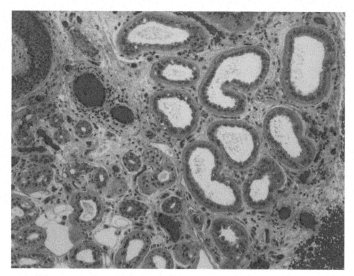

FIGURE 12-4. Normal eccrine gland.

Apocrine Glands These glands are found primarily in the axillae, groin, eyelids, and ears, as well as in the mammary and perineal regions.[3] The function of these glands is not well understood, but they are known to cause body odor when their secretions are excreted onto the skin due to the presence of bacteria that colonize the skin surface. Apocrine glands are composed of a secretory component located in the lower reticular dermis or the subcutis and a tubular duct linking the gland with the pilosebaceous follicle. The secretory portion is composed of eosinophilic cuboidal cells. Decapitation secretion may be observed with routine hematoxylin and eosin stains. The duct portion is similar in morphology to the eccrine duct.

Pilosebaceous Unit The pilosebaceous unit is composed of the hair follicle, hair shaft, arrector pili, and sebaceous glands [**Figure 12-5**]. The hair follicle is divided into three main segments: the infundibulum, the isthmus, and the inferior segment, or hair bulb.[1] The inferior segment extends from the base of the hair follicle to the insertion of the arrector pili muscle. The isthmus extends from the arrector pili muscle to the entrance of the sebaceous duct, and the infundibulum extends from the entrance of the sebaceous duct to the follicular orifice. There are five major components in the inferior segment of the hair follicle: the dermal hair papilla, the hair matrix, the hair, the inner root sheath, with Huxley and Henle layers, and the outer root sheath. The hair consists of the medulla, cortex, and hair cuticle. Hair follicle stem cells are located in the bulge, adjacent to entrance of the sebaceous duct. Destruction of the bulb plays an important role in cicatricial alopecia. Hair follicles are associated with sebaceous glands, which are present everywhere except on the palms and soles. The sebaceous glands are holocrine glands that secrete oily, lipid-rich secretions composed predominately of disintegrated cells into the hair follicle.[1] The arrector pili are composed of bundles of smooth muscle fibers that are controlled by the autonomic nervous system.

REGIONAL VARIATIONS IN SKIN HISTOLOGY

Glabrous skin is non–hair-bearing skin found on the palms and soles. Skin on the palms and soles has an additional eosinophilic acellular layer defined as the stratum lucidum. Pilosebaceous glands are absent, and the dermis contains encapsulated sense organs. For example, Pacinian corpuscles are lamellated structures found in the subcutaneous fat on the palms and soles and are responsible for sensing deep pressure and vibration. Meissner corpuscles are found primarily in the dermal papillae on hands, feet, and lips and are responsible for touch sensation. Hair-bearing skin has pilosebaceous units and lacks the encapsulated dermal sense organs found on glabrous skin. The size, structure, and density of hair follicles can vary depending on the body site. For example, large terminal follicles are present on the scalp and men's facial hair. Vellus hairs are smaller in diameter and shorter in length and are found on areas such as the forehead.[4]

SKIN PHYSIOLOGY IN SKIN OF COLOR

◼ PIGMENTATION

One of the most striking differences in skin of color is the varying degree of pigmentation seen in this population. As stated earlier, melanocytes are responsible for producing the cutaneous pigment, melanin, but there are no racial differences in the number of melanocytes present in skin.[3] The racial differences in pigmentation are mainly due to the number, size, and aggregation of melanosomes within the melanocyte and the keratinocyte.[3] People with skin of color, particularly those of African descent, tend to have large, nonaggregated melanosomes that absorb and scatter more energy, providing higher photoprotection in pigmented skin.[5] The number of melanocytes in normal skin is constant. The number and shape of melanosomes account for differences in skin color [**Figure 12-6**].

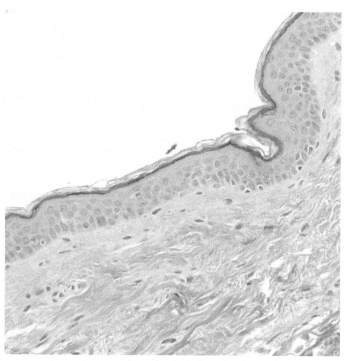

FIGURE 12-6. Pigmented skin at low power. The number of melanocytes in normal skin is constant. The number and shape of melanosomes account for differences in skin color.

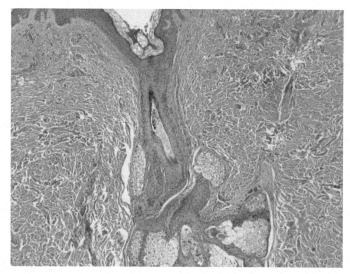

FIGURE 12-5. Pilosebaceous unit.

EPIDERMIS

Stratum Corneum The average stratum corneum thickness is similar between those of African descent and Caucasians, but studies suggest that the stratum corneum is more compact in the former. Studies have been performed demonstrating that removal of the stratum corneum in darker skin requires more cellophane tape strips than removal in Caucasian skin.[6-8] This finding may be a reflection of the greater intercellular cohesion present in darkly pigmented skin. The spontaneous desquamation rate of the stratum corneum in darker-skinned individuals is 2.5 times greater than that seen in Caucasians and Asians, which may account for the increased frequency of xerosis seen clinically in people of African descent.[5]

SKIN APPENDAGES

Eccrine Sweat Glands There are few differences in the number of eccrine sweat glands between races, but some functional differences are of note. One such difference was an increased sweating rate in Caucasians compared with dark skin of color Africans.[1] Furthermore, Africans had a lower concentration of salt in their sweat than Caucasians.[3]

Apocrine Sweat Glands Three limited studies suggest African Americans have larger apocrine glands in greater number and more turbid secretion.[3]

Sebaceous Glands One study showed that African Americans have larger sebaceous glands and higher sebum levels than whites.[3]

Hair Follicles There are distinctive differences in the hair follicles of individuals of African descent when compared with other races. These differences consist of hair pattern, elastic fiber and melanosome distribution, total hair density, and ultrastructure of the hair. Four hair patterns have been noted: straight, wavy, helical, and spiral, with spiral being the most largely represented in the skin of color population.[3] The follicles on the scalp and the hair are curved, but there are no discernible differences in the thickness of the cuticle and shape and size of scale and cortical cells between the hair of the African Americans and Caucasian Americans studied.[3] African Americans have fewer elastic fibers anchoring the hair follicles to the dermis. Melanosomes are distributed in both the outer root sheath and the bulb of vellus hairs. People of African descent have more heavily pigmented hair due to the presence of larger melanin granules. The ultrastructure of African American hair tends to be altered such that it has a tendency to form knots, longitudinal fissures, and splits along the hair shaft.

DERMIS

The major differences in the dermis of skin of color are present within its cellular components. There is an increase in quantity and size of fibroblasts that are either binucleated or multinucleated.[3] In addition, the collagen bundles present in the dermis of skin of color are smaller, more closely stacked, and run in a pattern parallel to the epidermis. Microscopic examination of people with darker skin of color reveals that the mast cells present in the dermis contain larger intracellular granules.[6]

Finally, it has been determined that African Americans and Hispanics have significantly more dermal papillae per area of facial skin than other racial groups.[9]

REFERENCES

1. Sternberg SS. *Histology for Pathologists.* 2nd ed. Philadelphia, PA: Lippincott Williams & Wilkins; 1997:25-43.
2. Hood AF, Kwan TH, Mihm MC, et al. *Primer of Dermatopathology.* 3rd ed. Philadelphia, PA: Lippincott Williams & Wilkins; 2002:3-15.
3. Taylor SC. Skin of color: biology, structure, function, and implications for dermatologic disease. *J Am Acad Dermatol.* 2002;46:S44.
4. Calonje E, Brenn T, Lazar A, McKee P. *McKee's Pathology of the Skin.* 4th ed. Beijing, China: Elsevier Saunders; 2012:1-31.
5. Berardesca W, Maibach H. Racial differences in skin pathophysiology. *J Am Acad Dermatol.* 1996;34:667-672.
6. Wesley NO, Maibach HI. Racial (ethnic) differences in skin properties: the objective data. *Am J Clin Dermatol.* 2003;4:843-860.
7. Rawlings AV. Ethnic skin types: are there differences in skin structure and function? *Int J Cosmet Sci* 2006;28:79-93.
8. Richards GM, Oresajo CO, Halder RM. Structure and function of ethnic skin and hair. *Dermatol Clin.* 2003;21:595-600.
9. Sugiyama-Nakagiri Y, Sugata K, Hachiya A, Osanai O, Ohuchi A, Kitahara T. Ethnic differences in the structural properties of facial skin. *J Dermatol Sci.* 2009;53:135-139.

CHAPTER 13

Genetics of Skin Diseases

Shirley B. Russell
Saundrett Arrindell
George P. Stricklin
Karen C. Broussard
Stella Bulengo
Jennifer Lee

KEY POINTS

- Differences in incidence and prevalence of disease in different racial and ethnic populations provide evidence for a genetic contribution to the etiology of a disorder.

- Familial clustering of disease and more frequent concordance of disease in monozygotic (MZ) than dizygotic twins provide further support for a genetic component.

- Less than 100% concordance in MZ twins as well as evidence for epigenetic modifications in disease support a strong environmental component in addition to the genetic contribution.

- Genome-wide linkage and gene association studies provide evidence for involvement of genes at specific chromosomal regions.

- Systemic lupus erythematosus (SLE), vitiligo, systemic sclerosis (SSc), sarcoidosis, and keloids are genetically complex, with multiple genetic loci and environmental triggers conferring risk for the disease and its severity.

- Autoimmune diseases including SLE, SSc, sarcoidosis, and vitiligo share some susceptibility loci at human chromosomal region 6p21, which contains genes of the major histocompatibility complex as well as many non–human leukocyte antigen loci involved in lymphocyte activation (B and T-cells), cytokine pathways, and host–microbe interactions. Sharing among subsets of autoimmune disease and network analysis of the functions of candidate genes may provide important information about disease pathogenesis and therapeutic strategies.

- In addition to shared genetic susceptibilities, some gene differences are observed mainly within a single disorder, within a single racial group, or within a group of patients with similar clinical symptoms.

- Problems in replicating genetic findings and in elucidating the genetic contribution to the pathogenesis of complex diseases are currently being addressed by analyzing results from different racial group separately; admixture mapping to identify association of specific disease-related variation with ancestry; association studies using panels of single-nucleotide polymorphisms (SNPs) from different racial populations; using subsets of patients with similar clinical symptoms; and using ordered subset analysis to obtain evidence for gene interaction (epistasis) between different genetic loci. To further refine findings from genome-wide association studies, where significant SNP associations often implicate more than one gene, comprehensive analysis of all gene variation at associated loci and functional studies are needed to identify specific gene involvement and causal mutations.

- The gene discovery process is an ongoing and dynamic one. Tables of specific genes and chromosomal regions require frequent updating, and the reader is referred to regularly updated resources including Online Mendelian Inheritance in Man (http://omim.org/) and the website for the National Human Genome Research Institute (http://www.genome.gov/) studies for the most current compilations.

Multiple types of evidence support a genetic contribution to human disease. Differences in incidence and prevalence in different racial and ethnic populations provide strong suggestive evidence for a genetic contribution to the etiology of a disorder. Although socioeconomic, behavioral, and environmental factors confound the identification and contribution of genetic factors, dissimilar frequencies of rare alleles and polymorphisms that associate with disease in different racial groups support a role for genetic factors. Gene admixture complicates assignment of individuals to a single group. Studies in multiple populations, using panels of ancestry informative markers (AIMs) and single-nucleotide polymorphisms (SNPs) with highly significant differences in allele frequency in different ancestral populations, have provided estimates of the degree of admixture of genes among different groups, from which the expected distribution of genes in an individual may be more accurately predicted[1-5] [**Table 13-1**]. Admixture mapping (AM) identifies gene variants involved in racial variation in disease risk and/or severity and is based on the idea that the different prevalence of a genetic disease in different populations is due to differences in frequency of predisposing genetic variants.[6] In admixed populations, these variants are expected to occur more often in chromosomal regions inherited from the ancestral population with the higher frequency of the disease. AM has been used in studies of several disorders that occur more frequently in individuals of African ancestry, including asthma,[7] type 2 diabetes,[8] nondiabetic end-stage kidney disease,[6] sarcoidosis,[9] and systemic lupus erythematosus (SLE).[10] Characterization of genetic contributions to disease occurrence and severity in racial populations can provide important diagnostic and prognostic information.

Familial clustering of disease and more frequent concordance of disease in monozygotic (MZ) than dizygotic (DZ) twins provide further support for a genetic component. Twin studies depend on the fact that MZ twins have virtually identical genomes (except for somatic mutation and contributions from mitochondrial inheritance), whereas DZ twins share, on average, only 50% of their genes. If pairs of MZ twins

develop a disease (concordance) more often than pairs of DZ twins, a genetic contribution is supported. Concordance of significantly less than 100% in MZ twin pairs is evidence for the contribution of both genetic and environmental factors. Epigenetic influences on the expression of autoimmune diseases and keloid formation are becoming better recognized.[10,11] Epigenetic variation refers to stable alterations in gene expression that do not involve changes in the primary DNA sequence. Cytosine methylation, histone modifications, and microRNAs are the major epigenetic mechanisms of this process that link variability in the expression of disease to various extrinsic factors, including exposure to drugs, pollutants, and infection.[11,12]

Great strides in clarifying the genetic contribution to disease in recent years have been facilitated by technologic advances in molecular biology needed for genome-wide linkage studies, characterization of small differences within genes, genome-wide testing of associations between particular gene variants and disease (genome-wide association studies [GWAS]),[13] and the dramatically decreased cost of genome sequencing. The human genome contains 3 billion base pairs and an estimated 22,000 protein-coding genes. The human genome sequence is essentially the same (>99.9%) in all people. Genetic diversity between individuals is attributable to the remaining 0.1%. A small variation in DNA sequence, such as a single nucleotide change in a rare mutation or an SNP, can be critical in determining whether an individual has a genetic predisposition to a disease and its severity. The human genome has at least 10 million SNPs. SNPs are usually biallelic. To qualify as an SNP, the minor allele must occur in at least 1% of the population. Because of a statistical phenomenon known as linkage disequilibrium (LD), in which multiple nonalleles occur together more frequently on the same chromosome than expected by chance, the genotype of one SNP allele, referred to as a tag SNP, provides information about the genotypes of other SNP alleles in a particular chromosome region. A group of SNPs in LD forms an LD block or haplotype. Identification of a tag SNP allows the imputation of other SNP alleles in the haplotype block and definition of a chromosomal region, which may contain multiple protein-coding genes. A successful GWAS depends on an appropriate selection of tag SNPs. A useful tool in selecting tag SNPs is HapMap, a database produced by the International HapMap Project that contains LD maps in several different populations, now expanded but originally European (CEU), West African (YRI), Han Chinese (CHB), and Japanese (JPT).[14] Although many haplotypes are common to different populations, differences exist in size and content, making knowledge about population substructure important. Of particular note is that the size of blocks is similar in the CEU, CHB, and JPT samples but is smaller in the YRI samples, reflecting the fact that the

TABLE 13-1   Admixture estimates for different populations[1]

Sample examined	No.	Population contribution assessed by structure (%)			
		European	African	Asian	Native American Indian
European American:				0.7	0.5
Chicago	39	98.4	0.4	0.9	1.3
Baltimore	39	97.5	0.4		
African American:					
Chicago	18	18.4	80.6	0.7	0.3
Pittsburgh	23	18.3	80.6	0.6	0.5
Baltimore	45	15.9	83.2	0.5	0.5
North Carolina	23	18.8	79.6	0.5	1.1
African:					
Senegal	46	2.8	95	1.6	0.6
Ghana	33	0.1	99.8	0.1	0.1
Cameroon	20	0.1	99.8	0.1	0.1
Botswana	21	1.2	98.4	0.3	0.1
Chinese:					
Cantonese	40	0.2	0.1	98.9	0.8
Amerindian:					
Mexican Zapotec	29	4.3	0.3	0.5	94.8

African population is much older.[15] Genetic mapping of SNPs has made it possible to trace migration of the human species, affording a window into the multifaceted genetic makeup of different populations.

The role of genetics in dermatologic disease has been evident for centuries. Most, if not all, disorders discussed here, notably SLE, vitiligo, systemic sclerosis (SSc), sarcoidosis, and keloids, are genetically complex, with multiple genetic loci and environmental triggers conferring risk for the disease and its severity. Even where an autosomal dominant pattern of inheritance has been observed in some families, reduced penetrance supports contributions by more than one gene, and variable expression within the same individual supports a role for environmental factors. Involvement of different genes in the etiology of a disease (locus heterogeneity) has been suggested by clinical heterogeneity in disease presentation and confirmed by genetic linkage to different chromosomal regions in different families and racial groups.

Autoimmune diseases, including but not limited to SLE, SSc, vitiligo, and sarcoidosis, arise from interactions between multiple genetic and environmental factors. Genome-wide linkage studies of autoimmune diseases have identified at least 30 chromosomal regions of overlap for different autoimmune diseases, suggesting shared susceptibility loci for these clinically related disorders.[16,17] Many autoimmune diseases share susceptibility loci on the short arm of chromosome 6 [**Figure 13-1**] at 6p21.3 [**Figure 13-2**]. This region contains genes of the major histocompatibility complex (MHC), including the highly polymorphic class I human leukocyte antigen (HLA) genes (B, C, and A), class II HLA genes (DR, DQ, and DP), genes in the class II region that code for components of the proteasome, and class III HLA genes (cytokines and complement proteins). Patterns of inheritance seen in some familial cases indicate a predisposition to autoimmune disease development rather than to a specific autoimmune disease.[18] The occurrence of different types of autoimmune diseases within a pedigree may be determined by additional genetic loci and environmental influences. GWAS have identified SNPs associated with particular autoimmune diseases, and microarray studies have identified clusters of genes that are differentially expressed in multiple autoimmune diseases, many of which are located in chromosomal regions that contain susceptibility loci for autoimmune disease.[19] This convergence of genetic linkage, gene association, and differences in gene expression at particular loci provides a strong basis for exploring the clinical significance of gene differences in different diseases and populations.

Identification of genes for genetically complex diseases is in a dynamic state, with many findings not replicated in subsequent studies. The failure to replicate is due to a number of factors, including the following: (1) different genes may cause the same disease in different racial populations; (2) different genes may cause different forms of disease characterized by different clinical features; (3) interactions between genes at different loci (epistasis) may influence whether a particular gene causes susceptibility to the disease; and (4) environmental factors mediated through epigenetic mechanisms may change the clinical phenotype. Consequently, an increasing number of gene linkage and gene association studies are taking genetic heterogeneity and gene interactions into account by analyzing results from different racial groups separately, by examining the role of specific genes in subsets of patients with a similar set of symptoms, by performing AM to identify associations of specific disease-related variation with ancestry,[6,9,10,20,21] by performing association studies using panels of SNPs from different racial populations,[22] and by using ordered subset analysis to obtain evidence for gene interaction between loci on different chromosomal regions.[23] To further refine findings from GWAS, where significant SNP associations often implicate more than one gene, comprehensive analysis of all gene variation at associated loci as well as functional studies are needed to identify specific gene involvement and causal mutations.[17]

SYSTEMIC LUPUS ERYTHEMATOSUS

SLE is a multisystem autoimmune disorder characterized by the deposition of autoantibodies leading to tissue injury in multiple organs, including but not limited to skin, heart, kidneys, brain, lungs, and joints.

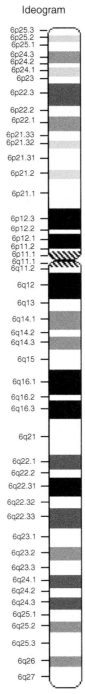

Ideogram

FIGURE 13-1. Ideogram of chromosome 6 (National Center for Biotechnology Information MapView). Many autoimmune diseases share susceptibility loci on the short arm of human chromosome 6 at region p21.3.

Genetic, epigenetic, and nongenetic factors, such as environmental and hormonal influences, affect disease expression, severity, and outcome. Evidence supporting a genetic predisposition to SLE is strong but complex.[24,25] The overall prevalence of SLE is estimated at 1 in 2000. Increased prevalence in certain populations and within families supports a genetic component. African Americans, Asians, and Hispanics have an increased incidence, estimated at 1 in 1000 African American women versus 1 in 4000 Caucasian American women. Ninety percent of cases occur in women, mainly of childbearing age, suggesting a hormonal influence in addition to conventional genetic factors.[26-28] Phenotype is strongly affected by race. African Americans and Hispanics experience more active, aggressive disease that occurs at a younger age.[29] Genetic admixture underscores the observation that Hispanic SLE patients of

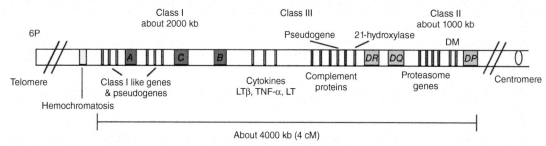

FIGURE 13-2. Major histocompatibility locus. Chromosomal region 6p21.3 contains the highly polymorphic class I human leukocyte antigen (HLA) genes (*B, C,* and *A*), class II HLA genes (*DR, DQ,* and *DP*), genes in the class II region that code for components of the proteasome, and class III HLA genes (cytokines and complement proteins).

Mexican and Central American ancestry have more severe disease than mainland Puerto Rican patients, although mainland Puerto Ricans have more cutaneous manifestations.[3] Better definition of studied populations is crucial; for example, studies in Hispanic American patients have shown that American Indian ancestry within this group predisposes to an increased overall incidence of SLE.[20] Familial aggregation and a high MZ-to-DZ twin concordance ratio support a genetic component. This ratio has been estimated at 10, with an MZ twin concordance rate between 24% and 58% and a DZ twin concordance rate between 2% and 5%, similar to that of nontwin siblings.[30,31] The MZ twin discordance can be at least partially explained by epigenetics. For example, Javierre et al[32] identified a consistent and distinct pattern of immune-related genes that were less methylated in the lupus-affected twin; a similar pattern was not found in studies of rheumatoid arthritis and dermatomyositis. The risk for a sibling is 20- to 40-fold higher than the risk for an unrelated person in the general population.[33]

Candidate gene association and genome-wide linkage studies have been used to detect multiple susceptibility genes and loci for SLE. GWAS[25,30,34-41] and targeted genome scans[42-48] using cohorts of SLE multiplex families (two or more affected individuals) of different races have detected numerous chromosomal regions that show evidence of linkage to SLE. Compilations of specific genes and chromosomal regions[49-51] require frequent updating; the reader is referred to regularly updated resources including Online Mendelian Inheritance in Man (OMIM; http://omim.org/) and the website of the National Human Genome Research Institute (http://www.genome.gov/). Perhaps the most prominent loci associated with SLE are the HLA, complement, and Fc-γ low-affinity receptor gene families. MHC genes *HLA-DRB1, HLA-DQA1, HLA-DQA2, HLA-DQB2,* and *HLA-DR3* located at 6p21.32-33, human low-affinity receptors *FcGR2A* and *FcGR3A* at 1q23, and deficiency of complement components C4 and C2 at 6p21, C1q at 1p36, and C1r/s at 12p13 are associated with increased risk of disease.[25,31,44,50-58] Individuals with a hereditary deficiency of C1q develop SLE at a young age with severe photosensitivity rash without respect to sex or race. A strong risk of developing rheumatic disease occurs in greater than 90% of cases with deficient C1q, 75% with deficient C4, and 10% with deficient C2. A hereditary deficiency of complement component C4A conferred a risk for SLE development in almost all racial groups evaluated. Variation in gene copy number has been recognized as a heritable source of susceptibility to complex genetic diseases. Low *FcGR3B* copy number has been associated with increased risk for autoimmune glomerulonephritis in a subset of SLE patients.[59] Reduced copy number of C4 is a risk factor for, and increased copy number is protective against, SLE in European Americans.[60] A risk haplotype upstream of the tumor necrosis factor (TNF) superfamily gene *TNFSF4* at chromosome 1q25, which increases expression of the gene, has been associated with increased risk for SLE.[61]

Numerous other genes and chromosomal loci have been significantly associated with lupus, although their individual contributions are quite modest. These may be usefully grouped into functional classes. In addition to the HLA, complement, and Fc-γ low-affinity receptor families discussed earlier, these groupings include T-cell signaling (eg, *PTPN22*

1p13; *STAT4* 2q32.3; *TNFSF4* 1q25.1), B-cell signaling (eg, *IL-10* 1q31-32; *BANK1* 4q24; *BLK* 8p23.1; *RASGRP3* 2p22.3), toll-like receptor (TLR)/interferon (IFN) signaling (eg, *IRF5* 7q32.1; *IRF7* 11p15.5; *IRF8* 16q24.1; *TYK2* 19p13.2; *STAT4* 2q32.3), inflammasome activation of interleukin (IL)-1β (*NLRP1* 17p3), cell cycle/apoptosis/cell metabolism (eg, *TNFAIP3* 6q23.3; *RASGRP3* 2p22.3; *UBE2LR* 22q), and transcriptional regulation (eg, *JAZF1* 7p15.2-p15.1; *UHRF1BP1* 6p21.31). The specific groupings and their contents vary among authors, and some genes remain in a miscellaneous grouping or are ascribed multiple roles.[49-51,62]

Some gene associations have been identified mainly in specific groups. An association with the programmed cell death-1 (*PD-1*) allele (2q37 linkage) is seen in people of European descent but not in African American families. A *PD-1* association in Spanish cases of lupus was found.[63-65] A study of SLE patients stratified for discoid lupus manifestations revealed linkage at 11p13 in African American families.[66] SLE susceptibility linkage at 12q24 was observed mainly in Hispanic and European families.[40] *ETS1* (11q24.3) and *WDFY4* (10q11.23) were reported as novel risk factors in Chinese.[67] An important SLE susceptibility gene, *SLEH1* at 11q14, was found in African Americans when pedigrees were stratified by the presence of antinucleolar autoantibodies[68] or hemolytic anemia.[69] When pedigrees were stratified for renal disease, three SLE susceptibility loci were identified: *SLEN1* at 10q22.3 in Caucasians and *SLEN2* at 2q34-35 and *SLEN3* at 11p15.5 in African Americans.[70,71] As reviewed by Lee and Bae,[72] there are groups of reliably associated loci with similar and distinct allelic frequencies across racial groups, loci that demonstrate allelic heterogeneity, and loci that appear to consistently show racial predilections. Recently, Molineros et al[10] showed *IFIH1* to be an important lupus susceptibility gene associated with apoptosis, inflammation, and autoantibody production. It was first identified in an African American population and appears to have been evolutionarily driven to a significantly increased level in European Americans. Large studies involving different racial groups and correcting for admixture are needed to better define useful susceptibility loci.

Overlap of SLE susceptibility loci with other autoimmune diseases is evident.[24,25] Candidate genes for multiple autoimmune diseases have been observed at chromosomal regions 1p13 (*P2PN22*), 2q37 (*PDCD1*), 2q32.2-q32.3 (*STAT4*), 2q33 (*CTLA4*), and 16q12 (*NOD2/CARD150*).[49] For example, cytotoxic T lymphocyte antigen-4 (*CTLA-4*) polymorphisms at chromosomal region 2q33 have been implicated in several types of autoimmunity, suggesting a role for *CTLA-4* as a general susceptibility gene for autoimmune diseases, including SLE.[73-75] Chromosomal regions 10q22.3, 2q34-q35, and 11p15.5 are seen in SLE with an increased risk for lupus nephritis,[70] 17p13 in SLE associated with vitiligo,[76] 11q14 in SLE associated with hemolytic anemia,[69] and 1q41 with thyroid-lupus autoantigen.[77]

Viewing susceptibility loci in functional terms suggests therapeutic approaches targeting gene networks rather than multiple discrete genes. Evidence that the type 1 IFN pathway plays a causal role in SLE has been provided by finding that several different functional variants of the gene for IFN regulatory factor 5 confer susceptibility for or protection against

SLE.[53] Recently, biologics have emerged to target B-lymphocyte stimulation (belimumab) and IFN-α(rontalizumab, sifalimumab) and IFN-α/β subtypes (Medi546).[78] Agents targeting B cells, T-cells, cytokines, and other immunomodulators are being examined; for a recent review, see Paz and Tsokos.[79] Ultimately, a personalized genomic approach may direct highly specific therapies for lupus.

VITILIGO

Vitiligo is a disorder of pigmentation characterized by the destruction of melanocytes due to a complex pathogenesis of genetic susceptibility, autoimmune destruction, biochemical defects, and environmental factors. Phenotypic variance is evident in the different clinical expressions of vitiligo, such as focal, vulgaris (generalized), universal, segmental, acrofacial, and mucosal. Vitiligo affects 0.1% to 2.0% of various populations.[80,81] In a survey of 2624 vitiligo probands (83% Caucasian) from North America and the United Kingdom, the frequency in males and females was equal. The prevalence of vitiligo was reported to be 0.19% in the Chinese Han people, the ethnic group representing greater than 90% of the Chinese population.[82] Evaluation of 2247 probands in this population revealed that age of onset with the highest prevalence was 10 to 14 years, as compared to a later age of onset of 20 to 24 years in U.S. females.[83] Distribution between Chinese males and females was equal. First-degree relatives had a 3- to 13-fold higher relative risk of developing vitiligo; the risk was two to four times higher for second-degree relatives.[82] A prevalence of 0.34% was seen in the French West Indies (Isle of Martinique), where 96% of the population is of African European descent (black Caribbean). The prevalence among relatives was 7%, and age of onset was much later (31 years).[84] A study of 357 Nigerian vitiligo patients showed a male-to-female ratio of 1:1.3, onset in the second and third decades of life, and a family history in 18% of probands.[85] The prevalence of vitiligo in the United States has been estimated at 1%. Studies in other countries have reported prevalences of 0.38% in Denmark, 1.13% in Surat, India, and 0.45% in Calcutta, India.[86]

Progress in defining a genetic component has depended on clearly defining the disorder. Consequently, most studies have focused on generalized vitiligo. Strong evidence for genetic factors in the pathogenesis of generalized vitiligo comes from studies of patients' close relatives.[87] Among Caucasians, the frequency in probands' siblings was 6.1%, approximately 18 times the population frequency, and 20% of probands had at least one affected first-degree relative, highly suggestive of a genetic component. There is a similar risk of generalized vitiligo in other first-degree relatives: 7.1% in Caucasians, 6.1% in Indo-Pakistanis, and 4.8% in Hispanics. A lower risk is seen in more distant relatives. Also, among Caucasians the mean age of onset is 21.5 years in patients from families in which multiple family members are affected,[83] but is 24.2 years in unselected (mainly sporadic) cases. Earlier disease onset in familial cases and a lower risk of disease with increased genetic distance from an affected family member are commonly observed features of polygenic disorders.[88] Although there is strong evidence for genetic factors in the pathogenesis of vitiligo, the concordance in MZ twins was only 23%, suggesting additional nongenetic triggers.[88] A role for an epigenetic contribution to vitiligo pathogenesis is supported by findings of increased DNA methylation in peripheral blood mononuclear cells of vitiligo patients associated with decreased IL-10 expression and a dominant CD8+ T-lymphocyte profile leading to melanocyte destruction.[89]

The association of vitiligo with other autoimmune diseases is well documented. In 23% of generalized vitiligo cases, there was an increase in frequency of six autoimmune disorders in probands and their first-degree relatives: vitiligo, autoimmune thyroid disease, pernicious anemia, Addison disease, SLE, and inflammatory bowel disease.[88] Additionally, associations with diabetes mellitus and alopecia areata have been documented.[90] Gene linkage and gene association studies have found susceptibility loci for vitiligo at chromosomal regions 1p31 (*AIS1*, autoimmune susceptibility 1), 1p13 (*PTPN22*), 6p21.3 (*HLA-DRB-1, HLA-DRB-4, HLA-DQB-1*), chromosome 7 (*AIS2*), chromosome 8 (*AIS3*), and 17p13 (*SLEV1* [*NALP1*]).[87,91-95] *NALP1*, now renamed *NLRP1* (nuclear localization leucine-rich-repeat protein), encodes a key regulator of the immune system that, as part of the *NLRP1* inflammasome, activates IL-1β and possibly other inflammatory pathways.[96,97] Linkage to *AIS1*, *AIS2*, and *NALP1* may predispose to vitiligo associated with susceptibility to autoimmune diseases, whereas linkage at *AIS3* is not noted for that association.[95] Although many of these linkage results have been confirmed in Caucasian populations, different linkage results have been obtained in Han Chinese families, suggesting that different genes may be involved in vitiligo pathogenesis in different populations.[87]

Over the past several years, GWAS have identified SNPs associated with vitiligo.[98-102] GWAS in Caucasians with generalized vitiligo detected SNPs in numerous MHC loci (6p21.3) and non-MHC loci, including *PTPN22* (1p13.2), *TYR* (11q14-q21), *FOXP1* (forkhead box T1; 3p13), *LPP* (3q28), *TSLP* (thymic stromal lymphopoietin; 5q22.1), *IL2RA* (IL-2 receptor α chain) (10p15.1), *XBP1* (22q12), and *CCR6*, among others. *CCR6* is close to the 6q27 association signal originally identified in an isolated Romanian village[103] and was the only shared non-MHC association seen in a Chinese GWAS.[101] Recently, in another GWAS in the Han Chinese, three novel susceptibility loci for vitiligo at 12q13.2, 11q23.3, and 10q22.1 were identified, and three loci previously associated with vitiligo in Caucasian populations at 3q28, 10p15.1, and 22q12.3 were confirmed in the Han Chinese, supporting shared as well as different disease susceptibilities in Chinese and Caucasian populations.

Melanocyte-specific factors also play a role in vitiligo genetics. Association with the *TYR* gene[98] directly relates to the expression of tyrosinase, the rate-limiting enzyme in the production of melanin, which is mutated in oculocutaneous albinism 1 (*OCA1*). Tyrosinase is thought to be an autoantigen presented on the surface of melanocytes for immune targeting.[104] Vitiligo-associated SNPs have also been identified within the *OCA2* region.[100] *OCA2* encodes a melanosomal membrane transporter and is mutated in oculocutaneous albinism type 2. Although no association between these genes and vitiligo has been seen in studies of the Chinese, the most significant association seen in a recent study is at 12q13.2, upstream of the promoter region of *PMEL*, a major melanocyte antigen that shows dramatically decreased expression in lesional skin.[102] Association with vitiligo of *TYR* and *OCA2* variants in Caucasians and with *PMEL* in Chinese supports a connection between these antigens and how the immune system sees and attacks melanocytes.

Although GWAS have increased our knowledge of genes involved with vitiligo and other complex diseases, they are limited by a variety of factors, including availability of relevant SNPs, phenotypic and genotypic heterogeneity, gene interactions, and the size of the study. Therefore, it is not surprising that important genes may not be identified in a particular GWAS. For example, *NLRP1* at 17p3 has repeatedly been associated with the risk of several autoimmune diseases, including vitiligo, SLE,[62] and SSc.[105] Analyses of hundreds of SNPs under the 17p3 peak, as well as sequencing around and within the *NLRP1* gene, have identified risk variants that associate with vitiligo and other autoimmune diseases.[106,107] Next-generation sequencing has also revealed that two high-risk haplotypes in the *NLRP1* gene increase IL-1β activation in normal individuals.[97] Thus GWAS are not currently capable of identifying all genes of interest. As exome and whole-genome sequencing becomes less expensive and more widely available, we may expect a dramatic increase in the identification of variant genes and gene networks that contribute to the pathogenesis of complex diseases such as vitiligo and other autoimmune diseases.

SYSTEMIC SCLEROSIS

SSc is a chronic systemic fibrotic disease. Although the defining characteristics of SSc are thickening of the skin and peripheral vascular abnormalities, the clinical phenotype varies from limited cutaneous involvement and Raynaud phenomenon to diffuse and life-threatening fibrosis of skin and visceral organs and very severe vascular abnormalities.

It is likely that genetic risk factors as well as environmental triggers lead to the onset of SSc. Three types of evidence support a genetic component in the pathogenesis of SSc. The first is variation in disease prevalence and incidence among ethnic and racial groups. Prevalence and severity are significantly higher in African Americans than in Caucasians[108] and lowest in Japanese.[109] An Oklahoma Choctaw Indian population has the highest reported prevalence, due, it is believed, to a founder effect.[110] The ancestry of the SSc patients in this population was traced to five founding families in the eighteenth century.[111,112] Second, SSc occurs significantly more frequently in families, with a positive family history being the strongest risk factor for the disease.[113] A recent large family study of Utah residents showed a significant increase of Raynaud phenomenon and other autoimmune disorders in first- and second-degree relatives.[114] Third, candidate polymorphisms and rare mutations have been identified that show a positive association with the disease, including genes for the class II HLA (6p21), TNF-α (12p13), IL-4 receptor a (16p12.1-p11.2), IL-8 receptor 2 (2q35), topoisomerase 1 (20q12), transforming growth factor β (TGF-β; 19q13.1), and connective tissue growth factor (CTGF; 6q23-27).[115-118] Several susceptibility loci, including fibrillin (15q21) and *SPARC* (secreted protein, acidic and rich in cysteine; 5q31-33), were observed in the Oklahoma Choctaw Indian population referred to earlier.[115] In addition, studies have shown that epigenetics plays a role in SSc (eg, demethylation of CD40L leading to overexpression in SSc).[11] The combination of genetic association and gene linkage studies for regions of SSc susceptibility indicates that the disorder is multifactorial, with a number of contributing genetic loci, and is consistent with the view that some autoimmune rheumatic disorders share genetic associations. Recent GWAS showed strong risk factors in STAT4 and IRF5,[114] as well as PTPN22, BANK1, BLK, CD247, and TNFSF4.[119] Although there have been no reported differences in disease concordance between MZ and DZ twins, concordance for antinuclear and anticytoplasmic antibodies was significantly higher in MZ than in DZ twins (90% vs 40%).[120-122]

In addition to differences in disease prevalence in different racial and ethnic groups, certain clinical phenotypes may be unequally distributed. African Americans and Hispanics have a higher frequency of diffuse disease than European Americans.[123,124] There appears to be a higher prevalence of SSc renal crisis among African Americans, characterized by abrupt onset of severe uncontrolled hypertension and rapidly progressive oliguric renal failure with high renin levels.[125] A significantly lower proportion of Caucasians has diffuse skin involvement, digital pits and ulcers, and hypopigmentation/hyperpigmentation. A higher proportion has facial telangiectasias. Hypothyroidism is diagnosed more frequently in whites than in nonwhite Hispanics and appears to be absent in African Americans.[123]

At least some of these clinical differences may be attributed to differences in the type of autoantibodies produced.[126] Patients with SSc express a number of autoantibodies to nuclear antigens, each with its own clinical associations. These include anti-centromere antibodies (ACA), anti-topoisomerase 1 (ATA; Scl-70), anti-RNA polymerase I and III (anti-RNAPI and anti-RNAPIII), and anti-nucleolar antibodies (AnoA). Each SSc patient typically produces only one of these antibody types.[115,116,127] There is strong evidence from twin studies and from associations with MHC genes that the types of autoantibodies produced in SSc are influenced by hereditary factors and vary in different racial groups.[126] ACAs occur most frequently in Caucasians, with significantly lower frequency in Hispanic, African American, and Thai patients. They are strongly associated with limited cutaneous SSc, with a higher risk for calcinosis and ischemic digital loss and with a lower frequency of interstitial pulmonary fibrosis. Patients who are ACA positive have a lower mortality than those who are positive for ATA or AnoA. ATAs that are unique to SSc occur at higher frequency in Mexican American, African American, Native American, Thai, and Japanese patients.[128] Chinese patients also seem to have higher frequencies of ATA and anti-U1-ribonucleoprotein (U1RNP), which corresponds to higher risk of diffuse forms of SSc. Conversely, Chinese patients were lower in ACA and anti-RNAPIII.[129] ATAs are associated with fibrosing alveolitis

but not with scleroderma renal crisis. African American and Japanese patients with SSc had a significantly lower survival rate than Caucasians with ATAs. This may be explained by a higher frequency of progressive pulmonary interstitial fibrosis in these two groups.[130] In Chinese patients, pulmonary fibrosis was also strongly associated with ATA.[129] A particular class of AnoA, anti-fibrillarin/anti-U3-RNP (AFA), is found with higher frequency in SSc patients of African descent than in Caucasians, and is associated with diffuse skin involvement, gastrointestinal dysmotility, myositis, pulmonary hypertension, cardiac involvement, and renal disease.[117,123,126,131,132] African American patients with AFA also had younger age of onset and more severe vascular disease and digital ulcers.[133] However, AFA-positive patients appear to have less severe lung involvement.[133] Overproduction of the nucleolar protein fibrillarin has been reported in fibroblasts from scleroderma patients,[127] and decreased fibrillarin level has been shown to result in decreased collagen secretion.[134] Thus overproduction of fibrillarin may play a role in the very severe fibrosis seen in some scleroderma patients. Associations have been shown between particular class II MHC alleles and the type of autoantibodies made.[115] These findings, along with the results of twin studies, support a genetic influence on which class of autoantibodies will be produced. Because the autoantibody class produced appears to correlate with some of the phenotypic variability, further characterization of the genetic basis and functional significance of differences in autoantibody production and the distribution of relevant alleles in different individuals and populations may help to identify, prevent, and treat different forms of scleroderma.

SARCOIDOSIS

Sarcoidosis is an autoimmune systemic granulomatous disease associated with an accumulation of CD4+ T-cells.[135] Although its etiology has not been determined, hypothetical causative agents include infectious organisms and noninfectious environmental agents, including metals and organic and inorganic dusts, and autoantigens.[22,136,137] Pulmonary involvement occurs in most cases, but any organ system may be involved, most commonly skin, eye, heart, liver, and nervous system. In addition to heterogeneous manifestations, the disease lacks a precise definition, and clinical overlap with other diseases and insensitive and nonspecific diagnostic tests lead to misclassification. The frequency of sarcoidosis varies in different parts of the world, likely due to differences in environmental exposure, surveillance methods, and predisposing HLA alleles and other genetic factors. In northern European countries, the frequency has been estimated at 5 to 40 cases per 100,000 people. In Japan, the annual incidence ranges from 1 to 2 cases per 100,000, and in the United States, the prevalence in African Americans is approximately three times higher than in European Americans (35.5 cases per 100,000 vs 10.9 cases per 100,000).[138]

A genetic component in the pathogenesis of sarcoidosis is supported by the following: (1) variation in disease prevalence and incidence among racial groups; (2) the fact that relatives of individuals with sarcoidosis are more likely to have the disease[115,139]; and (3) gene linkage and gene association studies.[115,140] Further support for a genetic contribution to sarcoidosis comes from twin studies in which concordance in MZ twins was 14.8% compared with 1.2% concordance in DZ twins.[141] As seen for other autoimmune diseases, the low concordance in MZ twins and association with a variety of environmental triggers (see above) support a strong environmental component.

Candidate genes for sarcoidosis include loci that influence immune regulation, T-cell function, antigen presentation or recognition and polymorphisms in class I and class II HLA loci, and genes for immunoregulatory cytokines, growth factors, and angiotensin-converting enzyme.[115,142] Of particular note are polymorphisms in HLA class II genes located in the MHC and mutations in the butyrophilin-like gene (BTNL2) at human chromosome region 6p21-22 in Caucasians, African Americans, and Japanese.[22,138,140,142-144] Significant differences have been observed in the distribution of HLA class II alleles between African Americans and Caucasians. The HLA *DRB1*1501* allele increases risk in Caucasians but is protective in African Americans.[145] Other allelic forms are associated with different clinical phenotypes, including eye and bone marrow involvement in African Americans and hypercalcemia in whites.[145] Specific polymorphisms in HLA class II genes may interact with environmental exposures in determining susceptibility to sarcoidosis.[146]

Prior to 2006, two genome scans for linkage were reported, one in German families[147] and the other in African Americans.[148] Several linkage peaks were seen in the German study, with the highest signal at 6p21 and other peaks of interest at chromosome locations 1p22, 3p21, 7q36, and 9q33 and on the long arm of the X chromosome. In the African American study, linkage was detected at 2p25, 5q11, 5q35, 9q34, 11p15, 20q13, and 3p14-11. Although not all of these linkage peaks have been confirmed, in an admixture study using families from a population of African American families with sarcoidosis, it was found that the families fell into two groups, the first contributing to observed linkage peaks at 1p22, 3p21-14, 11p15, and 17q21 and the second group contributing to peaks at 5p13-15 and 20q13, whereas both sets of families contributed to peaks at 2p25, 5q11, 5q35, and 9q34-11.[21] Another admixture study of unrelated African American cases and controls identified several ancestry associations for sarcoidosis, some with increased African ancestry and some with increased European ancestry.[9] Of special interest were associations with particular clinical phenotypes such as pulmonary fibrosis, which is more prevalent in individuals of African ancestry.[114,149,150]

Recently, several GWAS done in European and African origin populations have further identified shared and race-specific alleles.[22,151-157] In several Caucasian GWAS, SNPs associated with sarcoidosis were located at 6p21.32-33, a region that contains MHC and *BTLN2* genes; 6p12.1 containing *RAB23* and several other genes; 10p12.2; and new risk loci in the German population at 11q13.1 and 12q13-3-q14. Of particular note is a susceptibility locus, *ANXA11* (10q22.3-q23.1) that was initially observed in several European GWAS.[154,156,158] *ANXA11* is a member of the annexin family, a group of calcium-dependent phospholipid proteins that play a role in cell division, endo- and exocytosis, and apoptosis.[159,160] *ANXA11* has been reported to give rise to autoantibodies in several autoimmune disorders including antiphospholipid syndrome, SLE, rheumatoid arthritis, and SSc.[161] A recent GWAS study[157] comparing *ANXA11* variation in African Americans and European Americans found a major susceptibility locus of *ANXA11* (rs1049550) in both populations. However, additional SNPs seen only in the African American population were more significant in patients classified as having radiographically persistent fibrotic lung disease. These investigators also identified an additional independent locus at the minor A allele of SNP rs1860052 and found that it was associated with a protective effect on sarcoidosis in African Americans. This protective SNP is described in the 1000 Genomes Project as having an allele frequency of only 2% in African Americans and 11% in European Americans. Most recently, in a GWAS of African and European origin Americans, Adrianto et al[22] reported shared associations including several class II HLA genes (*DRA*, *DRB5*, and *DRB1*), *BTNL2* (different SNPs in the African and Caucasian populations), and *ANXA11*. They also identified a significant association between sarcoidosis and a previously unreported locus, *Notch4*, in African Americans. *Notch4* is a member of the notch family of receptor proteins that regulate many aspects of embryonic development, T-cell–mediated immune responses, and cell proliferation and apoptosis.[114] *Notch4* is highly expressed in lung and has been reported to contribute to the pathogenesis of asthma, lung arteriovenous shunts, neonatal lupus, multiple sclerosis and SSc, and other immune-related disorders.[22] Other recent studies in different populations have identified an *SLC11A1* gene polymorphism (2q35) associated with sarcoidosis in a Turkish population[162] and genetic variation in a TLR gene cluster (4p14) *TLR10-TLR1-TLR6* that influences disease course in a population in the Netherlands.[163] Although studies have pointed to plausible gene candidates, further work is needed to validate associations with specific genes and to elucidate their role in the pathogenesis of sarcoidosis and how these findings may aid in the diagnosis, treatment, and prognosis of this multisystem, granulomatous disease.

KELOIDS

Keloids are benign collagenous tumors of the dermis that form during a prolonged wound-healing process.[164,165] A prolonged period of fibroblast proliferation and an elevated rate of collagen synthesis relative to normal wound healing characterize keloid formation. The genetic predisposition to form keloids is found predominantly in people of African and Asian descent. The key alteration(s) responsible for the pathologic processes resulting in keloid formation has not been identified, and there is no curative treatment for this disorder. Keloid formation is one of a group of fibroproliferative diseases characterized by an exaggerated response to injury that occur at higher frequency or with more severe manifestations in people of African ancestry. These diseases include hypertension,[166] nephrosclerosis,[167] SSc,[108] sarcoidosis,[135] asthma,[168] and uterine fibroma.[169] It has been suggested[166,167,170-172] that common genetic factors may contribute to their unusual racial distribution.

A strong genetic component for keloid formation is supported by the occurrence of keloids at different frequencies in different racial populations. Keloids have been estimated to occur in approximately 1 in 30 African Americans and approximately 1 in 625 of the overall U.S. population.[173] In a study of 14 pedigrees with familial keloids, the inheritance pattern was consistent with an autosomal dominant trait with incomplete penetrance and variable expression.[174] Earlier reports provided evidence for both autosomal dominant[175] and autosomal recessive inheritance.[176]

Several studies have sought to identify the genetic basis of keloids. In one African American family, linkage was detected between keloid formation and chromosome region 14q22-q23.[177] In two other families, linkage to 2q23 (Japanese) and 7p11 (African American) was shown.[164] In a recent GWAS in a Japanese population, four SNP loci in three chromosomal regions (1q41, 3q22.3-q23, and 15q21.3) showed significant association with keloid formation.[178] The limited data from these studies suggest genetic complexity, involving contributions of multiple susceptibility loci. Microarray studies indicating altered expression of multiple genes at or close to these regions in keloid fibroblasts suggest candidate genes for further study.[170] Additional GWAS and AM approaches will be necessary to more fully define genetic variation responsible for keloid formation and the genetic mechanisms that account for its increased prevalence in individuals of African and Asian ancestry. Although some cases of keloid formation may be due to somatic mutation,[179] multiple keloids in the same individual and evidence for a multicellular origin of keloids[180-182] argue against somatic mutation as the primary event and suggest that an environmental factor present during wound healing triggers abnormal gene expression in genetically susceptible individuals. Evidence for an epigenetically altered program in fibroblasts cultured from keloids includes persistence of altered gene expression over the culture lifetime, an altered pattern of DNA methylation, and histone acetylation. Additionally, reversal of some of the phenotypic characteristics of keloids by trichostatin A, an inhibitor of histone deacetylation, has been observed.[183,184]

CONCLUSION

SLE, vitiligo, SSc, sarcoidosis, and keloids, commonly observed diseases in patients with skin of color, are genetically complex, with multiple genetic loci and environmental triggers conferring risk for the disease and its severity.

Autoimmune diseases including SLE, SSc, sarcoidosis, and vitiligo share some susceptibility loci at human chromosomal region 6p21, which contains genes of the MHC as well as many non-HLA loci involved in lymphocyte activation (B and T-cells), cytokine pathways, and host–microbe interactions. Overall, identifying genetic susceptibility and genes for specific disorders in skin of color populations is an ongoing, complicated, and dynamic process. Updates may be obtained from the National Human Genome Research Institute website (http://www.genome.gov/) for the most current compilations of genes.

REFERENCES

1. Smith MW, Patterson N, Lautenberger JA, et al. A high-density admixture map for disease gene discovery in african americans. *Am J Hum Genet.* 2004;74:1001-1013.

2. Parra EJ, Marcini A, Akey J, et al. Estimating African American admixture proportions by use of population-specific alleles. *Am J Hum Genet.* 1998;63:1839-1851.

3. Vila LM, Alarcon GS, McGwin G Jr, et al. Early clinical manifestations, disease activity and damage of systemic lupus erythematosus among two distinct US Hispanic subpopulations. *Rheumatology (Oxford).* 2004;43:358-363.

4. Galanter JM, Fernandez-Lopez JC, Gignoux CR, et al. Development of a panel of genome-wide ancestry informative markers to study admixture throughout the Americas. *PLoS Genet.* 2012;8:e1002554.

5. Qu HQ, Li Q, Xu S, et al. Ancestry informative marker set for Han Chinese population. *G3 (Bethesda).* 2012;2:339-341.

6. Winkler CA, Nelson GW, Smith MW. Admixture mapping comes of age. *Annu Rev Genomics Hum Genet.* 2010;11:65-89.

7. Flores C, Ma SF, Pino-Yanes M, et al. African ancestry is associated with asthma risk in African Americans. *PLoS ONE.* 2012;7:e26807.

8. Cheng CY, Reich D, Haiman CA, et al. African ancestry and its correlation to type 2 diabetes in African Americans: a genetic admixture analysis in three U.S. population cohorts. *PLoS ONE.* 2012;7:e32840.

9. Rybicki BA, Levin AM, McKeigue P, et al. A genome-wide admixture scan for ancestry-linked genes predisposing to sarcoidosis in African-Americans. *Genes Immun.* 2011;12:67-77.

10. Molineros JE, Maiti AK, Sun C, et al. Admixture mapping in lupus identifies multiple functional variants within IFIH1 associated with apoptosis, inflammation, and autoantibody production. *PLoS Genet.* 2013;9:e1003222.

11. Lu Q. The critical importance of epigenetics in autoimmunity. *J Autoimmun.* 2013;41:1-5.

12. Hughes T, Sawalha AH. The role of epigenetic variation in the pathogenesis of systemic lupus erythematosus. *Arthritis Res Ther.* 2011;13:245.

13. National Human Genome Research Institute. GWAS catalog. http://www.genome.gov/gwastudies/. Accessed January 15, 2015.

14. Altshuler DM, Gibbs RA, Peltonen L, et al. Integrating common and rare genetic variation in diverse human populations. *Nature.* 2010;467:52-58.

15. Nussbaum RL, McInnes RR, Willard HF. *Thompson & Thompson Genetics in Medicine.* 7th ed. Philadelphia, PA: Saunders Elsevier; 2007.

16. Becker KG. The common genetic hypothesis of autoimmune/inflammatory disease. *Curr Opin Allergy Clin Immunol.* 2001;1:399-405.

17. Zenewicz LA, Abraham C, Flavell RA, Cho JH. Unraveling the genetics of autoimmunity. *Cell.* 2010;140:791-797.

18. Shamim EA, Miller FW. Familial autoimmunity and the idiopathic inflammatory myopathies. *Curr Rheumatol Rep.* 2000;2:201-211.

19. Aune TM, Parker JS, Maas K, Liu Z, Olsen NJ, Moore JH. Co-localization of differentially expressed genes and shared susceptibility loci in human autoimmunity. *Genet Epidemiol.* 2004;27:162-172.

20. Molineros JE, Kim-Howard X, Deshmukh H, Jacob CO, Harley JB, Nath SK. Admixture in Hispanic Americans: its impact on ITGAM association and implications for admixture mapping in SLE. *Genes Immun.* 2009;10:539-545.

21. Thompson CL, Rybicki BA, Iannuzzi MC, Elston RC, Iyengar SK, Gray-McGuire C. Reduction of sample heterogeneity through use of population substructure: an example from a population of African American families with sarcoidosis. *Am J Hum Genet.* 2006;79:606-613.

22. Adrianto I, Lin CP, Hale JJ, et al. Genome-wide association study of African and European Americans implicates multiple shared and ethnic specific loci in sarcoidosis susceptibility. *PLoS ONE.* 2012;7:e43907.

23. Gaffney PM, Langefeld CD, Graham RR, et al. Fine-mapping chromosome 20 in 230 systemic lupus erythematosus sib pair and multiplex families: evidence for genetic epistasis with chromosome 16q12. *Am J Hum Genet.* 2006;78:747-758.

24. Rhodes B, Vyse TJ. General aspects of the genetics of SLE. *Autoimmunity.* 2007;40:550-559.

25. Wong M, Tsao BP. Current topics in human SLE genetics. *Springer Semin Immunopathol.* 2006;28:97-107.

26. Hochberg MC. The epidemiology of sysemic lupus erythematosus. In: Wallace DJ, Hahn BH, Quismorio FP, eds. *Dubois' Lupus Erythematosus.* Baltimore, MD: Williams & Wilkins; 1997:49-65.

27. Rus VHA. Systemic lupus erythematosus. In: Silman AJHM, ed. *Epidemiology of Rheumatic Diseases.* Oxford, United Kingdom: Oxford University Press; 2001:123-140.

28. Smith-Bouvier DL, Divekar AA, Sasidhar M, et al. A role for sex chromosome complement in the female bias in autoimmune disease. *J Exp Med.* 2008;205:1099-1108.

29. Uribe AG, McGwin G Jr, Reveille JD, Alarcon GS. What have we learned from a 10-year experience with the LUMINA (Lupus in Minorities; Nature vs. nurture) cohort? Where are we heading? *Autoimmun Rev.* 2004;3:321-329.

30. Cantor RM, Yuan J, Napier S, et al. Systemic lupus erythematosus genome scan: support for linkage at 1q23, 2q33, 16q12-13, and 17q21-23 and novel evidence at 3p24, 10q23-24, 13q32, and 18q22-23. *Arthritis Rheum.* 2004;50:3203-3210.

31. Shen N, Tsao BP. Current advances in the human lupus genetics. *Curr Rheumatol Rep.* 2004;6:391-398.

32. Javierre BM, Hernando H, Ballestar E. Environmental triggers and epigenetic deregulation in autoimmune disease. *Discov Med.* 2011;12:535-545.

33. Wandstrat A, Wakeland E. The genetics of complex autoimmune diseases: non-MHC susceptibility genes. *Nat Immunol.* 2001;2:802-809.

34. Gaffney PM, Kearns GM, Shark KB, et al. A genome-wide search for susceptibility genes in human systemic lupus erythematosus sib-pair families. *Proc Natl Acad Sci U S A.* 1998;95:14875-14879.

35. Moser KL, Neas BR, Salmon JE, et al. Genome scan of human systemic lupus erythematosus: evidence for linkage on chromosome 1q in African-American pedigrees. *Proc Natl Acad Sci U S A.* 1998;95:14869-14874.

36. Gaffney PM, Ortmann WA, Selby SA, et al. Genome screening in human systemic lupus erythematosus: results from a second Minnesota cohort and combined analyses of 187 sib-pair families. *Am J Hum Genet.* 2000;66:547-556.

37. Gray-McGuire C, Moser KL, Gaffney PM, et al. Genome scan of human systemic lupus erythematosus by regression modeling: evidence of linkage and epistasis at 4p16-15.2. *Am J Hum Genet.* 2000;67:1460-1469.

38. Lindqvist AK, Steinsson K, Johanneson B, et al. A susceptibility locus for human systemic lupus erythematosus (hSLE1) on chromosome 2q. *J Autoimmun.* 2000;14:169-178.

39. Shai R, Quismorio FP Jr, Li L, et al. Genome-wide screen for systemic lupus erythematosus susceptibility genes in multiplex families. *Hum Mol Genet.* 1999;8:639-644.

40. Nath SK, Quintero-Del-Rio AI, Kilpatrick J, Feo L, Ballesteros M, Harley JB. Linkage at 12q24 with systemic lupus erythematosus (SLE) is established and confirmed in Hispanic and European American families. *Am J Hum Genet.* 2004;74:73-82.

41. Koskenmies S, Lahermo P, Julkunen H, Ollikainen V, Kere J, Widen E. Linkage mapping of systemic lupus erythematosus (SLE) in Finnish families multiply affected by SLE. *J Med Genet.* 2004;41:e2-e5.

42. Tsao BP, Cantor RM, Grossman JM, et al. PARP alleles within the linked chromosomal region are associated with systemic lupus erythematosus. *J Clin Invest.* 1999;103:1135-1140.

43. Tsao BP, Cantor RM, Kalunian KC, et al. Evidence for linkage of a candidate chromosome 1 region to human systemic lupus erythematosus. *J Clin Invest.* 1997;99:725-731.

44. Moser KL, Gray-McGuire C, Kelly J, et al. Confirmation of genetic linkage between human systemic lupus erythematosus and chromosome 1q41. *Arthritis Rheum.* 1999;42:1902-1907.

45. Criswell LA, Moser KL, Gaffney PM, et al. PARP alleles and SLE: failure to confirm association with disease susceptibility. *J Clin Invest.* 2000;105:1501-1502.

46. Graham RR, Langefeld CD, Gaffney PM, et al. Genetic linkage and transmission disequilibrium of marker haplotypes at chromosome 1q41 in human systemic lupus erythematosus. *Arthritis Res.* 2001;3:299-305.

47. Magnusson V, Lindqvist AK, Castillejo-Lopez C, et al. Fine mapping of the SLEB2 locus involved in susceptibility to systemic lupus erythematosus. *Genomics.* 2000;70:307-314.

48. Johanneson B, Lima G, von Salome J, Alarcon-Segovia D, Alarcon-Riquelme ME. A major susceptibility locus for systemic lupus erythemathosus maps to chromosome 1q31. *Am J Hum Genet.* 2002;71:1060-1071.

49. Tsokos GC. Systemic lupus erythematosus. *N Engl J Med.* 2011;365:2110-2121.

50. Cui Y, Sheng Y, Zhang X. Genetic susceptibility to SLE: recent progress from GWAS. *J Autoimmun.* 2013;41:25-33.

51. Connolly JJ, Hakonarson H. Role of cytokines in systemic lupus erythematosus: recent progress from GWAS and sequencing. *J Biomed Biotechnol.* 2012;2012:798924.

52. Nath SK, Kilpatrick J, Harley JB. Genetics of human systemic lupus erythematosus: the emerging picture. *Curr Opin Immunol.* 2004;16:794-800.

53. Graham RR, Ortmann WA, Langefeld CD, et al. Visualizing human leukocyte antigen class II risk haplotypes in human systemic lupus erythematosus. *Am J Hum Genet.* 2002;71:543-553.

54. Magnusson V, Johanneson B, Lima G, Odeberg J, Alarcon-Segovia D, Alarcon-Riquelme ME. Both risk alleles for FcgammaRIIA and FcgammaRIIIA are susceptibility factors for SLE: a unifying hypothesis. *Genes Immun.* 2004;5:130-137.

55. Ghebrehiwet B, Peerschke EI. Role of C1q and C1q receptors in the pathogenesis of systemic lupus erythematosus. *Curr Dir Autoimmun.* 2004;7:87-97.

56. Manderson AP, Botto M, Walport MJ. The role of complement in the development of systemic lupus erythematosus. *Annu Rev Immunol.* 2004;22:431-456.

57. Slingsby JH, Norsworthy P, Pearce G, et al. Homozygous hereditary C1q deficiency and systemic lupus erythematosus. A new family and the molecular basis of C1q deficiency in three families. *Arthritis Rheum.* 1996;39:663-670.

58. Haywood ME, Hogarth MB, Slingsby JH, et al. Identification of intervals on chromosomes 1, 3, and 13 linked to the development of lupus in BXSB mice. *Arthritis Rheum.* 2000;43:349-355.

59. Fanciulli M, Norsworthy PJ, Petretto E, et al. FCGR3B copy number variation is associated with susceptibility to systemic, but not organ-specific, autoimmunity. *Nat Genet.* 2007;39:721-723.

60. Yang Y, Chung EK, Wu YL, et al. Gene copy-number variation and associated polymorphisms of complement component C4 in human systemic lupus erythematosus (SLE): low copy number is a risk factor for and high copy number is a protective factor against SLE susceptibility in European Americans. *Am J Hum Genet.* 2007;80:1037-1054.

61. Graham DS, Graham RR, Manku H, et al. Polymorphism at the TNF superfamily gene TNFSF4 confers susceptibility to systemic lupus erythematosus. *Nat Genet.* 2008;40:83-89.

62. Pontillo A, Girardelli M, Kamada AJ, et al. Polimorphisms in inflammasome genes are involved in the predisposition to systemic lupus erythematosus. *Autoimmunity.* 2012;45:271-278.

63. Prokunina L, Castillejo-Lopez C, Oberg F, et al. A regulatory polymorphism in PDCD1 is associated with susceptibility to systemic lupus erythematosus in humans. *Nat Genet.* 2002;32:666-669.

64. Ferreiros-Vidal I, Gomez-Reino JJ, Barros F, et al. Association of PDCD1 with susceptibility to systemic lupus erythematosus: evidence of population-specific effects. *Arthritis Rheum.* 2004;50:2590-2597.

65. Prokunina L, Padyukov L, Bennet A, et al. Association of the PD-1.3A allele of the PDCD1 gene in patients with rheumatoid arthritis negative for rheumatoid factor and the shared epitope. *Arthritis Rheum.* 2004;50:1770-1773.

66. Nath SK, Namjou B, Kilpatrick J, et al. A candidate region on 11p13 for systemic lupus erythematosus: a linkage identified in African-American families. *J Investig Dermatol Symp Proc.* 2004;9:64-67.

67. Yuan YJ, Luo XB, Shen N. Current advances in lupus genetic and genomic studies in Asia. *Lupus.* 2010;19:1374-1383.

68. Sawalha AH, Namjou B, Nath SK, et al. Genetic linkage of systemic lupus erythematosus with chromosome 11q14 (SLEH1) in African-American families stratified by a nucleolar antinuclear antibody pattern. *Genes Immun.* 2002;3(Suppl 1):S31-S34.

69. Kelly JA, Thompson K, Kilpatrick J, et al. Evidence for a susceptibility gene (SLEH1) on chromosome 11q14 for systemic lupus erythematosus (SLE) families with hemolytic anemia. *Proc Natl Acad Sci U S A.* 2002;99:11766-11771.

70. Quintero-Del-Rio AI, Kelly JA, Kilpatrick J, James JA, Harley JB. The genetics of systemic lupus erythematosus stratified by renal disease: linkage at 10q22.3 (SLEN1), 2q34-35 (SLEN2), and 11p15.6 (SLEN3). *Genes Immun.* 2002;3(Suppl 1):S57-S62.

71. Quintero-del-Rio AI, Kelly JA, Garriott CP, et al. SLEN2 (2q34-35) and SLEN1 (10q22.3) replication in systemic lupus erythematosus stratified by nephritis. *Am J Hum Genet.* 2004;75:346-348.

72. Lee HS, Bae SC. What can we learn from genetic studies of systemic lupus erythematosus? Implications of genetic heterogeneity among populations in SLE. *Lupus.* 2010;19:1452-1459.

73. Hudson LL, Rocca K, Song YW, Pandey JP. CTLA-4 gene polymorphisms in systemic lupus erythematosus: a highly significant association with a determinant in the promoter region. *Hum Genet.* 2002;111:452-455.

74. Fernandez-Blanco L, Perez-Pampin E, Gomez-Reino JJ, Gonzalez A. A CTLA-4 polymorphism associated with susceptibility to systemic lupus erythematosus. *Arthritis Rheum.* 2004;50:328-329.

75. Liu MF, Wang CR, Lin LC, Wu CR. CTLA-4 gene polymorphism in promoter and exon-1 regions in Chinese patients with systemic lupus erythematosus. *Lupus.* 2001;10:647-649.

76. Nath SK, Kelly JA, Namjou B, et al. Evidence for a susceptibility gene, SLEV1, on chromosome 17p13 in families with vitiligo-related systemic lupus erythematosus. *Am J Hum Genet.* 2001;69:1401-1406.

77. McKusick V. Online Mendelian Inheritance in Man. http://omim.org/. Accessed January 15, 2015.

78. Bronson PG, Chaivorapol C, Ortmann W, Behrens TW, Graham RR. The genetics of type I interferon in systemic lupus erythematosus. *Curr Opin Immunol.* 2012;24:530-537.

79. Paz Z, Tsokos GC. New therapeutics in systemic lupus erythematosus. *Curr Opin Rheumatol.* 2013;25:297-303.

80. Hann S, Nordlund JJ. *Vitiligo.* Oxford, United Kingdom: Blackwell Science; 2000.

81. Bolognia J, Nordlund, JJ, Ortonne, J-P. Vitiligo vulgaris. In: Nordlund J, Boissy RE, Hearing VJ, King RA, Ortonne J-P, eds. *The Pigmentary System.* New York, NY: Oxford University Press; 1998.

82. Zhang XJ, Liu JB, Gui JP, et al. Characteristics of genetic epidemiology and genetic models for vitiligo. *J Am Acad Dermatol.* 2004;51:383-390.

83. Laberge G, Mailloux CM, Gowan K, et al. Early disease onset and increased risk of other autoimmune diseases in familial generalized vitiligo. *Pigment Cell Res.* 2005;18:300-305.

84. Boisseau-Garsaud AM, Garsaud P, Cales-Quist D, Helenon R, Queneherve C, Claire RC. Epidemiology of vitiligo in the French West Indies (Isle of Martinique). *Int J Dermatol.* 2000;39:18-20.

85. Onunu AN, Kubeyinje EP. Vitiligo in the Nigerian African: a study of 351 patients in Benin City, Nigeria. *Int J Dermatol.* 2003;42:800-802.

86. Kovacs SO. Vitiligo. *J Am Acad Dermatol.* 1998;38:647-666; quiz 667-648.

87. Spritz RA. The genetics of generalized vitiligo and associated autoimmune diseases. *Pigment Cell Res.* 2007;20:271-278.

88. Alkhateeb A, Fain PR, Thody A, Bennett DC, Spritz RA. Epidemiology of vitiligo and associated autoimmune diseases in Caucasian probands and their families. *Pigment Cell Res.* 2003;16:208-214.

89. Zhao M, Gao F, Wu X, Tang J, Lu Q. Abnormal DNA methylation in peripheral blood mononuclear cells from patients with vitiligo. *Br J Dermatol.* 2010;163:736-742.

90. Grimes PE, Halder RM, Jones C, et al. Autoantibodies and their clinical significance in a black vitiligo population. *Arch Dermatol.* 1983;119:300-303.

91. Fain PR, Gowan K, LaBerge GS, et al. A genomewide screen for generalized vitiligo: confirmation of AIS1 on chromosome 1p31 and evidence for additional susceptibility loci. *Am J Hum Genet.* 2003;72:1560-1564.

92. Dunston GM, Halder RM. Vitiligo is associated with HLA-DR4 in black patients. A preliminary report. *Arch Dermatol.* 1990;126:56-60.

93. Arcos-Burgos M, Parodi E, Salgar M, et al. Vitiligo: complex segregation and linkage disequilibrium analyses with respect to microsatellite loci spanning the HLA. *Hum Genet.* 2002;110:334-342.

94. Orozco-Topete R, Cordova-Lopez J, Yamamoto-Furusho JK, Garcia-Benitez V, Lopez-Martinez A, Granados J. HLA-DRB1*04 is associated with the genetic susceptibility to develop vitiligo in Mexican patients with autoimmune thyroid disease. *J Am Acad Dermatol.* 2005;52:182-183.

95. Spritz RA, Gowan K, Bennett DC, Fain PR. Novel vitiligo susceptibility loci on chromosomes 7 (AIS2) and 8 (AIS3), confirmation of SLEV1 on chromosome 17, and their roles in an autoimmune diathesis. *Am J Hum Genet.* 2004;74:188-191.

96. Bruey JM, Bruey-Sedano N, Luciano F, et al. Bcl-2 and Bcl-XL regulate proinflammatory caspase-1 activation by interaction with NALP1. *Cell.* 2007;129:45-56.

97. Levandowski CB, Mailloux CM, Ferrara TM, et al. NLRP1 haplotypes associated with vitiligo and autoimmunity increase interleukin-1beta processing via the NLRP1 inflammasome. *Proc Natl Acad Sci U S A.* 2013;110:2952-2956.

98. Jin Y, Birlea SA, Fain PR, et al. Variant of TYR and autoimmunity susceptibility loci in generalized vitiligo. *N Engl J Med.* 2010;362:1686-1697.

99. Birlea SA, Jin Y, Bennett DC, et al. Comprehensive association analysis of candidate genes for generalized vitiligo supports XBP1, FOXP3, and TSLP. *J Invest Dermatol.* 2011;131:371-381.

100. Jin Y, Birlea SA, Fain PR, et al. Genome-wide association analyses identify 13 new susceptibility loci for generalized vitiligo. *Nat Genet.* 2012;44:676-680.

101. Quan C, Ren YQ, Xiang LH, et al. Genome-wide association study for vitiligo identifies susceptibility loci at 6q27 and the MHC. *Nat Genet.* 2010;42:614-618.

102. Tang XF, Zhang Z, Hu DY, et al. Association analyses identify three susceptibility loci for vitiligo in the Chinese Han population. *J Invest Dermatol.* 2013;133:403-410.

103. Birlea SA, Gowan K, Fain PR, Spritz RA. Genome-wide association study of generalized vitiligo in an isolated European founder population identifies SMOC2, in close proximity to IDDM8. *J Invest Dermatol.* 2010;130: 798-803.

104. Spritz RA. Six decades of vitiligo genetics: genome-wide studies provide insights into autoimmune pathogenesis. *J Invest Dermatol.* 2012;132: 268-273.

105. Dieude P, Guedj M, Wipff J, et al. NLRP1 influences the systemic sclerosis phenotype: a new clue for the contribution of innate immunity in systemic sclerosis-related fibrosing alveolitis pathogenesis. *Ann Rheum Dis.* 2011;70:668-674.

106. Jin Y, Mailloux CM, Gowan K, et al. NALP1 in vitiligo-associated multiple autoimmune disease. *N Engl J Med.* 2007;356:1216-1225.

107. Jin Y, Birlea SA, Fain PR, Spritz RA. Genetic variations in NALP1 are associated with generalized vitiligo in a Romanian population. *J Invest Dermatol.* 2007;127:2558-2562.

108. Mayes MD, Lacey JV Jr, Beebe-Dimmer J, et al. Prevalence, incidence, survival, and disease characteristics of systemic sclerosis in a large US population. *Arthritis Rheum.* 2003;48:2246-2255.

109. Tamaki T, Mori S, Takehara K. Epidemiological study of patients with systemic sclerosis in Tokyo. *Arch Dermatol Res.* 1991;283:366-371.

110. Zhou X, Tan FK, Wang N, et al. Genome-wide association study for regions of systemic sclerosis susceptibility in a Choctaw Indian population with high disease prevalence. *Arthritis Rheum.* 2003;48:2585-2592.

111. Vaughn SE, Kottyan LC, Munroe ME, Harley JB. Genetic susceptibility to lupus: the biological basis of genetic risk found in B cell signaling pathways. *J Leukoc Biol.* 2012;92:577-591.

112. Tan FK, Stivers DN, Foster MW, et al. Association of microsatellite markers near the fibrillin 1 gene on human chromosome 15q with scleroderma in a Native American population. *Arthritis Rheum.* 1998;41:1729-1737.

113. Arnett FC, Cho M, Chatterjee S, Aguilar MB, Reveille JD, Mayes MD. Familial occurrence frequencies and relative risks for systemic sclerosis (scleroderma) in three United States cohorts. *Arthritis Rheum.* 2001;44: 1359-1362.

114. Broen JC, Coenen MJ, Radstake TR. Genetics of systemic sclerosis: an update. *Curr Rheumatol Rep.* 2012;14:11-21.

115. du Bois RM. The genetic predisposition to interstitial lung disease. Proceedings and Abstracts of the 44th Annual Thomas Petty Aspen Lung Conference: Pulmonary Genetics, Genomics, Gene Therapy. *Chest.* 2002;121:1S-110S.

116. Sato H, Lagan AL, Alexopoulou C, et al. The TNF-863A allele strongly associates with anticentromere antibody positivity in scleroderma. *Arthritis Rheum.* 2004;50:558-564.

117. Johnson RW, Tew MB, Arnett FC. The genetics of systemic sclerosis. *Curr Rheumatol Rep.* 2002;4:99-107.

118. Fonseca C, Lindahl GE, Ponticos M, et al. A polymorphism in the CTGF promoter region associated with systemic sclerosis. *N Engl J Med.* 2007;357:1210-1220.

119. Romano E, Manetti M, Guiducci S, Ceccarelli C, Allanore Y, Matucci-Cerinic M. The genetics of systemic sclerosis: an update. *Clin Exp Rheumatol.* 2011;29(2 Suppl 65):S75-S86.

120. Feghali-Bostwick CA. Genetics and proteomics in scleroderma. *Curr Rheumatol Rep.* 2005;7:129-134.

121. Assassi S, Arnett FC, Reveille JD, Gourh P, Mayes MD. Clinical, immunologic, and genetic features of familial systemic sclerosis. *Arthritis Rheum.* 2007;56:2031-2037.

122. Mayes MD, Trojanowska M. Genetic factors in systemic sclerosis. *Arthritis Res Ther.* 2007;9(Suppl 2):S5.

123. Reveille JD, Fischbach M, McNearney T, et al. Systemic sclerosis in 3 US ethnic groups: a comparison of clinical, sociodemographic, serologic, and immunogenetic determinants. *Semin Arthritis Rheum.* 2001;30: 332-346.

124. Mayes MD. Scleroderma epidemiology. *Rheum Dis Clin North Am.* 2003;29:239-254.

125. Prisant LM, Loebl DH, Mulloy LL. Scleroderma renal crisis. *J Clin Hypertens (Greenwich).* 2003;5:168-170, 176.

126. Cepeda EJ, Reveille JD. Autoantibodies in systemic sclerosis and fibrosing syndromes: clinical indications and relevance. *Curr Opin Rheumatol.* 2004;16:723-732.

127. Zhou X, Tan FK, Xiong M, et al. Systemic sclerosis (scleroderma): specific autoantigen genes are selectively overexpressed in scleroderma fibroblasts. *J Immunol.* 2001;167:7126-7133.

128. Arnett FC. HLA and autoimmunity in scleroderma (systemic sclerosis). *Int Rev Immunol.* 1995;12:107-128.

129. Wang J, Assassi S, Guo G, et al. Clinical and serological features of systemic sclerosis in a Chinese cohort. *Clin Rheumatol.* 2013;32:617-621.

130. Kuwana M, Kaburaki J, Arnett FC, Howard RF, Medsger TA Jr, Wright TM. Influence of ethnic background on clinical and serologic features in patients with systemic sclerosis and anti-DNA topoisomerase I antibody. *Arthritis Rheum.* 1999;42:465-474.

131. Tormey VJ, Bunn CC, Denton CP, Black CM. Anti-fibrillarin antibodies in systemic sclerosis. *Rheumatology (Oxford).* Oct 2001;40:1157-1162.

132. Arnett FC, Reveille JD, Goldstein R, et al. Autoantibodies to fibrillarin in systemic sclerosis (scleroderma). An immunogenetic, serologic, and clinical analysis. *Arthritis Rheum.* 1996;39:1151-1160.

133. Sharif R, Fritzler MJ, Mayes MD, et al. Anti-fibrillarin antibody in African American patients with systemic sclerosis: immunogenetics, clinical features, and survival analysis. *J Rheumatol.* 2011;38:1622-1630.

134. Lefevre F, Garnotel R, Georges N, Gillery P. Modulation of collagen metabolism by the nucleolar protein fibrillarin. *Exp Cell Res.* 2001;271:84-93.

135. Rybicki BA, Maliarik MJ, Major M, Popovich J Jr, Iannuzzi MC. Epidemiology, demographics, and genetics of sarcoidosis. *Semin Respir Infect.* 1998;13:166-173.

136. Moller DR, Chen ES. What causes sarcoidosis? *Curr Opin Pulm Med.* 2002;8:429-434.

137. Oswald-Richter KA, Drake WP. The etiologic role of infectious antigens in sarcoidosis pathogenesis. *Semin Respir Crit Care Med.* 2010;31:375-379.

138. Iannuzzi MC, Rybicki BA, Teirstein AS. Sarcoidosis. *N Engl J Med.* 2007;357:2153-2165.

139. Rybicki BA, Iannuzzi MC, Frederick MM, et al. Familial aggregation of sarcoidosis. A case-control etiologic study of sarcoidosis (ACCESS). *Am J Respir Crit Care Med.* 2001;164:2085-2091.

140. Iannuzzi MC, Rybicki BA. Genetics of sarcoidosis: candidate genes and genome scans. *Proc Am Thorac Soc.* 2007;4:108-116.

141. Sverrild A, Backer V, Kyvik KO, et al. Heredity in sarcoidosis: a registry-based twin study. *Thorax.* 2008;63:894-896.

142. Rybicki BA, Walewski JL, Maliarik MJ, Kian H, Iannuzzi MC. The BTNL2 gene and sarcoidosis susceptibility in African Americans and whites. *Am J Hum Genet.* 2005;77:491-499.

143. Suzuki H, Ota M, Meguro A, et al. Genetic characterization and susceptibility for sarcoidosis in Japanese patients: risk factors of BTNL2 gene polymorphisms and HLA class II alleles. *Invest Ophthalmol Vis Sci.* 2012;53:7109-7115.

144. Valentonyte R, Hampe J, Huse K, et al. Sarcoidosis is associated with a truncating splice site mutation in BTNL2. *Nat Genet.* 2005;37:357-364.

145. Rossman MD, Thompson B, Frederick M, et al. HLA-DRB1*1101: a significant risk factor for sarcoidosis in blacks and whites. *Am J Hum Genet.* 2003;73:720-735.

146. Iannuzzi MC, Maliarik MJ, Poisson LM, Rybicki BA. Sarcoidosis susceptibility and resistance HLA-DQB1 alleles in African Americans. *Am J Respir Crit Care Med.* 2003;167:1225-1231.

147. Schurmann M, Reichel P, Muller-Myhsok B, Schlaak M, Muller-Quernheim J, Schwinger E. Results from a genome-wide search for predisposing genes in sarcoidosis. *Am J Respir Crit Care Med.* 2001;164:840-846.

148. Iannuzzi MC, Iyengar SK, Gray-McGuire C, et al. Genome-wide search for sarcoidosis susceptibility genes in African Americans. *Genes Immun.* 2005;6:509-518.

149. Judson MA, Baughman RP, Thompson BW, et al. Two year prognosis of sarcoidosis: the ACCESS experience. *Sarcoidosis Vasc Diffuse Lung Dis.* 2003;20:204-211.

150. Swigris JJ, Olson AL, Huie TJ, et al. Sarcoidosis-related mortality in the United States from 1988 to 2007. *Am J Respir Crit Care Med.* 2011;183:1524-1530.

151. Fischer A, Nothnagel M, Schurmann M, Muller-Quernheim J, Schreiber S, Hofmann S. A genome-wide linkage analysis in 181 German sarcoidosis families using clustered biallelic markers. *Chest.* 2010;138:151-157.

152. Fischer A, Schmid B, Ellinghaus D, et al. A novel sarcoidosis risk locus for Europeans on chromosome 11q13.1. *Am J Respir Crit Care Med.* 2012;186:877-885.

153. Franke A, Fischer A, Nothnagel M, et al. Genome-wide association analysis in sarcoidosis and Crohn's disease unravels a common susceptibility locus on 10p12.2. *Gastroenterology.* 2008;135:1207-1215.

154. Hofmann S, Fischer A, Nothnagel M, et al. Genome-wide association analysis reveals 12q13.3-q14.1 as new risk locus for sarcoidosis. *Eur Respir J.* 2013;41:888-900.

155. Hofmann S, Fischer A, Till A, et al. A genome-wide association study reveals evidence of association with sarcoidosis at 6p12.1. *Eur Respir J.* 2011;38:1127-1135.

156. Hofmann S, Franke A, Fischer A, et al. Genome-wide association study identifies ANXA11 as a new susceptibility locus for sarcoidosis. *Nat Genet.* 2008;40:1103-1106.

157. Levin AM, Iannuzzi MC, Montgomery CG, et al. Association of ANXA11 genetic variation with sarcoidosis in African Americans and European Americans. *Genes Immun.* 2013;14:13-18.

158. Li Y, Pabst S, Kubisch C, Grohe C, Wollnik B. First independent replication study confirms the strong genetic association of ANXA11 with sarcoidosis. *Thorax.* 2010;65:939-940.

159. Fatimathas L, Moss SE. Annexins as disease modifiers. *Histol Histopathol.* 2010;25:527-532.

160. Xavier RJ, Rioux JD. Genome-wide association studies: a new window into immune-mediated diseases. *Nat Rev Immunol.* 2008;8:631-643.

161. Jorgensen CS, Levantino G, Houen G, et al. Determination of autoantibodies to annexin XI in systemic autoimmune diseases. *Lupus.* 2000;9:515-520.

162. Akcakaya P, Azeroglu B, Even I, et al. The functional SLC11A1 gene polymorphisms are associated with sarcoidosis in Turkish population. *Mol Biol Rep.* 2012;39:5009-5016.

163. Veltkamp M, van Moorsel CH, Rijkers GT, Ruven HJ, Grutters JC. Genetic variation in the Toll-like receptor gene cluster (TLR10-TLR1-TLR6) influences disease course in sarcoidosis. *Tissue Antigens.* 2012;79:25-32.

164. Marneros AG, Norris JE, Watanabe S, Reichenberger E, Olsen BR. Genome scans provide evidence for keloid susceptibility Loci on chromosomes 2q23 and 7p11. *J Invest Dermatol.* 2004;122:1126-1132.

165. Niessen FB, Spauwen PH, Schalkwijk J, Kon M. On the nature of hypertrophic scars and keloids: a review. *Plast Reconstr Surg.* 1999;104:1435-1458.

166. Dustan HP. Does keloid pathogenesis hold the key to understanding black/white differences in hypertension severity? *Hypertension.* 1995;26:858-862.

167. August P, Suthanthiran M. Transforming growth factor beta and progression of renal disease. *Kidney Int Suppl.* 2003;87:S99-S104.

168. Nickel R, Beck LA, Stellato C, Schleimer RP. Chemokines and allergic disease. *J Allergy Clin Immunol.* 1999;104:723-742.

169. Flake GP, Andersen J, Dixon D. Etiology and pathogenesis of uterine leiomyomas: a review. *Environ Health Perspect.* 2003;111:1037-1054.

170. Smith JC, Boone BE, Opalenik SR, Williams SM, Russell SB. Gene Profiling of keloid fibroblasts shows altered expression in multiple fibrosis-associated pathways. *J Invest Dermatol.* 2008;128:1298-1310.

171. Russell SB, Trupin JS, Myers JC, et al. Differential glucocorticoid regulation of collagen mRNAs in human dermal fibroblasts. Keloid-derived and fetal fibroblasts are refractory to down-regulation. *J Biol Chem.* 1989;264:13730-13735.

172. Catherino WH, Leppert PC, Stenmark MH, et al. Reduced dermatopontin expression is a molecular link between uterine leiomyomas and keloids. *Genes Chromosomes Cancer.* 2004;40:204-217.

173. Barrett J. Keloid. In: Bergsma D, ed. *Birth Defect Compendium.* Baltimore, MD: Williams & Wilkins; 1973:553.

174. Marneros AG, Norris JE, Olsen BR, Reichenberger E. Clinical genetics of familial keloids. *Arch Dermatol.* 2001;137:1429-1434.

175. Bloom D. Heredity of keloids. *N Y State Med J.* 1956;56:511-519.

176. Omo-Dare P. Genetic studies on keloid. *J Natl Med Assoc.* 1975;67:428-432.

177. Davis KD, Garcia M, Phillips JA III, et al. Detection of a critical interval for a familial keloid locus on chromosome 14q22-q23 in an African-American pedigree. *Am J Hum Genet.* 2000;67:A21.

178. Nakashima M, Chung S, Takahashi A, et al. A genome-wide association study identifies four susceptibility loci for keloid in the Japanese population. *Nat Genet.* 2010;42:768-771.

179. Saed GM, Ladin D, Olson J, Han X, Hou Z, Fivenson D. Analysis of p53 gene mutations in keloids using polymerase chain reaction-based single-strand conformational polymorphism and DNA sequencing. *Arch Dermatol.* 1998;134:963-967.

180. Chevray PM, Manson PN. Keloid scars are formed by polyclonal fibroblasts. *Ann Plast Surg.* 2004;52:605-608.

181. Moulton-Levy P, Jackson CE, Levy HG, Fialkow PJ. Multiple cell origin of traumatically induced keloids. *J Am Acad Dermatol.* 1984;10:986-988.

182. Trupin JS, Williams JM, Hammons J, Russell JD. Multicellular origin of keloids. *Fifth International Conference on Birth Defects.* 1977;121.

183. Russell SB, Russell JD, Trupin KM, et al. Epigenetically altered wound healing in keloid fibroblasts. *J Invest Dermatol.* 2010;130:2489-2496.

184. Diao JS, Xia WS, Yi CG, et al. Trichostatin A inhibits collagen synthesis and induces apoptosis in keloid fibroblasts. *Arch Dermatol Res.* 2011;303:573-580.

Biology of Hair

Sotonye Imadojemu
John Seykora

KEY POINTS

- Embryologic development of hair follicles is the same for all races, with the important exception of the distribution of melanin along the hair follicle of individuals of African descent.
- The shapes of hair follicles and the hair shaft differ based on race.
- The amino acid structure of hair is consistent across all racial groups.
- Textured hair of individuals of African descent is more susceptible to breakage (lower tensile strength) than Asian or Caucasian hair.
- As measured by the number of hair follicles in a 4-mm punch biopsy specimen, Asian and textured African hair is less dense than Caucasian hair.
- Textured African hair swells less than either Asian or Caucasian hair when in contact with water and has a decreased moisture content.

INTRODUCTION

Hair serves many useful biologic functions such as protection against physical and chemical damage; insulation against heat loss, desiccation, and overheating; and dispersion of eccrine and apocrine gland secretions. It also has a particular psychosocial importance in our society, especially with regard to sex, class, and racial distinctions. Diseases and disturbances in hair (eg, excessive hair growth or loss or deformity) cause significant morbidity in affected individuals.

ANATOMY OF THE HAIR FOLLICLE [FIGURE 14-1]

The hair follicle and shaft reveal a complex architecture that is made of many distinct structures. There are three main types of hair follicles: lanugo, vellus, and terminal. These follicles each demonstrate similar microanatomic features. The dermal papilla, a mesenchymal derivative, interacts with the hair matrix, which is of ectodermal origin.[1-3] The interaction between the dermal papillae and the hair matrix controls hair growth and differentiation. The bulb is the lowermost portion of the hair follicle and contains the proliferating matrix cells; these cells produce the hair shaft and all epithelial compartments of the hair follicle and shaft except the outer root sheath.[3]

The hair shaft consists of three cell lineages: the cuticle, cortex, and medulla. These three layers contribute to the appearance of the shaft by regulating its structure. In addition, the structure of hair influences attributes such as light absorption, reflection, and refraction.[2] The cuticle, composed of flattened cells, forms the hair surface. It protects the shaft from weathering. Cuticular damage causes the hair shaft to fracture, split, and break. The cortex is the multicelluar compartment and the site of keratinization. It is composed of hair-specific intermediate filaments and associated proteins and is essential for shaft rigidity.[1] The medulla is centrally located within the cortex of terminal hair; it is often absent in vellus hair.[3]

The hair shaft is encompassed by the inner root sheath and the outer root sheath. The inner root sheath is composed of three distinct layers: the inner root sheath cuticle, the Huxley layer, and the Henle layer.[3] As the matrix cells differentiate and migrate upward and outward, they are compressed into their final configuration by the rigid inner root sheath. It was thought that the configuration of the inner root sheath determined hair shape, but recent evidence suggests hair shape is programmed from the anagen hair bulb, particularly the degree of axial asymmetry in the

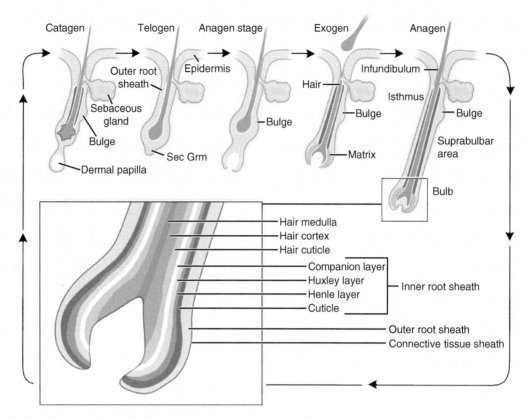

FIGURE 14-1. Hair follicle cycling and hair anatomy. Sec Grm, secondary germ. (Reproduced with permission from Goldsmith LA, et al. Fitzpatrick's Dermatology in General Medicine. 8th ed. New York, NY: McGraw-Hill; 2012.)

hair matrix.[4] The outer root sheath surrounds the inner root sheath and provides an important barrier function delineating the hair follicle from the dermis. The bulge portion of the outer root sheath, located at the insertion of the arrector pili muscle, contains epithelial and melanocytic stem cells responsible for regenerating follicles in the anagen stage of the hair cycle.[1,5] Additionally, cell populations within the outer root sheath have the ability to differentiate into sebaceous glands and epidermis and migrate out of the follicle and regenerate the epidermis after injury.[1,3] Melanocytes, Langerhans cells, and Merkel cells are also found in the outer root sheath and play their part in certain functions of the hair follicle. The pigment of the hair shaft is produced by melanocytes mixed in among the matrix cells.[1]

STRUCTURAL PROTEINS IN THE HAIR FOLLICLE

Keratins are the major structural component of the hair follicle and shaft. They are divided into type I (acidic) and type II (neutral to basic) keratins. Together, the two types of keratin form keratin intermediate filaments through heterodimerization.[3] Keratins are subclassified into epithelial, or soft, keratins and hair, or hard, keratins. Hair keratins are only expressed in highly keratinized tissues, such as the hair shaft and nails. The epithelial keratins are widely expressed in the epithelia of various tissues.[3] Hair keratins have a higher sulfur content in the N- and C-terminal regions compared with epithelial keratins. This plays an important role in the high degree of cross-linking with hair keratin–associated proteins.[3]

The hair shaft is a highly keratinized structure formed within the hair follicle. When trichocytes, the specific epithelial cells in the hair shaft, pass through the keratinizing zone, keratinization occurs and the rigid hair shaft is generated. Hair keratins are the major structural component of the hair shaft. Seventeen functional hair keratin genes have been identified. These genes are abundantly expressed in the hair shaft.[3] WNT/β-catenin signaling has been shown to regulate the expression of hair keratin genes, along with Msx2, Foxn1, and Hoxc13.[3] Epithelial

keratins are expressed in the outer root sheath, companion layer, inner root sheath, and hair shaft medulla.[3]

Desmosomes are another important structure in the hair follicle. Desmosomes are critical to cell–cell adhesion in epithelial structures. Desmosomes anchor the keratin intermediate filaments to the cell membrane and connect cells to one another, thereby maintaining tissue integrity by incorporating with the keratin intermediate filament cytoskeleton.[3] The desmosome cadherin family, which is composed of desmogleins and desmocollins, is the major structural component of the desmosome.[3] Desmoglein 4 is expressed in the hair shaft, including the keratinizing zone. The expression of desmoglein 4 is regulated by transcription factors like LEF1, Hoxc13, and Foxn1, which also control the expression of hair keratins in differentiating trichocytes.

MORPHOGENESIS OF THE HAIR FOLLICLE

Roughly 5 million hair follicles cover the human body at birth, and no additional follicles are formed after birth.[1] The precise spacing, distribution, and future phenotype of hair follicles are established by genes that are expressed very early in follicle morphogenesis.[1] During embryogenesis, the formation of hair follicles is determined by the reciprocal interaction of the epithelium and underlying mesenchymal dermal cells.[1,3]

It is thought that the first signal to initiate formation of the hair follicle originates in the dermis. Activation of the WNT signaling pathway is believed to be essential for initiating this dermal signal.[1,6] The overlying epithelial cells receive this signal, leading to a cascade of activation of ectodysplasin A and ectodysplasin A receptor (EDA/EDAR) signaling in the epithelium, subsequent epithelial WNT signaling, and activation of bone morphogenetic protein (BMP) signaling.[2,6] This then leads to the formation of a placode, which is a thickening of columnar cells.[3] An epithelial WNT signal from the placode causes clustering of underlying mesenchymal cells, forming a dermal condensate.[6] The epidermal placode eventually envelopes the dermal condensate, which then becomes the hair follicle dermal papilla after receiving a second dermal signal regulated by WNT, platelet-derived growth factor A, and sonic hedge-hog.[1,6] The epithelial cells then proliferate and differentiate into the distinct layers of the hair follicle and shaft.[3] Morphogens such as sonic hedgehog and WNT, together with intracellular signaling molecules such as β-catenin and lymphoid-enhancer factor 1, influence the maturation of new hair follicles.[1]

HAIR FOLLICLE CYCLE

Hair follicles perpetually cycle through three stages: anagen (growth), catagen (involution), and telogen (rest). The length of the hair cycle is proportional to the length of hair. For example, the anagen phase in human hair follicles of the scalp ranges from 2 to 8 years, which can produce a relatively long hair shaft, whereas the hair of the eyebrow has a cycle length of 2 to 3 months, which results in short hairs.[1] During the hair cycle, the lower two-thirds of the hair follicle undergoes dynamic changes in structure and is thus called the cycling portion.[3] The upper one-third, or permanent portion, of the hair follicle does not change its structure during the hair cycle. Insulin-like growth factor 1 and fibroblast growth factor (FGF) 7 have important roles in hair follicle cycling. They are produced by the hair follicle dermal papilla and have receptors on the overlying matrix cells.[1]

The anagen (growth) stage recapitulates hair follicle development in that the formation of the new lower follicle begins with migration and proliferation of stem cells and their progeny from the bulge, mediated by interactions between the dermal papilla and the overlying follicular epithelium.[1] The follicle grows downward as the cells migrate to form the matrix at the base of the hair follicle. The matrix cells rapidly proliferate and differentiate into the distinct cell layers of the follicle and shaft.[3] Anagen appears to be regulated by FGF5, which has been shown to be expressed just before the end of anagen.[1] In fact, mouse mutants that lack FGF5 have an extended anagen phase with hair that is 50% longer than normal, called the *angora phenotype*, which is responsible for the long-hair phenotype of angora cats.[1] However, one could posit that FGF5 is not the only mediator of the cessation of anagen phase because the hair follicles in these mice do eventually transition from the anagen to catagen phase. Epidermal growth factor receptors (EGFRs) are also involved in the cessation of anagen as evidenced by the fact that mice with nonfunctional EGFR have a prolonged anagen phase.[1]

The catagen phase sees the hair follicle complete a highly controlled process of involution-mediated apoptosis or programmed cell death of the follicular keratinocyte.[1] Follicular melanogenesis also ceases as follicular melanocytes undergo apoptosis. Near the end of catagen, the dermal papilla condenses and moves upward underneath the hair follicle bulge. Interestingly, if the dermal papilla does not reach the bulge during the catagen stage, the follicle stops cycling and the hair is permanently lost, as seen in mice with mutations in the *hairless* gene.[1]

During the telogen or resting stage, the hair shaft matures into a club hair and is encased by the permanent portion of the hair follicle.[1,3] The hair is eventually shed from the follicle during combing or shampooing. Telogen stage usually lasts for 2 to 3 months before anagen is initiated and the cycle is repeated. About 5% to 15% of scalp hair follicles are in the telogen phase at any point in time. Approximately 50 to 150 scalp hairs are shed each day. This shedding may be an active regulated process or a passive event. The active process of club hair shedding has been suggested as a distinct phase of the hair cycle, called the exogen phase.

MODULATORS OF HAIR CYCLE AND GROWTH

Estrogens, glucocorticoids, retinoids, thyroid hormones, prolactin, and growth hormones modulate hair growth. However, the greatest modulators of hair growth are the androgens. Testosterone and dihydrotestosterone, an active metabolite, act through androgen receptors in the dermal papilla by increasing the size of the hair follicles in the androgen-dependent areas of the beard or, alternatively, miniaturizing the hair follicles as seen in androgenetic alopecia.[1] Estrogens prolong the anagen stage. The sudden withdrawal of estrogen in the postpartum period can result in telogen effluvium.

Exogenous modulators of hair growth include finasteride, dutasteride, and minoxidil. Finasteride blocks type II 5-α-reductase (5AR), which is predominantly located in the genitalia as well as the inner root sheath follicles, thereby inhibiting androgen-mediated follicle miniaturization, prolonging the anagen stage in androgen-dependent scalp follicles, and converting vellus follicles to terminal follicles. Dutasteride is a dual (type I and type II) 5AR and, as such, has the same mechanism as finasteride. However, dutasteride may be more efficacious than finasteride because type I 5AR is located mainly in the skin, including hair follicles and sebaceous glands.[7-9] Minoxidil also prolongs the anagen stage and converts vellus follicles to terminal follicles.[1]

Hair follicles are the most richly innervated component of the skin. The bulge region is especially rich in nerve endings.[1] Merkel cells produce nerve growth factor that may control the proliferation of follicles. The study of hair follicles in the catagen phase reveals several neurotrophins and their receptors that inhibit hair growth.[1]

RACIAL VARIATIONS IN HAIR

The hair of people of Asian descent is typically straight and round in cross-section[10] [**Table 14-1**]. The hair of those of African descent is usually helical, coiled, or spiraled and is flattened in cross-section.[10] The hair of those of European descent is generally straight, wavy, or curly and is ovoid or round in cross-section.[11] The hair fibers of people of African descent show the greatest percentage of section variability, with regular restrictions of the cross-section along the fiber. This is in contrast with Asian and Caucasian hair.[10]

Despite these racial differences in morphology, only one biochemical difference in hair along racial lines has been described. Researchers have analyzed the variance in amino acid composition from members of African, Asian, and Caucasian descent and have found no significant alterations in the hair from different racial groups.[12,13] X-ray analysis of the keratin structure of hair of people of African, Asian, and Caucasian descent did not reveal any difference in the structure of the keratin.[10] It has also been shown that the sulfur-containing proteins thought to be important for stabilizing the keratin structure and tensile strength of hair are the same across different racial groups.[14] Additionally, the distribution of these cystine-rich sulfur-containing proteins is the same across racial groups.[15]

A racial difference in hair lipids has recently been described. Hair lipids account for about 1% of the chemical content of hair and are composed of fatty acids, cholesterol sulfate, ceramides, and cholesterol. Integral hair lipids are located in the cell membrane complex of the hair cuticle. They maintain hair integrity with their qualities of hydrophobicity, moisturization, and stiffness.[16] Asian hair appears to have higher levels of integral hair lipids than hair from African and

TABLE 14-1	Summary of characteristics of hair of various racial groups				
Race	Morphology	Hair lipid content	Tensile strength	Density	Growth rate
European descent	Straight, wavy, or curly; ovoid or round cross-section	Low	High	High	Medium
African descent	Helical, coiled, or spiraled; flattened cross-section	Low, but high squalene content	Low	Low	Low
Asian descent	Straight; round cross-section	High	High	Low	High

Caucasian individuals. Hair from those of African descent has higher levels of squalene but lower lipid content compared with hair from those of Asian and Caucasian descent. Ji et al[16] demonstrated that lipid content is depleted after ultraviolet (UV) A and UVB exposure, but Asian hair samples, with high lipid content, suffered less damage, suggesting that lipid content is protective against damage from UV light.

Although there are few data to support differences in the chemical structure of hair between various racial groups, differences in how hair from people in the three major racial groups behaves under various conditions and stresses have been described. Franbourg et al[10] performed investigations of radial swelling of hair in water and response to mechanic stress. Using a specific Palmer device developed in their laboratory, the investigators measured the initial diameter of a 3-mm-long hair sample from people of African, Asian, and Caucasian descent. They then introduced a drop of distilled water to the hair and observed the evolution of the diameter of the hair fiber as the water was absorbed. They found that African hair appeared to have the lowest radial swelling rate, whereas Asian and Caucasian hair appeared to have similar higher rates of swelling. This difference cannot be explained by any differences in the keratin structure of hair, because no difference in protein structure has been described. The authors suggest that the difference in radial swelling in water may be due to differences in lipids in fiber composition, which has not yet been well studied.

Franbourg et al[10] tested the tensile strength of hair from the three major racial groups. In dry conditions (45% relative humidity), the investigators found that the African hair fibers displayed lower breaking stress and breaking elongation than Asian and Caucasian hair, suggesting that African hair is more fragile than Asian and Caucasian hair. The authors posit that this difference in fragility may be due to the geometric and morphologic differences in hair based on racial origin.[10] Khumalo et al[15] argue that the apparent fragility of African hair is due to significantly increased structural damage such as breaks, partial breaks, knots, and longitudinal splits from external trauma from grooming practices among those of African descent, rather than from inherent weakness of the fibers. It has been shown that African hair was more likely to form longitudinal fissures along the hair shaft and had a higher proportion of knot formation, which was never and rarely observed, respectively, in Caucasian and Asian hair.[17] The investigators posit that the physical effect of washing and combing may increase knotting by stretching out the coils, which then causes them to interlock when they spring back.[17]

Finally, hair density also appears to differ between racial groups. A retrospective analysis of healthy scalp hair density by race revealed that African Americans have a significantly lower mean density of hair follicles compared with other groups (22.4 vs 35.5 per transverse section of a 4-mm punch biopsy, respectively).[18] Using a noninvasive technique called phototrichogram, Loussouarn et al[19] found that Caucasian hair is more dense than Asian hair and African hair (mean ± standard deviation [SD]: 226 ± 73, 175 ± 54, and 161 ± 50 hairs/cm², respectively). These investigators also found differences in the percentage of hair in the telogen phase across different racial groups. Africans tended to have higher telogen counts than Asians and Caucasians (mean ± SD: 14% ± 9%, 12% ± 7%, and 12% ± 8%, respectively).[19] Finally, despite high interindividual variability, African hair grew more slowly than Caucasian hair, which grew more slowly than Asian hair (mean ± SD: 280 ± 50, 367 ± 56, and 411 ± 43 μm/d, respectively).[19]

REFERENCES

1. Paus R, Cotsarelis G. The biology of hair follicles. *N Engl J Med.* 1999;341:491-497.
2. Schlake T. Determination of hair structure and shape. *Semin Cell Dev Biol.* 2007;18:267-273.
3. Shimomura Y, Christiano AM. Biology and genetics of hair. *Annu Rev Genomics Hum Genet.* 2010;11:109-132.
4. Thibaut S, Gaillard O, Bouhanna P, Cannell DW, Bernard BA. Human hair shape is programmed from the bulb. *Br J Dermatol.* 2005;152:632-638.
5. Nishimura EK, Granter SR, Fisher DE. Mechanisms of hair graying: incomplete melanocyte stem cell maintenance in the niche. *Science.* 2005;307:720-724.
6. Millar SE. Molecular mechanisms regulating hair follicle development. *J Invest Dermatol.* 2002;118:216-225.
7. Chen W, Zouboulis CC, Orfanos CE. The 5 alpha-reductase system and its inhibitors: recent development and its perspective in treating androgen-dependent skin disorders. *Dermatology.* 1996;193:177-184.
8. Thiboutot D, Harris G, Iles V, Cimis G, Gilliland K, Hagari S. Activity of the type 1 5 alpha-reductase exhibits regional differences in isolated sebaceous glands and whole skin. *J Invest Dermatol.* 1995;105:209-214.
9. Sato T, Sonoda T, Itami S, Takayasu S. Predominance of type I 5 alpha-reductase in apocrine sweat glands of patients with excessive or abnormal odor derived from apocrine sweat (osmidrosis). *Br J Dermatol.* 1998;139:806-810.
10. Franbourg A, Hallegot P, Baltenneck F, Toutain C, Leroy F. Current research on ethnic hair. *J Am Acad Dermatol.* 2003;48:S115-S119.
11. Lindelof B, Forslind B, Hedblad M. Human hair form: morphology revealed by light and scanning electron microscopy and computer aided three-dimensional reconstruction. *Arch Dermatol.* 1988;124:1359-1363.
12. Gold RJM, Schriver CR. The amino acid composition of hair from different racial origins. *Clin Chima Acta.* 1971;33:465-466.
13. Hrdy D, Baden HP. Biochemical variation of hair keratins in man and non-human primates. *Am J Phys Anthropol.* 1973;39:19-24.
14. Dekio S, Jidoi J. Hair low-sulfur protein composition does not differ electrophoretically among different races. *J Dermatol.* 1988;15:393-396.
15. Khumalo NP, Dawber RPR, Ferguson DJP. Apparent fragility of African hair is unrelated to the cystine-rich protein distribution: a cytochemical electron microscopic study. *Exp Dermatol.* 2005;14:311-314.
16. Ji JH, Park TS, Lee JH, et al. The ethnic differences of the damage of hair and integral hair lipid after ultra violet radiation. *Ann Dermatol.* 2013;25:54-60.
17. Khumalo NP, Dawber RPR, Ferguson DJP. What is normal black African hair? A light and scanning electron-microscope study. *J Am Acad Dermatol.* 2000;43:814-820.
18. Sperling LC. Hair density in African Americans. *Arch Dermatol.* 1999;135:656-658.
19. Loussouarn G, El Rawadi C, Genain G. Diversity of hair growth profiles. 2005;44(Suppl 1):6-9.

Biology of Nails

Richard K. Scher
Gisela Torres Bonilla
Nicole DeYampert

KEY POINTS

- Nail matrix melanocytes in skin of color contain mature melanosomes that produce nail plate pigmentation.
- Melanonychia in multiple nails reduces but does not eliminate the probability of melanoma.
- Although melanoma of the nail unit is uncommon in skin of color, acral locations, including nails, occur disproportionately more frequently.
- Over 90% of melanonychias arise from the distal rather than the proximal nail matrix.
- Melanomas are more frequent in the great toe and thumb than in other digits.
- Most melanomas arising from melanonychia striata are in situ melanomas.

The nail unit is composed of the matrix, plate, bed, proximal and lateral nail folds, and hyponychium [**Figure 15-1**]. The nail develops from an ingrowth of the epidermis into the dermis during gestational week 9, and the nail unit is fully developed at week 15 and then continues to grow throughout life. Because the nail unit lies immediately above the periostium of the distal phalanx, disorders of the nail and bone can affect each other. The shape of the distal phalangeal bone also determines the shape and transverse curvature of the nail. The nail functions

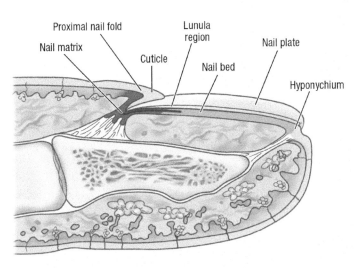

FIGURE 15-1. Basic anatomy of the nail unit.

to protect the distal phalanges and to increase tactile sensation. Toenails protect the distal toenail and aid in pedal biomechanics.

EMBRYOLOGY

The development of the digits, nails, and nail folds occurs early in embryonic development [**Table 15-1**]. Individual digits are developing by the eighth week of gestation.[1] The nail develops during the ninth embryonic week from the same primitive epidermis that gives rise to hair, sweat glands, and the stratum corneum. At week 10, the primary nail field is developed. Proximal and lateral nail folds develop during weeks 13 and 14. The nail plate covers the majority of the nail bed at week 17. From week 20 to birth, the nail unit and digit grow in unison.

NAIL MATRIX

Nail matrix keratinocytes divide in the basal cell layer; they keratinize in the absence of a granular layer. The site of keratinization of nail matrix onychocytes can be clearly distinguished in histologic sections as an eosinophilic area where cells show fragmentation of their nuclei and condensation of their cytoplasm. The maturation and differentiation of nail matrix keratinocytes occur along a diagonal axis that is distally oriented. Thus keratinization of the proximal nail matrix cells produces the dorsal nail plate, and keratinization of the distal nail matrix cells produces the intermediate plate [**Table 15-2**].

In culture, nail matrix keratinocytes are larger and have a greater proliferation rate than epidermal keratinocytes. At the ultrastructural level, nail matrix cells contain a higher euchromatin:heterochromatin ratio and a lower nucleus:cytoplasm ratio than epidermal keratinocytes.[2] Both soft and hard keratins are produced by the nail matrix keratinocytes.[3] Soft keratins are produced by the dorsal matrix in bovine hoofs, whereas the ventral matrix produces mainly hard keratins, with a small population of keratinocytes coexpressing both hard and soft keratins. In humans, the proximal nail matrix is composed of soft keratins K10, K14, K16, K17, K1, K5, and K6. The distal matrix contains soft keratins K10, K14, K20, K1, and K5 and the hard keratin Ha1.[4]

TABLE 15-1   Nail embryology

	Gestational development (week)
Digits	8
Nail	9
Primary nail field	10
Nail folds	13, 14
Nail plate	17

TABLE 15-2   Nail matrix and plate formation

Proximal matrix	Upper nail plate
Intermediate matrix	Intermediate nail plate
Distal matrix	Lower nail plate

When cultured in serum-containing medium, nail matrix cells produced an outgrowth of epithelium and a spontaneous migration phenomenon associated with a tendency to stratify in a semilunar area that resembles the architecture of the nail matrix.[2] The pluristratified epithelium showed characteristic markers of nail differentiation. Cultures of nail matrix cells have been a useful model to study the biology of the nails, including structure, nail disease, and effects of drugs.

MELANOCYTES

It has been demonstrated that melanocytes densely populate the nail matrix [**Figure 15-2 and Table 15-3**]. The number of melanocytes ranges from 208 to 576 cells/mm².[5] Melanocytes are most prominent in the distal matrix. Melanocytes of the proximal matrix have been described as being in a single compartment of largely dormant cells. The distal matrix is composed of a dormant and an active component.[5] The dopa-positive melanocytes in the distal areas are larger and more dendritic than those in proximal areas.[6] Active melanocytes in the distal matrix result in longitudinal melanonychia. A study in Japanese patients showed dopa-staining melanocytes in the lower two to four layers of the nail matrix epithelium.[6]

There is considerable debate as to whether melanocytes are present in the nail bed. In a study using tyrosinase-related protein-1 (TRP-1) staining, the density of nail bed melanocytes was found to be 45 melanocytes/mm².[7] Nail matrix melanocytes in patients with skin of color contain mature melanosomes that produce melanin [**Table 15-4**]. In nails of Japanese individuals, melanocytes containing melanosomes were seen regularly in the dorsal, apical, and ventral matrices.[8] These melanocytes contained all gradations of maturing melanosomes, the majority being an immature variety with visible longitudinal cristae and transverse striations. Transferred melanosomes were seen regularly within the keratinocytes. The melanosomes were either mature and dense or immature and half filled with dense melanin. In nails of black individuals, most of the melanosomes were mature and dense. Transferred melanosomes also were mature.[8] The nail matrix of Caucasian patients lacks mature melanosomes but has premelanosomes, as well as stage I and stage II melanosomes. Although the Caucasian nail is not pigmented, pigmentation of the nail plate in a horizontal or longitudinal band has been reported to occur in response to an increased plasma melanocyte-stimulating hormone.[8]

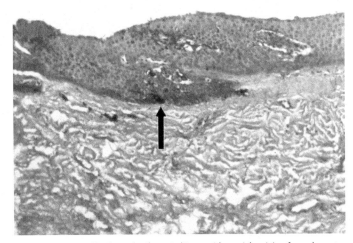

FIGURE 15-2. Histology of nail matrix biopsy with special staining for melanocytes (*arrow*).

TABLE 15-3	Nail matrix melanocytes
Distal matrix	Longitudinal melanonychia; larger, more dendritic melanocytes
Proximal matrix	Single compartment, largely dormant melanocytes

Nail matrix melanocytes differ from melanocytes elsewhere in the skin in that they are located primarily in the distal matrix and suprabasal layers.[6] In the nail matrix, the melanocytes are less dense and more frequently dormant than in the epidermis.[9] Because the nail matrix is covered by the nail plate and the nail fold at the proximal areas, these melanocytes are presumed not to be stimulated by ultraviolet (UV) radiation. It has been postulated that this is the reason the population of dopa-positive melanocytes is fewer in the nail matrix than in the epidermis.

Melanin in the nail plate is composed of granules derived from nail matrix melanocytes. Longitudinal melanonychia may be a benign phenomenon, particularly in African American patients [**Figure 15-3**]. Studies have reported that 77% of skin of color individuals will have melanonychia by age 20 and almost 100% by age 50.[10] A study of a Japanese population revealed a 10% to 20% prevalence of longitudinal melanoncyhia.[11] Unlike darker-skinned individuals and Japanese, in Caucasians, subungual pigmented lesions have a greater likelihood of being malignant.[12]

LANGERHANS CELLS AND MERKEL CELLS

Langerhans cells are found predominantly in the suprabasal layers of the nail matrix epithelium. They are more common in the proximal rather than the distal nail matrix. However, Langerhans cells may be seen occasionally within the basal layer of the nail matrix epithelium. There are fewer numbers of antigen-presenting Langerhans cells in the nail matrix compared with skin, which may explain the higher susceptibility of development of verrucae on this site.[13] Merkel cells also have been demonstrated in the nail matrix. The density of Merkel cells has been shown to decrease with age because these cells are more numerous in fetal than in adult nails.[14]

LUNULA (DISTAL MATRIX)

The lunula is the convex margin of the matrix, which can be visualized through the nail plate. It is most commonly visible on the thumbs and the great toes, although the proximal nail fold may conceal the lunula. The lunula is the area where the nail plate is least adherent.

NAIL BED

The nail bed epithelium is comprised of two to five cell layers. Keratinization occurs without formation of a granular layer. Few or no melanocytes have been found in the nail bed. The nail bed epithelium is adherent to the nail plate, causing it to remain attached to the nail plate after nail avulsion. After nail avulsion, the nail bed may develop a granular layer. Nail bed has been estimated to contribute to one-fifth of nail thickness and mass. The ventral nail plate is formed by a horny layer produced by keratinization of the nail bed.[15] On histologic examination, the ventral portion is identified by its eosinophilic appearance.

TABLE 15-4	Nail matrix melanosomes	
Race/Ethnicity	Percentage with melanonychia	Type of melanosomes in matrix
Japanese	11.4%	Immature and mature melanosomes
African	77%	Mature and dense melanosomes
Caucasian	Rare	Premelanosomes

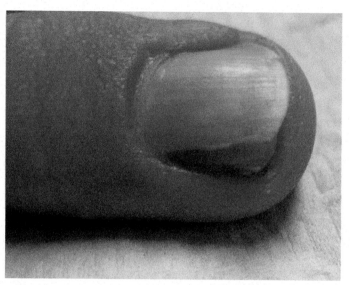

FIGURE 15-3. Melanonychia striata on right index finger of an African American patient.

HYPONYCHIUM

The epithelium of the hyponychium is equivalent to the epithelium of the volar skin, with both a granular and a thick cornified layer being present. Anatomically, it is defined as the cutaneous margin underlying the free edge of the nail, bordered distally by the distal groove at the point where the nail plate separates from the dorsal digit.

FOLDS

The dorsal portion of the proximal nail fold corresponds to the skin of the dorsal digit. The proximal nail fold contains sweat glands but lacks pilosebaceous units. It is densely innervated; thus inflammation of this area causes severe pain. The ventral portion of the nail fold continues proximally with the germinative matrix and covers approximately one-fourth of the nail plate. The border between the proximal nail fold and the nail matrix can be established histologically at the site of disappearance of the granular layer.

The horny layer of the proximal nail fold forms the eponychium, which is firmly attached to the superficial nail plate and prevents separation of the nail plate from the nail fold. The integrity of the eponychium is essential for maintaining homeostasis and minimizing the likelihood of infection.

The epithelium of the proximal nail fold contains a granular layer. Structurally, the dermis of the proximal nail fold contains superficial capillaries that are arranged in regular loops. These capillaries can provide useful information about microvascular alterations and assist in the diagnosis of connective tissue disorders[16] [**Figure 15-4**].

PLATE

The nail plate is composed of onychocytes, compacted keratinized epithelial cells. The plate covers both the nail bed and matrix. The nail plate is curved along both the longitudinal and transverse axes. This allows it to be embedded into the nail folds at its proximal and lateral margin, thus providing strong attachment. The curvature of the toenail is greater than that of the fingernail. The upper surface of the nail plate is smooth and may have a variable number of longitudinal ridges that increase with age.[17] The ventral surface also has longitudinal ridges that correspond to complementary grooves on the upper aspect of the nail bed. The nail plate gains thickness and density as it grows distally. A thick nail plate may imply a long intermediate matrix. This stems from the process whereby the longitudinal axis of the intermediate matrix becomes the vertical axis of the nail plate.[18] The proximal regions of

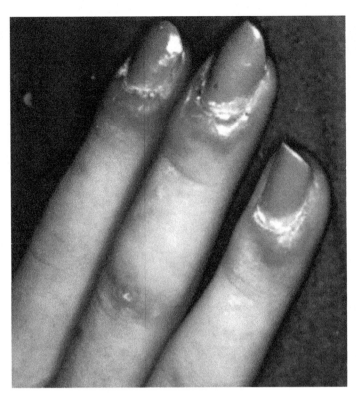

FIGURE 15-4. Inflammation and dilated capillaries at proximal nail folds of a patient with dermatomyositis.

matrix produce the dorsal nail plate, and the distal matrix produces the ventral nail plate.

The dorsal plate has a relatively high calcium, phospholipid, and sulfhydryl group content. It has little acid phosphatase activity and is physically hard. The phospholipid content may provide some water resistance.[19] The intermediate nail plate shares a similar chemical composition as the dorsal nail plate, except that it has a high acid phosphatase activity, probably corresponding to the number of retained nuclear remnants. There are many disulfide bonds (few bound sulfhydryl groups). It also contains phospholipids and calcium. The intermediate plate cells are eosinophilic and move both upward and forward with nail growth. The nail plate has been found to have a superficial dry compartment and a deep humid one. Corneocytes of the dorsal nail plate are joined laterally by spaced deep interdigitations. The interdigitations are more frequent in the deeper parts of the nail plate.

VASCULAR SUPPLY/INNERVATION

The nail unit has an abundant blood supply provided by four lateral digital arteries. The palmar digital arteries provide the main blood supply to the fingers. The nail fold is supplied by a superficial arcade. The distal and subungual arcades, arising from an anastomosis of the palmar arch and the dorsal nail fold, supply the subungual region. Glomus bodies contain nerve endings and arteriovenous anastomoses that regulate capillary circulation. The glomus bodies are found predominately in the dermis, with a density varying from 90 to 500/mm².[20] Their typical length is 300 μm. They are particularly important in maintaining blood supply to the periphery in cold weather. Pared digital nerves give rise to the cutaneous sensory nerves, which have a parallel course to the digital vessels. There is a very high density of nerve endings in the nail folds.

CHEMICAL PROPERTIES

The onychocytes of the nail are composed primarily of keratins. The keratins are low-sulfur filamentous proteins with a parallel orientation. Because of this orientation, the nail is more susceptible to transverse

fractures. The keratins are embedded in nonkeratin proteins, which are rich in sulfur, glycine, and tyrosine. The hardness of the nail plate is secondary to the hard keratins. From 80% to 90% of the nail keratins are hard hairlike keratins. The soft skinlike keratins comprise the remaining 10% to 20%.[21]

The normal water content of the nail ranges from 7% to 18% compared with 15% to 25% in the epidermis. Most of the water is localized to the intermediate nail plate, which has been found to be 1000 times more permeable to water than the skin.[22,23] The porosity of the nail causes the nail to be readily hydrated and dehydrated. When the percentage of water decreases below 7%, the nail becomes brittle; when the water content rises above 30%, it becomes opaque and soft.[24] The nail also contains trace organic elements, including iron, zinc, and calcium. These elements do not contribute to the hardness of the nail. The total fat content of the nail plate varies from 0.1% to 5%, in comparison with the stratum corneum, which has 10% fat content.[20] The primary lipid in the nail is cholesterol.

PHYSICAL PROPERTIES

The physical properties of the nail plate are hardness, strength, and flexibility. The presence of hard keratins and cystine-rich high-sulfur proteins determines the hardness of the nail. The strength is attributed to the curved axis in the longitudinal and transverse orientations and the firm adhesion of the onychocytes.[25] The maximum elastic stress of the nail has been found to be 420 to 880 kg/cm².[26] The flexibility is a consequence of its water content.

The ultrastructural character of the nail plate varies in each of its three layers.[22] The dorsal nail plate contains flat onychocytes with a shorter diameter perpendicular to the nail plate surface. Intermediate plate cell adhesion is provided by desmosomes and interdigitations of the cell membranes. The ventral nail plate is very thin and composed of soft keratins. The ventral nail plate provides firm attachment to the underlying nail bed.

NAIL GROWTH

Fingernails grow at 3 mm per month versus 1 mm per month for toenails, leading to a complete replacement of the fingernails in 6 months and of toenails in 12 to 18 months.[23] Because of this slow rate of growth, diseases of the nail matrix require a significant period of time to become apparent. The rate of nail growth is typically greatest during the second and third decades. After age 50, the rate of nail growth decreases sharply.[27] Many conditions have been associated with either increased or decreased rate of growth. Slow rate of growth is associated with fever, onychomycosis, malnutrition, and the yellow nail syndrome. Accelerated growth has been associated with pregnancy, hyperthyroidism, psoriasis, and pityriasis rubra pilaris. The nail's slow rate of growth allows evaluation of pathologic events that have occurred in the past.[28,29] One such change is the development of Beau lines, which are the result of a disturbance of the normal nail matrix growth.

REFERENCES

1. Sellheyer K, Nelson P. The concept of the onychodermis (specialized nail mesenchyme): an embryological assessment and a comparative analysis with the hair follicle. *J Cutan Pathol.* 2013;40:463-471.
2. Picardo M, Tosti A, Marchese C, et al. Characterization of cultured nail matrix cells. *J Am Acad Dermatol.* 1994;30:434-440.
3. Kitahara T, Ogawa H. Coexpression of keratins characteristic of skin and hair differentiation in nail cells. *J Invest Dermatol.* 1993;100:171-175.
4. DeBerker D, Wojnarowsha F, Sviland L, et al. Keratin expression in the normal nail unit: markers of regional differentiation. *Br J Dermatol.* 2000;142:89-96.
5. Tosti A, Cameli N, Piraccini B, et al. Characterization of nail matrix melanocytes with anti-PEP1, anti-PEP8, TMH-1, and HMB-45 antibodies. *J Am Acad Dermatol.* 1994;31:193-196.

6. Higashi N. Melanocytes of nail matrix and nail pigmentation. *Arch Dermatol.* 1968;97:570-574.

7. Perrin C, Michelis JF, Pisani A, Ortonne JP. Anatomic distribution of melanocytes in normal nail unit: an immunohistochemical investigation. *Am J Dermatolpathol.* 1997;19:462-467.

8. Hashimoto K. Ultrastructure of the human toenail: I. Proximal nail matrix. *J Invest Dermatol* 1971;56:235-246.

9. Higashi N, Saito T. Horizontal distribution of the dopa-positive melanocytes in the nail matrix. *J Invest Dermatol.* 1969;53:163-165.

10. Monash S. Normal pigmentation in the nails of the Negro. *Arch Dermatol.* 1932;25:876-881.

11. Kawamura T. Pigmentation longitudinalis striata unguium and pigmentation of the nail plate in Addison's disease. *Jpn J Dermatol.* 1958;68:10.

12. Baran R, Kechijian P. Longitudinal melanonychia (melanonychia striata): diagnosis and management. *J Am Acad Dermatol.* 1989;21:1165-1175.

13. Ito T, Ito N, Saathoff M, et al. Immunology of the human nail apparatus: the nail matrix is a site of relative immune privilege. *J Invest Dermatol.* 2005;125:1139-1148.

14. Moll I, Moll R. Merkel cells in ontogenesis of human nails. *Arch Dermatol Res.* 1993;285:366-371.

15. Johnson M. Nail is produced by the normal nail bed: a controversy resolved. *Br J Dermatol.* 1991;125:27-29.

16. Hahn M, Heubach T, Steins A. Hemodynamics in nailfold capillaries of patients with systemic scleroderma: synchronous measurement of capillary blood pressure and red blood cell velocity. *J Invest Dermatol.* 1998;110:982-985.

17. Tosti A, Piraccini BM. Biology of nails and nail disorders. In: Goldsmith LA, Katz SI, Gilchrest BA, Paller AS, Leffell DJ, Wolff K, eds. *Fitzpatrick's Dermatology in General Medicine.* 8th ed. New York, NY: McGraw-Hill Medical; 2012:1009-1030.

18. DeBerker D, Mawhinney B, Sviland L. Quantification of regional matrix nail production. *Br J Dermatol.* 1996;134:1083-1086.

19. Lee DY, Park JH, Shin HT, Jang KT, Shim JS. Immunohistochemical study of epithelial markers in longitudinal and transverse sections of the human nail unit. *Clin Exp Dermatol.* 2012;37:688-689.

20. Dawber RPR, deBerker DAR, Baran R. Science of the nail apparatus. In: Baran R, Dawber RPR, deBerker DAR, eds. *Diseases of the Nails and Their Management.* Oxford, England: Blackwell Science; 2001:1-47.

21. Lynch MH, O'Guin W, Hardy C, et al. Acidic and basic hair/nail ("hard") keratins: their colocalization in the upper cortical and cuticle cells of the human hair follicle and their relationship to "soft" keratins. *J Cell Biol.* 1986;103:2593-2606.

22. Jemec GBE, Serup J. Ultrasound structure of the human nail plate. *Arch Dermatol.* 1989;125:643-646.

23. Spruit D. Measurement of water vapor loss through human nail in vivo. *J Invest Dermatol.* 1971;56:359-361.

24. Runne U, Orfanos CE. The human nail: structure, growth and pathologic changes. *Curr Probl Dermatol.* 1981;9:102-149.

25. Finlay AY, Frost P, Keith AD. Assessment of factors influencing flexibility of human fingernail. *Br J Dermatol.* 1980;10:357-365.

26. Young RW. Strength of fingernails. *J Invest Dermatol.* 1965;44:358-360.

27. Bean WB. Nail growth: 30 years observation. *Arch Intern Med.* 1974;134:497-502.

28. Zaiac MN, Walker A. Nail abnormalities associated with systemic pathologies. *Clin Dermatol.* 2013;31:627-649.

29. Geyer AS, Onumah N, Uyttendaele H, Scher RK. Modulation of linear nail growth to treat diseases of the nail. *J Am Acad Dermatol.* 2004;50:229-234.

CHAPTER 16

Biology of Wounds and Wound Care

Richard A.F. Clark
A. Paul Kelly

KEY POINTS

- Chronic wounds are becoming an increasing problem among all races.

- The basic biology of wound healing applies to skin of light and dark color.

- Certain pathologic processes are more common in skin of color, such as keloids and postinflammatory hyperpigmentation.

- Diversity in skin color can pose a challenge in assessing patients with wounds.

INTRODUCTION

Diversity in skin color can pose a challenge in assessing patients with wounds. For example, erythema is difficult to detect in patients with darker pigmented skin.[1] It is important that healthcare practitioners understand the differences between lighter [**Figure 16-1**] and darker [**Figure 16-2**] pigmented skin.[2] Bennett[1] defines darker pigmented skin coloration as skin that does not blanch when pressure is applied over a bony prominence [**Figure 16-3**], irrespective of the patient's race or ethnicity. Failure to detect signs of inflammation or nonblanching erythema may lead to the development of a life-threatening wound infection.

The skin is the largest organ in the body whose primary function is to serve as a protective barrier against the environment. Other important functions of the skin include fluid homeostasis, thermoregulation, immune surveillance, sensory detection, and healing. Loss of the integrity the skin due to injury or illness compromises its protective function and, when the loss is extensive, may result in significant disability or even death. It is estimated that in 1996, there were 35.2 million cases of significant skin loss (U.S. figures) that required major therapeutic intervention.[3] Of these, approximately 5 million wounds became chronic.

This chapter covers the basic biology of wound healing, and elucidates different types of wounds, their assessments, treatment and special issues for patients with skin of color.

WOUND TYPES AND THEIR THERAPY

Often the etiology of cutaneous wounds stems from a mixture of both intrinsic and extrinsic factors. An example of an intrinsic factor is the genodermatosis, epidermolysis bullosa disorders which predisposes to skin disruption from minor insults such as friction. More mechanistically complex intrinsic conditions, such as venous insufficiency or diabetes mellitus, alter skin architecture and/or its physicochemical properties, leading to ulceration and nonhealing states that are often precipitated by minor trauma. Every year in the United States, there are approximately 2 million cases of chronic diabetic ulcers, many of which eventually necessitate amputation. Pressure ulcers and leg ulcers, including venous ulcers, affect another 3 million people in the United States with treatment costs as high as $8 billion annually.[4] Arterial obstruction

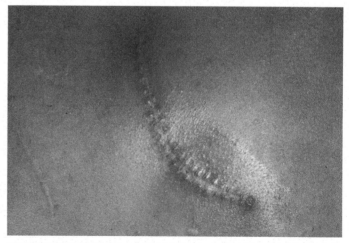

FIGURE 16-1. Incision line on lighter-pigmented skin; notice the pinkness of the postoperative site.

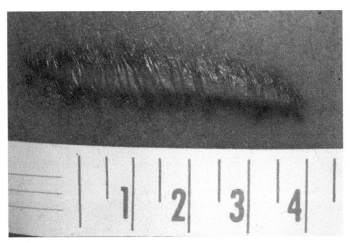

FIGURE 16-2. Four weeks after an incision, a slight hypertrophic scar has developed on the medium-color pigmented skin. The borders of the incision are hyperpigmented, and the center of the incision is hypopigmented.

is another important intrinsic factor. Extrinsic factors, such as high, chronic doses of glucocorticoids (prednisone) and/or anticancer therapy or diets insufficient in nutrients and/or vitamins, particularly vitamin C, may lead to abnormalities of skin structure or function that predispose to wounds and poor healing. Other extrinsic factors that complicate healing of wounds of all types include foreign body contamination and bacterial colonization, infection, and biofilm formation. All of these factors must be taken into consideration and remediated for proper healing.

The depth of skin wounds greatly impacts the skin's ability to heal rapidly and possibly without scarring. Intraepidermal wounds and wounds at the dermal–epidermal junction have the greatest possibility of healing rapidly and without scarring because there is no need for granulation tissue. Wounds that extend into the dermis tend to heal more slowly. Slow healing and the potential for severe scarring are partially dependent on the depth and extent of dermal injury. Mid-dermal wounds have a limited ability to contract and therefore are unlikely to form hypertrophic scars or scar contractions. In addition, the epidermis can initially regenerate from epidermal cells of hair follicles and other appendages.[5] Full-thickness wounds with loss of dermis and epidermis leave no structures from which the epidermis can regenerate. In addition, the lack of residual dermis leads to marked wound contraction that is associated with overgrowth of fibrous tissue. This increased scar formation leads to lack of skin flexibility, which can result in severe deformity.

The types of insults that cause skin wounds include sharp or blunt trauma, thermal or electrical injury, and cold injury. The most common cause of significant skin loss is thermal injury, which accounts for an estimated 1 million emergency department visits per year.[6] In

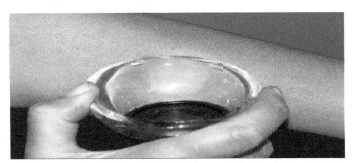

FIGURE 16-3. A glass applied to the skin shows blanching erythema on lighter-pigmented skin. In contrast, in darker-pigmented skin, the blanching would be difficult, if not impossible, to see.

2011, a survey estimated the U.S. market for advanced wound care products, including biological and synthetic dressings, at approximately $3 billion. This market is expected to increase significantly as the American population ages and becomes more susceptible to underlying causes of chronic wounds.[7,8] The quality-of-life tolls of chronic wounds are extremely high.

Over the past two decades, extraordinary advances in cellular and molecular biology have greatly expanded our understanding of the basic biological processes involved in acute wound healing and the pathobiology of chronic wounds.[9,10] One recombinant growth factor, platelet-derived growth factor-BB (rPDGF-BB; Regranex, Ortho-McNeil), and several skin substitutes (eg, *dermal substitutes*: Integra Matrix Wound Dressings, Integra LifeSciences; AlloDerm, LifeCell; OASIS Wound Matrix, Healthpoint; Dermagraft and TransCyte, Advanced BioHealing; and *epidermal/dermal substitutes*: Apligraf, Organogenesis; Orcel, Forticell Bioscience; Tissuetech, Fidia Advanced Biopolymers) have reached the marketplace for second-line therapy of recalcitrant ulcers.[11] These therapeutic interventions have added to the clinician's ability to promote skin healing, but they have not had the impact that was predicted. Regardless of the advanced wound care product, the ideal goal would be to regenerate tissues where both the structural and functional properties of the wounded tissue are restored to the levels prior to injury. In contrast to adult wounds, embryonic wounds undergo complete regeneration, terminating in a scarless repair.[12,13] Thus, investigators are now using morphogenetic cues including hair development[14,15] to develop engineered constructs capable of tissue regeneration.[16,17]

SPECIAL WOUND-HEALING ISSUES WITH SKIN OF COLOR

The biologic processes of wound healing are essentially the same in patients regardless of skin color. However, people with darker skin do have a higher incidence of keloids than lighter-skinned individuals for reasons that are presently not understood.[18] Furthermore, the additional activity of melanogenesis in people of color leads to more perceivable dyschromia. Thus, postinflammatory hypopigmentation and hyperpigmentation is more obvious in the healed wounds in patients with darker skin.

A keloid is defined as an abnormal, persistent proliferation of fibrous scar tissue that grows beyond the original margins of a scar.[19] In contrast, hypertrophic scars usually resolve with time and do not grow beyond the boundaries of the original wound. The pathology of keloids is characterized by hyalinized collagen, nonflattened epidermis, nonfibrotic papillary dermis, and a tonguelike advancing edge of hyalinized collagen under normal epidermis.[20] Although some consider the presence of α-smooth muscle actin as a distinguishing feature of hypertrophic scars, the study by Lee et al[20] demonstrated that keloids had a 45% expression, whereas hypertrophic scars had a 70% expression. The underlying etiology (or etiologies) of keloids is not understood. The dearth of fundamental knowledge about keloids has been partly secondary to lack of clarity in distinguishing keloids from hypertrophic scars.[19] Nevertheless, recent progress has been made in genomics[21,22] and molecular biology.[23-26] To date, it appears that the predisposition to keloid formation is polygenomic and the molecular mechanisms at play during keloid formation are multifactorial. In the meantime, treatment of keloids has not advanced much beyond intradermal injections with glucocorticoids, which remain the mainstay of therapy; however, some interesting thoughts on treatment have appeared in the past few years.[27,28]

Although delayed wound closure and/or increased inflammation are often touted as the cause of hyperpigmentation and hypopigmentation of wound sites, the mechanism(s) of these phenomena are poorly understood and seldom investigated.[29] Despite the lack of understanding pathobiology in these conditions, both surgical and nonsurgical treatments have advanced. Postburn hyperpigmentation of the fingers has been successfully treated with split-thickness plantar grafts, whereas postburn hypopigmentation has been treated with noncultured melanocyte-keratinocyte transplantation.[30] In other conditions of dyschromia, including nonburn scars, ablative and nonablative fractional thermolysis has been found to be beneficial.[31] With fractional photothermolysis, the microscopic, pixilated pattern of wounding in the dermis results in significant skin pigmentary and textural improvements without the adverse effects of prolonged wound healing. Skin-lightening therapy and cosmetics have garnered a bad reputation secondary to their overuse for general skin lightening.[32,33]

BASIC BIOLOGY OF WOUND REPAIR

Wound repair is not a simple linear process, but rather an integration of dynamic interactive processes involving soluble mediators, formed blood elements, the extracellular matrix (ECM), and parenchymal cells. Unencumbered, these wound repair processes follow a specific time sequence and can be temporally categorized into three major groups: inflammation, tissue formation, and tissue remodeling. The three phases of wound repair, however, are not mutually exclusive but rather overlapping in time. The reader is referred to *The Molecular and Cellular Biology of Wound Repair*[34] for a more detailed discussion of the many processes involved in wound healing.

■ INFLAMMATION

Severe tissue injury causes blood vessel disruption with concomitant extravasation of blood constituents. Blood coagulation and platelet aggregation generate a fibrin-rich clot that plugs severed vessels and fills any discontinuity in the wounded tissue. While the blood clot within vessel lumen reestablishes homeostasis, the clot within a wound space acts as a growth factor reservoir and provides a provisional matrix for cell migration.

The primary cell types involved in the overall process of inflammation are platelets, neutrophils, and monocytes. Upon injury, successful reestablishment of homeostasis depends on platelet adhesion to interstitial connective tissue, which leads to their aggregation, coagulation, and activation. Activated platelets release several adhesive proteins to facilitate their aggregation, chemotactic factors for blood leukocytes, and multiple growth factors[9,10] to promote new tissue formation.

Of the two primary phagocytic leukocytes, neutrophils and monocytes, neutrophils arrive first in large numbers due to their abundance in circulation. Infiltrating neutrophils cleanse the wounded area of foreign particles, including bacteria. If excessive microorganisms or indigestible particles have lodged in the wound site, neutrophils will probably cause further tissue damage as they attempt to clear these contaminants through the release of enzymes and toxic oxygen products. When particle clearance has been completed, generation of granulocyte chemoattractants ceases, and the remaining neutrophils become recede.

Transition Between Inflammation and Repair Whether neutrophil infiltrates resolve or persist, monocyte accumulation continues, stimulated by selective monocyte chemoattractants.[34] Besides promoting phagocytosis and debridement, adherence to ECM also stimulates monocytes to undergo metamorphosis into inflammatory or reparative macrophages. Because cultured macrophages produce and secrete the peptide growth factors interleukin-1 (IL-1), platelet-derived growth factor-BB (PDGF-BB), transforming growth factor alpha (TGF-α), transforming growth factor beta (TGF-β), and fibroblast growth factor (FGF), presumably wound macrophages also synthesize these protein products.[35] Although neutrophils and macrophages have a critical role in fighting infection and macrophages can contribute growth factors to the wound, it has become increasingly clear that too much inflammation may be harmful.[36] In fact, from knock-out and knock-down experiments, it is evident that wounds in some situations heal faster with fewer inflammatory cells, especially if microorganism invasion is avoided by some other means.[37]

■ REEPITHELIALIZATION

Reepithelialization of a wound begins within hours after injury by the movement of epithelial cells from the surrounding epidermis over the denuded surface. Rapid reestablishment of the epidermal surface and its permeability barrier prevents excessive water loss and reduces time of exposure to bacterial infections, which decreases the morbidity and mortality of patients who have lost a substantial amount of skin surface. If a wide expanse of the epidermis is lost, epidermal cells regenerate from stem cells in pilosebaceous follicles.[38] Migrating epithelial cells markedly alter their phenotype by retracting their intracellular filaments, dissolving most of their desmosomes, and forming peripheral actin filaments (which facilitate cell movement).[34] These migrating cells also undergo dissolution of their hemidesmosomal links between the epidermis and the dermis. All these phenotypic alterations provide epithelial cells with the needed lateral mobility for migration over the wound site. Migrating epidermal cells possess a unique phenotype that is distinct from both the terminally differentiated keratinocytes of normal (stratified) epidermis and the basal cells of stratified epidermis. It is now appreciated that the signals that control wound healing in the adult animal are similar to those that control epithelial fusion during embryogenesis.[39]

If the basement membrane is destroyed by injury, epidermal cells migrate over a provisional matrix of fibrin(ogen), fibronectin, tenascin, and vitronectin as well as stromal type I collagen.[40] Wound keratinocytes express cell surface receptors for fibronectin, tenascin, and vitronectin, which belong to the integrin superfamily.[41] In addition, α2β1 collagen receptors, which are normally disposed along the lateral sides of basal keratinocytes, redistribute to the basal membrane of wound keratinocytes as they come in contact with type I collagen fibers of the dermis. Whereas β1 integrins are clearly essential for normal reepithelialization,[42] it is not clear which subtype is essential. It is most likely that there is a redundancy in the requirement for α5β1 and α2β1 in reepithelialization.

The migrating wound epidermis does not simply transit over a wound eschar, but rather dissects through the wound, separating the fibrin/fibronectin-rich eschar and desiccated dermis containing denatured collagen from underlying viable tissue.[43] The path of dissection appears to be determined by the array of integrins expressed on the migrating epidermal cells. Keratinocytes do not express αvβ3, the integrin receptor for fibrinogen/fibrin and denatured collagen, in vitro or in vivo.[43] Thus, keratinocytes do not have the capacity to interact with these matrix proteins. Furthermore, fibrinogen or fibrin appears to inhibit epidermal cell interactions with fibronectin; hence, migrating wound epidermis avoids the fibrin/fibronectin-rich clot and migrates along the type I collagen–rich wound edge via the α2β1 collagen receptor until it meets the fibronectin-rich granulation tissue and then proceeds to migrate over this newly forming tissue via the α5β1 receptor.

ECM degradation is clearly required for the dissection of migrating wound epidermis between the collagenous dermis and the fibrin eschar and probably depends on epidermal cell production of collagenase, plasminogen activator, and stromelysin. Plasminogen activator activates collagenase (matrix metalloproteinase-1 [MMP-1]) as well as plasminogen and thus facilitates the degradation of interstitial collagen and provisional matrix proteins. Interestingly, keratinocytes in direct contact with collagen greatly increase the amount of MMP-1 they produce compared with that produced when they reside on a laminin-rich basement membrane or purified laminin.[44] The migrating epidermis of superficial skin ulcers and burn wounds, in fact, expresses high levels of MMP-1 mRNA in areas where it presumably comes in direct contact with dermal collagen.[45]

One to 2 days after injury, epithelial cells at the wound margin begin to proliferate. Although the exact mechanism is still not clear, both proliferation and migration of epithelial cells may be triggered by the absence of neighboring cells at the wound margin (the *free-edge effect*). The free-edge effect in the wound epidermis may be secondary to modulation of cadherin junctions as described for V-cadherins during angiogenesis.[46] In fact, studies indicate that epidermal desmosomes lose their hyperadhesiveness, and cadherins switch from E-cadherins to P-cadherins at the wound edge.[47] Other possibilities, not exclusive of the former, are a release of autocrine or paracrine growth factors that induce epidermal migration and proliferation and/or increased expression of growth factor receptors. Although some growth factors, such as insulin-like growth factor (IGF), may come from the circulation and thereby act as a hormone, other growth factors, such as heparin-binding epidermal growth factor (HB-EGF) and FGF-7 (also called keratinocyte growth factor [KGF]) are secreted from macrophages and dermal parenchymal cells, respectively, and act on epidermal cells through a paracrine pathway.[48] In contrast, TGF-α and TGF-β originate from keratinocytes themselves and act directly on the producer cell or adjacent epidermal cells in an autocrine or juxtacrine fashion. Many of these growth factors have been shown to stimulate reepithelialization in animal models.[9] Furthermore, lack of growth factors or their receptors in knock-out mice supports the hypothesis that growth factor activation of keratinocytes is required for optimal epidermal migration and/or proliferation during normal wound healing.[49] In fact, it has been demonstrated that JNK is a key signal transduction factor responsible for "resetting" the epidermal program from differentiation to proliferation, and possibly migration.[50]

As reepithelialization progresses, basement membrane proteins reappear in a very ordered sequence from the margin of the wound inward in a zipper-like fashion.[9] Epidermal cells revert to their normal phenotype, once again firmly attaching to the reestablished basement membrane through hemidesmosomal proteins, α6β4 integrin, and 180-kDa bullous pemphigoid antigen,[51] and to the underlying neodermis through type VII collagen fibrils.[52]

■ GRANULATION TISSUE

New stroma, often called *granulation tissue*, begins to form approximately 4 days after injury. The name derives from the granular appearance of newly forming tissue when it is incised and visually examined. Numerous new capillaries endow the neostroma with its granular appearance. Macrophages, fibroblasts, and blood vessels move into the wound space as a unit that correlates well with the biologic interdependence of these cells during tissue repair. Macrophages and ingrowing parenchymal cells provide a continuing source of cytokines necessary to stimulate fibroplasia and angiogenesis, fibroblasts construct the new ECM necessary to support cell ingrowth, and blood vessels carry the oxygen and nutrients necessary to sustain cell metabolism. Recently, the importance of oxygenation has been reemphasized.[53] The quantity and quality of granulation tissue depend on biologic modifiers present, the activity level of target cells, and the ECM environment. As mentioned in the section on inflammation, the arrival of peripheral blood monocytes and their activation to macrophages establish conditions for continual synthesis and release of growth factors. In addition and perhaps more importantly, injured and activated parenchymal cells can synthesize and secrete growth factors. For example, migrating wound epidermal cells produce vascular endothelial growth factor (VEGF), TGF-β, and PDGF-BB, to which endothelial cells and fibroblasts respond, respectively. The provisional ECM also promotes granulation tissue formation by positive feedback regulation of integrin ECM receptor expression.[54] Once fibroblasts and endothelial cells express the appropriate integrin receptors, they invade the fibrin/fibronectin-rich wound space [Figure 16-2]. Although it has been recognized for many years that the ECM modulates cell differentiation by signal transduction from ligation of ECM receptors, more recently it has become evident that the force and geometry of the ECM influence cell behavior and differentiation.[55-57]

Fibroplasia Components of granulation tissue derived from fibroblasts including the cells themselves and the ECM are collectively known as fibroplasia. Growth factors, especially PDGF and TGF-β, in concert with the provisional matrix molecules,[54] presumably stimulate fibroblasts of the periwound tissue to proliferate, express appropriate

integrin receptors, and migrate into the wound space. Many of these growth factors are released from macrophages or other tissue cells[9,10]; however, fibroblasts themselves can produce growth factors to which they respond in an autocrine fashion.[58] Multiple complex interactive biologic phenomena occur within fibroblasts as they respond to wound cytokines including the induction of additional cytokines and modulation of cytokine receptor number or affinity. In vivo studies support the hypothesis that growth factors are active in wound repair fibroplasia. Several studies have demonstrated that PDGF, connective tissue growth factor (CTGF), TGF-α, TGF-β, HB-EGF, and FGF family members are present at sites of tissue repair.[59-62] Furthermore, purified and recombinant-derived growth factors have been shown to stimulate wound granulation tissue in normal and compromised animals,[9] and a single growth factor may work both directly and indirectly by inducing the production of other growth factors in situ.[63]

Structural molecules of the early ECM, coined *provisional matrix*,[64] contribute to tissue formation by providing a conduit for cell migration (fibronectin),[65] low impedance for cell mobility (hyaluronic acid),[66] a reservoir for cytokines,[67] and direct signals to the cells through integrin receptors.[41] Fibronectin appearance in the periwound environment and the expression of fibronectin receptors appear to be critical rate-limiting steps in granulation tissue formation.[68] In addition, a dynamic reciprocity between fibroblasts and their surrounding ECM creates further complexity.[69] That is, fibroblasts affect ECM through new synthesis, deposition, and remodeling,[70] whereas the ECM affects fibroblasts by regulating their function including their ability to synthesize, deposit, remodel, and generally interact with the ECM.[54,71] Thus, the reciprocal interactions between ECM and fibroblasts dynamically evolve during granulation tissue development.

As fibroblasts migrate into the wound space, they initially penetrate the blood clot composed of fibrin and lesser amounts of fibronectin and vitronectin. Fibroblasts may require fibronectin in vivo for movement from the periwound collagenous matrix into the fibrin/fibronectin-laden wound space, as they do in vitro for migration from a three-dimensional collagen gel into a fibrin gel.[65] Fibroblasts bind to fibronectin through receptors of the integrin superfamily. The Arg-Gly-Asp-Ser (RGDS) tetrapeptide within the cell-binding domain of these proteins is critical for binding to the integrin receptors α3β1, α5β1, αvβ1, αvβ3, and αvβ5. In vivo studies have shown that the RGD-dependent, fibronectin receptors α5β1 and αvβ3 are upregulated on periwound fibroblasts the day prior to granulation tissue formation and on early granulation tissue fibroblasts as they infiltrate the provisional matrix-laden wound.[54] In contrast, the non–RGD-binding α1β1 and α2β1 collagen receptors were either suppressed or did not appear to change appreciably.[54,72] Both in vitro PDGF and TGF-β can stimulate fibroblasts to migrate and can upregulate integrin receptors. For example, fibronectin- or fibrin-rich environments promote the ability of PDGF to increase α5β1 and α3β1, but not α2β1, by increasing mRNA stability and steady-state levels.[54] The opposite is true in a collagen-rich environment. These data suggest that the type of integrin induced by PDGF stimulation depends on the ECM context and suggests a positive feedback between ECM and ECM receptors. Thus, growth factors, such as PDGF and TGF-β, in the context of provisional matrix ECM, appear responsible for inducing a migrating fibroblast phenotype.

Movement into a cross-linked fibrin blood clot or any tightly woven ECM may also necessitate active proteolysis to cleave a path for migration. A variety of fibroblast-derived enzymes in conjunction with serum-derived plasmin are potential candidates for this task, including plasminogen activator, interstitial collagenase-1 and -3 (MMP-1 and MMP-13, respectively), the 72-kDa gelatinase A (MMP-2), and stromelysin (MMP-3). In fact, high levels of immunoreactive MMP-1 have been localized to fibroblasts at the interface of granulation tissue with eschar in burn wounds,[45] and many stromal cells stain for MMP-1 and MMP-13 in chronic ulcers.[73] Whereas TGF-β downregulates proteinase activity, PDGF stimulates the production and secretion of these proteinases.[74] From elegant knock-out mouse studies, it is clear that the plasminogen activating system is critical for clearing fibrin clot from the wound.[75] In addition, single knock-out of MMP-8 (also called collagenase-2) adversely affected cutaneous wound repair,[76] and double knock-out of MMP-13 (also called collagenase-3) and plasminogen activator created more delay of healing compared with single knock-out of plasminogen activator.[77] Thus, although there is great overlap in MMP function in tissue repair, their activity is clearly necessary for proper healing of cutaneous wounds.

When fibroblasts have completed their migration into the wound site, they switch their major function to protein synthesis.[70] Thus, the migratory phenotype is supplanted by a profibrotic phenotype characterized by decreased $\alpha3\beta1$ and $\alpha5\beta1$ provisional matrix receptors, increased $\alpha2\beta1$ collagen receptors, and collagen synthesis.[54,70] The fibronectin-rich provisional matrix is gradually supplanted with a collagenous matrix.[70,71] Under these conditions, PDGF, which is still abundant in these wounds,[78] stimulates extremely high levels of $\alpha2\beta1$ collagen receptor, but not $\alpha3\beta1$ or $\alpha5\beta1$ provisional matrix receptors, supporting the contention that the ECM provides a positive feedback for integrin expression.[54] TGF-β observed in wound fibroblasts at this time[71] probably induces the great quantities of collagen produced.[79] Because IL-4 also can induce a modest increase in type I and III collagen production,[80] IL-4–producing mast cells present in healing wounds, as well as fibrotic tissue, may contribute to collagen matrix accumulation at these sites.

Once abundant collagen matrix is deposited in the wound, fibroblasts decrease collagen synthesis despite the presence of TGF-β.[71] Both in vitro and in vivo studies suggest that γ-interferon may downregulate collagen production.[81] In addition, collagen matrix itself can suppress both fibroblast proliferation and fibroblast collagen synthesis.[71,82] In contrast, a fibrin or fibronectin matrix has little or no suppressive effect on the mitogenic or synthetic potential of fibroblasts.[71,83]

Although the attenuated fibroblast activity in collagen gels is not associated with cell death, many fibroblasts in day 10 healing wounds develop pyknotic nuclei,[84] a cytologic marker for apoptosis or programmed cell death, as well as other signs of apoptosis. These results in cutaneous wounds and other results in lungs and kidney suggest that apoptosis is the mechanism responsible for the transition from a fibroblast-rich granulation tissue to a relatively acellular scar.[85] Although signals for wound fibroblast apoptosis have not been elucidated, fibroplasia in wound repair is clearly tightly regulated, whereas, in fibrotic diseases such as keloids, morphea, and scleroderma, these processes become dysregulated. Recent evidence suggests that fibroblast apoptotic signals in keloids are disrupted.[86]

Neovascularization Fibroplasia would halt if neovascularization failed to accompany the newly forming complex of fibroblasts and ECM. The process of new blood vessel formation is called angiogenesis.[87] Many soluble factors that stimulate angiogenesis in wound repair have been elucidated.[88] Angiogenic activity can be recovered from activated macrophages as well as epidermal cells, fibroblasts, endothelial cells, and numerous tumor cells.[89] Most biologically important angiogenic molecules have probably been identified and include VEGF, FGF-1 and FGF-2, TGF-α, TGF-β, TNF-α, platelet factor-4 (PF-4), angiogenin, angiotropin, angiopoietin, IL-8, PDGF, and low-molecular-weight substances including bioactive peptides, low oxygen tension, biogenic amines, lactic acid, and nitric oxide (NO).[9,10] Some of these factors, however, are intermediaries in a single angiogenesis pathway; for example, TNF-α induces PF-4 that stimulates angiogenesis through NO.[90] Even more important, low oxygen tension stabilizes hypoxia inducible factor-1α (HIF-1α), which induces increased expression of VEGF.[91] To emphasize the complexity of the interactions, not all growth factors within a family stimulate angiogenesis equally. For example, of four VEGF isoforms (VEGF-A, -B, -C, and -D) and three receptors (VEGFR1/Flt-1, VEGFR2/KDR/Flk-1, and VEGFR3), VEGF-A does not interact with VEGFR1 and VEGFR2 equally and the signal transduction stimulated is not the same.[92] Furthermore, VEGF-C and VEGF-D stimulate lymphangiogenesis, rather than angiogenesis, through VEGFR3.

Another complexity is that different growth factors affect blood vessel development at different stages. For example, VEGF-A stimulates nascent sprout angiogenesis, whereas angiopoietin induces blood vessel maturation.[93]

Angiogenesis cannot be directly related to proliferation of cultured endothelial cells because endothelial cell migration is also required. In fact, Folkman and Shing[94] postulated that endothelial cell migration can induce proliferation. If true, endothelial cell chemotactic factors may be critical for angiogenesis. Some factors, however, have both proliferative (mitogenic) and chemotactic (motogenic) activities; for example, PDGF[95] and EGF[96] are motogenic and mitogenic for dermal fibroblasts, whereas VEGF is motogenic and mitogenic for endothelial cells.[97]

Besides growth factors and chemotactic factors, an appropriate ECM is also necessary for angiogenesis. Three-dimensional ECM protein gels provide a more natural environment for cultured endothelial cells than monolayer protein coats,[88] as is true for many other cultured cells.[98] Not surprisingly, different ECM proteins induce differential cell responses. For example, laminin-containing gels in the absence of growth factors induce human umbilical vein and dermal microvascular cells to produce capillary-like structures within 24 hours of plating.[99] In contrast, type I collagen does not induce angiogenesis without contributing factors.[100] Together, these studies suggest that the ECM plays an important role in angiogenesis. Consonant with this hypothesis, angiogenesis in the chick chorioallantoic membrane is dependent on the expression of $\alpha v\beta3$, an integrin that recognizes fibrin and fibronectin, as well as other provision matrix proteins.[101] Furthermore, in porcine cutaneous wounds, $\alpha v\beta3$ is expressed on capillary sprouts as they invade the fibrin clot.[35] In fact, in vitro studies demonstrate that $\alpha v\beta3$ can promote endothelial cell migration on provisional matrix proteins.[102]

Given the information outlined above, a series of events leading to angiogenesis can be hypothesized. Substantial injury causes tissue-cell destruction and hypoxia. Potent angiogenesis factors such as FGF-1 and FGF-2 are released secondary to cell disruption,[103] whereas VEGF is induced by hypoxia. Proteolytic enzymes released into the connective tissue degrade ECM proteins. Specific fragments from collagen, fibronectin, and elastin, as well as many phylogistic agents, recruit peripheral blood monocytes to the injured site, where these cells become activated macrophages that release more angiogenesis factors. Certain angiogenic factors, such as FGF-2, stimulate endothelial cells to release plasminogen activator and procollagenase. Plasminogen activator converts plasminogen to plasmin and procollagenase to active collagenase, and in concert, these two proteases digest basement membrane constituents.

The fragmentation of the basement membrane allows endothelial cells to migrate into the injured site in response to FGF and other endothelial cell chemoattractants. To migrate into the fibrin/fibronectin-rich wound, endothelial cells express $\alpha v\beta3$,[101] as well as $\alpha v\beta5$ integrin.[104] Newly forming blood vessels first deposit a provisional matrix containing fibronectin and proteoglycans but ultimately form basement membrane. TGF-β may induce endothelial cells to produce the fibronectin and proteoglycan provisional matrix as well as assume the correct phenotype for capillary tube formation. FGF and other mitogens such as VEGF stimulate endothelial cell proliferation, resulting in a continual supply of endothelial cells for capillary extension. Capillary sprouts eventually branch at their tips and join to form capillary loops through which blood flow begins. New sprouts then extend from these loops to form a capillary plexus. Angiopoietin[105] and perienodothelial cell (pericytes) recruitment[106] are important for maturation and stabilization of the newly formed capillaries.

Within a day or two after removal of angiogenic stimuli, capillaries undergo regression as characterized by mitochondrial swelling in the endothelial cells at the distal tips of the capillaries, platelet adherence to degenerating endothelial cells, vascular stasis, endothelial cell necrosis, and ingestion of the effete capillaries by macrophages. It is fairly clear that thrombospondin[107] and other ECM molecules are good candidate ligands for controlling endothelial cell apoptosis.[108]

WOUND CONTRACTION AND EXTRACELLULAR MATRIX ORGANIZATION

During the second and third weeks of healing, fibroblasts begin to assume a myofibroblast phenotype characterized by large bundles of actin-containing microfilaments disposed along the cytoplasmic face of the plasma membrane and the establishment of cell–cell and cell–matrix linkages.[70,109] In some,[84] but not all,[70] wound situations, myofibroblasts express smooth muscle actin. Importantly, TGF-β can induce cultured human fibroblasts to express smooth muscle actin and may also be responsible for its expression in vivo.[110]

Myofibroblast appearance corresponds to the initiation of connective tissue compaction and wound contraction. These cells link to ECM proteins through α5β1 for fibronectin[70] and α1β1 and α2β1 for collagen[111] and to each other through direct adherens junctions.[70] Fibroblast α2β1 receptors are markedly upregulated in 7-day wounds,[54] a time when a new collagenous matrix is accumulating and fibroblasts are beginning to align with collagenous fibrils through cell–matrix connections.[70] New collagen bundles in turn have the capacity to join end-to-end with collagen bundles at the wound edge and to ultimately form covalent crosslinks among themselves and with the collagen bundles of the adjacent dermis.[112] These cell–cell, cell–matrix, and matrix–matrix links provide a network across the wound whereby the traction of myofibroblasts on their pericellular matrix can be transmitted across the wound to effect wound contraction.[113]

Cultured fibroblasts dispersed within a hydrated collagen gel provide an in vitro model of wound contraction.[114] When serum is added, contraction of the collagen matrix occurs over the course of a few days. Via time-lapse microphotography, collagen condensation appears to result from a "collection of collagen bundles" executed by fibroblasts as they extend and retract pseudopodia attached to collagen fibers.[115] The transmission of these traction forces across the in vitro collagen matrix depends on two linkage events: fibroblast attachment to the collagen matrix through the α2β1 integrin receptors[116] and crosslinks between the individual collagen bundles.[117] This linkage system probably plays a significant role in the in vivo situation of wound contraction as well. In addition, cell–cell adhesions appear to provide an additional means by which the traction forces of the myofibroblast may be transmitted across the wound matrix.[109] Gap junctions between wound fibroblasts probably provide the mechanism for contraction control across the cell population.[118]

F-actin bundle arrays, cell–cell and cell–matrix linkages, and collagen crosslinks are all facets of the biomechanics of ECM contraction. The contraction process, however, needs a cytokine signal. For example, cultured fibroblasts mixed in a collagen gel contract the collagen matrix in the presence of serum, PDGF, or TGF-β. Because TGF-β, but not PDGF, persists in dermal wounds during the time of tissue contraction, it is the most likely candidate for the stimulus of contraction.[9] Nevertheless, it is possible that both PDGF and TGF-β signal wound contraction—one more example of the many redundancies observed in the critical processes of wound healing. In summary, wound contraction represents a complex and masterfully orchestrated interaction of cells, ECM, and cytokines.

Collagen remodeling during the transition from granulation tissue to scar is dependent on continued collagen synthesis and collagen catabolism. The degradation of wound collagen is controlled by a variety of collagenase enzymes from macrophages, epidermal cells, and fibroblasts. These collagenases are specific for particular types of collagens, but most cells probably contain two or more different types of these enzymes.[119] Three MMPs have been described that have the ability to cleave native collagen: MMP-1 or classic interstitial collagenase, which cleaves types I, II, III, XIII, and X collagens; neutrophil collagenase (MMP-8); and a novel collagenase that is prominent in chronic wounds (MMP-13).[73] Currently, it is not clear which interstitial collagenases are

critical in the remodeling stage of human wound repair. For example, no wound healing defect was observed in mice deficient of MMP-13[120]; however, a double knock-out of MMP-13 and the plasminogen activating system created an additional delay of healing compared with knock-out of only the plasminogen activating system.[77] These findings are likely attributable to the redundancy of nature.

Cytokines such as TGF-β, PDGF, IL-1, and the ECM itself clearly play an important role in the modulation of collagenase and tissue inhibitor of metalloproteinase (TIMP) expression in vivo. Interestingly, type I collagen induces MMP-1 expression through the α2β1 collagen receptor while suppressing collagen synthesis through the α1β1 collagen receptor.[121] Type I collagen also induces expression of α2β1 receptors[54]; thus, collagen can induce the receptor that signals a collagen degradation-remodeling phenotype. Such dynamic, reciprocal cell–matrix interactions appear to occur generally during tissue formation and remodeling processes such as morphogenesis, tumor growth, and wound healing.[98]

Wounds gain only about 20% of their final strength by the third week, during which time fibrillar collagen has accumulated relatively rapidly and has been remodeled by myofibroblast contraction of the wound. Thereafter, the rate at which wounds gain tensile strength is slow, reflecting a much slower rate of collagen accumulation. In fact, the gradual gain in tensile strength has less to do with new collagen deposition than further collagen remodeling with formation of larger collagen bundles and an accumulation of intermolecular crosslinks. Nevertheless, wounds fail to attain the same breaking strength as uninjured skin. At maximum strength, a scar is only 70% as strong as intact skin.

CHRONIC WOUNDS

Acute wounds are those that heal through the routine processes of inflammation, tissue formation, and remodeling, which occur in a timely fashion. As discussed earlier, these processes may overlap temporally. However, prolonged continuance of any of these reparative processes may result in the formation of a chronic wound. Chronic wounds are often associated with underlying pathological conditions that contribute to impaired healing. Venous leg ulcers and diabetic foot ulcers are common examples of chronic wounds caused or accentuated by an underlying disorder; whereas the former are induced by insufficient venous flow that results in increased blood pressure in the lower limb and, therefore, increased vascular permeability, the latter are caused by peripheral neuropathy that leads to abnormal load distribution on the foot surface and decreased sensation.[122] Subsequently, these abnormalities cause a loss of tissue viability, suboptimal local tissue permeability, and an elevated and sustained inflammatory response.

Purple ulcers caused by an effusion of blood under the skin, may be treated less seriously than they should be, especially in patients with darker pigmented skin, in whom they are difficult to identify. However, they represent full-thickness skin loss; biopsy reveals hemorrhage and early gangrenous changes. The skin may be intact or the epidermis "brushed" off, exposing a discolored area. This can rarely be reversed[32] [**Figures 16-4 and 16-5**].

ASSESSING WOUNDS

A problem for clinicians when assessing patients with darker-pigmented skin is the lack of specific guidance. However, the literature addresses general assessment of pressure ulcers, burns, and leg ulcers. Although pressure ulcer assessment tools are mostly designed for risk assessment rather than ulcer assessment,[123] a new assessment tool has been recently tested for pressure ulcer prognosis.[124] Burn injury assessment is concerned with level and extent of injury, which relates to healing prognosis and scarring.[125] Leg ulcer assessment[126] has also been related to prognosis.[127] Nevertheless, there is no written standard for wound assessment of darker-pigmented individuals.

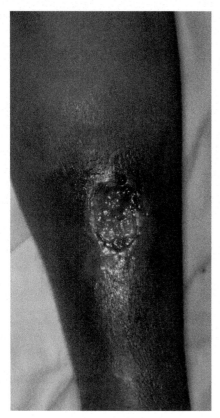

FIGURE 16-4. Purple leg ulcer caused by an effusion of blood under the skin.

As part of a comprehensive wound assessment, it is accepted practice to make a total patient assessment, including other health issues and lifestyle. It is important to know, for example, that patients have diabetes, which makes them more prone to foot and leg ulcers. The assessment and patient history should be thoroughly documented. Equally important is to document wound progress, either in writing or pictures. This is the only way to evaluate the effectiveness of treatment interventions.[128]

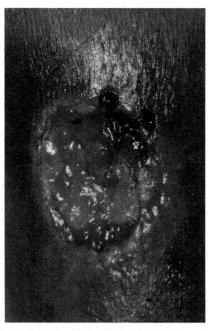

FIGURE 16-5. Purple leg ulcer (Close-up view of the leg for illustrative purpose).

GENERAL WOUND EXAMINATION

At a minimum, wound assessment should include a thorough patient examination, evaluation of the wound type, and wound characteristics such as location, size, depth, exudate, and tissue type.

Visually assessing the wound should determine its type, location, size, depth, exudate, and tissue type. The next step is a thorough physical examination of the wound and its surrounding skin. The skin surrounding a wound can provide valuable information for ongoing evaluations and future wound care management. When palpated, skin should quickly return to its original state. A slow return may indicate dehydration or be the effect of aging. Soft tissue may indicate an underlying infection. Tense skin may indicate lymphedema and cellulitis.

It is also important to assess the entire integument, not just of the wound site, looking for lesions, bruising, absence of hair, shiny skin, callus formation, and hypertrophic and keloid scars, which are more prevalent in darker-pigmented skin, as mentioned earlier. In addition, in patients with darker-pigmented skin, it is harder to detect signs of venous insufficiency such as hemosiderin deposits, characterized by the reddish-brown color as seen on the lower legs of lighter-pigmented patients with venous ulcers, ankle flare, and atrophy blanche. In such cases, patient history becomes the key to diagnosis. Skin assessment can also reveal the classic signs of arterial ulcers: hair loss, weak or absent pulses, and thin, shiny, and taut skin.

SPECIAL GUIDELINES FOR WOUND ASSESSMENT IN DARKER-PIGMENTED SKIN

Color Adjacent skin color can signal disruptions in circulation related to injury or infection. These can be diagnosed easily in lighter pigmented skin. Pressing on the area closes the capillaries, causing a blanching in lighter pigmented skin [Figure 16-3]; the color returns to normal when pressure is released.[1] Erythema is characteristic of many skin conditions, including pressure ulcers. The change in normal skin color results from the dilation of capillaries near the skin's surface and usually lasts about 2 to 5 days from the time of injury. Nonblanching erythema in lighter-pigmented skin is redness that does not disappear within 20 minutes of removing pressure. Nonblanching erythema signals erythrostasis in the capillaries and venules and hemorrhage.[2]

Erythema is more difficult to diagnose in darker-pigmented skin. Inflammation may show as a darker hue, rather than redness, often a violaceous gray [**Figures 16-6 and 16-7**]. Another complicating factor noted by Sussman[129] is differentiating inflammation from the darkening of the skin caused by hemosiderin staining. Hemosiderin staining usually occurs close to the wound edges, whereas injury-related color changes usually extend out a considerable distance and are accompanied by the other signs of inflammation.

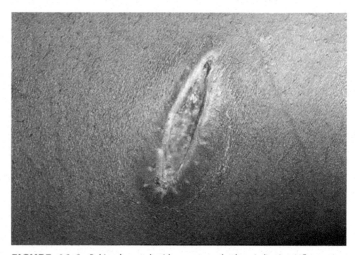

FIGURE 16-6. Dehisced wound with grey wound edges indicating inflammation. (Reproduced with permission from Knoop KJ, Stack LB, Storrow AB: Atlas of Emergency Medicine. 3rd edition. New York: McGraw-Hill; 2010. Photo contributor: Alan B. Storrow, MD.)

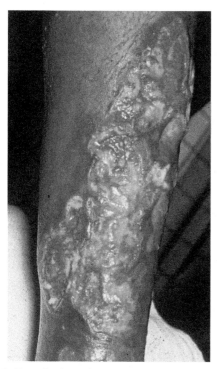

FIGURE 16-7. Venous leg ulcer with grey wound edges indicating inflammation.

Sussman[129] offers the following guidelines for assessing the extent of inflammation/trauma in darker-pigmented skin:

- Use natural light or halogen light, not fluorescent light.
- Outline the margins of color change on the surrounding skin with a marking pen.
- Select a reference point for future measures.
- Calculate the area of color change (as described for all length-by-width measurements).

Scarring As the epidermis migrates over the wound, the area covered with epithelium is pearly or silvery and shiny. In darker-pigmented skin, the color of the epithelium will be tonally related to normal skin, but as with scar tissue in lighter skin, it will be different from the surrounding undamaged epidermis [Figure 16-2]. As stated previously, hypertrophic scarring and keloids, which are abnormalities associated with the maturation phase of healing, occur more frequently in patients with darker skin. Hypertrophic scars usually regress completely in a year to 18 months, whereas keloids may grow larger over time[130] [**Figures 16-8 and 16-9**].

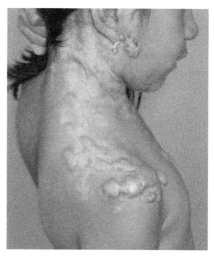

FIGURE 16-9. Scarification from a thermal burn on the posterior neck and upper back of a young Hispanic girl showing both keloids and hypertrophic scars.

Hypertrophic scars occur directly after initial repair, tend to follow the line of the incision, and are more common in young patients. Careful placing of incisions along Langer lines (incisions are made in natural creases) and fine suture material can help patients to avoid excessive scar formation.[130]

Keloid scars, by definition, are larger than the wound itself and, even if the scar is excised, the keloid scar is likely to recur. Keloid scars may appear sometime after healing and range from red to dark brown. The scars are prominent and continue to grow and spread, invading surrounding healthy tissue, whereas hypertrophic scars do not[130] [Figures 16-8 and 16-9]. Darker-pigmented skin is more likely to develop keloid scarring than lighter skin. Although the reasons are not fully understood, melanocyte-stimulating hormone (MSH) may be linked to keloid formation.[131] Perhaps a better understanding of melanocyte responses to wounding may suggest ways to prevent posthealing keloids as well as pigmentary disturbances and thus avoid the necessity for further surgical intervention [**Figures 16-10 and 16-11**].

An updated summary of chronic wound care can be found in the third edition of *Comprehensive Dermatologic Drug Therapy* edited by S.E. Wolverton.[132] Most of the basic cutaneous surgical techniques are the same for darker- and lighter-pigmented skin and are described in other chapters of this textbook. However, certain disorders requiring cutaneous surgery either occur more frequently in darker-pigmented

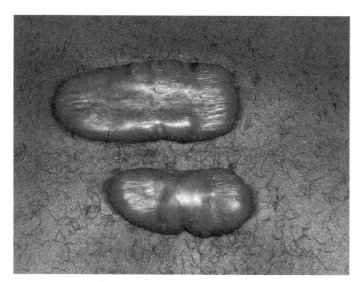

FIGURE 16-8. Horizontal keloids on the chest of a darker-pigmented man.

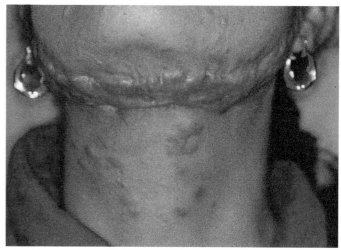

FIGURE 16-10. Ear-to-ear keloid formation secondary to an excisional surgery on a Hispanic woman.

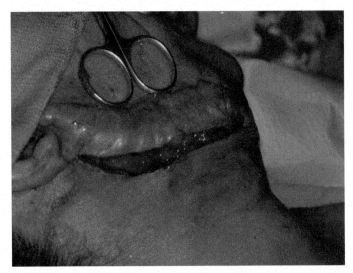

FIGURE 16-11. Keloidectomy of the patient in Figure 16-10. The patient was injected with corticosteroids at the time of excision and then four times every 2 weeks postoperatively to prevent recurrence.

patients or may require special surgical adaptations. These disorders include:

- Keloids
- Acne keloidalis
- Hidradenitis suppurativa
- Punch grafts for the vitiligo repigmentation
- Dermatosis papulosa nigra
- Dermabrasion

CONCLUSION

Medicine in general and dermatology specifically must place a greater emphasis on quality wound care for all patients, and attention needs to be focused on darker-pigmented patients as well. We emphasize that patients should not go undiagnosed because of the color of their skin. Subsequent research in education, wound healing, and pressure ulcers must include patients with darker-pigmented skin.

REFERENCES

1. Bennett MA. Report of the task force on the implications for darker pigmented intact skin in the prediction and prevention of pressure ulcers. *Adv Wound Care.* 1995;8:34-35.
2. Mehendale F, Martin P. The cellular and molecular events of wound healing: melanocytes. In: Falanga V, ed. *Cutaneous Wound Healing.* London, United Kingdom: Martin Dunitz; 2001:28-29.
3. Bickers DR, Lim HW, Margolis D, et al. The burden of skin diseases: 2004 a joint project of the American Academy of Dermatology Association and the Society for Investigative Dermatology. *J Am Acad Dermatol.* 2006;55:490-500.
4. Supp DM, Boyce ST. Engineered skin substitutes: practices and potentials. *Clin Dermatol.* 2005;23:403-412.
5. Marneros AG, Norris JE, Watanabe S, et al. Genome scans provide evidence for keloid susceptibility loci on chromosomes 2q23 and 7p11. *J Invest Dermatol.* 2004;122:1126-1132.
6. American Burn Association. Burn incidence and treatment in the United States: 2011 fact sheet. http://www.ameriburn.org/resources_factsheet.php. Accessed January 16, 2013.
7. Grinnell F, Lamke CR. Reorganization of hydrated collagen lattices by human skin fibroblasts. *J Cell Sci.* 1984;66:51-63.
8. BCC Research. Markets for advanced wound care technologies. http://www.giiresearch.com/report/bc219298-markets-advanced-wound-care-technologies.html. Accessed January 16, 2013.
9. Singer AJ, Clark RA. Cutaneous wound healing. *N Engl J Med.* 1999;341:738-746.
10. Gurtner GC, Werner S, Barrandon Y, et al. Wound repair and regeneration. *Nature.* 2008;453:314-321.
11. Zeng Q, Macri LK, Prasad A, et al. Skin tissue engineering. In: Ducheyne P, Healy KE, Hutmacher DW, et al, eds. *Comprehesive Biomaterials.* New York, NY: Elsevier; 2011:103-125.
12. Redd MJ, Cooper L, Wood W, et al. Wound healing and inflammation: embryos reveal the way to perfect repair. *Philos Trans R Soc Lond B Biol Sci.* 2004;359:777-784.
13. Martin P, Parkhurst SM. Parallels between tissue repair and embryo morphogenesis. *Development.* 2004;131:3021-3034.
14. Ito M, Yang ZX, Andl T, et al. Wnt-dependent de novo hair follicle regeneration in adult mouse skin after wounding. *Nature.* 2007;447:316-320.
15. Chuong CM. Regenerative biology: new hair from healing wounds. *Nature.* 2007;447:265-266.
16. Lyubimova A, Garber JJ, Upadhyay G, et al. Neural Wiskott-Aldrich syndrome protein modulates Wnt signaling and is required for hair follicle cycling in mice. *J Clin Invest.* 2010;120:446-456.
17. Lee LF, Jiang TX, Garner W, et al. A simplified procedure to reconstitute hair-producing skin. *Tissue Eng Part C Methods.* 2011;17:391-400.
18. Yedomon GH, Adegbidi H, Atadokpede F, et al. Keloids on dark skin: a consecutive series of 456 cases. *Med Sante Trop.* 2012;22:287-291.
19. Atiyeh BS, Costagliola M, Hayek SN. Keloid or hypertrophic scar: the controversy: review of the literature. *Ann Plast Surg.* 2005;54:676-680.
20. Lee JY, Yang CC, Chao SC, et al. Histopathological differential diagnosis of keloid and hypertrophic scar. *Am J Dermatopathol.* 2004;26:379-384.
21. Zhang X. Genome-wide association study of skin complex diseases. *J Dermatol Sci.* 2012;66:89-97.
22. Marneros AG, Norris JEC, Watanabe S, et al. Genome scans provide evidence for keloid susceptibility loci on chromosomes 2q23 and 7p11. *J Invest Dermatol.* 2004;122:1126-1132.
23. Smith JC, Boone BE, Opalenik SR, et al. Gene profiling of keloid fibroblasts shows altered expression in multiple fibrosis-associated pathways. *J Invest Dermatol.* 2008;128:1298-1310.
24. Syed F, Sherris D, Paus R, et al. Keloid disease can be inhibited by antagonizing excessive mTOR signaling with a novel dual TORC1/2 inhibitor. *Am J Pathol.* 2012;181:1642-1658.
25. Halim AS, Emami A, Salahshourifar I, et al. Keloid scarring: understanding the genetic basis, advances, and prospects. *Arch Plast Surg.* 2012;39:184-189.
26. Russell SB, Russell JD, Trupin KM, et al. Epigenetically altered wound healing in keloid fibroblasts. *J Invest Dermatol.* 2010;130:2489-2496.
27. Syed F, Bayat A. Superior effect of combination vs. single steroid therapy in keloid disease: a comparative in vitro analysis of glucocorticoids. *Wound Repair Regen.* 2013;21:88-102.
28. Viera MH, Caperton CV, Berman B. Advances in the treatment of keloids. *J Drugs Dermatol.* 2011;10:468-480.
29. Ruiz-Maldonado R, Orozco-Covarrubias ML. Postinflammatory hypopigmentation and hyperpigmentation. *Semin Cutan Med Surg.* 1997;16:36-43.
30. Moon SH, Lee SY, Jung SN, et al. Use of split thickness plantar skin grafts in the treatment of hyperpigmented skin-grafted fingers and palms in previously burned patients. *Burns.* 2011;37:714-720.
31. Tierney EP, Hanke CW. Review of the literature: treatment of dyspigmentation with fractionated resurfacing. *Dermatol Surg.* 2010;36:1499-1508.
32. Skin-lightening cosmetics: frequent, potentially severe adverse effects. *Prescrire Int.* 2011;20:209-213, 215.
33. Mistry N, Shapero J, Kundu RV, et al. Toxic effects of skin-lightening products in Canadian immigrants. *J Cutan Med Surg.* 2011;15:254-258.
34. Clark RAF. Wound repair: overview and general considerations. In: Clark RAF, ed. *The Molecular and Cellular Biology of Wound Repair.* New York, NY: Plenum Press; 1996:3-50.
35. Clark RA, Tonnesen MG, Gailit J, et al. Transient functional expression of alphaVbeta 3 on vascular cells during wound repair. *Am J Pathol.* 1996;148:1407-1421.
36. Martin P, Leibovich SJ. Inflammatory cells during wound repair: the good, the bad and the ugly. *Trends Cell Biol.* 2005;15:599-607.
37. Ashcroft GS, Yang X, Glick AB, et al. Mice lacking Smad3 show accelerated wound healing and an impaired local inflammatory response. *Nat Cell Biol.* 1999;1:260-266.
38. Cotsarelis G. Epithelial stem cells: a folliculocentric view. *J Invest Dermatol.* 2006;126:1459-1468.
39. Jacinto A, Martinez-Arias A, Martin P. Mechanisms of epithelial fusion and repair. *Nat Cell Biol.* 2001;3:E117-E123.
40. Yamada KM, Clark RAF. Provisional matrix. In: Clark RAF, ed. *Molecular and Cellular Biology of Wound Repair.* New York, NY: Plenum Press; 1996:51-93.

41. Huttenlocher A, Horwitz AR. Integrins in cell migration. *Cold Spring Harb Perspect Biol.* 2011;3:a005074.

42. Grose R, Hutter C, Bloch W, et al. A crucial role of beta 1 integrins for keratinocyte migration in vitro and during cutaneous wound repair. *Development.* 2002;129:2303-2315.

43. Kubo M, Van de Water L, Plantefaber LC, et al. Fibrinogen and fibrin are anti-adhesive for keratinocytes: a mechanism for fibrin eschar slough during wound repair. *J Invest Dermatol.* 2001;117:1369-1381.

44. Petersen MJ, Woodley DT, Stricklin GP, et al. Enhanced synthesis of collagenase by human keratinocytes cultured on type I or type IV collagen. *J Invest Dermatol.* 1990;94:341-346.

45. Stricklin GP, Nanney LB. Immunolocalization of collagenase and TIMP in healing human burn wounds. *J Invest Dermatol.* 1994;103:488-492.

46. Dejana E. Endothelial adherens junctions: implications in the control of vascular permeability and angiogenesis. *J Clin Invest.* 1996;98:1949-1953.

47. Koizumi M, Matsuzaki T, Ihara S. Expression of P-cadherin distinct from that of E-cadherin in re-epithelialization in neonatal rat skin. *Dev Growth Differ.* 2005;47:75-85.

48. Werner S. Keratinocyte growth factor: a unique player in epithelial repair processes. *Cytokine Growth Factor Rev.* 1998;9:153-165.

49. Grose R, Werner S. Wound-healing studies in transgenic and knockout mice. *Mol Biotechnol.* 2004;28:147-166.

50. Gazel A, Banno T, Walsh R, et al. Inhibition of JNK promotes differentiation of epidermal keratinocytes. *J Biol Chem.* 2006;281:20530-20541.

51. Litjens SH, de Pereda JM, Sonnenberg A. Current insights into the formation and breakdown of hemidesmosomes. *Trends Cell Biol.* 2006;16:376-383.

52. El Ghalbzouri A, Hensbergen P, Gibbs S, et al. Fibroblasts facilitate re-epithelialization in wounded human skin equivalents. *Lab Invest.* 2004;84:102-112.

53. Ueno C, Hunt TK, Hopf HW. Using physiology to improve surgical wound outcomes. *Plast Reconstr Surg.* 2006;117:59S-71S.

54. Xu J, Clark RA. Extracellular matrix alters PDGF regulation of fibroblast integrins. *J Cell Biol.* 1996;132:239-249.

55. Discher DE, Janmey P, Wang YL. Tissue cells feel and respond to the stiffness of their substrate. *Science.* 2005;310:1139-1143.

56. Vogel V, Sheetz M. Local force and geometry sensing regulate cell functions. *Nat Rev Mol Cell Biol.* 2006;7:265-275.

57. Ingber DE. Tensegrity II. How structural networks influence cellular information processing networks. *J Cell Sci.* 2003;116:1397-1408.

58. Pardoux C, Derynck R. JNK regulates expression and autocrine signaling of TGF-beta1. *Mol Cell.* 2004;15:170-171.

59. Pierce GF, Tarpley JE, Yanagihara D, et al. Platelet-derived growth factor (BB homodimer), transforming growth factor-beta 1, and basic fibroblast growth factor in dermal wound healing. Neovessel and matrix formation and cessation of repair. *Am J Pathol.* 1992;140:1375-1388.

60. Werner S, Peters KG, Longaker MT, et al. Large induction of keratinocyte growth factor expression in the dermis during wound healing. *Proc Natl Acad Sci U S A.* 1992;89:6896-6900.

61. Marikovsky M, Breuing K, Liu PY, et al. Appearance of heparin-binding EGF-like growth factor in wound fluid as a response to injury. *Proc Natl Acad Sci U S A.* 1993;90:3889-3893.

62. Grotendorst GR, Duncan MR. Individual domains of connective tissue growth factor regulate fibroblast proliferation and myofibroblast differentiation. *Faseb J.* 2005;19:729-738.

63. Mustoe TA, Pierce GF, Morishima C, et al. Growth factor-induced acceleration of tissue repair through direct and inductive activities in a rabbit dermal ulcer model. *J Clin Invest.* 1991;87:694-703.

64. Clark RA, Lanigan JM, DellaPelle P, et al. Fibronectin and fibrin provide a provisional matrix for epidermal cell migration during wound reepithelialization. *J Invest Dermatol.* 1982;79:264-269.

65. Greiling D, Clark RA. Fibronectin provides a conduit for fibroblast transmigration from collagenous stroma into fibrin clot provisional matrix. *J Cell Sci.* 1997;110:861-870.

66. Toole BP. Proteoglycans and hyaluronan in morphogenesis and differentiation. In: Hay ED, ed. *Cell Biology of the Extracellular Matrix.* New York, NY: Plenum Press; 1991:305-341.

67. Macri L, Silverstein D, Clark RA. Growth factor binding to the pericellular matrix and its importance in tissue engineering. *Adv Drug Deliv Rev.* 2007;59:1366-1381.

68. McClain SA, Simon M, Jones E, et al. Mesenchymal cell activation is the rate-limiting step of granulation tissue induction. *Am J Pathol.* 1996;149:1257-1270.

69. Schultz GS, Davidson JM, Kirsner RS, et al. Dynamic reciprocity in the wound microenvironment. *Wound Repair Regen.* 2011;19:134-148.

70. Welch MP, Odland GF, Clark RA. Temporal relationships of F-actin bundle formation, collagen and fibronectin matrix assembly, and fibronectin receptor expression to wound contraction. *J Cell Biol.* 1990;110:133-145.

71. Clark RA, Nielsen LD, Welch MP, et al. Collagen matrices attenuate the collagen-synthetic response of cultured fibroblasts to TGF-beta. *J Cell Sci.* 1995;108:1251-1261.

72. Gailit J, Xu J, Bueller H, et al. Platelet-derived growth factor and inflammatory cytokines have differential effects on the expression of integrins alpha 1 beta 1 and alpha 5 beta 1 by human dermal fibroblasts in vitro. *J Cell Physiol.* 1996;169:281-289.

73. Vaalamo M, Mattila L, Johansson N, et al. Distinct populations of stromal cells express collagenase-3 (MMP-13) and collagenase-1 (MMP-1) in chronic ulcers but not in normally healing wounds. *J Invest Dermatol.* 1997;109:96-101.

74. Circolo A, Welgus HG, Pierce GF, et al. Differential regulation of the expression of proteinases/antiproteinases in fibroblasts. Effects of interleukin-1 and platelet-derived growth factor. *J Biol Chem.* 1991;266:12283-12288.

75. Bugge TH, Kombrinck KW, Flick MJ, et al. Loss of fibrinogen rescues mice from the pleiotropic effects of plasminogen deficiency. *Cell.* 1996;87:709-719.

76. Gutierrez-Fernandez A, Inada M, Balbín M, et al. Increased inflammation delays wound healing in mice deficient in collagenase-2 (MMP-8). *FASEB J.* 2007;21:2580-2591.

77. Juncker-Jensen A, Lund LR. Phenotypic overlap between MMP-13 and the plasminogen activation system during wound healing in mice. *PLoS One.* 2011;6:e16954.

78. Pierce GF, Tarpley JE, Tseng J, et al. Detection of platelet-derived growth factor (PDGF)-AA in actively healing human wounds treated with recombinant PDGF-BB and absence of PDGF in chronic nonhealing wounds. *J Clin Invest.* 1995;96:1336-1350.

79. Roberts AB, Sporn MB, Assoian RK, et al. Transforming growth factor type beta: rapid induction of fibrosis and angiogenesis in vivo and stimulation of collagen formation in vitro. *Proc Natl Acad Sci U S A.* 1986;83:4167-4171.

80. Postlethwaite AE, Holness MA, Katai H, et al. Human fibroblasts synthesize elevated levels of extracellular matrix proteins in response to interleukin 4. *J Clin Invest.* 1992;90:1479-1485.

81. Granstein RD, Murphy GF, Margolis RJ, et al. Gamma-interferon inhibits collagen synthesis in vivo in the mouse. *J Clin Invest.* 1987;79:1254-1258.

82. Grinnell F. Fibroblasts, myofibroblasts, and wound contraction. *J Cell Biol.* 1994;124:401-404.

83. Tuan TL, Song A, Chang S, et al. In vitro fibroplasia: matrix contraction, cell growth, and collagen production of fibroblasts cultured in fibrin gels. *Exp Cell Res.* 1996;223:127-134.

84. Desmouliere A, Redard M, Darby I, et al. Apoptosis mediates the decrease in cellularity during the transition between granulation tissue and scar. *Am J Pathol.* 1995;146:56-66.

85. Desmouliere A, Badid C, Bochaton-Piallat ML, et al. Apoptosis during wound healing, fibrocontractive diseases and vascular wall injury. *Int J Biochem Cell Biol.* 1997;29:19-30.

86. Linge C, Richardson J, Vigor C, et al. Hypertrophic scar cells fail to undergo a form of apoptosis specific to contractile collagen-the role of tissue transglutaminase. *J Invest Dermatol.* 2005;125:72-82.

87. Madri JA, Sankar S, Romanic AM. Angiogenesis. In: Clark RAF, ed. *The Molecular and Cellular Biology of Wound Repair.* New York, NY: Plenum Press; 1996:355-372.

88. Tonnesen MG, Feng X, Clark RA. Angiogenesis in wound healing. *J Investig Dermatol Symp Proc.* 2000;5:40-46.

89. Cao Y. Tumor angiogenesis and molecular targets for therapy. *Front Biosci.* 2009;14:3962-3973.

90. Montrucchio G, Lupia E, de Martino A, et al. Nitric oxide mediates angiogenesis induced in vivo by platelet-activating factor and tumor necrosis factor-alpha. *Am J Pathol.* 1997;151:557-563.

91. Andrikopoulou E, Zhang X, Sebastian R, et al. Current insights into the role of HIF-1 in cutaneous wound healing. *Curr Mol Med.* 2011;11:218-235.

92. Olsson AK, Dimberg A, Kreuger J, et al. VEGF receptor signalling—in control of vascular function. *Nat Rev Mol Cell Biol.* 2006;7:359-371.

93. Eklund L, Olsen BR. Tie receptors and their angiopoietin ligands are context-dependent regulators of vascular remodeling. *Exp Cell Res.* 2006;312:630-641.

94. Folkman J, Shing Y. Angiogenesis. *J Biol Chem.* 1992;267:10931-10934.

95. Senior RM, Huang JS, Griffin GL, et al. Dissociation of the chemotactic and mitogenic activities of platelet-derived growth factor by human neutrophil elastase. *J Cell Biol.* 1985;100:351-356.

96. Chen PK, Gupta K, Wells A. Cell movement elicited by epidermal growth factor receptor requires kinase and autophosphorylation but is separable from mitogenesis. *J Cell Biol.* 1994;124:547-555.

97. Zachary I. VEGF signalling: integration and multi-tasking in endothelial cell biology. *Biochem Soc Trans.* 2003;31:1171-1177.

98. Nelson CM, Bissell MJ. Of extracellular matrix, scaffolds, and signaling: tissue architecture regulates development, homeostasis, and cancer. *Annu Rev Cell Dev Biol.* 2005;22:287-309.

99. Kubota Y, Kleinman HK, Martin GR, et al. Role of laminin and basement membrane in the morphological differentiation of human endothelial cells into capillary-like structures. *J Cell Biol.* 1988;107:1589-1598.

100. Addison CL, Nör JE, Zhao H, et al. The response of VEGF-stimulated endothelial cells to angiostatic molecules is substrate-dependent. *BMC Cell Biol.* 2005;6:38.

101. Brooks PC, Clark RA, Cheresh DA. Requirement of vascular integrin alpha v beta 3 for angiogenesis. *Science.* 1994;264:569-571.

102. Leavesley DI, Schwartz MA, Rosenfeld M, et al. Integrin beta 1- and beta 3-mediated endothelial cell migration is triggered through distinct signaling mechanisms. *J Cell Biol.* 1993;121:163-170.

103. Ku PT, D'Amore PA. Regulation of basic fibroblast growth factor (bFGF) gene and protein expression following its release from sublethally injured endothelial cells. *J Cell Biochem.* 1995;58:328-343.

104. Weis SM, Cheresh DA. V integrins in angiogenesis and cancer. *Cold Spring Harb Perspect Med.* 2011;1:a006478.

105. Singh H, Tahir TA, Alawo DO, et al. Molecular control of angiopoietin signalling. *Biochem Soc Trans.* 2011;39:1592-1596.

106. Ribatti D, Nico B, Crivellato E. The role of pericytes in angiogenesis. *Int J Dev Biol.* 2011;55:261-268.

107. Koch AE, Polverini PJ, Kunkel SL, et al. Interleukin-8 as a macrophage-derived mediator of angiogenesis. *Science.* 1992;258:1798-1801.

108. Cheresh DA, Stupack DG. Regulation of angiogenesis: apoptotic cues from the ECM. *Oncogene.* 2008;27:6285-6298.

109. Hinz B, Pittet P, Smith-Clerc J, et al. Myofibroblast development is characterized by specific cell-cell adherens junctions. *Mol Biol Cell.* 2004;15:4310-4320.

110. Gabbiani G. The myofibroblast in wound healing and fibrocontractive diseases. *J Pathol.* 2003;200:500-503.

111. Ignatius MJ, Large TH, Houde M, et al. Molecular cloning of the rat integrin alpha 1-subunit: a receptor for laminin and collagen. *J Cell Biol.* 1990;111:709-720.

112. Birk DE, Zycband EI, Winkelmann DA, et al. Collagen fibrillogenesis in situ: fibril segments are intermediates in matrix assembly. *Proc Natl Acad Sci U S A.* 1989;86:4549-4553.

113. Hinz B. Masters and servants of the force: the role of matrix adhesions in myofibroblast force perception and transmission. *Eur J Cell Biol.* 2006;85:175-181.

114. Carlson MA, Longaker MT. The fibroblast-populated collagen matrix as a model of wound healing: a review of the evidence. *Wound Repair Regen.* 2004;12:134-147.

115. Bell E, Sher S, Hull B, et al. The reconstitution of living skin. *J Invest Dermatol.* 1983;81:2S-10S.

116. Schiro JA, Chan BM, Roswit WT, et al. Integrin alpha 2 beta 1 (VLA-2) mediates reorganization and contraction of collagen matrices by human cells. *Cell.* 1991;67:403-410.

117. Woodley DT, Yamauchi M, Wynn KC, et al. Collagen telopeptides (cross-linking sites) play a role in collagen gel lattice contraction. *J Invest Dermatol.* 1991;97:580-585.

118. Follonier L, Schaub S, Meister JJ, et al. Myofibroblast communication is controlled by intercellular mechanical coupling. *J Cell Sci.* 2008;121:3305-3316.

119. Mott JD, Werb Z. Regulation of matrix biology by matrix metalloproteinases. *Curr Opin Cell Biol.* 2004;16:558-564.

120. Hartenstein B, Dittrich BT, Stickens D, et al. Epidermal development and wound healing in matrix metalloproteinase 13-deficient mice. *J Invest Dermatol.* 2006;126:486-496.

121. Langholz O, Röckel D, Mauch C, et al. Collagen and collagenase gene expression in three-dimensional collagen lattices are differentially regulated by alpha 1 beta 1 and alpha 2 beta 1 integrins. *J Cell Biol.* 1995;131:1903-1915.

122. Mustoe TA, O'Shaughnessy K, Kloeters O. Chronic wound pathogenesis and current treatment strategies: a unifying hypothesis. *Plast Reconstr Surg.* 2006;117:35S-41S.

123. Webster J, Coleman K, Mudge A, et al. Pressure ulcers: effectiveness of risk-assessment tools. A randomised controlled trial (the ULCER trial). *BMJ Qual Saf.* 2011;20:297-306.

124. Sanada H, Iizaka S, Matsui Y, et al. Clinical wound assessment using DESIGN-R total score can predict pressure ulcer healing: pooled analysis from two multicenter cohort studies. *Wound Repair Regen.* 2011;19:559-567.

125. Bezuhly M, Fish JS. Acute burn care. *Plast Reconstr Surg.* 2012;130:349e-358e.

126. Lazarus GS, Cooper DM, Knighton DR, et al. Definitions and guidelines for assessment of wounds and evaluation of healing. *Arch Dermatol.* 1994;130:489-493.

127. Margolis DJ, Berlin JA, Strom BL. Risk factors associated with the failure of a venous leg ulcer to heal. *Arch Dermatol.* 1999;135:920-926.

128. Baranoski S, Ayello EA. Wound assessment. In: Baranoski S, Ayello EA, eds. *Wound Care Essentials: Practice Principles.* New York, NY: Lippincott Williams & Wilkins; 2004:79-90.

129. Sussman C. Chapter 4: assessment of the skin and wound. In: Sussman C, Bates-Jensen B, eds. *Wound Care: A Collaborative Practice Manual for Physical Therapists and Nurses.* Aspen, CO: Aspen Publication; 1998:85-122.

130. Kelly AP. Update on the management of keloids. *Semin Cutan Med Surg.* 2009;28:71-76.

131. Stanisz H, Seifert M, Tilgen W, et al. Reciprocal responses of fibroblasts and melanocytes to alpha-MSH depending on MC1R polymorphisms. *Dermatoendocrinol.* 2011;3:259-265.

132. Kandula S, Ramachandran SM, Clark RA. Chapter 50: products for the care of chronic wounds. In: Wolverton SE, ed. *Comprehensive Dermatologic Drug Therapy.* New York, NY: Elsevier; 2013:584-592.

CHAPTER 17 — Biology of the Oral Mucosa

Yi-Ling Lin
Carol A. Bibb

KEY POINTS

- The oral mucosa is similar to the skin with respect to ectodermal derivation, histologic features of stratified squamous epithelium and underlying connective tissue, and significant barrier functions.

- The key differences between oral mucosa and skin include the moist environment of the oral cavity influenced by saliva, the presence of a biofilm of microorganisms, the mechanical and chemical stresses of mastication and diet, the presence of teeth, and the specialized sensory function of the taste buds on the tongue.

- The oral epithelium has two maturation phases: nonkeratinized and keratinized, with regional differences in the oral cavity determined by function.

- Nonkeratinized epithelium, termed *lining mucosa*, appears moist and flexible and is located on the labial and buccal mucosae, soft palate, floor of the mouth, and ventral surface of the tongue.

- Keratinized epithelium, termed *masticatory mucosa*, is typically parakeratinized but may be orthokeratinized. It appears rubbery and immobile and is located on the hard palate, attached gingiva, and dorsum of the tongue.

- The epithelium on the dorsum of the tongue is subcategorized as specialized mucosa due to the presence of taste buds on the papillae of the anterior two-thirds of the dorsal surface.

- Physiologic pigmentation is a common normal finding in the oral cavity of persons of color.

INTRODUCTION

This chapter describes the normal oral mucosa as a foundation for understanding the common oral diseases described in Chapters 56 and 57.

The oral mucosa is the lining of the oral cavity, continuous with the skin at the vermilion border of the lips. It has several similarities with skin, including derivation from ectoderm, histologic features of stratified squamous epithelium and underlying connective tissue, and significant barrier functions.

The clinician should also keep in mind important differences between the skin and oral mucosa. The first is the environment to which the oral mucosa is exposed. This environment is influenced by saliva, a variable population of microorganisms, the mechanical stresses of mastication, and chemical effects of diet. Unlike skin, oral mucosa contains minor salivary glands, which contribute to the moist environment. It does not contain skin appendages such as sweat glands and hair follicles, although sebaceous glands can be found in the oral mucosa and are called Fordyce granules (described later). Oral mucosa is coated with a plethora of bacteria, both pathogens and nonpathogens, collectively referred to as *bacterial biofilm*.[1-3] The second major difference is the unique presence of teeth that have erupted through the oral mucosa and have a specialized junction located between the crown and root with the critical function of sealing the supporting tissues of the tooth from the oral environment. The third significant difference is the specialized sensory function of the taste buds located on the tongue.

STRUCTURE OF ORAL MUCOSA

Oral mucosa consists of a surface epithelium supported by fibrous connective tissue (lamina propria). Submucosa is not always present, and when it is present, there is no muscularis mucosae separating it from the lamina propria.

ORAL EPITHELIUM

Oral mucosa is covered by stratified squamous epithelium, composed of the same cell types as those in the skin, including keratinocytes, melanocytes, Langerhans cells, and Merkel cells. Keratinocytes constitute the major cell population, and it is important to recognize that the number of melanocytes in oral mucosa is consistent in all races. Therefore, the physiologic pigmentation in the oral cavity, commonly seen in persons of color (described later), is due to increased melanocyte activity and decreased breakdown of melanosomes.

Oral epithelium follows two maturation patterns: nonkeratinization and keratinization [**Figure 17-1**]. Nonkeratinized epithelium is present on the alveolar, labial, and buccal mucosae; the soft palate; the floor of the mouth; and ventral tongue. It consists of the basal layer (stratum basale), the prickle cell layer (stratum spinosum), the intermediate layer (stratum intermedium), and the superficial layer (stratum superficiale), and has no granular cell layer. The keratinized epithelium on the oral mucosa is mostly parakeratinized; however, the epithelium can undergo orthokeratinization, and this change is considered normal. Keratinized epithelium is present on the hard plate, dorsal tongue, and attached gingiva. Keratinized epithelium is composed of the basal layer, the prickle cell layer, the granular layer (stratum granulosum), and the keratinized layer (stratum corneum). In parakeratinized epithelium, the keratinized layer contains nuclei, and the granular cell layer is difficult to identify under the light microscope. This is in contrast to the absence of nuclei of the keratinized layer and the prominent granular cell layer in orthokeratinized epithelium.

There are considerable differences in the thickness of oral epithelia in different locations of the oral cavity. Nonetheless, oral epithelium, regardless of its keratinization status, is thicker than epidermis. Although the thickness and keratinization status of the epithelium are determined by genetic factors, they can be influenced by local factors from the environment. For example, chronic irritation on the buccal mucosa caused by chewing and biting turns a nonkeratinized epithelium into a keratinized type, producing the linea alba (described later) adjacent to the occlusal plane (biting surfaces) of the posterior teeth.

LAMINA PROPRIA

Similar to the dermis of skin, the lamina propria is located beneath the oral epithelium and serves as the connective tissue support structure for the oral mucosa. It consists of cells (fibroblasts, macrophages, mast

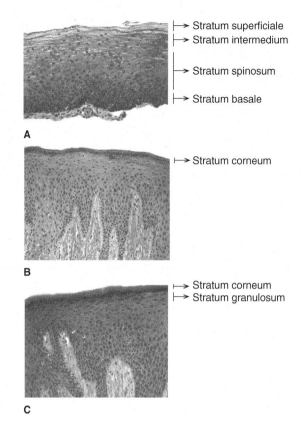

FIGURE 17-1. Hematoxylin and eosin photomicrographs of oral epithelium. **(A)** Nonkeratinized epithelium contains stratum intermedium but no stratum corneum or stratum granulosum. **(B)** Parakeratinized epithelium contains nuclei in the stratum corneum, and the stratum granulosum is difficult to identify. There is no stratum intermedium. **(C)** Orthokeratinized epithelium contains no nuclei in the stratum corneum, and the stratum granulosum is prominent. There is no stratum intermedium.

cells, and inflammatory cells), blood vessels, nerves, fibers, and ground substance. The most common cell type is the fibroblast. Similar to the surface epithelium, there is also regional variation in the lamina propria.

SALIVARY GLANDS

In oral mucosa, there are numerous minor salivary glands [**Figure 17-2**] located in or beneath the mucosa with short ducts opening directly onto the surface. Their secretion is mainly mucous in nature except for the serous Von Ebner glands in the tongue. There are also three major salivary glands—parotid, submandibular, and sublingual glands—located adjacent to but outside the oral cavity. All salivary glands contribute to the moist environment of the oral cavity.

REGIONAL DIFFERENCES IN ORAL MUCOSA

The oral cavity is divided into the vestibule and the oral cavity proper [**Figure 17-3A**]. The vestibule is limited by the gingiva and the teeth medially and by the labial and buccal mucosae laterally. The palate and tongue are the most prominent structures in the oral cavity proper. The oral mucosa can be classified as lining, masticatory, and specialized depending on location and function. Each type has characteristic clinical and histologic features.

Lining mucosa characterizes the alveolar, labial, and buccal mucosae; the soft palate; the floor of the mouth; and ventral surface of the tongue. Clinically, lining mucosa is moist, flexible, and compressible. Histologically, it is composed of nonkeratinized stratified squamous epithelium with a relatively smooth interface with the underlying lamina propria, which contains abundant elastin fibers. Masticatory mucosa is found on the hard palate and attached gingiva [**Fgure 17-3B**], regions subject to

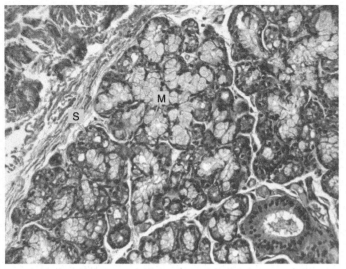

FIGURE 17-2. Hematoxylin and eosin photomicrograph of minor salivary glands. Most minor glands are mucous (M) or have a small serous (S) component, as shown here.

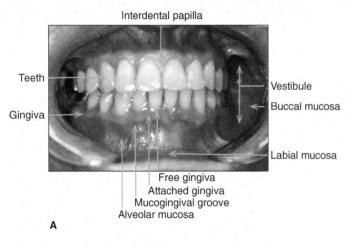

A

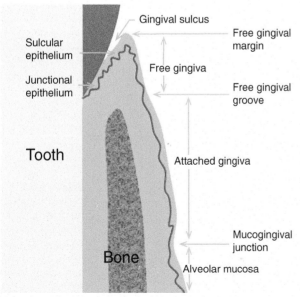

B

FIGURE 17-3. Anatomy of oral cavity and gingiva. **(A)** Oral cavity. Vestibule (shown here) is limited by the gingiva and the teeth medially and by the labial and buccal mucosae laterally. **(B)** Gingiva, attached to the underlying bone.

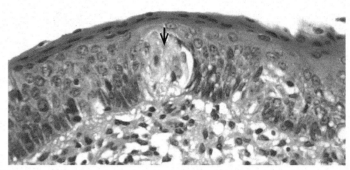

FIGURE 17-4. Hematoxylin and eosin photomicrograph of specialized mucosa (tongue) showing a taste bud (*arrow*).

masticatory stress. It is attached directly to the periosteum of the underlying bone and clinically appears rubbery and immobile. Histologically, it is composed of keratinized stratified squamous epithelium with prominent rete pegs and connective tissue papillae providing a strong interface. Specialized mucosa is found on the dorsal and lateral surfaces of the tongue. It is categorized as specialized mucosa due to the presence of taste buds [**Figure 17-4**].

LIP AND VERMILION BORDER

The external margin of the lips, that is, the transition zone between mucous membrane and skin, is known as the vermilion border [**Figure 17-5**]. It is pink to brown in color, hairless, and covered by a thin, dry epithelium. The vermilion border is clearly defined except in advanced age or with chronic sun exposure.

BUCCAL AND LABIAL MUCOSAE

Both buccal and labial mucosae are covered by a nonkeratinized epithelium, and the buccal epithelium is thicker. Both contain numerous minor salivary glands that occasionally produce a pebbly appearance. On the buccal mucosa near the second maxillary molar tooth is the parotid papilla [**Figure 17-6**], which is an elevation containing the opening of the Stensen duct from the parotid gland. Buccal mucosa is the most common site for Fordyce granules, which are sebaceous glands that appear clinically as pale yellow spots [**Figure 17-7**]. They also can be present in other oral mucosae, and it is estimated that three quarters of adults have Fordyce granules. The linea alba is also a common finding on the buccal mucosa [Figure 17-6]. It is a horizontal white line present at the level of the occlusal plane of the adjacent teeth, resulting from hyperkeratinization due to chronic mechanical irritation.

HARD AND SOFT PALATE

The hard palate is covered by a thin keratinized epithelium. The mucosa of the hard palate is firmly attached to the underlying bone, rendering

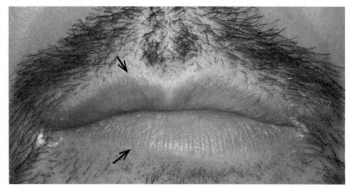

FIGURE 17-5. Vermillion border, indicated by *arrows*, is the external margin of the transitional zone between mucous membrane and skin.

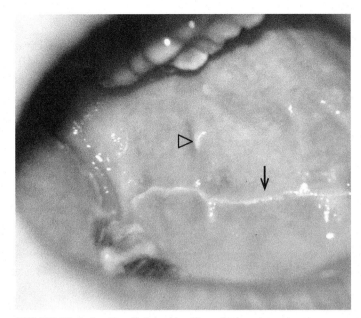

FIGURE 17-6. Parotid papilla (*triangle*) and linear alba (*arrow*).

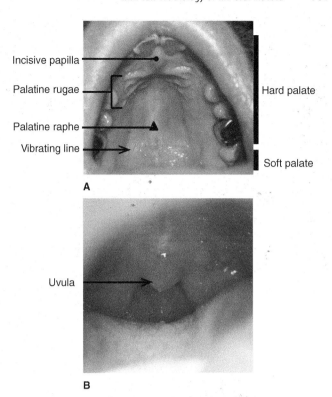

FIGURE 17-8. Anatomy of palate. (**A**) Hard palate: incisive papilla (*circle*), palatine rugae (*bracket*), palatine raphe (*triangle*), and vibrating line (*arrow*). (**B**) Soft palate: uvula (*arrow*).

it slightly paler than the rest of the oral mucosae [**Figure 17-8A**]. The incisive papilla is located in the anterior portion of the hard palate immediately behind the two central maxillary incisors. Adjacent and posterior to the incisive papilla, ridges called palatine rugae radiate laterally. The palatine raphe is a slightly elevated ridge that runs from the incisive papilla to the soft palate in the midline. Minor salivary glands are also found bilaterally and off the midline in the posterior third of the hard palate. The excretory ducts of these glands appear as small umbilicated papules.

The soft palate lies posterior to the hard palate beginning at the vibrating line [Figure 17-8A]. The soft palate has no bone support and is covered by a thin, nonkeratinized epithelium. It is rich in blood vessels; hence, it is redder than the hard palate. Minor salivary glands are also found in the soft palatal mucosa. The uvula is a conical projection from the posterior edge of the middle of the soft palate [**Figure 17-8B**].

GINGIVA AND ALVEOLAR MUCOSA

Anatomically, gingiva is divided into free marginal gingiva and attached gingiva by the free marginal groove, both covered by thick keratinized epithelium [Figure 17-3A]. From the upper border of the free gingiva, the interdental papillae emerge with their characteristic triangular shape

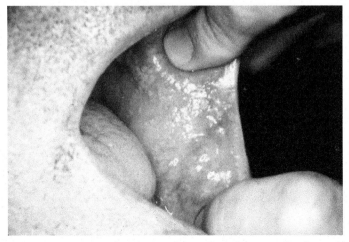

FIGURE 17-7. Fordyce granules are sebaceous glands that appear clinically as pale yellow spots on buccal mucosa.

occupying the spaces between the teeth. The marginal end of the gingiva folds over the tooth surface and attaches itself to the tooth below the gingival border. The gingival sulcus is the space between a tooth and gingiva [**Figure 17-3B**]. It is lined by sulcular epithelium from the base to the free gingival margin. The base is lined by the junctional epithelium, which surrounds the tooth like a collar. Both junctional and sulcular epithelia are nonkeratinized, and junctional epithelium is very thin, consisting of only two to five cell layers. The depth of the sulcus in a healthy individual varies from 1 to 3 mm. The attached gingiva extends from the free gingival groove to the beginning of the alveolar crest and is continuous with the alveolar mucosa, which is covered by a nonkeratinized epithelium [Figure 17-3B]. The mucogingival junction is identified by a slight indentation, called the mucogingival groove, and also by the color from the paler pink of the gingiva to the bright pink of the alveolar mucosa due to differences in the keratinization status [Figure 17-3A]. The gingiva is the most frequent site of occurrence of physiologic oral melanin pigmentation[4] [**Figure 17-9**], and the incisor area has the highest rate, which decreases considerably in the posterior areas.[5] Clinically, it manifests as multifocal or diffuse melanin pigmentation. Pigmentation varies in prevalence among different races, and dark-skinned people have a higher prevalence of oral pigmentation, although this phenomenon is not confined to those of African descent.[6,7]

TONGUE

The mucosa of the dorsum of the tongue is covered by a thick epithelium exhibiting lingual papillae with keratinized and nonkeratinized surfaces. It binds directly to the underlying muscle and has the thickest epithelium in the oral cavity. The tongue is divided into two parts by a V-shaped groove, the sulcus terminalis (terminal groove) [**Figure 17-10A**]. The anterior two-thirds of the tongue is derived from the ectoderm and is the functional, or tasting, portion of the tongue. The posterior third is derived from the endoderm; it is the lymphatic portion because it contains the lingual tonsils.

The anterior two-thirds of the dorsal tongue is covered by densely arranged filiform papillae with scattered fungiform papillae, giving this area a rough, white appearance [**Figure 17-10B**]. The filiform papillae

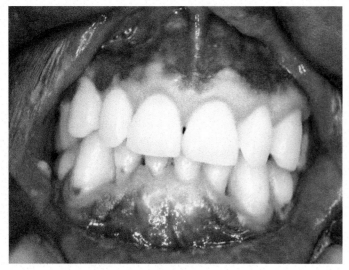

FIGURE 17-9. Physiologic pigmentation in the gingiva.

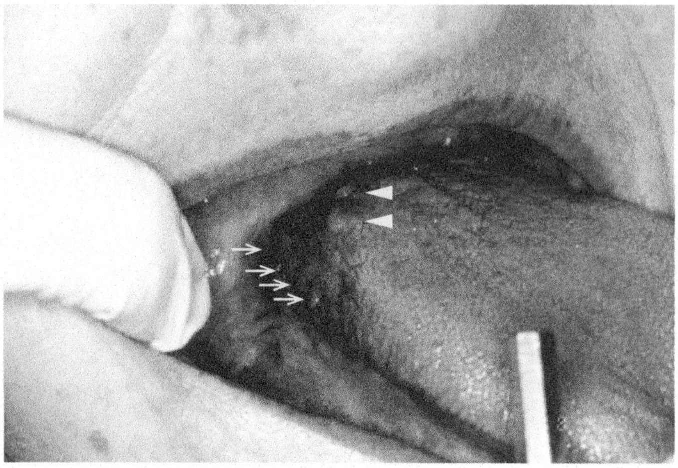

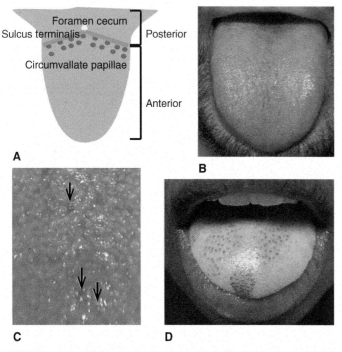

FIGURE 17-11. Circumvallate papillae (*triangles*) and foliate papillae and lingual tonsils (*arrows*).

are hairlike, are covered by a keratinized epithelium, and appear white. The fungiform papillae are smooth and round, are covered by non-keratinized epithelium, and appear red [**Figure 17-10C**]. Brown or black accumulation of melanin pigmentation has been reported in the fungiform papillae in African Americans and other people with skin of color [**Figure 17-10D**]. Adjacent and anterior to the sulcus terminalis are 10 to 12 round and flat circumvallate papillae [Figure 17-10A and **Figure 17-11**]. They are covered by nonkeratinized epithelium and converge at the angle of the V at the site of the foramen cecum, which represents the site of origin of the thyroid gland. Von Ebner glands, the only serous glands of the minor salivary glands, are present beneath the circumvallate papillae. Foliate papillae are found on the posterior lateral surface of the tongue [Figure 17-11]. They resemble leaves, and the surface is not keratinized. Lingual tonsils are found immediately beneath

the foliate papillae. The tongue is the primary organ of taste, and all but filiform papillae contain taste buds.

The ventral tongue is covered by a thin, nonkeratinized epithelium and contains a plexus of veins. Sublingual administration of drugs is an ideal route for introducing certain medications to the body. This is due to the thin surface and rich vascularity that allows direct access of the medication to the cardiovascular system, avoiding drug degradation by bypassing the gastrointestinal tract. The lingual frenulum is located in the midline of the floor of the mouth, extending from the mandibular gingiva to the ventral surface of the tongue [**Figure 17-12**].

◼ FLOOR OF THE MOUTH

The floor of the mouth is covered by a thin, nonkeratinized epithelium and is a continuation of the ventral lingual mucosa on one side, whereas on the other side, it is reflected onto the gingiva. The openings of the submandibular and sublingual glands are seen as elevated, crater-like structures (sublingual caruncles) at each side of the lingual frenum [Figure 17-12]. The sublingual folds are elevations seen at each side of the midline produced by the sublingual glands.

TURNOVER OF ORAL MUCOSA

Epithelial homeostasis is maintained by constant cell production in the deeper layers and loss of cells from the surface. In general, lining mucosa has a higher turnover rate than masticatory mucosa, and the average cell cycle time of oral epithelium is around 63 hours (between 2.5 and 3 days).[8] Oral epithelium has a faster turnover rate than skin, which serves as an important protective mechanism limiting colonization and invasion of microorganisms adherent to the mucosal surface.[9] These relative turnover times have clinical significance in the context of healing and repair of the oral tissues.

FIGURE 17-10. (A) Tongue anatomy: sulcus terminalis (*blue line*), foramen cecum (*yellow circle*), and circumvallate papillae (*red circle*). **(B)** Dorsal tongue. **(C)** Fungiform papillae (*arrows*) appear red and are scattered among densely packed filiform papillae. **(D)** Pigmented fungiform papillae.

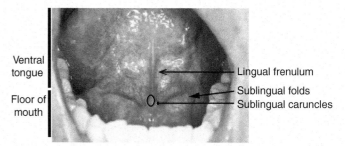

FIGURE 17-12. Ventral tongue and floor of mouth.

REFERENCES

1. Duncan MJ. Genomics of oral bacteria. *Crit Rev Oral Biol Med.* 2003;14:175-187.
2. Wada K, Kamisaki Y. Roles of oral bacteria in cardiovascular diseases—from molecular mechanisms to clinical cases: involvement of *Porphyromonas gingivalis* in the development of human aortic aneurysm. *J Pharmacol Sci.* 2010;113:115-119.
3. Aas JA, Paster BJ, Stokes LN, Olsen I, Dewhirst FE. Defining the normal bacterial flora of the oral cavity. *J Clin Microbiol.* 2005;43:5721-5732.
4. Dummett CO, Barens G. Oromucosal pigmentation: an updated literary review. *J Periodontol.* 1971;42:726-736.
5. Tamizi M, Taheri M. Treatment of severe physiologic gingival pigmentation with free gingival autograft. *Quintessence Int.* 1996;27:555-558.
6. Mishiro Y, Ogihara K, Zhang Y, Hu D. Gingival pigmentation in preschool children of Chengdu, West China. *J Pedod.* 1990;14:150-151.
7. Gorsky M, Buchner A, Fundoianu-Dayan D, Aviv I. Physiologic pigmentation of the gingiva in Israeli Jews of different ethnic origin. *Oral Surg Oral Med Oral Pathol.* 1984;58:506-509.
8. Thomson PJ, Potten CS, Appleton DR. Mapping dynamic epithelial cell proliferative activity within the oral cavity of man: a new insight into carcinogenesis? *Br J Oral Maxillofac Surg.* 1999;37:377-383.
9. Squier CA, Kremer MJ. Biology of oral mucosa and esophagus. *J Natl Cancer Inst Monogr.* 2001;29:7-15.

CHAPTER 18

Acute Effects of Light on Skin

Virginia J. Reeder

Henry W. Lim

KEY POINTS

- Different wavelengths of solar radiation stimulate a diverse range of biologic effects within human skin.
- Biologic responses of skin to solar radiation are variable not only by the dose and wavelength of the radiation itself, but also by the phototype of the skin absorbing the radiation.
- For a biologic process in the skin to result from exposure to solar radiation, there must be a chromophore within the exposed skin capable of absorbing the wavelengths of the incident solar radiation.
- Acute effects of solar radiation on human skin include: erythema, pigment darkening, epidermal cell proliferation, vitamin D synthesis, and immunomodulation.

The studies of Sir Isaac Newton in the seventeenth century and his discovery of the visible light spectrum are recognized as a turning point in photobiology.[1] More than a century later, Sir William Herschel and Johann Ritter furthered the understanding of optical radiation with their discoveries of infrared and ultraviolet (UV) radiation, respectively.[2,3] In the intervening centuries, investigations into the properties of solar radiation have focused primarily on the UV spectrum. More recently, however, interest has arisen concerning the impact of visible light and infrared radiation. The acute effects of exposure to solar radiation, which will be reviewed in this chapter, include erythema, pigment darkening, epidermal cell proliferation, vitamin D synthesis, and immunomodulation.

Biologic responses of human skin to optical radiation vary by the dose and wavelength of the radiation as well as by the phototype of the skin absorbing the radiation.[4,5] Radiation is the transfer of energy via particles (photons) and waves that propagate through space.[6] The energy of each photon has an inverse relationship to its wavelength, which is the best predictor of the biologic impact that radiation will have on the skin.[5] There are three possible ways by which electromagnetic radiation can interact with the skin: reflection, scattering, or

absorption.[6] Reflection occurs when the radiation bounces off of the surface of the skin. When reflected, there is no biological impact, but this phenomenon can be used to gain information about the topography of the skin surface, and it allows the retina to perceive the color of the skin.[6] Scatter occurs when the direction of the radiation wave propagation is physically altered by interaction with components of the skin. Shorter wavelength radiation is more likely to scatter, which means that shorter wavelengths are less likely to penetrate to deeper portions of any substrate, including the skin.[6] This is the reason why the shortest wavelength UV rays, UVC, do not reach the surface of the earth because they are absorbed in the atmosphere. Radiation that is not reflected or scattered may be absorbed by molecules (known as chromophores) in the skin.[6] When radiation is absorbed by molecules within the skin, the energy of the photons is transferred to these molecules.[5] This energy may then be processed in one of three ways: the energy may drive biologic reactions within the skin; the energy may be released as heat; or the energy may be released as longer wavelength radiation, a process called fluorescence or phosphorescence.[6] Each molecule within the skin has the capacity to absorb a unique range of radiation wavelengths, which is determined by the chemical and molecular structure of the molecule itself.[5] The wavelengths that are likely to be absorbed by a particular chromophore are called its absorption spectrum.[5] Without chromophores that can absorb radiation, photobiologic events cannot occur.[6]

SOLAR RADIATION

UV radiation comprises the 100- to 400-nm portion of the spectrum emitted by the sun. UV is further subdivided by wavelength into three spectral regions: UVA, UVB, and UVC. This convention was first introduced in the 1930s, and these spectral regions of UV were initially based on which wavelengths were able to pass through various filters rather than on the biologic effects the UV might have upon human skin. UVA was defined as 315 to 400 nm, UVB as 280 to 315 nm, and UVC as less than 280 nm.[5,7] Currently, these remain the official definitions of the spectral regions of UV radiation according to the Commission Internationale de l'Eclairage (CIE). However, in photobiology, the convention has become to divide UV by the biologic activity of the wavelengths.[5] For the purposes of this chapter, we will use the conventions of photomedicine: UVA, 320 to 400 nm, UVB, 290 to 320 nm, and UVC, 200 to 290 nm.[5] In recognition of the fact that the biologic properties of short-wavelength UVA are closer to those of UVB, UVA is now divided into two spectral regions: UVA1 (340 to 400 nm) and UVA2 (320 to 340 nm).[5]

Solar radiation that reaches the surface of the earth encompasses the wavelengths from 290 to 4000 nm[6] [**Table 18-1**]. Thus, little to no UVC radiation reaches the surface of the earth except perhaps at very high altitudes.[5] It has been estimated that UV radiation constitutes approximately 7% of terrestrial solar radiation, with 5% being UVB and 95%

TABLE 18-1   Components of sunlight

Component	Wavelength (nm)	Composition of sunlight at earth's surface
Ultraviolet (UV) radiation	100–400	7%
UVC	200–290	
UVB	290–320	
UVA	320–400	
UVA2	320–340	
UVA1	340–400	
Visible light	400–760	39%
Infrared radiation (IR)	760–1,000,000	54%
IR-A	760–1400	
IR-B	1400–3000	
IR-C	3000–100,000	

TABLE 18-2 Skin phototypes

Phototype	Ability to tan	Propensity to sunburn
I	None	Always
II	With difficulty	High
III	Medium tan	Moderate
IV	Dark tan	Low
V	Tans very easily	Very low
VI	Tans very easily	Exceedingly low

UVA.[8] Thirty-nine percent of visible light reaches the earth's surface, which comprises a higher proportion than UV.[8,9] Visible light, between 400 and 760 nm, is defined as the spectrum of electromagnetic radiation that can be appreciated by the retina.[5] At different wavelengths within this spectrum, the human eye will perceive light as various colors, from blue (shortest wavelength) to red (longest wavelength).[5] Infrared radiation (IR) is defined as electromagnetic radiation with wavelengths from 760 nm to 1 mm.[8,10] IR radiation has been estimated to make up 54% of the solar radiation that reaches the surface of the earth; it imparts the sensation of warmth upon exposure to the skin. IR is divided into IR-A (760 to 1400 nm), IR-B (1400 to 3000 nm), and IR-C (3000 nm to 1 mm).[11] Another commonly used and very similar division for IR uses slightly different terminology: near IR (760 to 3000 nm), middle IR (3000 to 30,000 nm), and far IR (30,000 nm to 1 mm).[11] In this chapter, we will use the IR-A, IR-B, and IR-C subclassification.

SKIN TYPE

The most widely used classification of skin types, Fitzpatrick skin phototypes, is based on susceptibility of individuals to sunburn, as well as the constitutive color of the skin [**Table 18-2**]. Sunburn, or erythema, is predominantly caused by UVB and, to a lesser extent, UVA2. Constitutive skin color is a reflection of the ratio of the type (eumelanin or pheomelanin) and the amount of melanin present in the skin.[12,13] It should be emphasized that the differences in skin color and response to solar radiation are not due to differences in the number of melanocytes in the skin but rather to differences in the number, size, and distribution of melanin containing pigment granules known as melanosomes that are produced by melanocytes, as well as the type of melanin that is contained within the melanosomes.[12,13]

ACUTE EFFECTS OF SOLAR RADIATION: MOLECULAR MECHANISMS

With its longer wavelengths, UVA is able to penetrate more deeply into the skin than UVB. The majority of UVA radiation reaches the dermis of the skin, whereas the majority of UVB is absorbed in the epidermis with only a small fraction reaching the dermis.[14-16] Nevertheless, because of the close interaction between the epidermis and the dermis, both UVA and UVB radiation have major biologic effects on the skin.[14] DNA serves as a primary chromophore for UVB, but it can also absorb UVA.[14,17-21] DNA is located in living skin cells, all of which are located beneath the protective stratum corneum layer of the epidermis. The stratum corneum reflects and scatters some of the radiation, predominantly the shorter wavelengths, that reaches the surface of the skin. It is estimated that the wavelength most efficient at reaching and being absorbed by DNA is around 313 nm, which is included in the UVB spectrum.[14] The most common result of UV absorption by DNA is the formation of cyclobutane pyrimidine dimers (CPDs),[14] with thymine dimers being a specific type of CPD. Exposure to both UVB and UVA is now known to generate CPD formation. Other end products are pyrimidine (6-4) pyrimidone photoproducts[14] and Dewar valence isomers, which are isomers of pyrimidine (6-4) pyrimidone products.[22,23] CPDs have been

reported to be 20 to 40 times more likely to be formed than any other photoproduct.[24] CPDs are also thought to be the most mutagenic of the direct photoproducts and, if not repaired correctly, may lead to carcinogenesis or cell death.[25]

The primary chromophore for UVA remains unknown. However, it is known that exposure to UVA results in the generation of reactive oxygen species (ROS), which alter the chemical structure of DNA, lipids, and proteins.[25,26] When ROS interacts with DNA, the most common end product is 8-oxo-7,8-dihydro-2'-deoxyguanosine (8-oxodG), which results from oxidation of the 8 position of guanine.[14] ROS also induces alteration of membrane lipids, which increases phospholipase activity and prostaglandins.[27] UVA may also react with melanin to produce ROS that generates breaks in DNA.[28] In comparison to UVB, UVA produces relatively more indirect, oxidative damage to DNA.[25] However, when looking at the effects of UVA on DNA independently, it is worth mentioning that UVA produces three to six times more CPDs than 8oxodG.[29] It is thought that UVB likely produces ROS as well but at proportionally far less quantities than UVA; there are few empirical data in this area.[25] Exposure to UVA also results in the release of nitric oxide into the skin.[30-32] Suschek et al[32] demonstrated that exposure to UVA can increase nitric oxide serum levels by 40%.

UV radiation affects cells through other chromophores in addition to DNA, such as melanin and urocanic acid. Tryptophan, tyrosine, and other aromatic amino acids are chromophores for UVB radiation and represent a mechanism by which UVB affects cellular proteins.[5] 7-Dehydrocholesterol is also a chromophore for UVB, which, as we will discuss further, plays an important role in the synthesis of vitamin D.[5]

Visible light, being of longer wavelengths than UV, is less prone to scatter and is thus able to penetrate more deeply into the skin. Chromophores for visible light include porphyrins, β-carotene, melanin, riboflavin, hemoglobin, bilirubin, and water.[33] However, there is much less information regarding the specific processes and mediators induced through the absorption of visible light by these molecules. It is known that visible light contributes greatly to the amount of indirect DNA damage occurring via oxidative mechanisms.[34] An ex vivo study specifically investigating free radical formation after exposure to solar radiation noted that visible light was responsible for 33% of the ROS formed and UVA was responsible for 67%.[35] Another study noted that wavelengths between 400 and 500 nm induce about 10% of the total oxidative damage that occurs in cells following exposure to sunlight.[36]

Because photon energy is inversely proportional to wavelength, even the shortest wavelength of IR has only about a third of the energy associated with UVB radiation.[8] Although IR makes up approximately half of incident solar radiation reaching human skin, IR has not been studied as thoroughly as UV.[37,38] Because longer wavelength IR is strongly absorbed by water in the epidermis, the depth of penetration in the skin for IR decreases with increasing wavelength.[11] Thus, within the IR spectrum, in contrast to UV, shorter wavelengths penetrate more deeply into the skin. Although a small amount of IR-A, the shortest wavelength IR, is absorbed in the epidermis, nearly half is absorbed in the dermis and 17% penetrates into the deeper subcutaneous tissues. It has been estimated that 65% of IR-A reaches the dermis or deeper tissues.[38] Only a small amount of IR-B penetrates into the dermis and subcutaneous tissues because the majority is absorbed in the epidermis, and 100% of IR-C is absorbed in the epidermis.[11] Due to its long wavelength, IR-A penetrates more deeply into the skin than any of the spectral regions of sunlight.[38] Because the majority of the terrestrial IR is in the IR-A range, it is estimated that IR-A composes approximately one-third of the solar radiation experienced by human skin.[39] Although all absorbed solar radiation is capable of producing some heat, absorbed IR is more prone to increasing skin temperature than other portions of this spectrum.[11] Exposure to IR may generate a sensation in the skin ranging from warmth to the pain like that associated with a thermal burn.[11] Of note, the thermal effects of IR are correlated to the irradiance (ie, rate of delivery of energy) rather than the dose.[40] Similar to UVA, exposure to IR can induce the release of nitric oxide stores in the skin.[41]

TABLE 18-3	Components of sunlight and erythema			
	UVB radiation	UVA radiation	Visible light	IR
Onset of erythema	Immediate possible in light-skinned individuals. More common: delayed onset with peak between 6 and 24 hours.	Immediate. Some studies report a second peak between 6 and 24 hours.	Immediate, only in darker-skinned individuals. No erythema in fairer-skinned individuals.	Immediate.
Resolution of erythema	Up to 2 weeks in light skin types. Up to 72 hours for darker skin types.	Most studies report biphasic response with immediate erythema resolving within 4 hours. Delayed erythema fades after 24 hours.	Within 2 hours.	Within 1 hour.

Abbreviations: IR, infrared radiation; UV, ultraviolet.

ERYTHEMA

Acute exposure to any portion of the spectrum of solar radiation, including UV, visible light, or IR, may result in erythema of the skin, which is commonly known as sunburn [Table 18-3]. Sunburn is associated not only with erythema but also with tenderness, warmth, and swelling of the skin.[42] The severity of the sunburn is typically directly proportional to the amount of energy absorbed by the skin. Total energy delivered to the skin is equivalent to the dose delivered multiplied by the time period over which the dose is administered, which is a concept known as the law of reciprocity.[42] Thus, higher doses of radiation over shorter periods of time are equivalent to lower doses continuously delivered over longer periods of time.[42] When larger amounts of body surface area are sunburned, affected individuals may experience systemic symptoms, including fever, headache, nausea, or vomiting.[42] Although it may be difficult to perceive erythema in those individuals with skin of color, the symptoms of sunburn are similar among people with different skin types.[43] The dose of UV exposure required to produce these symptoms is, however, variable by skin type.[43]

Although UVB comprises only about 0.5% of the solar radiation that reaches the surface of the earth, it is the primary component responsible for the acute erythema following exposure to sunlight.[8,10] UVB is approximately 1000 times more effective at producing erythema than UVA.[42,44] A study of the action spectrum of formation of thymidine dimers in individuals with skin types II and III showed a peak at 300 nm in the upper layer of living epidermis. The action spectrum for the 6-4 photoproducts is not known but is suspected to be similar to that for the thymidine dimers.[25] The erythema action spectrum in these skin types is similar to the action spectrum for thymidine dimer formation, supporting the concept that DNA is the major chromophore for erythema.[17] CPDs and the 6-4 photoproducts trigger the release of various inflammatory mediators, including cytokines, histamine, kinins, eicosanoids, and other chemotactic factors, resulting in the clinically observed changes of erythema, warmth, and tenderness.[27,42] It is possible for the erythema induced by UVB to be seen immediately in skin types I and II.[42] However, the more typical response to UVB is a delayed erythema that peaks somewhere between 6 and 24 hours after exposure.[42,45,46] The persistence of erythema due to UVB is variable by skin type, with erythema in lighter-skinned individuals lasting for up to 2 weeks.[46] Those with darker skin types may experience resolution of erythema by 72 hours after exposure.[47]

As previously mentioned, UVA is far less erythemogenic than UVB and requires much higher doses to produce this effect on the skin. Shorter wavelength UVA (UVA2) behaves in a fashion similar to UVB and may cause some erythema via direct DNA damage with formation of CPDs and thymine dimers.[42] Longer UVA wavelengths (UVA1) are known to result in indirect damage to DNA via oxidative mechanisms but are thought to also cause some direct damage to DNA by using DNA as a chromophore.[48] In a recent study, UVA1 was shown to produce CPDs but, interestingly, did not produce thymine dimers.[48] Additionally, in patients with comparable amounts of erythema resulting from exposure to UVA1 versus UVB, it was noted that UVA1 produced fewer dimers located deeper within the skin, whereas UVB produced more dimers located more superficially within the skin.[48] UVA, particularly

UVA1, produces erythema only at very high doses and is more likely to produce erythema in fairer-skinned individuals.[18,49] Mahmoud et al[9] specifically investigated the effects of UVA1 on individuals with different skin types and noted that there was no erythema in response to UVA1 in all skin types at doses up to 60 J/cm^2.[9] With dosing high enough to induce erythema, both monophasic and biphasic erythema have been reported following exposure to UVA. Studies reporting a biphasic response describe an immediate erythema that quickly resolves and is followed by a delayed erythema that peaks within minutes to hours.[50-52] The immediate erythema is reported to fade at least partially prior to the development of a delayed response that peaks within 6 to 24 hours.[46,51] Other studies report a monophasic response to UVA with development of immediate erythema.[53,54] In a study of individuals with skin types II and III, Kaidbey and Kligman[54] described a monophasic response to UVA with the erythema developing immediately after exposure. The threshold dose for erythema induction was 13 J/cm^2, and at this dose, the erythema was transient. Larger doses produced more intense erythema that persisted for longer durations of time. This was directly proportional to dosing with higher fluences resulting in longer duration of erythema.[54] At the highest doses administered, the erythema persisted unchanged for longer than 24 hours, but the investigators did not note a biphasic response.[54] Another study noted that peak erythema for both UVA1 and broadband UVA was within 1 hour after exposure.[53] In addition to the erythemogenic effects of CPDs previously discussed, UVA, and to a lesser extent, UVB also contribute to the sunburn response via production of ROS, which also induce inflammatory mediators such as prostaglandins.[27]

High fluencies in the visible light spectrum can also induce an immediate erythema.[9,33,55] Until recently, one difficulty with investigations into the effects of visible light has been the need for a light source that emits radiation falling only within the visible light portion of the electromagnetic spectrum. Even some filtered light sources designed with the goal of emitting wavelengths only between 400 and 700 nm are not 100% effective at blocking all UV and IR components. One study exposed 20 subjects with skin types II to IV to visible light and noted an immediate erythema that faded by 24 hours after the exposure.[56] Notably, in this study, the filter used allowed longer UVA wavelengths to be present in the filtered light source.[9,56] The authors speculated that the erythema induced by visible light might be created via thermal mechanisms.[56] Mahmoud et al[9] used a light source emitting 98.3% visible light on individuals with type V or VI skin and noted an immediate central pigment darkening with a surrounding ill-defined halo of erythema. Because this study used a more effective filter, there were less IR and UV components, so these results likely better represent the true effects of visible light than the first study, whose report of the 24-hour duration of the immediate erythema may have been influenced by the UVA1 component. Mahmoud et al[9] found that the immediate erythema associated with visible light exposure faded over the course of 90 to 120 minutes and that the intensity of the erythema was proportional to the dose of visible light administered. Interestingly, in the same study, administration of equivalent and greater doses of visible light to individuals with type II skin showed that, even at much higher fluences, no erythema could be elicited in these fairer-skinned subjects.[9] The authors postulated that the absorption of visible light by melanin may produce heat.[9] Individuals with skin of color have more melanin and therefore may generate more heat in response to absorption of visible light. This thermal energy may lead to vasodilation of vessels in the subpapillary plexus of the deeper dermis, which manifests as erythema.[9]

IR absorbed in the epidermis results in an increase in skin temperature, which can produce thermal pain and injury.[40] Several studies have documented acute erythema following exposure of the skin to IR, which has been described as appearing within 1 minute of irradiation.[57] Pujol and Lecha[57] treated 24 subjects with skin types II and III with IR and noted an immediate erythema that extended outside of the boundaries of the area that was treated with the radiation. They also found that this erythema was nearly imperceptible at 10 minutes following exposure and totally resolved within 1 hour.[57] It is unclear whether this immediate erythema represents a thermal response or a vasodilatory response, or perhaps a combination of both phenomena. It has been noted that when the skin reaches approximately 40°C, local vasodilator responses are activated to promote skin cooling, which protects the skin from thermal injury.[10] This vasodilation may result in the appearance of erythema. Another study looked at the effects of IR-A in mice and found that although the temperature of the skin increased, there was no measurable erythema at doses between 30 and 60 J/cm[2].[58] The skin temperature of the mice reached an average maximum of 31.2°C ± 1.3°C, which may not have been high enough to activate a vasodilator response and returned to baseline within 30 minutes following the irradiation with IR.[58] Histologic examination of the mouse skin after irradiation showed no inflammatory changes such as inflammatory cell infiltrate or edema.

Another study exposed 28 individuals to a light source emitting 90% broad-spectrum IR and 10% visible light and found that higher doses ranging between 187 and 295 J/m[2] were required to induce erythema, which was described as being reticular in pattern.[59] In 27 of the 28 subjects, the erythema was immediate and monophasic and faded within 4 hours, but in one subject, a biphasic erythema was noted.[59] Histologic studies of the skin of these subjects were significant for perivascular degranulated mast cells and dilated vessels.[59] Similar in concept to the minimal erythema dose (MED) for UV radiation, Pujol and Lecha[57] came up with a standard IR dose based on the immediate erythema they noted following irradiation with IR, which they called the *minimal response dose* (MRD). Lee et al[10] later argued that this MRD lacked consistency and promoted the use of a new standard unit, which they termed the *minimal heating dose* (MHD).[10] These authors note that erythema following IR is variable by the radiation dose and wavelength and thus cannot be considered as a reliable comparator for determination of IR irradiation dosing between individuals. They describe the MHD as the point at which the skin temperature stops changing when being irradiated with a constant wavelength at a given irradiance. They found that as long as the skin temperature was above 41°C, MHD was constant and independent of radiation dose.[10] They found no relationship between the MHD and erythema or the amount of melanin in the skin.[10] Ultimately, current investigations support a thermal etiology of the immediate erythema following exposure to IR, and there has been no systematic investigation into whether the effects of IR vary among the various skin types.

PIGMENTATION

Exposure to solar radiation results in darkening of skin pigment. All components of solar radiation reaching the earth's surface contribute to the process except for IR [**Table 18-4**]. Darkening of skin pigment can be divided temporally into distinct stages, including immediate pigment darkening (IPD), persistent pigment darkening (PPD), and delayed tanning (DT).[60] IPD and PPD are the result of redistribution and oxidation of the melanin that already exists within the skin and do not represent production of new melanin, whereas DT is the result of new melanogenesis.[60] IPD appears immediately following exposure to solar radiation and disappears within minutes to an hour following the exposure.[9,42,61,62] IPD is observed more dramatically in individuals with darker skin type, who have more melanin present in the skin. IPD can occur following

TABLE 18-4   Components of sunlight and pigmentation

UVB	UVA2	UVA1	Visible light
All skin types: Erythema followed by delayed tanning	Fairer skin types: Erythema followed by delayed tanning Darker skin types: IPD (gray color) followed by PPD	IPD (gray color) followed by PPD	IPD (brown color) followed by PPD

Abbreviations: IPD, immediate pigment darkening; PPD, persistent pigment darkening; UV, ultraviolet.

exposure to UVA and visible light. Whereas UVB is known to be more erythemogenic than UVA, UVA is much more effective at producing pigment darkening than UVB.[42,63] Although UVA1 produces IPD in all individuals, the response to exposure to UVA2 varies by skin type. Particularly in fairer-skinned individuals, UVA2 produces erythema without pigment darkening, whereas in individuals with darker skin types, there is IPD without erythema.[42] In general, the biologic behavior of UVA2 is similar to UVB, and the erythemogenic effects are more pronounced in those with lighter skin.[42]

The peak action spectrum in the UV range for IPD is 340 nm.[9,33,42,61] The dose of UVA required to induce IPD is variable by skin type, with some studies reporting threshold doses of 1 to 2 J/cm[2].[61,64] The IPD induced by UVA will fade within minutes unless the UVA dose is at least 10 J/cm[2], in which case the IPD may last for up to 1 to 2 hours before fading.[63] The IPD induced by UVA is typically gray in color.[9,42] IPD induced by visible light has been described as being dark brown in color and as being more sustained in intensity and duration than the IPD from UVA.[9] Several studies have investigated which wavelengths within the visible light spectrum might be responsible for inducing IPD. One study reported that visible light produced IPD only from 400 to 470 nm.[62] Another study, using a visible light source that contained some long-wave UVA, reported that the peak IPD response to visible light occurred at wavelengths between 380 and 500 nm.[52]

PPD appears between 2 and 24 hours following exposure to solar radiation and is again the result of redistribution and oxidation of the melanin that already exists.[33] PPD may last for days and may blend into the course of development of DT.[9,33,60] Exposure to UVA and visible light can result in PPD. Although the specific mechanism for PPD remains unknown, it has been speculated that UV and visible light use the same intermediates and pathway in producing this effect.[64] Visible light and UVA have similar efficacy in producing IPD, but UVA is 25 times more efficient at producing PPD than visible light.[64] However, it is important to keep in mind that there is proportionally more visible light than UVA reaching the surface of the earth. Mahmoud et al[9] estimate that there is 15 times more visible light than UVA in solar radiation. On a clear day at sea level, it is estimated that a person spending approximately 1 hour in direct sunlight would receive a dose of approximately 20 J/cm[2] of UVA and 300 J/cm[2] of visible light.[9] At these doses, Mahmoud et al[9] found that the PPD and DT induced by UVA1 faded within 2 weeks, whereas similar responses induced by visible light showed no signs of fading at 2 weeks after exposure, which was the conclusion of the observation period.

DT is the result of production of new melanin, which is thought to be induced by repair of DNA damage.[42] UVA, UVB, and visible light are all capable of inducing DT. A study investigating the action spectrum for melanogenesis found the peak to be at 290 nm.[65] Importantly, however, the intensity and duration of DT can be affected by skin type, wavelength, and dose.[63] UVB is more effective at producing DT than UVA, but DT resulting from UVA lasts longer than DT from UVB exposure.[63] UVB-induced DT may last up to 3 months, whereas UVA-induced DT may last up to 5 to 6 months.[53,66] Because UVA penetrates more deeply than UVB, UVA is capable of increasing the melanin content deeper within the epidermis, whereas UVB induces melanogenesis in more superficial epidermal cells that are lost more quickly due to physiologic shedding.[53,63] The dose of UV radiation needed to induce DT is dependent on skin type, with darker-skinned individuals requiring higher doses to induce this response.[67] The overall increase in pigment, however, is not correlated with skin type, and for individuals of all skin types, the absolute increase in pigment shows a direct correlation with UV exposure such that increasing doses of UV result in increasing amounts of DT.[66-68] UVB-induced pigmentation always represents DT and is always preceded by erythema.[42,43,63] Compared to broadband UVB, DT induced by narrowband UVB has a quicker onset, with a peak between 3 and 6 days; a shorter duration, with resolution by 1 month; and less intensity.[53] Broadband UVB-induced DT peaks by 4 to 7 days, resolves by 3 months, and is more intense.[53] UVA2 is capable of producing effects similar to UVB in that it is more erythemogenic than UVA1.[42] Particularly in fairer-skinned individuals, UVA2 produces erythema followed by DT in a similar fashion to UVB, whereas in individuals with darker skin types, IPD without erythema occurs followed later by DT.[42] UVA1 and visible light both produce pigment darkening that can persist for up to several weeks. Mahmoud et al[9] note a redistribution of melanin seen by diffuse reflectance spectroscopy following UVA1 and visible light, but there is no documentation of melanogenesis following exposure to UVA1 radiation and visible light.

EPIDERMAL CELL PROLIFERATION

Epidermal hyperplasia is an acute response to exposure to solar radiation [Table 18-5]. This response is protective against further exposure to sunlight.[69-71] Some investigators proposed that epidermal thickening, particularly thickening of the stratum corneum, may be more photoprotective than melanogenesis.[72,73] This is controversial, however, with other data indicating that melanogenesis induced by prior solar radiation exposure offers more photoprotection than stratum corneum thickening.[74] Radiation with UVB has been shown to cause an initial decrease in epidermal cellular proliferation followed by a rebound increase in cellular hyperproliferation.[75] This rebound hyperproliferation of epidermal cells is thought to be a result of an initial inhibition of DNA synthesis due to UVB-induced DNA damage to the cells and a rebound increased rate of DNA synthesis following DNA repair.[75,76] UVB is the best studied of the solar radiation spectrum with regard to its effect on epidermal cell proliferation. Histologic exam of UVB irradiated skin in individuals with type II skin demonstrates that exposure to UVB radiation at MED stimulates an increase in thickness of the epidermis within 24 hours following exposure.[77]

The effect of UVA radiation on epidermal thickness is more controversial. One study showed that exposure to UVA radiation in individuals with type II skin at the MED did not induce a significant change in epidermal thickness within the same time frame.[77] Another study in individuals with type I or II skin, however, showed that at doses 2.5 times the MED delivered 3 times weekly for 3 weeks, UVA did result in an increased epidermal thickness, including specifically an increase in the stratum corneum thickness.[71]

There have not been any investigations into the acute effects of visible light on epidermal proliferation, but there have been limited studies on the impact of IR on this process. A study in mice demonstrated that epidermal proliferation was reversibly decreased following a single exposure to IR-A.[58] The authors noted that the initial response to IR and UVB radiation at a cellular level is very similar, with initial decrease in cellular proliferation. After UVB exposure, however, there is a rebound hyperproliferation following the initial decreased proliferation, whereas after IR exposure, there is a biphasic decrease in proliferation. The initial reduction following IR occurred between 5 hours and 1 day after

irradiation, and the second reduction occurred at 5 days after irradiation. Proliferation of epidermal cells returned to baseline by 14 days after the IR irradiation.[58] The authors postulated that IR exposure retards the cell cycle but is not damaging enough to cause injury to the cellular DNA.[58] Without actual DNA damage, there is no subsequent DNA repair, which is thought to stimulate an increase in DNA synthesis and cell proliferation. Ultimately, it is known that exposure to solar radiation induces changes in epidermal cell proliferation with increased epidermal thickening, particularly increased stratum corneum thickness, following UV exposure and decreased epidermal cell proliferation following exposure to IR. No studies have been conducted on whether epidermal cell proliferation induced by solar radiation is variable by skin type. There have been investigations into baseline epidermal and dermal variations among skin types. Epidermal thickness, stratum corneum thickness, and corneocyte size are thought to be unrelated to skin type.[78-80] There does seem to be some variation in the number of cell layers in the stratum corneum, with individuals of African descent having more cell layers than Caucasian individuals.[79] Further investigation into acute epidermal responses to solar radiation among various skin types are needed to determine whether skin type plays any role in this response.

VITAMIN D SYNTHESIS

Vitamin D_3, or cholecalciferol, is a hormone that plays a crucial role in regulating the concentrations of calcium and phosphorus within the human body.[81] UVB (300 ± 5 nm) is the action spectrum of vitamin D_3 synthesis [Figure 18-1]. 7-Dehydrocholesterol (7-DHC) is also known as provitamin D_3.[81] It is a vitamin D precursor and is found within keratinocytes.[82] 7-DHC is also a chromophore for UVB.[5] When 7-DHC absorbs UVB radiation, previtamin D_3 is formed.[81] At body temperature, previtamin D_3 isomerizes to form active vitamin D_3. However, if the previtamin D_3 product absorbs UVB, then it isomerizes to form lumisterol and tachysterol, neither of which are active in the regulation of calcium or phosphate levels.[83] Vitamin D_3 is formed in the cell membrane of keratinocytes. After formation, it exits the keratinocytes and moves to the dermal capillary bed where it is bound by vitamin D–binding protein.[81,84] Active vitamin D_3 is photolabile, so if it remains in the skin and is not protein bound, it is converted to the metabolically inactive products, 5,6-*trans*-vitamin D_3, supersterol I, and supersterol II.[81] Thus, although UVB is essential to the formation of vitamin D_3 in the skin, there are several mechanisms by which excessive UVB exposure self-limits the amount of active vitamin D_3 that is formed.[81]

Individuals with skin of color are known to be at risk for vitamin D insufficiency.[85,86] One study has noted that there was no association between skin pigmentation and vitamin D levels following controlled exposure to UVB radiation.[87] Most evidence, however, does suggest an inverse relationship between increasing skin pigmentation and vitamin D_3.[88] Following equivalent doses of UVB exposure, another study demonstrated that serum cholecalciferol levels were lower in individuals with more pigmented skin.[89] An investigation into baseline vitamin D levels in Americans by race found that whites had the highest level, followed by Mexican Americans and then African Americans.[90] East Asians and South Asians are reported to have lower levels than Europeans.[91]

IMMUNE EFFECTS

Exposure to solar radiation can induce immunomodulation [Table 18-6]. This has been supported by extensive research and provides the rationale for the use of phototherapy as a therapeutic regimen for many disorders of the skin. UV radiation decreases the number and alters the morphology and function of Langerhans cells in the skin.[25,92] Additionally, keratinocytes produce and secrete tumor necrosis factor-α (TNF-α) following exposure to UV radiation.[92] UV irradiation decreases cell-mediated immune responses to contact sensitizing antigens.[92] Some of the documented events following exposure to UVB radiation include the formation of CPDs and *trans*- to *cis*-urocanic acid (UCA) isomerization in the stratum corneum.[93] It has been suggested that

TABLE 18-5	Components of sunlight and epidermal proliferation	
UVB	UVA	IR
Increase in epidermal proliferation and thickness	Increase in epidermal proliferation and thickness	Biphasic decrease in epidermal proliferation

Abbreviations: IR, infrared radiation; UV, ultraviolet.

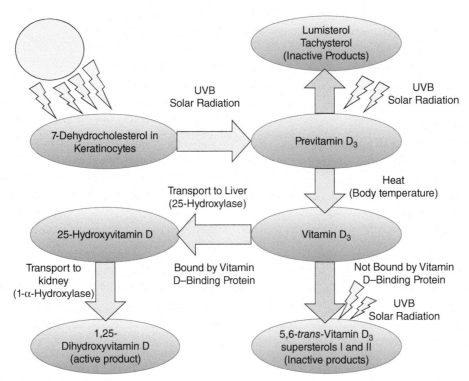

FIGURE 18-1. Vitamin D synthesis. UV, ultraviolet.

trans-UCA, which is naturally occurring in the stratum corneum, is a chromophore for UVB radiation and that its isomer, *cis*-UCA, is the molecule responsible for some of the immunosuppressive effects that follow UVB exposure.[92] However, studies have shown inconsistent effects of *cis*-UCA in inducing changes in contact sensitivity suppression in skin, which is a known effect of UVB irradiation on the skin.[92,94] The action spectrum for contact sensitivity suppression induced by UV radiation and the action spectrum for UCA photoisomerization are also not the same.[95] There is evidence that through its CPD products, DNA may be the chromophore that results in the suppression of contact hypersensitivity induced by UVB radiation.[95] UVB is also thought to affect innate immunity by decreasing the activity of natural killer cells.[96-98] This inhibition of natural killer cells is thought likely to be the effect of *cis*-UCA because it can be reproduced without UV exposure when *cis*-UCA is independently introduced to the skin without UV radiation.[98] When administered with the exogenous photosensitizer psoralen, UVA radiation was shown to induce similar inhibitory effect on natural killer cells.[98]

The primary mechanism for UVA-induced immunosuppression in the epidermis is thought to be related to its production of ROS.[99] UVA and UVB have been demonstrated to have different peak action spectra for immunosuppression, so it is likely that they have different primary chromophores and mechanisms for inducing immunosuppression.[100]

The peak action spectrum for UVA-induced immunosuppression is at 370 nm, which is in the UVA1 spectrum.[100] There is suggestion that exposure of the skin to UV radiation may have some systemic immunosuppressive effects, which may affect internal organs, but the mechanism behind this is unclear, and it is thought that the chromophores for this effect are different than those that mediate the immunosuppression seen in the epidermis following UV radiation.[101] It is known that visible light exposure results in the formation of ROS in a fashion similar to exposure to UVA1.[102]

There has been limited investigation into the acute effects of IR on immune responses in the skin. The investigation of Danno and Sugie[58] into the effects of IR-A on mice skin implies that there is an immediate immunosuppression in the epidermis following the irradiation. They noted that IR induces a decrease in Langerhans cell density, which was greatest at 3 days after irradiation and was nearly returned to baseline by 14 days after irradiation.[58] They also noted morphologic changes in the existing Langerhans cells and decreased local contact sensitivity responses, which were returned to baseline by 14 days following the irradiation.[58] They found no evidence to support a systemic immunosuppressive response induced by IR irradiation.[58]

Ultimately, all forms of solar radiation, aside from visible light, have been shown to affect the immune function of the skin; however, there has been little investigation into the effect of skin type on these

TABLE 18-6	Components of sunlight and immunomodulation		
Component	UVB	UVA	IR
Mechanisms	Formation of CPDs Isomerization of *trans*- to *cis*-urocanic acid	Generation of ROS	Unknown
Effects	Decrease in number and changes in function of Langerhans cells Inhibition of natural killer cells TNF-α secretion	Decrease in number and changes in function of Langerhans cells Inhibition of natural killer cells	Decrease in number and changes in function of Langerhans cells
Time course	Effects seen by 24 hours; peak at 48 hours	Effects seen by 48 hours and resolve by 72 hours after exposure	Resolves within 14 days

Abbreviations: CPD, cyclobutane pyrimidine dimer; IR, infrared radiation; ROS, reactive oxygen species; TNF-α, tumor necrosis factor-α; UV, ultraviolet.

phenomena. Because melanin is a neutral density filter, higher melanin content in dark-skinned individuals would be expected to result in less penetration of photons from exposure to sunlight; this is consistent with the clinical observation of less erythema, photoaging, and photocarcinogenesis observed in this group of individuals. A study investigating the relationship between UCA isomers and other factors such as skin type, pigmentation, and MED in individuals with types I to IV skin demonstrated no correlation between UCA isomer levels and these factors.[103] Future studies are needed to ascertain the differences in immunomodulation induced by exposure to solar radiation by skin type and to assess the effects of visible light on immune function.

REFERENCES

1. Newton I. A new theory about light and colours. *Phil Trans R Soc Lond.* 1672;6:3075-3087.
2. Ritter JW. *Physisch-Chemische Abhandlungen.* Vol 2. Leipzig, Germany; 1801.
3. Herschel W. Experiments on the refrangibility of invisible rays of the sun. *Phil Trans R Soc Lond.* 1800;90:255-326.
4. Jackson BA. Lasers in ethnic skin: a review. *J Am Acad Dermatol.* 2003;48 (6 Suppl):S134-S138.
5. Diffey BL, Kochevar IE. Basic principles of photobiology. In: Lim HW, Honigsmann H, Hawk JL, eds. *Photodermatology.* New York, NY: Informa Healthcare USA; 2007:15-27.
6. Lui H, Anderson RR. Radiation sources and interaction with skin. In: Lim HW, Honigsmann H, Hawk JL, eds. *Photodermatology.* New York, NY: Informa Healthcare USA, Inc; 2007:29-40.
7. Coblentz WW. The Copenhagen Meeting of the Second International Congress on Light. *Science.* 1932;76:412-415.
8. Kochevar IE, Pathak MA, Parrish JA. Photophysics, photochemistry and photobiology. In: Freederber IM, Eisen AZ, Wolff K, eds. *Fitzpatrick's Dermatology in General Medicine.* New York, NY: McGraw Hill; 1999:220-229.
9. Mahmoud BH, Ruvolo E, Hexsel CL, et al. Impact of long-wavelength UVA and visible light on melanocompetent skin. *J Invest Dermatol.* 2010;130:2092-2097.
10. Lee HS, Lee DH, Cho S, Chung JH. Minimal heating dose: a novel biological unit to measure infrared irradiation. *Photodermatol Photoimmunol Photomed.* 2006;22:148-152.
11. Schieke SM, Schroeder P, Krutmann J. Cutaneous effects of infrared radiation: from clinical observations to molecular response mechanisms. *Photodermatol Photoimmunol Photomed.* 2003;19:228-234.
12. Alaluf S, Heath A, Carter N, et al. Variation in melanin content and composition in type V and VI photoexposed and photoprotected human skin: the dominant role of DHI. *Pigment Cell Res.* 2001;14:337-347.
13. James WD, Elston DM, Berger TG, Andrews GC. *Andrews' Diseases of the Skin: Clinical Dermatology.* 11th ed. London, United Kingdom: Saunders Elsevier; 2011.
14. Garmyn M, Yarosh DB. The molecular and genetic effects of ultraviolet radiation exposure on skin cells. In: Lim HW, Honigsmann H, Hawk JL, eds. *Photodermatology.* New York, NY: Informa Healthcare USA; 2007:41-51.
15. Young AR, Potten CS, Chadwick CA, Murphy GM, Hawk JL, Cohen AJ. Photoprotection and 5-MOP photochemoprotection from UVR-induced DNA damage in humans: the role of skin type. *J Invest Dermatol.* 1991;97:942-948.
16. Everett MA, Yeargers E, Sayre RM, Olson RL. Penetration of epidermis by ultraviolet rays. *Photochem Photobiol.* 1966;5:533-542.
17. Young AR, Chadwick CA, Harrison GI, Nikaido O, Ramsden J, Potten CS. The similarity of action spectra for thymine dimers in human epidermis and erythema suggests that DNA is the chromophore for erythema. *J Invest Dermatol.* 1998;111:982-988.
18. Matsumura Y, Ananthaswamy HN. Short-term and long-term cellular and molecular events following UV irradiation of skin: implications for molecular medicine. *Expert Rev Mol Med.* 2002;4:1-22.
19. Agar N, Young AR. Melanogenesis: a photoprotective response to DNA damage? *Mutat Res.* 2005;571:121-132.
20. Sutherland JC, Griffin KP. Absorption spectrum of DNA for wavelengths greater than 300 nm. *Radiat Res.* 1981;86:399-409.
21. Matsunaga T, Hieda K, Nikaido O. Wavelength dependent formation of thymine dimers and (6-4) photoproducts in DNA by monochromatic ultraviolet light ranging from 150 to 365 nm. *Photochem Photobiol.* 1991;54:403-410.
22. Chadwick CA, Potten CS, Nikaido O, Matsunaga T, Proby C, Young AR. The detection of cyclobutane thymine dimers, (6-4) photolesions and the Dewar photoisomers in sections of UV-irradiated human skin using specific

antibodies, and the demonstration of depth penetration effects. *J Photochem Photobiol B.* 1995;28:163-170.
23. Clingen PH, Arlett CF, Roza L, Mori T, Nikaido O, Green MH. Induction of cyclobutane pyrimidine dimers, pyrimidine(6-4)pyrimidone photoproducts, and Dewar valence isomers by natural sunlight in normal human mononuclear cells. *Cancer Res.* 1995;55:2245-2248.
24. Yoon JH, Lee CS, O'Connor TR, Yasui A, Pfeifer GP. The DNA damage spectrum produced by simulated sunlight. *J Mol Biol.* 2000;299:681-693.
25. Seite S, Fourtanier A, Moyal D, Young AR. Photodamage to human skin by suberythemal exposure to solar ultraviolet radiation can be attenuated by sunscreens: a review. *Br J Dermatol.* 2010;163:903-914.
26. Cooke MS, Olinski R, Loft S. Measurement and meaning of oxidatively modified DNA lesions in urine. *Cancer Epidemiol Biomarkers Prev.* 2008;17:3-14.
27. Hruza LL, Pentland AP. Mechanisms of UV-induced inflammation. *J Invest Dermatol.* 1993;100:35S-41S.
28. Noonan FP, Zaidi MR, Wolnicka-Glubisz A, et al. Melanoma induction by ultraviolet A but not ultraviolet B radiation requires melanin pigment. *Nat Commun.* 2012;3:884.
29. Courdavault S, Baudouin C, Charveron M, Favier A, Cadet J, Douki T. Larger yield of cyclobutane dimers than 8-oxo-7,8-dihydroguanine in the DNA of UVA-irradiated human skin cells. *Mutat Res.* 2004;556:135-142.
30. Paunel AN, Dejam A, Thelen S, et al. Enzyme-independent nitric oxide formation during UVA challenge of human skin: characterization, molecular sources, and mechanisms. *Free Radic Biol Med.* 2005;38:606-615.
31. Oplander C, Volkmar CM, Paunel-Gorgulu A, et al. Whole body UVA irradiation lowers systemic blood pressure by release of nitric oxide from intracutaneous photolabile nitric oxide derivates. *Circ Res.* 2009;105:1031-1040.
32. Suschek CV, Oplander C, van Faassen EE. Non-enzymatic NO production in human skin: effect of UVA on cutaneous NO stores. *Nitric Oxide.* 2010;22:120-135.
33. Mahmoud BH, Hexsel CL, Hamzavi IH, Lim HW. Effects of visible light on the skin. *Photochem Photobiol.* 2008;84:450-462.
34. Liebel F, Kaur S, Ruvolo E, Kollias N, Southall MD. Irradiation of skin with visible light induces reactive oxygen species and matrix-degrading enzymes. *J Invest Dermatol.* 2012;132:1901-1907.
35. Haywood R. Relevance of sunscreen application method, visible light and sunlight intensity to free-radical protection: A study of ex vivo human skin. *Photochem Photobiol.* 2006;82:1123-1131.
36. Kielbassa C, Roza L, Epe B. Wavelength dependence of oxidative DNA damage induced by UV and visible light. *Carcinogenesis.* 1997;18:811-816.
37. Schroeder P, Calles C, Benesova T, Macaluso F, Krutmann J. Photoprotection beyond ultraviolet radiation: effective sun protection has to include protection against infrared A radiation-induced skin damage. *Skin Pharmacol Physiol.* 2010;23:15-17.
38. Holzer AM, Athar M, Elmets CA. The other end of the rainbow: infrared and skin. *J Invest Dermatol.* 2010;130:1496-1499.
39. Calles C, Schneider M, Macaluso F, Benesova T, Krutmann J, Schroeder P. Infrared A radiation influences the skin fibroblast transcriptome: mechanisms and consequences. *J Invest Dermatol.* 2010;130:1524-1536.
40. Piazena H, Kelleher DK. Effects of infrared-A irradiation on skin: discrepancies in published data highlight the need for an exact consideration of physical and photobiological laws and appropriate experimental settings. *Photochem Photobiol.* 2010;86:687-705.
41. Lohr NL, Keszler A, Pratt P, Bienengraber M, Warltier DC, Hogg N. Enhancement of nitric oxide release from nitrosyl hemoglobin and nitrosyl myoglobin by red/near infrared radiation: potential role in cardioprotection. *J Mol Cell Cardiol.* 2009;47:256-263.
42. Honigsmann H. Erythema and pigmentation. *Photodermatol Photoimmunol Photomed.* 2002;18:75-81.
43. Kollias N, Malallah YH, al-Ajmi H, Baqer A, Johnson BE, Gonzalez S. Erythema and melanogenesis action spectra in heavily pigmented individuals as compared to fair-skinned Caucasians. *Photodermatol Photoimmunol Photomed.* 1996;12:183-188.
44. Sunlight, ultraviolet radiation, and the skin excerpts: NIH consensus statement. *Md Med J.* 1990;39:851-852.
45. Farr PM, Diffey BL. The erythemal response of human skin to ultraviolet radiation. *Br J Dermatol.* 1985;113:65-76.
46. Ibbotson SH, Farr PM. The time-course of psoralen ultraviolet A (PUVA) erythema. *J Invest Dermatol.* 1999;113:346-350.
47. Kollias N, Baqer A, Sadiq I. Minimum erythema dose determination in individuals of skin type V and VI with diffuse reflectance spectroscopy. *Photodermatol Photoimmunol Photomed.* 1994;10:249-254.

48. Tewari A, Sarkany RP, Young AR. UVA1 induces cyclobutane pyrimidine dimers but not 6-4 photoproducts in human skin in vivo. *J Invest Dermatol.* 2012;132:394-400.

49. Applegate LA, Scaletta C, Treina G, Mascotto RE, Fourtanier A, Frenk E. Erythema induction by ultraviolet radiation points to a possible acquired defense mechanism in chronically sun-exposed human skin. *Dermatology.* 1997;194:41-49.

50. Diffey BL, Farr PM, Oakley AM. Quantitative studies on UVA-induced erythema in human skin. *Br J Dermatol.* 1987;117:57-66.

51. Parrish JA, Anderson RR, Ying CY, Pathak MA. Cutaneous effects of pulsed nitrogen gas laser irradiation. *J Invest Dermatol.* 1976;67:603-608.

52. Pathak MA, Fanselow DL. Photobiology of melanin pigmentation: dose/response of skin to sunlight and its contents. *J Am Acad Dermatol.* 1983;9:724-733.

53. Suh KS, Roh HJ, Choi SY, et al. A long-term evaluation of erythema and pigmentation induced by ultraviolet radiations of different wavelengths. *Skin Res Technol.* 2007;13:360-368.

54. Kaidbey KH, Kligman AM. The acute effects of long-wave ultraviolet radiation on human skin. *J Invest Dermatol.* 1979;72:253-256.

55. Maddodi N, Jayanthy A, Setaluri V. Shining light on skin pigmentation: the darker and the brighter side of effects of UV radiation. *Photochem Photobiol.* 2012;88:1075-1082.

56. Porges SB, Kaidbey KH, Grove GL. Quantification of visible light-induced melanogenesis in human skin. *Photodermatol.* 1988;5:197-200.

57. Pujol JA, Lecha M. Photoprotection in the infrared radiation range. *Photodermatol Photoimmunol Photomed.* 1992;9:275-278.

58. Danno K, Sugie N. Effects of near-infrared radiation on the epidermal proliferation and cutaneous immune function in mice. *Photodermatol Photoimmunol Photomed.* 1996;12:233-236.

59. Schulze HJ, Schmidt R, Mahrle G. Infrared erythema. *Zeitschrift fur Hautkrankheiten.* J 1985;60:938-944.

60. Rhodes LE, Lim HW. The acute effects of ultraviolet radiation on the skin. In: Lim HW, Honigsmann H, Hawk JL, eds. *Photodermatology.* New York, NY: Informa Healthcare USA, Inc; 2007:75-89.

61. Routaboul C, Denis A, Vinche A. Immediate pigment darkening: description, kinetic and biological function. *Eur J Dermatol.* 1999;9:95-99.

62. Rosen CF, Jacques SL, Stuart ME, Gange RW. Immediate pigment darkening: visual and reflectance spectrophotometric analysis of action spectrum. *Photochem Photobiol.* 1990;51:583-588.

63. Sklar LR, Almutawa F, Lim HW, Hamzavi I. Effects of ultraviolet radiation, visible light, and infrared radiation on erythema and pigmentation: a review. *Photochem Photobiol Sci.* 2013;12:54-64.

64. Ramasubramaniam R, Roy A, Sharma B, Nagalakshmi S. Are there mechanistic differences between ultraviolet and visible radiation induced skin pigmentation? *Photochem Photobiol Sci.* 2011;10:1887-1893.

65. Parrish JA, Jaenicke KF, Anderson RR. Erythema and melanogenesis action spectra of normal human skin. *Photochem Photobiol.* 1982;36:187-191.

66. Ravnbak MH, Philipsen PA, Wiegell SR, Wulf HC. Skin pigmentation kinetics after exposure to ultraviolet A. *Acta Derm Venereol.* 2009;89:357-363.

67. Ravnbak MH, Wulf HC. Pigmentation after single and multiple UV-exposures depending on UV-spectrum. *Arch Dermatol Res.* 2007;299:25-32.

68. Ravnbak MH, Philipsen PA, Wiegell SR, Wulf HC. Skin pigmentation kinetics after UVB exposure. *Acta Derm Venereol.* 2008;88:223-228.

69. Casetti F, Miese A, Mueller ML, Simon JC, Schempp CM. Double trouble from sunburn: UVB-induced erythema is associated with a transient decrease in skin pigmentation. *Skin Pharmacol Physiol.* 2011;24:160-165.

70. Svobodova A, Vostalova J. Solar radiation induced skin damage: review of protective and preventive options. *Int J Radiat Biol.* 2010;86:999-1030.

71. Pearse AD, Gaskell SA, Marks R. Epidermal changes in human skin following irradiation with either UVB or UVA. *J Invest Dermatol.* 1987;88:83-87.

72. Schmalwieser AW, Wallisch S, Diffey B. A library of action spectra for erythema and pigmentation. *Photochem Photobiol Sci.* 2012;11:251-268.

73. Gniadecka M, Wulf HC, Mortensen NN, Poulsen T. Photoprotection in vitiligo and normal skin. A quantitative assessment of the role of stratum corneum, viable epidermis and pigmentation. *Acta Derm Venereol.* 1996;76:429-432.

74. Sheehan JM, Potten CS, Young AR. Tanning in human skin types II and III offers modest photoprotection against erythema. *Photochem Photobiol.* 1998;68:588-592.

75. Epstein JH, Fukuyama K, Fye K. Effects of ultraviolet radiation on the mitotic cycle and DNA, RNA and protein synthesis in mammalian epidermis in vivo. *Photochem Photobiol.* 1970;12:57-65.

76. Epstein WL, Fukuyama K, Epstein JH. Early effects of ultraviolet light on DNA synthesis in human skin in vivo. *Arch Dermatol.* 1969;100:84-89.

77. Gambichler T, Rotterdam S, Tigges C, Altmeyer P, Bechara FG. Impact of ultraviolet radiation on the expression of marker proteins of gap and adhesion junctions in human epidermis. *Photodermatol Photoimmunol Photomed.* 2008;24:318-321.

78. Rawlings AV. Ethnic skin types: are there differences in skin structure and function? *Int J Cosmet Sci.* 2006;28:79-93.

79. Weigand DA, Haygood C, Gaylor JR. Cell layers and density of Negro and Caucasian stratum corneum. *J Invest Dermatol.* 1974;62:563-568.

80. Corcuff P, Lotte C, Rougier A, Maibach HI. Racial differences in corneocytes. A comparison between black, white and oriental skin. *Acta Derm Venereol.* 1991;71:146-148.

81. Holick MF. McCollum Award Lecture, 1994: vitamin D—new horizons for the 21st century. *Am J Clin Nutr.* 1994;60:619-630.

82. Gupta R, Dixon KM, Deo SS, et al. Photoprotection by 1,25 dihydroxyvitamin D3 is associated with an increase in p53 and a decrease in nitric oxide products. *J Invest Dermatol.* 2007;127:707-715.

83. Holick MF, MacLaughlin JA, Doppelt SH. Regulation of cutaneous previtamin D3 photosynthesis in man: skin pigment is not an essential regulator. *Science.* 1981;211:590-593.

84. Holick MF, MacLaughlin JA, Clark MB, et al. Photosynthesis of previtamin D3 in human skin and the physiologic consequences. *Science.* 1980;210:203-205.

85. Harris SS, Dawson-Hughes B. Seasonal changes in plasma 25-hydroxyvitamin D concentrations of young American black and white women. *Am J Clin Nutr.* 1998;67:1232-1236.

86. Armas LA, Dowell S, Akhter M, et al. Ultraviolet-B radiation increases serum 25-hydroxyvitamin D levels: the effect of UVB dose and skin color. *J Am Acad Dermatol.* 2007;57:588-593.

87. Bogh MK, Schmedes AV, Philipsen PA, Thieden E, Wulf HC. Vitamin D production after UVB exposure depends on baseline vitamin D and total cholesterol but not on skin pigmentation. *J Invest Dermatol.* 2010;130:546-553.

88. Vanchinathan V, Lim HW. A dermatologist's perspective on vitamin D. *Mayo Clin Proc.* 2012;87:372-380.

89. Matsuoka LY, Wortsman J, Haddad JG, Kolm P, Hollis BW. Racial pigmentation and the cutaneous synthesis of vitamin D. *Arch Dermatol.* 1991;127:536-538.

90. Bischoff-Ferrari HA, Dietrich T, Orav EJ, Dawson-Hughes B. Positive association between 25-hydroxy vitamin D levels and bone mineral density: a population-based study of younger and older adults. *Am J Med.* 2004;116:634-639.

91. Gozdzik A, Barta JL, Weir A, et al. Serum 25-hydroxyvitamin D concentrations fluctuate seasonally in young adults of diverse ancestry living in Toronto. *J Nutr.* 2010;140:2213-2220.

92. Moodycliffe AM, Kimber I, Norval M. The effect of ultraviolet B irradiation and urocanic acid isomers on dendritic cell migration. *Immunology.* 1992;77:394-399.

93. Kim TH, Moodycliffe AM, Yarosh DB, Norval M, Kripke ML, Ullrich SE. Viability of the antigen determines whether DNA or urocanic acid act as initiator molecules for UV-induced suppression of delayed-type hypersensitivity. *Photochem Photobiol.* 2003;78:228-234.

94. el-Ghorr AA, Norval M. A monoclonal antibody to cis-urocanic acid prevents the ultraviolet-induced changes in Langerhans cells and delayed hypersensitivity responses in mice, although not preventing dendritic cell accumulation in lymph nodes draining the site of irradiation and contact hypersensitivity responses. *J Invest Dermatol.* 1995;105:264-268.

95. Reeve VE, Ley RD, Reilly WG, Bosnic M. Epidermal urocanic acid and suppression of contact hypersensitivity by ultraviolet radiation in Monodelphis domestica. *Int Arch Allergy Immunol.* 1996;109:266-271.

96. Schacter B, Lederman MM, LeVine MJ, Ellner JJ. Ultraviolet radiation inhibits human natural killer activity and lymphocyte proliferation. *J Immunol.* 1983;130:2484-2487.

97. Hersey P, Magrath H, Wilkinson F. Development of an in vitro system for the analysis of ultraviolet radiation-induced suppression of natural killer cell activity. *Photochem Photobiol.* 1993;57:279-284.

98. Gilmour JW, Vestey JP, George S, Norval M. Effect of phototherapy and urocanic acid isomers on natural killer cell function. *J Invest Dermatol.* 1993;101:169-174.

99. Halliday GM, Byrne SN, Damian DL. Ultraviolet A radiation: its role in immunosuppression and carcinogenesis. *Semin Cutan Med Surg.* 2011;30:214-221.

100. Damian DL, Matthews YJ, Phan TA, Halliday GM. An action spectrum for ultraviolet radiation-induced immunosuppression in humans. *Br J Dermatol.* 2011;164:657-659.

101. Halliday GM, Damian DL, Rana S, Byrne SN. The suppressive effects of ultraviolet radiation on immunity in the skin and internal organs: implications for autoimmunity. *J Dermatol Sci.* 2012;66:176-182.

102. Hoffmann-Dorr S, Greinert R, Volkmer B, Epe B. Visible light (>395 nm) causes micronuclei formation in mammalian cells without generation of cyclobutane pyrimidine dimers. *Mutat Res.* 2005;572:142-149.

103. de Fine Olivarius F, Wulf HC, Therkildsen P, Poulsen T, Crosby J, Norval M. Urocanic acid isomers: relation to body site, pigmentation, stratum corneum thickness and photosensitivity. *Arch Dermatol Res.* 1997;289:501-505.

CHAPTER 19
Chronic Effects of Light on Skin

Richard H. Huggins
Dakara Rucker Wright
Lawrence S.W. Khoo
Henry W. Lim

KEY POINTS

- The chronic effects of ultraviolet (UV) radiation are photoaging and photocarcinogenesis.

- Photoaging is greatly influenced by the amount of melanin, its composition, and its distribution.

- In darker skin of color, photoaging is typically not evident until the fifth or sixth decade.

- Photoaging in Asians presents more often as pigmentary changes and less often as wrinkling.

- Hispanics are an extremely heterogeneous group with widely varied photoaging phenotypes.

- Because of the protective effects of melanin, individuals with skin of color are less prone to develop UV-associated skin cancers compared with fair-skinned individuals.

CHRONIC EFFECTS OF ULTRAVIOLET RADIATION

Photoaging and photocarcinogenesis are the primary long-term effects of chronic ultraviolet (UV) radiation (UVR) on skin.

PHOTOAGING

Photoaging, or dermatoheliosis, is distinct from intrinsic aging. Intrinsic skin aging is due to the passage of time, whereas photoaging results from damage to the skin from UVR superimposed on intrinsically aged skin. Intrinsically aged skin appears lax, dry, and pale with fine wrinkles and is prone to the development of benign neoplasms. In contrast, photoaged skin is coarser, rougher, leathery, inelastic with deep wrinkles, and telangiectatic. In addition, pigmentary changes consist of persistent constitutive hyperpigmentation, irregular hyperpigmentation, reticular hyperpigmentation (poikiloderma of Civatte), guttate hypomelanosis, freckling, and/or solar lentigines. Open comedones (Favre-Racouchot syndrome), sebaceous hyperplasia, and erosive pustulosis may also be present in photodamaged skin. Irregular hyperpigmented macules ("sunburn freckles") can develop as early as several months after a sunburn. Repeated exposure to suberythemogenic UVR has the potential to change the morphology of acquired melanocytic nevi with increased size, darker color, and dermoscopic patterns that simulate melanoma in situ.[1] Photoaged skin loses resilience and elasticity and has increased fragility and decreased capacity for wound healing. Histologically, there can be acanthosis or atrophy, loss of polarity, cellular atypia in the epidermis, and increased melanin in keratinocytes, especially in skin of color. In the dermis, reduced anchoring fibrils, loss of mature collagen, basophilic collagen degeneration, elastosis, increased ground substance and, in skin of color, increased number of large, densely melanin-packed melanophages may be seen.[2] Additionally, there is an increase in the numbers of mast cells, histiocytes, fibroblasts, and mononuclear cells, although in the epidermis, there are decreased numbers of Langerhans cells.[3]

Both UVA and UVB can induce photoaging. However, UVA plays a more significant role due to its greater average depth of penetration into the dermis, increased abundance in terrestrial sunlight (5% UVB, 95% UVA), and persistent irradiance throughout the day and year. Studies also demonstrated that exposure of human skin to suberythemogenic doses of UVA alone resulted in stratum corneum thickening, Langerhans cell depletion, and dermal inflammatory infiltrates with deposition of lysozyme on the elastic fibers. This suggests that frequent casual exposure to sunlight containing primarily UVA eventually may result in dermal collagen and elastin damage, contributing to photoaging. UVA increases the cross-linking of collagen fibers, rendering dermal collagen more resistant to degradation, whereas UVB renders collagen more susceptible to enzymatic degradation.[4] In a human study using a solar simulator with emission spectra of 47% UVB, 27% UVA, and 26% visible and near-infrared, one single exposure to 0.5 minimal erythema dose was shown to induce increased levels of matrix metalloproteinases (MMPs) in keratinocytes and connective tissue.[5] Studies using reconstructed skin in vitro containing live fibroblasts in a dermal matrix and differentiated epidermis showed that UVA induced fibroblast apoptosis in the upper dermis and secretion of MMPs, whereas UVB affected epidermal cells, giving rise to cyclobutane pyrimidine dimers and sunburn cells (apoptotic keratinocytes).[4] Interestingly, infrared radiation (760 nm to 1 mm) contributes, independently and in conjunction with UVR, to photoaging.[6]

On a molecular level, UV irradiation directly activates cell surface receptors, partly through reactive oxygen species (ROS), which in turn initiates intracellular signaling. This results in activation of a nuclear transcription complex, AP-1, which is composed of proteins c-Jun and c-Fos. Increased AP-1 blocks the effects of the transforming growth factor-β (TGF-β) cytokine on its receptors, thus inhibiting collagen transcription.[4] The aforementioned AP-1 may be involved in this process because increased AP-1 activity has been shown to result in increased levels of several MMPs that degrade collagen. MMP-8 (collagenase) from UV-induced neutrophilic infiltration further exacerbates matrix degradation. Tissue inhibitors of metalloproteinases are also upregulated, but not to a sufficient enough extent to completely block cumulative dermal collagen damage. Collagen degradation products not only reduce the integrity of the skin, but also prevent new collagen synthesis.[4]

Not only do ROS damage the dermal matrix, but they also damage mitochondrial DNA (mtDNA). Photoaged skin has more mtDNA mutations than sun-protected skin, which leads to poor mitochondrial function and further accumulation of ROS as a result of a dysfunctional respiratory chain system.[4] Telomeres may also play a role in photoaging of the skin. Telomeres protect the chromosome from degradation or fusion; they also serve as a biological clock. Older epidermal cells and dermal fibroblasts have shorter terminal sequences or telomeres because DNA polymerase cannot replicate the final base pairs of each chromosome. Therefore, these older cells are less protected from the damage caused by repeated UVR or prolonged exposure to ROS, which results in accelerated cellular senescence.[4] The hallmark of aged nondividing cells is lipofuscin, a yellow-brown granular pigment that is the result of an accumulation of oxidized, cross-linked proteins that were not degraded by proteasomes. Proteasomes are known to have diminished activity in aging human keratinocytes and fibroblasts.[1]

PHOTOAGING IN SKIN OF COLOR

Histologically, there are few differences in the structure of skin between races. However, skin of color appears to be protected from many of the effects of UVR that are seen in Caucasian skin. For example, when exposed to equivalent doses of UVR, DNA damage that was observed throughout the epidermis and the papillary dermis in light, intermediate, and tanned skin was limited to the suprabasal portion of the epidermis in brown or dark skin.[7] Although there is some variation in the dermal fibroblast quantity and function and there are small differences in the epidermal and dermal thicknesses and compositions, it is evident that the key factor protecting skin of color from UVR is melanin.[8] In vitro studies examining the extent of DNA damage resulting from UVR reveal an inverse relationship between melanin concentration and depth of photodamage.[9] It should be noted that there are no differences between racial groups in the number of melanocytes per unit area of the skin. However, studies have shown that ethnic groups with darker skin (African and Indian) have nearly twice as much melanin compared with those with lighter skin (European, Chinese, and Mexican). Lighter skin has been found to contain up to three times the proportion of the more lightly colored pheomelanin compared with the darker eumelanin.[10,11] In addition, melanin in skin of color is distributed in widely dispersed, densely melanin-packed melanosomes, and this appears to be just as important for its photoprotective effect as the amount of melanin present.[2,12] Lastly, there is a degree of variance in the diameter of melanosomes between African Americans ($1.44 \pm 0.67 \times 10^{-2}$ μm^2), Asians ($1.36 \pm 0.15 \times 10^{-2}$ μm^2), and Caucasians ($0.94 \pm 0.48 \times 10^{-2}$ μm^2).[13]

Photoaging, which is a major sign of photodamage, is greatly influenced by the amount of melanin, its composition, and its distribution.[14] Individuals of color display a decreased susceptibility to photodamage. As a result, although all races experience photoaging, in skin of color, these changes develop at more advanced ages [**Figure 19-1**]. In general, people with skin of color tend to develop photoaging 10 to 20 years later and to a far lesser extent than their Caucasian counterparts.[15] In evaluating the extent of facial wrinkling across ethnic groups in Los Angeles, California, Rawlings[16] found the following order of decreasing wrinkle severity: Caucasian > Hispanic > African American > East Asian.[16] The typical signs of photoaging in skin of color vary by skin type. In more lightly complexioned skin of color (Fitzpatrick skin types III and IV), lentigines, keratosis, rhytids, telangiectasia, and loss of elasticity are commonly observed.[15] Photoaging develops earlier and to a greater extent in lighter-complexioned individuals. Increasing unevenness of skin tone and loss of subcutaneous fat are more characteristic of photoaging in darker skin of color (Fitzpatrick skin types IV to VI).[15] We will discuss photoaging in specific racial and ethnic groups in the following sections.

Dark Skin of Color Dark skin of color appears to be significantly protected from actinic damage. It is estimated that the epidermis of black skin has an inherent sun protective factor (SPF) of 13.4 compared with the SPF of 3.3 associated with Caucasian skin.[17] This translates to mean dermal UVB transmissions of 5.7% in blacks compared with 29.4% in Caucasians. There is an even larger discrepancy in the corresponding mean UVA transmissions of 17.5% and

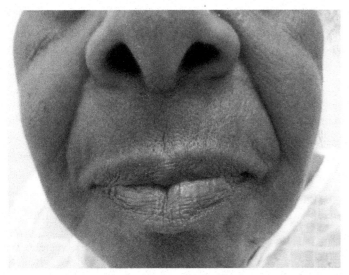

FIGURE 19-1. Photoaging in a 79-year-old African American female. Note the relative lack of wrinkling and dyspigmentation.

55.5% for black and Caucasian skin, respectively.[17] As a result of the natural photoprotection of skin of color compared with lighter skin, in vitro studies have shown decreased photodamage in darker skin of color. When comparing the histology of 45- to 50-year-old Caucasian and African American subjects in Tucson, Arizona, samples of sun-exposed skin from the African American subjects showed only a fraction of the photodamage observed in the corresponding Caucasian skin samples. Additionally, the dermal elastic fibers in the African American sun-exposed skin samples appeared similar to samples taken from photoprotected areas of Caucasian skin.[18] It has been well documented that both the epidermis and dermis of African American skin are spared from a significant proportion of the actinic damage that equally irradiated Caucasian skin is subject to.[19-21] The increased quantity of melanin as well as the distinct packaging and distribution of melanin in dark skin of color appear to be central to this photoprotection. Cultured melanocytes from African American skin have been shown to produce twice as much melanin as those obtained from Caucasian skin.[16] Darker skin also shows increased levels of tyrosinase-related protein-1, a key enzyme in melanogenesis, compared with Mexican and Caucasian skin.[22] In addition, compared with the clusters of melanosomes found in white skin, melanosomes in black skin are more widely dispersed, further aiding in their absorption of UVR.[12] Although the absorption of UVR by the stratum corneum is similar between white and black skin, because of the differences in melanin discussed earlier, in black skin, UVR absorption in the malpighian layers exceeds that of the stratum corneum and is the primary site of UVR absorption in this group.[17] There are also differences in the dermis of individuals with skin of color that have photoaging implications. Compared with Caucasians, African Americans (along with Asians) possess a thicker and more compact dermis.[19-21] Additionally, the dermis of older skin of color individuals contains less elastotic tissue and more fiber fragments, hypertrophied multinucleated fibroblasts, and macrophages, which may suggest more biosynthesis, degradation, and turnover than is appreciated in older fairer-skinned individuals.[2]

Due to the histologic differences discussed in the previous paragraph, skin of color patients do not show signs of photoaging as early or to the same extent as their Caucasian counterparts. The fact that, in the United States, many skin of color individuals prefer to have untanned skin and therefore do not actively seek to tan as frequently as American Caucasians do may also contribute to this difference. Nonetheless, evidence of photoaging is not typically observed in blacks until the fifth or sixth decade.[23] Skin of color individuals with lighter complexions tend to develop more significant photoaging than those who are dark-skinned. In addition, African Americans seem to experience more photoaging than Africans and Afrocaribbeans, which may reflect the heterogenous genetic background of Americans of African descent.[24]

Darker-skinned individuals display enhanced maintenance of skin laxity relative to Caucasians.[16] This is supported by a clinical study in which a device was used to compare recovery and viscoelasticity between sun-exposed and photoprotected skin across different groups. Black subjects displayed similar parameters between exposed and unexposed sites, whereas Hispanic and white subjects showed discrepancies between the sites.[25] The decreased facial wrinkling observed in skin of color relative to fairer skinned individuals appears to be a related phenomenon and may be a result of the thicker, more compact dermis and/or the increased dermal biological activity, which were discussed earlier.[2,15] Other signs of photoaging frequently observed in skin of color include mottled pigmentation and development of dermatosis papulosa nigra. Exaggerated facial laxity with sagging of the malar fat pads toward the nasolabial folds can also be observed in older subjects with skin types IV to VI.[24]

Asian Skin Asians also experience diminished dermatoheliosis compared with Caucasians. In this group, signs of photoaging may not become apparent until the age of 50 years.[26] Exceptions include more fair-skinned Asians who live in areas of intense sun exposure, such as portions of Southeast Asia, in whom photoaging can become apparent by 40 years of age.[27] In addition to any structural difference in the skin that may account for their relative photoprotection, Asians as a whole avoid sun exposure because milky white complexions are widely regarded as beautiful.[28] Parasols, long-sleeved clothing, hats, and sunscreens are often used in this group to minimize tanning. The Asian population can be subcategorized into East and Southeast Asians (including Chinese, Japanese, Koreans, Singaporeans, Malaysians, and Thais) and South Asians (including Indians and Pakistanis). Among East and Southeast Asians, signs of photoaging are primarily pigmentary changes, including solar lentigines, seborrheic keratoses (SKs), and mottled hyperpigmentation.[24] Sun-related hyperpigmentation, increasing presence of SKs, and dermatosis papulosa nigra lesions are common features of dermatoheliosis among South Asians.[24] American Asians actually develop age-related pigmentary changes at a decreased rate relative to other skin of color groups in the United States, but their appearance can still be a significant cosmetic concern in this group.[16] Among Japanese women living further south in Japan and, as a result, receiving 1.5 times as much UVR as women in northern Japan, a significantly greater number of larger facial wrinkles, more hyperpigmentation, more yellow skin, a rougher skin texture, and reduced stratum corneum hydration were observed.[29] Photoaging in Asians presents more often as pigmentary changes and less often as wrinkling.[30,31]

SKs are some of the more common pigmentary changes observed in this group. These lesions are the major pigmentary lesion seen in Asian men [**Figure 19-2**].[32] The number of SKs is directly proportional to age, with a mean overall prevalence of 78.9% in 40-year-olds, 93.9% in 50-year-olds, and 98.7% in Asians over the age of 60 years.[33] Sunlight exposure has been shown to be an independent risk factor for the development of SKs in Asians, with a greater size and number of these lesions developing in chronically sun-exposed skin than in more photoprotected skin. As would be expected, these lesions are concentrated on the face, followed by the dorsal hands.[33]

Although classically wrinkling has not been associated with photoaging among Asians, recent studies have shown the development of rhytids to be a prominent feature of the sun-induced aging process of skin in this group.[30-32] Although present in both sexes, Chung et al[32] found facial wrinkling to be more severe among women. Taking into consideration the effects of the possible confounders of age and sex, Asians exposed to more than 5 hours of daily sunlight exhibited a 4.8 times greater likelihood of developing wrinkling compared with Asian women receiving 1 to 2 hours of sun exposure per day.[32] The pattern of wrinkling in Asians is quite different from that of Caucasians. Whereas wrinkling in Caucasian skin is usually finer and predominantly affects the cheeks and crow's feet area, among Asians, wrinkles are usually deeper and thicker and more commonly affect the forehead

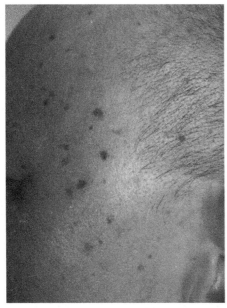

FIGURE 19-2. Photoaging in an Asian male. Note numerous pigmented seborrheic keratoses on temple and cheek.

and the perioral region in addition to the periorbital region.[28] A study examining the prevalence of rhytids across different locations of the face revealed involvement in the following order: eye areas > lower eyelid > upper eyelid > cheek > forehead > mouth area > nasolabial grooves > glabella.[34] The development of facial wrinkling is also far less severe in Asians when compared to Caucasians. Moderate to severe wrinkling is observed to develop 10 to 20 years later in Asians than in Caucasians.[35] A study comparing Caucasian females in Cincinnati, Ohio, to Japanese women showed decreased wrinkle and facial sagging scores in the Asian cohort. As with African Americans, Asian skin has been found to have a thicker, more compact dermis than Caucasians, possibly explaining this difference.[15]

Hispanic Skin Photoaging is the third most common reason Hispanic individuals present to the dermatologist, accounting for 16.8% of Hispanic dermatology visits.[36] The Hispanic diaspora is composed of individuals with varying degrees of European and Native American backgrounds. As such, this is an extremely heterogeneous ethnic group with expectedly varied photoaging phenotypes. More fair-skinned Hispanics, such as those of European descent, photoage similarly to darker-skinned Caucasians, primarily with fine wrinkling.[2,24] The fine wrinkling and mottled pigmentation that are frequently observed in photoaged Asians are often apparent in older, more darkly complexioned Hispanics.[2] Individuals in the hot climates of Mexico and Central and South America fit into this subset because they may present with Fitzpatrick skin type IV or V. The most significant dermatoheliosis among Hispanics can be observed in individuals who have labored in outdoor occupations for many years, and these individuals can display particularly deep wrinkling.[23]

PHOTOCARCINOGENESIS

UVR suppresses the skin's immune system in a localized (direct) and systemic manner (at a distant unirradiated site).[36] Clinical examples of UV immunosuppression are the reactivation of herpes simplex infections after solar exposure or the increased risk of certain skin cancers in chronically immunosuppressed solid organ transplant patients.[37,38] Previously, it was thought that mainly UVB induces immunosuppression, but UVA radiation may also play a role by inducing oxidative damage.[39,40] The chromophores responsible for initiating the skin's immune modulation and downstream signaling in response to UVR have not been completely elucidated but are presumed to be nuclear DNA and urocanic acid (UCA), which is found in the stratum corneum. UVR increases a variety of pro- and anti-inflammatory mediators. In particular, tumor necrosis factor-a, interleukin-1β, and the eicosanoid, prostaglandin E_2, may be involved in stimulating the migration of Langerhans cells out of the epidermis, resulting in diminished antigen presentation function and reduced immunosurveillance. UVR can also stimulate T-suppressor cells or T-regulatory cells and inhibit the activity of natural killer cells involved in innate immunity and tumor suppression.[38]

Both UVB and UVA are capable of inducing DNA damage, although through different mechanisms. UVB is most efficient in inducing DNA damage through the formation of cyclobutane pyrimidine dimers, and pyrimidine (6-4) pyrimidone photoproducts. UVA radiation produces DNA damage mainly through indirect mechanisms. UVA induces the generation of single oxygen, hydrogen peroxide, and superoxide radicals. However, it should be noted that the action spectra in inducing DNA damage in mammalian cells by UVB and UVA are not mutually exclusive.[41] Although UVA predominately induces DNA damage through generation of ROS, in vivo, UVA has been shown to also induce pyrimidine dimer formation in human skin.[42] UVB is also known to induce oxidative damage on the DNA [**Table 19-1**].

UV exposure has been associated with the development of actinic keratoses, squamous cell carcinomas (SCCs), basal cell carcinomas (BCCs), and possibly melanomas. Because melanin acts as a natural UV filter, skin of color has the dual benefit of decreased actinic DNA damage as well as reduced UV-induced immunosuppression, together

TABLE 19-1 UV-Induced DNA damage
Predominant effects of UVB
Cyclobutane pyrimidine dimers
Thymine-thymine
Cytosine-thymine
Thymine-cytosine
Cytosine-cytosine
Pyrimidine (6-4) pyrimidone photoproducts
Thymine-cytosine (6,4) dimers
Cytosine-cytosine (6,4) dimers
Thymine-thymine (6,4) dimers
Predominant effects of UVA
Generation of reactive oxygen species
8-Hydroxy-2'-deoxyguanosine

Abbreviation: UV, ultraviolet.

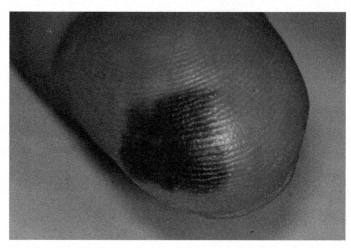

FIGURE 19-4. Acral lentiginous melanoma in a Hispanic patient.

greatly contributing to the decreased rates of skin cancer in skin of color. The incidence of SCC in the U.S. Caucasian population has been reported to be 17 to 150 per 100,000 women and 30 to 360 per 100,000 men. This can be starkly contrasted with the SCC incidences of 13.8 to 32.9 per 100,000 in U.S. Hispanics, 3 per 100,000 in U.S. individuals with dark skin of color, and 2.6 to 2.9 per 100,000 in Chinese Asians.[43] Caucasian men have the highest incidence of BCC at 250 per 100,000 population, while Caucasian women have been reported to have an incidence of 212 per 100,000. The reported incidences of BCC per 100,000 population in dark skin of color men (1), dark skin of color women (2), Chinese men (6.4), Chinese women (5.8), Japanese men and women (16.5 to 25), U.S. Hispanic men (91 to 171), and U.S. Hispanic females (50 to 113) are notably lower.[43] **Figure 19-3** is an image of a BCC in skin of color. Far less prevalent than the other cutaneous malignancies in the Caucasian population, melanoma incidences of 31.6 and 19.9 per 100,000 men and women, respectively, were reported in the Surveillance, Epidemiology, and End Results (SEER) data from 2005 to 2009.[44] The SEER data for melanoma incidence rates per 100,00 population for the same time span are substantially lower in blacks (1.1 in men, 0.9 in women), Asians/Pacific Islanders (1.6 in men, 1.2 in women), and Hispanics (4.7 in men, 4.6 in women). **Figure 19-4** shows the acral lentiginous subtype of melanoma in dark skin, which is the subtype most frequently seen in those with skin of color. For more in-depth discussion of SCC, BCC, and melanoma in skin of color, please refer to Chapters 44 to 46.

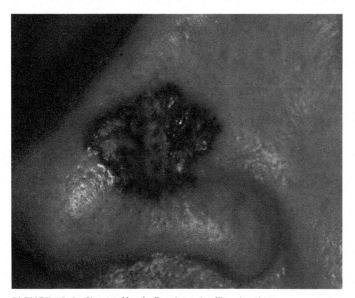

FIGURE 19-3. Pigmented basal cell carcinoma in a Hispanic patient.

CONCLUSION

This chapter has summarized the chronic cutaneous effects of UVR in general and its impact on patients with skin of color in particular. Due to the effects of melanin, individuals with skin of color are less likely to develop UV-associated skin cancers and photoaging compared with fair-skinned individuals. In skin of color, photoaging is typically not evident until the fifth or sixth decade. Photoaging in Asians presents as pigmentary changes and facial wrinkling. Hispanics are an extremely heterogeneous ethnic group with widely varied photoaging phenotypes.

REFERENCES

1. Calzavara-Pinton P, Ortel B. Pigmentation after solar radiation. In: Giacomoni PU, ed. *Biophysical and Physiological Effects of Solar Radiation on Human Skin*. Vol 10. Melville, NY: RSC Publishing; 2007:65-97.
2. Halder R, Richards G. Photoaging in patients of skin of color. In: Rigel D, Weiss R, Lim H, Dover J, eds. *Photoaging*. New York, NY: Marcell Dekker, Inc; 2004:55-63.
3. Wlaschek M, Tantcheva-Poor I, Naderi L. Solar UV irradiation and dermal photoaging. *J Photochem Photobiol B*. 2001;63:41-51.
4. Yaar M. The chronic effects of ultraviolet radiation on the skin: photoaging. In: Lim H, Honigsmann H, Hawk J, eds. *Photodermatology*. New York, NY: Informa Healthcare USA, Inc; 2007:92-106.
5. Fisher GJ, Wang ZQ, Datta SC, Varani J, Kang S, Voorhees JJ. Pathophysiology of premature skin aging induced by ultraviolet light. *N Engl J Med*. 1997;337:1419-1428.
6. Schieke S, Schroeder P, Krutmann J. Cutaneous effects of infrared radiation: from clinical observations to molecular response mechanisms. *Photodermatol Photoimmunol Photomed*. 2003;19:228-234.
7. Del Bino S, Sok J, Bessac E, Bernerd F. Relationship between skin response to ultraviolet exposure and skin color type. *Pigment Cell Res*. 2006;19:606-614.
8. Taylor SC. Skin of color: biology, structure, function, and implications for dermatologic disease. *J Am Acad Dermatol*. 2002;46(2 Suppl):S41-S62.
9. Yamaguchi Y, Takahashi K, Zmudzka B, et al. Human skin responses to UV radiation: pigment in the upper epidermis protects against DBA damage in the lower epidermis and facilitates apoptosis. *FASEB J*. 2006;20:1486-1488.
10. Alaluf S, Heath A, Carter N, et al. Variation in melanin content and composition in type V and VI photoexposed and photoprotected human skin: the dominant role of DHI. *Pigment Cell Res*. 2001;14:337-347.
11. Alaluf S, Atkins D, Barrett K, Blount M, Carter N, Heath A. Ethnic variation in melanin content and composition in photoexposed and photoprotected human skin. *Pigment Cell Res*. 2002;15:112-118.
12. Tadokoro T, Kobayashi N, Zmudzka BZ, et al. UV-induced DNA damage and melanin content in human skin differing in racial/ethnic origin. *FASEB J*. 2003;17:1177-1179.
13. Thong HY, Jee SH, Sun CC, Boissy RE. The patterns of melanosome distribution in keratinocytes of human skin as one determining factor of skin colour. *Br J Dermatol*. 2003;149:498-505.

14. Nielsen KP, Zhao L, Stamnes JJ, Stamnes K, Moan J. The importance of the depth distribution of melanin in skin for DNA protection and other photobiological processes. *J Photochem Photobiol B*. 2006;82:194-198.

15. Kundu RV, Halder RM. Evaluation of the ethnic skin patient presenting for cosmetic procedures. In: Alam M, Bhatia AC, Kundu RV, Yoo SS, Chan HH, eds. *Cosmetic Dermatology for Skin of Color*. New York, NY: McGraw-Hill Medical; 2009:12-15.

16. Rawlings AV. Ethnic skin types: are there differences in skin structure and function? *Int J Cosmet Sci*. 2006;28:79-93.

17. Kaidbey KH, Agin PP, Sayre RM, Kligman AM. Photoprotection by melanin—a comparison of black and Caucasian skin. *J Am Acad Dermatol*. 1979;1:249-260.

18. Burgess CM. Special considerations in African American skin. In: Alam M, Bhatia AC, Kundu RV, Yoo SS, Chan HH, eds. *Cosmetic Dermatology for Skin of Color*. New York, NY: McGraw-Hill Medical; 2009:163-168.

19. Halder RM. The role of retinoids in the management of cutaneous conditions in blacks. *J Am Acad Dermatol*. 1998;39:S98-S103.

20. Montagna W, Kirchner S, Carlisle K. Histology of sun-damaged human skin. *J Am Acad Dermatol*. 1989;21:907-918.

21. Montagna W, Carlisle K. The architecture of black and white facial skin. *J Am Acad Dermatol*. 1991;24:929-937.

22. Alaluf S, Barrett K, Blount M, Carter N. Ethnic variation in tyrosinase and TYRP1 expression in photoexposed and photoprotected human skin. *Pigment Cell Res*. 2003;16:35-42.

23. Halder RM, Ara CJ. Skin cancer and photoaging in ethnic skin. *Dermatol Clin*. 2003;21:725-732.

24. Munavalli GS, Weiss RA, Halder RM. Photoaging and nonablative photorejuvenation in ethnic skin. *Dermatol Surg*. 2005;31:1250-1260.

25. Berardesca E, de Rigal J, Leveque JL, Maibach HI. In vivo biophysical characterization of skin physiological differences in races. *Dermatologica*. 1991;182:89-93.

26. Goh SH. The treatment of visible signs of senescence: the Asian experience. *Br J Dermatol*. 1990;122:105-109.

27. Kotrajaras R, Kligman AM. The effect of topical tretinoin on photodamaged facial skin: the Thai experience. *Br J Dermatol*. 1993;129:302-309.

28. Chung JH. Photoaging in Asians. *Photodermatol Photoimmunol Photomed*. 2003;19:109-121.

29. Hillebrand GG, Miyamoto K, Schnell B, Ichihashi M, Shinkura R, Akiba S. Quantitative evaluation of skin condition in an epidemiological survey of females living in northern versus southern Japan. *J Dermatol*. 2001;27(Suppl 1): S42-S52.

30. Griffiths CE, Wang TS, Hamilton TA, Voorhees JJ, Ellis CN. A photonumeric scale for the assessment of cutaneous photodamage. *Arch Dermatol*. 1992;128:347-351.

31. Larnier C, Ortonne JP, Venot A, et al. Evaluation of cutaneous photodamage using a photographic scale. *Br J Dermatol*. 1994;130:167-173.

32. Chung JH, Lee SH, Youn CS, et al. Cutaneous photodamage in Koreans: influence of sex, sun exposure, smoking, and skin color. *Arch Dermatol*. 2001;137:1043-1051.

33. Kwon OS, Hwang EJ, Bae JH, et al. Seborrheic keratosis in the Korean males: causative role of sunlight. *Photodermatol Photoimmunol Photomed*. 2003;19:73-80.

34. Tsukahara K, Takema Y, Kazama H, et al. A photographic scale for the assessment of human facial wrinkles. *J Soc Cosmet Chem*. 2000;51:127-140.

35. Chan HH, Jackson B. Laser treatment in ethnic skin. In: Lim H, Honigsmann H, Hawk J, eds. *Photodermatology*. New York, NY: Informa Healthcare USA, Inc; 2007:417-432.

36. Sanchez MR. Cutaneous diseases in Latinos. *Dermatol Clin*. 2003;21:689-697.

37. Schwartz T. Photoimmunosuppression. *Photodermatol Photoimmunol Photomed*. 2002;18:141-145.

38. Perna J, Mannix M, Rooney J, Notkins A, Straus S. Reactivation of latent herpes simplex virus infection by ultraviolet light: a human model. *J Am Acad Dermatol*. 1987;17:473-478.

39. Rhodes L, Lim H. Acute effects of ultraviolet radiation on the skin. In: Lim H, Honigsmann H, Hawk J, eds. *Photodermatology*. New York, NY: Informa Healthcare USA, Inc; 2007:76-89.

40. Kullavanijaya P, Lim H. Photoprotection. *J Am Acad Dermatol*. 2005;52:937-958.

41. Kielbassa C, Roza L, Epe B. Wavelength dependence of oxidative DNA damage induced by UV and visible light. *Carcinogenesis*. 1997;18:811-816.

42. Young AR, Potten CS, Nikaido O, et al. Human melanocytes and keratinocytes exposed to UVB or UVA in vivo show comparable levels of thymine dimers. *J Invest Dermatol*. 1998;111:936-940.

43. Gloster HM Jr, Neal K. Skin cancer in skin of color. *J Am Acad Dermatol*. 2006;55:741-760.

44. National Cancer Institute. SEER Stat Fact Sheets: melanoma of the skin. http://seer.cancer.gov/statfacts/html/melan.html#incidence-mortality. Accessed February 18, 2013.

CHAPTER

20

Nuances in Skin of Color

A. Paul Kelly

Karen A. Heidelberg

KEY POINTS

- Visual observation can be more useful than sophisticated technology in distinguishing abnormalities from common nuances of skin of color.

- Futcher lines, abrupt color demarcations on the flexor surface of the upper arm, are common among adults with skin of color, although rare in infants.

- In children, hair lines, characterized by an abrupt linear demarcation between the darker, lateral, lanugo hair-containing area of the arm and the medial non-hairy area, occur in a similar pattern as Futcher lines.

- Forearm and thigh lines, less common than Futcher lines and often hard to distinguish, are seldom mentioned in the literature.

- Linea nigra and linea alba demarcations of the trunk are common among patients with darker skin of color.

- Although not found in infants, palmar and plantar hyperpigmentation becomes more common in older patients.

- Infants with darker skin of color frequently have localized areas of hyperpigmentation.

- Hyperpigmentation of the oral mucosa and sclera, although common in adults, is not found in young children, but infants often have a lip discoloration that disappears quickly.

- Melanonychia striata, common in older adults, is rare in young children, suggesting trauma as the usual cause, although melanoma must be considered.

- Idiopathic guttate hypomelanosis, characterized by hypopigmented patches primarily on the anterior leg, is more common in older patients.

- Mongolian spots that present in Native American, Asian, and African American infants may not appear in the classic lumbosacral region but rather on the hip.

Skin, our largest organ, is a window of human biology and pathology. Yet too often, clinical observation is undervalued on the assumption that it will add nothing to information obtained by light or electron microscopy, immunofluorescent techniques, and other more sophisticated investigative approaches. Additionally, until recently, dermatology has focused on Caucasian skin. Now, however, it is beginning to focus on skin of color as a definitive area of study. This chapter focuses on visual observations of several skin nuances in individuals with skin of color, particularly in people with darker pigmentation. Many such nuances have not been described previously or were called abnormal, even though they were common to a large percentage of people with more darkly pigmented skin [**Figure 20-1, A and B**].

Dramatic shifts in worldwide demographics are anticipated throughout the twenty-first century and beyond. For example, in 2013, Hispanics, Asians, and African Americans composed 37% of the American population. By 2060, they will represent more than half of the population in the United States.[1]

Although Niedelman's article, *Abnormalities of Pigmentation in the Negro*, was published over 60 years ago,[2] and Kelly[3] and Johnson[4] have since better defined these norms, confusion remains as to what is normal and abnormal when evaluating skin of color. This chapter will clearly elucidate and discuss cutaneous variants in skin of color.

PIGMENTARY DEMARCATION LINES

FUTCHER LINES

Futcher lines were described by Futcher[5] as an abrupt linear demarcation on the flexor surface of the upper arm; the medial side was lighter in color than the lateral side. However, in 1913, Matsumoto[6] was the first to report this finding. Other Japanese authors also described this demarcation line, and their findings were summarized by Ito,[7] who reported that it was present in 43% of the Japanese and 10 times more often in females. Maruya, cited by Miura,[8] screened more than 1300 Japanese individuals and found the line in 39% of females and 23% of males. Vollum[9] observed it in 26% of Jamaican children aged 1 to 11 years, but unlike the Japanese reports, there was no male/female difference. James et al[10] described six types of pigmentary demarcation lines, of which type A lines corresponded to the classic Futcher lines. They found a 44% incidence of type A lines, with a higher incidence in female patients. Selmanowitz and Krivo[11] reported that 37% of 100 patients with darker skin of color had this type of pigmentary demarcation on the arm, with an approximately equal sex ratio.

To localize Futcher lines anatomically, they have been divided into quadrants. The upper outer surface is quadrant 1, counterclockwise on the left and right arms. Most demarcations occur in quadrant 1. The next most common is quadrant 2, where the lines are more proximal and often continue for a short distance along the posterior auxiliary fold [**Figure 20-2A**].

A study performed at King Drew Medical Center (KDMC; Los Angeles, CA) indicated that more than 50% of the darker-pigmented patients examined had this abrupt color change bilaterally, whereas less than 10% had it unilaterally.[3] There was no correlation of unilateral lesions with the dominant hand or body build. There was no significant variation in the frequency of these lines in males and females, except in senior citizens, in whom demarcation lines were found in 20% fewer males. Futcher demarcation lines averaged approximately 10 cm in length. There was no correlation of these lines with skin color. Anatomically, Futcher lines follow no definite muscle, nerve, or blood vessel, although they have been associated with the biceps muscle, division of the C8 and T1, and course of the cephalic vein, respectively [**Figure 20-2B**].[5]

HAIR LINES

Infants with darker-pigmented skin seldom demonstrate Futcher lines. Most, however, display a hair line in a similar pattern as Futcher lines and characterized by an abrupt linear demarcation [**Figure 20-3**]. Since there is a definite hair line in approximately the same percentage of infants as Futcher lines in adults, a possible explanation for the lines is that the larger or more numerous hair follicles impart a darker color to the skin. This is further illustrated by the often abrupt demarcation between the dark sideburn areas in infants and the lighter brown skin anterior and posterior to this future hair-bearing area [**Figure 20-4, A and B**].

A hair line appeared on quadrant 1 of the arm in 50% of the KDMC darker-pigmented infants, and 80% of these had a concomitant line

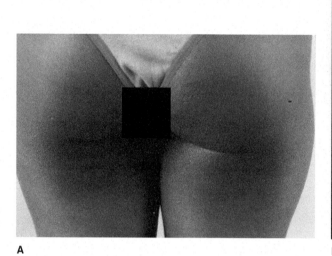

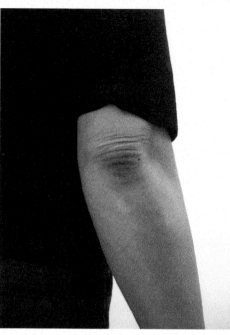

A   B

FIGURE 20-1. (A) and (B) A larger percentage of people with darker skin display hyperpigmentation as part of their normal skin color (Used with permission from Karen Heidelberg, MD, USA.)

extending from the upper back, above the axillae, and down the proximal third of quadrant 2 of the arm.[3] This divided the arm into two separate colors without the blending that is usually observed on the dorsal (exterior) aspect of the arm in children and adults. Because this demarcation is usually on the ventral surface of the arm on the one side, it should not represent Voigt lines separating the ventral from the dorsal aspect of the body, as discussed by Matsumoto[6] and Wasserman.[12]

FOREARM LINES

Forearm lines, a color demarcation on the medial aspect of the forearm, were present in 60% of males and 75% of females in the KDMC study.[3] More than 50% of males had only one forearm involved, and this was

usually on the dominant side. A few of these demarcations seemed to be continuations of Futcher lines, although most had no connection. No mention was made of this demarcation by James et al.[10] This may be due to the fact that although the incidence is high, the lines are often hard to discern.

THIGH LINES

Thigh lines or according to James et al., type B lines[10] [**Figure 20-5**] were present in approximately one quarter of the darker-pigmented males and females examined, and two-thirds of those examined had concomitant Futcher lines.[3] They were most often present on the posteromedial aspect of the thigh. Thigh lines seemed to follow the area innervated

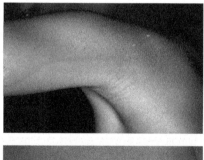

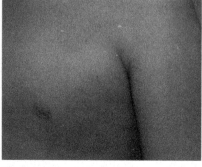

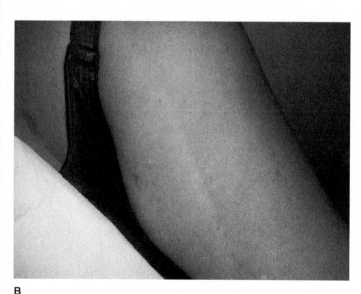

A   B

FIGURE 20-2. (A) and (B) Futcher lines. Four quadrants are present on left and right arms. Note the demarcations on each arm. (B: Used with permission from Karen Heidelberg, MD, USA.)

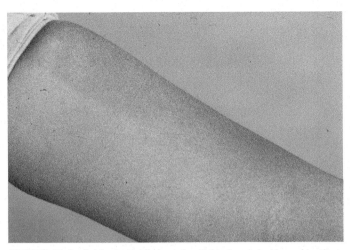

FIGURE 20-3. Hair line in skin of color male, which is characterized by an abrupt linear demarcation between the darker, lateral, lanugo hair-containing area of the arm and the medial nonhairy area.

by the anterior femoral cutaneous nerve (I1, I2, I3) medially and the posterior femoral cutaneous nerve (S1, S2, S3) laterally. Some people with thigh lines had extensions across the popliteal area onto the calf, sometimes extending to the medial aspect of the ankle. Although the incidence in males and females was the same, more females had bilateral thigh demarcations.

▮ LEG DEMARCATION LINES

Leg demarcation lines are either not reported or seldom mentioned in previous articles on skin lines. This line may be an extension of the thigh line, and sometimes, it is the only demarcation on the lower extremity. The most likely reason that these leg and thigh lines have seldom been described by other investigators and are considered a rarity is the phenomenon of "ashiness." When dark skin is dry, especially in cold weather, it seems to be covered with grayish bran-like scales, termed *ash*. The legs are especially prone to ashiness, which most likely

masks most linear demarcations. Because the leg demarcation is not as vivid as that of the arm, wiping the leg with a wet cloth or applying an emollient cream or an oil preparation before examining the leg for lines is imperative. In the KDMC study,[3] leg demarcations usually extended from the popliteal fossa to the medial ankle, being most prominent above the calf. There was no difference in the incidence according to age, sex, or body build with the exception of infants, who had questionable hair line demarcations on the thighs and legs. Hair lines on their lower extremities occurred in approximately the same configurations and frequency (30%) as in adults with true lower extremity linear cutaneous demarcations.

James et al[13] reported two women who developed lower extremity linear demarcations (type B lines) during pregnancy. Furthermore, 14% of mothers with darker skin of color claimed that they first noted these lines during pregnancy.[13] Fulk[14] also supported this observation.

MIDTRUNK DEMARCATIONS

Cutaneous linea nigra and linea alba are interesting skin markings occurring in patients. Two-thirds of all patients with darker skin of color examined at KDMC had linea nigra, a dark line extending from the suprapubic area to the umbilicus.[3] There was no variation of the midtrunk demarcation based on age or sex. These demarcations ranged from 1 to 14 cm in length and from 1 to 8 mm in width. Usually these lines extended from the umbilicus to the suprapubic area, although 20% of patients had the line extending to a supraumbilical location [**Figure 20-6**]. The longest line was 9 cm above the umbilicus. There were no subjects in whom the linea nigra was located only in a supraumbilical position.

Cutaneous linea alba, also termed midline hypopigmentation, is a vertical hypopigmented demarcation in or near the midsagittal line that may begin on one side of the trunk, cross the midline, and continue in a vertical direction on the opposite side [**Figure 20-7**]. Niedelman[2] mentioned but did not elaborate on this line. Selmanowitz and Krivo[15] found a linea alba in 43% of males and 33% of females with darker skin of color. In contrast, the KDMC evaluations showed a greater than 60% occurrence in both sexes, with a slightly higher incidence in males. Linea alba

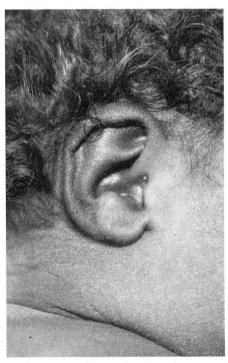

A

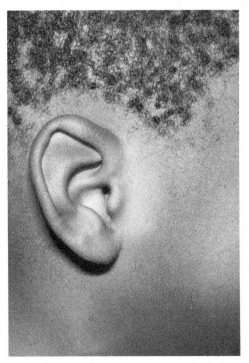

B

FIGURE 20-4. (A) and (B) Infants with darker skin of color showing an abrupt demarcation between the dark sideburn area and the lighter brown anterior and posterior areas.

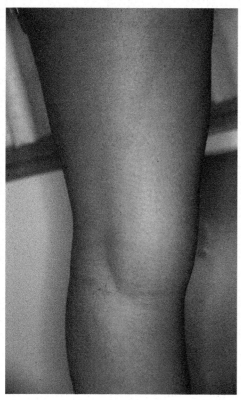

FIGURE 20-5. A type B thigh line demarcation in a patient with darker skin of color.

appeared anywhere from the dorsal aspect of the manubrium to the umbilicus. However, none extended below the umbilicus. Size ranged from 2 mm to 2 cm in diameter and from 4 to 25 cm in length. Linea alba corresponds to the type C lines that James et al[10] found in 36% of their patients with darker skin of color (44% male, 20% female). Others found these lines in approximately 40% of their patients with darker skin of color, with a slight male predominance.[15,16]

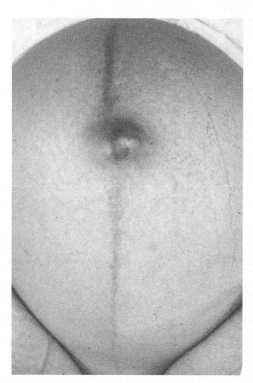

FIGURE 20-6. Linea nigra, a dark line extending from the suprapubic area to the umbilicus.

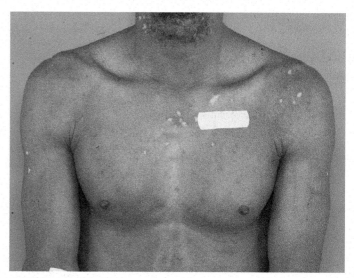

FIGURE 20-7. Cutaneous linea alba is a vertical hypopigmentation in or near the midsagittal line that often starts on one side, crosses the midline, and then moves down the opposite side.

It is unknown why the upper half of the anterior trunk would have a hypopigmented ventral midline demarcation and the lower anterior trunk a hyperpigmented demarcation. One plausible explanation is that melanocytes, migrating in a dorsal to ventral direction from the neutral crest origin, do not always complete their journey in the upper, wider chest region and come together to the point of supersaturation on the lower abdominal area due to its smaller girth. Skin color, sex, and body build did not seem to have any influence on the presence or absence of these ventral linear color demarcations.

A broad area of midback vertical hypopigmentation (type D lines[10]) was found in 3 of 50 infants and 5 of 100 adults.[3] The lines are often hard to discern, and the incidence is not sufficient to be considered common in people with darker skin of color.

Bilateral hypopigmented macules (type E lines)[10] were found in 12% of the KDMC patients, with a slight male predominance.[3] Selmanowitz and Krivo[15] found a 16% incidence, with male patients having twice the incidence of females, whereas James et al[10] reported a 13% incidence with an equal sex ratio. Because these are not linear demarcations but bilateral hypopigmented macules, it is sometimes difficult to differentiate the changes from postinflammatory hypopigmentation or pityriasis alba.

Futcher also described a midchest demarcation;[17] this has also been seen in patients at KDMC [**Figure 20-8**].[3] The frequency of the

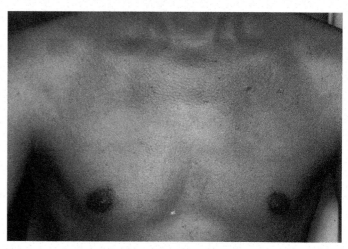

FIGURE 20-8. Futcher line with midchest demarcation.

demarcation makes it difficult to determine whether there is any association with age, sex, body type, skin color, or disease.

PALMAR AND PLANTAR HYPERPIGMENTATION

Palmar and plantar hyperpigmentation is a common finding in adults with darker skin of color [**Figure 20-9, A–E**]. A study at KDMC revealed that hyperpigmented macules and patches of the palms were present in 35% of examined adults with darker skin of color and in more than 50% of those over the age of 50, but were absent in infants with darker skin of color.[3] The youngest patient in the KDMC study demonstrating palmar hyperpigmentation was 4 years old. None of the examined infants with darker skin of color had plantar hyperpigmentation, whereas it was present in more than 70% of patients with darker skin of color over the age of 50. Because hyperpigmentation of neither the palms nor the soles is present at birth, trauma leading to postinflammatory changes may be the

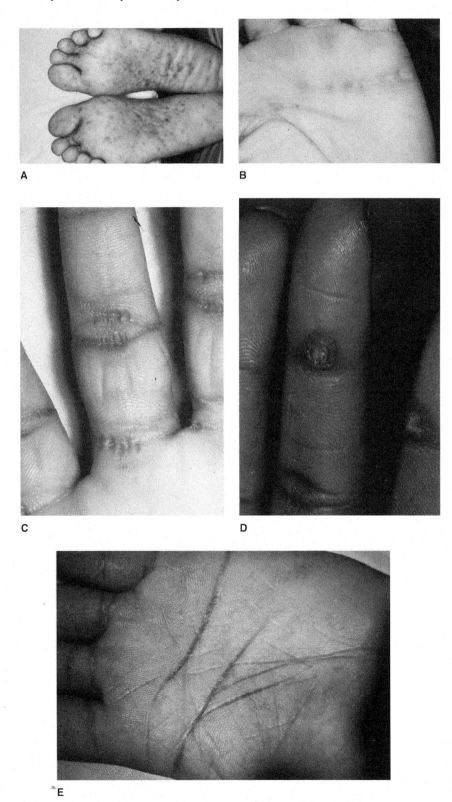

FIGURE 20-9. (A–D) Hyperpigmentation of soles and palms and punctate keratosis of palmar creases in adults with darker skin of color over the age of 50 years. **(E)** Hyperpigmentation of the palms in a Nigerian man. (E: Used with permission from Felix Oresanya, MD, Lagos, Nigeria.)

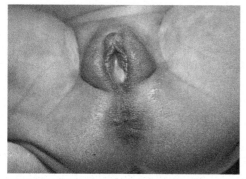

FIGURE 20-10. Hyperpigmentation of genitourinary region in an infant with skin of color.

precipitating factor. Going barefooted as a child did not seem to explain with any predictability the presence or absence of plantar hyperpigmentation.

PUNCTATE KERATOSIS OF PALMAR CREASES

Patients with darker skin of color often develop keratotic plugs in their palmar and finger creases. When the plugs are removed, shallow pits are left [Figure 20-9, A–E]. Some patients have involvement of the sole but only to a lesser degree. Atopy and manual labor are associated with this skin abnormality, but the exact cause is unknown. Therapy is usually not needed; however, if the plugs become painful, daily use of 40% urea cream is usually a successful therapy.

LOCALIZED HYPERPIGMENTATION IN INFANTS

Infants with darker skin of color have localized areas of hyperpigmentation. This phenomenon is not mentioned in any dermatology textbooks, including the *Atlas of Black Dermatology*.[18] The usual areas of involvement are the helix of the ears [Figure 20-4, A and B], lips, fingernail and toenail matrix areas, penis, scrotum, vulva, nipples, umbilicus, axillae, and anal orifice [**Figure 20-10**]. Between 60% and 85% of all infants with darker skin of color have these localized areas of darkness. There was no correlation with skin color, sex, or body build. Finger, toe, nail matrix, nipple, penis, scrotum, and vulvar hyperpigmentation seems to persist for the duration of one's life, whereas earlobe and axillary hyperpigmentation seems to disappear during the first year of life, whether the infant is exposed to sunlight or not. The rest of the skin seems to get darker, and the dark areas seem to get somewhat lighter.

It is difficult to explain why the ears (with 1400 ± 80 melanocytes/mm^2) and not the cheeks (with 2310 ± 150 melanocytes/mm^2)[18] are darker at birth. In some cultures, these dark areas are used to predict the ultimate skin color of the baby—that is, the color he or she will have as an adult.

MUCOUS MEMBRANE HYPERPIGMENTATION

Oral mucous membrane hyperpigmentation is common in darker-pigmented patients of all ages. Hyperpigmentation of the lips is common in older people with darker skin of color but is not completely absent in younger patients [**Figure 20-11, A and B**]; however, in the KDMC study, deep grayish to violaceous, dry discoloration of the lips, especially the upper lip, was found in 60% of infants examined.[3] It seemed to start at the lower or inner aspect of the free margin of the lips and progress inward approximately 5 to 7 mm. The discoloration clears within a few weeks of life without residual cutaneous markings. Search of the dental, otolaryngology, and dermatology literature failed to reveal any mention of this nuance. One possible explanation is lip sucking in utero.

Hyperpigmentation of the gums appeared in 25% of infants, and less than 10% had hyperpigmentation of the buccal mucosa. The severity and frequency of oral pigmentation seem to increase with age. Almost 80% of patients with darker skin of color over the age of 65 will have

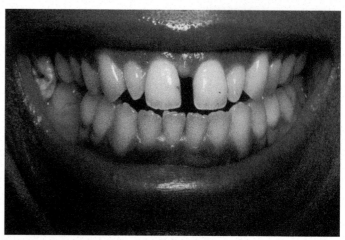

A

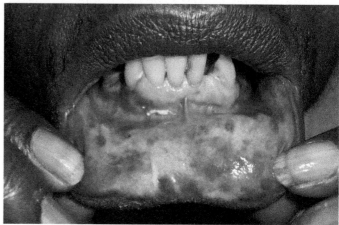

B

FIGURE 20-11. **(A)** In a darker-pigmented younger adult, the hyperpigmentation of the mucous membrane of the gum is not as extensive as in older adults. **(B)** Mucous membrane hyperpigmentation of the gum in a darker-pigmented adult over the age of 65 years. (B: Used with permission from Karen Heidelberg, MD, USA.)

some type of oral mucous membrane hyperpigmentation, with the gums and lips being the areas most commonly involved.

An absence of scleral pigmentation was noted in all the infants with darker skin of color and children younger than 5 years of age. Scleral (actually the overlying conjunctiva) pigmentation seems to start in that portion of the conjunctiva exposed to sunlight and other elements, such as wind, heat, cold, and airborne particles. Over 80% of the adults with darker skin of color examined at KDMC had conjunctival pigmentation.[3] Brown discoloration was the most common, but reddish brown, red, and yellowish brown discolorations also were noticed. Males had a higher incidence than females, suggesting that environmental exposure may be a contributing factor.

MELANONYCHIA STRIATA

Between 50% and 90% of senior citizens with darker skin of color have at least one fingernail with a vertical linear streak (ie, longitudinal melanonychia or melanonychia striata) [**Figure 20-12, A–C**]. The youngest patient with melanonychia striata identified at KDMC was 6 years of age, but melanonychia striata is found primarily in adults.[3] This suggests trauma, either acute or chronic, as the etiologic agent, especially because the thumb and/or index finger were involved most often. There seems to be no association of melanonychia with any systemic diseases; however, melanoma must be ruled out. Involvement of one nail with a width of 6 mm or more and variegation in color are features of longitudinal melanonychia secondary to malignant melanoma.

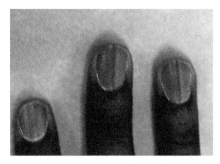

A

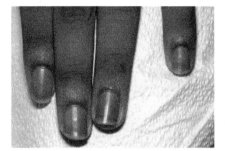

B

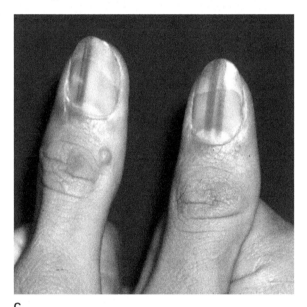

C

FIGURE 20-12. (A and B) Linear melanonychia striata in senior citizens with skin of color. **(C)** Linear melanonychia in a person with skin of color from Brazil. (B: Used with permission from Karen Heidelberg, MD, USA; C: Used with permission from Marcia Ramos-e-Silva, MD, Rio de Janeiro, Brazil.)

IDIOPATHIC GUTTATE HYPOMELANOSIS

Idiopathic guttate hypomelanosis (IGH) is an overt pigmentary nuance in patients with darker skin of color. Although present in fairer-skinned individuals, it is often difficult to discern.[19] In individuals with very darkly pigmented skin, the initial lesions are often yellow-brown in color. It is characterized by asymptomatic, hypopigmented, polygonal macules or patches (1 to 20 mm in diameter with an average diameter of 4 mm) and primarily affects the anterior legs.

The incidence of IGH varies according to age. It is present in more than 90% of senior citizens with darker skin of color, with the legs, thighs, abdomen, arms, and back involved, in decreasing order [**Figure 20-13**]. It appears to begin earlier in females and is rare in

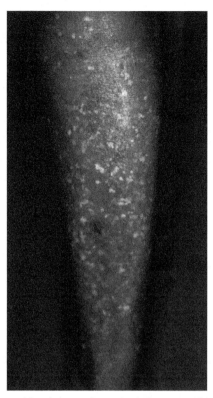

FIGURE 20-13. Idiopathic guttate hypomelanosis lesions are yellow-brown, asymptomatic hypopolymacules. The patches occur primarily on the anterior legs as can be seen in this older patient with darker skin of color.

children and young adults.[20] Patients with IGH do not have an increased susceptibility to other pigmentary disorders.

CIRCUMSCRIBED DERMAL MELANOCYTOSIS (MONGOLIAN SPOTS)

Circumscribed dermal melanocytosis, originally termed Mongolian spots, consists of dark blue-gray macules [**Figure 20-14, A and B**]. The patches are present at birth and usually regress during childhood. They occur in 98% of African American infants, 90% of Native American infants, 81% of Asian American infants, 40% to 70% of Hispanic infants, and 10% of Caucasian infants. Usually found on the buttocks, the color of the patches are uniform, and there are no significant visible changes in the epidermis.

Circumscribed dermal melanocytosis is a perfect example of how clinical observation has led to erroneous assumptions before cause and incidence are delineated. Erwin Balz, a German professor of internal medicine, was teaching in Tokyo, Japan in the early 1930s when he observed blue spots on the buttocks of Japanese children and named them "Mongolian spots," thinking them a characteristic of Mongolians.[21] When Buntaro Adachi found the same spot in a Caucasian child, he insisted that it should be called a "child spot" instead. Initially, the Japanese believed that the spot was caused by bleeding in the fetus.[22] It is now known that the Mongolian spot is caused by the arrest of melanocytes in the dermis as they migrate from the neural crest to the epidermis during the eleventh to fourteenth weeks of gestation.[21,22]

The KDMC study demonstrated that the frequency of Mongolian spots was approximately the same in babies with darker skin of color with skin colors ranging from very fair to very dark.[3] They were most noticeable in medium-brown infants and often difficult to detect in very dark babies. In 18% of cases, the Mongolian spots were not in the classic lumbosacral area; approximately half of these were located on the hips. The maximum number of lesions present in any infant was seven. As the KDMC study indicates, 92% incidence is similar to that reported by other authors.[22,23]

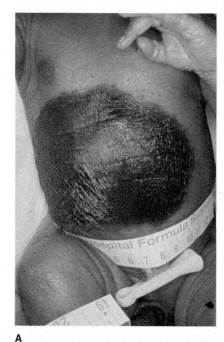

A

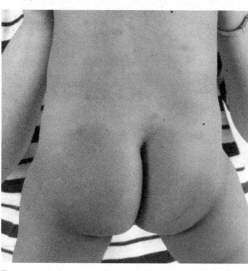

B

FIGURE 20-14. (A) Large Mongolian spot on the abdomen of a darkly pigmented infant. **(B)** Mongolian spots on the buttocks of an infant.

CONCLUSION

There are many skin nuances in individuals of color that are not readily recognized by physicians or are mistaken for abnormalities. As physicians continue to treat a growing population of patients with skin of color, it is important to recognize skin colorations that are normal variances. Patients then can be reassured that the colorations are indeed normal, and potentially unnecessary procedures may be avoided.

REFERENCES

1. U.S. Census Bureau. U.S. Census Bureau projections show a slower growing, older, more diverse nation a half century from now. https://www.census.gov/newsroom/releases/archives/population/cb12-243.html. Accessed January 18, 2013.
2. Niedelman ML. Abnormalities of pigmentation in the Negro. *Arch Dermatol.* 1945;51:1-9.
3. Kelly AP. Nuances of black skin: study performed at King Drew Medical Center (KDMC). Presented at the National Medical Association Section on Dermatology; New Orleans, LA; 1974.
4. Johnson SAM. The black skin: norms and abnorms. *Cutis.* 1978;22:332-336.
5. Futcher PH. A peculiarity of pigmentation of the upper arm of Negroes. *Science.* 1938;88:570-571.
6. Matsumoto S. Ueber eine eigentiiml. Über eine eigentümliche pigmentverteilung an den voigtschen linien. *Arch Dermat u Syph.* 1913;118:157.
7. Ito K. The peculiar demarcation of pigmentation along the so-called Voigt's lines among the Japanese. *Dermatol Int.* 1965;4:45-47.
8. Miura O. On the demarcation lines of pigmentation observed among Japanese on inner sides of their extremities and on the anterior and posterior sides of their medial regions. *Tohoku J Exp Med.* 1951;54:135-140.
9. Vollum DI. Skin markings in Negro children from the West Indies. *Br J Dermatol.* 1972;86:260-263.
10. James WD, Carter JM, Rodman OG. Pigmentary demarcation lines: a population survey. *J Am Acad Dermatol.* 1987;16:584-590.
11. Selmanowitz VJ, Krivo JM. Pigmentary demarcation lines. Comparison of Negroes with Japanese. *Br J Dermatol.* 1975;93:371-377.
12. Wasserman HP. Peculiar pigment-division along Voigt's line in a European and in a Xhosa woman. *Dermatologica.* 1967;135:461-464.
13. James WD, Meltzer MC, Guill MA, et al. Pigmentary demarcation lines associated with pregnancy. *J Am Acad Dermatol.* 1984;11:438-440.
14. Fulk CS. Primary disorders of hyperpigmentation. *J Am Acad Dermatol.* 1984;10:1-16.
15. Selmanowitz J, Krivo JM. Hypopigmented markings in negroes. *Int J Dermatol.* 1973;12:229-235.
16. Kisch B, Nasuhoglu A. A mediosternal depigmentation line in Negroes. *Exp Med Surg.* 1953;11:265-267.
17. Futcher PH. The distribution of pigmentation on the arm and thorax of man. *Bull Johns Hopkins Hosp.* 1940;67:372-373.
18. Rosen T, Martin S. *Atlas of Black Dermatology.* Boston, MA: Little, Brown and Company; 1981.
19. Whitehead WJ, Moyer DG, Vander Ploeg DE. Idiopathic guttate hypomelanosis. *Arch Dermatol.* 1966;94:279-281.
20. Treadwell PA. Dermatoses in newborns. *Am Fam Physician.* 1997;56:443-450.
21. Muraoka K. On the Mongolian spot in the Japanese. *Acta Anat Jpn.* 1931;3:1371-1390.
22. Kikuchi I. What is a Mongolian spot? *Int J Dermatol.* 1982;21:131-133.
23. Brennemann J. The sacral or so-called "Mongolian" pigment spots of earliest infancy and childhood, with especial references to their occurrence in the American Negro. *Am Anthropol.* 1907;9:12-30.

CHAPTER
21

Normal and Pathological Skin Lesions

Sharona Yashar
Jennifer Haley
Leslie Robinson-Bostom
Nianda Reid

KEY POINTS

- Pigmentary demarcation lines are normal boundaries of the skin that represent a transition between levels of melanin pigment in the skin corresponding to dermatomal innervation.

- Longitudinal melanonychia is a normal pattern of nail pigmentation seen in patients with skin of color. It is important to differentiate normal nail pigmentation from malignant melanocytic proliferations and extraneous pigment deposition.

- Physiologic pigmentation of the oral mucosa is commonly seen in patients with skin of color.

- Erythema dyschromicum perstans is seen more often in people with skin of color.

- Lability of pigment in the darker-skinned population causes dramatic changes in skin color after inflammatory processes of the skin.

- Many common dermatologic conditions manifest with follicular or papular lesions in dark-skinned individuals.

- Keloidal scarring is common in patients with skin of color.

NORMAL VARIATIONS IN SKIN OF COLOR

The skin can provide diagnostic evidence of either local or systemic disease. Therefore, when evaluating pigmentation, it is important to understand and recognize normal variants.[1] Knowledge of normal variations in skin is crucial in the evaluation and management of patients with skin of color because there are a number of skin lesions that represent physiologic variants. Historically, the lack of recognition of benign variations in dark skin has led to unnecessary treatment and potentially poor results. These lesions fall into pigmentary and nonpigmentary categories.[2]

PIGMENTARY VARIANTS

PIGMENTARY DEMARCATION LINES

Pigmentary demarcation lines are normal boundaries of the skin that represent a transition between darker and lighter melanin pigment distribution corresponding to dermatomal innervation by spinal nerves. There are six types of pigmentary demarcation lines based on anatomic location[3] [**Table 21-1**]. In one study, 79% of African American women and 75% of African American men had at least one pigmentary demarcation line. These lines may be present at birth, arise later in life, or occur during pregnancy.[4]

Type A lines, also termed *Voigt (Futcher) lines*, are sharply demarcated, frequently bilateral lines of pigmentation found at the anterolateral junction of the upper arms [**Figure 21-1**]. The change from darker to lighter pigment occurs at the junction of the extensor to flexor surface of the arm. Type B lines occur at the posteromedial aspect of the lower legs and often arise during pregnancy.[5] Up to 14% of black women present with type B lines during pregnancy.[4] Other pigmentary demarcation lines occur on the spine, chest, legs [**Figure 21-2**], and face.[6] Type E demarcation lines are also referred to as *midline hypopigmentation*. Midline hypopigmentation occurs over the anterior aspect of the central and midsternal chest and consists of hypopigmented linear or oval macules. There may be an autosomal dominant inheritance pattern of this condition.[2] The differential diagnosis includes ash leaf macules of tuberous sclerosis, postinflammatory hypopigmentation, idiopathic guttate hypomelanosis, vitiligo, seborrheic dermatitis, and tinea versicolor.[7]

The etiology of pigmentary demarcation lines is unclear. Genetic and hormonal influences have been proposed for type B pigmentary demarcation lines. Compression of peripheral nerves between S1 and S2 by the pregnant uterus may also be a factor.[8] Although reported, pigmentary demarcation lines in Caucasian patients are rare. Skin biopsy shows increased pigmentation in the basal keratinocytes of the epidermis without an inflammatory infiltrate or increase in melanocytes.[5]

Pigmentary demarcation lines represent a change in the amount of melanin pigment in the skin and should be differentiated from the rare condition of acquired dermal melanocytosis, in which there is an increase in melanocytes in the dermis. These lesions appear as blue-gray patches on the face, trunk, or extremities and may also appear during pregnancy.[9]

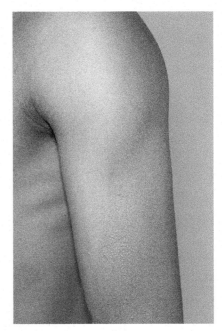

FIGURE 21-1. Futcher line of demarcation on the arm.

NAIL PIGMENTATION

Another frequent pigmentary variant in skin of color is nail pigmentation. Longitudinal melanonychia is defined as a longitudinal band of brown or black pigment in the nail[10] [**Figure 21-3**]. Longitudinal melanonychia often occurs as an acquired condition in pigmented skin, and there is often a history of trauma. Over 50% of African Americans over age 50 have at least one nail involved. The degree of nail pigmentation is increased in patients with darker skin. Histologically, there is increased melanin in the matrix and nail plate. The differential diagnosis includes melanocytic nevus, malignant melanoma, and pigmentation due to infection, drugs, chemicals, or postradiation changes. Malignant longitudinal melanonychia (melanoma) is usually wider than 5 mm[10]; it is associated with brown discoloration at the nail fold at the base of the melanonychia (Hutchinson sign). Recently, dermoscopy has become an increasingly helpful tool in the diagnosis of nail pigment. A grayish

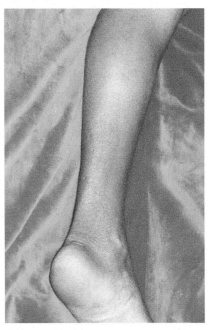

FIGURE 21-2. Demarcation line on the posteromedial aspect of the lower leg.

TABLE 21-1	Pigmentary demarcation lines	
Type	Location	Pigment
A	Anterolateral upper arms, pectoral area	Hyperpigmented
B	Posteromedial aspect of lower legs	Hyperpigmented
C	Vertical line in presternal area	Hypopigmented
D	Posteromedial area of spine	Hyperpigmented
E	Chest from midthird of clavicle to peri-areolar skin	Hypopigmented
F	Straight or curved convex line on the face	Hyperpigmented

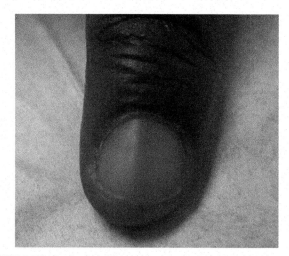

FIGURE 21-3. Longitudinal melanonychia.

background and thin, regular gray lines are common characteristics of nail pigmentation in skin of color,[11] whereas longitudinal black lines of subungual melanoma tend to be irregular in color, spacing, thickness, and parallelism.

ORAL PIGMENTATION

There may be substantial variations in the color of healthy oral mucosa. Physiologic pigmentation of the oral mucosa is common in darker skin types and may be influenced by physical, hormonal, and chemical factors.[12,13] Oral pigmentation is seen commonly on the gingivae, hard palate, buccal mucosa, and tongue in darker skin types and varies in color from light brown to blue discoloration[12] [**Figure 21-4**]. This physiologic pigmentation is due to greater melanocytic activity rather than a greater number or size of melanocytes.[13,14] The gingiva is the most common intraoral site of pigment.[15] Lesions appear as a bilateral, well-demarcated, ribbon-like, dark brown bands that usually spare the marginal gingiva, an important feature that helps to distinguish them from other pathologic causes of pigmentation, such as Addison disease.[16] In contrast, pigmentation of the buccal mucosa, hard palate, lips, and tongue may appear as less well-demarcated brown patches. In contrast to nail pigmentation, the association between the frequency of oral mucosal pigmentation and darker skin pigment is not as clear. Some observers have suggested that the degree of pigmentation may be partially related to mechanical, chemical, and physical stimulation, which can increase melanin production.[17,18]

The differential diagnosis for oral mucosal pigmentation is broad. Oral pigmentation has been classified as endogenous or exogenous, localized or generalized, melanin-based or non–melanin-based, and

TABLE 21-2	Classification of oral pigmentation
Localized pigmentation	
Amalgam tattoo	
Graphite tattoo	
Nevus	
Melanotic macule	
Melanoacanthoma	
Kaposi sarcoma	
Epithelioid oligomatosis	
Verruciform xanthoma	
Melanoma	
Generalized pigmentation	
Genetic	
Physiologic	
Peutz-Jeghers syndrome	
Laugier-Hunziker syndrome	
Spotty pigmentation	
Carney syndrome	
Leopard syndrome	
Lentiginosis profuse	
Hemochromatosis	
Neurofibromatosis	
Wilson disease	
Endocrine	
Addison disease	
Albright syndrome	
Acanthosis nigricans	
Pregnancy	
Hyperthyroidism	
Drugs	
Antimalarials	
Antimicrobials	
Minocycline	
Amiodarone	
Chlorpromazine	
Zidovudine	
Ketoconazole	
Methyldopa	
Busulfan	
Menthol	
Contraceptive pills	
Other	
Smoking	
Heavy metals	
Human immunodeficiency virus	
Nutritional deficiency	
Benign vascular tumors	

benign or malignant [**Table 21-2**]. One must always distinguish the normal variation of oral pigmentation from melanoma, melanocytic nevi, postinflammatory changes, contact dermatitis, smoker's melanosis, secondary syphilis, and drug or heavy metal ingestion. Physiologic oral pigmentation usually appears in infancy and darkens with puberty.[16] Systemic disease or exogenous influence must be suspected when pigmentation develops or darkens rapidly in adulthood.[16] Melanoma in the oral cavity is rare and has a poor prognosis.[19] Peutz-Jeghers syndrome is a genetic disorder defined by intestinal hamartomas and mucocutaneous lentigines. Oral pigmented macules are usually found on the lower lip and buccal mucosa and rarely on the upper lip, tongue, palate, and gingiva.[17] Laugier-Hunziker syndrome presents with longitudinal melanonychia and benign hyperpigmented macules of the lips, buccal mucosa, and genitalia.[20] Smoker's melanosis is directly related to tobacco use and represents a benign focal pigmentation of the oral mucosa.[21,22] Lesions present as multiple brown pigmented macules less than 1 cm in diameter at the attached labial anterior gingival and interdental papillae

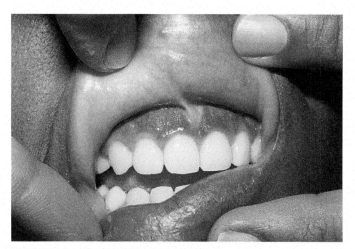

FIGURE 21-4. Oral pigmentation involving the gingiva.

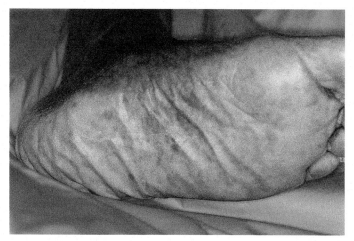

FIGURE 21-5. Plantar hyperpigmented macules.

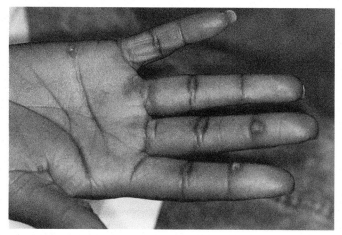

A

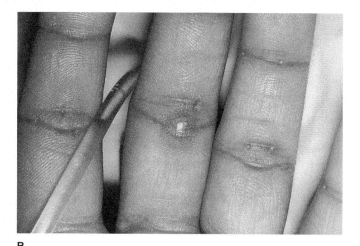

B

FIGURE 21-6. **(A) and (B)** Punctate keratoses on palms and fingers.

of the mandible.[17] Antimalarial agents induce oral pigmentation that is characterized by a slate gray color.

PALMAR AND PLANTAR HYPERPIGMENTED MACULES

Hyperpigmented macules on the palms and soles are another normal pigmentary variant in skin of color. These lesions vary in size and shape and may be sharp or ill-defined with a reticulated appearance [**Figure 21-5**]. They must be distinguished from similar-appearing lesions of secondary syphilis, tinea nigra, lentigines, nevi, and melanoma.

NONPIGMENTARY VARIANTS

PUNCTATE KERATOSES OF THE PALMS AND SOLES

Most often occurring in the creases of the palms and soles, punctate keratoses are 1- to 5-mm discrete comedo-like keratinous plugs [**Figure 21-6, A and B**]. This condition can be acquired as a result of repetitive trauma; however, autosomal dominant inheritance has been reported.[23] Punctate keratoses are a benign normal variant seen most often in black patients. A personal or family history of atopy has been reported in up to 80% of patients with keratosis palmaris et plantaris.[23] Histologically, punctate keratoses show hyperkeratosis and parakeratosis overlying a pyknotic, vacuolated epidermis and some spongiosis in the basal layer. Occlusion of glands may be present. Keratosis punctata palmaris et plantaris must be differentiated from the palmar pits of nevoid basal cell carcinoma syndrome, in which lesions tend to spare the creases. There is still some debate as to whether punctate keratoses are a variant of hyperkeratosis follicularis et parafollicularis in cutem penetrans (Kyrle disease).[23] In perforating disorders such as Kyrle disease, keratotic papules with central plugs are seen on the extremities.

ORAL LEUKOEDEMA

Leukoedema is a benign, pearly, gray-white discoloration of the buccal mucosa that is present as a normal variant in many skins of color. It may develop at any age and is usually asymptomatic.[24] Leukoedema is seen in as many as 90% of black adults and, although less prominent, in half the Caucasian population.[24] Tobacco smoking and chewing may enhance the white appearance and size of the lesions. Leukoedema is characterized histologically by intracellular edema and vacuolated epithelial cells with some pyknosis.[25] The epithelium is hyperplastic with elongated rete ridges. Treatment for leukoedema is unnecessary, and there is no malignant potential. The differential diagnosis includes white sponge nevus, leukoplakia, oral lichen planus, frictional keratosis, smokeless tobacco keratosis, and Witkop syndrome (scalp hair normal to thin, hypodontia of secondary teeth, normal sweating, and prolonged retention of primary teeth).

PEARLY PENILE PAPULES

Pearly penile papules are benign, dome-shaped papules found on the corona of the glans penis. They vary in size (ranging from 1 to 2 mm in width and up to 4 mm in length), color (pink, white, yellowish, or translucent), and shape (dome, acuminate, or annular). In most cases, they are asymptomatic and are found incidentally. A higher incidence has been reported in blacks and in uncircumcised men.[26-28] Histologically, pearly penile papules resemble angiofibromas with prominent orthokeratosis, hypergranulosis, ectatic vessels, and stellate fibroblasts with dermal fibrosis.[29] The clinical differential diagnosis includes condylomata acuminata, ectopic sebaceous glands, and lichen nitidus.[29] No treatment is necessary, but ablative methods such as cryotherapy and carbon dioxide laser have been tried with equivocal results.[30,31]

COMMON SKIN DISORDERS SEEN PREDOMINANTLY IN DARKER SKIN

Several reports have examined the rates of common skin disorders in pigmented skin. **Table 21-3** shows the common skin diagnoses seen in black, Latino American, Arab American, and South Asian American populations in the United States.[32-35] The most common skin disorders seen in skin of color include acne and eczematous dermatitis.

Acne lesions in skin of color include papules, pustules, comedones, and numerous hyperpigmented macules with a higher percentage of keloidal scarring (up to 54.1%) [**Figure 21-7**].[36] Halder et al[37] showed that comedonal lesions biopsied from African American females showed marked inflammation, including polymorphonuclear leukocytes, in

TABLE 21-3 Common skin conditions reported in Black, Hispanic, Asian, and Arab groups in the United States

Blacks[a]		Hispanics[b]		Arabs[c]		South Asians[d]	
Acne	27.7%	Acne	20.7%	Acne	37.7%	Acne	37.0%
Eczematous dermatitis	23.4%	Eczematous dermatitis	19.3%	Eczematous dermatitis	25.5%	Eczematous dermatitis	22.0%
Pigmentary disorders	9.0%	Photoaging	16.8%	Fungal infection	20.0%	Fungal infection	20.0%
Seborrheic dermatitis	6.5%	Tinea/onychomycosis	9.9%	Condyloma/warts	20.0%	Condyloma/warts	8.0%
Alopecia	5.3%	Melasma	8.2%	Melasma	14.5%	Moles	8.0%
Fungal infections	4.3%	Condyloma/warts	7.1%	Keloid	10.7%		
Condyloma/warts	2.4%	Hyperpigmentation	6%	Psoriasis	4.7%		
Tinea versicolor	2.2%	Seborrheic keratosis	4.5%	Vitiligo	2.0%		
Keloids	2.1%	Acrochordon	4.2%				
Pityriasis rosea	2.0%	Seborrheic dermatitis	3.2%				
Urticaria	2.0%	Alopecia	2.3%				
		Psoriasis	0.8%				

[a]Halder RM, Roberts CI, Nootheti PK. Cutaneous diseases in the black races. *Dermatol Clin.* 2003;21:679-687, ix.

[b]Sanchez MR. Cutaneous diseases in Latinos. *Dermatol Clin.* 2003;21:689-697.

[c]El-Essawi D, Musial J, Hammad A, Lim H. A survey of skin disease and skin-related issues in Arab Americans. *J Am Acad Dermatol.* 2007;56:933-938.

[d]Shah SK, Bhanusali DG, Sachdev A, Geria AN, Alexis AF. A survey of skin conditions and concerns in South Asian Americans: a community based study. *J Drugs Dermatol.* 2011;10:524-528.

contrast to comedonal lesions in white skin, which did not show significant inflammation. This may account for why acne in darker skin commonly results in postinflammatory hyperpigmentation.[37]

Melasma is another very frequent and distressing pigmentary disorder that occurs in people with skin of color.[38] Hormonal causes, ultraviolet (UV) radiation, and lability of melanocytes may be influential etiologic factors [**Figure 21-8**].[39]

In addition to common skin disorders seen in all skin types, there are several dermatoses that are far more frequent in darker skin. One well-known example is actinic prurigo seen in Native Americans and the Mestizo population in Latin America.[40] Actinic prurigo is an idiopathic photodermatosis that affects the sun-exposed skin, resulting in erythematous papules, nodules, and lichenified plaques.[41] Cheilitis of the lower lip is common. Conjunctivitis and pterygium formation have also been reported.[42] Its onset is usually in childhood, and there is a 2:1 to 4:1 ratio of females to males affected.[43,44] The differential diagnosis for actinic prurigo includes polymorphous light eruption, atopic dermatitis with photosensitivity, and chronic actinic dermatitis.

Histopathologic characteristics of actinic prurigo include hyperkeratosis, ortho- or parakeratosis, regular acanthosis, and a dense lymphocytic inflammatory infiltrate in the superficial dermis. There is usually a lack of deep inflammatory infiltrate, periadnexal involvement, and solar elastosis. The dense lymphoplasmacytic infiltrate may be lichenoid or form follicles or germinal centers. In addition, numerous eosinophils are usually present. It has been proposed that the prevalence of actinic prurigo in certain racial groups is a reflection of certain genetic predisposition. There are several reports of human leukocyte antigen (HLA) associations with actinic prurigo, including HLA-A24 and HLA-Cw4 in Cree Indians from Saskatchewan, Canada[45]; HLA-Cw4 in Chimila Indians from Colombia[46]; and HLA-DR4, HLA-A28, and HLA-B39 in Mexicans.[47]

Erythema dyschromicum perstans (ashy dermatosis) is an uncommon, idiopathic skin condition that appears in the first few decades of life and consists of asymptomatic blue-gray patches of varying size over the trunk, extremities, and neck, with early lesions reported to have an advancing erythematous border.[33] This disease is common in people with dark skin, particularly in women of South Asian or Latin descent.[48,49] The differential diagnosis includes lichen planus pigmentosus, melasma, idiopathic eruptive macular pigmentation, fixed drug eruptions, mastocytosis, macular amyloidosis, and postinflammatory hyperpigmentation.[50]

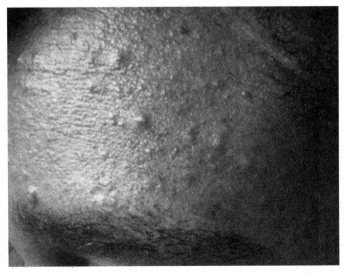

FIGURE 21-7. Acne vulgaris.

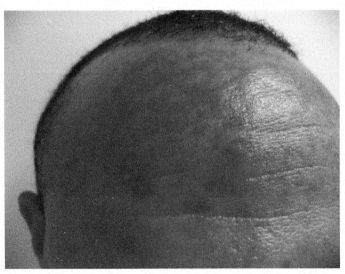

FIGURE 21-8. Facial melasma.

The histopathologic findings from the active border include increased pigmentation of the basal layer of the epidermis, vacuolar alteration of the basement membrane, and a mild perivascular lymphohistiocytic infiltrate with melanophages. A range of predisposing factors for erythema dyschromicum perstans has been revealed, including ingestion of ammonium nitrate,[51] nematode-induced intestinal parasitosis, use of oral contrast media, and contact with chemicals such as the pesticide chlorothalonil and cobalt.[52-55] Although the exact immunologic basis of erythema dyschromicum perstans has not been elucidated, a recent study performed in the Mexican population pointed to a higher association of HLA-DR4 (DRB1*0407) in this condition.[56]

CUTANEOUS REACTION PATTERNS

Both hereditary and environmental factors contribute to the appearance and incidence of certain dermatoses in skin of color. Hereditary factors likely include pigmentary differences, as well as other, yet to be identified key differences in immunology. Environmental factors that are important in altering skin disease include nutrition, emotions, socioeconomic status, hygiene, and occupation. In addition to the unequal prevalence of certain dermatologic and systemic disorders in individuals with dark skin, there is also a predisposition to develop atypical reaction patterns to common dermatoses. Some cutaneous reaction patterns seen more commonly in skin of color include follicular, annular, papular, granulomatous, keloidal, fibromatous, and ulcerative patterns.[7]

LABILITY OF PIGMENT

Pigmentary disorders are a significant concern in individuals with Fitzpatrick skin types IV to VI. The lability of pigment in this population causes dramatic change in skin color after inflammatory or bullous diseases characterized by postinflammatory hypopigmentation or hyperpigmentation [**Figure 21-9**].[34] Although the exact mechanism of postinflammatory pigment change is not known, the normal release of inflammatory mediators and cytokines from inflammatory cells has specific effects on melanocyte biology.[57] Leukotriene B_4, prostaglandins D_2 and E_2, endothelins, interleukin-1 and -6, and tumor necrosis factor-α have been shown to increase melanogenesis, whereas leukotriene C_4 may decrease melanogenesis and also cause movement of melanocytes.[58] Postinflammatory pigment change is often more dramatic in dark skin and may persist for an extended period of time compared with similar inflammatory conditions in lighter skin (Fitzpatrick skin types I to III).

FOLLICULAR AND PAPULAR REACTIONS

Dark-skinned individuals may develop follicular or papular reactions to many common dermatoses. This may be a result of yet unknown factors that cause an affinity for the pilar apparatus [**Figure 21-10**]. Follicular tinea versicolor, papular pityriasis rosea, papular lichen planus, and follicular eczema are seen more frequently in black individuals. Disseminate and recurrent infundibulofolliculitis is a variant of follicular eczema that presents as recurrent, pruritic, follicular-based papules on the neck, trunk, and proximal extremities. Black adults tend to develop a papular variant of lichen simplex chronicus.[59] Sarcoidosis may be papular, lichenoid, or verrucous. Secondary syphilis may be pruritic and present in a papular or follicular distribution.[1] Dermatosis papulosa nigra, histologically identical to seborrheic keratosis, presents as small 1- to 5-mm papular lesions on the face in up to 70% of black individuals.[60]

VESICULOBULLOUS DISEASES

Bullous lichen planus,[61,62] papulovesicular pityriasis rosea,[63] and bullous secondary syphilis have been reported in patients with skin of color. In addition, acropustulosis of infancy and transient neonatal pustular melanosis tend to occur more commonly in black children.[64]

GRANULOMATOUS LESIONS

There is a propensity to develop granulomatous reactions in dermatoses in skin of color. Sarcoidosis has been reported more commonly in black individuals. In a recent study, the risk of sarcoidosis among the African American population was three to four times greater than among Caucasians in the United States. Familial clustering was also found, indicating a certain genetic susceptibility. Familial sarcoidosis is more frequent among African Americans (17%) than among Caucasians (6%). Sarcoidosis may present as hypopigmented or hyperpigmented, papular, nodular, plaquelike, and ichthyosiform lesions.[65] Secondary syphilis,[66] rosacea, and seborrheic dermatitis may present as granulomatous lesions as well.[8]

KELOIDAL REACTIONS

Keloid scarring occurs in all races but has been reported to occur more frequently in skin of color. It has been reported to arise 3 to 18 times more often in black individuals than in white individuals[67] and to be more common in the Chinese population in Asia.[68] Although not fully understood, keloidal scarring occurs through the interaction between fibroblasts and cytokines that serve to aid the production of excessive collagen and inhibit the degradation of the extracellular matrix components.[69] In addition, keloid fibroblasts overexpress several growth factors including transforming growth factor-β and insulin-like growth factor-1, thereby contributing to increased collagen production and

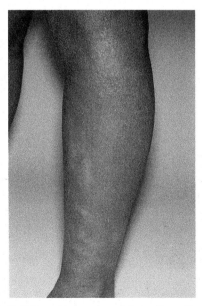

FIGURE 21-9. Postinflammatory hypopigmentation and hyperpigmentation on the leg.

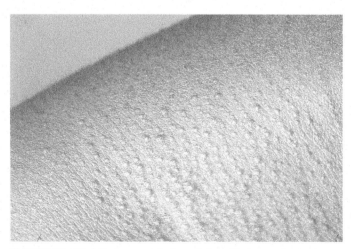

FIGURE 21-10. Follicular accentuation in atopic dermatitis.

greater resistance to apoptosis.[69] Studies show that fibroblasts are larger and binucleated or multinucleated in the skin of black persons.[70] Several etiologic factors for keloids have been proposed, including trauma, infection, abnormal metabolism of melanocyte-stimulating hormone, physiologic hyperactivity of the pituitary gland (eg, during puberty and pregnancy), genetic and familial disorders, and malnutrition; theories suggesting an immunologic basis for keloid formation have also been proposed.[71-76] However, the exact mechanism through which there is a higher incidence of keloidal scarring in darker-skinned individuals is still unknown.

REFERENCES

1. Alexis AF, Sergay AB, Taylor SC. Common dermatologic disorders in skin of color: a comparative practice study. *Cutis.* 2007;80:387-394.
2. Henderson AL. Skin variations in blacks. *Cutis.* 1983;32:376-377.
3. Amichai B, Grunwald MH. Pigmentary demarcation lines of pregnancy. *Eur J Obstet Gynecol Reprod Biol.* 2006;131:239-240.
4. James WD, Carter JM, Rodman OG. Pigmentary demarcation lines: a population survey. *J Am Acad Dermatol.* 1987;16:584-590.
5. Bonci A, Patrizi A. Pigmentary demarcation lines in pregnancy. *Arch Dermatol.* 2002;138:127-128.
6. Malakar S, Dhar S. Pigmentary demarcation lines over the face. *Dermatology.* 2000;200:85-86.
7. McLaurin CI. Cutaneous reaction patterns in blacks. *Dermatol Clin.* 1988;6:353-362.
8. Ozawa H, Rokugo M, Aoyama H. Pigmentary demarcation lines of pregnancy with erythema. *Dermatology.* 1993;187:134-136.
9. Rubin AI, Laborde SV, Stiller MJ. Acquired dermal melanocytosis: appearance during pregnancy. *J Am Acad Dermatol.* 2001;45:609-613.
10. Haneke E, Baran R. Longitudinal melanonychia. *Dermatol Surg.* 2001;27:580-584.
11. Ronger S, Touzet S, Ligeron C, et al. Dermoscopic examination of nail pigmentation. *Arch Dermatol.* 2002;138:1327-1333.
12. Gaeta GM, Satriano RA, Baroni A. Oral pigmented lesions. *Clin Dermatol.* 2002;20:286-288.
13. Cicek Y, Ertas U. The normal and pathologic pigmentation of oral mucous membrane: a review. *J Contemp Dent Pract.* 2003;15:76-86.
14. Kauzman A, Pavone M, Blanas N, et al. Pigmented lesions of the oral cavity: review, differential diagnosis, and case presentations. *J Can Dent Assoc.* 2004;70:682-683.
15. Ozbayrak S, Dumlu A, Ercalik-Yalcinkaya S. Treatment of melanin-pigmented gingiva and oral mucosa by CO_2 laser. *Oral Surg Oral Med Oral Pathol Oral Radiol Endod.* 2000;90:14-15.
16. Eisen D. Disorders of pigmentation in the oral cavity. *Clin Dermatol.* 2000;18:579-587.
17. Cicek Y, Ertas U. The normal and pathological pigmentation of oral mucous membrane: a review. *J Contemp Dent Pract.* 2003;4:76-86.
18. Dummett C. Clinical observation on pigment variations in healthy oral tissues in the Negro. *J Dent Res.* 1945;24:7-13.
19. Gloster HM Jr, Neal K. Skin cancer in skin of color. *J Am Acad Dermatol.* 2006;55:741-760.
20. Moore RT, Chae KA, Rhodes AR. Laugier and Hunziker pigmentation: a lentiginous proliferation of melanocytes. *J Am Acad Dermatol.* 2004;50:S70-S74.
21. Dummett CO. Oral tissue color changes, part I. *Quintessence Int Dent Dig.* 1979;10:39-45.
22. Araki S, Murata K, Ushio K, et al. Dose-response relationship between tobacco consumption and melanin pigmentation in the attached gingiva. *Arch Environ Health.* 1983;38:375-378.
23. Anderson W, Elam M, Lambert C. Keratosis punctata and atopy: report of 31 cases with a prospective study of prevalence. *Arch Dermatol.* 1984;120:884-890.
24. Martin JL. Leukoedema: an epidemiological study in whites and African-Americans. *J Tenn Dent Assoc.* 1997;77:18-21.
25. Martin JL. Leukoedema: a review of the literature. *J Natl Med Assoc.* 1992;84:938-940.
26. Rehbein HM. Pearly penile papules: incidence. *Cutis.* 1977;19:54-57.
27. Glicksman JM, Freeman RG. Pearly penile papules: a statistical study of incidence. *Arch Dermatol.* 1966;93:56-59.
28. Neinstein LS, Goldenring J. Pink pearly papules: an epidemiologic study. *J Pediatr.* 1984;105:594-595.
29. Agrawal SK, Bhattacharya SN, Singh N. Pearly penile papules: a review. *Int J Dermatol.* 2004;43:199-201.
30. McKinlay JR, Graham BS, Ross EV. The clinical superiority of continuous exposure versus short-pulsed carbon dioxide laser exposures for the treatment of pearly penile papules. *Dermatol Surg.* 1999;25:124-126.
31. Korber A, Dissemond J. Pearly penile papules. *CMAJ.* 2009;181:397.
32. El-Essawi D, Musial J, Hammad A, Lim H. A survey of skin disease and skin-related issues in Arab Americans. *J Am Acad Dermatol.* 2007;56:933-938.
33. Sanchez MR. Cutaneous diseases in Latinos. *Dermatol Clin.* 2003;21:689-697.
34. Halder RM, Roberts CI, Nootheti PK. Cutaneous diseases in the black races. *Dermatol Clin.* 2003;21:679-687, ix.
35. Shah SK, Bhanusali DG, Sachdev A, Geria AN, Alexis AF. A survey of skin conditions and concerns in South Asian Americans: a community-based study. *J Drugs Dermatol.* 2011;10:524-528.
36. Taylor SC, Fran Cook-Bolden F, Rahman Z, et al. Acne vulgaris in skin of color. *J Am Acad Dermatol.* 2002;46:S98-S106.
37. Halder RM, Brooks HL, Callender VD. Acne in ethnic skin. *Dermatol Clin.* 2003;21:609-615, vii.
38. Grimes PE, Stockton T. Pigmentary disorders in blacks. *Dermatol Clin.* 1988;6:271-281.
39. Grimes PE. Melasma: etiologic and therapeutic considerations. *Arch Dermatol.* 1995;131:1453-1457.
40. Cornelison RL Jr. Cutaneous diseases in Native Americans. *Dermatol Clin.* 2003;21:699-702.
41. Zuloaga-Salcedo S, Castillo-Vazquez M, Vega-Memije E, et al. Class I and class II major histocompatibility complex genes in Mexican patients with actinic prurigo. *Br J Dermatol.* 2007;156:1074-1075.
42. Fletcher DC, Romanchuk KG, Lane PR. Conjunctivitis and pterygium associated with the American Indian type of polymorphous light eruption. *Can J Ophthalmol.* 1988;23:30-33.
43. Lane PR, Hogan DJ, Martel MJ, et al. Actinic prurigo: clinical features and prognosis. *J Am Acad Dermatol.* 1992;26:683-692.
44. Birt AR, Davis RA. Hereditary polymorphic light eruption of American Indians. *Int J Dermatol.* 1975;14:105-111.
45. Sheridan DP, Lane PR, Irvine J, et al. HLA typing in actinic prurigo. *J Am Acad Dermatol.* 1990;22:1019-1023.
46. Bernal JE, Duran de Rueda MM, Ordonez CP, et al. Actinic prurigo among the Chimila Indians in Colombia: HLA studies. *J Am Acad Dermatol.* 1990;22:1049-1051.
47. Hojyo-Tomoka T, Granados J, Vargas-Alarcon G, et al. Further evidence of the role of HLA-DR4 in the genetic susceptibility to actinic prurigo. *J Am Acad Dermatol.* 1997;36:935-937.
48. Convit J, Piquero-Martin J, Perez RM. Erythema dyschromicum perstans. *Int J Dermatol.* 1989;28:168-169.
49. Novick NL, Phelps R. Erythema dyschromicum perstans. *Int J Dermatol.* 1985;24:630-633.
50. Pandya AG, Guevara IL. Disorders of hyperpigmentation. *Dermatol Clin.* 2000;18:91-98, ix.
51. Jablonska S. Ingestion of ammonium nitrate as a possible cause of erythema dyschromicum perstans (ashy dermatosis). *Dermatologica.* 1975;150:287-291.
52. Stevenson JR, Miura M. Erythema dyschromicum perstans (ashy dermatosis). *Arch Dermatol.* 1966;94:196-199.
53. Lambert WC, Schwartz RA, Hamilton GB. Erythema dyschromicum perstans. *Cutis.* 1986;37:42-44.
54. Penagos H, Jimenez V, Fallas V, et al. Chlorothalonil, a possible cause of erythema dyschromicum perstans (ashy dermatitis). *Contact Dermatitis.* 1996;35:214-218.
55. Zenorola P, Bisceglia M, Lomuto M. Ashy dermatosis associated with cobalt allergy. *Contact Dermatitis.* 1994;31:53-54.
56. Correa MC, Vega Memije E, Vargas-Alarcón G. HLA-DR association with the genetic susceptibility to develop ashy dermatosis in Mexican Mestizo patients. *J Am Acad Dermatol.* 2007;56:617-620.
57. Morelli JG, Norris DA. Influence of inflammatory mediators and cytokines on human melanocyte function. *J Invest Dermatol.* 1993;100:191S-195S.
58. Morelli JG, Kincannon J, Yohn JJ, et al. Leukotriene C_4 and TGF-α are stimulators of human melanocyte migration in vitro. *J Invest Dermatol.* 1992;98:290-295.
59. Brauner G. Cutaneous diseases in the black races. In: Demis DJ, Dobson RL, McGuire J, eds. *Dermatology.* New York, NY: Harper & Row; 1975:1704-1733.
60. Grimes PE, Arora S, Minus HR, et al. Dermatosis papulosa nigra. *Cutis.* 1983;32:385-386, 392.
61. Huang C, Chen S, Liu Z, et al. Familial bullous lichen planus (FBLP): pedigree analysis and clinical characteristics. *J Cutan Med Surg.* 2005;9:217-222.
62. Mora RG, Nesbitt LT Jr, Brantley JB. Lichen planus pemphigoides: clinical and immunofluorescent findings in four cases. *J Am Acad Dermatol.* 1983;8:331-336.

63. Miranda SB, Lupi O, Lucas E. Vesicular pityriasis rosea: response to erythromycin treatment. *J Eur Acad Dermatol Venereol.* 2004;18:622-625.
64. Laude TA. Approach to dermatologic disorders in black children. *Semin Dermatol.* 1995;14:15-20.
65. Griffiths CE, Leonard JN, Walker MM. Acquired ichthyosis and sarcoidosis. *Clin Exp Dermatol.* 1986;11:296-298.
66. Green KM, Heilman E. Secondary syphilis presenting as a palisading granuloma. *J Am Acad Dermatol.* 1985;12:957-960.
67. Louw L. Keloids in rural black South Africans, part 1: general overview and essential fatty acid hypotheses for keloid formation and prevention. *Prostaglandins Leukot Essent Fatty Acids.* 2000;63:237-245.
68. Alhady SM, Sivanantharajah K. Keloids in various races: a review of 175 cases. *Plast Reconstr Surg.* 1969;44:564-566.
69. Louw L. The keloid phenomenon: progress toward a solution. *Clin Anat.* 2007;20:3-14.
70. Montagna W, Carlisle K. The architecture of black and white facial skin. *J Am Acad Dermatol.* 1991;24:929-937.
71. Murray JC, Pollack SV, Pinnell SR. Keloids: a review. *J Am Acad Dermatol.* 1981;4:461-470.
72. Chait LA, Kadwa MA. Hypertrophic scars and keloids: cause and management—current concepts. *S Afr J Surg.* 1988;26:95-98.
73. Lawrence WT. In search of the optimal treatment of keloids: report of a series and a review of the literature. *Ann Plast Surg.* 1991;27:164-178.
74. Tritto M, Kanat IO. Management of keloids and hypertrophic scars. *J Am Podiatr Med Assoc.* 1991;81:601-605.
75. Darzi MA, Chowdri NA, Kaul SK, et al. Evaluation of various methods of treating keloids and hypertrophic scars: a 10-year follow-up study. *Br J Plast Surg.* 1992;45:374-379.
76. Tuan TL, Nichter LS. The molecular basis of keloid and hypertrophic scar formation. *Mol Med Today.* 1998;4:19-24.

CHAPTER 22 Dermatosis Papulosa Nigra

Marcia J. Glenn
Wendy E. Roberts

KEY POINTS

- Dermatosis papulosa nigra (DPN) is a common skin disorder in many patients with skin of color.
- DPN are benign pigmented papules that appear on the face, neck, and trunk.
- There is a genetic predilection, with a family history of DPN reported by at least 50% of affected individuals.
- DPN is rare in childhood and the number and size of lesions increase with age.
- The pathology of DPN is similar to that of seborrheic keratosis.
- DPN has a chronic progressive course.
- DPN can be treated electively by simple excision electrodesiccation or laser.

Dermatosis papulosa nigra (DPN) is a condition where benign, darkly pigmented papules appear primarily on the face, neck, and trunk of women and men with skin of color worldwide.[1] DPN is often called pigmented papules, skin tags, or flesh moles. The incidence of DPN is reported to be as high as 70% in the African American population and up to 50% among family members of affected patients [**Figure 22-1**].[2,3]

A retrospective study of 1000 Afro-Caribbean subjects ranked DPN as a common finding.[4] In Africa, 40% of the population over the age of 30 has DPN.[1,5] Similar lesions have been described in Asians, Hispanic, and Latin Americans [**Figure 22-2**], although the exact incidence is unknown.[2,6,7]

The development of DPN in children, although rare, has been reported.[8] It is chronic and progressive in adults. Although DPN is generally asymptomatic, the papules can become pruritic and burning.[9] Treatment is often pursued to enhance cosmetic appearance.

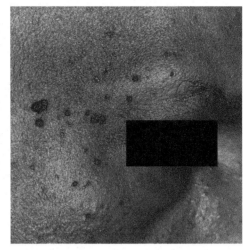

FIGURE 22-1. A man with skin type VI with periocular and temple pigmented papules.

ETIOLOGY AND PATHOGENESIS

Castellani[2] reported the first case of DPN in 1925, but the exact etiology remains uncertain. It is speculated that DPN is derived from an epidermal nevus or a hamartoma with follicular origin or from a nevoid developmental defect of the pilosebaceous follicles.[10-12] The preponderance of DPN within certain families suggests a strong genetic predilection.[11] Niang et al[13] suggest that the sun may be an etiopathogenic factor in the increase in lesions in the African population.

CLINICAL FINDINGS

DPN may begin as early as the first decade of life.[8] However, these small, darkly pigmented papules usually begin in adolescence and progress slowly over the years, peaking in number in the sixth decade.[11] The average age of onset is 22 years.[12] DPN has been reported to have between a 1:1 and 2:1 female-to-male ratio of incidence.[1] Family history of DPN is reported by at least 50% of those with DPN.[9] Approximately

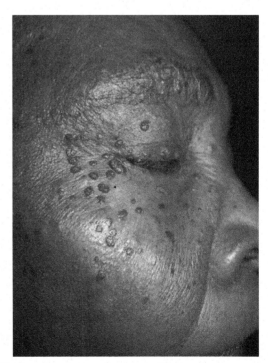

FIGURE 22-2. Dermatosis papulosa nigra on a Hispanic woman.

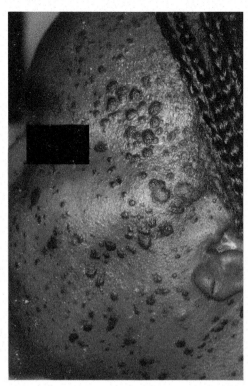

FIGURE 22-3. African American woman with numerous 0.5- to 1-mm pigmented papules predominantly in the photo-exposed malar area.

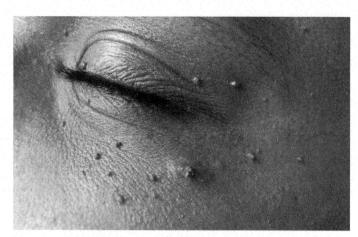

FIGURE 22-5. Asian female with dermatosis papulosa nigra located in the malar area. (Used with permission from Dr. Siew Eng Choon, Malaysia.)

25% of patients with facial lesions will also have lesions in other locations on the body. Although most people with DPN are generally asymptomatic and present primarily with a cosmetic dilemma, some individuals pursue removal because of symptoms, including pruritus, burning, and tenderness.[10-12]

Darker and deeper skin hues evidence more DPN.[1] Lesions are seldom or never described on white skin and are less frequently described on lighter skin than on darker skin.[1,3] Of note, however, is that with the nonwhite populations approaching an incidence of 50%, due in part to multiracial skin types, DPN cases in the future may be seen in skin that appears phenotypically white but that has the genotype of a darker skin of color.

Over time, the pigmented papules become more numerous, may enlarge, and often flatten in occluded areas [**Figures 22-3 and 22-4**].[12]

In a prospective study of DPN cases in Dakar, Senegal, 67% of patients had 50 to 100 lesions, and in 27% of the patients the lesions coalesced to form plaques.[13] Some papules are smooth and round, and others are filiform, projectile, or keratotic. The face is the most common location of DPN, predominantly the malar and temple areas [**Figure 22-5**]. The neck and trunk [**Figure 22-6**] are also frequently affected areas.[14] Scaling, crusting, and ulcerations are not features of DPN.[15]

One interesting case has been reported that involved an explosive eruption of DPN in a 42-year-old woman with skin of color, which was coincident with symptomatic iron deficiency anemia. Lesions quickly progressed from her face to the trunk. One remarkable feature was the 'Christmas tree' pattern of pigmented papules on her back [**Figure 22-7**]. Subsequent workup revealed an ascending colon adenocarcinoma.[16,17] A biopsy was consistent with the diagnosis of DPN.

PATHOLOGY

Usually, DPN is diagnosed clinically. If there is any doubt, a skin biopsy can be performed. The histopathology of DPN can be described as a collision neoplasm of seborrheic keratosis and acrochordon. The features consistent with seborrheic keratosis are hyperkeratosis, acanthosis, and a marked hyperpigmentation of the basal layer.[18,19] The features of acrochordons are the polypoid shape and papillomatosis. Keratin-filled

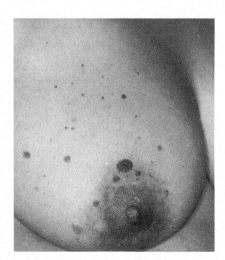

FIGURE 22-4. Small, medium, and large pigmented papules on a breast. This area is usually covered by a brassiere.

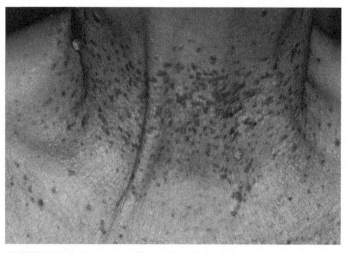

FIGURE 22-6. Numerous small-to medium-sized smooth pigmented papules on the neck of an African American man.

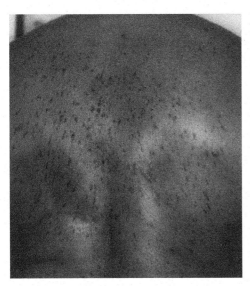

FIGURE 22-7. An example of a 'Christmas tree' distribution of pigmented papules on the trunk of a man with dark skin.

invaginations of the epidermis may be present. DPN usually has an acanthotic pattern with thick interwoven tracts of epidermis, but it may also have a reticulated pattern consisting of a double row of basaloid cells.[18] On a molecular level, *FGFR3* and *PIK3CA* mutations have been reported to be involved in the pathogenesis of seborrheic keratosis. In an analysis of 7 lesions done to determine whether DPN and stucco keratosis were of similar origin as seborrheic keratosis, results indicated that *FGFR3* and *PIK3CA* mutations were involved in the pathogenesis of both stucco keratosis and DPN. The results of this small pilot study would indicate a shared common genetic background.[19,20]

LABORATORY AND OTHER TESTS

The Leser-Trélat sign is the association of malignancy with numerous eruptive seborrheic keratoses.[18] Routine cancer screening, especially for colon and breast cancer, may be advisable with the sudden onset of a large number of DPN lesions, as seen with seborrheic keratosis.[19,20]

DIFFERENTIAL DIAGNOSIS

A biopsy may be helpful in differentiating clinical mimickers of DPN, such as:

- Acrochordons
- Seborrheic keratosis
- Verruca vulgaris
- Melanocytic nevi

COMPLICATIONS

DPN is cosmetically troublesome, especially when the papules obscure clear complexions and facial features and increase in number and even size in some instances.[20] If one theorizes that the lesions are a variant of seborrheic keratosis in patients with skin of color, large and sudden eruptions may foretell internal malignancy, and patients with this history should receive the appropriate workup.[18]

PROGNOSIS/PREVENTION

The lesions of DPN increase in number and sometimes size with age, peaking in the sixth decade.[1] A positive family history is likely in 50% to 90% of those affected.[1] Because the lesion itself is benign, the medical

TABLE 22-1   Treatment options for Dermatosis Papulosa Nigra
First-line therapies
• Electrodesiccation depletes water and blood supply to the lesion by the electrical generation of heat.
• Scissor/shave excision removes a surface growth off.
• Cryotherapy sprays liquid nitrogen to freeze the growth.
Second-line therapies
• Laser, including carbon dioxide, erbium-doped yttrium aluminium garnet (Er:YAG), 532 diode, and potassium titanyl phosphate lasers causes light-specific destruction of tissue.
• Curettage scrapes off the growth.

interventions should not provide more risk than the disease process itself. In a prospective study done in Senegal, lesions were primarily photodistributed, which implicates the sun as a provocateur of the condition.[13] With the possible exception of screening the skin from the sun, preventative measures do not exist.

Treatment of DPN is elective, and a conservative approach minimizes dyschromia (eg, hyperpigmentation or hypopigmentation), scarring (eg, hypertrophic or keloidal), and pain resulting from aggressive therapy [**Table 22-1**].[21] Lidocaine prilocaine cream, topical lidocaine cream, or intralesional 1% lidocaine with or without epinephrine provides simple and uncomplicated anesthesia for the procedures outlined as a first- or second-line treatment.[22-24] First-line therapies are inexpensive and efficient surgical options for medical providers practiced in the treatment of skin of color, and include electrodessication and Gradle or iris excision.[22,23] Second-line therapies such as laser treatment are more costly but may have a benefit in patient comfort.[24] In a recent study evaluating electrodessication versus pulse dye laser versus curettage for the treatment of DPN, there were no clinical outcome differences. Half of the patients in the study, however, preferred electrodessication, stating that it was less painful than laser treatment.[25]

A plan should be discussed with the patient prior to treatment, in order to manage expectations. This includes discussion of how many sessions are required for near 100% clearance. With severe cases, the DPN removal may take two to three sessions or longer. Multiple treatments are often needed because of the advent of new lesions or the incomplete resolution of any particular existent lesion [**Figures 22-8 and 22-9**].

Aggressive electrodessication and/or curettage may create a permanent change in the pigment or may result in scar formation. When using electrodessication, a low-energy setting should be selected and the lesion should be touched lightly to avoid direct heat contact with the underlying epidermis.[23] On dark skin of color, loss or deposition of color may result from all removal techniques, and the patient should be forewarned that postinflammatory hypopigmentation is temporary and normal skin color will return within 2 weeks. Skillful and careful treatment with liquid nitrogen is essential to remove DPN in darker skin types, because such treatment may result in permanent and disfiguring hypopigmentation. Risk of hypertrophic scarring or keloid formation should be assessed before any cold steel ablation.[25]

Aftercare includes the avoidance of ultraviolet A light (use of sun protection factor is mandatory) and exfoliants or irritating topical preparations, including retinoids and glycolic or salicylic acids, which may promote postinflammatory pigmentary changes. Petrolatum-based ointments, with or without antibiotic properties, may be used after the procedure. No difference has been found in the efficacy or safety of one preparation versus another.[26]

CONCLUSION

DPN is a common benign skin disorder in people with dark skin of color worldwide. The diagnosis is made clinically by appearance and by noting the distribution of the small, darker pigmented papules on the face,

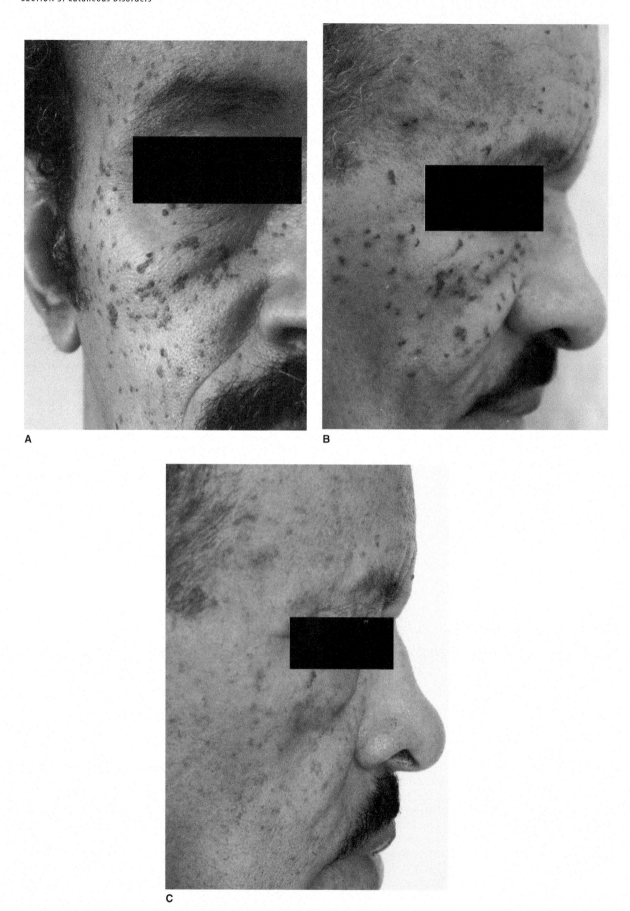

FIGURE 22-8. Professor A. Paul Kelly, MD, dermatologist and co-editor of this book, with facial dermatosis papulosa nigra **(A)** prior to removal, **(B)** 4 days after removal, and **(C)** after finishing the removal treatment.

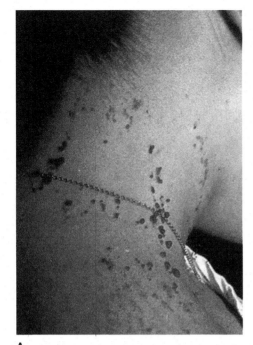

A

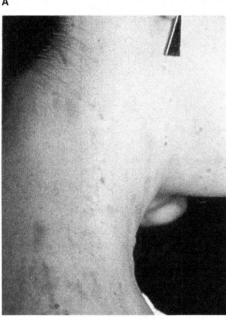

B

FIGURE 22-9. (A) Asian female patient with dermatosis papulosa nigra prior to treatment. **(B)** After electrodessication treatment. (Used with permission from Dr. Joyce Lim, Singapore.)

neck, and trunk. These darker papules range from 1 to 5 mm. Approximately 75% of people with skin of color may be affected with DPN. Onset is usually after childhood and peaks near 60 years of age. Lesions have a familial predilection in 50% of the patients. Seborrheic keratosis and DPN lesions are histologically indistinguishable, and nevi or fibroepithelial polyps can also resemble DPN. The course of the development of DPN is chronic and progressive. An eruptive variant may correlate with malignancy. DPN is rarely symptomatic. Electrodessication, scissor/shave excision, and cryotherapy are first-line treatments, whereas laser and curettage are second-line treatments. Patients may elect to use these cosmetic treatments in order to remove their DPN 'flesh moles.'

REFERENCES

1. Grimes PE, Arora S, Minus HR, et al. Dermatosis papulosa nigra. *Cutis.* 1983;32:385-386, 392.
2. Castellani A. Observations on some diseases of Central America. *J Trop Med Hyg.* 1925;28:1-14.
3. Shaheedi M, Naseh-Ghafoori H. Dermatosis papulosa nigra in a white female and her family members. http://www.ams.ac.ir/AIM/0253/0253197.htm. Accessed December 27, 2012.
4. Dunwell P, Rose A. Study of the skin disease spectrum occurring in an Afro-Caribbean population. *Int J Dermatol.* 2003;42:287-289.
5. Van Hees C, Naffs B. Dermatosis papulosa nigra. Common skin diseases in Africa: an illustrated guide. http://web.squ.edu.om/med-Lib/MED_CD/E_CDs/health%20development/html/clients/skin/index.htm. Accessed December 27, 2012.
6. Lee CS, Lim HW. Cutaneous diseases in Asians. *Dermatol Clin.* 2003;214:669-677.
7. Sanchez MR. Cutaneous diseases in Latinos. *Dermatol Clin.* 2003;21:689-697.
8. Babapour R, Leach J, Levy H. Dermatosis papulosa nigra in a young child. *Pediatr Dermatol.* 1993;10:356-358.
9. Davis EC, Callender VD. Postinflammatory hyperpigmentation: a review of the epidemiology, clinical features, and treatment options in skin of color. *J Clin Aesthet Dermatol.* 2010;3:20-31.
10. Woodhouse JG, Tomecki KJ. Common benign growths. In: Carey WD, ed. *Cleveland Clinic: Current Clinical Medicine 2010.* 2nd ed. Philadelphia, PA: Saunders Elsevier; 2010.
11. Michael JC, Seale ER. Dermatosis papulosa nigra. *Arch Dermatol Syph.* 1929;20:629-639.
12. Champion RH, Burton JL, Ebling F, et al. *Rook/Wilkinson/Eblings Textbook of Dermatology.* 6th ed. Oxford, United Kingdom: Blackwell Publishing; 1998:2413-2415.
13. Niang SO, Kane A, Diallo M, et al. Dermatosis papulosa nigra in Dakar, Senegal. *Int J Dermatol.* 2007;46:4522S-4527S.
14. Karuturi S. Dermatosis papulosa nigra. http://www.imnotebook.com/content/dermatosis-papulosa-nigra. Accessed December 13, 2012.
15. Visual DX. Dermatosis papulosa nigra. http://see.visualdx.com/diagnosis/dermatosis_papulosa_nigra. Accessed January 30, 2013.
16. Morand JJ, Lightburn EE. Characteristics of genetically pigmented skins. *Bull Soc Pathol Exot.* 2003;96:394-400.
17. Nowfar-Rad M. Dermatosis papulosa nigra. http://emedicine.medscape.com/article/1056854-overview. Accessed December 27, 2012.
18. Schwartzberg J. Eruptive dermatosis papulosa nigra as a possible sign of internal malignancy. *Int J Dermatol.* 2007;46:186S-187S.
19. Hafner C, Landthaler M, Mentzel T, et al. FGFR3 and PIK3CA mutations in stucco keratosis and dermatosis papulosa nigra. *Br J Dermatol.* 2010;162:508-512.
20. Balin AK. Seborrheic keratosis. http://emedicine.medscape.com/article/1059477-overview. Accessed July 4, 2012.
21. Kauh YC, McDonald JW, Rapaport JA, et al. A surgical approach for dermatosis papulosa nigra. *Int J Dermatol.* 1983;22:590-592.
22. Joshi S, Suh KY, Roopal Y, et al. Comparison of electrodessication and KTP laser for treatment of dermatosis papulosa nigra. *J Am Acad Dermatol.* 2008;58:2800.
23. Carter EL, Coppola CA, Baranti FA. Formulation prior to electrodesiccation of dermatosis papulosa nigra. *Dermatol Surg.* 2006;32:1-6.
24. Jackson B. Lasers in ethnic skin: a review. *J Am Acad Dermatol.* 2003;8:5134-5138.
25. Garcia MS, Azari R, Eisen DB. Treatment of dermatosis papulosa nigra in 10 patients: a comparison trial of electrodesiccation, pulsed dye laser, and curettage. *Dermatol Surg.* 2010;36:1968-1972.
26. Taylor SC, Averyhart AN, Heath CR. Postprocedural wound-healing efficacy following removal of dermatosis papulosa nigra lesions in an African American population: a comparison of a skin protectant ointment and a topical antibiotic. *J Am Acad Dermatol.* 2011;64:S30-S35.

| CHAPTER | # Seborrheic Dermatitis |
| 23 | Adam Whittington
Roopal V. Kundu |

KEY POINTS

- Seborrheic dermatitis is a common concern among patients with skin of color.
- The clinical features of seborrheic dermatitis depend on the age of the individual, his or her Fitzpatrick skin type, and the presence or absence of concurrent systemic illnesses.
- In addition to the scaly appearance, lesions of seborrheic dermatitis in skin of color may be hypopigmented, hyperpigmented, or erythematous.
- Treatment options are numerous but should be adjusted to the hair-grooming practices of the individual.

Seborrheic dermatitis is a chronic papulosquamous condition affecting the scalp, face, and trunk. It is a superficial inflammatory disease that can occur as an isolated condition in the sebum-rich areas of the scalp or in conjunction with other common disorders such as blepharitis, acne vulgaris, and rosacea. Certain systemic illnesses have been associated with seborrheic dermatitis, particularly acquired immunodeficiency syndrome (AIDS) and Parkinson disease.[1-4] Seborrheic dermatitis may also be seen in patients who have received psoralen with ultraviolet A therapy.[5]

The exact etiology of seborrheic dermatitis is unknown; however, some of the theorized causative factors include production of sebum by the sebaceous glands, *Malassezia globosa* yeast species, and a genetic susceptibility for an inflammatory response.[6] Clinically, seborrheic dermatitis is easily recognized. However, findings may differ based on the Fitzpatrick skin type of the affected individual. Treatment options are numerous but should be adjusted for individuals with a Fitzpatrick skin type of IV to VI, based on their hair grooming practices. Treatment is usually successful in controlling the symptoms and the clinical manifestations of the disease; however, a cure is rarely attained.

EPIDEMIOLOGY

The occurrence of seborrheic dermatitis in the general population is reported to be 3% to 5%.[7] The condition can affect people of all ages. There are two age categories with distinct increases in the rate of occurrence: infancy and the fourth through fifth decades of life. Males are affected by seborrheic dermatitis more often than females [**Figure 23-1**], and African American populations are affected more frequently than fairer-skinned populations.[8] An increased incidence is found in human immunodeficiency virus (HIV)-positive patients or those with AIDS, with estimates ranging from 20% to 83%.[9-11] Higher rates of occurrence have also been found in individuals with Parkinson disease,[3,4] familial amyloidosis with polyneuropathy,[12] trisomy 21 genetic disorder,[13] anorexia nervosa,[14] increased stress levels,[9] and chronic alcohol consumption [**Table 23-1**].[15]

ETIOLOGY

The exact etiology of seborrheic dermatitis is unknown. Although, it is possible that seborrheic dermatitis is multifactorial in nature. Possible cofactors include the *Malassezia* yeast species,[6,16,17] increased sebum and lipid levels,[18,19] an impaired skin barrier,[17] activation of the complement pathway,[17] and T-cell depression.[17,20,21]

The presence of the lipophilic *Malassezia* species of yeast is a contributing factor in seborrheic dermatitis.[16] This is supported by the fact

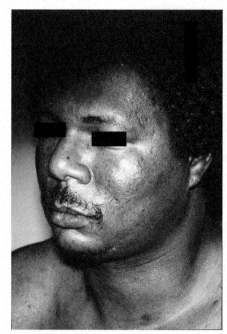

FIGURE 23-1. A male patient with Fitzpatrick skin type V with annular thin papules along the nasolabial folds.

that fluconazole (50 mg/d) has been found to effectively remove a high percentage of the *Malassezia* species, in addition to producing a clinical improvement in the symptoms of seborrheic dermatitis.[22] Also, a recurrence of the clinical findings has been linked to an increase in the growth of lipophilic yeast. However, *Malassezia* yeast alone is not sufficient to cause seborrheic dermatitis, because these yeast species are also found in individuals without this skin disease.[6,16]

In addition to the *Malassezia* yeast species, a genetic susceptibility is needed to produce the disease. Historically, the elevated sebum and lipid levels in individuals with seborrheic dermatitis have gained attention as possible factors. The increased lipid content in the skin of some African Americans, compared with Caucasians, could account for the higher rate of this skin disease within the African American community.[19] Similarly, increased sebum has been documented in individuals with Parkinson disease and has also been found in newborns.[18] Newborn infants have large and active sebaceous glands, perhaps explaining 'cradle cap,' which is seen frequently among the African American population.

Another potential cofactor includes depressed T-cell function, which could lead to the increased growth of *Malassezia* yeast and may account for the high incidence of seborrheic dermatitis in AIDS patients.[23] Likewise, it is accepted that seborrheic dermatitis often parallels AIDS severity.[21] An increase in natural killer cell activation has been reported,[17,23] as well as increased complement activation.[17] This could potentially lead to the inflammation found in cases of seborrheic dermatitis.

Additionally, neuroleptic medications have been implicated in inducing or aggravating cases of seborrheic dermatitis. When associated with neuroleptic-induced parkinsonism, haloperidol and chlorpromazine have been associated with an increased incidence of this skin disease.[4,24]

TABLE 23-1 Disorders commonly associated with seborrheic dermatitis
Anorexia nervosa
Chronic alcohol consumption
Familial amyloidosis with polyneuropathy
HIV/AIDS
Parkinson disease
Trisomy 21 genetic disorder

Abbreviations: AIDS, acquired immunodeficiency syndrome; HIV, human immunodeficiency virus.

TABLE 23-2	Clinical patterns of seborrheic dermatitis
Patient group	Pattern/location
Infants	'Cradle cap' and 'napkin' dermatitis
Adults	Areas with facial hair (such as the eyebrows, mustache, and eyelid margins)
General	Skin flexures (such as the nasolabial folds, postauricular folds, axillae, and groin)
HIV/AIDS	Extensive adult clinical findings, blepharitis, and superinfections

Abbreviations: AIDS, acquired immunodeficiency syndrome; HIV, human immunodeficiency virus.

CLINICAL FEATURES

The clinical features of seborrheic dermatitis depend on the age of the individual, his or her Fitzpatrick skin type, and the presence or absence of concurrent systemic illnesses [**Table 23-2**]. Manifestations of seborrheic dermatitis in newborn infants include scaling, crusting, and skin that is oily in appearance. This constellation of clinical findings when occurring on the scalp, is referred to as 'cradle cap' and is likely related to an overproduction of sebum [**Figure 23-2**]. Scales of

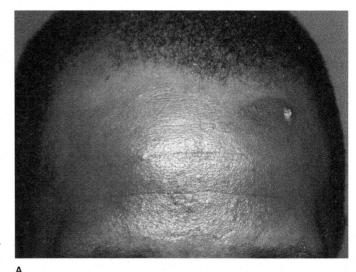

A

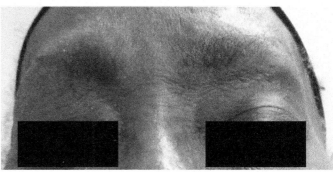

B

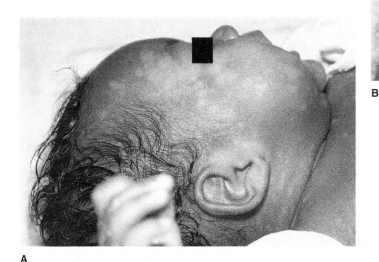

A

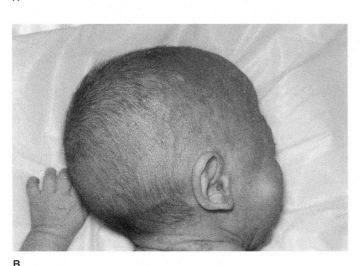

B

FIGURE 23-2. Seborrheic dermatitis can affect infants. (**A**) An infant with Fitzpatrick skin type IV with facial seborrheic dermatitis-related hypopigmentation. (**B**) An infant displaying extensive 'cradle cap.'

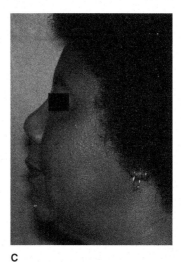

C

FIGURE 23-3. (**A**) Hyperpigmented annular plaque on the lateral forehead. (**B**) Erythematous, finely scaled, thin plaques extending from the eyebrows onto the upper eyelids. (**C**) Annular hyperpigmented patches along the nasal ala, cheek, and chin.

seborrheic dermatitis are often located throughout the scalp but can also be located on the face, chest, groin, neck, ears, and eyelids [**Figure 23-3**]. The clinical findings in Fitzpatrick skin types IV to VI can be different based on the reduced visible erythema of the involved skin. The skin may be either hypopigmented or hyperpigmented. Severe and generalized seborrheic dermatitis in infancy may represent Leiner disease, an exfoliative disorder that occurs in combination with anemia, diarrhea, immunodeficiency, and concomitant bacterial and candidal infections.

Clinical findings of seborrheic dermatitis in the adult population vary by the location of involvement. Common locations include the scalp, face, chest, axillae, and submammary, groin, and gluteal areas. The involvement of the face and head is most prominent around the eyebrows, perinasal skin, postauricular areas, ears, and eyelids. The face and scalp may be either dry and flaky with white scales or greasy with a crusty appearance. The disease may extend from the frontal scalp onto the upper forehead. In Fitzpatrick skin types IV to VI, the skin is often hypopigmented beneath the scale [**Figure 23-4**]. The perinasal and postauricular skin can appear hypopigmented, hyperpigmented, or erythematous. Inner ear scaling may be obvious and will include the aural canals [**Figure 23-5**]. Infrequently, bacterial superinfection can occur. Chest, axilla, groin, and gluteal involvement is usually scaly with hypopigmentation or erythema beneath the scales.

HIV/AIDS patients have clinical findings that are similar to those of other adults with seborrheic dermatitis. However, the skin involvement is often more extensive. Blepharitis can occur, as well as occlusion of the meibomian glands, resulting in scaling and a burning sensation on the eyelids. Physicians should note that erythema of the eyelids may not be as obvious in patients with darker skin. Axillary, extremity, and groin involvement is often diffuse. Bacterial, candidal, and dermatophyte superinfections may also be present. The involved skin is often more visibly inflamed in those who are immunocompromised. Plaques on the torso and extremities appear moist with erythema, which may be visible even in patients with darker skin.

HISTOPATHOLOGY

The histologic findings of seborrheic dermatitis are consistent with those of other forms of spongiotic dermatitis and include marked spongiosis, acanthosis, and hyperkeratosis. Classic findings also include parakeratosis, neutrophilic infiltrate, and scale crust at the opening of the hair follicle's infundibulum, in addition to psoriasiform hyperplasia of the epidermis. Furthermore, some degree of elongation of the epidermal ridges is often present. The histologic differential diagnosis includes psoriasis. However, psoriasis can be distinguished by an absence of spongiosis. The histologic findings of seborrheic dermatitis in immunocompetent patients are different than those in patients with AIDS [**Table 23-3**].[25] In the latter group of patients, there are superficial perivascular infiltrates of plasma cells, neutrophils, leukocytoclasia, and keratinocyte necrosis.[25]

ASSOCIATED SYSTEMIC ILLNESSES

The prevalence and severity of seborrheic dermatitis in HIV/AIDS patients have been well documented,[1,2] although the etiology is still undetermined. There is an increased presence of the *Malassezia* species and an increased prevalence of immunologic dysfunction inherent to this systemic illness. It is estimated that 43% of newly diagnosed HIV/AIDS patients are African American and approximately 20% are Latino.[26] Therefore, the significance of this skin disease in these communities should be noted.

Parkinson disease is a chronic progressive neurologic disorder characterized by tremors, rigidity, bradykinesia, and a disturbance of the gait and posture. Many cutaneous clinical findings have been reported, including seborrheic dermatitis and hyperhidrosis. Although the etiology remains elusive, the mechanisms suggested include increased sebum excretion rate in Parkinson patients and a possible induction by the use of chronic neuroleptic medications.[4,18,24]

DIFFERENTIAL DIAGNOSIS

The differential diagnosis for seborrheic dermatitis can be separated by the aforementioned distinct age groups that are primarily affected by this skin disease. Skin eruptions in infancy may represent a variety of infections, or dermatitides. These include contact dermatitis, atopic

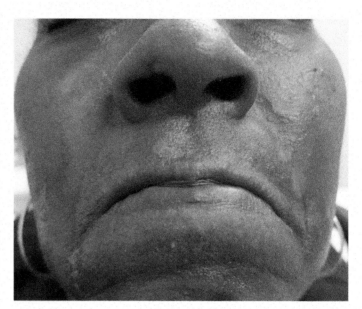

FIGURE 23-4. Annular hypopigmented and erythematous plaques macules along the nasolabial folds extending to the lips.

dermatitis, tinea capitis, tinea faciei, candidiasis, multiple carboxylase deficiency, biotin-responsive dermatitis, scabies, impetigo, and psoriasis [**Table 23-4**]. Fungal and bacterial cultures, skin biopsies, family history, and laboratory studies can help to distinguish between these conditions.

The differential diagnosis for adults includes psoriasis, pityriasis rosea, contact dermatitis, systemic lupus erythematosus, atopic dermatitis, candidiasis, rosacea, impetigo, tinea versicolor, and sarcoidosis [**Table 23-4**]. Fungal and bacterial cultures, skin biopsies, and laboratory studies may be performed if necessary.

GROOMING PRACTICES

The treatment of scalp seborrheic dermatitis in patients with skin of color requires an understanding of the known biological differences in skin and hair between Fitzpatrick skin types IV to VI. Equally important

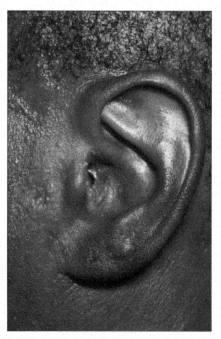

FIGURE 23-5. Scaling and crusting of the inner aural canal.

TABLE 23-3 Histopathologic differences between aids-associated seborrheic dermatitis and classic seborrheic dermatitis

Type	Differences
Classical seborrheic dermatitis	Spongiotic dermatitis and neutrophils at the infundibulum of hair follicles
AIDS-associated seborrheic dermatitis	Necrotic keratinocytes within the epidermis, perivascular infiltrates of the plasma cells, and neutrophils

Abbreviation: AIDS, acquired immunodeficiency syndrome.

is a familiarity with the hairstyling practices and the cultural standards of hair care within certain racial groups. Treatment recommendations can be aligned with these cultural practices to enhance patient compliance.

The textured hair found in many African Americans is biologically similar to, but morphologically different from, Caucasian hair. It is oval in shape, flat, and elliptically shaped in the cross-section.[28] This textured hair grows from a curved hair follicle and appears curly. It has a reduced moisture content and is therefore inherently drier than Caucasian hair.[28,29] The tensile strength is lower, and the hair's spiral form makes it more difficult for sebum to be distributed along the hair's length.[27] These factors lead to increased hair breakage.[29] Therefore, the frequency of hair washing in this group is usually limited to once weekly or every other week, in order to decrease the hair's loss of moisture and its fragility.

Hairstyling practices in African American women are quite varied; however, approximately 80% are believed to have chemically straightened hair. The chemical relaxers used are sodium (pH 10 to 14), guanine, and potassium hydroxide. Ammonium thioglycolate (pH 9.4 to 9.6) is also used occasionally. These ingredients break the cysteine disulfide bonds so as to straighten each hair strand. The chemical straightening process may lead to increased hair breakage when compared with non chemically treated hair.[30]

Hot combing is a styling technique that straightens textured hair without the use of chemicals. A pomade or oil-based hair product is applied to the hair, followed by the application of a heated comb that may reach temperatures greater than 150°F. The straight hairstyle achieved will revert back to its original curly texture if the hair becomes wet (including if moistened by perspiration). Therefore, patients are likely to wash and hot comb their hair once every 2 weeks.

Natural hairstyles are seen primarily among African American men and a small but increasing number of women. Tight braiding of the hair, either in cornrows or individual braids (with or without additional synthetic or human hair), may be maintained for extended periods of time without washing or releasing tension from the hair. Dreadlocks are achieved by allowing the natural hair to twist, knot, and become matted over time. Washing the hair is discouraged, although cleaning the scalp with a nonconditioning soap is recommended. Another common hairstyle in the African American community is a weave. This is where human or synthetic hair is woven into the base of the natural hair, either by being sown with a thread or bonded to the scalp with glue. Recently, a study of 201 African American women suggested that hair extensions are associated with an increased rate of seborrheic dermatitis.[31]

These popular hairstyles within the African American population have several common features. The styles are maintained for extended periods of time, ranging from 1 week to 1 month. Loss of the style occurs with hair washing, which necessitates restyling; frequent washing and restyling often results in hair breakage. Thus, consideration must be given when instructing the patient about the frequency of hair washing with a medicated shampoo. The possibility that this shampoo may further dry out the patient's hair should also be considered, in addition to the role that the medicated substances may play in reverting a straight hairstyle.

Asian hair has a round hair shaft, resulting in hair strands that appear straight. The hair shaft of this type of hair has the largest diameter, with a circular geometry, when compared with African American and Caucasian hair.[28] The hair has a higher tensile strength than white or African American hair and is typically dark in color. Hairstyling methods are used to tighten the hair and create curls. Ammonium and hydrogen peroxide are used to bleach Asian hair and may be combined with other agents to perm the hair. Other methods used to curl the hair include hot curling irons, as well as mousses and gels in combination with heated dryers. All of these hairstyles and styling agents may lead to dry hair and increased hair fragility. Therefore, some Asians use coconut oil or milk to condition the hair and reduce fragility.

The hair and styling preferences of Latinos depend on the individual's hair texture. Latinos may have hair that is morphologically similar to textured African American hair, or they may have hair that is identical to the straight or curly hair of Caucasian individuals. Patients with hair that is similar to textured African American hair may use some or all of the previously discussed methods to achieve a desired appearance and to maximize manageability. The most commonly used method is to chemically straighten the hair. A high percentage of Latino individuals have brown or black hair and many use hydrogen peroxide to bleach their hair or use permanent hair dyes. Both of these processes can lead to increased fragility. In contrast, Latino hair that is morphologically similar to Caucasian hair will have a similar moisture content. These individuals will often need to wash their hair frequently to reduce the oily appearance of the hair.

Native American hair is morphologically similar to Caucasian hair. Therefore, the hair has an intermediate diameter and cross-section compared with African American and Asian hair.[28] The hair has more moisture and decreased fragility compared with African American hair.[28]

TREATMENT

Seborrheic dermatitis can be controlled with several different topical agents, some of which are described in the following sections. A summary of some of these products is provided in **Table 23-5**.

▨ TOPICAL STEROIDS

Nonfluorinated topical steroids, which address the inflammatory nature of the disorder, are effective in the treatment of scalp, facial, and truncal seborrheic dermatitis. The steroid vehicle is very important when selecting the treatment for scalp seborrheic dermatitis in patients who have textured hair. Solutions and gels are often considered to be too drying for textured hair, especially hair that has been chemically straightened. Steroid ointments or oils may be preferred for chemically or hot comb straightened hair, braided hair, or natural hair in African Americans

TABLE 23-4 Differential diagnosis of seborrheic dermatitis in children[27] and adults[3,7]

Children	Adults
Contact dermatitis	Psoriasis
Atopic dermatitis	Pityriasis rosea
Tinea capitis	Contact dermatitis
Tinea faciei	Systemic lupus erythematosus
Candidiasis	Atopic dermatitis
Multiple carboxylase deficiency	Candidiasis
Biotin-responsive dermatitis	Rosacea
Scabies	Impetigo
Impetigo	Tinea versicolor
Psoriasis	Sarcoidosis

or Afro-Latinos. However, ointments and oils are inappropriate for those with dreadlocks because they inhibit the locking process. Steroid foams, lotions, shampoos, and gels are generally useful for the natural, nonchemically treated hair of Asians, Native Americans, and Latinos. These vehicles do not give the hair an oily appearance. Steroid foams may be acceptable in chemically straightened hair for individuals who do not wish to use oil-based products.[32] Low- and middle-potency steroid creams and lotions are useful for the treatment of facial and body seborrheic dermatitis. High-potency steroid products are discouraged due to the risk of hypopigmentation and/or atrophy, which may be particularly disfiguring in patients with Fitzpatrick skin types IV to VI.

TOPICAL ANTIFUNGAL AGENTS

Ketoconazole is a broad-spectrum antifungal agent that can be used to decrease *Malassezia* species. This broad-spectrum cream also treats *Candida albicans* and most dermatophytes. Ketoconazole is effective in the treatment of facial and truncal seborrheic dermatitis in infants and adults. It is acceptable for individuals with Fitzpatrick skin types IV to VI because it does not lead to hypopigmentation. Ketoconazole 2% shampoo is also effective for scalp disease in all skin types. However, the results of shampoo use are often delayed in patients who shampoo their hair less frequently. The use of ketoconazole shampoo has also been noted to exacerbate the dryness of chemically treated hair, which can lead to increased hair breakage. Shampoo use should be limited to once weekly and combined with moisturizing conditioners.[33] Ciclopirox 1% cream and shampoo can treat superficial dermatophyte infections, as well as inhibiting the growth of *Malassezia* and *Candida* species. This medication has anti-inflammatory properties that allow it to be effective against seborrheic dermatitis.[19] The shampoo must not be used too frequently and should be combined with moisturizing conditioners to prevent the overdrying and breakage of chemically treated hair. Selenium sulfide has both antifungal and antiseborrheic properties.[34] This product is available as a 1%, 2.25%, or 2.5% shampoo and is effective against *Malassezia* fungi. Its frequency of use must be reduced in chemically treated hair. Finally, patients should be instructed to apply medicated shampoos onto the scalp, wait for 5-10 minutes and rinse out without lathering the hair. Follow with a conditioning shampoo to lather the hair.

TOPICAL IMMUNOMODULATORS

Topical tacrolimus and pimecrolimus have been reported to show antifungal activity.[34] Although they are not currently approved by the U.S. Food and Drug Administration (FDA) for the treatment of seborrheic dermatitis, these agents are being used increasingly for this purpose. The use of these agents avoids the potential side effects associated with topical corticosteroids, as shown in a 12-week study comparing hydrocortisone ointment and tacrolimus. Tacrolimus 0.1% ointment was applied less frequently but showed analogous improvement of clinical features to hydrocortisone 1%.[35] Another trial of tacrolimus 0.1% ointment in patients with seborrheic dermatitis demonstrated a 70% or greater clearance of the seborrheic dermatitis.[36] A randomized, double-blind, vehicle-controlled, 4-week trial tested the efficacy of pimecrolimus cream for the treatment of facial seborrheic dermatitis. The results revealed that pimecrolimus 1% cream is an effective and well-tolerated treatment for moderate to severe facial seborrheic dermatitis. The trial revealed that, in some cases, efficacy was noted after only 2 weeks of treatment.[37]

An open-label pilot trial of pimecrolimus 1% cream was performed for 16 weeks to treat seborrheic dermatitis in five African American adults with associated hypopigmentation.[36,38] All subjects in the study noted a marked decrease in the severity of the seborrheic dermatitis, as well as an improvement in the hypopigmentation.

OTHER INGREDIENTS

Zinc pyrithione is noted to be effective against *Malassezia* fungi species.[34] It is an active ingredient in many medicated shampoos and conditioners, and comes in a variety of concentrations ranging from 0.25% to

TABLE 23-5	Treatments for seborrheic dermatitis
Medication	**Brand names[a]/vehicles**
Topical steroids	Maximum strength Scalpicin Scalp Itch medication and several creams, foams, ointments, oils, and shampoos
Selenium sulfide	Exsel shampoo, Fostex medicated cream, Head & Shoulders shampoo, Selsun Blue shampoo, and Vichy Dercos shampoo
Lithium succinate	Ointment
Ketoconazole	Nizoral cream and shampoo
Ciclopirox olamine	Loprox cream, lotion, and shampoo
Zinc pyrithione	AXE shampoo/conditioner, Clear shampoo/conditioner, Denorex shampoo, DermaZinc DHS zinc shampoo, Folicure products, Garnier Fructis products, Head & Shoulders shampoo, Kenra products, Noble Formula products, Pantene Pro-V shampoo, Suave products, Theraplex Z products, and Zincon shampoo
Coal tar	Denorex Extra Strength shampoo, DHS Tar shampoo, Duplex T products, Herald Tar shampoo, Ionil T shampoo, MG217 medicated ointment, Millcreek Botanicals products, Mushatt's creams, Neutrogena T/Gel shampoo, Pentrax medications, Pert Plus shampoo/conditioner, Polytar shampoo, Reme-T shampoo, Tarsum shampoo/gel, Tegrin shampoo, Theraplex T shampoo, and Walgreens T Plus shampoo
Salicylic acid	Beta Sal medicated shampoo, Denorex Shampoo, DHS Sal shampoo, Ionil Plus shampoo, Neutrogena T/Sal shampoo, Baker Cummins P&S shampoo, SAL3 soap, Scalpicin medication, Walgreens SheaMoisture Organic African Black Soap, Sebulex shampoo, Walgreens T Plus shampoo, X-Seb T products, and Zema lotion
Sodium sulfacetamide	OVACE gel, shampoo, and wash
Olive/mineral oil	Several lotions, oils, and shampoos
Topical immunomodulators	Pimecrolimus and Tacrolimus
Sulfur	Glover's medicated shampoo and oil, JASON shampoo, SAL3 soap, and Sulfur8 Medicated Conditioner
Metronidazole	Several creams, gels, and lotions
Azelaic acid	Several creams and gels
Tea tree oil	Max Green Alchemy shampoo, Pura D'or shampoo, and various castile (olive-based) soaps and oils
Capillus	Several creams, gels, and shampoos
Naftifine	Several gels
Pine tar	Elorac Inc. Packer's pine tar soap and Grandpa's Soap Company Wonder Pine Tar Shampoo/Pine Tar Conditioner
No specific active ingredient	Promiseb topical creams

[a]The names of products mentioned in this table are trademarks owned by their respective manufacturers.

2%. For facial involvement, a 0.25% spray is available. A facial cleansing bar with 2% zinc is also effective.[34] A recent study showed no evidence of tachyphylaxis with long-term zinc-based treatment.[39]

Treatment with coal tar preparations has been considered a mainstay of therapy for seborrheic dermatitis. Shampoos contain either 0.4% or 0.5% of the active ingredient. Limiting factors include the odor of the preparation, the reduced frequency of shampoo use in some groups, and the concern about possible carcinogenesis due to the polycyclic aromatic hydrocarbons.

Sodium sulfacetamide is available in a 10% face wash and a 10% scalp foam and gel. The lack of alcohol in the scalp foam allows for less drying and breakage when used on chemically treated hair. Sulfur-containing shampoos and soaps have been used as treatment due to their antimicrobial and keratinolytic properties.[40]

Salicylic acid 3% shampoos are available and beneficial, with the same limitations as noted for all antiseborrheic shampoos.[17] An olive oil or mineral oil compress with warm water is helpful for loosening the crusts and scabs that form on the scalps of infants. This can be combined with a baby shampoo or a low-potency steroid for a quicker response. A novel nonsteroidal topical cream with antifungal and anti-inflammatory actions, approved by the FDA for managing seborrheic dermatitis, has shown a similar efficacy to corticosteroid creams and was more effective at preventing relapses.[41]

Lithium succinate is a topical ointment that has also been used for treatment. This medication interferes with the free fatty acids that are instrumental in the growth of *Malassezia* fungi.[10] Due to its antibacterial and antifungal properties, tea tree oil, an essential oil, has also been used to treat seborrheic dermatitis.[40,42] Tea tree oil may be more accepted by patients who are looking for an organic or alternative treatment. Azelaic acid, a therapy used for the treatment of rosacea, is now being used to treat seborrheic dermatitis due to its antimicrobial properties and sebosuppressive activity.[17] Metronidazole 1% gel has been shown to be effective in the treatment of facial seborrheic dermatitis.[43,44] Although it has not been well characterized in studies, pyridoxine has also been suggested as a treatment option.[42]

CONCLUSION

Seborrheic dermatitis is a common cutaneous disorder in patients with skin of color. In addition to the characteristic scaling of the face and scalp, postinflammatory changes are common. The distinctive structure of the hair and culturally based hair- and scalp-grooming practices drive the acceptability of different treatments for seborrheic dermatitis. An avoidance of shampoos and topical products that dry the hair is important for patients who suffer from lack of moisture in their hair. Medications that avoid potential side effects such as atrophy and telangiectasias are also preferable; these can include antifungal agents. Finally, a reliance on topical agents in acceptable vehicles, such as foam, oils, and/or ointments, is important.

REFERENCES

1. Mahe A, Simon F, Coulibaly S, et al. Predictive value of seborrheic dermatitis and other common dermatoses for HIV infection in Bamako, Mali. *J Am Acad Dermatol*. 1996;34:1084-1086.
2. Rosatelli JB, Machado AA, Roselina AM. Dermatoses among Brazilian HIV+ patients: correlation with the evolutionary phases of AIDS. *Int J Dermatol*. 1997;36:729-734.
3. Naldi L, Rebora A. Seborrheic dermatitis. *N Engl J Med*. 2009;360:387-396.
4. Binder RL, Jonelis FJ. Seborrheic dermatitis in neuroleptic-induced parkinsonism. *Arch Dermatol*. 1983;119:473-475.
5. Tegner E. Seborrheic dermatitis of the face induced by PUVA treatments. *Acta Derm Venereol*. 1983;63:335-339.
6. Dawson TL Jr. *Malassezia globosa* and *restricta*: a breakthrough understanding of the etiology and treatment of dandruff and seborrheic dermatitis through whole-genome analysis. *J Investig Dermatol Symp Proc*. 2007;12:15-19.
7. Selden S. Seborrheic dermatitis. www.emedicine.medscape.com/article/1108312-overview#aw2aab6b2b4aa. Accessed December 23, 2012.
8. Pierce HE. Treatment of seborrheic dermatitis in the Negro scalp. *J Natl Med Assoc*. 1966;58:345-346.
9. Schwartz RA, Janusz CA, Janniger CK. Seborrheic dermatitis: an overview. *Am Fam Physician*. 2006;74:125-130.
10. Cuelenaere C, Debersaques J, Kint A. Use of topical lithium succinate in the treatment of seborrheic dermatitis. *Dermatology*. 1992;184:194-197.
11. Sampaio AL, Mameri AC, Vargas TJ, et al. Seborrheic dermatitis. *An Bras Dermatol*. 2011;86:1061-1071.
12. Rocha N, Velho G, Horta M, et al. Cutaneous manifestations of familial amyloidotic polyneuropathy. *J Eur Acad Dermatol Venereol*. 2005;19:605-607.
13. Ercis M, Balci S, Atakan N. Dermatological manifestations of 71 Down syndrome children admitted to a clinical genetics unit. *Clin Genet*. 1996;50:317-320.
14. Strumia R. Dermatologic signs in patients with eating disorders. *Am J Clin Dermatol*. 2005;6:165-173.
15. Rao GS. Cutaneous changes in chronic alcoholics. *Indian J Dermatol Venereol Leprol*. 2004;70:79-81.
16. Pechère M, Krischer J, Remondat C, et al. *Malassezia* spp carriage in patients with seborrheic dermatitis. *J Dermatol*. 1999;26:558-561.
17. Bikowski J. Facial seborrheic dermatitis: a report on current status and therapeutic horizons. *J Drugs Dermatol*. 2009;8:125-133.
18. Mastrolonardo M, Diaferio A, Logroscino G. Seborrheic dermatitis, increased sebum excretion, and Parkinson's disease: a survey of (im)possible links. *Med Hypotheses*. 2003;60:907-911.
19. Chosidow O, Maurette C, Dupuy P. Randomized, open-labeled, noninferiority study between ciclopiroxolamine 1% cream and ketoconazole 2% foaming gel in mild to moderate facial seborrheic dermatitis. *Dermatology*. 2003;206:233-240.
20. Ashbee HR, Ingham E, Holland KT, et al. Cell-mediated immune response to *Malassezia furfur* serovars A, B, and C in patients with pityriasis versicolor, seborrheic dermatitis and controls. *Exp Dermatol*. 1994;3:106-112.
21. Parry ME, Sharpe GR. Seborrheic dermatitis is not caused by an altered immune response in *Malassezia* yeast. *Br J Dermatol*. 1998;139:254-263.
22. Zisova LG. Fluconazole and its place in the treatment of seborrheic dermatitis: new therapeutic possibilities. *Folia Med (Plovdir)*. 2006;48:39-45.
23. Bergbrant IM, Johansson S, Robbins D, et al. An immunological study in patients with seborrheic dermatitis. *Clin Exp Dermatol*. 1991;16:331-338.
24. Binder RL, Jonelis FJ. Seborrheic dermatitis: a newly reported side effect of neuroleptics. *J Clin Psychiatry*. 1984;45:125-126.
25. Soeprono FF, Schinella RA, Cockerell CJ, et al. Seborrheic-like dermatitis of acquired immunodeficiency syndrome. A clinicopathologic study. *J Am Acad Dermatol*. 1986;14:242-248.
26. Department of Health and Human Services, Office of Minority Health. HIV/AIDS Data/Statistics. www.minorityhealth.hhs.gov/templates/browse.aspx?lvl=3&lvlid=70. Accessed December 28, 2012.
27. Williams ML. Differential diagnosis of seborrheic dermatitis. *Pediatr Rev*. 1986;7:204-211.
28. Franbourg A, Hallegot P, Baltenneck F, et al. Current research on ethnic hair. *J Am Acad Dermatol*. 2003;48:S115-S119.
29. de Sá Dias TC, Baby AR, Kaneko TM, et al. Relaxing/straightening of Afro-ethnic hair: historical overview. *J Cosmet Dermatol*. 2007;6:2-5.
30. McMichael AJ. Hair breakage in normal and weathered hair: focus on the black patient. *J Investig Dermatol Symp Proc*. 2007;12:6-9.
31. Wright DR, Gathers R, Kapke A, et al. Hair care practices and their association with scalp and hair disorders in African American girls. *J Am Acad Dermatol*. 2011;64:253-262.
32. George YA, Ravis SM, Gottlieb J, et al. Betamethasone valerate 0.12% in a foam vehicle for scalp seborrheic dermatitis in African Americans. *Cosmet Dermatol*. 2002;15:25-29.
33. McMichael AJ. Scalp and hair disorders in African American patients: a primer of disorders and treatments. *Cosmet Dermatol*. 2003;16(Suppl 3): 37-41.
34. Johnson BA, Nunley JR. Treatment of seborrheic dermatitis. *Am Fam Physician*. 2000;61:2703-2710.
35. Papp KA, Papp A, Dahmer B, et al. Single-blind, randomized controlled trial evaluating the treatment of facial seborrheic dermatitis with hydrocortisone 1% ointment compared with tacrolimus 0.1% ointment in adults. *J Am Acad Dermatol*. 2012;67:11-15.
36. Meshkinpour A, Sun J, Weinstein G. An open pilot study using tacrolimus ointment in the treatment of seborrheic dermatitis. *J Am Acad Dermatol*. 2003;49:145-147.
37. Warshaw EM, Wohlhuter RJ, Liu A, et al. Results of a randomized, double-blind vehicle-controlled efficacy trial of pimecrolimus cream 1% for the treatment of moderate to severe facial seborrheic dermatitis. *J Am Acad Dermatol*. 2007;57:257-264.
38. Gupta AK, Bluhm R, Cooper EA, et al. Seborrheic dermatitis. *Dermatol Clin*. 2003;21:401-412.
39. Schwartz JR, Rocchetta H, Asawanonda P, et al. Does tachyphylaxis occur in long-term management of scalp seborrheic dermatitis with pyrithione zinc-based treatments? *Int J Dermatol*. 2009;48:79-85.
40. Waldroup W, Scheinfeld N. Medicated shampoos for the treatment of seborrheic dermatitis. *J Drugs Dermatol*. 2008;7:699-703.
41. Elewski B. An investigator-blind, randomized, 4-week, parallel-group, multicenter pilot study to compare the safety and efficacy of a nonsteroidal cream

(promiseb topical cream) and desonide cream 0.05% in the twice-daily treatment of mild to moderate seborrheic dermatitis of the face. *Clin Dermatol.* 2009;27:S48-S53.

42. Morelli V, Calmet E, Jhingade V. Alternative therapies for common dermatologic disorders, part 1. *Prim Care.* 2010;37:269-283.

43. Siadat AH, Iraji F, Shahmoradi Z, et al. The efficacy of 1% metronidazole gel in facial seborrheic dermatitis: a double blind study. *Indian J Dermatol Venereol Leprol.* 2006;72:266-269.

44. Zip CM. Innovative use of topical metronidazole. *Dermatol Clin.* 2010;28:525-534.

CHAPTER 24 Psoriasis

Amy Geng
Charles McDonald

KEY POINTS

- Psoriasis occurs worldwide and its prevalence differs among racial groups. Certain racial groups may also be more genetically predisposed to develop psoriasis.

- Higher prevalences seem to be found in Scandinavia (3% to 4.8%), Malaysia (4% to 5%), East Africa (1.25% to 3%), and South Africa (4% to 5%), and lower prevalences are seen in West Africans (0.3% to 0.8%), African Americans (0.45% to 1.3%), Southeast Asians (0.4% to 2.3%), Indians and East Asians (~0.3%), and the indigenous populations of the Americas (nearly absent).

- The clinical features of psoriasis are similar across racial groups; however, darker skin phototypes show a tendency toward violaceous plaques, gray scale, and postinflammatory dyspigmentation.

- The treatment of psoriasis is similar across racial groups. Traditional medicine is used by certain populations.

Psoriasis is a chronic, immune-mediated, inflammatory, and hyperproliferative disease of the skin that presents in a number of clinical forms that are similar across racial groups. The onset of the disease and its severity are strongly influenced by age and genetics, and may be provoked by a variety of factors such as physical injury to the skin, systemic drugs, infections, and emotional stress. Psoriasis is a systemic disease process and is associated with inflammatory arthritis, cardiovascular disease, and metabolic syndrome. The incidence of psoriasis is worldwide in distribution, but its prevalence varies by racial groups and geography. The treatment of psoriasis varies minimally among this groups.

EPIDEMIOLOGY

Psoriasis appears to be most prevalent in northern European populations, particularly in Scandinavians, in whom the peak prevalence approaches 5%. Elsewhere in Europe, the prevalence ranges from 0.7% to 2.9%. In the United States, it ranges from 1.4% to 3.2%. Psoriasis is observed less frequently in people with darker skin phototypes. Differences in psoriasis prevalence may be due to differences in genetics and environmental exposures. It should be noted that with the exception of a few studies in India, China, Japan, the African continent, and among African Americans, large-scale, population-based studies of the prevalence of psoriasis in people with skin of color have yet to be reported. There are very few published studies on psoriasis in Native Americans and the Latin American populations of North, Central, and South America. In addition, studies vary in methodologies and sample sizes. **Table 24-1** summarizes the available data.

Data from Southeast Asia show that the prevalence of psoriasis ranges from 0.5% to 2.3% in India, and 4% to 5% in Malaysia; it is about 0.4%

in Sri Lanka.[1] In Japan, China, and the Pacific Islands, prevalence rates are much lower and range from 0.05% to 0.47%.[2-6]

Psoriasis has not been found in the Samoan and Australian aboriginal populations. Psoriasis is also rare to nonexistent in the native Andean population of South America; there were no cases found in a 1962 comprehensive dermatologic survey (n = 26,000), but a few cases of both psoriasis and psoriatic arthritis were recently reported from a single clinic.[7] Whether this reflects nonindigenous heritage is unknown.

On the African continent, a number of studies show that psoriasis prevalence varies widely with geographic location. In several western African countries—Nigeria, Angola, Mali, and Senegal—prevalence rates range from 0.3% to 0.8%; these rates are substantially below those of most European populations.[8] In northern, southern, and eastern Africa, psoriasis prevalence approaches that found in Europe, 1.3% to 3%. Considerable discussion has centered around data showing marked similarities in psoriasis prevalence in African Americans (0.7% to 1.4%) and people in western Africa.[8-11] Historically, most African Americans trace their origins to western Africa, the center of the African slave trade, which may explain why they share similar rates of psoriasis prevalence. However, the present-day African American population may be an amalgamation of multiple groups including Native Americans, Europeans, and Africans, perhaps accounting for the intermediate prevalence of psoriasis in the African American population, between that of the western African and the overall U.S. population; this assumption remains speculative and requires further population-level genetic research.

IMMUNOPATHOLOGY AND GENETICS

Historically, psoriasis was characterized as a disease that occurred principally as a result of epidermal cell hyperplasia and dermal inflammation. The attributed characteristics were based on the histopathologic features found in a typical psoriatic plaque, rapid cell replication, and the reduced cell transit time within the epidermis. The epidermis in a psoriatic plaque is hyperplastic, and there is incomplete maturation of epidermal cells above the germinative cell area. Abnormalities of the cutaneous vasculature can also be seen, particularly within the upper dermis. There is an increased number of inflammatory cells in the dermis, such as dendritic cells, lymphocytes, polymorphonuclear leukocytes, and macrophages, as well as T-cells in the epidermis.

In more recent decades, it became clear that the major players of the dermal cell population in psoriasis were activated T-cells. These cells are capable of inducing changes within dermal structures that both initiate and maintain the disease state. A cascade of events from a complex interaction between environmental and genetic factors causes the activation of dendritic cells, which in turn stimulate T-cells. T-cells are attracted to the endothelium of the cutaneous vasculature and travel through the vessel wall into the dermis. Once inside the dermis, activated T-cells induce changes in keratinocytes, vascular endothelial cells, and other inflammatory cells of the dermis, including other T-lymphocytes, macrophages, and dendritic cells. The secretion of a number of protein cytokines (especially type I interferons, interferon-γ, tumor necrosis factor-α [TNF-α] interleukin-17A, and interleukin-22) by these varied cell types induces changes in epidermal keratinocytes that lead to the formation and maintenance of the psoriatic lesion.

Psoriasis develops as part of an overall increased innate immune response with polygenetic origins. Some authors have theorized that the increased risk of infections from industrialization and urbanization helped select for polymorphisms associated with increased innate immune responses. They further hypothesize that various populations have been subjected to these evolutionary pressures to different degrees and thus have corresponding differences in the prevalence of psoriasis.[12]

Classic linkage and genome-wide association studies of various populations worldwide have identified many genetic polymorphisms associated with psoriasis. There is clearly heterogeneity of these psoriasis susceptibility genes among different populations. Although some genes

TABLE 24-1 Prevalence of psoriasis: ethnic and geographic comparison

Country or ethnicity	% of dermatology patients with psoriasis	% of overall population with psoriasis	Details
Arctic Kasach'ye[75]		11.8	
Norway[75]		3–4.8	
Norway, Lapp[76]		1.4 (n = 2963)	
Norway[77]		1.1, 1.4, 1.4	
Norway[78]		4.2	
Sweden[77]		2.0	
Denmark[77]		2.8	
Faroe Islands[79]		2.8	
United Kingdom[77]		0.8, 1.5, 1.9	
Scotland[77]		0.7	
Ireland[78]	5.5		
Germany[80]		2.3–2.5	
Italy[77]		2.9	
Italy, Sardinia[81]		0.9	
Spain[77]		1.4	
Yugoslavia[77]		1.6	
Croatia[78]		1.6	
Russia, European[77]		0.7	
Former Soviet Union[78]		2.0	
Central Europe		1.5	
Egypt[8]		3.0	
Kuwait[78]	3.1		
Uganda[8]	2.8 (n = 3371)		African black
Kenya[8]	1.9 (n = 1230)		African black
Ethiopia[8]	1.3 (n = 6580)		African black
Nigeria, Northern[9]	0.8 (n = 9806)		
Nigeria[8]	0.5 (n = 1156)		African black
Senegal[8]	0.6 (n = 45,000)		Ethnicity not reported
Mali[78]	0.1		
Angola[78]	0.3		
East Africa[78]	0.7		
Tanzania[78]	3.0		
South Africa[8]		4.0–5.0	
United States, overall[8,82,83]		1.4–4.6, 2.2, 3.2	
United States, Caucasian[8,9]		2.5, 2.5	
United States, African American[8,9,75]		1.3, 1.3, 0.5–0.7	
Canada[78]	4.7		
Mexico[78]		3.0	
Jamaica[84]	6.0 (n = 1000)		95% Afro-Caribbean 0.8% Caucasian 1.4% Indian 1.4% Chinese
Brazil[8,78]	0.7 (n = 3140), 1.3		35% Mestizo 25% European 40% African black
Venezuela[78]	2.0		
Paraguay[78]	4.2		
Japan, China, Pacific Islands[2-6]		0.1–0.5	
China[5,6,85]		0.3–0.5	Male > female
Taiwan[23]		0.2	0.23 male > 0.16 female
Japan[4]		0.3–1.2	
Malaysia[1]		4.0–5.0	
India[1,86]		0.5–2.8	
Sri Lanka[1]		0.4 (n = 1366)	
Australia, Caucasian[79]		2.3–6.6	
Native North American		Nearly absent	
Native South American (Andean)[84]		Nearly absent	Previously thought to be nonexistent (n = 26,000), now with reported cases
Samoa[84]		No cases reported	
Alaskan Eskimos[78]		Nearly absent	
Australia, Aborigine		No cases reported (n = 3000)	

have been found to be associated with psoriasis across many different populations, other genes are associated with psoriasis only for certain populations.

The most important genetic locus seems to be *PSORS1*, which may account for 35% to 50% of the heritability of psoriasis.[13] *PSORS1* is located in the major histocompatibility complex (MHC), which encodes for human leukocyte antigens (HLAs). HLA-Cw6 is felt to be the strongest risk factor in fairer-skinned psoriatic patients, in whom 50% to 80% have the HLA-Cw6 allele.[14] In contrast, only 17% of Chinese patients with psoriasis carry HLA-Cw6.[15] However, the HLA-Cw6 allele in Chinese patients is still correlated with a greater risk of psoriasis and more severe disease; in one study, 18.6% of Taiwanese psoriasis patients had the allele versus 6.6% of control individuals.[16-18]

In one study from northern India, HLA-Cw6 showed a very strong correlation with psoriasis.[19] In contrast, although the prevalence of psoriasis is higher in eastern Africa than in western Africa, the distribution of HLA-Cw6 in eastern Africa does not differ appreciably from that in western Africa. In addition, although the prevalence of HLA-Cw6 is higher in black Africans (15.1%) than in Caucasians (9.6%), the prevalence of psoriasis in Africa overall is lower than in European countries.[20]

Psoriatic spondyloarthritis is often associated with HLA-B27. In Europeans, the prevalence of HLA-B27 in patients with psoriatic arthritis is 40% to 50% versus 8% in the general population. In Japan, HLA-B27 prevalence is low (>1%), and the incidence of spondyloarthropathy is also exceedingly low;[21] HLA-B51 has been implicated in a few cases of psoriatic arthritis in Japan.[22]

CLINICAL MANIFESTATIONS

There are very few published studies that document the specific clinical features of psoriasis in various populations. Based on case reports and other experiential data, psoriasis appears to present similarly across skin types. In this section, the general clinical manifestations of psoriasis and the available data regarding any specific variations are described.

The clinical onset of nonpustular psoriasis occurs during two peak age ranges. Early-onset disease peaks around the second decade, at the age of 16 for females and 20 for males. Late-onset disease peaks at ages 57 to 60. This bimodal distribution for age of onset appears to hold true for most groups. However, one large population-based study in Taiwan found an increased prevalence at age 70 and above.[23]

The primary lesion in psoriasis patients with lighter skin is a red, scaling papule that further develops into a red, scaling plaque with sharply demarcated peripheral borders [**Figures 24-1 to 24-3**]. The scale is silvery white. Plaques are often localized to the elbows, knees, scalp, umbilicus, and intergluteal fold. In patients with dark skin, the distribution is similar, but the papules and plaques are usually violaceous with a gray

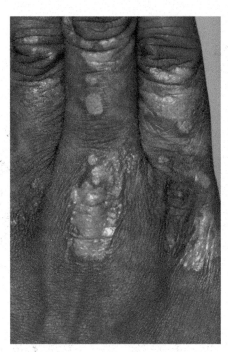

FIGURE 24-2. Chronic plaque psoriasis. Well-demarcated salmon-pink papules and plaques on the dorsum of the hand and fingers of an Asian patient. (Courtesy of the National Skin Centre, Singapore.)

scale [**Figures 24-4 to 24-7**]. Intertriginous involvement may manifest as smooth, pink to violaceous plaques depending on the underlying skin color [**Figure 24-8**] or as hypertrophic plaques with scale [**Figure 24-9**]. On the palms and soles, well-demarcated lesions with a pink to red hue may contain collections of sterile pustules and, at times, thick scale [**Figure 24-10**]. Enlarging plaques may expand to encompass more than 50% of the body's surface area [**Figure 24-11**]. External trauma, including rubbing, scratching, or scrubbing of the skin, leads to long-term maintenance of the individual psoriatic plaque; this is known as the Koebner phenomenon. Plaques may resolve with postinflammatory hypopigmentation and/or hyperpigmentation [**Figure 24-12**].

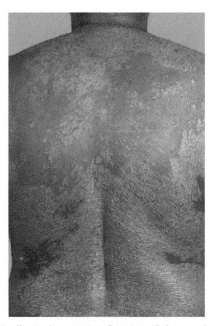

FIGURE 24-3. Chronic plaque psoriasis. Extensive well-demarcated salmon-pink scaly plaques on the back of an Asian patient. (Courtesy of the National Skin Centre, Singapore.)

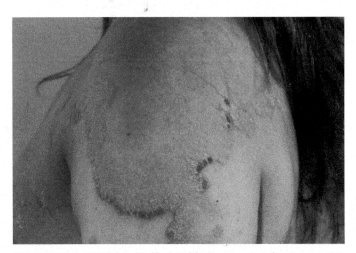

FIGURE 24-1. With lighter skin, like that of this Hispanic patient, the primary psoriatic lesions are salmon-pink or red plaques with silver-white scale.

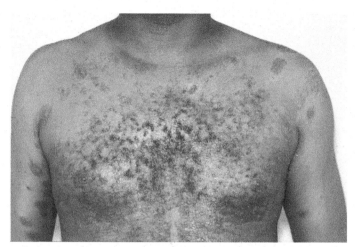

FIGURE 24-4. In patients with darker skin, like this African American patient, the papules and plaques are violaceous with gray scale.

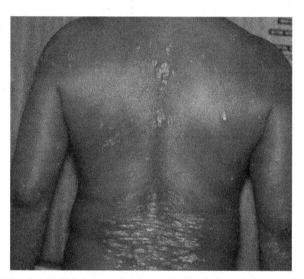

FIGURE 24-5. Well-demarcated pink to violaceous papules and plaques with scale located on the back of an African American patient with psoriasis.

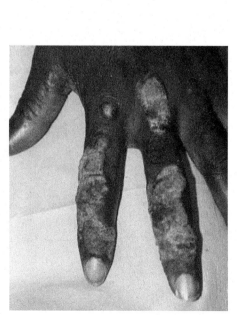

FIGURE 24-6. This African American patient had violaceous plaques with thick, micaceous, gray scale on the dorsal fingers.

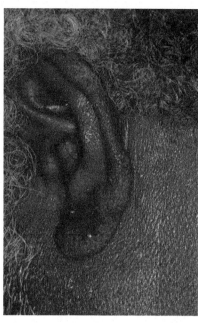

FIGURE 24-7. Well-demarcated violaceous plaques with gray scale on the helix of the ear of an African American patient.

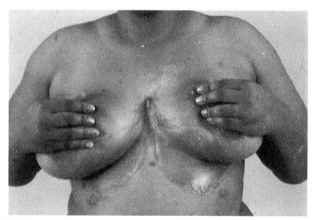

FIGURE 24-8. Intertriginous involvement manifested as smooth violaceous plaques in this African American patient.

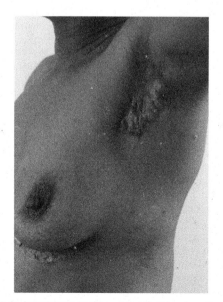

FIGURE 24-9. Intertriginous involvement manifested as hypertrophic, violaceous plaques with white scale on this African American patient.

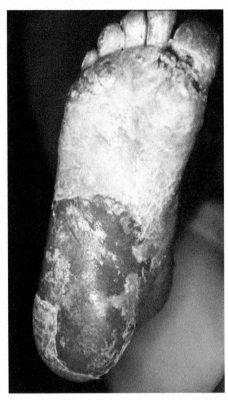

FIGURE 24-10. Plantar foot psoriasis with thick, micaceous scale on an African American patient.

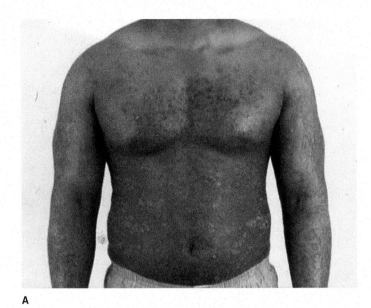

A

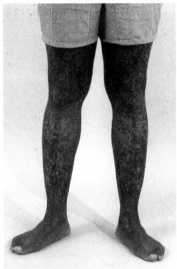

B

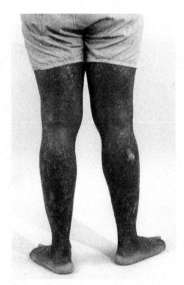

C

FIGURE 24-11. (A–C) Enlarging plaques may expand and coalesce to encompass a large proportion of the body's surface area. This African American patient had psoriasis involving the chest, arms, abdomen, back, and legs.

The classic form of guttate psoriasis presents with large numbers of small, red- to salmon-colored papules and plaques that may be covered with a very fine silvery scale. In darker skin with guttate psoriasis, violaceous and gray colors predominate [**Figure 24-13**]. This type of psoriasis often occurs with an explosive or rapid onset, primarily in young patients, and its onset is frequently associated with upper respiratory infections such as viral or streptococcal pharyngitis. Guttate psoriasis is often noted as the initial episode of psoriasis.

Pustular psoriasis is characterized by the development of groups of macroscopic sterile pustules located at the periphery of stable plaques, or it may erupt spontaneously in the absence of identifiable psoriatic lesions. Generalized pustular psoriasis presents with large clusters or sheets of pustules on a fiery red base and usually represents a very serious, potentially fatal presentation of disease. High fevers, chills, and a peripheral leukocytosis accompany the acute onset of pustules. Generalized pustular psoriasis may be lethal in improperly diagnosed and treated patients. Severe cases of pustular psoriasis such as generalized pustular psoriasis are often seen in patients with extensive psoriasis who have been treated with systemic or intensive and prolonged topical corticosteroids. Pustular psoriasis of a less severe nature also may occur as a primary manifestation of palmoplantar psoriasis. The characteristic lesion may present initially on the inner sole of the foot, eventually spreading to engulf the entire foot or hand. The distinction between palmoplantar pustular psoriasis and dyshidrotic eczema may be difficult to make [**Figures 24-14 and 24-15**].

Erythrodermic psoriasis may present at any time during the course of psoriasis. It manifests as diffuse, generalized redness of the skin associated with extensive scaling. The skin feels warm to touch, and the patient's body temperature becomes quite erratic. Cutaneous blood flow increases, initiating a stream of abnormal metabolic events that result in a severely ill patient. The sudden withdrawal of long-term systemic or intensive topical corticosteroid treatment often serves as the trigger for developing erythrodermic psoriasis.

Nail changes are relatively common in psoriasis. They are quite characteristic and often diagnostic yet bear no relationship to the severity of psoriasis. Pitting of the nail is the most common finding, followed by

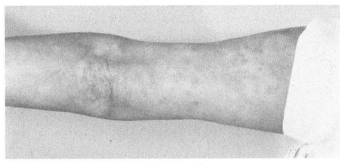

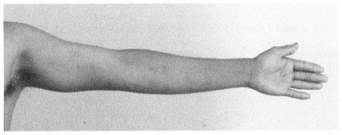

FIGURES 24-12. Plaques may resolve with postinflammatory (**A**) hypopigmentation and/or (**B**) hyperpigmentation.

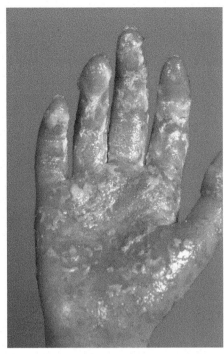

FIGURE 24-14. Pustular psoriasis may occur as a primary manifestation of palmoplantar psoriasis. In this Asian patient, the characteristic pustular and crusted erosions spread to engulf the hand and fingers. (Courtesy of the National Skin Centre, Singapore.)

leukonychia and longitudinal grooves and ridges. Often a reddish brown discoloration of the nail bed results in the appearance of a characteristic 'oil drop' sign. Subungual hyperkeratosis may also be observed. The number of nails affected varies.

There are a few studies describing the clinical characteristics of psoriasis in skin of darker phototypes. In a study of 1220 psoriatic patients in India, 93% had plaque-type psoriasis, followed by pustular, guttate, erythrodermic, nail, flexural, and arthropathic types of psoriasis.[24] In this case series, the extent of disease in patients was mild, involving less than 25% of body surface area. Most patients described their lesions as relatively asymptomatic with minor pruritus and burning, and postinflammatory hyperpigmentation was observed more commonly than hypopigmentation. In this study, only a few of the Indian patients admitted to having cosmetic embarrassment from their skin lesions.

In a similar study from Sri Lanka, 5% to 10% of patients identified specific triggers of psoriasis; these included sore throat, pregnancy or parturition, and chloroquine use. Other less common precipitating factors such as chickenpox, diarrhea, alcohol use, and mental stress also were identified.[25]

Nail involvement in Indian and Sri Lankan patients with psoriasis varied from 14% to 56%, and pitting of the nail was the most commonly

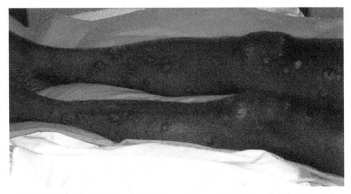

FIGURE 24-13. In darker skin with guttate psoriasis, violaceous and gray colors predominate.

reported nail change. Fewer than 1% of patients had psoriasis limited to the nails.[25]

Studies from India also have described a higher incidence of palmoplantar psoriasis. Predisposing factors are likely to include trauma from manual labor, the practice of wearing open-toed slippers, and the Indian custom of walking barefoot.[26] A survey of 28,628 Japanese patients with psoriasis revealed that the vast majority had plaque-type psoriasis vulgaris (86%), followed by guttate psoriasis (2.8%), psoriatic arthritis (1.0%), generalized pustular psoriasis (0.9%), psoriatic erythroderma (0.8%), and localized pustular psoriasis (0.5).[27]

In African American and Native American patients, there appears to be little difference in the clinical presentation of psoriasis compared with other skin phototypes; most patients seem to have classic plaque-type disease. The course of the disease has been described as "mild," with only a few reported cases of erythrodermic psoriasis. In a survey of dermatologists in the United States, respondents reported slightly different manifestations of disease in African Americans, such as more dyspigmentation, less erythema, and thicker plaques.[28]

In a 1967 study by Verhagen and Koten of 1230 Kenyan patients, the prevalence of psoriasis was 2.6%.[29] The diagnosis was established using the same criteria used in Western countries. In contrast to the hyperpigmentation seen in the Indian and Sri Lankan populations, Verhagen and Koten described "hypopigmentation as an outspoken feature in African skin" during both active disease and in residual lesions.[29] Psoriasis has been reported to cause hair loss in a few children in Nigeria.[30]

Some racial differences in psoriasis were found using data from the Etanercept Assessment of Safety and Effectiveness (EASE) trial. At baseline, Caucasians had the longest disease duration (19 years) and the lowest percentage of body surface area (BSA) involvement (28%). Asians had the highest percentage of BSA involvement (41%). The Dermatology Life Quality Index (DLQI) score was lowest (best quality of life) for Caucasians (12.0) at baseline and highest for Hispanics/Latinos (14.6). The BSA involvement at week 12 was reduced by more than 50% for all groups but remained higher for Asians (17%) than for Caucasians (13%) and African Americans (13%). The mean DLQI score for Asians (5.2) was higher than for Caucasians (3.5) and Hispanics/Latinos (3.8).[31]

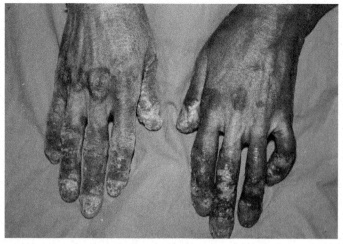

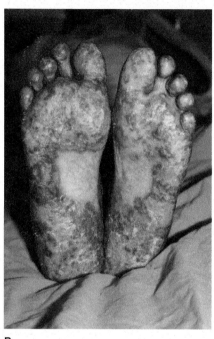

B

FIGURE 24-15. (A) and (B) In this African American patient with palmoplantar psoriasis, yellow-brown macules and sterile pustules became confluent in areas, causing extensive scale, crust, and nail loss.

In contrast with studies in populations of European descent, several studies in Asia have found an increased prevalence of psoriasis in males. These include large studies in China,[6] Taiwan,[23] and Japan,[27] as well as smaller studies in India,[32] Malaysia, and Bangladesh.[33]

In Taiwan, a population-based cohort study of 3686 psoriasis patients revealed an increased risk of cancer (hazard ratio, 1.66), including cancers of the urinary bladder, skin, oropharynx/larynx, liver/gallbladder, and colon/rectum. Ultraviolet B (UVB) (but not psoralen and ultraviolet A [PUVA] or oral medications) appeared to reduce the risk of cancer (adjusted hazard ratio, 0.52).[34] Also in Taiwan, a population-based cohort study found an association between psoriasis and chronic obstructive pulmonary disease.[35]

In a series of 12 patients with hypertrophic or verrucous psoriasis, a rarely reported histologic subtype of psoriasis, the populations were as follows: Caucasian (n = 8), Hispanic (n = 3), and African (n = 1).[36] A single case of erythrodermic verrucous psoriasis was reported in an African American.[37]

PSORIATIC ARTHRITIS

Psoriatic arthritis is an inflammatory arthritis associated with psoriasis. The histologic picture in affected joints of patients with psoriatic arthritis shows similar features to those found in the skin of patients with psoriasis. Moll and Wright classify psoriatic arthritis into five subgroups: (1) asymmetric oligoarticular arthritis, found in over 70% of patients with arthritis and characterized by the typical 'sausage-shaped digits'; (2) symmetric metacarpophalangeal joint involvement; (3) distal interphalangeal joint involvement, producing the pathognomonic 'swan neck' deformity; (4) arthritis mutilans, characterized by extensive bone resorption; and (5) spondylitis/sacroiliitis or spondyloarthropathy. The age of onset peaks at about 40 years, and onset is often acute. A few cases of acute-onset psoriatic arthritis have been observed in young female patients with a degree of severity that required long-term treatment with antineoplastic agents (McDonald CJ, unpublished data).

The geoepidemiology of psoriatic arthritis remains an area of study because the criteria used for evaluating arthritis vary widely among physicians and studies. Prevalence rates are not determined with equivalent data, and thus comparisons among populations may not be accurate. Overall, psoriatic arthritis seems more prevalent in Europe and North and South America and less prevalent in Africa and Asia, especially in Japan. Genetic studies have found differences in the genes associated with psoriatic arthritis in different populations.[38]

In Latin America, the Iberoamerican Registry of Spondyloarthritis registered patients from Argentina, Brazil, Costa Rica, Chile, Mexico, Peru, Uruguay, Venezuela, Spain, and Portugal. Compared with other Western countries, patients with psoriatic arthritis from this registry were older at the time of the study visit, at onset of symptoms, and at diagnosis of spondyloarthritis; had longer mean disease duration from onset of symptoms to diagnosis; and were more likely to have dactylitis, nail involvement, enthesitis, and peripheral arthritis in lower and upper extremities.[39]

The prevalence of psoriatic arthritis in the Indian psoriatic population is lower (4%) than in the U.S. psoriatic population (10%). In a case-controlled study of 80 patients with psoriasis in Singapore, Indians were twice as likely to have psoriatic arthritis than Han Chinese patients.[40] Authors in India, Singapore, and Malaysia have noted that patients with psoriasis of Indian descent are more likely to develop psoriatic arthritis than patients of other Asian populations.[40,41]

PSORIASIS AND METABOLIC SYNDROME

Metabolic syndrome is a combination of risk factors (central obesity, hypertension, dyslipidemia, and insulin resistance) that is associated with cardiovascular disease, stroke, and type 2 diabetes. Several organizations have suggested slightly different criteria for metabolic syndrome; the International Diabetes Federation (a consensus definition by several countries) definition is central obesity (defined as waist circumference with group specific values) and any two of the following: (1) raised triglycerides: >150 mg/dL (1.7 mmol/L), or specific treatment for this lipid abnormality; (2) reduced high-density lipoprotein cholesterol: <40 mg/dL (1.03 mmol/L) in males, <50 mg/dL (1.29 mmol/L) in females, or specific treatment for this lipid abnormality; (3) raised blood pressure (BP): systolic BP >130 mm Hg or diastolic BP >85 mm Hg, or treatment of previously diagnosed hypertension; and (4) raised fasting plasma glucose (FPG): >100 mg/dL (5.6 mmol/L), or previously diagnosed type 2 diabetes. If FPG is >5.6 mmol/L or 100 mg/dL, an oral glucose tolerance test is strongly recommended but is not necessary. If body mass index is >30 kg/m², central obesity can be assumed, and waist circumference does not need to be measured.

Several population-based studies have suggested a relationship between psoriasis and metabolic syndrome. Although the prevalence of metabolic syndrome is variable among populations, overall there seems to be an increased prevalence of metabolic syndrome in patients with psoriasis in most countries. One of two studies from Korea did not find an association between metabolic syndrome and psoriasis; however, the study described some limitations, including using a predominance of young patients and using telephone interviews to define metabolic syndrome instead of laboratory data. The authors noted that metabolic syndrome seemed to be associated with older patients with more severe plaque-type disease. From Taiwan, one of two studies did not find an association between metabolic syndrome and psoriasis, possibly due to missing data for lipid profiles and body mass index.

In a U.S. study, the occurrence rate of occlusive vascular episodes was substantially greater in psoriatic patients than in patients without psoriasis, and psoriasis itself appeared to be a significant predisposing factor for cardiovascular disease. Females with psoriasis tended to experience more venous and less arterial disease than males, and there did not appear to be any variation in cardiovascular disease.[42]

TREATMENT OF PSORIASIS

The treatment of psoriasis seems to be similar across various populations. The therapies used worldwide include topical and systemic glucocorticosteroids, calcipotriene, anthralins, tar, topical and oral retinoids, phototherapy (including PUVA, narrowband UVB [nb-UVB] and broadband UVB, and the 308 nm excimer laser), and immunosuppressive systemic medications. Biological agents are used primarily in developed countries due to cost issues.

Complementary and alternative medicine (CAM) is used by 51% of patients with psoriasis in the United States and Great Britain,[43,44] and in certain populations, the prevalence of CAM use may be higher. Although the evidence for efficacy is preliminary, patients expect dermatologists to be able to provide some basic information regarding CAM and psoriasis.

In a study of 28,628 psoriatic patients in Japan, topical corticosteroid use was the most common treatment modality (68%). Topical vitamin D derivatives were used rarely (2.4%). Phototherapeutic regimens included use of topical PUVA (12%), systemic PUVA (8%), and nb-UVB. PUVA is contraindicated in psoriasis patients who are pregnant or lactating (0.5%). Systemic regimens included, most commonly, herbal medicine (14%), followed by etretinate (7.6%), nonsteroidal anti-inflammatory drugs (4.4%), oral corticosteroids (4.1%), methotrexate (2.8%), cyclosporine (1.6%), and other antineoplastic medications (1.4%).

Phototherapy may be relatively unpopular among Asian patients due to a cultural aversion to tanning. A tanned complexion is considered a sign of having to perform manual outdoor labor and is considered undesirable. Asian patients have been reported to complain about unwanted tanning from phototherapy,[45] and one should consider the issue of compliance when prescribing phototherapy in this population.

To avoid unwanted tanning from phototherapy, one study suggests using PUVA twice weekly versus thrice weekly, which did not change efficacy as measured by the psoriasis area and severity index score. For nb-UVB, twice-weekly dosing may be effective, but longer treatment courses are required. A recent study suggests that in darker-skinned individuals, suberythrogenic doses of nb-UVB are as effective as erythrogenic doses.[46]

Female patients of certain ethnic populations may be averse to exposing parts of their body; some authors have suggested using lightweight cotton gowns with increased UV dosages.

Several traditional Chinese herbal products have been shown to be effective in the treatment of psoriasis through anti-inflammatory and/or immunosuppressive properties, including indirubin, *Tripterygium wilfordii* Hook, and *Tripterygium hypoglaucum* Hutch. Side effects include gastrointestinal symptoms, myelosuppression, and elevated liver function tests.[47-58] *T. wilfordii* Hook was used to good effect in 638 patients with psoriatic arthritis, 16 patients with pustular psoriasis, and 5 patients with erythrodermic psoriasis.[16,59,60]

Salvia miltiorrhiza radix is commonly used for dermatologic disorders including psoriasis. Tanshinone IIA, an active component, inhibits keratinocyte growth by causing cell cycle arrest and apoptosis in mice.[61]

Indigo naturalis oil extract can be used topically for plaque psoriasis as well as nail psoriasis, including pustular psoriasis of the nail. This herb inhibits keratinocyte proliferation, TNF-α–induced vascular cell adhesion molecule-1, and superoxide anion and elastase release by neutrophils.

Another traditional Chinese herb, *Radix angelicae dahuricae*, has been used topically with ultraviolet A (UVA) for a psoralen-like effect. *R. angelicae dahuricae* contains imperatorin, isoimperatorin, and alloimperatorin, which, like psoralens, are furocoumarins. Psoriasis clearance rates were similar between *R. angelicae dahuricae* with UVA versus PUVA, but with fewer side effects.[62-64] *R. angelicae pubescentis* also has been used successfully with UVA.[65]

Traditional Chinese medicine (TCM) usually involves the use of multiple herbs simultaneously, but there are very few studies of multiple-agent TCM treatment of psoriasis. Notably, a study of 801 patients with psoriasis found a 50% to 85% response rate in patients treated with a mixture of five herbs (*rhizoma sparganii*, *rhizoma zedoariae*, *herba serissae*, *resina boswelliae*, and *myrrha*).[66]

Acupuncture is also used for psoriasis. In a case series of 61 patients with refractory psoriasis, 50% had complete to near-complete clearance and 33% had partial improvement with acupuncture.[67] In contrast, a Swedish study reported no difference between patients treated with TCM-indicated points and patients treated with sham points.[68] Note, however, that the use of sham points may itself have a physiologic effect and thus is not usually considered to be an adequate control.[69]

In India, the overall cost–benefit ratio of treatments becomes an important factor in treatment decisions, especially for a chronic disease like psoriasis. Coal tar is still considered to be the most useful topical agent because the cost is nearly 25 times less than that of calcipotriol.[70] Anthralin and topical steroids are also cost-effective options and are used for localized disease.[71] In extensive psoriasis, methotrexate is the drug of choice in India primarily because of its affordability and relatively few associated side effects. Hydroxyurea is used as a second-line agent for patients who are intolerant of methotrexate. Retinoids are not used, likely due to their associated teratogenic effects.

Alternative therapeutic regimens have implemented Ayurvedic or herbal therapy in treating psoriasis and psoriatic arthritis. Neem oil (from the Neem tree, *Azadirachta indica*) has been used for treating localized plaque psoriasis primarily because of its emollient properties.[72] This inexpensive oil removes scale from thickened psoriatic plaques and also functions as an anti-inflammatory agent. Its properties, like those of coal tar, are enhanced when used with ultraviolet light. Turmeric (*Curcuma longa*) is another inexpensive alternative topical agent for psoriasis. This mustard-yellow, fragrant powder is made from the stems of a ginger root-like plant and is used most often in curry powder. Outside the kitchen, turmeric is prized for its anti-inflammatory and powerful antioxidant properties. This powder can be mixed with water or aloe vera gel to form a paste that can be applied directly to psoriatic skin lesions. Curcumin modulates many molecular targets, including nuclear factor-κB, inducible nitric oxide synthase, TNF-α, interleukin-1, and interleukin-6.[73]

An Ayurvedic herbal remedy for psoriasis is *chakramadha tailam*, which is a formulation containing *Cassia tora*. It is applied topically, and has been shown to reduce epidermal thickness in rats with UVB-induced psoriasis.[74] Other herbs used for psoriasis include *Ficus hispida*, *Aloe vera*, and *Psoralea corylifolia*, which contains psoralens.

Another Ayurvedic therapy is the practice of *snehapanam*, in which medicated *ghee* (clarified butter) or specific herbal oils are combined and consumed by the patient over a 2-week period in increasing quantities. This process is designed to purify the blood and is thought to heal the body in conditions such as psoriasis and psoriatic arthritis.

Stress can exacerbate psoriasis and is an important factor to address especially in refractory cases of psoriasis. Complementary and alternative therapies such as TCM and Ayurvedic medicine emphasize the importance of lifestyle in the management of psoriasis. Practices such as yoga, tai chi, and meditation are encouraged to achieve a state of mental well-being and thus contribute holistically to the management of psoriasis.

CONCLUSION

Psoriasis occurs worldwide, but there is scant research characterizing the disease in individual racial and cultural groups. Overall, the prevalence of psoriasis seems to be lower in certain populations, including certain populations of Africa, East Asia, India, and Samoa and indigenous populations of the Americas. Some data suggest that racial differences in the genetic predisposition to develop psoriasis may exist. Although clinical manifestations may differ slightly, the treatment of psoriasis seems to be similar among various populations, although certain cultures have developed unique treatment regimens, including cost-effective therapies and herbal medicine. There is a need for additional studies of psoriasis skin of color populations.

REFERENCES

1. Raychauduri SP, Farber EM. The prevalence of psoriasis in the world. *J Eur Acad Dermatol Venerol.* 2001;15:16-17.
2. Yip SY. The prevalence of psoriasis in the Mongoloid race. *J Am Acad Dermatol.* 1984;10:965-968.
3. Cheng L, Zhang SZ, Xiao CY, et al. The A5.1 allele of the major histocompatibility complex class I chain-related gene A is associated with psoriasis vulgaris in Chinese. *Br J Dermatol.* 2000;143:324-329.
4. Aoki T. Psoriasis in Japan. *Arch Dermatol.* 1971;104:328-329.
5. Lin XR. Psoriasis in China. *J Dermatol.* 1993;20:746-755.
6. Ding X, Wang T, Shen Y. Prevalence of psoriasis in China: a population-based study in six cities. *Eur J Dermatol.* 2012;22:663-7.
7. Toloza S, Vega-Hinojosa O, Chandran V, et al. Psoriasis and psoriatic arthritis in Peruvian aborigines: a report from the GRAPPA 2011 annual meeting. *J Rheumatol.* 2012;39:2216-2219.
8. Farber EM, Nall L. Psoriasis in the tropics: epidemiologic, genetic, clinical, and therapeutic aspects. *Dermatol Clin.* 1994;12:805-816.
9. Gelfand JM, Stern RS, Nijsten T, et al. The prevalence of psoriasis in African-Americans: results from a population-based study. *J Am Acad Dermatol.* 2005;52:23-26.
10. Jacyk WK. Psoriasis in Nigerians. *Trop Geogr Med.* 1981;33:139-142.
11. Leder RO, Farber EM. The variable incidence of psoriasis in sub-Saharan Africa. *Int J Dermatol.* 1997;36:911-919.
12. Bos J. Psoriasis, innate immunity, and gene pools. *J Am Acad Dermatol.* 2007;56:468-471.
13. Nestle FO, Kaplan DH, Barker J. Psoriasis. *N Engl J Med.* 2009;361:496-509.
14. Wuepper KD, Coulter SN, Haberman A. Psoriasis vulgaris: a genetic approach. *J Invest Dermatol.* 1990;95:2S-4S.
15. Cao K, Song FJ, Li HG, et al. Association between HLA antigens and families with psoriasis vulgaris. *Chin Med J.* 1993;6:132-135.
16. Tsai TF, Hu CY, Tsai WL, et al. HLA-Cw6 specificity and polymorphic residues are associated with susceptibility among Chinese psoriatics in Taiwan. *Arch Dermatol Res.* 2002;294:214-220.
17. Chang YT, Tsai SF, Lee DD, et al. A study of candidate genes for psoriasis near HLA-C in Chinese patients with psoriasis. *Br J Dermatol.* 2003;148:418-423.
18. Fan X, Yang S, Sun L, et al. Comparison of clinical features of HLA-Cw*0602-positive and -negative psoriasis patients in a Han Chinese population. *Acta Derm Venereol.* 2007;87:335-340.
19. Rani R, Narayan R, Fernandez-VinMa A, et al. HLA-B and C alleles in psoriasis in patients in North India. *Tissue Antigens.* 1998;51:618-622.
20. Ouédraogo DD, Meyer O. Psoriatic arthritis in Sub-Saharan Africa. *Joint Bone Spine.* 2012;79:17-19.
21. Hukuda S, Minami M, Saito T, et al. Spondyloarthropathies in Japan: nationwide questionnaire survey performed by the Japan Ankylosing Spondylitis Society. *J Rheumatol.* 2001;28:554-559.
22. Yamamoto T, Yokozeki H, Nishioka K. Psoriasis arthropathy and HLA-B51: report of 5 cases. *J Dermatol.* 2005;32:606-610.
23. Chang Y, Chen T, Liu P, et al. Epidemiological study of psoriasis in the national health insurance database in Taiwan. *Acta Derm Venereol.* 2009;89:262-266.
24. Kaur I, Handa S, Kumar B. Natural history of psoriasis: study from the Indian subcontinent. *J Dermatol.* 1997;24:230-234.
25. Gunawardena DA, Gunawardena KA, Vasanthanathan NS, Gunawardena JA. Psoriasis in Sri Lanka: a computer analysis of 1366 cases. *Br J Dermatol.* 1978;98:85-96.

26. Kumar B, Saraswat A, Kaur I. Palmoplantar lesions in psoriasis. *Acta Dermatol Venerol.* 2002;82:192-195.
27. Kawada A, Tezuka T, Nakamizo Y, et al. A survey of psoriasis patients in Japan from 1982-2001. *J Dermatol Sci.* 2003;31:59-64.
28. McMichael A, Vachiramon V, Guzmán-Sánchez D, et al. Psoriasis in African-Americans: a caregivers' survey. *J Drugs Dermtol.* 2010;11:478-482.
29. Verhagen AR, Koten JW. Psoriasis in Kenya. *Arch Dermatol.* 1967;96:39-41.
30. Nnoruka E, Obiagboso I, Maduechesi C. Hair loss in children in South-East Nigeria: common and uncommon cases. *Int J Dermatol.* 2007;46(Suppl):18-22.
31. Shah S, Arthur A, Yang Y, et al. A retrospective study to investigate racial and ethnic variations in the treatment of psoriasis with etanercept. *J Drugs Dermatol.* 2011;10:866-872.
32. Asokan N, Prathap P, Ajithkumar K, et al. Pattern of psoriasis in a tertiary care teaching hospital in south India. *Indian J Dermatol.* 2011;56:118-119.
33. Islam M, Paul H, Zakaria S, et al. Epidemiological determinants of psoriasis. *Mymensingh Med J.* 2011;20:9-15.
34. Chen Y, Wu C, Chen T, et al. The risk of cancer in patients with psoriasis: a population-based cohort study in Taiwan. *J Am Acad Dermatol.* 2011;65:84-91.
35. Chiang Y, Lin H. Association between psoriasis and chronic obstructive pulmonary disease: a population-based study in Taiwan. *J Eur Acad Dermatol Venereol.* 2012;26:59-65.
36. Khalil FK, Keehn CA, Saeed S, Morgan MB. Verrucous psoriasis: a distinctive clinicopathologic variant of psoriasis. *Am J Dermatopathol.* 2005;27:204-207.
37. Curtis A, Yosipovitch G. Erythrodermic verrucous psoriasis. *J Dermatolog Treat.* 2012;23:215-218.
38. Tam LS, Leung YY, Li EK. Psoriatic arthritis in Asia. *Rheumatology.* 2009;48:1473-1477.
39. Espinoza L, Toloza S, Valle-Onate R, et al. Global partnering opportunities and challenges of psoriasis and psoriatic arthritis in Latin American: a report from the GRAPPA 2010 annual meeting. *J Rheumatol.* 2012;39:445-447.
40. Thumboo J, Tham SN, Tay YK. Patterns of psoriatic arthritis in Orientals. *J Rheumatol.* 1997;24:1949-1953.
41. Tey H, Ee H, Tan A, et al. Risk factors associated with having psoriatic arthritis in patients with cutaneous psoriasis. *J Dermatol.* 2010;37:426-430.
42. McDonald CJ, Calabresi P. Psoriasis and occlusive vascular disease. *BMD.* 1978;99:469-475.
43. Fleischer AB, Feldman SR, Rapp SR, et al. Alternative therapies commonly used within a population of patients with psoriasis. *Cutis.* 1996;58:216-220.
44. Clark CM, Mckay RA, Fortune DG, et al. Use of alternative treatments by patients with psoriasis. *Br J Gen Pract.* 1998;48:1873-1874.
45. Choe YB, Rim JH, Youn JI. Quantitative assessment of narrow-band UVB induced tanning during phototherapy in Korea. *Photodermatol Photoimmunol Photomed.* 2002;18:127-130.
46. Syed Z, Hamzavi I. Role of phototherapy in patients with skin of color. *Semin Cutan Med Surg.* 2011;30:184-189.
47. Prieto JM, Recio MC, Giner RM, et al. Influence of traditional Chinese anti-inflammatory medicinal plants on leukocyte and platelet functions. *J Pharm Pharmacol.* 2003;55:1275-1282.
48. Koo J, Desai R. Traditional Chinese medicine in dermatology. *Dermatol Ther.* 2003;16:98-105.
49. Wang MX, Wang HL, Lui WS, et al. Study of the therapeutic effect and pharmacological action of indirubin in treating psoriasis. *Chin J Dermatol.* 1982;15:157-160.
50. Lu YT. Treating 159 cases of psoriasis vulgaris with pilulae Indigo naturalis compositae. *Chin J Integr Tradit West Med.* 1989;9:558.
51. Yuan ZZ, Yuan X, Xu ZX. An observation on the therapeutic effect of Indigo naturalis in 46 cases of psoriasis. *J Tradit Chin Med.* 1982;23:43.
52. Chen LZ. Treating 23 cases of psoriasis with indirubin tablets. *J Clin Dermatol.* 1981;10:157-158.
53. Ling MW, Chen DY, Zhu YX, et al. Treatment of 26 cases of psoriasis with indirubin. *J Clin Dermatol.* 1982;11:131-132.
54. Yan SF. A clinical observation of treating 43 cases of psoriasis with indirubin. *Yunnan J Tradit Chin Med.* 1982;2:21.
55. Lin XR, Yang CM, Yang GL, et al. Treatment of psoriasis with meisoindigo. *J Clin Dermatol.* 1989;18:29-30.
56. Yang CM, Lin XR, Yang GL, et al. A study of the treatment of psoriasis with meisoindigo. *J Clin Dermatol.* 1989;18:295-297.
57. Chen NQ, Dai ZH, Wang LZ. An observation of the effectiveness of N-acetylindirubin in treating psoriasis. *J Clin Dermatol.* 1988;17:328.
58. Xie ZZ. Treatment of psoriasis with pilulae Indigo naturalis compositae. *J Tradit Chin Med.* 1984;25:39-40.
59. Guan F, Wong DH. Treatment of psoriasis with *Tripterygium wilfordii* Hook. *J Clin Dermatol.* 1981;10:91-93.

60. Zhang JY. Treating 148 cases of psoriasis vulgaris with *Tripterygium wilfordii* Hook. *J Clin Dermatol.* 1982;11:118.

61. Li F, Xu R, Zeng Q, et al. Tanshinone IIA inhibits growth of keratinocytes through cell cycle arrest and apoptosis: underlying treatment mechanism of psoriasis. *Evid Based Complement Alternat Med.* http://dx.doi.org/10.1155/2012/927658.

62. Zhang GW, Li SB, Wang HJ, et al. Inhibition of Chinese herb medicine, *Angelica dahurica* (Benth et Hook) and UVA synthesis of DNA of lymphocytes in vitro. *Chin J Dermatol.* 1980;13:138-140.

63. Zhang GW. [Treatment of psoriasis by photochemotherapy: A comparison between the photosensitizing capsule of *Angelica dahurica* and 8-MOP.] *Zhonghua Yi Xue Za Zhi.* 1983;63:16-19.

64. Shi SY, Xu S, Yian YP. A therapeutic evaluation of *Tripterygium wilfordii* Hook in the treatment of 19 cases of psoriatic arthritis. *J Clin Dermatol.* 1988;17:294-296.

65. Li FQ. Cases suffering from psoriasis treated with traditional Chinese medicine *Angelicae tuhuo* and long wave ultraviolet. *Chin J Phys Ther.* 1983;6:144-145.

66. Lin CH, Wang HY. Comparison of long term clinical effects of microcirculation modulation traditional drugs and ethylene diamine tetraacetylimide in the treatment of psoriasis. *J Clin Dermatol.* 1988;17:125-130.

67. Liao SJ, Liao TA. Acupuncture treatment for psoriasis: a retrospective case report. *Acupunct Electrother Res.* 1992;17:195-208.

68. Jerner B, Skogh M, Vahlquist A. A controlled trial of acupuncture in psoriasis: no convincing effect. *Acta Derm Venereol.* 1997;77:154-156.

69. Streitberger K, Kleinhenz J. Introducing a placebo needle into acupuncture research. *Lancet.* 1998;352:364-365.

70. Sharma V, Kaur I, Kumar B. Calcipotriol versus coal tar: a prospective randomized study in stable plaque psoriasis. *Int J Dermatol.* 2003;42:834-838.

71. Agarwal R, Saraswat A, Kaur I, et al. A novel liposomal formulation of dithranol in psoriasis: preliminary results. *J Dermatol Treat.* 2002;13:119-122.

72. Subapriya R, Nagini S. Medicinal properties of Neem leaves: a review. *Curr Med Chem Anticancer Agents.* 2005;5:149-156.

73. Shishodia S, Sethi G, Agarwal BB. Curcumin: getting back to the roots. *Ann NY Acad Sci.* 2005;1056:206-217.

74. Singhal M, Kansara N. Cassia tora Linn cream inhibits ultraviolet-B-induced psoriasis in rats. *ISRN Dermatol.* 2012;2012:346510.

75. Farber EM, Nall ML. Epidemiology of psoriasis: natural history and genetics. In: Roenigk HH, Maibach HI, eds. *Psoriasis.* 3rd ed. New York, NY: Marcel Dekker; 1998:107-158.

76. Falk E, Vandbakk O. Prevalence of psoriasis in a Norwegian Lapp population. *Acta Derm Venereol Suppl (Stockh).* 1993;182:6-9.

77. Parisi R, Symmons D, Griffiths C, et al. Global epidemiology of psoriasis: a systematic review of incidence and prevalence. *J Invest Dermatol.* 2013;133:377-385.

78. Cimmino M. Epidemiology of psoriasis and psoriatic arthritis. *Reumatismo.* 2007;59(Suppl 1):19-24.

79. Lomholt G. Prevalence of skin diseases in a population: a census study from the Faroe Islands. *Danish Med Bull.* 1964;11:1-7.

80. Augustin M, Glaeske G, Schäfer I, et al. Processes of psoriasis healthcare in Germany: long-term analysis of data from the statutory health insurances. *J Dtsch Dermatol Ges.* 2012;10:648-655.

81. Sardu C, Cocco E, Mereu A, et al. Population based study of 12 autoimmune diseases in Sardinia, Italy: prevalence and comorbidity. *PLoS One.* 2012;7:e32487.

82. Stern RS, Nijsten T, Feldman SR, et al. Psoriasis is common, carries a substantial burden even when not extensive, and is associated with widespread treatment dissatisfaction. *J Investig Dermatol Symp Proc.* 2004;9:136-139.

83. Kurd S, Gelfand J. The prevalence of previously diagnosed and undiagnosed psoriasis in US adults: results from NHANES 2003-2004. *J Am Acad Dermatol.* 2009;60:218-224.

84. Campalani E, Barker JN. The clinical genetics of psoriasis. *Curr Genomics.* 2005;6:51-60.

85. Li R, Sun J, Ren L, et al. Epidemiology of eight common rheumatic diseases in China: a large-scale cross-sectional survey in Beijing. *Rheumatology (Oxford).* 2012;51:721-729.

86. Dogra S, Yadav S. Psoriasis in India: prevalence and pattern. *Indian J Dermatol Venereol Leprol.* 2010;76:595-601.

CHAPTER 25

Pityriasis Rosea

Dwana R. Shabazz

KEY POINTS

- Pityriasis rosea (PR) is a self-limiting papulosquamous dermatosis that is found in all Fitzpatrick skin types (I to VI), with some distinct presentations in patients with skin of color.

- PR is associated with drugs (barbiturates, metronidazole, terbinafine, isotretinoin, gold, and clozapine), vaccinations (hemagglutinin 1 neuraminidase 1 [H1N1]), and viruses (human herpes virus [HHV]-6, HHV-7, and HHV-8).

- The etiology of PR is unclear. However, antiviral therapies are proving to be effective in decreasing the duration and severity of this condition.

INTRODUCTION

Pityriasis rosea (PR) is an acute, self-limiting papulosquamous dermatosis that is thought to have a viral origin. It occurs over a broad age range, most often between the ages of 10 and 35 years, and rarely before the age of 2. The peak occurrence is during the spring and fall seasons. It usually has a classic clinical presentation, is asymptomatic, and undergoes spontaneous resolution in 6 to 10 weeks.

PR is found worldwide without a racial predilection. In an overview of disorders more commonly seen in patients with skin of color, PR was listed as occurring in about 2% of patients[1] [**Table 25-1**].

The incidence of PR has been decreasing. This may be due to its self-limiting nature, which could result in cases of PR never coming to the attention of a physician. Furthermore, dermatologists are usually the second or third physician a patient sees for the diagnosis and treatment of PR. By this point, the condition has often cleared up and the patient is seeking to determine the cause of the dermatosis, and/or the patient has healed but has been left with postinflammatory dyspigmentation (often in the form of hyperpigmentation).

Because PR may differ clinically in those with skin of color, in comparison with patients who have Fitzpatrick skin types I to III, it is important to highlight the clinical differences. It is also necessary to note the effects of certain treatment options for patients with skin of color.

PATHOGENESIS

PR is thought to be due to a virus or bacterium. Most of the literature points to a viral etiology.[2] Human herpes virus (HHV)-6 and HHV-7 are the two viruses most closely associated with PR, although this correlation is inconclusive.

HHV-6 belongs to the *Roseolovirus* genus and is closely homologous with HHV-7; thus HHV-7 belongs to the same genus. HHV-6 is widespread in the population and persists, often in a latent state, in its hosts' monocytes and bone marrow progenitor cells and as a chronic infection of the salivary glands.[2] It is this infection of the salivary glands that is thought to be the mode of transmission for HHV-6.[2] In support of the close association between the two viruses, it has been reported that an infection with HHV-7 can lead to the reactivation of HHV-6

TABLE 25-1 General information on pityriasis rosea

- Pityriasis rosea occurs in 2% of dermatology patients with skin of color.
- Onset is usually between the ages of 10 and 35 years.
- Spontaneous resolution occurs in 6 to 10 weeks.

TABLE 25-2   Viral etiology of pityriasis rosea
• The peak occurrence is in spring and fall, which supports a viral origin.
• Human herpes virus (HHV)-6 is closely associated.
• HHV-7 is also closely associated.

from latency.[2] HHV-6 causes ballooning and induces apoptosis in the uninfected cluster of differentiation 4 (CD4) T-helper cells.[2] In addition, HHV-6 causes the enhancement of natural killer T-cell activity, the suppression of peripheral blood mononuclear cell proliferation, and the induction of many cytokines.[2]

Approximately 95% of the human population is seropositive for HHV-6. As a result, a positive viral culture for HHV-6 does not necessarily correspond to a clinically relevant infection, due to the large number of asymptomatic carriers.

HHV-7 is also prevalent worldwide. The primary infection of this virus occurs in childhood, but at a later age than HHV-6 infections. HHV-7 shares its mode of infection with HHV-6, by showing a latency in the peripheral blood T-cells and a persistent infection of the salivary glands. HHV-7 is prone to reactivation. Less is known about the pathogenicity of HHV-7, but it is thought to be the primary causative agent of PR, with HHV-6 having a close association. However, there is no definitive proof that these viruses are the pathogenesis of PR.

Both HHV-6 and HHV-7 are associated with a febrile illness and exanthem subitum (roseola infantum), which has a characteristic rash. Although viruses are not a proven cause, patients with PR may experience a fever as a prodrome and a classic exanthem that resolves spontaneously and peaks in the spring and fall. Therefore, this supports a viral etiology [**Table 25-2**].

Many other studies have been done to resolve the controversy regarding the exact cause of PR; however, definitive conclusions cannot be drawn as a result of some of these studies.[3-5] This is due to limitations such as their sample size and the fact that they were not randomized controlled studies. For example, a study was done with 34 Kaposi sarcoma–negative, immunocompetent patients with PR. The results of this study showed that HHV-8 was detected by DNA sequencing in 20% of the cases; however, the small sample size is not sufficient to prove that HHV-8 was the definitive causative agent.[5]

With the recent increase in hemagglutinin 1 neuraminidase 1 (H1N1) cases, it is interesting to note a case of pandemic H1N1 that was associated with PR.[6] In another case, a patient developed PR after receiving the H1N1 vaccine.[7] However, it is still unclear whether H1N1 was the primary cause in these two cases, or whether H1N1 triggered the reactivation of other viral causes.[6] The latter theory is supported by studies carried out in 2009 and 2010 claiming that the skin manifestations of PR are a reactive response, rather than an actual infection of the skin cells.[8,9]

There have been reports of several drugs causing PR, or rashes that look quite similar to this condition. These reports show that when PR has been induced by medication, it presents in a more atypical pattern, has a longer course, and is more resistant to treatment. Some of the implicated drugs include arsenic, barbiturates, bismuth, captopril, clonidine, D-penicillamine, interferon-α, isotretinoin, metronidazole, gold, omeprazole, and terbinafine[10] [**Table 25-3**].

TABLE 25-3   Medication-induced pityriasis rosea
Medication-induced pityriasis rosea (PR) displays:
• An atypical clinical pattern
• Slower resolution
• Greater resistance to treatment
Drugs that can induce PR include gold, arsenic, barbiturates, bismuth, captopril, terbinafine, D-penicillamine, interferon-α, metronidazole, isotretinoin, and omeprazole.

CLINICAL PRESENTATION

Medical textbooks illustrate a classic cutaneous exanthem of salmon- or rose-colored papules and plaques in PR patients with Fitzpatrick skin types I to III [**Figure 25-1**]. However, in patients with skin of color, the lesions are usually violaceous or gray in color [**Figure 25-2** and **Table 25-4**]. Following a fever, and a respiratory tract infection in some patients, a herald patch, or 'mother patch,' can arise. This is seen in 50% to 90% of patients with PR [**Figure 25-3** and **Table 25-5**]. About 1 to 2 weeks later, a generalized secondary rash develops, consisting of oval plaques with a collarette scale. The scale usually occurs on the inner border of the plaque and points to the center of the lesion [**Figure 25-4**]. The secondary rash develops along the Langer lines and has been characterized as occurring in a 'Christmas tree' distribution on the trunk [**Figure 25-5**] and a 'school of minnows' pattern on the flank [**Figure 25-6**]. The sun-exposed areas of the body are seldom involved. In patients with dark skin of color, the lesions are more papular, and the papules often have small necrotic-like centers [**Figure 25-7**]. These patients also have a more follicular accentuation [**Figure 25-8**], and the lesions usually occur in an inverse pattern, involving the face, neck, axilla, groin, and lower abdomen[11] [**Figure 25-9**]. African American children are particularly predisposed to the papular variant, which is also prevalent in Hispanic children [**Figure 25-10**].

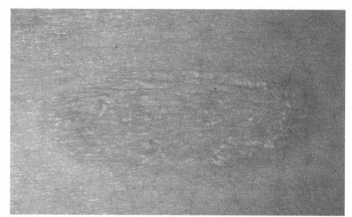

A

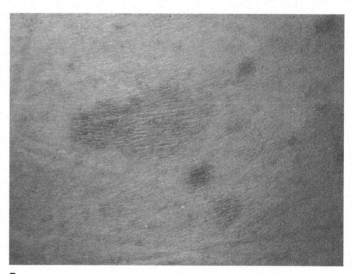

B

FIGURE 25-1. (A) A classic salmon-colored pityriasis rosea lesion. **(B)** Rose-colored pityriasis rosea lesions.

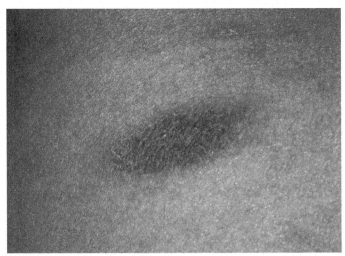

A

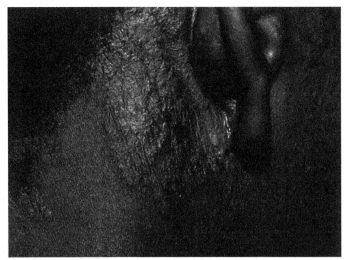

FIGURE 25-3. A violaceous herald patch on the right posterior auricular area.

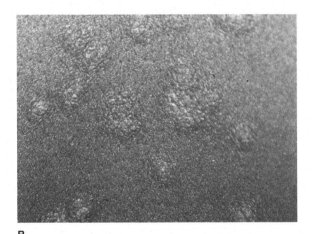

B

FIGURE 25-2. (A) A violaceous plaque in an African American patient with pityriasis rosea. **(B)** Gray plaques in a pityriasis rosea patient with darker skin of color.

with ashy dermatosis, other lichenoid reactions, or Kaposi sarcoma, or it can be seen in the setting of human immunodeficiency virus infection. Many annular eruptions may resemble PR, such as pityriasis alba, nummular eczema, seborrheic dermatitis, and tinea. Inverse papular PR can be difficult to distinguish from Gianotti-Crosti syndrome. Secondary syphilis may imitate papular or scaly plaque PR [**Figure 25-12**]; thus, the Venereal Disease Research Laboratory (VDRL) test titer should be checked when considering PR as a diagnosis.

In diagnosing PR, it is important to note that the herald patch may be absent, or it may appear as multiple lesions. The secondary lesions may be located on the extremities with little truncal involvement. Focal lesions may also appear, especially in children. Oral, purpuric, vesicular, and pustular forms of PR are sometimes present in children. The patient's palms and soles may be involved, and it may be difficult to distinguish from secondary syphilis. PR is usually diagnosed clinically. However, in some of the atypical variants, PR may be difficult to diagnose.

PATHOLOGY

The histologic findings of PR are nonspecific. There is a decrease or absence of the granular layer, acanthosis, spongiosis, a superficial dermal infiltrate of lymphocytes, extravasated erythrocytes extending to the epidermis, and parakeratosis. The parakeratosis is often focal and in mounds. In a micropapular variant in patients with dark skin of color, there are often triangular mounds of parakeratosis that look tilted with respect to the underlying epidermis.[13] Focal spongiosis occasionally progresses to vesiculation. In older lesions, the perivascular infiltrate is often superficial and deep, with less spongiosis and more epidermal hyperplasia. This makes it difficult to distinguish between psoriasis and lichen planus.[14]

Patients with PR can experience pruritus, which occurs occasionally on the palms and is rarely generalized [**Figure 25-11**]. In a study assessing the quality of life in children with PR, the majority of the children were only minimally itchy; thus their school life, other daily activities, and sleep were not greatly affected.[12] PR usually resolves spontaneously in 6 to 10 weeks, although in some instances, it may last for 4 to 5 months. In patients with skin of color, resolution often occurs with postinflammatory hyperpigmentation, although it occasionally results in postinflammatory hypopigmentation. In rare cases, the scalp, eyelids, penis, and oral mucosa are also involved.

If PR persists beyond 3 months, the diagnosis must be reconsidered. The 'Christmas tree' distribution of lesions on the trunk can be confused

TABLE 25-4	Clinical presentation of pityriasis rosea-Fitzpatrick skin types	
Characteristics	I–III	IV–VI
Color of lesions	Rose or salmon	Gray or violaceous
Location	Predominance truncal	Predominance on the extremities
Scale	Collarette scales	Central scales
Special features	Central hyperpigmentation seldom seen	Central necrotic-like hyperpigmentation

TABLE 25-5	Four clinical features of pityriasis rosea
1.	An initial plaque (herald patch) lasts 6 to 10 weeks, occurs 1 to 14 days (or longer) before other lesions may appear and heals with postinflammatory hyperpigmentation darker skin of color
2.	Characteristic individual lesions include collarette scale
3.	Lesions along lines of cleavage may form in a 'School of minnows' or a 'Christmas tree' pattern
4.	Papules with central necrotic-like hyperpigmentation occur especially on the extremities in children with dark skin of color

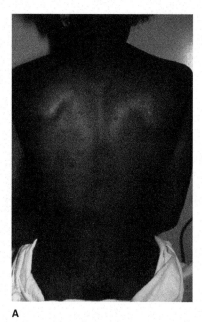

A

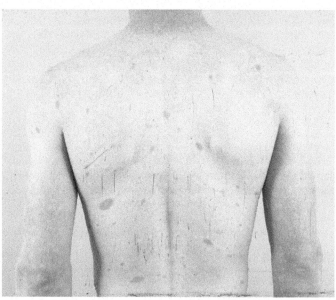

B

FIGURE 25-4. **(A)** Secondary pityriasis rosea rash with several residual patches with collarette scale. **(B)** Secondary lesions with several residual herald patches in a Hispanic man. The color is a dark erythema, somewhat intermediate between the rose- or salmon-colored lesions commonly seen in patients with Fitzpatrick skin types I to III, and the violaceous or gray lesion often seen in patients with darker skin of color.

MANAGEMENT

PR is self-limiting; thus, treatment is usually not necessary. When treatment is given to a patient with PR, it is often for the symptomatic relief of the pruritus, for which medium-strength topical steroids and/or antihistamines are prescribed. Intramuscular or oral corticosteroids given early may help to prevent postinflammatory hyperpigmentation, especially in patients with skin of color.[11] This usually attenuates the lesions in 2 to 3 weeks, but systemic corticosteroids may exacerbate the other symptoms of PR. In a severe vesicular form, PR can be treated with dapsone. Ultraviolet B (UVB) radiation has been shown to decrease the severity of the disease but does not ease the accompanying pruritus.[15] The combination of UVB treatment and a topical corticosteroid may make this mode of therapy more effective. Because UVB can cause postinflammatory

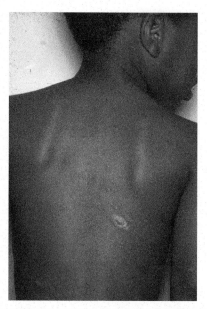

FIGURE 25-5. A 'Christmas tree' pattern of pityriasis rosea lesions on the back.

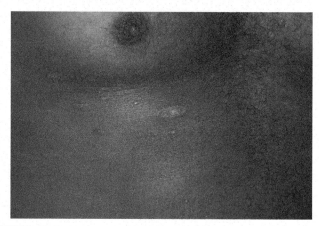

FIGURE 25-6. Pityriasis rosea lesions appearing as a herald patch with narrow linear lesions on the flank chest (the 'school of minnows' pattern).

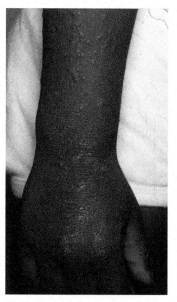

FIGURE 25-7. Papular lesions on the dorsum of the hands and forearms, many with necrotic-like centers.

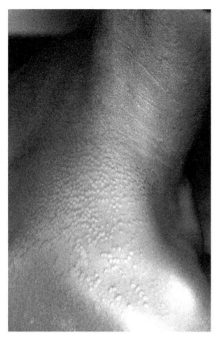

FIGURE 25-8. A male with follicular pityriasis rosea.

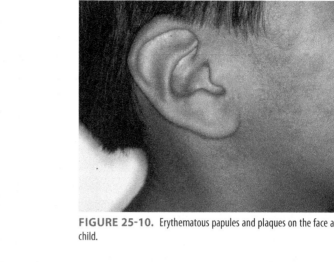

FIGURE 25-10. Erythematous papules and plaques on the face and neck of a Hispanic child.

hyperpigmentation, it may not be the treatment of choice for patients with skin of color.

Studies have shown that erythromycin may be effective in treating PR. In one study, 73% of the PR patients (out of 45 total patients) treated with erythromycin (250 mg/d) achieved a complete clearance in 2 weeks;[16] spontaneous remission usually takes at least 6 weeks.

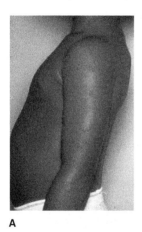

A

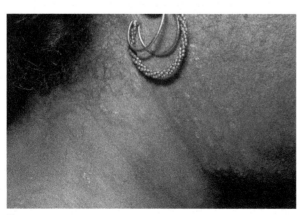

B

FIGURE 25-9. **(A)** Papules on the arms and chest of a boy with darker skin of color. **(B)** Pityriasis rosea lesions on the face and neck of a woman with darker skin of color.

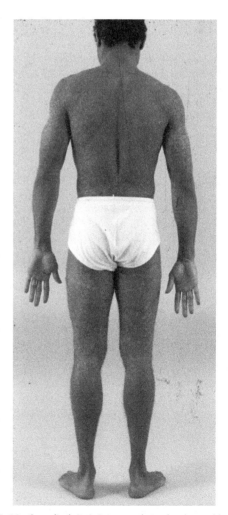

FIGURE 25-11. Generalized pityriasis rosea on the trunk and extremities of a man with darker skin of color.

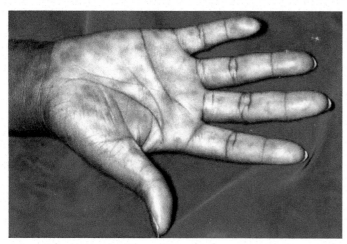

FIGURE 25-12. Palmar lesions of secondary syphilis.

Because many organisms are sensitive to erythromycin, confounding factors have to be identified. As a result, this medication is not a definitive therapy for patients with PR. In fact, a recent article by Rasi et al[17] found that oral erythromycin is ineffective in the treatment of PR.

Recently, there has been research into the role of acyclovir in the treatment of PR, although this is not yet conclusive. Because HHV-6, HHV-7, and now HHV-8 have been implicated as potential causes of PR, using antiviral therapy may reduce the severity and duration of the condition. Acyclovir is not the most sensitive agent to treat HHV-6 and HHV-7, but it is the safest. A number of studies have shown that high doses of acyclovir, given to patients in the first week after their onset of PR, have been effective in clearing PR lesions.[18-20] However, another study indicates that low doses of acyclovir may induce responses in the first 3 weeks of treatment.[21] Although there is debate as to how much acyclovir can be beneficial, given its low side effect profile, consideration should be taken when prescribing this medication in very extensive and/or symptomatic PR cases[21] [**Table 25-6**].

CONCLUSION

PR occurs over a wide age range, usually between the ages of 10 and 35 years and is found in individuals with all skin phototypes. PR has some unique features in patients with skin of color, and physicians should be aware of

the distinct effects that PR treatment options could have on patients with Fitzpatrick skin types IV to VI.

Due to PR's self-limiting nature, treatment is not usually necessary; however, therapy can be given to relieve symptoms of pruritus. Topical steroids and/or antihistamines are often the first line of treatment. In patients with skin of color, intramuscular or oral corticosteroids given early may help to prevent postinflammatory hyperpigmentation. UVB in conjunction with a topical corticosteroid is another treatment option, but UVB can cause postinflammatory hyperpigmentation, so it is not advised for patients with darker skin of color.

Erythromycin is used to treat PR in some instances; however, physicians should note that studies are not conclusive on the efficacy of this medication. Acyclovir is a new potential PR treatment that is proving to be beneficial. Although there is still a debate over the dosage, acyclovir has minimal side effects and, therefore, should be considered in severe cases of PR.

REFERENCES

1. Halder RM, Nootheti PK. Ethnic skin disorders overview. *J Am Acad Dermatol.* 2003;48:S143-S148.
2. Araujo DT, Berman B, Weinstein A. Human herpesviruses 6 and 7. *Dermatol Clin.* 2002;20:301-306.
3. Chuh AA. The association of pityriasis rosea with cytomegalovirus, Epstein-Barr virus and parvovirus B19 infections: a prospective case control study by polymerase chain reaction and serology. *Eur J Dermatol.* 2003;13:25-28.
4. Parija M, Thappa DM. Study of role of streptococcal throat infection in pityriasis rosea. *Indian J Dermatol.* 2008;53:171-173.
5. Prantsidis A, Rigopoulos D, Papatheodorou G, et al. Detection of human herpesvirus 8 in the skin of patients with pityriasis rosea. *Acta Derm Venereol.* 2009;89:604-606.
6. Mubki TF, Bin Dayel SA, Kadry R. A case of pityriasis rosea concurrent with the novel influenza A (H1N1) infection. *Pediatr Dermatol.* 2011;28: 341-342.
7. Chen JF, Chiang CP, Chen YF, et al. Pityriasis rosea following influenza (H1N1) vaccination. *J Chin Med Assoc.* 2011;74:280-282.
8. Drago F, Broccolo F, Rebora A. Pityriasis rosea: an update with a critical appraisal of its possible herpesviral etiology. *J Am Acad Dermatol.* 2009;61:303-318.
9. Rebora A, Drago F, Broccolo F. Pityriasis rosea and herpesvirus: facts and controversies. *Clin Dermatol.* 2010;28:497-501.
10. Bjornberg A, Tegner E. Pityriasis rosea. In: Freedberg IM, Eisen AZ, Wolff K, et al, eds. *Fitzpatrick's Dermatology in General Medicine.* 6th ed. New York, NY: McGraw-Hill; 2003:445-450.
11. Halder RM, Roberts CI, Nootheti PK. Cutaneous diseases in the black races. *Dermatol Clin.* 2003;21:679-687.
12. Chuh AA. Quality of life in children with pityriasis rosea: a prospective case control study. *Pediatr Dermatol.* 2003;20:474-478.
13. Brady SP. Parakeratosis. *J Am Acad Dermatol.* 2004;50:77-84.
14. Ackerman AB. *Histologic Diagnosis of Inflammatory Skin Disease.* Philadelphia, PA: Lea & Febiger; 1978:335-351.
15. Leenutaphong V, Jiamton S. UVB phototherapy for pityriasis rosea: a bilateral comparison study. *J Am Acad Dermatol.* 1995;33:996-999.
16. Sharma PK, Yadav TP, Gautam RK, et al. Erythromycin in pityriasis rosea: a double-blind, placebo-controlled clinical trial. *J Am Acad Dermatol.* 2000;42:241-244.
17. Rasi A, Tajziehchi L, Savabi-Nasab S. Oral erythromycin is ineffective in the treatment of pityriasis rosea. *J Drugs Dermatol.* 2008;7:35-38.
18. Drago F, Vecchio F, Rebora A. Use of high-dose acyclovir in pityriasis rosea. *J Am Acad Dermatol.* 2006;54:82-85.
19. Ehsani A, Esmaily N, Noormohammadpour P, et al. The comparison between the efficacy of high dose acyclovir and erythromycin on the period and signs of pitiriasis rosea. *Indian J Dermatol.* 2010;55:246-248.
20. Amatya A, Rajouria EA, Karn DK. Comparative study of effectiveness of oral acyclovir with oral erythromycin in the treatment of pityriasis rosea. *Kathmandu Univ Med J.* 2012;10:57-61.
21. Rassai S, Feily A, Sina N, et al. Low dose of acyclovir may be an effective treatment against pityriasis rosea: a random investigator-blind clinical trial on 64 patients. *J Eur Acad Dermatol Venereol.* 2011;25:24-26.

TABLE 25-6	Pityriasis rosea therapy
Treatment	Results/comments
Intramuscular or oral corticosteroids	Attenuates dermatosis but must be used early in the disease process.
UVB radiation and topical treatment	UVB treatment should be used in conjunction with a topical corticosteroid. UVB treatment can cause postinflammatory hyperpigmentation, so it is not optimal for patients with darker skin of color.
Erythromycin, 250 mg qid	Complete clearance is usually achieved in 2 weeks, but there is some controversy over its role in the treatment of pityriasis rosea.[17]
Acyclovir	There is a debate over the most effective dosage for acyclovir. It should be considered for extensive and/or symptomatic cases, because it has a low side effect profile.

Note. Pityriasis rosea is self-limiting; therefore, treatment is usually not necessary. When treatment is given, it is often for the symptomatic relief of pruritus.

Abbreviations: UVB, ultraviolet B; qid, four times a day.

Lichen Planus and Lichen Nitidus

Khari H. Bridges

KEY POINTS

- Lichen planus is an autoimmune inflammatory mucocutaneous condition affecting the skin, mucosal surfaces, scalp, or nails.

- Evidence suggests that lichen planus is due to altered self-antigens on basal keratinocytes, a process that appears to be multifactorial.

- Lichen planus has a multitude of clinical variants, including some actinic variants that occur in darker skin types.

- Lichen nitidus is characterized by clusters of numerous, tiny, discrete, skin-colored, uniform, pinhead-sized papules.

- Histology of lichen nitidus reveals a 'ball and claw' arrangement.

- There is an actinic variant of lichen nitidus that occurs predominantly in people with more darkly pigmented skin.

LICHEN PLANUS

Lichen planus (LP) is an autoimmune inflammatory mucocutaneous condition that can affect the skin, oral mucosa, scalp, or nails. LP is often idiopathic but at times may be linked to drugs (eg, penicillamine, gold, angiotensin-converting enzyme [ACE] inhibitors, antimalarials, or quinidine) or viral infections (especially hepatitis C virus [HCV] infection). Topical steroids are used to treat localized LP, whereas systemic steroids and other modalities are used to treat patients with generalized LP.[1]

EPIDEMIOLOGY

LP affects from 0.22% to 1% of the adult population,[2] whereas oral LP (OLP) affects 1% to 4%.[3] There is no apparent racial predisposition. Worldwide incidence varies from 0.29% in those of African descent to 0.1% to 1% in East Indians.[4] Two-thirds of patients develop the disease between the ages of 30 and 60 years.[5] There is a slight predominance in women, although some authors report women being affected twice as often as men.[1,4,5] Women tend to develop the disease later in life in comparison to men (sixth vs fourth decade).[2] There may be a small genetic component to LP because 1% to 2% of cases are familial.[6]

OLP may be found in 50% to 75% of cases of cutaneous LP.[7,8] Cutaneous LP is found in 10% to 20% of OLP cases. Of patients with LP of any form, 25% will have solely mucosal involvement.[8]

PATHOGENESIS

A growing body of evidence suggests that LP represents a T-cell–mediated autoimmune process directed against basal keratinocytes that express altered self-antigens on their surfaces.[8] How these altered self-antigens arise appears to be multifactorial.

The role of viruses has been investigated to explain the origin of antigens in the generation of effector T-cells with cytotoxic potential. HCV is one of the suspected viruses. Several case-control studies have found that HCV is more prevalent in LP populations than in controls by 4% to 38%.[6,9] Conversely, it has been reported that 5% of all HCV patients have LP.[6] HCV is believed to be more commonly associated with OLP than cutaneous LP. Moreover, HCV RNA has been found in 93% of OLP lesions via the polymerase chain reaction technique.[10] Other suspected viruses include transfusion transmitted virus and human herpes virus 6.[11,12]

Medications also play a role in some lichenoid reactions. Although any drug can cause a lichenoid reaction, some are more likely to do so than others. β-blockers, ACE inhibitors, nonsteroidal anti-inflammatory drugs, antimalarials, quinidine, hydrochlorothiazide, gold, and penicillamine are the classic agents known to cause lichenoid eruptions.

The interval to onset can be anywhere from 10 days to several years. When a lichenoid drug reaction is suspected, discontinuation of the drug is recommended, if at all possible.

Contact allergens, specifically metals in dental restorations or constructions such as mercury, copper, and gold, have been linked to the induction or exacerbation of OLP. About 94% of these patients improved after removal of the sensitizing material.[13]

Lichenoid eruptions also have been observed in association with autoimmune liver disease, myasthenia gravis, thymoma, and ulcerative colitis.[4] LP also has been reported in association with underlying malignancy.[14]

A murine model of LP has been established by employing autoreactive T-cells, which respond to self-major histocompatibility complex class II antigens on macrophages and Langerhans cells. The result is induction of LP-like skin lesions with histologic changes similar to LP or lichenoid skin diseases.[15] CD8+ T-cells make up a large proportion of the inflammatory infiltrate, especially in older LP lesions.[15]

After an antigen-presenting cell presents a cross-reactive antigen to an antigen-specific naive T-cell, the T-cell elaborates tumor necrosis factor (TNF)-α and interferon (IFN)-γ. These cytokines upregulate E-selectin and subsequently intercellular adhesion molecule-1 (ICAM-1) in endothelial cells, facilitating migration of T-cells across the endothelium and into the dermis.[8]

IFN-γ also induces elaboration of C-X-C motif chemokines (CXCL)10, CXCL9, and CXCL11, which bind to chemokine receptor 3 (CXCR3). CXCR3 has been found to be consistently expressed by the majority of CD4+ and CD8+ dermal T-cells and natural killer (NK) cells and is thought to also function in the activation, recruitment, and maintenance of these effector cells.[16]

Both T-helper (T_H) 1 and T_H2 subsets elaborate chemokines and cytokines in a mixed pro- and anti-inflammatory cytokine profile. The balance between these profiles determines the clinical behavior of the disease.[17]

Apoptosis of keratinocytes is likely to occur through cross-linking of the Fas receptor expressed on the keratinocytes with the Fas ligand expressed by CD8+ T-cells and possibly NK cells. An additional T-cell cytotoxic effect on keratinocytes is mediated by perforin and granzymes. IFN-γ and TNF-α, which have been found in high concentrations in LP lesions, can induce keratinocyte expression of ICAM-1, thus facilitating this latter T-cell–keratinocyte interaction.[18] IFN-γ and TNF-β also may function to enhance expression of apoptosis-associated proteins in keratinocytes.

CLINICAL FEATURES

LP is classically described as small, polygonal, violaceous, flat-topped papules that may coalesce into plaques [**Figure 26-1**]. There may be

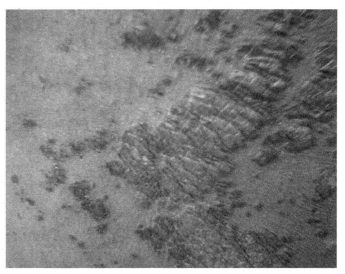

FIGURE 26-1. Polygonal, violaceous, planar papules and plaques of lichen planus.

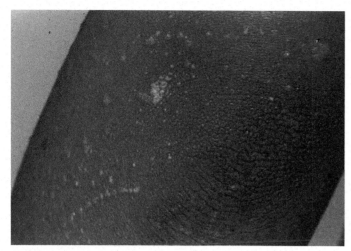

FIGURE 26-2. Lichen planus, an umbilicated clinical variant, also exhibiting the Koebner phenomenon.

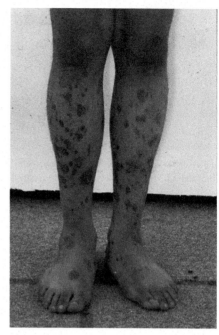

FIGURE 26-4. Lichen planus characteristically involving the anterior shins.

umbilication [**Figure 26-2**]. The surface is shiny or transparent, with a network of fine white lines called Wickham striae. Wickham striae are usually prominent on the oral mucosa of those with darker skin. There may be small gray-white puncta that correspond to focal thickening of the granular layer. The Koebner (isomorphic) phenomenon is commonly seen [**Figure 26-2**].

Most frequently involved sites are the flexor surfaces of the wrists and forearms [**Figure 26-3**], the dorsal surfaces of the hands, and the anterior aspect of the lower legs [**Figure 26-4**]. The oral mucosa is affected in over half of patients[8] [**Figure 26-5**]. Lesions begin as pinpoint papules and expand to 0.5- to 1.0-cm plaques.[6] They are characterized by the six P's: pruritic, polygonal, planar, purple papules, and plaques.[1] In skin of color, the classic purple may appear as black, gray, brown, or violaceous. When an exacerbation of LP occurs, it usually takes 2 to 16 weeks to reach maximal spread.[19]

LP is classically a spasmodic, intensely pruritic condition. The itching sensation may feel out of proportion to the localized appearance of the disease. However, scratching causes pain, and many patients rub rather than scratch, resulting in few visible excoriations.[6]

There are many deviations from this classic description. Variants include the following:

- Acute LP, in which eruptive lesions occur most often on the trunk.
- Annular LP, which occurs in 10% of patients with lesions with central inactivity or involution.

- Atrophic LP, which describes resolving lesions of LP, usually on the lower leg.
- Bullous LP, in which lesions exhibit blisters within long-standing plaques, evidenced histologically by exaggerated Max Joseph spaces.
- Hypertrophic LP, in which lesions present with thick hyperkeratotic plaques [**Figures 26-6 and 26-7**].
- Lichen planopilaris, a follicular variant that can result in scarring alopecia of the scalp and includes the Graham-Little subvariant, characterized by the clinical triad of spinous follicular lesions, mucocutaneous LP, and alopecia.
- LP pemphigoides, which manifests as bullae in previously uninvolved skin of patients with LP and is characterized by circulating immunoglobulin G autoantibodies against *BPAG2* (type XVII collagen).
- Linear LP, in which linear lesions occur spontaneously rather than by isomorphic phenomenon, and is found along Blaschko lines.
- LP/lupus erythematosus overlap syndrome, which describes patients with characteristics of both disorders.
- Nail LP, characterized by nail thinning, ridging, fissuring, or pterygium formation; 20-nail dystrophy represents a subvariant of nail LP.

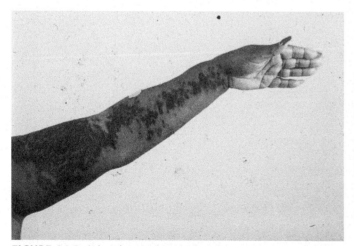

FIGURE 26-3. Lichen planus involving the flexor forearm and wrist of a darkly pigmented individual.

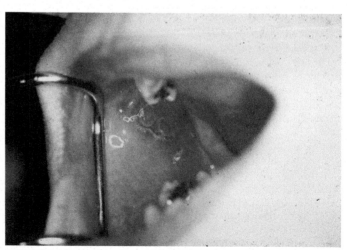

FIGURE 26-5. Oral lichen planus of the buccal mucosa.

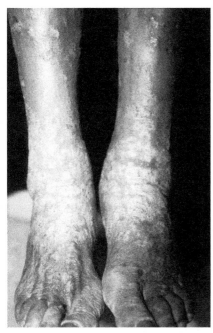

FIGURE 26-6. Hypertrophic lichen planus of the anterior shins and ankles.

- Oral LP, more common in women than men, which has varying morphologies, including an asymptomatic white, reticular variant on the buccal mucosa [**Figure 26-8**]; erosive or bullous variants can result in severe pain.
- Ulcerative LP, seen within palmoplantar lesions of LP, which consists of bullae and causes permanent loss of the toenails.[8]

The actinic variant of LP, as well as LP pigmentosus, will be discussed later in this chapter. This variant is found more often in people with darkly pigmented skin.

OLP occurs in approximately 50% to 75% of patients with cutaneous LP. Lesions can be reticulate without symptoms, atrophic, or ulcerated and very painful, with involvement of the buccal mucosa or the gingiva.[7] The ulcerative form is the most common, occurring in just under half of patients with OLP. Reticulate lesions occur in about a third of patients, whereas 20% have atrophic lesions.[6] The ulcerative form also can occur

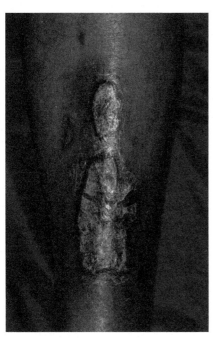

FIGURE 26-7. Hypertrophic lichen planus of the anterior shins.

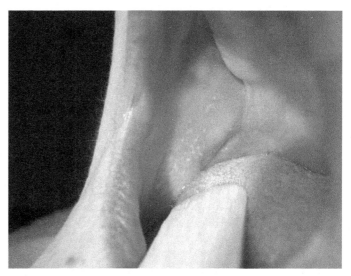

FIGURE 26-8. Oral lichen planus, reticulate variant.

in vulvovaginal-gingival syndrome and is characterized by gingival involvement in conjunction with vulvar and vaginal ulcerative lesions.[6]

Chronic ulcerative lesions, especially oral lesions, carry a risk of developing into squamous cell carcinoma (SCC).[8] It is important to monitor oral and genital LP for that possibility.[1] Approximately 0.5% of cutaneous LP patients develop oral SCC, and 1% of OLP patients develop SCC over a 3-year period. Erosive mucosal LP should be considered a premalignant condition, and the threshold to biopsy of suspicious lesions should be very low.[6]

Nail LP occurs in approximately 10% of patients. The 20-nail dystrophy variant involves all nails but not the skin.[7] Nail LP can cause multiple types of dystrophy, including ridging, distal splitting, thinning, subungual hyperkeratosis, pterygium formation [**Figure 26-9**], and loss of the nail.[1]

Lichen planopilaris, affecting the scalp, presents as alopecia with keratotic follicular papules. It can progress to scarring alopecia if left untreated.[1] This can manifest as *pseudopelade,* described poetically as "footprints in the snow."[19]

■ PATHOLOGY

The lichenoid tissue pattern is characterized by hyperkeratosis, wedge-shaped hypergranulosis, 'saw-toothed' acanthosis, and dyskeratotic epidermal basal cell damage, which is seen as Civatte bodies (also known as colloid, cytoid, or hyaline bodies) and is associated with a massive band-like infiltration of mononuclear cells at the dermal-epidermal junction.[1]

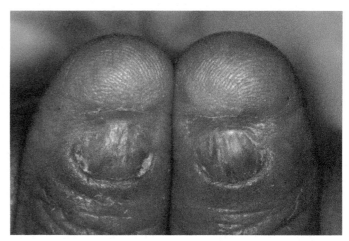

FIGURE 26-9. Pterygium formation in lichen planus involving the nails.

Vacuolar damage to the basal layer can become confluent and result in small separations at the dermal-epidermal junction (Max Joseph spaces).[8] If more than focal parakeratosis is present, LP cannot be diagnosed on histologic grounds.[20] OLP more commonly shows parakeratosis, and the epidermis is often atrophic.[8]

TREATMENT

LP is largely a self-limiting disease. Spontaneous remission occurs in most patients in approximately 1 year.[1] More specifically, more than 50% of cases resolve within 6 months, and 85% resolve after 1 year.[19] OLP, on the other hand, lasts for an average of 5 years.[19,21] However, ulcerative LP rarely resolves spontaneously.[21] Fewer than 3% of patients with OLP have spontaneous remission within 5 years. Hypertrophic LP has the worst prognosis of all, lasting an average of 8 years. The duration of LP variants has the following order: generalized < cutaneous < mucocutaneous < mucous < hypertrophic = lichen planopilaris.[22]

For more rapid improvement, topical steroids are the first-line therapy for localized disease. Intralesional steroids may be effective for resistant lesions or hyperkeratotic LP. OLP can be treated with a steroid mixed in an adhesive vehicle. Systemic corticosteroids are helpful in patients with generalized involvement. Although systemic steroids relieve symptoms in the short term, they are not recommended for long-term therapy. They are not known to shorten the duration of the disease,[1] although one study has shown a reduction in median time to clearance with their use.[23] The usual dose of prednisone is 15 to 20 mg daily for 2 to 6 weeks, with tapering if indicated. Triamcinolone, 50 to 60 mg intramuscularly every 3 weeks, helps for severe LP but must be tapered gradually to prevent rebound.

Steroid-sparing therapies including the following:

- Acitretin, a systemic retinoid, 30 mg daily for 8 weeks. Due to the teratogenicity of this drug, it is typically reserved for men and women incapable of producing children (eg, postmenopausal women, or those having undergone tubal ligation or a hysterectomy).[1]

- Topical tacrolimus and pimecrolimus, both calcineurin inhibitors, are effective for oral and genital LP.[7,24]

- Low-molecular-weight heparin, 3 mg subcutaneously every week for 4 to 6 weeks, is reported to be very effective for skin and reticulated oral lesions due to the immunomodulatory and antilymphoproliferative effects at low doses.[25]

- Psoralen with ultraviolet A (PUVA), griseofulvin, dapsone, and hydroxychloroquine also have been reported anecdotally to be effective for steroid-resistant LP.[1] Griseofulvin is especially effective for erosive OLP.[2] Hydroxychloroquine, 200 to 400 mg daily for 6 months, has been reported to give an excellent response in OLP.[6,26]

- For women with vulvovaginal syndrome, corticosteroids can be delivered in a vaginal bioadhesive glycerin-based moisturizer.[6]

- Cyclosporine, 1 to 6 mg daily, may be effective in patients with recalcitrant LP resistant to steroid and retinoid therapy.

- Oral antihistamines can reduce the pruritus associated with LP.[8]

Recrudescence of LP occurs in approximately 15% to 20% of patients.[22] In skin of color, LP usually causes prominent postinflammatory hyperpigmentation.

The following two sections discuss variants of LP seen in darker-pigmented skin.

LICHEN PLANUS ACTINICUS

Lichen planus actinicus (LPA), also known as actinic LP, LP subtropicus, LP tropicus, lichenoid melanodermatitis, and summertime actinic lichenoid eruption, is a photodistributed variant of LP. It has a predilection for darker-skinned individuals, especially in subtropical climates, and in individuals of Middle Eastern, African, or Asian descent.[6,27] Sun exposure appears to be a triggering factor. The lateral aspect of the forehead is the most common site of presentation. Most outbreaks occur during the spring or summer, followed by remission in the winter.

LPA has an earlier age of onset and a longer course than classic LP. There is a female preponderance. In contrast to classic LP, pruritus, scaling, nail involvement, and Koebner phenomenon are frequently absent.[6,27]

Several morphologic patterns have been described, including: annular hyperpigmented plaques, most commonly located on the dorsum of the fingers and hands, with increased hyperpigmentation at the center of the plaque; melasma-like patches with hyperpigmented patches on the face and neck ranging from 5 mm to 5 cm; dyschromic papules measuring 2 to 3 mm with small central keratotic plugs on the posterior neck and dorsum of the hands; and classic lichenoid papules/plaques that are violaceous in sun-exposed areas.[27]

The histopathology of LPA is consistent with classic LP.[27] In addition, there is melanin incontinence with the presence of dermal melanin, which corresponds to the typical blue-gray hyperpigmentation.[6] There are several treatments available for LPA. Some cases remit spontaneously with sun avoidance and the use of sunblock. Some cases require more aggressive therapy with hydroxychloroquine or intralesional corticosteroids. Acitretin, combined with topical corticosteroids, has resulted in complete resolution of lesions without recurrence. Bismuth, Grenz rays, arsenicals, and topical steroids under occlusion have produced varied results. There are no reports of PUVA, isotretinoin, systemic corticosteroids, cyclosporine, or dapsone being successful in LPA treatment.[27]

LICHEN PLANUS PIGMENTOSUS

Lichen planus pigmentosus (see Chapter 30) occurs in Latin Americans and others with darkly pigmented skin. It manifests as asymptomatic dark brown macules or patches in sun-exposed areas and flexural folds. Histology reveals an atrophic epidermis, vacuolar alteration of the basal cell layer, a sparse lymphocytic lichenoid infiltrate, and pigment incontinence. This type of lichenoid dermatosis may be a case of phenotypic overlap with erythema dyschromicum perstans (ashy dermatosis).[28]

LICHEN NITIDUS

EPIDEMIOLOGY

Lichen nitidus (LN) is a somewhat rare disease; hence, adequate epidemiologic data are difficult to obtain. Although it seems to affect dark-skinned individuals more than light-skinned individuals, studies do not show any predilection according to sex, race, or age. There is a rare generalized variant of LN that predominates in females.[8] Rare familial cases of LN do occur.[6]

CLINICAL FEATURES

LN is characterized by clusters of numerous, asymptomatic, discrete, skin-colored, uniform, pinhead-sized papules [**Figure 26-10**]. Papules are

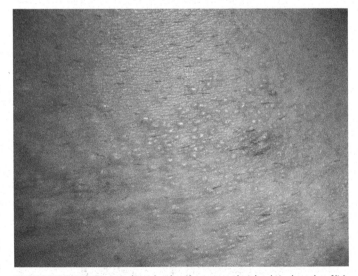

FIGURE 26-10. Discrete, skin-colored, uniform, grouped, pinhead-sized papules of lichen nitidus.

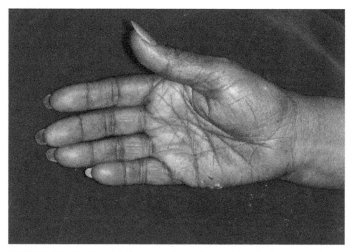

FIGURE 26-11. Lichen nitidus papules have a flat top with a shiny surface.

flat-topped with a shiny surface [**Figure 26-11**]. Papules in dark-skinned individuals tend to be hypopigmented, but sometimes are hyperpigmented. Lesions are usually found on the flexor aspects of the upper extremities, dorsal hands [**Figure 26-12**], chest, abdomen, and genitalia. Nails are involved in approximately 10% of cases, exhibiting pitting, rippling, ridging, fissuring, and increased longitudinal linear striations. The Koebner reaction is seen in LN. Generalized LN can exhibit coalescence of the papules into plaques. Oral lesions, Wickham striae, nail lesions, and palmar lesions are somewhat rare.

PATHOLOGY

LN is characterized by parakeratosis, an absence or thinning of the granular layer, with epidermal atrophy. Often there is vacuolar change of the basal cell layer with melanin incontinence and/or hyperplastic rete ridges that surround a well-circumscribed dermal infiltrate consisting of lymphocytes, epithelioid cells, and Langhans giant cells in a 'ball and claw' arrangement. The infiltrate is typically confined to the width of two to three dermal papillae.[8,29]

TREATMENT

Most cases spontaneously resolve in 1 to 3 years, with treatment largely guided by symptoms. Oral antihistamines and topical steroids can relieve the pruritus sometimes associated with LN, whereas topical tacrolimus has proven effective anecdotally in children.

Although most cases of LN are asymptomatic and resolve without sequelae, in cases where the lesions are generalized, persistent, cosmetically undesirable, or pruritic, alternative treatment may be warranted.

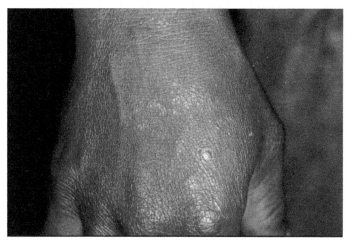

FIGURE 26-12. Lichen nitidus lesions can be found on the dorsal hands.

Narrowband ultraviolet B (UVB) phototherapy plus a topically applied steroid has proven effective in one study for patients who could not tolerate other therapies.[30] For children, who tend to be more sensitive to PUVA, narrowband UVB has yielded a positive response after three treatments and complete resolution of symptoms after fewer than 20 treatments.[30]

There are anecdotal reports of improvement with PUVA, acitretin, itraconazole, and dinitrochlorobenzene.[31,32] However, PUVA is contraindicated for children. Low-dose cyclosporin has also proven successful. In one case where the onset of LN came after exposure to *Mycobacterium tuberculosis* and, subsequently, a Japanese lacquer tree, the patient's LN responded well to the antituberculous agent oral isoniazid.[33]

ACTINIC LICHEN NITIDUS

Actinic LN, similar to LN, has been reported in Middle Easterners and others with darkly pigmented skin. The lesions are clinically and histologically similar to LN, posing a diagnostic challenge to dermatologists. The lesions occur in sun-exposed areas of the dorsal region of the hands, extensor forearms, and posterior neck.

Lesions typically respond to sun protection, but topical steroids can be added when there is resistance.[6] One case study reported success in treating actinic LP using topical 0.1% pimecrolimus cream.[34] The majority of cases clear spontaneously in several months to a year. In an occasional patient, however, actinic LN may persist for a lifetime. Patients usually heal with postinflammatory pigmentary changes or scars.

REFERENCES

1. Katta R. Lichen planus. *Am Fam Physician*. 2000;61:3319-3324.
2. Boyd AS, Neldner KH. Lichen planus. *J Am Acad Dermatol*. 1991;25:593-619.
3. Scully C, Beyli M, Ferreiro MC, et al. Update on oral lichen planus: etiopathogenesis and management. *Crit Rev Oral Biol Med*. 1998;9:86-122.
4. Scully C, el-Kom M. Lichen planus: review and update on pathogenesis. *J Oral Pathol*. 1985;14:431-458.
5. Silverman S, Gorsky M, Luzada-Nur F. A prospective follow-up study of 570 patients with oral lichen planus: persistence, remission, and malignant association. *Oral Surg Oral Med Oral Pathol*. 1985;60:30-34.
6. Odom RB, James WD, Berger TG, eds. *Andrews' Diseases of the Skin: Clinical Dermatology*. 9th ed. Philadelphia, PA: WB Saunders; 2000:266-280.
7. DermNet NZ. Lichen planus. http://dermnetnz.org/scaly/lichen-planus.html. Accessed March 13, 2013.
8. Shiohara T, Kano Y. Lichen planus and lichenoid dermatoses. In: Bolognia JL, Jorizzo JL, Rapini RP, et al, eds. *Dermatology*. London, United Kingdom: Mosby (Elsevier); 2003:175-184, 186-188.
9. Conklin RJ, Blasberg B. Oral lichen planus. *Dermatol Clin*. 1987;5:663-673.
10. Nagao Y, Kameyama T, Sata M. Hepatitis C virus RNA detection in oral lichen planus tissue. *Am J Gastroenterol*. 1998;93:850.
11. Rodriguez-Inigo E, Arrieta JJ, Casqueiro M, et al. TT virus detection in oral lichen planus lesions. *J Med Virol*. 2001;64:183-189.
12. Requena L, Kutzner H, Escalonilla P, et al. Cutaneous reactions at sites of herpes zoster scars: an expanded spectrum. *Br J Dermatol*. 1998;138:161-168.
13. Usman A, Kimyai-Asadi A, Stiller MJ, et al. Lichenoid eruption following hepatitis B vaccination: first North American case report. *Pediatr Dermatol*. 2001;18:123-126.
14. Helm TN, Camisa C, Liu AY, et al. Lichen planus associated with neoplasia: a cell-mediated immune response to tumor antigen? *J Am Acad Dermatol*. 1994;30:219-224.
15. Shiohara T, Moriya N, Nagashima M. Induction and control of lichenoid tissue reactions. *Springer Semin Immunopathol*. 1992;13:369-385.
16. Flier J, Boorsma DM, van Beek PJ, et al. Differential expression of CXCR3 targeting chemokines CXCL10, CXCL9, and CXCL11 in different types of skin inflammation. *J Pathol*. 2001;194:398-405.
17. Simark-Mattsson C, Bergenholtz G, Jontell M, et al. Distribution of interleukin-2, -4, -10, tumour necrosis factor-alpha and transforming growth factor-beta mRNAs in oral lichen planus. *Arch Oral Biol*. 1999;44:499-507.
18. Yasukawa M, Ohminami H, Arai J, et al. Granule exocytosis, and not the Fas/Fas ligand system, is the main pathway of cytotoxicity mediated by alloantigen-specific CD4(+) as well as CD8(+) cytotoxic T-lymphocytes in humans. *Blood*. 2000;95:2352-2355.

19. Chuang TY, Stitle L. Lichen planus. www.emedicine.com/DERM/topic233. htm. Accessed January 12, 2013.

20. Prieto BG, Casal M, McNutt NS. Lichen planus-like keratosis: a clinical and histological reexamination. *Am J Surg Pathol.* 1993;17:259-263.

21. Mignogna MD, Muzio LL, Russo LL, et al. Oral lichen planus: different clinical features in HCV-positive and HCV-negative patients. *Int J Dermatol.* 2000;39:134-139.

22. Tompkins JK. Lichen planus: a statistical study of forty-one cases. *Arch Dermatol.* 1955;71:515-519.

23. Cribier B, Frances C, Chosidow O. Treatment of lichen planus: an evidence-based medicine analysis of efficacy. *Arch Dermatol.* 1998;134:1521-1530.

24. Rozycki TW, Rogers RS 3rd, Pittelkow MR, et al. Topical tacrolimus in the treatment of symptomatic oral lichen planus: a series of 13 patients. *J Am Acad Dermatol.* 2002;46:27-34.

25. Stefanidou MP, Ioannidou DJ, Panayiotides JG, et al. Low molecular weight heparin: a novel alternative therapeutic approach for lichen planus. *Br J Dermatol.* 1999;141:1040-1045.

26. Eisen D. Hydroxychloroquine sulfate (Plaquenil) improves oral lichen planus: an open trial. *J Am Acad Dermatol.* 1993;28:609-612.

27. Meads SB, Kunishige J, Ramos-Caro FA, et al. Lichen planus actinicus. *Cutis.* 2003;72:377-381.

28. Vega ME, Waxtein L, Arenas R, et al. Ashy dermatosis versus lichen planus-pigmentosus: a controversial matter. *Int J Dermatol.* 1992;31:87-88.

29. Lapins NA, Willoughby C, Helwig EB. Lichen nitidus: a study of forty-three cases. *Cutis.* 1978;21:634-637.

30. Do MO, Kim MJ, Kim SH, et al. Generalized lichen nitidus successfully treated with narrow-band UVB phototherapy: two cases report. *J Korean Med Sci.* 2007;22:163-166.

31. Chen W, Schramm M, Zouboulis CC. Generalized lichen nitidus. *J Am Acad Dermatol.* 1997;36:360-361.

32. Kano Y, Otake Y, Shiohara T. Improvement of lichen nitidus after topical dinitrochlorobenzene application. *J Am Acad Dermatol.* 1998;39:305-308.

33. Kubota Y, Kiryu H, Nakayama J. Generalized lichen nitidus successfully treated with an antituberculous agent. *Br J Dermatol.* 2002;146:1081-1083.

34. Ezzedine K, Simonart T, Vereecken P, et al. Facial actinic lichen planus following the Blaschko's lines: successful treatment with topical 0.1% pimecrolimus cream. *J Eur Acad Dermatol Venereol.* 2009;23:458-459.

CHAPTER 27	# Atopic Dermatitis and Other Eczemas

Aanand N. Geria
Andrew F. Alexis

KEY POINTS

- Atopic dermatitis (AD) is a common inflammatory skin disorder that may affect individuals of any age, sex or race.

- Genetic, environmental, and cultural factors likely contribute to differences in the prevalence of AD in skin of color populations compared with lighter-skinned individuals of European descent.

- Erythema, which is the clinical hallmark of inflammation in the skin, is more difficult to detect in darker-skinned individuals.

- Postinflammatory hyper- and hypopigmentation are of particular concern in patients with skin of color.

- Follicular prominence is a characteristic presentation of AD in patients of African descent and is rarely seen in Fitzpatrick skin types I to III.

- As with other skin types, the mainstay of treatment of AD in patients with skin of color involves recommended bathing practices and the judicious use of emollients, topical corticosteroids, and calcineurin inhibitors.

Atopic dermatitis (AD) is a common inflammatory skin disease that may affect individuals of any age, sex or race.[1,2] It arises most commonly in childhood or infancy and is characterized by a chronic, relapsing course. Although the etiology of AD is not completely understood, genetic and environmental factors are thought to play important roles in its pathogenesis. The diagnosis of AD is based on a constellation of clinical features, which includes a chronic pruritic eruption that usually involves the flexural skin and occurs in conjunction with numerous associated features, such as an early age of onset and a personal or family history of atopy (ie, asthma, hay fever, and/or AD). Variations in clinical presentation, frequency, cultural perception, and response to treatment can be seen among individuals of different racial groups.

EPIDEMIOLOGY

The epidemiologic data pertaining to AD in non-Caucasian populations are limited. To illustrate this point, less than 60% of AD studies published in the United States in the last decade reported patients' races. Of these studies, the subject population included 62.1% white, 18.0% black, 6.9% Asian, and 2.0% Hispanic individuals.[3]

Several population studies have demonstrated considerable geographical and racial variations in the prevalence of AD.[4-6] Based on incompletely understood environmental factors, AD appears to be more common in industrialized nations and urban settings than in developing countries and rural communities.[7] Population surveys in northern Europe, the United States, and Japan have reported prevalence rates of 15.6%, 17.2%, and 21%, respectively, whereas a prevalence of 8.5% was reported in a recent study from southeastern Nigeria.[8-11] However, with increased urbanization and the adoption of Western lifestyles, the prevalence of AD appears to be on the rise in developing countries, as it is in more industrialized nations.[11]

Several epidemiologic studies have shown AD to be more common in individuals with skin of color compared to Caucasians. A prospective, 12-month observational study of 182 babies born in Australia found that AD developed in 21%, 44%, and 17% of the Caucasian, Chinese, and Vietnamese infants, respectively. Because both the Caucasian and Chinese infants were of similar socioeconomic backgrounds, genetic differences likely played a role in the different incidence rates. In contrast, because the Vietnamese infants were of a different socioeconomic background but of the same racial group as the Chinese infants, environmental factors may have contributed more than genetic factors to this difference in incidence.[6]

Analysis of the 2003 National Survey of Children's Health found that having darkly pigmented skin was significantly associated with a higher prevalence of eczema.[12] Likewise, London-born black Caribbean children had a prevalence of AD almost twice that of their Caucasian counterparts.[5] However, a study of Indian and Caucasian preschool children in Leicester, United Kingdom, failed to show any differences in the prevalence of AD.[13] A prospective cohort study by Moore et al[14] evaluated the perinatal predictors of AD occurring in the first 6 months of life. In this U.S.-based study of 1005 mothers and their infants, infants born to either Asian mothers or mothers with darkly pigmented skin were more than twice as likely to be diagnosed with AD than infants born to Caucasian mothers. However, among infants born to Hispanic mothers, an increased risk for AD was not found. The increased risk of AD among infants born to Asian mothers or darkly pigmented mothers persisted after controlling for potential confounding variables, including socioeconomic status and infant feeding patterns.[14]

Reasons for these observed differences in prevalence may be based at least in part on variations in genetic and environmental factors; however, the differences in research methodologies between epidemiologic studies must be considered when comparing prevalence rates among populations. Further research into the epidemiology of AD among non-Caucasian populations is warranted.

PATHOPHYSIOLOGY

The exact pathophysiology of AD is not entirely understood but it is thought to involve a complex interplay between barrier dysfunctions, allergies, microbes, and autoimmunity. A deficiency in the production of ceramides and filaggrin (FLG) results in an impaired cornified envelope allowing for water loss and the decreased cohesion of the *stratum corneum*.[15] The compromised epidermis is then more susceptible to the penetration of exogenous allergens and irritants into the skin.[16] The epicutaneous sensitization incites a T-cell–mediated response. Initially, a type 2 helper T-cell (T_H2) cytokine profile predominates in acute lesions but switches to a type 1 helper T-cell (T_H1) profile in chronic lesions, due to interleukin-12 production by the eosinophils.[17] The decreased production of antimicrobial peptides such as defensins and cathelicidins may predispose lesions to *Staphylococcus aureus* colonization, with subsequent recognition by Toll-like receptor 2 on the keratinocytes, thereby prompting an inflammatory response.[18] In addition, the structural similarities between the exogenous allergens and self-proteins expressed by the keratinocytes and endothelial cells may lead to the development of circulating immunoglobulin E (IgE) autoantibodies in some patients.[19,20]

GENETICS

Genetic factors are thought to play an important role in conferring susceptibility to AD among individuals. Few studies have evaluated the racial variations in gene expression with regard to AD. However, some studies have yielded variable associations between candidate susceptibility genes and AD in different populations.

It has been shown that African American children begin to show signs of atopic diathesis as early as 2 years of age. Indeed, a birth cohort study from Detroit, Michigan, showed that African American children were more likely than Caucasian children to have at least one positive skin prick test (21.7% vs 11.0%) and at least one specific IgE test of ≥0.35 IU/mL (54.0% vs 42.9%) from a panel of 10 allergens, as well as higher total IgE levels (23.4 IU/mL vs 16.7 IU/mL). The associations did not vary after adjusting for household income, environmental variables (such as dog, cat, and cockroach allergens in house dust), or breastfeeding.[21]

An association between atopic eczema/dermatitis syndrome (AEDS) and a variant of the gene encoding chymase (*CMA1*)—a *Bst XI* polymorphism (–1903G/A) on the long arm of chromosome 14 (at 14q11.2)—has been reported previously in a Japanese population.[22] Because mast cell inflammatory mediators, such as tryptase and chymase, are important factors in the pathophysiology of AD and asthma, mast cell chymase has been considered a strong candidate gene for atopy and atopic disease.[22] However, a small study in Italy failed to demonstrate an association between the –1903G/A polymorphism and AEDS.[23]

FLG loss-of-function (*FLG* null) mutations have been associated with an increased risk of AD. Such mutations were found in 27.5% and 5.8% of Caucasian and African American subjects, respectively, but the effects of these mutations were similar in the two groups.[24] Work has also been done looking at the importance of unique *FLG* gene mutations in Asian populations.[25-27] Although these data are limited, they suggest that there may be variable patterns of gene expression among different racial, and/or geographic groups. Further study will be necessary to elucidate the potential role of skin of color in conferring genetic susceptibility to AD.

ENVIRONMENTAL AND CULTURAL FACTORS

Environmental factors likely contribute to observed differences in the prevalence of AD in skin of color populations compared with lighter-skinned individuals of European descent. Some authors have suggested that migration is an increased risk factor for AD. A study in New Zealand found higher rates of AD among migrant populations, possibly due to new or increased allergen exposure after migration or exposure to new environmental triggers associated with urbanization.[28] Another study from New Zealand and its territory of Tokelau—a small group of islands in the South Pacific—found a higher prevalence of AD among Tokelauan children who had migrated to New Zealand compared with the children who had remained in Tokelau.[29] However, another study in Italy found that eczema was less frequent in immigrant children than in local

children and that eczema incidences were lower in children born to foreign parents.[30]

Variations in infant feeding patterns, antigen exposures, and climactic factors may contribute to the differences in AD prevalence among different populations. Moreover, cultural differences in diet and household environmental exposures may influence the prevalence patterns of AD in different racial groups. Cultural practices—including bathing habits, the use of harsh soaps or astringents, or the use of topical home remedies—may also contribute to racial variations in disease severity. Further study of the role of the environmental and cultural factors in AD is necessary.

CLINICAL PRESENTATION

The clinical presentation of AD in individuals with skin of color is distinguished by a number of specific features. Most notably, erythema, which is the clinical hallmark of inflammation in the skin, is more difficult to detect in darker-skinned individuals. Although this phenomenon is true for all inflammatory diseases of the skin, it is particularly notable in eczematous conditions. In individuals with skin of color, acute, subacute, and chronic stages of AD present with various degrees of hyperpigmentation; depending on the skin type, the erythema may be subtle or imperceptible compared to patients with lighter skin [**Figure 27-1**]. For this reason, special attention should be given to

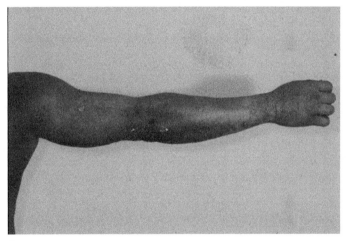

A

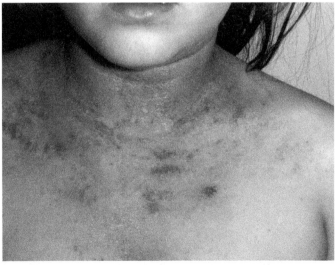

B

FIGURE 27-1. Atopic dermatitis with (**A**) erythema, lichenification, and focal depigmentation in a patient with darker-skin of color compared with (**B**) a Hispanic female with lighter skin of color.[30]

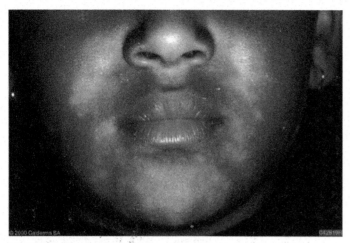

FIGURE 27-2. Postinflammatory hypopigmentation.

recognizing the subtle signs of cutaneous inflammation in darker skin so that the severity of the eczema is not underestimated.

Additionally, postinflammatory hyper- and hypopigmentation are of particular concern in patients with skin of color [**Figure 27-2**]. Typically, AD resolves with pigmentary changes that can last from several weeks to many months. Often this depigmentation can be of equal or greater concern to the patient than the dermatitis itself, particularly among patients with skin of color. Therefore, it is important to recognize and treat AD early to minimize or prevent long-term postinflammatory pigment abnormalities.

Lastly, follicular prominence is a characteristic presentation of AD in patients of African descent [**Figure 27-3**] rarely seen in types I to III skin. In some patients, multiple 1- to 3-mm follicular papules may be the sole feature of AD. As such, typical morphologic features of eczema, including lichenification, erythema, crusting, and scales, may be absent [**Figure 27-4**]. However, lichenification without follicular prominence can also be seen in darker-skinned patients, as it is in Caucasians or individuals with light skin of color [**Figure 27-5**]. In addition, a lichenoid presentation of AD was reported in 16% of African Americans patients in an inner city practice.[31] The clinical nuances of AD in individuals with skin of color are outlined in **Table 27-1**.

Racial variations in the disease severity of AD have been reported. In a longitudinal survey of children with AD in the United Kingdom, those with darker skin of color were found to be almost six times more likely to develop severe AD than their counterparts with lighter skin, after adjusting for erythema.[32] Of note, without adjusting for erythema scores, no statistically significant difference was found, suggesting that the reliance on measuring erythema in darkly pigmented skin can mask

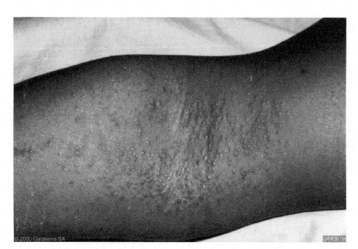

FIGURE 27-3. Follicular prominence.

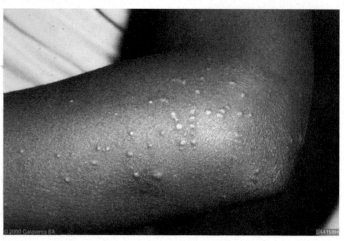

A

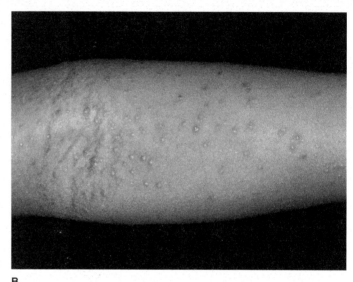

B

FIGURE 27-4. Discrete papules without lichenification on an (**A**) African American patient and (**B**) Hispanic male. (**B**: Image appears with permission from VisualDx.)

disease severity in AD. Further evaluation of potential racial differences in AD severity in other populations is warranted.

OTHER ECZEMAS IN PATIENTS WITH SKIN OF COLOR

Other eczematous variants such as nummular, asteatotic, and dyshidrotic eczema are also frequently seen in individuals with skin of color. Similar to AD, these conditions may resolve with postinflammatory hyperpigmentation [**Figure 27-6**]. Differences in epidemiology, clinical presentation, and responses to treatment for these conditions have not been formally studied but appear to be similar across racial groups. Nevertheless, cultural variations in the use of emollients, ointments, astringents, and harsh soaps, as well as frequency of bathing, can potentially lead to differences in the prevalence and severity of eczematous conditions in different populations.

TREATMENT CONSIDERATIONS

The clinical management of AD in darker-skinned individuals varies only slightly from that for other skin types. As with other skin types, the mainstay of treatment of AD in individuals with skin of color involves recommended bathing practices, the judicious use of emollients, and prescribed courses of topical corticosteroids and calcineurin inhibitors.

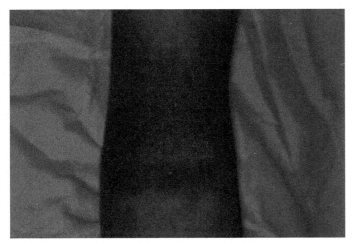

A

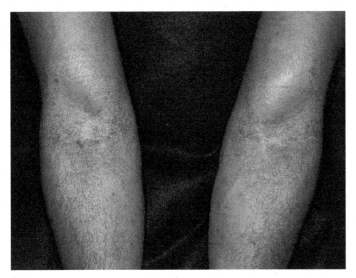

B

FIGURE 27-5. Lichenification on an (**A**) African American patient and (**B**) Hispanic male. (**B:** Images appears with permission from VisualDx.)

■ RECOMMENDED BATHING PRACTICES AND EMOLLIENTS

Long baths or showers with hot water should be avoided; rather, bathing should be limited to less than 5 minutes with water that is warm or lukewarm. The skin should be dabbed dry, leaving some residual moisture, after which a strong emollient should be promptly applied. Bathing recommendations for AD patients with skin of color are summarized in **Table 27-2**.

■ TOPICAL STEROIDS

Patients, or the parents of any young patients, need to be informed that pigmentary changes can persist long after the eczema is treated, and as a result, topical steroids should not be continued in areas where only postinflammatory dyspigmentation remains. Patients and parents of child patients should be reassured that hyper- or hypopigmentation will eventually resolve in most cases. However, in cases of complete

TABLE 27-1	Clinical nuances of atopic dermatitis in skin of color

Erythema is more subtle: it may appear as skin darkening or have a violaceous hue due to the optical effects of melanin.

Postinflammatory hyper- and hypopigmentation is more common.

Follicular accentuation, particularly in patients of African descent.

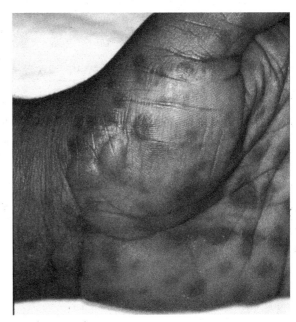

FIGURE 27-6. Dyshidrotic eczema with postinflammatory hyperpigmentation.

depigmentation from severe AD, resolution may not occur. It is important not to cause any additional hypopigmentation by using potent topical corticosteroids.

■ PROBIOTIC SUPPLEMENTATION

A recent systematic review has shown that probiotic supplementation in mothers and infants may be helpful in preventing the development and reducing the severity of AD. In particular, *Lactobacillus rhamnosus* GG was effective in the long-term prevention of AD development. Supplementation with prebiotics and blackcurrant seed oil (a combination of γ-linolenic acid and ω-3 fatty acids) was additionally shown to be effective in reducing the development of AD. The use of γ-linolenic acid reduced the severity of AD.[33]

HEALTHCARE UTILIZATION

Even though treatment among various racial groups is similar, a study by Janumpall et al found that individuals with very dark skin of color and Asians/Pacific Islanders were almost three and seven times more likely, respectively, to seek medical care for their AD than their fairer-skinned counterparts.[34] These differences were not due to the trends of greater overall healthcare utilization; patients with fairer skin had a greater number of *per capita* visits for all medical and dermatologic conditions during the same time period than patients with very dark skin of color or Asians/Pacific Islanders. Racial disparities in patient education, as well as the differential cultural responses to AD, may contribute to the observed differences in healthcare utilization for patients with AD.

TABLE 27-2	Bathing recommendations for atopic dermatitis patients with skin of color

Limit bathing to less than 5 minutes and use warm or lukewarm water.

Limit soap use to the axillae and groin.

Avoid harsh soaps and detergents.

Avoid vigorous scrubbing with washcloths, bars, or loofahs.

Pat dry after bathing and apply liberal amounts of a bland emollient while the skin is still damp.

Avoid using rubbing alcohol, hydrogen peroxide, or triple-antibiotic ointments.

'Black soap' may have a drying effect on the skin, and alternatives should be considered.

It is unclear to what extent, if any, the results of this study reflect the racial differences in the prevalence and/or severity of AD.

REFERENCES

1. Gawkrodger DJ. Racial influences on skin disease. In: Champion RH, Burton JL, Burns DA, et al, eds. *Rook/Wilkinson/Ebling Textbook of Dermatology.* 6th ed. Oxford, United Kingdom: Blackwell Science Ltd; 1998:3239-3258.

2. National Institute of Arthritis and Musculoskeletal and Skin Diseases. Handout on health: atopic dermatitis. www.niams.nih.gov/Health_Info/atopic_dermatitis/default.asp#b. Accessed January 26, 2014.

3. Hirano SA, Murray SB, Harvey VM. Reporting, representation, and subgroup analysis of race and ethnicity in published clinical trials of atopic dermatitis in the United States between 2000 and 2009. *Pediatr Dermatol.* 2012;29:749-755.

4. The International Study of Asthma and Allergies in Childhood (ISAAC) Steering Committee. Worldwide variation in prevalence of symptoms of asthma, allergic rhinoconjunctivitis, and atopic eczema: ISAAC. *Lancet.* 1998;351:1225-1232.

5. Williams HC, Pembroke AC, Forsdyke H, et al. London-born black Caribbean children are at increased risk of atopic dermatitis. *J Am Acad Dermatol.* 1995;32:212-217.

6. Mar A, Tam M, Jolley D, et al. The cumulative incidence of atopic dermatitis in the first 12 months among Chinese, Vietnamese, and Caucasian infants born in Melbourne, Australia. *J Am Acad Dermatol.* 1999;40:597-602.

7. Diepgen TL. Atopic dermatitis: the role of environmental and social factors, the European experience. *J Am Acad Dermatol.* 2001;45:S44-S48.

8. Schultz Larsen F, Diepgen T, Svensson A. The occurrence of atopic dermatitis in north Europe: an international questionnaire study. *J Am Acad Dermatol.* 1996;34:760-764.

9. Laughter D, Istvan JA, Tofte SJ, et al. The prevalence of atopic dermatitis in Oregon school children. *J Am Acad Dermatol.* 2000;43:649-655.

10. Sugiura H, Umemoto N, Deguchi H, et al. Prevalence of childhood and adolescent atopic dermatitis in a Japanese population: comparison with the disease frequency examined 20 years ago. *Acta Derm Venereol.* 1998;78:293-294.

11. Nnoruka EN. Current epidemiology of atopic dermatitis in south-eastern Nigeria. *Int J Dermatol.* 2004;43:739-744.

12. Shaw TE, Currie GP, Koudelka CW, et al. Eczema prevalence in the United States: data from the 2003 National Survey of Children's Health. *J Invest Dermatol.* 2011;131:67-73.

13. Neame RL, Berth-Jones J, Kurinczuk JJ, et al. Prevalence of atopic dermatitis in Leicester: a study of methodology and examination of possible ethnic variation. *Br J Dermatol.* 1995;132:772-777.

14. Moore MM, Rifas-Shiman SL, Rich-Edwards JW, et al. Perinatal predictors of atopic dermatitis occurring in the first six months of life. *Pediatrics.* 2004;113:468-474.

15. Hansson L, Bäckman A, Ny A, et al. Epidermal overexpression of stratum corneum chymotryptic enzyme in mice: a model for chronic itchy dermatitis. *J Invest Dermatol.* 2002;118:444-449.

16. Cork MJ, Robinson DA, Vasilopoulos Y, et al. New perspectives on epidermal barrier dysfunction in atopic dermatitis: gene-environment interactions. *J Allergy Clin Immunol.* 2006;118:3-21.

17. Homey B, Steinhoff M, Ruzicka T, et al. Cytokines and chemokines orchestrate atopic skin inflammation. *J Allergy Clin Immunol.* 2006;118:178-189.

18. Cardona ID, Cho SH, Leung DY. Role of bacterial superantigens in atopic dermatitis: implications for future therapeutic strategies. *Am J Clin Dermatol.* 2006;7:273-279.

19. Mittermann I, Aichberger KJ, Bünder R, et al. Autoimmunity and atopic dermatitis. *Curr Opin Allergy Clin Immunol.* 2004;4:367-371.

20. Aichberger KJ, Mittermann I, Reininger R, et al. Hom s 4, an IgE-reactive autoantigen belonging to a new subfamily of calcium-binding proteins, can induce Th cell type 1-mediated autoreactivity. *J Immunol.* 2005;175:1286-1294.

21. Wegienka G, Havstad S, Joseph CL, et al. Racial disparities in allergic outcomes in African Americans emerge as early as age 2 years. *Clin Exp Allergy.* 2012;42:909-917.

22. Iwanaga T, McEuen A, Walls AF, et al. Polymorphism of the mast cell chymase gene (*CMA1*) promoter region: lack of association with asthma but association with serum total immunoglobulin E levels in adult atopic dermatitis. *Clin Exp Allergy.* 2004;34:1037-1042.

23. Pascale E, Tarani L, Meglio P, et al. Absence of association between a variant of the mast cell chymase gene and atopic dermatitis in an Italian population. *Hum Hered.* 2001;51:177-179.

24. Margolis DJ, Apter AJ, Gupta J, et al. The persistence of atopic dermatitis and filaggrin (FLG) mutations in a US longitudinal cohort. *J Allergy Clin Immunol.* 2012;130:912-917.

25. Enomoto H, Noguchi E, Iijima S, et al. Single nucleotide polymorphism-based genome-wide linkage analysis in Japanese atopic dermatitis families. *BMC Dermatol.* 2007;7:5.

26. Nomura T, Sandilands A, Akiyama M, et al. Unique mutations in the filaggrin gene in Japanese patients with ichthyosis vulgaris and atopic dermatitis. *J Allergy Clin Immunol.* 2007;119:434-440.

27. Enomoto H, Hirata K, Otsuka K, et al. Filaggrin null mutations are associated with atopic dermatitis and elevated levels of IgE in the Japanese population: a family and case-control study. *J Hum Genet.* 2008;53:615-621.

28. Clayton T, Asher MI, Crane J, et al. Time trends, ethnicity and risk factors for eczema in New Zealand children: ISAAC Phase Three. *Asia Pac Allergy.* 2013;3:161-178.

29. Waite DA, Eyles EF, Tonkin SL, et al. Asthma prevalence in Tokelauan children in two environments. *Clin Allergy.* 1980;10:71-75.

30. Marcon A, Cazzoletti L, Rava M, et al. Incidence of respiratory and allergic symptoms in Italian and immigrant children. *Respir Med.* 2011;105:204-210.

31. Allen HB, Jones NP, Bowen SE. Lichenoid and other clinical presentations of atopic dermatitis in an inner city practice. *J Am Acad Dermatol.* 2008;58:503-504.

32. Ben-Gashir MA, Hay RJ. Reliance on erythema scores may mask severe atopic dermatitis in black children compared with their white counterparts. *Br J Dermatol.* 2002;147:920-925.

33. Foolad N, Brezinski EA, Chase EP, et al. Effect of nutrient supplementation on atopic dermatitis in children: a systematic review of probiotics, prebiotics, formula, and fatty acids. *JAMA Dermatol.* 2013;149:350-355.

34. Janumpally SR, Feldman SR, Gupta AK, et al. In the United States, blacks and Asian/Pacific Islanders are more likely than whites to seek medical care for atopic dermatitis. *Arch Dermatol.* 2002;138:634-637.

CHAPTER 28

Allergic Contact Dermatitis

Vincent DeLeo

KEY POINTS

- Environmental, cultural, occupational, genetic, individual, and racial differences are important in the study of contact dermatitis.

- Two important differences in skin physiology that determine the relationship between skin of color and contact dermatitis are barrier function and percutaneous absorption.

- Allergic contact dermatitis (ACD) in patients with skin of color could be more commonly associated with lichenification and hyperpigmentation than the vesicular, papular, and erythematous response often seen in Caucasians.

- Interpreting the results of a patch test in patients with skin of color is more difficult, particularly given the challenge of detecting erythema. This leads to an underestimation of ACD in skin of color.

Contact dermatitis is an altered state of skin reactivity induced by exposure to an external agent. Certainly, sex, age, and environmental, occupational, and genetic factors are thought to be important in the study of contact dermatitis. However, the effect of contact dermatitis on people with skin of color has been studied less frequently. One of the most frequent pathologic manifestations of the skin is contact dermatatitis.[1] It is divided into two basic types depending on the nature of the underlying etiologic mechanism: irritant and allergic [**Figure 28-1**].

In the United States, the prevalence of contact dermatitis is estimated to be between 1.5% and 5.4%, and it is the third most common reason that a patient consults a dermatologist.[2] The frequency of allergic contact dermatitis (ACD) is hard to determine exactly. Of 4913 patients patch

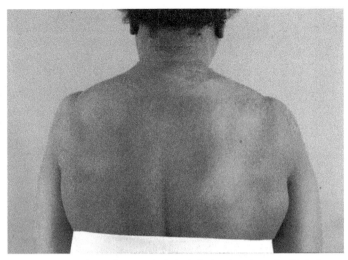

FIGURE 28-1. Contact dermatitis on the back of a female patient with skin of color.

tested in the North American Contact Dermatitis Group study, 69% had at least one positive allergic reaction and 15.4% had irritant contact dermatitis (ICD).[3] Similar results were found in a retrospective study in Kansas, which found that 68.6% of patients had at least one positive allergic reaction.[4] However, over a 15-year cohort study, incidence rates of contact allergy and ACD were 13.4% and 7.8%, respectively.[5] The real prevalence of the disease is unknown because it is frequently misdiagnosed as other kinds of eczema.[6] ACD is therefore an important dermatologic disease with considerable morbidity and economic impact.

ICD occurs when a chemical agent induces direct damage to the skin and produces inflammation without the classic 'allergic' mechanism. The clinical manifestations can be subtle, such as a stinging sensation on exposure, or marked, such as severe chemical burns. The timing of the reaction varies according to exposure—usually occurring within a short period of minutes for a single exposure and within days or weeks for multiple exposures. Most irritant reactions seen in the clinic are of moderate severity, and are due to cumulative insult with mildly toxic substances, such as ordinary soap and water.[2]

ACD occurs when contact with a specific allergen or a closely related chemical substance elicits an immunologic inflammatory response in the allergic individual, usually between 24 and 72 hours after reexposure [**Figure 28-2**]. A dose-response relationship exists for both allergens and irritants but is more important in the irritant reaction. The presence or combination of more irritants or allergens potentially influences the allergenicity of a substance.[7,8]

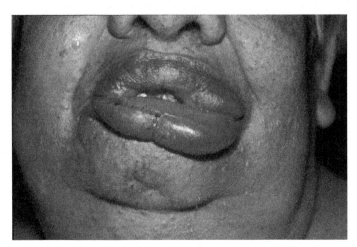

FIGURE 28-2. An allergic immunologic inflammatory response to lip gloss in a patient with skin of color.

Clinically, ACD is inflammation of the skin manifested by varying degrees of erythema, edema, and vesiculation in its acute form, but it may also present as a subacute or chronic eczematous process. A diagnosis of ACD may be suspected based on clinical and historic grounds but can only be diagnosed definitively through the use of the patch test procedure. In patch testing, small quantities of the allergens are applied to the skin for a fixed duration, and the skin is examined 2 to 4 days later for the presence of eczematous changes.

In a study by Reduta et al,[9] the most frequent allergens were as follows: nickel sulfate ($NiSO_4$), cobalt chloride, fragrance mix, potassium dichromate, balsam of Peru, neomycin, p-phenylenediamine (PPDA), quarternium-15, detreomycin, and budesonide.

The ability of the offending agent to cause contact dermatitis depends on both the nature of the allergen/irritant and the skin's condition. The severity of the symptoms depends on exogenous and endogenous factors. Exogenous factors include the chemical and physical properties of the substance and the frequency of application. Endogenous factors include age, sex, preexisting skin diseases, skin sensitivity, genetics, and probably skin of color.[10]

RACIAL DIFFERENCES IN SKIN PHYSIOLOGY AND PATHOPHYSIOLOGY

Differences in physiology and pathophysiology have been described in patients with skin of color. The literature supports a difference in epidermal melanin content and melanosome distribution in people with skin of color compared with fair-skinned individuals.[11] Other studies have shown differences in hair structure and fibroblast size and structure between skin of color and fair skin.[12,13]

It is probable that the two most significant differences in skin physiology in determining the relationship between skin color and contact dermatitis are barrier function and percutaneous absorption. Studies done on the percutaneous absorption of chemicals into the skin have, in many cases, shown that skin of color is generally more impervious than Caucasian skin, although this is not true in all cases. Wedig and Maibach[14] observed 30% less absorption of dipyrithione in subjects with skin of color versus Caucasian subjects.[14] Similarly, Astner et al[15] evaluated the variability of skin responses to a common household irritant among different groups and found that significant differences in the cutaneous irritant response suggested the superior barrier function of African American or darkly pigmented skin. Lotte et al[16] also looked at all three races and found a slight increase in absorption among Asian patients and a slight decrease in absorption in patients with skin of color compared with the Caucasian patients. Additional studies used transepidermal water loss (TEWL) as a measure of the skin's barrier function in terms of the evaporation potential for water. Kompaore et al[17] compared TEWL among Caucasians, patients with skin of color, and Asians and found significantly increased values in patients with skin of color and Asians compared with Caucasians. Reed et al[18] used TEWL and found that subjects, regardless of race, who had lighter-pigmented skin had a more easily perturbed barrier function and a longer recovery time.

Overall, these findings suggest a reduced degree of penetration by a chemical into skin of color, and an increase in barrier function of those with darker skin[18]; both may help to explain the reduced irritant and allergic response discussed later in this chapter.

CLINICAL PRESENTATION

A very common type of skin allergy, ACD is a cell-mediated (type IV) immunologic response driven by T-lymphocytes in response to allergenic small molecules (haptens).[19] Heavy metals, fragrances, preservatives, and topical medications make up the main classes of causative agents.[9,20] However, the overall incidence of ACD is less than that of ICD, which causes 8 out of 10 cases of contact dermatitis.[21]

Detecting the occurrence of contact dermatitis in different patients presents the first challenge. When a diagnosis of ACD is suspected, Fisher[22] pointed out that the manifestation in patients with skin of color

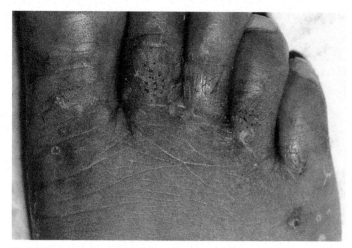

FIGURE 28-3. Contact dermatitis on the dorsum of the toes and foot of an African American male with skin type IV to V.

may be different from that in fairer-skinned patients; the dermatitis is more commonly associated with lichenification and hyperpigmentation in individuals with skin of color versus the vesicular, papular, erythematous response usually seen in Caucasians [**Figure 28-3**]. In addition, some of the difficulty in diagnosing ACD in skin of color arises from the perception of erythema, which is an end point in determining contact dermatitis through patch testing.[22] The interpretation of patch test results in skin of color is more difficult given the challenge of detecting erythema,[23] which may potentially lead to an underestimation of ACD among these individuals.

SUSCEPTIBILITY IN SKIN OF COLOR

Data on the differences regarding susceptibility to ACD in different skin color groups are sparse, largely because few investigators are willing or able to knowingly sensitize test subjects in order to prospectively study the etiology and mechanisms of the development of ACD. In the past, however, several studies were performed looking at the induction of contact dermatitis among different races. Two such studies have shown a reduced sensitivity for individuals with skin of color versus Caucasians. Rostenberg and Kanof[24] studied both individuals with skin of color and Caucasian subjects to determine the incidence of induced sensitization to dinitrochlorobenzene (DNCB) and paranitrosodimethylaniline (PNDA). Each material was tested at a concentration of 1%, which was applied openly to a uniform area of skin. One month following the exposure, the subjects were challenged with the chemical to determine if sensitization had occurred. If no sensitization was present, the process was repeated up to four times in an attempt to induce sensitization.[24]

The two chemicals differed in their ability to sensitize, with DNCB being the less potent sensitizer. With DNCB, the cumulative incidence of sensitization increased gradually, with an increasing number of Caucasian subjects showing positive responses at each treatment. In contrast, sensitization to PNDA occurred more rapidly, although in a similar way to DNCB, among Caucasians. The cumulative incidence in Caucasian subjects grew more rapidly, showing that subjects with skin of color were more resistant than Caucasians to induced sensitization by these chemicals.[24]

These results were corroborated 25 years later by Kligman,[25] who compared the response of subjects with skin of color and Caucasian subjects to several commonly encountered skin allergens. Kligman[25] studied the induction of sensitization to PPDA, monobenzyl ether of hydroquinone, penicillin A, NiSO$_4$, penicillin G (Pen G), and neomycin sulfate (NEO) between fair-skinned people and people with darker skin of color. In this study, the sensitization rates of the weak allergens were statistically higher in those with fairer skin than in those with skin of

color. However, the strongest contact allergen, Pen G, showed little difference in the response between these groups. From these results, Kligman[25] concluded that darker skin of color is less responsive to the exogenous insult than fairer skin, possibly as a result of the difference in the ability of a substance to penetrate through darker skin of color versus fairer skin.

In contrast, the North American Contact Dermatitis Group reported information on contact dermatitis in approximately 10,000 patients; 10.5% identified themselves as having darker skin of color.[26] These patients had all received patch testing between 1992 and 1998. The percentage of patients with positive patch test results was similar between patients with darker skin of color and patients with fairer skin. Additionally, the sites of the dermatitis were similar between the groups. The hands, feet, and face were affected most commonly. The most common allergen was nickel, with a comparable response rate between the groups. The skin of color population was found to have a higher incidence of contact dermatitis to PPDA, a hair dye allergen, than the Caucasian population [**Figure 28-4**]. The rates of sensitization in this study were extremely high for the skin of color population, ranging from 7.8% to 10.6%. Along with the response to NiSO$_4$, this was the highest response rate of any allergen tested in the skin of color group.[26] Similar high rates of sensitization and a predominance among individuals with skin of color were reported in a study on a smaller group of patients by Dickel et al.[27] Fisher[28] had previously reported PPDA to be the most common sensitizer in patients with skin of color receiving patch testing.

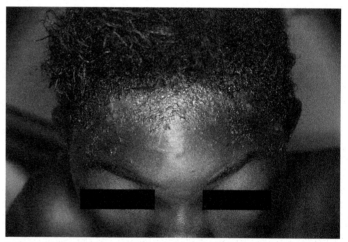

A

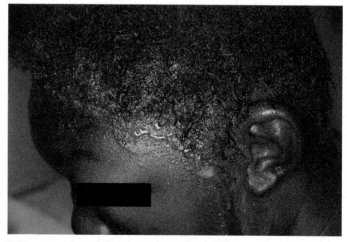

B

FIGURE 28-4. Contact dermatitis to *p*-phenylenediamine on the scalp of an African American female with skin type IV to V, (**A**) front and (**B**) side views.

Although it is possible that biological and genetic distinctions were contributors to these differences in incidences of reaction to the hair dye allergen PPDA, it is more likely that cultural differences leading to different exposure patterns played a larger role. Dickel et al[27] examined the possibility that racial differences in acetylator genotype and phenotype might explain the higher rates of sensitization to PPDA in the skin of color population. PPDA-sensitive patients could theoretically have differences in their ability to acetylate *N*-acetyltransferase 1 or 2, and that such difference in the acetylation of PPDA could result in a higher or lower allergenicity to PPDA. However, this reasoning alone would not explain differences in the sensitization rates between patients with skin of color and fairer-skinned patients because those two groups have been shown in the past to have similarly high proportions of slow acetylators. Therefore, it is more likely that the differences in PPDA sensitization rates are related to differences in the exposure pattern of the two races.

This component of hair dye, PPDA, is found in higher concentrations in the darker shades of dye that are commonly used by African Americans or those with very tightly coiled hair. Therefore, the exposure is not necessarily due to the amount of hair dye used but rather the concentration used, leading to higher sensitization rates. Another possibility is that the sensitivity shown by patients with skin of color represents a cross-sensitization to other chemically related substances that are most often used to treat diseases in African American patients, such as thiazide diuretics and oral antidiabetic drugs. However, if this were the case, one would expect to find a higher level of sensitization in similarly related allergens, such as benzocaine, which is not the case.[27]

The incidence of ACD among different groups living within the same community was examined in over 400 patients in West Yorkshire, England. The study aimed to compare patients with Fitzpatrick skin types I to IV and patients from India, Pakistan, and Bangladesh with skin type V.[29] Although the results found that fewer patients from the Indian subcontinent had positive reactions compared with the European patients (44% vs 56%, respectively), the study found no significant differences in the contact allergens responsible between the two groups.[29] Fairhurst and Shah[29] concluded that the lower incidence of positive patch tests among the Indian subcontinent group could be explained by differing exposure to contact allergens and is not necessarily evidence of skin color variability in susceptibility. Additionally, a study by Sharma and Chakrabarti[30] concluded that the European standard series of patch testing was suitable for detecting ACD in India.

Epidemiologic studies, however, are by definition retrospective and cannot be controlled for exposure. The assumptions made here are that exposure is equivalent among groups and that there is no difference between patients with skin of color and those with fairer skin in terms of sensitization to allergens. However, in reality, to say that exposures are[24,25] equivalent is an extremely large assumption.

These studies are only able to monitor the elicitation phase, whereas the historical studies, such as those by Rostenberg and Kanof[24] and Kligman,[25] were able to examine the actual sensitization process of ACD in naïve patients. Those studies show that in experimentally controlled conditions, patients with skin of color actually show significantly less sensitivity to the induction of sensitization.[24,25]

Although the literature comparing the sensitivity to ACD in Caucasians and patients with skin of color is limited, the literature on other racial comparisons is even more scarce. Ni et al[20] found that PPDA, nickel, fragrance, mercury, and rubber chemicals are common allergens in Chinese patients with hand eczema; these are similar to the common allergens found by Reduta et al.[9] A study on Thai patients found that the most frequent allergens were potassium dichromate, followed by $NiSO_4$, fragrance mix, and cobalt chloride.[31] Rapaport[32] found that Japanese patients tend to show a more severe allergic reaction to standard cosmetic ingredients than Caucasians but not a higher incidence. However, the limited data that these studies provide are incomplete because there is no report as to the materials tested. In retrospective studies of patch test subjects in Singapore, Goh[33,34] found no difference in the incidence

of ACD among Chinese, Malays, and Indians within the indigenous population.

Therefore, according to the minimal data available, there is a possible decreased susceptibility among patients with skin of color, but no other racial differences in the susceptibility to ACD have been found.

IMPACT OF CULTURAL AND OCCUPATIONAL PRACTICES

In addition to genetic and biological differences and exposure rates playing a role in the occurrence of contact dermatitis, cultural practices are important as well. ACD to PPDA can be found in other individuals due to their exposure patterns as well. Black henna, used as a ceremonial skin decoration in the Middle East, North Africa, and the Indian subcontinent, has been found to contain the dye PPDA. Several case reports of ACD after receiving a henna tattoo have been published. Although ACD due to lawsone (*Lawsonia inermis*), the major allergen in henna, is rare, subjects who experienced the reactions nevertheless almost always had a history of permanent hair dye use in the past, and all reacted positively to a PPDA patch test.[35-37]

Occupation also plays a role; occupational contact dermatitis, including ACD, is one of the most frequently seen occupational diseases.[38] For example, increased prevalence of positive skin reactions to PPDA have been found in hairdressers, and to chromate in metal and construction workers [**Figure 28-5**].[20] Chromate is a very common sensitizer for individuals living in industrialized countries.[39] Additionally, a large number of contact dermatitis cases have resulted from the repeated exposure of the hands to soaps, cleansers, and detergents; latex allergies are particularly common among healthcare workers.[39] Therefore, it is important that dermatologists perform thorough patch testing and take a detailed patient history, including details of what the patient may handle on a daily basis, to determine the causative agents of the allergic reaction.

There may also be preferences in certain beauty and healthcare products among different groups. Formaldehyde and related formaldehyde-releasing preservatives, although sometimes found in the industrial setting, are allergens primarily found in cream-based moisturizers and shampoos. These chemicals have been shown to have a higher rate of sensitization in patients with fairer skin than in those with skin of color. The hypothesis for this finding is that the Caucasian population tends to use more cream-based products, whereas individuals with skin of color tend to prefer more oil-based products, although this may not necessarily be the case. Nevertheless, lower exposure in the skin of color

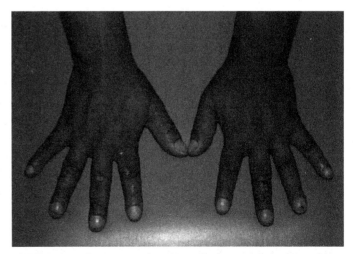

FIGURE 28-5. Irritant contact dermatitis on the dorsum of the hands in an African American cement worker. This occurred as a reaction to the chromium in the cement manufacturing process.

population would lead to lower sensitization rates. However, a decrease in sensitization to chemicals found in similar products has not been demonstrated.[28,40] Conflicting data on several other products, such as quaternium-15 and NEO, signal the fact that additional work is required in this area. For example, a retrospective study of over 600 patients found that there was a statistically significant decrease of positive patch test results for neomycin over 6 consecutive years.[41]

NEED FOR MORE SKIN OF COLOR GROUPS IN CLINICAL TESTS

Clinical testing is important to understand ACD among different skin color groups. However, there is a predominance of volunteers of Caucasian decent for skin safety testing. The question then arises as to whether clinical laboratories underestimate the ability of skin care and pharmaceutical products to cause contact dermatitis in non-Caucasian populations. This is an area that warrants additional research.[42,43]

CONCLUSION

ACD in patients with skin of color poses a challenge to clinicians and researchers. Current data on the differences in susceptibility to ACD among a range of skin color groups have been inconclusive. Research suggests both an increased and decreased susceptibility of skin of color to ACD. Overall, demographic and clinical data support the idea that the prevalence among different skin color groups is the same. However, reports have shown differences in the types of allergens that different groups are sensitive to. Given the sparse amount of data and the conflicting studies on contact dermatitis in subjects with skin of color, additional investigation is clearly required. These studies should be based on certain variables, including environmental, cultural, occupational, genetic, individual, and racial differences.

REFERENCES

1. Worm M. Allergic contact dermatitis beyond IL-1β-role of additional family members. *Exp Dermatol.* 2014;23:151-152.
2. Taylor JS, Amado A. Contact dermatitis and related conditions. www.clevelandclinicmeded.com/medicalpubs/diseasemanagement/dermatology/contact-dermatitis-and-related-conditions/. Accessed February 15, 2014.
3. Pratt MD, Belsito DV, DeLeo VA, et al. North American Contact Dermatitis Group patch-test results, 2001-2002 study period. *Dermatitis.* 2004;15:176-183.
4. Saripalli YV, Achen F, Belsito DV. The detection of clinically relevant contact allergens using a standard screening tray of twenty-three allergens. *J Am Acad Dermatol.* 2003;49:65-69.
5. Mortz CG, Bindslev-Jensen C, Andersen KE. Prevalence, incidence rates and persistence of contact allergy and allergic contact dermatitis in The Odense Adolescence Cohort Study: a 15-year follow-up. *Br J Dermatol.* 2013;168:318-325.
6. Statescu L, Branisteanu D, Dobre C, et al. Contact dermatitis: epidemiological study. *Maedica (Buchar).* 2011;6:277-281.
7. Pedersen LK, Johansen JD, Held E, et al. Augmentation of skin response by exposure to a combination of allergens and irritants: a review. *Contact Dermatitis.* 2004;50:265-273.
8. Smith HR, Basketter DA, McFadden JP. Irritant dermatitis, irritancy and its role in allergic contact dermatitis. *Clin Exp Dermatol.* 2002;27:138-146.
9. Reduta T, Bacharewicz J, Pawłoś A. Patch test results in patients with allergic contact dermatitis in the Podlasie region. *Postepy Dermatol Alergol.* 2013;30:350-357.
10. Krob HA, Fleischer AB Jr, D'Agostino R Jr, et al. Prevalence and relevance of contact dermatitis allergens: a meta-analysis of 15 years of published T.R.U.E. test data. *J Am Acad Dermatol.* 2004;51:349-353.
11. Alaluf S, Atkins D, Barrett K, et al. Ethnic variation in melanin content and composition in photoexposed and photoprotected human skin. *Pigment Cell Res.* 2002;15:112-118.
12. Taylor SC. Skin of color: biology, structure, function, and implications for dermatologic disease. *J Am Acad Dermatol.* 2002;46:S41-S62.
13. Richards GM, Oresajo CO, Halder RM. Structure and function of ethnic skin and hair. *Dermatol Clin.* 2003;21:595-600.
14. Wedig JH, Maibach HI. Percutaneous penetration of dipyrithione in man: effect of skin color (race). *J Am Acad Dermatol.* 1981;5:433-438.
15. Astner S, Burnett N, Rius-Díaz F, et al. Irritant contact dermatitis induced by a common household irritant: a noninvasive evaluation of ethnic variability in skin response. *J Am Acad Dermatol.* 2006;54:458-465.
16. Lotte C, Wester RC, Rougier A, et al. Racial differences in the in vivo percutaneous absorption of some organic compounds: a comparison between black, Caucasian and Asian subjects. *Arch Dermatol Res.* 1993;284:456-459.
17. Kompaore F, Marty JP, Dupont C. In vivo evaluation of the stratum corneum barrier function in blacks, Caucasians and Asians with two noninvasive methods. *Skin Pharmacol.* 1993;6:200-207.
18. Reed JT, Ghadially R, Elias PM. Skin type, but neither race nor gender, influence epidermal permeability barrier function. *Arch Dermatol.* 1995;131:1134-1138.
19. Gober MD, Gaspari AA. Allergic contact dermatitis. *Curr Dir Autoimmun.* 2008;10:1-26.
20. Ni C, Dou X, Chen J, et al. Contact sensitization in Chinese patients with hand eczema. *Dermatitis.* 2011;22:211-215.
21. National Health Services (NHS) Choices. Contact dermatitis. www.nhs.uk/conditions/eczema-(contact-dermatitis)/Pages/Introduction.aspx. Accessed February 15, 2014.
22. Fisher AA. Contact dermatitis in black patients. *Cutis.* 1977;20:303-309, 316.
23. Riordan B, Sprigle S, Linden M. Testing the validity of erythema detection algorithms. *J Rehabil Res Dev.* 2001;38:13-22.
24. Rostenberg A Jr, Kanof NM. Studies in eczematous sensitizations: I. A comparison between the sensitizing capacities of two allergens and between two different strengths of the same allergen and the effect of repeating the sensitizing dose. *J Invest Dermatol.* 1941;4:505-516.
25. Kligman AM. The identification of contact allergens by human assay: 3. The maximization test: a procedure for screening and rating contact sensitizers. *J Invest Dermatol.* 1966;47:393-409.
26. North American Contact Dermatitis Group. Epidemiology of contact dermatitis in North America: 1972. *Arch Dermatol.* 1973;108:537-540.
27. Dickel H, Taylor JS, Evey P, et al. Comparison of patch test results with a standard series among white and black racial groups. *Am J Contact Dermat.* 2001;12:77-82.
28. Fisher AA. New advances in contact dermatitis. *Int J Dermatol.* 1977;16:552-568.
29. Fairhurst DA, Shah M. Comparison of patch test results among white Europeans and patients from the Indian subcontinent living within the same community. *J Eur Acad Dermatol Venereol.* 2008;22:1227-1231.
30. Sharma VK, Chakrabarti A. Common contact sensitizers in Chandigarh, India: a study of 200 patients with the European standard series. *Contact Dermatitis.* 1998;38:127-131.
31. Boonchai W, Iamtharachai P, Sunthonpalin P. Prevalence of allergic contact dermatitis in Thailand. *Dermatitis.* 2008;19:142-145.
32. Rapaport MJ. Patch testing in Japanese subjects. *Contact Dermatitis.* 1984;11:93-97.
33. Goh CL. Contact sensitivity to topical medicaments. *Int J Dermatol.* 1989;28:25-28.
34. Goh CL. Prevalence of contact allergy by sex, race and age. *Contact Dermatitis.* 1986;14:237-240.
35. Mohamed M, Nixon R. Severe allergic contact dermatitis induced by paraphenylenediamine in paint-on temporary "tattoos." *Australas J Dermatol.* 2000;41:168-171.
36. Läuchli S, Lautenschlager S. Contact dermatitis after temporary henna tattoos: an increasing phenomenon. *Swiss Med Wkly.* 2001;131:199-202.
37. Le Coz CJ, Lefebvre C, Keller F, et al. Allergic contact dermatitis caused by skin painting (pseudotattooing) with black henna, a mixture of henna and p-phenylenediamine and its derivatives. *Arch Dermatol.* 2000;136:1515-1517.
38. Holness DL. Occupational skin allergies: testing and treatment (the case of occupational allergic contact dermatitis). *Curr Allergy Asthma Rep.* 2014;14:410.
39. ClinicalKey, Elsevier, Inc. Contact dermatitis. www.clinicalkey.com/topics/dermatology/contact-dermatitis.html. Accessed February 15, 2014.
40. Deleo VA, Taylor SC, Belsito DV, et al. The effect of race and ethnicity on patch test results. *J Am Acad Dermatol.* 2002;46:S107-S112.
41. Duarte IA, Tanaka GM, Suzuki NM, et al. Patch test standard series recommended by the Brazilian Contact Dermatitis Study Group during the 2006-2011 period. *An Bras Dermatol.* 2013;88:1015-1018.
42. Robinson MK, Perkins MA, Basketter DA. Application of a 4-h human patch test method for comparative and investigative assessment of skin irritation. *Contact Dermatitis.* 1998;38:194-202.
43. Epstein AM. Healthcare in America: still too separate, not yet equal. *N Engl J Med.* 2004;351:603-605.

Photosensitivity

Patricia Oyetakin-White
Elma D. Baron

KEY POINTS

- Photosensitive disorders are cutaneous diseases caused by an abnormal reaction to ultraviolet or visible light.
- The differences in quality and quantity of melanin pigmentation between skin types play a role in the prevalence of photosensitivity between racial groups.
- A diagnosis of photosensitivity involves a detailed history, clinical examination of sun-exposed areas and sun-protected areas, phototesting, photopatch testing, and photoprovocation testing.
- Treatment plans should emphasize photoprotection, symptomatic relief, and phototherapy or systemic medications when indicated.

INTRODUCTION

Sunlight is important for human life because it plays a key role in psychological well-being and physiologic systems.[1] The solar radiation that reaches the earth's surface is in the electromagnetic spectrum with wavelengths greater than 290 nm. This includes ultraviolet (UV) B (290 to 320 nm), UVA (320 to 400 nm), visible light (400 to 760 nm), and infrared radiation (760 nm to 1 mm). Fortunately, the more damaging higher energy short wavelengths, UVC (<290 nm), are absorbed by the ozone layer and atmosphere and do not reach the earth's surface.[2] When UV interacts with the skin, the electromagnetic waves are absorbed, reflected, or scattered.

Photosensitivity is a term that refers to a group of skin diseases induced or exacerbated by UV or visible light. Photosensitivity is synonymous with photodermatosis, and these terms are sometimes used interchangeably. Photosensitive disorders can be classified into four categories: (1) primary or immunologically mediated disorders, (2) drug- and chemical-induced disorders, (3) photoaggravated disorders, and (4) inherited disorders with defective DNA repair or with chromosomal instability [**Table 29-1**].[3,4]

SKIN PIGMENTATION AND PHOTOSENSITIVITY

Skin color is dependent on the number, type, and distribution of melanin pigment granules, hemoglobin, and carotenoids.[5] Melanocytes located in the basal epidermis produce melanin pigment granules within specialized organelles called melanosomes and then transfer them to neighboring keratinocytes via dendritic processes.[6] The photoprotective property of melanins is attributed to their ability to absorb and scatter UV light, converting it into a less harmful form of energy, thermal heat. They are located in the supranuclear region of melanocytes and keratinocytes to protect DNA from UV damage.[7] The amount of melanocytes between races is approximately the same; however, the quantity and quality of the melanin pigments account for phenotypic racial differences.[6]

Melanocytes produce two chemically distinct types of melanin pigments, the brownish black eumelanin and the reddish yellow pheomelanin.[8] Both types are significantly increased in photoexposed compared with photoprotected skin.[9] The eumelanin-to-pheomelanin ratio is higher in darker skin than in lighter skin, and the amount of eumelanin has been shown to be approximately two-fold higher in African and Indian skin types compared with Mexican, Chinese, and European skin types.[9] Eumelanin is also effective at scavenging free radicals produced by UV light,[10,11] whereas pheomelanin has been shown to generate hydroxyl radicals and superoxide anions that contribute to oxidative DNA damage.[12,13] Pheomelanin also increases the release of histamine following UV light exposure, which contributes to the erythema and edema seen in lighter-skinned individuals.[7] These qualities

TABLE 29-1	Four categories of photosensitive disorders

1. Immunologically mediated
   Actinic prurigo
   Chronic actinic dermatitis
   Hydroa vacciniforme
   Solar urticaria
   Polymorphous light eruption

2. Drug- and chemical-induced
   Exogenous agents
      Phototoxicity
      Photoallergy
   Endogenous agents
      Porphyrias
      Pellagra

3. Photoaggravated
   Acne vulgaris
   Atopic dermatitis
   Bullous pemphigoid
   Carcinoid syndrome
   Darier disease
   Dermatomyositis
   Disseminated superficial actinic porokeratosis
   Erythema multiforme
   Grover disease
   Lichen planus
   Lupus erythematosus
   Pemphigus
   Pityriasis rubra pilaris
   Psoriasis
   Reticular erythematous mucinosis
   Rosacea
   Seborrheic dermatitis
   Viral infections

4. Inherited disorders with defective DNA repair or with chromosomal instability
   Ataxia-telangiectasia
   Bloom syndrome
   Cockayne syndrome
   Hailey-Hailey disease
   Hartnup disease
   Kindler syndrome
   Rothmund-Thomson syndrome
   Trichothiodystrophy
   Xeroderma pigmentosum

Source: Adapted with permission from Santoro FA, Lim HW. Update on photodermatoses, Semin Cutan Med Surg 2011 Dec;30(4):229-238.[4]

of pheomelanin likely contribute to the higher rates of photosensitivity and photodamage seen in lighter-skinned individuals.

CLINICAL EVALUATION

It is important to take a detailed medical history when evaluating photosensitivity. Emphasis should be placed on the sun exposure history in relationship to the development of the skin lesions. The age of the affected individual is helpful for arriving at a differential diagnosis because some diseases are more likely to manifest in infancy and early childhood (eg, juvenile spring eruption, congenital erythropoietic porphyria) versus adulthood (eg, chronic actinic dermatitis (CAD), drug-induced photosensitivity).[3,14] Information about family history, seasonal variations in the winter and summer months, time intervals between sun exposure and development of lesions, duration of the eruption and systemic symptoms, and the effect of window glass are helpful factors in determining the diagnosis.[14,15]

Physical examination should focus on the morphology and distribution of the lesions. Severe eruptions tend to occur on sun-exposed areas of the skin: forehead, cheeks, lateral and posterior neck, dorsum of hands, and extensor aspects of forearms. Areas of relative sun protection, such as the nasolabial folds, postauricular area, upper eyelids, and superior pinna of the ear, should be examined because these areas are relatively spared in photosensitive disorders unlike the presentation in patients with airborne allergic dermatitis.[3] Laboratory evaluations and skin biopsies may be necessary to arrive at the diagnosis.

PHOTOTESTING AND PHOTOPATCH TESTING

Phototesting is performed to confirm photosensitivity and to determine the specific wavelengths that elicit a cutaneous reaction. Photoprotected areas of skin, such as the back or abdomen, are exposed to increasing doses of UVB, UVA, and/or visible radiation.[3] The exposed areas should be evaluated immediately (to detect solar urticaria) and 24 hours later (to assess the minimal erythema dose [MED]). Evaluations at later time points may be necessary when considering delayed erythema reactions such as in photosensitive lupus erythematosus (LE). The minimal erythema dose (MED) is the lowest dose of UVA (MED-A), UVB (MED-B), or visible light that causes visually detectable erythema uniformly covering the entire irradiated area. Photoprovocation testing is repeated irradiation of an area of skin over 3 to 4 consecutive days to induce lesions in polymorphous light eruption (PMLE) and photosensitive LE.[16]

As seen in **Table 29-2**, results from phototesting will be normal or decreased depending on the disease process.[3,4] A recent retrospective study by Que et al[17] showed that 68% of patients with suspected photosensitivity will have normal MED-A, MED-B, and visible light results. A majority of the patients with normal MEDs were diagnosed with PMLE, photoallergic (contact) dermatitis, photodistributed dermatitis, photoexacerbated atopic dermatitis, and solar urticaria. Their results also confirm what is known about phototesting in solar urticaria, where development of hives occurs within minutes of phototesting but normal MEDs are observed in 24 hours. Phototesting in patients with skin of color will depend on the skin phototype of constitutive pigmented areas of skin. Diagnosis and management of patients with darker skin types (Fitzpatrick skin types IV, V, and VI) may prove challenging because of the difficulty in evaluating erythema to determine the MED in some individuals.[18] A study by Wee et al[19] found increasing MED values for darker skin types (II, III, IV, V, and VI) in Chinese, Malay, and Indian individuals but significant overlap between the different phototypes. Objective constitutional skin color assessment and quantification of MED significantly differentiated skin types I, IV, and V in Colombian high school children, but this combined approach was not effective for skin types II and III.[20]

When photoallergic contact dermatitis is suspected, photopatch testing is performed by applying a panel of common photoallergens to two uninvolved areas of back skin. Then, 24 hours later, one of the areas is irradiated with UVA (10 J/cm² or 50% of MED-A, whichever is lower) and the other area is left unexposed. Evaluation of both skin sites is performed at 48 hours after the photoallergen application. Comparison

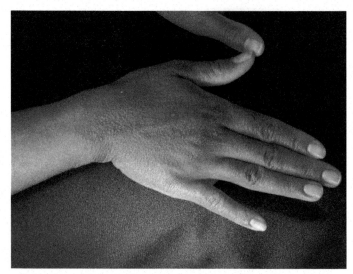

FIGURE 29-1. Polymorphous light eruption in a skin of color patient. Pin-head papules on dorsum of hand. (Used with permission from Henry W. Lim, MD, Henry Ford Hospital, Detroit, MI).

of the reactions between the unirradiated and irradiated sites will help distinguish between photoallergic contact dermatitis, allergic contact dermatitis, or allergic contact dermatitis with photoaggravation.

POLYMORPHOUS LIGHT ERUPTION (PMLE)

PMLE is a common acquired immune-mediated photosensitivity disorder and is often referred to as "sun poisoning." The rash occurs hours after UV light exposure. It is most severe in the spring or early summer and gradually resolves as the summer progresses, a process attributed to photoadaptation, or hardening. The term polymorphous refers to the variability in the appearance of the skin lesions between individuals. The lesions develop as symmetric nonscarring, mild pruritic, erythematous papules, papulovesicles, vesicles, plaques, or nodules on sun-exposed areas of skin [**Figure 29-1**].[21] The distribution of the lesions includes the dorsum of the hands and forearms, the 'V' area of the neck, and the malar region of the face. All skin types are affected by PMLE; however, the clinical presentation in darker skin types (IV to VI) has been described as the pinpoint papular variant, which appears as multiple pinpoint skin-colored papules that often mimics lichen nitidus [**Figure 29-2**].[22] A study from Singapore in Chinese, Malay, Indian, and Cambodian individuals diagnosed with PMLE found that 29.6% of all the phototested patients had the pinpoint papular variant.[23]

The prevalence of PMLE is estimated at 10% to 20%[22] and first appears in the second and third decades of life. Females are affected

TABLE 29-2	Phototesting and photopatch testing results			
Disorder	MED-A	MED-B	Visible light	Photopatch test
Polymorphous light eruption	Normal or ↓ in 15%–30%	Normal or ↓ in 15%–30%	Normal	Negative
Chronic actinic dermatitis	Normal or ↓	Normal or ↓	Normal or ↓	Positive or negative
Solar urticaria	Normal *Immediate urticaria that resolves in 24 hours*	Normal *Immediate urticaria that resolves in 24 hours*	Normal *Immediate urticaria that resolves in 24 hours*	Negative
Hydroa vacciniforme	↓	Normal or ↓	Normal	
Actinic prurigo	Normal or ↓	Normal or ↓	Normal	
Photoallergy	Normal or ↓	Normal	Normal	Positive
Phototoxicity	Normal or ↓	Normal	Normal	Negative

Abbreviations: MED, minimal erythema dose; A, ultraviolet A; B, ultraviolet B.

Source: Adapted with permission from Santoro FA, Lim HW. Update on photodermatoses, Semin Cutan Med Surg 2011 Dec;30(4):229-238.[4]

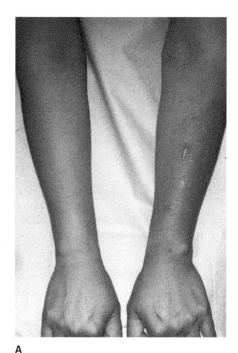

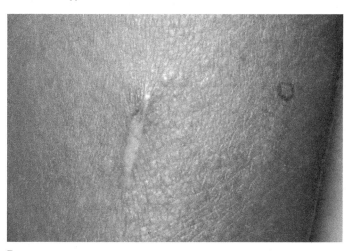

FIGURE 29-2. Pinpoint papular polymorphous light eruption. **(A)** Skin-colored pinpoint papules involving the dorsal forearms. **(B)** Skin-colored pinpoint papules.

photoprovocation testing may be performed to confirm the diagnosis. Histopathology will show edema, focal spongiosis, and small vesicles in the epidermis.[21] As mentioned earlier, most patients with PMLE have normal MEDs; however, photoprovocation testing can elicit lesions in 60% of patients.[4] The action spectrum of PMLE is usually in the UVA range rather than the UVB range.[27]

Management of PMLE begins with a detailed explanation of the diagnosis to the patient and comprehensive counseling about photoprotection strategies involving the use of appropriate clothing, sun avoidance, and application of broad-spectrum sunscreens with adequate UVA protection. First-line therapy for acute eruptions includes topical corticosteroids, which may help clear mild to moderate attacks, and a short course of systemic corticosteroids for more severe episodes. Patients with frequent episodes in the summer may benefit from prophylactic phototherapy and hardening of the skin with narrowband UVB (NB-UVB). UVB hardening has been shown to significantly normalize UV-induced migration of Langerhans cell and neutrophils in PMLE patients.[30] Phototherapy should begin in the early spring three times a week for 15 sessions, starting at 70% MED and increased as tolerated by 10% to 20% each session.[4] Other therapies include antimalarials, β-carotene, nicotinamide, ω-3 polyunsaturated fatty acids, *Escherichia coli* filtrate, and oral *Polypodium leucotomos* extract, but large clinical trials validating the safety and efficacy of these interventions have not been done.[21]

CHRONIC ACTINIC DERMATITIS

CAD is an immunologically mediated disease with a contact dermatitis-like delayed-type hypersensitivity reaction against sunlight-induced endogenous cutaneous allergens.[27] The exact etiology of CAD remains unknown. Clinically the lesions appear as pruritic, lichenified eczematous eruptions involving sun-exposed skin [**Figures 29-3 and 29-4**]. The reaction can be more severe in summer months or after prolonged exposure to sunlight. The most common areas affected are the face, back of the neck, forearms, and dorsal arms. This disorder is commonly thought to affect more males than females and those ≥50 years old[31]; however, a recent study by Que et al[32] showed that the diagnosis of CAD at a North American institution was common in younger females with skin types IV to VI and older males with skin types I to III.[32] Recent studies have suggested an increase in the incidence of photosensitive disorders due to climate change factors such as irradiance and duration of sunlight.[33,34] A study by Kyu-Won et al[35] showed that the increase in the duration of sunshine from

two to three times more often than males, and one-sixth of the affected patients report a positive family history.[24] Although most studies report a higher incidence in lighter skin types (I to III) compared with darker skin types (IV to V), a 2007 study by Kerr and Lim[25] showed a statistically significant difference in rate of 67.4% in African Americans versus 41.1% in fairer-skinned individuals.

Recent studies suggest that the pathogenesis is related to a type IV delayed-type hypersensitivity reaction where UV irradiation induces antigen formation in the skin.[26] The failure of normal UV-induced immunosuppression in photosensitive individuals likely leads to the immunologic response.[27] In normal skin, CD1a⁺ Langerhans cells migrate from the epidermis upon UV exposure, which is one of the phenomena that contribute to immune suppression. However, in PMLE skin, these cells are still present 48 and 72 hours after exposure to six MEDs of UV light.[28] A study by Schornagel et al[29] showed decreased neutrophil infiltration in PMLE skin following UVB exposure.

Diagnosis is usually based on history and clinical findings; therefore, laboratory tests and skin biopsies are not usually performed. In atypical cases, lupus serology, porphyrin screening, biopsy, phototesting, and

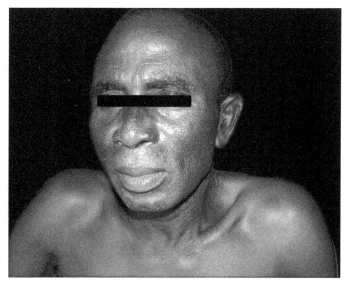

FIGURE 29-3. Chronic actinic dermatitis. Hyperpigmentation and lichenification involving the face and anterior neck. (Used with permission from Frances Ajose, MD.)

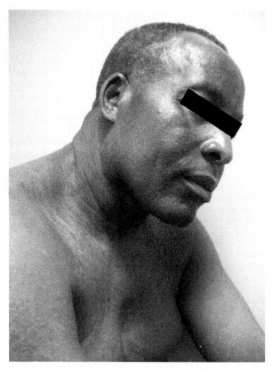

FIGURE 29-4. Chronic actinic dermatitis. Hyperpigmentation and lichenification involving the face, anterior neck, and chest. (Used with permission from Frances Ajose, MD.)

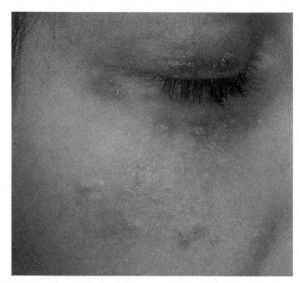

FIGURE 29-5. Actinic prurigo. Erythematous papules and erosions on eyelid and cheek. (Used with permission from Henry W. Lim, MD, Henry Ford Hospital, Detroit, MI).

2000 to 2008 in a region in South Korea correlated with an increase in the incidence of CAD.

CAD is diagnosed based on three criteria: (1) persistent eczematous eruptions mostly affecting sun-exposed areas with or without infiltrated papules and plaques, (2) histopathology showing chronic eczematous changes with or without a dermal infiltrate composed of lymphocytes and macrophages, and (3) phototesting showing decreased MED to UVA, UVB, or visible light.[36] Although the pathogenesis of CAD is not fully understood, the populations of lymphocyte cells in affected skin suggest a delayed-type hypersensitivity reaction to a sun-induced skin allergen. Other contact allergens that have been suggested to contribute to the pathogenesis include sesquiterpene lactones, colophony, and fragrances.[37] However, a recent study by Chew et al[38] demonstrated a significant decline in positive reactions to a sesquiterpene lactone mix in patch- and photopatch-tested CAD patients. These authors also showed a significant increase in positive patch tests to nonfragrance consumer allergens, particularly p-phenylenediamine. In the previously mentioned Korean study by Kyu-Won et al,[35] positive patch tests and photopatch tests were seen in 80.4% and 68.6% of CAD patients, respectively. Positive photopatch test reactions were seen with balsam of Peru, promethazine hydrochloride (HCl), chlorpromazine HCl, and a perfume mix.

Treatment of CAD involves strict avoidance of UV and/or visible light and relevant contact allergens. Photoprotection with clothing and application of broad-spectrum UVA and UVB sunscreens is also important. Topical or sporadic oral corticosteroids and emollients are helpful in managing this difficult-to-treat disease.[37] Topical calcineurin inhibitors such as tacrolimus and pimecrolimus have also been used in some cases. Patients with more severe resistant disease may respond to NB-UVB hardening; however, oral and topical corticosteroids should be given before NB-UVB exposure. Systemic therapies include azathioprine, hydroxychloroquine, mycophenolate mofetil, and cyclosporine.[37]

ACTINIC PRURIGO

Actinic prurigo (AP) is an acquired chronic photosensitivity of unknown etiology that usually begins in childhood. It is more common in Mestizo populations of Latin American countries. The term Mestizo refers to people with mixed Indian and European ancestry. AP is also seen in Native American Indians and Inuit peoples in Canada and the United States. It has been described under may names: solar dermatitis, Guatemalan cutaneous syndrome, solar prurigo, light-sensitive eruption in American Indians, hereditary PMLE of American Indians, and PMLE (prurigo type).[3] However, AP is the most commonly accepted term by dermatologists. Affected individuals have a pruritic sensation a few hours after sun exposure that leads to the development of the cutaneous lesions.

AP begins around the age of 4 to 5 and affects females more than males in a 2:1 ratio. In a 2012 study of children evaluated at a photobiology center in the United Kingdom, the prevalence of AP was found to be 9.6%.[39] The pathogenesis of AP is an abnormal immune response in genetically predisposed individuals. A high association with HLA-A24, HLA-Cw4, and HLA-DR4 (DRB1*0407) has been shown.[3] Langerhans cells from patients with AP were resistant to UV-induced immunosuppression, unlike normal individuals.[40]

Clinically, AP presents as symmetric, pruritic, erythematous papules or nodules and crusts and lichenified plaques due to chronic scratching. Lesions are distributed on the face, ears, forearms, hands, legs, and feet. An important feature is mucosal involvement, which is quite common and manifests as acute cheilitis of the lips [**Figure 29-5**] and conjunctivitis and photophobia of the eyes. Treatment of AP includes photoprotection, topical and systemic corticosteroids, antihistamines, antimalarials, phototherapy, and thalidomide.[41] Thalidomide (50 to 100 mg/d) is the most effective therapy, with excellent response of skin and lip lesions in 1 to 2 months.

SOLAR URTICARIA

Solar urticaria is a rare acquired photosensitivity characterized by skin erythema and wheals within a few minutes of sun exposure that resolve within 24 hours. It is more common in females, with a peak age of onset in the fourth or fifth decade. Disease prevalence ranges from 0.08% of patients with urticaria to 7% to 17.8% of patients diagnosed with photosensitivity.[42] The 2007 study by Kerr and Lim[25] showed a prevalence of 2.2% in African Americans versus 8% in fairer-skinned individuals. Pathogenesis is related to a type I immunoglobulin E-mediated hypersensitivity reaction to photoinduced skin allergens. The wheals that appear are located in sun-exposed skin and are associated with pruritus.

Photoprovocation testing usually settles the diagnosis, and the areas should be evaluated within 30 minutes of UV or visible light exposure. Symptomatic relief of acute eruptions is achieved with oral antihistamines, topical corticosteroids, and cool compresses, although response

TABLE 29-3 Differentiating features of phototoxic and photoallergic reactions

Feature	Phototoxicity	Photoallergy
Reaction with first exposure	Yes	No
Incidence	High	Low
Incubation period necessary after first exposure	No	Yes
Amount of agent required for photosensitivity	Large	Small
Onset of eruption after exposure	Minutes to hours	24–48 hours
Cross-reactivity with other agents	Rare	Common
Clinical changes	Similar to sunburn	Varied morphology
Distribution	Exposed skin only	Exposed skin, may spread to unexposed
Covalent binding with carrier protein	No	Yes
Development of persistent light reaction	No	Yes
Relative concentration of drug necessary for reaction	High	Low

Source: Adapted with permission from Lankerani L, Baron ED: Photosensitivity to exogenous agents, J Cutan Med Surg 2004 Nov-Dec;8(6):424-431.[43]

to therapy is variable. Skin hardening with UVA phototherapy is commonly used. Occasionally, lifestyle and work schedule changes need to be implemented to cope with the disease.

DRUG- AND CHEMICAL-INDUCED PHOTOSENSITIVITY

There are various topical and systemic agents that have been shown to be potent photosensitizers upon interaction with UV or visible light. They can cause phototoxic or photoallergic reactions in the skin [**Table 29-3**].[43]

Phototoxic reactions are irritant reactions that occur within minutes to hours of light exposure. The mechanism of phototoxicity involves three steps: (1) the agent must reach viable cells in the skin, (2) the action spectrum of light must penetrate the skin, and (3) light must be absorbed by the photosensitizing agent.[43] When the photosensitive substance interacts with UV light, formation of reactive oxygen species is induced, which causes damage through the oxidation of cellular components (lipids, nucleic acids, and proteins).[43] The phototoxicity is usually immediate and clinically manifests as an exaggerated sunburn on exposed areas of skin. Common topical and systemic phototoxic agents are listed in **Tables 29-4 and 29-5**[43]. Clinically, phototoxic reactions in sun-exposed areas appear as severe sunburn disproportionate to the amount of UV exposure. Erythema, edema, and blisters are common features, whereas pseudoporphyria, photo-onycholysis, slate-gray hyperpigmentation, and lichenoid eruptions are less commonly seen. Associated symptoms include pain, tenderness, burning, or prickling. Hyperpigmentation is a common result and may persist for several months after clearance of the acute reaction. Hyperpigmentation is common in darker skin types and may persist for months to years. Phototoxic reactions cause significant damage to the epidermis and dermis with necrotic keratinocytes, spongiosis, edema, vasodilation, and infiltration of inflammatory cells seen on histopathology. Removal of the offending photosensitive agent leads to resolution of the clinical findings.

Photoallergic reactions occur due to a cell-mediated delayed hypersensitivity reaction to a UV-induced allergen. Following UV light exposure, the offending allergen binds with carrier proteins that act as antigens that induce an immune response in the skin. Reexposure to the allergen and the inciting UV action spectrum will result in a delayed

hypersensitivity reaction. Common topical and systemic phototoxic agents are listed in **Table 29-6**[43]. Sensitized individuals develop pruritic, eczematous eruptions resembling contact dermatitis within 24 to 48 hours after reexposure. Histopathology is similar to that of allergic contact dermatitis with epidermal spongiosis. Similar to phototoxic reactions, resolution is seen with removal of the offending agent.

TABLE 29-4 Topical agents that may induce cutaneous phototoxicity

Dyes	Topical agents
Brilliant lake red R	Tretinoin
Methylene blue	Benzocaine
Acridine orange	Hydrocortisone
Rose bengal (used in ophthalmologic examinations)	Coal tar and derivatives
Neutral red	Coumarin and derivatives (occurs naturally in plants, fruits, and vegetables; used in perfumes and cosmetics; used for topical photochemotherapy)
Fluorescein	
Disperse blue 35	
Eosin	Benzydamine
	Ketoprofen
	Methoxsalen
Topical antiseptic and antifungal agents	**Essential oils**
B-Bromo-4-chlorosalicylanilide	Bergamot oil
Tetrachlorosalicylanilide	Oils of citron
Hexachlorophene	lavender
Buclosamide	lime
Erythromycin	sandalwood
	cedar

Source: Adapted with permission from Lankerani L, Baron ED: Photosensitivity to exogenous agents, J Cutan Med Surg 2004 Nov-Dec;8(6):424-431.[43]

TABLE 29-5 Commonly encountered systemic phototoxic agents

Antianxiety drugs	**Anticancer drugs**
Alprazolam	Fluorouracil
Chlordiazepoxide	Dacarbazine
Antidepressants	Methotrexate
Tricyclics	Vinblastine
Desipramine	**Antifungal**
Imipramine	Griseofulvin
Antimalarials	**Cardiac**
Chloroquine	Amiodarone
Quinine	Quinidine
Antimicrobials	**Diuretics**
Quinolones	Furosemide
Ciprofloxacin	Thiazides
Enoxacin	**Food additives**
Ofloxacin	Sulfites
Sulfonamides	**Hypoglycemics**
Tetracyclines	Sulfonylureas
Demeclocycline	Tolbutamide
Doxycycline	Tolazamide
Minocycline	Glyburide
Tetracycline	Acetohexamide
Trimethoprim	**Hypolipidemics**
Retinoids	Bezafibrate
Isotretinoin	Clofibrate
Acitretin	Fenofibrate
Furocoumarins	Fibric acid derivatives
Psoralens	**Nonsteroidal anti-inflammatory drugs**
	Piroxicam
	Propionic acid derivative
	Ibuprofen
	Ketoprofen
	Naproxen
	Celecoxib

Source: Adapted with permission from Lankerani L, Baron ED: Photosensitivity to exogenous agents, J Cutan Med Surg 2004 Nov-Dec;8(6):424-431.[43]

TABLE 29-6	Most common groups of topical and systemic photoallergens

Antibacterials	**Sunscreens**
Tetrachlorosalicylanilide	Benzophenone-3
Dibromosalicylanilide	Benzophenone-4
Tribromosalicylanilide	Padimate O
Hexachlorophene	Padimate A
Chlorhexidine	Para-aminobenzoic acid
Triclosan	Homosalate
Bithionol	Avobenzone
Antifungals	Menthyl anthranilate
Fenticlor	**Fragrances**
Buclosamide	Musk ambrette
Bamipine/bromochlorosalicylanilide	6-Methylcoumarin
Others	Sandalwood oil
Ketoprofen	
Promethazine	
Quinidine	
Thiourea	
Chlorpromazine hydrochloride	
Clioquinol	
Olaquindox	

Source: Adapted with permission from Lankerani L, Baron ED: Photosensitivity to exogenous agents, J Cutan Med Surg 2004 Nov-Dec;8(6):424-431.[43]

CUTANEOUS PORPHYRIAS

Porphyrias are a group of inherited or acquired metabolic disorders caused by specific enzyme deficiencies in the heme biosynthesis pathway.[44] Heme is required for synthesis of hemoglobin and cytochromes in the bone marrow and liver. Enzyme deficiencies lead to accumulation of intermediate molecules in the pathway that have cutaneous and/or neurologic manifestations. The porphyrias are classified in two major categories: (1) acute or inducible porphyrias and (2) chronic or cutaneous porphyrias.[45] **Table 29-7** lists the pathogenesis and clinical features of the porphyrias;[4,45] cutaneous porphyrias will be discussed in more detail below. The acute porphyrias cause neurovisceral symptoms, abdominal pain, constipation, and weakness. Chronic or cutaneous porphyrias lead to porphyrin accumulation in the skin, red blood cells, and hepatocytes. The porphyrins act as photosensitizers as they absorb light, particularly in the Soret band region (400 to 410 nm), which leads to singlet oxygen formation and tissue damage.[46] It is important to note that this action spectrum lies in the visible light region; therefore, patients will report photosensitivity even without outdoor sunlight exposure.

Porphyria cutanea tarda (PCT) is the most common type of porphyria in humans, with an estimated incidence of approximately 1 in 25,000 in the United States.[45] It is due to a deficiency of the uroporphyrinogen decarboxylase (UROD) enzyme. Risk factors for PCT include alcohol abuse, hepatitis C virus infection, human immunodeficiency virus infection, estrogen intake, and hereditary hemochromatosis (*HFE* gene mutation). The prevalence of PCT is significantly less in African Americans than in Caucasians.[25] This is likely due to the autosomal recessive *HFE* gene mutation found more commonly in fairer-skinned individuals of European descent. PCT usually presents in the fourth to fifth decade of life with vesicles, bullae, blisters, and sores on traumatized sun-exposed skin, particularly the dorsal hands and forearms [**Figure 29-6**]. The vesicles and bullae rupture to form slow-healing crusts that often lead to hypo- or hyperpigmentation and/or sclerotic changes. Hypertrichosis is another common feature seen in these patients. Histopathology reveals subepidermal blistering [**Figure 29-7**] and thickened vascular walls.

The three types of PCT are all associated with reduced UROD activity: (1) type I (sporadic); (2) type II (familial); and (3) type III. Type I (sporadic) PCT is the most common form of PCT and is usually caused by acquired deficiency of hepatic UROD activity but normal erythrocyte UROD activity. Type II (familial) PCT is seen in approximately 20% of patients with an inherited autosomal dominant mutation that decreases erythrocyte and hepatic UROD activity to approximately 50%. Type II PCT is a rare familial form with normal erythrocyte UROD activity

TABLE 29-7	Classification and characteristics of porphyrias		
		Enzyme deficiency	Clinical findings
Acute or inducible porphyrias			
Acute intermittent porphyria		Porphobilinogen deaminase	AD Acute neurovisceral attacks No photosensitivity
δ-ALA dehydratase deficiency porphyria		δ-ALA dehydratase	AR Acute neurovisceral attacks
Hereditary coproporphyria		Coproporphyrinogen oxidase	AD Acute neurovisceral attacks Erythema and blistering
Variegate porphyria		Protoporphyrinogen oxidase	AD Acute neurovisceral attacks
Chronic or cutaneous porphyrias			
Congenital erythropoietic porphyria		Uroporphyrinogen III cosynthase	AR Onset in infancy Vesicles, bullae, erosions, ulcers, scarring, hyperpigmentation, hypertrichosis, mutilation Hemolytic anemia, and hepatosplenomegaly Deposits in bones and teeth
Erythropoietic protoporphyria		Ferrochelatase	AD or AR Onset in childhood Erythema, edema, purpura, skin thickening, and waxy scars Liver damage in 10%
Hepatoerythropoietic porphyria		Uroporphyrinogen decarboxylase	AR Onset in infancy Severe photosensitivity; vesicles, bullae, skin fragility, erosions, crusts, milia, scarring, and hypertrichosis Liver damage
Porphyria cutanea tarda		Uroporphyrinogen decarboxylase	AD or some develop acquired variant Onset in fourth to fifth decades of life Moderate to severe photosensitivity; skin fragility, vesicles, bullae, skin fragility, erosions, crusts, milia, scarring, and hypertrichosis Liver damage

Abbreviations: AD, autosomal dominant; δ-ALA, δ-aminolevulinic acid; AR, autosomal recessive.

Source: Adapted with permission from Lambrecht RW, Thapar M, Bonkovsky HL. Genetic aspects of porphyria cutanea tarda, Semin Liver Dis Feb 2007;27(1):99-108.[45]

and decreased hepatic UROD activity. In addition to cutaneous findings, diagnosis can be confirmed by elevated uroporphyrins and fecal porphyrins. Management involves avoidance of aggravating factors (eg, alcohol, estrogen, or certain medications) and strict photoprotection with clothing and sunscreens to block visible light. Periodic phlebotomies are beneficial for decreasing disease episodes and decreasing hepatic iron stores. Deferoxamine can also be used for this purpose. Antimalarials are also used to chelate porphyrins and facilitate their urinary excretion.

Erythropoietic protoporphyria, the second most commonly encountered cutaneous porphyria, is caused by a defect in ferrochelatase, which is the last enzyme in the heme biosynthetic pathway. It usually presents by 2 years of age with photosensitivity symptoms of skin pain, burning, stinging, and itching within minutes of sun or visible light exposure. The lesions clinically consist of erythema, petechiae, purpura, and fissures. Unlike PCT, skin fragility and blisters are not common findings.[47] Swelling resembling angioedema may be present. Multiple episodes

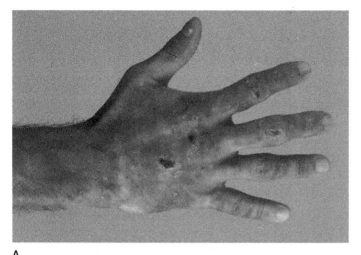

A

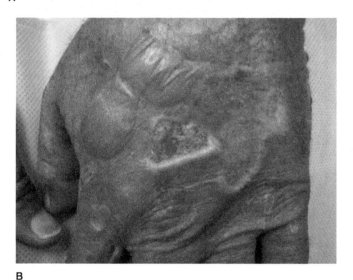

B

FIGURE 29-6. Porphyria cutanea tarda. **(A)** Skin fragility, erosions, and crusting of the dorsal right hand. **(B)** Tense blisters on the dorsal left hand.

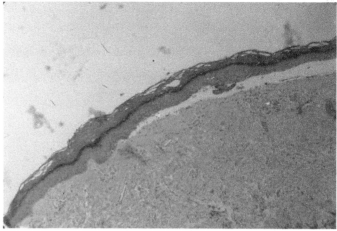

A

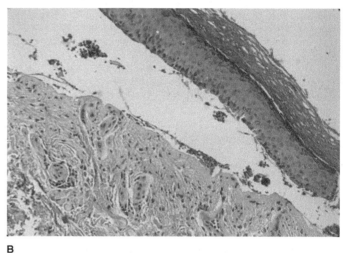

B

FIGURE 29-7. Histopathology of porphyria cutanea tarda. **(A)** Low-power magnification showing intradermal blister formation. **(B)** High-power magnification showing blister formation.

of photosensitivity may lead to scarring, lichenification, and leathery pseudovesicles of the dorsal hands, forearms, and interphalangeal joints [**Figure 29-8**]. Histopathology shows capillary basement membrane thickening and hyalinization. Approximately 20% to 30% of affected individuals will have liver dysfunction signaled by elevations of the liver enzymes, and 5% will have severe liver disease requiring liver transplantation.[48] There is also an increased incidence of gallstone formation in patients with erythropoietic protoporphyria.

Treatment of erythropoietic protoporphyria includes photoprotection with clothing and barrier sunscreens with zinc oxide or titanium dioxide. β-Carotene has been used, but response rates vary. Other treatment modalities include antihistamines, cysteine, N-acetylcysteine, and NB-UVB phototherapy. Afamelanotide is a synthetic analog of α-melanocyte–stimulating hormone that promotes melanin production and skin pigmentation, and studies have shown improved tolerance to sunlight with this therapy.[49] Regular monitoring of liver function is essential, and hepatic complications of erythropoietic protoporphyria should be treated with cholestyramine. Liver transplantation should be considered in advanced disease.

XERODERMA PIGMENTOSUM

Xeroderma pigmentosum (XP) is a rare autosomal recessive disease caused by defective nucleotide excision repair (NER) mechanisms. It is characterized by severe photosensitivity, lentigines, and early

development of ocular and cutaneous malignancies. Chronic sun exposure leads to poikilodermatous skin changes with hypo- and hyperpigmentation [**Figure 29-9**].[50] Clinical symptoms occur in early childhood with severe acute reactions to minimal sunlight exposure and skin cancers occurring within the first two decades of life. Abnormalities can be seen in any tissue exposed to sunlight. XP is caused by a defect in one of the seven XP genes, *XP-A* to *XP-G*, which are involved in the NER pathway. The prevalence is estimated at 1 in 1 million in Europe and the

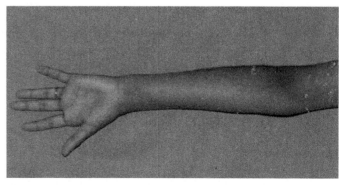

FIGURE 29-8. Erythropoietic protoporphyria. Lichenification and pseudovesicles involving the flexor forearm.

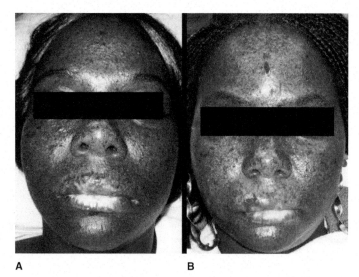

A   **B**

FIGURE 29-9. (A and B) Xeroderma pigmentosum. A 34-year-old African American woman with poikiloderma and mottled hypo- and hyperpigmentation. (Reproduced with permission from Orosco RK, Wang T, Byrne PJ. Xeroderma pigmentosum in an African-American. *ORL J Otorhinolaryngol Relat Spec.* 2011;73:162-165.)

United States.[51] Cases have been reported worldwide, including in Japan, North Africa, Nigeria, and Zimbabwe.[52,53] XP is more common in populations where consanguineous marriages are commonly practiced. This is demonstrated in the black Mayotte population in the Indian Ocean, which has a high incidence rate of 1 in 5000.[54]

An early diagnosis is important for disease management to facilitate the early detection and treatment of neoplasms. Clinical findings can be confirmed by laboratory assays showing defective DNA repair and skin fibroblast hypersensitivity to UV exposure. Sun protection education emphasizing coverage of all body surfaces with protective clothing, glasses, and wide-brim hats, as well as the daily use of sunscreens is very important. Patients should be monitored closely with interdisciplinary care including dermatologists, ophthalmologists, and pediatricians.

REFERENCES

1. Reichrath J. Skin cancer prevention and UV-protection: how to avoid vitamin D-deficiency? *Br J Dermatol.* 2009;161(Suppl 3):54-60.
2. de Gruijl FR. Skin cancer and solar UV radiation. *Eur J Cancer.* 1999;35:2003-2009.
3. Lim H, Honigsmann H, Hawk J. *Photodermatology.* New York, NY: Informa Healthcare; 2007.
4. Santoro FA, Lim HW. Update on photodermatoses. *Semin Cutan Med Surg.* 2011;30:229-238.
5. Stamatas GN, Zmudzka BZ, Kollias N, et al. Non-invasive measurements of skin pigmentation in situ. *Pigment Cell Res.* 2004;17:618-626.
6. Ito S, Wakamatsu K. Quantitative analysis of eumelanin and pheomelanin in humans, mice, and other animals: a comparative review. *Pigment Cell Res.* 2003;16:523-531.
7. Kadekaro AL, Kavanagh RJ, Wakamatsu K, et al. Cutaneous photobiology. The melanocyte vs. the sun: who will win the final round? *Pigment Cell Res.* 2003;16:434-447.
8. Thody AJ, Higgins EM, Wakamatsu K, et al. Pheomelanin as well as eumelanin is present in human epidermis. *J Invest Dermatol.* 1991;97:340-344.
9. Alaluf S, Atkins D, Barrett K, et al. Ethnic variation in melanin content and composition in photoexposed and photoprotected human skin. *Pigment Cell Res.* 2002;15:112-118.
10. Bustamante J, Bredeston L, Malanga G, et al. Role of melanin as a scavenger of active oxygen species. *Pigment Cell Res.* 1993;6:348-353.
11. Tada M, Kohno M, Niwano Y. Scavenging or quenching effect of melanin on superoxide anion and singlet oxygen. *J Clin Biochem Nutr.* 2010;46:224-228.
12. Mitra D, Luo X, Morgan A, et al. An ultraviolet-radiation-independent pathway to melanoma carcinogenesis in the red hair/fair skin background. *Nature.* 2012;491:449-453.

13. Wenczl E, Van der Schans GP, Roza L, et al. (Pheo)melanin photosensitizes UVA-induced DNA damage in cultured human melanocytes. *J Invest Dermatol.* 1998;111:678-682.
14. Murphy GM. Diseases associated with photosensitivity. *J Photochem Photobiol B.* 2001;64:93-98.
15. Tuchinda C, Srivannaboon S, Lim HW. Photoprotection by window glass, automobile glass, and sunglasses. *J Am Acad Dermatol.* 2006;54:845-854.
16. Nyberg F, Skoglund C, Stephansson E. Early detection of epidermal dust-like particles in experimentally UV-induced lesions in patients with photosensitivity and lupus erythematosus. *Acta Derm Venereol.* 1998;78:177-179.
17. Que SK, Brauer JA, Soter NA, et al. Normal minimal erythema dose responses in patients with suspected photosensitivity disorders. *Photodermatol Photoimmunol Photomed.* 2012;28:320-321.
18. Mehta RV, Shenoi SD, Balachandran C, et al. Minimal erythema response (MED) to solar simulated irradiation in normal Indian skin. *Indian J Dermatol Venereol Leprol.* 2004;70:277-279.
19. Wee LK, Chong TK, Quee DK. Assessment of skin types, skin colours and cutaneous responses to ultraviolet radiation in an Asian population. *Photodermatol Photoimmunol Photomed.* 1997;13:169-172.
20. Sanclemente G, Zapata JF, Garcia JJ, et al. Lack of correlation between minimal erythema dose and skin phototype in a Colombian scholar population. *Skin Res Technol.* 2008;14:403-409.
21. Honigsmann H. Polymorphous light eruption. *Photodermatol Photoimmunol Photomed.* 2008;24:155-161.
22. Kontos AP, Cusack CA, Chaffins M, et al. Polymorphous light eruption in African Americans: pinpoint papular variant. *Photodermatol Photoimmunol Photomed.* 2002;18:303-306.
23. Chiam LY, Chong WS. Pinpoint papular polymorphous light eruption in Asian skin: a variant in darker-skinned individuals. *Photodermatol Photoimmunol Photomed.* 2009;25:71-74.
24. Morison WL, Stern RS. Polymorphous light eruption: a common reaction uncommonly recognized. *Acta Derm Venereol.* 1982;62:237-240.
25. Kerr HA, Lim HW. Photodermatoses in African Americans: a retrospective analysis of 135 patients over a 7-year period. *J Am Acad Dermatol.* 2007;57:638-643.
26. Norris PG, Hawk JL. Polymorphic light eruption. *Photodermatol Photoimmunol Photomed.* 1990;7:186-191.
27. Smith E, Kiss F, Porter RM, et al. A review of UVA-mediated photosensitivity disorders. *Photochem Photobiol Sci.* 2012;11:199-206.
28. Kolgen W, Van Weelden H, Den Hengst S, et al. CD11b+ cells and ultraviolet-B-resistant CD1a+ cells in skin of patients with polymorphous light eruption. *J Invest Dermatol.* 1999;113:4-10.
29. Schornagel IJ, Sigurdsson V, Nijhuis EH, et al. Decreased neutrophil skin infiltration after UVB exposure in patients with polymorphous light eruption. *J Invest Dermatol.* 2004;123:202-206.
30. Janssens AS, Pavel S, Out-Luiting JJ, et al. Normalized ultraviolet (UV) induction of Langerhans cell depletion and neutrophil infiltrates after artificial UVB hardening of patients with polymorphic light eruption. *Br J Dermatol.* 2005;152:1268-1274.
31. Lim HW, Morison WL, Kamide R, et al. Chronic actinic dermatitis. An analysis of 51 patients evaluated in the United States and Japan. *Arch Dermatol.* 1994;130:1284-1289.
32. Que SK, Brauer JA, Soter NA, et al. Chronic actinic dermatitis: an analysis at a single institution over 25 years. *Dermatitis.* 2011;22:147-154.
33. Abarca JF, Casiccia CC, Zamorano FD. Increase in sunburns and photosensitivity disorders at the edge of the Antarctic ozone hole, southern Chile, 1986-2000. *J Am Acad Dermatol.* 2002;46:193-199.
34. Diffey B. Climate change, ozone depletion and the impact on ultraviolet exposure of human skin. *Phys Med Biol.* 2004;49:R1-R11.
35. Kyu-Won C, Chae-Young L, Yeong-Kyu L, et al. A Korean experience with chronic actinic dermatitis during an 18-year period: meteorological and photoimmunological aspects. *Photodermatol Photoimmunol Photomed.* 2009;25:286-292.
36. Hawk JL, Magnus IA. Chronic actinic dermatitis—an idiopathic photosensitivity syndrome including actinic reticuloid and photosensitive eczema [proceedings]. *Br J Dermatol.* 1979;101(Suppl 17):24.
37. Hawk JL. Chronic actinic dermatitis. *Photodermatol Photoimmunol Photomed.* 2004;20:312-314.
38. Chew AL, Bashir SJ, Hawk JL, et al. Contact and photocontact sensitization in chronic actinic dermatitis: a changing picture. *Contact Dermatitis.* 2010; 62:42-46.
39. Rizwan M, Haylett AK, Richards HL, et al. Impact of photosensitivity disorders on the life quality of children. *Photodermatol Photoimmunol Photomed.* 2012;28:290-292.

40. Torres-Alvarez B, Baranda L, Fuentes C, et al. An immunohistochemical study of UV-induced skin lesions in actinic prurigo. Resistance of Langerhans cells to UV light. *Eur J Dermatol.* 1998;8:24-28.

41. Daldon PE, Pascini M, Correa M. Case for diagnosis. Actinic prurigo. *An Bras Dermatol.* 2010;85:733-735.

42. Botto NC, Warshaw EM. Solar urticaria. *J Am Acad Dermatol.* 2008;59:909-920.

43. Lankerani L, Baron ED. Photosensitivity to exogenous agents. *J Cutan Med Surg.* 2004;8:424-431.

44. Puy H, Gouya L, Deybach JC. Porphyrias. *Lancet.* 2010;375:924-937.

45. Lambrecht RW, Thapar M, Bonkovsky HL. Genetic aspects of porphyria cutanea tarda. *Semin Liver Dis.* 2007;27:99-108.

46. Sarkany RP. Making sense of the porphyrias. *Photodermatol Photoimmunol Photomed.* 2008;24:102-108.

47. Michaels BD, Del Rosso JQ, Mobini N, et al. Erythropoietic protoporphyria: a case report and literature review. *J Clin Aesthet Dermatol.* 2010;3:44-48.

48. Balwani M, Bloomer J, Desnick R. Erythropoietic protoporphyria, autosomal recessive. *GeneReviews.* September 27, 2012.

49. Harms JH, Lautenschlager S, Minder CE, et al. Mitigating photosensitivity of erythropoietic protoporphyria patients by an agonistic analog of alpha-melanocyte stimulating hormone. *Photochem Photobiol.* 2009;85:1434-1439.

50. Orosco RK, Wang T, Byrne PJ. Xeroderma pigmentosum in an African-American. *ORL J Otorhinolaryngol Relat Spec.* 2011;73:162-165.

51. Kleijer WJ, Laugel V, Berneburg M, et al. Incidence of DNA repair deficiency disorders in western Europe: xeroderma pigmentosum, Cockayne syndrome and trichothiodystrophy. *DNA Repair (Amst).* 2008;7:744-750.

52. Ahmed H, Hassan RY, Pindiga UH. Xeroderma pigmentosum in three consecutive siblings of a Nigerian family: observations on oculocutaneous manifestations in black African children. *Br J Ophthalmol.* 2001;85:110-111.

53. Chidzonga MM, Mahomva L, Makunike-Mutasa R, et al. Xeroderma pigmentosum: a retrospective case series in Zimbabwe. *J Oral Maxillofac Surg.* 2009;67:22-31.

54. Cartault F, Nava C, Malbrunot AC, et al. A new XPC gene splicing mutation has lead to the highest worldwide prevalence of xeroderma pigmentosum in black Mahori patients. *DNA Repair (Amst).* 10;10:577-585.

CHAPTER 30

Erythema Dyschromicum Perstans (Ashy Dermatosis) and Related Disorders

Degambar D. Banodkar
Pravin Degambar Banodkar
Kruti Pravin Banodkar
Priyanka G. K. Banodkar

KEY POINTS

- Erythema dyschromicum perstans (EDP) primarily affects Latin Americans but is also seen in darker-pigmented people and Asians; it is rarely seen in non-Hispanic Caucasians.

- EDP is also known as *dermatitis cenicienta* ("ashy dermatosis"), *los cenicientos* ("the ashy ones"), and erythema chronicum figuratum melanodermicum, and pintoid.

- The pathogenesis is elusive, and often no etiologic cause can be assigned to the disease.

- EDP is characterized by asymptomatic, progressive, and often symmetrically distributed hyperpigmented macules and patches.

- Modest success has been reported with clofazimine and dapsone therapy.

SYNONYMS

- Erythema dyschromicum perstans
- Ashy dermatosis
- Dermatosis cenicienta

- Erythema chronicum figuratum melanodermicum
- Pintoid

INTRODUCTION

Erythema dyschromicum perstans (EDP) is a chronic, acquired, rare pigmentary disorder most commonly reported in Hispanics, but it also occurs worldwide, especially in those with darker-pigmented skin.

This condition was first reported by Ramirez in El Salvador in 1957.[1] He called these patients *los cenicientos*, meaning "ashy ones." In Spanish, the word *cenicienta* refers to the folklore character Cinderella, who had an ash-dirtied face due to constantly sitting close to the fireplace at home.[2] It is also known as ashy dermatosis because of the ashy gray color exhibited by the Tyndall effect due to pigment incontinence in the dermis. The term erythema dyschromicum perstans was coined by Venezuelan physician Marion Sulzberger to highlight the word *erythema* because an erythematous border is observed in the early lesions and also to suggest the variety and persistence of the dyschromia.[3,4] In South Africa, EDP is also referred to as erythema chronicum figuratum melanodermicum.

Although EDP is a distinct entity, little progress has been made in elucidating its pathogenesis or finding effective treatments. In the past, many considered it a controversial entity and regarded it as a form of lichen planus or lichen planus actinicus.[5-7] A proposed clinical classification has been devised, dividing ashy dermatosis from EDP, with the former lacking the erythematous borders, and then adding a third category for simulators such as the lichen planus variety and medication-induced melanodermas.[8]

CLINICAL PRESENTATION

Individuals with Fitzpatrick skin types III to VI are predominantly affected. Most diagnosed patients are Latin American; however, the disease has been described in Asians and darker-pigmented people, but rarely in non-Hispanic Caucasians. It has been reported in most regions of the world. There is no clear sex predilection, although several reviews relate a slightly higher incidence in women.[4,9,10] The disease predominantly affects adults between the second and third decades of life but can occur at any age, including in prepubertal children as young as 2 years of age [**Table 30-1**].[11]

The onset of the disease is insidious, and it usually spreads widely before patients seek medical treatment.[10] The classic clinical presentation is characterized by the rapid eruption of asymptomatic (rarely pruritic), progressive, and often symmetrically distributed hyperpigmented macules and patches in shades that range from slate gray to lead-colored to silvery brown in different individuals[12] [**Figures 30-1 to 30-3**]. The lesions may be round, oval, or more commonly polycyclic, and gradually extend peripherally. They develop over nearly any body part but more commonly arise on the torso and proximal upper extremities, followed by the neck and face, and spread over weeks or months.[13] The oral and genital mucosa, scalp, nails, palms, and soles are excluded. This distinction is useful for differentiating this entity from lichen planus, which

TABLE 30-1 Clinical presentation of erythema dyschromicum perstans

Affects adults between second and third decades of life

Insidious onset

Characterized by asymptomatic, progressive, and often symmetrical macules and patches, ranging in color from slate gray to silvery brown

Lesions may be round, oval, or more commonly polycyclic and tend to extend peripherally

Commonly occurs on torso and proximal upper extremities

Early lesions display a slightly elevated 1- or 2-mm erythematous margin that resolves by the time the patient seeks dermatologic care

Although the pigmentation is recalcitrant, it resolves by itself in some patients, but is more frequently found in pediatric patients

FIGURE 30-1. Classic erythema dyschromicum perstans in a woman on her lumbosacral area with characteristically bluish gray-hued pigmented patches.

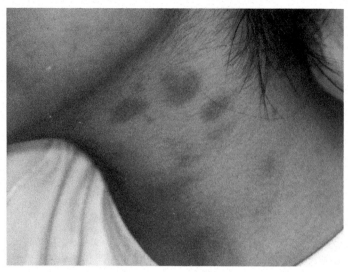

FIGURE 30-3. Round and oval lesions, in a typical grayish brown color, on the neck of a young female patient with erythema dyschromicum perstans.

frequently involves mucosal surfaces, and secondary syphilis, which commonly affects the palms and soles.[14] The eruption can become considerably widespread and involve a large surface area of the body, leading to considerable cosmetic disfigurement and contributing to profound psychological stress.[11-14]

Early lesions may display a slightly elevated, 1- to 2-mm erythematous margin, indicating that a fleeting inflammatory process leads to the subsequent long-standing pigmentary alteration.[9-14] When present, this finding is particularly helpful in establishing a diagnosis and provides the most characteristic histopathologic changes to confirm the clinical impression, but often the erythema has resolved by the time the patient seeks dermatologic care.[10,12-15]

An incontinentia pigmenti pattern with ashy-colored linear and reticulate patches involving Blaschko lines on the chest, back, and abdomen has been described in the literature.[15] Yokozeki et al[16] described unilateral ashy dermatosis distributed along Blaschko lines in the first reported case in 2005. Since then, many cases of unilateral EDP have been reported, and unilateral eruptions may represent resolving linear lichen planus pigmentosus.[16,17] Cases of ashy dermatosis with concomitant vitiligo or lichen planopilaris are rare.

A recent series described the findings in 14 children and found an additional 25 children reported in the literature.[11] No trigger factors were identified. Compared with adults, resolution of pigmentation occurs more frequently in children, with half of pediatric cases experiencing eventual improvement over 2 to 3 years.[11,18]

PATHOGENESIS AND PRECIPITATING FACTORS

The pathogenesis of the disease remains elusive. Anecdotally reported precipitating factors include exposure to the fungicide chlorothalonil during fumigation of banana plantations, intestinal whipworm infection (for which effective eradication resulted in lesional remission), orally administered radiographic contrast media, ingestion of ammonium nitrate, chronic hepatitis C or human immunodeficiency virus infections, endocrinopathies, occupational cobalt allergy in plumbers, and intentional ingestion of the fertilizer ammonium nitrite by a truant youth [**Table 30-2**].[4,13] However, in most cases, no apparent cause could be demonstrated, and the etiologic importance of most of these factors is disputable. Some have proposed that EDP is not a specific disease entity, but that the lesions constitute a variant of postinflammatory hyperpigmentation and represent the end stage of a nonspecific inflammatory response.[19]

However, immunopathologic investigations of active EDP implicate the role of immune modulation. It has been proposed that an aberrant immune response targeting basal cell layer antigens may initiate the disease process. Miyagawa et al[8] detected increased expression of intercellular adhesion molecule-1 (ICAM-1) and major histocompatibility complex class II molecules (human leukocyte antigen-DR) within the basal cell layer.[8] Ia antigen expression of keratinocytes and pronounced OKT5 and OKT6 staining of Langerhans cells have been demonstrated. In addition, the presence of thrombospondin receptor CD36 has been identified in the strata *spinosum* and granulosum of EDP lesional skin.

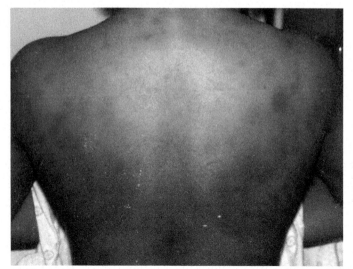

FIGURE 30-2. Classic erythema dyschromicum perstans on the back area of a patient with slate gray to lead-colored, symmetrically distributed, hyperpigmented macules and patches.

TABLE 30-2	Pathogenesis and precipitating factors of erythema dyschromicum perstans

- Pathogenesis still remains elusive
- Precipitating factors anecdotally reported include the following:
  1. Exposure to fungicide chlorothalonil
  2. Intestinal whipworm infections
  3. Oral administration of radiographic contrast media
  4. Ingestion of ammonium nitrate
  5. Chronic hepatitis C infection
  6. Human immunodeficiency virus infection
  7. Endocrinopathies
  8. Cobalt allergies
  9. Ingestion of ammonium nitrite
- Immune modulation targeting basal cell layer antigens has been implicated

This is ordinarily absent in normal skin but characteristically found in inflammatory cutaneous diseases.[20]

DIAGNOSIS

The diagnosis of EDP relies predominantly on clinical observation and is only supported by nonpathognomonic histopathologic features.[12] The main benefit of a biopsy is usually the exclusion of other diagnoses in consideration rather than confirmation of the diagnosis of ashy dermatosis. Examination of the inflamed, active border reveals mild basal cell layer vacuolar degeneration with occasional scattered colloid bodies, hyperkeratosis, a prominent granular layer, and minimal focal parakeratosis.[10] The superficial dermis may be edematous and shows a mild to moderate, often patchy lichenoid infiltrate of lymphocytes and histiocytes intermingled with melanophages that extends minimally to the mid-dermis, where the pattern is more perivascular.[14] The infiltrate contains both helper/inducer and suppressor/cytotoxic lymphocytes. There is also prominent pigment incontinence in the upper dermis with variable basal cell hypermelanosis. Plasma cells and eosinophils are inconspicuous. In contrast, biopsies from older patches show compact hyperkeratosis and histologic features consistent with postinflammatory dermal hyperpigmentation, including a scant perivascular mononuclear infiltrate with numerous melanin-laden macrophages in the dermis.[12]

The vacuolization of the epidermal basal cells in early lesions suggests that the basal cell layer is a principal target, with the resulting pigment incontinence contributing to the characteristic ashy-gray color. Such a finding has triggered the hypothesis that an aberrant immune response targeting basal cell layer antigens incites the disease process. Inflammation is less severe than that seen in lichen planus but may extend more deeply.[13] Immunofluorescence is similar to that seen in lichen planus, namely, colloid bodies with possible immunoglobulin (Ig) M or IgG deposition with complement and fibrin occasionally located at the interface.[13]

DIFFERENTIAL DIAGNOSIS

The differential diagnosis includes a number of eruptions with increased pigmentation [**Table 30-3**]. Some of these diseases can be difficult to differentiate clinically and even histopathologically from EDP even by healthcare providers with experience in pigmentary disorders. A common practice is to clinically diagnose any ashy-colored eruption as EDP; however, this hue may be produced by a number of factors, including the depth of the melanin in the dermis or deposits of metal salts. Although most of these eruptions are merely disfiguring, more serious diseases, such as urticaria pigmentosa and pigmented cutaneous T-cell lymphoma, need to be considered. The presence of the Darier sign in the former and of scaling in the latter helps to exclude ashy dermatosis, but microscopic skin examination is reassuring and valuable in confirming the correct diagnosis.

■ POSTINFLAMMATORY HYPERPIGMENTATION

Postinflammatory hyperpigmentation is the most common pigmentary problem in skin of color (see Chapter 52). Although seemingly omnipresent in dark tan to brown skin, hyperpigmentation also commonly develops after the active stages of inflammatory or infectious skin diseases or trauma in persons with Fitzpatrick skin type III from Hispanic, Native American, Middle Eastern, and Asian backgrounds. Melanogenesis and pigment incontinence are further exacerbated by scratching or rubbing. Notably, the erythema may be unappreciable on visual inspection, so early inflammatory lesions may not be detected by the patient or even the physician.[21]

Although many skin diseases produce demarcated patches and plaques that can heal with increased pigmentation, the ones more frequently misdiagnosed clinically as EDP include pityriasis rosea, nummular eczema, contact dermatitis, lichen planus, drug eruptions, syphilis, and pityriasis lichenoides chronica. Histopathologic examination can help to exclude these diseases if the classic changes of the causative dermatosis are present or if there is absence of dermal melanophages. An important consideration in formulating the treatment plan is that melanogenesis can be sustained for weeks after clinical resolution of inflammation, indicating that there may be value in continuing anti-inflammatory therapy even after signs of inflammation are no longer detectable. Ultraviolet (UV) light worsens and perpetuates hyperpigmentation, so the use of sunblock or UV-protective clothing is essential. Untreated, pigmentation can persist for many months, especially if there is a dermal component.

■ PITYRIASIS ROSEA

Pityriasis rosea is a common benign erythematous papulosquamous disease (see Chapter 25). An initial oval or round, larger, salmon-colored patch with dark red edges (the herald patch) often appears days or weeks prior to involvement of the trunk and proximal extremities. The lesions may appear gray on patients with darker skin shades. However, the eruption usually consists of small, oval patches or barely raised plaques of uniform size with a circumferential collar of fine scale. The lesions are oriented in a 'Christmas tree' pattern with their long axes following the lines of cleavage. The incidence increases in the spring and fall. Typically, the face is spared. Another differentiation is that pruritus is present in 75% of patients, whereas EDP is nearly always asymptomatic. However, in about 20% of patients, the eruption is atypical and more challenging diagnostically. These variants are more common in persons with skin of color. In some of these cases, the lesions may erupt predominantly on the extremities or in the axillae or groin. The lesions may be large (gigantic), urticarial, vesicular, pustular, purpuric, or erythema multiforme-like. The natural history of pityriasis rosea is spontaneous resolution in approximately 6 weeks, in contrast to the persistent hyperpigmentation of ashy dermatosis.

In children with darker-pigmented skin, the clinical presentation of pityriasis rosea differs in several ways from the classical textbook descriptions. Facial involvement is seen in 30% of those with pityriasis, and the scalp is scalier 8% more often than cases described in the Caucasian population. The disease process resolves in nearly 50% of patients within 2 weeks. Residual postinflammatory hyperpigmentation is observed in nearly 48% of patients, whereas hypopigmentation is seen in 29% of patients, especially the papular and papulovesicular varieties.[22]

Many authors have reported cases of idiopathic eruptive macular hyperpigmentation (IEMP) following pityriasis rosea. They consider it an atypical form of pityriasis rosea and have proposed it be considered pigmentogenes pityriasis rosea.[23-25]

■ LICHEN PLANUS PIGMENTOSUS

Lichen planus actinicus (see Chapter 26), also known as lichen planus tropicus, lichen planus subtropicus, and summertime actinic lichenoid dermatitis, is often considered synonymous with lichen planus pigmentosus. However, there are features in lichen planus pigmentosus that permit differentiation. This rare condition preferentially affects children and young adults. Most important among its symptoms are the predominance of lesions over areas exposed to UV light, a tendency to remit in winter, the presence of erythema in some lesions at the time of diagnosis, and the absence of lesions from intertriginous areas.[26]

TABLE 30-3	Differential diagnosis of related disorders

Postinflammatory hyperpigmentation
Lichen planus pigmentation
Pityriasis rosea
Idiopathic eruptive macular pigmentation
Drug-induced pigmentation
Friction melanosis
Macular amyloidosis
Linear atrophoderma of Moulin
Confluent and reticulate papillomatosis (Gougerot-Carteaud syndrome)
Prurigo pigmentosa
Acquired relapsing Blaschko dermatitis

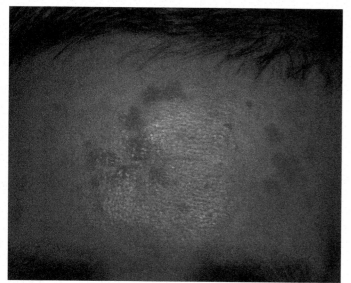

FIGURE 30-4. Lichen planus presenting with erythematous papules and plaques on the forehead.

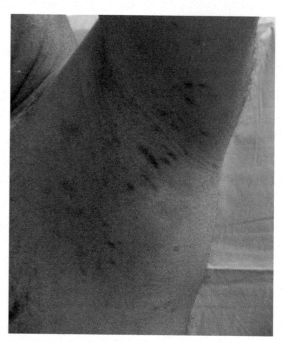

FIGURE 30-5. Violaceous macules and papules that rapidly became deeply pigmented, characteristic of lichen planus pigmentosus.

Four morphologic patterns have been reported: annular, dyschromic, plaque-like, and pigmented.[26] In the annular form, the lesions are ringlike erythematous papules and plaques that become pigmented. In addition to the histologic changes characteristic of lichen planus, there is significant pigment incontinence [**Figure 30-4**]. The dyschromic type is characterized by small, white, angular papules that coalesce into plaques on the neck and dorsum of the hands. In the classic plaquelike type, the lesions are those of lichen planus, but the distribution is predominantly over sun-exposed areas. Notably, severe pruritus, the Koebner phenomenon, and mucous membrane involvement are not common features of lichen planus actinicus. Lichen planus pigmentosus predominates in Latin American, Middle Eastern, Asian, and other persons with Fitzpatrick skin types III to V. The eruption consists of oval and round macules and small patches that develop insidiously on sun-exposed body regions, usually the face (especially the preauricular area and temples) and neck and uncommonly the trunk and upper extremities.[27] The lesions can become diffuse. The color is usually brown, but in darker skin shades, the hue may be gray-brown or slate gray. The lesions are pruritic in over half of the patients affected. Reticulate and perifollicular patterns also have been described. In one patient, there was progressive diffuse darkening of the entire face. Flexural involvement over the axilla, inframammary folds, and occasionally the groin is present in some patients, and the lesions may be limited to intertriginous areas, prompting the term lichen planus pigmentosus inversus[28] [**Figure 30-5**]. Antecedent erythema is reportedly absent. The palms and soles are spared, but lesions may arise on the mucous membranes. Bluish-black pigmentation diffusely present bilaterally over the buccal mucosa and lateral borders of the tongue has been described, but it is not certain if these changes simply represent common pigmentation patterns in dark-skinned patients. The eruption is symmetric in approximately 90% of patients and is limited to 10% or less of the body's surface area in two-thirds of patients, although occasionally, the lesions may involve more than 50% of the skin's surface.[27]

Linear lichen planus pigmentosus, the combined type of lichen planus pigmentosus and linear lichen planus, is rare. Pigmented macules and patches appear in a zosteriform pattern that seems to follow the lines of Blaschko. The clinical features are similar to those of EDP but can be distinguished first by the characteristic distribution and second by the older mean age at onset (commonly the fourth to fifth decades for lichen planus pigmentosus vs the second to third decades for EDP), and lastly, by the coexistence of classic lichen planus lesions in up to 20% of patients.[27] The course is characterized by exacerbations and remissions that occasionally are accompanied by pruritus. Histopathologic changes consist of a usually perivascular rather than lichenoid mononuclear dermal infiltrate with numerous melanophages in the papillary dermis.

Beneath the epidermis, there are densely aggregated eosinophilic bodies surrounded by periodic acid–Schiff stain (PAS)-positive remnant basement membrane with vacuolar degeneration of the basal layer. The eosinophilic bodies are immunoreactive with keratin, and it has been suggested that they represent the denatured epidermal rete ridge damaged by apoptotic changes. Hyperkeratosis and epidermal thinning are present in some cases.

IDIOPATHIC ERUPTIVE MACULAR PIGMENTATION

IEMP is a pigmentary dermatosis of unknown etiology and is clinically characterized by asymptomatic brown-black benign macules and patches usually affecting the neck, trunk, and proximal extremities. It occurs in young patients aged 1 to 31 years and affects both sexes equally. The pigmentation does not require any specific treatment and is known to resolve on its own after several months. It mimics the diagnosis of lichen planus pigmentosus, EDP, mastocytosis, and postinflammatory hyperpigmentation. Histologically, it shows papillomatosis of the dermis with prominent pigmentation of the basal layer without any significant dermal infiltration.

In 1978, Degos et al[29] were the first to propose the term IEMP to designate the pigmented dermatosis that they and other authors had observed but that had been previously published under different terms. Most of these cases were published in the French literature.[29-32] However, de Galdeano et al[33] were the first to publish five cases of IEMP in the English literature in 1996, and many have followed since.

The pathogenesis of this condition still remains unclear. Sun or light exposure is not important because most of the lesions occur on photo-protected areas. Hormonal factors may be involved in increased production of the pigment because most of the patients are children and young adults.[33] Clinically there is no inflammation; however, the histopathologic analysis favors a subclinical focal interface inflammation process. Histologically the most common features are epidermal thickening with irregular basal cell pigmentation and discrete pigmentary incontinence with mild inflammation with focal lichenoid changes. The histology is similar at different times in the evolution of the disease. Ultrastructure investigations of IEMP show numerous mature melanosomes in the basal cell and suprabasal keratinocytes and macrophages containing clustered melanosomes, but no vacuolar pattern of the basal cell layer, discontinuity of the basal lamina, colloid bodies, or a lichenoid infiltrate that might indicate a diagnosis of lichen planus pigmentosus or EDP.[32,34]

According to de Galdeano et al,[33] the following criteria should be fulfilled to diagnose IEMP:

1. Eruption of brownish, nonconfluent, asymptomatic macules involving the trunk, neck, and proximal extremities in children and adolescents

2. The absence of preceding inflammatory lesions

3. No previous drug exposure

4. Basal cell layer hyperpigmentation of the epidermis and prominent dermal melanophages without visible basal layer damage or lichenoid inflammatory infiltrate

5. A normal mast cell count

IEMP can be differentiated from drug eruptions and postinflammatory pigmentation by a lack of history of medication intake or the absence of clinical manifestions of previous dermatosis affecting the dermoepidermal interface, such as lichen planus, lichenoid reactions, and erythema multiforme. A normal number of mast cells and an absence of Darier signs excludes mastocytosis. In EDP, the macules are an ashy color that tend to coalesce and have a raised erythematous border.

DRUG-INDUCED PIGMENTATION

Drug-induced pigmentation represents 10% to 20% of cases of acquired hyperpigmentation.[35] The most common drug eruptions that resemble EDP in darker-skinned persons are fixed drug, erythema multiforme, lichenoid, photosensitive, pityriasis rosea-like, or eczematous reactions. The pathogenesis depends on the agent, and the disorder may result from increased synthesis or incontinence of melanin, tissue deposition of the drug, synthesis of drug-induced pigments, or deposits of iron after a nonspecific cutaneous inflammation[35]. Lesions are frequently worsened by sun exposure.[35] The most frequently implicated drugs are nonsteroidal anti-inflammatory drugs, antimalarial agents, amiodarone, cytotoxic drugs, heavy metals, psychotropic drugs, and tetracyclines. Minocycline usually causes pigmentation on the face (especially over areas of prior inflammation, such as acne), blue-gray pigmentation on the pretibial areas and forearms, or a generalized darkening of the skin that is accentuated on sun-exposed areas. The pigmentation can be diffuse or patchy and may affect the nail beds, sclerae, conjunctivae, and oral mucosa. It has been reported that 4% of persons whose cumulative dose exceeds 100 g develop pigmentation.[35] The antimalarial agents chloroquine and hydroxychloroquine can cause a blue-black pigmentation that usually affects the face and anterior aspects of the lower legs. Clofazimine induces a diffuse reddish brown discoloration that accentuates inflammatory lesions. The photosensitive reaction associated with amiodarone can produce a slate-gray pigmentation in some patients. Widespread flagellate pigmented patches can be induced by bleomycin [**Figure 30-6**]. Other therapeutic agents that are notoriously implicated

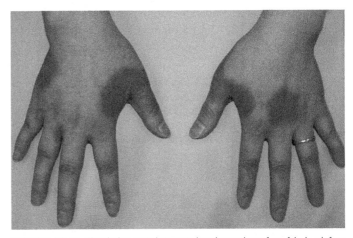

FIGURE 30-7. Sharply demarcated pigmented patches on the surface of the hands from a fixed drug eruption.

in patients with pigmentary alterations include carbamazepine, chlorpromazine, thioridazine, zidovudine, busulfan, cyclophosphamide, doxorubicin, bismuth, silver, and gold.

The characteristic lesion of a fixed drug eruption is a single (or multiple), circular or oval, erythematous, edematous, barely raised, occasionally centrally vesiculating plaque that becomes pigmented on any body region but preferentially on the hands [**Figure 30-7**], feet, and trunk. There may be stinging or, itching. Plaques commonly develop on the oral and genital mucosae, and mucous membranes may be the only region affected. In the nonpigmented variant, the lesions resolve in 2 to 3 weeks without residual hyperpigmentation. However, the disease also can present as pigmented patches that recur at fixed sites. The pigmentation becomes darker and larger with each recurrence. There is predilection for Blaschko lines, and a linear variant has been reported.[36] Morphologic variants include morbilliform, scarlatiniform, multiforme, eczematous, urticarial, and nodular forms. The eruption may be localized, generalized, bullous, or bullous necrotizing. Lesions erupt from 30 minutes to 8 hours after administration of the offending drug; however, they may rarely develop even in the absence of medications. Although this presentation is not characteristic, this reaction should be considered in the evaluation of any patient with discrete, demarcated hyperpigmentation.

Mizukawa and Shiohara[37] described a patient who was initially diagnosed as having EDP. However, on immunohistochemical biopsy evaluation, intraepidermal T-cells were identified between basal and suprabasal keratinocytes, suggesting a fixed drug eruption. The patient suffered recurrence even after the presumed culpable drug, theophylline, was withheld. The most frequently responsible drugs include the muscle relaxant chlorzoxazone, antibacterials (especially sulfonamides), nonsteroidal anti-inflammatory drugs (particularly piroxicam and mefenamic acid), β-blockers, carbamazepine, theophylline, and nifedipine.[37] It has been proposed that the drug induces tumor necrosis factor-α–dependent keratinocyte ICAM-1 expression in lesional skin, which, in turn, stimulates the activation of T-cells that cause selective damage to the epidermis. Recently, it has been suggested that expansion of interleukin-10–producing CD4+ and CD8+ T-cells may be responsible for the spontaneous resolution of the reaction.[38]

MACULAR AMYLOIDOSIS

Macular amyloidosis is a pruritic eruption consisting of dusky-brown or slate-gray macules symmetrically distributed over the upper back and, in some patients, the arms. It has a characteristic reticulated or rippled pattern of pigmentation. The deposits contain amyloid P (a nonfibrillar protein that is identical to serum plasma globulin and inhibits the activity of elastase) and altered keratins. The amyloid is either secreted by disrupted epidermal cells in the basal layer or is the end product of filamentous degeneration of necrotic epidermal cells that have been

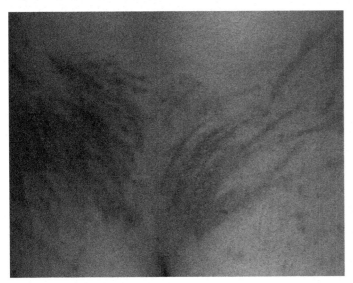

FIGURE 30-6. Pigmented streaks from a bleomycin reaction.

transformed by macrophages. The deposits are readily demonstrated with stains such as Congo red, PAS, and crystal violet.

FRICTION MELANOSIS

The lesions of friction melanosis can be either single or multiple, irregular, ill-defined, smooth, hyperpigmented patches secondary to repeated frictional trauma with rough materials such as scrub pads, loofahs, nylon towels, brushes, horse hair gloves, and tight clothing or caps [**Figure 30-8**]. It is found in obese people, similarly to intertrigo, on such areas as the upper thighs where skin rubs skin. It has also been reported in some non-obese individuals of Jewish faith; the lesions appeared as a result of the rigid backrests that rub against the lower back during the swaying activity associated with *Torah* study or *davening* (also known as Davener dermatosis). The pigmentation may be uniform or mottled. Cases may occur due to rubbing against stretch benches during exercise. These lesions develop more commonly in young adults. The prevalent areas involved are the clavicular zones, acromion, thyroid cartilage, vertebral spines, scapular and suprascapular areas, elbow and epicondyles, ulnar styloid, ulnar aspect of the forearms, forehead, and lateral aspect of the distal thighs.[39] When amyloid is present histologically, the condition is considered to be a form of macular amyloidosis, but amyloid deposits are not seen histologically in many patients (only 40% in one study).[40] Because in some cases amyloid may be seen in subsequent biopsies, it may appear reasonable to consider this entity as a variant of macular amyloidosis. Furthermore, in one study, amyloid was present in all cases under electron microscopy.[40] However, in contrast to the former, the lesions of friction melanosis are invariably asymptomatic and persist for longer than the typical 3- to 5-year duration of macular amyloidosis.

LINEAR ATROPHODERMA OF MOULIN

Linear atrophoderma of Moulin presents with discrete, hyperpigmented, well-demarcated patches that may be slightly depressed and follow Blaschko lines.[41] Early in the course, the atrophic changes may be subtle and not easy to detect clinically. Establishing a diagnosis can be particularly challenging because the only changes present may be irregular hyperpigmentation of the basal epidermis without dermal atrophy, pigment incontinence, inflammation, or alteration of connective tissue.[41] In some reported cases, depending on the stage of evolution, variable findings, such as a perivascular mononuclear infiltrate, sclerosis with thick collagen, decreased elastic fibers, and psoriasiform changes with hyperkeratosis and acanthosis, have been observed.

The contrast between normal and involved skin can be emphasized with an incisional biopsy across the border from lesional to clinically unaffected skin. The lesions first appear during childhood or adolescence and occasionally in early adulthood. Telangiectatic and inflammatory variants have been documented, and some have considered the entity as a linear variant of idiopathic atrophoderma of Pasini and Pierini, with 'cliff-drop' edges that distinguish affected and unaffected skin. The differential diagnosis includes pigmented skin conditions that appear in linear distribution or follow Blaschko lines. These include linear lichen planus pigmentosus, linear morphea, Goltz syndrome, linear and whorled nevoid hypermelanosis, a linear epidermal nevus, stage 3 of incontinentia pigmenti, X-linked reticulate pigmentary disorder, and a linear fixed or lichenoid drug eruption.

CONFLUENT AND RETICULATE PAPILLOMATOSIS

Confluent and reticulate papillomatosis, also known as Gougerot-Carteaud syndrome, involves 1- to 5-mm gray-brown, papillated, hyperkeratotic, barely raised papules that form plaques that become confluent centrally and reticulated at the periphery [**Figure 30-9**]. The first lesions usually appear in the intermammary area, chest, and midback. Subsequent lesions may develop in the neck, axillae, and upper abdomen. The disease is significantly more prevalent in people with darker pigmentation and in young women. Skin biopsies of involved skin show acanthosis, papillomatosis, hyperkeratosis, and an increased number of melanosomes in the stratum corneum. Most cases are sporadic, but familial cases have been described. A role for *Malassezia furfur,* which is frequently cultured from lesions, has been proposed. Some of these patients respond to antifungal therapy, raising speculation that the disease is a variant of pityriasis versicolor on seborrheic areas. However, other patients do not respond to antifungals but to minocycline or azithromycin, and yet others are therapeutically recalcitrant and require tazarotene or systemic retinoids.[42]

PRURIGO PIGMENTOSA

Prurigo pigmentosa is a recurrent inflammatory dermatosis characterized by pruritic, urticarial, erythematous papules and occasionally papulovesicles and vesicles arranged in reticular pattern and symmetrically distributed on the back, neck, and chest. The lesions heal within days, resulting in a retiform hyperpigmentation. Most reported cases have been young Japanese women, and the eruption is more common in the spring and summer. One case was caused by an allergy to chrome in a detergent[43]. Skin biopsy of early lesions shows a superficial perivascular infiltrate with neutrophils that invade the epidermis. Spongiosis, ballooning, and necrotic keratinocytes are present.[43] In late lesions, the infiltrate assumes a patchy lichenoid pattern with more eosinophils and

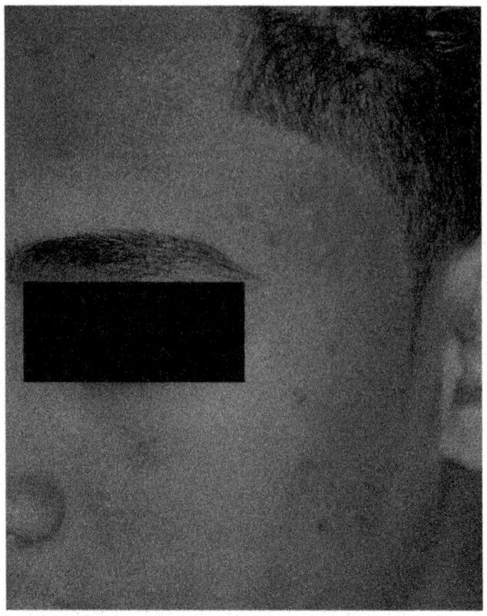

FIGURE 30-8. Friction melanosis on the face and neck as a result of rubbing with an exfoliative scrubber.

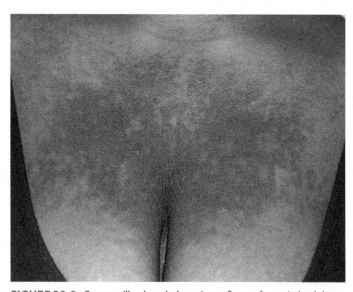

FIGURE 30-9. Brown papillated papules becoming confluent to form reticulated plaques on the chest in confluent and reticulate papillomatosis (Gougerot-Carteaud syndrome).

lymphocytes than neutrophils. There is epidermal vesiculation and, in some cases, vacuolar alteration at the dermal-epidermal junction. In the later stage, the epidermis becomes hyperplastic, parakeratotic, and studded with melanin, with melanophages appearing in the dermis.[43] Immunofluorescence is invariably negative. Notably, minocycline or doxycycline is usually effective in resolving symptoms as well as the pigmentation. Dapsone can be used in unresponsive cases.

ACQUIRED RELAPSING BLASCHKO DERMATITIS

Acquired relapsing Blaschko dermatitis presents with acquired, hyperpigmented, unilateral, occasionally scaly papules that become confluent and form plaques in a linear arrangement on the trunk and neck and heal spontaneously. Variants with papulovesicles and involvement of the palms and soles have been described. The lesions form a 'V' shape over the spine and an 'S' shape on the lateral and anterior aspects of the trunk because Blaschko lines assume these configurations over these areas due to movements of the skin during embryogenesis.[44] The eruption relapses, particularly during times of stress. On histopathologic examination, there is a superficial perivascular infiltrate of lymphocytes and eosinophils.[44] The epidermis is hyperplastic, and spongiosis and mounds of parakeratosis are present. Systemic corticosteroids have been found to be effective.

TREATMENT

EDP is a chronic, persistent, and rather resistant disorder and has no established therapy. It may persist unchanged for years, although some cases eventually resolve over a period of time, especially in prepubescent children. In a series of four patients followed up for 2 years in Finland, three showed spontaneous resolution.[45]

Many therapeutic modalities have been attempted without any satisfactory results. These include UV exposure, UV avoidance, antibiotics, antihistamines, griseofulvin, chemical peels, antibiotics, local and systemic corticosteroids, vitamins, isoniazid, chloroquine, and psychotherapy. The use of narrowband UVB phototherapy has been successful in a few patients.[46] A low-potency topical steroid applied twice a day to the affected areas may be used, with or without a 4% hydroquinone cream for the hyperpigmentation.[47] However, the most successful systemic treatment with modest response has been reported with clofazimine and dapsone in a few cases [**Table 30-4**].

In one series of eight patients,[48] seven had a good or excellent response to clofazimine administered either at 100 mg every other day to patients weighing less than 40 kg or at 100 mg every day to patients weighing more than 40 kg. This regimen was continued for 3 months and then reduced to 200 mg/wk and 400 mg/week, respectively. The one remaining patient had only a marginal response. One study found some improvement in early cases, but no cures were reported. This medication seems to have a valuable effect on the inflammatory phase of EDP.[49]

Clofazimine may be of some modest benefit via its anti-inflammatory and immunomodulatory effects.[50] The drug was found to reduce the expression of intercellular adhesion and lymphocyte activation molecules and decreased the mononuclear cell infiltrate. In seeming

contradiction, clofazimine exerts both proinflammatory and antiinflammatory effects. It serves as a hypochlorous acid forager, decreasing neutrophilic inflammation, and modifies monocytes and lymphoid cell function. Specifically, Piquero-Martin et al[51] found that clofazimine improved skin coloration, which correlated with attenuation of venous blood CD4:CD8 ratios.[51] Some have suggested that the drug's induction of a diffuse red-brown coloration helps to mask the pigmented lesions of EDP.

Dapsone also has been investigated in a few series and is reported to hasten resolution of pigmentation.[52] Because of the unavailability of clofazimine in some countries, dapsone has become a more popular treatment. Its effectiveness is possibly mediated through an immunomodulatory effect. Kontochristopoulos et al[53] reported regression of active disease, improvement of pigmentation, and cessation of the disease process with dapsone continued from 2 to 3 months. An adult dose of 100 mg daily is administered for at least 8 to 12 weeks.[53] Recently a large study by Hossain et al[54] was carried out on a total of 30 patients aged 20 to 60 years who had ashy dermatosis. All of the patients were diagnosed clinically with diagnosis confirmed by histopathologic examination. The patients were given dapsone 100 mg daily for 3 months, and follow-up was done for the next 3 months. Of 30 patients, 2 patients (6.66%) showed excellent response, 7 patients (23.33%) showed good response, 8 patients (26.66%) showed fair response, 8 patients (26.66%) showed poor response, and the remaining 5 patients (16.66%) did not show any response clinically. Thus, improvement was shown in 25 patients (83.33%), whereas 5 patients (16.66%) showed no improvement at all. This study suggests that dapsone has significant efficacy and is a treatment option in EDP. In an earlier report, a patient from Turkey was also described as responding remarkably well to treatment with dapsone.[52]

UV phototherapy is also known to help in the treatment of EDP. The photoimmunologic effects of UV phototherapy by the suppression of immune function and reduction in proinflammatory cytokines assist by exerting potent anti-inflammatory effects. UV phototherapy provides camouflage, which hides the dermal pigmentation by stimulating pigment production. In addition to hyperpigmentation, UV phototherapy also induces thickening of the stratum corneum and apoptosis of T-lymphocytes, which causes a decrease in the lichenoid inflammatory infiltrate that often is observed in active areas of EDP.[55] Narrowband UVB phototherapy has been used recently in the treatment of other lichenoid pigmentary disorders with success.[56] Therefore, it was proposed that UV light is an excellent and viable treatment option for patients with this difficult-to-treat disorder of pigmentation.

Hydroquinone and chemical peels are usually ineffective because the melanin deposition is found too deep in the dermis to achieve therapeutic concentrations.

Laser treatments have been disappointing. Nonablative 1550-nm fractional laser therapy was found to be ineffective for EDP and postinflammatory hyperpigmentation in a pilot study by Kroon et al.[57] The Neodymium-doped yttrium aluminium garnet (Nd:YAG) laser has been tested for the treatment of postinflammatory hyperpigmentation and melasma, also with disappointing results, and is not recommended in the treatment of ashy dermatosis.[58] Other lasers, like Q-switched ruby (694-nm), Q-switched Nd:YAG (1064-nm), and Q-switched alexandrite (755-nm) lasers, have also yielded disappointing results.

REFERENCES

1. Ramírez CO. *Los Cenicientos: Problema Clínico: Report of the First Central American Congress of Dermatology.* Vols 5-8. San Salvador, El Salvador: CACD; 1957:122-130.
2. Ramírez CO. The ashy dermatosis (erythema dyschromicum perstans): epidemiological study and report of 139 cases. *Cutis.* 1967;3:244-247.
3. Convit J, Kerdel-Vegas F. Erythema dyschromicum perstans a hitherto undescribed skin disease. *J Invest Dermatol.* 1961;36:457-462.
4. Schwartz RA. Erythema dyschromicum perstans: the continuing enigma of Cinderella or ashy dermatosis. *Int J Dermatol.* 2004;43:230-232.
5. Berger RS, Hayes TJ, Dixon SL. Erythema dyschromicum perstans and lichen planus: are they related? *J Am Acad Dermatol.* 1989;21:438-442.

TABLE 30-4 Treatment of erythema dyschromicum perstans

First line
- Topical low-potency corticosteroids
- Emollients
- Dapsone
- Clofazimine

Second line
- Narrowband ultraviolet B therapy

Other (anecdotal)
- Systemic corticosteroids
- Chloroquine
- Vitamins
- Isoniazid

6. Kark EC, Litt JZ. Ashy dermatosis: a variant of lichen planus? *Cutis.* 1980;25:631-633.

7. Naidorf KF, Cohen SR. Erythema dyschromicum perstans and lichen planus. *Arch Dermatol.* 1982;118:683-685.

8. Miyagawa S, Komatsu M, Oluchi T. Erythema dyschromicum perstans: immunopathologic studies. *J Am Acad Dermatol.* 1989;20:882-886.

9. Osswald SS, Proffer LH, Sartori CR. Erythema dyschromicum perstans: a case report and review. *Cutis.* 2001;68:25-28.

10. Pandya AG, Guevara IL. Disorders of hyperpigmentation. *Dermatol Clin.* 2000;18:91-98.

11. Torrelo A, Zaballos P, Colmenero I, et al. Erythema dyschromicum perstans in children: a report of 14 cases. *J Eur Acad Dermatol Venereol.* 2005;19:422-426.

12. Sanchez MR. Cutaneous diseases in Latinos. *Dermatol Clin.* 2003;21:689-697.

13. Dominguez-Soto L, Hojyo–Tomoka T, Vega M, et al. Pigmentary problems in the tropics. *Dermatol Clin.* 1994;12:777-784.

14. Sanchez MR. Dermatologic disease in Hispanics/Latinos. In: Halder R, ed. *Dermatology and Dermatological Therapy of Pigmented Skin.* Boca Raton, FL: CRC Press; 2005:357-384.

15. Vega ME, Waxtein L, Arenas R, et al. Ashy dermatosis and lichen planus pigmentosus: a clinicopathologic study of 31 cases. *Int J Dermatol.* 1992;31:90-94.

16. Yokozeki H, Ueno M, Komori K, et al. Multiple linear erythema dyschromicum perstans (ashy dermatosis) in the lines of Blaschko. *Dermatology.* 2005;210:356-357.

17. Akagi A, Ohnishi Y, Tajima S, et al. Linear hyperpigmentation with extensive epidermal apoptosis: a variant of linear lichen planus pigmentosus? *J Am Acad Dermatol.* 2004;50:S78-S80.

18. Silverberg NB, Herz J, Wagner A, et al. Erythema dyschromicum perstans in prepubertal children. *Pediatr Dermatol.* 2003;20:398-403.

19. Convit J, Piquero-Martin J, Perez RM. Erythema dyschromicum perstans. *Int J Dermatol.* 1989;28:168-169.

20. Baranda L, Torres-Alvarez B, Cortes-Franco R, et al. Involvement of cell adhesion and activation molecules in the pathogenesis of erythema dyschromicum perstans (ashy dermatosis): the effect of clofazimine therapy. *Arch Dermatol.* 1997;133:325-329.

21. Taylor SC. Enhancing the care and treatment of skin of color: I. The broad scope of pigmentary disorders. *Cutis.* 2005;76:249-255.

22. Amer A, Fischer H, Li X. The natural history of pityriasis rosea in black American children: how correct is the "classic" description? *Arch Pediatr Adolesc Med.* 2007;161:503-506.

23. Dupre A, Christol B, Albarel N, et al. Pigmentation eruptive maculeuse eruptive idiopathique. *Ann Dermatol Venereol.* 1980;107:413-417.

24. de Galdeano SC, Léauté-Labrèze C, Bioulac-Sage P, et al. Idiopathic eruptive macular pigmentation: report of five patients. *Pediatr Dermatol.* 1996;13:274-277.

25. Jang KA, Choi JH, Sung KS, et al. Idiopathic eruptive macular pigmentation: report of 10 cases. *J Am Acad Dermatol.* 2001;44:351-353.

26. Meads SB, Kunishige J, Ramos-Caro FA, et al. Lichen planus actinicus. *Cutis.* 2003;72:377-381.

27. Kanwar AJ, Dogra S, Handa S, et al. A study of 124 Indian patients with lichen planus pigmentosus. *Clin Exp Dermatol.* 2003;28:481-485.

28. Pock L, Jelinkova L, Drlik L, et al. Lichen planus pigmentosus-inversus. *J Eur Acad Dermatol Venereol.* 2001;15:452-454.

29. Degos R, Civatte J, Belaich S. La pigmentation maculeuse eruptive idiopathique. *Ann Dermatol Venereol.* 1978;105:177-182.

30. Blasco GF, de Unamuno P, Armijo M. Idiopathic eruptive macular pigmentation. *Actas Dermo-Sifiliogr.* 1979;70:639-644.

31. Dupre A, Christol B, Albarel N, et al. Pigmentation eruptive maculeuse idiophatique—au décours dún pityriasis rosé de Gibert. *Ann Dermatol Venereol.* 1980;107:413-417.

32. Plantin P, Le Berre A, Le Roux P, et al. Pigmentation maculeuse eruptive idiopathique. *Arch Fr Pediatr.* 1993;50:607-608.

33. de Galdeano CS, Leaute-Labreze C, Bioulac-Sage P, et al. Idiopathic eruptive macular pigmentation: report of five patients. *Pediatr Dermatol.* 1996;13:274-277.

34. Jang KA, Choi JH, Sung KS, et al. Idiopathic eruptive macular pigmentation: report of 10 cases. *J Am Acad Dermatol.* 2001;44:351-335.

35. Dereure O. Drug-induced skin pigmentation: epidemiology, diagnosis and treatment. *Am J Clin Dermatol.* 2001;2:253-262.

36. Megahed M, Reinauer S, Scharffetter-Kochanek K, et al. Acquired relapsing self-healing Blaschko dermatitis. *J Am Acad Dermatol.* 1994;31:849-852.

37. Mizukawa Y, Shiohara T. Fixed drug eruption presenting as erythema dyschromicum perstans: a flare without taking any medications. *Dermatology.* 1998;197:383-385.

38. Sehgal VN, Srivastava G. Fixed drug eruption (FDE): changing scenario of incriminating drugs. *Int J Dermatol.* 2006;45:897-908.

39. Al-Aboosi M, Abalkhail A, Kasim O, et al. Friction melanosis: a clinical, histologic, and ultrastructural study in Jordanian patients. *Int J Dermatol.* 2004;43:261-264.

40. Siragusa M, Ferri R, Cavallari V, et al. Friction melanosis, friction amyloidosis, macular amyloidosis, and towel melanosis: many names for the same clinical entity. *Eur J Dermatol.* 2001;11:545-548.

41. Miteva L, Nikolova K, Obreshkova E. Linear atrophoderma of Moulin. *Int J Dermatol.* 2005;44:867-869.

42. Davis MD, Weenig RH, Camilleri MJ. Confluent and reticulate papillomatosis (Gougerot-Carteaud syndrome): a minocycline-responsive dermatosis without evidence for yeast in pathogenesis. A study of 39 patients and a proposal of diagnostic criteria. *Br J Dermatol.* 2006;154:287-293.

43. Boer A, Misago N, Wolter M, et al. Prurigo pigmentosa: a distinctive inflammatory disease of the skin. *Am J Dermatopathol.* 2003;25:117-129.

44. Megahed M, Reinauer S, Scharffetter-Kochanek K, et al. Acquired relapsing self-healing Blaschko dermatitis. *J Am Acad Dermatol.* 1994;31:849-852.

45. Palatsi R. Erythema dyschromicum perstans. A follow-up study from northern Finland. *Dermatologica.* 1977;155:40-44.

46. Tlougan BE, Gonzalez ME, Mandal RV, et al. Erythema dyschromicum perstans. *Dermatol Online J.* 2010;16:17.

47. Muñoz C, Chang AL. A case of Cinderella: erythema dyschromicum perstans (ashy dermatosis or dermatosis cinecienta. *Skinmed.* 2011;9:63-64.

48. Schwartz RA. Erythema dyschromicum perstans treatment and management. http://emedicine.medscape.com/article/1122807-treatment. Accessed March 27, 2013.

49. Dermaamin. Erythema dyschromicum perstans. http://www.dermaamin.com/site/atlas-of-dermatology/5-e/465-erythema-dyschromicum-perstans-----.pdf. Accessed March 27, 2013.

50. Stratigos AJ, Katsambas AD. Optimal management of recalcitrant disorders of hyperpigmentation in dark-skinned patients. *Am J Clin Dermatol.* 2004;5:161-168.

51. Piquero-Martin J, Perez-Alfonzo R, Abrusci V, et al. Clinical trial with clofazimine for treating erythema dyschromicum perstans: evaluation of cell-mediated immunity. *Int J Dermatol.* 1989;28:198-200.

52. Bahadir S, Cobanoglu U, Cimsit G, et al. Erythema dyschromicum perstans: response to dapsone therapy. *Int J Dermatol.* 2004;43:220-222.

53. Kontochristopoulos G, Stavropoulos P, Pantelos D. Erythema dyschromicum perstans: response to dapsone therapy. *Int J Dermatol.* 1998;37:790-799.

54. Hossain MS, Bhuian I, Wahab A, et al. Outcome of dapsone in the treatment of ashy dermatosis. *Med Coll.* 2012;4:18-12.

55. Honigsmann H, Schwarz T. Ultraviolet therapy. In: Bolognia JL, Jorizzo JL, Schaffer JV, et al, eds. *Dermatology.* 2nd ed. New York, NY: Mosby Elsevier Limited; 2008:2053.

56. Kocaturk E, Kavala M, Zindanci I, et al. Narrowband UVB treatment of pigmented purpuric lichenoid dermatitis (Gougerot-Blum). *Photodermatol Photoimmunol Photomed.* 2009;25:55.

57. Kroon MW, Wind BS, Meesters AA, et al. Non-ablative 1550 nm fractional laser therapy not effective for erythema dyschromicum perstans and postinflammatory hyperpigmentation: a pilot study. *J Dermatolog Treat.* 2012;23:339-344.

58. Mosher TB, Fitzpatrick TB. Hypomelanoses and hypermelanoses. In: Freedberg IM, ed. *Fitzpatrick's Dermatology in General Medicine.* 5th ed. New York, NY: McGraw-Hill; 1999:996-1009.

CHAPTER 31

Amyloidosis

Richard S. Mizuguchi
Allen G. Strickler

KEY POINTS

- Amyloidosis is the deposition of amyloid, a group of unrelated proteins, in the extracellular space of various organs and tissues of the body.

- Amyloidosis is divided into primary systemic and localized cutaneous types.

- Primary cutaneous amyloidosis is subdivided into nodular, macular, and lichen types.

- Individuals with skin of color, particularly Asians, Arabs, and South Americans, appear to be predisposed to developing lichen amyloidosis.
- A review of common dermatologic diagnoses lists lichen amyloidosis as one of the 12 most common skin disorders affecting those of Asian ethnicity.
- The treatment options for amyloidosis are palliative, not curative, and alleviate the symptoms of pruritus.

INTRODUCTION

The term amyloid was coined in 1838 by Schleiden, a German botanist, to describe cellulose-like substances in plants.[1] *Amyloidosis* refers to the deposition of amyloid, a group of unrelated proteins in the extracellular space of various organs and tissues of the body, which leads to a pathologic change. Eosinophilic amorphous substances are seen through the use of a light microscope, and amyloid subtypes are composed of 7.5- to 10-nm-wide linear, nonbranching tubular fibrils. These are arranged in a meshwork pattern,[2] and each fibril has a β-pleated sheet configuration. However, the quaternary structure of these amyloids is not yet understood.[3]

Several classifications of amyloidosis exist. The original classification system divides the condition into primary or secondary types of either systemic or localized amyloidosis. Another more recent classification scheme designates amyloidosis as either acquired or hereditary. The clinical subtype will depend on the type of amyloid fibril protein that is deposited.

Systemic amyloidosis can be primary (AL) or secondary (AA). It can also be associated with other processes such as hemodialysis.[4] In primary systemic amyloidosis, the type of amyloid deposited is the immunoglobulin variable fragment designated as AL amyloid.[4,5] Serum amyloid A deposition is the cause of systemic AA amyloidosis. This form is typically associated with chronic inflammatory conditions such as Crohn disease, rheumatoid arthritis, dermatomyositis, cystic fibrosis, and lupus.[4] The skin can be variably affected in systemic amyloidosis. The cutaneous signs, which are more indicative of systemic involvement, include hemorrhages, waxy papules that are pruritic and/or hemorrhagic, macroglossia, and lesions resembling scleroderma.[6]

Like systemic amyloidosis, localized amyloidosis can be primary or secondary, but this form only affects a single tissue type. It can be deposited either in a diffuse manner or as discrete tumor-like formations.[7] Primary localized amyloidosis can affect tissues such as the heart, breast, lung, or urinary tract. Secondary localized amyloidosis can manifest in the cornea (due to inflammatory conditions such as syphilis), the thyroid (due to medullary thyroid cancer), or the skin (due to primary skin tumors).[4,8,9]

Localized cutaneous amyloidosis affects only the skin and can be subdivided into nodular, macular, lichenoid (papular), or secondary categories. Macular amyloidosis and lichen amyloidosis are thought to be different clinical manifestations of the same disease and both types can be seen in the same patient. This coexistent condition is termed biphasic amyloidosis. Secondary cutaneous amyloidosis is a result of amyloid deposition due to the presence of another primary skin condition. Some of these conditions include sweat gland tumors, dermatofibroma, pilomatrixoma, seborrheic keratosis, basal cell carcinoma, Bowen disease, actinic keratosis, and solar elastosis induced by psoralen and ultraviolet A (PUVA) therapy.[7]

Freudenthal first introduced the term lichen amyloidosis in 1930.[10] Individuals with skin of color, particularly Asians and Southeast Asians, Arabs, and South Americans, seem to be predisposed to developing localized cutaneous amyloidosis, especially lichen amyloidosis.[11-16] A review of common dermatologic diagnoses lists lichen amyloidosis as one of the 12 most common skin disorders affecting those of Asian ethnicity [**Table 31-1**]. The remainder of this chapter will include a discussion of primary cutaneous macular and nodular amyloidosis. However, the main focus will be on primary cutaneous lichen amyloidosis, as this is the form that more often affects patients with Fitzpatrick skin types III and IV.

TABLE 31-1 Common dermatologic diagnoses in Asian patients

Percentage	Diagnosis
20.4	Xerosis
19.3	Pruritus
16.8	Nummular dermatitis
14.2	Dyshidrosis
9.9	Atopic dermatitis
7.1	Melasma
4.5	Photodermatoses
4.2	Psoriasis
3.2	Vitiligo
2.3	Lichen amyloidosis (South Asian)
0.8	Nevus of Ito
2.0	Nevus of Ota

Source: Data from Halder R, Nootheti P. Ethnic hair and skin: what is the state of the science. *J Am Acad Dermatol.* 2003;48:S143-S148.

PATHOGENESIS

Many factors have been implicated as possible etiologic factors in lichen amyloidosis[17-21] [**Table 31-2**]. In primary localized cutaneous amyloidosis of the lichen and macular types, it is thought that the amyloid is derived from keratin peptides of an epidermal origin. These peptides are formed secondary to the necrotic keratinocytes.[22,23] The antikeratin antibodies are used to confirm the keratin epitopes of primary cutaneous amyloidosis.[22,24-30]

The exact mechanism of amyloid formation in lichen and macular amyloidosis is unknown and remains controversial. The presence of cytokeratins in primary cutaneous amyloidosis supports Hashimoto's fibrillar body theory of amyloidogenesis.[31] The theory proposes that epidermal basal keratinocytes are transformed into amyloid proteins. The cells that undergo apoptosis accumulate tonofilaments and form colloid bodies. These bodies are then modified by histiocytes and fibroblasts to form amyloid deposits.[31] This theory is supported by histologic[32] and ultrastructural[23] studies that demonstrate the transitional forms between keratinocytes and amyloids. The amyloidosis fibrillar body theory is further supported by the sequential changes in the antigenic profile from basal keratinocytes to amyloids, through cytoid bodies.[33] Further substantiating this theory are studies showing that amyloids, colloid bodies, and isolated keratin filaments can bind to amyloid P components and vitronectin.

In an alternative theory, Yamagihara et al[34] suggest that disrupted basal keratinocytes produce and secrete precursor proteins at the epidermal–dermal interface. This theory, known as the secretion theory, has been supported by ultrastructural evidence of a *lamina densa* disruption above the amyloid deposits in lichen amyloidosis.[35] Electron microscopic evidence of a *lamina densa* disruption, above the amyloid deposits, was found in patients with lichen and macular amyloidosis.[23] The deposits contained basement membrane antigens, such as types IV and VII collagen, laminin, a *lamina densa*-like substance, and a low dose antigen-1, which is a basement membrane component.[35]

The amyloid deposition in primary cutaneous nodular amyloidosis is quite different from that in the macular and lichen types. It is composed of κ and λ immunoglobulin light chains of the AL type.[36] The deposition typically occurs in the dermis, the small vessels of the dermis, and the

TABLE 31-2 Possible etiologic factors for lichen amyloidosis[15-19]

Prolonged friction (eg, from use of back scratchers)
Genetic predisposition
Epstein-Barr virus
Human immunodeficiency virus infection
Environmental factors

subcutaneous tissue.[36] In this form of amyloidosis, there is a definitive absence of cytokeratins, in contrast to the macular and lichen forms.[36]

CLINICAL PRESENTATION

Lichen amyloidosis is characterized by the multiple firm, discrete, hyperpigmented and hyperkeratotic, scaly papules that sometimes coalesce to form plaques [**Figure 31-1**]. Pruritus is a prominent feature of lichen amyloidosis. The sites of predilection are the shins or other extensor surfaces of the extremities.[37] Bullous lesions have been described in patients with lichen amyloidosis.[38] However, the bullous lesions are seen more frequently in those with systemic amyloidosis. Generalized lichen amyloidosis occurs very infrequently.[39,40]

Macular amyloidosis presents as pruritic pigmented macules and/or plaques often seen on the upper back, but sometimes on other areas of the trunk extremities.[6] An associated reticulated or rippled pigmentation

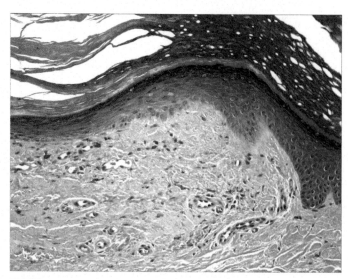

FIGURE 31-2. Using a hematoxylin and eosin stain, this figure shows hyperkeratosis with a thinning of the epidermis. In the papillary dermis, amyloid deposits are seen, as well as a sparse perivascular lymphohistiocytic infiltrate.

may also be visible.[41] Nodular amyloidosis is typified by grouped or solitary waxy nodules, with associated atrophic dermis and telangiectasias.[6]

A familial form of primary cutaneous amyloidosis occurs rarely. In all reported cases, inheritance was autosomal dominant. Although most families had skin of color,[42-46] there have also been reports of families with Fitzpatrick skin types I and II who had this form of amyloidosis.[47-51] Therefore, skin phototypes III and IV may not be a predisposing factor in familial macular and lichen amyloidosis.

PATHOLOGY

The amyloid deposits are restricted primarily to the papillary dermis and may displace the rete ridges. The epidermis above the deposits may show acanthosis or thinning and hyperkeratosis. There are often perivascular lymphohistiocytic infiltrates, as well as pigment incontinence [**Figure 31-2**].

Amyloid deposits can be better visualized through the use of special stains, and Congo red stain is the most effective. When this stain is combined with polarized light, amyloid deposits emit a characteristic apple-green birefringence. There are a variety of other histologic stains that may also be successful in staining amyloid deposits[52-55] [**Table 31-3**].

TREATMENT

Lichen and macular amyloidosis are chronic skin disorders that do not respond to any single treatment modality. The treatment options are palliative, not curative, and alleviate the symptoms of pruritus rather than removing the amyloid deposits [**Table 31-4**]. Possible precipitating and/or aggravating factors, such as chronic friction induced by scratching and rubbing, should be avoided.[56] In mild cases, topical corticosteroids (with or without occlusion) and intralesional corticosteroids are the first line of treatment.[57] The addition of a keratolytic agent, such as urea or salicylic acid, may also be beneficial. It has been shown that calcipotriol is effective in the treatment of lichen amyloidosis.[54] Tacrolimus has also been reported to have a beneficial effect.[58]

Dimethyl sulfoxide (DMSO) has been known as an effective treatment for both lichen and macular amyloidosis, although there are some refractory cases.[53,54,59] Application of DMSO 50% or 100% solutions will resolve pruritus. However, the reported side effects include irritant dermatitis and contact dermatitis/urticaria.[54] Phototherapy with ultraviolet B (UVB) and photochemotherapy (PUVA) should be considered in patients who do not respond to topical therapy.[55]

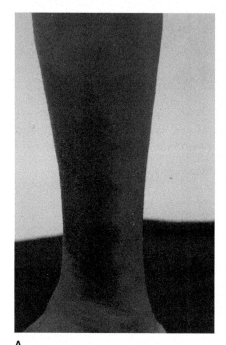

A

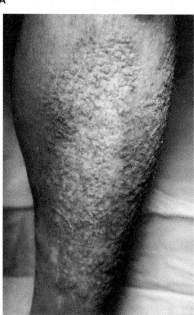

B

FIGURE 31-1. (A and B) Lichen amyloidosis displaying hyperpigmented and hyperkeratotic scaly papules coalescing into plaques on patients with darker skin of color.

TABLE 31-3	Histologic stains for amyloid deposits[48-50]

Highman's crystal and methyl violet

Benhold's Congo red

Orange G

Cotton dyes (Pagoda red, RIT® Scarlet No. 5, RIT® Cardinal Red No. 9)

Thiazole dye

Triphenylmethane dye

Periodic acid–Schiff

Sirius red

As is the case with topical therapy, systemic therapy may be beneficial for some patients, but not all. It has been reported that systemic retinoids, specifically acitretin, have improved the pruritus of lichen amyloidosis and resulted in a flattening of the skin lesions.[60,61] Cyclosporine has also been shown to be effective.

Surgical options include dermabrasion[62] and removal of the amyloid deposits in the epidermis with a scalpel.[63,64] However, potential side effects must be considered when using such therapies.[65] Frequency-doubled Q-switched neodymium-doped yttrium aluminium garnet (Nd:YAG) laser treatment has been used with some success. It is less invasive than dermabrasion or surgical removal via scalpel and perhaps should be tried before more invasive treatment modalities are pursued.[66] Hyperpigmentation may limit the usefulness of lasers, and a test spot should be done prior to treatment. The physical treatment modalities, such as electrodessication, split-thickness skin graft, removal via scalpel, and use of a carbon dioxide (CO_2) laser, are the mainstays of nodular amyloidosis treatment.[67] Despite successful treatment, recurrence is still common.[62,67]

Lichen amyloidosis is thought to be purely a cutaneous disease. As such, therapy has been directed at relieving the symptoms of pruritus. Some surgical techniques are directed toward removing the amyloid deposits from the dermis, although pain and discomfort, as well as hospitalization, may limit the usefulness of these options.

CONCLUSION

Amyloidosis is divided into primary systemic and localized cutaneous (nodular, macular, or lichen) types. Individuals with skin of color appear to have a predisposition for developing localized cutaneous amyloidosis.

The treatment options for lichen and macular amyloidosis are palliative, not curative, with most of the potential treatments aimed at alleviating the patients' symptoms of pruritus, rather than removing the amyloid deposits or the cutaneous manifestations of the disease.

For mild cases, topical corticosteroids and intralesional corticosteroids are most commonly prescribed. In addition, a keratolytic agent can be added to alleviate the visual changes of the disease. Other topical therapy options include calcipotriol, tacrolimus, or DMSO. DMSO is known to be effective in treating both lichen and macular amyloidosis. However, the reported side effects include irritant and contact dermatitis/urticaria, and it is often difficult to find a pharmacy where one can purchase DMSO for patient use.

TABLE 31-4	Treatment of lichen amyloidosis[45-47,51-59,68,69]

Remove precipitating and/or aggravating factors

Topical corticosteroids (with or without occlusion)

Intralesional corticosteroids

Keratolytic agents (urea or salicylic acid)

Calcipotriol

Tacrolimus

Dimethyl sulfoxide

Phototherapy with ultraviolet B and photochemotherapy (psoralen with ultraviolet A)

Systemic retinoids (acitretin)

Cyclosporine

Dermabrasion

Removal via scalpel

Q-switched neodymium-doped yttrium aluminium garnet laser

If a patient does not respond to topical treatment, either phototherapy with UVB or photochemotherapy with PUVA should be considered. A further option for treatment is dermabrasion or removal via scalpel of the amyloid deposits in the epidermis. Frequency-doubled Q-switched Nd:YAG laser treatment has proven to be beneficial. It should be tried before dermabrasion or removal via scalpel, because it is less invasive than these therapies and less likely to result in scarring. Physicians should note that lasers can cause hyperpigmentation, and a test spot should be done prior to treatment, particularly for patients with darker skin of color.

Physical treatment modalities include electrodessication, a split-thickness skin graft, removal via scalpel, and the use of a CO_2 laser. These methods are often initially successful; however, the results are frequently only temporary.

REFERENCES

1. Kyle RA, Gertz MA. Primary systemic amyloidosis: clinical and laboratory features in 474 cases. *Semin Hematol.* 1995;32:45-59.
2. Breathnach SM. Amyloid and amyloidosis. *J Am Acad Dermatol.* 1988;18:1-16.
3. Lambert WC. Cutaneous deposition disorders. In: Farmer ER, Hood AF, eds. *Pathology of the Skin.* Norwalk, CT: Appleton & Lange; 1990:432-450.
4. Georgiades CS, Neyman EG, Barish MA, et al. Amyloidosis: review and CT manifestations. *Radiographics.* 2004;24:405-416.
5. Rosenzweig M, Landau H. Light chain (AL) amyloidosis: update on diagnosis and management. *J Hematol Oncol.* 2011;4:47.
6. Schreml S, Szeimies RM, Vogt T, et al. Cutaneous amyloidoses and systemic amyloidoses with cutaneous involvement. *Eur J Dermatol.* 2010;20:152-160.
7. Westermark P. Localized AL amyloidosis: a suicidal neoplasm? *Ups J Med Sci.* 2012;117:244-250.
8. Hill JC, Maske R, Bowen RM. Secondary localized amyloidosis of the cornea associated with tertiary syphilis. *Cornea.* 1990;9:98-101.
9. Lee YS, Fong PH. Secondary localized amyloidosis in trichoepithelioma. A light microscopic and ultrastructural study. *Am J Dermatopathol.* 1990;12:469-478.
10. Wong CK. History and modern concepts (cutaneous amyloidosis). *Clin Dermatol.* 1990;8:1-6.
11. Black MM, Wilkinson DS. Metabolic and nutritional disorders: amyloid and amyloidosis of the skin. In: Rook A, Wilkinson DS, Ebling FJG, et al, eds. *Textbook of Dermatology.* 5th ed. Oxford, United Kingdom: Blackwell Scientific; 1992:2333-2344.
12. Kibbi AG, Rubeiz NG, Zaynoun ST, et al. Primary localized cutaneous amyloidosis. *Int J Dermatol.* 1992;31:95-98.
13. Wong CK. Lichen amyloidosis: a relatively common skin disorder in Taiwan. *Arch Dermatol.* 1974;110:438-440.
14. Looi LM. Primary localized cutaneous amyloidosis in Malaysians. *Aust J Dermatol.* 1991;32:39-44.
15. Ollague W, Ollague J, Ferretti H. Epidemiology of primary cutaneous amyloidosis in South America. *Clin Dermatol.* 1990;8:25-29.
16. Tan T. Epidemiology of primary cutaneous amyloidoses in southeast Asia. *Clin Dermatol.* 1990;8:20-24.
17. Halder R, Nootheti P. Ethnic hair and skin: what is the state of the science. *J Am Acad Dermatol.* 2003;48:S143-S148.
18. Weyers W, Weyers I, Bonczkowitz M, et al. Lichen amyloidosis: a consequence of scratching. *J Am Acad Dermatol.* 1997;37:923-928.
19. Chang YT, Liu HN, Wong CK, et al. Detection of Epstein-Barr virus in primary cutaneous amyloidosis. *Br J Dermatol.* 1997;136:823-826.
20. Vaghjimal A, Ahmad H, Soto NE, et al. Lichen amyloidosis in an HIV-infected patient: a case report and review of the literature. *Acta Derm Venereol.* 1998;78:399.
21. Buezo GF, Peñas PF, Daudén Tello E, et al. Lichen amyloidosis and human immunodeficiency virus infection. *Dermatology.* 1995;191:56-58.
22. Goller MM, Cohen PR, Duvic M. Lichen amyloidosis presenting as a papular pruritus syndrome in a human-immunodeficiency-virus-infected man. *Dermatology.* 1997;194:62-64.
23. Maeda H, Ohta S, Saito Y, et al. Epidermal origin of the amyloid in localized cutaneous amyloidosis. *Br J Dermatol.* 1982;106:345-351.
24. Kumakiri M, Hashimoto K. Histogenesis of primary localized cutaneous amyloidosis: sequential change of epidermal keratinocytes to amyloid via filamentous degeneration. *J Invest Dermatol.* 1979;73:150-162.
25. Huilgol SC, Ramnarain N, Carrington P, et al. Cytokeratins in primary cutaneous amyloidosis. *Australas J Dermatol.* 1998;39:81-85.

26. Yoneda K, Watanabe H, Yanagihara M, et al. Immunohistochemical staining properties of amyloids with anti-keratin antibodies using formalin-fixed, paraffin-embedded sections. *J Cutan Pathol.* 1989;16:133-136.

27. Ortiz-Romero PL, Ballestin-Carcavilla C, Lopez-Estebaranz JL, et al. Clinicopathologic and immunohistochemical studies on lichen amyloidosis and macular amyloidosis. *Arch Dermatol.* 1994;130:1559-1560.

28. Kobayashi H, Hashimoto K. Amyloidogenesis in organ-limited cutaneous amyloidosis: an antigenic identity between epidermal keratin and skin amyloid. *J Invest Dermatol.* 1983;80:66-72.

29. Norén P, Westermark P, Cornwell GG, et al. Immunofluorescence and histochemical studies of localized cutaneous amyloidosis. *Br J Dermatol.* 1983;108:277-285.

30. Masu S, Hosokawa M, Seiji M. Amyloid in localized cutaneous amyloidosis: immunofluorescence studies with anti-keratin antiserum especially concerning the difference between systemic and localized cutaneous amyloidosis. *Acta Derm Venereol Suppl.* 1981;61:381-384.

31. Kitano Y, Okada N, Kobayashi Y, et al. A monoclonal anti-keratin antibody reactive with amyloid deposit of primary cutaneous amyloidosis. *J Dermatol.* 1987;14:427-429.

32. Hashimoto K. Progress on cutaneous amyloidosis. *J Invest Dermatol.* 1984;82:1-3.

33. Black MM, Jones EW. Macular amyloidosis: a study of 21 cases with special reference to the role of the epidermis in its histogenesis. *Br J Dermatol.* 1971;84:199-209.

34. Eto H, Hashimoto K, Kobayashi H, et al. Differential staining of cytoid bodies and skin-limited amyloids with monoclonal anti-keratin antibodies. *Am J Pathol.* 1984;116:473-481.

35. Yamagihara M, Kitajima Y, Yaoita H, et al. Ultrastructural observation of the relationship between amyloid filaments and half desmosomes in macular amyloidosis. *J Cutan Pathol.* 1980;7:213.

36. Horiguchi Y, Fine JD, Leigh IM, et al. Lamina densa malformation involved in histogenesis of primary localized cutaneous amyloidosis. *J Invest Dermatol.* 1992;99:12-18.

37. Souza Júnior JD, Schettini RA, Tupinambá WL, et al. Localized primary cutaneous nodular amyloidosis: case report. *An Bras Dermatol.* 2011;86: 987-990.

38. Wang WJ. Clinical features of cutaneous amyloidoses. *Clin Dermatol.* 1990;8:13-19.

39. Khoo BP, Tay YK. Lichen amyloidosis: a bullous variant. *Ann Acad Med Singapore.* 2000;29:105-107.

40. Tursen U, Kaya TI, Dusmez D, et al. Case of generalized lichen amyloidosis. *Int J Dermatol.* 2003;42:649-651.

41. Yalçin B, Artüz F, Toy GG, et al. Generalized lichen amyloidosis associated with chronic urticaria. *Dermatology.* 2003;207:203-204.

42. Vijaya B, Dalal BS, Sunila, et al. Primary cutaneous amyloidosis: a clinicopathological study with emphasis on polarized microscopy. *Indian J Pathol Microbiol.* 2012;55:170-174.

43. Ozaki M. Familial lichen amyloidosis. *Int J Dermatol.* 1984;23:190-193.

44. Rajagopalan K, Tay CH. Familial lichen amyloidosis: report of 19 cases in 4 generations of a Chinese family in Malaysia. *Br J Dermatol.* 1972;87:123-129.

45. Porto JA, Posse FA. Amiloidosecutaneagenuina familial. *Bol da Soc Brasil Dermatol E Sif.* 1960;35:102-103.

46. De Souza AR. Amiloidosecutaneabohlosa familial: observacao de 4 casos. *Rev Hosp Clin Fac Med Sao Paolo.* 1963;18:413-417.

47. De Pietro WP. Primary familial cutaneous amyloidosis: a study of HLA antigens in a Puerto Rican family. *Arch Dermatol.* 1981;117:639-642.

48. Hartshorne ST. Familial primary cutaneous amyloidosis in a South African family. *Clin Exp Dermatol.* 1999;24:438-442.

49. Sagher F, Shanon J. Amyloidosis cutis. Familial occurrence in three generations. *Arch Dermatol.* 1963;87:171-175.

50. Vasily DB, Bhatia SG, Uhlin SR. Familial primary cutaneous amyloidosis: clinical, genetic, and immunofluorescent studies. *Arch Dermtaol.* 1978;114:1173-1176.

51. Newton JA, Jagjivan A, Bhogal B, et al. Familial primary cutaneous amyloidosis. *Br J Dermatol.* 1985;112:201-208.

52. Bergamo F, Annessi G, Ribuffo M, et al. Familial lichen amyloidosis. *Chron Dermatol.* 1997;6:959-961.

53. Highman B. Improved methods for demonstrating amyloid in paraffin sections. *Arch Pathol (Chic).* 1946;41:559-562.

54. Kobayashi T, Yamasaki Y, Watanbe T, et al. Extensive lichen amyloidosis refractory to DMSO. *J Dermatol.* 1995;22:755-758.

55. Ozkaya-Bayazit E, Kavak A, GüngÖr H, et al. Intermittent use of topical dimethyl sulfoxide in macular and papular amyloidosis. *Int J Dermatol.* 1998;37:949-954.

56. Jin AG, Por A, Wee LK, et al. Comparative study of phototherapy (UVB) vs photochemotherapy (PUVA) vs topical steroids in the treatment of primary cutaneous lichen amyloidosis. *Photodermatol Photoimmunol Photomed.* 2001;17:42-43.

57. Hashimoto K, Ito K, Kumakiri M, et al. Nylon brush macular amyloidosis. *Arch Dermatol.* 1987;123:633-637.

58. Khoo B, Tay Y, Goh C. Calcipotriol ointment vs betamethasone 17-valerate ointment in the treatment of lichen amyloidosis. *Int J Dermatol.* 1999;38:539-541.

59. Castanedo-Cazares JP, Lepe V, Moncada B. Lichen amyloidosis improved by 0.1% topical tacrolimus. *Dermatology.* 2002;205:420-421.

60. Pandhi R, Kaur I, Kumar B. Lack of effect of dimethylsulfoxide in cutaneous amyloidosis. *J Dermatolog Treat.* 2002;13:11-14.

61. Hernández-Núñez A, Daudén E, Moreno de Vega MJ, et al. Widespread biphasic amyloidosis: response to acitretin. *Clin Exp Dermatol.* 2001;26: 256-259.

62. Reider N, Sepp N, Fritsch P. Remission of lichen amyloidosis after treatment with acitretin. *Dermatology.* 1997;194:309-311.

63. Wong CK. Treatment (cutaneous amyloidosis). *Clin Dermatol.* 1990;8:108-111.

64. Behr FD, Levine N, Bangert J. Lichen amyloidosis associated with atopic dermatitis: clinical resolution with cyclosporine. *Arch Dermatol.* 2001;137:553-555.

65. Teraki Y, Katsuta M, Shiohara T. Lichen amyloidosis associated with Kimura's disease: successful treatment with cyclosporine. *Dermatology.* 2002;204:133-135.

66. Harahap M, Marwali MR. The treatment of lichen amyloidosis. A review and a new technique. *Dermatol Surg.* 1998;24:251-254.

67. Liu HT. Treatment of lichen amyloidosis (LA) and disseminated superficial porokeratosis (DSP) with frequency-doubled Q-switched Nd:YAG laser. *Dermatol Surg.* 2000;26:958-962.

68. Bozikov K, Janezic T. Excision and split thickness skin grafting in the treatment of nodular primary localized cutaneous amyloidosis. *Eur J Dermatol.* 2006;16:315-316.

69. Prophet EB, Mills B, Arrington JB, et al. *Laboratory Methods in Histotechnology.* Washington, DC: Armed Forces Institute of Pathology; 1992.

70. Yanagihara M, Mehregan AH, Mehregan DR. Staining of amyloid with cotton dyes. *Arch Dermatol.* 1984;120:1184-1185.

CHAPTER 32	**Acquired Bullous Diseases**
	Chia-Chun Ang
	Victoria Werth

KEY POINTS

- The causes of acquired bullous diseases are multiple and can be broadly differentiated based on the age of onset and the chronicity of the disease.

- Autoimmune blistering diseases can be challenging to diagnose and treat.

- Potential issues that will affect management of autoimmune bullous diseases in patients with skin of color include a difference in prevalence of specific autoimmune bullous diseases, disease presentation, postinflammatory dyspigmentation and scarring, and for some, access to care.

- Large multicenter controlled trials are needed to show differences in response to treatment, if any, between patients with skin of color and Caucasian patients with autoimmune bullous diseases.

INTRODUCTION

Cutaneous blisters appear because of disruption of the desmosomal or hemidesmosomal cell junctions or because of cytolysis of keratinocytes. The differential diagnoses are diverse, and the epidemiology and presentation of cutaneous blisters can be different in patients with darker skin. Advances in treatment have improved the outlook for patients with chronic blistering diseases such as autoimmune blistering diseases and hereditary epidermolysis bullosa, but these treatments can be expensive, require regular monitoring and follow-up, and may not be routinely available. The main concern for patients with skin of color is cosmetically significant postinflammatory hyper- and hypopigmentation as well as potential cutaneous scarring after resolution of the blistering disease.

In this chapter, we will present an approach to diagnosing blistering diseases. We will then focus on the epidemiology, clinical presentation, diagnosis, and treatment of autoimmune blistering diseases and highlight the recent literature involving African, Hispanic, and Asian patient populations.

APPROACH TO BLISTERING DISEASES

An approach to diagnosing blistering diseases is to consider the age of the patient and the tempo of the clinical presentation [**Figures 32-1 and 32-2**].

Blistering genodermatoses are rare and present predominantly during childhood. Epidermolysis bullosa (EB) is due to an inherited defect of structural components of basal keratinocytes (such as hemidesmosomal proteins, keratins 5 and 14, desmoplakin, and plakophillin) and demonstrates varying severity of skin and extracutaneous involvement.[1-4] Some types of EB present in older children and can be mistaken for acquired blistering diseases. These include localized EB simplex with palmoplantar bulla, late-onset junctional EB, or dystrophic EB pruriginosa. Other causes of inherited childhood blistering diseases include cutaneous porphyrias[5] and epidermolytic ichthyosis.[6] Although inherited blistering diseases predominantly present in childhood, the most frequent cause of blistering in children is still from acquired causes [Figure 32-1].

Acquired blistering diseases are the predominant form of blistering disease seen in adults [Figure 32-2]. Important clues can often be gleaned from a comprehensive history and physical examination, whereas histologic and immunofluorescence examination of lesional skin can help to confirm the diagnosis of autoimmune blistering diseases[7,8] [**Tables 32-1 and 32-2**].

AUTOIMMUNE BLISTERING DISEASE

Autoimmune blistering diseases are caused by pathogenic autoantibodies that target proteins in the desmosomal and hemidesmosomal complex, leading to intraepidermal (pemphigus group of diseases) or subepidermal (pemphigoid group of diseases) blisters, respectively.

▨ PEMPHIGUS FOLIACEUS, PEMPHIGUS VULGARIS, AND THEIR VARIANTS

Pemphigus is caused by autoantibodies directed against members of the desmosome cell junction in the skin and mucous membranes.[9] Autoantibodies directed against desmoglein 1 (Dsg 1) are found in pemphigus foliaceus and its variants (pemphigus erythematosus and fogo selvagem), desmoglein 3 (Dsg 3) antibodies are found in mucosal-dominant pemphigus vulgaris and its variant pemphigus vegetans, whereas both Dsg 1 and Dsg 3 antibodies are found in mucocutaneous pemphigus vulgaris. Acantholysis is postulated to occur from steric hindrance by the antibodies on the desmoglein adhesion sites and disruption of normal desmoglein homeostasis through intracellular signaling that occurs after binding of antibodies to its targets.[9] Antibodies targeting other keratinocyte cell surface proteins have also been discovered, and an alternative theory of "apoptolysis" has been proposed to explain the pathogenesis of pemphigus.[10] The level in the epidermis where acantholysis occurs is explained by the desmoglein compensation theory.[11] Certain human leukocyte antigen (HLA) haplotypes[12] and potential environmental triggers[13] have been associated with pemphigus. Pemphigus can be triggered by multiple drugs[14] containing a thiol, phenol, or neither group in its chemical structure. The actual mechanism that leads

to loss of tolerance to desmoglein proteins and subsequent autoantibody formation is still an area of research.

Fogo selvagem (endemic pemphigus foliaceus) has been reported in South American countries (Brazil, Colombia, Venezuela, Peru, Ecuador, and Paraguay) and Tunisia. It tends to affect children and young adults and shows geographic clustering of cases, being more common in rural Brazil and disappearing with urbanization. Exposure to novel insect antigens that cross-react with Dsg 1 after bites from black flies (*Simulium* species) or other hematophagous insects in rural areas is postulated to lead to a loss of tolerance for Dsg 1 in predisposed individuals with particular HLA-DR allele associations, with subsequent formation of pathogenic immunoglobulin (Ig) G4 antibodies targeting the extracellular domains (EC1 and EC2) of Dsg 1.[15-17]

Pemphigus is usually less common than bullous pemphigoid and affects middle-age patients. Pemphigus vulgaris is usually more commonly seen than pemphigus foliaceus. Pemphigus vegetans, pemphigus erythematosus, and fogo selvagem are rare. In the United Kingdom,[18] the incidence of pemphigus vulgaris was 0.7 per 100,000 person-years, whereas the incidence of bullous pemphigoid was 4.3 per 100,000 person-years. The mean age of presentation of pemphigus vulgaris was 71 years, and 66% of patients were female. In the United States,[19] pemphigus disorders accounted for an age-adjusted mortality rate of 0.023 per 100,000 persons per year, and 90.2% of deaths occurred in patients older than age 65 years. Comparatively, in Turkey,[20] the estimated annual incidence of pemphigus was 0.18 per 100,000 inhabitants, with a mean age at onset of 48 years and a male-to-female ratio of 1:1.64. Pemphigus vulgaris was the most common subtype seen. In Tunisia,[21] Iran,[22] and Kuwait,[23] pemphigus was more common than bullous pemphigoid. Other published epidemiologic studies are from India,[24] Taiwan,[25] Thailand,[26] Japan,[27] South Africa,[28] Korea,[29] and Singapore.[30]

Patients with pemphigus vulgaris commonly present with oral mucosal erosions [**Figure 32-3**]. Desquamative gingivitis[31] and involvement of other mucosa (ocular,[32] otorhinolaryngeal,[33,34] esophageal,[35] or anogenital mucosa[36,37]) can occur as an initial or concurrent presentation in pemphigus vulgaris, leading to considerable morbidity. Careful history taking can suggest extraoral mucosal involvement and should be done as part of the routine clinical assessment.

The typical skin lesions of mucocutaneous pemphigus vulgaris are flaccid blisters or erosions with overlying crust that heal with hyperpigmentation in skin of color [**Figure 32-4**]. The blister can be produced in clinically uninvolved skin by lateral pressure (Nikolsky sign) or direct pressure over an intact bulla (Asboe-Hansen sign). Impairment of the skin barrier with fluid loss and secondary infection were common causes of death for these patients previously when there was no effective treatment, and they can still occur in patients who lack access to care because of socioeconomic reasons. Pemphigus vegetans presents with pustules and vegetative plaques involving the scalp, face, and intertriginous areas. Pemphigus vulgaris can involve the nails[38] and result in loss of hair.[39] Atypical clinical presentations include bilateral foot ulcers,[40] macroglossia,[41] and vesiculopustular eruption on the hands and feet.[42]

Pemphigus foliaceus is characterized by erosions with overlying cornflake-like scales in the face, scalp, and upper trunk with no mucosal involvement [**Figure 32-5**]. Nikolsky sign can be elicited on perilesional skin. Uncommon presentations include erythroderma,[43] seborrheic keratosis-like lesions,[44] and psoriasiform lesions.[45] Senear-Usher syndrome (pemphigus erythematosus) presents with erythematous scaly plaques on the malar cheeks reminiscent of the malar rash of acute cutaneous lupus and has a characteristic immunofluorescence finding [Table 32-1]. Fogo selvagem (endemic pemphigus foliaceus) is clinically identical to pemphigus foliaceus and less commonly presents with annular exfoliative plaques, erythroderma, diffuse hyperpigmentation (involving lesional and nonlesional skin), or keratotic lesions.[15] Drug-induced pemphigus can present as pemphigus foliaceus or pemphigus vulgaris. Patients can go into remission if the offending drug is identified and stopped. Pemphigus herpetiformis refers to the erythematous urticated plaques with herpetiform vesicles seen in either pemphigus vulgaris or pemphigus foliaceus. Pemphigus vulgaris has been occasionally

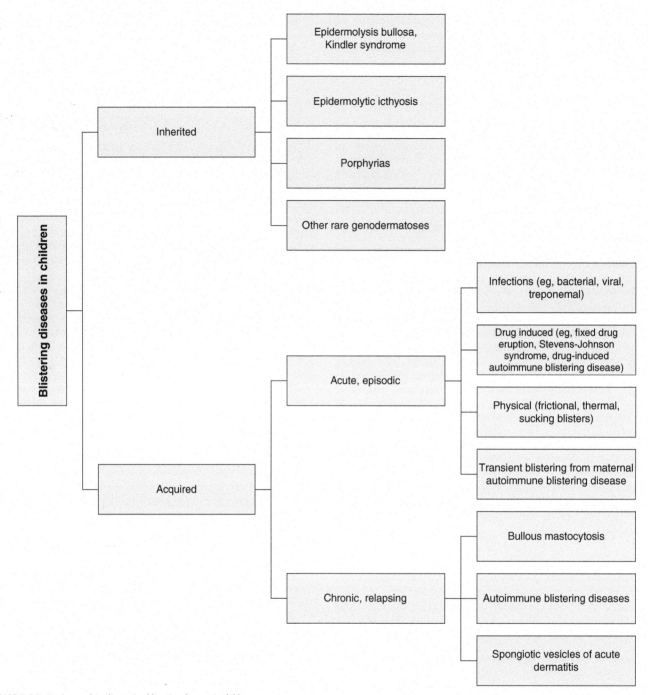

FIGURE 32-1. Approach to diagnosing blistering diseases in children.

reported to evolve to pemphigus foliaceus during treatment, whereas the reverse is less common.[46] This may be due to preferential suppression of autoantibody production against Dsg 1.

The diagnosis can be confirmed on histology by biopsy from fresh lesions, direct immunofluorescence (DIF) on perilesional normal-appearing skin, or indirect immunofluorescence (IIF) with a patient's sera [Table 32-1]. For IIF, monkey esophagus is a more sensitive substrate for detecting Dsg3 autoantibodies, whereas guinea pig esophagus is a more sensitive substrate for detecting Dsg 1 autoantibodies.[47] Commercial enzyme-linked immunosorbent assay (ELISA) systems allow quantification of circulating anti-Dsg 1 and anti-Dsg 3 antibodies to distinguish the different pemphigus subtypes and to monitor disease activity.[48] In some patients, the anti-Dsg antibody titers can remain elevated despite the patient being in clinical remission.[49] This can be due

to the detection of nonpathogenic anti-Dsg antibodies that remains in circulation during clinical remission.

Pemphigus causes significant morbidity, can be fatal, and affects quality of life.[50] The goal of treatment is to achieve clinical remission with the least treatment-related side effects. This can be done through a three-pronged approach:

1. Topical therapy and wound care, including treatment of secondary skin infections

2. Systemic therapy to induce and maintain clinical remission

3. Peer emotional support with help from local disease support groups[51]

Topical glucocorticoids, topical calcineurin inhibitors, or petrolatum jelly can be applied to uninfected erosions. Purulent lesions can be cleaned with regular soaks with diluted potassium permanganate

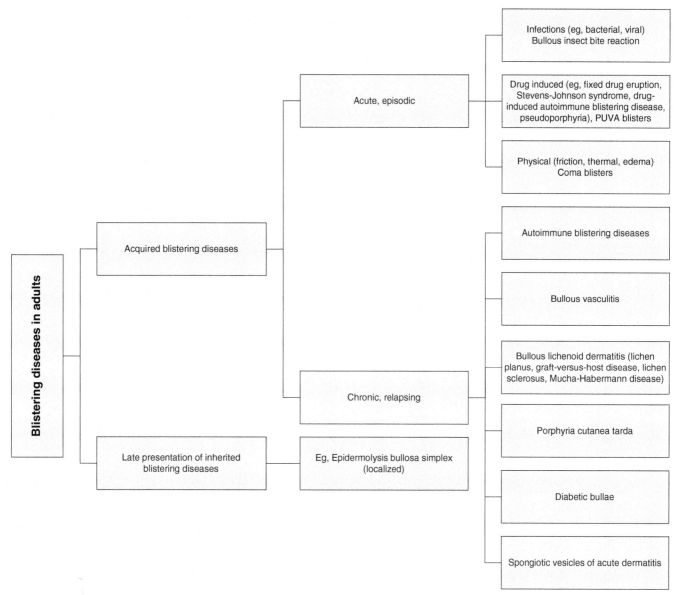

FIGURE 32-2. Approach to diagnosing blistering diseases in adults. PUVA, psoralen plus ultraviolet A.

solution as an astringent, dressed with antibiotic ointment or petroleum jelly, or covered with a silver-impregnated nonadherent dressing. An empirical course of systemic antibiotics is appropriate in the setting of extensive impetiginized skin lesions, and herpes simplex infection should be suspected and treated especially when mucosal erosions do not respond to immunosuppressive therapy. Patients with oral erosions benefit from a diet with a soft consistency and maintenance of oral hygiene with regular application of antiseptic or antibacterial/anticandidal mouthwash. Local mucosal therapy with topical anesthetic agents or topical glucocorticoids in an adhesive paste formulation is a useful adjunct to systemic glucocorticoids or immunosuppressive therapy. Consultation with a dentist, otorhinolaryngologist, or gastroenterologist may be necessary if other mucosal surfaces are involved.

Many systemic medications for the treatment of pemphigus are used off-label, and treatment recommendations are based on case series, uncontrolled clinical trials, small controlled clinical trials, consensus, and expert opinion. The assessment of disease extent, severity, and treatment response had not been standardized for many earlier studies, making direct comparison difficult. A Cochrane Review[52] of the literature prior to October 2008 on the treatment of pemphigus identified 11 studies, but the results of the analysis were limited by the small sample sizes and overall low statistical quality of the studies reviewed. A consensus statement by a panel of world experts[53] was published in 2008 to define disease end points in pemphigus. Scoring systems,[54] such as the Autoimmune Bullous Skin Disorder Intensity Score and Pemphigus Disease Area Index, are validated and available currently. These would assist in the design and conduct of multicenter controlled clinical trials to assess systemic treatment for pemphigus.

Multiple treatment guidelines have been published in the last 10 years.[55-62] The treatment regimen used should be individualized to the severity of pemphigus, efficacy of treatment, potential side effects in relation to the patient's health status, availability, and cost. Using a treatment regimen of prednisone and conventional adjuvants (azathioprine, cyclosporine, cyclophosphamide, dapsone, or gold), Herbst and Bystryn[63] were able to achieve complete long-lasting remission (defined as no evidence of disease for at least 6 months while not receiving systemic therapy) in 25% of their cohort 2 years after diagnosis, 50% in 5 years, and 75% in 10 years. Patients with mild to moderate disease at onset and a rapid response to therapy were more likely to achieve complete long-lasting remission.

Anti-CD20 antibody (rituximab) has been used since 2003[64] as salvage therapy in treatment-resistant pemphigus[65] or, rarely, as first-line

TABLE 32-1	Histologic and immunofluorescence features of intraepidermal autoimmune blistering diseases		
	Histologic findings	Immunofluorescence findings	Main target antigens
Pemphigus foliaceus	Intraepidermal blister with acantholysis in the upper epidermis, dermal mixed inflammatory cell infiltrate	DIF: Intercellular IgG, may be more intense in the upper epidermis IIF human skin: Intercellular IgG Desmoglein 1 ELISA positive, desmoglein 3 ELISA negative	Desmoglein 1
Pemphigus erythematosus	Similar to pemphigus foliaceus	DIF: Intercellular IgG with lupus band IIF human skin: Intercellular IgG and ANA	Desmoglein 1
Endemic pemphigus (fogo selvagem)	Similar to pemphigus foliaceus	Similar to pemphigus foliaceus	Desmoglein 1
Pemphigus vulgaris	Suprabasilar cleft with acantholysis and tomb-stoning of basal keratinocytes; dermal inflammatory cell infiltrate with eosinophils	DIF: Intercellular IgG, may be more intense in the lower epidermis IIF monkey esophagus: Intercellular IgG Mucocutaneous pemphigus vulgaris: Desmoglein 1 ELISA positive, desmoglein 3 ELISA positive Mucosal pemphigus vulgaris: Desmoglein 1 ELISA negative, desmoglein 3 ELISA positive	Desmoglein 3 ± desmoglein 1
Pemphigus vegetans	Suprabasilar acantholysis, acanthosis and papillomatosis, intraepidermal microabscesses, intense dermal inflammatory cell infiltrate with eosinophils	Similar to pemphigus vulgaris	Desmoglein 3 ± desmoglein 1
Paraneoplastic pemphigus	Suprabasilar acantholysis, necrotic and dyskeratotic keratinocytes, lymphocytic exocytosis, basal vacuolar degeneration or lichenoid lymphocytic inflammatory infiltrate in the dermis	DIF: Intercellular and BMZ IgG, can be negative IIF rat bladder: Intercellular IgG, can be negative Desmoglein 1, desmoglein 3, and BP230 ELISA can be positive ELISA of N-terminal fragment of envoplakin positive Immunoprecipitation or Western blotting	Envoplakin, periplakin, desmoglein 3
IgA pemphigus	Acantholytic clefts and neutrophilic pustules localize to the subcorneal region in SPD IgA pemphigus and to the midepidermis in the IEN IgA pemphigus	DIF: Intercellular IgA > IgG or C3 IIF human skin or monkey esophagus: Intercellular IgA, may be negative	Desmocollin 1 in SPD IgA pemphigus
Drug-induced pemphigus	Histologically similar to pemphigus vulgaris or pemphigus foliaceus, with presence of eosinophils in some cases	DIF and IIF findings follow either pemphigus foliaceus (66%) or pemphigus vulgaris (33%) or are negative (rarely)	Desmoglein 1 (66%), desmoglein 3 (33%) Non–immune-mediated acantholysis (rarely)

Abbreviations: ANA, antinuclear antibody; BMZ, basement membrane zone; DIF, direct immunofluorescence; ELISA, enzyme-linked immunosorbent assay; IEN, intraepidermal neutrophilic; Ig, immunoglobulin; IIF, indirect immunofluorescence; SPD, subcorneal pustular dermatosis.

therapy,[66] often with impressive treatment outcomes. In a retrospective single-center review[67] of adjuvant rituximab in 31 patients with pemphigus unresponsive or contraindicated to conventional systemic therapy, 58% of patients achieved complete remission on no or minimal therapy, with a median duration of remission of 19 months. These patients were given rituximab significantly earlier in the course of disease compared to patients who did not achieve complete remission. The benefit from early use of rituximab and the optimal dose and dosing interval require confirmation by multicenter controlled clinical trials. Optimism with rituximab use should be tempered by the risk from life-threatening infections, venous thromboembolism, late-onset neutropenia,[68] infusion-related hemolytic anemia,[69] and other yet unknown long-term complications, as well as cost.

Our approach to the treatment of pemphigus vulgaris and pemphigus foliaceus is presented here. Appropriate treatment-specific screening tests before and at intervals during treatment should be performed to monitor for potential treatment-related side effects. Oral glucocorticoids are the cornerstone of therapy for pemphigus. Lower doses of oral prednisone (0.5 mg/kg/d) can be started for milder disease, whereas higher doses of oral prednisone (≥1 mg/kg/d) are required for severe or rapidly progressing disease. Other adjuvant steroid-sparing agents are usually introduced concurrently because these require 4 to 6 weeks to take effect. Anti-inflammatory adjuvant agents such as dapsone or tetracycline antibiotics are used for less extensive, steroid-responsive pemphigus vulgaris and pemphigus foliaceus. Immunosuppressive adjuvant agents such as azathioprine, mycophenolate mofetil, or methotrexate are used in patients with moderate to severe disease to allow weaning of oral glucocorticoids and

maintenance of remission. Dapsone can be added in maintenance-phase pemphigus vulgaris to allow further tapering of oral glucocorticoids.[70] Repeated courses of intravenous immunoglobulin or oral cyclophosphamide can be considered as adjuvant maintenance therapy in patients with recalcitrant pemphigus who have failed more conventional therapies. Pulsed intravenous steroid therapy or high-dose intravenous immunoglobulin infusion can be used to gain control of severe or recalcitrant disease, but oral glucocorticoids and adjuvant immunosuppressive agents are required to maintain remission. Rituximab can be used as salvage therapy in patients with treatment-resistant disease, but we are increasingly favoring its use as a first-line steroid-sparing agent in patients with severe pemphigus. Systemic corticosteroids or other adjuvant agents are still required for the initial 2 to 3 months after infusion before rituximab takes effect.

▋ IgA PEMPHIGUS

IgA pemphigus is rare and presents as annular vesicles and pustules on erythematous plaques on the intertriginous regions, trunk, and proximal extremities.[71] Mucosal involvement is rarely reported. Two subtypes are recognized: subcorneal pustular dermatosis (SPD) and intraepidermal neutrophilic (IEN) type IgA pemphigus. The autoantibodies target desmocollin 1 in SPD-type IgA pemphigus,[72] whereas the antigenic target for IEN-type IgA pemphigus is still unknown. Malignancy has been reported to occur with IgA pemphigus.[73,74] The histologic and immunofluorescence features are highlighted in Table 32-1. Prednisone, dapsone, isotretinoin, acitretin, mycophenolate, and adalimumab have been used to treat IgA pemphigus in case reports.[71]

TABLE 32-2 Histologic and immunofluorescence features of subepidermal autoimmune blistering diseases

	Histologic findings	Immunofluorescence findings	Main target antigens
Bullous pemphigoid (BP)	Prebullous phase: eosinophilic spongiotic dermatitis Bullous phase: subepidermal blister, dermal inflammatory cell infiltrate with eosinophils	DIF: Linear IgG and C3 at BMZ IIF salt split skin: predominant epidermal (roof) binding IgG BP180 NC16a ELISA positive in 75%–90% of patients BP230 ELISA positive in 50%–70% of patients, useful in diagnosis of BP only in patients with positive DIF and negative BP180 ELISA	BP180 NC16a domain (type XVII collagen/BPAG2)
Pemphigoid gestationis (PG)	Similar to bullous pemphigoid	DIF: linear C3 ± IgG at BMZ IIF salt split skin: Epidermal binding C3 >> IgG Complement fixing IgG demonstrable with modified IIF technique BP180 NC16a ELISA positive in 90% of patients	BP180 NC16a domain
Mucous membrane pemphigoid (MMP)	Subepidermal blister with a lymphohistiocytic infiltrate and plasma cells; dermal fibrosis is seen in advanced lesions	DIF: Linear deposits of IgG, IgA, and C3 at BMZ IIF salt split skin: Anti-BP180, α6 integrin, and β4 integrin antibodies bind the epidermal side; anti-laminin-332 binds the dermal side; may be negative or at very low titer BP180 NC16a ELISA may be positive	Laminin 332, α6β4 integrin, BP180
Linear IgA bullous dermatosis (LABD)	Subepidermal blister with neutrophilic or eosinophilic dermal inflammatory infiltrate	DIF: linear deposits of IgA at BMZ, occasionally IgG, IgM, or C3 at BMZ IIF salt split skin: epidermal > dermal > mixed binding IgA BP180 NC16a ELISA may be positive	Shed ectodomains of BP180 (LAD-1/120 kDa, 97 kDa)
Dermatitis herpetiformis (DH)	Subepidermal blister with neutrophilic microabscesses at the dermal papilla	DIF: Granular IgA deposits at dermal papillae; rarely continuous BMZ IgA staining. IIF monkey esophagus: endomysium binding IgA ELISA for antitissue or epidermal transglutaminase IgA	Epidermal and tissue transglutaminase
Epidermolysis bullosa acquisita (EBA)	Basal vacuolar alteration or frank subepidermal blister; dermal inflammatory infiltrate may be present or minimal	DIF: Linear homogenous IgG ± C3, IgM, or IgA at BMZ IIF salt split skin: Dermal binding IgG; may be negative Immunoblotting or ELISA for type VII collagen antibody	Type VII collagen
Bullous systemic lupus erythematosus (BSLE)	Subepidermal blister with neutrophils in the papillary dermis (DH or LABD like); histologic features of cutaneous lupus are absent	DIF: Linear or granular IgG, IgM, IgA, C3, fibrinogen at BMZ IIF salt split skin: negative or dermal binding IgG	Type VII collagen
Anti-laminin γ1 (p200) pemphigoid	Subepidermal blister with neutrophilic or eosinophilic dermal inflammatory infiltrate	DIF: Linear IgG and C3 at BMZ IIF salt split skin: Dermal binding IgG Western blotting or ELISA for laminin γ1 antibody	Laminin γ1

Abbreviations: BMZ, basement membrane zone; DIF, direct immunofluorescence; ELISA, enzyme-linked immunosorbent assay; Ig, immunoglobulin; IIF, indirect immunofluorescence.

■ PARANEOPLASTIC PEMPHIGUS

Paraneoplastic pemphigus (PNP) is one of five possible clinical manifestations of a distinct neoplasia-associated multiorgan inflammatory reaction known as paraneoplastic autoimmune multiorgan syndrome (PAMS). It is characterized by humoral and cellular immune response

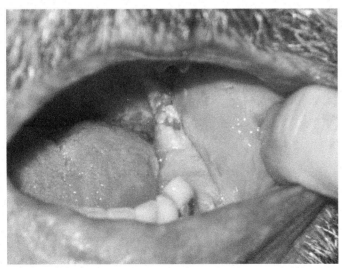

FIGURE 32-3. Erosions on the buccal and palatal mucosa in a patient with pemphigus vulgaris.

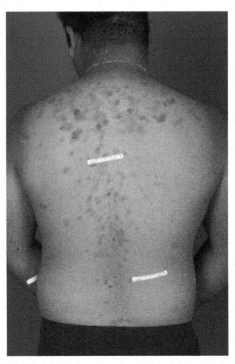

FIGURE 32-4. Postinflammatory hyperpigmented macules on the back of an Asian patient with pemphigus vulgaris.

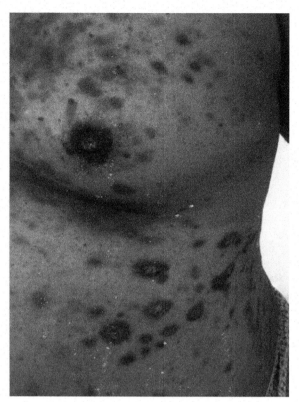

FIGURE 32-5. Hyperpigmented macules with overlying hyperkeratotic scale on the trunk of an African American patient with pemphigus foliaceus.

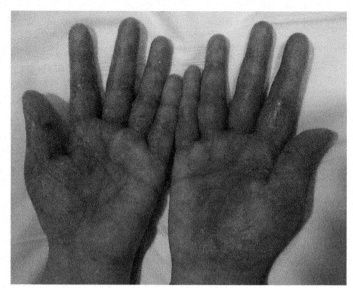

FIGURE 32-6. Violaceous scaly plaques on the palms of an Asian patient with paraneoplastic pemphigus.

to epithelial cell junction proteins, especially to the plakin family of cytoskeletal linking proteins.[75-79] PNP/PAMS is uncommon, with an estimate of 450 cases published in the literature up until 2011.[79] PNP/PAMS composed 0.2% of 1402 patients seen over 10 years in a bullous diseases research center in Iran.[22] The most common neoplasm described in childhood[80] and Chinese patients[81] with PNP/PAMS is Castleman disease. Hematologic and lymphoproliferative diseases account for the majority of malignancies described with adult PNP/PAMS in the Western literature, whereas carcinomas and sarcomas are less common.[82]

Nguyen et al[77] classified PAMS into five clinicopathologic subtypes: pemphigus-like (PNP), bullous pemphigoid-like, erythema multiforme-like, graft-versus-host disease-like, and lichen planus-like presentation. Recalcitrant stomatitis that extends to the vermillion lip is the hallmark of PNP/PAMS. Other mucosal surfaces can be involved. Involvement of the bronchial lining can lead to obstructive lung disease, respiratory failure, and death from constrictive bronchiolitis (bronchiolitis obliterans).[83,84] Skin lesions can appear as tense blisters, scattered or extensive erosions mimicking toxic epidermal necrolysis, targetoid erythematous plaques, violaceous plaques, and erythroderma [**Figure 32-6**]. The mortality rate of PNP/PAMS has been reported as 68%[85] to 90%,[83] and death was due to infections, progression of underlying neoplasia, or respiratory failure from bronchiolitis obliterans.[83,85] Erythema multiforme-like skin lesions with extensive mucocutaneous involvement predicted a worse outcome in a French case series.[85]

The histology of PNP/PAMS depends on the clinical subtype seen. The presence of anti-plakins and other autoantibodies characteristic of this disease can be demonstrated through DIF, IIF on rat bladder substrate, ELISA, immunoprecipitation, or immunoblotting [Table 32-1]. In patients who received rituximab as part of their treatment protocol for chronic lymphocytic leukemia or non-Hodgkin lymphoma, autoantibodies can be absent[86] or develop later in the course of disease.[87] A combination of clinical, histopathologic, and immunologic features is required to diagnose PNP/PAMS.[75,76,79] Treatment is difficult and requires a multidisciplinary approach with the oncologist and pulmonologist. Management of the underlying tumor may not alter the course

of PNP/PAMS. Multiple immunosuppressive treatment regimens are used to suppress the autoimmune inflammatory response driving PNP/PAMS,[75-79] with variable efficacy. Placebo-controlled trials should ideally be performed to look at the efficacy of treatment, but this is hampered by the rarity of the condition and the high morbidity and mortality of these patients.

■ BULLOUS PEMPHIGOID AND ITS VARIANTS (LICHEN PLANUS PEMPHIGOIDES, PEMPHIGOID GESTATIONIS)

Bullous pemphigoid (BP), lichen planus pemphigoides (LPP), and pemphigoid gestationis (PG) are caused by autoantibodies targeting type XVII collagen (BP180/BPAG2) on the hemidesmosome, of which the immunodominant epitope is the noncollagenous 16-A domain.[88,89] Binding of the antibodies leads to an inflammatory cascade that includes complement activation, mast cell degranulation, infiltration of neutrophils and eosinophils, production of proteinases, and degradation of BP180 and other extracellular matrix proteins leading to dermalepidermal separation. Antibodies against BP antigen 1 (BPAG1/BP230) can be found in BP and PG but are not directly pathogenic. BP180 is expressed in the placental amniotic epithelium.[90] In women with PG, BP180 is presented to the maternal immune system on aberrantly expressed major histocompatibility complex (MHC) class II peptides in the placenta and leads to a loss of tolerance. The resulting immune response and IgG autoantibodies cross-react with BP180 in the skin and lead to blistering.[91] Estrogens and progesterone have a modulating effect on the maternal immune system, which accounts for flares of PG during menstruation and while taking hormonal contraception.[91] Certain HLA haplotypes have been associated with BP[92] and PG.[91,93] Medications (spironolactone and phenothiazine), poor health, and neuropsychiatric conditions such as dementia, Parkinson disease, and unipolar and bipolar disorders were found to be associated with a higher risk of BP.[94] Other medications reported to induce BP include furosemide, phenacetin, penicillamine, terbinafine, antibiotics, angiotensin-converting enzyme inhibitors,[95] and dipeptidyl peptidase IV inhibitors plus metformin.[96] A drug history will be useful to exclude possible drug-induced pemphigoid, because this is potentially reversible with discontinuation of the medication. BP has also been reported to be triggered by radiotherapy, phototherapy, trauma, and burns.

BP affects middle-age to elderly adults and rarely children. It is usually more common relative to pemphigus. In the United Kingdom,[18] the incidence of BP was 4.3 per 100,000 person-years and has increased over time. The median age at presentation was 80 years, and 61% of patients were female. In France,[97] the estimated incidence of BP was 21.7 cases per million persons per year, increasing to 162 cases per million per year in patients over 70 years. In the United States,[19] BP accounted for an age-adjusted mortality rate of 0.028 per 100,000 persons per year. Mortality rates were significantly higher in individuals with darker skin of color and females and showed an increasing trend over time. However, no difference was seen between the expected mortality of BP patients relative to age-matched controls in another study from the United States.[98] The risk of death for patients with BP in the United Kingdom[18] was double, in Switzerland[99] triple, and in France[97] six times greater than that of the control population. BP was the most common autoimmune bullous disease seen in Singapore[100] and affected mostly Chinese patients. The estimated incidence was 7.6 per million persons per year, with a mean age of onset of 77 years. Surprisingly, BP was less common than pemphigus and accounted for 23.6% of cases seen in a Tunisian dermatology department,[21] 11.6% of cases seen in the Bullous Diseases Research Center in Tehran, Iran,[22] and 22% of cases seen in the National Dermatology Center in Kuwait.[23] PG has an incidence of 1 in 50,000 pregnancies with no racial predilection.[91]

Early lesions, or prebullous BP, appear as pruritic, excoriated, eczematous or urticated papules or plaques. BP may remain at this stage for weeks or months to years and may be unresponsive to topical steroid therapy. The established lesions of BP appear as pruritic, large, tense blisters arising on normal skin or inflamed urticated plaques [**Figure 32-7**]. Nikolsky sign is negative. Erosions, crusting, and impetiginization are seen in older lesions. Healing results in pigmentary changes and occasionally milia. Oral mucosal involvement occurs in about 10% to 30% of patients; involvement of other mucosal surfaces is rare. Nail involvement is occasionally seen.[38]

Clinical variants of BP include localized pemphigoid (pretibial, peristomal, periumbilical, on amputation stumps or paralyzed limbs), acral dyshidrosiform pemphigoid, vesicular pemphigoid, pemphigoid nodularis, flexural pemphigoid vegetans, and erythrodermic pemphigoid.[101] These presentations can mimic other dermatoses, and a high index of suspicion for BP in older patients is necessary. LPP refers to BP occurring in patients with lichen planus and should be distinguished from bullous lichen planus secondary to blistering from an intense lichenoid inflammation on existing lichen planus lesions. BP in children is rare and can occur in infancy (infantile BP) or in childhood with a predilection for acral skin and genitalia mucosa (childhood localized vulval or penile BP).[102-104] On rare occasions, patients with pemphigus can transition to BP or have concurrent BP.[105,106] PG usually occurs in the second or third trimester of pregnancy and less commonly in the immediate postpartum period. Pruritic urticated polycyclic plaques and

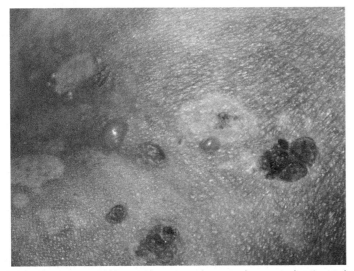

FIGURE 32-7. Tense blisters arising on an erythematous plaque, crusted erosions, and postinflammatory hypopigmented macules on the trunk of an Asian patient with bullous pemphigoid. (Used with permission from Dr. Shan-Xian Lee, Changi General Hospital, Singapore.)

blisters appear in the periumbilical region and elsewhere. These skin lesions usually improve before delivery, only to flare in the postpartum period. PG usually resolves after a period of time postpartum, but can recur in subsequent pregnancies or with hormonal contraceptives or menstruation. PG has been reported to occur with hydatidiform moles, trophoblastic tumors, and choriocarcinoma. Up to 10% of babies born to mothers with PG can develop self-limiting urticated plaques and blisters as a result of passive transfer of maternal autoantibodies.[91]

Patients with BP have different histologic features depending on the stage of disease at time of biopsy [Table 32-2]. The diagnosis should be confirmed by the presence of pathogenic antibodies on DIF, IIF on 1 mol/L of salt split skin, and ELISA testing using commercially available kits for antibodies targeting the NC16a domain of BP180 or the C-terminal domain of BP230[107] [Table 32-2]. False-positive BP180 NC16a ELISA testing in patients without immunobullous disease[107] or false-negative BP180 NC16a ELISA testing in patients with BP[108] can occur. This emphasizes the point that confirmation of disease requires clinical, pathologic, and immunofluorescence correlation. Once the diagnosis is confirmed, BP180 NC16a ELISA can be used to monitor disease activity.[107] For patients in clinical remission, a high titer of anti-BP180 ELISA and, to a lesser extent, a positive DIF performed on the day of cessation of systemic corticosteroids put them at higher risk of relapse within 12 months of cessation of therapy.[109] Several factors[110,111] predict a poor outcome in BP: old age, poor premorbid state as measured by Karnofsky score, low serum albumin, and use of high doses of glucocorticoids.

The goal of treatment in BP is to achieve clinical remission with the least treatment-related side effects. Topical therapy and wound care, peer support, and systemic therapy are essential components of the treatment plan. Similar to pemphigus, many systemic medications for the treatment of BP are used off-label, and previously, there has been a lack of good-quality controlled studies, standardized disease end points, and severity measures. In 2012, an international panel of experts published a set of guidelines on disease end points and severity measures (Bullous Pemphigoid Disease Area Index)[112] to assist in the conduct of controlled clinical trials. A Cochrane Review in 2010 on the treatment of BP[113,114] reviewed 10 randomized controlled trials with different quality of design, follow-up duration, and potential biases. The conclusions drawn include the following: use of potent topical steroids is effective and safe, lower doses of systemic steroids (0.5 mg/kg/d) are safe and effective in moderate BP, and adjuvant agents (plasma exchange, azathioprine, mycophenolate mofetil, tetracycline, and nicotinamide) in BP may be beneficial but require further study. Multiple other treatments (topical tacrolimus, dapsone, doxycycline, leflunomide, rituximab, omalizumab, intravenous immunoglobulin, and immunoadsorption/immunoapheresis) have been used in BP, but their real efficacy requires confirmation by controlled trials. Various treatment guidelines have been published for BP.[115-121] The treatment of PG is reviewed elsewhere[91,122] and will not be discussed further.

Patients with BP tend to be old and have multiple comorbidities with potential drug interactions. Use of systemic agents must be balanced with the potential for harm. Our approach is to use potent topical steroids or topical tacrolimus for BP with limited skin involvement. For moderately severe BP, we will commence oral prednisone at 0.5 mg/kg/d. Anti-inflammatory agents such as tetracycline and niacinamide or dapsone can be added if patients are unable to reduce the dose of oral prednisone or have poor response to it. For severe BP, immunosuppressive adjuvants (azathioprine, mycophenolate mofetil, or methotrexate) can be started concurrently with oral prednisone. Intravenous immunoglobulin can be used to induce or maintain remission in treatment-resistant cases or when there are contraindications to other therapy, but adjuvant agents are still required to prevent a rebound of disease before the next infusion.

MUCOUS MEMBRANE PEMPHIGOID

Mucous membrane pemphigoid[123,124] (MMP) refers to a group of rare subepidermal blistering diseases in the elderly, affecting the mucosa and less commonly the skin, leading to erosions and disabling scarring of the affected mucosa. The incidence of MMP was 1 per million persons per year in France[125] and 2 per million persons per year in Germany.[126] In comparison, MMP is extremely rare in Singapore[100] and accounted for 0.7% of autoimmune bullous diseases diagnosed in Iran,[22] 1.1% in Tunisia,[21] and 14% in Uganda.[127] The incidence in dermatology literature may be underreported because patients can present to other specialties for their site-specific complaints. Three variants are defined: anti-epiligrin MMP (anti–laminin-332 antibody), ocular MMP (anti-integrin β4 subunit antibody), and oral MMP (anti-BP180 NC16a and anti-BP180 C-terminal region or anti-integrin α6 subunit antibody). Mucosal-predominant epidermolysis bullosa acquisita (anti-collagen VII NC1 domain antibody) has a similar presentation to MMP. The pathogenesis of these rare disorders is still under research. The factors triggering a loss of tolerance to these hemidesmosomal proteins are unknown, but certain HLA subtypes are associated with MMP. Blistering occurs through inflammatory or noninflammatory pathways after antibody binding.[123]

Painful erosions can occur in the oral, ocular, nasal, laryngeal, esophageal,[35] and anogenital mucosa. Healing occurs with scarring and stenosis, affecting the function of the mucosal surfaces involved. Life-threatening airway obstruction and blindness are the most severe complications of MMP. Skin involvement is rare. Tense blisters appear on the head, neck, and upper torso preferentially, and heal with scarring, dyspigmentation, and milia. Scarring alopecia can occur.[39] MMP presenting with blisters in the head and neck with minimal mucosal involvement has been termed Brunsting-Perry pemphigoid. The histologic and immunofluorescence features are summarized in Table 32-2. The course of the disease is often chronic and progressive despite treatment. Patients with anti–laminin-332 (anti-epiligrin) MMP have a 6.8-fold relative risk of developing a solid organ cancer.[128] The time interval between onset of anti–laminin-332 MMP and cancer was estimated to be 14 months.[129] Patients with anti–laminin-332 MMP should receive age-appropriate cancer screening. The treatment regimen is tailored to the risk of scarring and involves a multidisciplinary approach using systemic and topical immunosuppressive agents with the aims of controlling symptoms and preserving function.[124,130]

EPIDERMOLYSIS BULLOSA ACQUISITA

Epidermolysis bullosa acquisita (EBA) is a rare subepidermal blistering disorder and can affect both adults and children.[131] The incidence in France[125] was 0.17 to 0.26 per million per year, whereas in Germany,[126] it was 0.5 per million per year. EBA forms a very low proportion of patients with autoimmune blistering disorders in Iran[22] (0.5%), Kuwait[23] (2.3%), Uganda[127] (5%), and Singapore[100] (6%). A report from France[132] noted a high proportion of black people of African descent (54%) with EBA in their cohort. They tended to be younger, had increased mortality, and had a higher frequency of the HLA-DRB1*15:03 allele.[132] Association with the HLA-DR2 allele was also found in black and white EBA patients and bullous systemic lupus erythematosus patients previously.[133] Autoantibodies to type VII collagen are postulated to cause blistering by interfering with the structure or function of type VII collagen or initiating an inflammatory cascade disrupting the dermoepidermal junction.[131]

EBA has a heterogeneous clinical presentation.[131,134] The mechanobullous presentation is similar to dystrophic EB with blisters and atrophic scarring (with risk of nail loss, scarring alopecia, mitten deformities, dyspigmentation, and milia) affecting trauma-prone areas of the body [**Figure 32-8**]. A phenotype similar to BP, linear IgA bullous dermatosis or MMP can also be seen. The histologic and immunofluorescence findings are summarized in Table 32-2. An ELISA system has recently been developed as a research tool to aid diagnosis of EBA.[135] Reported associations with EBA include inflammatory bowel disease, amyloidosis, and lymphoma. EBA can be chronic and refractory to treatment. Patients should actively protect the skin from trauma. Because of its rarity, there are no randomized controlled therapeutic trials to date. Multiple systemic anti-inflammatory, immunosuppressive, and immunomodulating treatment agents have been tried with varying results.[131,134]

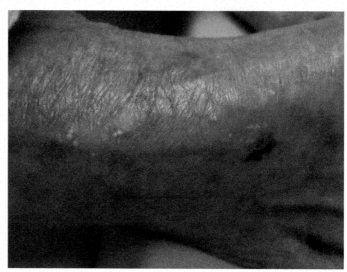

FIGURE 32-8. Two clusters of milia on the dorsum of the right foot in an Asian patient with epidermolysis bullosa acquisita.

BULLOUS SYSTEMIC LUPUS ERYTHEMATOSUS

Bullous systemic lupus erythematosus[136] (BSLE) is an extremely rare autoimmune blistering disease due to autoantibodies against type VII collagen, seen in the setting of active systemic lupus erythematosus (SLE). It can present with tense cutaneous blisters or vesicles particularly on sun-exposed skin. Mucous membrane involvement can occur with blisters and erosions. The histologic and immunofluorescence features are summarized in Table 32-2. It can be responsive to treatment with dapsone, although prednisone or other systemic immunosuppressive agents may be needed if the skin blistering is severe or if other SLE symptoms necessitate this treatment.

ANTI-LAMININ γ1 PEMPHIGOID

Anti-laminin γ1 pemphigoid or anti-p200 pemphigoid is a newly described autoimmune subepidermal bullous disease.[137,138] Antibody against the extracellular matrix glycoprotein laminin γ1 was discovered in 2009,[139] but its pathogenicity remains to be determined.[140] More than 70 cases had been diagnosed in Japan and Germany by 2010.[138] It affects adults, with a male predominance. An underlying history of psoriasis can sometimes be elicited.[137] Lesions resembling BP, linear IgA bullous dermatosis, or dermatitis herpetiformis can be seen, with occasional mucosal involvement. Histology and immunofluorescence findings resemble EBA, BSLE, and MMP [Table 32-2]. Although these conditions can sometimes be differentiated based on clinical features, definite diagnosis depends on demonstration of the p200 antigen by immunoblotting or ELISA, which may not be routinely available. Treatment is based on case reports and case series.[138]

LINEAR IgA BULLOUS DERMATOSIS

Linear IgA bullous dermatosis (LABD) is uncommon in adults, although it is the predominant cause of autoimmune blistering diseases in children together with dermatitis herpetiformis.[141-143] The incidence of LABD was 29 new cases a year in France[125] and 1 per million people per year in Germany,[126] behind BP, MMP, and PG. In Uganda,[127] the proportion of patients with LABD was higher, at 18% of all blistering diseases, probably due to its younger population. LABD forms a small proportion of all autoimmune blistering diseases in Tunisia[21] (6.3%), Iran[22] (0.4%), Kuwait[23] (7%), and Singapore[100] (3%). Association with HLA Cw7, B8, and DR3 in British and black South African patients was described.[144] The antigenic targets in LABD include the 120-kDa and 97-kDa shed ectodomain of type XVII collagen (BP180), BP180 NC16a domain, BP230, type VII collagen, LAD285, and others. Binding of IgA antibodies to these targets activates an inflammatory cascade with neutrophil infiltration and subsequent blistering. Medications (especially vancomycin) have been associated with inducing adult LABD, although the veracity of these associations has been challenged.[145] Associations have also been described with malignancies, inflammatory bowel diseases, autoimmune conditions, and infections.

Childhood LABD[146,147] presents with itchy or painful blisters commonly located on the lower body and perineum. Urticated polycyclic plaques with central healing and peripheral tense blisters (string of pearls sign) are classic for childhood LABD. Adult LABD presents with tense blisters or herpetiform vesicles arising on normal skin or urticated plaques, similar to BP or dermatitis herpetiformis.[147,148] Atypical presentations (erythema multiforme,[149] Stevens-Johnson syndrome,[150] toxic epidermal necrolysis,[151] and morbiliform[152] and localized[153] forms) are possible with drug-induced LABD. Mucosal involvement can be seen. Histologic and immunofluorescence features are highlighted in Table 32-2. Most patients respond to dapsone. Other anti-inflammatory or immunosuppressive agents can be used if dapsone is contraindicated.[147,154,155] Remission is seen in most adult LABD after a few years and before puberty in childhood LABD.

DERMATITIS HERPETIFORMIS

Dermatitis herpetiformis (DH) is a unique autoimmune blistering disease where the autoantibody targets epidermal transglutaminases instead of the hemidesmosomal proteins.[156,157] It is seen in patients of northern European descent, less commonly in Asians, and rarely in African Americans. Patients with DH have underlying gluten hypersensitivity with subclinical to mild celiac disease. In genetically predisposed individuals with HLA-DQ8 or HLA-DQ2 haplotypes, intestinal tissue transglutaminase modifies gliadin in gluten into an autoantigen, resulting in T-cell stimulation and an inflammatory response against gliadin and tissue transglutaminase–gliadin complexes. IgA autoantibodies against tissue transglutaminases cross-react with epidermal transglutaminases and are deposited as immune complexes in the dermal papillae, leading to an inflammatory response with subepidermal blister formation. Patients present with itchy excoriated papules on the elbows, knees, buttocks, shoulders, back, and scalp. Palmoplantar purpura is uncommon but specific for DH. Symptoms and signs of celiac disease and malabsorption can occur, and these issues should be co-managed with a gastroenterologist. Associations with other organ-specific autoimmune diseases, non-Hodgkin lymphomas, splenic atrophy, partial IgA deficiency, neurologic involvement, and iodine sensitivity have been reported. The evaluation includes skin biopsy for histology and DIF studies [Table 32-2], IIF looking for antiendomysial antibodies, and ELISA testing for IgA anti-tissue or anti-epidermal transglutaminase antibodies. ELISA testing for IgG anti-transglutaminase or anti-endomysial antibodies can be used if patients have IgA deficiency. Existing guidelines suggest screening for associated diseases such as autoimmune thyroid diseases, insulin-dependent diabetes mellitus, other autoimmune diseases, and splenic atrophy.[157] Patients with symptomatic DH respond rapidly to dapsone, but clinical remission is possible only with a lifelong gluten-free diet.

CONCLUSION

In this chapter, we have presented an approach to diagnosing blistering diseases, followed by a concise review of the more complex subject of autoimmune blistering diseases. Some clinical issues that can be faced in skin of color include difficulty in discerning erythema and disfiguring postinflammatory dyspigmentation. Patients may present late in the course of their disease because of unsuccessful attempts at cure with traditional or alternative medications or from a lack of access to care. Although there is an increasing amount of published literature regarding the epidemiology of autoimmune blistering diseases in skin of color, it is difficult to discern differences in response to treatment, if any, between skin of color populations and the Caucasian population without large, multicenter, controlled trials.

REFERENCES

1. Fine JD, Eady RA, Bauer EA, et al. The classification of inherited epidermolysis bullosa (EB): report of the Third International Consensus Meeting on Diagnosis and Classification of EB. *J Am Acad Dermatol*. 2008;58:931-950.
2. Fine JD, Mellerio JE. Extracutaneous manifestations and complications of inherited epidermolysis bullosa: part I. Epithelial associated tissues. *J Am Acad Dermatol*. 2009;61:367-384.
3. Fine JD, Mellerio JE. Extracutaneous manifestations and complications of inherited epidermolysis bullosa: part II. Other organs. *J Am Acad Dermatol*. 2009;61:387-402.
4. Lai-Cheong JE, Tanaka A, Hawche G, et al. Kindler syndrome: a focal adhesion genodermatosis. *Br J Dermatol*. 2009;160:233-242.
5. Puy H, Gouya L, Deybach JC. Porphyrias. *Lancet*. 2010;375:924-937.
6. Oji V, Tadini G, Akiyama M, et al. Revised nomenclature and classification of inherited ichthyoses: results of the First Ichthyosis Consensus Conference in Sorèze 2009. *J Am Acad Dermatol*. 2010;63:607-641.
7. Schmidt E, Zillikens D. Modern diagnosis of autoimmune blistering skin diseases. *Autoimmun Rev*. 2010;10:84-89.
8. Mutasim DF, Adams BB. Immunofluorescence in dermatology. *J Am Acad Dermatol*. 2001;45:803-822.
9. Amagai M, Stanley JR. Desmoglein as a target in skin disease and beyond. *J Invest Dermatol*. 2012;132:776-784.
10. Grando SA. Pemphigus autoimmunity: hypotheses and realities. *Autoimmunity*. 2012;45:7-35.
11. Mahoney MG, Wang Z, Rothenberger KL, et al. Explanation for the clinical and microscopic localization of lesions in pemphigus foliaceus and vulgaris. *J Clin Invest*. 1999;103:461-468.
12. Sinha AA. The genetics of pemphigus. *Dermatol Clin*. 2011;29:381-391.
13. Mashiah J, Brenner S. Medical pearl: first step in managing pemphigus—addressing the etiology. *J Am Acad Dermatol*. 2005;53:706-707.
14. Brenner S, Goldberg I. Drug-induced pemphigus. *Clin Dermatol*. 2011;29:455-457.
15. Aoki V, Sousa JX Jr, Diaz LA; Cooperative Group on Fogo Selvagem Research. Pathogenesis of endemic pemphigus foliaceus. *Dermatol Clin*. 2011;29:413-418.
16. Zenzo GD, Zambruno G, Borradori L. Endemic pemphigus foliaceus: towards understanding autoimmune mechanisms of disease development. *J Invest Dermatol*. 2012;132:2499-2502.
17. Qian Y, Jeong JS, Maldonado M, et al. Cutting edge: Brazilian pemphigus foliaceus anti-desmoglein 1 autoantibodies cross-react with sand fly salivary LJM11 antigen. *J Immunol*. 2012;189:1535-1539.
18. Langan SM, Smeeth L, Hubbard R, et al. Bullous pemphigoid and pemphigus vulgaris: incidence and mortality in the UK: population based cohort study. *BMJ*. 2008;337:a180.
19. Risser J, Lewis K, Weinstock MA. Mortality of bullous skin disorders from 1979 through 2002 in the United States. *Arch Dermatol*. 2009;145:1005-1008.
20. Bozdag K, Bilgin I. Epidemiology of pemphigus in the western region of Turkey: retrospective analysis of 87 patients. *Cutan Ocul Toxicol*. 2012;31:280-285.
21. Zaraa I, Kerkeni N, Ishak F, et al. Spectrum of autoimmune blistering dermatoses in Tunisia: an 11-year study and a review of the literature. *Int J Dermatol*. 2011;50:939-944.
22. Daneshpazhooh M, Chams-Davatchi C, Payandemehr P, et al. Spectrum of autoimmune bullous diseases in Iran: a 10-year review. *Int J Dermatol*. 2012;51:35-41.
23. Nanda A, Dvorak R, Al-Saeed K, et al. Spectrum of autoimmune bullous diseases in Kuwait. *Int J Dermatol*. 2004;43:876-881.
24. Kanwar AJ, De D. Pemphigus in India. *Indian J Dermatol Venereol Leprol*. 2011;77:439-449.
25. Huang YH, Kuo CF, Chen YH, et al. Incidence, mortality, and causes of death of patients with pemphigus in Taiwan: a nationwide population-based study. *J Invest Dermatol*. 2012;132:92-97.
26. Kulthanan K, Chularojanamontri L, Tuchinda P, et al. Clinical features and course of pemphigus in Thai patients. *Asian Pac J Allergy Immunol*. 2011;29:161-168.
27. Tanikawa A, Amagai M. Pemphigus treatment in Japan. *Dermatol Clin*. 2011;29:685-686.
28. Aboobaker J, Morar N, Ramdial PK, et al. Pemphigus in South Africa. *Int J Dermatol*. 2001;40:115-119.
29. Seo PG, Choi WW, Chung JH. Pemphigus in Korea: clinical manifestations and treatment protocol. *J Dermatol*. 2003;30:782-788.

30. Goon AT, Tan SH. Comparative study of pemphigus vulgaris and pemphigus foliaceus in Singapore. *Australas J Dermatol.* 2001;42:172-175.

31. Lo Russo L, Fierro G, Guiglia R, et al. Epidemiology of desquamative gingivitis: evaluation of 125 patients and review of the literature. *Int J Dermatol.* 2009;48:1049-1052.

32. Daoud YJ, Cervantes R, Foster CS, et al. Ocular pemphigus. *J Am Acad Dermatol.* 2005;53:585-590.

33. Kavala M, Altıntaş S, Kocatürk E, et al. Ear, nose and throat involvement in patients with pemphigus vulgaris: correlation with severity, phenotype and disease activity. *J Eur Acad Dermatol Venereol.* 2011;25:1324-1327.

34. Mahmoud A, Miziara ID, Costa KC, et al. Laryngeal involvement in pemphigus vulgaris: a proposed classification. *J Laryngol Otol.* 2012;126:1041-1044.

35. Hokama A, Yamamoto Y, Taira K, et al. Esophagitis dissecans superficialis and autoimmune bullous dermatoses: a review. *World J Gastrointest Endosc.* 2010;2:252-256.

36. Malik M, Ahmed AR. Involvement of the female genital tract in pemphigus vulgaris. *Obstet Gynecol.* 2005;106:1005-1012.

37. Malik M, El Tal AE, Ahmed AR. Anal involvement in pemphigus vulgaris. *Dis Colon Rectum.* 2006;49:500-506.

38. Tosti A, André M, Murrell DF. Nail involvement in autoimmune bullous disorders. *Dermatol Clin.* 2011;29:511-513.

39. Miteva M, Murrell DF, Tosti A. Hair loss in autoimmune cutaneous bullous disorders. *Dermatol Clin.* 2011;29:503-509.

40. Tan HH, Tay YK. An unusual case of pemphigus vulgaris presenting as bilateral foot ulcers. *Clin Exp Dermatol.* 2000;25:224-226.

41. Milgraum SS, Kanzler MH, Waldinger TP, et al. Macroglossia. An unusual presentation of pemphigus vulgaris. *Arch Dermatol.* 1985;121:1328-1329.

42. Gurgen J, Dorton D. Unusual case of pemphigus vulgaris mimicking localized pustular psoriasis of the hands and feet. *Cutis.* 2010;86:138-140.

43. Nousari HC, Moresi M, Klapper M, et al. Nonendemic pemphigus foliaceus presenting as fatal bullous exfoliative erythroderma. *Cutis.* 2001;67:251-252.

44. Bagheri MM, Alagheband M, Memar OM, et al. Pemphigus foliaceus presenting as eruptive seborrheic keratosis and responding to oral gold treatment. *J Drugs Dermatol.* 2002;1:333-334.

45. Grekin SJ, Fox MC, Gudjonsson JE, et al. Psoriasiform pemphigus foliaceus: a report of two cases. *J Cutan Pathol.* 2012;39:549-553.

46. Ng PP, Thng ST. Three cases of transition from pemphigus vulgaris to pemphigus foliaceus confirmed by desmoglein ELISA. *Dermatology.* 2005;210:319-321.

47. Sabolinski ML, Beutner EH, Krasny S, et al. Substrate specificity of anti-epithelial antibodies of pemphigus vulgaris and pemphigus foliaceus sera in immunofluorescence tests on monkey and guinea pig esophagus sections. *J Invest Dermatol.* 1987;88:545-549.

48. Cheng SW, Kobayashi M, Kinoshita-Kuroda K, et al. Monitoring disease activity in pemphigus with enzyme-linked immunosorbent assay using recombinant desmogleins 1 and 3. *Br J Dermatol.* 2002;147:261-265.

49. Kwon EJ, Yamagami J, Nishikawa T, et al. Anti-desmoglein IgG autoantibodies in patients with pemphigus in remission. *J Eur Acad Dermatol Venereol.* 2008;22:1070-1075.

50. Chee SN, Murrell DF. Pemphigus and quality of life. *Dermatol Clin.* 2011;29:521-525.

51. Murrell DF, Werth VP, Segall J, et al. The International Pemphigus and Pemphigoid Foundation. *Dermatol Clin.* 2011;29:655-657.

52. Martin LK, Werth VP, Villanueva EV, et al. A systematic review of randomized controlled trials for pemphigus vulgaris and pemphigus foliaceus. *J Am Acad Dermatol.* 2011;64:903-908.

53. Murrell DF, Dick S, Ahmed AR, et al. Consensus statement on definitions of disease, end points, and therapeutic response for pemphigus. *J Am Acad Dermatol.* 2008;58:1043-1046.

54. Daniel BS, Hertl M, Werth VP, et al. Severity score indexes for blistering diseases. *Clin Dermatol.* 2012;30:108-113.

55. Frew JW, Martin LK, Murrell DF. Evidence-based treatments in pemphigus vulgaris and pemphigus foliaceus. *Dermatol Clin.* 2011;29:599-606.

56. Strowd LC, Taylor SL, Jorizzo JL, et al. Therapeutic ladder for pemphigus vulgaris: emphasis on achieving complete remission. *J Am Acad Dermatol.* 2011;64:490-494.

57. Bystryn JC, Rudolph JL. Pemphigus. *Lancet.* 2005;366:61-73.

58. Harman KE, Albert S, Black MM; British Association of Dermatologists. Guidelines for the management of pemphigus vulgaris. *Br J Dermatol.* 2003;149:926-937.

59. Tsuruta D, Ishii N, Hashimoto T. Diagnosis and treatment of pemphigus. *Immunotherapy.* 2012;4:735-745.

60. Kasperkiewicz M, Schmidt E, Zillikens D. Current therapy of the pemphigus group. *Clin Dermatol.* 2012;30:84-94.

61. Singh S. Evidence-based treatments for pemphigus vulgaris, pemphigus foliaceus, and bullous pemphigoid: a systematic review. *Indian J Dermatol Venereol Leprol.* 2011;77:456-469.

62. Tirado-Sánchez A, León-Dorantes G. Treatment of pemphigus vulgaris. An overview in Mexico. *Allergol Immunopathol (Madr).* 2006;34:10-16.

63. Herbst A, Bystryn JC. Patterns of remission in pemphigus vulgaris. *J Am Acad Dermatol.* 2000;42:422-427.

64. Herrmann G, Hunzelmann N, Engert A. Treatment of pemphigus vulgaris with anti-CD20 monoclonal antibody (rituximab). *Br J Dermatol.* 2003;148:602-603.

65. Feldman RJ, Ahmed AR. Relevance of rituximab therapy in pemphigus vulgaris: analysis of current data and the immunologic basis for its observed responses. *Expert Rev Clin Immunol.* 2011;7:529-541.

66. Craythorne EE, Mufti G, DuVivier AW. Rituximab used as a first-line single agent in the treatment of pemphigus vulgaris. *J Am Acad Dermatol.* 2011;65:1064-1065.

67. Lunardon L, Tsai KJ, Propert KJ, et al. Adjuvant rituximab therapy of pemphigus: a single-center experience with 31 patients. *Arch Dermatol.* 2012;148:1031-1036.

68. Rios-Fernández R, Gutierrez-Salmerón MT, Callejas-Rubio JL, et al. Late-onset neutropenia following rituximab treatment in patients with autoimmune diseases. *Br J Dermatol.* 2007;157:1271-1273.

69. Li WW, Chen XX, Yu J, et al. Haemolytic anaemia following rituximab treatment in a patient with pemphigus vulgaris. *Br J Dermatol.* 2009;161:205-206.

70. Werth VP, Fivenson D, Pandya AG, et al. Multicenter randomized, double-blind, placebo-controlled, clinical trial of dapsone as a glucocorticoid-sparing agent in maintenance-phase pemphigus vulgaris. *Arch Dermatol.* 2008;144:25-32.

71. Tsuruta D, Ishii N, Hamada T, et al. IgA pemphigus. *Clin Dermatol.* 2011;29:437-442.

72. Hashimoto T, Kiyokawa C, Mori O, et al. Human desmocollin 1 (Dsc1) is an autoantigen for the subcorneal pustular dermatosis type of IgA pemphigus. *J Invest Dermatol.* 1997;109:127-131.

73. Petropoulou H, Politis G, Panagakis P, et al. Immunoglobulin A pemphigus associated with immunoglobulin A gammapathy and lung cancer. *J Dermatol.* 2008;35:341-345.

74. Aste N, Fumo G, Pinna AL, et al. IgA pemphigus of the subcorneal pustular dermatosis type associated with monoclonal IgA gammopathy. *J Eur Acad Dermatol Venereol.* 2003;17:725-727.

75. Anhalt GJ, Kim SC, Stanley JR, et al. Paraneoplastic pemphigus. An autoimmune mucocutaneous disease associated with neoplasia. *N Engl J Med.* 1990;323:1729-1735.

76. Camisa C, Helm TN. Paraneoplastic pemphigus is a distinct neoplasia-induced autoimmune disease. *Arch Dermatol.* 1993;129:883-886.

77. Nguyen VT, Ndoye A, Bassler KD, et al. Classification, clinical manifestations, and immunopathological mechanisms of the epithelial variant of paraneoplastic autoimmune multiorgan syndrome: a reappraisal of paraneoplastic pemphigus. *Arch Dermatol.* 2001;137:193-206.

78. Billet SE, Grando SA, Pittelkow MR. Paraneoplastic autoimmune multiorgan syndrome: review of the literature and support for a cytotoxic role in pathogenesis. *Autoimmunity.* 2006;39:617-630.

79. Czernik A, Camilleri M, Pittelkow MR, et al. Paraneoplastic autoimmune multiorgan syndrome: 20 years after. *Int J Dermatol.* 2011;50:905-914.

80. Mimouni D, Anhalt GJ, Lazarova Z, et al. Paraneoplastic pemphigus in children and adolescents. *Br J Dermatol.* 2002;147:725-732.

81. Zhang J, Qiao QL, Chen XX, et al. Improved outcomes after complete resection of underlying tumors for patients with paraneoplastic pemphigus: a single-center experience of 22 cases. *J Cancer Res Clin Oncol.* 2011;137:229-234.

82. Kaplan I, Hodak E, Ackerman L, et al. Neoplasms associated with paraneoplastic pemphigus: a review with emphasis on non-hematologic malignancy and oral mucosal manifestations. *Oral Oncol.* 2004;40:553-562.

83. Nousari HC, Deterding R, Wojtczack H, et al. The mechanism of respiratory failure in paraneoplastic pemphigus. *N Engl J Med.* 1999;340:1406-1410.

84. Maldonado F, Pittelkow MR, Ryu JH. Constrictive bronchiolitis associated with paraneoplastic autoimmune multi-organ syndrome. *Respirology.* 2009;14:129-133.

85. Leger S, Picard D, Ingen-Housz-Oro S, et al. Prognostic factors of paraneoplastic pemphigus. *Arch Dermatol.* 2012;148:1165-1172.

86. Cummins DL, Mimouni D, Tzu J, et al. Lichenoid paraneoplastic pemphigus in the absence of detectable antibodies. *J Am Acad Dermatol.* 2007;56:153-159.

87. Bennett DD, Busick TL. Delayed detection of autoantibodies in paraneoplastic pemphigus. *J Am Acad Dermatol.* 2007;57:1094-1095.

88. Ujiie H, Nishie W, Shimizu H. Pathogenesis of bullous pemphigoid. *Dermatol Clin.* 2011;29:439-446.

89. Di Zenzo G, Calabresi V, Grosso F, et al. The intracellular and extracellular domains of BP180 antigen comprise novel epitopes targeted by pemphigoid gestationis autoantibodies. *J Invest Dermatol.* 2007;127:864-873.

90. Huilaja L, Hurskainen T, Autio-Harmainen H, et al. Pemphigoid gestationis autoantigen, transmembrane collagen XVII, promotes the migration of cytotrophoblastic cells of placenta and is a structural component of fetal membranes. *Matrix Biol.* 2008;27:190-200.

91. Semkova K, Black M. Pemphigoid gestationis: current insights into pathogenesis and treatment. *Eur J Obstet Gynecol Reprod Biol.* 2009;145:138-144.

92. Zakka LR, Reche P, Ahmed AR. Role of MHC class II genes in the pathogenesis of pemphigoid. *Autoimmun Rev.* 2011;11:40-47.

93. Shornick JK, Jenkins RE, Artlett CM, et al. Class II MHC typing in pemphigoid gestationis. *Clin Exp Dermatol.* 1995;20:123-126.

94. Bastuji-Garin S, Joly P, Lemordant P, et al: French Study Group for Bullous Diseases. Risk factors for bullous pemphigoid in the elderly: a prospective case-control study. *J Invest Dermatol.* 2011;131:637-643.

95. Lee JJ, Downham TF 2nd. Furosemide-induced bullous pemphigoid: case report and review of literature. *J Drugs Dermatol.* 2006;5:562-564.

96. Skandalis K, Spirova M, Gaitanis G, et al. Drug-induced bullous pemphigoid in diabetes mellitus patients receiving dipeptidyl peptidase-IV inhibitors plus metformin. *J Eur Acad Dermatol Venereol.* 2012;26:249-253.

97. Joly P, Baricault S, Sparsa A, et al. Incidence and mortality of bullous pemphigoid in France. *J Invest Dermatol.* 2012;132:1998-2004.

98. Parker SR, Dyson S, Brisman S, et al. Mortality of bullous pemphigoid: an evaluation of 223 patients and comparison with the mortality in the general population in the United States. *J Am Acad Dermatol.* 2008;59:582-588.

99. Cortés B, Marazza G, Naldi L, et al; Autoimmune Bullous Disease Swiss Study Group. Mortality of bullous pemphigoid in Switzerland: a prospective study. *Br J Dermatol.* 2011;165:368-374.

100. Wong SN, Chua SH. Spectrum of subepidermal immunobullous disorders seen at the National Skin Centre, Singapore: a 2-year review. *Br J Dermatol.* 2002;147:476-480.

101. Joly P, Tanasescu S, Wolkenstein P, et al. Lichenoid erythrodermic bullous pemphigoid of the African patient. *J Am Acad Dermatol.* 1998;39:691-697.

102. Fisler RE, Saeb M, Liang MG, et al. Childhood bullous pemphigoid: a clinicopathologic study and review of the literature. *Am J Dermatopathol.* 2003;25:183-189.

103. Martinez-De Pablo MI, González-Enseñat MA, Vicente A, et al. Childhood bullous pemphigoid: clinical and immunological findings in a series of 4 cases. *Arch Dermatol.* 2007;143:215-220.

104. Mirza M, Zamilpa I, Wilson JM. Localized penile bullous pemphigoid of childhood. *J Pediatr Urol.* 2008;4:395-397.

105. Sami N, Ahmed AR. Dual diagnosis of pemphigus and pemphigoid. Retrospective review of thirty cases in the literature. *Dermatology.* 2001;202:293-301.

106. Recke A, Rose C, Schmidt E, et al. Transition from pemphigus foliaceus to bullous pemphigoid: intermolecular B-cell epitope spreading without IgG subclass shifting. *J Am Acad Dermatol.* 2009;61:333-336.

107. Schmidt E, della Torre R, Borradori L. Clinical features and practical diagnosis of bullous pemphigoid. *Dermatol Clin.* 2011;29:427-438.

108. Mariotti F, Grosso F, Terracina M, et al. Development of a novel ELISA system for detection of anti-BP180 IgG and characterization of autoantibody profile in bullous pemphigoid patients. *Br J Dermatol.* 2004;151:1004-1010.

109. Bernard P, Reguiai Z, Tancrède-Bohin E, et al. Risk factors for relapse in patients with bullous pemphigoid in clinical remission: a multicenter, prospective, cohort study. *Arch Dermatol.* 2009;145:537-542.

110. Rzany B, Partscht K, Jung M, et al. Risk factors for lethal outcome in patients with bullous pemphigoid: low serum albumin level, high dosage of glucocorticosteroids, and old age. *Arch Dermatol.* 2002;138:903-908.

111. Joly P, Benichou J, Lok C, et al. Prediction of survival for patients with bullous pemphigoid: a prospective study. *Arch Dermatol.* 2005;141:691-698.

112. Murrell DF, Daniel BS, Joly P, et al. Definitions and outcome measures for bullous pemphigoid: recommendations by an international panel of experts. *J Am Acad Dermatol.* 2012;66:479-485.

113. Kirtschig G, Middleton P, Bennett C, et al. Interventions for bullous pemphigoid. *Cochrane Database Syst Rev.* 2010;10:CD002292.

114. García-Romero MT, Werth VP. Randomized controlled trials needed for bullous pemphigoid interventions. *Arch Dermatol.* 2012;148:243-246.

115. Patton T, Korman NJ. Bullous pemphigoid treatment review. *Expert Opin Pharmacother.* 2006;7:2403-2411.

116. Roujeau JC, Ingen-Housz-Oro S, Leroux C, et al. Treatment of bullous pemphigoid and pemphigus. The French experience, 2009 update. *G Ital Dermatol Venereol.* 2009;144:333-338.

117. Schmidt E, Zillikens D. The diagnosis and treatment of autoimmune blistering skin diseases. *Dtsch Arztebl Int.* 2011;108:399-405.

118. Khandpur S, Verma P. Bullous pemphigoid. *Indian J Dermatol Venereol Leprol.* 2011;77:450-455.

119. Daniel BS, Borradori L, Hall RP 3rd, et al. Evidence-based management of bullous pemphigoid. *Dermatol Clin.* 2011;29:613-620.

120. Venning VA, Taghipour K, Mohd Mustapa MF, et al. British Association of Dermatologists' guidelines for the management of bullous pemphigoid 2012. *Br J Dermatol.* 2012;167:1200-1214.

121. Culton DA, Diaz LA. Treatment of subepidermal immunobullous diseases. *Clin Dermatol.* 2012;30:95-102.

122. Intong LR, Murrell DF. Pemphigoid gestationis: current management. *Dermatol Clin.* 2011;29:621-628.

123. Kourosh AS, Yancey KB. Pathogenesis of mucous membrane pemphigoid. *Dermatol Clin.* 2011;29:479-484.

124. Chan LS, Ahmed AR, Anhalt GJ, et al. The first international consensus on mucous membrane pemphigoid: definition, diagnostic criteria, pathogenic factors, medical treatment, and prognostic indicators. *Arch Dermatol.* 2002;138:370-379.

125. Bernard P, Vaillant L, Labeille B, et al. Incidence and distribution of subepidermal autoimmune bullous skin diseases in three French regions. Bullous Diseases French Study Group. *Arch Dermatol.* 1995;131:48-52.

126. Bertram F, BrÖcker EB, Zillikens D, et al. Prospective analysis of the incidence of autoimmune bullous disorders in Lower Franconia, Germany. *J Dtsch Dermatol Ges.* 2009;7:434-440.

127. Mulyowa GK, Jaeger G, Kabakyenga J, et al. Autoimmune subepidermal blistering diseases in Uganda: correlation of autoantibody class with age of patients. *Int J Dermatol.* 2006;45:1047-1052.

128. Egan CA, Lazarova Z, Darling TN, et al. Anti-epiligrin cicatricial pemphigoid and relative risk for cancer. *Lancet.* 2001;357:1850-1851.

129. Sadler E, Lazarova Z, Sarasombath P, et al. A widening perspective regarding the relationship between anti-epiligrin cicatricial pemphigoid and cancer. *J Dermatol Sci.* 2007;47:1-7.

130. Kourosh AS, Yancey KB. Therapeutic approaches to patients with mucous membrane pemphigoid. *Dermatol Clin.* 2011;29:637-641.

131. Gupta R, Woodley DT, Chen M. Epidermolysis bullosa acquisita. *Clin Dermatol.* 2012;30:60-69.

132. Zumelzu C, Le Roux-Villet C, Loiseau P, et al. Black patients of African descent and HLA-DRB1*15:03 frequency overrepresented in epidermolysis bullosa acquisita. *J Invest Dermatol.* 2011;131:2386-2393.

133. Gammon WR, Heise ER, Burke WA, et al. Increased frequency of HLA-DR2 in patients with autoantibodies to epidermolysis bullosa acquisita antigen: evidence that the expression of autoimmunity to type VII collagen is HLA class II allele associated. *J Invest Dermatol.* 1988;91:228-232.

134. Lehman JS, Camilleri MJ, Gibson LE. Epidermolysis bullosa acquisita: concise review and practical considerations. *Int J Dermatol.* 2009;48:227-235.

135. Saleh MA, Ishii K, Kim YJ, et al. Development of NC1 and NC2 domains of type VII collagen ELISA for the diagnosis and analysis of the time course of epidermolysis bullosa acquisita patients. *J Dermatol Sci.* 2011;62:169-175.

136. Sebaratnam DF, Murrell DF. Bullous systemic lupus erythematosus. *Dermatol Clin.* 2011;29:649-653.

137. Dilling A, Rose C, Hashimoto T, et al. Anti-p200 pemphigoid: a novel autoimmune subepidermal blistering disease. *J Dermatol.* 2007;34:1-8.

138. Dainichi T, Koga H, Tsuji T, et al. From anti-p200 pemphigoid to anti-laminin gamma1 pemphigoid. *J Dermatol.* 2010;37:231-238.

139. Dainichi T, Kurono S, Ohyama B, et al. Anti-laminin gamma-1 pemphigoid. *Proc Natl Acad Sci U S A.* 2009;106:2800-2805.

140. Vafia K, Groth S, Beckmann T, et al. Pathogenicity of autoantibodies in anti-p200 pemphigoid. *PLoS One.* 2012;7:e41769.

141. Kenani N, Mebazaa A, Denguezli M, et al. Childhood linear IgA bullous dermatosis in Tunisia. *Pediatr Dermatol.* 2009;26:28-33.

142. Aboobaker J, Wojnarowska FT, Bhogal B, et al. Chronic bullous dermatosis of childhood—clinical and immunological features seen in African patients. *Clin Exp Dermatol.* 1991;16:160-164.

143. Sansaricq F, Stein SL, Petronic-Rosic V. Autoimmune bullous diseases in childhood. *Clin Dermatol.* 2012;30:114-127.

144. Collier PM, Wojnarowska F, Welsh K, et al. Adult linear IgA disease and chronic bullous disease of childhood: the association with human lymphocyte antigens Cw7, B8, DR3 and tumour necrosis factor influences disease expression. *Br J Dermatol.* 1999;141:867-875.

145. Fortuna G, Salas-Alanis JC, Guidetti E, et al. A critical reappraisal of the current data on drug-induced linear immunoglobulin A bullous dermatosis: a real and separate nosological entity? *J Am Acad Dermatol.* 2012;66:988-994.

146. Mintz EM, Morel KD. Clinical features, diagnosis, and pathogenesis of chronic bullous disease of childhood. *Dermatol Clin.* 2011;29:459-462.
147. Fortuna G, Marinkovich MP. Linear immunoglobulin A bullous dermatosis. *Clin Dermatol.* 2012;30:38-50.
148. Venning VA. Linear IgA disease: clinical presentation, diagnosis, and pathogenesis. *Dermatol Clin.* 2011;29:453-458.
149. Tonev S, Vasileva S, Kadurina M. Depot sulfonamid associated linear IgA bullous dermatosis with erythema multiforme-like clinical features. *J Eur Acad Dermatol Venereol.* 1998;11:165-168.
150. Cummings JE, Snyder RR, Kelly EB, et al. Drug-induced linear immunoglobulin A bullous dermatosis mimicking Stevens-Johnson syndrome: a case report. *Cutis.* 2007;79:203-207.
151. Waldman MA, Black DR, Callen JP. Vancomycin-induced linear IgA bullous disease presenting as toxic epidermal necrolysis. *Clin Exp Dermatol.* 2004;29:633-636.
152. Billet SE, Kortuem KR, Gibson LE, et al. A morbilliform variant of vancomycin-induced linear IgA bullous dermatosis. *Arch Dermatol.* 2008;144:774-778.
153. Walsh SN, Kerchner K, Sangüeza OP. Localized palmar vancomycin-induced linear IgA bullous dermatosis occurring at supratherapeutic levels. *Arch Dermatol.* 2009;145:603-604.
154. Ng SY, Venning VV. Management of linear IgA disease. *Dermatol Clin.* 2011;29:629-630.
155. Mintz EM, Morel KD. Treatment of chronic bullous disease of childhood. *Dermatol Clin.* 2011;29:699-700.
156. Bolotin D, Petronic-Rosic V. Dermatitis herpetiformis. Part I. Epidemiology, pathogenesis, and clinical presentation. *J Am Acad Dermatol.* 2011;64:1017-1024.
157. Bolotin D, Petronic-Rosic V. Dermatitis herpetiformis. Part II. Diagnosis, management, and prognosis. *J Am Acad Dermatol.* 2011;64:1027-1033.

CHAPTER 33	# Keloids

A. Paul Kelly
Ardeshir Bayat

KEY POINTS

- Keloid disease is a significant clinical problem for patients with skin of color.
- Keloid scars are overgrowths of dense fibrous tissue which develop as a result of a cutaneous injury and invade the healthy tissue in the area surrounding the injury.
- Hypertrophic scars are also overgrowths of fibrous tissue, but in contrast to keloids, they usually stay within the confines of the precipitating cutaneous injury.
- Keloids differ from hypertrophic scars in their metabolic activity and collagen turnover.
- Many theories have been advanced to explain the etiology of keloids, although none have been substantiated. However, it can be said that there is a familial tendency of keloid susceptibility. This hereditary tendency is more common in patients with skin of color.
- Although keloids may be found anywhere on the body, they tend to have a regional predilection, occurring most often on the ears, anterior chest, upper back, and shoulders.
- Although rare, keloids may develop on the genitalia, palms and soles, mucous membranes, tongue, and even cornea.

INTRODUCTION

Synonyms for Keloids include:

- *Cheloide*
- Keloid disease
- Keloidal scar
- Raised dermal scarring
- Excessive scar tissue
- Abnormal wound healing

Keloids are common, hyperproliferative, reticular, dermal lesions of unknown etiopathogenesis that often occur in genetically susceptible individuals. Keloid scars develop as a result of an overgrowth of scar tissue beyond the site of the original skin injury (no matter how minor) such as surgical incisions, traumatic wounds, vaccination sites, burns, chickenpox, acne, or even minor scratches. Keloids are more common in people with skin of color, such as African Americans.

Although keloids are clinically benign (not neoplastic), they can behave in an aggressive manner and are often psychologically and/or socially devastating for patients. Keloids represent an overgrowth of dense, fibrous tissue that develops as a result of even the most minor form of cutaneous injury. Hypertrophic scars usually stay within the confines of the precipitating injury, whereas keloids invade the surrounding noninjured normal skin. Additional clinical and histologic characteristics distinguish keloid scars from hypertrophic scars [**Table 33-1**]. However, the medical literature regarding hypertrophic scars and keloid scars is often confusing because many lesions that are keloid-like are mislabeled as hypertrophic scars or vice versa. Additionally, some patients have both kinds of scars caused by the same traumatic incident. Clinical studies often lump the two disorders together, thus leading to the dissemination of incorrect information, which is a practical concern when evaluating the therapeutic response.[1,2]

Keloids and hypertrophic scars are thought to be produced by an overgrowth of fibrous tissue, which is always secondary to some form of injury (eg, lacerations, surgical incisions, ear piercings, vaccinations, herpes zoster, acne lesions, insect bites, or burns). There are, however, reports of a small percentage of patients who develop so-called spontaneous keloids—that is, keloids with no known antecedent trauma or injury. These types of lesions occur most often in patients with a family history of keloids and are usually located in the mid-sternal area. Except for burn patients, most keloids occur in the second or third decade of life, although they can occur any time between infancy and old age.[3,4]

Hypertrophic scars usually develop rapidly after a cutaneous injury or trauma, whereas keloids develop slowly but continue to enlarge for months to years. In most instances, hypertrophic scars regress with

TABLE 33-1	A comparison of keloids and hypertrophic scars	
Characteristics	Keloids	Hypertrophic scars
Stays in confines of injury	No	Yes
Precipitated by trauma	Not always	Yes
Area of occurrence	Area of little motion	Area of motion
Growth	For extended period	Regresses in time
Symptomatic	Usually	Usually
Response to treatment	Poor	Good
Sodium	Normal	Decreased
Magnesium	Increased	Decreased
Calcium	Increased	Decreased
Mucinous ground substance	Abundant	Scarce
Fibroblasts	Few	Numerous
Foreign-body reactions	None	Frequent
Luxol fast blue collagen stain	Reddish	Blue
Mast cells	Increased	Increased
Pathogenesis	Unknown	Unknown
Contain myofibroblasts	No	Yes
Alanine transaminase	Increased	Normal

therapy, in contradistinction to keloids, which often recur during therapy or when the therapy is discontinued.

HISTORY

Jean Louis Alibert (1768–1837), one of the principal founders of French dermatology, proposed the word *cheloide* (derived from the Greek *chele,* meaning "crab's claw," and *-oid,* meaning "like") in 1806, which he had originally called *cancroide* [**Figure 33**-1].[5] Alibert later changed the name to *cheloid* to avoid confusion with cancer and its connotations. In 1825, he wrote a chapter entitled, "*Les cancroides ou keloids,*" using for the first time the word that would be adopted by American, English, and German dermatologists.[6] Even though Alibert was the first to describe the clinical characteristics of keloids, Retz had, according to Kaposi, in 1790 already described a cicatricial tumor of the skin, which he thought was of spontaneous origin, under the name *darte de graisse.*[7] In 1835, Hawkins described lesions that may have been keloids, and Macpherson added to the early literature on keloids.[8,9]

The first recorded description of keloid-like scars appears in the *Edward Smith Surgical Papyrus:* "The existence of swelling on his breast, large, spreading, and hard, touching them is like touching a ball of wrappings."[10]

Also, the Yorubas recorded their awareness of keloids 10 centuries before Alibert and Retz. Omo-Dare[11] described some of these observations on the character and presentation of keloids. The Yorubas knew, for example, that keloids frequently appeared in the same family but that not all members of the family were affected. They knew that there was a time interval between the infliction of the trauma that produced a keloid and the appearance of the lesion. Local customs of facial marking and earlobe perforation were usually performed toward the end of the first week of life. However, if there was a delay in the scarification process, according to a Yoruba saying, facial marks made in adolescence and adult life might then develop into keloids. The Yorubas also knew that once a lesion appeared, it grew and had no effective therapy except when "the Divine Power is suitably appropriated to intervene in bringing about its resolution."[11]

In 1854, Addison introduced the term true keloids (arising spontaneously) and labeled Alibert's lesions false keloids (those arising at sites of trauma).[12] The lesions he described were probably morphea or scleroderma, and his nomenclature of true keloids and false keloids should be discarded.[13]

Although originally thought to occur only in humans, lesions similar to keloids have been reported in horses, cattle, dogs, and on the feet of vultures and eagles.[14] However, even though these animals may form keloid-like scars, they are not good models for studying wound repair because the excessive collagen deposited in animals is reabsorbed when the tissue insult ceases.[15]

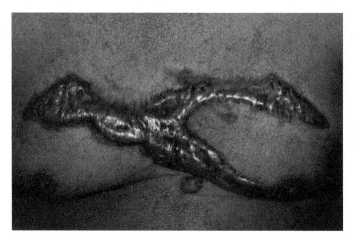

FIGURE 33-1. A crab-like keloid in the mid-sternal region of an African American man. Jean Louis Alibert (1768–1837) proposed the word cheloide (derived from the Greek *chele,* meaning "crab's claw," and *-oid,* meaning "like") in 1806.

TABLE 33-2	Epidemiology

- Incidence varies according to population studied
  - Low of 0.09% in England
  - High of 16% in Zaire
  - People with skin of color affected 5–16 times more often than lighter-skinned people
  - Asians and Hispanics fall in between these reported incidences
- The average age of onset is 22–23 years old
  - Onset after puberty
  - Young skin more taut due to greater rate of collagen synthesis

EPIDEMIOLOGY

Due to numerous variables, such as the anatomic location, type of trauma, race, age, and gender, the reported incidence of keloids in the general population ranges from a high of 16% in Zairean adults to a low of 0.01% in English Caucasian adults [**Table 33**-2].[1] People with dark skin of color develop keloids more often than those with fairer skin; however, the reported incidence ratio between the two groups ranges from 2:1 to 19:1 (in dark-skinned individuals vs light-skinned individuals, respectively).[16,17] Fox found keloids in 3 of 8382 light-skinned patients and in 76 out of 11,486 dark-skinned patients.[17] Matas reported a dark-skinned to light-skinned ratio of 9:1.[18,19] Additionally, Geschickter and Lewis[20] reported a ratio of 6:1, and Cosman et al[14] reported a ratio of 3:1.

In Aruba, however, where more than 3% of children have keloids, the children of Polynesian ancestry with keloids outnumber the dark-skinned children who have keloids. Also, in West Malaysia, the lighter-skinned Chinese appear to be slightly more prone to keloid formation than the darker-skinned Indians and Malays.[21] Arnold et al[22] found that in Hawaii, keloids are five and three times more common in Japanese and Chinese individuals, respectively, than in Caucasians. It has been reported that Europeans living in the tropics are more likely to develop keloids than those living in more temperate zones, although there has been no subsequent documentation of this observation.[23] The question of why people with skin of color develop keloids and hypertrophic scars more often than fairer-skinned individuals has inspired many theories, none of which have been accepted as the sole reason. An interesting theory advanced by Bohrod[24] was based on the principle of long-term social and religious mores of scarification, which, in turn, determined genetic predisposition.

The male-to-female incidence has been reported to be equal by some investigators, whereas others have reported that the incidence is greater in females.[25] Cosman et al[14] found that the average age of patients at the time of initial treatment was 25.8 years, and the median age at onset was 22.3 years in women and 22.6 years in men. Although it is extremely rare, the onset of keloids and hypertrophic scars has been noted in children before their first birthday, as well as in septuagenarians.

ETIOLOGY

◼ TRAUMA

Many theories have been advanced to explain the etiology of keloids [**Table 33**-3]. In most patients, trauma is the main, if not the only, precipitating factor. The trauma may take many different forms, such as simple scratches, abrasions, insect bites, vaccinations, acne papules, chickenpox lesions, surgical procedures, chemical burns, or thermal

TABLE 33-3	Proposed etiology of keloids

- Trauma
- Skin tension
- Infection
- Endocrine factors
- Genetic predisposition

burns. Because most people sustain cutaneous trauma, especially on the feet, without developing keloids, and because some keloids arise spontaneously on nontraumatized areas, one may summarize that there is most likely another predisposing variable(s) or factors(s) other than trauma itself that leads to keloid formation.[4,26]

SKIN TENSION

Increased skin tension has been cited as the reason for keloids occurring after surgery.[25,27,28] Cutting across Langer lines, with a resulting increase in skin tension, has also been suggested. An increased predisposition to developing keloid scars has been observed in certain anatomic sites that are under increased mechanical tension, such as the development of butterfly-shaped keloid scars that occur in the mid-sternal region.[29,30]

Increased skin tension can also cause coiffure keloids, which form, in a few cases, on the scalp in response to the tightly braided hairstyles that are found in many parts of Africa and that are increasing in popularity in the United States and worldwide.[31]

SEBUM

Yagi et al[32] introduced the sebum autoimmune mechanism concept of keloid formation. They postulated that after cutaneous trauma, functioning sebaceous glands may secrete sebum intradermally. The sebum then acts as an antigen, initiating an autoimmune granulomatous response that may lead to keloid formation. These authors cite the virtual absence of keloids on the palms, soles, forehead, and lips, areas that are essentially devoid of sebaceous glands, as further evidence of their theory.

FOREIGN BODY

Some investigators have suggested that it is a foreign-body reaction, or the presence of suture debris or dirt in wounds, that stimulates the formation of keloids and not the trauma itself.[26] Others have also proposed that inert material or natural products such as damaged collagen or keratin are causative stimuli.[33]

CUTANEOUS INFECTIONS

Infections, either bacterial or viral, have been implicated as a contributing factor in the formation of keloids [Table 33-4]. One of the earliest opinions was that tubercle bacilli caused keloids.[34]

However, in later studies on keloid patients, not one was found to have clinical evidence of tuberculosis, and the number of positive tuberculin reactions was within the normal population range.[34,35] Keloids may appear after chickenpox or herpes zoster infections and after smallpox vaccinations. In the past, there were many inferences that syphilis promoted keloid growth, but of more than 100 patients with keloids, only one was found to have syphilis.[1,17]

ENDOCRINE FACTORS

Keloid formation has been associated with endocrinologic factors, but there is still no definite proof that such factors are of major importance. The thymus, parathyroid, ovaries, thyroid, and pituitary glands, alone or in combination, have been incriminated.[36] Acromegalics and pregnant women have demonstrated a marked susceptibility to keloid formation.[34,37] There seems to be a greater incidence of keloids when hyperpigmentation is associated with hyperthyroidism, pregnancy, or puberty.[38] It has been postulated that in all of the preceding conditions, there is an excessive secretion of melanocyte-stimulating hormone (MSH) and the increased sensitivity of melanocytes to MSH. This may explain why people with skin of color, whose melanocytes may be more reactive to MSH, have a higher incidence of keloids than those with lighter skin

TABLE 33-4   Infections associated with keloids
• Viral infections—higher incidence of keloids after herpes zoster and chickenpox
• Bacterial infections—in the past, tuberculosis and syphilis incriminated; now, no evidence that infections precipitate keloid formation

TABLE 33-5   Factors suggesting an association between keloids and melanocytes
• Not reported in albinos
• Patients with keloids developed vitiligo
• Keloids regressed in vitiliginous areas
• May form with secretion of melanocyte-stimulating hormone
• Face, neck, deltoid area
• Presternal area, earlobes

[Table 33-5].[39] Evidence for this supposition is purely circumstantial; keloids are rare on the palms and soles, where the concentration of melanocytes is minimal.

Residues of the thymus gland have been reported in several patients with keloids.[40] Other investigators mention that the thymus may be involved in keloid formation, but to date, there has been no proof of this association.[35]

Hyperthyroidism was mentioned as a possible cause of keloid formation by Justice[41] after keloids were induced in hyperthyroid patients by irritating their skin with "excitant pharmacologic substances," the activity of which was slight. Asboe-Hansen[27] reported that young patients who underwent a thyroidectomy for Graves disease were apt to form keloids in the surgical wound, and after the injection of the thyroid extract. Also, it has been reported that hard fibrous patches, which were probably keloids, regressed in a female patient after a unilateral resection of the thyroid gland on that side.[42]

Although Asboe-Hansen[27] reported that the blood calcium level in most patients with keloids was within normal limits, Pautrier and Zorn[43] found an elevated serum calcium concentration in 9 of 12 patients with keloids, each of whom was noted to have elevated calcium levels in all of the keloid tissues. Farndon[44] observed that, during a parathyroidectomy on a patient, if the surgical incision curves down onto the sternum, then keloid formation is more likely.

Pituitary secretions have been held responsible for keloid formation, especially since acromegalics have been reported to have an increased susceptibility of developing keloids. This phenomenon was attributed to the action of growth hormones, which stimulate the formation of new connective tissues, especially collagen fibrils. Keloids seem to be more common in acromegalics and seem to grow more rapidly in pregnancy and puberty, times when there is physiologic hyperactivity of the pituitary gland.[37]

The suggestion of pituitary involvement in keloid formation has also been based on the fact that there is an association with increased pigmentation in states of increased pituitary activity (eg, pregnancy and puberty); increased pigmentation is based on an increased production of MSH by the pituitary gland.[37]

Ovarian function has also been associated with keloids: for instance, in the formation of keloids during puberty, the development of keloid growth during pregnancy, and the spontaneous resolution of keloids after menopause.[45] Geschickter and Lewis[20] reported increased estrogen content in keloids, which further supports the ovarian influence, but their findings are somewhat suspect as the results were obtained by assaying an earlobe keloid that had been preserved in formaldehyde for 1 to 3 years. Solomons[46] found that the suppression of the ovaries did not alter keloid growth. In addition, Vargas,[47] attempting to produce uterine fibroids by administering estrogen to monkeys, was not able to produce cutaneous keloids. The observation that scars and keloids tend to grow during pregnancy supports a pituitary-ovarian influence on keloid formation.[37]

Because keloids seldom occur before puberty, the sex hormones may play an important role in their formation. Sex hormone levels have been found to differ between keloids and the clinically normal surrounding skin and between keloids and hypertrophic scars. Personen et al[48] found that the diffusion of progesterone from the culture medium into the tissue is most effective in keloids, with normal skin being the second most effective; hypertrophic scars and the skin surrounding keloids proved ineffective in taking up progesterone.

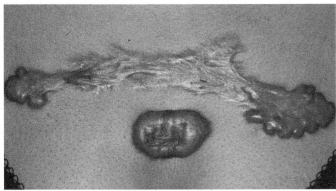

FIGURE 33-2. Keloids in the mid-chest area of an African American woman. Additional evidence favoring the role of androgens in keloid formation is that keloids have a predilection for the chest and upper back, which have an increased rate of dihydrotestosterone metabolism.

Ford et al[49] found that keloids have a high level of androgen binding, whereas estrogen and progesterone receptor binding was essentially undetectable in any of the keloid tissues from males or in the keloid tissue from some females. They also found that the level of androgen binding in the skin adjacent to keloids was elevated, whereas the level in skin adjacent to hypertrophic scars was only 0.1% of that found in keloids.[49]

Mustafa and Abdel-Fattah[37] postulated that estrogen plays a causative role in keloid formation based on a single case of a keloid that enlarged during pregnancy. However, they did not mention that maternal circulating androgens increase during pregnancy, especially in patients carrying a male fetus, nor did they mention the gender of the fetus. Additional evidence favoring the role of androgens is that keloids have a predilection for the chest, upper back, and neck regions, all of which have an increased rate of dihydrotestosterone metabolism [**Figures 33-2 to 33-4**].[50]

A South African study suggests that nutritional inadequacy, most notably the low intake of calcium, may lead to abnormal collagen production and be a factor in keloid formation.[51] However, malnutrition with protein deficiency seems to decrease fibroplasias.[52,53] Bowesman[54] suggested that adequate nutrition is necessary for keloid formation. Keloid formation is uncommon in patients with acquired immunodeficiency syndrome.[55]

The relationship between hypertrophic scars and hormonal factors is a subject that needs more research to make definitive determinations.[1,56,57]

FAMILIAL GENETIC FACTORS

Keloids have a definite familial predisposition, especially in those with multiple lesions.[1,57-60] Approximately one third of keloid patients have a

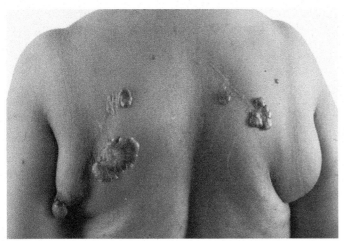

FIGURE 33-3. Keloids on the upper back of an African American woman.

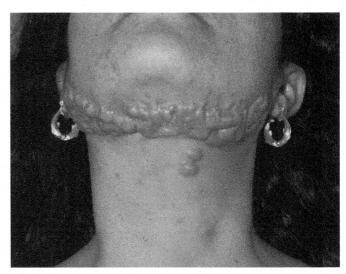

FIGURE 33-4. Keloids on the anterior neck of a Hispanic woman; this area is uncommon for the formation of keloids.

first-degree relative with keloids. Also, clinical experience indicates that familial predisposition is more common in dark-skinned individuals. Both autosomal recessive and autosomal dominant patterns of inheritance have been reported.[1] Bloom[3] also mentioned some studies in the German literature that describe congenital keloids, two cases of which were in identical twins.

Therefore, familial predisposition, high prevalence in certain populations, and frequent occurrence in twins suggest a strong genetic component to keloid susceptibility. Nevertheless, no single causative gene or genes have been identified and confirmed to be solely responsible for the genetic susceptibility to keloid formation.[61]

Numerous approaches have attempted to address and better understand the genetics of keloid scarring, and these include the determination of inheritance patterns, performance of linkage studies, case-control association studies, whole-genome gene expression and micro ribonucleic acid (RNA) microarrays, and comparative genomic hybridization studies.[62]

It is apparent that a varied inheritance pattern (predominantly autosomal dominant) is identified in most keloid families. There is also evidence of a weak linkage found in certain loci on chromosomes 2q23 and 7p11. In addition, several human leukocyte antigen (HLA) alleles (HLA-DRB1*15, HLA-DQA1*0104, HLA-DQB1*0501, and HLA-DQB1*0503) have been shown to be associated with keloids.[60,63-65]

Copy number variations (CNVs) in genes have been associated with several human diseases including common skin disorders. CNVs have been found to be present in the genome of keloid patients and may contribute to the development of keloids.[66] In particular, chromosome 6p21.32 (targeting HLA-DRB5) was found to be significantly associated with keloid formation in a Caucasian population ($P < 0.001$). The presence of HLA-DRB5 was associated with the HLA-DRB1*15 status.[66]

Inflammatory responses in keloid patients have pointed to the HLA system as a viable target for investigating disease etiology.[66] Frequencies of the HLA class I alleles A*01, A*03, A*25, B*07, Cw*08:02, HLA-DQA1, and HLA-DQB1 were analyzed in patients with skin of color, including 165 keloid patients and 119 healthy controls of Jamaican Afro-Caribbean origin. There were no statistically significant differences in allele frequency between the keloid patients and the controls. Additionally, characteristics of the keloid patients, including gender, family history, and multiple- or single-site scarring, did not show any significant allele-disease association.[67]

The incidence of keloids in an Italian population was found to be greater in those with HLA-B14 and HLA-BW16 antigens, whereas studies by Cohen et al and other researchers have noted a general HLA-A and HLA-B antigen pattern in patients with keloids.[58,68-70]

CLINICAL FINDINGS

CLINICAL CHARACTERISTICS

There are several clinical findings that distinguish keloids and hypertrophic scars [**Table 33-6**].[68,57,70-72] Although keloids may be found anywhere on the body, they tend to have a regional predilection, which occurs most often on the ears [**Figure 33-5**], the chest, upper back, and shoulders [**Figures 33-6 to 33-8**]. The latter three areas have increased skin tension, and keloids in these locations seem to arise with minimal trauma, are usually flatter with broader bases than keloids elsewhere, and respond less favorably to all modes of therapy. Keloids can occur from head to toe and at all locations in between [**Figures 33-9 and 33-10**]. Keloids on the shoulder and back tend to grow larger compared to keloids elsewhere [**Figure 33-11**]. Abdominal keloids, although rare in men, are common in darker-pigmented women who have had cesarean sections, hysterectomies, or other types of abdominal laparoscopic surgery. Darker-pigmented men who shave tend to develop keloids more often in the facial hair regions than those who do not shave [**Figure 33-12**]. There seems to be greater involvement in the flanks in women than in men [**Figure 33-13**].[73,74]

The areas less commonly associated with the formation of keloids include the face [**Figure 33-14**], neck [Figure 33-4], arms, wrist [**Figure 33-15**], and lower extremities. Mid-sternal lesions are often quite tender [**Figures 33-16 to 33-18**]. Although rare, keloids may develop on the eyelids, genitalia, palms, soles, mucous membranes, tongue, and corneas.[75] Lesions on the extremities can be very taut [**Figures 33-19 to 33-21**].[34] Keloids are rare on the oral mucosa.[1] There have been two known cases of keloids on the penis, one secondary to circumcision and the other from another form of trauma.[76,77] There are some lesions that resemble keloids clinically but that are epidermal cysts of the earlobe [**Figure 33-22**], lipomas of the earlobe [**Figure 33-23**], and linear xanthomas [**Figure 33-24**].[39]

CLINICAL COURSE AND PROGNOSIS

Keloids present as exaggerated scar tissue growths, extending past the areas of trauma, and once present, tend to continue to enlarge. Sometimes keloids are invaded by squamous cell carcinoma [**Figure 33-25**].[78,79] In contrast, hypertrophic scars are limited to the traumatized area and regress spontaneously in 12 to 18 months [**Figure 33-26**]. Both types of lesions are usually asymptomatic, but keloids may be tender, painful, and pruritic, or cause a burning sensation. However, cosmetic concern is the main reason patients seek medical intervention. Keloids range in consistency from soft and doughy to rubbery and hard. They project above the level of surrounding skin but rarely extend into the underlying subcutaneous tissue. Even though the overlying epidermis is thinned from pressure, they seldom ulcerate.[73]

Oluwasanmi[23] reported that most keloids occur within a year of the injury or disease that incited their formation, although approximately 20% develop 1 to 24 years after the first recognizable injury. The lag period is usually much shorter in lesions that recur after excision.

Initial lesions are often erythematous, become brownish red and then pale in the center as they age, and are often darker at the outer border. They are usually void of hair follicles. Once they are present, the clinical course varies. Most continue to grow for weeks to months, and others may continue to grow for years. The growth is usually slow, but keloids

TABLE 33-6	Clinical findings of keloidal and hypertrophic scars
Keloids	**Hypertrophic scars**
• Invade clinically normal skin	• Limited to traumatized area
• May continue to grow for the patient's life, often resistant to therapy	• Usually regress spontaneously in 12–18 months
• Erythematous borders indicate continuing growth	• Usually respond to therapy
• Pruritic, painful, burning	• Rarely grow after 2–3 months
	• Usually asymptomatic

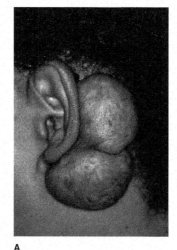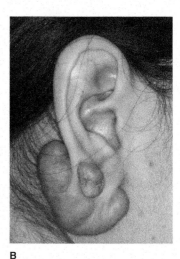

A   B

FIGURE 33-5. (A) Two large keloids of the left posterior earlobe of an African American woman. **(B)** Keloids also occur in lighter-skinned patients such as this Hispanic woman.

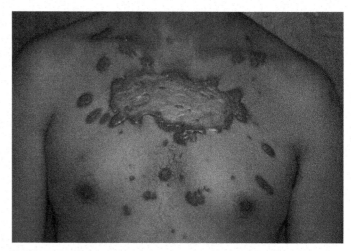

FIGURE 33-6. Regional predilection of keloids on the chest of a lighter-pigmented man.

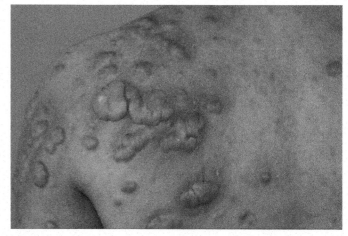

FIGURE 33-7. Regional predilection of keloids on the upper back and shoulders of a Hispanic man.

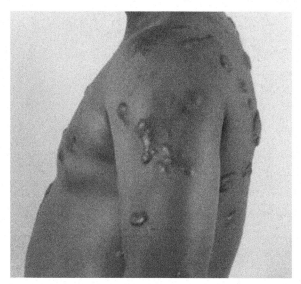

FIGURE 33-8. Regional predilection of keloids on the upper back and shoulders on an African American man.

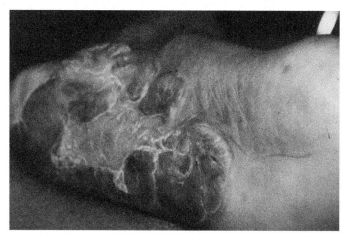

FIGURE 33-10. Keloids on the sole of the left foot; it is uncommon for keloids to occur on the feet.

will sometimes enlarge rapidly, tripling their size in months. Once they stop growing, keloids are usually asymptomatic and remain stable or involute slightly. They rarely regress spontaneously. Spontaneous regression is usually associated with advanced age; it has been reported that one keloid regressed after being present for 40 years.[73]

Keloids may range in size from papules a few millimeters in diameter to football-sized or larger tumors. Those on the ears, neck, and abdomen tend to be pedunculated, whereas those on the central chest and extremities are usually raised with a flat surface, with the base often being wider than the top. Most are round, oval, or oblong with regular margins; however, some have claw-like configurations with irregular borders. Most patients present with one or two keloids, but a few patients, especially those with spontaneous keloids, have multiple lesions, as do those who develop keloids secondary to acne or chickenpox.[34]

The malignant transformation of keloids is rare, and reported cases are poorly documented. Most patients had undergone some type of radiation therapy prior to the development of malignancy.[78] According to Stout,[79] a keloid will never develop into malignant hyperplasia; when a carcinoma does develop within a keloid, it is not a malignant degeneration of the keloid but rather of the overlying epidermis. Thus, no case has yet been reported of an unequivocally malignant change in an unirradiated keloid. Not only do keloids seem to resist malignancy, but they also seem to be spared in most generalized dermatoses.

PATHOGENESIS

COLLAGEN SYNTHESIS

Electron microscopic studies by Gueft[80] revealed that keloid collagen fibers are thinner and have irregularities of cross-striations, suggesting that keloid collagen is immature.[80] Studies of thermal contraction have demonstrated that, initially, keloid collagen acts like young tissue, which, once formed, proceeds to age the same way as any other newly synthesized collagen.[81]

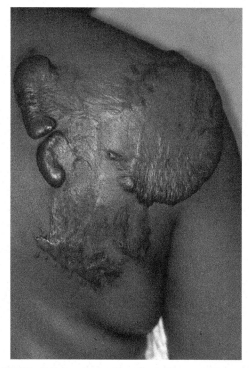

FIGURE 33-11. Keloids on the shoulder and back often grow to be larger than keloids elsewhere. As can be seen in the image, the medial border of the keloid is violaceous, which means that the keloid is still enlarging.

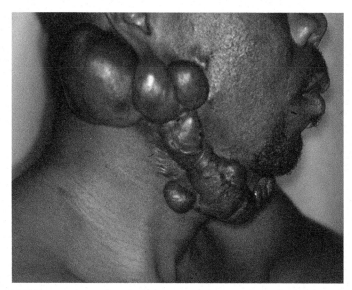

FIGURE 33-9. Large keloid on the head and neck of an African American man.

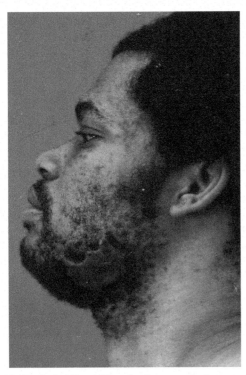

FIGURE 33-12. Darker-skinned African American men who shave can often develop keloids in the beard areas; the coarsely curled hair may act as an irritant in the formation of keloids.

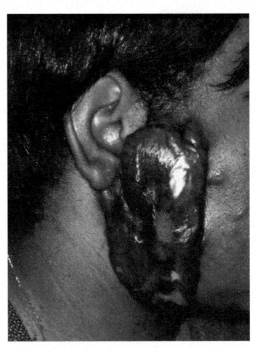

FIGURE 33-14. The face is a less commonly involved area for the formation of keloids.

Harris and Sjoerdsma[82] found that the water content of keloid tissue is uniformly higher than that of the clinically normal skin of the same patients, and there is no correlation between the water content and the age of the lesion. Additional findings were that the soluble collagen content and the alpha-to-beta ratio (single-polypeptide chains:double-peptide chains) are increased in all keloids. The collagen concentration in keloids is normal, but it is lower in recently formed scars. Early hypertrophic scars have the same collagen profile as keloids, whereas those more than 87 months old have the same collagen content as normal skin.[83]

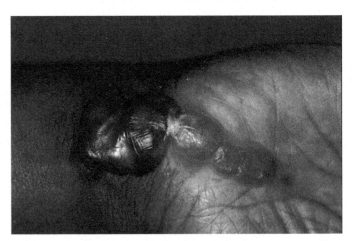

FIGURE 33-15. The wrist is a less commonly involved area for the formation of keloids.

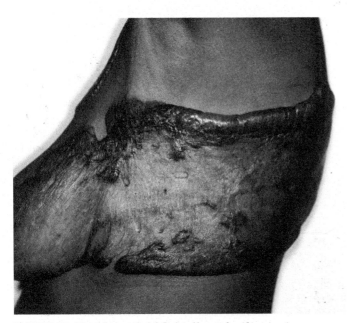

FIGURE 33-13. Keloids on the left flank and breast of an African American woman.

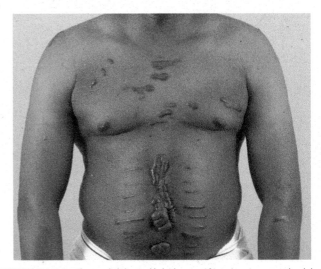

FIGURE 33-16. Chest and abdominal keloids on an African American man; the abdominal keloids were secondary to abdominal surgery.

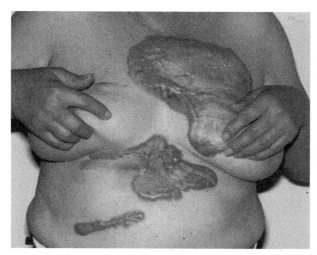

FIGURE 33-17. Chest, breast, and abdominal keloids on a Hispanic woman.

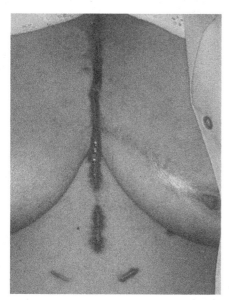

FIGURE 33-18. Keloids on the mid-chest of an Asian American woman, secondary to cardiac surgery.

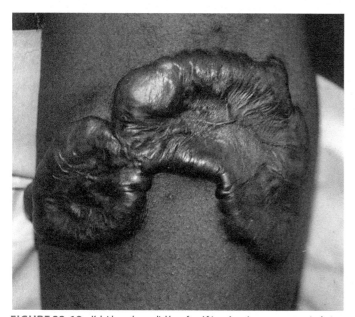

FIGURE 33-19. Keloids on the medial leg of an African American man; extremity lesions are usually quite taut, and this is an uncommon area for the formation of keloids.

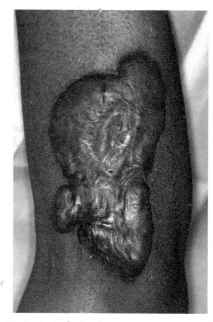

FIGURE 33-20. Proximal right forearm keloids on an African American man; extremity lesions are usually quite taut.

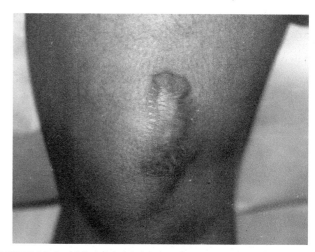

FIGURE 33-21. Keloid of the left thigh of an African American man. This keloid had a reddish center that was biopsied and proved to be sarcoidosis.

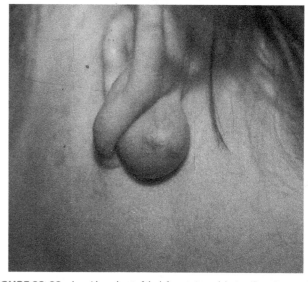

FIGURE 33-22. An epidermal cyst of the left posterior earlobe in a Hispanic woman.

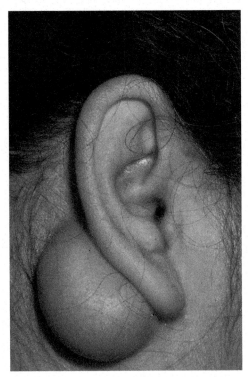

FIGURE 33-23. A lipoma of the right posterior earlobe in a Hispanic woman.

◼ FIBRONECTIN

Fibronectin is a glycoprotein synthesized by fibroblasts and an integral factor in fibroblast aggregation. Kischer and Hendrix[84] found that the immunofluorescence reaction of fibronectin is intense in hypertrophic scars and keloids and reflects exactly the conformation of the nodular structure, especially in the upper and middle reticular dermis. The investigators noted the intense reactivity of fibronectin in the hypertrophic

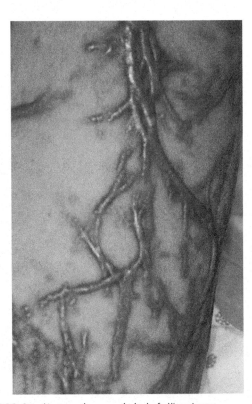

FIGURE 33-24. Linear xanthomas on the back of a Hispanic man.

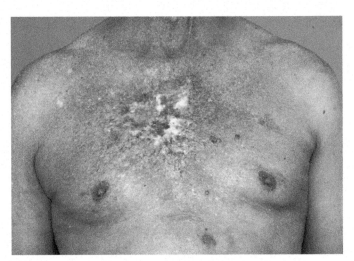

FIGURE 33-25. An African American man who developed squamous cell carcinoma in the mid-chest area, secondary to radiation treatment of a large chest keloid.

scar and keloid cultures, but little or none in the normal skin cultures, suggesting that fibroblasts cultured from keloids and hypertrophic scars may be synthesizing more fibronectin than those from normal dermis.[83-85]

Keloid formation seems to be a function of the rate of collagen synthesis or degradation, yet does not resemble the conditions involving a change in either collagen synthesis (eg, active scleroderma, pulmonary fibrosis, liver cirrhosis, and synovial tissue proliferation in the inflammatory stages of rheumatoid arthritis) or collagen degradation (eg, cartilage destruction in rheumatoid arthritis, epidermolysis bullosa dystrophica, and hormonal disturbances such as hyperthyroidism, hyperparathyroidism, and Paget disease of bone). Keloids have an exuberance of dermal proliferation composed mostly of bands of collagen that have increased hyaluronic acid (HA) and sulfated glycosaminoglycans.[86]

Keloid lesions have a significantly reduced HA content and also show altered HA organization patterns compared with unscarred skin and normal scars. Tumor necrosis factor-stimulated gene-6 levels, a known HA family molecule, are significantly reduced within keloid lesions compared with the dermis of unscarred skin ($P = 0.017$).[87] An altered expression of hyaluronan synthase and hyaluronidase messenger RNA may affect HA distribution in keloid disease compared with normal skin.[88]

There are 25 types of collagen, of which type I and type III are found in the skin. The bulk of skin collagen, as well as that of bones and tendons, is type I, which contains two identical alpha chains designated alpha 1 and a third chain called alpha 2. Type III collagen is composed

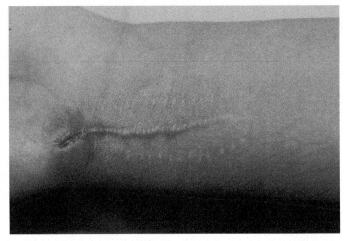

FIGURE 33-26. Linear hypertrophic scar on the wrist.

of three chemical features, which are relatively high levels of hydroxyproline and lysine plus some cystine. Type III accounts for more than half of the total collagen in fetal skin but less than 20% in adult skin.[86,89]

In light of the preceding, one might surmise that keloids have an increase in type I collagen, especially since this type is more resistant to proteolysis than type III.[90,91] However, studies by Clore et al[92] showed no significant difference in the percentage of type III collagen synthesized by fresh keloid biopsies compared with normal dermis. Likewise, there was no significant difference in the percentage of type III collagen synthesized by keloid fibroblasts compared with normal fibroblasts.[93] However, fibroblasts from different sites in keloid tissue, such as the perilesional site (on the margin) compared with the intralesional and extralesional sites, show differential apoptosis and contraction. Additionally, early versus later cell culture passages display differential collagen expression. Fibroblasts from the growing margin of the keloid scars have a higher production of collagen I and III compared with other lesional sites. Additionally, the temporal extension of the cell passage affects collagen production. Clinically these findings may influence the selection and interpretation of extended cell passages and provide future direction for lesional site-specific therapy in keloid scars.[94]

It has been suggested that the increased collagen accumulation in keloids does not appear to result from increased fibroblast proliferation, because fibroblasts are sparse on the histologic section of older, developing lesions, and the keloid DNA content is the same as in normal dermis. McCoy and Cohen[95] have found that sera from keloid patients do not contain a factor that significantly modifies the in vitro growth kinetics or collagen synthesis of keloid-derived or normal dermal fibroblasts.

Other studies by McCoy et al[96] have demonstrated that altered collagen synthesis by keloid fibroblasts is not related to abnormal cell growth. Keloid fibroblasts did not exhibit markedly shortened in vitro life spans compared with normal dermal fibroblasts under routine culture conditions. Under sparse growth conditions, however, the keloid fibroblasts appeared to lose replicative capacities earlier than normal skin fibroblasts.[97]

An examination of the collagenase produced by explants from normal skin, hypertrophic scars, and keloids cultured in vitro revealed no significant differences in either the amount of the enzyme produced or in the nature of that enzyme. The principal site of collagenase production in keloid specimens appeared to be, as in normal skin, the upper dermal or epidermal layer, with minimal production occurring in the lower fibrous or nodular areas.[98] On the other hand, an examination of the activity of the enzyme collagen synthesis revealed that it is markedly elevated in both keloids and hypertrophic scars compared with normal scars and normal skin, suggesting that the rate of collagen biosynthesis is increased in both abnormal scar types in vitro.[98]

Although collagen synthesis is significantly increased in keloids, collagen degradation (ie, collagenase activity) is also the same or increased compared with that in normal skin and normal scar formation. It would seem as if this increase in collagenase would counterbalance the increase in collagen synthesis. However, Oliver et al[99] found a third factor that influences the collagen production–destruction activity in keloids: tissue α-globulins.[99] Serum α-globulins are known inhibitors of skin collagenase. Patients with keloids have normal serum α-globulins but an increased deposition of the α-globulin α_1-antitrypsin and α_2-macroglobulin in the keloid tissue. Investigations by Oliver et al[99] postulate that this increased deposition may, in turn, inhibit the activity of collagenase, causing a decrease in the rate of collagen degradation. In addition, these authors found that women taking oral contraceptives had elevated serum levels of α-globulins, a phenomenon that may explain why pregnant women sometimes experience a growth of existing keloids or hypertrophic scars.[99,100]

Completing the collagenase-α-globulin picture is the phenomenon of intralesional steroids causing keloids to become smaller. After intralesional triamcinolone acetonide injections, there is usually a reduction in the size of a keloid as well as a significant reduction of the α_1-antitrypsin deposits.[101] These findings suggest that α-globulins may be involved in abnormal scar formation and that the triamcinolone acetonide may

remove collagenase inhibitors, thereby allowing activation of the collagenase with subsequent breakdown and reabsorption of the excessive collagen.[93]

LABORATORY TESTS

TISSUE CULTURES

In 1935, Tuma[102] published the first report on tissue culture techniques in the study of keloids. Almost 25 years later, Conway et al[103] found three morphologically distinct cell types in keloid tissue cultures. The most abundant was a small, highly spindle-shaped cell with a high metabolic rate, which was called the type I fibroblast. The second type, several times greater in volume with many fine cytoplasmic processes extending from its surface, was called the type II fibroblast. The type II fibroblasts migrated more slowly than type I cells and contained a larger number of mitochondria and larger nuclei. The third cell type appeared to be essentially normal fibroblasts.

Conway et al[103] postulated that the type I cell is responsible for the production of the fibrous matrix and the type II cell for absorption of the matrix. This theory is even more plausible in view of the observation that older keloids, both stable and regressing, show a preponderance of cells with abnormally large nuclei (type II fibroblasts) in contrast to recently developed keloids, which usually produce an exuberant growth of type I fibroblasts in tissue culture.

Keloid scars contain distinct subpopulations of mesenchymal-like stem cells (MLSCs). Cells positive for CD13, CD29, CD44, and CD90 were found to be significantly higher in the top and middle compartments of keloid scars ($P <0.05$) compared with the extralesional skin, where cells positive for CD34, CD90, and CD117 (representing hematopoietic stem cells) predominated. A unique population of CD34+ cells (cells positive for CD13, CD29, CD34, CD44, and CD90) were found in keloid scars and in extralesional skin. Fluorescence-activated cell sorting and quantitative polymerase chain reaction analysis showed that many of the mesenchymal stem cell markers were progressively downregulated and all of the hematopoietic stem cell markers were lost during the extended keloid fibroblast culture process.[104] There are distinct subpopulations of hematopoietic and nonhematopoietic cells whereby MLSCs reside in keloid scars, and hematopoietic stem cells accumulate extralesionally. Future therapy for keloids may have to differentially target both stem cell populations to deprive these tumors of their regenerative cell pools.

Mucin-like changes have been demonstrated in keloids. However, the condition is not a true endogenous mucinosis and differs histochemically from cutaneous mucinosis. These patients had previously undergone corticosteroid injections, and the interaction of the steroids within the fibrous tissue probably produced these histologic changes.[105] Other histopathologic findings include one case of keloid calcification and one case of pseudomelanoma.[106,107]

HISTOPATHOLOGY

Because keloids and hypertrophic scars have clinical similarities, histopathologic differentiation between them is difficult.[108] Some investigators claim that no clear distinction can be made between the lesions, whereas others have found definite morphologic differences.[109] Blackburn and Cosman[100] reported that keloids have conspicuous bundles of thick, glassy, faintly refractile, pale-staining collagen—a feature absent from hypertrophic scars. In addition, keloid tissue usually has abundant mucinous ground substance, few fibroblasts, and no foreign-body reactions, whereas hypertrophic scars have scarce mucinous ground substance, numerous fibroblasts, and frequent foreign-body reactions.[110]

Another difference between keloids and hypertrophic scars is that Luxol fast blue stains normal collagen blue and keloid collagens reddish. Keloids that develop in skin defects (eg, burns and cuts) do not have a normal papillary dermis, whereas so-called spontaneous keloids and those that develop from old acne lesions are separated from the epidermis by a fairly normal papillary dermis.[111]

Early forms of fibroblasts persist longer in keloids than in normal scar tissue. In normal wound healing, connective tissue elements regress after the third week, whereas in keloids, fibroblasts proliferate around the neovascular formations to form dense masses of collagen. This process can continue for months to years, thus determining the size of the keloids.[112]

Craig et al[113] reported that, in keloid tissue, as in normal skin, mast cells are present only in the dermis and never in the epidermis. However, unlike normal skin, where the mast cells are located primarily around the adnexal tissue in the superficial dermis, keloid mast cells occur throughout the dermis, interspersed among collagen bundles. Although the concentration of mast cells in the keloid dermis is not appreciably different from that in normal skin, the much thicker dermis of a keloid suggests a greater total mast cell number under a given epidermal area.[113]

New elastic tissue formation is often a feature of normal scar tissue formation but not of keloids, which are also deficient in or devoid of lymphatics. Normal lymphatic function is associated with the presence of elastic tissue; lymphatics are not able to function without it.[114]

Keloids have an exuberance of dermal proliferation composed mostly of bands of collagen glycosaminoglycans.[26] Chemical analysis shows the activity of α-naphthyl acid phosphatase to be greater in keloids than in normal skin. The enzymes of the Embden-Meyerhof glycolytic pathway, and of other systems relating carbohydrate to amino acid and fatty acid metabolism, are more active in keloids and hypertrophic scars than in normal skin. Because of their high water content, collagen fibrils in keloids are bound to HA until they reach maturity.[26] A significant increase in alanine transaminase is found in keloids but not in hypertrophic scars.[115]

Keloids differ from hypertrophic scars in osmotic pressure, metabolic activity, and collagen turnover, as reflected in the local concentrations of sodium, magnesium, and calcium, respectively. Keloids have a higher content of water and soluble collagen than normal skin. They are deficient in lymphatics and associated elastic fibers. These qualities are true of early hypertrophic scars as well, but after 7 months, the two diverge as hypertrophic scars normalize their water and collagen content. Sodium, a measure of osmotic pressure, is normal in keloids and decreased in hypertrophic scars, whereas magnesium, a measure of metabolic activity, is increased in keloids but decreased in hypertrophic scars. Calcium, which reflects collagen metabolism, is increased in keloids and decreased in hypertrophic scars.[116]

T-cells and macrophages are increased in keloid scars and are thought to contribute to its pathogenesis. In particular, T-cells, B cells, degranulated and mature mast cells (co-expressing OX40 ligand), and alternative macrophages (M2) are all significantly increased in intralesional and perilesional keloid scar sites compared with normal skin and scar tissue ($P < 0.05$). The increased number and activity of mast cells and M2 may implicate inflammation in the fibrotic process in keloid scar tissue. Additionally, in one study, 15% of keloid cases showed the presence of distinctive lymphoid aggregates called keloid-associated lymphoid tissue (KALT), which resembled mucosa-associated lymphoid tissue.[117] It may perpetuate inflammatory stimuli that promote keloid growth. KALT, mast cells, and M2 are promising novel targets for future keloid scar therapy.

DIFFERENTIAL DIAGNOSIS

The following are differential diagnoses that could be confused with keloids[118]:

- Hypertrophic scar
- Lipoma
- Dermatofibrosarcoma protuberans
- Dermatofibroma
- Squamous cell carcinoma
- Fibromatosis

Keloids are usually distinctive enough not to be confused with other cutaneous lesions, although sometimes hypertrophic scars may

TABLE 33-7 Keloid preventative measures
• Withhold ear piercing or elective cosmetic surgery from known keloid-formers
• Avoid tattoos
• Close surgical wounds with normal tension
• Avoid making cross-joint spaces
• Avoid mid-chest incisions
• Educate the patient on postoperative care

be difficult to rule out. As mentioned previously, hypertrophic scars remain within the bounds of the initial injury, are not claw-like, and often regress spontaneously.[35] Allergic contact dermatitis secondary to gold earrings may produce keloid-like lesions on the earlobes, but a histopathologic study of these lesions shows a dense infiltration of lymphoid cells, plus the formation of lymphoid follicles, rather than dense collagen tissue.[71,119-121]

TREATMENT

The first rule of keloid therapy is prevention [**Table 33-7**]. Withhold nonessential cosmetic surgeries from known keloid-formers, close all surgical wounds with minimal tension, make sure that incisions do not cross joint spaces, avoid mid-sternal incisions, and, when making incisions, follow the skin creases if possible. Known keloid-formers should apply pressure with a gradient elastic garment or other apparatus for 4 to 6 months after burns, surgical procedures, or major skin trauma.

No single therapeutic modality is best for all keloids [**Table 33-8**]. The type of therapy depends on the location, size, and depth of the lesion; age of the patient; and past responses to treatment. Treatment can be frustrating for both the patient and the physician. Excision of the lesion is actually the least important part of treatment; the patient's compliance in the postoperative therapy is by far the most important factor.[122] The lack of uniform treatment guidelines, with no foolproof protocol for physicians to follow, is the crux of the problem regarding keloids. In fact, even the optimal time to start treatment is currently unknown.[73]

■ STEROID INJECTIONS

The treatment of choice for most earlobe keloids, and those in locations other than the mid-sternal region, is corticosteroid injections [**Tables 33-9 to 33-11**]. Steroid injections should be given every 2 to 3 weeks at least four times prior to the surgery. The diagnosis and treatment of keloids remain basically the same irrespective of the patient's skin color.[63,64]

Here are a few therapeutic recommendations:

1. *Procedures to decrease the pain from injections:*

   - Prior to the injection of intralesional steroids, the keloid should be covered with a topical anesthetic such as a eutectic mixture of one-half (2%) lidocaine and one-half prilocaine, to help the patient withstand the pain of the injection. This topical anesthesia should be applied an hour before surgery and occluded with a very thin plastic wrap. The lidocaine does not relieve the initial pain of injection, but does allow multiple injections with minimal discomfort and prevents most postinjection pain.

   - Another way of making steroid injections less painful is to pretreat the keloid with liquid nitrogen, and then allow a 10- to 15-second thaw time. This causes tissue edema, making the injection into the keloid much easier. Allowing more than a 25-second thaw time will

TABLE 33-8 Treatment of keloids
• No one therapeutic modality is best for all keloids.
• Standard treatment includes intralesional steroids, surgical excision, pressure, radiation, lasers, cryosurgery, and other medical therapies.
• Polytherapy is more successful than monotherapy.
• Excision alone has a 45%–100% recurrence rate.

TABLE 33-9   Intralesional steroid injections

- Inject triamcinolone acetonide (40 mg/mL) with maximum amount of 1–1.5 mL
  - Any dose of triamcinolone acetonide greater than 3 mg/mL may cause hypopigmentation that may last 6–12 months
- Use a small-bore (27- or 29-gauge) needle because it does not clog as often as large-bore needles
- Inject where the skin is wrinkled (pinch the skin for more wrinkling)
  - Epidermal-dermal plane is easier to find
  - Atrophy also may occur at injection site(s), usually lasting 6–12 months
  - For preoperative anesthesia and keloid inhibition, inject a mixture of half 40 mg/mL triamcinolone acetonide and half 2% lidocaine
  - Corticosteroids delay wound healing
  - Wait 2–3 weeks before removing sutures, except for the face, where 10 days are sufficient
- Following surgical removal with corticosteroid injections is the most common procedure
  - Wait 2 weeks after suture removal to avoid wound dehiscence
  - Give corticosteroid to postoperative site every 2–3 weeks
- Freeze with liquid nitrogen (N_2) for 10–15 seconds for easier injection
  - Liquid N_2 also provides some anesthesia and edema
- Inject every 2–3 weeks before surgery
  - To ease injection pain, apply 2% lidocaine and 2% prilocaine cream thickly under occlusion 1 hour prior to injection
- Inject inflammatory border surrounding keloid

TABLE 33-10   Multiple complications with the use of systemic corticosteroids in the treatment of keloids

- Severe infections
- Hyperglycemia (not usual)
- Edema
- Osteonecrosis
- Myopathy
- Peptic ulcer disease
- Hypokalemia
- Osteoporosis
- Euphoria
- Psychosis
- Myasthenia gravis
- Growth suppression
- Abrupt discontinuation may cause an adrenal crisis

TABLE 33-11   Intralesional interferon-α-2b

- Inject 1 million units per linear centimeter of the postoperative site
- Repeat 1–3 weeks later
- Warn patients about flu-like symptoms
  - Premedicate with 500–1000 mg of acetaminophen
  - Taken every 6 hours in the evening for pain for 2 days
- 18% recurrence with interferon-α-2b
- 51%–100% recurrence with surgery only

often cause hypopigmentation; triamcinolone acetonide injections in strengths of 3 mg/mL or stronger may also cause hypopigmentation of the injected area for 6 to 12 months. Patients need to be informed of this possibility.

2. *Needle injection procedure:*
   - Because the keloids are often hard, one method of injecting the steroid is to insert the needle deep into the keloid. Slowly remove the needle while injecting the keloid until reaching the dermal–epidermal junction. In this way, the steroid can be injected more easily into the keloid. It is recommended to use a small 27-gauge needle, because larger-bore needles may behave like a punch biopsy.
   - Sometimes the base of the keloid is so fibrotic that it is almost impossible to inject. In these cases, insert a large-bore needle into the keloid, and inject the triamcinolone acetonide solution as the needle is slowly withdrawn.

3. *Intralesional steroid mixture for keloid therapy:*
   - Triamcinolone acetonide should be mixed in equal parts: 10 and 40 mg/mL. If the keloid is large enough to require multiple injections, a dilution of the 10 mg/mL solution can be mixed with an equal part of 2% lidocaine.
   - If the response to the triamcinolone acetonide injections is minimal to absent after two or three injections, or if the keloids have been

injected previously with the same concentration of triamcinolone acetonide without improvement, then a higher concentration of the steroid is recommended, for example, full-strength triamcinolone acetonide (40 mg/mL).

- Use a Luer-Lok needle or fixed-needle insulin syringe to prevent the needle from separating from the syringe during the injection. To prevent clogging, use nothing larger than a 27-gauge needle for either dosage of triamcinolone acetonide. The 40 mg/mL dosage sometimes puddles in the injected sites, forming superficial xanthoma-like deposits that may have to be removed for optimal cosmetic results.

4. *Using a small curette:* For easy removal of the steroid, use a small curette, or make a nick in the skin and use a strong suction apparatus.

5. *Procedures to prevent leakage/atrophy:*
   - The steroid solution is under great pressure and often leaks out. To prevent leaking, paint the area around the needle site with a tincture of benzoin, and cover it with a piece of waterproof tape immediately after withdrawing the needle.
   - Inject only the base of the keloid or the lesion itself, not the surrounding tissue; injecting the surrounding areas may cause normal tissue to atrophy and the keloid to sink down to skin level without becoming flat or softer.

6. *Be sure to inform patients that:*
   - The initial injection usually produces no visible change in the keloid but often makes it softer and alleviates most symptomology.
   - The steroid injections will not narrow the scar, even if it completely flattens.[120,122-126]

The effect of corticosteroids on collagen synthesis and degradation is not completely understood, but it is known that corticosteroids seem to work better in early keloids. This may be because only the younger fibroblasts can be induced by steroids to produce collagenase.[127] Older cells appear not to respond to steroids with collagenase production. In addition, cortisol administration in rats causes a rapid disappearance of collagen from the dermis, whereas prednisone, cortisone, and deoxycorticosterone are without effect. This difference indicates that the β-hydroxyl group present in prednisone, cortisol, and triamcinolone acetonide is necessary to exert the effect and may explain why triamcinolone acetonide injections are helpful in reducing the size of keloids.[123-126]

Approximately 50% of patients with keloids are considered nonresponders (or steroid-resistant) with no consensus or indicators in detecting steroid-sensitive patients. In view of the undesirable side effects, uncertainty in timing, and regularity of steroid treatment, it is important to identify responders and nonresponders to target treatment more effectively. Ud-Din et al[128] developed a scar injection pro forma to capture a detailed history, focusing on the symptoms and signs (redness, appearance, contour, texture, distortion, and severity) associated with keloids. The cause, site, number of keloid scars, and scar recurrence were recorded while the lesions were injected on a monthly basis. A detailed description of the response to steroid injection was documented, and photographs were taken. Patients were classified as steroid responders if they showed improvement in symptoms and signs within 3 months. There was a statistically significant correlation between patients with higher contour scores of keloids prior to treatment ($P = 0.013$) and the frequency of injections ($P = 0.003$). Thus, the odds of being a responder were greater for patients with more than one injection and with higher contour scores. This preliminary case series provided early evidence in enabling identification of steroid responders versus nonresponders within a 3-month period.[128] Potentially painful injections, their subsequent side effects, the unnecessary continuation of a redundant therapy and the need for subsequent follow-ups can all be avoided if keloid nonresponders are not subjected to steroid treatment.

Current use of corticosteroid injections is partially beneficial with a significant recurrence rate. Additionally, the efficacy of different steroids, alone or in combination, as opposed to monotherapy in treating keloids remains unclear. Syed and Bayat[129] compared the single and combined efficacy of glucocorticoids—dexamethasone, triamcinolone acetonide, and methylprednisolone—on primary keloid and normal skin fibroblasts at the cellular, protein, and messenger RNA levels in vitro.[129] They demonstrated that cytotoxicity to steroids was dose dependent. Cell spreading, attachment, and proliferation were significantly reduced by methylprednisolone and triamcinolone acetonide (P <0.05). The migration and invasion properties of the keloid fibroblasts were significantly inhibited by methylprednisolone and triamcinolone acetonide (P <0.05), compared with dexamethasone. At both the protein and messenger RNA levels, the keloid-associated fibrotic markers were significantly decreased by methylprednisolone and triamcinolone acetonide (P <0.05), compared with dexamethasone. However, the vascular endothelial growth factor expression was significantly decreased by dexamethasone (P = 0.01), compared with triamcinolone acetonide and methylprednisolone. Methylprednisolone and triamcinolone acetonide caused significant apoptosis (P <0.04), whereas dexamethasone inhibited the ultraviolet-induced apoptosis and upregulated survivin. The blocking of the glucocorticoid receptor by RU486 inhibited the cytoprotective property of dexamethasone and the apoptotic properties of triamcinolone acetonide and methylprednisolone. Combined treatment with dexamethasone and triamcinolone acetonide, as well as dexamethasone and methylprednisolone, significantly induced apoptosis (P <0.05). In conclusion, this is the first study to report the efficacy of three well-known steroids on keloid fibroblasts and suggest that a combination of steroids may be superior to using a single steroid in the treatment of keloids.

SURGERY

If there is no significant regression of the keloid tissue after four injections, or if the keloid no longer responds to further injections, surgery is recommended [**Figure 33-27**]. The surgical method differs according to the size and location of the lesions:

1. For keloids with a narrow base (<1 cm in diameter), a simple excision followed by an undermining of the base and closure with interrupted sutures will suffice. Before closure, the base of the operative site should be injected with Kenalog-40 so that the earliest fibroblasts are exposed to steroids. Alternatively, surgical anesthesia can be provided with one-half 2% lidocaine and one-half triamcinolone acetonide (40 mg/mL) mixed together.

2. For posterior pedunculated earlobe keloids, for which cosmetic appearance is not important, shaving followed by pressure hemostasis is a simple and efficient method of removal.

3. For large, nonpedunculated earlobe keloids and keloids with wide bases (>1 cm in diameter) on other parts of the body, removal is more complex. First, a half-moon incision, approximately one fifth of the size of the lesion, is made from one border onto the part of the keloid with the smoothest and flattest-looking surface. The remaining part of the keloid should then be excised, and the tip of the saved epidermis and superficial dermis carefully dissected from the underlying white glistening fibrous tissue mass. Triamcinolone acetonide (40 mg/mL) should be injected into the base of the surgical site. The overlying skin should then be approximated to the undermined borders of the excision with 6-0 nylon interrupted sutures. The sutures should be left in for 10 to 14 days because earlier removal may cause wound dehiscence. This slow healing is the consequence of the steroid injection. A week after suture removal, the postoperative site should be injected with triamcinolone acetonide (10 mg/mL) every 2 weeks. In most cases, four postoperative injections are sufficient to prevent recurrence [**Figure 33-28**].

4. In patients in whom the overlying skin is not smooth enough to be used as a cover for the excised tissue, a tissue expander may be inserted so that the keloid can be excised and then closed several months later.[73]

Keloid disease is known to show variable clinical behavior in response to surgical excision, and there is no clinicopathologic classification that predicts such varied behavior. A study in 2010 by Tan et al[130] showed the effect of excision margins and other histopathologic characteristics on keloid prognosis. A detailed histopathologic examination of all tissue samples identified keloid border or margin characteristics, which were classified into circumscribed (borders clearly demarcated) and infiltrative (borders not clearly demarcated and not easily definable). The specific histologic findings were correlated with keloid recurrence, which revealed that incomplete peripheral and deep excision margins as well as infiltrative borders were associated with higher 1-year reported recurrence rates (P <0.001, P <0.001, and P <0.05, respectively).[131] This study has provided evidence that incomplete surgical excision is associated with higher recurrence, and this may justify the practice of routine histopathologic reporting of keloid excision margins.

PRESSURE

Another adjunct for preventing recurrence is the use of a pressure-gradient garment on the postoperative site for at least 12 hours a

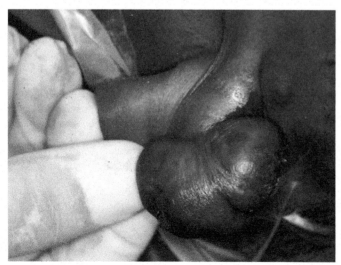

FIGURE 33-27. A surgically removed keloid.

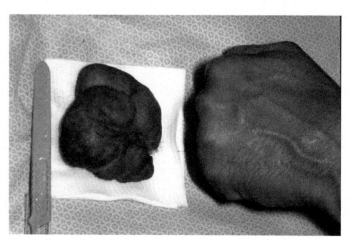

FIGURE 33-28. A surgically removed keloid approximately the size of a man's fist.

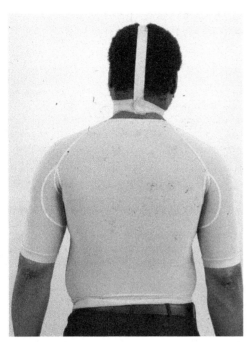

FIGURE 33-29. A pressure-gradient garment that helps to prevent recurrence of treated keloids.

day—although 20 hours is preferable—for 4 to 6 months [**Figure 33-29**]. For earlobe keloids, special pressure earrings or devices may be used. The proposed mechanism of action is outlined in **Table 33-12**.[131-133]

RADIATION THERAPY

For patients with mid-chest keloids or a history of keloid recurrence after surgery, radiation therapy is an adjunct modality. A dose of 2.50 Gy is given immediately after surgery, followed by four more treatments at weekly intervals. Other regimens include a single dose of 10 Gy the day after surgery or 3 Gy the day after surgery and then every other day thereafter for a total of three treatments.

Fisher and Storck[134] treated more than 300 patients with radiotherapy alone. In a 20-year follow-up, they found that radiotherapy was most effective when used within the first 5 months of keloid formation. Their total dose ranged from 8 to 24 Gy over a period of 2 to 5 months. They noted better results with postoperative keloids, lacerations, and infections than with scars from burns, scalds, and caustics. More intensive studies by van den Brank and Minty[72] concluded that primary irradiation of early keloids that are still cellular, well-vascularized, and growing may cause some resolution if more than 10 Gy is given. They found no merit in fractionating the doses. When treating older keloids, primary radiation alone failed to cause resolution, although it did relieve symptoms such as pruritus. Doses of 10 Gy or more may cause atrophy of the irradiated area or radionecrosis, leading to more keloid formation.

Additionally, van den Brank and Minty[72] demonstrated that preoperative radiation was unsatisfactory for reducing keloids, and because of the rapid recovery from radiation, there may be superregeneration. Postoperative radiation within 48 hours of surgery was the most effective technique in their series; the optimal dose was between 10 and 15 Gy. They advocated a margin of 0.5 cm of normal skin. This dose caused atrophy of the subcutaneous tissues, which eventually may lead to squamous cell carcinoma.[72]

TABLE 33-12 Keloid pressure treatment

- Start pressure garments 1 week after suture removal
- Reduces size and thickness of keloids
- Reduces intralesional mast cells
- Reduces histamine production
- Combine with a class I steroid

Other investigators, after protecting the surrounding skin with putty containing bismuth, found that 5 Gy every 5 days, starting on the first postoperative day, for four doses, prevents recurrence.[135,136] Shaffer et al[137] evaluated 13 studies of keloids treated with radiation, with a total of 2225 patients having 2592 keloidal scars. They concluded that although all the studies were retrospective and uncontrolled, it appeared that radiation after surgical excision prevented recurrence of keloidal scars in approximately 75% of patients at a 1-year follow-up. The most frequently used treatment was superficial X-rays of 9 cGy or greater in fractions given within 10 days of surgery.[137]

Young children with keloids either should not be irradiated or, if they are, the metaphyses should be shielded to prevent retardation of bone growth. Even doses of less than 4 Gy may cause growth retardation.[26]

LASER TREATMENT

Abergel et al[138] reported the successful treatment of keloids with the neodymium-doped yttrium aluminium garnet (Nd:YAG) laser. However, the authors of this chapter have found that laser therapy (carbon dioxide or Nd:YAG) alone does not prevent keloid recurrence. It must be combined with intralesional steroids during surgery and every 2 to 3 weeks, with four treatments per week. In addition, pressure therapy should be used as an adjunct to prevent recurrence. A study evaluating the 585-nm pulsed-dye laser for the treatment of keloidal scars demonstrated efficacy in reducing subjective symptoms, color, and height of the scars.[139]

OTHER TREATMENTS

Silicone gel and other dressings [**Table 33-13**] have been evaluated in 12 studies involving 538 patients with keloidal or hypertrophic scars. Treatment was applied for at least 12 hours. Although most of the studies involved hypertrophic scars, in the one with keloidal scars, 34% of the scars showed flattening after 6 months of continuous gel use.[140]

Ligatures may be used for pedunculated keloids when surgery or corticosteroid injections are either contraindicated or refused by the patient. A 4-0 nonabsorbable suture should be tied tightly around the base of the lesion, and a new one applied every 2 to 3 weeks. The sutures will gradually cut into and strangulate the keloid, eventually causing it to fall off. An interesting past custom in the southern part of the United States was to tie the hair of a horse's mane around the keloid instead of a suture.[73]

Topical tretinoin applied twice a day may alleviate pruritus and other keloid symptoms and may cause various degrees of regression. This method seems to be even more effective when combined with a potent topical steroid.[141]

In addition, there have been small studies or case reports using several other modalities. Ultraviolet A1 radiation has been reported to soften and flatten keloids.[142,143] Onwukwe[144] had success with surgical excision combined with methotrexate. Methotrexate induces folic acid deficiency, resulting in poor collagen formation. Methotrexate (15 to 20 mg) should be given orally in a single dose every 4 days, starting a week prior to surgery, and continued for 3 to 4 months after the postoperative site is healed.

Oral medications such as asiatic acid, penicillamine, colchicine, and β-aminopropionitrile have been combined with surgical excision to prevent recurrence. Numerous other topical, physical, and systemic modalities have been advocated but have either been unsuccessful or proved less effective than those mentioned earlier.[73,74] Imiquimod is a topical therapeutic agent that behaves as an immune response modulator by inducing interferon-α; interluken-1, interluken-6, and interluken-8; and tumor necrosis factor-α. In a small 13-patient study by Berman

TABLE 33-13 Miscellaneous treatments for keloids

- Silicone gel sheeting, flurandrenolide tape, or cosmetic pad
  - Start 1 week after suture removal
- Pentoxifylline (400 mg) 3 times a day
  - Limited success

and Kaufman,[125] imiquimod cream was applied to the postoperative site daily for 8 weeks, starting immediately after surgery. Some of these patients experienced marked irritation and had to discontinue the medication for 3 to 6 days. Imiquimod should not be used on postoperative incision sites, flaps, grafts, large wounds, and wounds under tension for 4 to 6 weeks because they may splay or dehisce. Also, over half of the patients using imiquimod will develop hyperpigmentation of the treated areas.[124]

Photodynamic therapy (PDT) uses light to activate a photosensitizer localized in diseased tissues. Two recent case studies and in vitro studies on keloid-derived fibroblasts indicate the potential use of PDT in treating keloids.[145-147] In 2013, Ud-Din et al[148] showed the effect of PDT in 20 keloid patients who were divided into three groups: those with existing keloid scars, those after surgical debulking, and those after total surgical excision. Patients underwent three treatments of PDT at weekly intervals. The methyl aminolevulinate photosensitizer was applied 3 hours prior to the PDT, administered at 37 J/cm^2. Noninvasive measures provided quantitative data for pliability, hemoglobin, melanin, collagen, and flux. Pain and pruritus scores were measured, and patients were monitored for keloid recurrence. All patients had reduced pain and pruritus scores. Hemoglobin flux ($P = 0.032$), collagen ($P = 0.066$), and hemoglobin levels ($P = 0.060$) decreased from week 1 to 3 in all except one patient, and pliability increased significantly ($P = 0.001$). Increases in pliability were significantly related to decreases in flux ($P = 0.001$). Only one patient with a keloid in a stress-prone anatomic location experienced recurrence. None of the other patients showed recurrence at a 9-month follow-up. Minimal side effects were reported. In conclusion, PDT reduces scar formation in keloids, evidenced by decreased blood flow, increased pliability, and decreased collagen and hemoglobin levels. These findings indicate potential utility of PDT in the treatment of keloids.

CONCLUSION

Keloids are benign fibrous growths that result from an abnormal connective tissue response in certain predisposed individuals. Those with dark skin form keloids more often than those with light skin, but the reason for this difference is not known. Trauma, foreign-body reactions, infections, and endocrine dysfunction have all been proposed as precipitating factors. Keloids are found most commonly on the earlobes, shoulders, upper back, and mid-chest. They extend past the area of trauma and, once present, tend to remain stable. Although sometimes pruritic, painful, or tender, they are usually asymptomatic. Keloids often arise during pregnancy, grow more rapidly during pregnancy, and are more common after puberty. The Yoruba people of West Africa believe that piercing before puberty may prevent keloid formation. Estrogen increases serum α-globulins, which are collagenase inhibitors. Histologically, although there have been many therapeutic modalities, most have had limited success. The most commonly used therapeutic approach is a combination of cryotherapy, intralesional steroid injections, surgical excision, and pressure devices.

REFERENCES

1. Datubo-Brown DD. Keloids: a review of the literature. *Br J Plast Sur.* 1990;43:70-77.
2. Atiyeh BS, Costagliola M, Hayek SN. Keloid or hypertrophic scar: The controversy: Review of the literature. *Ann Plast Surg.* 2005;54:676-680.
3. Bloom D. Heredity of keloids: a review of the literature and report of a family with multiple keloids in five generations. *N Y State J Med.* 1975;56:511-519.
4. Yedomon GH, Adegbidi H, Atadokpede F, et al. Keloids on dark skin: a consecutive series of 456 cases. *Med Sante Trop.* 2012;22:287-291.
5. Alibert JLM. *Description des maladies de la peau: Observées à l'Hôspital Saint Louis, et exposition des meilleures méthodes suivies pour leur traitement.* Paris, France: Barrois l'Aîné et Fils; 1806:113.
6. Alibert JL. *Description des maladies de la peau: Observées à l'Hôpital Saint Louis, et Exposition des Meilleures Méthodes Suivies Pour Leur Traitement.* 2nd ed. Brussels, Belgium: Auguste Wahlen; 1825:34.
7. Kaposi M. Keloid. In: von Hebra F, Kaposi M, eds. *On Diseases of the Skin Including the Exanthema.* London, United Kingdom: New Sydenham Society; 1874:272.
8. Hawkins C. Cases of warty tumors in cicatrices. *Med Chir Trans.* 1835;19:19-34.
9. Macpherson J. On tumors of cicatrices. *London Med Gaz.* 1844;35:348.
10. Breasted JH. *The Edwin Smith Surgical Papyrus*, Vol 1: *Hieroglyphic Translation and Commentary.* Chicago, IL: University of Chicago Press; 1930:403-406.
11. Omo-Dare P. Yoruban contribution to the literature on keloids. *J Natl Med Assoc.* 1973;65:367-406.
12. Addison T. On the keloid of Alibert, and on true keloid. *Med Chir Trans.* 1854;37:27-47.
13. Addison T. On the keloid of Alibert and on true keloid. In: Shelley WB, Crissey JT, Stokes JH, eds. *Classics in Clinical Dermatology with Biographical Sketches.* Springfield, IL: Charles C Thomas Publisher; 1953:93-94.
14. Cosman B, Crikelair FG, Ju MC. The surgical treatment of keloids. *Plast Reconstr Surg.* 1961;27:335-345.
15. Cohen IK, McCoy BJ. Keloid: biology and treatment. In: Dineen P, Hildick-Smith G, eds. *The Surgical Wound.* Philadelphia, PA: Lea & Febiger; 1981:123-131.
16. Brenizer AG. Keloid formation in the Negro. *Ann Surg.* 1915;61:83-87.
17. Fox H. Observations on skin diseases in the American Negro. *J Cutan Dis.* 1908;26:67-79.
18. Matas R. The surgical peculiarities of the Negro. *Transact Am Surg Assoc.* 1896;14:483-610.
19. Hazen HH. Personal observations upon skin diseases in the American Negro. *J Cutan Dis.* 1914;32:705-712.
20. Geschickter CF, Lewis D. Tumors of connective tissue. *Am J Cancer.* 1935;25:630-655.
21. Alhady SM, Sivanantharajah K. Keloids in various races: a review of 175 cases. *Plast Reconstr Surg.* 1969;44:564-566.
22. Arnold HL. Keloids. In: Maddon S, ed. *Current Medical Management.* 2nd ed. St. Louis, MO: Mosby; 1975:194.
23. Oluwasanmi JO. Keloids in the African. *Clin Plast Surg.* 1974;1:179-195.
24. Bohrod MG. Keloids and sexual selection: a study in the racial distribution of disease. *Arch Derm Syphilol.* 1937;36:19-25.
25. Ketchum LD, Cohen IK, Masters FW. Hypertrophic scars and keloids: a collective review. *Plast Reconstr Surg.* 1974;53:140-154.
26. Al-Attar A, Mess S, Thomassen JM, et al. Keloid pathogenesis and treatment. *Plast Reconstr Surg.* 2006;117:286-300.
27. Asboe-Hansen G. Hypertrophic scars and keloids: etiology, pathogenesis, and dermatologic therapy. *Dermatologica.* 1960;120:178-184.
28. Kelly AP. *An Etiological Update on Keloids.* National Medical Association, Section on Dermatology, Lecture in San Antonio, TX, August 1, 1999.
29. Bayat A, Arscott G, Ollier WE, et al. Description of site-specific morphology of keloid phenotypes in an Afrocaribbean population. *Br J Plast Surg.* 2004;57:122-133.
30. Suarez E, Syed F, Alonso-Rasgado T, et al. Up-regulation of tension-related proteins in keloids: knockdown of Hsp27, α2β1-integrin, and PAI-2 shows convincing reduction of extracellular matrix production. *Plast Reconstr Surg.* 2013;131:158e-173e.
31. Bayles MA. Coiffure keloids. *Br J Dermatol.* 1972;86:415-416.
32. Yagi KI, Dafalla AA, Osman AA. Does an immune reaction to sebum in wounds cause keloid scars? Beneficial effect of desensitisation. *Br J Plast Surg.* 1979;32:223-225.
33. Ginarte M, Peteiro C, Toribio J. Keloid formation induced by isotretinoin therapy. *Int J Dermatol.* 1999;38:228-229.
34. Koonin AJ. The aetiology of keloids: a review of the literature and a new hypothesis. *S Afr Med J.* 1964;38:913-916.
35. Garb J, Stone MJ. Keloids: review of the literature and a report of eighty cases. *Am J Surg* 1942;58:315-335.
36. Lorber B. Are all diseases infectious? *Ann Intern Med.* 1996;125:844-851.
37. Moustafa MF, Abdel-Fattah MA, Abdel-Fattah DC. Presumptive evidence of the effect of pregnancy estrogens on keloid growth: case report. *Plast Reconstr Surg.* 1975;56:450-453.
38. Kelly AP, Zheng P, Johnson BL. Mast cells and keloid formation. *J Invest Dermatol.* 1996;106:838-841.
39. Diegelmann RF, Bryant CP, Cohen IK. Tissue alpha-globulins in keloid formation. *Plast Reconstr Surg.* 1977;59:418-423.
40. Glucksmann A. Local factors in the histogenesis of hypertrophic scars. *Br J Plast Surg.* 1951;4:88-103.
41. Justice J. Beobachtungen und experimente zur ätiologie des keloids. *Arch Dermatol Syph.* 1919;197:274.

42. Allan JC, Keen P. The management of keloid in the South African Bantu. *S Afr Med J.* 1954;28:1034-1037.

43. Pautrier LM, Zorn R. Calcemie: teneur en calcium de la peau dans les chéloides et les acnés chéloidiennes. *Bull Soc Fr Dermatol Syphiligr.* 1931;38:953-961.

44. Farndon JR. Postoperative complications of parathyroidectomy. In: Holzheimer RG, Mannick JA, eds. *Surgical Treatment: Evidence-Based and Problem-Oriented.* Munich, Germany: Zuckschwerdt; 2001. http://www.ncbi.nlm.nih.gov/books/NBK6967/. Accessed July 31, 2013.

45. Myśliwska J, Trzonkowski P, Bryl E, et al. Lower interleukin-2 and higher serum tumor necrosis factor levels are associated with perimenstrual, recurrent, facial herpes simplex infection in young women. *Eur Cytokine Netw.* 2000;11:397-406.

46. Solomons B Jr. Keloids and their treatment. *Practitioner.* 1952;168:465-472.

47. Vargas L Jr. Attempt to induce formation of fibroids with estrogens in the castrated female Rhesus monkey. *Bull Johns Hopkins Hosp.* 1943;73:23-28.

48. Personen S, Rintala A, Soivio A, et al. On the [4-^{14}C] progesterone metabolism of keloid and hypertrophic scar: a preliminary report. *Scand J Plast Reconstr Surg.* 1976;10:173-176.

49. Ford LC, Kind DF, Lagasse LD, et al. Increased androgen binding in keloids: a preliminary communication. *J Dermatol Surg Oncol.* 1983;9:545-547.

50. Cohen IK, Diegelmann RF, Keiser HR. Collagen metabolism in keloid and hypertrophic scar. In: Longacre JJ, ed. *The Ultrastructure of Collagen.* Springfield, IL: Charles C Thomas Publisher; 1973:199-212.

51. Louw L, Dannhauser A. Keloids in rural black South Africans. Part 2: dietary fatty acid intake and total phospholipid fatty acid profile in the blood of keloid patients. *Prostaglandins Leukot Essent Fatty Acids.* 2000;63:247-253.

52. Edgerton MT Jr, Hanrahan EM, Davis WB. Use of vitamin E in the treatment of keloids. *Plast Reconstr Surg (1946).* 1951;8:224-233.

53. Kobak MW, Benditt EP, Wissler RM, et al. Relationship of protein deficiency to experimental wound healing. *Surg Gynecol Obstet.* 1947;85:751-756.

54. Bowesman C. *Surgery and Clinical Pathology in the Tropics.* Edinburgh, United Kingdom: E & S Livingstone; 1960:798.

55. Discussions with Wilbert Jordan, MD, Director of the OASIS Clinic, Los Angeles County Department of Health Services, Martin Luther King Jr. Multi-Service Ambulatory Care Center, Los Angeles, CA.

56. Lee JY, Yang CC, Chao SC, et al. Histopathological differential diagnosis of keloid and hypertrophic scar. *Am J Dermatopathol.* 2004;26:379-384.

57. Marneros AG, Norris JE, Olsen BR, et al. Clinical genetics of familial keloids. *Arch Dermatol.* 2001;137:1429-1434.

58. Cohen IK, McCoy BJ, Mohanakumar T, et al. Immunoglobulin, complement, and histocompatibility antigen studies in keloid patients. *Plast Reconstr Surg.* 1979;63:689-695.

59. Bayat A, Bock O, Mrowietz U, et al. Genetic susceptibility to keloid disease and hypertrophic scarring: transforming growth factor beta1 common polymorphisms and plasma levels. *Plast Reconstr Surg.* 2003;111:535-543.

60. Bayat A, Walter JM, Bock O, et al. Genetic susceptibility to keloid disease: mutation screening of the TGFbeta3 gene. *Br J Plast Surg.* 2005;58:914-921.

61. Shih B, Bayat A. Genetics of keloid scarring. *Arch Dermatol Res.* 2010;302:319-339.

62. Brown JJ, Bayat A. Genetic susceptibility to raised dermal scarring. *Br J Dermatol.* 2009;161:8-18.

63. Brown JJ, Ollier WE, Thomson W, et al. Positive association of HLA-DRB1*15 with keloid disease in Caucasians. *Int J Immunogenet.* 2008;35:303-307.

64. Brown JJ, Ollier W, Thomson W, et al. Positive association of HLA-DRB1*15 with Dupuytren's disease in Caucasians. *Tissue Antigens.* 2008;72:166-170.

65. Brown JJ, Ollier WE, Arscott G, et al. Association of HLA-DRB1* and keloid disease in an Afro-Caribbean population. *Clin Exp Dermatol.* 2010;35:305-310.

66. Shih B, Bayat A. Comparative genomic hybridisation analysis of keloid tissue in Caucasians suggests possible involvement of HLA-DRB5 in disease pathogenesis. *Arch Dermatol Res.* 2012;304:241-249.

67. Ashcroft KJ, Syed F, Arscott G, et al. Assessment of the influence of HLA class I and class II loci on the prevalence of keloid disease in Jamaican Afro-Caribbeans. *Tissue Antigens.* 2011;78:390-396.

68. Laurentaci G, Dioguardi D. HLA antigens in keloids and hypertrophic scars. *Arch Dermatol.* 1977;113:1726.

69. Halim AS, Emami A, Salahshourifar I, et al. Keloid scarring: understanding the genetic basis, advances and prospects. *Arch Plast Surg.* 2012;39:184-189.

70. Mowlem R. Hypertrophic scars. *Br J Plast Surg.* 1951;4:113-120.

71. Psillakis JM, de Jorge FB, Sucena RC, et al. Water and electrolyte content of normal skin, scars and keloid. *Plast Reconstr Surg.* 1971;47:272-274.

72. van den Brank HA, Minty CC. Radiation in the management of keloids and hypertrophic scars. *Br J Surg.* 1960;47:595-605.

73. Kelly AP. Keloids. *Dermatol Clin.* 1988;6:413-424.

74. Kelly AP. Update on the management of keloids. *Semin Cutan Med Surg.* 2009;28:71-76.

75. Lahav M, Cadet JC, Chirambo M, et al. Corneal keloids: a histopathological study. *Graefes Arch Clin Exp Ophthalmol.* 1982;218:256-261.

76. Körmöczy I. Enormous keloid (?) on a penis. *Br J Plast Surg.* 1978;31:268-269.

77. Parsons RW. A case of keloid of the penis. *Plast Reconstr Surg.* 1966;37:431-432.

78. Perez CA, Lockett MA, Young G. Radiation therapy for keloids and plantar warts. *Front Radiat Ther Oncol.* 2001;35:135-146.

79. Stout AP. Fibrosarcoma, the malignant tumor of fibroblasts. *Cancer.* 1948;1:30-63.

80. Gueft B. Keloids. *Trans Electron Microsc Soc Am.* 1965;23:5.

81. Rasmussen DM, Wakim KG, Winkelmann RK. Isotonic and isometric thermal contraction of human dermis: (3) scleroderma and cicatrizing lesions. *J Invest Dermatol.* 1964;43:349-355.

82. Harris ED Jr, Sjoerdsma A. Collagen profile in various clinical conditions. *Lancet.* 1966;2:707-711.

83. Tuan TL, DiCesare P, Cheung D, et al. Keloids and hypertrophic scars. In: Nimni ME, Kang AH, eds. *Collagen: Pathobiochemistry.* Boca Raton, FL: CRC Press; 1991:125-136.

84. Kischer CW, Hendrix MJ. Fibronectin (FN) in hypertrophic scars and keloids. *Cell Tissue Res.* 1983;231:29-37.

85. Kischer CW, Wagner HN Jr, Pindur J, et al. Increased fibronectin production by cell lines from hypertrophic scar and keloid. *Connect Tissue Res.* 1989;23:279-288.

86. Babu M, Diegelmann R, Oliver N. Fibronectin is overproduced by keloid fibroblast during abnormal wound healing. *Mol Cell Biol.* 1989;9:1642-1650.

87. Tan KT, McGrouther DA, Day AJ, et al. Characterization of hyaluronan and TSG-6 in skin scarring: Differential distribution in keloid scars, normal scars and unscarred skin. *J Eur Acad Dermatol Venereol.* 2011;25:317-327.

88. Sidgwick GP, Iqbal SA, Bayat A. Altered expression of hyaluronan synthase and hyaluronidase mRNA may affect hyaluronic acid distribution in keloid disease compared with normal skin. *Exp Dermatol.* 2013;22:377-379.

89. Cohen IK, Keiser HR, Sjoerdsma A. Collagen synthesis in human keloid and hypertrophic scar. *Surg Forum.* 1971;22:488-489.

90. Tuan TL, Nichter LS. The molecular basis of keloid and hypertrophic scars formation. *Mol Med Today.* 1998;4:19-24.

91. Bettinger DA, Yager DR, Diegelmann RF, et al. The effect of TGF-β on keloid fibroblast proliferation and collagen synthesis. *Plast Reconstr Surg.* 1996;98:827-833.

92. Clore JN, Cohen IK, Diegelmann RF. Quantitative assay of types I and III collagen synthesized by keloid biopsies and fibroblasts. *Biochim Biophys Acta.* 1979;586:384-390.

93. Uitto J, Perejda AJ, Abergel RP, et al. Altered steady-state ratio of type I/III procollagen mRNAs correlates with selectively increased type I procollagen biosynthesis in cultured keloid fibroblasts. *Proc Natl Acad Sci U S A.* 1985;82:5935-5939.

94. Syed F, Ahmadi E, Iqbal SA, et al. Fibroblasts from the growing margin of keloid scars produce higher levels of collagen I and III compared with intralesional and extralesional sites: clinical implications for lesional site-directed therapy. *Br J Dermatol.* 2011;164:83-96.

95. McCoy BJ, Cohen IK. Effects of various sera on growth kinetics and collagen synthesis by keloid and normal dermal fibroblasts. *Plast Reconstr Surg.* 1981;67:505-510.

96. McCoy BJ, Galdum J, Cohen IK. Effects of density and cellular aging on collagen synthesis and growth kinetics in keloid and normal skin fibroblast. *In Vitro.* 1982;18:79-86.

97. Calderon M, Lawrence WT, Banes AJ. Increased proliferation of keloid fibroblasts wounded in vitro. *J Surg Res.* 1996;61:343-347.

98. García-Ulloa AC, Arrieta O. Tubal occlusion causing infertility due to an excessive inflammatory response in patients with predisposition for keloid formation. *Med Hypotheses.* 2005;65:908-914.

99. Oliver N, Babu M, Diegelmann R. Fibronectin gene transcription is enhanced in abnormal wound healing. *J Invest Dermatol.* 1992;99:579-586.

100. Blackburn WR, Cosman B. Histologic basis of keloid and hypertrophic scar differentiation: clinicopathologic correlation. *Arch Pathol.* 1966;82:65-71.

101. Craig RD. Collagen biosynthesis in normal human skin, normal and hypertrophic scar and keloid. *Eur J Clin Invest.* 1975;5:69-74.

102. Tuma W. Quelques experiences sur la culture des keloids humaines in vitro. *C R Assoc Anat.* 1935;30:507.

103. Conway H, Gillette RW, Findley A. Observation on the behavior of human keloids in vitro. *Plast Reconstr Surg.* 1959;24:229-237.

104. Iqbal SA, Syed F, McGrouther DA, et al. Differential distribution of hae-matopoietic and nonhaematopoietic progenitor cells in intralesional and extralesional keloid: do keloid scars provide a niche for nonhaematopoietic mesenchymal stem cells? *Br J Dermatol.* 2010;162:1377-1383.

105. Santa Cruz DJ, Ulbright TM. Mucin-like changes in keloids. *Am J Clin Pathol.* 1981;75:18-22.

106. Redmond WJ, Baker SR. Keloidal calcification. *Arch Dermatol.* 1983;119:270-272.

107. Hiss Y, Shafir R. "Pseudomelanoma" in a keloid. *J Dermatol Surg Oncol.* 1978;4:938-939.

108. Uitto J, Lichtenstein JR. Defects in the biochemistry of collagen in diseases in connective tissue. *J Invest Dermatol.* 1976;66:59-79.

109. Cohen IK, McCoy BJ, Mohanakumar T, et al. Immunoglobulin, comple-ment, and histocompatibility antigen studies in keloid patients. *Plast Recon-str Surg.* 1979;63:689-695.

110. Boyce DE, Ciampolini J, Ruge F, et al. Inflammatory cell subpopulations in keloid scars. *Br J Plast Surg.* 2001;54:511-516.

111. Mehregan AH. *Pinkus' Guide to Dermatohistopathology.* 4th ed. New York, NY: Appleton-Century-Crofts; 1986:537.

112. Mancini RE, Quaife JV. Histogenesis of experimentally produced keloids. *J Invest Dermatol.* 1962;38:143-181.

113. Craig SS, DeBlois G, Schwartz LB. Mast cells in human keloid, small intes-tine, and lung by an immunoperoxidase technique using a murine mono-clonal antibody against tryptase. *Am J Pathol.* 1986;124:427-435.

114. Crockett DJ. Regional keloid susceptibility. *Br J Plast Surg.* 1964;17:245-253.

115. Bhangoo KS, Quinlivan JK, Connelly JR. Elastic fibers in scar tissue. *Plast Reconstr Surg.* 1976;57:308.

116. King GD, Salzman FA. Keloid scars: analysis of 89 patients. *Surg Clin North Am.* 1970;50:595-598.

117. Bagabir R, Byers RJ, Chaudhry IH, et al. Site-specific immunophenotyping of keloid disease demonstrates immune upregulation and the presence of lymphoid aggregates. *Br J Dermatol.* 2012;167:1053-1066.

118. Halder RM, Roberts CI, Nootheti PK, et al. Dermatologic disease in blacks. In: Halder R, ed. *Dermatology and Dermatological Therapy of Pigmented Skins.* Boca Raton, FL: Taylor & Francis Group; 2006:405-435.

119. Fisher AA. Allergic dermal contact dermatitis due to gold earrings. *Cutis.* 1987;39:473-475.

120. Iwatsuki K, Yamada M, Takigawa M, et al. Benign lymphoplasia of the earlobes induced by gold earrings: immunohistologic study on the cellular infiltrates. *J Am Acad Dermatol.* 1987;16:83-88.

121. Niessen FB, Spauwen PH, Schalkwijk J, et al. On the nature of hypertrophic scars and keloids: a review. *Plast Reconstr Surg.* 1999;104:1435-1458.

122. Viera MH, Amini S, Valins W, et al. Innovative therapies in the treatment of keloids and hypertrophic scars. *J Clin Aesthet Dermatol.* 2010;3:20-26.

123. Berman B, Flores F. Recurrence rates of excised keloids treated with postop-erative triamcinolone acetonide injections or interferon-afla-2b injections. *J Am Acad Dermatol.* 1997;37:755-757.

124. Berman B, Kaufman J. Pilot study of the effect of postoperative imiquimod 5% cream on the recurrence rate of excised keloids. *J Am Acad Dermatol.* 2002;47:S209-S211.

125. Fitzpatrick RE. Treatment of inflamed hypertrophic scars using intralesional 5-FU. *Dermatol Surg.* 1999;25:224-232.

126. Bodokh I, Brun P. Treatment of keloids with intralesional bleomycin. *Ann Dermatol Venereol.* 1996;123:791-794.

127. Houck JC, Sharma VK, Carillo A. Control of cutaneous collagenolysis. In: Weber G, ed. *Advances in Enzyme Regulation.* Vol 8. New York, NY: Per-gamon Press; 1970:269-278.

128. Ud-Din S, Bowring A, Derbyshire B, et al. Identification of steroid sensitive responders versus non-responders in the treatment of keloid disease. *Arch Dermatol Res.* 2013;305:423-432.

129. Syed F, Bayat A. Superior effect of combination vs. single steroid therapy in keloid disease: a comparative in vitro analysis of glucocorticoids. *Wound Repair Regen.* 2013;21 88-102.

130. Tan KT, Shah N, Pritchard SA, et al. The influence of surgical excision mar-gins on keloid prognosis. *Ann Plast Surg.* 2010;64:55-58.

131. Brent B. The role of pressure therapy in the management of earlobe keloids: preliminary report of a controlled study. *Ann Plast Surg.* 1978;1:579-581.

132. Lawrence WT. Treatment of earlobe keloids with surgery plus adjuvant intra-lesional verapamil and pressure earrings. *Ann Plast Surg.* 1996;37:167-169.

133. Snyder GB. Button compression for keloids of the lobule. *Br J Plast Surg.* 1974;27:186-187.

134. Fischer E, Storck H. X-ray treatment of keloids. *Schweiz Med Wochenschr.* 1957;87:1281-1285.

135. Arnold HL Jr, Grauer FH. Keloids: etiology, and management by excision and intensive prophylactic radiation. *Arch Dermatol.* 1959;80:772-777.

136. Borok TL, Bray M, Sinclair I, et al. Role of ionizing irradiation for 393 keloids. *Int J Radiat Oncol Biol Phys.* 1998;15:865-870.

137. Shaffer JJ, Taylor SC, Cook-Bolden F. Keloidal scars: a review with a critical look at therapeutic options. *J Am Acad Dermatol.* 2002;46:S63-S97.

138. Abergel RP, Dwyer RM, Meeker CA, et al. Laser treatment of keloids: a clinical trial and an in vitro study with Nd:YAG laser. *Lasers Surg Med.* 1984;4:291-295.

139. Alster TS, Williams CM. Treatment of keloid sternotomy scars with 585 nm flashlamp-pumped pulsed-dye laser. *Lancet.* 1995;345:1198-1200.

140. Mercer NS. Silicone gel in the treatment of keloid scars. *Br J Plast Surg.* 1989;42:83-87.

141. Janssen de Limpens AM. The local treatment of hypertrophic scars and keloids with topical retinoic acid. *Br J Dermatol.* 1980;103:319-323.

142. Asawananda P, Khoo LSW, Fitzpatrick TB, et al. UV-A1 for keloid. *Arch Dermatol.* 1999;135:348-349.

143. Hannuksela-Svahn A, Grandal OJ, Thorstensen T, et al. UVA1 for treatment of keloids. *Acta Derm Venereol.* 1999;79:490.

144. Onwukwe MF. Surgery and methotrexate for keloids. *Schoch Lett.* 1978;28:4.

145. Mendoza J, Sebastian A, Allan E, et al. Differential cytotoxic response in keloid fibroblasts exposed to photodynamic therapy is dependent on pho-tosensitiser precursor, fluence and location of fibroblasts within the lesion. *Arch Dermatol Res.* 2012;304:549-562.

146. Nie Z, Bayat A, Behzad F, et al. Positive response of a recurrent keloid scar to topical methyl aminolevulinate-photodynamic therapy. *Photodermatol Photoimmunol Photomed.* 2010;26:330-332.

147. Sebastian A, Allan E, Allan D, et al. Addition of novel degenerate electrical waveform stimulation with photodynamic therapy significantly enhances its cytotoxic effect in keloid fibroblasts: first report of a potential combination therapy. *J Dermatol Sci.* 2011;64:174-184.

148. Ud-Din S, Thomas G, Morris J, et al. Photodynamic therapy: an innovative approach to the treatment of keloid disease evaluated using subjective and objective non-invasive tools. *Arch Dermatol Res.* 2013;305:205-214.

CHAPTER 34 Acne Keloidalis Nuchae

A. Paul Kelly
Ardeshir Bayat

KEY POINTS

- Acne keloidalis nuchae (AKN) initially presents as a folliculitis that often develops into keloid-like papules and plaques.

- AKN occurs in patients with darkly pigmented skin of color with coarse, curly hair, usually after puberty.

- Although the older literature implies that AKN only occurs in males, it can also occur in females.

- Therapy can be medical, surgical, or a combination of both.

- Excision with second-intention healing is the optimal surgical modal-ity, but the cosmetic outcome can vary.

- The application of a class I or II topical corticosteroid is the recog-nized standard medical therapy.

- Long-pulse diode laser or long-pulse neodymium-doped yttrium aluminium garnet (Nd:YAG) laser therapy may significantly improve some AKN lesions.

- Initiating treatment as early as possible achieves the best results and improves the likelihood of controlling the disease.

SYNONYMS

- Acne keloidalis nuchae

- Dermatitis papillaris capillitii

- Keloidal folliculitis

- Sycosis nuchae
- Folliculitis keloidalis nuchae
- Folliculitis nuchae scleroticans
- Nuchal keloid acne
- Keloid acne
- Folliculitis keloidalis
- Folliculitis barbae traumatica
- Sycosis framboesiformis
- Lichen keloidalis nuchae

INTRODUCTION

Acne keloidalis nuchae (AKN) refers to the formation of keloid-like papules and/or plaques on the occipital scalp and posterior neck almost exclusively in darker-pigmented men with coarse, curly hair.[1,2] It usually starts after puberty as an acute folliculitis and perifolliculitis that becomes chronic. As the disease progresses, the papules enlarge to form keloid-like plaques. Associated scarring alopecia is common in the involved scalp area.

AKN was first described by Kaposi in 1869 as dermatitis papillaris capillitii, one of the older synonyms for AKN.[3] This name was based on the anatomic location of acne keloidalis; the capillitium is the suboccipital portion of the skin. Three years later, Bazin named the disorder acne keloidalis, a designation that still prevails today.[4]

The older literature implies that AKN only occurs in males, but we now know that it can occur in females, with a male-to-female ratio of approximately 20:1.[5] Although, AKN is found predominately in darker-pigmented men with coarse, curly hair, the next most common group with AKN is Hispanics followed by Asians; Caucasians develop it least often.[6]

ETIOLOGY AND PATHOGENESIS

The exact cause of AKN is unknown. It does not represent acne vulgaris, nor is it a true keloid. AKN lesions are not comedonal in comparison to acne lesions. Acute folliculitis and perifolliculitis usually precede AKN, followed by chronic folliculitis and then AKN. Systemic antibiotics may cure the folliculitis but do not soften or clear the existing keloid-like lesions. AKN may respond to systemic steroid therapy.[6]

George et al[6] found that 15% of their patients had a family history of AKN. As in pseudofolliculitis barbae (PFB), shaving short, tightly curled hair, which is common among darker-pigmented men, and then having the new hair growth curve back to penetrate the skin may be the precipitating factors. The same precipitating factors are thought to occur in women with curving of new tightly curled hair into the skin.[7] Additional factors include continuous irritation from shirt collars, chronic low-grade folliculitis, and an autoimmune process.[8]

Goette and Berger[9] presented histologic evidence that AKN is a transepithelial elimination disorder similar to perforating folliculitis, whereas Sperling et al[10] found histologic evidence that AKN is a form of scarring alopecia. These findings negate an association between PFB and AKN.

Burkhart and Burkhart[11] reported that AKN represents a variant form of lichen simplex chronicus with fibrotic keloid scarring rather than acne mechanica, as proposed by Knable et al.[12] George et al[6] suggested that AKN is associated with the male gender, seborrheic constitution, early reproduction years, and increased fasting blood testosterone concentrations. Increased mast cell density and dilatation of the dermal capillaries are features that may predispose AKN to form on the vascular prominent occipital location.

The use of antiepileptic drugs, causing an increased number of mast cells in the occipital region, and the use of cyclosporine for renal transplant patients both have been cited as causes of AKN. Azurdia et al[13] reported cases of three Caucasian men who developed AKN lesions on the occipital scalp and nuchal neck after treatment with cyclosporine following organ transplantation. Also, AKN-like lesions have been reported on the scalp of an epileptic patient on diphenylhydantoin and carbamazepine. The lesions resolved when the drugs were discontinued.[14]

These proposed precipitating factors for AKN suggest that the etiology of AKN may be multifactorial.

PATHOLOGY

Histologically, AKN is characterized by follicular and perifollicular inflammation that changes in composition during the evolution of the lesions. Initially, the infiltrate is composed of neutrophils and lymphocytes. In 1942, Fox[15] reported that mast cells were predominant in AKN. This finding is significant because mast cells are also increased in keloids and other fibrosing disorders. Mast cells are not increased in darker-pigmented men with coarse, curly hair unless they have fibrotic disease. The folliculitis begins at the upper third of the hair follicle. Herzberg et al[16] found that the follicular lymphocyte infiltrate contained mixed B- and T-cell populations and that the plasma cell immunoglobulins were of a polyclonal nature.

Sebaceous glands are markedly diminished or absent in all stages of folliculitis. In more advanced lesions, hair follicles are disrupted, and broken hair fragments are surrounded by granulomatous inflammation. Dermal fibrosis and scars are seen at this stage and resemble the collagen fibers in scar tissue rather than those in true keloids.[4]

One follicle can show several stages of inflammation at a given point in time. The lower portion of the follicle, including the matrix, is usually spared until later in the disease process. The shaft that guides the hairs to the surface is lost in the inflammatory process, and these hair fragments proliferate beneath fibrotic tissue and are surrounded by a foreign body response, producing the tufted hairs seen late in the disease process. Tufted hair folliculitis or polytrichia hairs are characterized by several to 20 or more hairs emerging from a single follicular opening or from large follicular pustules.[9] These hairs have separate follicles in the lower dermis, but the inflammation and scar tissue higher in the dermis seem to cause the amalgamation of hairs into one follicle [**Figure 34-1**].

■ LABORATORY STUDIES

Other than histopathology, there are no specific tests for AKN. Bacterial cultures should be taken intermittently for any pustular or draining lesions. If pathogens are found, the patient should be treated with the appropriate antibiotics.

CLINICAL FINDINGS

AKN begins after puberty as firm, dome-shaped papules 2 to 4 mm in diameter on the nape of the neck or the occipital scalp [**Figures 34-2 to 34-4**]. Pustules also may be present in the same areas, but they are

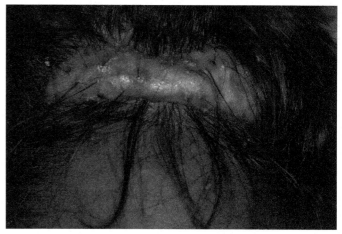

FIGURE 34-1. A large keloidal hairless plaque with tufted hairs producing doll-like hair on the upper border.

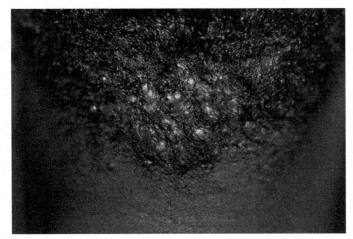

FIGURE 34-2. All stages of acne keloidalis pustules, dome-shaped papules, and plaques.

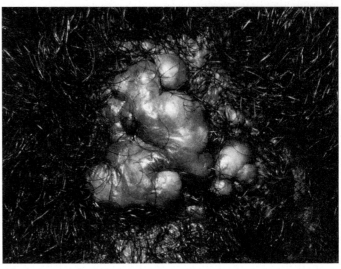

FIGURE 34-4. Small to large dome-shaped keloid nodules on the posterior occipital area.

usually short-lived because the tops are sometimes scratched off as a result of pruritus of the involved area, or they are traumatized when the hair is combed or brushed. In contradistinction to acne, comedones are not present.

As the disease progresses, more papules may appear, and those already present may enlarge. Some coalesce to form keloid-like plaques, which are usually arranged in a horizontal band-like fashion involving the occipital scalp. The plaques are most often only a few centimeters in diameter but sometimes cover the majority of the occipital scalp. Large lesions are usually hairless, and their upper border is often fringed with tufted hairs appearing like doll's hair, as in Figure 34-1. Scarring alopecia and subcutaneous abscesses with draining sinuses also may be present.

The early papular lesions are usually asymptomatic, but the pustular ones are often pruritic and may be painful. Also, larger plaques are usually more painful than smaller ones. Chronic lesions with abscesses and sinuses may emit an odorous discharge. Even though many lesions are asymptomatic, their appearance is often a cause of tremendous cosmetic concern to the patient.

One explanation for the development of AKN provided by Herzberg et al[16] is based on extensive transverse microscopy-histochemistry and electron microscopic analysis. These researchers described the hypothetical sequence of inflammatory events that takes place in AKN. The acute inflammation, whether it begins in the sebaceous gland or elsewhere in the region of the deep infundibular or isthmus levels, is a cause or the result of a weakened follicular wall at these levels. This enables the release of hair shafts into the surrounding dermis. The 'foreign' hairs incite further acute and chronic granulomatous inflammation, which manifests clinically as a papular lesion. Fibroblasts lay down collagen,

and scars form in the region of inflammation. Distortion and occlusion of the follicular lumen by fibrosis lead to hair retention in the inferior follicle and further smoldering granulomatous inflammation and scarring. The scar and granulomatous inflammation manifest clinically as scars and plaques.[16] Interestingly, little can be added to Adamson's clinical description of AKN written in 1914:

> The eruption occurs on the back of the neck in the form of a raised transverse band at the lower margin of the hairy scalp. The band is usually dusky red in color, smooth and firm to the touch in fact, of keloidal aspect and consistence. It is hairless except at its upper margin, which is abrupt, broken in nodules and fringed with hair tufts, like aigrettes, or the bunches of bristles in a brush. There may be pustules or crusted nodules here and there along the upper border. The lower margin slopes gradually to the normal skin. Usually there are no comedones or follicular pustules of acne when the patient comes under observation, and there may or may not be a history of acne on youthful faces. Often the patient complains of itching at the site of eruption.[17]

DIFFERENTIAL DIAGNOSIS

A diagnosis of AKN can be made when the following criteria are fulfilled:

- Keloid-like plaques [**Figure 34-5**]
- Scarring alopecia

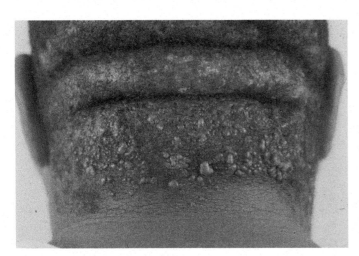

FIGURE 34-3. Numerous papular lesions on the nuchal areas of a darker-pigmented man with coarse, curly hair.

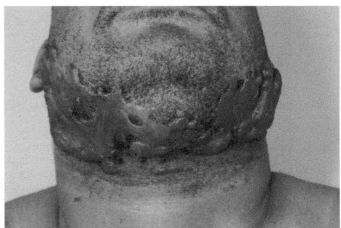

FIGURE 34-5. A diagnosis of acne keloidalis nuchae can be made from keloid-like plaques such as those pictured in the beard of this African American man.

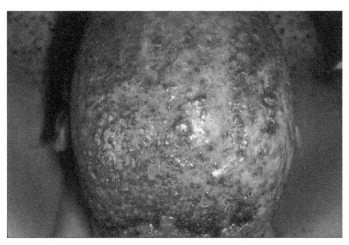

FIGURE 34-6. Acute folliculitis infection can be the precursor to acne keloidalis nuchae (AKN). It can be difficult differentiate from a diagnosis of AKN.

- Acute folliculitis infection [**Figure 34-6**]
- Perifolliculitis
- Chronic folliculitis and perifolliculitis

Because the presentation of AKN is often classic, in most cases, there is no need for a differential diagnosis, but perifolliculitis capitis *abscedens et suffodiens*, folliculitis, sarcoidosis, and nevus sebaceous of Jadassohn must be ruled out.

COMPLICATIONS

Although AKN is a medically benign dermatosis, it can be socially or psychologically debilitating to patients (**Figure 34-7**). In addition, patients with AKN can develop squamous cell carcinoma secondary to radiation therapy or keloid-like lesions.

CLINICAL COURSE AND PROGNOSIS

The course of the disease is usually chronic and often leads to hair follicle destruction and polytrichoid hairs (3 to 20 hairs coming out of one follicle).[18] The only reported case of familial AKN involved a father and all three of his sons, but not his two daughters.[19] It is rare for AKN to develop before adolescence or after the age of 50. Darker-pigmented

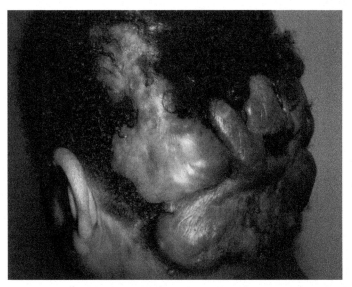

FIGURE 34-7. A darker-pigmented man with coarse, curly hair with several large keloid-like lesions covering most of the occipital scalp. Such lesions can be socially or psychologically debilitating to patients.

men with coarse, curly hair seem to have an earlier age of onset of AKN. If the lesions are treated early enough, the prognosis is good for a near complete recovery.[20]

PREVENTION

Patients at risk of developing AKN should be made aware that their actions may precipitate the onset of the disorder. Avoidance of the use of a razor or clippers on the edge of the occipital hairline and of tight-fitting shirts, hats, or other clothing that continuously rubs the posterior hairline is important. However, once a lesion appears, the rapid initiation of therapy will likely minimize the chance of developing large disfiguring lesions.[1]

TREATMENT

Dermatologists should be aware that certain medications have been associated with the development of AKN, particularly cyclosporine. Unfortunately, there is no one therapeutic modality that cures AKN except systemic corticosteroids, which may stop the lesional activity and cause a partial or near complete regression of any AKN lesions. However, when systemic corticosteroids are discontinued, the lesions typically return in weeks to months, and long-term oral corticosteroids are not recommended because chronic therapy may lead to many complications, especially adrenal suppression and brittle bones.[1]

▦ TOPICAL THERAPY

Topical therapy is sometimes effective in attenuating AKN:

- A class I or II corticosteroid gel (eg, betamethasone dipropionate or desoximetasone) or clobetasol foam can be applied twice daily[21]
- A corticosteroid gel combined with retinoic acid gel applied every night can relieve symptoms and help flatten existing lesions
- For pustules and other evidence of infection, topical clindamycin or mupirocin should be applied twice daily until the pustules abate and the inflammation subsides
- Imiquimod can be applied daily for 5 days, followed by 2 days off, for a total of 8 weeks

▦ MINOR INVASIVE THERAPIES

The following treatments often attenuate AKN but usually are not curative.

Intralesional Corticosteroids Injections

- Intralesional injections of a mixture of one-half 10 mg/mL triamcinolone acetonide and one-half 40 mg/mL may be administered, using an insulin syringe with a 29-gauge needle performed at 3-week intervals.
- *Note:* It is important to inform the patient that he or she may develop hypopigmentation or dermal atrophy, lasting 12 to 18 months, at the injection site as well as on the surrounding healthy skin.

Excision of Papules

- Removal of individual papules with a hair transplant punch may be performed, leaving the postoperative site to close by second-intention healing or primary closure with sutures.
- *Note:* A technique by which the punch extends deep into the subcutaneous tissue and past the deepest layer of the hair follicle will decrease recurrence of the lesion. Removal of only the superficial portion of the papule is associated with a much higher incidence of recurrence.

De-roofing Smaller Lesions

- The removal of the superficial portion or top of each papule using a scalpel with local anesthetic, followed by cauterization of the base of the lesion, is an acceptable treatment. The de-roofed wound site may be allowed to close by second-intention healing or, rarely, with sutures.

- *Note:* The de-roofing excision should extend past the deepest layer of the ingrown hair follicle, into the subcutaneous tissue, because superficial removal is likely to have a higher incidence of recurrence.

Laser Therapy

- Laser therapy (carbon dioxide or Nd:YAG) has proven successful in some patients. Indeed, Esmat et al[22] reported that laser hair depilation can significantly improve the chronic aspects of AKN. Initiating treatment as early as possible achieves the best results, and the progression of the disease can be stopped if followed by regular sessions for maintenance.

- Preliminary studies show that long-pulse diode laser therapy or long-pulse Nd:YAG lasers may be successful in removing trapped hairs, which then may attenuate the *nidus* of AKN.[23]

Cryotherapy

- Cryotherapy is a useful therapy for some patients.
- The AKN lesions are frozen for ≥20 seconds, allowed to thaw, and then frozen again for ≥20 seconds.
- Morbidity, which includes discomfort and drainage, is greater than with other modalities.
- When the freeze–thaw time is greater than 25 seconds, the melanocytes are destroyed, and the treated areas often become hypopigmented and may remain so for 12 to 18 months.

■ SURGICAL REMOVAL OF LARGE LESIONS

Large linear lesions up to 1 cm in diameter may be excised and closed using a horizontal ellipse with 4-0 sutures. Often the postoperative site may later splay to the diameter of the initial excision, so it is advisable to close the operative site without flexing the posterior neck. When it is necessary to flex the neck to close the excisional defect, the patient will spend a week or more looking upward. Under such tension, the resulting scar splays, often to the size of the amount of area removed and frequently creating an area of alopecia as large as the initial defect. Gloster[24] recommends treating extremely large lesions with multiple-stage excisions.

■ OTHER PROCEDURES FOR REMOVAL OF LARGE LESIONS

For large lesions that do not respond to medical treatment or minor surgical intervention, the area of AKN can be excised to the fascia or to the deep subcutaneous tissue and left to heal secondarily.[25] The technique is as follows:

- For optimal healing, excise the posterior scalp using a horizontal ellipse that includes the posterior hairline and extends to the muscle fascia or deep subcutaneous tissue [**Figures 34-8 and 34-9**].

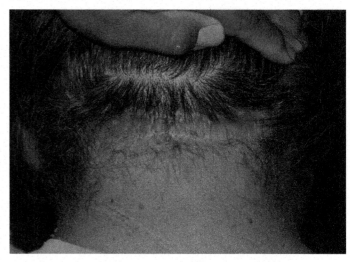

FIGURE 34-9. One month after second-intention healing of the man in Figure 34-8.

- Tie off or cauterize bleeding vessels, and then apply pressure to the postoperative site for 10 to 15 minutes and then reevaluate for bleeding.
- Apply a topical antibiotic ointment on the day of the procedure and then twice daily after cleaning the wound with saline.
- *Note:* Do not inject corticosteroids until wound healing (reepithelialization) is completed because it can prevent wound contraction.
- A nonhorizontal elliptic excision will result in a poor cosmetic result if (1) the excision extends above the occipital notch; (2) the lower border of the excision is above the posterior hairline; and/or (3) intralesional steroids are used prior to complete wound healing [**Figures 34-10 and 34-11**].

POSTOPERATIVE CONSIDERATIONS

The postoperative site usually heals in 8 to 12 weeks. A 10-day course of a broad-spectrum antibiotic (eg, erythromycin, cephalosporin, or tetracycline) should begin immediately after surgery. Once healing has occurred, apply a retinoic acid and corticosteroid gel preparation nightly. Note that excision with grafting is usually not a viable option because it may result in an atrophic non–hair-bearing area.

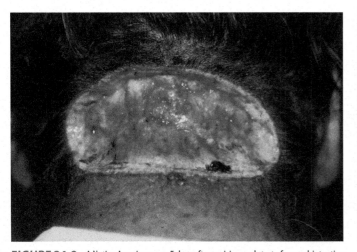

FIGURE 34-8. A Native American man 5 days after excision and start of second-intention healing. This case shows that people with straight hair also can develop acne keloidalis nuchae.

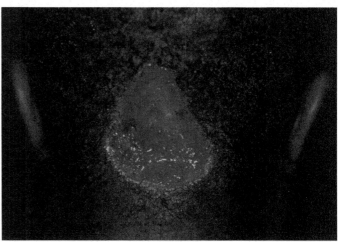

FIGURE 34-10. After excision of an acne keloidalis lesion that was done in a nonelliptical fashion above the posterior hairline and not below the hair follicles.

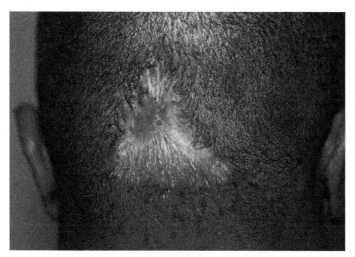

FIGURE 34-11. Poor healing in the patient in Figure 34-10 due to direction, depth, and excision above the hairline.

PATIENT PREPARATION FOR SURGERY

- Before surgery, instruct the patient and his or her caregiver to clean the postoperative site twice daily with saline and then apply an antibiotic ointment.
- Show the patient and caregiver photographs of the stages of healing to facilitate understanding of the process.
- Explain the level of discomfort or pain that may occur postoperatively and that acetaminophen should be sufficient to relieve it.

CONCLUSION

Although the causes of AKN are still uncertain, there are effective and helpful treatments including topical agents, minor invasive techniques, laser therapy, and excision. Surgery using a horizontal elliptical excision below the hair follicles, with second-intention healing, results in the postoperative site healing completely within 3 months. Second-intention healing often results in a good to excellent cosmetic result [**Table 34-1**].

TABLE 34-1 Overview of acne keloidalis
First reported by Kaposi in 1869
Most common synonyms
• Acne keloidalis nuchae
• Folliculitis keloidalis
• Acne keloid
Etiology and pathogenesis
• Found mainly in darkly pigmented men with coarse, curly hair
• Occurs after puberty or before the age of 50
• Starts as chronic folliculitis of the posterior scalp and neck
• Probably related to close shaving and irritation from tight shirt collars or caps
Differential diagnosis
• Folliculitis
• Acne vulgaris
• Keloid
• Nevus sebaceous
Treatment
• Intralesional corticosteroids
• Liquid nitrogen
• Laser therapy: Long-pulse diode laser therapy or long-pulse Nd:YAG
• Excise with second-intention closure. Long-pulse diode laser therapy or long-pulse Nd:YAG lasers significantly improve acne keloidalis nuchae lesions, when used in conjunction with intralesional corticosteroids
• Starting treatment as early as possible achieves the best results and improves the likelihood of controlling the disease.

REFERENCES

1. Bayat A, Arscott G, Ollier WER, et al. Description of site-specific morphology of keloid phenotypes in an Afrocaribbean population. *Br J Plast Surg.* 2004;57:122-133.
2. Kelly AP. Acne keloidalis nuchae. http://emedicine.medscape.com/article/1072149-overview. Accessed January 27, 2015.
3. Kaposi M. Über diesogennante Framboesia und mehrere andere Arten von papillären Neubildungen der Haut. *Arch Dermatol Syphilol.* 1869;1:382-423.
4. Cosman B, Wolff M. Acne keloidalis. *Plast Reconstr Surg.* 1972;50:25-30.
5. Dinehart SM, Tanner L, Mallory SB, et al. Acne keloidalis in women. *Cutis.* 1989;44:250-252.
6. George AO, Akanji AO, Nduka EU, et al. Clinical, biochemical and morphologic features of acne keloidalis in a black population. *Int J Dermatol.* 1993;32:714-716.
7. Ogunbiyi A, George A. Acne keloidalis in females: case report and review of literature. *J Natl Med Assoc.* 2005;97:736-738.
8. Salami T, Omeife H, Samuel S. Prevalence of acne keloidalis nuchae in Nigerians. *Int J Dermatol.* 2007;46:482-484.
9. Goette DK, Berger TG. Acne keloidalis nuchae: a transepithelial elimination disorder. *Int J Dermatol.* 1987;26:442-444.
10. Sperling LC, Homoky C, Pratt L, et al. Acne keloidalis is a form of primary scarring alopecia. *Arch Dermatol.* 2000;136:479-484.
11. Burkhart CG, Burkhart CN. Acne keloidalis is lichen simplex chronicus with fibrotic keloidal scarring. *J Am Acad Dermatol.* 1998;39:661.
12. Knable AL, Hanke CW, Gonin R. Prevalence of acne keloidalis nuchae in football players. *J Am Acad Dermatol.* 1997;37:570-574.
13. Azurdia RM, Graham RM, Weismann K, et al. Acne keloidalis in Caucasian patients on cyclosporin following organ transplantation. *Br J Dermatol.* 2000;143:465-467.
14. Malberbe WDF. Dermatome dermaplaning and sycosis nuchae excision. *Clin Plast Surg.* 1977;4:289-296.
15. Fox H. Folliculitis keloidalis a better term than dermatitis papillaris capillittii. *Arch Dermatol Syphilol.* 1942;55:112-113.
16. Herzberg AJ, Dinehart SM, Kerns BJ, et al. Acne keloidalis. Transverse microscopy, immunohistochemistry, and an electron microscopy. *Am J Dermatopathol.* 1990;12:109-121.
17. Adamson HG. Dermatitis papillaris capillitti (Kaposi): acne keloid. *Br J Dermatol.* 1914;26:2669-2683.
18. Luz Ramos M, Muñoz-Pérez MA, Ports A, et al. Acne keloidalis and tufted hair folliculitis. *Dermatology.* 1997;194:71-73.
19. D'Souza P, Iyer VK, Ramam M. Familial acné keloidalis. *Acta Dermatol Venerol.* 1998;78:382.
20. Kelly AP. Lecture given at National Medical Association Annual Meeting: Update on AKN. National Medical Association Annual Meeting, Atlanta, GA, 2008.
21. Callender VD, Young CM, Haverstock CL, et al. An open label study of clobetasol propionate 0.05% and betamethasone volerate 0.12% foams in the treatment of mild to moderate acne keloidalis. *Cutis.* 2005;75:317-321.
22. Esmat SM, Abdel Hay RM, Abu Zeid OM, et al. The efficacy of laser-assisted hair removal in the treatment of acne keloidalis nuchae; a pilot study. *Eur J Dermatol.* 2012;22:645-650.
23. Shah GK. Efficacy of diode laser for treating acne keloidalis nuchae. *Indian J Dermatol Verol Leperol.* 2005;71:31-34.
24. Gloster HM Jr. The surgical management of extensive cases of acne keloidalis nuchae. *Arch Dermatol.* 2000;136:1376-1379.
25. Glenn MJ, Bennett RG, Kelly AP. Acne keloidalis nuchae: treatment with excision and second-intention healing. *J Am Acad Dermatol.* 1995;33:243-246.

Drug Eruptions

CHAPTER 35

Temitayo A. Ogunleye

KEY POINTS

- Cutaneous drug eruptions are one of the most common signs of adverse drug reaction.
- Certain types of drug eruptions may occur with increased frequency in various racial groups as elucidated by recent pharmacogenetic studies.
- Cutaneous adverse drug reactions vary greatly in clinical findings and symptoms.
- A systematic approach to identifying drug eruptions including a complete medication history and recognition of reaction patterns on clinical examination are important in determining the causative medication.
- Early withdrawal of suspected medications is essential, along with supportive care and case-dependent appropriate treatment.

INTRODUCTION

Cutaneous eruptions are one of the most common signs of adverse drug reaction.[1] Drug reactions are estimated to occur with a prevalence of 2% to 3% in hospitalized patients, and 1 in every 1000 patients has a serious cutaneous drug reaction.[1-3] Reactions may range from common exanthematous eruptions to life-threatening conditions, and may be limited to the skin or, alternatively, have multiorgan system involvement. In patients with darker skin, clinical findings may be subtle and more difficult to diagnose. In addition, recent research in pharmacogenomics has identified skin of color populations who may be at greater risk for certain types of cutaneous drug reactions. In this chapter, we discuss pertinent clinical findings in various drug eruptions and some important differences that may be seen in patients with skin of color.

CLINICAL FEATURES IN SKIN OF COLOR

Drug eruptions in skin of color populations differ little in progression, diagnosis, and treatment. Minor differences in clinical presentation include subtleties in discerning early erythema in drug eruptions, differences in quality of erythema, and posteruption sequelae. In patients with darker skin tones, initial areas of erythema may be difficult to visualize and may have a darker purple hue. In addition, postinflammatory hyperpigmentation may be a more significant cosmetic issue in patients with skin of color compared with lighter populations, even in seemingly mild eruptions.

PHARMACOGENETICS

The emerging field of pharmacogenetics has played a major role in identifying patients and population groups that are at increased risk for developing certain types of adverse cutaneous reactions. For example, pharmacogenetic studies have linked human leukocyte antigen (HLA) B*5701 allele to the abacavir hypersensitivity syndrome.[4] This allele is found in 5% to 7% of Caucasian (including Hispanic) populations; 5% to 20% of Indian populations; <2% of Chinese, Korean, and Thai populations, and <1% of African populations.[4] It is believed that HLA-B*5701 has a high correlation with abacavir hypersensitivity in both African Americans and Caucasians in North America, with unclear significance in other populations.[5-8] Although these studies elucidate the requirement for the presence of this allele, 45% of patients who carry HLA-B*5701 do not develop this syndrome.[6] This suggests that this allele is necessary but not sufficient for the reaction to occur.

Identification of HLA alleles that may increase the risk of certain drug eruptions can influence prescribing practices and subsequently decrease their incidence. Studies evaluating the occurrence of Stevens-Johnson syndrome and other drug reactions help to highlight the importance of considering race when prescribing medications, in order to avoid adverse cutaneous drug eruptions [**Tables 35-1 and 35-2**].[9]

PATIENT APPROACH

EXANTHEMATOUS ERUPTIONS

Exanthematous drug eruptions, also known as morbilliform or maculopapular eruptions, are the most common type of cutaneous drug eruption (accounting for 40% of drug reactions), followed by urticaria and angioedema.[10-12] Morbilliform eruptions typically begin 7 to 14 days after institution of the medication, but may also begin a few days after discontinuation of the medication. Lesions consist of pink to red macules that coalesce, with involvement of the trunk and subsequent progression peripherally onto the limbs [**Figure 35-1 and 35-2**]. In patients with darker skin hues, redness may be difficult to visualize, with erythema manifesting as a purplish discoloration [**Figure 35-3**]. Mucous membranes are classically spared. Pruritus is a common feature,

TABLE 35-1	Reported genetic biomarkers for anticonvulsants and allopurinol-induced cutaneous drug reactions		
Causative drug	HLA-B	Population	Cutaneous reaction
Carbamazepine	*1502	Han Chinese (Taiwan)	SJS/TEN
		Han Chinese (Hong Kong)	
		Thai	
		Indians	
Carbamazepine	*1511	Japanese	SJS/TEN
Phenytoin	*1502	Han Chinese (Taiwan)	SJS/TEN
		Thai	
Lamotrigine	*1502	Han Chinese (Taiwan)	SJS
Oxcarbazepine	*1502	Han Chinese (Taiwan)	SJS
Allopurinol	*5801	Han Chinese (Taiwan)	SJS/TEN or DRESS
		Thai	SJS/TEN
		Caucasians	
		Japanese	

Abbreviations: DRESS, drug reaction with eosinophilia and systemic symptoms; HLA, human leukocyte antigen; SJS, Stevens-Johnson syndrome; TEN, toxic epidermal necrolysis.

Source: Adapted with permission from Aihara M. Pharmacogenetics of cutaneous adverse drug reactions. *J Dermatol.* 2011;38:246-254.

TABLE 35-2	Reported genetic markers for antiretroviral medications		
Causative medication	HLA	Population	Cutaneous reaction
Abacavir	B*5701	Caucasian	Hypersensitivity syndrome
		African origin	
		Japanese	
Nevirapine	B*3505	Thai	Hypersensitivity syndrome
	Cw8	Japanese	Hypersensitivity syndrome
		Sardinian	
	B14	Sardinian	Hypersensitivity syndrome

Abbreviation: HLA, human leukocyte antigen.

Source: Adapted with permission from Aihara M. Pharmacogenetics of cutaneous adverse drug reactions. *J Dermatol.* 2011;38:246-254.

TABLE 35-3	Approach to the patient with suspected drug eruption

Complete history
    Date of onset of the eruption
    Time interval between drug introduction and skin eruption
        Full medication list (discontinued, active) used in last 2 weeks to 6 months,
        including herbal medications, vitamins, and illicit drugs with start/end dates
Physical examination
        All skin; oral, genital, ocular, and anal mucosa; and lymph nodes
        Determination of the type of primary lesion and the distribution of lesions
        Associated signs and symptoms
Testing and other inquiry
        Skin biopsy if indicated
        Laboratory evaluations (CBC, CMP, vasculitis and/or connective tissue disease evalu-
        ation, etc.)
        Perform literature search to determine most likely agent(s)
Discontinuation of suspected nonessential medications
Provide appropriate treatment and/or supportive care

Abbreviations: CBC, complete blood count; CMP, complete metabolic panel.

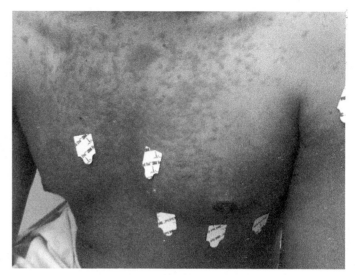

FIGURE 35-2. Morbilliform drug eruption. (Used with permission from Lisa Pappas-Taffer, MD.)

and low-grade fever may be present. Resolution of the eruption consists of fading erythema and may be followed by scaling or desquamation.

Common causative medications include penicillins, sulfonamides, cephalosporins, nonnucleoside reverse transcriptase inhibitors, and antiepileptic medications.[1] Drug–viral enhancement of these eruptions, such as that which can occur after treatment of a patient with infectious mononucleosis with penicillins, increases this risk several fold, from a range of 4% to 13% to a range of 60% to 100%.[13] Similar drug–viral interactions occur in patients with human immunodeficiency virus (HIV) who take sulfonamide antibiotics. The major differential diagnosis includes a viral exanthem, and the two may be difficult to distinguish.

Drug Reaction with Eosinophilia and Systemic Symptoms Hypersensitivity syndrome, or drug reaction with eosinophilia and systemic symptoms (DRESS), is characterized by an exanthematous eruptions accompanied by internal organ involvement. The incidence of this reaction is estimated to be 1 in 1000 to 1 in 10,000 exposures to drugs

such as anticonvulsants. This condition typically begins 2 to 6 weeks after exposure to the suspected medications such as antiepileptic drugs (phenytoin, carbamazepine, phenobarbital), sulfonamides, nevirapine, abacavir, minocycline, or allopurinol. The pathogenesis of this eruption is complex, with factors such as slow acetylation and reactivation of human herpes viruses, including Epstein-Barr virus and human herpesvirus (HHV) 6 and 7.[14] In fact, the detection of HHV-6 reactivation has been recently proposed as a diagnostic marker for DRESS.[14]

Fever and a morbilliform eruption are the most common symptoms. Pustular variants rarely occur [**Figure 35-4**]. The face, upper trunk, and extremities are common areas of involvement, with facial edema as a frequent additional finding. Lymphadenopathy is often present, with arthralgia/arthritis sometimes occurring. Visceral involvement can be serious and life threatening. Hepatitis is the most common visceral involvement, with fulminant hepatitis being a frequent cause of death

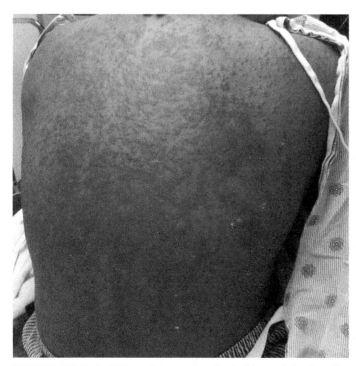

FIGURE 35-1. Morbilliform drug eruption. (Used with permission from Lisa Pappas-Taffer, MD.)

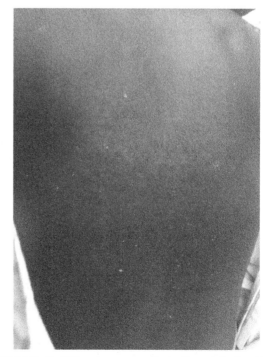

FIGURE 35-3. Morbilliform drug eruption. (Used with permission from Lisa Pappas-Taffer, MD.)

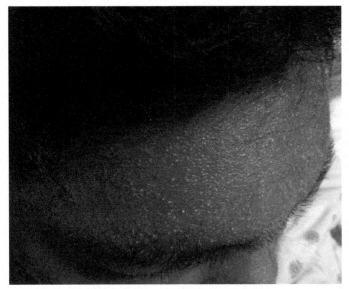

FIGURE 35-4. Pustular variant of drug reaction with eosinophilia and systemic symptoms. (Used with permission from Lisa Pappas-Taffer, MD.)

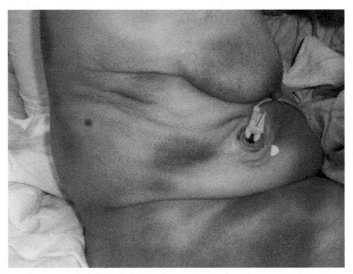

FIGURE 35-5. Fixed drug eruption.

in these patients. However, almost any organ system may be involved, with reports of thyroiditis, pneumonitis, myocarditis, nephritis, and central nervous system infiltration. As the name indicates, prominent eosinophilia is a characteristic feature. Atypical lymphocytosis may also be seen. The reaction may continue for several weeks or months after discontinuation of the offending medication, and immunosuppressive therapy for several months is frequently necessary.

Acute Generalized Exanthematous Pustulosis Acute generalized exanthematous pustulosis (AGEP) is an acute febrile drug eruption characterized by sterile non–follicular-based pustules, arising on an erythematous base. It begins on the face or intertriginous areas but can generalize within a few hours. Associated signs and symptoms include lymphocytosis, edema of the face and hands, purpura, vesicles, bullae, erythema multiforme-like lesions, and mucous membrane involvement.[15] AGEP can arise as early as 2 days after starting the offending medication (commonly β-lactam and macrolide antibiotics, calcium channel blockers, and antimalarials) and resolves with generalized desquamation occurring 1 to 2 weeks after the start of the eruption. Differential diagnosis includes acute pustular psoriasis of von Zumbusch, as well as toxic epidermal necrolysis in severe cases. These entities can usually be differentiated via medication history and pathologic findings. Discontinuation of the medication and liberal emollient use and topical steroids are typically sufficient for therapy.

URTICARIAL ERUPTIONS

Urticaria is characterized by transient erythematous and edematous papules, or wheals, with associated pruritus. Wheals typically last for a few hours but less than 24 hours. Lesions vary in size and number, may occur at any location on the body, and resolve without residua. Associated findings include angioedema, or deep dermal/subcutaneous/submucosal swelling of the face and, less commonly, extremities or genitalia. Severe cases are associated with anaphylaxis accompanied by hypotension and tachycardia, which may be fatal.

Angioedema occurs in 1 to 2 per 1000 new users of angiotensin-converting enzyme (ACE) inhibitors.[16] ACE inhibitor-induced angioedema may begin shortly after the start of the medication or may occur after years of use. African Americans and those with a history of idiopathic angioedema are at increased risk for developing ACE inhibitor-induced angioedema.[17]

Urticarial reactions secondary to drugs are usually immunoglobulin (Ig) E-mediated immediate hypersensitivity reactions and cause reactions within minutes of reexposure to the offending medication. Immunologic-mediated reactions are most commonly caused by antibiotics, especially the penicillins and cephalosporins, and less often tetracyclines and sulfonamides. Nonsteroidal anti-inflammatory drugs (NSAIDS) and radiocontrast dyes are causes of nonimmunologic or anaphylactoid urticarial eruptions. In these types of reactions, histamine/inflammatory mediator release is not induced by IgE but by other mediators.

FIXED DRUG ERUPTIONS

Fixed drug eruptions consist of erythematous or dark purple, round patches that may have a dusky or bullous center [**Figure 35-5**]. They usually appear within 24 hours of exposure to the inciting medication. Lesions recur in the same location upon subsequent exposure to the medication, with possible new areas of involvement developing. Fixed drug eruptions commonly occur on the genitals, lips, hands, and feet, but they may occur elsewhere on the body. Patients may be asymptomatic or complain of burning, stinging, or pain, especially with mucosal or bullous lesions. The eruption resolves over the course of a few days or weeks, but often leaves residual postinflammatory hyperpigmentation. The nonpigmented variant, commonly associated with pseudoephedrine, consists of large erythematous plaques that heal without residual pigmentation.

Many medications have been associated with fixed drug eruption; however, common offenders include barbiturates, tetracyclines, NSAIDS, sulfonamides, and carbamazepine. Patch testing may be helpful in elucidating the causative medication.

OTHER BULLOUS ERUPTIONS

Linear IgA Bullous Dermatosis Linear IgA bullous dermatosis is a rare autoimmune mucocutaneous blistering disease typically consisting of tense vesicles and bullae appearing in an annular configuration on the trunk and extremities. It can, however, be heterogeneous in its presentation, with morphology mimicking erythema multiforme, bullous pemphigoid, and dermatitis herpetiformis. Both drug-induced and idiopathic linear IgA bullous dermatosis are clinically and histologically indistinguishable from one another and are characterized immunohistopathologically by a subepithelial blister and linear deposition of IgA on direct immunofluorescence along the basement membrane zone. The primary distinguishing factor between the two entities is spontaneous remission of the eruption after discontinuation of the responsible medication. Vancomycin is the most commonly described inciting medication, with an incidence rate of 46.2% of all cases reviewed in a recent article.[18] Other medications that cause linear IgA bullous dermatosis include captopril and trimethoprim/sulfamethoxazole.[18] Mean time to reaction ranges from 2 days to 2 weeks for vancomycin, but has been described with continuous use of trimethoprim/sulfamethoxazole that was begun 26 months before the eruption began.[19] Complete clinical resolution after the discontinuation of the offending drug may only be seen in approximately 50% of cases.[18] Immunosuppressive therapy may be necessary to induce remission.

Drug-Induced Bullous Pemphigoid Drug-induced bullous pemphigoid (BP) is typified by large, tense bullae on an erythematous base, although the eruption may be polymorphic and mimic other drug-induced diseases such as erythema multiforme/Stevens-Johnson syndrome, fixed drug eruption, porphyria cutanea tarda, and eczematous disorders.[20] The most common drugs implicated in drug-induced BP are furosemide and captopril. Features that may distinguish drug-induced BP from BP include younger age and mucous membrane involvement. In addition, overlap of clinical and immunohistologic features of pemphigoid and pemphigus may suggest a drug-induced variant.[21-23] Spontaneous remission or resolution after short-term immunosuppressive treatment may also favor drug etiology.[24] However, some cases of drug-induced BP may require prolonged immunosuppressive therapy, because it is thought that in these patients, the drug may have triggered the idiopathic form of the disease.

Drug-Induced Pemphigus Drug-induced or drug-triggered pemphigus is a bullous eruption indistinguishable from the idiopathic form. Clinical findings congruent with a diagnosis of pemphigus foliaceus are more common than those of pemphigus vulgaris.[24,25] Physical findings may include scaly, crusted erosions on an erythematous base, in a seborrheic distribution, consistent with a diagnosis of pemphigus foliaceus. However, findings of pemphigus vulgaris, including flaccid, fragile blisters occurring on skin and mucosal surfaces, may occur. Pruritus and burning are common complaints in pemphigus foliaceus subtypes, whereas pain is more commonly described in pemphigus vulgaris subtypes, although overlap is common.

Many of the causative drugs contain thiol groups (-SH), and common medications include penicillamine, captopril, and gold. Nonthiol drugs containing sulfur in their molecular structure may undergo changes to form active thiol groups and include penicillins, cephalosporins, and piroxicam.[26,27] The incubation period to the start of the eruption ranges from 2 weeks to 6 months.[27] Up to 50% of cases may remit spontaneously upon discontinuation of the offending medication, whereas others may require immunosuppressive therapy.

LICHENOID ERUPTIONS

Lichenoid drug eruptions do not differ clinically from traditional lichen planus. Purple polygonal plaques scattered on the trunk and extremities are present, although mucous membranes and nails are usually spared [**Figure 35-6**]. However, unlike other drug eruptions, the reaction may begin 2 months to 2 years after beginning the medication. Lichenoid eruptions may require several months or years to resolve. Similar to lichen planus, they often resolve with postinflammatory hyperpigmentation. Offending medications include penicillamine and antihypertensive drugs such as captopril and β-blockers.

DRUG-INDUCED LUPUS ERYTHEMATOSUS

Drug-induced systemic lupus erythematosus (SLE) is dominated by systemic symptoms such as fever, arthritis, myalgias, and serositis occurring in association with antihistone antibodies, and only rarely displays cutaneous findings.[28] Medications typically implicated in this condition include hydralazine, procainamide, isoniazid, and D-penicillamine.

Drug-induced subacute cutaneous lupus erythematosus (SCLE) is typified by erythematous, annular and/or scaly plaques occurring mainly in sun-exposed areas in association with Ro/SS-A autoantibodies [**Figure 35-7**]. This entity is clinically and immunohistopathologically indistinguishable from the native form.[29] Common inciting medications

include thiazide diuretics, calcium channel blockers, and allylamine antifungals (such as terbinafine). Thiazide diuretics and calcium channel blockers tend to have the longest incubation period before onset of the cutaneous reaction, with a range of 6 months to 5 years.[30-32] Allylamine antifungal reactions occur more quickly, as early as 5 weeks after medication initiation.[33,34] The overwhelming majority of cases resolve upon discontinuation of the offending medication.

PHOTOTOXIC AND PHOTOALLERGIC REACTIONS

Phototoxic Reactions Phototoxic reactions are far more common than photoallergic reactions. They can occur in any person who receives sufficient amounts of ultraviolet radiation and/or visible light and the offending medication. They typically require higher doses of the medication and can occur on the first administration of the drug. Clinically, an exaggerated sunburn response is seen in sun-exposed areas, followed by hyperpigmentation. Hyperpigmentation may persist for several months after the initial reaction and, especially in darker-skinned populations, may be the only noted feature, as initial erythema may have been minimal. Areas of sparing may include upper eyelids, submental region, postauricular skin, scalp, flexural areas, palms, and soles.

Photo-onycholysis, characterized by separation of the nail plate from the nail bed, and pseudoporphyria, characterized by bullae in sun-exposed areas, are uncommon presentations of phototoxicity.

The drugs most commonly associated with phototoxic reactions are the tetracyclines, especially doxycycline and demeclocycline, NSAIDs, fluoroquinolones, amiodarone, psoralens, and phenothiazines. Removal of the offending agent results in resolution of the reaction, although sequelae such as hyperpigmentation may be longer lasting.

However, voriconazole, a broad-spectrum antifungal, has recently been associated with photosensitivity and photoaging, with sequelae that continue long after discontinuation of the medication.[35] Patients with voriconazole-induced phototoxicity treated for over 1 year have been observed to have increased incidence of aggressive squamous cell carcinoma in sun-exposed sites.[36] This association of skin cancer and more than 1 year of treatment with voriconazole warrants close follow-up of these patients.

Photoallergic Reactions Photoallergic reactions occur as a result of cell-mediated hypersensitivity. Ultraviolet radiation is necessary to convert the drug into an immunologically active compound. As a result, the reaction does not appear on first exposure, but requires a sensitization period before signs and symptoms develop. Even in sensitized individuals, the onset of the eruption may take 24 to 72 hours after the administration of the drug and exposure to light. Clinical manifestations include eczematous patches, usually confined to sun-exposed sites, although unexposed sites may be involved. Rarely, lichenoid reactions may occur. Acute reactions may be vesicular, whereas chronic reactions have predominant findings of erythema, scaling, and lichenification.

Thiazide diuretics; sulfonamide antibiotics; sunscreen ingredients such as para-aminobenzoic acid (PABA), cinnamates, and benzophenones; and NSAIDs are common causes of photoallergic reactions. Rapid discontinuation of the culprit medication can lead to resolution of the rash, but symptoms may take months to resolve. Chronic exposure may lead to persistent light reactions, where symptoms continue despite discontinuation of the medication and the disease continues to flare with light exposure. These patients would be included in the chronic actinic dermatitis spectrum. Treatment includes topical corticosteroids, physical barriers, and strict photoprotection, with broad-spectrum sunscreen use.

DRUG-INDUCED PIGMENTARY CHANGES

Drug-induced pigmentation may occur via several mechanisms, including the induction of melanin production, deposition of drug products in skin, or postinflammatory changes [**Figure 35-8**]. Hyperpigmentation may be more pronounced in sun-exposed areas, as is seen in reactions caused by amiodarone, chlorpromazine, desipramine, and silver.[37]

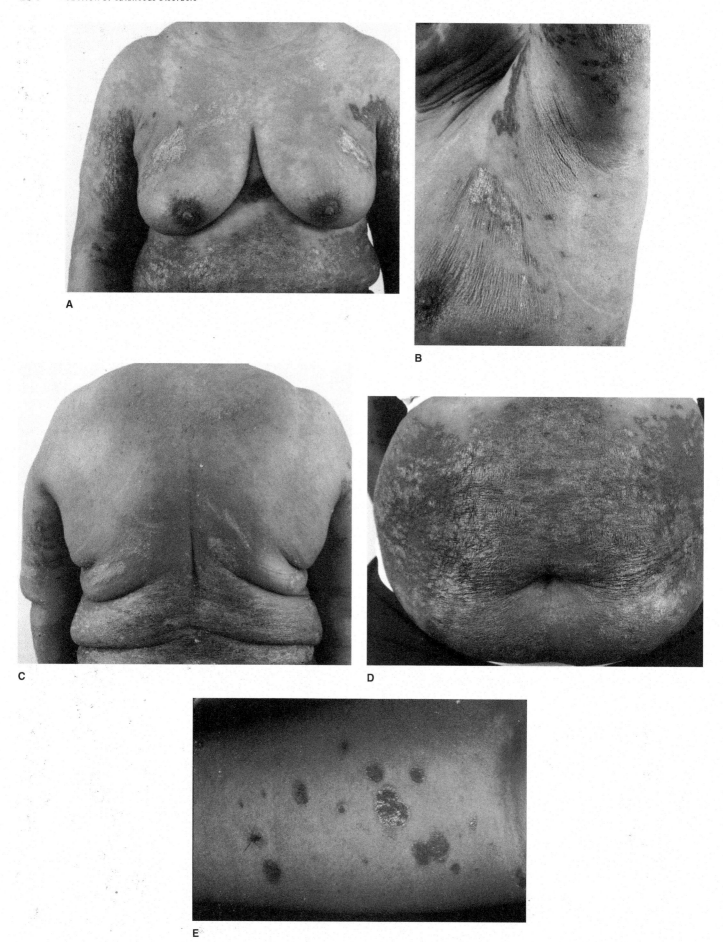

FIGURE 35-6. **(A–E)** Lichenoid drug eruption. (**E:** Used with permission from William D. James, MD.)

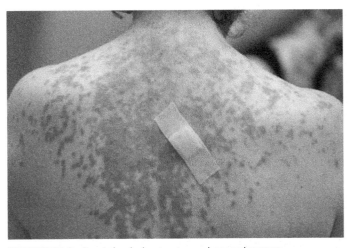

FIGURE 35-7. Drug-induced subacute cutaneous lupus erythematosus.

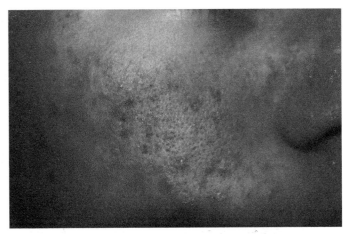

FIGURE 35-9. Minocycline pigmentation within acne scars.

Amiodarone may cause an overall slate gray discoloration, in addition to golden brown pigmentation in sun-exposed areas. Desipramine has been associated with a slate gray pigmentation, and silver may cause blue-black pigmentation in sun-exposed areas. Clofazimine causes violet-brown to blue-gray discoloration in areas of inflammation and diffuse reddish discoloration of the skin and conjunctivae.

Minocycline is a common cause of pigmentary abnormalities that are divided into four types.[38] Type I is characterized by blue-black discolorations in scars or areas of inflammation, including those from acne [**Figure 35-9**]. Type II consists of blue-gray patches on the anterior legs. Diffuse muddy brown discoloration more prominent in sun-exposed areas typifies type III. Type IV consists of circumscribed blue-gray pigmentation concentrated within acne scars on the back.

Topical hydroquinone is a rare cause of pigmentation in the form of exogenous ochronosis. It manifests as gray-brown or blue-black macules in hydroquinone-exposed regions, typically in sun-exposed regions [**Figure 35-10**]. Risk factors include darker skin, lack of sun protection, skin irritation and vigorous friction, and hydroquinone concentrations greater than 3% for a period longer that 6 months, although there have been reports of exogenous ochronosis with the use of 2% concentrations for less than 6 months.[39,40]

Discontinuation of the inciting medication halts the progression in most cases, but discoloration, especially in cases of pigment/metal deposition, may take months or years for complete resolution. In many cases, complete spontaneous resolution will not occur. Treatment with laser therapy may be helpful, but early recognition and discontinuation of the offending medication are critically important.

VASCULITIS

Idiopathic small-vessel vasculitis occurs with greater frequency than drug-induced cases, which account for 10% of all cases. Clinical findings of purpuric papules and plaques, sometimes termed *palpable purpura*, are found mostly on the lower extremities [**Figure 35-11**]. Urticarial lesions, ulcers, nodules, pustules, and hemorrhagic blisters may also be found [**Figure 35-12**]. Extracutaneous findings are occasionally observed including fever, malaise, arthralgia, myalgia, and weight loss. Some research suggests that more severe organ involvement may develop in patients when the causal drug is not withdrawn quickly,[41] but, in general, the clinical course is mild. The kidney is the most commonly involved organ, but rapidly progressive glomerulonephritis is uncommon.[42] Renal findings vary widely and may include hematuria, proteinuria, and elevated serum creatinine.[43] Pulmonary manifestations are rare, with possible intra-alveolar hemorrhage and subsequent cough, dyspnea, and hematoptysis.[44]

Vasculitis usually occurs 7 to 21 days after drug administration. Causative medications include minocycline; allopurinol; hydralazine; anti-tumor necrosis factor-α agents such as adalimumab, etanercept, and infliximab; and antithyroid drugs such as propylthiouracil and methimazole.[45] Antineutrophil cytoplasmic antibody-positive vasculitis

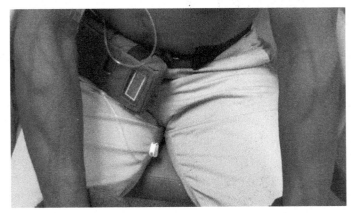

FIGURE 35-8. Supravenous hyperpigmentation secondary to peripheral intravenous fluorouracil treatment. This is thought to be a result of extravasation of the cytotoxic agent, causing epidermal basal hyperpigmentation and dermal melanin incontinence.

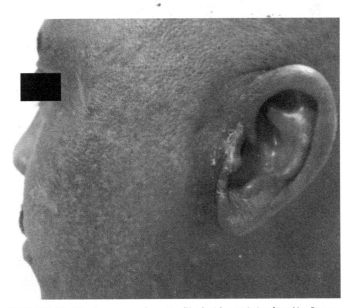

FIGURE 35-10. Exogenous ochronosis. (Used with permission from Lisa Pappas-Taffer, MD.)

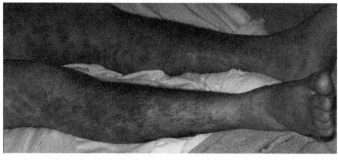

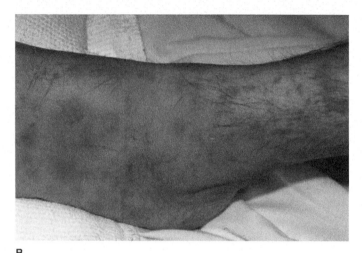

FIGURE 35-11. **(A and B)** Drug-induced leukocytoclastic vasculitis.

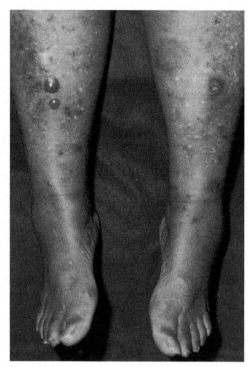

FIGURE 35-12. Bullous leukocytoclastic vasculitis. (Used with permission from William D. James, MD.)

with antimyeloperoxidase antibodies has been associated with several drugs, including propylthiouracil, hydralazine, and minocycline. Treatment includes discontinuation of the offending medication and use of immunosuppressive medications in patients with serious systemic effects.

STEVENS-JOHNSON SYNDROME AND TOXIC EPIDERMAL NECROLYSIS

Stevens-Johnson syndrome (SJS)/toxic epidermal necrolysis (TEN) is considered to be one of the most serious drug-induced skin reactions. This life-threatening, adverse cutaneous drug reaction spectrum is characterized by mucocutaneous necrosis and extensive tenderness, erythema, and skin sloughing. The reaction is caused by a wide range of medications, and early discontinuation of the causative drug is of paramount importance. Medications commonly associated with SJS/TEN include allopurinol, sulfa medications, NSAIDs, barbiturates, carbamazepine, antiretroviral medications, and antiepileptic drugs such as phenytoin and lamotrigine.

SJS/TEN has an incidence of approximately one to seven cases per million people per year.[3,46] Groups thought to be at increased risk include immunocompromised patients especially patients with HIV/acquired immunodeficiency syndrome (AIDS).[47] SJS and TEN most often begin 4 to 28 days after the initiation of the causative agent. Initial symptoms include fever, stinging of eyes, and pain with swallowing that may precede cutaneous symptoms by a few days. Patients then develop erythematous to dusky purpuric, irregularly shaped macules that coalesce to larger patches that start on the trunk and spread to the neck, face, and extremities. Spontaneous epidermal detachment may occur, indicative of the full-thickness epidermal necrosis noted on

histopathology. Epidermal detachment may also be elicited to reveal a positive Nikolsky sign, by exerting tangential pressure on dusky areas of involvement.

Cases are categorized based on the percentage of total body surface area with epidermal detachment: <10% body surface area epidermal detachment in SJS, 10% to 30% in SJS/TEN overlap, and >30% in TEN. Mucosal involvement is nearly ubiquitous, with painful erosions possible on the lip, oral cavity, conjunctiva, nasal cavity, urethra, vagina, gastrointestinal tract, and/or respiratory tract[48] [**Figures 35-13 and 35-14**]. Progression can occur very quickly over the course of a few hours or days with large areas of total body surface involvement.

Mortality rates range from 25% to 50% (average, 25% to 35%) for patients with TEN; the mortality rate is 5% for patients with SJS.[49,50] In patients with TEN, the SCORTEN [**Table 35-4**][51] is a prognostic scoring

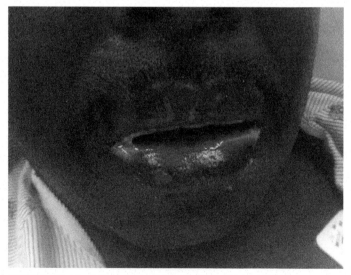

FIGURE 35-13. Oral mucosal involvement in Stevens-Johnson syndrome/toxic epidermal necrolysis. (Used with permission from Lisa Pappas-Taffer, MD.)

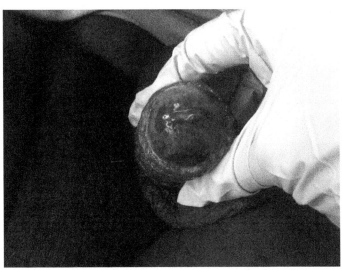

FIGURE 35-14. Genital mucosal involvement in Stevens-Johnson syndrome/toxic epidermal necrolysis. (Used with permission from Lisa Pappas-Taffer, MD.)

TABLE 35-4	SCORTEN: A prognostic scoring system for patients with toxic epidermal necrolysis[51]		
Risk factor		0 Points	1 Point
Age		<40	>40
Associated malignancy		No	Yes
Heart rate (bpm)		<120	>120
Total body surface area involvement on day 1		<10%	>10%
Serum urea level (mg/dL)		<27	>27
Serum bicarbonate level (mEq/L)		<20	<20
Serum glucose level (mg/dL)		<250	>250
Number of risk factors (points)		% Mortality	
0-1		3.2	
2		12.1	
3		35.8	
4		58.3	
≥5		90	

system that can be used to predict outcome. Immediate discontinuation of the causative medication is crucial, and supportive care is a mainstay of treatment. Immunosuppressive therapy with corticosteroids or intravenous Ig is controversial but can be effective in select cases.[52-56]

Healing of areas of involvement begins in a few days after halting of the process, with complete healing in approximately 3 weeks. Sequelae such as symblepharon, entropion, vaginal synechiae, phimosis, scarring, or dyspigmentation may occur. A multidisciplinary approach to patient care is necessary to decrease morbidity, with consultations from appropriate specialties based on areas of involvement.

DRUG REACTIONS IN HIV INFECTION

Patients with HIV comprise a special group of patients at risk for drug eruptions. Immune dysregulation likely plays a role, with cutaneous adverse reactions being one of the most common toxicities associated with antiretroviral medications.[57] In 2009, African Americans accounted for 14% of the U.S. population but composed 44% of all new HIV infections.[58] Latinos accounted for 20% of new HIV infections in the United States while representing only 16% of the U.S. population.[59] When population size is taken into account, in 2005, American Indians and Alaska Natives ranked third in rates of HIV/AIDS diagnosis, after African Americans and Latinos.[60] Given this disproportionate incidence in these populations and the widespread use of antiretroviral treatment, it is important to recognize the range of cutaneous effects that may occur [**Table 35-5**].

TREATMENT

General management of cutaneous drug eruptions includes discontinuation of the causative medication. In many cases, several medications are suspected, and all nonessential medications are therefore discontinued. If the suspected medication is necessary, no other alternative exists, and the reaction is relatively mild, the causative drug may be continued with management of symptoms. For mild eruptions, topical steroids, antihistamines, and emollients are appropriate treatment modalities. More serious eruptions may require immunosuppressive therapy after discontinuation of the inciting agent as well as supportive and wound care. Avoidance of repeat exposure to the causative medication is recommended and is absolutely necessary in more serious reactions.

TABLE 35-5	Common adverse cutaneous reactions of antiretroviral therapy for HIV[60,61]		
Adverse cutaneous effect	Associated medication	Findings	Associated findings/notes
Lipodystrophy syndrome	NRTI (stavudine, didanosine) PI (eg, atazanavir, ritonavir, indinavir) Less commonly NNRTI (efavirenz)	Loss of fat in the face, limbs, and buttocks with accumulation of buffalo hump, abdominal visceral fat, and gynecomastia	Insulin resistance, hyperinsulinemia, hyperglycemia, dyslipidemia
Nail and mucocutaneous hyperpigmentation	Zidovudine	Longitudinal brown or blue bands or diffuse brown or blue discoloration	Darker-skinned patients have more intense hyperpigmentation
Hypersensitivity syndrome	Abacavir, nevirapine	Morbilliform eruption; occasional urticarial, erythema multiforme-like lesions	Requires 2 of 5 symptoms: fever, rash, GI disturbances, constitutional symptoms, respiratory symptoms; associated with certain HLA subtypes (see Table 35-3)
Retinoid-like effects	Indinavir	Alopecia, cheilitis, xerosis, paronychia	
Stevens-Johnson syndrome/toxic epidermal necrolysis	NNRTI (eg, nevirapine, efavirenz, etravirine)	Widespread epidermal necrosis with mucocutaneous findings	Associated with certain HLA subtypes (see Table 35-3)
Morbilliform eruptions	Has been described with many antiretroviral medications, particularly nevirapine	Erythematous papules and patches on face, trunk, extremities	

Abbreviations: HIV, human immunodeficiency virus; HLA, human leukocyte antigen; NNRTI, nonnucleotide reverse transcriptase inhibitors; NRTI, nucleotide reverse transcriptase inhibitors; PI, protease inhibitors;

REFERENCES

1. Bigby M, Jick S, Jick H, Arndt K. Drug-induced cutaneous reactions. A report from the Boston Collaborative Drug Surveillance Program on 15,438 consecutive inpatients, 1975 to 1982. *JAMA.* 1986;256:3358-3363.
2. Bigby M. Rates of cutaneous reactions to drugs. *Arch Dermatol.* 2001;137: 765-770.
3. Roujeau JC, Stern RS. Severe adverse cutaneous reactions to drugs. *N Engl J Med.* 1994;331:1272-1285.
4. Hughes AR, Mosteller M, Bansal AT, et al. Association of genetic variations in HLA-B region with hypersensitivity to abacavir in some, but not all, populations. *Pharmacogenomics.* 2004;5:203-211.
5. Sun HY, Hung CC, Lin PH, et al. Incidence of abacavir hypersensitivity and its relationship with HLA-B*5701 in HIV-infected patients in Taiwan. *J Antimicrob Chemother.* 2007;60:599-604.
6. Saag M, Balu R, Phillips E, et al. High sensitivity of human leukocyte antigen-b*5701 as a marker for immunologically confirmed abacavir hypersensitivity in white and black patients. *Clin Infect Dis.* 2008;46:1111-1118.
7. Zucman D, Truchis P, Majerholc C, Stegman S, Caillat-Zucman S. Prospective screening for human leukocyte antigen-B*5701 avoids abacavir hypersensitivity reaction in the ethnically mixed French HIV population. *J Acquir Immune Defic Syndr.* 2007;45:1-3.
8. Sadiq ST, Pakianathan M. Uncertainties of routine HLA B*5701 testing in black African HIV cohorts in the UK. *Sex Transm Infect.* 2007;83:181-182.
9. Aihara M. Pharmacogenetics of cutaneous adverse drug reactions. *J Dermatol.* 2011;38:246-254.
10. Stubb S, Heikkila H, Kauppinen K. Cutaneous reactions to drugs: a series of in-patients during a five-year period. *Acta Derm Venereol.* 1994;74: 289-291.
11. Kauppinen K, Stubb S. Drug eruptions: causative agents and clinical types. A series of in-patients during a 10-year period. *Acta Derm Venereol.* 1984;64:320-324.
12. Crowson AN, Brown TJ, Magro CM. Progress in the understanding of the pathology and pathogenesis of cutaneous drug eruptions: implications for management. *Am J Clin Dermatol.* 2003;4:407-428.
13. Breathnach SM, Hintner H. *Adverse Drug Reactions and the Skin.* Oxford, United Kingdom: Blackwell Scientific Publications; 1992.
14. Tohyama M, Hashimoto K, Yasukawa M, et al. Association of human herpesvirus 6 reactivation with the flaring and severity of drug-induced hypersensitivity syndrome. *Br J Dermatol.* 2007;157:934-940.
15. Roujeau JC, Bioulac-Sage P, Bourseau C, et al. Acute generalized exanthematous pustulosis. Analysis of 63 cases. *Arch Dermatol.* 1991;127:1333-1338.
16. Hedner T, Samuelsson O, Lunde H, Lindholm L, Andren L, Wiholm BE. Angio-oedema in relation to treatment with angiotensin converting enzyme inhibitors. *BMJ.* 1992;304:941-946.
17. Brown NJ, Ray WA, Snowden M, Griffin MR. Black Americans have an increased rate of angiotensin converting enzyme inhibitor-associated angioedema. *Clin Pharmacol Ther.* 1996;60:8-13.
18. Fortuna G, Salas-Alanis JC, Guidetti E, Marinkovich MP. A critical reappraisal of the current data on drug-induced linear immunoglobulin A bullous dermatosis: a real and separate nosological entity? *J Am Acad Dermatol.* 2012;66:988-994.
19. Polat M, Lenk N, Kurekci E, Oztas P, Artuz F, Alli N. Chronic bullous disease of childhood in a patient with acute lymphoblastic leukemia: possible induction by a drug. *Am J Clin Dermatol.* 2007;8:389-391.
20. Vassileva S. Drug-induced pemphigoid: bullous and cicatricial. *Clin Dermatol.* 1998;16:379-387.
21. Troy JL, Silvers DN, Grossman ME, Jaffe IA. Penicillamine-associated pemphigus: is it really pemphigus? *J Am Acad Dermatol.* 1981;4:547-555.
22. Velthuis PJ, Hendrikse JC, Nefkens JJ. Combined features of pemphigus and pemphigoid induced by penicillamine. *Br J Dermatol.* 1985;112:615-619.
23. Rasmussen HB, Jepsen L V, Brandrup F. Penicillamine-induced bullous pemphigoid with pemphigus-like antibodies. *J Cutan Pathol.* 1989;16:154-157.
24. Ruocco V, Sacerdoti G. Pemphigus and bullous pemphigoid due to drugs. *Int J Dermatol.* 1991;30:307-312.
25. Brenner S, Bialy-Golan A, Ruocco V. Drug-induced pemphigus. *Clin Dermatol.* 1998;16:393-397.
26. Wolf R, Tamir A, Brenner S. Drug-induced versus drug-triggered pemphigus. *Dermatologica.* 1991;182:207-210.
27. Brenner S, Wolf R, Ruocco V. Drug-induced pemphigus. I. A survey. *Clin Dermatol.* 1993;11:501-505.
28. Sontheimer RD, Maddison PJ, Reichlin M, Jordon RE, Stastny P, Gilliam JN. Serologic and HLA associations in subacute cutaneous lupus erythematosus, a clinical subset of lupus erythematosus. *Ann Intern Med.* 1982;97:664-671.
29. Lowe G, Henderson CL, Grau RH, Hansen CB, Sontheimer RD. A systematic review of drug-induced subacute cutaneous lupus erythematosus. *Br J Dermatol.* 2011;164:465-472.
30. Reed BR, Huff JC, Jones SK, Orton PW, Lee LA, Norris DA. Subacute cutaneous lupus erythematosus associated with hydrochlorothiazide therapy. *Ann Intern Med.* 1985;103:49-51.
31. Brown CW Jr, Deng JS. Thiazide diuretics induce cutaneous lupus-like adverse reaction. *J Toxicol Clin Toxicol.* 1995;33:729-733.
32. Darken M, McBurney EI. Subacute cutaneous lupus erythematosus-like drug eruption due to combination diuretic hydrochlorothiazide and triamterene. *J Am Acad Dermatol.* 1988;18:38-42.
33. Lorentz K, Booken N, Goerdt S, Goebeler M. Subacute cutaneous lupus erythematosus induced by terbinafine: case report and review of literature. *J Dtsch Derm Ges.* 2008;6:823-827.
34. Kasperkiewicz M, Anemuller W, Angelova-Fischer I, Rose C, Zillikens D, Fischer TW. Subacute cutaneous lupus erythematosus associated with terbinafine. *Clin Exp Dermatol.* 2009;34:e403-e404.
35. Santoro FA, Lim HW. Update on photodermatoses. *Semin Cutan Med Surg.* 2011;30:229-238.
36. Cowen EW, Nguyen JC, Miller DD, et al. Chronic phototoxicity and aggressive squamous cell carcinoma of the skin in children and adults during treatment with voriconazole. *J Am Acad Dermatol.* 2010;62:31-37.
37. Gould JW, Mercurio MG, Elmets CA. Cutaneous photosensitivity diseases induced by exogenous agents. *J Am Acad Dermatol.* 1995;33:551-556.
38. Mouton RW, Jordaan HF, Schneider JW. A new type of minocycline-induced cutaneous hyperpigmentation. *Clin Exp Dermatol.* 2004;29:8-14.
39. Charlin R, Barcaui CB, Kac BK, Soares DB, Rabello-Fonseca R, Azulay-Abulafia L. Hydroquinone-induced exogenous ochronosis: a report of four cases and usefulness of dermoscopy. *Int J Dermatol.* 2008;47:19-23.
40. Bongiorno MR, Arico M. Exogenous ochronosis and striae atrophicae following the use of bleaching creams. *Int J Dermatol.* 2005;44:112-115.
41. Morita S, Ueda Y, Eguchi K. Anti-thyroid drug-induced ANCA-associated vasculitis: a case report and review of the literature. *Endocr J.* 2000;47:467-470.
42. Dobre M, Wish J, Negrea L. Hydralazine-induced ANCA-positive pauci-immune glomerulonephritis: a case report and literature review. *Renal Fail.* 2009;31:745-748.
43. John R, Herzenberg AM. Renal toxicity of therapeutic drugs. *J Clin Pathol.* 2009;62:505-515.
44. Yamauchi K, Sata M, Machiya J, et al. Antineutrophil cytoplasmic antibody positive alveolar haemorrhage during propylthiouracil therapy for hyperthyroidism. *Respirology.* 2003;8:532-535.
45. Radic M, Kaliterna DM, Radic J. Drug-induced vasculitis: a clinical and pathological review. *Neth J Med.* 2012;70:12-17.
46. Letko E, Papaliodis DN, Papaliodis GN, Daoud YJ, Ahmed AR, Foster CS. Stevens-Johnson syndrome and toxic epidermal necrolysis: a review of the literature. *Ann Allerg Asthma Immunol.* 2005;94:418-436.
47. Chan HL. Observations on drug-induced toxic epidermal necrolysis in Singapore. *J Am Acad Dermatol.* 1984;10:973-978.
48. Hazin R, Ibrahimi OA, Hazin MI, Kimyai-Asadi A. Stevens-Johnson syndrome: pathogenesis, diagnosis, and management. *Ann Med.* 2008;40:129-138.
49. Roujeau JC, Guillaume JC, Fabre JP, Penso D, Flechet ML, Girre JP. Toxic epidermal necrolysis (Lyell syndrome). Incidence and drug etiology in France, 1981-1985. *Arch Dermatol.* 1990;126:37-42.
50. Revuz J, Penso D, Roujeau JC, et al. Toxic epidermal necrolysis. Clinical findings and prognosis factors in 87 patients. *Arch Dermatol.* 1987;123:1160-1165.
51. Bastuji-Garin S, Fouchard N, Bertocchi M, Roujeau JC, Revuz J, Wolkenstein P. SCORTEN: a severity-of-illness score for toxic epidermal necrolysis. *J Invest Dermatol.* 2000;115:149-153.
52. Tripathi A, Ditto AM, Grammer LC, et al. Corticosteroid therapy in an additional 13 cases of Stevens-Johnson syndrome: a total series of 67 cases. *Allerg Asthma Proc.* 2000;21:101-105.
53. Schneck J, Fagot JP, Sekula P, Sassolas B, Roujeau JC, Mockenhaupt M. Effects of treatments on the mortality of Stevens-Johnson syndrome and toxic epidermal necrolysis: a retrospective study on patients included in the prospective EuroSCAR Study. *J Am Acad Dermatol.* 2008;58:33-40.
54. Prins C, Kerdel FA, Padilla RS, et al. Treatment of toxic epidermal necrolysis with high-dose intravenous immunoglobulins: multicenter retrospective analysis of 48 consecutive cases. *Arch Dermatol.* 2003;139:26-32.
55. Mittmann N, Chan B, Knowles S, Cosentino L, Shear N. Intravenous immunoglobulin use in patients with toxic epidermal necrolysis and Stevens-Johnson syndrome. *Am J Clin Dermatol.* 2006;7:359-368.
56. Shortt R, Gomez M, Mittman N, Cartotto R. Intravenous immunoglobulin does not improve outcome in toxic epidermal necrolysis. *J Burn Care Rehabil.* 2004;25:246-255.

57. Carr A, Cooper DA. Adverse effects of antiretroviral therapy. *Lancet.* 2000;356:1423-1430.

58. Centers for Disease Control and Prevention. HIV among African Americans. http://www.cdc.gov/hiv/topics/aa/index.htm. Accessed January 1, 2013.

59. Centers for Disease Control and Prevention. HIV among Hispanics and Latinos. http://www.cdc.gov/hiv/latinos/index.htm. Accessed January 1, 2013.

59. Centers for Disease Control and Prevention. HIV/AIDS among American Indians and Alaska Natives. http://www.cdc.gov/hiv/resources/factsheets/aian.htm. Accessed January 1, 2013.

60. Introcaso CE, Hines JM, Kovarik CL. Cutaneous toxicities of antiretroviral therapy for HIV: part II. Nonnucleoside reverse transcriptase inhibitors, entry and fusion inhibitors, integrase inhibitors, and immune reconstitution syndrome. *J Am Acad Dermatol.* 2010;63:563-570.

61. Introcaso CE, Hines JM, Kovarik CL. Cutaneous toxicities of antiretroviral therapy for HIV: part I. Lipodystrophy syndrome, nucleoside reverse transcriptase inhibitors, and protease inhibitors. *J Am Acad Dermatol.* 2010;63:542-549.

CHAPTER 36

Tattoo, Body Piercing, and Scarification

Jennifer David
Susan C. Taylor

KEY POINTS

- Tattoos, piercings, and scarifications are forms of body modification that date back thousands of years.

- Trends in tattooing have shifted from abstract images obtained for religious and ceremonial purposes, to the depiction of literal images that are often the result of a random, impulsive act.

- It is estimated that 13% of the American population has at least one tattoo and 35% have piercings.

- In the United States, tattoo pigments are classified as cosmetics and are approved only for topical use under the Food, Drug, and Cosmetic Act of 1938; these pigments are not for intradermal injection.

- Common reactions to both tattoos and piercings include infection (viral and bacterial), hypersensitivity reactions, localization of various dermatoses, and scarring.

TATTOOS AND SCARIFICATION

BACKGROUND

For centuries, humans have adorned themselves with various forms of body art. Practices such as tattooing, scarification, branding, piercing, and body painting are performed to express individualism, mark rites of passage, substantiate group membership, and serve as ritualistic symbols [**Figure 36-1**].

The term tattoo comes from the Tahitian word *tatau* meaning "to mark."[1,2] Tattooing is a form of body modification that typically uses needles to inject pigment into the dermal layer of the skin. However, there are various types of tattoos ranging from temporary henna tattoos and body painting to the permanent decorative and makeup tattoos using the dermal injection of pigment.

Numerous tombs have been unearthed revealing mummies with intact tattoos and, interestingly, pictures on the walls of the tomb that depict humans with tattoos. Ancient tattoos such as Egyptian, Aboriginal, and Japanese, are generally abstract and primarily composed of geometric shapes, dots, and lines that have personal or nonfigurative meanings. Māori culture in New Zealand traditionally attributes spiritual and cultural significance to certain words, images, and patterns, as all cultures do. *Ta moko*, traditional Māori tattooing, often on the face, is a *taonga* (treasure) to Māori for which the purpose and applications

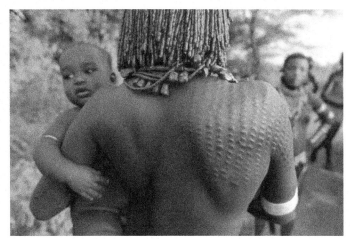

FIGURE 36-1. Scarification on an Ethiopian woman. (Used with permission from Jodi Cobb/National Geographic Creative.)

are sacred [**Figure 36-2**]. Every *moko* contains ancestral/tribal messages specific to the wearer. These messages tell the story of the wearer's family and tribal affiliations and the wearer's place in these social structures. A *moko's* message would also contain the wearer's 'value' by way of their genealogy and their knowledge and standing in their social level. *Ta moko* as an art form declined during the twentieth century; however, recently it has been revived as an important art form among Māori that is worn as an expression of cultural pride and integrity.[3] This is in contrast to modern Western tattooing practices that tend to use literal images such as flowers, butterflies, and trademarked animated characters.[4,5] Many attribute this shift in representation as a reflection of the current Western society's focus on consumerism.[4-6]

Body painting is the application of paint onto the skin with special pens, yielding a temporary tattoo. Although the paint is applied topically to the skin, the pigments in the paint penetrate the superficial layers of the stratum corneum resulting in a tattoo that persists for 1 or 2 days and then easily washes off.[6] Henna (mehndi) is a form of body painting that has been used around the world for more than 3000 years.[5] Leaves from the henna bush (*Lawsonia inermis*) are ground and formed into a

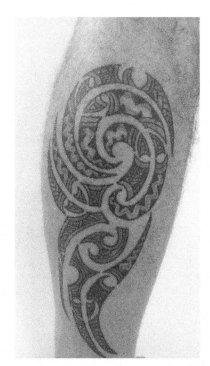

FIGURE 36-2. *Ta moko,* traditional Māori tattooing, on the calf of a man. (Used with permission from Nassir Masoud.)

paste that is painted on the skin. After setting for a few hours, the henna penetrates into the superficial epidermal layer.[6] Henna tattoos typically last for about 3 weeks.

EPIDEMIOLOGY

Tattoos are very popular today, with an estimated 13% of the American population and 3% to 5% of the remainder of Western society having at least one tattoo. Recent studies show that people with skin of color, including Hispanics, comprise the majority of the tattooed population in the United States.[7-9]

Laumann and Derick[7] conducted a prevalence study in 2006 where random digit dialing technology was used to obtain a national probability sample of 500 subjects (253 women and 247 men) ranging in age from 18 to 50 years. The demographics of the respondents were 79% Caucasian, 12% African American, and 9% Hispanic; of these, 24% had tattoos. Among each group, 28% of African Americans, 38% of Hispanics, 36% of the individuals who identified themselves as "other," and 22% of Caucasians had at least one tattoo.[7] Of the tattooed respondents, 98% had acquired their tattoos within the United States, with the majority of those having been obtained in a tattoo shop or studio. A total of 32 tattooed respondents (26%) had either tattooed themselves or had someone else perform the tattooing in a location other than a studio.[7]

As tattoos have become more mainstream, the age at which individuals obtain them has decreased. A cross-sectional study sampled high school students (n = 2101) from eight states and questioned them regarding their interest in tattooing[10]. The age of the participants ranged from 14 to 18 years. Of those, 10% had tattoos and 55% expressed an interest in tattooing. The tattoos were commonly performed in the ninth grade, but there were reports of children as young as 8 years old receiving tattoos. More than half of the subjects were female. Permanent markings and bloodborne diseases were reasons respondents gave for refraining from tattooing, yet 55% (n = 1159) expressed an interest in tattooing.[10] Given the permanent nature of tattoos, it is important for adolescents to be educated on the long-term implications of their decision to obtain one.

TATTOO PIGMENT

In the United States, ink pigments are classified as cosmetics and are approved only for topical use under the Food, Drug, and Cosmetic Act of 1938, and not for intradermal injection.[11-13] Tattoo pigments are composed of inorganic and organic pigments [**Table 36-1**]. The pigment is inoculated into the dermal layer permanently and is encapsulated in the fibrous tissue, thus becoming less reactive histologically.[6] However, occasional immunologic reactions occur if sensitivity to a component of the pigment is present. Even when purchased through a manufacturer, the composition of tattoo ink is highly variable and frequently unsterile, leading to an increased risk of allergic reactions and/or infections.

TABLE 36-1	Tattoo pigments
Black	India ink, carbon, iron oxide, logwood extract, magnetite (sensitizing additive agent dibutyl phthalate and cytotoxic agent 9-fluorenone)
Red	Mercury sulfide (cinnabar), cadmium selenide (cadmium red), sienna (red ochre, ferric hydrate, and ferric sulfate), azo dyes, hematite
Yellow	Cadmium sulfide (cadmium yellow), ochre, curcumin yellow, azo dyes, limonite, anthraquinone
Green	Chromium oxide (casalis green), hydrated chromium sesquioxide (guignet green), malachite green, lead chromate, ferric ferrocyanide, curcumin green, phthalocyanine dyes (copper salts with yellow coal tar dyes)
Blue	Cobalt aluminate (azure blue), phthalocyanine, ferric ferrocyanide, indigoid
Violet	Manganese violet, indigoid
White	Titanium dioxide, zinc oxide, corundum

TABLE 36-2	Adverse effects of tattooing[14,15,17-19]
Allergic contact dermatitis
Photoallergic dermatitis
Granulomatous and lichenoid skin changes
Pseudolymphomatous skin changes
Bacterial infections: impetigo, erysipelas, tuberculosis cutis, atypical mycobacterium, syphilis, leprosy, furunculosis
Viral infections: warts, molluscum contagiosum, herpes simplex, herpes zoster, rubella, viral hepatitis, and human immunodeficiency virus

ADVERSE REACTIONS

There is a direct correlation between the increased popularity of tattoos and the increased incidence of adverse events.[13] Common reactions to permanent tattoos include infection (viral and bacterial), hypersensitivity reactions, localization of various dermatoses, and benign or malignant tumors [**Table 36-2** and **Figure 36-3**].

Hypersensitivity reactions have been documented for the most commonly used tattoo pigments such as dichromate (green), cobalt (blue), cadmium (yellow), and mercury salt (red) based pigments.[14] Certain pigments are associated with specific reactions. For example, mercury sulfide (cinnabar) is classically associated with granulomatous, lichenoid, and pseudolymphomatous reactions. However, it is imperative to rule out sarcoidosis when granulomatous lesions appear in a tattoo. Cadmium sulfide (cadmium yellow) is known for causing phototoxic reactions, whereas chromium oxide (casalis green) causes an eczematous rash.[13,14] Topical steroids are a good first-line agent for treating allergic reactions; however, if the rash is unresponsive or worsens, biopsy and further workup should be performed.

Infections are usually transmitted during unsanitary tattoo procedures or via contaminated inks. Transmission of bloodborne or dermatologic pathogens is possible if the tattoo needle is not sterilized or the skin surface is improperly cleansed.[11,13-15] There has been a recent increase in the incidence of tattoo-related *Mycobacterium chelonae* infections, and in 2012, the Centers for Disease Control and Prevention (CDC) conducted a full investigation after numerous reports of *M. chelonae*-infected tattoos were reported across the United States[16].

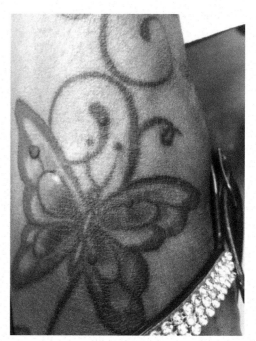

FIGURE 36-3. An African American woman presented with verrucous papules 3 weeks after obtaining a tattoo. Biopsy confirmed the diagnosis of verrucous vulgaris, and the patterns of lesions suggests inoculation from contaminated black ink.

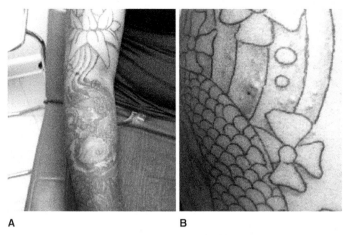

FIGURE 36-4. (A) and (B) An African American female presented with scattered pink and violaceous papules 2 weeks after obtaining a new tattoo. Biopsy and culture results confirmed the rash to be a *Mycobacterium chelonae* infection.

M. chelonae is a nontuberculosis, rapidly growing (Runyon group IV) *mycobacterium* found in municipal tap water, soil, plant material, and aerosols. Direct inoculation of *M. chelonae* into tattoos is typically secondary to contaminated diluted ink. Patients will typically present with persistent inflammation or pink, red, or violaceous papules and/ or plaques 1 to 2 weeks after receiving a tattoo. The CDC investigation concluded that the infections were associated with use of the same nationally distributed, prediluted gray ink[16]. Once cultures confirm an *M. chelonae* infection, patients should be started on antibiotic therapy with clarithromycin [**Figure 36-4**].[17]

Henna tattoos, when performed using natural pigment from the henna bush, do not typically cause allergic reactions. The color spectrum of the natural extract ranges from dark red to brown. To produce black shades, additional pigments must be added, with the most common additive being *p*-phenylenediamine (PPD), a common allergen.[6] Reported reactions to black henna tattoos containing PPD include keloids, persistent leukoderma, severe bullous contact dermatitis, and lichenoid reactions.[18]

REMOVAL

Most people acquire tattoos at a young age and often during adulthood want them removed for personal, occupational, or social reasons [**Figure 36-5**].[13,15] Depending on the size and location of the tattoo, removal via surgical excision is an effective method. However, in most cases, this is not a realistic option if the area is large or an individual is prone to keloidal scarring. Mechanical abrasion, cryosurgery, and the application of caustic chemicals are additional methods for tattoo removal. Historically, these methods have been effective in removing tattoo pigments from the skin but can also lead to substantial inflammation and subsequent scarring. Over the past few decades, the advancement of laser technology has accelerated the success rate of permanent tattoo removal. Early tattoo removal lasers, the normal-mode ruby (694 nm), argon (488 to 514 nm), or carbon dioxide (10,600 nm) lasers, were effective at targeting and ablating tattoo pigment. However, they also caused significant thermal damage to surrounding tissue and subsequent scarring. Currently, the nanosecond Q-switched ruby, Q-switched neodymium-doped yttrium aluminium garnet (Nd:YAG, 1064 and 532 nm), Q-switched alexandrite (755 nm), and flash lamp pulsed dye laser (510 nm) are effective in lightening a variety of ink colors with minimal thermal damage to surrounding tissue. Because melanin is a competing chromophore, when selecting a laser treatment and treating tattoos with Q-switched lasers, a patient's skin color must be taken into consideration. Patients with darker skin tones are best treated with the Nd:YAG laser because the longer wavelength affords better relative sparing of the epidermis, thus causing less hyperpigmentation and scarring.

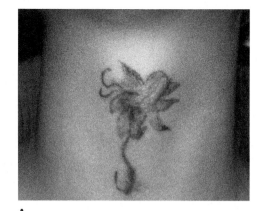

A

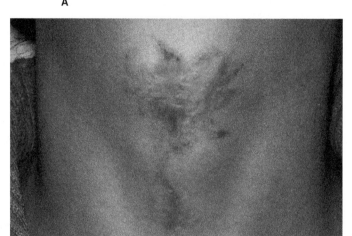

B

FIGURE 36-5. (A) Tattoo on the neck of an Asian male before laser treatment. **(B)** Results of tattoo removal after three Q-switched alexandrite laser therapy sessions. (Used with permission from Dr. Zhong Lu, Dermatology Department, Huashan Hospital, Fudan University, Shanghai, China.)

When treating patients with skin of color with the ruby or alexandrite lasers, lowering the fluence helps minimize thermal damage. Clearance of tattoos may require anywhere from 5 to 12 treatments, spaced 6 to 8 weeks apart.[13,19]

SCARIFICATION AND BRANDING

BACKGROUND

Scarification (also referred to as cicatrization) is a form of body modification that involves burning, scratching, etching, or superficially cutting designs, pictures, or words into the skin. Irritants may be rubbed to produce a permanent raised scar.[5,7] It is a common practice in certain regions of Africa where scarification patterns identify a person as belonging to a particular tribe or ethnic group.[7]

Branding is a specific type of scarification process that involves burning the skin with heat, lasers, or an electrocautery device to imprint a specific pattern onto the skin. Strike branding uses heated metal, whereas cold branding involves the use of metal immersed in liquid nitrogen.[7] In the United States, strike branding is a common practice among certain African American college fraternities where it is a part of their initiation rituals. A hot iron in the shape of a fraternity's Greek insignia is imprinted onto the member's skin, serving as a symbol of life-long loyalty and membership.

EPIDEMIOLOGY

Although less common in the United States, scarification is still common in West Africa. In 2010, questionnaires were administered to 143 adult

Nigerians to study the practice and complications of scarification in their country.[20] Respondents included 44 males (30.8%) and 99 females (69.2%) with a mean age of 21.4 years. The majority (n = 104; 72.7%) of the respondents had a tertiary education, whereas only six (4.2%) had no formal education at all. Of that total, 117 of the respondents (81.8%) knew about scarification and 73 (51.0%) had had scarification at one time or another. Consent was given by only 20 (14.0%) before they were given scarifications. Scarifications were performed by native/traditional doctors in 23 respondents (16.1%), whereas 25 (17.5%) were performed by the subjects' fathers, 12 (8.4%) by mothers, and 9 (6.3%) by uncles.[20]

A razor blade was the most commonly used instrument for scarification in 60 of the respondents (42.0%), whereas a knife was used in 13 (9.1%).[20] In the respondents, 33 scarifications (23.1%) were administered with a single-use instrument, whereas 30 (21.0%) were performed using an instrument shared with 2 or more individuals. Religion and education did not appear to affect scarification practices. The reasons given for scarifications included protection from evil in 30 (41.1%), treatment for febrile convulsion in 6 (8.2%), and treatment for epilepsy in 3 (4.1%).[19]

Although branding and scarification are practiced among certain subcultures within the United States, there is a lack of statistical data available to reveal its prevalence.

ADVERSE REACTIONS

Scarification and branding carry the risk of developing local and systemic infections. Depending on the method used (such as rubbing of caustic chemicals), allergic reactions are possible. Hypertrophic scaring and keloid formation are the most common adverse reactions, and this practice should be avoided in individuals with known history of keloid formation.[6]

BODY PIERCING

BACKGROUND

Body piercing is another ancient form of body modification. It involves puncturing or cutting the skin to create an opening for implanting jewelry. It has been practiced in almost every society and is commonly associated with ritual ceremonies and religious rites of passage.[6,7] Mummified bodies with pierced ears have been discovered, including the oldest mummified body discovered to date, the 5300-year-old Otzi, the Iceman, discovered in a glacier in Austria. Otzi was also found to have multiple tattoos.[9] Interestingly, at the same time that piercings can be culturally binding, they may also be a means of rebellion, particularly for adolescents in Western cultures.[6,7] The soft area of the earlobes, the mouth, and the nose are some of the most common sites for piercings.[7]

EPIDEMIOLOGY

The aforementioned 2006 study by Laumann and Derick also found that in the 18- to 50-year-old age group, 35% of respondents reported having had piercings[7]. Of those with piercings, 19% of men and 49% of women had soft earlobe piercings and 8% of men and 21% of women had piercings in other parts of the body. Most body piercings were performed in a professional parlor or shop, although 14 people had done at least one on themselves, and another nine respondents had had someone else do a body piercing somewhere other than in a professional studio.[7]

ADVERSE REACTIONS

The risk of infection secondary to piercing depends on the hygiene regimens in place, experience of the practitioner, and the customer's aftercare. Local infections caused by *Staphylococcus aureus* or group A streptococci are common and require removal of the piercing in addition to antibiotic therapy.[6,21] Allergic reaction to nickel sulfate-containing jewelry is very common and can elicit eczematous reactions and even granulomatous lesions.[6,21] Other complications that are more prevalent in the skin of color population are hypertrophic scars and keloids [**Figure 36-6**]. Keloids are predominantly seen after earlobe piercing but may occur at any pierced site on the body (see Chapter 33, Keloids).

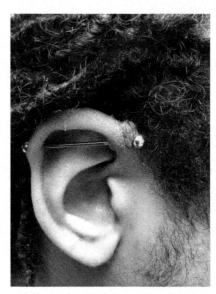

FIGURE 36-6. African American male patient with a keloid on the inner and outer surface of the ear helix. The keloid was first noticed 2 months after obtaining the industrial-style ear piercing.

REFERENCES

1. Sanders CR. *Customizing the Body: The Art and Culture of Tattooing.* Philadelphia, PA: Temple University Press; 1989.
2. Caplan J, ed. *Written on the Body: The Tattoo in European and American History.* Princeton, NJ: Princeton University Press; 2000.
3. Best E. The Uhi-Maori, or native tattooing instruments. *J Polynesian Soc.* 1904;13:166-172.
4. Johnson FJ. Tattooing: mind, body and spirit. The inner essence of the art. *Sociol View.* 2007;23:45-61.
5. Bell S. Tattooed: a participant observer's exploration of meaning. *J Am Cult.* 1999;22;53-58.
6. Kaatz M, Elsner P, Bauer A. Body-modifying concepts and dermatologic problems: tattooing and piercing. *Clin Derm.* 2008;23:2635-2644.
7. Laumann AE, Derick AJ. Tattoos and body piercings in the United States: a national data set. *J Am Acad Dermatol.* 2006;55:413-421.
8. Braverman PK. Body art: piercing, tattooing, and scarification. *Adolesc Med Clin.* 2006;17:505-519.
9. Brown KM, Perlmutter P, McDermott RJ. Youth and tattoos: what school health personnel should know. *J Sch Health.* 2000;70:355-360.
10. Armstrong ML, Murphy KP. Tattooing: another adolescent risk behavior warranting health education. *Appl Nurs Res.* 1997;10:181-189.
11. Carlson VP, Lehman EJ, Armstrong M. Tattooing regulations in U.S. states, 2011. *J Environ Health.* 2012;75:30-37.
12. U.S. Food and Drug Administration. Tattoos and permanent makeup. http://www.fda.gov/Cosmetics/ProductsIngredients/Products/ucm108530.htm. Accessed December 6, 2012.
13. Mayers LB, Judelson DA, Moriarty BW, et al. Prevalence of body art (body piercing and tattooing) in university undergraduates and incidence of medical complications. *Mayo Clin Proc.* 2002;77:29-34.
14. Jacob CI. Tattoo-associated dermatoses: a case report and review of the literature. *Dermatol Surg.* 2002;28:962-965.
15. Kluger N. Cutaneous complications related to permanent decorative tattooing. *Exp Rev Clin Immunol.* 2010;6:363-371.
16. Centers for Disease Control and Prevention (CDC). Tattoo-associated nontuberculous mycobacterial skin infections—multiple States, 2011–2012. *MMWR Morb Mortal Wkly Rep.* 2012; 61: 653-656.
17. Drage LA, Ecker PM, Orenstein R, et al. An outbreak of *Mycobacterium chelonae* infection in tattoos. *J Am Acad Dermatol.* 2010;62:501-506.
18. Gunasti S, Aksungur V. Severe inflammatory and keloidal, allergic reaction due to para-phenylenediamine in temporary tattoos. *Indian J Dermatol Venereol Leprol.* 2010;76:165-167.
19. Bernstien E. Laser treatments of tattoos. *Clin Dermatol.* 2006;24:43-55.
20. Babatunde OP, Oyeronke AE. Scarification practice and scar complications among the Nigerian Yorubas. *Indian J Dermatol Venereol Leprol.* 2010;76:571-572.
21. Hesse RW Jr. *Jewelry Making Through History: An Encyclopedia (Handicrafts Through World History).* Westport, CT: Greenwood Publishing Group; 2007:71.

CHAPTER 37

Hair Care Practices: Complications, Treatments, and Prevention

Chemene R. Quinn
Mobolaji Opeola

KEY POINTS

- African hair is five times more difficult to comb, is more fragile, and has a lower stress requirement for breaking than Caucasian or Asian hair.
- It is estimated that 80% of African American women use chemical relaxers and/or thermal instruments to straighten their hair. The type and extent of use will vary based on intraracial curl pattern differences.
- Specialized grooming products and procedures are needed to ensure that African hair maintains its cosmetic value.
- There are no biochemical differences among African, Caucasian, and Asian hair types.
- In men and women with African hair, many scalp dermatoses and alopecias are associated with hair care practices.
- Dermatologists should be knowledgeable about the various styling methods and cultural attitudes of patients with textured hair to avoid recommending treatments that may cause further damage.

Hair care in patients with skin of color can prove to be perplexing to even the most seasoned dermatologist. The variations in hair textures, grooming practices, cultural identity, and even terminology can be overwhelming during a limited office visit.

Human hair is categorized into three groups: African, Asian, and Caucasian. There are no biochemical differences among African, Asian, and Caucasian hair types.[1,2] Many women and men with African hair spend a great deal of time and money grooming their hair; some visit hair salons as often as once or twice weekly. Hair care is a multi-billion dollar industry.[3,4]

This chapter will outline and discuss hair care practices, with a focus on the patient of African ancestry. A summation of practical hair care guidelines for clinical reference is provided in **Table 37-1**.

PHENOTYPE OF AFRICAN HAIR

Because the hair phenotype varies from tightly coiled in sub-Saharan Africa to very straight in northern areas, individuals whose ancestors hailed from the African continent now form a mosaic of other racial groups.[5,6] The degree of curl in 'virgin' (untreated) African hair varies tremendously, from almost none at all to tightly coiled hair through which a comb cannot be drawn [**Figure 37-1**].[7] Porter et al have shown that as hair becomes curlier in appearance, it has a lower curve diameter, extends less when strained, and is more susceptible to breakage.[8] These findings suggest that the mechanical fragility of hair increases with higher degrees of curl [**Table 37-2**].[8]

Due to the fact that hair texture is not uniform among those of African ancestry, basic hair care practices vary based on the phenotype or the degree of tightness of the curl, as determined by the curve diameter.

STRUCTURAL PROPERTIES

Studies suggest that African hair has a lower radial swelling rate/percentage upon exposure to water, but the hair composition and structure do not differ for the three racial types of hair.[1,2,9] African hair is described as excessively curly, possessing an elliptical or flattened shape in cross-section, and with spiral curls in its tertiary structure.

The intraracial variability of this elliptical shape is increased in African hair; in the 'twist' regions, hair of African origin displays a wide variety of shapes [**Table 37-3**].[10,11] The tensile properties of excessively curly hair indicate that it has a lower strain value at breaking point compared with straight hair.[12] This means that it takes less strain for African hair to reach its breaking point, and thus the hair will break more easily. African hair has a tendency to form knots, as well as longitudinal fissures and splits along the hair shaft.[13] This complex shaft structure ensures the need for specialized grooming products and procedures to ensure that the hair maintains its cosmetic value.[7]

MAINTENANCE TECHNIQUES

CUTTING AND TRIMMING

African hair grows more slowly and breaks more often than Asian or Caucasian hair.[10] Combing the hair can increase the number of fractures and breaks in natural, virgin hair as it grows longer. African hair tends to develop a high static charge when combed in a dry state, and combed natural hair can remain short for many years without ever being cut.[5,7] The constant formation of knots will cause hair to break when combed [**Figure 37-2**]. A 'steady state' of daily breakage and equivalent new growth can be reached independently.[5] Females with African hair may have tightly coiled hair and may also be averse to cutting their hair because of the natural 'daily haircut' due to breakage.

The act of straightening hair or allowing it to 'lock' may be the only way for some patients to realize the true anagen phase length potential of their textured African hair. African hair with relaxers, dreadlocks, and twist styles may reach increased lengths and show decreased breakage rates. A small study by Whisenant and Taylor[14] found that frequent shampooing and trimming were associated with hair damage in African hair. Yet excessive damage from styling practices may increase the need to cut damaged hair; this may warrant further investigation.[14]

Despite these conflicting data, it may be wise to instruct patients with African hair to trim their hair every 8 to 12 weeks to minimize distal breakage and maximize luster and style maintenance.

CLEANSING

Hair cleansing needs differ between straight hair and African hair. African hair has significantly lower water content than Caucasian or Asian hair and does not become coated with sebum secretion as naturally as straight hair. Tightly coiled hair naturally stands away from the scalp; therefore, increased sebum can increase styling ease.[7,13] Cleansing agents targeted to populations with African hair may contain mild amphoteric detergents, detangling agents, silicone-based materials, quaternary ammonium compounds, and cationic polymers that will not aggravate the scalp.[12,15]

TABLE 37-1	Hair care recommendations for individuals with African hair

Practical hair care recommendations for patients with African hair
- Cleanse hair every 1–2 weeks. Chemicals (eg, chlorine) should be washed out daily.
- Use cleansers and conditioners formulated for the hair texture (coarse, dry, or damaged hair); carefully evaluate products marketed solely for African hair.
- Avoid the application of direct heat to the hair more than two times a week.
- Do not apply heat to dirty hair or hair layered with styling products.
- For styling purposes, air dry or wet set hair rather than blow drying it.
- Hair should be trimmed every 8–12 weeks.
- Establish open communication with stylists in the local area.
- Use emollients on the hair shafts only.
- Excessive scalp irritation, burns, or hair breakage should be evaluated promptly by a dermatologist knowledgeable in African hair types.

Additional recommendations based on styling choices
Chemically altered hair
- Schedule a professional touch-up no more than every 6–8 weeks.
- Use non–lye-based chemical relaxers.
- Avoid scalp manipulation prior to chemical treatments.
- Highlights, cellophanes, and colors should be done by a professional stylist to avoid damage to the hair shafts.
- Only visit licensed cosmetologists for chemical treatments.
- Promptly seek medical attention for alopecia, burns, or persistent scalp irritation.

Braids, weaves, locks, plaits, and cornrows
- Avoid styles that put tension/traction on the hair.
- Use emollients on the hair shafts only.
- Use 'no damage' hair hosiery instead of rubber bands.
- The volume and weight of hair extensions should not be excessive.
- Remove and replace braids every 4–6 weeks.

◼ CONDITIONING

Heavier conditioning products are required to overcome the higher static charge of African hair.[16] Conditioners are used to ease the process of both wet and dry combing; to smooth, seal, and realign damaged areas; to provide protection against thermal and mechanical procedures; and to improve the hair's appearance and tactile sensation.[12]

◼ COMPLICATIONS/TREATMENTS/PREVENTION

Shampooing Women with African hair who shampoo their hair twice weekly or more often have a higher rate of damage to the hair shaft; therefore, shampooing can be limited to once every 1 to 2 weeks.[14] Conditioning shampoos marketed to people with damaged, chemically treated, or color-treated hair can decrease breakage for patients with

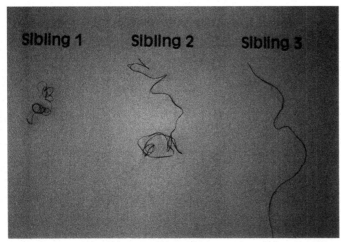

FIGURE 37-1. The intraracial variability of the curl degree is shown here in three siblings with unprocessed virgin hair.

TABLE 37-2	Phenotype of African hair

African hair becomes curlier in appearance when:
- It has a lower curve diameter.
- It extends less when strained.
- It is more susceptible to breakage.

The mechanical fragility of African hair increases with higher degrees of curl.

African hair. It has been shown that those containing sphinganine-derived ceramide (ie, C18-dhCer) bind to and protect both virgin and chemically treated African hair from excessive breakage.[17] Excessive exposure to chemicals such as the chlorine in pool water should be avoided or washed from the hair on a daily basis if necessary, despite the preceding recommendation, and a conditioning agent should be applied to prevent breakage.

Women with hairstyles such as weaves, relaxers, curly perms, Jheri curls, or braids sometimes opt to shampoo even less frequently so that their hair will not revert back to its natural state. However, this is not recommended and can promote seborrhea, increase the risk of fungal infection, and result in an unpleasant odor.[18] Conditions such as seborrhea, tinea capitis, and psoriasis will necessitate more frequent washing and are explained in more detail in Chapters 23, 24, and 38.

Conditioners, Moisturizers, Scalp Oils, and Pomades Many patients will describe the process of moisturizing as greasing or basting the scalp. Generally, the hair is sectioned with a comb in small parts, and a moisturizing agent is applied directly to the exposed scalp and proximal hair shafts. Subsequently, the agent is left in the hair and not washed out. Moisturizing the hair in this way enables the patient to comb their hair without having to tug or pull, movements that often result in breakage. Because the water content of African hair is slightly less than that of Caucasian hair, most patients with African hair will make use of a daily grooming agent.[7,12]

Wet hair shafts should be coated with a conditioning agent; furthermore, to decrease breakage, a wide-tooth comb [**Figure 37-3**] or fingertips should be used to comb the hair, starting at the ends and advancing proximally.

The overuse of moisturizers can lead to pomade acne involving the forehead [**Figure 37-4**], scalp oil folliculitis, chronic oil folliculitis, and seborrheic dermatitis. Patients should avoid products that are vegetable oil- or petrolatum-based, or contain high-melting hydrocarbons.[19-21]

Newer agents containing less occlusive agents are recommended, such as those containing cyclomethicone or dimethicone.[22] Moisturizers should be applied to the entire hair shaft and not to the scalp. Patients should be questioned regarding scalp irritation or pruritus, and evaluation of the scalp should be performed if patients continue to apply pomades directly to the scalp.

STYLING TECHNIQUES

◼ THERMAL STRAIGHTENING

Blow drying refers to the process of drying wet hair with repetitive combing while using a hair dryer to direct air toward the hair at varying degrees

TABLE 37-3	Structural properties of African hair

- African hair has a lower radial swelling rate, which depends on the percentage of exposure to water.
- The composition and structure are the same for the three types of hair.
- African hair is described as excessively curly, possessing an elliptical or flattened shape in cross-section and with spiral curls in its tertiary structure.
- There is intraracial variability of the elliptical shape of the hair; this variability is increased in African hair.
- At the 'twist' regions, African hair has a wide variety of shapes.

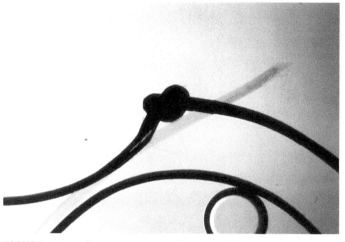

FIGURE 37-2. A knot forming in a fiber of African hair. Passing a comb through knots will fracture the hair.

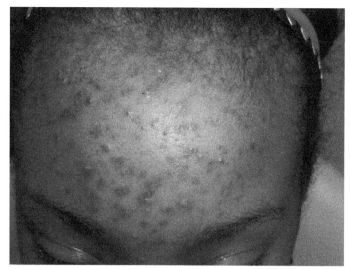

A

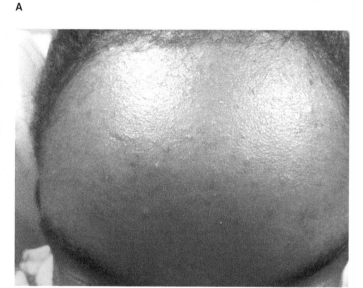

B

FIGURE 37-4. Multiple closed comedones of pomade acne on the forehead from hair lubricant use. Before **(A)** and after **(B)** the cessation of the pomades with treatment using topical and oral medications.

of heat. It is used to straighten hair, prepare it for pressing (see below), and style it. Alternative drying methods, such as air drying or wet setting, decrease the chance of breakage; however, despite aggressive use, these styling methods may not achieve or maintain the desired styling effect, and it may be hard to convince patients to use these methods instead.

Commonly called pressing or hot combing, thermal straightening is the process of straightening the hair using high heat (~350°F), oils, and metal implements. Flat irons, marcel irons, and curling irons are implements heated by marcel stoves or electrical heat [**Figure 37-5**]. These instruments are used for the styling of virgin or chemically processed hair. Daily use of these methods can contribute to excessive dryness, bubble hairs, proximal trichorrhexis nodosa, weathering, trichoptilosis, and chronic breakage.[23]

The straightening effect of thermal styling is temporary, due to the temporary rearrangement of hydrogen and disulfide bonds within the hair shaft, and will be reversed with water exposure.[4]

Complications/Treatments/Prevention Hair pressing should not be done more than two times a week, and it is not recommended to press hair that has not been properly cleansed and conditioned prior to the application of heat. Patients with African hair have a high incidence of repeating and layering hair care products on a daily basis and a lower frequency of shampooing; these practices can increase the hair's flammability.[24] Proximal breakage may occur, and a foul odor may emanate from hair when it has not been cleansed prior to heat thermal styling.

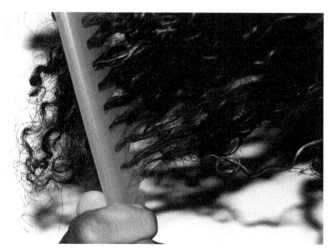

FIGURE 37-3. Wide-tooth combs or fingers can decrease breakage from combing.

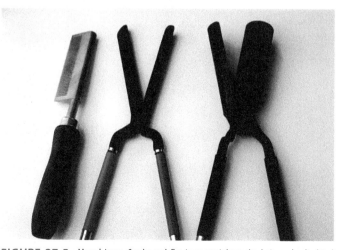

FIGURE 37-5. Marcel irons. Combs and flat-irons straighten the hair, and cylindrical devices are then used to curl the straightened hair.

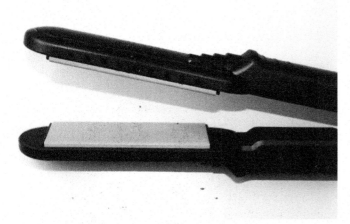

FIGURE 37-6. Heat-controlled negative-ion ceramic-plated irons with automatic shut-down features can be safer and easier to use and give the hair a smoother finish.

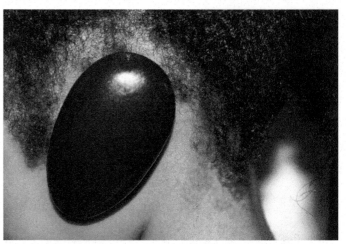

A

Hairline breakage and thinning may result from the excessive use of thermal implements which are used to maintain straightness in the face of daily perspiration and water exposure.[4]

It is impractical to counsel every patient to discontinue the use of all thermal devices. Newer ceramic irons, which generate negative ions, now possess adjustable temperature controls, and devices with automatic shut-down features in case of overheating are recommended to replace pressing combs [**Figure 37-6**]. These irons, as with other thermal devices, should not be used on damp hair. Communication with hair care professionals in the region can aid patients in learning healthy styling behavior.

Scalp, ear, and neck burns are commonly seen in patients who use thermal styling agents and devices [**Figure 37-7**]. Exposure to extreme heat should be avoided by using protective devices, which can be purchased at beauty supply stores [**Figure 37-8**]. Local treatment may be necessary to prevent scarring, keloids, and infections.

■ CHEMICAL RELAXATION/LANTHIONIZATION

Mistakenly called perms, chemical relaxers have been used for decades by many males and females of African descent, and a total of 70% of African American females use chemical relaxers. Chemical relaxers straighten the hair shaft using chemicals that alter the hair's natural texture; with this technique, the hair will not revert to its virgin state upon exposure to water.

Chemical relaxers containing sodium, potassium, or guanidine hydroxides straighten by affecting the cysteine disulfide bonds of the

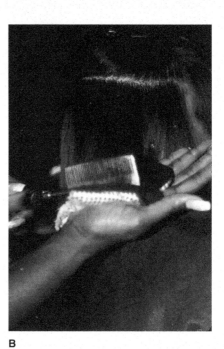

B

FIGURE 37-8. Ear protectors (**A**) and handheld devices (**B**) should be used in salons to protect both the client and stylist from burns during thermal styling.

hair.[25] Sodium hydroxide (lye-based) relaxers are used mainly in salons, whereas other relaxers (non–lye-based) are popular for home use. It is widely believed by stylists and patrons that lye-based relaxers have a better straightening effect. Lye-based relaxers have more irritation potential, are cheaper and easier to use, and are preferred by stylists for perceived relaxer performance. However, recent laboratory results have indicated that non–lye-based (guanidine-based) cream-finished products show greater efficacy over lye-based products.[26]

Japanese straightening and relaxing systems can be harsh on African hair, because they often require thermal processing on damp hair. Caution should be used if applying a Japanese straightening system to African type hair.

Numerous 'comb thru' or S-curl texturizers are marketed to those with African hair type, especially men, children, and those with sensitive scalps. The results are less permanent, and the settings on these texturizers can be controlled for the desired curl relaxation. Chemicals such as sulfites, lithium hydroxide, and guanidine are the active ingredients in these non–lye-based products. With these techniques, the hair shaft is not completely straightened, which allows for a looser curl and a more manageable style.[27]

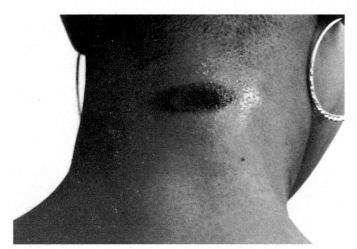

FIGURE 37-7. Thermal burn after the use of a curling iron.

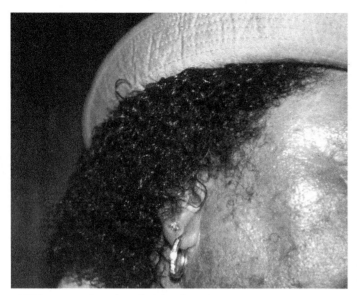

FIGURE 37-9. Jheri curls need a daily curl activator to maintain the style, which can be messy and give a greasy appearance to the hair.

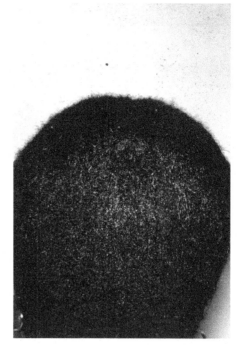

FIGURE 37-10. Chronic proximal hair breakage in an adult woman with skin of color.

Jheri curls or curly perms [**Figure 37-9**] use ammonium thioglycolate with a lotion; the hair is wrapped on rollers to relax the curl, and then is reset in a curly or wavy pattern. Both styles can be maintained with a glycerin-based lotion moisturizer or a spray curl activator; however, these are generally messy and labor intensive. A daily leave-in conditioner can be recommended as a more elegant alternative.

The curly shape of hair is programmed from the bulb (the lowermost section of the root of the hair) and is formed from a 'shape-memory' material. Touch-ups to new growth are necessary to maintain the style as the hair grows; the regular reapplication of any of the previously mentioned relaxers to new growth can prevent texture differences that may predispose hair to breakage at areas of textural transition.[28]

Complications/Treatments/Prevention A total of 73% of women with African hair complain of breakage, trichoptilosis (where the hairs are covered with feather-like projections), and dryness caused by chemical treatments [**Figure 37-10**].[29-31] Touch-ups should be applied no more than every 8 to 12 weeks to minimize breakage and the advent of relaxer-induced alopecia and to decrease scalp irritation.[32]

Patients who use chemical relaxers should be counseled to avoid scalp irritants or manipulation prior to receiving touch-ups. Requesting a copy of the patient's salon 'relaxer record' can aid in making recommendations when damage to the scalp has occurred [**Table 37-4**]. It has been suggested that repetitive scalp irritation and burns may play a role in fibrosis and inflammation of the scalp associated with cicatricial and noncicatricial alopecia, although more research is necessary to confirm the association.[33-35] Using a sebum production tester, a noninvasive method to examine molecular events, Tackey and Holloway Barbosa revealed that although hair is the target of chemical relaxers, sensory irritation of the scalp occurs and this irritation may be both cytokine-mediated and neurogenic.[36] A study in South Africa found that relaxers are associated with reduced cystine bonds, which is in turn associated with fragile, damaged hair.[37]

KERATIN TREATMENTS AND BRAZILIAN BLOWOUTS

■ FORMALDEHYDE-CONTAINING KERATIN STRAIGHTENING AGENTS

Keratin hair treatments are promoted as smoothing treatments that work to repair the damage caused by chemical treatments and that can be used on chemically relaxed hair. The keratin hair-straightening treatment consists of using naturally occurring hydrolyzed keratin that then rapidly diffuses into the hair cortex to react with hair keratin. The amino acids that make up the hydrolyzed keratin are cross-linked to the hair keratin by cross-linking agents such as formaldehyde or its derivatives, formalin or methylene glycol.[38,39]

In a salon, the keratin treatment is applied to the hair in small sections, and then the hair is blow-dried and a flat iron is used to seal the keratin onto the hair [**Figure 37-11**]. The client must then wait at least 72 hours before getting their hair wet, washing their hair, or going swimming, to avoid reversing the process. Additionally, during this time, the hair cannot be pulled back in any way, for instance with clips, ponytail holders, hats, or sunglasses.[40] To maintain the treatment, only sodium sulfate-free shampoos and hair care products should be used.[40] This may prove difficult in patients with scalp conditions that require topical applications of medication and therapeutic shampoos. It may be difficult to ensure that the patient receives and uses a sodium sulfate-free product, particularly with the current rise of generic substitutions. Keratin hair treatments have a natural reversion process as the treatment washes out of the hair in 3 to 5 months.

Keratin hair treatments can be applied to already chemically relaxed hair because the treatments do not break the disulfide bonds but claim to infuse keratin into the cuticle.[40] This is especially useful for patients who routinely use chemical relaxers to straighten hair. Chemical relaxers can cause significant damage to hair and will result in overprocessing if reapplied to previously processed hair.[37]

To date, keratin hair treatments have assisted many patients in recovering from breakage and have encouraged the discontinuation of relaxers that can damage the hair and potentially cause inflammation, leading to scalp disorders.[37]

■ NON–FORMALDEHYDE-CONTAINING KERATIN STRAIGHTENING AGENTS

Recently introduced to the market, non–formaldehyde-containing keratin straightening products are said to have comparable results to products with formaldehyde. The main ingredients are hydrolyzed keratin with a combination of glyoxyloyl carbocysteine, glyoxyloyl keratin amino acids, silicone derivatives, and fatty acids.[38,41]

TABLE 37-4	Relaxer record

Name_____   Tel _____

Address _____ City _____ State _____ Zip Code _____

Description of hair

FORM	LENGTH	TEXTURE	POROSITY	
☐ wavy	☐ short	☐ coarse	☐ soft	☐ very ☐ less
☐ curly	☐ medium	☐ medium	☐ silky	☐ moderate ☐ least
☐ extra curly	☐ long	☐ fine	☐ wiry	☐ normal ☐ resistant
				☐ lightened

Condition

☐ virgin	☐ retouched	☐ dry	☐ oily	☐ lightened

Tinted with _____

Previously relaxed with (name of relaxer) _____

☐ Original sample of hair enclosed

Type of relaxer or straightener

☐ whole head	☐ re-touch
☐ relaxer _____ strength	☐ straightener _____ strength

Results

☐ good	☐ poor	☐ sample of relaxed hair enclosed	☐ not enclosed
Date	Operator	Date	Operator

_____   _____

_____   _____

_____   _____

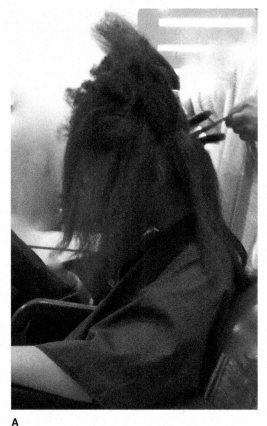
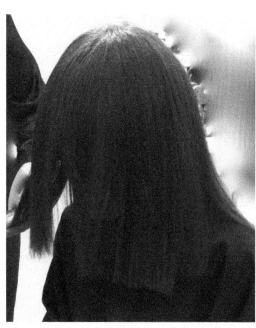

A   **B**

FIGURE 37-11. Keratin treatment is applied to the hair in small sections and blown dry. A flat iron is then used to seal the keratin onto the hair. Before **(A)** and after **(B)** the treatment.

Complications/Treatments/Prevention The U.S. Food and Drug Administration (FDA) and the Occupational Safety and Health Administration have scrutinized the formaldehyde levels in keratin treatments. The Brazilian Blowout® treatment was singled out by the FDA as a danger due to the high levels of formaldehyde; yet, despite these concerns, the treatment is still widely available and extremely popular. A settlement was reached in 2012 between the Attorney General of the State of California and the manufacturer of Brazilian Blowout® products that will require the company to warn consumers and hair stylists that two of its most popular hair-smoothing products emit formaldehyde gas.[42] Products causing the following symptoms should be reported to the FDA: eye and nervous system disorders, respiratory tract problems, chest pain, vomiting, and rashes.

The authors recommend a patch test of the product prior to treatment and warn against use in patients with known sensitivities to formaldehyde and their releasing agents.[43] Despite these warnings, the proper use of keratin-based products, especially those without high formaldehyde levels, has been revolutionary in assisting patients suffering from hair breakage and in decreasing the need for damaging styling agents.

NONPROCESSED OR NATURAL STYLING

AFROS

Afros are a natural hairstyle in which the hair is unprocessed and allowed to grow radially from the head [**Figure 37-12**]. Moisturizers and oils are needed to maintain this style. With the Afro style, the hair is not combed with a standard comb, but rather a 'pick' or fingers are used for daily maintenance. The style is most often worn by men with African hair. The frequency of the Afro style in women may increase as they get older; this may be due to lifestyle changes, retirement, alopecias, hair breakage, or financial constraints.[25] Many middle-aged women with African hair who have adopted an Afro express an acceptance and understanding of their hair type that they did not have in their youth, and those no longer in the work force feel less pressure for "hair assimilation."

LOCKS, TWISTS, AND DREADLOCKS

Twisting of the hair can help to minimize the bulk of thick hair and redefines the hair shaft's natural curl, making the hair more manageable. Two pieces of hair are twisted around one another to form the twist [**Figure 37-13**]. Locks, which are irreversible, are formed when uncombed hair tangles and mats into clusters. There are several lock styles, including free-form, wrapping, and sisterlocks.[44]

MISCELLANEOUS STYLING

Various molding techniques (eg, finger waving, freezing, and wrapping) are used to create hairstyles ranging from a tight hold to a freeze hold

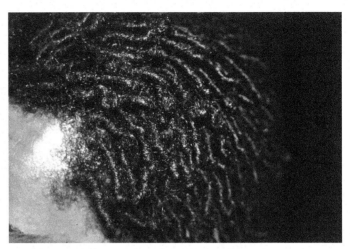

FIGURE 37-13. A man with skin of color with a twist style.

[**Figure 37-14**]. The fixatives used are balanced with plasticizers such as propylene glycol or glycerin. Styling gels and/or spritzers are often used to achieve and maintain these styles; these may contain upward of 64% of SD-40 alcohol by weight and should be avoided because this can cause increased hair shaft dryness and breakage.[13]

HAIR EXTENSIONS AND HAIR WEAVES

Braids (also called plaits) and micro-braids are styles created by interlocking three or more pieces of hair to create a three-dimensional section that extends from the head [**Figure 37-15**]. Hair braiding can be done with or without hair extensions, which are packaged bulks of synthetic or human hairs that are then integrated with the existing hair at the scalp. Braiding hair with extensions involves interweaving small to micro-sections of the natural hair with the hair extensions to give an appearance of longer hair. Braiding can also be done with cornrows, which are stationary braids that lay flat on the scalp. Cornrows and plaits are used commonly under wigs, with weave styles, and for children. Many women adopt a braid style when implementing an exercise program to avoid styling dilemmas.[45]

Another form of hair extensions is termed hair weaving. Hair weaving has become extremely popular recently in all segments of society. Weaves are commonly worn by entertainers and reality show stars; as a result, the everyday use of weaves for African American females has exploded. Many are unable to afford high-quality weaves and suffer from traction and other related forms of hair loss. Human hair is very expensive

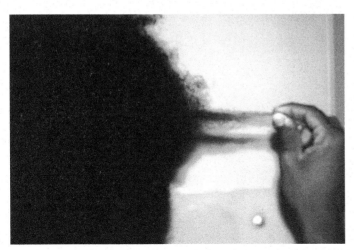

FIGURE 37-12. An example of the Afro style; extending the curled hairs reveals the actual length.

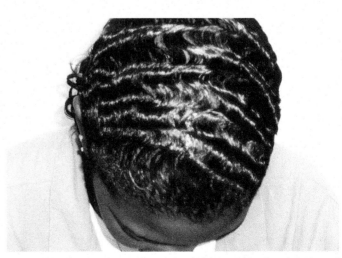

FIGURE 37-14. A woman with skin of color with a "freeze hold" style and complaints of alopecia. However, the molded hairstyle made a clinical scalp examination impossible.

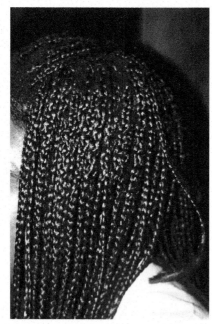

FIGURE 37-15. A woman with skin of color with individual braids.

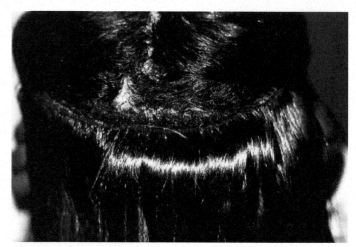

FIGURE 37-16. A woman with skin of color with a weave style sewn onto braided cornrows to add volume and length.

and has become an expensive commodity. Hair weaving can be done for aesthetic, therapeutic, or prosthetic reasons. Many women believe that a weave style will help their hair grow, cover balding areas, or add thickness to their hair.[44] Dermatologists should therefore determine the reasons behind a patient's decision to wear hair extensions; although the decision may often be purely aesthetic, it could indicate that the patient is attempting to cover up existing hair loss.[46]

Hair extensions may be held into place by different methods, such as sewing, gluing, or braiding [**Table 37-5**]. With thread weaving, the scalp hair is plaited into several cornrows and wefts of hair extensions are then sewed onto the rows of natural hair at the scalp [**Figure 37-16**]. Fusion or micro-ring extensions are performed by twisting small sections of approximately 25 natural hairs at the base and then attaching a small weft of the extension hair weave with an adhesive or micro-rings. Another alternative technique is to bond the hair weaves where adhesives are applied to the weft of hair extensions and attached to the scalp or at the base of the hair. Another common method is to use clip-in hair extensions, which have hair clips at the base of the hair extension that can be attached to the natural hair near the scalp.

Wigs can be used to reduce the frequency of heat application and chemicals and also to avoid general damage to the hair at the scalp. However, there are several methods to secure wigs onto the scalp that can further harm the scalp hair. The chronic use of wig clips on thinning temporal scalp hair can worsen alopecia. Lace wigs (shafts of hair extensions attached to a lace net wig cap) are becoming increasing popular among celebrities as well as the average woman, because they allow for convenient and versatile hairstyling. Unfortunately, these lace wigs are often attached to the scalp with a strong adhesive that can result in hair loss around the perimeter of the hair during removal [**Figure 37-17**].

Complications/Treatments/Prevention Traction folliculitis and resulting traction alopecia are found commonly in patients with African hair who wear tight hairstyles, such as twists, locks, weaves,

ponytails, braids, and extensions, or those who use hair rollers [**Figures 37-18 and 37-19**].[47,48] The loosening of these styles can prevent long-term alopecia. Patients should be counseled to avoid hairstyles that are too tight and to loosen their hair overnight as the style permits. Contact or irritant dermatitis due to adhesive/glue products (acrylates) and hair extensions can complicate weave styling. To maintain healthy scalp hair and avoid traction alopecia, braided or weaved-in hair extensions should be applied with as little traction as possible, and the direction of the braided hair should be changed frequently.[49]

SPECIAL CONSIDERATIONS FOR MEN WITH AFRICAN HAIR

Men with skin of color have a wide variety of hair care practices that include most, if not all, of the earlier mentioned processes. Men's hair is often subjected to the following processes and styles: shaving; cornrows; twisting; braiding; an Afros or dreadlocks; chemically treated for complete straightening or straightened partially with an S-curl texturizer; and, rarely, hair extensions. Most men with African hair maintain a short buzz haircut or will sometimes even shave their entire head. To this end, some younger men experiment with shaving patterns into the scalp hair.

Originally created as protective garments for the hair, wave caps or do-rags [**Figure 37-20**] are worn by men with African hair to physically relax the curl and maintain the hair overnight. Do-rags are also used to

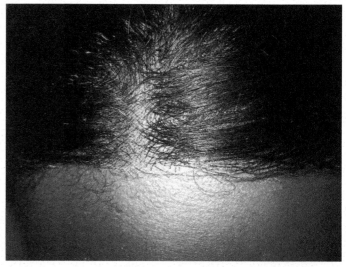

FIGURE 37-17. Lace wigs attached to the scalp, with a strong adhesive, can result in hair loss around the perimeter of the hair during removal.

TABLE 37-5	Hair extension techniques
Braiding/cornrows	
Threading hair weaves	
Bonding hair weaves	
Fusion/micro-ring hair extensions	
Clip-in hair extensions	

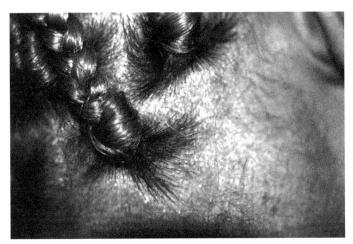

FIGURE 37-18. Traction folliculitis, erythematous papules, and pustules at areas of tension.

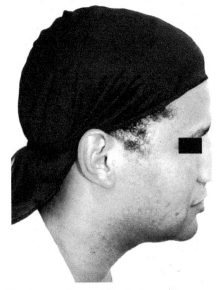

FIGURE 37-20. Do-rag use by a man with skin of color.

maintain neat braid styles in people of both genders with African hair. Often, a petrolatum-based pomade or wave-enhancing cream can be applied to help control the curl tightness.

An uncommon practice for some men with African hair is a tattoo micropigmentation process, which involves tattooing a brown-colored pigment on the scalp to give the illusion of hair.

COMPLICATIONS/TREATMENTS/PREVENTION

The use of creams and pomades under a do-rag or other occluding headwear can cause pomade acne and irritant dermatitis, as well as spread infection and exacerbate seborrhea. It is important to instruct patients to clean the headgear and to use breathable or mesh fabric to minimize these complications.

Some men with African hair use chemicals to relax, not straighten, the natural curl of their hair. A minority may use chemicals and thermal instruments to achieve straight hair and to lengthen the hair. Similar recommendations should be given for hair maintenance as for female patients with such styles.

Due to constant shaving of tightly curled hair, men with skin of color are prone to developing acne keloidalis nuchae (see Chapter 34).

SPECIAL CONSIDERATIONS FOR PEDIATRIC HAIR

Braids/plaits are common in young girls with African hair, and although boys with African hair usually wear the Afro style cropped short, braids and cornrows are increasing in popularity for them as

well [**Figure 37-21**]. Numerous products are increasingly being marketed for children of African descent that promise straighter and more manageable hair. Chemical relaxers are used quite frequently in the pediatric population, and some patients may be subjected to these as early as 3 years of age.

COMPLICATIONS/TREATMENTS/PREVENTION

The frequency of hair loss in young women is growing. Women with African hair are particularly susceptible to hair breakage from infancy through adolescence. These young women are at risk of haphazard hair maintenance, experimentation, aversion to hair trimming, and the frequent use of homemade chemical and thermal hair products by unlicensed stylists. Chronic proximal hair breakage is common in children when the chemical relaxers used are not maintained properly [**Figure 37-22**]. More than 70% of adult women with African hair admit to the use of hot combs in childhood, and 51% recall experiencing scalp burns as a child.[50]

As mentioned earlier, braids and cornrows with sufficient tension can cause traction folliculitis and alopecia [**Figure 37-23**]. It is recommended that hair be loosened each night and that the part pattern be changed frequently to decrease the chance of breakage and thinning. To minimize damage and traction alopecia, products such as Girl No

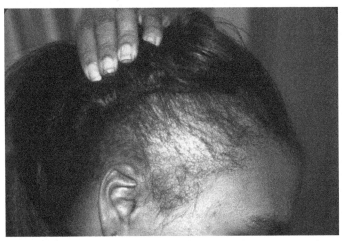

FIGURE 37-19. Traction alopecia from the prolonged weaving of hair.

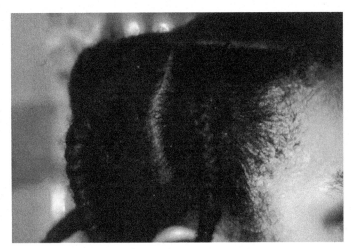

FIGURE 37-21. A child with skin of color wearing plaits (braids).

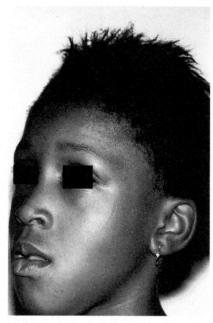

FIGURE 37-22. Chronic hair breakage from relaxer use in a female child with skin of color.

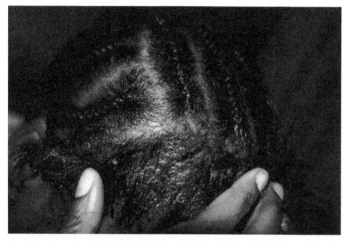

A

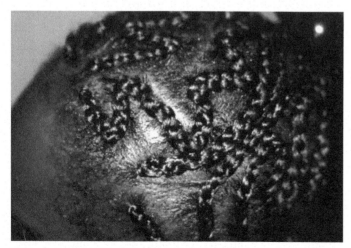

B

FIGURE 37-23. (A and B) Traction alopecia in children with skin of color with cornrows.

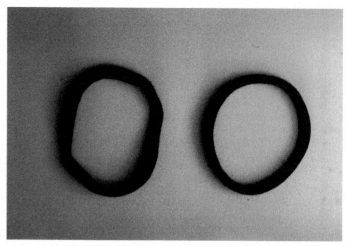

FIGURE 37-24. Hair bands without metal implements can decrease the tension on the scalp and prevent hair shaft breakage.

Damage® Hair Ties can be used to gather and hold sectioned hair in place [**Figure 37-24**].[51] Rubber bands and bands with metal implements should be avoided.

Physicians and dermatologists should discourage the use of chemical styling agents in pediatric patients due to the risks of chemical burns, contact dermatitis, inconsistent hair grooming routines, greater susceptibility to fungal infections, and possible cultural identity issues. The authors also strongly discourage the use of weaves in the pediatric population due to the previously mentioned complications and the subsequent self-esteem issues that may result.

REFERENCES

1. Lindelöf B, Forslind B, Hedblad MA, Kaveus U. Human hair form. Morphology revealed by light and scanning electron microscopy and computer aided three-dimensional reconstruction. *Arch Dermatol.* 1988:124:1359-1363.
2. Dekio S, Jidoi J. Hair low-sulfur protein composition does not differ electrophoretically among different races. *J Dermatol.* 1988;15:393-396.
3. Callender VD, McMichael AJ, Cohen GF. Medical and surgical therapies for alopecias in black women. *Dermatol Ther.* 2004;17:164-176.
4. Grimes PE, Davis LT. Cosmetics in blacks. *Dermatol Clin.* 1991;9:53-68.
5. Khumalo NP. African hair morphology: macrostructure to ultrastructure. *Int J Dermatol.* 2005;44:10-12.
6. Taylor SC. As simple as black and white? *J Am Acad Dermatol* 2006;54: 1070-1071.
7. Draelos ZD. Understanding African-American hair. *Dermatol Nurse.* 1997;9:227-231.
8. Porter CE, Diridollou S, Holloway Barbosa V. The influence of African-American hair's curl pattern on its mechanical properties. *Int J Dermatol.* 2005;44:4-5.
9. Franbourg A, Hallegot P, Baltenneck F, et al. Current research on ethnic hair. *J Am Acad Dermatol.* 2003;48:S115-S119.
10. Loussouarn G. African hair growth parameters. *Br J Dermatol.* 2001;145: 294-297.
11. Wickett RR. Presentation. L'Oréal's 1st International Symposium on Ethnic Skin and Hair, Chicago, IL, 2001.
12. Syed AN. Ethnic hair care products. In: Johnson DH, ed. *Hair and Hair Care.* Vol 17. New York, NY: Marcel Dekker; 1997:235-259.
13. Taylor SC. Skin of color: biology, structure, function, and implications for dermatologic disease. *J Am Acad Dermatol.* 2002;46:S41-S62.
14. Whisenant K, Taylor SC. Presentation. L'Oréal's 2nd International Symposium on Ethnic Skin and Hair: New Directions in Research, Chicago, IL, 2003.
15. Draelos ZD. *Hair Care: An Illustrated Dermatologic Handbook.* Oxon, United Kingdom: Taylor & Francis; 2005:25-39.
16. Jachowicz J, Wis-Surel G, Garcia ML. Relationship between trichoelectric charging and surface modifications of human hair. *J Soc Cosmet Chem.* 1985; 36:189-212.
17. Bernard BA, Franbourg A, François AM, et al. Ceramide binding to African-American hair fibre correlates with resistance to hair breakage. *Int J Cosmet Sci.* 2002;24:1-12.

18. Silverberg NB, Weinberg JM, DeLeo VA. Tinea capitis: focus on African American women. *J Am Acad Dermatol.* 2002;46:S120-S124.

19. Bhate K, Williams HC. Epidemiology of acne vulgaris. *Br J Dermatol.* 2013; 168:474-485.

20. Plewig G, Fulton JE, Kligman AM. Pomade acne. *Arch Dermatol.* 1970;101:580-584.

21. Draelos ZD. Hair serum dimethicone zaps static, smooths cuticle. http://dermatologytimes.modernmedicine.com/dermatology-times/news/modernmedicine/modern-medicine-now/hair-serum-dimethicone-zaps-static-smooths. Accessed June 2, 2013.

22. Coley MK, Alexis AF. Managing common dermatoses in skin of color. *Semin Cutan Med Surg.* 2009;28:63-70.

23. Brown VM, Crounse RG, Abele DC. An unusual new hair shaft abnormality: "bubble hair." *J Am Acad Dermatol.* 1986;15:1113-1117.

24. Cannel D. Cosmetic/pharmaceutical research: development, safety, and efficacy of ethnic products. L'Oréal's 3rd International Symposium on Ethnic Skin and Hair: Advancing the Scientific Frontier, Chicago, IL, 2005.

25. McMichael AJ. Hair and scalp disorders in ethnic populations. *Dermatol Clin.* 2003;21:629-644.

26. Bryant H, Yang GY, Holloway Barbosa V. Lye versus no-lye relaxers: comparison of laboratory results and end-user perceptions. L'Oréal's 3rd International Symposium on Ethnic Skin and Hair: Advancing the Scientific Frontier, Chicago, IL, 2005.

27. Pro-line International. Products. http://www.webplusbeauty.com/2125a0000.html. Accessed August 27, 2012.

28. Joyner M. Hair care in the black patient. *J Pediatr Health Care.* 1988;2:281-287.

29. Halder RM. Hair and scalp disorders in blacks. *Cutis.* 1983;32:378-380.

30. Bulengo-Ransby SM, Bergfeld WF. Chemical and traumatic alopecia from thioglycolate in a black woman: a case report with unusual clinical and histologic findings. *Cutis.* 1992;49:99-103.

31. Miller JJ. Relaxer-induced alopecia. *Am J Contact Dermat.* 2001;12:238-239.

32. Thibaut S, Bernard BA. The biology of hair shape. *Int J Dermatol.* 2005;44:2-3.

33. Nicholson AG, Harland CC, Bull RH, et al. Chemically induced cosmetic alopecia. *Br J Dermatol.* 1993;128:537-541.

34. Nnoruka EN. Hair loss: is there a relationship with hair care practices in Nigeria? *Int J Dermatol.* 2005;44:13-17.

35. Swee W, Klontz KC, Lambert LA. A nationwide outbreak of alopecia associated with the use of a hair-relaxing formulation. *Arch Dermatol.* 2000;136:1104-1108.

36. Tackey RN, Holloway Barbosa V. Molecular response in the scalp after application of relaxer to the hair. L'Oréal's 3rd International Symposium on Ethnic Skin and Hair: Advancing the Scientific Frontier, Chicago, IL, 2005.

37. Khumalo NP, Stone J, Gumedze F, et al. "Relaxers" damage hair: evidence from amino acid analysis. *J Am Acad Dermatol.* 2010;62:402-408.

38. Weathersby C, McMichael A. Brazilian keratin hair treatment: a review. *J Cosmet Dermatol.* 2013;12:144-148.

39. Drahl C. Hair straighteners: cross-linkers, redox chemistry, or high pH, all in the name of beauty. *Chem Eng News.* 2010;88:54.

40. Kertain Complex. Home page. http://www.keratincomplex.com. Accessed June 2, 2013.

41. KeraLuxe. Home page. http://kera-luxe.com. Accessed June 2, 2013.

42. Office of the Attorney General. Attorney General Kamala D. Harris Announces Settlement Requiring Honest Advertising over Brazilian Blowout Products. http://oag.ca.gov/news/press-releases/attorney-general-kamala-d-harris-announces-settlement-requiring-honest. Accessed August 27, 2013.

43. Stylenet. Brazilian keratin treatment consumer agreement form. http://stylenet.com/cf/tag4hair/Keratin%20Consent%20Form.pdf. Accessed August 27, 2013.

44. Ferrell P, Rackley L, eds. *Let's Talk Hair: Every Black Woman's Personal Consultation for Healthy Growing Hair.* Vol 1. Washington, DC: Cornrows & Co; 1996.

45. Hall RR, Francis S, Whitt-Glover M, et al. Hair care practices as a barrier to physical activity in African American women. *JAMA Dermatol.* 2013;149:310-314.

46. Weaver SM. *Dr. Weaver's Black Hair Loss Guide: How to Stop Thinning Hair and Avoid Permanent Baldness.* Tucson, AZ: Wheatmark Inc.; 2013.

47. Rucker Wright D, Gathers R, Kapke A, et al. Hair care practices and their association with scalp and hair disorders in African American girls. *J Am Acad Dermatol.* 2011;64:253-262.

48. Ntuen E, Stein SL. Hairpin-induced alopecia: case reports and a review of the literature. *Cutis.* 2010;85:242-245.

49. Roseborough IE, McMichael AJ. Hair care practices in African-American patients. *Semin Cutan Med Surg.* 2009;28:103-108.

50. Cook-Bolden F. Enlist hair stylists in stopping traction alopecia. *Skin Allergy News.* 2002;33:45.

51. Scünci. Girl No Damage® hair ties. http://www.scunci.com/products.php?products_id=524. Accessed August 27, 2013.

CHAPTER 38

Alopecia

Temitayo A. Ogunleye
Chemene R. Quinn
Amy McMichael

KEY POINTS

- Alopecia is classified as cicatricial or noncicatricial.

- Classification of cicatricial alopecia is often confusing and controversial.

- Central centrifugal cicatricial alopecia (CCCA) is responsible for more cases of cicatricial alopecia than all other forms in African American women.

- Prompt diagnosis and aggressive treatments of alopecias are warranted to halt progression of disease and salvage viable hair follicles.

- Many disorders have overlapping clinical and histologic features.

- Scalp biopsy and histopathologic evaluation are strongly recommended for diagnosing alopecia in skin of color patients.

- Medical therapy and education on proper hair care practices are imperative in the treatment of alopecia.

INTRODUCTION

Alopecia is the fifth most common dermatologic diagnosis in African American patients, and severe central alopecia affects 5.6% of African American women.[1-3] A systematic approach to the diagnosis of alopecia in the skin of color patient population is necessary to allow for adequate and appropriate treatment of disease. Alopecias can be subdivided into cicatricial (also known as scarring) and nonscarring subcategories, although overlap may occur. The diagnostic hallmark clinically distinguishing between these types of alopecia is the loss of follicular ostia in cicatricial alopecia, which may be typified by increased interfollicular distance on physical examination. Careful history and physical examination, as well as laboratory testing and/or biopsy, may be necessary for definitive diagnosis. Treatment should be based on clinical and histopathology results.

APPROACH TO THE PATIENT WITH ALOPECIA

The evaluation of the patient with alopecia must be comprehensive and include the following:

- Complete hair history including: onset of hair loss, loss of the full hair shaft versus hair breakage, localized versus diffuse, symptoms (itching, pain, burning, tenderness), recent illnesses/stressors (eg, death of loved one)

- Discussion of hair care practices: relaxers (frequency of use, type of relaxer), frequency of heat use, frequency of washing/conditioning, styles (braids, weaves, locks, tight ponytails)

- Full pertinent medical history should be obtained, including: history of menstrual cycle regularity/flow, history of medications (new, dose changes, herbal), history of anemia or thyroid disease

- Clinical examination of scalp and all hair-bearing areas

- Laboratory testing as indicated

- Histopathologic evaluation

PRIMARY CICATRICIAL ALOPECIAS

Cicatricial alopecia represents a poorly understood group of disorders characterized by a common final pathway of replacement of the hair follicle structure by fibrous tissue.[4] The North American Hair Research Society (NAHRS) classifies the primary cicatricial alopecias by histopathologic findings: lymphocytic, neutrophilic, mixed, and nonspecific.[4] Sperling[5] identified five distinct pathologic forms of scarring alopecia:

TABLE 38-1	Sperling's scarring alopecia classification
Chronic cutaneous lupus	
Lichen planopilaris	
Dissecting cellulites	
Acne keloidalis nuchae (folliculitis keloidalis)	
Central centrifugal scaring alopecia	

chronic cutaneous lupus, lichen planopilaris, dissecting cellulitis, acne keloidalis nuchae, and central centrifugal cicatricial alopecia (CCCA)[5] [**Table 38-1**]. Overlapping clinical and histopathologic features may lead to difficulty in distinguishing diagnoses, such that these entities often are included in the differential diagnoses of the other. We will discuss these five types of cicatricial alopecia in further detail as they pertain to darker-skinned populations.

CENTRAL CENTRIFUGAL CICATRICIAL ALOPECIA

EPIDEMIOLOGY, ETIOLOGY, AND PATHOGENESIS

CCCA is a poorly understood lymphocytic cicatricial alopecia seen commonly in women of African descent and less commonly in men. CCCA is thought to be responsible for more cases of scarring alopecia than all other forms in this population,[6] although no formal incidence or prevalence data are available. Formerly called *hot comb alopecia* or *follicular degeneration syndrome*, this disorder is not well defined, and the cause is still unknown. It has been proposed that the application of heat via hot combs or hooded dryers, hairstyles that pull too tightly on the scalp, harsh chemical treatments that damage the hair shaft, and family history contribute to the pathogenesis of CCCA.[7] However, recent studies have not consistently elucidated any core causes of CCCA, making a multifactorial etiology more likely.

CLINICAL FINDINGS

History Onset of disease is typically in the third to fifth decade, with patients occasionally having several years of activity before hair loss is noted. Many patients are asymptomatic, adding to the sometimes insidious nature of this condition. Some patients may complain of signs and symptoms such as paresthesia of the scalp described as a "pins and needles" sensation, itching, tenderness, hair breakage,[8] and pain. More inflammatory types of this form of hair loss may demonstrate scaling, pustules, or crusting.[9]

Physical Examination The early stage of the disease is characterized by central hair breakage, perifollicular hyperkeratosis, erythema, and thinning. Papules and pustules may be present [**Figures 38-1 and 38-2**]. CCCA is progressive and advances centrifugally to the

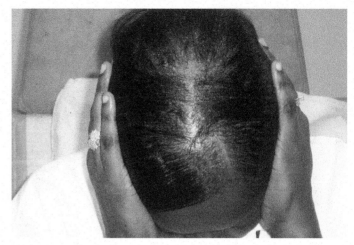

FIGURE 38-2. Moderate central centrifugal scarring alopecia.

surrounding areas. Many patients do not seek immediate medical care, and a common later presentation is a smooth scalp devoid of hair follicles at the vertex.[10] Mottled dyspigmentation with hypo- or hyperpigmented macules and characteristic loss of follicular ostia are common findings [**Figure 38-3**].

Laboratory Histopathology is widely believed to be due to premature desquamation of the inner root sheath (IRS). Horenstein and colleagues found that premature desquamation of the IRS is seen in a variety of cicatricial alopecias and cannot be used alone as a defining feature of CCCA.[6,11] The early stage exhibits a lichenoid infiltrate of lymphocytes separated from markedly thinned infundibulum by a prominent zone of alopecia.[12]

PROGNOSIS/CLINICAL COURSE

Many patients present with end-stage disease, and there is no definitive treatment regimen. For patients with earlier disease, the condition is thought to be chronic and progressive, if untreated.

TREATMENT

Prospective, controlled studies are needed to aid in effective treatment regimens. Price[13] recommends treatment based on histopathologic classification (ie, lymphocytic, neutrophilic, mixed). Aggressive treatment is warranted in the early stage of CCCA to halt progression, salvage viable hair follicles, and treat symptoms. Intralesional scalp injections of triamcinolone (7.5 to 10 mg/mL) every 6 to 8 weeks for six to eight cycles are helpful if tolerated by the patient [**Figure 38-4**]. This is typically coupled with topical high-potency corticosteroids applied daily for

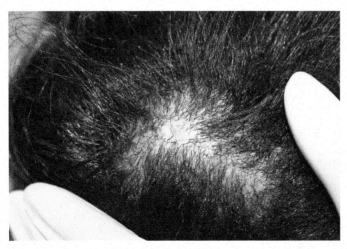

FIGURE 38-1. Early central centrifugal scarring alopecia.

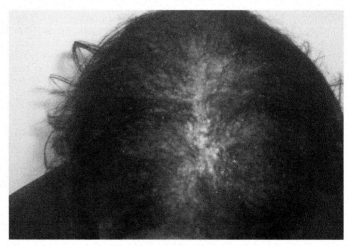

FIGURE 38-3. Late (end-stage) central centrifugal scarring alopecia.

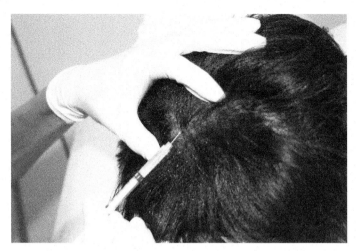

FIGURE 38-4. Intralesional scalp injection of triamcinolone acetate directly into scalp may halt progression in early disease.

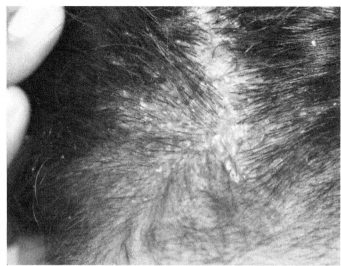

FIGURE 38-5. Hispanic patient on antiepileptic medication (diphenylhydantoin) showing folliculitis keloidalis.

2 to 4 weeks and then tapered to a few times weekly. In patients with more inflammatory disease, oral antibiotics such as tetracyclines (minocycline or doxycycline) or hydroxychloroquine may be useful for their anti-inflammatory properties.[13] Antidandruff shampoo used to treat any scaling is a common adjunctive treatment. Minoxidil 2% or 5% solution or foam can be helpful as an adjuvant therapy to prolong anagen cycling for viable hairs and promote regrowth of miniaturized hairs.[14] Minimizing traumatic hair care practices, such as excessive heat to affected areas of the scalp and tight hairstyles, may also be helpful in limiting the progression of the disease.

End Stage Hair transplants are an option and can be offered to patients when feasible. Patients should be medically managed and have stable disease for at least 6 months.[15] A test area can be performed with a 3- to 4-month wait time to evaluate for response.[15] Punch grafting for cicatricial alopecia can be used to optimize follicle survival due to less likely survival in scar tissue.[16] The risk of hypertrophic scars, keloids, and hyperpigmentation should be discussed with patients prior to surgery. The risk of keloids and hypertrophic scars can be reduced by prophylactic use of a mid-potency corticosteroid immediately postoperatively and a 2-week course of high-potency corticosteroid after suture removal.[16]

ACNE KELOIDALIS NUCHAE (Folliculitis Keloidalis)

▓ EPIDEMIOLOGY, ETIOLOGY, AND PATHOGENESIS

Acne keloidalis nuchae (AKN) was first described by Kaposi as *dermatitis papillaris capillitii*, and later Bazin coined the name *acne keloidalis nuchae*.[17,18] AKN is an acute folliculitis and perifolliculitis that becomes chronic and progresses into a primary cicatricial alopecia, occurring most commonly in African American men after puberty.[19] Onset prior to puberty or after age 50 years is extremely rare.[19] AKN represents 0.45% to 0.7% of dermatoses affecting patients of African origin.[19,20] No known cause of AKN has been elucidated, but there has been one case report of familial AKN, and one study found that 15% of AKN patients had a family history of AKN.[21,22]

Precipitating factors in AKN include constant irritation from shirt collars, chronic low-grade folliculitis, seborrhea, and hair grooming techniques.[23,24] Diphenylhydantoin and carbamazepine can produce folliculitis keloidalis-like lesions that resolve at cessation of therapy [**Figures 38-5 and 38-6**].

▓ CLINICAL FINDINGS

History The typical patient describes lesions that begin after a close haircut or appear gradually in the occipital scalp and posterior part of the neck, seemingly without precipitation. A thorough history should include duration of disease, frequency of flares, past therapeutic treatments and response, and hair grooming techniques.[19]

Physical Examination Firm, dome-shaped follicular and perifollicular papules on the nape of the neck and occipital scalp are typical findings [**Figure 38-6**]. Over time, the papules may coalesce into keloidal plaques with a bandlike distribution at or below the posterior hairline, with areas of polytrichia [**Figure 38-7**]. However, the condition can involve the entire scalp, leading to permanent alopecia[25,26] [**Figure 38-8**].

Laboratory and Other Tests Bacterial cultures and sensitivities from any pustular or draining lesions should be taken intermittently if there is no appropriate response to therapy. If pathogens are present, appropriate antibiotics should be prescribed. Potassium hydroxide (KOH) with fungal culture and assessment for cervical lymphadenopathy should be performed as clinically indicated and for nonresponsive cases.[27] Histopathologic evaluation is recommended for atypical presentations. Early papular lesions show chronic lymphocytic folliculitis.[6]

▓ DIFFERENTIAL DIAGNOSIS

- Dissecting cellulitis
- Tinea capitis
- Acne vulgaris
- Acneiform eruptions

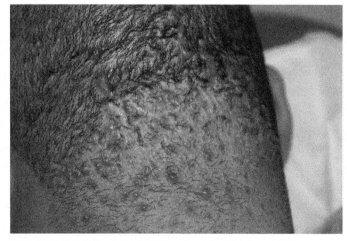

FIGURE 38-6. Folliculitis keloidalis in a male patient of Caucasian and African descent.

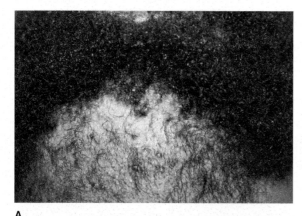

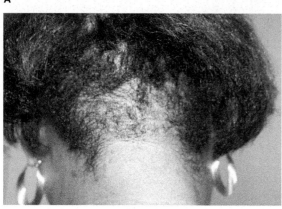

FIGURE 38-7. **(A)** Female patient with bandlike distribution of keloidalis folliculitis. **(B)** Female patient with folliculitis keloidalis and secondary infection.

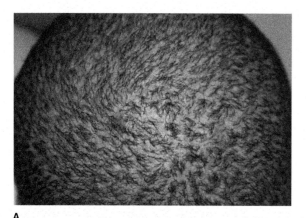

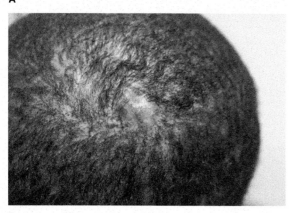

FIGURE 38-8. **(A)** Folliculitis keloidalis involving the entire scalp. **(B)** Keloidal scar at vertex scalp with long-term disease.

- Folliculitis
- Seborrheic dermatitis
- Traumatic keloids
- Folliculitis decalvans

COMPLICATIONS

- Secondary infection
- Disfiguring keloids
- Extension of disease

PROGNOSIS/CLINICAL COURSE

Large lesions can be painful and cosmetically unacceptable. Abscess and sinus formation are possible and may emit a foul odor. Coexistence of other forms of cicatricial alopecia may be observed.

TREATMENT [TABLE 38-2]

Medical There is no one therapeutic modality that cures AKN, and combination therapy is favored. Superpotent corticosteroids can be applied twice a day for 2 weeks and then tapered to a mid-potency agent for maintenance.[28] Corticosteroids in a foam or spray vehicle may be more cosmetically acceptable than creams, but the vehicle should be the patient's choice. Kelly[29] suggests that retinoic acid and a class II or III corticosteroid cream or gel base may be more effective than class I or II corticosteroids alone.

For control of pustules and inflammation, topical clindamycin (foam, gel, lotion, or solution) can be applied twice daily until the lesions subside. If there is no improvement, a bacterial culture and appropriate systemic antibiotics may be initiated. Large abscesses or draining sinuses may require a short course (7 to 10 days) of oral prednisone given concomitantly with systemic antibiotics. Treatment with imiquimod (Aldara) cream monotherapy for 5 days and then 2 days off for 8 weeks or in combination with pimecrolimus has been described.[29,30]

Intralesional steroid injections (10 to 40 mg/mL) administered directly into papules and plaques at 4- to 6-week intervals can be effective.[31] Patients should be warned that the injection sites may become hypopigmented, which may last for 6 to 12 months. An application of lidocaine-prilocaine cream or other topical anesthetic mixture under plastic film occlusion 2 hours prior to injection decreases the pain of injections.

Laser hair removal therapy (Nd:YAG or diode) has been successful for some patients. It is used to reduce hair growth and inflammation, and hair density will be permanently reduced.[32-34] Postoperative intralesional triamcinolone injections (10 mg/mL every 2 to 3 weeks) help to prevent recurrence.[35]

Cryotherapy also has proven to be successful in some patients. The area is frozen for 20 seconds, allowed to thaw, and then is frozen again a minute later. The morbidity (discomfort and drainage) is greater than with other modalities, and the treated site often becomes hypopigmented and may remain so for 12 to 18 months. When the thaw time is more than 25 seconds, melanocytes are destroyed, and

TABLE 38-2	Treatment of keloidalis folliculitis/acne keloidalis nuchae*
Superpotent corticosteroid gel or foam.	
Retin-A, Tazorac, and a class II–III corticosteroid.	
If infection suspected, start topical clindamycin foam, gel, or lotion.	
For abscesses and draining sinuses, prescribe a course of prednisone and antibiotics.	
Imiquimod.	
Intralesional steroid injections.	
Laser therapy—carbon dioxide, Nd:YAG, or diode.	
Adjunctive laser hair removal.	
Cryotherapy.	

*No one therapeutic modality will cure keloidalis folliculitis.

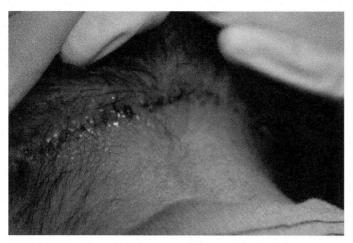

FIGURE 38-9. Excision with primary closure of folliculitis keloidalis.

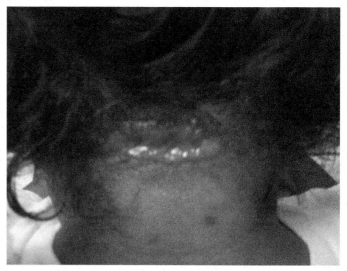

FIGURE 38-11. Excision and secondary-intention healing (4 weeks postoperatively).

the treated area often becomes hypopigmented, especially in patients with dark skin.[19]

Surgical Excision with primary closure is a surgical treatment modality for the management of extensive cases of AKN, and extremely large lesions may require excision in multiple stages.[36] Kelly recommends a horizontal ellipse for excision of larger linear lesions (1 cm or less in diameter) with primary closure. The base of the excision should extend below the hair follicles, and closure of the postoperative site should be done with 4-0 silk sutures[19,30] [**Figure 38-9**].

Excision with healing by secondary intention is an excellent option for large lesions that do not respond to medical therapy[37,38] [**Figures 38-10 to 38-12**]. A carbon dioxide (CO_2) laser in cutting mode has been successful in excising large plaques. Care must be taken to cut below the level of the hair follicles to the deep subcutaneous tissue, and the wound is left to heal by secondary intention.[35,39] Excision with grafting is not as cosmetically acceptable and is not recommended.[19]

PREVENTION

The first line of therapy is prevention. Patients should be counseled on preventative measures. Avoidance of close shaving at the hairline, tight-fitting shirts, helmets, or other possible irritation to the scalp is essential to prevent disease progression. As with all cicatricial alopecias, prompt and aggressive treatment should be initiated to prevent loss of viable hair follicles and to lower the chance of developing larger lesions.

DISSECTING CELLULITIS OF THE SCALP

EPIDEMIOLOGY, ETIOLOGY, AND PATHOGENESIS

This chronic inflammatory disorder of the scalp is most commonly seen in African American men in the second to fourth decades, although it is occasionally seen in females, Hispanics, Caucasians, and Asians.[40,41] There is an association with acne conglobata, hidradenitis suppurativa, and pilonidal cysts, known collectively as the *follicular occlusion tetrad*. The common pathogenesis is a destruction of hair follicles and hair follicle retention.

CLINICAL FINDINGS

History/Physical Examination Dissecting cellulitis is characterized by painful nodules, purulent discharge, burrowing interconnecting abscesses, and cicatricial alopecia. Boggy areas with pustules, nodules, discharge swelling, and patchy hair loss are seen [**Figure 38-13**]. Cerebriform configurations can be a late-term result resembling cutis verticis gyrata.

Laboratory and Other Tests Bacterial cultures and sensitivity or fungal cultures from any pustular or draining lesions should be taken if superinfection is suspected. If pathogens are present, appropriate antimicrobials should be prescribed.

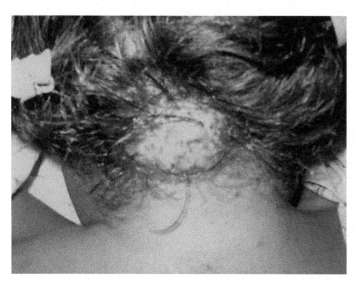

FIGURE 38-10. Excision and secondary-intention healing (preoperative).

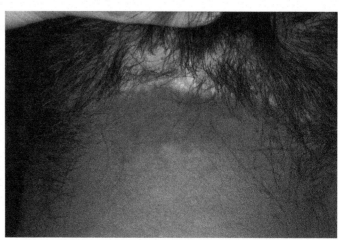

FIGURE 38-12. Excision and secondary-intention healing (4 months postoperatively).

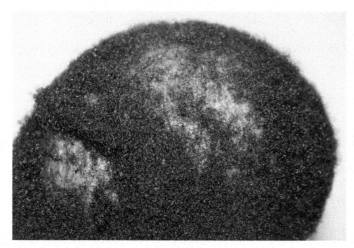

FIGURE 38-13. Dissecting cellulitis of the scalp.

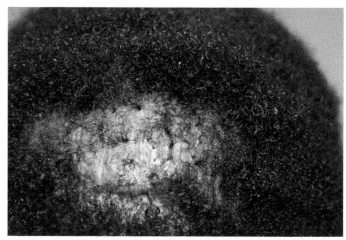

FIGURE 38-14. Tufted folliculitis. Fully developed lesions have up to 8 to 14 hairs emerging from an apparently common dilated follicular opening.

DIFFERENTIAL DIAGNOSIS

- Tinea capitis
- Hidradenitis suppurativa
- Folliculitis
- Folliculitis decalvans
- Cutis verticis gyrata

COMPLICATIONS

Hair loss can become permanent, and hypertrophic scars and keloids can develop on the scalp. Marjolin ulcers are possible in areas of chronic inflammation.

TREATMENT

Treatment of dissecting cellulitis is tailored to the extent and location of disease. Therapeutic modalities include:

- Topical corticosteroids
- Intralesional corticosteroids
- Systemic corticosteroids[42]
- Antibiotics
- Dapsone
- Isotretinoin[43,44]
- Oral zinc[41]
- External-beam radiation-induced epilation
- Incision and drainage
- Laser-assisted hair epilation
- CO_2 laser[45]
- Wide surgical excision with split-thickness grafting[46]

PREVENTION

Scalp hygiene for mild to limited cases and prompt treatment to salvage viable hair follicles constitute prevention strategies.

FOLLICULITIS DECALVANS

EPIDEMIOLOGY, ETIOLOGY, AND PATHOGENESIS

Folliculitis decalvans is a form of recurrent, patchy, painful folliculitis of the scalp causing scarring and hair loss. *Staphylococcus aureus* has been implicated as an etiologic agent.[47] Sperling et al[48] contend that pustules of folliculitis decalvans are a manifestation of either bacterial superinfection or an intense immune response to degenerating follicular components, and they classified folliculitis decalvans as a subset of CCCA. This condition affects men and women from young adulthood to middle age.

CLINICAL FINDINGS

Physical Examination Early lesions consist of small areas of perifollicular erythema and pustules. The process extends centrifugally, resulting in patches of cicatricial alopecia. Fully developed lesions consist of tufts of hair with 8 to 14 hairs emerging from an apparently common dilated follicular opening[49] [**Figure 38-14**]. These tufted follicles are a late-stage feature that can be seen with a variety of inflammatory alopecias including chronic cutaneous lupus, dissecting cellulitis of the scalp, and AKN.[50]

Laboratory and Other Tests Bacterial cultures and sensitivity should be performed when pustules are present. KOH and fungal cultures should be performed from noninflamed sites at baseline if nonresponsive to therapy and prior to use of systemic corticosteroids.

DIFFERENTIAL DIAGNOSIS

- Kerion (tinea capitis)
- Dissecting cellulitis
- Folliculitis
- AKN
- Lichen planopilaris (follicular)

COMPLICATIONS

- Secondary infection with abscesses and draining sinuses
- Disfiguring keloids
- Cicatricial alopecia
- Tufted folliculitis

PROGNOSIS/CLINICAL COURSE

Treatment, as in most cicatricial alopecias, is difficult. Patients should be counseled that there is no treatment for the permanent eradication of the disease.

TREATMENT

Treatment with oral rifampicin 300 mg twice daily and oral clindamycin 300 mg twice daily for 10 weeks has been shown to lead to significant improvement and no further extension of lesions.[13] Patients treated with oral clindamycin should be warned about the risk for pseudomembranous colitis. Due to the rapid emergence of resistance, it is not advisable to use rifampicin alone.[47] Depending on patient tolerance, clindamycin may be substituted with oral ciprofloxacin, 750 mg twice daily, or cephalexin, 500 mg four times daily, or doxycycline, 100 mg twice daily, along with rifampicin.[13] Those who are *Staphylococcus* carriers should have their nasal area treated with mupirocin.[13] Fusidic acid and zinc have been reported to be effective in a limited number of patients.[51]

PREVENTION

Scalp hygiene for mild to limited cases and prompt treatment to salvage viable hair follicles are prevention strategies.

LICHEN PLANOPILARIS, FRONTAL FIBROSING ALOPECIA, AND FIBROSING ALOPECIA IN A PATTERN DISTRIBUTION

EPIDEMIOLOGY, ETIOLOGY, AND PATHOGENESIS

The prevalence of lichen planopilaris (LPP) and its clinical variants is not known. Classic LPP is usually seen in women with a mean age of 50 years,[52] although men may be affected, and Caucasians are more commonly affected than individuals of color. Research suggests the role of the peroxisome proliferator-activated receptor-γ (PPAR-γ) in the pathogenesis of LPP. PPAR-γ is required for maintenance of a functional epithelial stem cell compartment in murine hair follicles.[53] The targeted deletion of PPAR-γ leads to skin findings that resemble LPP, and subsets of LPP patients demonstrate gene expression changes that indicate a defect in lipid metabolism and peroxisome biogenesis.[53] This new knowledge has had treatment implications with the recent use of PPAR-γ agonists (eg, thiazolidinediones) in certain subsets of patients.[54]

CLINICAL FINDINGS

Physical Examination LPP is a Cicatricial alopecia with characteristic perifollicular erythema and perifollicular scale at the margins of the areas of alopecia [**Figure 38-15**]. A positive pull test of anagen hairs is commonly present at the margin, indicating disease activity. Fifty percent of patients with LPP lack evidence of lichen planus at sites other than the scalp.

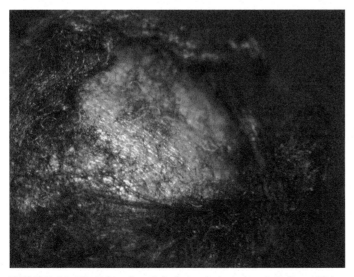

FIGURE 38-15. Lichen planopilaris. Patient had no systemic findings of lichen planus.

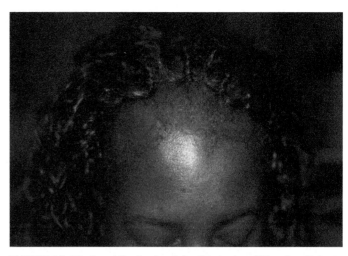

FIGURE 38-16. Frontal fibrosing alopecia is a clinical variant of lichen planopilaris.

Frontal fibrosing alopecia is a progressive subtype that affects postmenopausal women, although the pathogenesis seems to be unrelated to hormone replacement status.[55] It is characterized by a band of frontal/frontoparietal hair alopecia and a marked decrease or complete loss of the eyebrows [**Figure 38-16**].

Fibrosing alopecia in a pattern distribution is considered to be a variant of LPP that presents with rapidly progressive hair loss of the central scalp of women and men with underlying pattern hair loss.[56] Clinical findings are similar to LPP, located on the central scalp, with perifollicular scale, atrophy, and erythema. The overall picture appears as a mixed cicatricial and nonscarring alopecia, with evidence of pattern hair loss also possibly noted. Biopsy diagnosis is most helpful in suspected cases.

Laboratory and Other Tests

- Histopathologic examination
- Hepatitis panel

DIFFERENTIAL DIAGNOSIS

- Central centrifugal scarring alopecia
- Chronic cutaneous lupus
- Folliculitis decalvans
- End-stage cicatricial alopecia of various inflammatory alopecias
- Sarcoidosis
- Androgenetic alopecia
- Traction alopecia

PROGNOSIS/CLINICAL COURSE

Many patients develop hair, nail, and/or mucous membrane lesions similar to LPP lesions. The lesions of LPP may involute spontaneously or go on for years. Mehregan et al[57] reported that the average duration is 18 months.

TREATMENT

The goal of treatment is to control symptomology and halt the progression of the disease. High-potency topical and intralesional corticosteroids are the mainstay of treatment for primary symptoms and have a positive effect on hair regrowth in the active perimeter of the alopecic patch.[57] Additional therapies that may be used based on the amount of inflammation and/or involvement, as well as the rapidity of progression, are briefly reviewed below.

- Tetracyclines
- Hydroxychloroquine 200 mg twice daily[13]

- Mycophenolate mofetil 0.5 g twice daily and increased to 1 g twice daily for 5 months[13]
- Cyclosporine 3 to 5 mg/kg/d (usually 300 mg/d)[13,58]
- Finasteride (2.5 mg/d) showed an arrest in the progression of the disease in frontal fibrosing alopecia.[59]
- Thalidomide[60]
- Pioglitazone
- Scalp reduction and hair transplants can be used during the inactive stage.

CHRONIC CUTANEOUS LUPUS

▧ EPIDEMIOLOGY

Chronic cutaneous lupus erythematosus occur more frequently in African American women and is a cause of secondary alopecia (cicatricial) [**Figure 38-17**]. Discoid lupus erythematosus is a form of chronic lupus erythematosus that commonly affects the scalp and results in cicatricial alopecia. Females are more commonly affected than males with age of onset typically 20 to 40 years.[61] Only 5% to 10% of adults with discoid lupus erythematosus develop systemic lupus erythematous. The incidence of alopecia areata in patients with lupus erythematosus is increased in comparison to the general population.[62,63]

▧ CLINICAL FINDINGS

Physical Examination Annular lesions with central hypopigmentation and/or erythema and peripheral hyperpigmentation are common in discoid lupus erythematosus. Follicular plugging is typically seen, sometime referred to as "carpet tacking." Active lesions may be tender and itchy and may worsen after ultraviolet exposure.[64] Areas of involvement typically include the scalp, but it may occur on any part of the body, especially sun-exposed areas.

Laboratory Findings Scalp biopsies are often diagnostic. A thorough history and physical examination with antinuclear antibodies, complete blood count, and urinalysis should be carried out in every patient diagnosed with discoid lupus erythematosus.

▧ TREATMENT

Treatment of lupus may include oral corticosteroids, and for localized cutaneous disease, topical or intralesional corticosteroids can be very effective. Hydroxychloroquine and other systemic agents such as azathioprine, chlorambucil, methotrexate, and cyclosporine have been used with varying results.

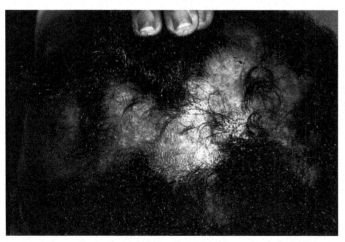

FIGURE 38-17. Scarring alopecia in a African American woman with discoid lupus erythematosus.

▧ PREVENTION

Patients with lupus should be counseled regarding the need for strict photoprotective measures. Tobacco use should be avoided while on hydroxychloroquine therapy.

NONSCARRING ALOPECIAS

TRACTION ALOPECIA

▧ EPIDEMIOLOGY, ETIOLOGY, AND PATHOGENESIS

Traction alopecia (TA) is seen with increased prevalence in African American men, women, and children [**Figure 38-18**]. African American hairstyling techniques can predispose this population to hair shaft damage from traction.[1,65] Weaves, braids, locks, cornrows, rubber band use, and other styles can predispose patients to TA. Early disease presents as a folliculitis and, if the traction is sustained, can progress to cicatricial alopecia.[15]

▧ CLINICAL FINDINGS

Physical Examination Perifollicular papules and pustules may be present at symmetric areas of traction. The bitemporal area is described most commonly [**Figure 38-19**]. The entire scalp may be involved, and this is dictated by the hairstyling technique. Hair casts can be seen with severe cases of traction, and vellus hairs are spared [**Figure 38-20**].

Histopathology The acute stage is reversible and resembles a mild form of trichotillomania.[50] Fibrosis in the area where terminal follicles were located with a normal number of vellus hairs is considered diagnostic for irreversible (late) TA.[27]

▧ DIFFERENTIAL DIAGNOSIS

- Ophiasis (alopecia areata)
- Androgenetic hair loss (female- and male-pattern hair loss)
- CCCA
- Tinea capitis

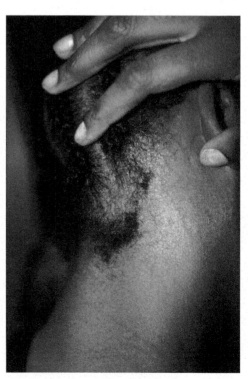

FIGURE 38-18. Early traction alopecia in a child.

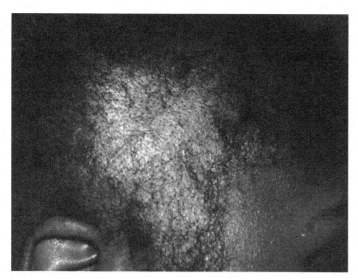

FIGURE 38-19. Late traction alopecia.

TREATMENT

Patients with TA should avoid styles that promote traction. Topical antibiotics (eg, topical clindamycin) with a topical corticosteroid can be used for early papule lesions. Other treatments include:

- Oral antibiotics
- Topical minoxidil
- Intralesional corticosteroids

Follicular unit transplantation, rotation flaps, minigrafting, and micrografting are therapeutic options[15,66] [**Figures 38-21 and 38-22**].

PREVENTION

Educating patients on avoiding hair care practices that promote tension can be curative if the process is caught in early stages.

ANDROGENETIC ALOPECIA (MALE-/FEMALE-PATTERN HAIR LOSS)

EPIDEMIOLOGY, ETIOLOGY, AND PATHOGENESIS

Pattern hair loss is the most common type of hair loss in men and affects more than 55% of women over the age of 70.[67] This type of hair loss occurs in genetically susceptible individuals secondary to the presence of androgens at the level of the hair follicle. Androgen receptors

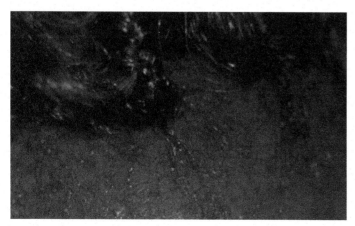

FIGURE 38-20. Peribulbar casts with extreme traction. Vellus hairs are attached to braid/weave style, worsening alopecia and contributing to complete hair loss.

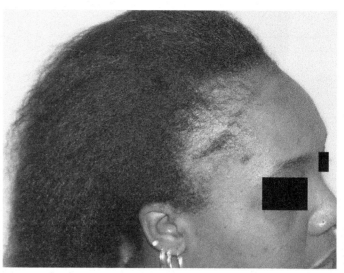

FIGURE 38-21. Hair transplant for traction alopecia (before). (Used with permission from Craig Ziering, MD.)

expressed within the dermal papilla and hair bulb bind testosterone, or dihydrotestosterone (DHT), which binds with a five-fold greater affinity than testosterone.[68] The conversion of testosterone to DHT is mediated by 5α-reductase (types 1 and 2), and the presence of DHT is thought to be required for pattern hair loss.[69] Androgen-sensitive hair follicles are located on the frontal and vertex scalp, accounting for the pattern noted in male-pattern hair loss.

Although androgens play a major a role in male-pattern hair loss, their role in female-pattern loss has not been clearly established. Female-pattern hair loss has been described in androgen insensitivity syndromes,[70] and although it can be associated with hyperandrogenic states, it often occurs in women with normal androgen levels. Estrogen signaling modifies androgen metabolism at the follicle and may explain the differences in male- and female-pattern hair loss.[71] The enzyme cytochrome P450 aromatase converts testosterone into estradiol and estrone, which reduces conversion of testosterone into DHT.[71,72] This enzyme is found in higher concentrations in the hair follicles of women, in particular the frontal and occipital scalp.[71,72] This may explain the preservation of the frontal hairline in women. In addition, woman have 40% fewer androgen receptors than men, and have 3 to 3.5 times less 5α-reductase than men.[71-73]

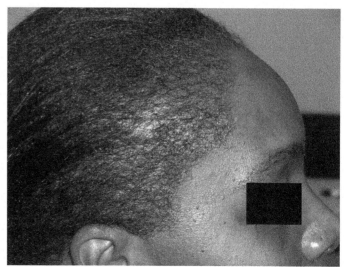

FIGURE 38-22. Hair transplant for traction alopecia (after). (Used with permission from Craig Ziering, MD.)

CLINICAL FINDINGS

History/Physical Examination In men, hair loss usually involves recession of the frontotemporal hairline, as well as nonscarring hair loss of the vertex of the scalp. Occipital scalp hair is retained. Women typically maintain the frontal hairline, with thinning on the vertex of the scalp, typified by widening of the central part. The Norwood-Hamilton classification system divides male-pattern hair loss into seven stages according to severity. The Ludwig classification divides female-pattern hair loss into three stages according to severity.

African American men may display different hair-loss patterns than Caucasian men. It has been observed that African American men predominantly exhibit scalp hair loss on the vertex of the scalp. A cicatricial alopecia presentation in African American men may be due to the biphasic nature or follicular dropout of pattern hair loss; this can also be an undiagnosed primary cicatricial alopecia.

Laboratory and Other Tests Pattern hair loss is usually diagnosed clinically by examination of hair and scalp. Biopsy may be considered in cases where clinical evidence of scarring alopecia is present. In women with other clinical findings of androgen excess such as hirsutism, menstrual abnormalities, or severe acne, laboratory analysis of dehydroepiandrosterone (DHEA) sulfate and testosterone may be obtained.

DIFFERENTIAL DIAGNOSIS

- Diffuse alopecia areata
- Telogen effluvium

TREATMENT

For Men and Women

- Minoxidil (2% to 5% lotion, solution, or foam applied one to two times daily)[68]
- Finasteride (1 to 5 mg by mouth daily)[74]
- Dutasteride (0.25 to 0.5 mg by mouth daily)
- Combination therapy (minoxidil and finasteride or dutasteride as above)
- Surgical—hair restoration
- Laser therapy (excimer laser, laser hair growth devices)
- Camouflage

For Women

- Spironolactone (100 to 200 mg orally per day)[75,76]
- Flutamide (62.5 to 250 mg orally once daily)[77,78]
- Combination therapy (ketoconazole 2% shampoo and finasteride as above)

Potential adverse events include impotence, decreased libido, breast tenderness and enlargement, and hypertrichosis. Additionally, pregnancy category D or X classification of some of these treatments necessitates discussion with patients.

ALOPECIA AREATA

EPIDEMIOLOGY, ETIOLOGY, AND PATHOGENESIS

Alopecia areata (AA) has a prevalence of 0.1% to 0.2%, with a lifetime prevalence of 1.7%.[79] Both women and men are equally affected, and AA is believed to affect all races equally.[79] Approximately 20% of all patients affected are children, and only 20% are above the age of 40.[80] The exact pathophysiology of AA remains unknown, but the most commonly accepted hypothesis is that AA is a T-cell–mediated autoimmune condition that occurs most frequently in genetically predisposed individuals.

CLINICAL FINDINGS

Physical Examination Typical areas of involvement are sharply demarcated, round, smooth, nonscarring patches of alopecia. Areas of involvement may be mildly inflamed clinically but are usually asymptomatic. Occasionally, symptoms such as burning, pain, or pruritus may occur. These patches are often found incidentally secondary to the asymptomatic nature of the hair loss. At the periphery of or within patches, exclamation point hairs (hairs that are tapered proximally and wider distally) may be found. The hair pull test may be positive at the periphery of active lesions.[81]

AA may be classified based on the amount and location of hair loss[81]:

- Patchy AA: partial loss of scalp hair
- AA totalis: total loss of scalp hair
- AA universalis: total loss of scalp and body hair
- AA ophiasis pattern: bandlike hair loss of the occipitotemporal scalp
- AA sisapho: bandlike hair loss of the frontotemporal scalp

Nail pitting is the most common nail finding[82,83] associated with AA, but other nail findings such as trachyonychia, thinning or thickening, koilonychias, or onychomadesis have been described.[81]

Associated Conditions Some autoimmune diseases occur with increased frequency with AA. Autoimmune thyroid disease is most commonly described, with an incidence of between 8% and 28%.[84] Although vitiligo occurs in only 1% of the general population, it occurs in about 3% to 9% of AA patients.[84]

Histopathology This diagnosis rarely requires biopsy for confirmation and can be made based on clinical findings. In cases where diagnosis is uncertain, biopsy may reveal a peribulbar lymphocytic infiltrate, likened to "a swarm of bees." In addition, a decrease in terminal hairs and increase in vellus hairs may be seen, with a ratio of 1.1:1 (normal is 7:1).

PROGNOSIS/CLINICAL COURSE

Extensive hair loss, ophiasis pattern, presence of other autoimmune disorders, nail involvement, and young age at first onset are poor prognostic factors and may indicate prolonged course.[85] However, the course is unpredictable, with up to 50% of patients recovering within a year without treatment.[81] Most patients (~85%) will have more than one episode of hair loss.[86]

DIFFERENTIAL DIAGNOSIS

- Male-/female-pattern hair loss
- Syphilis
- Trichotillomania
- Tinea capitis
- Telogen effluvium
- Frontal fibrosing alopecia

TREATMENT

- Topical corticosteroids
- Topical minoxidil
- Intralesional corticosteroids
- Anthralin (0.5% to 1.0% used as short contact therapy applied daily for 15 to 20 minutes initially and then washed off; contact time should be increased by 5 to 10 minutes weekly up to 1 hour, or until irritation occur)
- Topical immunotherapy (diphenylcyclopropenone, squaric acid dibutylester)
- Bimatoprost
- Phototherapy (psoralen with ultraviolet A [PUVA])

- Excimer laser
- Systemic therapies (oral glucocorticoids, sulfasalazine, cyclosporine, azathioprine, methotrexate)

CONCLUSION

The skin of color patient who presents with alopecia have a vexing clinical problem. Proper diagnostic techniques and use of current classification guidelines will aid the physician in determining appropriate treatment plans. Early diagnosis is the key to prevent loss of viable hair follicles.

REFERENCES

1. Halder RM. Hair and scalp disorders in blacks. *Cutis.* 1983;32:378-380.
2. Alexis AF, Sergay AB, Taylor SC. Common dermatologic disorders in skin of color: a comparative practice survey. *Cutis.* 2007;80:387-394.
3. Olsen EA, Callender V, McMichael A, et al. Central hair loss in African American women: incidence and potential risk factors. *J Am Acad Dermatol.* 2011;64:245-252.
4. Olsen EA, Bergfeld WF, Cotsarelis G, et al. Summary of North American Hair Research Society (NAHRS)-sponsored Workshop on Cicatricial Alopecia, Duke University Medical Center, February 10 and 11, 2001. *J Am Acad Dermatol.* 2003;48:103-110.
5. Sperling LC. Scarring alopecia and the dermatopathologist. *J Cutan Pathol.* 2001;28:333-342.
6. Sperling LC, Cowper SE. The histopathology of primary cicatricial alopecia. *Semin Cutan Med Surg.* 2006;25:41-50.
7. Dlova NC, Forder M. Central centrifugal cicatricial alopecia: possible familial aetiology in two African families from South Africa. *Int J Dermatol.* 2012;51(Suppl 1):17-20, 20-23.
8. Callender VD, Wright DR, Davis EC, Sperling LC. Hair breakage as a presenting sign of early or occult central centrifugal cicatricial alopecia: clinicopathologic findings in 9 patients. *Arch Dermatol.* 2012;148:1047-1052.
9. Martin ES, Elewski BE. Tinea capitis in adult women masquerading as bacterial pyoderma. *J Am Acad Dermatol.* 2003;49(2 Suppl Case Reports):S177-S179.
10. Quinn CKAP. Prevalence of undiagnosed hair and scalp disorders in African-American women presenting to an adult dermatology clinic. Presented at L'Oréal 2nd International Symposium: Ethnic Skin and Hair: New Directions in Research, Chicago, IL, 2003.
11. Horenstein MG, Simon J. Investigation of the hair follicle inner root sheath in scarring and non-scarring alopecia. *J Cutan Pathol.* 2007;34:762-768.
12. Deyampart NM, Taylor S. Central centrifugal alopecia. *J Am Acad Dermatol.* 2004;xx:90s.
13. Price VH. The medical treatment of cicatricial alopecia. *Semin Cutan Med Surg.* 2006;25:56-59.
14. Taylor S. Practical tips for managing hair disorders in African-American females. *Pract Dermatol.* 2006;3:25-27.
15. Callender VD, McMichael AJ, Cohen GF. Medical and surgical therapies for alopecias in black women. *Dermatol Ther.* 2004;17:164-176.
16. V. C. Hair transplant surgery in the treatment of alopecia in women of color. Presented at L'Oréal 2nd International Symposium: Ethnic Skin and Hair: New Directions in Research. Chicago, IL, 2003.
17. Kaposi M. Ueber die sogennante framboesia und mehrere andere arten von papillaren neubildungen der haut. *Arch Dermatol Syphilol.* 1869;1:382-423.
18. Cosman B, Wolff M. Acne keloidalis. *Plast Reconstr Surg.* 1972;50:25-30.
19. Satter EK. Acne keloidalis nuchae. *E-medicine Journal.* www.emedicine.com/derm/topic558.htm. Accessed May 30, 2006.
20. Adegbidi H, Atadokpede F, Do Ango-Padonou F, Yedomon H. Keloid acne of the neck: epidemiological studies over 10 years. *Int J Dermatol.* 2005;44(Suppl 1):49-50.
21. D'Souza P, Iyer VK, Ramam M. Familial acne keloidalis. *Acta Derm Venereol.* 1998;78:382.
22. George AO, Akanji AO, Nduka EU, Olasode JB, Odusan O. Clinical, biochemical and morphologic features of acne keloidalis in a black population. *Int J Dermatol.* 1993;32:714-716.
23. Khumalo NP, Jessop S, Ehrlich R. Prevalence of cutaneous adverse effects of hairdressing: a systematic review. *Arch Dermatol.* 2006;142:377-383.
24. Azurdia RM, Graham RM, Weismann K, Guerin DM, Parslew R. Acne keloidalis in caucasian patients on cyclosporin following organ transplantation. *Br J Dermatol.* 2000;143:465-467.
25. Grunwald MH, Ben-Dor D, Livni E, Halevy S. Acne keloidalis-like lesions on the scalp associated with antiepileptic drugs. *Int J Dermatol.* 1990;29:559-561.
26. Sellheyer K, Bergfeld WF. Histopathologic evaluation of alopecias. *Am J Dermatopathol.* 2006;28:236-259.
27. Sterling JB, Sina B, Gaspari A, Deng A. Acne keloidalis: a novel presentation for tinea capitis. *J Am Acad Dermatol.* 2007;56:699-701.
28. Callender VD, Young CM, Haverstock CL, Carroll CL, Feldman SR. An open label study of clobetasol propionate 0.05% and betamethasone valerate 0.12% foams in the treatment of mild to moderate acne keloidalis. *Cutis.* 2005;75:317-321.
29. Kelly AP. Pseudofolliculitis barbae and acne keloidalis nuchae. *Dermatol Clin.* 2003;21:645-653.
30. Barr J, Friedman A. Use of imiquimod and pimecrolimus cream in the treatment of acne keloidalis nuchae. *J Am Acad Dermatol.* 2005;52:590.
31. McMichael AJ. Scalp and hair disorders in African-American patients: a primer of disorders and treatments. *Cosmet Dermatol.* 2003;16:37-41.
32. McMichael AJ. Hair and scalp disorders in ethnic populations. *Dermatol Clin.* 2003;21:629-644.
33. Battle EF Jr, Hobbs LM. Laser-assisted hair removal for darker skin types. *Dermatol Ther.* 2004;17:177-183.
34. Valeriant M, Terracina FS, Mezzana P. Pseudofolliculitis of the neck and the shoulder: a new effective treatment with alexandrite laser. *Plast Reconstr Surg.* 2002;110:1195-1196.
35. Kantor GR, Ratz JL, Wheeland RG. Treatment of acne keloidalis nuchae with carbon dioxide laser. *J Am Acad Dermatol.* 1986;14(2 Pt 1):263-267.
36. Gloster HM Jr. The surgical management of extensive cases of acne keloidalis nuchae. *Arch Dermatol.* 2000;136:1376-1379.
37. Glenn MJ, Bennett RG, Kelly AP. Acne keloidalis nuchae: treatment with excision and second-intention healing. *J Am Acad Dermatol.* 1995;33(2 Pt 1):243-246.
38. Califano J, Miller S, Frodel J. Treatment of occipital acne keloidalis by excision followed by secondary intention healing. *Arch Facial Plast Surg.* 1999;4:308-311.
39. Jackson BA. Lasers in ethnic skin: a review. *J Am Acad Dermatol.* 2003;48(6 Suppl):S134-S138.
40. Stites PC, Boyd AS. Dissecting cellulitis in a white male: a case report and review of the literature. *Cutis.* 2001;67:37-40.
41. Kobayashi H, Aiba S, Tagami H. Successful treatment of dissecting cellulitis and acne conglobata with oral zinc. *Br J Dermatol.* 1999;141:1137-1138.
42. Adrian RM, Arndt KA. Perifolliculitis capitis: successful control with alternate-day corticosteroids. *Ann Plast Surg.* 1980;4:166-169.
43. Scerri L, Williams HC, Allen BR. Dissecting cellulitis of the scalp: response to isotretinoin. *Br J Dermatol.* 1996;134:1105-1108.
44. Schewach-Millet M, Ziv R, Shapira D. Perifolliculitis capitis abscedens et suffodiens treated with isotretinoin (13-cis-retinoic acid). *J Am Acad Dermatol.* 1986;15:1291-1292.
45. Glass LF, Berman B, Laub D. Treatment of perifolliculitis capitis abscedens et suffodiens with the carbon dioxide laser. *J Dermatol Surg Oncol.* 1989;15:673-676.
46. Bellew SG, Nemerofsky R, Schwartz RA, Granick MS. Successful treatment of recalcitrant dissecting cellulitis of the scalp with complete scalp excision and split-thickness skin graft. *Dermatol Surg.* 2003;29:1068-1070.
47. Powell JJ, Dawber RP, Gatter K. Folliculitis decalvans including tufted folliculitis: clinical, histological and therapeutic findings. *Br J Dermatol.* 1999;140:328-333.
48. Sperling LC, Solomon AR, Whiting DA. A new look at scarring alopecia. *Arch Dermatol.* 2000;136:235-242.
49. Annessi G. Tufted folliculitis of the scalp: a distinctive clinicohistological variant of folliculitis decalvans. *Br J Dermatol.* 1998;138:799-805.
50. Sperling LC. *An Atlas of Hair Pathology with Clinical Correlations.* New York, NY: Parthenon; 2003:23.
51. Abeck D, Korting HC, Braun-Falco O. Folliculitis decalvans. Long-lasting response to combined therapy with fusidic acid and zinc. *Acta Derm Venereol.* 1992;72:143-145.
52. Chiergato C, Zini A, Barba A, et al. Lichen planopilaris: report of 30 cases and review of the literature. *Int J Dermatol.* 2003;74:784-786.
53. Karnik P, Tekeste Z, McCormick TS, et al. Hair follicle stem cell-specific PPARgamma deletion causes scarring alopecia. *J Invest Dermatol.* 2009;129:1243-1257.
54. Harries MJ, Paus R. Scarring alopecia and the PPAR-gamma connection. *J Invest Dermatol.* 2009;129:1066-1070.
55. Kossard S, Lee MS, Wilkinson B. Postmenopausal frontal fibrosing alopecia: a frontal variant of lichen planopilaris. *J Am Acad Dermatol.* 1997;36:59-66.

56. Zinkernagel MS, Trueb RM. Fibrosing alopecia in a pattern distribution: patterned lichen planopilaris or androgenetic alopecia with a lichenoid tissue reaction pattern? *Arch Dermatol.* 2000;136:205-211.

57. Mehregan DA, Van Hale HM, Muller SA. Lichen planopilaris: clinical and pathologic study of forty-five patients. *J Am Acad Dermatol.* 1992;27(6 Pt 1): 935-942.

58. Mirmirani P, Willey A, Price VH. Short course of oral cyclosporine in lichen planopilaris. *J Am Acad Dermatol.* 2003;49:667-671.

59. Tosti A, Piraccini BM, Iorizzo M, Misciali C. Frontal fibrosing alopecia in postmenopausal women. *J Am Acad Dermatol.* 2005;52:55-60.

60. George SJ, Hsu S. Lichen planopilaris treated with thalidomide. *J Am Acad Dermatol.* 2001;45:965-966.

61. Wilson CL, Burge SM, Dean D, et al. Scarring alopecia in discoid lupus erythematosus. *Br J Dermatol.* 1992;126:307-314.

62. Werth VP, White WL, Sanchez MR, Franks AG. Incidence of alopecia areata in lupus erythematosus. *Arch Dermatol.* 1992;128:368-371.

63. Katta R, Nelson B, Chen D, Roenigk H. Sarcoidosis of the scalp: a case series and review of the literature. *J Am Acad Dermatol.* 2000;42:690-692.

64. Whiting DA. Cicatricial alopecia: clinicopathological findings and treatment. *Clin Dermatol.* 2001;19:211-215.

65. LoPresti P, Papa CM, Kligman AM. Hot comb alopecia. *Arch Dermatol.* 1968;98:234-238.

66. Earles RM. Surgical correction of traumatic alopecia marginalis or traction alopecia in black women. *J Dermatol Surg Oncol.* 1986;12:78-82.

67. Gan DC, Sinclair RD. Prevalence of male and female pattern hair loss in Maryborough. *J Invest Dermatol.* 2005;10:184-189.

68. Banka N, Bunagan MJ, Shapiro J. Pattern hair loss in men: diagnosis and medical treatment. *Dermatol Clin.* 2013;31:129-140.

69. Kaufman KD. Androgens and alopecia. *Mol Cell Endocrinol.* 2002;198:89-95.

70. Cousen P, Messenger A. Female pattern hair loss in complete androgen insensitivity syndrome. *Br J Dermatol.* 2010;162:1135-1137.

71. Sawaya ME, Price VH. Different levels of 5alpha-reductase type I and II, aromatase, and androgen receptor in hair follicles of women and men with androgenetic alopecia. *J Invest Dermatol.* 1997;109:296-300.

72. Shapiro J, Price VH. Hair regrowth. Therapeutic agents. *Dermatol Clin.* 1998;16:341-356.

73. Vierhapper H, Maier H, Nowotny P, Waldhausl W. Production rates of testosterone and of dihydrotestosterone in female pattern hair loss. *Metabolism.* 2003;52:927-929.

74. Drake L, Hordinsky M, Fiedler V, et al. The effects of finasteride on scalp skin and serum androgen levels in men with androgenetic alopecia. *J Am Acad Dermatol.* 1999;41:550-554.

75. Sinclair R, Wewerinke M, Jolley D. Treatment of female pattern hair loss with oral antiandrogens. *Br J Dermatol.* 2005;152:466-473.

76. Camacho-Martinez FM. Hair loss in women. *Semin Cutan Med Surg.* 2009;28:19-32.

77. Rogers NE, Avram MR. Medical treatments for male and female pattern hair loss. *J Am Acad Dermatol.* 2008;59:547-566.

78. Yazdabadi A, Sinclari R. Treatment of female pattern hair loss with the androgen receptor antagonist flutamide. *Australas J Dermatol.* 2011;52:132-134.

79. Safavi KH, Muller SA, Suman VJ, Moshell AN, Melton LJ III. Incidence of alopecia areata in Olmsted County, Minnesota, 1975 through 1989. *Mayo Clinic Proc.* 1995;70:628-633.

80. Lu W, Shapiro J, Yu M, et al. Alopecia areata: pathogenesis and potential for therapy. *Exp Rev Mol Med.* 2006;8:1-19.

81. Alkhalifah A, Alsantali A, Wang E, McElwee KJ, Shapiro J. Alopecia areata update. Part I. Clinical picture, histopathology, and pathogenesis. *J Am Acad Dermatol.* 2010;62:177-188.

82. Gandhi V, Baruah M, Bhattacharaya S. Nail changes in alopecia areata: incidence and pattern. *Indian J Dermatol Venereol Leprol.* 2003;69:114-115.

83. Kasumagic-Halilovic E, Prohic A. Nail changes in alopecia areata: frequency and clinical presentation. *J Eur Acad Dermatol Venereol.* 2009;23:240-241.

84. Seyrafi H, Akhiani M, Abbasi H, Mirpour S, Gholamrezanezhad A. Evaluation of the profile of alopecia areata and the prevalence of thyroid function test abnormalities and serum autoantibodies in Iranian patients. *BMC Dermatol.* 2005;5:11.

85. Lew B-L, Shin M-K, Sim W-Y. Acute diffuse and total alopecia: a new subtype of alopecia areata with a favorable prognosis. *J Am Acad Dermatol.* 2009;60:85-93.

86. Finner AM. Alopecia areata: clinical presentation, diagnosis, and unusual cases. *Dermatol Ther.* 2011;24:348-354.

CHAPTER 39

Pseudofolliculitis Barbae

A. Paul Kelly
Ana Maria Anido Serrano

KEY POINTS

- Pseudofolliculitis barbae (PFB) is a common dermatologic disorder of the hair follicles affecting people with skin of color who shave.

- Darkly pigmented men with coarse, tightly curled hair are especially affected by PFB.

- The primary lesions of PFB are papules and pustules in the beard area that cause cosmetic disfigurement, including scarring, postinflammatory hyperpigmentation, secondary infection, and keloid formation.

- Chronic PFB of the shaved areas may produce fine linear depressed scars, also known as grooves.

- The anterior neck, submandibular chin, and lower jaw are the next most common areas for PFB.

- Therapy for PFB with over-the-counter depilatories and/or specific shaving techniques has been used with success, as have topical combination creams.

- Hair-removal lasers and electrolysis increasingly are used for the treatment of PFB and are showing great effectiveness when used in combination with topical treatment.

SYNONYMS

- Shave bumps
- Razor bumps
- Barber's bumps
- Barber's itch
- Ingrown hairs
- Folliculitis barbae traumatica
- Sycosis barbae
- Pili incarnati
- Chronic scarring pseudofolliculitis of the Negro beard.

INTRODUCTION

Pseudofolliculitis barbae (PFB) is a common inflammatory skin problem affecting up to 60% of people with skin of color who have coarse, tightly curled hair and shave close to the skin[1] [**Figure 39-1**]. It can occur in any race and in either sex. In addition to the beard area, the pubic area [**Figure 39-2**], scalp, and legs also may develop PFB, particularly if they are shaved often.

Strauss and Kligman[2] coined the term pseudofolliculitis barbae in 1956. PFB is particularly troubling for affected men, especially those in the military,[3] law enforcement, or occupations that require workers to be clean shaven.

EPIDEMIOLOGY AND PATHOGENESIS

In a randomly sampled test population of 156 individuals at two U.S. Army hospitals in Germany, a much higher incidence of PFB was noted in the skin of color population (82%) as compared to the Caucasian population (18%).[4] These finding were felt to be within the previously reported PFB occurrence range of 45% to 85% in the skin of color population.[5] However, PFB can occur in any race and in either sex regardless of whether the person has dark pigmentation.[5]

The pathogenesis of this disorder has been shown to involve both transfollicular and extrafollicular penetration of the skin by a hair.

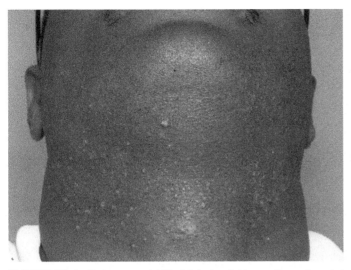

FIGURE 39-1. Moderate pseudofolliculitis barbae (with more than a dozen but less than 100 papules and pustules) of the chin and neck of a darkly pigmented man.

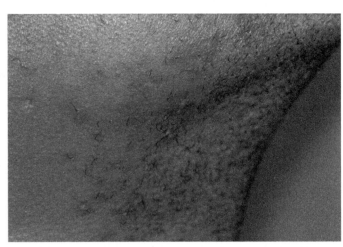

FIGURE 39-3. A darkly pigmented man with coarse, tightly curled hair and mild pseudofolliculitis barbae (fewer than a dozen papules) of the right anterior neck and cheek. Note the loop hairs that penetrate the skin.

With shaving, the razor produces short, sharp, and pointed hairs that penetrate the skin either in an extra- or transfollicular manner. Tightly curled hair is usually cut at an oblique angle, creating a sharp tip at the distal end that enables the hair to penetrate the skin 1 to 2 mm from where it exits the follicle. Once the hair penetrates the dermis, an inflammatory reaction ensues. Hair growth usually continues into the dermis, reaching a depth of 2 to 3 mm. In the dermis, it produces an even greater inflammatory reaction, manifested by pustules and papules. The hair reaches the length of 10 mm after a growth period of up to 6 weeks. At this point, a spring action occurs that pulls out the embedded tip.

Cutting the hair against the grain and pulling the skin taunt and then releasing can cause the hair to retract below the surface of the skin and then grow in a curved manner, piercing the follicular wall (transfollicular penetration). Inflammatory papules develop when the curving hair tips penetrate the hair follicle or the surrounding epidermis[5] [**Figure 39-3**]. Papules with hairs in the center may become infected. Complications from chronic PFB may result in hypertrophic scars [**Figure 39-4**] and keloids [**Figures 39-5 and 39-6**]. On occasion, cutaneous sarcoidosis may develop within the scarred areas.[6]

Through a family study and a large-scale investigation of 156 randomly sampled individuals affected and unaffected by PFB, it was

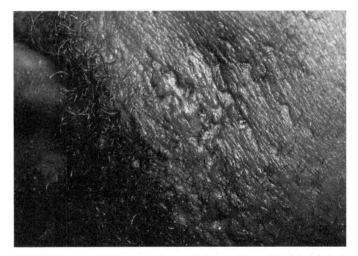

FIGURE 39-4. A darkly pigmented man with hypertrophic scarring of the left cheek secondary to chronic pseudofolliculitis barbae that he has had for more than 20 years. The patient also displays grooving, which can prevent the removal of hair with standard shaving techniques.

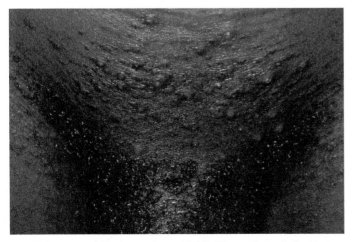

FIGURE 39-2. A darkly pigmented man with folliculitis secondary to shaving his suprapubic area.

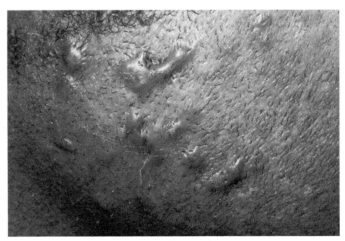

FIGURE 39-5. Small keloids secondary to pseudofolliculitis barbae in a man with skin of color.

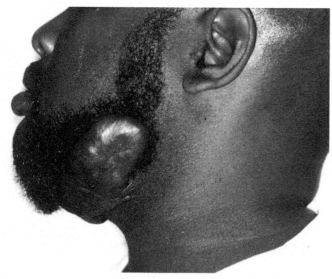

FIGURE 39-6. A large keloid secondary to pseudofolliculitis barbae on a darkly pigmented man's left cheek and submental area.

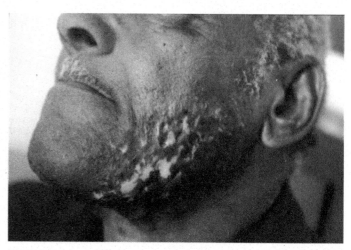

FIGURE 39-7. Moderate pseudofolliculitis barbae of the anterior neck of a darkly pigmented man; note the postinflammatory hypopigmentation.

demonstrated that an unusual single-nucleotide polymorphism, which gives rise to a disruptive Ala12Thr substitution in the 1A α–helical segment of the companion layer-specific keratin (K6hf) of the hair follicle, is partially responsible for the phenotypic expression and represents an additional genetic risk factor for the disorder.

A hair shaft is surrounded by several layers, including the outer root sheath (ORS), the companion layer, and the inner root sheath (IRS). The companion layer/IRS complex constitutes a functional tissue unit that tightly surrounds the hair shaft and serves to guide as well as stabilize the ascending hair. It is conceivable that mutations in the K6hf keratin may disturb both the mechanical integrity of companion layer cells and their firm attachment to the IRS and thus lead to a functionally compromised companion layer/IRS unit.

This compromised unit may no longer be able to tightly guide and protect the hair on its movement to the skin surface. With the PFB-associated curved hair follicle, both pressure and traction exerted on the skin by regular and close shaving may represent the mechanical stress that activates the deleterious nature of the K6hf Ala12Thr polymorphism. This may result in destabilized pointed hairs in the hair channel leaving the follicular orifice in a less than optimal manner and consequently growing back into concave skin areas of the submental or submandibular region.[4]

CLINICAL FINDINGS

The diagnosis of PFB is made on clinical grounds, based on the location and types of lesions present. There is general consensus among dermatologists that the diagnosis is easily made.[7] Erythematous, skin-colored, or hyperpigmented papules in a follicular distribution are the characteristic lesion of PFB.[8] Lesions range in size from 2 to 4 mm, and often the hair can be seen within the papule. Patients with chronic PFB may have grooved, linear, depressed patterns on the skin that occur as a result of parallel hair growth [Figure 39-4], preventing the removal of hairs by standard shaving techniques.

Pustules and papulopustules are thought to be secondary lesions that occur as a result of infection with *Staphylococcus epidermidis*. Pathogenic microorganisms, although less common, are sometimes recovered on culture and should be treated appropriately.

In a study by Perry et al,[8] 90.1% of patients reported hyperpigmentation, suggesting that postinflammatory hyperpigmentation is a major clinical finding in PFB. However, a few patients develop hypopigmentation in the areas of involvement [Figure 39-7]. The severity of PFB ranges from mild, with less than a dozen papules or

pustules, to severe, particularly on the neck of men and the chin of women[8] [Figures 39-8 to 39-10].

SYMPTOMS

A randomized, controlled study by Daniel et al[9] investigated the symptoms of a population of 90 male PFB subjects consisting of 69% African American, 30% Caucasian, and 1% multiracial subjects with a mean age of 38.8 years (± 10.9 years). In a questionnaire, the study participants reported four main symptoms that occurred after shaving. The intensity of the preshaving symptoms was not reported. The symptoms occurred either at each PFB papule or diffusely over the skin. The four primary symptoms associated with PFB were itching (61.11%), burning/stinging (67.78%), pain (1.11%), and cuts (33.33%).

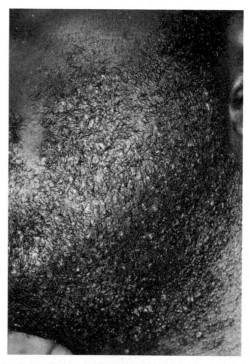

FIGURE 39-8. Profile of a darkly pigmented man with severe/chronic pseudofolliculitis barbae; present are numerous papulopustules, grooving, and postinflammatory hyperpigmentation of the left cheek. (Used with permission from Yvonne Knight, MD, Richmond, VA.)

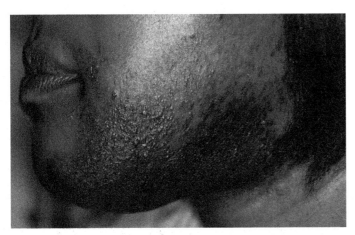

FIGURE 39-9. Moderate pseudofolliculitis barbae of the left cheek in a darkly pigmented woman with postinflammatory hyperpigmentation.

DIFFERENTIAL DIAGNOSIS

- Acne vulgaris
- Folliculitis
- Traumatic folliculitis
- Tinea barbae
- Sarcoidosis
- Keloids
- Hypertrophic scars

A distinguishing feature of PFB as compared to acne vulgaris is the absence of comedones. Also, acne is common on non–hair-bearing, nonshaved areas, unlike PFB. When cultured, the pustules that characterize folliculitis will be positive for bacteria, whereas only secondarily infected PFB lesions will have positive cultures. Traumatic folliculitis, also caused by shaving too closely, presents with inflammation of the follicle without evidence of infection and follicular penetration. Lesions of PFB are isolated, whereas those of tinea barbae are confluent and often unilateral. Although sycosis barbae papules may resemble PFB, Halder et al noted that shaving improves the condition but makes PFB worse.[7]

COMPLICATIONS

- Scarring
- Hyperpigmentation
- Hypopigmentation

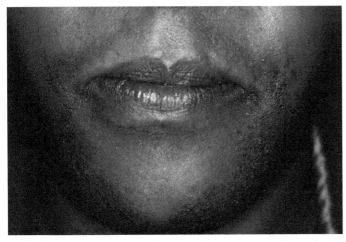

FIGURE 39-10. The female patient from Figure 39-9 showing pseudofolliculitis barbae with postinflammatory hyperpigmentation of the chin and medial cheeks.

- Hypotrophic scars
- Keloids
- Sarcoidal-like lesions

CLINICAL COURSE AND PROGNOSIS

The prognosis and clinical course of PFB may be variable. People with skin of color who have coarse, tightly curled hair and who shave have a greater susceptibility to PFB and there is a greater likelihood that the disease will worsen. Treatment plans, as discussed later in this chapter, are not fail-safe. The prognosis is not good unless the patient either stops shaving or has begun treatment early enough to stop the progression of PFB. The only 100% effective preventive measure is to discontinue shaving, which is not an alternative for many patients.

TREATMENT

Before initiating therapy, counsel patients on the cause of PFB, warning that the only complete cure is cessation of shaving or depilation.[10] However, if a patient must shave, instruct the patient on optimal shaving techniques. Ensure that the patient understands that the purpose of therapy is to control, not cure, PFB.

■ TOPICAL AGENTS

Glycolic Acid Perricone[11] published two studies that consisted of two placebo-controlled trials in 35 adult men. The results showed that glycolic acid lotion was significantly more effective than a placebo in treating PFB. There was over a 60% reduction in lesions on the treated side, which allowed daily shaving with little irritation. The author concluded that topical application of glycolic acid lotion is an effective therapy for PFB and allows the patient to resume a daily shaving regimen.

Tretinoin Kligman and Mills[12] studied the efficacy of a 0.05% solution of tretinoin applied nightly, which they evaluated in 11 early cases of moderately severe pseudofolliculitis of the beard and in 27 cases of pseudofolliculitis in older subjects, including some with long-standing cases of extreme severity. All had numerous papulopustules scattered on the neck and beard area. One fifth of the second group had severe disease with large indolent papules and much crisscross scarring.

Daily application of tretinoin was uniformly helpful for early-stage patients, producing good to excellent results within 8 weeks with reduction in papules, although without total resolution. A total of 19 out of 27 patients with moderate cases of long-standing PFB benefited to the same degree as those in the initial stages. Patients with severe PFB responded poorly, with four not responding and four having only slight improvement. Topically applied neomycin 0.5%, applied after the tretinoin to one side of the face of eight patients in the severe group, added no benefit to the result. Relapse occurred within 2 weeks after stopping treatment, although twice-weekly application resulted in sustained improvement in some of the younger subjects.[12]

Benzoyl Peroxide 5%/Clindamycin 1% Gel In a multicenter, double-blind pilot study performed by Cook-Bolden et al,[13] men with 16 to 100 combined papules and pustules on the face and neck were randomized to receive twice-daily benzoyl peroxide 5%/clindamycin 1% (BP/C) gel (n = 47) or vehicle (n = 41) for 10 weeks. A total of 68 (77.3%) of the participants were darker skin of color and were required to shave at least twice a week and use a standardized shaving regimen throughout the study. Clinical evaluations were performed at 2-week intervals.

The primary efficacy parameter was the percentage change from baseline in lesion counts. At weeks 2, 4, and 6, mean percentage reductions from baseline in combined papule and pustule counts were significantly greater with BP/C gel compared with vehicle ($P \leq 0.029$). Treatment differences in favor of active therapy were more pronounced in the subpopulations of darker skin of color patients, with least squares mean percentage reductions in papule and pustule counts ranging from 38.2% at week 2 to 63.9% at week 10. Study medication was well tolerated.[13]

■ OTHER TREATMENTS

There has been a limited amount of published data on shaving outcomes as they relate to clinically measurable PFB responses and patient satisfaction scoring. Current shaving recommendations for PFB include avoidance of shaving if possible and, when it is not possible, shaving with a singe-bladed razor in the direction of hair growth at least every 3 days. In a randomized, controlled trial of shaving methods on a population of 90 male PFB subjects (69% African American, 30% Caucasian, and 1% multiracial) by Daniel et al,[9] there were three treatment groups who were evaluated at baseline, week 6, and week 12: (1) 30 subjects in the control group shaved two to three times per week with a standard three-blade razor and standard gentle shaving products including soap, moisturizer, and basic shaving gel for sensitive skin; (2) 30 subjects in the daily standard group shaved daily with a five-blade razor and used the same gentle shaving products as the standard group; and (3) 30 subjects in the daily advanced group shaved daily with a five-blade razor and used advanced products including a pre-shaving facial wash, pre shaving gel, and post shaving lotion. The results revealed the following:

- Compared to baseline, there was a significant mean papule reduction detected for the control and daily advanced groups.

- Compared to baseline, there was a significant reduction in ingrown hairs for the control group and a directional reduction in the daily advanced group.

- The control group experienced significantly fewer ingrown hairs than both daily shaving groups (average reduction of 15 ingrown hairs from baseline).

- The control group experienced a significant baseline reduction in pustules and papules, and the daily advanced group had significant improvement in the baseline number of papules.

- The control and daily advanced groups experienced significant improvement in investigator-graded assessment of severity from baseline.

- From an objective standpoint of grading severity, daily shaving appeared as good as the more commonly recommended shaving regimen of two to three times per week.

- Subjective results revealed a better perceived response to treatment in the daily advanced versus the control group with less itching and burning/stinging in the daily advanced group compared with the daily standard and control groups, and patients seemed to have a more comfortable shaving experience with using the advanced product line.

- Increasing the number of blades was associated with a significant reduction in ingrown hair count and an improvement in investigator-graded severity scores and subjective response to treatment; however, there was a subjective increase in itching with increasing number of blades.

- Subjects who shaved against the grain had fewer papules.

Electrolysis is a somewhat tedious, long-term procedure in which a needle is inserted into the hair follicle, an electric current delivered, and the hair destroyed. In darkly pigmented patients with curved hair follicles, the standard electrolysis needle often penetrates the follicle before reaching and destroying the hair bulb. This may predispose to transfollicular penetration. Postinflammatory hyperpigmentation and mild scarring may result, especially in darkly pigmented patients.

Surgical depilation is a modality for permanent hair removal. Hage and Bowman[14] performed a retrospective review of the first 40 patients undergoing surgical depilation for PFB or local hirsutism of the face. Operations were performed from 1973 to 1988 on 4 males, 24 females, and 12 male-to-female transsexuals with a mean age of 33.6 years. Two patients were African American, and 38 were Caucasian. PFB was the presenting symptom in seven females, four males, and one transsexual. The surgery consisted of undermining the skin in all directions and

manually everting when making a submandibular incision. The hair roots were exposed and cut using serrated scissors. Postoperative pressure garments or injections of triamcinolone (to prevent scar formation) were instituted. In addition, some patients had electrical depilation to maximize results. This procedure is expensive, and scarring, including keloidal scars, can develop in patients.

Radiation resulting in temporary epilation can relieve the symptoms of PFB and provide an opportunity for the skin to improve before instituting other therapeutic modalities. Permanent epilation is contraindicated because of the high incidence of skin cancer, which may develop 10 to 25 years later.

When these procedures are not affordable or are impractical, other therapeutic measures are available to attenuate the disease while allowing the patient to shave. Except for mild cases, PFB requires medical intervention during the acute pustular phase, which is often painful and/or pruritic.

Cryotherapy in the form of a liquid nitrogen cryospray administered to cause a light peel is often helpful. A 10- to 15-second thaw time is usually sufficient. Freezing for longer than 25 seconds produces hypopigmentation, which may last 1 year or more.

Chemical peels, containing glycolic acid and other α-hydroxy acids, can be used to reduce hyperkeratosis of the follicular infundibulum and thickening of the stratum corneum.[11] This in turn allows the hair to grow out straighter and makes shaving easier. Topical or systemic antibiotics may be necessary to treat secondary infection.

Laser therapy also has proven effective, although in the past, it was considered controversial. Kauvar[15] claimed that more than 50% of darkly pigmented patients treated with a diode laser improved. Other researchers[16] reported a significant decrease in hair growth with long-pulsed diode laser treatment without signs of epidermal damage. Weaver and Sagaral[17] reported that the long-pulse neodymium-doped yttrium aluminium garnet (Nd:YAG) laser with continuous-contact cooling was a safe and effective means of treatment for PFB in both men and women with darker skin.[17] Ross et al[18] also agreed that the treatment of PFB in skin types IV, V, and VI with an Nd:YAG laser represented a safe and effective option for reducing papule formation. Because the long-pulsed Nd:YAG laser is more painful, the patient may need a topical anesthetic before therapy. The 810-diode laser seems better for lighter skin, and the 1064 nm Nd:YAG laser seems more appropriate for more darkly pigmented patients. Whatever type of laser is used, dyspigmentation, scarring, crusting, and blistering still may develop; however, the incidence is decreased and posttreatment side effects are reportedly low.[19]

New therapies using topical applications and lasers in combination are showing promising results. Xia et al[20] have shown that use of a combination of long-pulsed Nd:YAG laser and topical eflornithine hydrochloride significantly decreases hairs and inflammatory papules when compared to hair laser therapy alone.

Intense pulse light therapy (IPL) offers another line of treatment, although the effects are short-lived. In a study by Leheta[21] comparing Alexandrite laser therapy with IPL, it was found that both systems were effective, but that the Alexandrite laser was more effective at reducing the papules than IPL.

Historically, the management of PFB focused on home-based procedures like the modification of shaving procedures and the application of depilatory creams. Epilation and electrolysis were the mainstays for medical therapy. Fortunately, there are now more viable options to help patients with coarse curly hair. The new mainstay of therapy includes many treatment options that are less invasive and more effective.

The authors recommend the following therapeutic approach for PFB patients[10]:

1. Advise patients to discontinue shaving for 1 month for mild cases, 2 to 3 months for moderate cases, and 3 to 6 months for severe cases. During this shaving hiatus, beards can be trimmed with scissors or electric clippers to a minimum length of 1 cm. Inform the patient that the PFB probably will get worse initially after the first week of not shaving, when the shaved hairs are long enough to penetrate the skin, creating more lesions.

2. Apply a warm water, saline, or Burow's solution compress for 10 to 15 minutes three times a day to soothe the lesions, remove the crust, stop drainage secondary to inflammation, and soften the epidermis, allowing for the easier and earlier release of ingrown hairs.

3. After compressing and releasing the ingrown hairs, apply a topical hydrocortisone cream or lotion (for 3 to 4 weeks only) to the shaved area.

4. When secondary bacterial infection is present, prescribe a systemic antibiotic. In cases that do not improve with these steps, a therapeutic approach of a 5- to 10-day regimen of prednisone (40 to 60 mg/day) may be used, provided there are no contraindications. Shaving should not be resumed until all the inflamed lesions have cleared and all the ingrown hairs have been released.

For those who must shave, this author advises the following daily regimen:

1. Ingrown hairs should not be plucked because they may cause irritation or may grow and eventually penetrate the follicular wall.

2. Use electric clippers to remove as much preexisting beard hair as possible without causing irritation.

3. Wash the beard area with a washcloth and then massage with a soft tooth brush or polyester sponge.

4. Rinse the beard area to remove any remaining soap. Apply warm water compresses for approximately 5 minutes.

5. Use any brand of shaving cream, making sure not to let the lather dry. If for any reason it dries, reapply the lather before shaving.

6. Choose a sharp razor that cuts best without irritation. There are shavers on the market made especially for PFB, which interested patients can find through the Internet. Specific PFB foil-guarded razors have been reported to cause a significant reduction in the number of PFB lesions.[22] Electric shavers also seem to help those with mild to moderate PFB.

7. Shave with the grain of the hair, using short strokes while avoiding pulling the skin taut. Twice over one area is usually sufficient.

8. After shaving, rinse the face with warm tap water and then compress with cool water for approximately 5 minutes.

9. Use a magnifying mirror to search for any ingrown hairs. To release them gently, insert a toothpick under the loop or brush the beard area with a soft toothbrush.

10. Apply the most soothing and least irritating aftershave preparation. If burning or itching ensues, a topical hydrocortisone preparation can be used after the aftershave lotion.

11. In those areas where hair growth is haphazard (eg, the anterior neck and submandibular area), daily brushing of the beard often gives direction to the grain of the hair. Take care to avoid nicks and cuts to prevent traumatic folliculitis.

Those who find that shaving worsens their PFB or that shaving is too irritating may use chemical depilatories. The two basic types are barium sulfide and calcium thioglycolate preparations, both found in powder, lotion, cream, and paste forms. They work by lysing disulfide bonds in the hair. This results in hair with a softer, more brushlike tip, making extrafollicular and transfollicular penetration much more difficult.

Barium sulfide preparations must be mixed with water before being applied as a paste and often leave an odor. Calcium thioglycolate preparations can remain on the skin longer without causing irritation and do not have an offensive odor.

Because embedded hair tips are not affected by depilatories, it usually takes several weeks before an improvement is evident. Advise the patient before using a chemical depilatory to apply a small amount to a hair-bearing area on the forearm, leave it on for 5 to 10 minutes, and then wash it off with soap and water. If irritation develops on the test area within 48 hours, the depilatory should not be used on the face or on any area with PFB.

TABLE 39-1	Summary of pseudofolliculitis barbae (PFB)

First reported by Strauss and Kligman in 1956

The most common symptoms are shave bumps, razor bumps, or folliculitis

Etiology and pathogenesis:
- PFB is a chronic inflammatory disease that is caused by shaved hairs that have been cut at an oblique angle and subsequently grow back into the skin
- Found mainly in darkly pigmented men with coarse, tightly curled hair
- There is transfollicular and extrafollicular penetration

Clinical findings:
- Occurs after puberty but before age 50
- Foreign-body inflammatory reaction surrounding an ingrown hair
- Postinflammatory hyperpigmentation or keloids can result from PFB

Differential diagnosis:
- Folliculitis or acne vulgaris
- Sarcoidosis

Prevention and treatment:
- The only 100% effective preventative treatment is to discontinue shaving
- Electric shavers may help because they do not cut as close to the skin as manual blades
- Over-the-counter foil-guard safety razors may be a treatment option
- Although sometimes difficult for patients to tolerate, chemical depilatories can be used
- Electrolysis may not be effective on curved hair follicles

Complications:
- Once PFB grooves, scars, or hyperpigmentation appear, the skin does not return to normal
- Laser destruction of the hair follicles may cause scarring

One adjunct to shaving is topical tretinoin, especially early in the onset of the disease. It is thought to work by alleviating hyperkeratosis and toughening the skin.[12] The use of tretinoin does not alter the previously described shaving regimen.

Another product that can function as an adjunct for all of the previously mentioned therapeutic regimens is the eflornithine hydrochloride cream 13.8% described by Xia et al[20] used in combination with a laser. Eflornithine hydrochloride cream inhibits ornithine decarboxylase, a major enzyme involved in hair cell division, and slows the rate of hair growth. When used topically, it is applied twice a day and washed off 4 hours after application. Some patients, however, may develop irritant contact dermatitis as a result of use.

CONCLUSION

PFB is a disorder of the beard that affects a large number of individuals, particularly those who have coarse curly hair and shave. It also may develop in women and on any hair-bearing area that is closely and frequently shaved [**Table 39-1**]. The only permanent cures are growing the hair or depilation. All other treatments are aimed at controlling symptoms. An important part of the therapeutic regimen is patient education.

REFERENCES

1. Gottlieb JS, Skopit SE, Del Rosso JQ. Pseudofolliculitis barbae. www.aocd.org/skin/dermatologic_diseases/pseudofolliculitis.html. Accessed December 25, 2012.

2. Strauss JS, Kligman AM. Pseudofolliculitis of the beard. *AMA Arch Derm*. 1956;74:533-542.

3. Alexander AM, Delph WI. Pseudofolliculitis barbae in the military. A medical, administrative and social problem. *J Natl Med Assoc*. 1974;66:459-464, 479.

4. Winter H, Schissel D, Parry DAD, et al. An unusual Ala12Thr polymorphism in the 1A alpha-helical segment of the companion layer-specific keratin K6hf: evidence for a risk factor in the etiology of the common hair disorder pseudofolliculitis barbae. *J Invest Dermatol*. 2004;122:652-657.

5. Coley MK, Alexis AF. Dermatologic conditions in men of African ancestry. *Expert Rev Dermatol.* 2009;4:595.

6. Norton SA, Chesser RS, Fitzpatrick JE. Scar sarcoidosis in pseudofolliculitis barbae. *Mil Med.* 1991;156:369-371.

7. Halder RM, Roberts CI, Noothetic PK, Kelly AP. Dermatological disease in blacks. In: Halder RM, ed. *Dermatology and Dermatological Therapy of Pigmented Skin.* Boca Raton, FL: Taylor & Francis; 2004:405.

8. Perry P, Cook-Bolden FE, Rahman Z, et al. Defining pseudofolliculitis barbae in 2001: a review of the literature and current trends. *J Am Acad Dermatol.* 2002;46:3113-3119.

9. Daniel A, Gustafson CJ, Zupkosky PJ, et al. Shave frequency and regimen variation effects on the management of pseudofolliculitis barbae. *J Drugs Dermatol.* 2013;12:410-418.

10. Kelly AP. Pseudofolliculitis barbae. In: Arndt KA, LeBoit P, LeBiot PR, et al, eds. *Cutaneous Medicine and Surgery: An Integrated Program in Dermatology.* Philadelphia, PA: WB Saunders; 1996:499-502.

11. Perricone NV. Treatment of pseudofolliculitis barbae with topical glycolic acid: a report of two studies. *Cutis.* 1993;52:232-235.

12. Kligman AM, Mills OH. Pseudofolliculitis of the beard and topically applied tretinoin. *Arch Dermatol.* 1973;107:551-552.

13. Cook-Bolden FE, Barba A, Halder R, Taylor S. Twice-daily applications of benzoyl peroxide 5%/clindamycin 1% gel versus vehicle in the treatment of pseudofolliculitis barbae. *Cutis.* 2004;73(6 Suppl):18-24.

14. Hage JJ, Bowman FG. Surgical depilation for the treatment of pseudofolliculitis or local hirsutism of the face: experience in the first 40 patients. *Plast Reconstr Surg.* 1991;88:446-451.

15. Kauvar AN. Treatment of pseudofolliculitis with a pulsed infrared laser. *Arch Dermatol.* 2000;136:1343-1346.

16. Jackson BA, Junkins-Hopkins J. Long-pulse diode laser treatment for hair removal in dark skin: clinicopathologic correlation (abstract). Presented at Ethnic Hair and Skin: What Is the State of the Science Conference, Chicago, IL, September 29-30, 2001.

17. Weaver S, Sagaral E. Treatment of pseudofolliculitis barbae using a long-pulse Nd:YAG laser (abstract). Presented at Ethnic Hair and Skin: What Is the State of the Science Conference, Chicago, IL, September 29-30, 2001.

18. Ross EV, Cooke LM, Timko AL, et al. Treatment of pseudofolliculitis barbae in skin types IV, V, and VI with a long-pulsed neodymium:yttrium aluminum garnet laser. *J Acad Dermatol.* 2002;47:263-270.

19. Haedersdal M, Wulf HC. Evidence-based review of hair removal using lasers and light sources. *J Eur Acad Dermatol Venereol.* 2006;20:9-20.

20. Xia Y, Cho S, Howard RS, et al. Topical eflornithine hydrochloride improves the effectiveness of standard laser hair removal for treating pseudofolliculitis barbae: a randomized, double-blinded, placebo-controlled trial. *J Am Acad Dermatol.* 2012;67:694-699.

21. Leheta TM. Comparative evaluation of long pulse Alexandrite laser and intense pulsed light systems for pseudofolliculitis barbae treatment with one year of follow up. *Indian J Dermatol.* 2009;54:364-368.

22. Alexander AM. Evaluation of a foil-guarded shaver in the management of pseudofolliculitis barbae. *Cutis.* 1981;27:534-542.

- Lichen planus may cause irreversible scarring nail disease. Prompt treatment is imperative.

- Lichen planus and psoriasis may both exist as a primary nail disease without cutaneous disease.

- Psoriasis of the nail unit is difficult to treat primarily because of poor medication bioavailability.

- Onychomycosis is the most common nail disorder.

Examination of the nails is an important part of the dermatologic examination in every skin phototype. There are very few unique nail changes and nail diseases in patients with darker skin phototypes. Nail unit melanocytes are usually quiescent in all skin types, and the clinical appearance of nails of different skin phototypes is closer than perhaps any other cutaneous structure [**Figure 40-1**]. This chapter highlights the examination of nails in skin of color, featuring melanonychia and nail apparatus melanoma (NAM). Other common nail disorders including lichen planus, psoriasis, and onychomycosis will also be covered.

MELANONYCHIA

Melanonychia, or melanin-derived brown to black nail pigmentation, is an ambiguous clinical finding representing a diagnostic challenge for clinicians. Although the most serious disease of the nail unit, melanoma, presents with melanonychia in roughly two-thirds of cases, melanonychia also occurs as a result of other etiologies such as nail matrix melanocytic activation, benign nail matrix melanocytic hyperplasia, and nail invasion by melanin-producing pathogens.[1] In addition, other nail pathogens, exogenous substances, and subungual hemorrhage can cause nonmelanic brown to black nail pigmentation.[1-3]

Regrettably, patients with NAM are often initially misdiagnosed.[2] Due to diagnostic delays of an average of 2 years, NAM carries a poor prognosis, with reported 5- and 10-year survival rates of 30% and 13%, respectively.[4,5] Some experts also contend that melanomas of the nail unit are more aggressive malignancies that metastasize earlier than cutaneous melanoma, with worse survival rates, stage for stage and thickness for thickness, than cutaneous melanomas.[6,7] A thorough knowledge of the various causes of melanonychia and the use of a systematic approach when evaluating brown to black nail pigmentation may help prevent misdiagnosis and thereby improve prognosis.

PHYSIOLOGY

Nail plate melanin is primarily generated by nail matrix melanocytes.[2,8] Activated matrix melanocytes produce and then transfer

Nail Disorders

CHAPTER **40**

Julie Jefferson
Phoebe Rich

KEY POINTS

- Longitudinal melanonychia (LM) is common in darker skin types, usually as a result of melanocyte activation.

- Atypical LM may indicate nail apparatus melanoma (NAM).

- Evaluation of LM for NAM includes a detailed history and physical examination, examination of all 20 nails, use of dermoscopy, and often a nail matrix biopsy.

- NAM has a worse prognosis than its cutaneous counterpart in large part due to delayed diagnosis.

- Lichen planus commonly causes LM in persons of color.

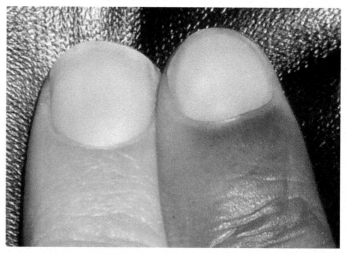

FIGURE 40-1. Skin phototype II (left) and V (right) index fingernails. The nail bed color is identical despite the different finger skin colors.

melanin-containing melanosomes by way of dendrites to differentiating nail matrix-derived onychocytes.[2,8] This process usually results in a longitudinal band of melanonychia, but rarely, total or transverse melanonychia can occur.[2,8,9] Importantly, melanonychia usually originates from the distal nail matrix.[2,8] Active (and dormant) distal nail matrix melanocytes lie in the first and second germinative layers, whereas most proximal nail matrix melanocytes lie dormant in the lower two to four germinative cell layers.[2,8] The etiologies of melanonychia can be divided into two broad categories: melanocytic activation and melanocytic hyperplasia (proliferation).[1-3]

MELANOCYTIC ACTIVATION

Melanocytic activation (also termed *functional melanonychia* or *melanocytic stimulation*) describes the process by which melanonychia results from increased melanic pigmentation of the nail matrix epithelium and nail plate without a concurrent increase in the number of melanocytes.[2] Persons with darker phototypes are predisposed to the activation and production of melanin.[10] Approximately 73% of adult cases of single-digit longitudinal melanonychia (LM) occur as a result of melanocytic activation.[2,11] There are many documented causes of this harmless melanocytic activation, including physiologic, local and regional, dermatologic, systemic, iatrogenic, and syndromic causes [**Table 40-1**].[2,12]

Physiologic Causes Physiologic causes of melanonychia include pregnancy and racial melanonychia.[2] Melanonychia is far more common in darkly pigmented individuals than Caucasians. Individuals with darkly pigmented skin such as African Americans, Hispanics, Asians, and Middle Easterners, often have multiple benign longitudinal pigmented bands in their nails, and the number and width frequently increase with age.[2,4,13] Nearly all African Americans develop one or more pigmented bands by 50 years of age [**Table 40-2**].[2]

Local and Regional Causes When melanonychia is associated with abnormalities of the nail plate or the periungual tissues, frictional trauma, onychotillomania, nail biting, and carpal tunnel syndrome should be explored as potential etiologies.[2,14] In particular, frictional melanonychia, an entity first described by Baran, is the most common cause of melanocytic activation for all races.[2,15] Hence, pigmented bands are most often located in the nails of digits used for grasping, such as the thumb, index finger, and middle finger, and in those digits prone to trauma, such as the great toe.[2] When melanonychia is symmetric and affects the lateral and external part of the fourth or fifth toenail and great toenail, repeated trauma from ill-fitting shoes or overriding toes is a probable cause [**Figure 40-2**].[2,15]

Dermatologic Causes Inflammation secondary to amyloidosis, chronic radiodermatitis, onychomycosis, paronychia, psoriasis, and lichen planus can cause melanocytic activation resulting in melanonychia.[2] Sometimes melanonychia is observed after an inciting inflammatory process has resolved because nails have a relatively slow growth rate compared to the surrounding skin.[2] In addition, melanocytic activation has been documented to occur in conjunction with a number of nonmelanocytic tumors and disorders including onychomatricoma,[16] Bowen disease,[17] myxoid pseudocyst,[13] basal cell carcinoma,[13] subungual fibrous histiocytoma,[13] verruca vulgaris,[13] and rarely subungual linear keratosis.[9,18]

Systemic Causes Systemic causes of melanocytic activation include acquired immunodeficiency syndrome (AIDS); alkaptonuria; the endocrine disorders Addison disease, Cushing syndrome, hyperthyroidism, and Nelson syndrome; graft-versus-host disease; hemosiderosis; hyperbilirubinemia; nutritional disorders; and porphyria.[2,13] Melanonychia secondary to systemic causes is generally characterized by multiple bands involving both fingernails and toenails. Melanonychia associated with AIDS, Addison disease, and nutritional disorders is regularly accompanied by mucosal and cutaneous pigmentation.[2,19]

Iatrogenic Causes Causes of iatrogenically induced melanocytic activation include medications (especially chemotherapeutic agents),[20-22]

TABLE 40-1	Causes of melanocytic activation

Physiologic Causes
Pregnancy
Racial melanonychia

Local and Regional Causes
Carpal tunnel syndrome
Frictional trauma
Nail biting
Onychotillomania
Occupational trauma

Dermatologic Causes
Amyloidosis
Basal cell carcinoma
Bowen disease
Chronic paronychia
Chronic radiation dermatitis
Lichen planus
Localized scleroderma
Myxoid pseudocyst
Onychomatricoma
Onychomycosis
Psoriasis
Subungual fibrous histiocytoma
Subungual linear keratosis
Systemic lupus erythematosus
Verruca vulgaris

Systemic Causes
Acquired immunodeficiency syndrome
Alkaptonuria
Endocrine disorders (acromegaly, Addison disease, Cushing syndrome, hyperthyroidism, Nelson syndrome)
Graft-versus-host disease (lichen planus-type changes accompanied by longitudinal melanonychia)
Hemosiderosis
Hyperbilirubinemia
Nutritional disorders
Porphyria

Iatrogenic Causes
Drugs
Electron beam therapy
Phototherapy
X-ray exposure

Syndromes
Laugier-Hunziker syndrome
Peutz-Jeghers syndrome
Touraine syndrome

Source: Data from Andre J, Lateur N. Pigmented Nail Disorders, Dermatol Clin 2006 Jul;24(3):329-339.[2]

X-ray exposure, phototherapy, and electron beam therapy[23] [**Figure 40-3 and Table 40-3**].[2] Particular presentations of melanonychia may vary significantly depending on the exposure, but several fingernails and toenails are usually involved.[2] Drug-induced melanonychia usually fades slowly following drug withdrawal.[2] Transverse melanonychia, while uncommon, most often occurs as a result of iatrogenic causes including the following: conventional radiographic therapy to treat hand dermatitis (used in the 1950s and 1960s),[24,25] psoralen with ultraviolet A (PUVA),[26-29] electron beam therapy,[23] infliximab,[30] zidovudine,[31] prolonged antimalarial therapy with amodiaquine, chloroquine, mepacrine, or quinacrine,[2,29,31] and chemotherapy with agents such as doxorubicin, bleomycin, cyclophosphamide, daunorubicin, dacarbazine, 5-fluorouracil, methotrexate,[23] and hydroxyurea.[29,32,33] Notably, transverse melanonychia associated with PUVA and electron beam therapy usually resolves following the

TABLE 40-2	Nail pigmentation in 296 people of African ancestry.[4]

- Pigmentation usually occurs in the form of longitudinal melanonychia (LM) and is a normal, common finding in most cases.
- Increasing age is associated with a higher prevalence LM, with increasing numbers of nails involved.
- There is no difference in the nail pigmentation between males and females.
- On each nail, there may be one or several bands, varying from thin to several millimeters wide.
- The bands vary in depth of color. The bands tends to be darker in persons with darker skin types.
- LM in these individuals may be present in any portion of the nail but most commonly occupies the central area or lateral margins.
- The pigment particles are found scattered throughout the onychocytes but are concentrated in the deeper layers (corresponding to the distal matrix).

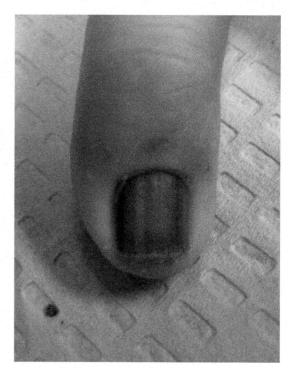

FIGURE 40-3. Melanonychia due to hydroxyurea therapy.

cessation of treatment.[23,26,29] Transverse brown to black nail pigmentation associated with the antimalarials amodiaquine, chloroquine, and mepacrine may be attributable to ferric acid dyschromia and/or melanin production.[2]

Syndrome-Associated Melanonychia Melanonychia associated with Peutz-Jeghers, Touraine, and Laugier-Hunziker syndromes typically involves multiple digits and occurs in conjunction with mucosal pigmented macules involving the lips and oral cavity.[2] Peutz-Jeghers and Touraine syndromes are autosomal dominant inherited disorders that typically manifest during childhood and are associated with intestinal polyposis and an increased risk for gastrointestinal and pancreatic malignancies, whereas Laugier-Hunziker syndrome is a chronic benign mucocutaneous syndrome that generally arises spontaneously in 20- to 40-year-old Caucasian adults.[2]

■ MELANOCYTIC HYPERPLASIA

Melanocytic hyperplasia is characterized by an increase in the number of matrix melanocytes.[2] Both benign and malignant causes exist.[2] Benign melanocytic hyperplasia can be subdivided into two categories:

- Lentigines, when nests of melanocytes are absent
- Nevi, when at least one melanocytic nest is present[2]

Lentigines occur far more often than nevi in adults, and nevi are observed far more often than lentigines in children [**Figures 40-4 and 40-5**]. Benign causes of melanocytic hyperplasia constitute 77.5% of cases of childhood melanonychia, and NAM occurs rarely in children.[2,34]

Nail matrix nevi primarily occur in the fingernails and most commonly involve the thumbnail. The majority of nevi are junctional, and nevi can be congenital or acquired.[1,2,8,31,32] Roughly half of nail matrix nevi are characterized by a band of over 3 mm in width, two-thirds by melanic brown-black pigmentation, and one-third by periungual

TABLE 40-3	Drugs thought to cause melanocytic activation
Nonchemotherapeutic medications	**Chemotherapeutic medications**
Adrenocorticotropic hormone	5-Fluorouracil
Amodiaquine	Bleomycin sulfate
Amorolfine	Busulfan
Arsenic	Cyclophosphamide
Chloroquine	Dacarbazine
Clofazimine	Daunorubicin hydrochloride
Clomipramine	Doxorubicin
Cyclines	Etoposide
Fluconazole	Hydroxyurea
Fluorides	Imatinib
Gold salts	Melphalan hydrochloride
Ibuprofen	Methotrexate
Ketoconazole	Nitrogen mustard
Lamivudine	Nitrosourea
Mepacrine	Tegafur
Mercury	
Melanocyte-stimulating hormone	
PCB	
Phenytoin	
Phenothiazine	
Psoralen	
Roxithromycin	
Steroids	
Sulfonamide	
Thallium	
Timolol	
Zidovudine	

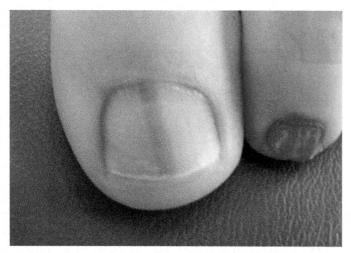

FIGURE 40-2. Frictional melanonychia of the great toe likely due to ill-fitting footwear.

Source: Adapted with permission from Andre J, Lateur N. Pigmented Nail Disorders, Dermatol Clin 2006 Jul;24(3):329-339.[2]

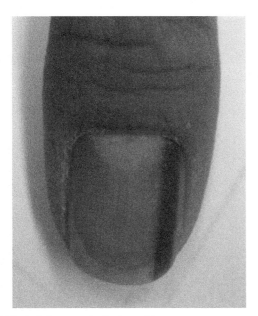

FIGURE 40-4. Nail apparatus lentigo in an adult.

melanic pigmentation.[2] However, nail matrix nevi may also appear as scarcely pigmented bands.[2,11,12,34,35]

Malignant melanocytic hyperplasia, or in situ or invasive melanoma, most commonly involves a thumbnail, index fingernail, or great toenail of a person aged 60 to 70 years [**Figure 40-6**].[2] Nearly 70% of these tumors are found on the thumb or hallux, perhaps because these digits represent a large proportion of the total amount of nail matrix tissue, perhaps because of trauma, or perhaps because of other, as of yet unexplained causes.[10,36-38] NAM tends to be asymptomatic. It is unlikely that ultraviolet (UV) exposure is extensively involved in the etiology.[10] The nail plate allows only a small amount of UVA penetration and blocks almost all UVB rays, so the nail bed receives very little of the damaging UV exposure.[10,39]

Men and women have nearly equal incidence of NAM.[40] Approximately 33% of melanomas in Native Americans,[1,41] 17% in Chinese,[1,42] 10% to 30% in Japanese,[1,43,44] 16% in Mexicans,[1,45] 15% to 25% in

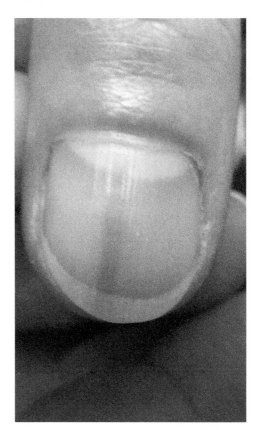

FIGURE 40-6. Nail apparatus melanoma in situ with in a middle-aged Caucasian adult.

African Americans,[1,46] and 1% to 3% in Caucasians[1,47-49] occur within the nail unit.[4,13] Because other forms of melanoma occur less often in more deeply pigmented people compared with Caucasians, the absolute incidence of NAM is quite similar.[1,2,50]

Although beyond the scope of this review, it is important to note that while melanonychia is the most common presentation of NAM, comprising roughly two-thirds of all cases, it is not the sole presentation.[1] Approximately one-quarter to one-third of all NAMs are amelanotic.[1] Alternatively, NAM may present as a subungual tumor, nail plate dystrophy, or inflammatory disease of the nail unit.[10] Bleeding is a late presentation.[10]

PATHOGEN-INDUCED MELANONYCHIA

As previously mentioned, certain pathogens involved in onychomycosis or paronychia can trigger an inflammatory response that in turn can cause melanocytic activation and melanonychia. Multiple fungi have been reported to cause LM, including *Trichophyton rubrum*,[51] *Fusarium solani*,[52] *Candida*,[53] *Exophiala dermatitidis*,[54] and *Wangiella dermatitidis*,[55] as well as black molds such as *Scytalidium dimidiatum*, *Aspergillus niger*, and *Alternaria alternata*.[1] In addition, certain dermatophyte strains, such as *T. rubrum* var. *nigricans*, and certain gramnegative pathogens such as *Proteus* mirabilis,[56] can produce melanin and infrequently present as a linear streak [**Figure 40-7**].[1] Several other organisms produce pigments other than melanin and can clinically present with linear brown to black nail dyschromia as well. However, it is important to note that secondary infections may mask changes of an underlying melanoma, making them more difficult to diagnose.[10]

CLINICAL APPROACH TO MELANONYCHIA

HISTORY

A detailed history with particular attention to the onset, progression, and any triggers of melanonychia should be obtained. It is ideal to have patients fill out a nail questionnaire concerning their occupation,

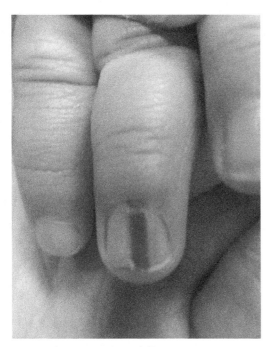

FIGURE 40-5. Nail apparatus nevus in a child.

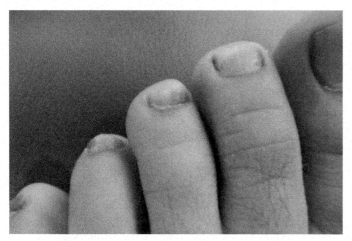

FIGURE 40-7. Melanonychia secondary to an infection with *Trichophyton rubrum* var. *nigricans*.

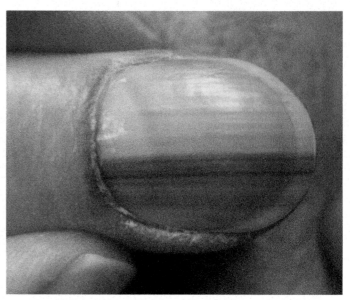

FIGURE 40-8. Nail apparatus melanoma in situ with Hutchinson sign.

hobbies, exposures to topical substances, digital trauma history, drug history, medical history, and family history prior to the visit because it provides patients with ample time to prepare thoughtful answers and also provides the physician with more time during the appointment to focus on key portions of the history. In general, NAM should be suspected in any patient with unexplained melanonychia with a history containing some of the following features:

- Involvement of a single digit (especially the thumb, great toe, or index finger)
- Development during the fourth decade of life or later
- Development in the setting of a history of digital trauma
- Development in the setting of a personal/family history of melanoma or dysplastic nevus syndrome
- Development in the setting of nail dystrophy
- Abrupt development or change (proximal widening or darkening)[1,4]

■ PHYSICAL EXAMINATION

During the initial examination, all 20 nails, skin, and mucous membranes should be evaluated under good lighting while keeping in mind all possible causes of brown to black nail pigmentation.

The following questions can help guide the initial nail examination:

- Are one or more nails involved?
- If multiple nails are involved, is one particular nail different from the rest or changing?
- Is the discoloration located on top of, within, or beneath the nail plate?
- Is the discoloration linear?
- Is the band darker or wider at the proximal end?
- Is the discoloration associated with nail plate dystrophy?

Exogenous Substances The possibility of linear nail pigmentation secondary to an exogenous substance on top of or beneath the nail plate should be ruled out. Notably, unlike NAM, a linear pigmented band produced by a nail pathogen is typically wider distally than proximally, indicating a distal rather than proximal (or matrix) origin, and occasionally exhibits pointed extensions proximally.[1,10] Infection can be confirmed by histopathologic examination and/or culture.[1]

Exogenous substances such as tar, tobacco, dirt, and potassium permanganate are usually located on top of the nail and follow the shape of the proximal nail fold rather than the lunula.[1,2] Additionally, exogenous substances grow out with the nail plate and can sometimes be simply scraped off.[1,2] In cases of suspected potassium permanganate staining, the manganese dioxide component can be reduced to a colorless compound with the application of 5% to 10% ascorbic acid.[1]

Subungual hematomas can occasionally present as a linear band.[1] For such cases, dermoscopy may help distinguish blood from melanin and is discussed later. A more invasive method of visualization involves punching a hole in the nail plate in the area of nail dyschromia and examining the underlying nail bed.[2,57] Additionally, the presence of blood can be confirmed with a positive pseudo-peroxidase reaction (Hemastix test).[1]

Hutchinson Sign Hutchinson sign is the extension of pigment from the matrix to the perionychium in association with NAM [**Figure 40-8**]. Evaluation for Hutchinson sign includes an examination of the proximal and lateral nail folds and eponychium. A true Hutchinson sign usually represents radial-growth-phase melanoma.[10] It is sometimes helpful in confirming the clinical diagnosis but is an inconsistent feature.[4,10] Melanoma can occur without Hutchinson sign, and pseudo-Hutchinson sign, or the presence or illusion of pigment in the perionychium, is associated with both benign and malignant conditions in the absence of melanoma [**Figure 40-9**].[2,4,58]

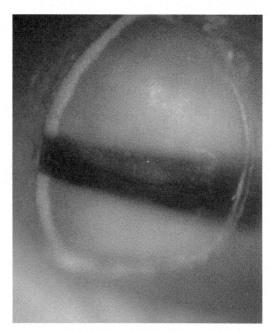

FIGURE 40-9. Nail apparatus nevus with pseudo-Hutchinson sign.

Dermoscopy Dermoscopy may provide clues when deciding whether a biopsy is necessary to evaluate for melanoma.[3,57] However, experts disagree on what dermoscopic findings are associated with benign etiologies versus NAM, and further studies are necessary. A study by Ronger et al[57] found that nail matrix nevi were significantly associated with the presence of regular lines and a brown coloration of the background, whereas nail apparatus lentigines, drug-induced pigmentation, and racial-type pigmentation were significantly associated with homogeneous longitudinal thin gray lines and gray background coloration.[3] In contrast, cases of NAM were significantly associated with the presence of irregular longitudinal lines (per parallelism, thickness, spacing, and color) and a brown coloration of the background [**Figure 40-10**].[3,57] The study also observed a micro-Hutchinson sign (a Hutchinson sign that is too small to be seen with the human eye) only in cases of melanoma, but this characteristic occurred so rarely that the study was unable to statistically evaluate for specificity.[3,57] Others have described dermoscopic Hutchinson sign on the hyponychium, with excellent sensitivity for melanoma, although the specificity was less accurate.[59]

In contrast to the skin, blood under the nail may show pseudopod formation, appearing like budding globules off of a darker red-black macule.[60] Johr and Izakovic[61] published a case series using dermoscopy for the evaluation of pigmentation of the nail unit. They found that color asymmetry (including black dots), irregular diffuse dark pigmentation, and (micro-) Hutchinson sign were important dermoscopic signs for melanoma.

Interestingly, dermoscopy of the free edge of the nail may help to identify the origin of a pigmented band and thereby facilitate preoperative mapping [**Figure 40-11**].[3,62] Distal matrix pigmentation, which accounts for approximately 90% of cases of LM, projects onto the undersurface of the free edge of the nail plate, whereas proximal matrix pigmentation projects onto the superficial surface of the nail plate.[10] This finding has important prognostic information because proximal matrix biopsies are more likely to leave a permanent dystrophy than distal matrix biopsies. If the location of the pigmented band cannot be determined simply by dermoscopic evaluation of the free edge, a distal nail clipping stained with Fontana Masson can reveal the matrix band origin.[3]

ABCs of Clinical Detection of NAM An ABCDEF mnemonic was created to aid the recall of certain key clinical features that should raise suspicion for the possibility of subungual melanoma.[63]

• **A:** *Age*—Subungual melanoma most commonly arises during the fifth to seventh decades of life, although it has been reported to occur in patients as young as 1 year old and as old as 90 years old.[63]

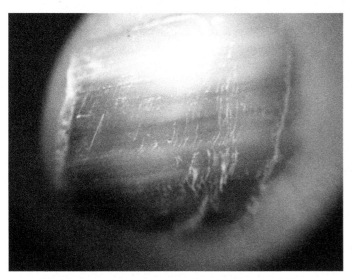

FIGURE 40-10. Dermoscopy of a nail apparatus melanoma in situ. Notice the presence of irregular longitudinal lines per color, spacing, thickness, and parallelism, and the brown coloration of the background.

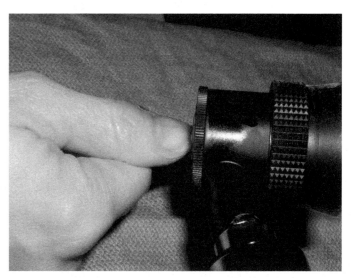

FIGURE 40-11. End-on dermoscopy allows localization of nail pigment to the superficial plate (proximal matrix origin) or undersurface of the plate (distal matrix origin).

• **B:** Subungual melanoma typically presents as a pigmented *band* with a breadth of over 3 mm and irregular or *blurred borders* that are composed of variegated shades of *brown to black*.[63]

• **C:** *Change*—A recent or sudden increase in the size of a pigmented band is comparable to the radial growth phase of a cutaneous melanoma.[63] A *change* in nail plate morphology is also concerning for melanoma.[63]

• **D:** Single-*digit* involvement, with the thumb and then great toe or index finger being most commonly involved.[63]

• **E:** *Extension* of pigment into the perionychium in association with melanoma (Hutchinson sign).[63]

• **F:** *Family* or personal history of melanoma and/or dysplastic nevus syndrome.[63]

BIOPSY OF MELANONYCHIA

A biopsy is often necessary to rule out melanoma.[3] A study by Di Chiacchio et al[64] found that the overall accuracy of dermatologists in the preoperative diagnosis of NAM in situ was low, ranging from 46% to 55%. The study also found that a dermatologist's level of expertise in nail disease did not statistically influence the correct diagnosis and that nail experts were no more accurate than nail novices.[64]

Although no formally adopted algorithm with guidelines for when to perform a biopsy exists, there are several suggested guiding principles.[4] In general, the threshold for biopsy should be low in fairer-skinned patients with unexplained melanonychia of a single digit. In contrast, for cases of multiple digits in a patient of any phototype, melanonychia should be closely monitored and biopsied if any suspicious features arise.[2,63]

When performing a biopsy, the entire origin of the pigment should be removed. Melanoma most often originates in the nail matrix (the most melanocyte-dense region of the nail unit), although every nail subunit contains melanocytes and hence may present with melanoma.[10]

The nail matrix biopsy, although a relatively safe and simple procedure when certain basic principles are followed, is associated with the greatest risk of scarring when compared to other biopsy locations within the nail unit.[65] A biopsy of the distal matrix is almost always preferred over a proximal matrix biopsy because any resultant scar, which clinically manifests as a thinned ridge, would lie on the undersurface of the nail plate.[4,65-68] Thinned ridges on the dorsal surface of the nail plate are easily traumatized because they catch on items such as clothing and are much more troublesome for the patient.[4]

To minimize any potential scarring, nail matrix excisional biopsies can be oriented transversely.[3,4,65] Moreover, full-thickness nail matrix biopsies larger than 3 mm can be sutured to achieve an optimal cosmetic result.[1,69]

The punch biopsy is generally reserved for LM less than 2.5 to 3 mm in width originating in the distal matrix.[1,3] A punch biopsy should be taken at the origin of the pigmented band and should extend to depth of the periosteum.[3,65] Punch biopsies are generally not recommended for evaluating pigmented lesions ≥3 mm in width (even if multiple punch biopsies are taken), because peripheral pigmentation may not be adequately sampled to rule out malignancy. Additionally, taking serial punch biopsies is associated with an increased risk of permanent nail dystrophy.[3]

The lateral longitudinal excision is best suited for biopsying large lesions with a high preoperative suspicion that are located in the lateral one-third of the nail. The lateral longitudinal excision technique samples all components of the nail unit including the nail matrix, nail bed, nail fold, and hyponychium.[1,3] The tangential (shave) excision is ideal for sampling a longitudinal pigmented band with a lower preoperative suspicion of melanoma.[1,41,70] The tangential technique, first described by Eckart Haneke in 1999, is less invasive than a transversely oriented matrix excision and is associated with minimal long-term dystrophy despite the increased width commonly associated with its use.[1,3,70] However, for any case with a high preoperative likelihood of invasive melanoma, a full-thickness nail matrix biopsy is necessary for prognosis determination because a tangential biopsy may not provide an accurate Breslow depth.[3]

DESCRIPTION OF BIOPSY TECHNIQUES

Regardless of the biopsy technique used, the nail plate should be partially or completely avulsed, or punched, to allow access to the primary biopsy site.[3] The nail plate can be sent for pathologic evaluation because it may contain important information as melanocytic pigmentation, blood, or even dematiaceous fungi.[3,70] Different tissue specimens should be submitted in formalin in separate containers for proper histologic processing.[3] If specimens are placed in the same container, they risk being mounted on the same slide, and in this way, deeper sections of one specimen can potentially sacrifice tissue from the other specimen.[3] Pathology requisition forms should specify that the tissue needs to be sliced longitudinally rather than transversely.[3]

The following are general guidelines that can be used when performing the lateral longitudinal excision and tangential excision techniques. Although experts often disagree on the finer points of these biopsy techniques, these general surgical guidelines are widely accepted.

Lateral Longitudinal Excision A number 10 or 15 scalpel blade can be used to cut through the skin and soft tissue down to the periosteum, proximally from a point halfway between the cuticle and the distal interphalangeal skin fold, 1 to 2 mm medial to the pigmented band, through the nail plate, and 3 to 4 mm past the hyponychium onto the digital tip.[3] The blade can then be reinserted laterally from the previous starting point, and the cut made so that the entire matrix horn is included.[3] The cut can then course into the nail sulcus and beyond to meet the end point of the first incision.[3] In this way, the incision is nearly elliptical [**Figure 40-12**].[3] The tissue specimen should be carefully removed and placed in formalin. Although the goal of this technique is to remove the entire lateral matrix horn, small matrix remnants are occasionally left behind and can cause subsequent postoperative cysts, spicules, and/or pain. To prevent this complication, lateral matrix pocket debridement with a small curette or a hemostat tip covered with gauze can be performed prior to tissue repair. Sutures can be placed to realign the proximal nail fold to the lateral nail fold and should remain in for 10 to 14 days.

Tangential Excision Using a number 15 blade, the pigment origin should be sampled with 1- to 2-mm margins using a shaving technique to produce a specimen less than 1 mm in thickness [**Figure 40-13**].[3] The specimen should not be placed directly into a formalin specimen

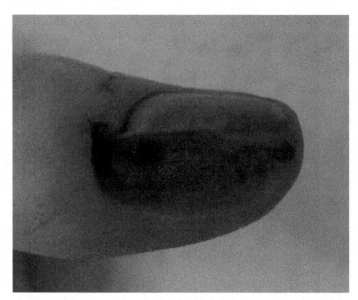

FIGURE 40-12. Defect following lateral longitudinal excision.

container because it is likely to roll and curl. Instead, it is recommended that the specimen be placed onto a piece of paper or cardboard or in a cassette prior to placing it in a formalin jar so that it remains flat, facilitating processing [**Figure 40-14**]. Repair of the remaining defect is straightforward. The nail plate can be replaced following the procedure to protect the nail bed.

HISTOPATHOLOGIC EVALUATION

In cases of onychomycosis, histology may show multiple fungal elements, including septate hyphae in dermatophyte infection, pseudohyphae and budding spores in yeast infection, and a number of elements with the range of nondermatophyte mold infections. Hemorrhage may be observed, although typical iron staining (such as Prussian blue) is negative in the nail plate. (The hemoglobin is not metabolized in the nail plate and hence not appreciated with this stain.) Instead, benzidine (for hemoglobin) is the preferred test for nail plate hemorrhage.[71]

In cases of melanonychia of matrix melanocyte origin, there are several possible histologic diagnoses. LM originating from the matrix

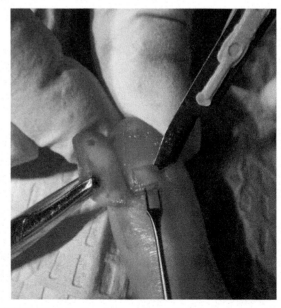

FIGURE 40-13. Following nail plate avulsion and lateral reflection, the origin of a pigmented band is being sampled using the tangential (shave) excision technique.

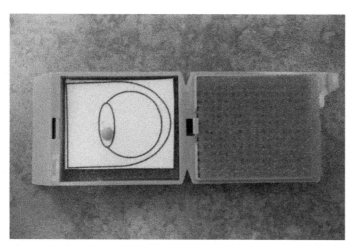

FIGURE 40-14. Biopsy specimen placed on a paper template within a cassette to facilitate pathologic examination.

without melanocytic hyperplasia has been termed *melanocytic activation or melanotic macule of the nail.*[72] Melanocytic hyperplasia may represent a lentigo, a nevus (most of which are of the junctional variety), melanoma in situ, or melanoma. Distinguishing lentigo from nevus may be difficult because nesting in matrix nevi may be inconspicuous; therefore, some prefer to label all benign matrix hyperplasia as nevus, eschewing the diagnosis of lentigo.[72]

Melanomas and melanomas in situ are characterized by poorly circumscribed proliferations of atypical melanocytes with varying degrees of upward growth. Single melanocytes predominate over nests. Nuclear enlargement with a coarse chromatin pattern is common. Mitoses vary but may not be prominent.[73] Nodular melanomas by definition lack a radial growth phase and grow vertically early in the disease. Unusually, melanoma may be associated with formation of cartilage and partly mineralized osteoid-like material.[74] This osteocartilaginous differentiation may delay or mask the diagnosis, particularly if radiologic studies are performed before or in place of tissue diagnosis.

All melanoma subtypes have been reported to present as NAM, although the acral lentiginous type has been observed the most, followed by the superficial spreading type. The diagnosis of NAM can be difficult for those unfamiliar with nail apparatus histology. The distribution and number of melanocytes in the nail matrix differ from those in other epithelium. Specifically, they may be found irregularly distributed basally or suprabasally, sometimes clustered in small groups of three to four cells.[75] Normal melanocytic nevi in children may even show potentially misleading features.[76] They may have large melanocytes with abundant cytoplasm and a dark, variably sized and shaped nucleus, occasionally showing spindle-shaped melanocytes or transepidermal migration of isolated melanocytes or even nests of melanocytes. Some nuclear atypia is considered by some to be present in benign nevi as well. The upward growth in nevi may be incorrectly interpreted as pagetoid scatter, leading to the misdiagnosis of melanoma in situ.[37] Immunohistochemistry may be helpful in ambiguous cases, but more traditional criteria, such as cellular morphology, necrosis, and mitotic activity, can be more crucial to diagnosing melanoma. S-100, HMB-45, Mart-1, and Melan-A are all accurate markers for cells of melanocytic origin.

Due to diagnostic delays, NAMs are significantly thicker than cutaneous melanomas at the time of diagnosis. The average Breslow depth ranges from 3.5 to 4.7 mm,[77,78] and 80% are deeper than 1.5 mm.[79] Approximately 60% to 70% are invasive to Clark level IV or V, and one-quarter of patients have lymph node or distant metastases at presentation.[79,80] Late changes and poor prognostic factors are disproportionately present at the time of diagnosis. One report of 46 patients showed 28% of tumors with ulceration, 11% with bony invasion, and 50% with nail destruction.[80] Historically, prognosis has been poor. In one study of 54 patients with 5-year follow-up, 26 patients died of disseminated

metastatic disease.[79] In most other series, all of which have been limited by the rarity of disease, the 5-year survival rates have been poor, ranging from 20% to 60%.[81] With more encouraging statistics, a study of NAM in Japanese patients compared survival rates in the time periods of 1969 to 1982 and 1983 to 1993.[82] The 5-year survival rate increased from 53% to 87% between these two time periods. The authors credited this dramatic progress to greater public awareness (and discovery of thinner melanomas) and to the introduction of improved chemotherapy.

Melanoma is viewed by many as a systemic disease, with an increased likelihood of widespread pathology related to tumor depth, ulceration, and perhaps tumor subtype or location. Quantifying the extent of melanoma is essential for determining appropriate treatment and for assessing prognosis. There are no current data to suggest a different approach to staging patients with NAM versus cutaneous melanoma. The most recent Tumor, Node, Metastasis (TNM) staging system published by the American Joint Committee on Cancer (AJCC)[83] reinforces that tumor depth (Breslow thickness) is the most important prognostic indicator in primary melanoma, with stratification cutoffs at ≤1 mm, 1.01 to 2 mm, 2.01 to 4 mm, and >4 mm. Microscopic ulceration is the next most significant adverse prognostic indicator. The number of lymph nodes involved supersedes size of lymph nodes as a negative factor. Indeed, the AJCC staging system incorporates micrometastases to the lymph node in its newest classification. Because this information may be gathered only through lymph node biopsy, current practice includes the use of sentinel lymph node biopsy for tumors at least 1 mm in depth as a staging technique, although its import at this point is theoretical; currently, there are no conclusive data that sentinel lymph node biopsy improves overall survival.[84] Most data do not support radiologic or lymph node staging for in situ melanomas or nonulcerated melanomas of less than 1 mm in depth, particularly if the Clark level is I to III. These recommendations may change with further data.

Over the past 20 years, there has been a movement toward smaller surgical margins for NAM.[85] Historically, digital (including nail unit) melanomas were treated with digital amputation from the level of the metacarpal/metatarsal bones.[80] More recently, there have been publications advocating more distal levels of amputation or simply excision with 1- to 2-cm margins, sparing amputation.[86] NAM in situ is treated adequately with total excision of all nail tissues without amputation.[87] For invasive tumors, some have proposed digit-sparing "functional" surgery, which encompasses en bloc excision of the nail unit and partial resection of the distal phalanx followed by three-dimensional histology to assure tumor-free resection margins.[86] A retrospective comparative analysis evaluated the survival rates between two groups of 31 patients, those with an amputation in or proximal to the distal interphalangeal joint and those with less radical "functional" surgery. The study showed no survival difference between the two groups at a median follow-up of 54 months.[86] Proponents of Mohs surgery have provided evidence of its usefulness in the therapy of NAM and NAM in situ.[88,89] Hence, local tumor removal with clear margins is advocated by all, but primary extirpation with wider rather than narrower margins has lost favor in the face of absent survival benefit.[85] Chemotherapeutic recommendations for NAM closely coincide with those for melanomas in other anatomic locations.

For all patients, regardless of their Breslow thickness or tumor specifications, careful follow-up for local recurrence, second primary tumors, and lymph node and distant metastasis is required for life.

LICHEN PLANUS

Lichen planus (LP) is a common inflammatory skin disease that affects approximately 1% of the U.S. population.[90] Approximately 10% to 25% of patients with LP have nail involvement, with a small proportion of them having nail disease in isolation.[91-94] LP of the nails occurs more commonly in the adult population and typically affects several or most nails.

LP may involve any or all subunits of the nail, including the bed, nail folds, and matrix, and may display protean signs. An understanding of the various possible presentations of nail unit disease is aided by comprehension of the different roles of nail subunits [**Table 40-4**].

TABLE 40-4	Presentation of nail lichen planus	
Ridging	Subungual hyperkeratosis	Wickham striae
Onychorrhexis	Hyperpigmentation	Hyperpigmentation
Pitting	Hypopigmentation	Hypopigmentation
Koilonychia		
Longitudinal erythronychia		
Leukonychia		
Onychauxis		
Nail plate thinning		
Trachyonychia		
Scarring		
Anonychia		
Pterygium		

Involvement of the nail matrix, which is responsible for nail plate production, is capable of producing a wide spectrum of plate abnormalities including longitudinal ridging, nail plate thinning, longitudinal fissuring, trachyonychia, and erythema of the lunula [**Figures 40-15 and 40-16**].[93] Nail bed disease may produce onycholysis, with nail bed hyperkeratosis presenting occasionally as a yellow discoloration.

In skin of color, LP varies in ways that are consistent with other cutaneous and nail diseases. Cutaneous erythema tends to be more violaceous and, for those unaccustomed to its examination, may appear subtle. Postinflammatory hyperpigmentation of the proximal nail fold and LM are more common in darker phototypes due to an increased likelihood of melanocytic activation.[95] Because the nail bed contains normally quiescent melanocytes and closely resembles the nail bed in other races, the changes are remarkably similar.

LP of the nails can be rapidly progressive, and up to 40% of patients develop permanent nail dystrophy in the forms of anonychia and dorsal pterygium (the extension and adherence of the proximal nail fold to the nail bed secondary to scarring of the nail matrix).[91,93] In particular, bullous LP of the nail unit represents a potential onychologic emergency, with rapid nail unit scarring and the development of dorsal pterygium.[10] Bullous LP of the nail unit classically presents with local pain.[10]

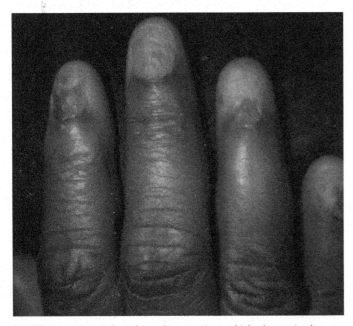

FIGURE 40-15. Lichen planus demonstrating multiple changes in the same patient: dorsal pterygium, nail plate thinning and ridging, and melanonychia (second fingernail).

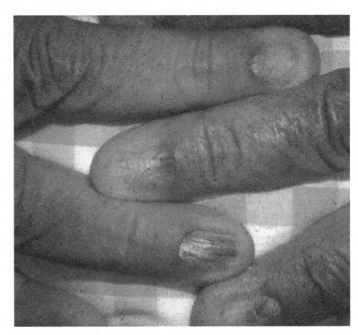

FIGURE 40-16. Lichen planus demonstrating multiple changes in the same patient: dorsal pterygium, anonychia, longitudinal ridging, and melanonychia (second nail from bottom).

LP is generally easy to diagnose by clinical examination alone, but if the diagnosis is questionable, a 3-mm punch biopsy of the nail matrix is usually conclusive.[93] A 3-mm punch biopsy of the nail bed may be necessary to distinguish between LP and psoriasis in some instances.[93]

Treatment of nail unit LP is no different in patients with skin of color. Treatment primarily consists of intralesional or systemic steroids, with systemic steroids preferred in cases that are rapidly progressive or involve more than three nails.[93]

Triamcinolone acetonide diluted to 2.5 to 5 mg/mL can be injected intradermally into the proximal and lateral nail folds, from which the solution can diffuse to the underlying matrix. Injection directly into the nail matrix is uncomfortable and unnecessary.[96] The steroid can be diluted with lidocaine and injected using a 30-gauge needle to reduce pain associated with its administration.[91] Additionally, a coolant spray applied to the area prior to the injection and the use of vibration during the injection can also help reduce associated discomfort.[91] Treatment is generally continued at monthly intervals until the proximal one-half of the nail appears normal, at which time injections can be tapered.

Recommendations for systemic therapy include oral prednisone 0.5 to 1 mg/kg/d (maximum 60 mg/d) for 4 to 6 weeks followed by a 4- to 6-week taper.[97] Alternatively, intramuscular injections of triamcinolone acetonide at a dose of 0.5 mg/kg may be given monthly for 3 to 6 months.[91,93,96]

Treatment of nail LP with topical or systemic corticosteroids has not been evaluated in randomized trials, and their use is based solely on clinical experience and limited evidence from small case series. In a study of 27 patients with nail LP treated with intramuscular or intralesional corticosteroids who were followed for more than 5 years (mean follow-up, 10 years), 9 patients (33.3%) did not respond to treatment, 18 (66.7%) were cured, and 11 (40.7%) relapsed.[96] In another study, 67 patients with histologically confirmed LP of the nails were treated with systemic and/or intralesional corticosteroids for 6 months.[98] Complete or substantial improvement was reported in 42 patients (63%).

In patients who do not respond to systemic or topical corticosteroids, treatment should be stopped after 6 months. Oral acitretin at a dose of 0.35 mg/kg/d may be an option in recalcitrant cases, although treatment with etretinate at dose of 0.35 mg/kg/d was found to be ineffective in a retrospective study by Piraccini et al.[96] The study also found that the addition of azathioprine 100 mg/d to systemic steroid therapy was ineffective.[96]

TABLE 40-5	Treatment of nail lichen planus

First line
Irritant-avoidance regimen
Intralesional corticosteroids
• 2.5–5 mg/mL triamcinolone, injected into the matrix, with treatments monthly until clear, then tapered gradually
Second line
Systemic corticosteroids
• 0.75–1.0 mg/kg/d prednisone continued for several weeks until clinical improvement is evident, then tapered gradually
Third line
Topical corticosteroids (potent, under occlusion)
Systemic retinoids
Systemic griseofulvin
Topical psoralen with ultraviolet A (PUVA)

It is important to note that trauma may worsen the disease (Koebner phenomenon) and that gentle nail care is important in any treatment; we recommend an irritant-avoidance regimen to all patients with nail unit LP.[99] **Table 40-5** lists treatments for moderate to severe LP divided into first-, second-, and third-line therapies.

PSORIASIS

Nail psoriasis is the most common nail disorder associated with a skin disease and occurs in over 50% of patients with cutaneous psoriasis and approximately 86% of patients with psoriatic arthritis.[91,93] However, the diagnosis of nail psoriasis can be challenging when psoriasis is limited to the nails, as is the case in 5% of patients.[91]

The clinical features of nail psoriasis vary depending on the portion of the nail unit involved.[91,93] Nail matrix involvement is characterized by nail pitting, crumbling, trachyonychia, leukonychia, and red spots in the lunula.[91,93] Nail pitting, the most common sign of nail psoriasis, indicates proximal nail matrix involvement and occurs when foci of parakeratotic cells leave the dorsal nail plate as it grows beyond the cuticle.[91,93] Psoriatic pits are typically irregular, deep, large, and randomly distributed within the nail plate.[93] Trachyonychia is due to excessive longitudinal ridging due to proximal nail matrix inflammation.[93] Leukonychia, occurs when psoriatic inflammation of the mid to distal nail matrix causes parakeratosis of the mid to ventral nail plate.[91,93] Mottled erythema of the lunula arises secondary to distal nail matrix inflammation.[91,93] Crumbling of the nail plate is a consequence of severe pitting due to diffuse psoriatic inflammation of the matrix[93] [**Figure 40-17**].

Psoriatic inflammation of the nail bed is associated with salmon patches (also termed *oil drops*), subungual hyperkeratosis, onycholysis, and splinter hemorrhages.[91,93] Salmon patches are characterized by irregular areas of yellow or pink discoloration in the nail bed as seen through the nail plate.[93] Subungual hyperkeratosis may be the only indication of psoriatic involvement of the toenails.[93] Splinter hemorrhages, which appear as longitudinal red or black lines under the nail plate, are typically seen in the fingernails.[91,93]

Psoriasis of the nail folds can resemble chronic paronychia and is often precipitated by treatment with systemic retinoids.[93,100] The Koebner phenomenon, or worsening of a particular condition in an area of recent trauma, is also seen within the nail unit.[91,93] Mycology is recommended for suspected cases of psoriatic nail disease that present similarly to onychomycosis with subungual hyperkeratosis and onycholysis, especially if disease is limited to the toenails.[91,93] Moreover, psoriatic nails are more susceptible to fungal infections.[93]

Treatment of nail unit psoriasis is no different in patients with skin of color. It requires patience because nails grow slowly and relapse is common.[91,93] Fortunately, psoriasis of the nails generally does not result in scarring, as opposed to psoriatic arthritis, which is erosive.[93] Nail matrix disease tends to be more responsive to therapy than nail bed disease. Topical calcipotriol or topical tazarotene may be used to treat nail bed

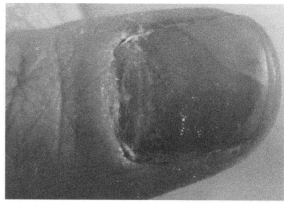

A

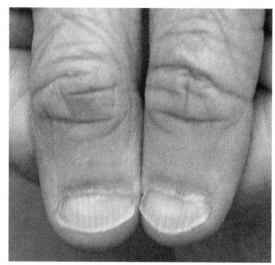

B

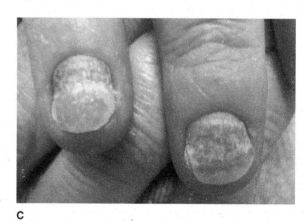

C

FIGURE 40-17. (A–C) Nail psoriasis characterized by pitting, onycholysis, subungual hyperkeratosis, oil spotting, and splinter hemorrhages.

hyperkeratosis, but success is variable due to poor medication bioavailability.[91,93] Topical therapy is not considered a treatment option for nail matrix psoriasis because topical medications cannot penetrate the overlying proximal nail fold and nail plate.[93] Topical superpotent steroids are rarely effective, even for nail bed psoriasis, and are associated with skin and bone atrophy with prolonged use.[93]

Monthly injections of 2.5 to 10 mg/mL of triamcinolone acetonide in the proximal and lateral nail folds is very effective for most cases.[91,93] Acitretin at a dose of 0.2 to 0.3 mg/kg/d is sometimes used for severe nail matrix and nail bed psoriasis in males and in females who agree to take adequate measures to prevent pregnancy.[91,93] Importantly, acitretin should not be dosed above 0.3 mg/kg/d because higher doses are associated with nail brittleness and paronychia and pyogenic granuloma formation.[93] Oral agents, such as methotrexate and cyclosporine, and biologic medications, such as infliximab and adalimumab, are used to treat nail psoriasis associated with cutaneous and/or arthritic involvement.[93] PUVA is not effective for nail psoriasis and may even worsen nail disease.[93] Because nail psoriasis frequently koebnerizes, gentle nail care with irritant avoidance is an important part of the treatment regimen.[99]

ONYCHOMYCOSIS

Onychomycosis, a fungal infection of the nail unit resulting in nail discoloration, thickening, and deformity, is the most common nail disorder that presents to the dermatologist's office, accounting for almost 50% of nail visits.[10,101] Millions of people suffer from this condition annually, and the incidence and prevalence of onychomycosis continue to increase worldwide.[101,102] Reportedly in Western countries, 10% of the general population, 20% of the population over 60 years of age, and possibly even 50% of individuals over age 70 have onychomycosis.[103] The prevalence of onychomycosis increases with age, seemingly due to peripheral vascular insufficiency, repeated nail trauma, longer exposure to pathogenic fungi, suboptimal immune function, and/or the inability to maintain good foot care.[102,104,105] Onychomycosis is also prevalent among persons suffering from immunodeficiency.[101,102] An estimated one-third of all diabetics and one-fourth of all patients infected with human immunodeficiency virus (HIV) have onychomycosis.[102,103] Other risk factors for onychomycosis include Down syndrome, use of communal bathing facilities, frequent environmental contact with pathogens, occlusive clothing and shoes, nail dystrophy, residing in a warm humid climate, tinea pedis, genetic predisposition, and residing with those who have onychomycosis.[101,102,106]

Although onychomycosis is not life-threatening, it may create sequelae that markedly impact the physical, functional, and psychosocial aspects of life.[101,102] Complications such as pain, cellulitis, and extensive dermatophytic infections may occur.[101] Patients frequently suffer from feelings of embarrassment, self-consciousness, anxiety, and/or depression because visible mycotic infections are often viewed as a sign of poor hygiene by others.[101]

Onychomycosis caused by dermatophyte fungi is called *tinea unguium*. The dermatophytes *T. rubrum* and *Trichophyton mentagrophytes* are the most commonly cited pathogens, but other dermatophytes including *Epidermophyton* species and *Microsporum* species are also frequently reported.[102,107] Nondermatophytes including *Candida albicans*, *Scytalidium dimidiatum*, *Scytalidium hyalinum*, and certain species of *Acremonium, Alternaria, Aspergillus, Fusarium, Onychocola,* and *Scopulariopsis* are implicated in 10% to 20% of cases, with a higher prevalence in humid climates.[107,108]

Zaias and colleagues have shown that the tendency to acquire distal subungual onychomycosis may be inherited in an autosomal dominant fashion with incomplete penetrance.[109,110] When children have the disorder, there is usually a parent with the disorder. The foot is a common reservoir for fungus.[111] According to Zaias and Rebell,[112] almost all individuals with onychomycosis have preceding tinea pedis. The pathogenic sequence of events leading up to tinea unguium involves repeated micro- or macrotrauma (eg, from tight shoes, high heels, stubbing the toe, exercise) that breaks the seal between the nail plate and the hyponychium or other periungual structure, allowing the fungus to enter the nail apparatus from the foot.[112] The pedal disease, however, may not present as obvious infection coexisting with the nail disease.[10] It is helpful when evaluating for the presence of tinea unguium to ask the patient if he or she knows of a past history (preceding nail involvement) of "athlete's foot" and to examine patients thoroughly and with use of magnification for coexisting tinea pedis.[10]

■ SUBTYPES

Onychomycosis is currently divided into four subtypes: distolateral subungual onychomycosis (DSO) [**Figure 40-18**], white superficial

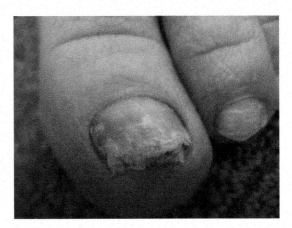

FIGURE 40-18. Distal subungual onychomycosis.

onychomycosis (WSO) [**Figure 40-19**], proximal subungual onychomycosis (PSO) [**Figure 40-20**], and *Candida* onychomycosis (CO).[113,114] The most common subtype, DSO, occurs when fungus invades the nail plate and nail bed by way of penetration of the distal or lateral margins.[102,108] The usual pathogen involved in DSO is *T. rubrum*.[10] WSO is the most common presentation observed in children and occurs when the fungus invades the nail plate directly from above yielding a nail surface characterized by powdery, white patchy discoloration.[102,108] In otherwise healthy individuals, *T. mentagrophytes* is the most commonly observed pathogen, whereas in the immunosuppressed population (ie, HIV population), *T. rubrum* is the most common etiology.[10] PSO, which occurs when the fungus invades the proximal margin embedded within the nail fold, is most prevalent in the immunodeficient population and is characterized by the appearance of infection from beneath the nail as it grows.[102,108] *T. rubrum* is the most common pathogen.[10] Disease progression often produces overlap variants of these presentations, and additional subtypes of onychomycosis have been proposed.[108,113]

CO is further divided into three subtypes based partly on route of invasion: initial paronychia with secondary plate invasion, distal onycholysis with secondary plate invasion, and direct nail plate invasion (seen in patients with chronic mucocutaneous candidiasis). The most common cause is *C. albicans*, which is isolated in 70% of cases, whereas *Candida parapsilosis, Candida tropicalis,* and *Candida krusei* are seen less frequently.[114,115]

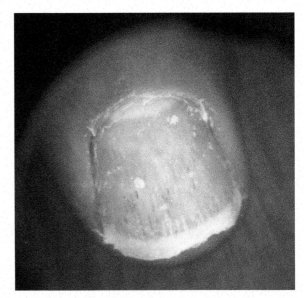

FIGURE 40-19. White superficial onychomycosis.

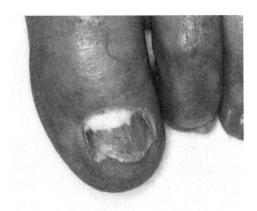

FIGURE 40-20. Proximal subungual onychomycosis.

DIAGNOSIS

Mycologic confirmation is critical for proper diagnosis and management because only about half of all dystrophic nails are due to fungal infection.[101] Certain nail dystrophies, including those attributed to psoriasis, eczematous conditions, senile ischemia (onychogryphosis), trauma, LP, periungual squamous cell carcinoma, and iron deficiency, are often clinically indistinguishable from onychomycosis.[107,108,113]

The following are considered definitive laboratory criteria for the diagnosis of onychomycosis: microscopic evidence of septate hyphae and/or arthroconidia using either potassium hydroxide (KOH) or Calcofluor white stains, positive fungal culture of nail clippings with subungual debris (or from surface debris in SWO), or positive histopathologic examination of nail clippings with periodic acid–Schiff (PAS) stain.[107,113] Although microscopy allows for diagnosis upon the initial visit, the fungus identified in the abnormal nails may be dead or a mere bystander not responsible for the actual nail pathology.[108] A positive culture may confirm fungal viability and also allow for its identification and determination of pathogenicity, but has poor sensitivity.[108,116,117] Although histopathologic examination of nail clippings with PAS stain is more sensitive than either KOH examination or fungal culture, the procedure is more expensive.[113,118] Like PAS, Calcofluor white stain possesses a higher sensitivity than KOH examination or fungal culture, but its use is limited because fluorescent microscopy is required for result interpretation.[117]

When nondermatophyte species are identified, it is often unclear whether or not they could be contributing to the clinical findings.[107,108] To diagnose nondermatophyte infection, the same organism must be isolated from sequential specimens, and correlation with direct microscopy and clinical changes is required.[107,108] Clinical criteria reported to be highly predictive of the diagnosis of onychomycosis include evidence of tinea pedis or tinea manuum, such as advancing scale between digits and/or redness with peripheral scaling and central clearing, or a history of tinea pedis or tinea manuum during the preceding year with noted nail discoloration.[108] If onychomycosis is suggested clinically, but routine laboratory testing produced only negative results, testing should be repeated.[107] If repeated testing continues to be negative, a nail-unit biopsy may be indicated to rule out other causes of nail dystrophy.[107]

KOH examination and fungal cultures are used commonly for diagnosis. A recent longitudinal study of 341 patients examined repeated KOH and culture results in onychomycosis patients who declined treatment to ascertain the accuracy of data obtained in the initial direct microscopic and culture studies used for and strongly relied upon in routine diagnosis.[119] Including dermatophyte and nondermatophyte molds, this study demonstrated that initial KOH and culture were 83.9% sensitive for indicating a true fungal etiology. Recent evidence suggests that nail plate clipping, histologic processing, and staining with PAS stain may be more sensitive (92%) than traditional KOH and culture technique when diagnosing onychomycosis.[120] Based on currently available data, both PAS and KOH plus culture are accepted diagnostic techniques, with comparable accuracy.

TREATMENT

Deciding whether or not to treat and how to treat onychomycosis involves several considerations including the certainty of diagnosis, patient comorbidities, efficacy, cost, and potential side effects of treatment.[108] All current therapeutic options are associated with a high rate of initial treatment failure or recurrence, and mycologic cure is not synonymous with clinical cure.[107,108,113] Even when treatment is effective, nails may continue to have an abnormal appearance. In 2007, Scher et al[107] defined cure for onychomycosis as total absence of clinical signs, or presence of negative microscopy and/or nail culture results with one or more of the following minor clinical criteria: (1) nail plate thickening secondary to a comorbid condition or (2) minimal distal subungual hyperkeratosis or onycholysis leaving less than 10% of the nail affected.

U.S. Food and Drug Administration (FDA)-approved oral agents shown to be effective in the treatment of onychomycosis through randomized controlled trials include terbinafine and itraconazole.[113] Although not currently FDA approved, once-weekly fluconazole has been found to be effective in patients with onychomycosis and may be particularly useful in patients with complicated medication regimens.[113,121] However, head-to-head trials have found once-weekly fluconazole to be neither as effective nor as cost-effective as terbinafine or itraconazole.[113,122-124] A meta-analysis revealed the following mycologic cure rates for dermatophyte onychomycosis in randomized controlled trials: terbinafine (76% ± 3%), itraconazole pulse therapy (63% ± 7%), itraconazole continuous therapy (59% ± 5%), and fluconazole (48% ± 5%).[125]

Terbinafine appears to be less effective against nondermatophytes such as *Candida* species than fluconazole, and many experts prefer to treat nondermatophyte infections with fluconazole rather than terbinafine. Both continuous and pulse regimens of itraconazole have been found to be effective in treating CO, but given its less favorable side effect profile, itraconazole is usually reserved in cases of fluconazole failure. Terbinafine and itraconazole appear to be effective against *Aspergillus* species and have limited efficacy versus *Scopulariopsis brevicaulis* and *Fusarium* species.[126,127]

Studies using FDA-approved, broad-spectrum, topical ciclopirox olamine 8% lacquer found that only 7% of patients attained disease-free, normal-appearing nails after 48 weeks of therapy, and only 4% of patients were able to maintain both clinical and mycologic cure 3 months after the completion of therapy.[18] In contrast, 40% to 60% of patients treated with oral terbinafine achieved complete cure at the end of the course of therapy.[128] Thus, topical therapy is typically reserved to treat patients in whom systemic treatment is contraindicated or declined or patients suffering from the white superficial subtype.[108] Topical therapy appears to be more effective when combined with vigorous filing of the upper surface of the nail.[108,129] Randomized trials have found no greater clinical efficacy of ciclopirox in combination with oral terbinafine compared with oral terbinafine alone.[113,130,131]

Preliminary data have been collected on several potential therapeutic modalities including infrared and near-infrared laser therapy,[132,133] photodynamic therapy,[134-136] iontophoretic delivery of topical medications,[137-140] and the use of medicated chest rubs containing eucalyptus oil, camphor, menthol, thymol, oil of turpentine, oil of nutmeg, and oil of cedar leaf.[141] Additional studies that support their efficacy are necessary before treatment with these agents can be recommended.[113] Surgery is generally used only in the treatment of an isolated nail infection or dermatophytoma (a collection of dermatophytes in solid form beneath the nail).[113]

In summary, certain nail disorders, including onychomycosis, LP, and psoriasis, occur in all individuals, including those with skin of color. Particular attention must be paid to LM, which is common in darker skin types; if atypical, it may indicate NAM. Evaluation of LM for NAM includes a detailed history and physical examination, examination of all 20 nails, use of dermoscopy, and often a nail matrix biopsy. Finally, it is important to note that NAM has a worse prognosis than its cutaneous counterpart in large part due to delayed diagnosis.

REFERENCES

1. Haneke E, Baran R. Longitudinal melanonychia. *Dermatol Surg.* 2001;27: 580-584.

2. Andre J, Lateur N. Pigmented nail disorders. *Dermatol Clin.* 2006;24:329-339.

3. Jellinek NJ. Nail matrix biopsy of longitudinal melanonychia: diagnostic algorithm including the matrix shave biopsy. *J Am Acad Dermatol.* 2007; 56:803-810.

4. Rich P. Chapter 149: nail surgery. In: Bolognia JL, Jorizzo JL, Rapini RP, eds. *Dermatology.* 2nd ed. New York, NY: Mosby; 2006:2260-2268.

5. Klausner JM, Inbar M, Gutman M, et al. Nail-bed melanoma. *J Surg Oncol.* 1987;34:208-210.

6. Quinn MJ, Thompson JE, Crotty K, et al. Subungual melanoma of the hand. *J Hand Surg (Am).* 1996;21:506-511.

7. Glat PM, Spector JA, Roses DF, et al. The management of pigmented lesions of the nail bed. *Ann Plast Surg.* 1996;37:125-134.

8. Perrin C, Michiels JF, Pisani A, et al. Anatomic distribution of melanocytes in normal nail unit: an immunohistochemical investigation. *Am J Dermatopathol.* 1997;19:462-467.

9. Baran R, Perrin C. Linear melanonychia due to subungual keratosis of the nail bed: report of two cases. *Br J Dermatol.* 1999;140:730-733.

10. Jellinek N, Daniel CR III. Chapter 38: nail disorders. In: Kelly AP, Taylor SC, eds. *Dermatology for Skin of Color.* 1st ed. New York, NY: McGraw Hill Medical; 2009:256-266.

11. Tosti A, Baran R, Piraccini BM, et al. Nail matrix nevi: a clinical and histopathological study of twenty-two patients. *J Am Acad Dermatol.* 1996;34:765-771.

12. Lateur N, Andre J. Melanonychia: diagnosis and treatment. *Dermatol Ther.* 2002;15:131-141.

13. Baran R, Kechijian P. Longitudinal melanonychia (melanonychia striata): diagnosis and management. *J Am Acad Dermatol.* 1989;21:1165-1175.

14. Aratari E, Regesta G, Rebora A. Carpal tunnel syndrome appearing with prominent skin symptoms. *Arch Dermatol.* 1984;120:517-519.

15. Baran R. Frictional longitudinal melanonychia: a new entity. *Dermatologica.* 1987;174:280-284.

16. Fayol J, Baran R, Perrin C, et al. Onychomatricoma with misleading features. *Acta Derm Venereol.* 2000;80:370-372.

17. Sass U, Andre J, Stene JJ, et al. Longitudinal melanonychia revealing an intraepidermal carcinoma of the nail apparatus: detection of integrated HPV-16 DNA. *J Am Acad Dermatol.* 1998;39:490-493.

18. Baran R, Haneke E. Tumours of the nail apparatus and adjacent tissues. In: Baran R, Dawber RPR, eds. *Diseases of the Nails and Their Management.* 2nd ed. Oxford, United Kingdom: Blackwell; 1994:417-496.

19. Cribier B, Leiva Mena M, Rey D, et al. Nail changes in patients infected with human immunodeficiency virus. *Arch Dermatol.* 1998;134:1216-1220.

20. Quinlan KE, Janiga JJ, Baran R, et al. Transverse melanonychia secondary to total skin electron beam therapy: a report of 3 cases. *J Am Acad Dermatol.* 2005;53:S112-S114.

21. Kar HK. Longitudinal melanonychia associated with fluconazole therapy. *Int J Dermatol.* 1998;37:719-720.

22. O'Branski EE, Russel EW, Prose NS, et al. Skin and nail changes in children with sickle cell anemia receiving hydroxyurea therapy. *J Am Acad Dermatol.* 2001;44:859-861.

23. Piraccini BM, Tosti A. Drug-induced nail disorders. Incidence, management and prognosis. *Drug Saf.* 1999;21:187-201.

24. Sutton R. Transverse band pigmentation of fingernails after x-ray therapy. *JAMA.* 1952;150:210-211.

25. Shelley W, Rawnsley H, Pillsbury D. Postirradiation melanonychia. *Arch Dermatol.* 1964;90:174-176.

26. Weiss E, Sayegh-Carreno R. PUVA-induced pigmented nails. *Int J Dermatol.* 1989;28:188-189.

27. Hann SK, Hwang SY, Park YK. Melanonychia induced by systemic photochemotherapy. *Photodermatol.* 1989;6:98-99.

28. Ledbetter LS, Hsu S. Melanonychia associated with PUVA therapy. *J Am Acad Dermatol.* 2003;48:S31-S32.

29. Naik RPC, Parameswara YR. 8-methoxypsoralen-induced nail pigmentation. *Int J Dermatol.* 1982;21:275-276.

30. Cunha AP, Resende C, Barros L, et al. Transverse melanonychia caused by the use of infliximab to treat refractory pyoderma gangrenosum (P23-28). *J Eur Acad Dermatol Venereol.* 2002;16:250.

31. Tosti A, Baran R, Dawber R. The nail in systemic diseases and drug-induced changes. In: Baran R, Dawber R, eds. *Diseases of the Nails and Their Management.* 2nd ed. Oxford, United Kingdom: Blackwell Scientific Publications; 1994:175-262.

32. Positano RG, DeLauro TM, Berkowitz BJ. Nail changes secondary to environmental influences. *Clin Podiatr Med Surg.* 1989;6:417-429.

33. Hernandez-Martin A, Ros-Forteza S, de Unamuno P. Longitudinal, transverse, and diffuse nail hyperpigmentation induced by hydroxyurea. *J Am Acad Dermatol.* 1999;41:333-334.

34. Goettmann-Bonvallot S, Andre J, Belaich S. Longitudinal melanonychia in children: a clinical and histopathologic study of 40 cases. *J Am Acad Dermatol.* 1999;41:17-22.

35. Leate-Labreze C, Bioulac-Sage P, Taieb A. Longitudinal melanonychia in children. A study of eight cases. *Arch Dermatol.* 1996;132:167-169.

36. Hinds MW. Anatomic distribution of malignant melanoma of the skin among non-Caucasians in Hawaii. *Br J Cancer.* 1979;40:497-499.

37. Banfield CC, Dawber RP. Nail melanoma: a review of the literature with recommendations to improve patient management. *Br J Dermatol.* 1999;141: 628-632.

38. Krull EA. Malignant melanoma. In: Krull EA, Baran R, Haneke E, eds. *Nail Surgery: A Text and Atlas.* Philadelphia, PA: Lippincott Williams & Wilkins; 2001:305-315.

39. Parker SG, Diffey BL. The transmission of optical radiation through human nails. *Br J Dermatol.* 1983;108:11-16.

40. Rigby HS, Briggs JC. Subungual melanoma: a clinicopathological study of 24 cases. *Br J Plast Surg.* 1992;45:275-278.

41. Black WC, Wiggins C. Melanoma among southwestern American Indians. *Cancer.* 1985;55:2899-2902.

42. Collins RJ. Melanomas in the Chinese of Hong Kong. Emphasis on volar and subungual sites Indians. *Cancer.* 1984;54:1482-1488.

43. Saida T, Ohshima Y. Clinical and histopathologic characteristics of the early lesions of subungual melanoma. *Cancer.* 1989;63:556-560.

44. Miura S, Jimbow K. Clinical characteristics of subungual melanoma in Japan, case report and questionnaire survey of 108 cases. *J Dermatol (Tokyo).* 1985;12:425-429.

45. Rodriguez-Cuevas S, Luna-Perez P. Subungual melanoma. Is elective regional lymph node dissection mandatory? *J Exp Clin Cancer Res.* 1993;12;173-178.

46. Thai KE, Young R, Sinclair RD. Nail apparatus melanoma. *Australas J Dermatol.* 2001;42:71-81.

47. Banfield CC, Redburn JC, Dawber RP. The incidence and prognosis of nail apparatus melanoma: a retrospective study of 105 patients in four English regions. *Br J Dermatol.* 1998;139:276-279.

48. Finley RK III, Driscoll DL, Blumenson LE, Karakousis CP. Subungual melanoma: an eighteen-year review. *Surgery.* 1994;116:96-100.

49. Paul E, Kleiner H, Bodeker RH. Epidemiologie und prognose subungualer melanome. *Hautarzt.* 1992;43:286-290.

50. Stevens NG, Liff JM, Weiss NS. Plantar melanoma: is the incidence of melanoma of the sole of the foot really higher in blacks than whites? *Int J Cancer.* 1990;45:691-693.

51. Perrin C, Baran R. Longitudinal melanonychia caused by *Trichophyton rubrum*: histochemical and ultrastructural study of two cases. *J Am Acad Dermatol.* 1994;31:311-316.

52. Lee HJ, Koh BK, Moon JS, et al. A case of melanonychia caused by *Fusarium solani. Br J Dermatol.* 2002;147:607-608.

53. Gautret P, Rodier MH, Kauffmann-Lacroix C, Jacquemin JL. Case report and review: onychomycosis due to *Candida parapsilosis. Mycoses.* 2000;43:433-435.

54. Hata Y, Naka W, Nishikawa T. A case of melanonychia caused by *Exophiala dermatitidis. Nippon Ishinkin Gakkai Zasshi.* 1999;40:231-234.

55. Matsumoto T, Matsuda T, Padhye AA, et al. Fungal melanonychia: ungual phaeohyphomycosis caused by *Wangiella dermatitidis. Clin Exp Dermatol.* 1992;17:83-86.

56. Agodi A, Stefani S, Corsaro C, et al. Study of a melanic pigment of *Proteus mirabilis. Res Microbiol.* 1996;147:167-174.

57. Ronger S, Touzet S, Ligeron C, et al. Dermoscopic examination of nail pigmentation. *Arch Dermatol.* 2002;138:1327-1333.

58. Baran R, Kechijian P. Hutchinson's sign: a reappraisal. *J Am Acad Dermatol.* 1996;34:87-90.

59. Kawabata Y, Ohara K, Hino H, Tamaki K. Two kinds of Hutchinson's sign, benign and malignant. *J Am Acad Dermatol.* 2001;44:305-307.

60. Haas N, Henz BM. Pitfall in pigmentation: pseudopods in the nail plate. *Dermatol Surg.* 2002;28:966-967.

61. Johr RH, Izakovic J. Dermatoscopy/ELM for the evaluation of nail-apparatus pigmentation. *Dermatol Surg.* 2001;27:315-322.

62. Braun RP, Baran R, Saurat JH, Thomas L. Surgical pearl: dermoscopy of the free edge of the nail to determine the level of nail plate pigmentation and the location of its probable origin in the proximal or distal nail matrix. *J Am Acad Dermatol.* 2006;55:512-513.

63. Levit EK, Kagen MH, Scher RK, et al. The ABC rule for clinical detection of subungual melanoma. *J Am Acad Dermatol.* 2000;42:269-274.

64. Di Chiaccio N, Hirata SH, Enokihara MY. Dermatologists' accuracy in early diagnosis of melanoma of the nail matrix. *Arch Dermatol.* 2010;146:382-387.

65. Rich P. Nail biopsy: indications and methods. *Dermatol Surg.* 2001;27: 229-234.

66. Haneke E. Chapter 1: surgical anatomy of the nail apparatus. In: Richert B, Di Chiaccio N, Haneke E, eds. *Nail Surgery.* New York, NY: Informa Healthcare; 2011:1-10.

67. Fleckman P. Chapter 3: structure and function of the nail unit. In: Scher RK, Daniel CR III, eds. *Nails: Diagnosis, Therapy, and Surgery.* Beijing, China: Elsevier Saunders; 2005:13-25.

68. DeBerker DAR, Mawhinney B, Sviland L. Quantification of regional matrix nail production. *Br J Dermatol.* 1996;134:1083-1086.

69. Moossavi M, Scher RK. Complications of nail surgery: a review of the literature. *Dermatol Surg.* 2001;27:225-228.

70. Haneke E. Operative therapie akraler und subungualer melanome. In: Rompel R, Petres J, eds. *Operative und Onkologische Dermatologie.* Berlin, Germany: Springer; 1999.

71. Hafner J, Haenseler E, Ossent P, et al. Benzidine stain for the histochemical detection of hemoglobin in splinter hemorrhage (subungual hematoma) and black heel. *Am J Dermatopathol.* 1995;17:362-367.

72. Husain S, Scher RK, Silvers DN, Ackerman AB. Melanotic macule of nail unit and its clinicopathologic spectrum. *J Am Acad Dermatol.* 2006;54: 664-667.

73. High WA, Quirey RA, Guillen DR, et al. Presentation, histopathologic findings, and clinical outcomes in 7 cases of melanoma in situ of the nail unit. *Arch Dermatol.* 2004;140:1102-1106.

74. Giele H, Hollowood K, Gibbons CL, et al. Subungual melanoma with osteocartilaginous differentiation. *Skeletal Radiol.* 2003;32:724-727.

75. Perrin C, Michiels JF, Pisani A, Ortonne JP. Anatomic distribution of melanocytes in normal nail unit: an immunohistochemical investigation. *Am J Dermatopathol.* 1997;19:462-467.

76. Goettmann-Bonvallot S, Andre J, Belaich S. Longitudinal melanonychia in children: a clinical and histopathologic study of 40 cases. *J Am Acad Dermatol.* 1999;41:17-22.

77. Park KG, Blessing K, Kernohan NM. Surgical aspects of subungual malignant melanomas. The Scottish Melanoma Group. *Ann Surg.* 1992;216:692-695.

78. Levit EK, Kagen MH, Scher RK, et al. The ABC rule for clinical detection of subungual melanoma. *J Am Acad Dermatol.* 2000;42:269-274.

79. Blessing K, Kernohan NM, Park KG. Subungual malignant melanoma: clinicopathological features of 100 cases. *Histopathology.* 1991;19:425-429.

80. Heaton KM, el-Naggar A, Ensign LG, et al. Surgical management and prognostic factors in patients with subungual melanoma. *Ann Surg.* 1994;219:197-204.

81. Spencer JM. Malignant tumors of the nail unit. *Dermatol Ther.* 2002;15: 126-130.

82. Kato T, Suetake T, Sugiyama Y, et al. Epidemiology and prognosis of subungual melanoma in 34 Japanese patients. *Br J Dermatol.* 1996;134:383-387.

83. Balch CM, Buzaid AC, Soong SJ, et al. Final version of the American Joint Committee on Cancer staging system for cutaneous melanoma. *J Clin Oncol.* 2001;19:3635-3648.

84. Johnson TM, Sondak VK, Bichakjian CK, Sabel MS. The role of sentinel lymph node biopsy for melanoma: evidence assessment. *J Am Acad Dermatol.* 2006;54:19-27.

85. O'Toole EA, Stephens R, Young MM, et al. Subungual melanoma: a relation to direct injury? *J Am Acad Dermatol.* 1995;33:525-528.

86. Moehrle M, Metzger S, Schippert W, et al. "Functional" surgery in subungual melanoma. *Dermatol Surg.* 2003;29:366-374.

87. Abimelec P, Dumontier C. Basic and advanced nail surgery: 2. Indications and complications. In: Scher RK, Daniel CR, eds. *Nails: Diagnosis, Therapy, Surgery.* 3rd ed. Philadelphia, PA: Elsevier Saunders; 2005:291-308.

88. Banfield CC, Dawber RP, Walker NP, et al. Mohs micrographic surgery for the treatment of in situ nail apparatus melanoma: a case report. *J Am Acad Dermatol.* 1999;40:98-99.

89. Brodland DG. The treatment of nail apparatus melanoma with Mohs micrographic surgery. *Dermatol Surg.* 2001;27:269-273.

90. Shiohara T, Kano Y. Lichen planus and lichenoid dermatoses. In: Bolognia J, Jorizzo J, Rapini R, eds. *Dermatology.* Vol 1. St. Louis, MO: Mosby; 2003: 175-198.

91. Rich P, Scher RK. Chapter 6: nail manifestations of cutaneous disease. In: *An Atlas of Diseases of the Nail.* New York, NY: Parthenon Publishing; 2003:51-59.

92. Scher RK. Lichen planus of the nail. *Dermatol Clin.* 1985;3:395-399.

93. Tosti A, Piraccini BM. Chapter 11: dermatological diseases. In: Scher RK, Daniel RC, eds. *Nails: Diagnosis, Therapy, and Surgery.* Beijing, China: Elsevier Saunders; 2005:105-121.

94. Tosti A, Peluso AM, Fanti PA, Piraccini BM. Nail lichen planus: clinical and pathologic study of 24 patients. *J Am Acad Dermatol.* 1993;28:724-730.

95. Juhlin L, Baran R. On longitudinal melanonychia after healing of lichen planus. *Acta Derm Venereol (Stockh).* 1990;70:183.

96. Piraccini BM, Saccani E, Starace M, et al. Nail lichen planus: response to treatment and long term follow-up. *Eur J Dermatol.* 2010;20:489-496.

97. Cribier B, Frances C, Chosidow O. Treatment of lichen planus. An evidence-based medicine analysis of efficacy. *Arch Dermatol.* 1998;134:1521-1530.

98. Goettmann S, Zaraa I, Moulonguet I. Nail lichen planus: epidemiological, clinical, pathological, therapeutic and prognosis study of 67 cases. *J Eur Acad Dermatol Venereol.* 2012;26:1304-1309.

99. Daniel CR III. Simple onycholysis. In: Scher RK, Daniel CR III, eds. *Nails: Diagnosis, Therapy, Surgery.* 3rd ed. Philadelphia, PA: Elsevier Saunders; 2005: 97-98.

100. Baran R. Retinoids and the nails. *J Dermatol Treat.* 1990;1:151-154.

101. Elewski BE. Onychomycosis: treatment, quality of life, and economic issues. *Am J Clin Dermatol.* 2000;1:19-26.

102. Kaur R, Kashyap B, Bhalla P. Onychomycosis: epidemiology, diagnosis, and management. *Indian J Med Microbiol.* 2008;26:108-116.

103. Thomas J, Jacobson GA, Narkowics CK, Perterson GM, Burnet H, Sharpe C. Toenail onychomycosis: an important global disease burden. *J Clin Pharm Ther.* 2010;35:497-519.

104. Elewski BE, Charif MA. Prevalence of onychomycosis in patients attending a dermatology clinic in northeastern Ohio for other conditions. *Arch Dermatol.* 1997;133:1172-1173.

105. Ghannoum MA, Hajjeh RA, Scher R, et al. A large-scale North American study of fungal isolates from nails: the frequency of onychomycosis, fungal distribution and antifungal susceptibility patterns. *J Am Acad Dermatol.* 2000;43:641-648.

106. Svejgaard EL, Nilsson J. Onychomycosis in Denmark: prevalence of fungal nail infection in general practice. *Mycoses.* 2004;47:131-135.

107. Scher R, Tavakkol A, Bact D, et al. Onychomycosis: diagnosis and definition of cure. *J Am Acad Dermatol.* 2007;56:939-944.

108. De Berker D. Fungal nail disease. *N Engl J Med.* 2009;360:2108-2116.

109. Faergemann J, Correia O, Nowicki R, Ro BI. Genetic predisposition: understanding underlying mechanisms of onychomycosis. *J Eur Acad Dermatol Venereol.* 2005;19:17-19.

110. Zaias N, Tosti A, Rebell G, et al. Autosomal dominant pattern of distal subungual onychomycosis caused by *Trichophyton rubrum. J Am Acad Dermatol.* 1996;34:302-304.

111. Daniel CR III, Jellinek NJ. The pedal fungus reservoir (editorial). *Arch Dermatol.* 2006;142:1344-1346.

112. Zaias N, Rebell G. Chronic dermatophytosis caused by *Trichophyton rubrum. J Am Acad Dermatol.* 1996;35:S17-S20.

113. Goldstein AO, Goldstein BG. Onychomycosis. In: Basow DS, ed. *UpToDate.* Waltham, MA: UpTpDate; 2011.

114. Cohen JL, Gupta AK, Scher RK, Pappert AS. Chapter 5: the nail and fungus infections. In: Elewski BE, ed. *Cutaneous Fungal Infections.* 2nd ed. New York, NY: Blackwell Science; 1998:119-153.

115. Andre J, Achten G. Onychomycosis. *Int J Dermatol.* 1987;26:481-490.

116. Denning DW, Evans EG, Kibbler CC, et al. Fungal nail disease: a guide to good practice (report of a Working Group of the British Society for Medical Mycology). *BMJ.* 1995;311:1277-1288.

117. Weinberg JM, Koestenblatt EK, Tutrone WD, et al. Comparison of diagnostic methods in the evaluation of onychomycosis. *J Am Acad Dermatol.* 2003;49:193-197.

118. Wilsmann-Theis D, Sareika F, Bieber T, et al. New reasons for histopathological nail-clipping examination in the diagnosis of onychomycosis. *J Eur Acad Dermatol Venereol.* 2011;25:235-237.

119. Summerbell RC, Cooper E, Bunn U, et al. Onychomycosis: a critical study of techniques and criteria for confirming the etiologic significance of non-dermatophytes. *Med Mycol.* 2005;43:39-59.

120. Weinberg JM, Koestenblatt EK, Tutrone WD, et al. Comparison of diagnostic methods in the evaluation of onychomycosis. *J Am Acad Dermatol.* 2003;49:193-197.

121. Scher RK, Breneman D, Rich P, et al. Once-weekly fluconazole (150, 300, or 450 mg) in the treatment of distal subungual onychomycosis of the toenail. *J Am Acad Dermatol.* 1998;38:S77.

122. Gupta AK. Pharmacoeconomic analysis of oral antifungal therapies used to treat dermatophyte onychomycosis of the toenails. A US analysis. *Pharmacoeconomics.* 1998;13:243-256.

123. Havu V, Heikkilä H, Kuokkanen K, et al. A double-blind, randomized study to compare the efficacy and safety of terbinafine (Lamisil) with fluconazole (Diflucan) in the treatment of onychomycosis. *Br J Dermatol.* 2000;142:97-102.

124. Salo H, Pekurinen M. Cost effectiveness of oral terbinafine (Lamisil) compared with oral fluconazole (Diflucan) in the treatment of patients with toenail onychomycosis. *Pharmacoeconomics.* 2002;20:319-324.

125. Gupta AK, Ryder JE, Johnson AM. Cumulative meta-analysis of systemic antifungal agents for the treatment of onychomycosis. *Br J Dermatol.* 2004;150:537-544.

126. Gupta A. Chapter 5: systemic antifungal agents. In: Wolverton SE, eds. *Comprehensive Dermatologic Drug Therapy.* 2nd ed. New York, NY: Saunders Elsevier; 2007:75-99.

127. Tosti A, Piraccini BM, Lorenzi S, et al. Treatment of non-dermatophyte mold and *Candida* onychomycosis. *Dermatol Clin.* 2003;21:491-497.

128. Epstein E. Fungus-free versus disease-free nails. *J Am Acad Dermatol.* 2004;50:151-152.

129. Tavakkol A, Fellman S, Kianifard F. Safety and efficacy of oral terbinafine in the treatment of onychomycosis: analysis of the elderly subgroup in Improving Results in Onychomycosis-Concomitant Lamisil and Debridement (IRON-CLAD), an open-label, randomized trial. *Am J Geriatr Pharmacother.* 2006;4:1-13.

130. Gupta AK, Onychomycosis Combination Therapy Study Group. Ciclopirox topical solution, 8% combined with oral terbinafine to treat onychomycosis: a randomized, evaluator-blinded study. *J Drugs Dermatol.* 2005;4:481-485.

131. Avner S, Nir N, Henri T. Combination of oral terbinafine and topical ciclopirox compared to oral terbinafine for the treatment of onychomycosis. *J Dermatolog Treat.* 2005;16:327-330.

132. Manevitch Z, Lev D, Hochberg M, et al. Direct antifungal effect of femtosecond laser on *Trichophyton rubrum* onychomycosis. *Photochem Photobiol.* 2010;86:476-479.

133. Landsman AS, Robbins AH, Angelini PF, et al. Treatment of mild, moderate, and severe onychomycosis using 870- and 930-nm light exposure. *J Am Podiatr Med Assoc.* 2010;100:166-167.

134. Watanabe D, Kawamura C, Masuda Y, et al. Successful treatment of toenail onychomycosis with photodynamic therapy. *Arch Dermatol.* 2008;144:19-21.

135. Piraccini BM, Rech G, Tosti A. Photodynamic therapy of onychomycosis caused by *Trichophyton rubrum*. *J Am Acad Dermatol.* 2008;59:S75.

136. Sotiriou E, Koussidou-Eremonti T, Chaidemenos G, et al. Photodynamic therapy for distal and lateral subungual toenail onychomycosis caused by *Trichophyton rubrum*: preliminary results of a single-centre open trial. *Acta Derm Venereol.* 2010;90:216-217.

137. Amichai B, Nitzan B, Mosckovitz R, Shemer A. Iontophoretic delivery of terbinafine in onychomycosis: a preliminary study. *Br J Dermatol.* 2010;162:46-50.

138. Amichai B, Mosckovitz R, Trau H, et al. Iontophoretic terbinafine HCL 1.0% delivery across porcine and human nails. *Mycopathologia.* 2010;169:343-349.

139. Nair AB, Kim HD, Chakraborty B, et al. Ungual and trans-ungual iontophoretic delivery of terbinafine for the treatment of onychomycosis. *J Pharm Sci.* 2009;98:4130-4140.

140. Derby R, Rohal P, Jackson C, et al. Novel treatment of onychomycosis using over-the-counter mentholated ointment: a clinical case series. *J Am Board Fam Med.* 2011;24:69-74.

141. Ramsewak RS, Nair MG, Stommel M, Selanders L. In vitro antagonistic activity of monoterpenes and their mixtures against 'toe nail fungus' pathogens. *Phytother Res.* 2003;17:376-379.

CHAPTER

41

Folliculitis

Kim Nichols
Miguel R. Sanchez

KEY POINTS

- Folliculitis is an inflammatory condition of the hair follicle that is caused by infection, physical injury, or chemical irritation.

- The most common type of folliculitis is infectious. This is usually secondary to *Staphylococcus aureus*, which is treated with topical or oral antibiotics.

- Staphylococcal folliculitis is particularly prevalent in the African American human immunodeficiency virus (HIV)-positive population.

- The noninfectious folliculitides are induced by drugs or chemicals, or they are activated mechanically.

- Eosinophilic folliculitis is a rare sterile folliculitis encompassing the classic Ofuji disease, HIV-associated eosinophilic folliculitis, and eosinophilic pustular folliculitis of infancy.

- Certain perifolliculocentric inflammatory disorders, such as pseudo-folliculitis barbae, acne keloidalis nuchae, and perifolliculitis capitis *abscedens et suffodiens,* although not true folliculitides, can often mimic folliculitis and are seen more often in African Americans.

SYNONYMS FOR FOLLICULITIS

- Pseudofolliculitis barbae (PFB)
- Tinea barbae
- Barber itch
- Gram-negative folliculitis
- Tufted hair folliculitis
- Perifolliculitis capitis *abscedens et suffodiens*
- Disseminated and recurrent infundibular folliculitis

INTRODUCTION

Folliculitis is a disease of the hair follicle that is usually caused by an infection. However, it can also be induced by irritation, chemical agents, medications, physical injury, or other factors that cause disruption and obstruction of the hair follicles and associated pilosebaceous units. The classification of folliculitis is complex, but this class of diseases is generally divided into infectious [**Table 41-1**] and noninfectious folliculitis and perifolliculitis [**Table 41-2**]. Perifolliculitis refers to inflammation in the perifollicular tissue and occasionally the adjacent reticular dermis. In addition to the classification of folliculitis according to its causative organism, this condition can also be designated as superficial or deep. Superficial folliculitis is when the upper portion of the hair follicle, the follicular infundibulum, is involved. Deep folliculitis is, when the inflammation extends into the isthmus and deeper portions of the follicle. In superficial folliculitis, the follicular inflammation is confined, leading to the formation of the characteristic clustered, 1- to 4-mm erythematous papule pustules that typically heal without scarring. This

type of folliculitis is usually seen in areas with terminal hair strands. Deep folliculitis is characterized by large, tender erythematous papules or nodules that can scar. The purulent material can extend into the subcutaneous tissue forming a large, deep mass or furuncle. Several infected follicles can coalesce to form a large mass or carbuncle.

Infectious folliculitis is the most common type of folliculitis and *Staphylococcus aureus* is by far the most common infectious agent causing folliculitis [**Figure 41-1A**]. In patients with skin of color, the lesions often heal with postinflammatory hyperpigmentation [**Figure 41-1B**]. Infectious folliculitis can also be caused by *Pseudomonas aeruginosa* and other Gram-negative bacteria, as well as by dermatophytes, *Pityrosporum, Candida, Demodex,* or a virus. Notably, secondary infectious folliculitis can be seen in perifollicular inflammatory disorders, such as acne keloidalis nuchae, PFB (see Chapter 39), and perifolliculitis capitis *abscedens et suffodiens,* which is also known as dissecting cellulitis. These conditions are far more prevalent in those with darker skin of color. Patients with dissecting cellulitis in particular also have a higher predilection for hidradenitis suppurativa, acne conglobata, and pilonidal sinus, which together constitute the follicular occlusion tetrad.

Folliculitis can also be noninfectious in origin. This is seen in the drug-related, eosinophilic, irritant-induced, and chemically induced types of folliculitis.

EPIDEMIOLOGY AND PATHOGENESIS

Folliculitis is a very common disorder in children and adults. There are no data to indicate a sexual predilection and it is thought to affect males and females equally. The overall incidence is increased in individuals who are obese, amputees, or immunocompromised, including those undergoing chemotherapy or those with diabetes mellitus, human immunodeficiency virus (HIV) infection, hypogammaglobulinemia, chronic granulomatous disease, or other diseases that suppress the immune system. The most important predisposing factors to the development of folliculitis are occlusion, friction, maceration, topical corticosteroids, and hyperhidrosis. The use of traction, occlusive wigs, and oils predisposes African Americans to folliculitis of the scalp.

The manipulation of the hair strands by shaving, waxing, or plucking can lead to traumatic folliculitis. Topical corticosteroids can induce folliculitis, especially when high-potency preparations, ointment vehicles, and occlusion are used. In addition, individuals with some pruritic skin diseases, such as atopic dermatitis, contact dermatitis, arthropod assault, and Darier disease, are prone to develop secondary folliculitis. Folliculitis may also develop in persons with infected abrasions, lacerations, surgical wounds, fistulas, and other breaks in the skin, as well as in those with bacterial infections, such as abscesses.

The infectious folliculitides often occur more frequently in particular populations or under specific conditions. For instance, because *S. aureus* is a normal inhabitant of the anterior nares in approximately 20% of adults, nasal carriers are prone to *S. aureus* folliculitis. *S. aureus* outbreaks are also common in athletes who wear occlusive clothing in hot, humid weather, share towels and athletic equipment, participate in contact sports, and shower in group facilities. *Pseudomonas* folliculitis is caused by colonization of hair follicles with certain strains of *P. aeruginosa* after exposure to contaminated water in hot tubs, whirlpools, swimming pools, water slides, and bathtubs. Gram-negative folliculitis develops in acne patients after prolonged antibiotic treatment. Tinea barbae is a fungal folliculitis that affects the mustache and beard areas of

285

TABLE 41-1	Common nonstaphylococcal infectious folliculitides
Type	Clinical features
Bacterial folliculitis	
Pseudomonas aeruginosa folliculitis	Develops after exposure to contaminated water in hot tubs, whirlpools, swimming pools, water slides, and bathtubs
Gram-negative folliculitis	Occurs at site of acne vulgaris, often on the face after long-term antibiotic therapy
Fungal folliculitis	
Tinea barbae	Due to *Trichophyton mentagrophytes* var. *mentagrophytes* or *T. verrucosum*; it is classically found in male farm workers
Majocchi granuloma	This is usually due to *Trichophyton rubrum*, and characteristically develops in women who shave their legs
Pityrosporum folliculitis	This often occurs in young adults in areas of occlusion and increased sweat production
Candida folliculitis	Usually associated with intertrigo in obese individuals and diabetics
Viral folliculitis	
Herpes simplex folliculitis	Herpes sycosis barbae is seen in men who shave with a history of recurrent facial herpes simplex infection
Follicular molluscum contagiosum	Often seen in association with immune suppression and shaving
***Demodex* folliculitis**	Often mistaken as rosacea

Sources: Data from Kelly AP. Folliculitis and the follicular occlusion triad. In: Bolognia JL, Jorizzo JL, Rapini RP, et al, eds. *Dermatology*. 1st ed. London, United Kingdom: Mosby; 2003:554;[9] and Lee PK, Zipoli MT, Weinberg AN, et al. Pyodermas: *Staphylococcus aureus, Streptococcus*, and other gram-positive bacteria. In: Freedberg IM, Eisen AZ, Wolff K, et al, eds. *Fitzpatrick's Dermatology in General Medicine*. 6th ed. New York, NY: McGraw-Hill; 2003:1860.[1]

men (usually farm workers) who are exposed to *Trichophyton*-carrying cattle and dogs. This condition, as well as Majocchi granuloma (caused by *Trichophyton rubrum*), herpetic folliculitis, and molluscum folliculitis, almost always occurs after shaving for both men and women.

STAPHYLOCOCCAL AND OTHER INFECTIOUS FOLLICULITIDES

■ CLINICAL FEATURES

S. aureus superficial folliculitis (Bockhart impetigo) is characterized by a grid-like grouping of papules or pustules on hair-bearing skin. It can occur on all body surfaces but is found most commonly on the head and neck (especially the perioral, scalp, and beard areas), upper trunk, axillae, groin, and buttocks. Folliculitis in an eyelash is called a hordeolum or sty. Folliculitis in the pubic and perianogenital area may be secondary to sexual transmission. The primary lesions are erythematous papules and fragile yellowish white dome-shaped pustules with central hairs (although the hair shaft is not always seen). Secondary changes include crusting, scale, and excoriations. Although they are often asymptomatic, the lesions can be pruritic, especially in occluded areas, but they usually heal without scarring. In most cases of superficial folliculitis, systemic symptoms are absent. In patients with darker skin of color, the classic erythema seen in those with a light skin color is often masked, and the lesions present as hyperpigmented pustules and papules.

Deep folliculitis involves the entire hair follicle, causing furuncles (boils), carbuncles, and sycoses. Furuncles are deep-seated erythematous nodules that can enlarge to up to 2 cm and become hard, painful, and fluctuant [**Figure 41-2**]. Over several days, they may undergo abscess formation, drain pus, and eventually rupture with a gradual diminution of pain and erythema. Furuncles usually evolve from superficial folliculitis in hair-bearing, occluded regions of the body. Carbuncles are red,

TABLE 41-2	Noninfectious folliculitis and perifollicultis
Superficial folliculitis	
Rosacea and perioral dermatitis	
Eosinophilic pustular folliculitis	
Toxic erythema of the newborn	
Follicular mucinosis	
Fox-Fordyce disease	
Infundibulofolliculitis	
Mechanical folliculitis	
Pruritic folliculitis of pregnancy	
Traumatic folliculitis	
Chemical folliculitis	
Deep folliculitis	
Acne conglobata	
Lupoid rosacea	
Keloidal acne of the neck	
Perforating folliculitis	
Superficial or deep folliculitis	
Acne vulgaris	
Halogenoderma	
Pseudofolliculitis	
Perifolliculitis	
Lichen planopilaris	
Keratosis pilaris	
Keratosis pilaris atrophicans	
Keratosis spinulosa	
Pityriasis rubra pilaris	
Phrynoderma	
Drug-induced perifolliculitis	
Perioral dermatitis	
Vitamin C deficiency	

Source: Data from Camacho F. Cicatricial alopecias. In: Camacho F, Montagna W, eds. *Trichology: Diseases of the Pilosebaceous Follicle*. Madrid, Spain: Aula Medica Group; 1997.[1a]

exquisitely tender masses of coalescing furuncles [**Figure 41-3**]. They can be associated with fever and malaise and may heal with prominent scarring.[1] They most often develop on the neck, back, and thighs. Sycosis barbae (also known as sycosis vulgaris or barber itch) is a chronic, recalcitrant eruption of follicular pustules with perifollicular inflammation, erythema, and crusting in the bearded/mustached areas [**Figure 41-4**]. It is caused by staphylococcal or dermatophytic infection and occurs only in postpubertal men who have begun shaving. The deeper, chronic, and scarring form of sycosis barbae is termed lupoid sycosis.[2] Sycosis barbae should be distinguished from tinea barbae, PFB, and herpetic sycosis. Tinea barbae is often unilateral and rarely affects the upper lip, but a clinical variant called mycotic sycosis closely resembles staphylococcal sycosis. PFB is not infectious, occurs mainly in African American men, and worsens with shaving.[3]

In herpes folliculitis, vesicles are present at some point during the disease course [**Figure 41-5**]. HIV-seropositive patients are especially prone to extensive and recurrent cases of staphylococcal folliculitis, furunculosis, and carbunculosis. *S. aureus* is the most common cutaneous bacterial pathogen because about half of all HIV-positive patients are nasal carriers. In one study, 54% of patients developed symptomatic *S. aureus* skin infection during the course of acquired immunodeficiency syndrome (AIDS).[4] In another recent multicenter longitudinal trial, the prevalence of skin disorders was compared in 2018 HIV-infected women and 557 HIV-uninfected women.[5] Not only were skin problems more frequent in HIV-infected women (63%), compared with HIV-uninfected women (44%), but HIV-infected women were also more likely to have more than two skin-related diagnoses. HIV infection was correlated with several specific skin conditions, including

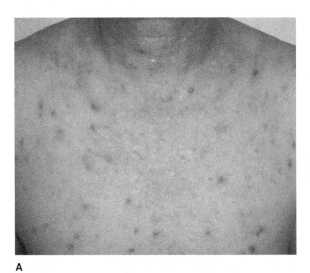

A

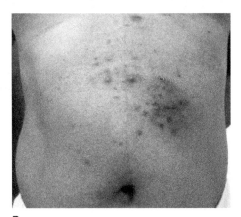

B

FIGURE 41-1. **(A)** Folliculitis on the chest of a Hispanic man. (Used with permission from Dr. Miguel Sanchez, New York University, Department of Dermatology.) **(B)** Superficial folliculitis with resulting disfiguring postinflammatory hyperpigmentation on the trunk of a male patient with skin of color. (Used with permission from the Ronald O. Perelman Department of Dermatology, New York University School of Medicine, NYU Langone Medical Center, New York.)

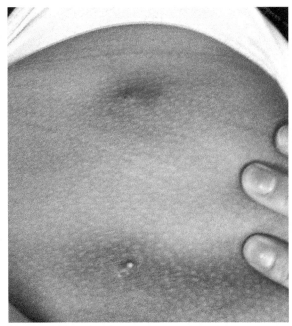

FIGURE 41-2. Furuncles on the thigh of a Hispanic woman. (Used with permission from the Ronald O. Perelman Department of Dermatology, New York University School of Medicine, NYU Langone Medical Center, New York.)

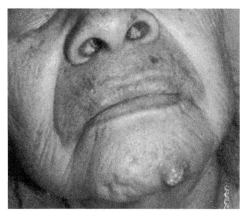

FIGURE 41-3. A Hispanic woman with a carbuncle on the chin consisting of a deep, exophytic, tender, red, fluctuant nodule composed of coalescing infected follicles. (Used with permission from the Ronald O. Perelman Department of Dermatology, New York University School of Medicine, NYU Langone Medical Center, New York.)

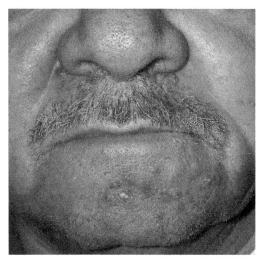

FIGURE 41-4. Culture-proven *Staphylococcus aureus* folliculitis of the beard area of a male patient. If left untreated, these lesions can progress to impetigo. (Used with permission from the Ronald O. Perelman Department of Dermatology, New York University School of Medicine, NYU Langone Medical Center, New York.)

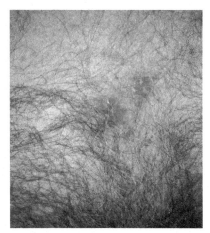

FIGURE 41-5. A case of biopsy-proven herpetic folliculitis. The presence of adjacent grouped vesicles is highly suggestive of the diagnosis. (Used with permission from the Ronald O. Perelman Department of Dermatology, New York University School of Medicine, NYU Langone Medical Center, New York.)

folliculitis. Notably, there was also an unexpected increased prevalence of skin conditions in HIV-positive African American women, compared with their Caucasian and Hispanic counterparts. The reasons for this racial predilection were unclear, but it was proposed that clinicians were less likely to identify lesions in patients with a lighter skin color.[5]

Pseudomonas folliculitis is a follicular infection of various strains of *P. aeruginosa* that is acquired in the contaminated water of whirlpools, swimming pools, and bathtubs, and, less commonly, after the use of bath sponges. It usually presents between 2 and 5 days after exposure, but can occur as late as 2 weeks afterward.[6] It is characterized by pruritic erythematous macules, papules, and pustules that occur most often under bathing suits and intertriginous areas. This is a clue that can help differentiate the lesions from arthropod bites. The eruption is self-limited and does not require treatment. It rarely scars, but in patients with skin of color, it may leave transient postinflammatory hyperpigmentation.

Gram-negative folliculitis is an infection of the hair follicles by Gram-negative bacilli and is usually seen in patients with acne vulgaris who have been treated with broad-spectrum antibiotics for prolonged periods of time, but it may also arise *de novo*. The condition occurred in less than 5% of acne subjects in two studies.[7,8] However, Gram-negative folliculitis should be suspected in patients with acne who are resistant to standard treatment or who experience a flare-up of pustular or cystic acne after being previously well controlled on antibiotics. The infection results from a disproportionate increase in the number of Gram-negative versus Gram-positive organisms in the anterior nares of these patients. In most cases, the ratio of organisms reverts to normal once antibiotics are discontinued. However, in a very small number of acne patients, usually those with an immune-mediated disease or with excessive moisture or seborrhea, Gram-negative organisms invade acne lesions and facial follicles. In some cases, superficial pustules develop around the nostrils and mouth, whereas in other cases, pustules and painful nodules develop in a malar distribution [**Figure 41-6**]. *Klebsiella, Escherichia,* and *Serratia* species tend to cause pustules, whereas *Proteus* species invade more deeply and also cause abscesses and cysts. *Aeromonas hydrophila* folliculitis has been associated with inflatable pools.

Nonstaphylococcal infectious folliculitides may not be clinically distinguishable from both the superficial and deep forms of *S. aureus* folliculitis. Therefore, they may require a culture, potassium hydroxide (KOH) test, or even a biopsy for diagnosis. However, a complete history and thorough physical examination will usually serve to narrow the microbial etiology. Table 41-1 summarizes the pathogens and clinical features of common nonstaphylococcal infectious folliculitides.

DIAGNOSIS

In practice, folliculitis is usually diagnosed clinically and treated empirically. However, in cases resistant to therapy, a Gram stain, culture, KOH test, or Tzanck smear may be required. A bacterial Gram stain and culture are performed by unroofing a pustular lesion and depositing the material on the cotton swab of a culture medium. Typically, the result shows the Gram-positive cocci of *S. aureus*, but it is often falsely negative.[9] In chronic cases of suspected staphylococcal folliculitis, a nasal culture should be performed to identify chronic nasal carriers. Viral cultures and Tzanck smears are performed to diagnose herpetic sycosis, showing the multinucleate giant cells characteristic of a herpetic infection. Because bacterial folliculitis can be complicated by concomitant mite infection, skin scrapings can be analyzed microscopically to look for *Demodex folliculorum*; however, again, false-negative results are common.

PATHOLOGY

Superficial folliculitis (also known as Bockhart impetigo) is characterized histologically by a subcorneal pustule at the follicular opening, surrounded by a dense inflammatory infiltrate predominated by neutrophils. A furuncle shows an area of perifollicular necrosis containing fibrinoid material and neutrophils. In chronic deep folliculitis (sycosis barbae and lupoid), the perifollicular infiltrate is mixed with neutrophils, lymphocytes, histiocytes, and plasma cells. This forms a large abscess that eventually destroys the hair follicle. In older lesions, granulation tissue with foreign body giant cells is seen surrounding the necrotic follicle. Eventually, as is the case in lupoid sycosis, fibrotic scar tissue can form.[10]

Similar histology is seen in *Pseudomonas* folliculitis with a disruption and often a rupture of the follicle by a dense polymorphic inflammatory infiltrate. In other infectious folliculitides, the biopsy can help to pinpoint the microbial etiology of lesions that clinically appear very similar. For example, in herpetic sycosis, the pathology will often show ballooning degeneration of the follicular epithelium and sebaceous cells with central eosinophilic inclusion bodies. *Pityrosporum* folliculitis is characterized by a monomorphic eruption of 2- to 4-mm itchy papules and pustules on the back, shoulders, chest, neck, and, less often, forehead and scalp [**Figure 41-7**]. KOH smears and periodic acid–Schiff (PAS) staining often reveals single-budding *Malassezia* yeasts and spores in the central and deep follicles [**Figure 41-8**].[11] *Candida* folliculitis is usually associated with intertrigo in obese individuals and diabetics. Facial

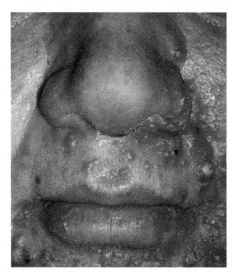

FIGURE 41-6. Gram-negative folliculitis consisting of perinasal and perioral pustules in a Hispanic woman on long-term doxycycline. The culture grew *Proteus mirabilis*. (Used with permission from the Ronald O. Perelman Department of Dermatology, New York University School of Medicine, NYU Langone Medical Center, New York.)

FIGURE 41-7. A close-up image of a relatively monomorphous eruption of follicular papules and pustules secondary to *Pityrosporum* folliculitis in a patient with skin of color. (Used with permission from the Ronald O. Perelman Department of Dermatology, New York University School of Medicine, NYU Langone Medical Center, New York.)

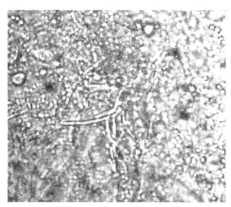

FIGURE 41-8. Multiple hyphae and spores in a spaghetti and meatball pattern in a potassium hydroxide (KOH) smear of the follicular contents from the patient pictured in Figure 41-7 with *Pityrosporum* folliculitis. (Used with permission from the Ronald O. Perelman Department of Dermatology, New York University School of Medicine, NYU Langone Medical Center, New York.)

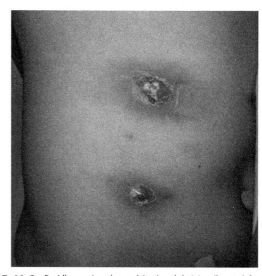

FIGURE 41-9. Rapidly growing ulcerated (top) and draining (bottom) furuncles with surrounding cellulitis on the flank secondary to culture-proven methicillin-resistant *Staphylococcus aureus*. Some follicular pustules are also present. (Used with permission from the Ronald O. Perelman Department of Dermatology, New York University School of Medicine, NYU Langone Medical Center, New York.)

lesions are rare and resemble acne rosacea or tinea barbae. *Demodex* folliculitis occurs predominately on the face, and the lesions are papulopustular or granulomatous. This condition should be considered in patients with atypical, treatment-unresponsive rosacea, especially when itching is present and there is scaling or mites with a white dot appearance at the base of the eyelid hairs. This diagnosis is commonly missed in individuals with skin of color.

☐ DIFFERENTIAL DIAGNOSIS

Although the infectious types of folliculitis can present similarly, a detailed history and examination of the lesions' morphology and body distribution can usually help in determining the etiology. The leading differential diagnoses for staphylococcal folliculitis include the noninfectious folliculitides (such as drug-induced, eosinophilic folliculitis, and PFB), acne vulgaris, miliaria, milia, pustular psoriasis, impetigo, steroid acne, intertrigo, tinea cruris, arthropod bites, and the many other conditions that can present with papulopustular eruptions. Most often in cases of folliculitis, the correct diagnosis can be made by the observation of the strictly perifollicular location of the papules and pustules and the lack of other associated primary lesions (such as comedones in acne vulgaris, scaly erythematous plaques in tinea cruris, and honey-crusted plaques in impetigo).

☐ TREATMENT

Mild cases of staphylococcal folliculitis are treated initially with antibacterial soaps and washes. It is recommended that affected areas be washed at least three times daily. In addition, topical benzoyl peroxide and topical antibiotics such as clindamycin may be used. For more severe cases of superficial folliculitis and for most cases of sycosis, empirical treatment with penicillinase-resistant oral antibiotics is indicated (such as a first-generation cephalosporin, azithromycin, or dicloxacillin). In cases where methicillin-resistant *S. aureus* (MRSA) is cultured, an appropriate MRSA antibiotic therapy should be used. For recurrent or recalcitrant folliculitis, 2% mupirocin ointment should be applied to the anterior nares to treat *S. aureus* nasal carriers.

For furuncles and carbuncles, treatment consists of local measures such as warm compresses and surgical drainage, along with the use of penicillinase-resistant antibiotics (or vancomycin if the MRSA is isolated) [**Figure 41-9**]. Prophylaxis against recurrences should include good personal hygiene, the use of hexachlorophene soap for bathing, and the topical use of mupirocin to the nares to eradicate colonization. In chronic furunculosis, extended courses of oral antibiotics, such as low-dose clindamycin or rifampin, have been used to eradicate the carrier state.

In all cases of staphylococcal folliculitis, care should also be taken to eliminate predisposing factors. The recommendations include the removal of occlusive clothes or dressings; the treatment of hyperhidrosis with frequent clothes changes, aluminum acetate soaks, and aluminum chloride solution; and the appropriate treatment and/or cure of concomitant preexisting dermatitides and skin injuries.

Pseudomonas folliculitis does not require treatment and resolves spontaneously. However, some patients require antipruritic treatment for their symptoms. In addition, care must be taken to properly clean and maintain the contaminated pools of water. For Gram-negative folliculitis, the most effective treatment is isotretinoin; however, in cases where isotretinoin cannot be used, certain Gram-negative bacteria–sensitive antibiotics can suppress the condition. *Pityrosporum* folliculitis is treated with an antiyeast shampoo or cream. However, if the condition is extensive and systemic, then triazole antifungals should be used. *Demodex* folliculitis responds to permethrin.

DRUG-, CHEMICAL-, AND MECHANICAL-INDUCED FOLLICULITIS

Drug-induced folliculitis is more common in acne-prone patients. It can develop within 2 weeks of starting a new medication, and its appearance and severity are usually dose- and duration-dependent. The eruptions resemble acne with monomorphic erythematous papules and pustules on the chest and back, but comedones are rarely present. Numerous medications have been implicated [**Table 41-3**]. Lithium can cause or exacerbate folliculitis, acne, and psoriasis, which are all conditions that are characterized by neutrophilic infiltration. In controlled studies, patients treated with lithium developed more cutaneous reactions than patients on other psychotropics, with a prevalence as high as 45%.[12] Studies have found alarmingly high rates of the use of anabolic steroids by young amateur athletes who take the steroids to improve their performance and by men who want to enhance their physical appearance [**Figure 41-10**]. The recently introduced tyrosinase kinase and epidermal growth factor inhibitors often cause follicular pustular eruptions of the torso, head, and face [**Figure 41-11**]. Corticosteroid-induced facial acneiform folliculitis is a problem in individuals with skin of color who use corticosteroids for bleaching purposes. In some patients, the eruption may be prevented with a prophylactic administration of tetracycline antibiotics.[13] For drug-induced folliculitis, discontinuing the medication, if possible, should be the first course of therapy. In addition, topical and oral antibiotics may facilitate more rapid resolution.

Numerous chemical irritants can cause folliculitis [Table 41-3], and although engineering and refinery workers experience a greater risk, it is estimated that over 1 million other types of workers in the United

TABLE 41-3 Partial list of agents reported to cause chemical-induced folliculitis
Medications
Celecoxib
Corticosteroids
Carbamazepine (eosinophilic folliculitis)
Corticotropin
Androgenic hormones
Bromides
Cyclosporine (also pseudofolliculitis barbae)
Chemotherapeutic agents
Cisplatin
Dactinomycin
Docetaxel
Methotrexate
Paclitaxel
Human epidermal growth factor receptor (EGFR) 1/EGFR inhibitors
Afatinib
Cetuximab
Dacomitinib
Erlotinib
Gefitinib
Vandetanib
Iodides
Isoniazid
Granulocyte colony-stimulating factor
Lithium
Non-EGFR targeting tyrosine kinase inhibitors
Dasatinib
Imatinib
Sorafenib
Sunitinib
Vaccinia vaccination
Chemicals
Coal tar distillates (creosote, pitch)
Crude petrolatum
Chlorinated hydrocarbons
Dioxins
Polychlorinated biphenyls
Industrial coolants and lubricants
Oils
Cutting oils
Diesel oil
Mineral oil
Wool fats
Paraffin
Pentachlorophenols
Pitch and asphalt
Triphenyl tin fluoride

States regularly use oils and greases at work. Exposure to these chemicals can lead to occupational acne and folliculitis through mechanical blockage of the pilosebaceous units. The treatment recommendations for chemical-induced folliculitis include the avoidance of occupational irritants, if possible, and frequent cleansing of the skin and washing of oil-soaked uniforms/clothing.[14]

For other workers, folliculitis occurs as a consequence of mechanical irritation. Wherever there is frictional trauma or occlusion, folliculitis

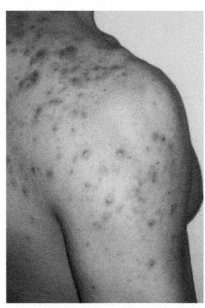

FIGURE 41-10. Folliculitis secondary to anabolic steroid use on the shoulders, back, and upper arms of a patient with skin of color. Although the eruption resembles acne vulgaris, there is an absence of comedones. (Used with permission from the Ronald O. Perelman Department of Dermatology, New York University School of Medicine, NYU Langone Medical Center, New York.)

can be seen. For example, truck drivers are prone to folliculitis of the buttocks and back, whereas football players have a high incidence of folliculitis underneath their padding and on their posterior scalp and neck, secondary to helmet irritation. Again, it is advised that patients wash their skin frequently and that tight, moist clothing be regularly changed.

EOSINOPHILIC FOLLICULITIDES

Eosinophilic folliculitis is a sterile type of papulopustular follicular eruption. There are three major types: (1) eosinophilic pustular folliculitis (EPF), (2) HIV/AIDS-associated eosinophilic folliculitis, and (3) EPF of infancy.

Classic EPF, also known as Ofuji disease, is a rare dermatosis of unknown etiology. This condition primarily affects young Asian men, especially from Japan. It is characterized clinically by recurrent pruritic follicular papules and pustules that coalesce to form annular plaques on the face, upper back, and upper extremities. Peripheral blood eosinophilia is usually seen. Histologically, infundibular eosinophilic pustules

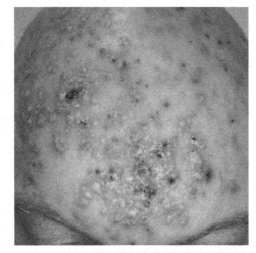

FIGURE 41-11. Pustular eruption of the forehead and scalp due to the epidermal growth factor receptor inhibitor rituximab. In addition to the face, there was also involvement of the chest, shoulders, and back. (Used with permission from the Ronald O. Perelman Department of Dermatology, New York University School of Medicine, NYU Langone Medical Center, New York.)

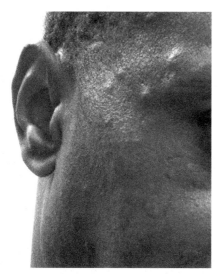

FIGURE 41-12. Human immunodeficiency virus-associated eosinophilic folliculitis on the face of a patient with skin of color. The lesions are pruritic and may resemble arthropod bites. (Used with permission from the Ronald O. Perelman Department of Dermatology, New York University School of Medicine, NYU Langone Medical Center, New York.)

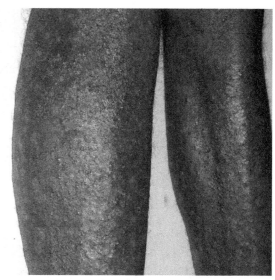

FIGURE 41-13. Relapsing pustular dermatitis on the leg of a patient with darker skin of color with a recurrent eruption of multiple follicular pustules, edema, and erosion. The culture grew *Staphylococcus aureus*. (Used with permission from the Ronald O. Perelman Department of Dermatology, New York University School of Medicine, NYU Langone Medical Center, New York.)

are the characteristic finding. The perifollicular infiltrate is mixed with eosinophils, lymphocytes, histiocytes, and mast cells. These mast cells are believed to be important in the pathogenesis of EPF because they are involved in the production of inflammatory mediators such as prostaglandin. For this reason, recent studies have shown that indomethacin, a potent prostaglandin inhibitor, is an effective treatment of EPF. Other reported therapies include ultraviolet B (alone or in conjunction with indomethacin), oral corticosteroids, minocycline, retinoids, and dapsone.[15]

HIV/AIDS-associated EPF (AIDS-EPF) is a pruritic eruption clinically similar but histologically different from classic EPF. In AIDS-EPF, the lesions remain discrete, and the eruption is more chronic. AIDS-EPF most often affects adult men with CD4+ counts of less than 300 cells/μL. The eruption consists of intensely pruritic perifollicular erythematous papules and pustules that are found on the head, neck, trunk, and proximal extremities. The intact lesions resemble small insect bites, but many are excoriated [**Figure 41-12**]. AIDS-EF can develop weeks after the initiation of antiretroviral therapy; in some reports, this is termed immune recovery inflammatory folliculitis, and it usually resolves in approximately 3 months. It has been postulated that a shift toward T-helper 2 immunity in the course of the HIV infection induces immunoglobulin E production and eosinophilia. This happens as an allergic response to an unknown antigen, possibly *Demodex*.[16] There is no definitive treatment for AIDS-EF. However, in addition to appropriate highly active antiretroviral therapy (HAART), topical and oral corticosteroids, ultraviolet B phototherapy, permethrin cream, and isotretinoin can be effective in certain cases.

EPF of infancy is a rare disorder affecting neonates in the first days to weeks of life, often within the first 24 hours. Clinically, it looks very similar to Ofuji disease, but it usually localizes mainly to the scalp and face. In infants of color, it is important to distinguish EPF from transient neonatal pustular melanosis and infantile acropustulosis, disorders that primarily affect children with darker skin of color. Physicians should reassure parents that EPF of infancy is a cyclic disease that is self-limiting and usually remits in the child's first few years of life.

OTHER FOLLICULITIS

Relapsing pustular dermatitis of the leg results in symmetric pustules that are mainly located on the pretibial area, occasionally with edema [**Figure 41-13**]. The condition was first reported in Nigerians under the term Nigerian shin disease or dermatitis cruris pustulosa et atrophicans.

It is probably precipitated by shaving and then applying occlusive oils and other inflammatory irritants. A superinfection with *S. aureus* may be responsible for the scarring and prolonged pigmentation that patients with this condition often experience.

Tufted hair folliculitis is a cicatricial folliculitis in which tufts of 5 to 15 hairs emerge from dilated follicular orifices, usually on the scalp [**Figure 41-14**]. The cause is unknown, but the changes represent an advanced stage of follicular injury following a deep follicular inflammation that may be caused by *S. aureus* infection. It could also potentially be caused by cicatricial inflammatory processes, including acne keloidalis, dissecting scalp cellulitis, folliculitis decalvans, and lichen planopilaris. *S. aureus* is frequently cultured from the follicles.

Recurrent and disseminated infundibulofolliculitis is an intermittently recurrent pruritic papulopustular follicular eruption on the

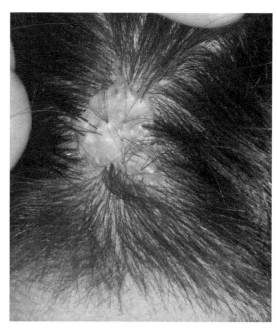

FIGURE 41-14. A case of tufted hair folliculitis on a keloidal scar caused by a scalp infection. (Used with permission from the Ronald O. Perelman Department of Dermatology, New York University School of Medicine, NYU Langone Medical Center, New York.)

trunk that occurs predominantly in African Americans in hot, humid environments. It is more common in atopic individuals, and many cases represent a follicular eczema.

Actinic folliculitis is very rare, occurs in sun-exposed areas, and has not been described in individuals with skin of color.

PERIFOLLICULOCENTRIC DISORDERS

Perifolliculocentric inflammatory disorders such as acne keloidalis nuchae, PFB, and perifolliculitis capitis *abscedens et suffodiens* (dissecting cellulitis) are not true folliculitides because they involve inflammation surrounding the hair follicles and do not directly involve the hair follicle. They are conditions that are more common in African Americans due to the inflammatory reaction caused by tightly curled hair reentering the perifollicular area. These conditions are discussed in detail in Chapters 34 and 39.

CONCLUSION

Folliculitis is a condition affecting the hair follicle. It is usually caused by an infection but can also be induced by irritation, chemical agents, medications, or physical injury. Folliculitis is a very common disorder in both children and adults, and staphylococcal folliculitis is particularly prevalent among those with darker skin of color who are HIV-positive.

Before treating any case of staphylococcal or infectious folliculitis, the patient should be instructed about eliminating all predisposing factors. This includes the removal of restrictive clothing or dressings; the treatment of hyperhidrosis with frequent clothing changes, aluminum acetate soaks, and aluminum chloride solution; and the appropriate treatment of skin conditions and injuries.

Mild cases of staphylococcal or infectious folliculitis should initially be treated with antibacterial soaps and washes, potentially in combination with topical benzoyl peroxide and topical antibiotics. For more severe cases, it is recommended that patients use an empirical treatment with penicillinase-resistant oral antibiotics.

The treatment of furuncles and carbuncles should include warm compresses and possibly surgical drainage, along with penicillinase-resistant antibiotics.

Pseudomonas folliculitis does not require treatment and resolves spontaneously. However, in some cases, antipruritic treatment is required for the patient's symptoms. The most effective treatment for Gram-negative folliculitis is isotretinoin. However, in cases where it cannot be used, certain Gram-negative bacteria–sensitive antibiotics can be beneficial. *Pityrosporum* folliculitis is treated with an antiyeast shampoo or cream, and permethrin can be used to treat *Demodex* folliculitis.

For drug-induced folliculitis, the offending medication must be discontinued, and topical and oral antibiotics can be prescribed to facilitate a more rapid resolution of the condition. The treatment of chemical- and mechanical-induced folliculitis includes the avoidance of these irritants, if possible, and frequent cleansing of skin and washing of clothing.

Recent studies have shown that indomethacin is an effective treatment for EPF. Other reported therapies for EPF include ultraviolet B, oral corticosteroids, minocycline, retinoids, and dapsone.[13]

There is no definitive treatment for HIV/AIDS-associated EPF. However, in certain cases, HAART, topical and oral corticosteroids, ultraviolet B phototherapy, permethrin cream, and isotretinoin can be effective.

REFERENCES

1. Lee PK, Zipoli MT, Weinberg AN, et al. Pyodermas: *Staphylococcus aureus, Streptococcus,* and other gram-positive bacteria. In: Freedberg IM, Eisen AZ, Wolff K, et al, eds. *Fitzpatrick's Dermatology in General Medicine.* 6th ed. New York, NY: McGraw-Hill; 2003:1856-1878.
1a. Camacho F., Cicatricial alopecias. In: Camacho F, Montagna W, eds. Trichology: Diseases of the Pilosebaceous Follicle. Madrid, Spain: Aula Medica Group; 1997.
2. Böni R, Nehrhoff B. Treatment of gram-negative folliculitis in patients with acne. *Am J Clin Dermatol.* 2003;4:273-276.
3. Bonifaz A, Ramírez-Tamayo T, Saúl A. Tinea barbae (tinea sycosis): experience with nine cases. *J Dermatol.* 2003;30:898-903.
4. Garman ME, Tyring SK. The cutaneous manifestations of HIV infection. *Dermatol Clin.* 2002;20:193-208.
5. Halder RM. Pseudofolliculitis barbae and related disorders. *Dermatol Clin.* 1998;6:407-412.
6. Berger RS, Seifert MR. Whirlpool folliculitis: a review of its cause, treatment, and prevention. *Cutis.* 1990;45:97-98.
7. Neubert U, Jansen T, Plewig G. Bacteriologic and immunologic aspects of gram-negative folliculitis: a study of 46 patients. *Int J Dermatol.* 1999;38:270-274.
8. Blankenship ML. Gram-negative folliculitis. Follow-up observations in 20 patients. *Arch Dermatol.* 1984;120:1301-1303.
9. Kelly AP. Folliculitis and the follicular occlusion triad. In: Bolognia JL, Jorizzo JL, Rapini RP, eds. *Dermatology.* 1st ed. London, United Kingdom: Mosby; 2003:554.
10. Lucas S. Bacterial disease. In: Elder D, Elenitsas R, Jaworsky C, et al, eds. *Lever's Histopathology of the Skin.* 8th ed. Philadelphia, PA: Lippincott Williams & Wilkins; 1997:461.
11. Assaf RR, Weil ML. The superficial mycoses. *Dermatol Clin.* 1996;14:57-67.
12. Yeung CK. Cutaneous adverse effects of lithium: epidemiology and management. *Am J Clin Dermatol.* 2004;5:3-8.
13. Bachet JB, Peuvrel L, Bachmeyer C, et al. Folliculitis induced by EGFR inhibitors, preventive and curative efficacy of tetracyclines in the management and incidence rates according to the type of EGFR inhibitor administered: a systematic literature review. *Oncologist.* 2012;17:555-568.
14. Peate WE. Occupational skin disease. *Am Fam Physician.* 2002;66:1025-1032.
15. Epstein EH Jr, Lutzner MA. Folliculitis induced by actinomycin D. *N Engl J Med.* 1969;281:1094-1096.
16. Ishiguro N, Shishido E, Okamoto R. Ofuji's disease: a report on 20 patients with clinical and histopathologic analysis. *J Am Acad Dermatol.* 2002;46:827-833.

CHAPTER 42

Acne Vulgaris

Nada Elbuluk
Jennifer David
Victoria Holloway Barbosa
Susan C. Taylor

KEY POINTS

- Acne vulgaris is a disorder that is seemingly common in skin of color populations, including those of African, Asian, and Latin descent.
- Although few studies examine possible differences in the pathogenesis of acne vulgaris in racial groups, it is likely that the pathogenesis is similar in all groups.
- Individuals with darker skin tones and acne frequently present with a chief complaint of hyperpigmentation, which is often referred to as dark marks, blemishes, scars, spots, discolorations, blotches, *descoloracions,* or *Mecheta.*
- Hyperpigmented macules may be the predominant lesions found in the skin of color patient with acne.
- Whereas comedonal acne occurs commonly in some skin of color individuals, nodulocystic acne is felt to occur less frequently in this population.
- By and large, treatment regimens for acne vulgaris in skin of color patients are similar to those for fairer-skinned patients, but it is important to avoid topical medications that lead to dryness or irritation and subsequent postinflammatory hyperpigmentation.
- Various methods can be used to improve tolerability to potentially drying topical agents for the skin of color patient.
- Oral agents, including antibiotics and retinoids, are effective for skin of color patients with acne.

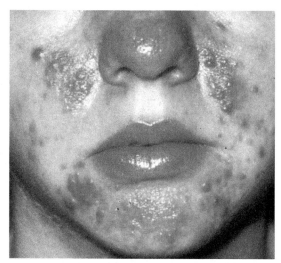

FIGURE 42-1. Acne vulgaris is a common skin disease seen from the preteen years through age 50.

- Procedural treatments including chemical peels, laser and light therapy, and surgical modalities can also be beneficial in providing adjuvant and/or combination therapy for acne vulgaris and its sequelae.

The diagnosis and treatment of acne vulgaris are a frequent reason for visits by patients to the dermatologist's office. This disease affects 40 to 50 million people in the United States, and it is commonly seen from the preteen years through age 50 in Caucasian patients [**Figure 42-1**].[1,2] Acne often has a negative psychological impact on patients and has been associated with anxiety, depression, social isolation, interpersonal difficulties, lower self-esteem and self-confidence, dissatisfaction with one's facial appearance, and fewer employment opportunities.[3-5] Furthermore, it may lead to permanent scarring. The U.S. Census estimates that by 2050, the skin of color population will constitute half of the U.S. population.[6] Given this demographic shift, dermatologists will be faced with increasing numbers of individuals of color with acne. Acne vulgaris patients with skin of color present with differences in the chief complaint, clinical presentation, precipitating and exacerbating factors, long-term sequelae, treatment, and subsequent adverse events [**Table 42-1**]. This chapter provides a comprehensive review and discussion of these differences.

EPIDEMIOLOGY

Acne vulgaris is a disorder that is seemingly common in skin of color populations, including those of African, Asian, and Latin descent.[4,7] Although exact information on the epidemiology of acne in skin of color patients is limited, healthcare utilization data provide an indication of the frequency with which patients seek healthcare for this inflammatory disorder. For the African American population, clinic and private practice visits for acne have been chronicled since the beginning of the

TABLE 42-1	Differences in acne vulgaris in skin of color populations compared to fairer-skinned populations

- Chief complaint is hyperpigmentation
- Cystic acne is an infrequent clinical presentation
- Pomade acne is a precipitating and exacerbating factor
- Long-term sequelae include scar formation, keloidal and ice pick scars
- Treatment protocols should include:
  - Concomitant treatment of hyperpigmentation
  - Avoidance of irritation
- Hyperpigmentation can be a treatment related adverse event

TABLE 42-2	National Ambulatory Medical Care Survey data (1993–2009) for percentage of acne visits[7]
Race/ethnicity	Percentage
Caucasians	14.8
African Americans	22.1
Asians or Pacific Islanders	18.7
Latinos	22.2

Source: Centers for Disease Control and Prevention. Center for Health Statistics Ambulatory HealthCare Data. www.cdc.gov/nchs/ahcd.htm. Accessed June 16, 2015.[7]

twentieth century. In 1908, Fox[8] reported that 4.6% of darker-skinned patients and 7.4% of fairer-skinned patients presented for treatment of acne. A more recent study evaluated the data from the National Ambulatory Medical Care Survey (NAMCS) from 1993 to 2009 and found that, in dermatology clinics, acne was the top diagnosis for African American, Hispanic, and Asian or Pacific Islander patients.[7,9] In comparison, acne was the second most common diagnosis among Caucasians [**Table 42-2**].[7,9] A hospital-based practice survey in New York of 1421 patients found that acne was the most common diagnosis made in both fairer-skinned patients (21.0%) and darker-skinned patients (28.4%), and dyschromia was the second most common diagnosis for darker-skinned patients.[10,11] A retrospective cohort study of health plan pediatric patients seen between 1997 and 2007 found that the most common diagnosis in all pediatric patients was acne (28.6%).[12] In Caucasian pediatric patients, acne was the most common diagnosis (29.9%), whereas in African American and Asians patients, it was the second most common diagnosis, at 27.5% and 22.2%, respectively. Similar statistics have been identified for European skin of color populations, with a 1996 survey from London, England, reporting acne as the primary cutaneous disease in 13.7% of patients.[13] In the skin of color African Caribbean population, the diagnosis of acne vulgaris was 29.21% in a practice survey from Kingston, Jamaica.[14] In Guadeloupe, 19.5% of African Caribbean patients presented with acne vulgaris compared with between 7.1% and 10.4% of Caucasians on the island.[15] In hospital-based studies of skin disease in Africa, the proportions of those with acne vulgaris was 4.6% in Ghana, 6.7% in Nigeria, and up to 17.5% in South Africa.[16]

Acne vulgaris is purportedly less common in the Asian population than in the Caucasian population.[17] However, it was the leading dermatologic diagnosis for Asians in the United States, occurring in 18.7% of these patients, as reported by the NAMCS for 1993 to 2009.[9] A more recent community-based study on South Asian Americans found that acne was the most common dermatologic diagnosis, affecting 37% of the patients.[18] The same study found that three of the top five most common patient concerns were uneven skin tone, dark spots, and acne at 21%, 18%, and 17%, respectively. Similarly, in Asia, the National Skin Center in Singapore indicated that acne was the second most common diagnosis among their patients, occurring in 10.9% of Asians, including 3.1% of the pediatric Asian population.[19]

A survey of Latino patients' visits to dermatologists in the United States demonstrated acne vulgaris to be the most common diagnosis in this population [**Figure 42-2**].[20] According to NAMCS, acne represented 22.2% of primary diagnoses in Latinos.[9] Another growing skin of color population is Arab Americans, who have a population of 3.5 million in the United States.[21] A study found that among Arab Americans, acne was the most common dermatologic diagnosis, affecting 37.7% of the population.[21] Patients' top concerns included uneven skin tone, skin discoloration, and acne at 56.4%, 55.9%, and 49.4%, respectively. In a Middle East pediatric population from Kuwait, acne was also a common diagnosis, comprising 10.5% of patients presenting for dermatologic care.[22]

As survey data indicate, acne vulgaris is a cutaneous disorder for which patients of color frequently seek dermatologic care. Therefore, it is important that healthcare providers fully understand this disease entity when serving the skin of color population.

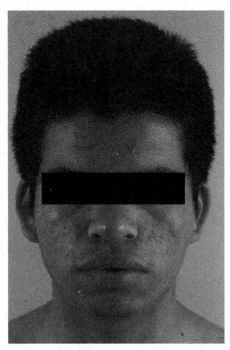

FIGURE 42-2. In the United States, acne vulgaris is the most common diagnosis in Latino patients, like this young man.

PATHOGENESIS

Although few studies examine possible differences in the pathogenesis of acne vulgaris in racial groups, it is likely that the pathogenesis is similar in all groups. Acne is a disease of the pilosebaceous follicle, with abnormal follicular keratinocyte desquamation resulting in the development of a follicular plug.[23] Androgen-stimulated increased sebum production and proliferation of the microorganism *Propionibacterium acnes* occur within the follicular plug.[23,24] An inflammatory response ensues through acting on toll-like receptor 2 (TLR-2) and stimulating the secretion of cytokines and interleukins (ILs) including IL-6, IL-8, and IL-12.[23,25]

There are no strong data that support differences in either the desquamation of the pilosebaceous epithelium or the proliferation of *P. acnes* between racial or ethnic groups. One study, which examined the microflora of facial skin in 30 African American and 30 Caucasian women, found a higher density of *P. acnes* in African American patients compared to Caucasian patients; however, the results were not statistically significant.[26] Data on differences in sebaceous gland size or activity as well as pore size have also been inconclusive. Nicolaides and Rothman[27] concluded that the production of sebum was greater in skin of color patients, but his methodology was deemed flawed. Kligman and Shelley[28] measured the surface sebum levels in five darker-skinned and five fairer-skinned subjects during a 4-hour time period and concluded that darker-skinned subjects had greater surface sebum levels than those with fairer skin. Forehead biopsies from two of the skin of color subjects with moderate or high levels of surface sebum showed they had appreciably larger sebaceous glands when compared with the biopsies from two fairer-skinned subjects who generated low amounts of sebum. Another more recent study found that sebum production was positively correlated with acne severity in African American, Asian, and Hispanic women, whereas pore size was positively correlated with acne in African American, Asian, and Continental Indian women.[29] However, other studies, including one by Grimes et al,[30] have evaluated differences in skin surface properties including sebum level, pH, moisture content, and barrier function and do not support this conclusion; they found no significant differences in sebum production between African American and Caucasian patients.[4,30]

Studies have also examined the stratum corneum of skin of color and found it to have more layers and to be more tightly packed than that of Caucasian skin. This difference was felt to potentially lead to differences in irritation potential among different races, with individuals with skin of color possibly having a stronger barrier to absorption and thus a higher threshold for irritation.[11,31-33] Other studies on absorption and barrier function have found conflicting results about skin irritability and cutaneous absorption in patients of different races.[11]

Genetic factors may also play a role in the pathogenesis of acne as shown by several recent studies. A study done on Chinese patients with severe acne found a possible association with the CYP17-34T/C polymorphism.[34] A different case-control study of a Chinese Han population found that the risk of acne vulgaris in a relative of a patient with acne vulgaris was significantly higher than for the relative of an unaffected individual, suggesting that familial factors may play an important role in determining an individual's susceptibility to developing acne.[35]

Geography and diet have also been implicated as possibly having a role in the pathogenesis of acne vulgaris. Some studies have shown that non-Westernized societies have a lower prevalence of acne.[36-39] This has often been tied to differences in diet, which suggest that the hyperinsulinemic diet in Western societies triggers an endocrine response that promotes unregulated tissue growth and enhanced androgen synthesis. This hypothesis was supported by the results of a study that found that Asian women from Los Angeles had a higher prevalence of acne than those from Japan, where the diet is known to be lower in total fat and sugar than in America.[29] Another study revealed the absence of acne vulgaris in individuals from any age group among Aché hunter-gatherers in Paraguay and Kitavan Islanders of Papua New Guinea, suggesting that Western diets may be contributing to the pathogenesis of acne and that a Paleolithic diet could be beneficial in acne prevention.[40,41] The effects of diet and geography on the pathogenesis of acne are still a controversial topic, and the effects of dietary modification on acne in a skin of color population are still not well known.

CLINICAL PRESENTATION

ACNE VULGARIS

The clinical presentation of acne vulgaris in skin of color patients often varies compared with that in fairer-skinned patients. Individuals with darker skin tones and acne frequently present with a chief complaint of hyperpigmentation, which they refer to as dark marks, blemishes, scars, spots, discolorations, blotches, *descoloracions*, or *Mecheta* [**Table 42-3**]. Hyperpigmented macules may be the predominant lesion found in the skin of color patient with acne [**Figure 42-3**]. Of the 313 patients studied at the Skin of Color Center in New York, hyperpigmented macules were seen in 65.3% of darker-skinned patients, 52.7% of Hispanic patients, and 47.4% of Asian patients, including Indians and Pakistanis[4] [**Table 42-4**]. Another study showed that hyperpigmentation and atrophic scarring were more prevalent in African Americans and Hispanics than in Asian, Continental Indian, and Caucasian women.[29] Patients with hyperpigmentation often seek treatment for the discoloration and view the active acne lesions as secondary or even unimportant. It is often a challenge for the dermatologist to persuade patients of the necessity of concurrent treatment of both the acne and the hyperpigmentation. It is important that any treatment regimen in this situation include a lightening agent as well as agents for the treatment of acne.

All the characteristic lesions of acne vulgaris may be seen in individuals with skin of color, including open and closed comedones, papules, pustules, nodules, and cysts [**Figure 42-4**]. A recent epidemiologic acne

TABLE 42-3	Terms frequently used for the chief complaint of hyperpigmentation
Dark marks	
Blemishes	
Discolorations	
Scars	
Spots	
Blotches	

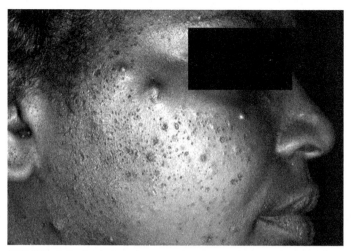

FIGURE 42-3. Papules, ice pick scars, pustules, open comedones, and postinflammatory hyperpigmentation in a patient with acne.

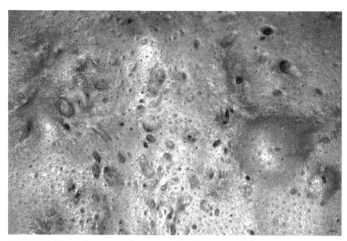

FIGURE 42-4. A patient with acne located on the upper back nodules, cysts, open and closed comedones, and hypertrophic scars can be seen.

study done on 2895 women found that clinical acne was more prevalent in African American (37%) and Hispanic women (32%) than in Continental Indian (23%), Caucasian (24%), and Asian (30%) women.[28] African Americans and Continental Indians showed equal prevalence of subtypes of acne, whereas for Asians, inflammatory acne was more prevalent than comedonal acne, and for Caucasians, comedonal acne was more prevalent than inflammatory acne.[28] Some studies have also supported the notion that nodulocystic acne is felt to occur less frequently in the skin of color population. Wilkins and Voorhees[42] examined the type of acne lesion present in 4000 incarcerated men and found that darker-skinned men had less nodulocystic acne (0.5%) than those who were fairer-skinned (5%). A Nigerian study found that of 418 students, the majority of students had mild acne, and none of the students had severe or nodulocystic acne.[16] The occurrence of nodulocystic acne in Latinos is comparable with that of Caucasians.[4] Taylor et al[4] reported at least one cystic lesion in 18% of African Americans, 25.5% of Hispanics, and 10.5% of Asians in a study of 313 individuals of color.

POMADE ACNE

In the skin of color population of African descent, hair care practices and product selection may have an impact on the clinical presentation of acne vulgaris. Comedonal acne involving the forehead and temples [**Figure 42-5**] due to hair pomade, also termed hair oil, grease, food, moisturizer, and styling agents, is not uncommon in this population.[3,4,43] [**Table 42-5**]. Hair pomades are products containing various types of oils, including olive, vegetable, mineral, castor, mink, tea tree, coconut, and other nut oils, that are applied to textured hair to improve manageability and styling. Clinically, pomade acne is characterized by multiple closed comedones and occasionally papulopustules in areas such as the forehead and temples, where the pomade seeps from the scalp. In a study conducted at the Skin of Color Center in New York, 46.2% of patients reported use of pomade or oil-based hair care products.[4] Hair oils and pomades are also used in the Arab American population, in addition to the use of natural products on the face including honey, sugar, olive oil, milk and cucumber, herbal mixtures, and Dead Sea clay.[21] Silicone-based products in a light liquid moisturizing vehicle should be recommended as an alternative to heavy, oil-based pomades.[25] Awareness of the cultural

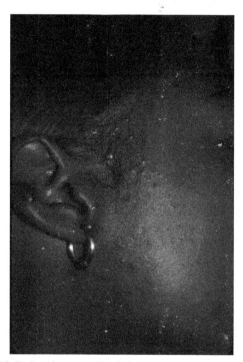

FIGURE 42-5. Pomade acne in a skin of color patient from the use of hair oils.

TABLE 42-5 Hair pomades

African Pride African Miracle Castor & Mink Oil

All Ways Natural Castor Oil Conditioning Hair Dress Formula for Maximum Shine and Body

Black n' Sassy Tea Tree Oil Triple Gro for Growth Condition & Healthy Hair

DAX Pomade with Lanolin Compounded with Vegetable Oils, Bergamot, Olive Oil, and Castor Oil

Doo Gro Mega Thick Growth Oil

Gabel's Lemon Pomade

Johnson Products Ultra Sheen Hair Food

Murray's Superior Hair Dressing Pomade

Vigorol Indian Hemp Hair & Scalp Conditioning Treatment

Soft Sheen Carson Sporting Wave Maximum Hold Pomade

L'Oreal Natures Therapy Mega Moisture Slick Moisturizing Pomade

D:Fl D:tails Pomade for Hold & Shine

Sebastian Collection Grease Pomade for Flexible Hold

KMS Hair Play Defining Pomade Medium, Flexible Control, High Shine

TABLE 42-4 Presence of hyperpigmented macules in a Skin of Color Center study[4]

Acne hyperpigmented macules	Percentage
African Americans	65.3
Hispanics	52.7
Asians	47.4

Source: Data from Taylor S. C., Cook-Bolden F, Rahman Z, et al. Acne vulgaris in skin of color. J Am Acad Dermatol. 2002;46:S98-S106.

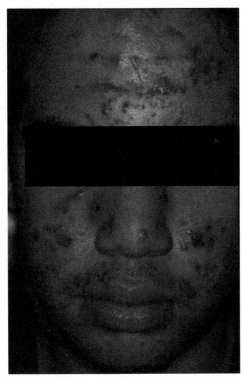

FIGURE 42-6. Acne conglobata is seen most commonly in men and is typically found on the face, as in this Hispanic patient.

differences in skin and hair practices among different skin of color populations is important when approaching treatment for acne and its sequelae in these populations.

ACNE CONGLOBATA

Another type of acne seen in skin of color is acne conglobata.[44] This form of acne is seen commonly in men and typically is found on the face [Figure 42-6], neck, chest, and back. Patients present with comedones, cysts, nodules, and abscesses with draining sinus tracts that may heal with scarring. When acne conglobata, hidradenitis suppurativa, and dissecting cellulitis are observed together, it is termed the follicular occlusion triad. This triad is not uncommon in the skin of color population.[44]

ACNE ROSACEA

Acne rosacea, which affects the facial pilosebaceous units, can also present in skin of color patients. In this population, this chronic disorder commonly presents with papules and or pustules in the central facial regions with an absence of comedones.[45,46] This is often coupled with increased capillary activity that leads to flushing and telangiectasia. The exact etiology is unknown; however, researchers believe it is likely due to a combination of hereditary and environmental factors. Triggers include alcohol, hot foods or drinks, spicy food, sunlight, temperature extremes, stress, exercise, hot baths, topical corticosteroids, and vasodilatory medications.[45,46] Acne rosacea can look very similar to inflammatory acne. There are four clinical subtypes of rosacea, and patients can simultaneously present with characteristics of more than one subtype [Table 42-6].[47] African American and Caribbean American patients are commonly diagnosed with the granulomatous subtype.[10,46-48] Flushing and facial erythema are usually the first presenting signs/symptoms of rosacea. These features are difficult to appreciate in darker-pigmented individuals; thus early cases with less obvious cosmetic disfigurement prompt fewer office visits from affected skin of color patients.[46] Unfortunately, this leads to a delay in diagnosing and treating early, less severe forms of the disease. In lieu of erythema, darker-skinned patients can present with increased sensitivity to skin care products as an early symptom. One should also be aware of the differential diagnoses for rosacea before initiating treatment [Table 42-7].

TABLE 42-6 Clinical subtypes or variants of rosacea

Subtype/variant	Features
Erythematotelangiectatic	• Persistent central facial erythema and flushing. Telangiectasia is common but not essential for the diagnosis.
Papulopustular	• Persistent central facial erythema with transient papules, pustules, or both in a central facial distribution.
Phymatous	• Thickened skin, irregular surface nodularities. • Phymatous rosacea occurs most commonly as rhinophyma but may appear elsewhere, including the chin, forehead, cheeks, and ears.
Ocular	• Watery or bloodshot appearance (interpalpebral conjunctival hyperemia), foreign-body sensation, burning, stinging, dryness, itching, light sensitivity, blurred vision, telangiectasia of the conjunctiva and lid margin, or periocular erythema. • Some patients may experience loss of vision as a result of corneal complications.
Granulomatous	• Firm, noninflammatory, monomorphous papules or nodules that typically occur on the cheeks and periorificial areas.

STEROID-INDUCED ACNE

Steroid-induced acne [Figure 42-7], which can sometimes be referred to as steroid rosacea, is also seen commonly in the skin of color community from use of bleaching products that contain corticosteroids.[10] These products can be purchased from other countries and illegally in the United States from many stores in major metropolitan cities. Many of these products contain high-potency corticosteroids, which can cause steroid-induced acne and/or perioral dermatitis. Up to 80% of African American patients with acne have been reported to use skin-bleaching products.[4] A Senegalese study on acne found that one of the most common predisposing factors for acne in their population was the use of depigmenting cosmetic products, which 38.7% of the women admitted to using.[49]

ACNE SCARRING

A sequelae of acne is acne scarring [Figure 42-8], which can affect up to 95% of patients, including people with skin of color.[50] The spectrum of scarring includes atrophic, ice pick, boxcar, rolling, hypertrophic, and keloidal scarring.[3,4,51] There are various factors underlying the scarring process including the initial severity of the acne, the extent of inflammation, and time lapsed prior to seeking medical treatment.[50] However, scarring is reportedly less prevalent in skin of color populations than in other racial groups, and this is felt to be related to the lower prevalence of nodulocystic acne in skin of color patients.[4] One study reported scarring in 5.9% of African American, 21.8% of Hispanic, and 10.5% of Asian/other patients.[4] When present, ice pick scarring is a sequela of facial acne; atrophic scarring is a sequela of chest, back, and jawline acne; and keloidal scarring is a sequela of chest, back, and jawline acne. One study found that keloidal scars were more frequent on the chest, back, and jawline of patients with skin type VI compared to those with skin types IV and V.[52] This was felt to be due to a stronger biological basis for African patients in the study to develop scars in contrast to patients from other regions with the same phenotype.[52] Given the long-lasting and devastating impact that keloidal scarring can have on patients, the risk of this type of scarring should motivate dermatologists to treat inflammatory acne early and aggressively in this patient population.

HISTOLOGY

When viewed histologically, patients with darker skin of color have been found to have greater inflammation than fairer-skinned patients within acne lesions despite a noninflammatory appearance clinically.[53] Halder et al[53] demonstrated that comedonal lesions exhibited striking inflammation with polymorphonuclear leukocyte infiltrates. Papular and pustular lesions included multinucleated giant cells that were dispersed

TABLE 42-7	Differential diagnoses of rosacea			
Diagnosis	Age of onset	Important factors	Location	Clinical appearance
Acne vulgaris	Puberty	Telangiectasia and flushing are absent	Face, chest, and back	Comedones, papules, pustules, and nodules in a sebaceous distribution
Systemic lupus erythematosus	2–40 years	Classic 'butterfly' rash	Face	Erythematous macular eruption on malar region of face
Steroid dermatitis	Any age	Associated with long-term use of potent topical steroids; no comedones	Face or any other areas of long-term potent topical steroid use	Severe dermatitis with erythema, papules, and pustules
Sarcoidosis (lupus pernio)	20–40 years	Most common in females with skin of color with longstanding pulmonary disease	Nose, cheeks	Lupus pernio is characterized by red to purple or violaceous, indurated plaques and nodules that usually affect the nose, cheeks, ears, and lips
Seborrheic dermatitis	Any age	African Americans and darker-skinned individuals are susceptible to annular seborrheic dermatitis	Face, scalp, and trunk	Erythematous patches with thick greasy scale

beyond the actual papule or pustule. The authors suggested that the inflammatory nature of these lesions is what leads individuals with darkly pigmented skin to develop postinflammatory hyperpigmentation on resolution of the acne.[53]

TREATMENT

GOAL OF ACNE THERAPY

By and large, treatment regimens for acne vulgaris in skin of color patients are similar to those for fairer-skinned patients. The goal of acne therapy is to reduce follicular hyperkeratosis, bacteria, sebum production, inflammation, and postinflammatory hyperpigmentation.[3,4] Achieving these goals necessitates an evaluation of the patient's skin type and potential for sensitivity, current skin regimen (including cleansing, toning, and moisturizing products), previous treatments, results, and

sequelae.[3] Taylor et al[4] have classified skin of color into three categories to assist in the selection of topical therapeutic agents:

1. Dry/sensitive skin and/or skin with a significant propensity to irritant reactions

2. Normal skin and/or skin with minimal propensity to irritant reactions

3. Oily skin and/or no propensity to irritant reactions

Selection of appropriate agents may be enhanced by taking skin type into consideration [Table 42-8]. For example, patients with dry skin are more likely to experience irritation secondary to topical medications, especially during the winter months or in areas of low humidity. Hence cream formulations are appropriate for this type of patient during the winter months, but a regimen may include a gel formulation during the hot and humid summer months.[4]

It is important to query the skin of color patient regarding over-the-counter (OTC) skin care product use. Toners and astringents containing

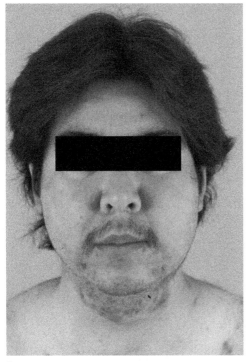
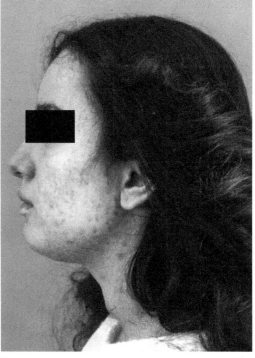

A   **B**

FIGURE 42-7. **(A)** Asian male on steroid therapy showing steroid-induced acne. **(B)** After the frequent use of topical steroids, this Latin American patient formed steroid-induced acne.

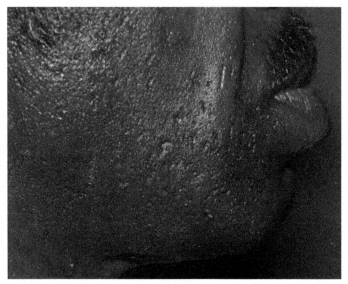

FIGURE 42-8. Postacne scarring in an African American patient.

witch hazel, alcohol, and other ingredients that are potentially drying may decrease the tolerability of topical medications. Moisturizing products containing oils, cocoa butter, shea butter, and petrolatum commonly used in this population may exacerbate acne.

TREATMENT OF ACNE VULGARIS

Treatment of acne vulgaris in skin of color populations includes OTC and prescription treatments that are designed to target the pathophysiologic mechanisms of acne. OTC agents are often mildly comedolytic and antimicrobial. Prescription therapy includes topical and systemic retinoids, topical and systemic antibiotics, and anti-inflammatory and hormonal agents.[4,54] Although all agents may be used in skin of color patients, these patients may be particularly susceptible to certain adverse events. Hence avoidance of contact irritant dermatitis is very important due to its potential for causing further hyperpigmentation. Additionally, consideration must be given to concomitant treatment of hyperpigmented macules.

TREATMENT OF ACNE ROSACEA

Treatments for acne rosacea overlap with many of the treatments for acne vulgaris. They include combinations of topical, oral, and/or procedural therapies.[45-48] Behavior modification is a valuable approach for prophylaxis, and patients should be counseled on avoiding rosacea triggers such as alcohol, spicy food, and extreme temperatures. When

following a treatment response for acne rosacea in patients with skin of color, one cannot rely on typical skin findings like erythema, flushing, or telangiectasia. Instead, patients may state that their skin feels irritated (burning or stinging) or warmer than usual. Topical medications include metronidazole, antibiotics, sulfur-based products, and azelaic acid. Oral antibiotics, including the tetracycline class and erythromycin, are used in rosacea primarily for their anti-inflammatory properties.[45-48] Isotretinoin can be used for severe cases of inflammatory rosacea.[45-48] Lasers and photodynamic therapy can also be used to treat the vascular component of rosacea, although studies using these modalities in skin types V and VI are limited.

TOPICAL THERAPY

TOPICAL THERAPEUTIC AGENTS

Topical therapeutic agents commonly prescribed for the treatment of acne vulgaris include benzoyl peroxide, azelaic acid, erythromycin, clindamycin, and retinoids. There are also numerous combination topical therapies including benzoyl peroxide–erythromycin, benzoyl peroxide–clindamycin, benzoyl peroxide–adapalene, and clindamycin-tretinoin [Table 42-8]. In the selection of topical agents for the treatment of acne, efficacy and tolerability of the agent are primary considerations. Secondary considerations include ability to treat or minimize hyperpigmented macules and maximizing penetration of other therapeutic agents.

BENZOYL PEROXIDE PREPARATIONS

Benzoyl peroxide preparations are available in various formulations, vehicles, and concentrations. These agents reduce the population of *P. acnes*, and there are no associated reports of resistance.[55] Formulations include cleansers, solutions, creams, pledgets, and gels with or without microspheres or ingredients such as urea, which may improve tolerability. Benzoyl peroxide preparations vary in concentration of the active ingredient from 2.5% to 10%, with higher concentrations potentially leading to excessive dryness and irritation. Higher concentrations are most appropriate for oilier skin. Although benzoyl peroxide preparations may bleach clothing, they have no bleaching or lightening effect on hyperpigmented macules.

Benzoyl peroxide may be combined with an antibiotic, such as erythromycin or clindamycin, or with a retinoid such as adapalene. The combination of benzoyl peroxide with antibiotics has been shown to be more effective in decreasing inflammatory and noninflammatory acne lesions than either agent alone.[56,57] As with benzoyl peroxide alone, combination products can also cause excessive dryness and irritation of skin of color. However, a recent study on efficacy and tolerability of clindamycin phosphate 1.2% and benzoyl peroxide gel in patients with moderate to severe

TABLE 42-8	**Compatibility of topical agents for skin of color**		
	Oily and/or no propensity to irritation	Normal and/or little propensity to irritation	Dry/sensitive and/or great propensity to irritation
Retinoid/retinoid analogue	Adapalene solution 0.1%, pledgets 0.1%, or gel 0.1% or 0.3%	Adapalene gel 0.1% or cream 0.1%	Adapalene cream 0.1% or gel 0.1%
	Tazarotene gel 0.05% or 0.1%	Tazarotene cream 0.1%	Tazarotene cream 0.05%
	Tretinoin gel 0.025% or 0.01%	Tretinoin cream 0.025% or microsphere 0.1%	Tretinoin cream 0.025% or microsphere 0.04%
Antibiotics	Clindamycin solution or pledgets	Clindamycin gel	Clindamycin lotion
	Erythromycin solution, pledgets, or gel	Erythromycin gel	Sulfacetamide lotion
	Benzoyl peroxide-erythromycin		
	Benzoyl peroxide-clindamycin		
Other	Azelaic acid	Azelaic acid	Benzoyl peroxide 2.5%–3%
	Benzoyl peroxide 6%–10%	Benzoyl peroxide 3%–6%	
	Salicylic acid 3%	Salicylic acid 3%	

Source: Adapted with permission from Taylor SC, Cook-Bolden F, Rahman Z, Strachan D. Acne vulgaris in skin of color. *J Am Acad Dermatol.* 2002;46:S98-S106.

acne found that Fitzpatrick skin types IV to VI were not more susceptible to cutaneous irritation from the combination product.[58] There was slightly more erythema reported in Fitzpatrick skin types I to III, and the efficacy and tolerability of the treatment were comparable between Fitzpatrick skin types I to III compared with types IV to VI. A study on the efficacy and safety of adapalene–benzoyl peroxide topical gel in 121 African American subjects with moderate acne found that compared with vehicle, after 12 weeks of treatment, subjects with skin of color had decreased counts of inflammatory and noninflammatory lesions as well as no cases of treatment-related postinflammatory hyperpigmentation.[59] Another study on adapalene–benzoyl peroxide gel also found that those with Fitzpatrick skin types I to III had higher rates of erythema than those with skin types IV to VI; however, it was noted that this result may have been related to difficulty in visualizing erythema in darker skin types.[60]

AZELAIC ACID

Azelaic acid is a dicarboxylic acid that has been shown to have mild anti-inflammatory and comedolytic effects, as well as activity as a tyrosinase inhibitor.[61] Efficacy in the treatment of inflammatory and noninflammatory acne, as well as in the treatment of hyperpigmentation, has been demonstrated.[62,63] Therefore, it is an agent that may address both of the components of active acne and hyperpigmentation in the skin of color patient. Dryness and irritation are potential adverse events with this agent. Finally, clinical experience has shown that the efficacy of azelaic acid is mild to, at most, moderate in the treatment of both acne and hyperpigmentation compared with other agents.

RETINOIDS

Retinoids are a preferred treatment for acne vulgaris in the skin of color population. The mechanisms of action of retinoids include inhibition of TLR-2 receptors, thus reducing inflammation; reduction of the formation of hyperproliferative keratins, thus reducing microcomedone formation; and inhibition of the AP-1 pathway, thus reducing inflammation and possibly scarring. Each of the three retinoids available in the United States—adapalene, tazarotene, and tretinoin—has been demonstrated to be effective in the treatment of both inflammatory and noninflammatory acne. Likewise, efficacy in the treatment of hyperpigmentation has been demonstrated with several of the retinoids, including 0.1% and 0.025% tretinoin cream, 0.1% adapalene gel, and 0.1% tazarotene cream.[64-70] These properties make the retinoids well suited for the concomitant treatment of both acne and hyperpigmentation in the skin of color population.

Retinoid dermatitis, characterized by dryness, peeling, and erythema of the skin, has been well described with the use of any retinoid or retinoid analogue. Both the concentration of the retinoid and its vehicle may have an impact on the dermatitis. Two of the retinoids—tazarotene and tretinoin—are formulated in multiple concentrations (0.05% and 0.1% for tazarotene and 0.025%, 0.0375%, 0.04%, 0.05%, 0.075%, 0.08% and 0.1% for tretinoin), with the lower concentrations having less potential for irritation. All three retinoids have cream formulations that are generally less drying than their gel formulations. Newer aqueous gel formulations and microsphere (microsponge) formulations, which allow for the controlled release of tretinoin, may also lead to less irritation and be better tolerated.[71] Overall, however, each of the retinoids still has the potential of causing irritation, dryness, and peeling of the skin, which may precipitate further hyperpigmentation. Goh et al[72] performed a study on a population of Chinese, Indian, Malay, and Caucasian patients, examining the cumulative irritation potential of adapalene gel 0.1% and tretinoin gel 0.025% and found that the adapalene gel was overall better tolerated when looking at differences in erythema, desquamation, dryness, stinging/burning, and pruritus. A newer combination product consisting of tretinoin 0.025% gel with clindamycin phosphate 1.2% was studied in all skin types and was found to lead to a greater reduction in acne lesions than clindamycin phosphate 1.2% gel alone.[73] It was also well tolerated even in darker skin types, with no dyspigmentation noted.[10,73]

TABLE 42-9 Methods to improve tolerability of drying topical agents

- Initiate treatment with the lowest concentration of the medication.
- Limit application initially to every other day.
- Begin treatment with a cream or lotion formulation.
- Apply a small amount of the medication (approximately a 'pea-sized' amount).
- Spread uniformly over a completely dry face.
- Avoid astringents, toners, harsh soaps, and cleansers.
- Use nondrying, gentle cleansers no more than twice daily.
- Use moisturizers before and/or after application of the topical agent.

There are various methods that can improve tolerability to potentially drying topical agents including retinoids [**Table 42-9**]. These include initiating treatment with the lower concentration of the agent, as well as with an every-other-day dosing schedule with a gradual increase to daily application.[3,4] Cream and lotion formulations of the topical medication are preferable for initiation of therapy. The use of moisturizing agents before and/or after application of the topical agent may improve tolerability but dilute the concentration of the active ingredient. The application of a small amount of the agent, approximately a 'pea-sized' amount, that is spread uniformly over a completely dry face is also recommended to improve tolerability. Avoidance of astringents, toners, and harsh soaps and cleansers is important, substituting nondrying and gentle cleansers.[4]

SODIUM SULFACETAMIDE AND OTHER AGENTS

Sodium sulfacetamide 10% is another topical agent that contains sulfur (1% to 5%) and can be used for treating acne.[10] It has several formulations including a topical suspension, cleanser, cleaning cloths, and a lotion. Dapsone is another topical agent; it comes in a 5% gel formulation and has both anti-inflammatory and antimicrobial effects. In skin of color patients, initiation of oral dapsone must await results of testing for glucose-6-phosphate dehydrogenase deficiency (G6PD). Studies have shown, however, that the risk for hemolytic anemia with topical dapsone 5% gel is very low in patients with G6PD deficiency, and therefore, it can be safely used for acne treatment in all patients.[48] Topical dapsone has also been shown to be safe and well tolerated when used in combination with adapalene or benzoyl peroxide.[74] However, providers should instruct their patients to avoid using topical dapsone immediately after benzoyl peroxide because this can cause a temporary orange or yellow discoloration of the skin.[75]

Another topical treatment that has been used in some European countries is nadifloxacin, which is a fluoroquinolone with broad-spectrum antibacterial activity and potent inhibition of proinflammatory cytokines and chemokines.[76] An 8-week split-face study done using 1% nadifloxacin cream in Korean patients with mild to moderate acne found that when compared with vehicle-treated skin, there was a significant decrease in inflammatory and noninflammatory acne lesions. Histopathologic examination showed decreased inflammation and IL-8 expression, and the treatment was determined to be safe, effective, and well tolerated in Asian subjects. Further studies are needed to determine its safety and efficacy in other skin of color populations.

Instituting therapy for hyperpigmentation along with acne treatment is not contraindicated in the skin of color patient. In addition to azelaic acid and the retinoids, which have been discussed, hydroquinone preparations containing 3% to 10% concentrations may be used in addition to a 2% OTC preparation.[4] Irritation is a possible side effect of higher concentrations of hydroquinone, and exogenous ochronosis can also occur with long-term use.

Sunscreen with a sun protection factor (SPF) of 15 or higher has also been suggested to be important in the daily regimen of skin of color patients.[4] Daily use of sunscreen can aid in the treatment of postinflammatory hyperpigmentation because it takes a longer period of time for this condition to resolve if the patient is continually exposed to ultraviolet radiation.

ORAL THERAPY

ORAL ANTIBIOTICS

The selection of oral antibiotics for the skin of color population does not vary greatly from that for the Caucasian population.[4] Antibiotics are used for their anti-inflammatory as well as bactericidal and static properties. Generally, adverse effects of oral antibiotics do not vary among racial backgrounds.[4] Options include the tetracycline family of medications, including tetracycline, doxycycline, and minocycline. In addition to the well-recognized adverse events of gastrointestinal distress, rashes, urticaria, and candidal vaginitis, hyperpigmentation and a lupus-like syndrome have been reported with the minocycline class of antibiotics. The latter two adverse effects may be of particular concern for the skin of color population, in whom lupus and hyperpigmentation are already common problems. Doxycycline can also cause photosensitivity.[10] Other oral antibiotics prescribed for the treatment of acne vulgaris include macrolides, such as erythromycin, as well as cefadroxil and trimethoprim-sulfamethoxazole.[10,54] Tetracyclines and macrolides work by inhibiting bacterial protein synthesis and have anti-inflammatory properties. Sulfonamides inhibit bacterial DNA synthesis. Antibiotic resistance by *P. acnes* is an emerging problem, with oral erythromycin displaying the most resistance, which is succeeded by clindamycin, tetracycline, and doxycycline.[56]

ISOTRETINOIN

Isotretinoin is an effective agent in the treatment of acne vulgaris because it targets all the pathophysiologic mechanisms of acne: sebum production, follicular hyperkeratinization, *P. acnes*, and inflammation. It is often reserved as the last treatment option for acne because of its potential adverse effects.[54,68]

Isotretinoin can be used safely in individuals with skin of color.[77] Between 1990 and 1997, 17% of acne visits resulted in treatment with isotretinoin.[78] According to IMS National Diagnosis and Therapeutic Index™ data, African Americans were seemingly prescribed isotretinoin less often than would be expected.[79] In 1999, only 2.4% of African Americans received treatment with isotretinoin, although 7.7% of African Americans presented to physicians with a diagnosis of acne vulgaris. In contrast, Hispanic and Asian isotretinoin prescriptions more closely reflected their office visits for acne vulgaris (4.9% prescriptions per 4.7% of Hispanic office visits and 4.4% prescriptions per 4.0% of Asian office visits).[79] A study by Fleischer et al[78] supports this finding, and the authors found that darker-skinned patients (3.9%) were less likely to be prescribed isotretinoin for acne treatment than fairer-skinned patients (93%).[78] Fleisher et al[78] postulated that the higher cost of the medication, lack of confidence in the healthcare system, opposing view of the risk-to-benefit ratio of treatment, or an overall decreased amount of visits to the dermatologist's office may account for the difference. This difference may also be related to fewer cases of nodulocystic acne occurring in the African American population compared to other skin of color populations.

HORMONAL THERAPY

Hormonal therapy can be used in women to combat the androgenetic stimulation of the sebaceous glands. Agents used include oral contraceptives and androgen receptor blockers (eg, spironolactone, flutamide, and cyproterone acetate).[3,24]

PROCEDURAL THERAPY

Various procedural treatments, including chemical peels, microdermabrasion, light and laser therapies, and surgery, have also been used as primary and/or adjuvant treatments for acne and the sequelae of acne including acne scarring and dyspigmentation [**Table 42-10**]. In recent years, there have been more studies evaluating the use of these modalities in skin of color populations.

TABLE 42-10 Procedural treatments for acne and acne sequelae

- Chemical peels
  - Glycolic acid 20%–70%
  - Salicylic acid 20%–30%
  - Salicylic-mandelic acid
  - Jessner solution
  - Modified phenol peels
- Lasers
  - Ablative
  - Nonablative
  - Fractional resurfacing
- Light therapies
  - Blue, red, and green
  - Intense pulsed
  - Photodynamic
  - Photopneumatic
- Surgical
  - Punch excision
  - Punch elevation
  - Dermabrasion
  - Subcutaneous incision
  - Filler injections
- Other
  - Bipolar radiofrequency
  - Sublative fractional bipolar radiofrequency

CHEMICAL PEELS

Chemical peels can be useful in acne patients, particularly those with hyperpigmentation and/or scarring. Glycolic acid in concentrations of 20% to 70% and salicylic acid (SA) in concentrations of 20% to 30% are used commonly.[10] Superficial chemical peeling can accelerate the removal of epidermal melanin and increase the penetration and potentially the efficacy of topical treatments for acne and dyspigmentation.[80] Glycolic acid, an α-hydroxy acid, induces epidermolysis, increases dermal collagen synthesis, and disperses the melanin in the basal layer.[10] It has also been shown to have an anti-inflammatory effect by being bactericidal against *P. acnes*.[81] SA, a β-hydroxy acid, has the added benefit of being lipophilic and comedolytic, which makes it a useful treatment for acne and dyspigmentation. It acts mainly on the superficial epidermis and sebaceous glands and induces keratolysis by disrupting intercellular lipid linkages between epithelioid cells.[10,82] Grimes[83] demonstrated improvement of acne in 67% of patients and in postinflammatory hyperpigmentation in 80% of patients treated with a series of five SA peels at 2-week intervals. A study done on Korean patients found that SA peels can also cause lightening of patient's normal skin as well as a decrease in erythema.[82]

Another commonly used chemical peel is Jessner's solution, which is a combination of resorcinol, SA, and lactic acid in ethanol that causes keratolysis by decreasing keratinocyte cohesion. Studies have shown that for acne treatment, Jessner's solution is most effective when used in combination with other peels.[81] Salicylic-mandelic acid (SMA) peels are a newer combination peel combining SA and mandelic acid, an α-hydroxy acid that penetrates the epidermis more slowly and uniformly, an advantage for treating patients with sensitive skin with severe acne and pigmentary issues. A study done in India on 44 patients (skin types IV to VI) comparing glycolic acid peels with SMA peels found that SMA peels had higher efficacy for most active acne lesions and hyperpigmentation.[84] SMA peels may also be a good alternative option to use in patients who have shown more resistance to other peels. Deeper chemical peels, such as phenol, although potentially more effective than superficial and medium-depth peels, should typically be avoided in darker skin types to avoid dyspigmentation and scarring. Recently newer modified phenol peels have been created that are meant to cause fewer side effects. A study was done on 11 Korean patients with acne scars who underwent treatment with a modified phenol peel, and 7 of the 11 patients had a 51% improvement in their acne scars; however, side effects of postinflammatory hyperpigmentation, hypopigmentation, prolonged erythema, keloids, and milia were observed.[85] Chemical peels should be used conservatively in the skin of color population to avoid the risk of adverse effects such as postinflammatory hyperpigmentation and scarring. Physicians should start at the lowest concentration and discontinue use of retinoids 1 week prior to treatment and 5 to 7 days after treatment.

LASER THERAPY

Laser therapy in relation to acne has involved laser skin resurfacing for treatment of acne scarring.[50] Laser resurfacing can be done with ablative, nonablative, and fractional laser technologies. The gold standard for skin resurfacing has traditionally been the ablative lasers, which include the carbon dioxide (CO_2) and erbium-doped yttrium aluminium garnet (Er:YAG) lasers. Use of these lasers can be associated with several adverse effects, particularly in the skin of color population. These include swelling, dyspigmentation, and prolonged postoperative erythema. Nonablative lasers, which include the 1320- and 1064-nm neodymium-doped yttrium aluminium garnet (Nd:YAG), 1450-nm diode, and 585-nm pulsed dye lasers, have also been used in the treatment of acne scarring with less downtime and side effects but generally lower efficacy. Fractional resurfacing lasers, which use a fractional approach of laser delivery to create microscopic zones of thermal damage with controlled width, depth, and densities, have also been used to improve acne scars through tissue ablation, immediate collagen shrinkage, and dermal collagen remodeling. This modality, however, has also been associated with high risks of hyperpigmentation in darker skin types.[86] With laser skin resurfacing, postinflammatory hyperpigmentation has been reported to occur in 68% to 100% of patients with darker skin (Fitzpatrick types IV to VI).[87]

A particular challenge in laser treatments in the skin of color population is the wide absorption spectrum of melanin, which ranges from 250 to 1200 nm and allows melanin to be targeted by all visible and near-infrared lasers.[87] Melanin in the basal layer of the epidermis can absorb nonspecific energy from a laser, which can lead to nonspecific thermal injury and subsequent adverse effects including dyspigmentation, textural changes, atrophy, and scarring. The absorption spectrum of melanin decreases with an increase in wavelength. This allows for lasers with longer wavelengths and deeper penetrations to be more safely and effectively used in the skin of color population. In general, conservative settings, with lower fluences and longer pulse durations, can help minimize tissue damage while allowing for effective treatment results. With fractional resurfacing, the rate of postinflammatory hyperpigmentation is directly proportional to the density of microthermal zones, and therefore, to lower the risk of postinflammatory hyperpigmentation, treatment levels should be lowered.[88] Longer treatment intervals can also help further reduce the risk of postinflammatory hyperpigmentation.[89] Care also needs to be taken to use cooling devices to prevent bulk heating and to avoid stacking laser pulses to avoid further scarring.[87,89] Further cooling of the skin can be provided through postoperative use of ice packs on treated areas. Patients should be educated to use sunscreen, SPF 30 or higher, both pre- and postoperatively. In general, for laser surgery in darker skin, the use of depigmenting agents preoperatively has not been found to decrease the incidence of hyperpigmentation, but it has been found to reduce rates of melanin production and speed reepithelialization postoperatively.[87]

Many studies on the use of lasers for acne scarring in skin of color have been done in the Asian population, and there are a limited number of studies in other skin of color populations. There are also few studies that provide histologic data on the effects of scar remodeling in patients of color. In a split-face Korean study with 18 patients with skin types IV or V, patients were treated for 14 weeks using the 585-nm pulsed dye laser and the 1064-nm Nd:YAG laser.[50] Both lasers were found to be effective treatment modalities for acne scarring, with ice pick scars responding better to pulsed dye laser treatment and boxcar scars responding to Nd:YAG treatment. Longer pulse durations for both lasers

were felt to provide a greater safety margin in darker-skinned patients. Adverse events included transient pain, erythema, and edema but no reports of dyspigmentation.

The 1450-nm diode laser, which works by heating the sebaceous gland and causing a decrease in sebum production and inflammatory acne lesions, has been shown to be effective in two clinical studies on Asian patients with skin types III to V.[90,91] Adverse effects in the study were few and included transient erythema and postinflammatory hyperpigmentation. The diode laser in combination with sublative fractional bipolar radiofrequency and bipolar radiofrequency has also been shown to be safe and effective in improving superficial and deep acne scars in skin types II to V.[92] The advantage of this combination is that radiofrequency energy is not absorbed by melanin, which makes it a good treatment option for patients with darker skin. Another study done using a 1320-nm Nd:YAG laser for atrophic acne scarring in Asians found that it was effective, but optimal treatment was only achieved when done in combination with intense pulsed light (IPL) and a surgical technique.[93] Side effects also included blistering and transient postinflammatory hyperpigmentation. Fractional ablative CO_2 laser resurfacing for acne scars has also been studied in several skin of color populations including Chinese and Thai.[86,94] In the study on Chinese patients, there was mild to moderate improvement after a single treatment; however, 55.5% and 11.1% of the patients experienced postinflammatory hyperpigmentation at 1 and 6 months after treatment, respectively.[94] The Thai population study found that at 6 months after treatment, 85% of the subjects had 25% to 50% improvement of their scars, with 92% of the subjects having mild postinflammatory hyperpigmentation that resolved in an average of 5 weeks.[86] Another study done on patients with skin types IV to VI using an Er:YAG fractionated laser for treatment of acne scars found that although patients did show clinical improvement, pain and postinflammatory hyperpigmentation were both significantly higher in darker skin.[95] Selection of the appropriate laser and use of conservative laser settings is essential in the use of lasers in the skin of color population for acne, acne scarring, and dyspigmentation.

LIGHT THERAPY

IPL, blue light therapy, and photodynamic therapy have also been used to treat acne. Blue light therapy involves targeting and killing fluorescent porphyrins within *P. acnes*.[10] A study on the use of blue light in Taiwanese patients (skin types III to IV) with acne found that it was successful in treating mild to moderate acne but caused a worsening of nodulocystic acne.[96] IPL, which is a polychromatic nonlaser light (400 to 1200 nm) that has been used to treat acne and acne scarring, is thought to have anti-inflammatory effects and can lead to photoinactivation of *P. acnes* and photothermolysis of the sebaceous glands. IPL can also improve atrophic scarring through inducing fibroblast activation and synthesis of new collagen and extracellular matrix components.[97] Studies have shown mixed results regarding the success of IPL, and some studies advocate for its use as part of a combination therapy instead of being a monotherapy.[10,98] A study on IPL combined with fractional CO_2 laser treatments in Chinese patients with inflammatory acne and scarring found that the majority of patients had a decrease in melanin, erythema, and skin sebum level after treatment.[97]

Photodynamic therapy, which uses a photosensitizer, targets bacteria by selectively inducing the porphyrin fluorescence of pilosebaceous units.[10] More recently, it has been considered an effective treatment option for patients with acne that has been refractory to conventional treatments and for those who are not appropriate candidates for isotretinoin. This treatment modality has been used with varying success in several Asian populations and in a case report of an African American female patient with moderate inflammatory acne.[99-101] Reported side effects have included transient hyperpigmentation, peeling, and scaling. Lastly, photopneumatic therapy is a newer acne treatment in which the skin is drawn into a handpiece allowing the mechanical removal of sebaceous material by suction pressure, followed by broadband light delivery to the treatment site.[10] The light delivery leads to bacterial destruction and has been shown to improve acne with only mild erythema as a side effect. This treatment, however, has not been well studied in the skin of color population.

Overall, light treatments for acne and acne sequelae including acne scarring and postinflammatory hyperpigmentation have shown varying degrees of success; however, studies in the skin of color population remain limited.[102] These treatments should be considered either as adjuvant or combination treatments to conventional treatments and should also be considered as an option for patients who have been recalcitrant to other acne treatments.

SURGICAL THERAPIES

Surgical procedures including punch excision, punch elevation, dermabrasion, subcutaneous incision (subcision), and filler injection have also been used for treatment of acne scarring. These treatments have provided varying results; some are suboptimal, whereas others have shown more efficacy, particularly when used in combination with other treatments.[50]

CONCLUSION

Acne vulgaris patients with skin of color present with differences in chief complaints, clinical presentations, precipitating and exacerbating factors, long-term sequelae, therapeutic needs, and adverse events. It is important for physicians to be culturally aware and sensitive to these differences in order to effectively treat acne vulgaris in skin of color patients.

REFERENCES

1. White GM. Recent findings in the epidemiologic evidence, classification, and subtypes of acne vulgaris. *J Am Acad Dermatol.* 1998;39:S34-S37.
2. Lookingbill DP. *Principles of Dermatology.* 3rd ed. Philadelphia, PA: Saunders; 2000.
3. Callender VD. Acne in ethnic skin: special considerations for therapy. *Dermatol Ther.* 2004;17:184-195.
4. Taylor SC, Cook-Bolden F, Rahman Z, et al. Acne vulgaris in skin of color. *J Am Acad Dermatol.* 2002;46:S98-S106.
5. Eichenfield LF, Krakowski AC. Moderate to severe acne in adolescents with skin of color: benefits of a fixed combination clindamycin phosphate 1.2% and benzoyl peroxide 2.5% aqueous gel. *J Drugs Dermatol.* 2012;11:818-824.
6. U.S. Census Bureau. Population projections–2009 population projections. https://www.census.gov. Accessed February 23, 2014.
7. Centers for Disease Control and Prevention. Center for Health Statistics Ambulatory HealthCare Data. www.cdc.gov/nchs/ahcd.htm. Accessed June 16, 2015.
8. Fox H. Observations on skin diseases in the Negro. *J Cutan Dis.* 1908;26:67-79.
9. Davis SA, Narahari S, Feldman SR. Top dermatologic conditions in patients of color: an analysis of nationally representative data. *J Drugs Dermatol.* 2012;11:466-473.
10. Davis EC, Callender VD. A review of acne in ethnic skin: pathogenesis, clinical manifestations, and management strategies. *J Clin Aesthet Dermatol.* 2010;3:24-38.
11. Alexis AF, Sergay AB, Taylor SC. Common dermatologic disorders in skin of color: a comparative practice survey. *Cutis.* 2007;80:387-394.
12. Henderson, MD, Abboud J, Cogan CM, et al. Skin-of-color epidemiology: a report of the most common skin conditions by race. *Pediatric Dermatol.* 2012;29:584-589.
13. Child FJ, Fuller LC, Higgins EM, et al. A study of the spectrum of skin disease occurring in a black population in southeast London. *Br J Dermatol.* 1999;141:512-517.
14. Dunwell P, Rose A. Study of the skin disease spectrum occurring in an Afro-Caribbean population. *Int J Dermatol.* 2003;42:287-289.
15. Mahe A, Mancel E. Dermatological practice in Guadeloupe (French West Indies). *Clin Exp Dermatol.* 1999;24:358-360.
16. Yahya H. Acne vulgaris in Nigerian adolescents: prevalence, severity, beliefs, perceptions, and practices. *Int J Dermatol.* 2009;48:498-505.
17. Lee CS, Lim HW. Cutaneous diseases in Asians. *Dermatol Clin.* 2003;21:669-677.
18. Shah SK, Bhanusali DG, Sachdev A. A survey of skin conditions and concerns in South Asian Americans: a community-based study. *J Drugs Dermatol.* 2011;10:524-528.
19. Churaty G, Goh CL, Koh SL. Pattern of skin diseases at the National Skin Center (Singapore) from 1989-1990. *Int J Dermatol.* 1992;31:555-559.
20. Sanchez MR. Cutaneous diseases in Latinos. *Dermatol Clin.* 2003;21:689-697.
21. El-Essawi D, Musial JL, Hammad A, et al. A survey of skin disease and skin-related issues in Arab Americans. *J Am Acad Dermatol.* 2007;56:933-938.
22. Nanda A, al-Hasawi F, Alsaleh QA. A prospective survey of pediatric dermatology clinic patients in Kuwait: an analysis of 10,000 cases. *Pedriatr Dermatol.* 1999;16:6-11.
23. Freedberg IM, Eisen AZ, Wolffet K, et al, eds. *Fitzpatrick's Dermatology in General Medicine.* New York, NY: McGraw-Hill; 2003.
24. Haider A, Shaw JC. Treatment of acne vulgaris. *JAMA.* 2004;292:726-735.
25. Davis EC, Callender VD. A review of acne in ethnic skin: pathogenesis, clinical manifestations, and management strategies. *J Clin Aesthet Dermatol.* 2010;3:24-38.
26. Warrier AG, Kligman AM, Harper RA, et al. A comparison of black and white skin using noninvasive methods. *J Soc Cosmet Chem.* 1996;47:229-240.
27. Nicolaides N, Rothman S. Studies on the chemical composition of human hair fat: II. The overall composition with regard to age, sex and race. *J Invest Dermatol.* 1953;21:9-14.
28. Kligman AM, Shelley WB. An investigation of the biology of the human sebaceous gland. *J Invest Dermatol.* 1958;30:99-125.
29. Perkins AC, Cheng CE, Hillebrand GG. Comparison of the epidemiology of acne vulgaris among Caucasian, Asian, Continental Indian and African American women. *J Eur Acad Dermatol Venereol.* 2011;25:1054-1060.
30. Grimes P, Edison BL, Green BA, et al. Evaluation of inherent differences between African American and white skin surface properties using subjective and objective measures. *Cutis.* 2004;73:392-396.
31. Robinson MK. Population differences in skin structure and physiology and the susceptibility to irritant and allergic contact dermatitis: implications for skin safety testing and risk assessment. *Contact Dermatitis.* 1999;41:65-79.
32. Taylor SC. Skin of color: biology, structure, function, and implications for dermatologic disease. *J Am Acad Dermatol.* 2002;46:S41-S62.
33. Richards GM, Oresajo CO, Halder RM. Structure and function of ethnic skin and hair. *Dermatol Clin.* 2003;21:595-600.
34. He L, Yang Z, Yu H. The relationship between CYP17-34T/C polymorphism and acne in Chinese subjects revealed by sequencing. *Dermatology.* 2006;212:338-342.
35. Xu SX, Wang HL, Fan X. The familial risk of acne vulgaris in Chinese Hans—a case-control study. *J Eur Acad Dermatol Venereol.* 2007;21:602-605.
36. Schaefer O. When the Eskimo comes to town. *Nutr Today.* 1971;6:8-16.
37. Steiner PE. Necropsies on Okinawans: anatomic and pathologic observations. *Arch Pathol.* 1946;42:359-380.
38. Bechelli LM, Haddad N, Pimenta WP, et al. Epidemiological survey skin diseases in schoolchildren living in the Purus Valley (Acre State, Amazonia, Brazil). *Dermatologica.* 1981;163:78-93.
39. Freyre EA, Rebaza RM, Sami DA, et al. The prevalence of facial acne in Peruvian adolescents and its relation to their ethnicity. *J Adolesc Health.* 1998;22:480-484.
40. Cordain L, Lindeberg S, Hurtado M, et al. Acne vulgaris: a disease of Western civilization. *Arch Dermatol.* 2002;138:1584-1590.
41. Melnik B. Diet in acne: further evidence for the role of nutrient signaling in acne pathogenesis. *Acta Derm Venereol.* 2012;92:228-231.
42. Wilkins JW Jr, Voorhees JJ. Prevalence of nodulocystic acne in white and Negro males. *Arch Dermatol.* 1970;102:631-634.
43. Plewig G, Fulton JE, Kligman AM. Pomade acne. *Arch Dermatol.* 1970;101:580-584.
44. Halder RM, Brooks HL, Callender VD. Acne in ethnic skin. *Dermatol Clin.* 2003;21:609-615.
45. Sanchez J, Somolinos AL, Almodóvar PI, et al. A randomized, double-blind, placebo-controlled trial of the combined effect of doxycycline hyclate 20-mg tablets and metronidazole 0.75% topical lotion in the treatment of rosacea. *J Am Acad Dermatol.* 2005;53:791-797.
46. Wolff K, Johnson RA, Suurmond D. Section 1. Disorders of sebaceous and apocrine glands. In: Wolff K, Johnson RA, Suurmond D, eds. *Fitzpatrick's Color Atlas & Synopsis of Clinical Dermatology.* 6th ed. New York, NY: McGraw-Hill; 2009.
47. Rosen T, Stone M. Acne rosacea in blacks. *J Am Acad Dermatol.* 1987;17:70-73.
48. Piette WW, Taylor S, Pariser D, et al. Hematologic safety of dapsone gel, 5% for the treatment of acne vulgaris. *Arch Dermatol.* 2008;144:1564-1570.

49. Kane A, Niang SO, Diagne AC. Epidemiologic, clinical, and therapeutic features of acne in Dakar, Senegal. *Int J Dermatol.* 2007;46:36-38.

50. Lee DH, Choi YS, Min SU. Comparison of a 585-nm pulsed dye laser and a 1064-nm Nd:Yag laser for the treatment of acne scars: a randomized split-face clinical study. *J Am Acad Dermatol.* 2009;60:801-807.

51. Bianconi-Moore A. Acne vulgaris in patients with skin of colour: special considerations. *Nurs Stand.* 2012;26:43-49.

52. Morrone A, Franco G, Valenzano M. Clinical features of acne vulgaris in 444 patients with ethnic skin. *J Dermatol.* 2011;38:405-408.

53. Halder RM, Holmes YC, Bridgeman-Shah S, et al. A clinicopathological study of acne vulgaris in black females. Abstracts for the 1996 Annual Meeting Society for Investigative Dermatology. *J Invest Dermatol.* 1996;106:888.

54. Lebwohl MG, Heymann WR, Berth-Jones J, et al. *Treatment of Skin Disease: Comprehensive Therapeutic Strategies.* St Louis, MO: Mosby; 2002:6-13.

55. Gollnick H, Cunliffe W, Berson D, et al. Management of acne: a report from a global alliance to improve outcomes in acne. *J Am Acad Dermatol.* 2006;49:S1-S67.

56. Leyden JJ. Topical treatment for the inflamed lesion in acne, rosacea, and pseudofolliculitis barbae. *Cutis.* 2004;73:4-5.

57. Leyden JJ. Antibiotic resistance in the topical treatment of acne vulgaris. *Cutis.* 2004;73:6-10.

58. Callender VD. Fitzpatrick skin types and clindamycin phosphate 1.2%/benzoyl peroxide gel: efficacy and tolerability of treatment in moderate to severe acne. *J Drugs Dermatol.* 2012;11:643-648.

59. Alexis AF, Johnson LA, Kerrouche N. Safety of adapalene-benzoyl peroxide topical gel in black subjects with moderate acne. *J Drugs Dermatol.* 2014;13:170-174.

60. Callender VD, Preston N, Osborn C. A meta-analysis to investigate the relation between Fitzpatrick skin types and tolerability of adapalene-benzoyl peroxide topical gel in subjects with mild or moderate acne. *J Clin Aesthetic Dermatol.* 2010;3:15-19.

61. Gollnick HP. Azelaic acid 15% gel in the treatment of acne vulgaris: combined results of two double-blind clinical comparative studies. *J Dtsch Dermatol Ges.* 2004;2:841-847.

62. Fitton A, Goa KL. Azelaic acid: a review of its pharmacological properties and therapeutic efficacy in acne and hyperpigmentary skin disorders. *Drugs.* 1991;41:780-798.

63. Balina LM, Graupe K. The treatment of melasma: 20% azelaic acid versus 4% hydroquinone cream. *Int J Dermatol.* 1991;30:893-895.

64. Bulengo-Ransby SM, Griffiths CE, Kimbrough-Green CK, et al. Topical tretinoin (retinoic acid) therapy for hyperpigmented lesions caused by inflammation of the skin in black patients. *N Engl J Med.* 1993;328:1438-1443.

65. Halder RM. The role of retinoids in the management of cutaneous conditions in blacks. *J Am Acad Dermatol.* 1998;39:S98-S103.

66. Jacyk WK. Adapalene in the treatment of African patients. *J Eur Acad Dermatol Venereol.* 2001;15:S37-S42.

67. Czernielewski J, Poncet M, Mizzi F. Efficacy and cutaneous safety of adapalene in black patients versus white patients with acne vulgaris. *Cutis.* 2002;70:243-248.

68. Tu P, Li GQ, Zhu XJ, et al. A comparison of adapalene gel 0.1% vs tretinoin gel 0.025% in the treatment of acne vulgaris in China. *J Eur Acad Dermatol Venereol.* 2001;15:S31-S36.

69. Zhu XJ, Tu P, Zhen J, Duan YQ. Adapalene gel 0.1%: Effective and well tolerated in the topical treatment of acne vulgaris in Chinese patients. *Cutis.* 2001;68:S55-S59.

70. Grimes P, Callender V. Tazarotene cream for postinflammatory hyperpigmentation and acne vulgaris in darker skin: a double-blind, randomized, vehicle-controlled study. *Cutis.* 2006;77:45-50.

71. Shah SK, Alexis AF. Acne in skin of color: practical approaches to treatment. *J Dermatol.* 2010;21:206-211.

72. Goh CL, Tang MB, Briantais P. Adapalene gel 0.1% is better tolerated than tretinoin gel 0.025% among healthy volunteers of various ethnic origins. *J Dermatol Treat.* 2009;20:282-288.

73. Callender VD, Young CM, Kindred CK, et al. Efficacy and safety of clindamycin phosphate 1.2% and tretinoin 0.025% gel for the treatment of acne and acne-induced post-inflammatory hyperpigmentation in patients with skin of color. *J Drugs Dermatol.* 2012;5:25-32.

74. Fleischer AB, Shalita A, Eichenfield, LF, et al. Dapsone gel 5% in combination with adapalene gel 0.1%, benzoyl peroxide gel 4% or moisturizer for the treatment of acne vulgaris: a 12-week, randomized, double-blind study. *J Drugs Dermatol.* 2010;9:33-40.

75. Aczone (dapsone) Gel, 5% [Package insert]. Irvine, CA: Allergan, Inc., March 2009.

76. Jung JY, Kwon HH, Yeom KB. Clinical and histological evaluation of 1% nadifloxacin cream in the treatment of acne vulgaris in Korean patients. *Int J Dermatol.* 2011;50:350-357.

77. Kelly AP, Sampson DD. Recalcitrant nodulocystic acne in black Americans: treatment with isotretinoin. *J Natl Med Assoc.* 1987;79:1266-1270.

78. Fleischer AB Jr, Simpson JK, McMichael A, et al. Are there racial and sex differences in the use of oral isotretinoin for acne management in the United States? *J Am Acad Dermatol.* 2003;49:662-666.

79. IMS. IMS National Diagnosis and Therapeutic Index, 1999. https://web01.imshealth.com/ndti/ndtilogin.aspx. Accessed February 4, 2015.

80. Coley MK, Alexis AF. Managing common dermatoses in skin of color. *Semin Cutan Med Surg.* 2009;28:63-70.

81. Salam A, Dadzie OE, Galadari H. Chemical peeling in ethnic skin: an update. *Br J Dermatol.* 2013;169:82-90.

82. Ahn HH, Kim I. Whitening effect of salicylic acid peels in Asian patients. *Dermatol Surg.* 2006;32:372-375.

83. Grimes PE. The safety and efficacy of salicylic acid chemical peels in darker racial ethnic groups. *Dermatol Surg.* 1999;25:18-22.

84. Garg VJ, Sinha S, Sarkar R. Glycolic acid peels versus salicylic-mandelic acid peels in active acne vulgaris and post-acne scarring and hyperpigmentation: a comparative study. *Dermatol Surg.* 2009;35:59-65.

85. Park JH, Choi YD, Kim SW. Effectiveness of modified phenol peel (Exoderm) on facial wrinkles, acne scars and other skin problems of Asian patients. *J Dermatol.* 2007;34:17-24.

86. Manuskiatti W, Triwongwaranat D, Varothai S, et al. Efficacy and safety of carbon-dioxide ablative fractional resurfacing device for treatment of atrophic scars in Asians. *J Am Acad Dermatol.* 2010;63:274-283.

87. Bhatt N, Alster TS. Laser surgery in dark skin. *Dermatol Surg.* 2008;34:184-195.

88. Sherling M, Friedman P, Adrian R, et al. Consensus recommendations on the use of erbium-doped 1,550 nm fractionated laser and its applications in dermatologic laser surgery. *Dermatol Surg.* 2010;36:461-469.

89. Chan HH, Manstein D, Yu CS, et al. The prevalence and risk factors of postinflammatory hyperpigmentation after fractional resurfacing in Asians. *Lasers Surg Med.* 2007;39:381-385.

90. Yeung CK, Shek SY, Yu CS, et al. Treatment of inflammatory facial acne with 1,450 diode laser in type IV to V Asian skin using an optimal combination of laser parameters. *Dermatol Surg.* 2009;35:593-600.

91. Yeung CK, Shek SY, Bjerring P, et al. A comparative study of intense pulsed light along or in combination with photodynamic therapy for the treatment of facial acne in Asian Skin. *Lasers Surg Med.* 2007;39:1-6.

92. Taub AF, Garretson CB. Treatment of acne scars of skin types II to V by sublative fractional bipolar radiofrequency and bipolar radiofrequency combined with diode laser. *J Clin Aesthet Dermatol.* 2011;4:18-27.

93. Chan HH, Lam L, Wong, DS, et al. Use of 1,320 Nd:Yag laser for wrinkle reduction and the treatment of atrophic acne scarring in Asians. *Lasers Surg Med.* 2004;34:98-103.

94. Chan NP, Ho SG, Yeung CY, et al. Fractional ablative carbon dioxide laser resurfacing for skin rejuvenation and acne scars in Asians. *Lasers Surg Med.* 2010;42:775-783.

95. Mahmoud BH, Srivastava D, Janiga JJ. Safety and efficacy of erbium-doped yttrium aluminum garnet fractionated laser for treatment of acne scars in type IV to VI skin. *Dermatol Surg.* 2010;36:602-609.

96. Oh SH, Ryu DJ, Han EC, et al. Effect of smooth pulsed light at 400 to 700 and 870 to 1,200 nm for acne vulgaris in Asian skin. *Dermatol Surg.* 2010;36:52-57.

97. Wang B, Wu Y, Luo J, et al. Combination of intense pulsed light and fractional CO2 laser treatments for patients with acne with inflammatory and scarring lesions. *Clin Exp Dermatol.* 2013;38:344-351.

98. Kawan S, Tachihara R, Kato T, et al. Effect of smooth pulsed light at 400 to 700 and 870 to 1,200 nm for acne vulgaris in Asian skin. *Dermatol Surg.* 36:52-57.

99. Itoh Y, Ninomiya Y, Tajima S, et al. Photodynamic therapy of acne vulgaris with topical δ- aminolevulinic acid and incoherent light in Japanese patients. *Br J Dermatol.* 2001;144:575-579.

100. Hong SB, Lee MH. Topical aminolevulinic acid-photodynamic therapy for the treatment of acne vulgaris. *Photodermatol Photoimmunol Photomed.* 2005;21:322-325.

101. Terrell S, Aires D, Schweiger ES. Treatment of acne vulgaris using blue light photodynamic therapy in an African-American patient. *J Drugs Dermatol.* 2009;8:669-671.

102. Huang L. A new modality for fractional CO2 laser resurfacing for acne scars in Asians. *Lasers Med Sci.* 2013;28:627-632.

CHAPTER 43

Hidradenitis Suppurativa

Virginia J. Reeder
Iltefat H. Hamzavi

KEY POINTS

- Hidradenitis suppurativa (HS) is a skin disease that may manifest as chronic, recurrent inflammatory nodules, abscesses, scarring, and/or fistulas that are incredibly painful.

- HS is thought to be more prevalent in individuals of African descent.

- HS patients report greatly decreased quality of life, and it should be recognized that this disease has not only physical but also social and emotional ramifications.

- Although primarily considered to be a disease of the skin, patients may be afflicted with a variety of associated systemic complications.

INTRODUCTION

Hidradenitis suppurativa (HS) is a chronic, recurrent inflammatory disease of the skin. It typically manifests as painful nodules and abscesses that can progress to form deep sinus tracts, fistulas, and severe scarring. This disease tends to affect areas of the body with apocrine gland–bearing tissue, including the groin, gluteal, axillary, and inframammary regions. For this reason, HS may also be referred to as *acne inversa*. HS lesions may chronically drain malodorous fluid, which can leave affected individuals uncomfortable and self-conscious. Cultures of fluid draining from HS lesions are classically described as being sterile, but a recent study demonstrated that cultures of deeper tissues following ablation of involved areas with a carbon dioxide laser were positive for coagulase-negative staphylococci, *Corynebacterium*, and α-hemolytic streptococci.[1] Pain from active lesions or restricted movement due to scarring can debilitate those affected. The pathogenesis of this disease process is not fully understood, and it can be quite difficult to treat. Inadequate treatments and incomplete comprehension of the disease process can leave both patients and physicians frustrated. Studies demonstrate that patients with this condition consistently report a significantly decreased quality of life,[2-6] even when compared with other conditions, such as psoriasis or atopic dermatitis, which are known to decrease quality of life.[2,6]

HISTORY

The first known descriptions and investigations into HS are attributed to the nineteenth century contemporary French physicians Velpeau, who is credited with first reporting a patient with this condition, and Verneuil, who later published several articles[7,8] providing the first conceptualization of this disease process as a discrete entity.[9] Because Verneuil was the first to study this disease in depth, HS is often called *Verneuil disease*. Due to the anatomic distribution of the disease, Verneuil believed that HS was associated with pathology of sweat glands. The disease has been frequently confused with simple infection of the skin, and its history is burdened with misunderstanding of HS as being an issue of inadequate personal hygiene and resulting misdiagnoses. Until the late twentieth century, even when recognized appropriately as HS, physicians continued to hypothesize that the disorder was associated with apocrine gland pathology.[10] In the 1990s, histologic studies helped show that the disease process likely emanates from the pilosebaceous unit rather than the apocrine glands.[11]

EPIDEMIOLOGY

There is a paucity of definitive data on prevalence for HS, with reported rates varying from 0.003% to 4% depending on the population surveyed.[12-15] There is evidence that the incidence of HS has been increasing in recent decades, which may account for some of the variability noted.[12] Additionally, it has been suggested that HS is more prevalent in people of African descent,[16] yet the majority of studies investigating prevalence of this disease are drawn from predominantly Western European and Caucasian populations.[12-14] This is perhaps another source of the differing data on the prevalence of the disease and demonstrates the need for further research in this area. Women are much more commonly affected than men at an estimated ratio of 3:1.[15,17] Onset is typically after puberty, with the average onset being in the third decade of life and the greatest prevalence being between ages 18 and 44 years.[15] One recent population-based study demonstrated that the highest incidence of HS is in women between the ages of 20 and 29.[12] Up to a third of patients have a family history of HS.[18]

PATHOGENESIS

As previously mentioned, HS was historically considered to be a disease associated with apocrine gland dysfunction. Although this disease does primarily affect skin bearing apocrine glands, it is currently thought that the apocrine glands themselves are not the primary source of the pathology. Several studies have convincingly demonstrated this concept.[11,19,20] One such study examined biopsy specimens and found that only 5% demonstrated primary involvement of the apocrine glands, and that only 12% demonstrated secondary involvement of the apocrine glands.[11] Histologic studies have also illuminated other key happenings including sebaceous gland atrophy, lymphocytic infiltration, and follicular plugging. Subsequent rupture of the follicles leads to spread of bacteria and keratin debris within the dermis and granuloma formation.[21] The abscesses of HS tend to be sterile, and the role of bacteria in the pathogenesis of the disease is uncertain.[22,23] Recent studies have focused on identifying an immune or inflammatory etiology for the disease, investigating the interleukin-12–interleukin-23 pathway[24] and abnormal expression of tumor necrosis factor-α (TNF-α)[25] as possible factors in HS pathogenesis. There is strong clinical evidence for the influence of sex hormones. The disease tends to present at menarche or adrenarche, and females often experience perimenstrual flares. Most patients, however, have normal androgen profiles.[26] This lends credence to the concept that the disease may emanate from the pilosebaceous unit as opposed to the apocrine glands because, in contrast to sebaceous glands, which are affected by sex hormones, apocrine glands are not androgen sensitive.[26] Identification of familial variants of HS with distinct autosomal dominant inheritance patterns has allowed for identification of a defect in the γ-secretase complex in a minority of HS patients with this inherited form of disease.[18] Although an exciting discovery, this mutation does not appear to be present in most patients with HS.[18] Identification of a specific defect may pave the way for therapeutic targets in the future and so will continue to be a focus of HS research.

CLINICAL FEATURES

The hallmarks of early HS are painful inflammatory nodules and abscesses that occur in apocrine-bearing skin folds such as the axillary, gluteal, inframammary, inguinal, and perineal regions. Double comedones, or comedones that have multiple openings through the skin surface, are often seen as well.[27] As the disease progresses, the abscesses rupture or coalesce and may eventually form sinus tracts and fistulae. Granulation tissue and hypertrophic scarring may form as well. If such scarring occurs, it often decreases range of motion of the extremities and can be debilitating. The diagnosis is typically clinical, and patients often experience delays in diagnosis due to confusion of the disease process with simple infection of the skin. Stress, perspiration, heat, and friction have been suggested as potential aggravating factors for the disease process, but the removal of these factors does not typically reverse the pathology.[9] A study surveying 110 HS patients evaluated the natural history of HS and found that the average duration of a lesion was 6.9 days, and the

TABLE 43-1	Sartorius grading system	
Criteria		Scoring
Anatomic region involved: axilla, groin, gluteal of other region, or inframammary region (left and/or right)		+ 3 points per region involved
Number and scores of lesions: abscesses, nodules, fistulae, scars (points added per lesion of all anatomic regions involved)		Fistulae = + 4; nodules = + 2; scars = + 1; others = + 1
The longest distance between two relevant lesions in each region		<5 cm = + 2; <10 cm = + 4; >10 cm = + 8
Are all lesions in each anatomic region clearly separated by normal skin?		If yes: + 0; if no: + 6.

Source: Data from Sartorius K, Lapins J, Emtestam L, Jemec GB. Suggestions for uniform outcome variables when reporting treatment effects in hidradenitis suppurativa. *Br J Dermatol.* 2003;149:211-213.

medium number of lesions per months was two.[9] Without treatment, most acute flairs were found to resolve within 7 to 10 days, but most patients noted that they had at least one painful lesion that persisted indefinitely even between flairs such that the pain never fully resolved.[9] Women frequently experience perimenstrual flairs and have been noted to experience improvement in disease during pregnancy as well as a great decrease in disease activity following menopause.[9,26,28-30] There are two clinical grading systems for assessing the severity of HS, which are helpful in documenting the progression of the disease process. The Sartorius grading system assigns a numerical score based on the anatomic regions involved, the number of lesions, the distance between lesions, and whether there is unaffected skin between lesions [**Table 43-1**].[31] Severity of HS may also be assessed using the Hurley staging system, which assesses disease severity based on lesion morphology [**Table 43-2 and Figure 43-1**].[32]

In addition to classification simply by disease severity, a recent study put forth an empirical subclassification based on association of clinical variables.[33] Patients were described as falling into "axillary-mammary," "gluteal," or "follicular" categories.[33] The axillary-mammary category encompasses the classic presentation of HS including lesions in the axillae and around the breast, a predominance of female patients, and higher body mass indices (BMIs).[33] The follicular classification is more likely to include men and include follicular lesions such as pilonidal cysts, severe acne, or epidermoid cysts.[33] The gluteal class members were more likely to be men, to have lower BMIs, to have more severe disease, and to have lesions in the gluteal region.[33] A separate population-based study also demonstrated that women were more likely to have axillary and upper torso lesions, whereas men were more likely to have lesions in the perineal or gluteal regions and more likely to have more severe disease.[12] Further investigation into these clinical subclassifications will be necessary to determine whether they will be generalizable to all patients with HS and whether they will be predictive of disease progression. This sort of clinical breakdown of HS is likely to further the understanding of the etiology, progression, and therapeutic responses of this disease. As more and more treatments for HS are available, there will be an increasing need for prediction of which patients are most likely to respond to each of the various therapeutic options.

A number of conditions are known to be associated with HS. Common associations include obesity, acne conglobata, acne vulgaris, Crohn disease, dissecting cellulitis of the scalp, and pilonidal disease.[34]

TABLE 43-2	Hurley staging system
Stage I: one or more abscesses with no cicatrization or sinus tract formation.	
Stage II: one or more widely separated abscesses that are recurrent and have cicatrization and/or sinus tract formation.	
Stage III: multiple interconnected abscesses and sinus tracts throughout an affected anatomic region.	

Source: Reproduced with permission from Roenigk RK, Roenigk HH (eds): *Dermatologic Surgery: Principles and Practice.* New York, NY: Marcel Dekker; 1989

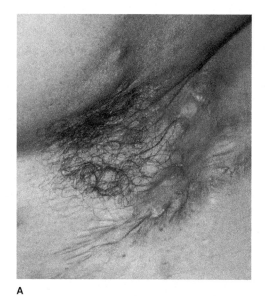

A

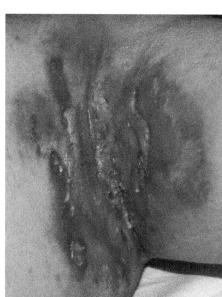

B

FIGURE 43-1. Axillary hidradenitis suppurativa illustrating the spectrum of disease severity as measured by Hurley stage. (**A**) Stage II. (**B**) Stage III.

Dissecting cellulitis of the scalp, pilonidal disease, acne conglobata, and HS are all disorders of follicular occlusion. Together, they are known as the follicular occlusion tetrad, and a patient who has one of these disease processes may also suffer from several of the other components of the tetrad.[35,36] There is also a strong association between obesity and HS.[12,37,38] HS patients are more likely to be obese than the general population, and increasing BMI has been correlated with increased disease severity but not definitively with causality.[37] It is unclear whether the obesity precedes HS and is a factor in the HS pathogenesis or whether the HS encourages obesity through increased systemic inflammation and/or increased tendency toward sedentary lifestyles due to pain and decreased range of motion. Similarly, smoking tobacco is another lifestyle factor that has been strongly associated with HS.[12,38,39] One population-based study found that 70% of HS patients had a lifetime history of smoking tobacco.[12] Less common but reported associations include acanthosis nigricans, Bazex-Dupré-Christol syndrome, Dowling-Degos disease, Fox-Fordyce disease, interstitial keratitis, keratitis-ichthyosis-deafness syndrome, pachyonychia congenita, PAPA (pyogenic arthritis, pyoderma gangrenosum, and acne) syndrome, pyoderma gangrenosum, reflex sympathetic dystrophy, SAPHO (synovitis, acne, pustulosis, hyperostosis, and osteitis) syndrome, and scrotal elephantiasis.[34]

Patients with HS consistently report a significantly decreased quality of life.[2-6] A study in Germany demonstrated that patients with HS suffer from profound disorders of sexual health and that women with HS are much more likely to have sexual dysfunction and distress than men with this disorder.[40] HS is prone to affecting intimate anatomic areas, which may result in much shame and embarrassment.[5] This may lead to avoidance of intimate relationships by those affected by this disorder. A study in Denmark revealed that the pregnancy and birth rates of females with HS were significantly lower than in females without the disease.[4] The same study showed that HS patients had a diminished perception of their overall health than the general population and that HS patients took more sick days from work than the general population.[4] Another study done in Denmark and the Netherlands reported decreased quality of life in HS patients even when compared to people with other dermatologic conditions such as atopic dermatitis and psoriasis.[6] Similar results were found in Poland, France, and Great Britain in terms of patients experiencing decreased quality of life scores even when compared to other chronic dermatologic conditions known to affect quality of life.[2,3,41]

In addition to the psychological morbidity, HS may have serious physical sequelae. Sinus tracts may develop that connect with the bowel, bladder, urethra, or rectum forming fistulae or possibly strictures. Chronic drainage from such fistulae can result in extensive skin breakdown, and fistulae may result in issues with voiding. Scarring may severely limit range of motion and leave those affected debilitated and unable to carry out activities or daily living [**Figure 43-2**]. The inflammation associated with chronic disease activity may result in anemia, secondary amyloidosis, hypoproteinemia, or nephrotic syndrome. Each

of these potential sequelae may individually be life threatening and demonstrates that HS is not merely a cutaneous malady, but is a disease process that may have serious systemic consequences with potential for morbidity and mortality.

Additionally, an association between HS and malignancy has been identified. One large retrospective study reviewed over 2000 cases and found that HS patients have a 50% increased risk of developing malignancy of some sort.[42] In particular, the risk of cutaneous squamous cell carcinoma (SCC) was increased in HS patients and was 4.6 times the risk of non-HS patients.[42] Other studies have similarly shown an increased incidence of cutaneous SCC in patients with HS.[43-47] The risk for SCC for males with HS has been found to be four times the risk for females with HS, and the majority of these malignancies occurred in the groin or gluteal regions.[45] A high mortality rate has been associated with these cutaneous SCCs in HS patients, with a reported 48% of patients dying within 2 years of diagnosis.[45]

HISTOLOGY

HS lesions may have some histologic variability depending on the stage of the lesion examined. Early lesions will demonstrate an inflammatory cell infiltrate in the lower dermis that may or may not extend in the subcutaneous tissue and hyperkeratosis and plugging of the pilosebaceous unit.[17] There is little primary involvement on the apocrine glands, but there is early atrophy of the sebaceous glands.[19] Stage II and III lesions may involve sinus tracts or frank abscesses. Sinus tracts are lined with squamous epithelium, which typically extends from an associated hair follicle, as well as keratinaceous debris. Later stage lesions show destruction of the hair follicle, granuloma formation, and an inflammatory infiltrate.[11,19,48]

DIFFERENTIAL DIAGNOSIS

The differential diagnosis for HS may depend on the stage of the disease. The erythema, nodules, and abscesses of early-stage HS may have to be distinguished from epidermoid cysts, furuncles, carbuncles, cellulitis, acne, or Bartholin abscesses. Due to the potential for sinus tracts and fistulas with later stage HS, disease processes that can cause this type of pathology should be considered, including actinomycosis, tuberculosis, lymphogranuloma venereum, granuloma inguinale, and Crohn disease.

TREATMENT

Although no treatments are universally or perfectly effective, there are a variety of options available for treating HS. Lifestyle modifications such as smoking cessation and weight loss are often the first recommendations due to the strong association with these factors and the minimal risk associated with making such changes. Additionally, patients may wear loose-fitting clothes to minimize friction in the intertriginous areas, which are often affected. Avoidance of moisture is recommended, and patients may use absorbent powders or aluminum chloride to achieve this effect.[16] Although the role of bacteria in the pathogenesis remains uncertain, antiseptic soaps and washes are generally recommended. Topical antibiotics, such as clindamycin 1%, either as a lotion or as a solution may also added to the therapeutic regimen early on in the disease process, and in a comparison between oral tetracycline and topical 1% clindamycin, the two therapies showed similar levels of improvement in HS symptoms.[49] Intralesional injection of steroids may be used for early inflammatory lesions.[16] If the disease is nonresponsive to these more conservative measures or has progressed beyond early-stage lesions, more aggressive treatment strategies may be used. There are currently no formal guidelines for more aggressive treatment of advanced disease, and there is not an overwhelming amount of evidence available from randomized controlled trials, so decisions on treatment are often made based on clinical experience.

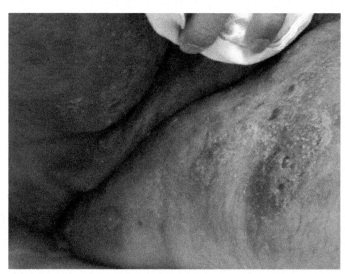

A

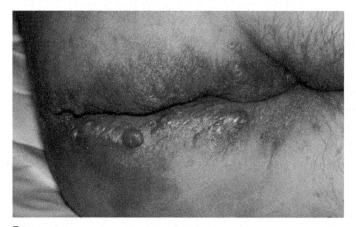

B

FIGURE 43-2. (A and B) Severe hidradenitis suppurativa may be incredibly painful and limit physical activity in affected individuals.

Medical treatments may include use of antibiotics, isotretinoin, anti-androgens, or immunosuppressive medications. Oral antibiotics are often the core of treatment of HS, but there is little high-quality evidence in the literature available for review.[34,50] A combination of clindamycin and rifampin twice daily for 10 weeks is one antibiotic regimen that is commonly used and has been investigated in several studies.[51,52] One study looked retrospectively at 14 patients who had this antibiotic regimen and found that 8 of these patients achieved remission and another 2 patients achieved remission when minocycline was used instead of clindamycin.[51] Another retrospective review showed that after 10 weeks, the disease severity, as measured by the Sartorius score, was significantly improved with this antibiotic regimen.[52] A third study retrospectively evaluated 34 patients who received this combination of oral antibiotics and determined that within 10 weeks of treatment, most patients had experienced the maximum benefit from this combination of antibiotics.[53] In all three of these studies, there was a subset of patients who withdrew due to adverse effects associated with treatment, which were primarily related to gastrointestinal upset.[51-53]

Dapsone has also been investigated as a treatment for HS.[54,55] A small retrospective review of five patients showed some improvement in HS but a requirement for maintenance therapy to continue the response.[54] Another retrospective review of 24 patients showed that only 38% experienced any improvement in symptoms and that, again, maintenance therapy was required to sustain the response.[55] Further investigations into the use of antibiotics for the treatment of HS are certainly needed to create evidence-based regimens for this disease process.

Retinoids have been theorized as a potential medical treatment for HS due to their efficacy in treating other follicular disorders such as acne, but studies of isotretinoin have shown disappointing results with poor efficacy.[56,57] Hormonal treatments such as antiandrogens have showed some promise in the treatment of HS,[58-61] primarily in female patients, but larger, randomized clinical trials are needed to evaluate efficacy. Another study investigated finasteride in seven patients with HS, including five females and two males, and found that six of the seven patients treated with this medication saw improvement in their disease.[60] One study retrospectively identified 64 female patients with HS and noted that antiandrogen therapy was associated with a 55% disease response rate, whereas antibiotic therapy only achieved a 26% disease response rate.[61] The same study also noted that 38% of female participants in the study had markers of polycystic ovarian syndrome.[61]

Metformin has also been used in a series of 25 patients who had previously failed more traditional therapies, including courses of oral antibiotics; 18 of these patients saw a significant decrease in Sartorius scores as well as improvement in quality of life scores.[62] For patients with severe disease, systemic immunosuppressives may be used with good results. There are reports of patients experiencing improvement in HS lesions with cyclosporine,[63-65] but treatment with methotrexate appears to demonstrate little benefit.[66] TNF-α inhibitors, including infliximab and etanercept, have shown promise in patients with HS.[67] A number of studies have investigated the use of infliximab for HS. Some studies have shown questionable response rates,[68,69] but the only study with grade A evidence demonstrated that more patients receiving infliximab experienced a greater than 50% reduction in symptoms than did patients receiving the placebo.[70] Etanercept has also been investigated for HS with numerous positive reports.[71-73] The only study with grade A evidence demonstrated no significant difference between the placebo and treatment groups.[67] There have been a few small studies investigating the use of adalimumab in the treatment of HS, but the results have not been consistent.[74,75] There has been only one prospective, double-blind, controlled study, and this study showed statistically significant improvement in the patients receiving adalimumab when compared to the patients receiving placebo, but there was no statistically significant difference between the two groups at 12 weeks of therapy.[76] One small prospective evaluation of five patients treated with efalizumab showed no improvement in symptoms.[77] Overall, the biologics with the most favorable outcomes in the treatment with HS are infliximab and etanercept, but there is a definite need for further studies into the use of these

medications for the treatment of HS. Recently, the TNF-alpha inhibitor and adalimumab have been approved by the FDA for the treatment of Hurley Stage II and Hurley Stage III HS.

Surgical options include use of laser surgery or excisional surgery. A number of studies have investigated use of the carbon dioxide laser and shown improvement in HS.[29,78-81] Multiple studies show that following treatment with the carbon dioxide laser, HS lesions resolve with little, if any, incidence of lesion recurrence.[29,78] Treatment with the carbon dioxide laser ultimately is effective in treating existing lesions but does not prevent the formation of de novo lesions. The Nd:YAG laser is also effective in treating existing HS lesions. A study investigating treatment of HS lesions with an Nd:YAG laser demonstrated an improvement of 65% after 3 months of treatment.[82] Surgical excision is often considered in the case of severe disease or scarring. Incision and drainage is not recommended because the lesions tend to recur,[83] but deroofing an abscess, marsupialization of a sinus tract, or performing a very limited localized excision of lesions may be effective surgical interventions.[84] Excisional surgery may use a primary closure or a gentamicin-soaked sponge followed primary closure, or the wound may be allowed to heal by secondary intention.[85] Radical excision is the most effective excisional surgical option for preventing recurrence of disease.[83] Other miscellaneous treatment options include photodynamic therapy[86] and radiation.[87,88]

Rambhatla et al[50] put forth a suggested evidence-based treatment approach based on systematic review of the literature regarding treatment options for HS. For Hurley stage I disease, topical clindamycin 1% and treatment of lesions with Nd:YAG laser are recommended therapeutic options. For stage II disease, a 10-week course of combination clindamycin and rifampin or three to four monthly treatments with Nd:YAG laser are suggested. If the disease progresses despite these therapies, or if the patient is unable to tolerate these treatments, escalation to use of a biologic medication is suggested, with infliximab being the treatment of choice. For Hurley stage III disease, a trial of the same treatment modalities mentioned for stage II disease is recommended. In the case of failure or unsatisfactory response, it is recommended that the patient be referred to a surgeon for evaluation for wide local excision of the affected area.[50] Ultimately, the therapeutic ladder should be reviewed on a case-by-case basis by the physician with each patient and the risks and benefits associated with each treatment discussed thoroughly before deciding on a treatment plan.

REFERENCES

1. Sartorius K, Killasli H, Oprica C, Sullivan A, Lapins J. Bacteriology of hidradenitis suppurativa exacerbations and deep tissue cultures obtained during carbon dioxide laser treatment. *Br J Dermatol*. 2012;166:879-883.
2. von der Werth JM, Jemec GB. Morbidity in patients with hidradenitis suppurativa. *Br J Dermatol*. 2001;144:809-813.
3. Matusiak L, Bieniek A, Szepietowski JC. Hidradenitis suppurativa markedly decreases quality of life and professional activity. *J Am Acad Dermatol*. 2010;62:706-708.
4. Jemec GB, Heidenheim M, Nielsen NH. Hidradenitis suppurativa—characteristics and consequences. *Clin Exp Dermatol*. 1996;21:419-423.
5. Esmann S, Jemec GB. Psychosocial impact of hidradenitis suppurativa: a qualitative study. *Acta Derm Venereol*. 2011;91:328-332.
6. Onderdijk AJ, van der Zee HH, Esmann S, et al. Depression in patients with hidradenitis suppurativa. *J Eur Acad Dermatol Venereol*. 2013;27:473-478.
7. Verneuil A. Etudes sur les tumeurs de la peau et quelques maladies des glands sudoripores. *Arch Gen Med*. 1854;4:447.
8. Verneuil A. Hypertrophie dune gland sudipare axillaire survenu a la suite dun abcestuberiforme de laisselle. *Gaz Hebd Med*. 1857;4.
9. von der Werth JM, Williams HC. The natural history of hidradenitis suppurativa. *J Eur Acad Dermatol Venereol*. 2000;14:389-392.
10. Schiefferdecker P. *Die Hautdrüsen des Menschen und der Säugetiere, ihre biologische und rassenanatomische Bedeutung, sowie die Muscularis sexualis*. Stuttgart, Germany: Schweizerbart; 1922.
11. Jemec GB, Hansen U. Histology of hidradenitis suppurativa. *J Am Acad Dermatol*. 1996;34:994-999.
12. Vazquez BG, Alikhan A, Weaver AL, Wetter DA, Davis MD. Incidence of hidradenitis suppurativa and associated factors: a population-based study of Olmsted County, Minnesota. *J Invest Dermatol*. 2013;133:97-103.

13. Jemec GB, Heidenheim M, Nielsen NH. The prevalence of hidradenitis suppurativa and its potential precursor lesions. *J Am Acad Dermatol.* 1996;35(2 Pt 1):191-194.

14. Lookingbill DP. Yield from a complete skin examination. Findings in 1157 new dermatology patients. *J Am Acad Dermatol.* 1988;18(1 Pt 1):31-37.

15. Cosmatos I, Matcho A, Weinstein R, Montgomery MO, Stang P. Analysis of patient claims data to determine the prevalence of hidradenitis suppurativa in the United States. *J Am Acad Dermatol.* 2013;68:412-419.

16. Amy McMichael ARC, Daniela Guzman-Sanchez, Paul Kelly A. Folliculitis and other follicular disorders. In: Bolognia J, ed. *Dermatology.* Vol 1, New York, NY: Elsevier Saunders; 2012.

17. Jemec GB. Clinical practice. Hidradenitis suppurativa. *N Engl J Med.* 2012;366:158-164.

18. Wang B, Yang W, Wen W, et al. Gamma-secretase gene mutations in familial acne inversa. *Science.* 2010;330:1065.

19. Yu CC, Cook MG. Hidradenitis suppurativa: a disease of follicular epithelium, rather than apocrine glands. *Br J Dermatol.* 1990;122:763-769.

20. Attanoos RL, Appleton MA, Douglas-Jones AG. The pathogenesis of hidradenitis suppurativa: a closer look at apocrine and apoeccrine glands. *Br J Dermatol.* 1995;133:254-258.

21. Xu LY, Wright DR, Mahmoud BH, Ozog DM, Mehregan DA, Hamzavi IH. Histopathologic study of hidradenitis suppurativa following long-pulsed 1064-nm Nd:YAG laser treatment. *Arch Dermatol.* 2011;147:21-28.

22. Jemec GB, Faber M, Gutschik E, Wendelboe P. The bacteriology of hidradenitis suppurativa. *Dermatology.* 1996;193:203-206.

23. Kurzen H, Kurokawa I, Jemec GB, et al. What causes hidradenitis suppurativa? *Exp Dermatol.* 2008;17:455-456.

24. Schlapbach C, Hanni T, Yawalkar N, Hunger RE. Expression of the IL-23/Th17 pathway in lesions of hidradenitis suppurativa. *J Am Acad Dermatol.* 2011;65:790-798.

25. Mozeika E, Pilmane M, Nurnberg BM, Jemec GB. Tumour necrosis factor-alpha and matrix metalloproteinase-2 are expressed strongly in hidradenitis suppurativa. *Acta Derm Venereol.* 2013;93:301-304.

26. Barth JH, Kealey T. Androgen metabolism by isolated human axillary apocrine glands in hidradenitis suppurativa. *Br J Dermatol.* 1991;125:304-308.

27. Habif TP. *Clinical Dermatology: A Color Guide to Diagnosis and Therapy.* St. Louis, MO: Mosby; 1985.

28. Fitzsimmons JS, Guilbert PR, Fitzsimmons EM. Evidence of genetic factors in hidradenitis suppurativa. *Br J Dermatol.* 1985;113:1-8.

29. Hazen PG, Hazen BP. Hidradenitis suppurativa: successful treatment using carbon dioxide laser excision and marsupialization. *Dermatol Surg.* 2010;36:208-213.

30. Jemec GB. The symptomatology of hidradenitis suppurativa in women. *Br J Dermatol.* 1988;119:345-350.

31. Sartorius K, Lapins J, Emtestam L, Jemec GB. Suggestions for uniform outcome variables when reporting treatment effects in hidradenitis suppurativa. *Br J Dermatol.* 2003;149:211-213.

32. Hurley H. *Axillary hyperhidrosis, Apocine Bromhidrosis, Hidradenitis Suppurativa, and Familial Benign Pemphigus: Surgical Approach.* New York, NY: Marcel Dekker; 1989.

33. Canoui-Poitrine F, Revuz JE, Wolkenstein P, et al. Clinical characteristics of a series of 302 French patients with hidradenitis suppurativa, with an analysis of factors associated with disease severity. *J Am Acad Dermatol.* 2009;61:51-57.

34. Alikhan A, Lynch PJ, Eisen DB. Hidradenitis suppurativa: a comprehensive review. *J Am Acad Dermatol.* 2009;60:539-561.

35. Chicarilli ZN. Follicular occlusion triad: hidradenitis suppurativa, acne conglobata, and dissecting cellulitis of the scalp. *Ann Plast Surg.* 1987;18:230-237.

36. Scheinfeld NS. A case of dissecting cellulitis and a review of the literature. *Dermatol Online J.* 2003;9:8.

37. Canoui-Poitrine F, Luc G, Juhan-Vague I, et al. Respective contribution of conventional risk factors and antihypertensive treatment to stable angina pectoris and acute coronary syndrome as the first presentation of coronary heart disease: the PRIME Study. *Eur J Cardiovasc Prev Rehabil.* 2009;16:550-555.

38. Sartorius K, Emtestam L, Jemec GB, Lapins J. Objective scoring of hidradenitis suppurativa reflecting the role of tobacco smoking and obesity. *Br J Dermatol.* 2009;161:831-839.

39. Konig A, Lehmann C, Rompel R, Happle R. Cigarette smoking as a triggering factor of hidradenitis suppurativa. *Dermatology.* 1999;198:261-264.

40. Kurek A, Peters EM, Chanwangpong A, Sabat R, Sterry W, Schneider-Burrus S. Profound disturbances of sexual health in patients with acne inversa. *J Am Acad Dermatol.* 2012;67:422-428.

41. Wolkenstein P, Loundou A, Barrau K, Auquier P, Revuz J. Quality of life impairment in hidradenitis suppurativa: a study of 61 cases. *J Am Acad Dermatol.* 2007;56:621-623.

42. Lapins J, Ye W, Nyren O, Emtestam L. Incidence of cancer among patients with hidradenitis suppurativa. *Arch Dermatol.* 2001;137:730-734.

43. Talmant JC, Bruant-Rodier C, Nunziata AC, Rodier JF, Wilk A. [Squamous cell carcinoma arising in Verneuil's disease: two cases and literature review]. *Ann Chir Plast Esthet.* 2006;51:82-86.

44. Malaguarnera M, Pontillo T, Pistone G, Succi L. Squamous-cell cancer in Verneuil's disease (hidradenitis suppurativa). *Lancet.* 1996;348:1449.

45. Maclean GM, Coleman DJ. Three fatal cases of squamous cell carcinoma arising in chronic perineal hidradenitis suppurativa. *Ann R Coll Surg Engl.* 2007;89:709-712.

46. Kurokawa I, Nishimura K, Yamanaka K, Mizutani H, Tsubura A, Revuz J. Cytokeratin expression in squamous cell carcinoma arising from hidradenitis suppurativa (acne inversa). *J Cutan Pathol.* 2007;34:675-678.

47. Altunay IK, Gokdemir G, Kurt A, Kayaoglu S. Hidradenitis suppurativa and squamous cell carcinoma. *Derm Surg.* 2002;28:88-90.

48. Kamp S, Fiehn AM, Stenderup K, et al. Hidradenitis suppurativa: a disease of the absent sebaceous gland? Sebaceous gland number and volume are significantly reduced in uninvolved hair follicles from patients with hidradenitis suppurativa. *Br J Dermatol.* 2011;164:1017-1022.

49. Jemec GB, Wendelboe P. Topical clindamycin versus systemic tetracycline in the treatment of hidradenitis suppurativa. *J Am Acad Dermatol.* 1998;39:971-974.

50. Rambhatla PV, Lim HW, Hamzavi I. A systematic review of treatments for hidradenitis suppurativa. *Arch Dermatol.* 2012;148:439-446.

51. Mendonca CO, Griffiths CE. Clindamycin and rifampicin combination therapy for hidradenitis suppurativa. *Br J Dermatol.* 2006;154:977-978.

52. Gener G, Canoui-Poitrine F, Revuz JE, et al. Combination therapy with clindamycin and rifampicin for hidradenitis suppurativa: a series of 116 consecutive patients. *Dermatology.* 2009;219:148-154.

53. van der Zee HH, Boer J, Prens EP, Jemec GB. The effect of combined treatment with oral clindamycin and oral rifampicin in patients with hidradenitis suppurativa. *Dermatology.* 2009;219:143-147.

54. Kaur MR, Lewis HM. Hidradenitis suppurativa treated with dapsone: a case series of five patients. *J Dermatolog Treat.* 2006;17:211-213.

55. Yazdanyar S, Boer J, Ingvarsson G, Szepietowski JC, Jemec GB. Dapsone therapy for hidradenitis suppurativa: a series of 24 patients. *Dermatology.* 2011;222:342-346.

56. Boer J, van Gemert MJ. Long-term results of isotretinoin in the treatment of 68 patients with hidradenitis suppurativa. *J Am Acad Dermatol.* 1999;40:73-76.

57. Soria A, Canoui-Poitrine F, Wolkenstein P, et al. Absence of efficacy of oral isotretinoin in hidradenitis suppurativa: a retrospective study based on patients' outcome assessment. *Dermatology.* 2009;218:134-135.

58. Mortimer PS, Dawber RP, Gales MA, Moore RA. A double-blind controlled cross-over trial of cyproterone acetate in females with hidradenitis suppurativa. *Br J Dermatol.* 1986;115:263-268.

59. Sawers RS, Randall VA, Ebling FJ. Control of hidradenitis suppurativa in women using combined antiandrogen (cyproterone acetate) and oestrogen therapy. *Br J Dermatol.* 1986;115:269-274.

60. Joseph MA, Jayaseelan E, Ganapathi B, Stephen J. Hidradenitis suppurativa treated with finasteride. *J Dermatolog Treat.* 2005;16:75-78.

61. Kraft JN, Searles GE. Hidradenitis suppurativa in 64 female patients: retrospective study comparing oral antibiotics and antiandrogen therapy. *J Cutan Med Surg.* 2007;11:125-131.

62. Verdolini R, Clayton N, Smith A, Alwash N, Mannello B. Metformin for the treatment of hidradenitis suppurativa: a little help along the way. *J Eur Acad Dermatol Venereol.* 2013;27:1101-1108.

63. Buckley DA, Rogers S. Cyclosporin-responsive hidradenitis suppurativa. *J R Soc Med.* 1995;88:289P-290P.

64. Rose RF, Goodfield MJ, Clark SM. Treatment of recalcitrant hidradenitis suppurativa with oral ciclosporin. *Clin Exp Dermatol.* 2006;31:154-155.

65. Bianchi L, Hansel K, Stingeni L. Recalcitrant severe hidradenitis suppurativa successfully treated with cyclosporine A. *J Am Acad Dermatol.* 2012;67:e278-e279.

66. Jemec GB. Methotrexate is of limited value in the treatment of hidradenitis suppurativa. *Clin Exp Dermatol.* 2002;27:528-529.

67. Blok JL, van Hattem S, Jonkman MF, Horvath B. Systemic therapy with immunosuppressive agents and retinoids in hidradenitis suppurativa: a systematic review. *Br J Dermatol.* 2013;168:243-252.

68. Usmani N, Clayton TH, Everett S, Goodfield MD. Variable response of hidradenitis suppurativa to infliximab in four patients. *Clin Exp Dermatol.* 2007;32:204-205.

69. Fardet L, Dupuy A, Kerob D, et al. Infliximab for severe hidradenitis suppurativa: transient clinical efficacy in 7 consecutive patients. *J Am Acad Dermatol.* 2007;56:624-628.

70. Grant A, Gonzalez T, Montgomery MO, Cardenas V, Kerdel FA. Infliximab therapy for patients with moderate to severe hidradenitis suppurativa: a randomized, double-blind, placebo-controlled crossover trial. *J Am Acad Dermatol.* 2010;62:205-217.

71. Adams DR, Yankura JA, Fogelberg AC, Anderson BE. Treatment of hidradenitis suppurativa with etanercept injection. *Arch Dermatol.* 2010;146: 501-504.

72. Giamarellos-Bourboulis EJ, Pelekanou E, Antonopoulou A, et al. An open-label phase II study of the safety and efficacy of etanercept for the therapy of hidradenitis suppurativa. *Br J Dermatol.* 2008;158:567-572.

73. Pelekanou A, Kanni T, Savva A, et al. Long-term efficacy of etanercept in hidradenitis suppurativa: results from an open-label phase II prospective trial. *Exp Dermatol.* 2010;19:538-540.

74. Amano M, Grant A, Kerdel FA. A prospective open-label clinical trial of adalimumab for the treatment of hidradenitis suppurativa. *Int J Dermatol.* 2010;49:950-955.

75. Blanco R, Martinez-Taboada VM, Villa I, et al. Long-term successful adalimumab therapy in severe hidradenitis suppurativa. *Arch Dermatol.* 2009;145:580-584.

76. Miller I, Lynggaard CD, Lophaven S, Zachariae C, Dufour DN, Jemec GB. A double-blind placebo-controlled randomized trial of adalimumab in the treatment of hidradenitis suppurativa. *Br J Dermatol.* 2011;165:391-398.

77. Strober BE, Kim C, Siu K. Efalizumab for the treatment of refractory hidradenitis suppurativa. *J Am Acad Dermatol.* 2007;57:1090-1091.

78. Lapins J, Marcusson JA, Emtestam L. Surgical treatment of chronic hidradenitis suppurativa: CO2 laser stripping-secondary intention technique. *Br J Dermatol.* 1994;131:551-556.

79. Lapins J, Sartorius K, Emtestam L. Scanner-assisted carbon dioxide laser surgery: a retrospective follow-up study of patients with hidradenitis suppurativa. *J Am Acad Dermatol.* 2002;47:280-285.

80. Finley EM, Ratz JL. Treatment of hidradenitis suppurativa with carbon dioxide laser excision and second-intention healing. *J Am Acad Dermatol.* 1996;34:465-469.

81. Madan V, Hindle E, Hussain W, August PJ. Outcomes of treatment of nine cases of recalcitrant severe hidradenitis suppurativa with carbon dioxide laser. *Br J Dermatol.* 2008;159:1309-1314.

82. Tierney E, Mahmoud BH, Hexsel C, Ozog D, Hamzavi I. Randomized control trial for the treatment of hidradenitis suppurativa with a neodymium-doped yttrium aluminium garnet laser. *Dermatol Surg.* 2009;35:1188-1198.

83. Ritz JP, Runkel N, Haier J, Buhr HJ. Extent of surgery and recurrence rate of hidradenitis suppurativa. *Int J Colorectal Dis.* 1998;13:164-168.

84. van der Zee HH, Prens EP, Boer J. Deroofing: a tissue-saving surgical technique for the treatment of mild to moderate hidradenitis suppurativa lesions. *J Am Acad Dermatol.* 2010;63:475-480.

85. Buimer MG, Ankersmit MF, Wobbes T, Klinkenbijl JH. Surgical treatment of hidradenitis suppurativa with gentamicin sulfate: a prospective randomized study. *Dermatol Surg.* 2008;34:224-227.

86. Gold M, Bridges TM, Bradshaw VL, Boring M. ALA-PDT and blue light therapy for hidradenitis suppurativa. *J Drugs Dermatol.* 2004;3(1 Suppl):S32-S35.

87. Frohlich D, Baaske D, Glatzel M. [Radiotherapy of hidradenitis suppurativa--still valid today?] *Strahlenther Onkol.* 2000;176:286-289.

88. Trombetta M, Werts ED, Parda D. The role of radiotherapy in the treatment of hidradenitis suppurativa: case report and review of the literature. *Dermatol Online J.* 2010;16:16.

CHAPTER 44

Melanomas

Carl V. Washington
Vineet Mishra
Seaver L. Soon

KEY POINTS

- The impact of melanoma varies considerably depending upon race, class, and ethnicity.
- There is an inverse relationship between the incidence of melanoma and skin color.
- Melanoma in African Americans and Asians most commonly occurs on palms, soles, and nail beds.
- Acral tumors constitute 30% to 70% of melanomas in African Americans, Asians, and Hispanics, whereas only 1% to 9% of Caucasians have acral melanomas.
- Subungual melanoma exhibits a preponderance in dark-skinned individuals.

INTRODUCTION

Melanoma represents a significant disease burden in the United States, with an estimated 89,474 new diagnoses in 2012 and a predicted 9180 deaths.[1] This impact varies considerably along the lines of race, class, and ethnicity as expressed in the broader social context, and as such, the relationship between these variables and melanoma outcome in minority populations is of clinical and social importance. Because melanoma is predominantly a cancer of white populations, it is perhaps expected that the majority of clinical research and public awareness campaigns promulgate the melanoma experience in Caucasians. This body of knowledge includes such risk factors as red hair, inability to tan, and propensity to freckle and to sunburn, as well as such prototypic clinical presentations as the irregular, changing pigmented lesion on the trunks of men and lower legs of women. Although important for the public health, these data may not be specifically relevant to the melanoma experience in people with skin of color and, furthermore, may inadvertently suggest that melanoma is not a health threat to these populations. U.S. Census data regarding increasing racial heterogeneity underscore the need for research focusing on the clinical and epidemiologic features of melanoma in various populations. By 2050, Hispanic, African, and Asian Americans will compose 24%, 15%, and 8% of the U.S. population, respectively, whereas Caucasians will compose approximately 50%.[2] Considering the time period from 2000 to 2050, these figures represent a population percentage increase of 188% for Hispanics, 71% for African Americans, 213% for Asian Americans, and only 7% for Caucasians.[2] Internationally, 20% of the world's melanoma occurs in black and Asian populations.[3] In coming years, knowledge of the clinical expression of melanoma in people with skin of color will become increasingly relevant for dermatologists and others interested in the health status of minorities. This chapter covers the epidemiology, clinical features, treatment, and prognosis of acral melanoma in various populations. The findings of our review suggest that the expression of melanoma in minority

populations is distinct from that in Caucasians and is typified by lower incidence rates, a characteristic anatomic distribution, advanced stage at presentation, and poorer overall prognosis.

An inverse relationship exists between melanoma incidence and degree of skin pigmentation. Incidence is highest among Caucasians, intermediate among Hispanics, and lowest among Asians and African Americans.[4-9] According to U.S. National Cancer Institute Surveillance, Epidemiology, and End Results (SEER) data, the U.S. melanoma incidence from 2005 to 2009 was 31.6 per 100,000 in Caucasians, 4.7 per 100,000 in Hispanics, 4.3 per 100,000 in Native Americans, 1.6 per 100,000 in Asian Americans, and 1.1 per 100,000 in African Americans.[1] SEER data (2000 to 2009) further depict rapidly increasing incidence rates among the lightest pigmented racial group (whites: 22.8 per 100,000 in 2000 vs 27.4 per 100,000 in 2009), whereas incidence rates in more darkly pigmented racial groups are comparatively stable (Hispanics: 4.2 per 100,000 in 2000 vs 3.8 per 100,000 in 2009; Native Americans: 3.4 per 100,000 in 2000 vs 3.8 per 100,000 in 2009; Asians: 1.9 per 100,000 in 2000 vs 1.7 per 100,000 in 2009; and African Americans: 0.8 per 100,000 in 2000 vs 1.1 per 100,000 in 2009).[1] The lower incidence observed in Hispanics, Asians, and Blacks most likely results from the protective effect of darker skin pigmentation. U.S. age-adjusted mortality rate (2005 to 2009) was 4.6 per 100,000 in whites, 1.0 per 100,000 in Hispanics, 1.7 per 100,000 in Native Americans, and 0.5 per 100,000 in blacks and Asians.[1] Thus, melanoma incidence and mortality vary significantly across racial or ethnic populations.

The preferred anatomic site and histologic subtype of melanoma similarly differs along the lines of race. Among elderly Caucasians, melanoma occurs predominately on the frequently sun-exposed head and neck with a high proportion of lentigo maligna subtype, whereas in young Caucasians, melanoma shows a predilection for the relatively sun-protected trunk in men and trunk and legs in women, with a greater representation of the superficial spreading melanoma subtype.[10] Melanoma distribution in Asians and blacks, by contrast, is weighted toward the sun-protected sites of the palms, soles, and nailbed.[11] An analysis of the California Cancer Registry (n = 18,855) reported that melanoma occurred on the lower extremity in only 9% of whites compared with 50% of blacks, 36% of Asians, and 20% of Hispanics.[7] It is of interest, however, that tumor distribution among Hispanics varies according to the degree of skin pigmentation: lightly pigmented Hispanics exhibit an anatomic distribution identical to whites, whereas darkly pigmented Hispanics exhibit a tumor distribution reminiscent of blacks.[8] Numerous studies report that the most common histologic subtype on the hands and feet is acral lentiginous melanoma.[7,12-20] Although often deemed interchangeable, the terms *acral lentiginous melanoma* and *acral melanoma* are not synonymous; acral lentiginous melanoma is a histologic designation, whereas acral melanoma is an anatomic designation. Acral melanoma thus encompasses both acral lentiginous melanoma and other histologic subtypes of melanoma (such as superficial spreading and nodular melanoma) that may arise in acral locations.

EPIDEMIOLOGY

ACRAL MELANOMA

Acral tumors constitute 30% to 70% of melanomas in black, Asian, and Hispanic populations and only 1% to 9% in Caucasians.[6,8,12,17,19,21-30] Large case series report that the mean age of presentation of acral melanoma is during the sixth decade of life, compared with the fifth decade for nonacral lesions.[27] The peak incidence of acral melanoma varies across different racial groups, with earlier incidence observed in more lightly pigmented groups. Reported peak incidence is in fourth to sixth decades for Hispanics[29,31,32]; in the sixth decade for Chinese,[33-35] Japanese,[26,36] and South Africans of mixed ancestry[37]; and in the seventh decade for Indians[38] and for American,[12,24,25,30,38-40] Carribean,[41] and South African[18] blacks. It is of interest that the absolute incidence of acral melanoma is almost identical between African and Caucasian Americans (1.7 per 100,000 and 2.0 per 100,000, respectively). The observed racial difference in acral melanoma prevalence results from the proportionally decreased occurrence of nonacral lesions in certain racial or ethnic populations.[42] The incidence of acral melanoma has further remained static over the past half-century, which contrasts sharply against the escalating rates of nonacral melanoma.[11,23,41,43]

This peculiar epidemiologic pattern of acral melanoma and its development on the infrequently sun-exposed sites of the palms and soles have historically suggested an etiologic role other than solar radiation.[5] Recent population-based studies in the United States, however, suggest a positive association between ultraviolet (UV) index and increasing incidence and mortality among black men (P <0.05), with a nonsignificant association observed among black women and Hispanics of both sexes.[6,11] Although preliminary, these results suggest that solar radiation may play a greater than expected role in the development of melanoma in darkly pigmented populations. Additional etiologic theories in acral melanoma include the effect of long-term chronic trauma on benign acral nevi (given the preponderance of acral melanoma on the pressure-bearing heel and ball of the foot)[44]; malignant transformation of unstable foci of acral melanocytes[45]; and the relative paucity of free radical–scavenging melanin on the palms and soles of people with skin of color.[3] None of these explanations appears satisfactory, however, and the pathogenetic sequence of acral melanoma should be considered unknown.

■ SUBUNGUAL MELANOMA

Like acral melanoma, subungual melanoma exhibits a preponderance in dark-skinned individuals. Subungual melanoma represents 15% to 20% of melanoma in African Americans,[46,47] 10% to 31% in Asians,[46,48-51] and 33% in Native Americans.[52] The peak incidence of subungual melanoma occurs in the fifth to seventh decades.[53] By contrast, results from the Sydney Melanoma Unit database (1950 to 1994) suggest that subungual melanoma accounts for 0.31% of melanoma in predominantly Caucasian populations (38 of 11,500 melanoma cases; all cases occurred in whites).[54]

CLINICAL FEATURES AND DIAGNOSIS

■ ACRAL MELANOMA

Acral melanoma in skin of color populations presents commonly as an asymmetric, enlarging, dark brown or black macule/patch with irregular, notched borders, variegated colors, and a diameter >6 mm[55] [**Figure 44-1**]. Although this description echoes the experience in Caucasians, reports in Hispanics highlight the appearance of flecked, gray-white areas in many tumors,[32] whereas reports in blacks underscore the presence of papillomatous, verrucous, or hyperkeratotic plaques[12] [**Figures 44-2 and 44-3**]. In case series reflecting the acral melanoma experience in Chinese,[33,35] Japanese,[26] Hispanics,[32] and American[12,20] and African blacks,[18,39] a significant proportion of tumors present with an unusually large surface area (generally >3 cm in diameter) and with signs of advanced local disease, including pain, crusting, bleeding, and nonhealing ulceration.

In terms of site distribution, case series in skin of color populations report predominance of plantar over palmar melanoma (approximate ratio, 17:1) and of palmoplantar lesions over subungual lesions (approximate ratio, 4:1).[26,27,29,32,33,35,56] Among volar lesions, the most common sites on the sole appear to be the heel and the ball of the foot, whereas no site predilection is obvious on the palm.[18,26,32,39,56] Melanoma of mucocutaneous surfaces is also proportionally more common in pigmented

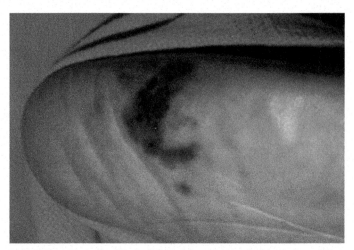

FIGURE 44-1. Acral melanoma. Ill-defined, asymmetric patch with irregular pigmentation on the heel of the foot.

than white populations (in which prevalence is <10%). In one series involving African Americans (n = 80), 44% of female subjects developed mucosal melanoma—including lip, palate, nasal, ocular, vulvar, vaginal, cervical, and anorectal surfaces—compared with only 10% of male subjects.[25] Oral, nasal, and ocular melanoma exhibited a favorable prognosis relative to cutaneous melanoma, whereas vulvovaginal and anorectal melanoma showed the worst prognosis. In addition to acral melanoma, women of African, and perhaps of other non-European, ancestry may be at increased risk of developing mucosal melanoma.[25]

One challenge in the dermatology of skin of color is the differentiation between benign pigmentation or melanocytic neoplasms and their malignant counterparts. Hyperpigmented macules of the palmoplantar

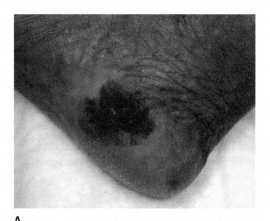

A

B

FIGURE 44-2. **(A)** Advanced acral melanoma. Irregular patch with central verrucous nodule on the heel of a foot. **(B)** Advanced acral melanoma. Long-standing patch with central nodule indicating vertical growth phase.

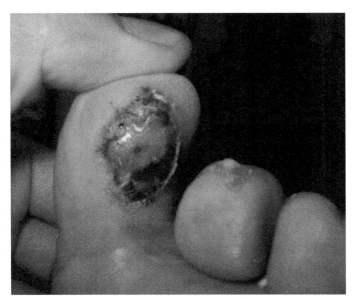

FIGURE 44-3. Advanced acral melanoma. Advanced tumor demonstrating ulceration, crusting, and bleeding.

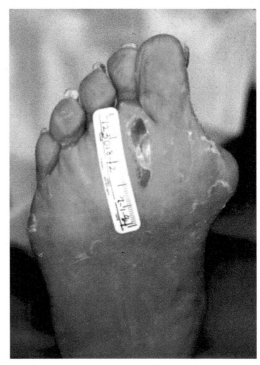

FIGURE 44-4. Acral lentiginous melanoma presenting as a callous. Note pigmentation of the skin along the lateral edge of the hyperkeratotic plaque.

creases, for example, occur in 60% of African American adults and may measure from 2 mm to several centimeters in diameter.[55] Acral nevi are also more common in darker-pigmented races. One series (n = 251) examining African Americans reported an average of eight nevi per patient, with only 2% of the population showing no nevi whatsoever. In this series, darkly pigmented blacks possessed fewer nevi and exhibited clustering of their nevi and increased mottled pigmentation on the palmoplantar surface.[56] By contrast, lightly pigmented blacks possessed more numerous nevi, with a greater proportion scattered over the body and relatively fewer on the palms and soles.[57] A Japanese series (n = 23,165) reported a 3% prevalence of plantar nevi, with a scattered distribution on the sole.[19]

Hyperpigmented macules of the palmoplantar creases, nevi, and mottled hyperpigmentation should not exhibit the classic morphologic features of acral melanoma. A diameter ≥7 mm has been proposed as a screening threshold for plantar melanoma in Asians, although smaller, biopsy-proven acral melanomas have been reported.[22,58] Additional considerations in the differential diagnosis of acral melanoma include angioma, hematoma, pyogenic granuloma, ulcer, and digital ischemia. One series of acral melanoma (n = 18) reported that 39% assumed the morphology of benign hyperkeratotic dermatoses, including large verruca, calluses, and dermatophyte infections[59] [**Figure 44-4**]. This hyperkeratotic acral melanoma variant may be associated with diagnostic delay and significantly poorer prognosis.[13,59,60] Lesions suspicious for melanoma require excisional biopsy or carefully planned incisional biopsy. Shave biopsies should be avoided because the thick stratum corneum of the palms and soles may result in failure to sample deeper, diagnostic pathology.

SUBUNGUAL MELANOMA

Subungual melanoma refers to melanoma of the nail bed and nail matrix. It presents clinically as a solitary brown or black longitudinal pigmented band of the nail (melanonychia striata) with irregular borders and variegated colors that increases in width to eventually involve the entirety of the nailbed[55] [**Figure 44-5**]. Hutchinson sign refers to pigment extension to the periungual skin and, when present, may increase the index of suspicion for melanoma [**Figure 44-6**]. Tumor progression to the vertical growth phase results in dystrophy, elevation, and eventually fracture of the nail plate, revealing a friable, ulcerated, and bleeding mass.[26,33,35,47,54] Among various populations, several studies indicate the predominance of hand over foot lesions, and of the thumbnail and great toenail over the nails of other digits.[26,27,33,50,54] As in acral

melanoma, the most common histologic pattern is acral lentiginous melanoma.[47,50,54,61]

Because misdiagnosis of early subungual melanoma is common, a Japanese study investigated the clinical features of early subungual melanoma (Clark level I and early Clark level II) to aid in early detection.[50] Melanonychia striata was the first sign of disease in all cases. Longitudinal pigment streaks, however, are present in approximately 11% of the general population in Japan[62] and in up to 100% of African Americans aged >50 years.[53] The following traits may help differentiate benign pigmented bands from those suspicious for subungual melanoma in skin of color populations: (1) onset after mid-adulthood, (2) diameter >6 mm, (3) variegated brown or homogenously black coloration, and (4) Hutchinson sign.[50] Rapid change may also be added to this list. It is of interest that, although Hutchinson sign is traditionally considered a marker of late disease, it was present in all five cases of in situ subungual melanoma in this series.[50]

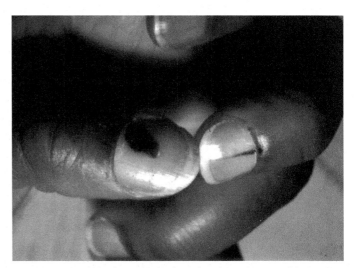

FIGURE 44-5. Early subungual melanoma. Early melanonychia striata of the third digit. Note coincidental subungual hematoma of the thumb.

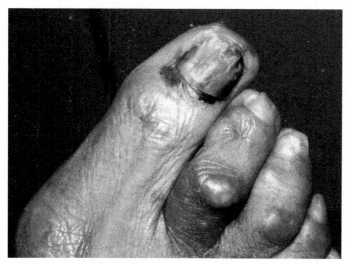

FIGURE 44-6. Subungual melanoma with Hutchinson sign. Subungual melanoma demonstrating pigment extension onto proximal and lateral nail folds, as well as the hyponychium.

Considerations in the differential diagnosis of melanonychia striata include lentigo and melanocytic nevus of the nail matrix or nail bed. Pigment bands of this origin, however, are rarely >4 mm in diameter; however, dysplastic or congenital nevi may attain or exceed this size. Systemic causes of nail pigmentation include Addison disease, Peutz-Jeghers syndrome, and ingestion of 5-fluorouracil, phenothiazines, silver, or arsenic.[50] Additional considerations include pyogenic granuloma, radiodermatitis, onychotillomania, squamous cell carcinoma, epithelioma cuniculatum, porocarcinoma, metastatic bronchogenic carcinoma, traumatic hematoma, and onychomycosis.[53] The most common misdiagnoses for subungual melanoma are hematoma and onychomycosis. Fortunately, a hematoma will migrate away from the proximal nail fold over a 4-week observation period, and in the case that this movement does not occur, a biopsy may be warranted.[63] In the same way, a 3- to 4-month course of antifungal therapy should yield a reassuring clear plane of nail at the proximal nail fold, and failure to respond to adequate antifungal treatment may warrant reconsideration of the diagnosis.[13]

TREATMENT

▇ ACRAL AND SUBUNGUAL MELANOMA

No randomized studies examining the outcome of acral melanoma in skin of color populations exist. Reported standard treatment for acral melanoma includes wide excision, with or without sentinel lymph node dissection (SLND) and adjuvant therapy. Excision on the plantar surface requires the construction of a durable and functional weight-bearing surface that simulates the normal anatomic structures that withstand pressure and shearing forces, while simultaneously allowing for satisfactory local disease control.[18] Where possible, preservation of a portion of the heel or ball of the foot to bear pressure while walking and of the fascia of the deep tendons as a base for skin grafting is recommended.[64] Most studies report excision with 3-cm margins down to the heel fat pad, small muscles, or plantar fascia of the sole, followed by defect closure using split-thickness skin graft.[17,39,63,65] Orthotic footwear should routinely be recommended to decrease sheer force and pressure on the graft site. Hyperkeratoses may develop at the interface between graft and normal skin but respond well to mechanical debridement.[17] In broad tumors, a 2-cm margin may be used to preserve functional, plantar weight-bearing surface, whereas primary amputation may be indicated in locally advanced disease with bony infiltration.[17] Sentinel lymph node biopsy may be offered to patients with tumor thickness >1 mm for staging purposes and to inform the decision to embark on adjuvant therapy.

Reported adjuvant treatments in U.S. blacks with acral melanoma include isolated limb perfusion with melphalan chemotherapy[66] and melanoma immunotherapy. Reported indications for regional limb perfusion include thicker primary acral melanoma (Breslow thickness >2 mm) and recurrent melanoma without visceral mestastasis.[12,17,39] One series involving black patients with stage I acral melanoma (n = 15) reported a survival benefit of excision and regional limb perfusion compared with excision alone (5-year survival: combined therapy, 72% vs excision, 23%; P <0.05); notably, the results of this approach in blacks compared favorably to the 5-year survival in Caucasians treated with the same regimen.[12] Another study (n = 185) in the United States on African Americans and Caucasian Americans reported a 5-year survival rate of 61% using adjuvant immunotherapy with irradiated melanoma cells, suggesting comparable efficacy to isolated limb perfusion.[27] The potential benefit of adjuvant interferon-α in metastatic melanoma is promising, but conflicting results in randomized studies suggest that its exact role remains to be elucidated.[67,68]

Similar to acral melanoma, treatment recommendations for subungual melanoma rely on the experience of large referral centers. The majority of these studies have been conducted in Caucasian populations, however, which raises the issue of whether they may be generalizable to people with skin of color. In the case of subungual melanoma, wide local excision is best achieved by amputation, with or without SLND and adjuvant therapy. For melanoma in situ, resection with 0.5- to 1.0-cm margins including the nail matrix and nail bed may be adequate; this approach may allow salvage of the digit.[50]

The precise level of amputation in subungual melanoma remains an area of contention, because it highlights the trade-off between preserving hand and foot function versus ensuring local disease control. One retrospective study (n = 38) compared functional versus ablative amputation for subungual melanoma in a Caucasian population.[54] This study defined functional amputation as one that retained finger contribution to hand function (eg, amputation distal to the neck of the proximal phalanx of the thumb or to the proximal interphalangeal [PIP] joint of the finger), whereas ablative amputation was defined as amputation proximal to these points and resulted in a digit unable to contribute to hand function. Recurrence analysis showed no difference between these options; therefore, these authors recommend amputation at the neck of the proximal phalanx of the thumb and at the level of the PIP joint of the finger to maximize hand function.[54] In advanced lesions extending to the proximal phalanx of the fingers or toes, ray amputation may be necessary.[39]

Whether choice of amputation level ultimately influences patient outcome is unclear. In fact, one series (n = 53) reported no difference in overall survival between subungual melanoma treated with or without amputation given that a high proportion of subungual melanomas present with metastatic disease.[27] It is reasonable to assume that the outcome of adjuvant therapies, including isolated limb perfusion, immunotherapy, interferon-α, and node dissection, should be comparable to that observed with acral melanoma; however, a precise estimate of outcome is unclear because most studies did not consider subungual melanoma in a subgroup analysis.[12,17,27,39,67,68]

Currently, the standard treatment for acral and subungual melanoma is surgical resection. As our understanding of the molecular genetics of melanoma improves, future therapeutics will likely become targeted for specific genetic subtypes. Although few studies have evaluated the molecular genetics of acral melanoma, *BRAF* mutations occur less frequently in acral compared to nonacral cutaneous melanoma. Recent data show that *BRAF* mutation frequencies range from approximately 10% to 20% in the acral subtype to >50% in melanomas located elsewhere on the skin.[69-71] BRAF protein is a member of the rapidly accelerated fibrosarcoma (RAF) family of serine/threonine kinases. It is an intermediary component of the mitogen-activated protein kinase (MAPK) pathway, which affects cell growth, survival, and differentiation. In contrast, *KIT* mutations are more frequently observed in acral and mucosal melanomas compared to other cutaneous subtypes.[72] KIT is a transmembrane receptor kinase. When bound to its ligand, activated KIT leads to downstream activation of the MAPK, PI3K-AKT1, and JAK signaling pathways involved in cell development, proliferation, survival, and migration.[73] Such findings imply that BRAF inhibitors may be less useful in acral melanomas, whereas KIT inhibitors may provide benefit.

Phase II trials of imatinib in patients with *KIT*-mutated melanomas have shown promising results. In one analysis (n = 43), Chinese patients harboring *KIT*-mutated melanomas were treated with imatinib and observed for up to 2 years with a median follow-up time of 1 year. While the median progression-free survival (PFS) was 3.5 months, the 6-month PFS rate was 36.6%. The cumulative rate of total disease control was 53.5%, with 23.3% and 30.2% of patients achieving partial response (PR) and stable disease (SD), respectively; 41.9% of patients demonstrated regression of tumor mass. While the 1-year overall survival (OS) rate was 51.0%, the median PFS and OS times for patients who had PR or SD versus disease progression were 9.0 months versus 1.5 months and 15.0 months versus 9.0 months, respectively.[74] Indeed, several case reports have described durable major responses with KIT inhibitors such as sorafenib, imatinib, sunitinib, nilotinib, and dasatinib in patients with melanoma harboring *KIT* mutations. The selection of an appropriate KIT inhibitor is dependent on the specific *KIT* mutation present. Certain *KIT* mutations, such as exon 11 and 13 kinase domain mutations, may demonstrate partial imatinib response, whereas exon 17 (D280Y) kinase domain mutation may predict imatinib resistance. In the latter case, sorafenib, a multikinase inhibitor, has been shown to provide 27% reduction in target tumors. Handolias et al[75] reported the palliative effects of KIT inhibitors in a case series wherein four patients received either sorafenib or imatinib depending on the *KIT* mutation present. All patients (n = 4) subsequently died from central nervous system (CNS) metastasis. It has been speculated that the progression of CNS disease is explained by the limited penetration of the KIT inhibitors into the brain.[75-79] Although deeper understanding of the molecular genetics of melanoma subtypes as well as the genetic differences between racial groups is needed, continued research will add to our fund of knowledge and allow for the development and implementation of more effective, targeted therapies.

PROGNOSIS

When compared with nonacral lesions, acral melanomas are associated with higher overall mortality, presumably because they occur in an area often overlooked by patients and physicians, leading to diagnostic delay and advanced stage at presentation.[13,27] Histologic subtype has no bearing on survival.[14] Acral melanoma in minority populations, however, carries an even graver prognosis when compared with Caucasian populations. Analysis of the California Cancer Registry noted that African Americans, Asians, and Hispanics were significantly more likely to have metastatic disease at diagnosis compared with whites. Among men, 15% of Hispanics, 13% of Asians, and 12% of blacks had metastatic disease at diagnosis, compared with only 6% of whites. Among women, 7% of Hispanics, 21% of Asians, and 19% of blacks had metastatic disease at diagnosis, relative to only 4% of whites. These differences are statistically and clinically significant.[7] Among U.S. blacks, SEER data (1986 to 1991) similarly report a three-fold increase in the proportion of blacks diagnosed with distant disease compared with whites (12% of blacks vs 4% of whites).[1]

Results of large case series involving acral melanoma speak to an analogous experience among blacks, Hispanics, and Asians internationally, characterized by advanced stage at presentation and poor overall survival. The aggregate experience among U.S. and African blacks is that acral melanoma typically presents as a thick lesion (mean Breslow thickness range, 2.75 to 7.10 mm), with a high proportion of histologic ulceration and of regional and distant metastases, and a dismal 20% to 30% 5-year survival.[12,17,18,20,30,39,40] By contrast, 5-year survival among contemporaneous whites ranges from 60% to 85%, a distinction that attained statistical significance in numerous studies.[20,24,27,30,40]

Among U.S. and South American Hispanics, acral melanoma similarly presents as a thick tumor (mean Breslow thickness, 5.5 mm),[32] with a high proportion of regional and distant metastases (approximate range, 20% to 40%), and a 23% to 66% 3-year survival rate.[29,32,56] It is of interest that one series in the U.S. Southeast (n = 54) reported a survival

advantage of Hispanics over non-Hispanic whites for both local and regional/distant metastatic disease; these authors suggested that the overall younger age of Hispanic patients may explain this finding.[31] The 5-year survival in acral melanoma among Chinese, Japanese, and East Indians is similar to blacks, ranging from 25% to 35%.[26,33-35,38,80] One Japanese study (n = 20), however, reported a 70% 5-year survival rate for acral melanoma.[36]

There is a paucity of data on the comparative survival of skin of color compared with Caucasian populations in subungual melanoma, and the majority of studies considering prognosis in darker-pigmented individuals consider that of subungual and acral melanoma in aggregate. Due largely to diagnostic delay, subungual melanoma in whites is associated with poor prognosis. Mean delay ranges from 9 to 23 months in approximately 50% of patients in reported series[53] and is complicated by the high proportion of amelanotic lesions (40% in the Sydney Melanoma Unit database).[54] In white populations, subungual melanoma is associated with a 55% overall 5-year survival rate (reported range, 16% to 76%).[54] Lesions present at an advanced stage (median thickness, 3.05 mm), with only 20% of subungual tumors presenting at stage I.[54] Nonetheless, one study (n = 3) of native Puerto Ricans reported a median Breslow thickness of 8.0 mm, with a mortality rate of 66% at 2 years.[32] All lesions in a Taiwanese study (n = 2) presented at Clark level III/IV and exhibited 100% mortality at 6 years.[35] A U.S. comparative study (n = 11) reported that U.S. blacks with subungual melanoma have a 3.5 times higher mortality rate than Caucasians, which remained significant even after controlling for stage and Clark level (suggesting that race may be an independent prognostic factor).[47]

The question of whether melanoma is a biologically more aggressive tumor in skin of color populations or whether race in fact serves as a proxy for social, cultural, and economic factors culminating in diagnostic delay and advanced tumor stage is unclear. Conflicting results have been noted in studies done in the US skin of color population, with some studies suggesting that race influences prognosis independent of tumor thickness and stage,[24,27] whereas others report that the prognostic importance of race becomes immaterial in face of regression analyses considering established prognostic indicators, such as Breslow thickness, ulceration, and stage.[20,30] One retrospective study in U.S. blacks (n = 79) examined melanoma outcome over three decades and reported a 35% 5-year survival rate in cohorts diagnosed before 1980, compared with a 49% 5-year survival rate in cohorts diagnosed between 1980 and 1989, reflecting increasing early patient presentation.[30] Earlier melanoma diagnosis and improved survival in more recent decades (1980s to 1990s) were similarly observed in population-based Japanese and Hispanic studies.[29,36] Another study involving 96 African Americans reported that aggressive surgical and adjuvant therapy in those patients with stage I disease amounted to a 78% 5-year survival, which is comparable to the outcome in Caucasian patients.[12] These studies provide encouraging evidence that the poor prognosis historically observed in persons of color may be a greater reflection of diagnostic delay and undertreatment rather than intrinsic tumor aggression and suggest that increased public and clinical awareness of melanoma in skin of color may continue the trend of improved prognosis.

CONCLUSION

As outlined in this chapter, the melanoma experience in people with skin of color is distinct from that in Caucasians and is characterized by decreased incidence, a characteristic anatomic distribution on the acral extremities, advanced stage at presentation, and overall poorer prognosis. Perhaps the most concerning of these features are the advanced presentation and poor survival in these populations from a tumor that is plainly visible and eminently curable in its early stages. Questioning why this occurs is fundamental to any effort to understand and to dismantle racial disparities in healthcare. In relation to dermatology, the concept of race encompasses both skin type and sociocultural beliefs and practices. Although evidence that race may be an independent prognosticator in acral and subungual melanoma exists,[24,27,47] other studies[20,30] as well as improving survival rates reported in more recent cohorts[29,36] suggest that the poor prognosis historically observed in people with skin of color may be a greater reflection of diagnostic delay rather than intrinsic tumor aggression. In fact, the American Anthropological Association argues in its Statement on Race that modern humans are a relatively homogenous species and that genetic data suggest as much variability between two people of the same racial group as between two people from any two different racial groups.[81] Thus, few biological differences should exist between large populations that are of explanatory relevance.[82,83]

Understanding race as a purely biological variable, divorced from its social and historical context, may oversimplify a public health issue that requires a broad perspective. Access to healthcare is one consideration. One study (n = 28,237) examining the effects of health insurance on early cancer detection reported a significant positive association between lack of health insurance and Medicaid insurance with late-stage melanoma diagnosis.[84] Socioeconomic variables alone, however, do not account for all racial health disparities; indeed, health inequalities exist even when universal access to healthcare is ensured.[72,83]

Public awareness campaigns that convey the unique features of melanoma in skin of color populations are necessary. Recent studies suggest a deficiency in the knowledge of African Americans and Hispanics regarding melanoma. According to a nationwide survey conducted by the American Academy of Dermatology, 75% of African Americans did not know the meaning of the word melanoma, compared with only 35% of whites ($P <0.05$).[85] A recent study in U.S. Hispanics demonstrated less awareness of melanoma, less awareness of skin cancer risk factors, and a decreased risk perception compared with non-Hispanic whites.[86] Shared beliefs, attitudes, and behaviors may manifest in particular health practices and illness profiles characteristic of a racial or cultural group. One study noted that both cultural and socioeconomic factors were able to account for the discrepancy in breast cancer mortality between African American and Caucasian women in the U.S., where neither was sufficient alone.[83] Perspective on such broad determinants of melanoma outcome in people with skin of color and attention to their unique clinical expression are necessary to improve the prognosis for these patients.

REFERENCES

1. Howlander N, Nonne AM, Krapcho M, et al. SEER Cancer Statistics Review, 1975-2009. Bethesda, MD: National Cancer Institute; 2012.
2. Anonymous. US interim projections by age, sex, race, and Hispanic origin. *US Census Bureau*. 2004. http://www.census.gov/population/projections/data/national/usinterimproj.html. Accessed February 6, 2015.
3. Armstrong B, Kricker A. How much melanoma is caused by sun exposure. *Melanoma Res*. 1993;3:395-401.
4. Crombie I. Racial differences in melanoma incidence. *Br J Cancer*. 1979;40:185-193.
5. Elder D. Melanoma and other specific nonmelanoma skin cancers. *Cancer*. 1995;75:245-256.
6. Hu S, Ma F, Collado-Mesa F, Kirsner R. UV radiation, latitude, and melanoma in Hispanics and blacks. *Arch Dermatol*. 2004;140:819-824.
7. Cress R, Holly E. Incidence of cutaneous melanoma among non-Hispanic whites, Hispanics, Asians and Blacks: an analysis of the California Cancer Registry data, 1988-93. *Cancer Causes Control*. 1997;8:246-252.
8. Bergfelt L, Newell G, Sider J. Incidence and anatomic distribution of cutaneous melanoma among United States Hispanics. *J Surg Oncol*. 1989;40:222-226.
9. Saxe N, Hoffman M, Krige J, Sayed R, King H, Hounsell K. Malignant melanoma in Cape Town, South Africa. *Br J Dermatol*. 1998;138:998-1002.
10. Weinstock M. Death from skin cancer among the elderly. *Arch Dermatol*. 1997;133:1207-1209.
11. Pennelo G, Devesa S, Gail M. Association of surface ultraviolet B radiation levels with melanoma and nonmelanoma skin cancer in United States Blacks. *Cancer Epidemiol Biomarkers Prev*. 2000;9:291-297.
12. Krementz E, Sutherland C, Carter R, Ryan R. Malignant melanoma in the American Black. *Ann Surg*. 1976;1976:533-542.
13. Bennett D, Wasson D, MacArthur J, McMillen M. The effect of misdiagnosis and delay in diagnosis on clinical outcome in melanoma of the foot. *J Coll Surg*. 1994;179:279-284.
14. Ridgeway C, Hieken T, Ronan S, Kim D, Das Gupta T. Acral lentiginous melanoma. *Arch Surg*. 1995;130:88-92.
15. Metzger S, Ellwanger U, Stroebel W, Schiebel U, Rassner G, Fierlbeck G. Extent and consequences of physician delay in the diagnosis of acral melanoma. *Melanoma Res*. 1998;8:181-186.
16. Kuchelmeister C, Schaumburg-Lever G, Garbe C. Acral cutaneous melanoma in Caucasians: clinical features, histopathology and prognosis in 112 patients. *Br J Dermatol*. 2000;143:275-280.
17. Hudson D, Krige J, Subbings H. Plantar melanoma: results of treatment in three populations. *Surgery*. 1998;124:877-882.
18. Hudson D, Krige J. Plantar melanoma in black South Africans. *Br J Surg*. 1993;80:992-994.
19. Kukita A, Ishihara K. Clinical features and distribution of malignant melanoma and pigmented nevi on the soles of the feet in Japan. *J Invest Dermatol*. 1989;92:210s-213s.
20. Bellows C, Belafsky P, Fortgang I, Beech D. Melanoma in African-Americans: trends in biological behavior and clinical characteristics over two decades. *J Surg Oncol*. 2001;78:10-16.
21. Reed R. *Acral Lentiginous Melanoma*. New York, NY: John Wiley & Sons, Inc.; 1976.
22. Wong T, Ohara K, Kawashima M, Sober A, Nogita T, Mihm M. Acral lentiginous melanoma (including in situ melanoma) arising in association with naevocellular nevi. *Melanoma Res*. 1996;6:241-246.
23. Dwyer P, Mackie R, Watt D, Aitchison T. Plantar malignant melanoma in a white Caucasian population. *Br J Dermatol*. 1993;128:115-120.
24. Reintgen D, McCarty K, Cox E, Seigler H. Malignant melanoma in black American and white American populations. *JAMA*. 1982;248:1856-1859.
25. Muchmore J, Mizuguchi R, Lee C. Malignant melanoma in American black females: an unusual distribution of primary sites. *J Am Coll Surg*. 1996;183:457-465.
26. Seiji M, Takematsu H, Hosokawa M, et al. Acral melanoma in Japan. *J Invest Dermatol*. 1983;80:56s-60s.
27. Slingluff C, Vollmer R, Seigler H. Acral melanoma: a review of 185 patients with identification of prognostic variables. *J Surg Oncol*. 1990;45:91-98.
28. Vayer A, Lefor A. Cutaneous melanoma in African Americans. *South Med J*. 1993;86:181-182.
29. Black W, Goldhahn R, Wiggins C. Melanoma within a southwestern Hispanic population. *Arch Dermatol*. 1987;123:1331-1334.
30. Crowley N, Dodge R, Vollmer R, Seigler H. Malignant melanoma in black Americans: a trend toward improved survival. *Arch Surg*. 1991;126:1359-1365.
31. Feun L, Raub W, Duncan R, et al. Melanoma in a southeastern Hispanic population. *Cancer Detect Prev*. 1994;18:145-152.
32. Vaszqez M, Ramos F, Sanchez J. Melanomas of volar and subungual skin in Puerto Ricans. *J Am Acad Dermatol*. 1984;10:39-45.
33. Collins R. Melanoma in the Chinese of Hong Kong: emphasis on volar and subungual sites. *Cancer*. 1984;54:1482-1488.
34. Chen Y-J, Wu C-Y, Chen J-T, Shen J-L, Chen C-C, Wang H-C. Clinicopathologic analysis of malignant melanoma in Taiwan. *J Am Acad Dermatol*. 1999;41:945-949.
35. Lin C-S, Wang W-J, Wong C-K. Acral melanoma: a clinicopathologic study of 28 patients. *Int J Dermatol*. 1990;29:107-112.
36. Kuno Y, Ishihara K, Yamazaki N, Mukai K. Clinical and pathological features of cutaneous malignant melanoma: a retrospective analysis of 124 Japanese patients. *Jpn J Clin Oncol*. 1996;26:144-151.
37. Swan M, Hudson D. Malignant melanoma in South Africans of mixed ancestry: a retrospective analysis. *Melanoma Res*. 2003;13:415-419.
38. Nair M, Varghese C, Mahadevan S, Cherian T, Joseph F. Cutaneous melanoma—clinical epidemiology and survival. *J Indian Med Assoc*. 1998;96:19-20, 28.
39. Krementz E, Reed R, Coleman W, Sutherland C, Carter R, Campbell M. Acral lentiginous melanoma: a clinicopathologic entity. *Ann Surg*. 1982;195:632-644.
40. Byrd K, Wilson D, Hoyler S, Peck G. Advanced presentation of melanoma in African Americans. *J Am Acad Dermatol*. 2004;50:21-24.
41. Garsaud P, Boisseau-Garsaud A, Ossondo M, et al. Epidemiology of cutaneous melanoma in French West Indies (Martinique). *Am J Epidemiol*. 1998;247:66-68.
42. Stevens N, Liff J, Weiss N. Plantar melanoma: is the incidence of melanoma of the sole of the foot really higher in blacks than whites? *Int J Cancer*. 1990;45:691-693.
43. Koh D, Wang H, Lee J, Chia K, Lee H, Goh C. Basal cell carcinoma, squamous cell carcinoma and melanoma of the skin: analysis of the Singapore Cancer Registry data 1968-97. *Br J Dermatol*. 2003;148:1161-1166.
44. Lewis M. Malignant melanoma in Uganda. *Br J Cancer*. 1967;21:483-495.

45. Lewis M, Johnson K. The incidence and distribution of pigmented naevi in Ugandan Africans. *Br J Dermatol.* 1968;80:362-366.

46. Baran R, Kechijian P. Longitudinal melanonychia (melanonychia striata): diagnosis and management. *J Am Acad Dermatol.* 1989;21:1165-1175.

47. O'Leary J, Berend K, Johnson J, Levin L, Seigler H. Subungual melanoma: a review of 93 cases with identification of prognostic variables. *Clin Orthop.* 2000;378:206-212.

48. Finley R, Driscoll D, Blumenson L, Karakousis C. Subungual melanoma: an eighteen year review. *Surgery.* 1994;116:96-100.

49. Kato T, Suetake T, Sugiyama T, Tabata N, Tagami H. Epidemiology and prognosis of subungual melanoma in 34 Japanese patients. *Br J Dermatol.* 1996;134:383-387.

50. Saida T, Oshima Y. Clinical and histopathological characteristics of the early lesions of subungual melanoma. *Cancer.* 1989;63:556-560.

51. Takematsu H, Obata M, Tomita Y, Kato T, Takahashi M, Abe R. Subungual melanoma. *Cancer.* 1985;55:2725-2731.

52. Black W, Wiggins C. Melanoma among southwestern Indians. *Cancer.* 1985;55:2899-2902.

53. Levit E, Kagen M, Scher R, Grossman M, Altman E. The ABC rule for clinical detection of subungual melanoma. *J Am Acad Dermatol.* 2000;42:269-274.

54. Quinn M, Thompson J, Crotty K, McCarthy W, Coates A. Subungual melanoma of the hand. *J Hand Surg.* 1996;1996:506-511.

55. Rahman Z, Taylor S. Malignant melanoma in African Americans. *Cutis.* 2001;67:403-404.

56. Panjota E, Llobet R, Roswit B. Melanoms of the lower extremity among native Puerto Ricans. *Cancer.* 1976;38:1420-1423.

57. Coleman W, Gately L, Krementz A, Reed R, Krementz E. Nevi, lentigines, melanomas in blacks. *Arch Dermatol.* 1980;116:548-551.

58. Saida T, Ishihara K, Tokuda Y. Effective detection of plantar malignant melanoma. *Int J Dermatol.* 1993;32:722-725.

59. Soon S, Solomon A, McAlpine B, Papadoupolous D, Washington C. Acral melanoma mimicking benign disease: the Emory experience. *J Am Acad Dermatol.* 2003;48:183-188.

60. Fortin P, Freiberg A, Rees R, Sondak V, Johnson T. Malignant melanoma of the foot and ankle. *J Bone Joint Surg Am.* 1995;77:1396-1403.

61. Blessing K, Kernohan N, Park K. Subungual malignant melanoma: clinicopathological features of 100 cases. *Histopathology.* 1991;19:425-429.

62. Kawamura T, Nishihara K, Kawasakiya S, Izumi T, Tanaka H. Pigmentatio longitudinalis striata unguium and the pigmentation of the nail in Addison's disease (abstract). *Jpn J Dermatol.* 1958;68:10.

63. Hughes L, Horgan K, Taylor B, Laidler P. Malignant melanoma of the hand and foot: diagnosis and management. *Br J Surg.* 1985;72:811-815.

64. Balch C. Excising melanoma: how wide is enough? And how to reconstruct. *J Surg Oncol.* 1990;44:135-136.

65. Shaw J, Koea J. Acral (volar-subungual) melanoma in Auckland, New Zealand. *Br J Surg.* 1988;75:69-72.

66. Krige J, King H, Strover R. Prophylactic hyperthermic limb perfusion in stage I melanoma. *Eur J Surg Oncol.* 1988;14:321-326.

67. Kirkwood J, Strawderman M, Ernstoff M, Smith T, Borden E, Blum R. Interferon alfa-2b adjuvant therapy of high-risk resected cutaneous melanoma: the Eastern Cooperative Oncology Group Trial EST 1684. *J Clin Oncol.* 1996;14:1-3.

68. Kirkwood J, Ibrahim J, Sondak V, et al. High- and low-dose interferon alfa-2b in high-risk melanoma: first analysis of intergroup trial E1690/S9111/C9190. *J Clin Oncol.* 2000;18:2444-2458.

69. Curtin JA, Fridlyand J, Kageshita T, et al. Distinct sets of genetic alterations in melanoma. *N Engl J Med.* 2005;353:2135-2147.

70. Maldonado JL, Fridlyand J, Patel H, et al. Determinants of BRAF mutations in primary melanomas. *J Natl Cancer Inst.* 2003;95:1878-1880.

71. Saldanha G, Potter L, DaForno P, et al. Cutaneous melanoma subtypes show different BRAF and NRAS mutation frequencies. *Clin Cancer Res.* 2006;12:4499-4505.

72. Torres-Cabala CA, Wang WL, Trent J, et al. Correlation between KIT expression and KIT mutation in melanoma: a study of 173 cases with emphasis on acral-lentiginous/mucosal type. *Mod Pathol.* 2009;22:1446-1456.

73. Grabbe J, Welker P, Dippel E, Czarnetzki BM. Stem cell factor, a novel cutaneous growth factor for mast cells and melanocytes. *Arch Dermatol Res.* 1994;287:78-84.

74. Guo J, Si L, Kong Y, et al. Phase II, open-label, single-arm trial of imatinib mesylate in patients with metastatic melanoma harboring c-Kit mutation or amplification. *J Clin Oncol.* 2011;29:2904-2909.

75. Handolias D, Hamilton AL, Salemi R, et al. Clinical responses observed with imatinib or sorafenib in melanoma patients expressing mutations in KIT. *Br J Cancer.* 2010;102:1219-1223.

76. Hodi FS, Friedlander P, Corless CL, et al. Major response to imatinib mesylate in KIT-mutated melanoma. *J Clin Oncol.* 2008;26:2046-2051.

77. Lutzky J, Bauer J, Bastian BC. Dose-dependent, complete response to imatinib and temozolomide in patients with metastatic melanoma with a K642E KIT mutation. *Pigment Cell Melanoma Res.* 2008;21:492-493.

78. Woodman SE, Trent JC, Stemke-Hale K, et al. Activity of dasatinib against L576P KIT mutant melanoma molecular, cellular, and clinical correlates. *Mol Cancer Ther.* 2009;8:2079-2085.

79. Minor DR, O'Day S, Kashani-Sabet M, et al. Sunitinib therapy for metastatic melanomas with KIT aberrations. *Proc Am Soc Clin Oncol.* 2010;28:8545.

80. Seiji M, Takahashi M. Acral melanoma in Japan. *Hum Pathol.* 1982;13:607-609.

81. Overby MM. AAA tells feds to eliminate "race." *Anthropol Newslett.* 1997;38:1-5.

82. Dressler W. Health in the African-American community: accounting for health inequalities. *Med Anthropol Q.* 1993;7:325-345.

83. Lannin D, Mathews H, Mitchell J, Swanson M, Swanson F, Edwards M. Influence of socioeconomic and cultural factors on racial differences in late-stage presentation of breast cancer. *JAMA.* 1998;279:1801-1807.

84. Roetzheim R, Pal N, Tennant C, et al. Effects of health insurance and race on early detection of cancer. *J Natl Cancer Inst.* 1999;91:1409-1415.

85. Anonymous. Survey of knowledge of and awareness about melanoma—United States, 1995. *MMWR.* 1996;45:346-349.

86. Pipitone M, Robinson J, Camara C, Chittineni B, Fisher S. Skin cancer awareness in suburban employees: a Hispanic perspective. *J Am Acad Dermatol.* 2002;47:118-123.

CHAPTER 45

Squamous Cell Carcinoma

Sheila M. Krishna
Algin B. Garrett

KEY POINTS

- Primary carcinoma of the skin is the most common form of cancer diagnosed in the United States, but the incidence in people with skin of color is reported as rare.

- Most squamous cell carcinomas (SCCs) in people with skin of color occur in non–sun-exposed areas; however, when SCC does occur in a sun-exposed area, the anatomic distribution is similar to that in Caucasians.

- SCC that occurs in sun-exposed skin has its origin in loss of the organized control of epidermal keratinocyte differentiation secondary to DNA damage as a direct result of ultraviolet light.

- The factors that are responsible for developing skin cancers in non–sun-exposed areas are unknown.

- Areas of chronic inflammation, chronic ulceration, and scarring are predisposed to the development of SCC.

INTRODUCTION

Most of the information regarding nonmelanoma skin cancer in skin of color reported in the U.S. literature focuses on disease incidence primarily in the African American population. The information is reported in the context of case reports or incidence studies from small groups. Information regarding the incidence of nonmelanoma skin cancer in other racial or ethnic groups, including Native Americans, Asians, and Hispanics, is sparse. The groups of people that constitute people with darker skin of color have grown considerably. Considering the changing demographics of the United States, to keep meaningful and accurate data, prospective research should recognize the population changes that are occurring. Larger population studies should be performed involving people with skin of color, which represents multiple ethnic and racial groups. U.S. Census information predicts that by the year 2050, the Caucasian population will be less than 50% of the total population.

This figure will continue to decline during the ensuing decades of continued immigration and assimilation in the United States.

MELANIN AND PHOTOPROTECTION

The reduced incidence of skin cancer in people with skin of color has been attributed to various factors. Montagna and Carlisle[1] have studied racial differences in melanin activity, fibroblast activity, and hair distribution on skin that may help to account for the reduced frequency of skin cancer in people with skin of color. Melanin, which is synthesized in melanosomes, is a known photoprotector in both animals and humans. It essentially creates a shield from the sun by absorbing and deflecting ultraviolet (UV) light.[2] The basal cell layer melanocyte is responsible for the production of melanin. There is no racial difference in the number of melanocytes.[3] The number of melanocytes may vary from one individual to the other and in different anatomic regions.[4] The variations in color that can be seen in individuals are attributed to the size and aggregation of melanosomes in the melanocyte and keratinocyte. The increased number and dispersion of stage IV melanosomes provide a measure of photoprotection.[2] Racial differences, as well as sun exposure, can affect the melanosome grouping. In African Americans with dark skin, melanosomes are large and nonaggregated, whereas in light-skinned African Americans, melanosomes are both large and nonaggregated and smaller and aggregated. Sun exposure also has been shown to change the pattern of melanosome distribution in Asian and Caucasian skin.[4,5] In addition to the role of melanin in photoprotection, the compactness or density of the keratinocyte layers also provides a measure of photoprotection.[6] The African American population is composed of a heterogeneous group with various shades of skin color; all the factors listed combine to provide an average sun protection factor of approximately 13.4.[2]

The relative safety from some of the effects of the sun is demonstrated by the comparatively low incidence of skin cancer in African Americans. However, there are changes that occur in melanin-laden skin that suggest that skin of color is not immune to photodamage. Kotrajaras and Kligman[7] demonstrated epidermal atypia and atrophy and both dermal collagen and elastin damage. The presence of these changes, which may be consistent with either damage from long-wavelength UV light or infrared radiation, suggests that melanin may be an efficient filter for shorter-wavelength UV light.

INCIDENCE

Primary carcinoma of the skin is the most common form of cancer diagnosed in the United States. Even though skin cancer is considered the most common form of cancer, the incidence in people with skin of color is reported as rare. McCall and Chen[8] reported a surprisingly high incidence of squamous cell carcinoma (SCC) in older African American females and suggest that the incidence may be higher than previously reported. The incidence of SCC involving the skin in Caucasian patients has been reported to be approximately 100 per 100,000 in women and 150 per 100,000 in men.[9] The incidence in African Americans is reported to be approximately 3.4 per 100,000.[10] There are very few incidence reports of skin cancer among other groups. Koh et al[11] report on the trends and differences of skin cancers in Chinese, Malays, and Indians living in Singapore. The incidence rate for SCC was 3.2 per 100,000 in men and 1.8 per 100,000 in women. The incidence rate for basal cell carcinoma (BCC) was 6.4 per 100,000 in men and 5.8 per 100,000 in women. Ichihashi et al[12] reported on age-adjusted incidence rates of BCC and solar keratosis in 4736 people in Kasai City. Two BCCs, 36 solar keratoses, and no SCCs were diagnosed in the group. It appears at least in the Asian population that BCCs are more common than SCCs.

SCC is the most commonly diagnosed skin cancer in African Americans.[13,14] Bang et al[15] reported that 34.1% of 126 African American patients were diagnosed with SCC, whereas 30.2% of the group was diagnosed with BCC. Fleming et al[16] reported on a small series of 58 African Americans with skin cancer. Thirty-eight cases of SCC and seven cases of BCC were diagnosed. Unlike BCCs, which occur commonly on sun-exposed skin, most SCCs in people with skin of color develop in non–sun-exposed areas. In a series reported by Howard University in 1988, 65% of the patients diagnosed with SCC had leg involvement, and 15% were diagnosed with anal SCC.[14] SCC involvement of the penis and scrotum also has been reported to occur in African Americans.[17-19]

PATHOGENESIS

The pathogenesis of SCC that occurs in sun-exposed skin has its origin in loss of the organized control of epidermal keratinocyte differentiation secondary to DNA damage as a direct result of UV light. The factors that are responsible for developing skin cancers in non–sun-exposed areas are unknown. Areas of chronic inflammation, chronic ulceration, and scarring are predisposed to the development of SCC. In these settings, normal cell differentiation and apoptosis of abnormal cells are altered, eventually producing the clonal expansion of a malignant cell line. The altered role of the *p53* gene in its response to cytotoxic stress may imperil the normal keratinocyte and predispose high-risk lesions to develop SCC.[20,21]

RISK FACTORS

The development of SCC has been linked to natural UV light exposure. UVB radiation is known to cause skin cancer. Phototherapy used to treat chronic skin diseases such as psoriasis has been shown to increase the risk of nonmelanoma skin cancer.[22] As mentioned previously, most SCCs in people with skin of color occur in non–sun-exposed areas; however, when SCC does occur in a sun-exposed area, the anatomic distribution is similar to that in Caucasians [**Figure 45-1**]. SCC develops in the following clinical settings in African Americans: chronic inflammation or scarring, burns, chronic infections, leg ulcers, albinism [**Figure 45-2**], lesions of chronic discoid lupus erythematosus [**Figure 45-3**], chronic radiation exposure [**Figure 45-4**], and vitiligo[14,23] [**Table 45-1**]. Other predisposing factors include cutaneous horns and scrotal ulcers. Chronic scars represent a significant risk for SCC and result in a higher rate of mortality.[24] Hubbell et al[25] reported on 175 cases of SCC involving the penis in darker skin of color patients. These authors reported a 15.4% overall mortality.

Actinic keratoses (AKs) are diagnosed more commonly in fair-skinned people and represent the most common precursor lesion for SCC on sun-exposed skin. AKs are rarely seen in African Americans and are diagnosed not infrequently in fair-skinned Asians.[11] In individuals who develop AKs, there is up to a 10% risk of developing SCC.[20]

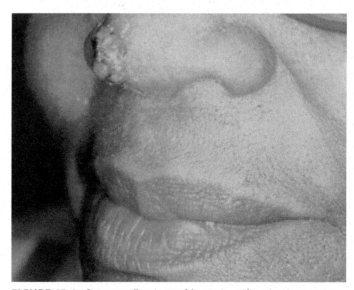

FIGURE 45-1. Squamous cell carcinoma of the nose in an African American woman.

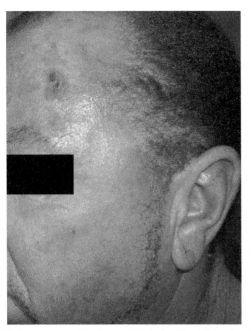

FIGURE 45-2. Squamous cell carcinoma of the forehead in an African American albino.

SCC in African Americans is generally considered to be a more aggressive disease with a poorer prognosis. Mora et al[24] reported an 18.4% mortality in 163 African Americans diagnosed with SCC of the skin. In their series, the face and leg were the most common sites of involvement. Fleming et al[16] reported a mortality rate of 29% in their series of African Americans with SCC. Weinstock[26] reported SCC as the skin cancer that is the major cause of death in African Americans. Not all reported series regarding SCC in AKs demonstrate comparatively decreased survival rates. Singh et al[27] reported on a series of 215 patients in a case-control study in which the presentation, course, and outcome of head and neck skin cancer in African Americans were studied. They showed that head and neck skin cancer is similar with regard

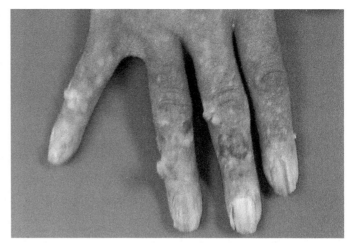

FIGURE 45-4. Squamous cell carcinoma secondary to chronic radiation exposure.

to presentation and distribution in white, Latin American, and African American patients. The study also showed that the cancers may be less aggressive in African Americans with appropriate treatment.

Several factors may contribute to the overall poor mortality and morbidity related to SCC in people with skin of color. The diagnosis is usually made at an advanced stage, possibly because of decreased accessibility to the healthcare system. In some instances, for unknown reasons, SCC has a more aggressive course in African Americans than in Caucasian patients with comparable disease. Often when the diagnosis of SCC is made, other associated diseases coexist and may make management of the advanced skin cancer more difficult.

ACTINIC KERATOSIS

As stated previously, an AK is a precursor lesion for SCC. The lesion usually occurs in a sun-exposed area and is usually rough in texture. The color may range from pale pink to erythematous, and occasionally, AKs may be pigmented. AKs are not found often in people with skin of color. They can be seen in Asians, Hispanics, and African Americans who have fair skin and are exposed to risk factors. A similar lesion can be seen in lesions of vitiligo or albinism and areas of depigmentation from a preexisting dermatitis, such as mycosis fungoides and discoid lupus erythematosus.

KERATOACANTHOMA

Keratoacanthoma is indistinguishable histologically from SCC. Generally it represents an epithelial tumor that grows rapidly over a period of approximately 6 weeks. The lesion may last for several weeks and then involute spontaneously. It usually appears as a solitary lesion and generally presents as a nodule with a crater-like center with a keratin plug. The lesion is rarely reported in people with skin of color.[28]

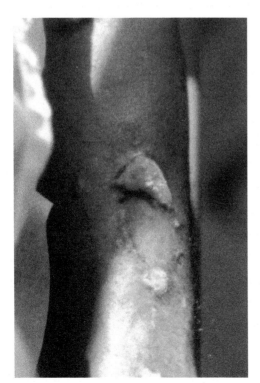

FIGURE 45-3. Squamous cell carcinoma developing in a chronic lupus erythematosus lesion.

TABLE 45-1	Risks factors for developing squamous cell carcinoma

- Chronic leg ulcers
- Chronic nonhealing wounds
- Discoid lupus erythematosus
- Lichen planus
- Ultraviolet light
- Vitiligo
- Ionizing radiation
- Oculocutaneous albinism
- Nevoid basal cell nevus syndrome
- Organ transplantation
- Acquired immunodeficiency syndrome
- Scrotal ulcers

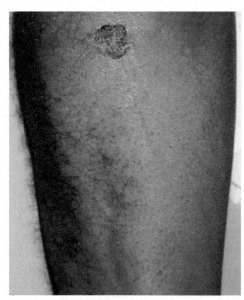

FIGURE 45-5. Bowen disease on the forearm of an African American man.

SQUAMOUS CELL CARCINOMA IN SITU

SCC in situ histologically represents involvement of the entire epidermal thickness with pleomorphic keratinocytes, which is seen in diseases such as Bowen disease and erythroplasia of Queyrat. Bowen disease is less commonly diagnosed in African Americans than other cutaneous malignancies.[14] Bowen disease presents as an erythematous solitary patch or plaque that may resemble eczema or psoriasis[29] [**Figures 45-5 and 45-6**]. Even though pigmented lesions are felt to be rare in Caucasian patients, the presence of pigment in lesions of Bowen disease in African American is common.

PROGNOSIS

Invasive SCC arising in areas of sun exposure [**Figure 45-7**] has a better prognosis than SCC that arises in non–sun-exposed areas. Aggressive behavior and local metastases occur more frequently in SCC arising in non–sun-exposed areas.[16,18] SCC of the nail bed has been reported to develop in African Americans and may be more common in females [**Figure 45-8**]. Bowen disease of the digits resembles verrucae or chronic paronychia and has been associated with human papillomavirus types 16 and 18.[29,30] SCC involving the mucosal skin has a greater tendency to metastasize and recur. Perianal SCC can arise in preexisting lesions such

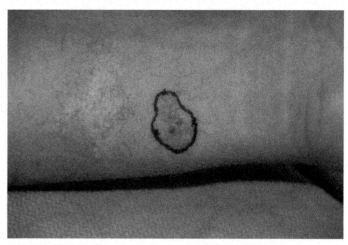

FIGURE 45-7. Squamous cell carcinoma of the forearm of a Hispanic female.

as perianal warts [**Figure 45-9**]. Anogenital lesions also can develop de novo [**Figure 45-10**].

SCC that presents in preexisting areas of disease such as a chronic leg ulcers or hidradenitis suppurativa or in areas of chronic scars may resemble the underlying disease. Such areas may appear not to respond to therapy or develop nonhealing ulcers or erosions. Invasive SCC can present as plaques, papules, and ulcers with induration. SCC should be excluded in the appropriate setting in which any of the preceding circumstances exist.

DIAGNOSIS AND THERAPY

SCC in an African American is potentially very aggressive and raises the possibility of an associated disease. Therefore, a detailed history and physical examination should be undertaken, and a biopsy of the suspicious lesion should be performed. The history should assess the duration of the lesion and history of prior treatment for preexisting skin cancer or preexisting skin disease. If indicated clinically, any evidence for immune deficiency should be evaluated. A physical examination

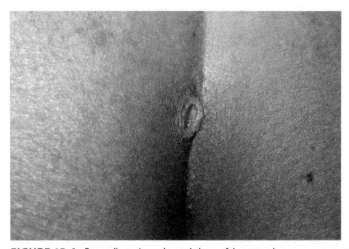

FIGURE 45-6. Bowen disease in an ulcerated plaque of the presacral area.

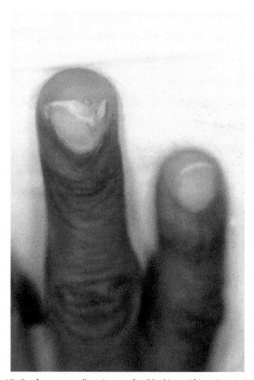

FIGURE 45-8. Squamous cell carcinoma of nail bed in an African American man.

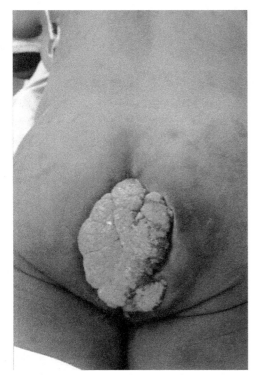

FIGURE 45-9. Squamous cell carcinoma developing in preexisting lesions such as perianal warts.

should be performed for local evaluation of the tumor and to assess the patient for the presence of lymphadenopathy.

The type of biopsy performed should be determined by the characteristics of the lesion. A shave biopsy can be performed on a relatively thin or superficial lesion. Thicker, more indurated plaques or tumors require a deeper punch or excisional biopsy.

The type of therapeutic intervention is determined by the histologic type of SCC, size of the tumor, location of the tumor, and presence or absence of metastatic disease [**Table 45-2**]. In thin lesions such as Bowen disease, a number of therapeutic options could be considered. The carbon dioxide laser has shown efficacy in the management of severe actinic cheilitis and in the treatment of superficial BCC, Bowen disease, and thin SCCs.[31,32] In addition to electrodessication with curettage and simple excision, both photodynamic therapy and topical 5-fluorouracil have proven to be efficacious in thin or superficial SCC.[33,34] Interferon-α and imiquimod both have been used in the management of SCCs. Intralesional interferon has been used to treat both SCC and BCC and has shown approximately an 80% cure rate in selected BCCs.[34] The use

TABLE 45-2	Treatments available for squamous cell carcinoma	
Medical	Surgical
5-Fluorouracil	Cryosurgery
Photodynamic therapy	Electrodesiccation and curettage
Imiquimod	Carbon dioxide laser
Interferon	Excision
Radiation therapy	Mohs micrographic surgery

of imiquimod in the management of BCCs has been approved recently. Its use in the treatment of SCC is currently under study, and its appears in selected lesions to be as effective as it is in the treatment of BCC.[35] Currently, imiquimod is not an approved drug for the treatment of cutaneous SCC.

For patients who have localized disease, excisional surgery and Mohs micrographic surgery are the primary forms of treatment. Aggressive management of the tumor is indicated because of the potential for SCC in people with skin of color to be more aggressive and have a higher rate of recurrence. If excisional surgery is undertaken, the tumor should be removed with adequate margins. The margins of the excision should be examined completely for evidence of residual disease. For tumors that are in cosmetically sensitive areas and that are considered high risk, Mohs micrographic surgery may be indicated. Large tumors involving the perianal region or tumors in areas of scarring or chronic ulceration require a wide local excision, often with complex repair.

Radiation therapy is used both as a primary form of therapy and as adjuvant therapy in the management of SCC, particularly of the head and neck. As adjuvant therapy, radiation is used when lymph nodes are positive, for the presence of perineural disease, and when residual disease is suspected after an excision or when clear margins are not established.

PATIENT PERSPECTIVES AND NONMELANOMA SKIN CANCER

Minorities often have greater morbidity and mortality than Caucasians from nonmelanoma skin cancer (NMSC), and African Americans in particular have higher cancer mortality than any other group in the United States.[36-38] Despite this, it has been shown in large studies that perception of skin cancer risk, along with other cancers, remains low in minority populations such as African Americans, Hispanics, and Asians.[39] In the Health Information National Trends Survey, African American and Hispanic patients were more likely to state that their risk of SCC was low, that behaviors do not lead to increased skin cancer risk, and that there is not much that can be done to lower skin cancer risk. Although it is accurate to state that the incidence of skin cancer is lower in these groups, it is not accurate to state that behavior modification cannot change skin cancer risk. Reduced exposure to UV radiation, scarring, trauma, and inflammation, all of which predispose to skin cancer, particularly in patients with skin of color, can reduce the incidence of skin cancer. Further, it is well established that use of sunscreen can prevent NMSC.[38] However, Summers et al[39] studied the patterns of sunscreen use in various populations and found that patients with skin of color had a lower likelihood of wearing sunscreen, even if they had a propensity for severe sunburn.[39] This could serve as a point for further education of skin cancer risk in these patient groups. Currently, it has been shown that of patients included in national dermatology screening and education programs over the past 15 years, only 1.2% have been patients with skin of color. Additionally, educational advertisements regarding skin cancer and sunscreen use are five times more common in magazines directed at patients with Caucasian skin.[40,41] Socioeconomic status and education level have also been shown to correlate with cancer risk, along with increased risk of NMSC and larger NMSCs. Further, lower skin cancer screening rates correlate with lower screening for other cancers, such as breast and colon, in patients with lower socioeconomic status

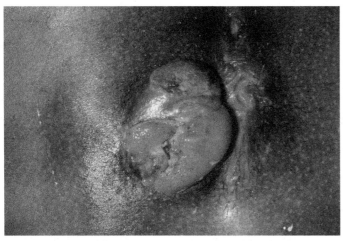

FIGURE 45-10. Anogenital squamous cell carcinoma also can develop de novo.

and education levels.[39] As the number of minority patients increases in the United States, it will be important to modify these perceptions and increase early detection of skin cancer in these populations.

REFERENCES

1. Montagna W, Carlisle K. The architecture of black and white facial skin. *J Am Acad Dermatol.* 1991;24:929-937.
2. Kaidbey KH, Agin PP, Sayre RM, et al. Photoprotection by melanin: a comparison of black and Caucasian skin. *J Am Acad Dermatol.* 1979;1:249-260.
3. Starkco RS, Pinkush. Quantitative and qualitative data on the pigment cell of adult human epidermis. *J Invest Dermatol.* 1957;28:33.
4. Toda K, Patnak MA, Parrrish A, et al. Alteration of racial differences in melanosome distribution in human epidermis after exposure to ultraviolet light. *Nat New Biol.* 1972;236:143-144.
5. Olson RL, Gaylor J, Everett MA. Skin color, melanin, and erythema. *Arch Dermatol.* 1973;108:541-544.
6. Freeman RG, Cockerell EG, Armstrong J. Sunlight as a factor influencing the thickness of epidermis. *J Invest Dermatol.* 1962;39:295-298.
7. Kotrajaras R, Kligman AM. The effect of topical tretinoin on photodamaged facial: the Thai experience. *Br J Dermatol.* 1993;129:302-309.
8. McCall CO, Chen SC. Squamous cell carcinoma of the legs in African-Americans. *J Am Acad Dermatol.* 2002;47:524-529.
9. Gray DT, Suman VJ, Su WPD, et al. Trends in the population-based incidence of squamous cell carcinoma of the skin first diagnosed between 1984 and 1992. *Arch Dermatol.* 1997;133:735-740.
10. Scotto J, Fears TR, Fraumeni JF Jr. Incidence of nonmelanoma skin cancer in the United States. NIH Report No. 83-243. Washington, DC: U.S. Government Printing Office; 1983.
11. Koh D, Wang H, Lee J, et al. Basal cell carcinoma, squamous cell carcinoma and melanoma of the skin: analysis of Singapore Cancer Registry data 1968–1997. *Br J Dermatol.* 2003;148:1161-1166.
12. Ichihashi M, Naruse K, Harada S, et al. Trends in nonmelanoma skin cancer in Japan. *Recent Results Cancer Res.* 1995;139:126-173.
13. Roenigk RK, Ratz JL, Bailin PL, et al. Trends in the presentation and treatment of basal cell carcinoma. *J Dermatol Surg Oncol.* 1986;12:860-865.
14. Halder RM, Bang KM. Skin cancer in African-Americans in the United States. *Dermatol Clin.* 1988;6:397-407.
15. Bang KM, Halder RM White JE, et al. Skin cancer in black Americans: a review of 126 cases. *J Natl Med Assoc.* 1987;79:51-58.
16. Fleming ID, Barnawell JR, Burlison PE, et al. Skin cancer in black patients. *Cancer.* 1975;33:600-605.
17. Rippentrop JM, Joslyn SA, Konety BR. Squamous cell carcinoma of the penis. *Cancer.* 2004;101:1357-1363.
18. Hubbell CR, Rabin VR, Mora RG. Cancer of the skin in blacks: V. A review of 175 black patients with squamous cell carcinoma of the penis. *J Am Acad Dermatol.* 1988;18:292-298.
19. McDonald MW. Carcinoma of scrotum. *Urology.* 1982;19:269-274.
20. Salasche SJ. Epidemiology of actinic keratoses and squamous cell carcinoma. *J Am Acad Dermatol.* 2000;44:S4-S7.
21. Glogau RG. The risk of progression to invasive disease. *J Am Acad Dermatol.* 2000;42:44-45.
22. Nijsten TEC, Stern RS. The increased risk of skin cancer is persistent after discontinuation of psoralen plus ultraviolet A: a cohort study. *J Invest Dermatol.* 2003;121:252-258.
23. Halder RM, Bridgeman-Shah S. Skin cancer in African-Americans. *Cancer.* 1995;75:667-673.
24. Mora RG, Perniciaro C, Lee B. Cancer of the skin in blacks: a review of 163 patients with cutaneous squamous cell carcinoma. *J Am Acad Dermatol.* 1981;5:535-543.
25. Hubbell CR, Rabin VR, Mora RG. Cancer of the skin in blacks: V. A review of 175 black patients with squamous cell carcinoma of the penis. *J Am Acad Dermatol.* 1988;18:292-298.
26. Weinstock MA. Nonmelanoma skin cancer mortality in the United States, 1969 through 1988. *Arch Dermatol.* 1993;129:1286-1290.
27. Singh B, Bhaya M, Shaha A, et al. Presentation, course and outcome of head and neck skin cancer in African-Americans: a case-control study. *Laryngoscope.* 1998;108:1159-1163.
28. Heyl T, Morrison JG. Keratoacanthoma in a Bantu. *Br J Dermatol.* 1975;93:699-700.
29. Preston DS, Stern RS. Nonmelanoma cancers of the skin. *N Engl J Med.* 1992;327:1649-1662.
30. Alam M, Ratner D. Cutaneous squamous cell carcinoma. *N Engl J Med.* 2001;344:975-983.
31. Karrer S, Szeimies RM, Hohenleutner U, et al. Role of laser and photodynamic therapy in the treatment of cutaneous malignancy. *Am J Clin Dermatol.* 2001;2:220-237.
32. Tantikun N. Treatment of Bowen's disease of the digit with carbon dioxide laser. *J Am Acad Dermatol.* 2000;43:1080-1083.
33. Morton CA, Whitehurst C, McColl JH, et al. Photodynamic therapy for large or multiple patches of Bowen disease and basal cell carcinoma. *Arch Dermatol.* 2001;137:319-324.
34. Miller SJ, Maloney ME, eds. *Cutaneous Oncology: Pathophysiology, Diagnosis, and Management.* Malden, MA: Blackwell Science; 1998:578-580.
35. Mackenzie-Wood A, Kossard S, de Launey J, et al. Imiquimod 5% cream in the treatment of Bowen's disease. *J Am Acad Dermatol.* 2001;44:462-470.
36. Wingo PA, Bolden S, Tong T, Parker SL, Martin LM, Heath CW Jr. Cancer statistics for African Americans, 1996. *CA Cancer J Clin.* 1996;46:113-125.
37. Gloster HM Jr, Neal K. Skin cancer in skin of color. *J Am Acad Dermatol.* 2006;55:741-760.
38. Weinstock MA. Nonmelanoma skin cancer mortality in the United States, 1969 through 1988. *Arch Dermatol.* 1993;129:1286-1290.
39. Buster K, You Z, Fouad M, et al. Skin cancer risk perceptions: a comparison across ethnicity, age, education, gender, and income. *J Am Acad Dermatol.* 2012;66:771-779.
40. Summers P, Bena J, Arrigain S, et al. Sunscreen use: non-Hispanic blacks compared with other racial and/or ethnic groups. *Arch Dermatol.* 2011;147:863-864.
41. Alexis AF, Rossi AM. Skin cancer in skin of color. *Cutis.* 2012;89:208-211.

CHAPTER	**Basal Cell Carcinoma**
46	Sheila M. Krishna Algin B. Garrett Seth B. Forman

KEY POINTS

- Although basal cell carcinoma (BCC) occurs less commonly in patients with skin of color compared with Caucasians, it remains an important and common diagnosis in patients with skin of color.

- BCCs classically present with a rolled border, telangiectasia, and erosions, but in patients with skin of color, the more common presentation consists of pigmented papules and nodules.

- Because BCCs are often pigmented, they can be mistaken for seborrheic keratoses, nevocellular nevi, or malignant melanomas.

- BCCs commonly present on the head and neck, but they may also appear in unusual locations such as the groin, scrotum, perianal region, and feet.

- It is important to do a complete skin examination in people with skin of color to ensure that a BCC is not overlooked.

- The approach to treating skin cancers in people with skin of color should be no different from treating patients with lighter skin.

INTRODUCTION

Basal cell carcinoma (BCC) is the most common malignancy found in humans. Its growth is driven by a distinct and well-defined biochemical pathway that has led to new insights into management and treatment. Although BCC does not have significant metastatic potential, it can lead to local destruction and disfigurement and present challenges in management, if unrecognized or untreated. While BCC has been described as uncommon in patients with skin of color, it remains the most common skin cancer in Hispanic, Japanese, and Chinese patients and the second most common skin cancer in blacks and Asian Indians.[1-4] Furthermore, patients with skin of color with skin cancer may be more likely to have greater morbidity and mortality associated with BCC than Caucasians.

INCIDENCE

The incidence of BCC in patients with skin of color varies with racial or ethnic group. BCC represents 65% to 75% of skin cancers in Caucasians, 20% to 30% of skin cancers in Asian Indians, 12% to 35% of skin cancers in African Americans,[1,3,5-7] and 2% to 8% of skin cancers in African blacks.[8,9] Beckenstein and Windle,[10] in a series from 1995, found that 1.8% (5 of 276) of skin cancers in African Americans were BCCs. The series by Fleming et al[5] noted that 12% (7 of 58) of all skin cancers in African Americans were BCCs. The study by Halder and Bang[1] from Howard University showed that 28.8% (38 of 103) of African American patients with skin cancer had a BCC. Altman et al[11] reported that 2.5% of all skin cancers in African Americans are BCCs.

The incidences of BCC per 100,000 population have been reported in nonblack patients as follows: Chinese men (6.4), Chinese women (5.8), Japanese (15 to 16.5), Japanese residents of Kauai, Hawaii (29.7), Japanese residents of Okinawa (26.1), New Mexican Hispanic women (113), New Mexican Hispanic men (171), southeastern Arizona Hispanic females (50), southeastern Arizona Hispanic males (91), Caucasian men (250), Caucasian women (212), and Caucasians in Kauai, Hawaii (185 to 340).[1,2,12-17] Although BCC occurs less commonly in patients with skin of color compared with Caucasians, it remains an important and common diagnosis in patients with skin of color.

PATHOGENESIS

Important insights into the pathogenesis of BCC have led to the development of novel targeted therapies for advanced BCC. BCC formation is driven by mutations in the sonic hedgehog (SHH) pathway, a signaling molecule that classically organizes dorsoventral limb patterning in vertebrates. In its native role, SHH binds to and inhibits patched (PTCH), a transmembrane protein receptor that functions as a tumor suppressor protein. PTCH inhibits the actions of smoothened (SMO), which subsequently activates GLI. GLI acts a nuclear transcription factor for several growth genes, which lead to unrestricted growth and tumorigenesis. Mutations in PTCH and SMO have been shown to be associated with the basal cell nevus syndrome and in sporadic BCCs. Mutations in PTCH have also been associated with esophageal squamous cell carcinoma, trichoepitheliomas, and transitional cell carcinomas of the bladder.[18] Sporadic PTCH mutations can be induced by ultraviolet radiation (UVR), but this effect is mitigated in patients with skin of color due to melanin photoprotection.

RISK FACTORS

BCC is primarily related to sustained, intensive exposure to UVR in all patients and occurs mainly on sun-exposed areas. In patients with skin of color, the effects of UVR are abrogated by the presence of melanin in the skin, which provides photoprotection. The incidence of BCC in patients with skin of color on sun-exposed and non–sun-exposed sites varies, and BCCs have appeared in unusual locations in both Caucasians and people with skin of color [**Table 46-1**].[10,11,19-23] Some studies suggest that the incidence of BCC on covered sites is the same for African Americans and Caucasians, whereas others demonstrate a higher percentage of BCCs on non–sun-exposed areas in African Americans as compared to those same areas in Caucasians. It has also been shown that 70% to 90% of BCCs occur on sun-exposed areas in African Americans, Japanese, and Asian Indians who develop BCC.[1-3] Halder and Bang[1] suggest that BCCs occur more often in sun-exposed areas, such as the head and neck [**Figures 46-1 and 46-2**]. However, Lesher et al[24] note in their series that 10% of BCCs in Caucasian patients occurred in covered, non–sun-exposed areas, whereas 24% of BCCs in African American patients occurred in covered, non–sun-exposed areas. Abreo and Sanusi[25] found that 88% (38 of 45) of BCCs occurred in the head and neck region of African American patients. In the series by Fleming et al,[5] 85.7% (six of seven) of the tumors were in sun-exposed areas. A series by White et al[7] found that

TABLE 46-1	Unusual locations of basal cell carcinomas

- Ankle
- Buttock
- Cervix
- Groin
- Nipple
- Plantar surface of the foot
- Scrotum
- Vulva

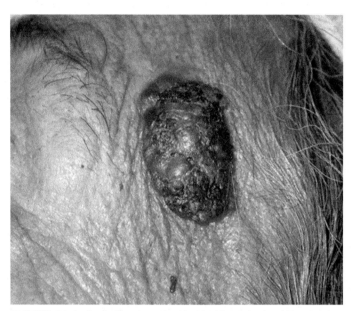

FIGURE 46-1. Basal cell carcinoma involving the left temple of an African American woman resembling a seborrheic keratosis.

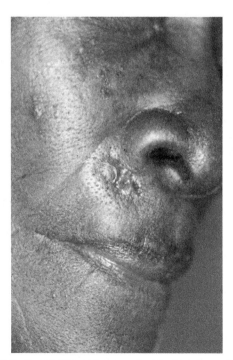

FIGURE 46-2. Pigmented basal cell carcinoma involving the right upper lip in an African American female.

TABLE 46-2	Syndromes with genetic predisposition for developing basal cell carcinoma

Nevoid basal cell carcinoma syndrome (Gorlin syndrome)
Oculocutaneous albinism
Xeroderma pigmentosum

54.5% (6 of 11) of BCCs diagnosed in African American patients were on covered, non–sun-exposed areas.

Overall, the data suggest that BCCs occur with greater frequency in the sun-exposed areas in people with skin of color. However, there is also evidence that a tumor may arise in covered, non–sun-exposed areas as well.

In addition to UVR, there are reports of BCCs developing in areas of chronic discoid lupus erythematosus lesions, areas previously treated with radiation, and stasis ulcers.[26,27] However, the effects of radiation are much greater in irradiated Caucasian patients, as compared to African American patients. Thermal and physical traumas, such as burns, have also been demonstrated to be important risk factors in the development of BCC in Asian Indians specifically, along with scarring and sun exposure.[3] Vitamin D has recently been examined for its role in cutaneous carcinogenesis. Although vitamin D deficiency is linked to skin cancer in vitro and in mouse models, the role of vitamin D in human skin cancer development is unclear, with studies showing both positive and neutral associations between vitamin D deficiency and skin cancer. However, it is well recognized that patients with skin of color, particularly African American and Hispanic patients, have greater difficulty synthesizing vitamin D from sunlight due to increased melanin, which absorbs the UVR needed for vitamin D production. This leads to a higher risk of vitamin D deficiency in darker-skinned patients, as has been shown in numerous observational studies. Therefore, the relationship between vitamin D and skin cancer in patients with skin of color may be of future clinical interest.[28]

Genetic syndromes can also contribute to the development of BCC in patients with skin of color. Gorlin syndrome (also known as nevoid BCC syndrome), oculocutaneous albinism, and xeroderma pigmentosum occur in skin of color populations.[29-32] These syndromes are associated with an increased incidence of all types of skin cancers, including BCCs. Hall et al[29] commented that less than 5% of cases of Gorlin syndrome occur in people with skin of color. Martin and Waisman[32] reported a case of an African American man with Gorlin syndrome who presented with his first BCC at age 77. Therefore, it may be prudent to look for other diagnostic criteria if one suspects Gorlin syndrome in a person of color (ie, palmar pits, frontal bossing, and odontogenic cysts). People with skin of color with oculocutaneous albinism are most likely to have type II oculocutaneous albinism, which is the expression of a mutation in the *P* gene.[33] Abreo and Sanusi[25] reported an albino patient with 12 separate primary BCCs. Itayemi et al[34] discussed an albino patient with a BCC metastasis to the cervical lymph nodes in their series. In the skin of color population, it is important to consider conditions predisposing a patient to develop BCC[35] [**Table 46-2**].

DIAGNOSIS

The diagnosis of BCC in patients with skin of color is made clinically and via pathology. Reports suggest that a clinical diagnosis of BCC is more difficult than a histopathologic one. Altman et al[11] commented that a BCC in people with skin of color may be misdiagnosed clinically as seborrheic keratosis, nevocellular nevus, or malignant melanoma. Halder and Bang[1] also remarked that a BCC may be confused for a nevus sebaceus. Beckenstein and Windle[10] reported a BCC that was initially misdiagnosed as a fungal infection.[10] A biopsy is the best and most definitive diagnostic test for a presumed BCC.

The histologic types of BCC in people with skin of color are similar to those seen in people with lighter skin. Various reports confirm the occurrence of nodular, morpheaform, superficial, adenoid, nodulocystic, and sclerosing types of BCC[11,24,25,36] [**Figures 46-3 and 46-4**]. The ulcerative

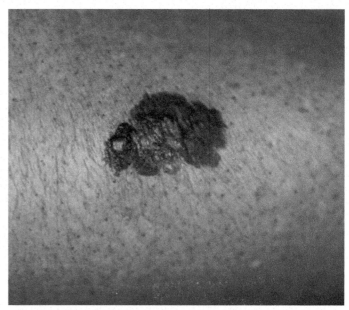

FIGURE 46-3. Pigmented basal cell carcinoma on the leg of an African American man.

type is discussed in many of the series and case reports concerning BCC in people with skin of color and is suggestive of a more aggressive course.[1,11,24] Altman et al[11] and Halder and Bang,[1] in two distinct series, commented that almost all BCCs are pigmented in people with skin of color. Hispanics, even those with fair skin, have a high incidence pigmented BCC [**Figure 46-5**]. In addition, Kidd et al[37] demonstrated greater carcinoembryonic antigen staining in BCCs in darker skin of color patients compared with Caucasians, which indicates an increased differentiation to follicular, eccrine, or sebaceous structures.

PROGNOSIS

A BCC excised with clear surgical margins provides an excellent prognosis. Complications arise when there is delay in diagnosis, resulting in locally aggressive tumor expansion or even metastasis. In contrast to

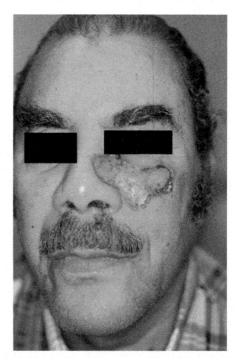

FIGURE 46-4. Sclerosing basal cell carcinoma on the left cheek of an African American man.

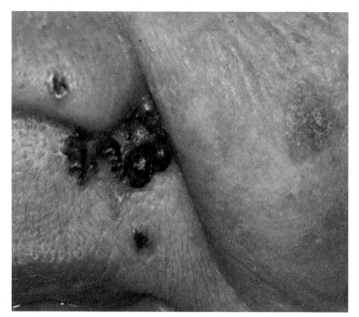

FIGURE 46-5. Basal cell carcinoma involving the left upper lip and nasal labial fold of a Hispanic woman.

SCC, BCC is not associated with increased morbidity in blacks compared with Caucasians, although case reports and series have described more aggressive BCC behavior in patients with skin of color.[1] Itayemi et al[34] in Nigeria reported that BCCs are most aggressive in people with skin of color. They reported two cases of tumors that were locally aggressive and destructive to the underlying bony structures. In the case report of Beckenstein and Windle,[10] a BCC was described as arising within a giant ulcer and spreading locally to the underlying vasculature.

Distant metastasis from BCCs of the scalp to cervical lymph nodes has been reported by Itayemi et al.[34] Lanehart et al[27] have reported a metastasis to the ipsilateral upper thigh from a primary tumor in a stasis ulcer. Recurrence of BCC in people with skin of color has not been widely reported in the literature.

SPECIAL CONSIDERATIONS

The occurrence of a BCC or even multiple BCCs in a person with darker skin of color should be reason for pause. Mora and Burris[6] noted in their series of 128 patients that 16.8% of patients with a BCC had a second primary malignancy elsewhere. Altman et al[11] found that one patient in their five-patient series had a second primary malignancy. In particular, darker skin of color women with BCC have been shown to be at increased risk for malignancy, particularly breast cancer. The authors suggested various mechanisms, such as abnormal DNA repair capacity, *p53* mutations, or higher levels of transurocanic acid in darker skin of color patients compared with Caucasian patients. Transurocanic acid is a photoreceptor that might induce immunosuppression, leading to decreased cancer surveillance and more rapid tumorigenesis.[38-44] **Table 46-3** lists the types of concurrent malignancies reported. SCC of the lung was the most frequently reported second primary malignancy in the series by Mora and Burris.[6] Therefore, it may be appropriate to perform an age-appropriate cancer screening on any patient who has at least one BCC.

TABLE 46-3   Concurrent second primary malignancies
Squamous cell carcinoma of the lung
Breast cancer
Cervical cancer
Prostate cancer
Uterine cancer

TREATMENT

The approach to a person with skin of color should not be different than that for a patient with light skin.[21] Management of a BCC should focus on complete extirpation of the tumor. Surgical techniques available to the practitioner include electrodesiccation and curettage, cryosurgery, excisional surgery with clear surgical margins, and Mohs micrographic surgery.[10,24,36,43] Other modalities in the treatment of BCC include photodynamic therapy, topical imiquimod, and laser surgery.[44] Newer modalities include targeted molecular therapy in the form of vismodegib, a small-molecule analog of the PTCH protein, which functions to inhibit SMO and thus decrease growth of the tumor. Vismodegib is currently approved for adults with metastatic BCC or with locally advanced BCC that has recurred following surgery or who are not candidates for surgery or radiation. Continued monitoring is essential because recurrence has been reported in up to 37.5% of patients in a series by Ademiluyi and Ijaduola.[30]

REFERENCES

1. Halder RM, Bang KM. Skin cancer in blacks in the United States. *Dermatol Clin.* 1988;6:397-405.
2. Koh D, Wang H, Lee J, Chia KS, Lee HP, Goh CL. Basal cell carcinoma, squamous cell carcinoma and melanoma of the skin: analysis of the Singapore Cancer Registry Data 1968-97. *Br J Dermatol.* 2003;148:1161-1166.
3. Dhir A, Orengo I, Bruce S, Kolbusz RV, Alford E, Goldberg L. Basal cell carcinoma on the scalp of an Indian patient. *Dermatol Surg.* 1995;21:247-250.
4. Kikuchi A, Shimizu H, Nishikawa T. Clinical and histopathological characteristics of basal cell carcinoma in Japanese patients. *Arch Dermatol.* 1996;132:320-324.
5. Fleming ID, Barnwell JR, Burlison PE, et al. Skin cancer in black patients. *Cancer.* 1975;3:600-605.
6. Mora R, Burris RG. Cancer in the skin of blacks: a review of 128 patients with basal cell carcinoma. *Cancer.* 1981;47:1456-1458.
7. White, JE, Strudwick WJ, Ricketts WN, et al. Cancer of the skin in Negroes: a review of 31 cases. *JAMA.* 1961;178:845-847.
8. Shapiro MP, Keen P, Cohen L. Skin cancer in the South African Bantu. *Br J Cancer.* 1953;7:45-57.
9. Oluwasanmi JO, Williams AO, Alli AF. Superficial cancer in Nigeria. *Br J Cancer.* 1969;23:714-728.
10. Beckenstein MS, Windle BH. Basal cell carcinoma in black patients: the need to include it in the differential diagnosis. *Ann Plast Surg.* 1995;35:546-548.
11. Altman A, Rosen T, Tschen JA, et al. Basal cell epithelioma in black patients. *J Am Acad Dermatol.* 1987;17:741-745.
12. Ichihashi M, Naruse K, Harada S, et al. Trends in nonmelanoma skin cancer in Japan. *Recent Results Cancer Res.* 1995;139:263-273.
13. Naruse K, Ueda M, Nagano T, Suzuki T. Prevalence of actinic keratoses in Japan. *J Dermatol Sci.* 1997;15:183-187.
14. Harris RB, Griffith K, Moon TE. Trends in incidence of nonmelanoma skin cancers in southeastern Arizona, 1985-1996. *J Am Acad Dermatol.* 2001;45:528-536.
15. Chuang TY, Reizner GT, Elpern DJ, Stone JL, Farmer ER. Nonmelanoma skin cancer in Japanese ethnic Hawaiians in Kauai, Hawaii: an incidence report. *J Am Acad Dermatol.* 1995;33:422-426.
16. Munyao TM, Othieno-Abinya NA. Cutaneous basal cell carcinoma in Kenya. *East Afr Med J.* 1999;76:97-100.
17. Miller DL, Weinstock MA. Nonmelanoma skin cancer in the United States: incidence. *J Am Acad Dermatol.* 1994;30:774-778.
18. Johnson RL. Human homolog of patched, a candidate gene for the basal cell nevus syndrome. *Science.* 1996;272:1668-1671.
19. Galinski AW. Plantar basal cell carcinoma: a case report. *J Foot Surg.* 1980;19:34-35.
20. Woods SG. Basal cell carcinoma in the black population. *Int J Dermatol.* 1995;34:517-518.
21. McDonald MW. Carcinoma of the scrotum. *Urology.* 1982;19:269-274.
22. Powers CN, Stastny JF, Frable WJ. Adenoid basal cell carcinoma of the cervix: a potential pitfall in cervicovaginal cytology. *Diagn Cytopathol.* 1996;14:172-177.
23. Morimoto SS, Gurevitch AW. Residents' corner: pedunculated pigmented basal-cell carcinoma on the buttock of a black man. *J Dermatol Surg Oncol.* 1985;11:115-117.
24. Lesher JL Jr, d'Aubermont PC, Brown VM. Morpheaform basal cell carcinoma in a young black woman. *J Dermatol Surg Oncol.* 1988;14:200-203.

25. Abreo F, Sanusi ID. Basal cell carcinoma in North American blacks. *J Am Acad Dermatol.* 1991;25:1005-1006.

26. Walther RR, Grossman ME, Troy JL. Basal cell carcinomas on the scalp of a black patient many years after epilation with x-rays. *J Dermatol Surg Oncol.* 1981;7:570-571.

27. Lanehart WH, Sanusi ID, Misra RP, et al. Metastasizing basal cell carcinoma originating in a stasis ulcer in a black woman. *Arch Dermatol.* 1983;119:587-591.

28. Tang JY, Fu T, Lau C, Oh DH, Bikle DD, Asgari MM. Vitamin D in cutaneous carcinogenesis: part II. *J Am Acad Dermatol.* 2012;67:817.

29. Hall J, Johnston KA, McPhillips JP, et al. Nevoid basal cell carcinoma syndrome in a black patient. *J Am Acad Dermatol.* 1998;38:363-365.

30. Ademiluyi SA, Ijaduola GT. Occurrence and recurrence of basal cell carcinoma of the head and neck in Negroid and albinoid Africans. *J Laryngol Otol.* 1987;101:1324-1328.

31. Kulkarni P, Brashear R, Chuang TY. Nevoid basal cell carcinoma syndrome in a person with dark skin. *J Am Acad Dermatol.* 2003;49:332-335.

32. Martin S, Waisman M. Basal cell nevus syndrome in a black patient. *Arch Dermatol.* 1978;114:1356-1357.

33. Centurion SA, Schwartz RA. Oculocutaneous albinism type 2. *Acta Dermatol Venereol.* 2003;12:32-36.

34. Itayemi SO, Abioye AA, Ogan O, et al. Aggressive basal cell carcinoma in Nigerians. *Br J Dermatol.* 1979;101:465-468.

35. Frank W, Morris D. Large basal cell carcinoma in a black patient. *Plast Reconstr Surg.* 1995;96:493-494.

36. Schwartz RA. Mutilating sclerosing basal cell epithelioma. *J Surg Oncol.* 1979;12:131-135.

37. Kidd MK, Tschen JA, Rosen T, Altman AR, Goldberg L. Carcinoembryonic antigen in basal cell neoplasms in black patients: an immunohistochemical study. *J Am Acad Dermatol.* 1989;21(5 Pt 1):1007-1010.

38. Troyanova P, Danon S, Ivanova T. Nonmelanoma skin cancer and risk of subsequent malignancies: a cancer registry based study in Bulgaria. *Neoplasma.* 2002;49:81-85.

39. Frisch M, Melbye M. New primary cancers after squamous cell skin cancer. *Am J Epidemiol.* 1995;41:916-922.

40. Rosenberg CA, Greenland P, Khandekar J, Loar A, Ascensao J, Lopez AM. Association of nonmelanoma skin cancer with second malignancy. *Cancer.* 2004;100:130-138.

41. Norval M. Effects of solar irradiation on the human immune system. In: Giacomoni PU, ed. *Sun Protection in Man.* Amsterdam, The Netherlands: Elsevier; 2001:91-113.

42. Staub F, Hoppe U, Sauermann G. Urocanic acid and its function in endogenous antioxidant defense and UV-protection in human skin (abstract). *J Invest Dermatol.* 1994;102:666.

43. Singh B, Bhaya M, Shaha A, et al. Presentation, course and outcome of head and neck skin cancer in African-Americans: a case-control study. *Layngoscope.* 1998;108:1159-1163.

44. Geisse J, Lindholm J, Golitz L, et al. Imiquimod 5% cream for the treatment of superficial basal cell carcinoma: results from two phase III, randomized, vehicle-controlled studies. *J Am Acad Dermatol.* 2004;50:722-733.

CHAPTER
47

Cutaneous T-Cell Lymphoma

Sharif Currimbhoy
Amit G. Pandya

KEY POINTS

- Cutaneous T-cell lymphoma (CTCL) refers to a group of non-Hodgkin lymphomas that primarily involve the skin.

- Mycosis fungoides (MF) represents the most common form of CTCL.

- The incidence and mortality rate of MF are higher in African Americans than in Caucasians, especially in African American females.

- Hypopigmented patches and plaques are not infrequently the presenting signs of MF in patients with skin of color.

- The age of onset is lower in patients with hypopigmented MF compared with nonhypopigmented disease.

- Treatment of CTCL includes topical nitrogen mustard, phototherapy, oral and systemic chemotherapy, and radiation therapy.

INTRODUCTION

Patients with skin of color comprise an important subset of those affected with cutaneous T-cell lymphoma (CTCL). CTCL refers to a group of non-Hodgkin lymphomas that primarily involve the skin and may later involve the lymph nodes, peripheral blood, and other organs. This group of lymphomas includes mycosis fungoides (MF) and Sézary syndrome. MF was first described in 1806 by the French dermatologist Alibert, who named the cutaneous nodules according to their mushroom-like appearance, even though fungi are not involved in the etiopathogenesis. MF usually presents with erythematous patches and scaly plaques, sometimes with an affinity for follicles.[1] Less common presentations include hypopigmented macules, pustules, bullae, keratoderma, granulomatous papules and nodules, slacked skin, and subcutaneous plaques.[2,3] Hypopigmented lesions are not infrequently the presenting sign of MF in patients with skin of color. Malignant cells have an affinity for the epidermis, allowing skin-directed therapy for most patients. More advanced stages of the disease are characterized by loss of this epidermal affinity. Sézary syndrome is the leukemic form of MF, characterized by generalized erythroderma, lymphadenopathy, and atypical T-cells located in the peripheral blood.

EPIDEMIOLOGY

According to Weinstock and colleagues,[4-7] the incidence of MF is 6.4 persons per million annually. The median survival is 9.7 years, but depends largely on the tumor-node-metastasis (TNM) stage at diagnosis. There was an estimated 3.2-fold rise in incidence of MF between 1969 to 1971 and 1984 but no further increase from 1984 to 1992. The cause of this increased incidence is unknown but may be the result of advances in diagnosis and improved reporting of new cases. Unlike other lymphomas, MF is more common in African Americans than Caucasians, with an incidence 1.6 times higher in African Americans than Caucasians.[5] In addition, the rate ratio for mortality is 2.4 times higher among African Americans than among Caucasians. On the other hand, the incidence in Asians and Hispanics is only 0.6 that of Caucasians. Early-onset MF, defined as patients with onset before age 40 years, has been seen more commonly in African American and Hispanic women. One study by Sun et al[8] found African American and Hispanic women to be twice as likely to present with early-onset MF compared with Caucasian women. Furthermore, African American women with early-onset MF had the highest rate of disease progression (38% vs only 10% and 5% for Caucasian and Hispanic women, respectively), as well as a significantly greater mortality.[8] The male-to-female incidence ratio of MF is 1.9:1, with a median age at presentation between 60 and 69 years old.[8] However, MF can occur in young patients as well.

ETIOLOGY

The cause of MF is unknown, but much research has been devoted to determining the mechanisms of disease progression. Normal lymphocytes that express the skin-homing protein cutaneous lymphoid antigen (CLA) are present in inflammatory infiltrates of the skin but not in other tissues. During lymphocyte activation in lymph nodes, the lymphocyte gains the ability to express CLA. The lymphocytes with CLA bind to endothelial cells that express E-selectin 1 on their cell surfaces to facilitate their extravasation into inflamed skin. Expression of CLA by malignant T-cells in CTCL helps to explain the skin localization of the disease.[9]

There have been a number of immunologic abnormalities associated with CTCL, including eosinophilia, increased immunoglobulin (Ig) E and IgA, decreased natural killer cell activity, and decreased T-cell response to mitogens. These changes have been attributed to an associated increase in T-helper 2 (T_H2)-associated cytokines, including interleukin (IL)-4, IL-5, IL-6, and IL-10.[10] In addition, patients with CTCL have abnormally high levels of soluble IL-2 receptors, thus decreasing the ability of IL-2 to drive a T_H1-mediated response against tumor cells.[11]

It has been suggested that CD8 lymphocytes are important in the survival of CTCL patients. According to Hoppe et al,[12] both T1 and T3 stage CTCL patients had a three-fold increase in mortality if they had only 0% to 15% CD8 T-cells in their skin biopsies compared with biopsies with more than 20% CD8 T-cells after a 6-year follow-up period. In addition, it has been observed that patients who responded favorably to treatment with extracorporeal photochemotherapy had lower CD4-to-CD8 T-cell ratios and high numbers of CD8 T-cells at the start of treatment.[13] Another marker to follow may be the erythrocyte sedimentation rate (ESR). A study by Hallermann et al[14] of 97 cases of patients with MF found a 100% 5-year survival rate in patients with a nonelevated ESR compared with a 52.83% 5-year survival rate in patients with an elevated ESR.

Since the advent of immunophenotyping, MF has been shown to consist primarily of epidermotropic malignant CD4 helper T-cells, with reactive CD8 and CD4 T-cells located mainly in the papillary dermis.[15,16] Occasionally, MF may have a predominant CD8 phenotype, especially in patients with hypopigmented lesions.[15,17]

CLINICAL PRESENTATION

The effect of external factors and infection on the development of MF and Sézary syndrome remains unknown. Environmental and occupational exposure to chemicals was once thought to play a role in MF, but this is not supported by data from a large, case-controlled study reported by Whittemore et al.[18] A viral etiology has been proposed, and human T-lymphotropic virus I (HTLV-I) has been found in the blood and skin lesions of some MF patients. Multiple infectious agents, including HTLV-I, cause prolonged antigenic stimulation, which may contribute to malignant transformation of T-cells.[19] However, other studies have failed to find such an association.[20,21]

Clinically, MF may present with nonspecific, slightly scaly skin lesions with nondiagnostic biopsies for months or years before a definitive diagnosis can be made, which is known as the premycotic phase, or pre-MF.[22,23] The eczematous form presents as a persistent, flat, red, pruritic lesion that is fixed in size. Parapsoriasis en plaque refers to small oval lesions with an erythematous to yellowish tint, fine scale, and a slightly wrinkled surface, found most often on the buttocks and thighs and ranging from 1 to 5 cm in diameter. Poikiloderma vasculare atrophicans is a term that refers to lesions with "cigarette paper" skin, telangiectasia, atrophy, and a mottled color. Patients with long-standing parapsoriasis-like lesions or poikiloderma vasculare atrophicans are more likely to develop MF. Even when the initial biopsies are negative, repeated biopsies should be performed in patients suspected of having MF. The patch stage of MF also presents as erythematous macules, sometimes with hyper- or hypopigmentation and slight scale [**Figures 47-1 and 47-2**]. Plaques are dusky red and scaly and may be round, oval, serpiginous, or arciform in shape. Plaque-stage lesions are usually more erythematous than patch-stage lesions [**Figure 47-3**]. Itching is variable and occasionally severe. If plaques occur in hair-bearing skin, alopecia may result and can be associated with follicular mucinosis on biopsy. The distribution ranges from solitary, isolated lesions to generalized involvement covering the majority of the skin surface area. Plaques can regress spontaneously, remain the same, or occasionally evolve into thicker tumors.[1,22,23]

Tumors of MF may arise from a preformed plaque or from erythematous or uninvolved skin [**Figure 47-4**]. When the tumors arise in plaques, they represent loss of epidermotropism and extension into the deep dermis. These tumors can ulcerate and may become secondarily infected, a common cause of morbidity in MF patients.

Generalized erythroderma in MF is usually accompanied by extreme pruritus and scaling [**Figures 47-5 and 47-6**]. The skin may be licheni-fied or atrophic, and plaques and tumors of MF also may be present on the background erythema. Lymphadenopathy is common in this form of CTCL. More advanced stages of CTCL are defined by involvement of the lymph nodes, peripheral blood, bone marrow, or other organs

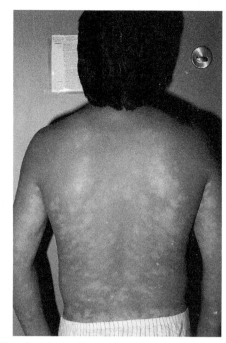

FIGURE 47-1. Hypopigmented mycosis fungoides in a Latin American patient.

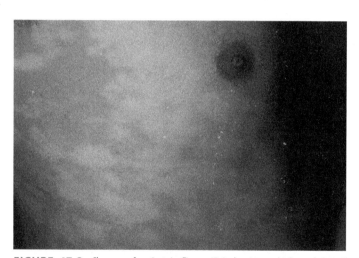

FIGURE 47-2. Close-up of patient in Figure 47-1 showing multiple oval-shaped hypopigmented macules

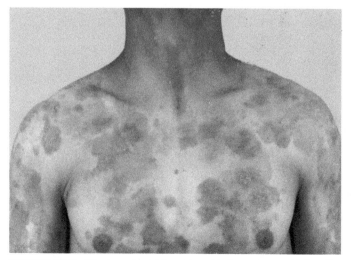

FIGURE 47-3. Thin plaques in an Asian patient with plaque-stage mycosis fungoides (stage IB).

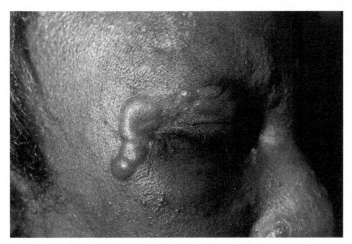

FIGURE 47-4. Tumor-stage cutaneous T-cell lymphoma (stage IIB) in an African American patient showing infiltrating tumor, erythema, and alopecia of the face.

[**Figures 47-7 to 47-9**]. Extensive skin involvement is a risk factor for developing extracutaneous skin disease. Whereas localized patch or plaque MF is unlikely to involve extracutaneous tissues, tumor or erythrodermic stages are often accompanied by lymphadenopathy. Visceral involvement is rare and may be a late finding, with the most commonly affected organs being the lungs, liver, spleen, and gastrointestinal tract.

The clinical picture of Sézary syndrome includes generalized erythroderma, lymphadenopathy, and circulating abnormal hyperconvoluted lymphoid cells (Sézary cells) in the peripheral blood. The number of cells that must be present to make a diagnosis varies between 5% and 20% of the total lymphocytes.[1] Patients can have all three components, or they may start with generalized erythroderma and then develop lymphadenopathy and peripheral blood involvement. Sézary syndrome has a worse prognosis than erythrodermic MF.

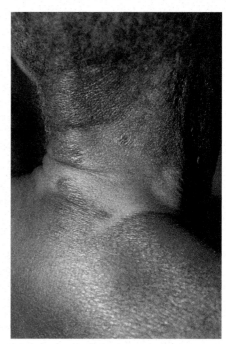

FIGURE 47-6. Close-up of posterior neck of patient in Figure 47-5.

DIFFERENTIAL DIAGNOSIS

MF can imitate many different skin diseases. The differential diagnosis includes atopic dermatitis, psoriasis, drug reactions, photodermatitis, parapsoriasis, neurodermatitis, nummular dermatitis, and tinea corporis. Less common mimickers include acanthosis nigricans, alopecia areata, dyshidrosis, erythema multiforme, perioral dermatitis, pigmented purpuric dermatitis, pityriasis alba, porokeratosis, palmoplantar pustulosis, sarcoidosis, and vitiligo. In patients who present with erythroderma, the differential diagnosis includes atopic dermatitis, contact dermatitis, drug eruption, and erythrodermic psoriasis.[24]

■ DIAGNOSIS

The single most important diagnostic tool for CTCL is the skin biopsy. A biopsy especially may be indicated in patients with skin of color who present with unusual areas of hypopigmentation. Classically, skin biopsy reveals a bandlike infiltrate involving the papillary dermis that consists of mononuclear cells with hyperchromatic, cerebriform nuclei without spongiosis. There is an infiltrate of atypical mononuclear cells in the epidermis (epidermotropism) that can form an intraepithelial aggregate

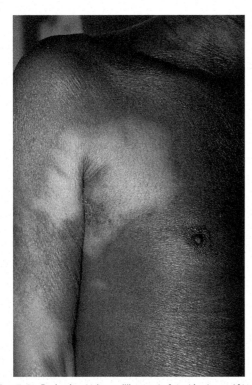

FIGURE 47-5. Erythrodermic (stage III) mycosis fungoides in an African American patient; note contrast between normal skin on lateral chest with involved skin on the remainder of the trunk.

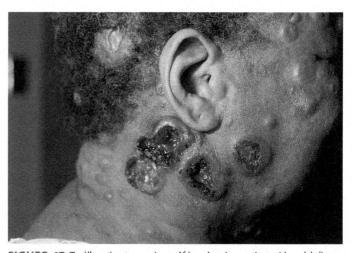

FIGURE 47-7. Ulcerating tumors in an African American patient with nodal disease (stage IVA).

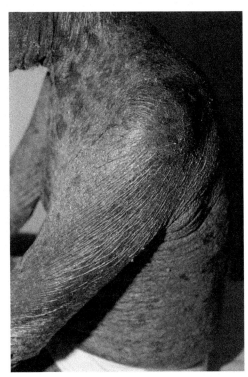

FIGURE 47-8. An African American patient with advanced, stage IVB disease with erythroderma, weight loss, and slack skin.

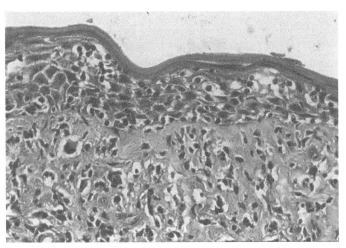

FIGURE 47-10. Histopathology of patch/plaque-stage mycosis fungoides showing multiple lymphocytes in the papillary dermis and epidermotropism. Note the small aggregates of lymphocytes in epidermis (Pautrier microabscesses).

CLASSIFICATION

Staging of MF/Sézary syndrome uses the TNM classification system [**Tables 47-1 and 47-2**].[25] The TNM classification for MF/Sézary syndrome was revised in 2007 by the International Society for Cutaneous Lymphomas and the European Organization for Research and Treatment of Cancer[25] to reflect advances in diagnostic tests that affect staging. Another category for high tumor burden with significant blood involvement with Sézary cells was added to the blood component of

known as a Pautrier microabscess [**Figure 47-10**]. Often, nonmalignant inflammatory cells are found in the dermis, presumably reacting to the malignant epidermal cells. Using electron microscopy, one can determine the nuclear contour index, which can be used to analyze the degree of lymphocyte nuclear folding and may be helpful to distinguish between MF and benign infiltrates.

Some patients with CTCL may develop nodal disease. In early stages of involvement, histologic examination of a lymph node affected by MF usually reveals small clusters of atypical cells with preserved nodal architecture. With more advanced disease, the clusters of atypical cells in the paracortical regions enlarge and can result in total effacement of the node.

Routine imaging in patients with small lesions or localized MF without lymphadenopathy is of low diagnostic yield and usually not performed. Patients with lymphadenopathy should have a lymph node biopsy. Physical examination and screening blood tests may reveal abnormalities that warrant further tests, such as computed tomography scanning or magnetic resonance imaging and bone marrow biopsy.

TABLE 47-1	Staging system for cutaneous lymphomas other than mycosis fungoides and Sézary syndrome

T (TUMOR)
- T1: solitary skin involvement
  - T1a: a solitary lesion <5-cm diameter
  - T1b: a solitary lesion >5-cm diameter
- T2: regional skin involvement: multiple lesions limited to one body region or two contiguous body regions[a]
  - T2a: all-disease-encompassing in a <15-cm diameter circular area
  - T2b: all-disease-encompassing in a >15- and <30-cm diameter circular area
  - T2c: all-disease-encompassing in a >30-cm diameter circular area
- T3: generalized skin involvement
  - T3a: multiple lesions involving 2 noncontiguous body regions
  - T3b: multiple lesions involving ≥3 body region

N (LYMPH NODE)
- N0: No clinical or pathologic lymph node involvement
- N1: Involvement of one peripheral lymph node region[b] that drains an area of current or prior involvement
- N2: Involvement of two or more peripheral lymph node regions[b] or involvement of any lymph node region that does not drain an area of current or prior skin involvement
- N3: Involvement of central lymph nodes

M (METASTASES)
- M0: No evidence of extracutaneous nonlymph node disease
- M1: Extracutaneous nonlymph node disease present

[a]Definition of body regions.

[b]Definition of lymph node regions is consistent with the Ann Arbor system: Peripheral sites: antecubital, cervical, supraclavicular, axillary, inguinal-femoral, and popliteal. C sites: mediastinal, pulmonary hilar, paraortic, iliac.

Source: Reproduced with permission from Goldsmith L, Katz S, Gilchrest B, et al. *Fitzpatrick's Dermatology in General Medicine,* 8th ed. New York, NY: McGraw-Hill; 2012.

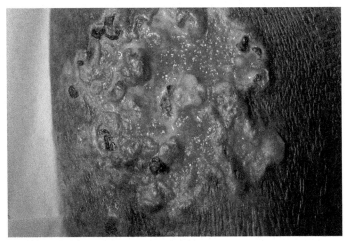

FIGURE 47-9. Close-up of ulcerated plaque from patient in Figure 47-8.

TABLE 47-2 Stage system for mycosis fungoides/Sézary syndrome

Stage	T (Tumor)	N (Lymph node)	M (Metastases)	B (Blood)
IA	T1	N0	M0	B0 or B1
IB	T2	N0	M0	B0 or B1
IIA	T1 or T2	N1 or N2	M0	B0 or B1
IIB	T3	N0-2	M0	B0 or B1
III	T4	N0-2	M0	B0 or B1
IIIA	T4	N0-2	M0	B0
IIIB	T4	N0-2	M0	B1
IVA1	T1-T4	N0-2	M0	B2
IVA2	T1-T4	N3	M0	B0-2
IVB	T1-T4	N0-N3	M1	B0-2

T1 = patch/plaque ≤10% of body surface; T2 = patch/plaque ≥10% of body surface; T3 = skin tumor(s); T4= erythroderma; N0 = normal nodes; N1= palpable nodes without clear histologic evidence of lymphoma [for N1 and N2, "a" or "b" may be added for either no (a) or detection (b) of a T-cell clone by Southern blot or PCR analysis]; N2 = palpable nodes, histologic evidence of lymphoma, node architecture preserved; N3 = palpable nodes with histologic evidence of lymphoma, effacement of node architecture; M0 = no visceral involvement; M1 = histologically confirmed visceral involvement. B0 = ≤5% Sézary cells (for B0 and B1, "a" or "b" may be added for either no (a) or detection (b) of a T-cell clone by Southern blot or PCR analysis); B1 = >5% Sézary cells but either less than 1.0 K/microL absolute Sézary cells or absence of a clonal rearrangement of the TCR or both; clonal rearrangement of the TCR in the blood and either 1.0 K/microL or more Sézary cells or one of the following two: (1) increased CD4+ or CD3+ cells with CD4/CD8 of ten or more or (2) increase in CD4+ cells with an abnormal phenotype (>40% CD4+/CD7- or >30% CD4+/CD26-).

Source: Reproduced with permission from Goldsmith L, Katz S, Gilchrest B, et al. *Fitzpatrick's Dermatology in General Medicine,* 8th ed. New York, NY: McGraw-Hill; 2012.

the TNM classification system due to poorer prognosis in patients with a higher number of circulating tumor cells. T0 was eliminated, and a better definition for evaluating plaques and patches was included. Revisions to the nodal section included elimination of the need to biopsy lymph nodes that are not clinically enlarged on examination and staging of clinically significant lymph nodes based on the National Cancer Institute–Veterans Administration histology classification or the Dutch system. The metastasis component largely remained unchanged with the exception of a better definition of peripheral organ involvement, including the spleen, liver, and bone marrow, based on diagnostic and clinical evaluation.

The extent and type of skin involvement and the presence of extracutaneous disease are the most important prognostic factors in MF. Patients with stage IA disease have an excellent prognosis, with life expectancy comparable with that of age-matched controls.[1] Patients with generalized patch and plaque disease without extracutaneous involvement (stage IB and IIA) have a median survival of 21.5 and 15.8 years, respectively.[26] When patients have tumors or generalized erythroderma (stage IIB or IIIA) without extracutaneous disease, they have a median survival of 4.7 years.[27] Patients with extracutaneous involvement in lymph nodes or viscera (stage IVA or IVB) have a median survival of only 3.8 and 1.4 years, respectively.[24] Transformation of MF or Sézary syndrome to a large-cell lymphoma is a poor prognostic sign.[1] Median survival from transformation is only 19 months and usually occurs less than 2 years from initial diagnosis of MF. Furthermore, young African American females with aggressive MF have been shown to have a high rate of mortality; thus, more aggressive therapies, such as allogeneic transplantation, should be considered in these patients.[8]

TREATMENT

Treatment for MF and Sézary syndrome can be divided into two categories: skin-directed and systemic therapies. Skin-directed therapy includes psoralens plus ultraviolet A (PUVA) photochemotherapy, ultraviolet B (UVB) phototherapy, topical therapy, and radiation therapy.

PUVA therapy is administered by taking oral 8-methoxypsoralens, which become activated when exposed to ultraviolet A (UVA) radiation in the 330- to 365-nm range. This drug can inhibit DNA and RNA synthesis by the formation of thymine adducts in the presence of UVA radiation. During the clearing phase, treatment is given three times per week, followed by a maintenance phase that ranges from once a week to once a month. PUVA therapy is generally restricted to patients with stage I and IIA disease. Side effects include nausea and actinic damage from UVA exposure, but PUVA is generally well tolerated.

A widely used skin-directed therapy is UVB phototherapy. Although broadband UVB was used in the past, currently, narrowband UVB (NB-UVB; 311 to 313 nm) is the most commonly used form. Advantages of NB-UVB compared with PUVA is its ease of administration, the lack of the acute side effect of nausea, and a much lower risk of actinic damage. However, because UVA used in PUVA does penetrate deeper into the skin compared to NB-UVB, PUVA should be strongly considered for patients with very dark skin and thick lesions. Treatment frequency of NB-UVB is similar to that described earlier for PUVA.

Topical therapy includes topical corticosteroids, topical retinoids, and topical chemotherapy. Topical corticosteroids frequently are used as adjunctive treatment along with PUVA or NB-UVB. The most widely used topical retinoid is bexarotene gel, applied one to four times daily. It causes significant irritation, which may limit the frequency of its application. Furthermore, it is cost prohibitive for most patients. Topical chemotherapy includes nitrogen mustard (mechlorethamine) and carmustine. Topical nitrogen mustard therapy is applied daily in solution or ointment form. However, at the time of this writing, the nitrogen mustard powder that is needed to prepare the solution is no longer available in the U.S. market, and a new formula of nitrogen mustard gel is now available. Major side effects include irritant and contact dermatitis and, rarely, squamous cell carcinomas and basal cell carcinomas. Topical carmustine has efficacy similar to nitrogen mustard but is associated with bone marrow suppression in some patients.

Radiation therapy is effective in treating CTCL, with localized radiation therapy for localized thick plaques or tumors and electron-beam radiation for generalized disease. Myelosuppression generally does not occur because less than 5% of the dose is delivered beyond 2 cm of the surface. Electron-beam therapy has response rates of 56% to 96% for stage IA to IIA disease, but it has a high relapse rate if no adjuvant therapy is given subsequently.[1] This therapy is used most often in MF patients with diffuse skin involvement, consisting of thick plaques and tumors, and patients with Sézary syndrome. Side effects include erythema, pain, swelling, hair and nail loss, and loss of sweat gland function. Most of these side effects are reversible, but telangiectasias and xerosis are the most common chronic adverse effects.

Extracorporeal photopheresis is a systemic therapy for CTCL in which patients' leukocytes are exposed extracorporeally to 8-methoxypsoralen and UVA and then returned to the patient. The reinfused cells stimulate a selective immune response against the malignant cells. This therapy is performed on 2 consecutive days every 2 to 4 weeks, after which maintenance therapy is given less often. Recent studies have found response rates ranging from 33% to 88% in patients with clinical stage IA to IIA disease.[27] However, because this is a treatment of circulating leukocytes, patients with peripheral blood involvement, particularly with Sézary syndrome with near-normal CD8 counts, and a short duration of advanced disease are the appropriate candidates for this treatment. Photopheresis has been used in conjunction with methotrexate, interferon-α, or oral bexarotene.

Systemic chemotherapy can be used in patients with refractory disease. Single-agent therapy can induce remission, but relapses are common. Agents showing the best results include methotrexate, pralatrexate, cyclophosphamide, cisplatin, etoposide, fludarabine, deoxycoformycin, bleomycin, doxorubicin, vincristine, and vinblastine. Combination chemotherapy also can be used for refractory disease but does not alter mortality when compared with skin-directed therapy or single-agent chemotherapy.[28]

Interferon-α (INF-α) is a commonly used agent in treating MF. In previously untreated patients with all stages of MF and Sézary syndrome, there is an overall response rate of 79%.[1] Adverse effects include fever, chills, myalgias, weight loss, and depression. Leukopenia, thrombocytopenia, and abnormal liver function tests also can occur.

Other novel, more targeted drug therapies are emerging such as histone deacetylase inhibitors, including vorinostat and romidepsin. This class of drugs prevents removal of acetyl modification to lysine residues, leading to a more open chromatin structure, which affects gene expression. They have been shown to cause cultured cancer cells to undergo arrest of growth, terminal differentiation, and apoptosis.[27] Other targeted novel therapies include pralatrexate and forodesine, which disrupt key enzymes in the gene synthesis of rapidly proliferating cancer cells.

HYPOPIGMENTED MYCOSIS FUNGOIDES

Several unique observations have been reported in patients with skin of color who have MF. As mentioned previously, the incidence and mortality rate of MF are higher in African Americans compared with Caucasians. Protection of the skin by melanin may allow tumor cells to avoid the therapeutic effects of natural UV light from the sun, which may be responsible for MF usually sparing sun-exposed areas. Unchecked, these cells may advance to tumors, which are more common in African Americans.

Hypopigmented MF is a unique clinical entity that is distinct from the hypopigmentation observed in resolving MF or MF associated with poikiloderma. Although early phases of MF most often present as erythematous, scaly plaques, it also can present with hypopigmented macules or patches with sharp borders and no erythema or scale, particularly in patients with skin of color.[29-31] Hypopigmented lesions can be the only manifestation of MF, or they can be associated with erythematous plaques or tumors. The age of onset is lower in patients with hypopigmented MF than in those who present with typical erythematous, scaly plaques. In addition, these patients tend to have a slower progression of their disease.

Histologically, the most consistent features of hypopigmented MF are reduced melanin granules in basal keratinocytes and melanocytes and lymphocytic epidermotropism.[16] Other features include Pautrier microabscesses and atypical cells.

The pathogenesis of hypopigmented MF remains unclear. In patients who possess a CD8+ phenotype, hypopigmentation may be due to the cytotoxic effect of atypical T-cells on melanocytes. Using electron microscopy, Breathnach et al[3] found abnormalities in the melanocytes, including swelling of cytoplasmic organelles, loss of mitochondrial cristae, dilatation of the rough endoplasmic reticulum, and cytoplasmic vacuolation. They found evidence of disordered melanogenesis, including the production of spherical, incompletely melanized melanosomes. These changes appeared to be a nonspecific response to cell injury associated with inflammation and may be due to ischemia secondary to disruption of epidermal architecture by edema.

The differential diagnosis of hypopigmented MF includes vitiligo, tinea versicolor, postinflammatory hypopigmentation, leprosy, pityriasis lichenoides chronica, and pityriasis alba. Biopsy is needed to correctly diagnose hypopigmented MF.

Hypopigmented MF usually responds well to PUVA or NB-UVB therapy,[31,32] but topical nitrogen mustard and carmustine also can induce complete remission and repigmentation.[30,33] Poor prognostic factors include association of hypopigmented macules with erythematous plaques or tumors and extensive body surface area involvement,[32] because these patients tend to relapse after therapy. Because most reported patients with hypopigmented MF have stage I disease without lymph node involvement, the prognosis is generally good.

ACKNOWLEDGMENTS

The authors would like to thank Halliday Craige McDonald for her contributions to the previous edition of this chapter.

REFERENCES

1. Siegel RS, Pandolfino T, Guitart J, et al. Primary cutaneous T-cell lymphoma: review and current concepts. *J Clin Oncol.* 2000;18:2908-2925.
2. Price NM, Fuks ZY, Hoffman TE. Hyperkeratotic and verrucous features of mycosis fungoides. *Arch Dermatol.* 1977;113:57.
3. Breathnach SM, McKee PH, Smith NP. Hypopigmented mycosis fungoides: report of five cases with ultrastructural observations. *Br J Dermatol.* 1982;106:643-649.
4. Weinstock MA, Horm JW. Mycosis fungoides in the United States: increasing incidence and descriptive epidemiology. *JAMA.* 1988;260:42-46.
5. Weinstock MA, Gardstein B. Twenty-year trends in the reported incidence of mycosis fungoides and associated mortality. *Am J Public Health.* 1999;89:1240-1244.
6. Weinstock MA, Reynes JF. The changing survival of patients with mycosis fungoides: a population-based assessment of trends in the United States. *Cancer.* 1999;85:208-212.
7. Criscione VD, Weinstock MA. Incidence of cutaneous T-cell lymphoma in the United States, 1973–2002. *Arch Dermatol.* 2007;143:854-859.
8. Sun G, Berthelot C, Li Y, et al. Poor prognosis in non-Caucasian patients with early-onset mycosis fungoides. *J Am Acad Dermatol.* 2009;60:231-235.
9. Herrick C, Heald P. Advances in clinical research: the dynamic interplay of malignant and benign T-cells in cutaneous T-cell lymphoma. *Dermatol Clin.* 1997;15:149-157.
10. Rook A, Heald P. The immunopathogenesis of cutaneous T-cell lymphoma. *Hematol Oncol Clin.* 1995;9:997-1010.
11. Drummer R, Posseckert G, Nestle F, et al. Soluble interleukin 2 receptors inhibit interleukin 2-dependent proliferation and cytotoxicity: Explanation for diminished natural killer cell activity in cutaneous T-cell lymphomas in vivo? *J Invest Dermatol.* 1992;98:50-54.
12. Hoppe RT, Medeiros LJ, Warnke RA, et al. CD8-positive tumor infiltrating lymphocytes influence the long-term survival of patients with mycosis fungoides. *J Am Acad Dermatol.* 1995;32:448-455.
13. Heald PW, Rook A, Perez M, et al. Treatment of erythrodermic cutaneous T-cell lymphoma patients with photopheresis. *J Am Acad Dermatol.* 1992;27:427-433.
14. Hallermann C, Niermann C, Fischer RJ, Schulze HJ. Erythrocyte sedimentation rate as an independent prognostic factor in mycosis fungoides. *Br J Dermatol.* 2012;166:873-874.
15. Izban KF, Hsi ED, Alkan S. Immunohistochemical analysis of mycosis fungoides on paraffin-embedded tissue sections. *Mod Pathol.* 1998;11:978-982.
16. Ralfkiaer E, Wollf-Sneedorff A, Thomsen K, et al. Immunophenotypic studies in cutaneous T-cell lymphomas: clinical implications. *Br J Dermatol.* 1993;129:655-659.
17. El Shabrawi-Caelen L, Cerroni L, Medeiros LJ, et al. Hypopigmented mycosis fungoides: frequent expression of a CD8+ T-cell phenotype. *Am J Surg Pathol.* 2002;26:450-457.
18. Whittemore AS, Holly EA, Lee IM, et al. Mycosis fungoides in relation to environmental exposures and immune response: a case-control study. *J Natl Cancer Inst.* 1989;81:1560.
19. Bonin S, Tothova SM, Barbazza R, Brunetti D, Stanta G, Trevisan G. Evidence of multiple infectious agents in mycosis fungoides lesions. *Exp Mol Pathol.* 2010;89:46-50.
20. Hall WW, Liu CR, Schneewind O, et al. Deleted HTLV-I provirus in blood and cutaneous lesions of patients with mycosis fungoides. *Science.* 1991;253:317-320.
21. Wood GS, Salvekar A, Schaffer J, et al. Evidence against a role for human T-cell lymphotrophic virus type I (HTLV-I) in the pathogenesis of American cutaneous T-cell lymphoma. *J Invest Dermatol.* 1996;107:301-307.
22. Hoppe RT, Wood GS, Abel EA. Mycosis fungoides and the Sézary syndrome: pathology, staging, and treatment. *Curr Prob Cancer.* 1990;14:293-371.
23. Habif TP. *Clinical Dermatology.* 4th ed. St Louis, MO: Mosby; 2004.
24. Zackheim HS, McCalmont TH. Mycosis fungoides: the great imitator. *J Am Acad Dermatol.* 2002;47:914-918.
25. Olsen E, Vonderheid E, Pimpinelli N, et al. Revisions to the staging and classification of mycosis fungoides and Sézary syndrome: a proposal of the International Society for Cutaneous Lymphomas (ISCL) and the cutaneous lymphoma task force of the European Organization of Research and Treatment of Cancer (EORTC). *Blood.* 2007;110:1713-1722.
26. Agar NS, Wedgeworth E, Crichton S, et al. Survival outcomes and prognostic factors in mycosis fungoides/Sézary syndrome: validation of the revised International Society for Cutaneous Lymphomas/European

Organisation for Research and Treatment of Cancer staging proposal. *J Clin Oncol.* 2010;28:4730-4739.

27. Lansigan F, Foss FM. Current and emerging treatment strategies for cutaneous T-cell lymphoma. *Drugs.* 2010;70:273-286.

28. Kaye FJ, Bunn PA Jr, Steinberg SM, et al. A randomized trial comparing combination electron-beam radiation and chemotherapy with topical therapy in the initial treatment of mycosis fungoides. *N Engl J Med.* 1989;321:1784-1790.

29. Ryan EA, Sanderson KV, Bartak P, et al. Can mycosis fungoides begin in the epidermis? A hypothesis. *Br J Dermatol.* 1973;88:419-429.

30. Stone ML, Styles AR, Cockerell CJ, et al. Hypopigmented mycosis fungoides: a report of 7 cases and review of the literature. *Cutis.* 2001;67:133-138.

31. Lambroza E, Cohen SR, Phelps R, et al. Hypopigmented variant of mycosis fungoides: demography, histopathology, and treatment of seven cases. *J Am Acad Dermatol.* 1995;32:987-993.

32. Ratnam KV, Pang BK. Clinicopathological study and five-year follow-up of 10 cases of hypopigmented mycosis fungoides. *J Eur Acad Dermatol Venereol.* 1994;3:505-510.

33. Zackheim HS, Epstein EH, Grekin DA, et al. Mycosis fungoides presenting as areas of hypopigmentation: a report of three cases. *J Am Acad Dermatol.* 1982;6:340-345.

CHAPTER

48

Disorders of Hypopigmentation

Ife J. Rodney
Justine Park
Doris Hexsel
Rebat M. Halder

KEY POINTS

- Hypopigmentation disorders are the third most common reason for patients with skin of color to seek dermatologic treatment. Dermatologists should know how to recognize and treat these conditions, with special sensitivity to their psychological aspects.

- The causes of hypopigmentation can be divided into two categories based on the pathogenesis: melanopenic and melanocytopenic. The causes can also be congenital or acquired.

- Hypopigmentation disorders can often be treated successfully with topical, oral, surgical, light- or laser-based techniques, either alone or in combination.

INTRODUCTION

Hypopigmentation and depigmentation disorders can be divided into two categories based on their pathogenesis: melanopenic or melanocytopenic. The melanopenic category refers to disorders of melanin pigment production by the melanocytes, whereas the melanocytopenic category refers to disorders that lead to a reduction in the numbers, or the complete absence, of melanocytes. Clinically, melanocytopenic macules are milky-white, due to the reflection of incident light. Under Wood lamp skin examination, they appear stark white in contrast to the surrounding skin. The skin undergoing melanopenic processes can be various degrees lighter than the normal skin color.

There are a number of disorders of hypopigmentation and depigmentation that are clinically relevant. Those that will be discussed in this chapter are tinea versicolor (TV), idiopathic guttate hypomelanosis (IGH), pityriasis alba (PA), postinflammatory hypopigmentation (PIH), piebaldism, and progressive macular hypomelanosis (PMH).

The incidence of some of these conditions, such as PA, is increased in individuals with skin of color, whereas others occur equally in Caucasians and those with skin of color. Hypopigmentation disorders are the third most common reason for patients with skin of color to seek dermatologic treatment.[1] These disorders are of great concern because of the marked contrast between the affected and normal skin, and they can be psychologically devastating. Dermatologists should know how to recognize and treat these conditions, with special sensitivity to their psychosocial effects on patients.

TINEA VERSICOLOR

CLINICAL FEATURES

TV, caused by the fungus *Pityrosporum ovale* (also known as *Microsporum furfur, Malassezia furfur,* or *Pityrosporum orbiculare*), is a superficial infection with a distinctive clinical appearance. It manifests as hypopigmented or hyperpigmented slightly scaly macules and patches that are an ivory to tan color and up to several centimeters in diameter. The lesions predominantly affect the sebaceous areas of the trunk, arms, neck, and face [**Figure 48-1**]. Patients sometimes present with follicular hypopigmentation, although there is no racial predilection [**Figure 48-2**].[2] The dyschromia that results from the infection is often more apparent in individuals with skin of color because of a greater contrast between the dyschromia and the patient's dark skin.

PATHOGENESIS

TV is classified as a melanopenic as well as melanocytopenic disorder. *P. ovale* is known to produce lipoxygenases that act on surface lipids, leading to the oxidization of oleic acid to azelaic acid. This dicarboxylic acid has been shown to inhibit tyrosinase and damage the melanocytes in tissue cultures.[3] It is also known that *P. ovale* acts on unsaturated fatty acids to produce lipoperoxidases. It is theorized that these lipoperoxidases are toxic to melanocytes and lead to depigmentation. In addition, ultrastructural studies have shown that the melanosomes in TV lesions are abnormally small.[4-6] Other authors postulate that the dispersion of ultraviolet (UV) light by a lipid-like material in the stratum corneum is responsible for the hypopigmentation.[7] Although the exact mechanism by which hypopigmentation occurs is unknown, it is certain that this effect is a result of an infection with *P. ovale*. The eradication of the organism results in repigmentation; however, this process is gradual and may take months for some patients.

HISTOLOGY

Histologic changes are mild and consist of hyperkeratosis and mild acanthosis. In the superficial dermis, a slight perivascular lymphohistiocytic infiltrate may be present. The stratum corneum contains round budding yeast and short septate hyphae. In the hypopigmented lesions of TV, there is a decreased pigmentation of the basal layer, with reduced numbers of smaller melanosomes in both the melanocytes and keratinocytes.[8]

DIAGNOSIS

If the diagnosis is in question, using a potassium hydroxide (KOH) preparation on the skin can be confirmatory; the skin will have a 'spaghetti and meatballs' appearance, representing the hyphae and spores. Physicians can also perform a Wood lamp examination, where a positive result will result in the hypopigmented skin having a greenish hue [**Figure 48-3**].

TREATMENT

Treatment can be initiated with topical antifungal shampoos, creams, or lotions that include selenium sulfide, terbinafine, or imidazoles. Alternatively, pulsed systemic antifungal therapy with oral ketoconazole, fluconazole, or itraconazole may be used. Oral terbinafine is not effective. Patients should be informed that recurrence is common and that the repigmentation process can be slow. Monthly prophylactic doses may be helpful for patients who have relapsed. A common regimen is the use of 2.5% selenium sulfide lotion or 2% ketoconazole shampoo applied to the affected area for 10 to 15 minutes before rinsing. This is usually implemented daily for a week and then followed by weekly maintenance applications for a month. Thereafter, a monthly maintenance application

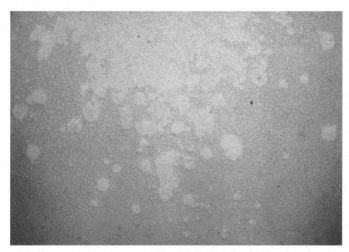

FIGURE 48-1. Tinea versicolor on the trunk of a patient with skin of color.

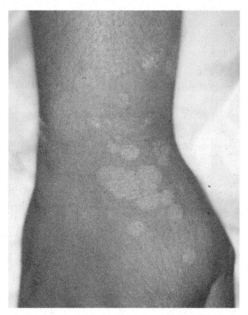

FIGURE 48-2. Tinea versicolor with follicular hypopigmentation on the hand of a patient with skin of color.

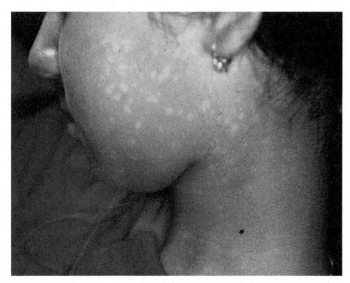

FIGURE 48-3. Tinea versicolor on the face and neck of a patient with skin of color. Under Wood lamp skin examination, the hypopigmented skin is fluorescent with a greenish hue.

is often successful. Persistent PIH can be treated with topical or oral psoralen plus ultraviolet A (PUVA) light or tar emulsion therapy.

IDIOPATHIC GUTTATE HYPOMELANOSIS

CLINICAL FEATURES

IGH is a very common acquired leukoderma of unknown etiology that occurs in individuals with all Fitzpatrick skin types, but is more apparent in those with darker skin of color.[9] The number of lesions increases with the patient's age, and IGH is more common in patients over the age of 70 years. In one study, 80% of the 452 IGH patients examined were 70 years old or older.[10] An apparent female predominance is possibly the result of a heightened cosmetic concern among women which may lead to more women seeking treatment for the condition as opposed to men.

Typically, the lesions are small, multiple, symmetric, discrete, circumscribed, and asymptomatic porcelain-white macules.[11] They are usually located on the extensor surfaces of the patient's arms and legs [**Figures 48-4 and 48-5**]. IGH occasionally affects an individual's trunk and, rarely, their face. The surface is smooth and is not scaly or atrophic. The lesions are usually 0.5 to 6 mm in diameter, but in some cases, they may be up to 2.5 cm. Once formed, the lesions do not enlarge or coalesce,[12] and spontaneous repigmentation has not been observed. Vellus hair within the lesions is usually not depigmented.[13]

PATHOGENESIS

The exact pathogenesis of IGH is unclear, but genetic factors, trauma, and autoimmunity have been suggested as potential causative factors. IGH is classified as both a melanopenic and melanocytopenic process. There is decreased tyrosinase activity and staining of melanin,[11,14,15] as well as a decreased number of melanocytes, which is demonstrated by electronic microscopy.[11] There seem to be two main forms of IGH:

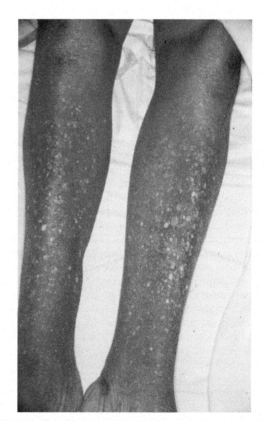

FIGURE 48-4. Idiopathic guttate hypomelanosis is a very common acquired leukoderma of unknown etiology that occurs in patients of all races and skin types but is more apparent in individuals with skin of color. The photograph shows a case of idiopathic guttate hypomelanosis on the legs of a patient with skin of color.

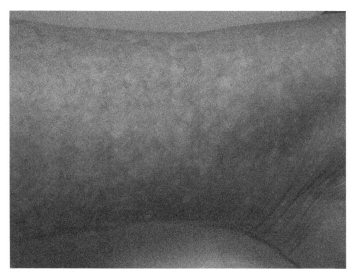

FIGURE 48-5. A Latina woman with skin of color displaying idiopathic guttate hypomelanosis on the ankle. (Used with permission from Marcia Ramos-e-Silva, School of Medicine and University Hospital, Federal University of Rio De Janeiro, Brazil.)

(1) actinic IGH, in which sunlight is thought to play a role because the lesions are most commonly distributed over sun-exposed areas of the body, and (2) hereditary IGH, which affects individuals with darker skin of color on sun-protected areas like the trunk. The role of ultraviolet light in the pathogenesis of IGH is supported by a study by Kaya et al,[16] in which a patient with mycosis fungoides developed widespread IGH during narrow-band ultraviolet B (NB-UVB) therapy.

HISTOLOGY

The histology of IGH shows that there is a flattening of the dermal-epidermal junction, with a marked reduction of melanin granules in the basal and suprabasal layers. The melanin granules that are present are irregularly distributed.[11] There is also a significant reduction in the number of 3,4-dihydroxyphenylalanine (dopa)-positive melanocytes.[17]

TREATMENT

Treatment is not necessary, although the appearance of the IGH lesions is a common concern for many patients, particularly those with skin of color. Patients should be reassured that the lesions usually remain small in size and do not coalesce. Because sun exposure may be a precipitating factor for individuals with IGH, sunbathing is discouraged and sunscreens and physical barriers should be used. Unfortunately, there is no consistently effective treatment yet available; however, options include cryotherapy, intralesional corticosteroids, topical calcineurin inhibitors, topical and oral PUVA, skin grafts, and localized superficial dermabrasion.[18-20] Cosmetic camouflage products can also be used to conceal the lesions.

Cryotherapy is the most frequently used treatment for patients with IGH. It is thought that the irritation and inflammation of the epidermis by cryotherapy stimulate a subsequent migration of melanocytes from the surrounding normally pigmented skin.[19] Because melanocytes are sensitive to freezing by liquid nitrogen, the risk of leukoderma, as well as postinflammatory hyperpigmentation, should be discussed with the patient. However, it has been shown that 3 to 5 seconds of cryotherapy with liquid nitrogen can be effective in treating IGH.[21] In a study by Ploysangam et al,[19] IGH lesions were frozen with liquid nitrogen. A histologic examination of the repigmenting lesions was then performed, which demonstrated the reappearance of dopa-positive melanocytes. The number of dopa-positive melanocytes was significantly greater in the repigmented areas than in the untreated lesions but was still decreased in comparison to normal skin.[19]

Hexsel[20] showed that localized dermabrasion was an effective, safe, fast, and inexpensive treatment modality. It does not require anesthesia,

and patients are able to immediately return to their regular activities. The objective is to put pressure on the dermabrader, so that it reaches the papillary dermis, without causing bleeding. It is then recommended that the skin be exposed to sunlight after the procedure. This stimulates a migration of melanocytes from the follicular epithelium to the healing skin, favoring repigmentation.[20]

Falabella et al[10] described the treatment of IGH with skin grafts and intralesional triamcinolone; this treatment had limited success, although the follow-up evaluations did not extend beyond 6 months. Also, in some cases, when normally pigmented skin was grafted onto the IGH lesions, the grafts then also became depigmented.[10]

PITYRIASIS ALBA

CLINICAL FEATURES

Pityriasis alba (PA) was first described by Fox[22] in 1923 and is a common self-limiting eczematous disorder. It presents as multiple, hypopigmented, round to oval patches with indistinct margins and fine white scales, usually occurring on an individual's face, neck, and trunk [**Figures 48-6 and 48-7**].[23] PA mostly affects young children and adolescents of all races, but it is most common in children with Fitzpatrick skin types IV to VI, as well as children of Hispanic or Asian origin.[24] Both genders are equally affected. This condition is more noticeable in those with darker skin of color and becomes more apparent during the summer months.

The relationship between PA and atopic dermatitis was first suggested by Watkins[25] in 1961, and PA is now regarded as a minor feature of atopic dermatitis. In the general population, the prevalence is estimated at 1%, but for atopic individuals, it is 32%.[26]

Initially, lesions consist of erythematous macules or patches, which then fade over a few weeks, and result in ill-defined hypopigmented patches with a whitish, dry, scaly surface. The border of these lesions may be slightly raised and erythematous. However, most patients present after the erythema has already faded and they are left with the

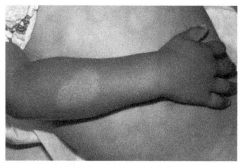

A

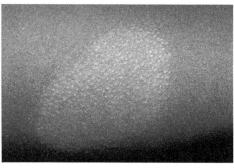

B

FIGURE 48-6. Pityriasis alba on the arm of a child with skin of color, from (**A**) afar and (**B**) close-up. Pityriasis alba is a common eczematous disorder that presents as multiple, hypopigmented, round to oval patches with indistinct margins and a fine white scale. It is more noticeable in children with darker skin of color.

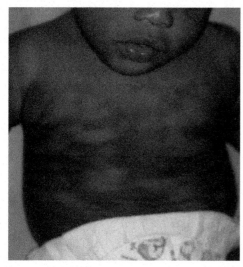

FIGURE 48-7. Pityriasis alba on the body of an infant. This condition affects young children and adolescents of all races but is most common in patients with Fitzpatrick skin types IV to VI.

remaining hypopigmentation with scaling. Although PA is generally asymptomatic, some patients complain of mild pruritus or burning. Lesions are frequently symmetrically distributed on the malar region of the face and vary in size from 5 to 30 mm. Less often, they may be found on the upper extremities and shoulders. A follicular accentuation, especially on the arms, is often seen. Although most patients have only two or three lesions, some can have as many as 20 lesions.

There are several variations of PA. Extensive PA consists of widespread and symmetric involvement of the skin on the trunk by numerous round, nonscaly hypopigmented patches.[27,28] It is an asymptomatic dermatosis that is usually seen in adults. Because there is no preceding erythema and patients give no history of atopy, some authors consider this to be a distinct entity.

Pigmenting PA may present as bluish hyperpigmentation surrounded by scaly hypopigmentation. The bluish pigment is due to the melanin deposition in the dermis. These lesions appear on the face; in up to 65% of affected patients, they may be associated with a superficial dermatophyte infection.[29]

PATHOGENESIS

The pathogenesis of PA is unclear, but several mechanisms have been proposed. It may be best characterized as an eczematous dermatitis related to atopy,[30,31] which results in hypomelanosis after the inflammation has subsided. This hypomelanosis may be related to an impaired pigment transfer from melanocytes to keratinocytes. Also, light and electron microscopy demonstrate a reduced number of melanocytes and a decrease in the size and number of melanosomes, within both melanocytes and keratinocytes.[32]

Xerosis, which may result from frequent bathing and hot showers, is often associated with both PA and atopic dermatitis.[27] This is explained by the reduced water-holding capacity of the stratum corneum in PA compared with healthy skin.[33]

Other proposed mechanisms include nutritional and vitamin deficiencies.[26,34,35] In particular, it has been shown that patients with PA have low serum levels of copper,[36] which is a cofactor for the enzyme tyrosinase, needed for melanin synthesis. Therefore, a copper deficiency may play a role in this condition.

HISTOLOGY

Histologically, the appearance of PA is nonspecific, showing a chronic spongiotic dermatitis with a disruption of melanin pigmentation in the skin's basal layer.[32]

DIAGNOSIS AND DIFFERENTIAL DIAGNOSIS

PA can imitate an array of other inflammatory skin conditions that are associated with PIH. However, these can usually be easily distinguished based on their clinical presentation, a histologic examination, or simple procedures like KOH preparation or the use of a Wood lamp skin examination.

The differential diagnosis includes TV, tinea faciei, vitiligo, nevus depigmentosus, nevus anemicus, hypopigmented mycosis fungoides and hypopigmentation secondary to leprosy, nummular eczema, psoriasis, or the use of topical corticosteroids. When lesions are extrafacial, pityriasis lichenoides chronica should be considered.

TREATMENT

PA is a self-limiting disease that usually remains stable for months or years but then resolves spontaneously at puberty. However, treatment should be attempted, particularly in those with darker skin of color, because the hypopigmentation may be striking. Treatment involves gentle skin care and emollients such as petroleum jelly or 12% ammonium lactate lotion, which lessens the dryness and irritation of the skin. Patients should also be advised to avoid hot baths and to limit their sun exposure, in order to minimize the disparity between the color of their affected and nonaffected skin.

Other reportedly effective modalities include those used to stimulate melanogenesis, such as tar emulsions, topical steroids, and topical or oral PUVA. Tar emulsions, applied twice daily, may be very beneficial, because tar alone is melanogenic without the addition of UV light.[37] It is available commercially as a 6% cream and may also be compounded as 5% liquor carbonis detergens in a variety of vehicles, such as acid mantle cream, or in combination with a low-potency topical steroid. Patients, particularly children, should be cautious of sun exposure with the use of tar-containing products.

Topical corticosteroids, with low potency for the face and medium potency for the body, have been used with some success. Because PA is considered a mild eczematous dermatitis, it is logical that topical corticosteroids may relieve the pruritus and inflammation associated with the disorder. As always, physicians must weigh the risks and benefits of any therapy before initiating the treatment, keeping in mind that children are more susceptible to the effects of topical medications.

Topical and oral PUVA are treatment alternatives for PA.[32] Patients are usually treated with topical PUVA once every week. The patient is exposed to UVA light at a starting dose of 0.5 J approximately 30 minutes after the application of 0.1% methoxsalen cream. This dose is then increased by 0.3 J on a weekly basis until repigmentation occurs; however, this must be before there is any resulting erythema or burning of the lesions. Oral PUVA is used for more widespread lesions.

Another treatment option is 311-nm NB-UVB phototherapy, which may be used with starting doses varying from 75 to 200 mJ/cm[2], depending on the skin phototype. This is subsequently increased by 20% at each treatment. The treatments are usually given two to three times per week.

Topical calcineurin inhibitors such as pimecrolimus and tacrolimus are a further therapeutic option for treating PA.[38]

POSTINFLAMMATORY HYPOPIGMENTATION

CLINICAL FEATURES

PIH is a common end result of cutaneous inflammation. This normal biological response in human skin is more noticeable and distressing in individuals with darker skin of color, and it accounts for a significant number of visits to dermatologists. Many conditions can lead to PIH, including papulosquamous diseases such as atopic dermatitis, seborrheic dermatitis, and psoriasis; vesiculobullous disorders; inflammatory diseases such as acne, lichen planus, and pityriasis lichenoides chronica; connective tissue diseases such as lupus erythematosus; and mycosis fungoides [**Figures 48-8 to 48-10**]. The size and shape of the hypopigmented lesions usually correlate with the distribution and configuration

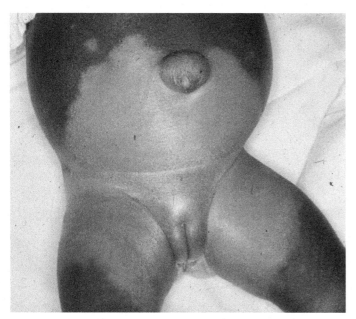

FIGURE 48-8. Postinflammatory hypopigmentation secondary to diaper dermatitis in an infant with darker skin of color.

of the original inflammatory dermatosis, and the color ranges from hypopigmentation to depigmentation. Complete depigmentation can be seen in cases of severe atopic dermatitis and discoid lupus erythematosus. At times, pigmentary changes can coexist with the original inflammatory lesions, which makes the diagnosis straightforward. However, in some conditions, the inflammatory phase is not always present, and the hypopigmentation may be the only feature. Thus, repeated examinations are required to identify the primary inflammatory dermatosis.

PIH can sometimes be seen after the use of therapeutic interventions such as topical retinoids, benzoyl peroxide, liquid nitrogen, and laser therapies, or after trauma to the skin. Minimal hypopigmentation usually resolves within a few weeks, but severe cases of hypopigmentation and depigmentation may be permanent, or it may take years for the repigmentation process to occur.

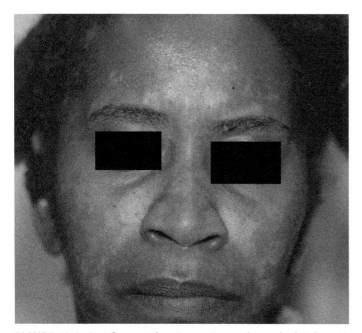

FIGURE 48-9. Postinflammatory hypopigmentation secondary to seborrheic dermatitis on the face of a patient with darker skin of color.

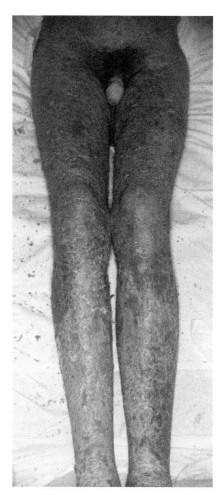

FIGURE 48-10. Postinflammatory hypopigmentation secondary to psoriasis in a male with darker skin of color.

■ PATHOGENESIS

The variation in individuals' responses to cutaneous inflammation or trauma is not well understood. Melanocytes can react with an increased, normal, or decreased melanin production rate in response to cutaneous inflammation or trauma. In cases of PIH, there is a decrease in the melanin production rate, resulting in clinically apparent light areas.[39] Melanogenesis is a complex process, which includes melanin synthesis, transport, and release to keratinocytes. It is controlled by multiple cytokines and inflammatory mediators (such as interferon-γ, tumor necrosis factor [TNF]-α, TNF-β, and interleukin [IL]-6 and IL-7) acting on the melanocytes, keratinocytes, and fibroblasts. Through the release of these mediators, cutaneous inflammation may cause an aberration of melanogenesis.[40,41] Other proposed theories for the loss or blockage of the melanosome transfer process include epidermal edema and rapid cell turnover.

There may also be a melanocyte cell-surface expression of intercellular adhesion molecule-1 induced by these inflammatory mediators. The theory is that this may lead to leukocyte-melanocyte attachments, with the final result being the destruction of 'innocent bystander' melanocytes. The severe inflammation leading to the death of melanocytes may result in permanent pigmentary changes.

■ HISTOLOGY

The histopathologic findings are nonspecific and include decreased epidermal melanin, mild superficial lymphohistiocytic infiltrate, and melanophages in the upper dermis. There may also be histologic evidence of the underlying disorder. Even specimens that show nonspecific findings are useful in that they may exclude many dermatoses that present with hypopigmentation, such as sarcoidosis, leprosy, and mycosis fungoides.

DIAGNOSIS AND DIFFERENTIAL DIAGNOSIS

The diagnosis for PIH is generally based on a patient's history and physical examination. PIH can be distinguished from melanocytopenic conditions, such as vitiligo and piebaldism, with the use of a Wood lamp. In these melanocytopenic diseases, the hypopigmentation is accentuated with the Wood lamp. However, this technique is sometimes not helpful in patients with skin of color due to optical factors.[42]

The differential diagnosis of PIH also includes PA, PMH, pityriasis versicolor, leprosy, sarcoidosis, a hypopigmented variant of mycosis fungoides, and hypopigmentation from medication, especially potent topical corticosteroids and intralesional corticosteroids. These conditions can be differentiated by their clinical findings (such as epidermal changes, induration, the presence of scales, and the lesions' distribution) and a histopathologic examination.[43,44]

TREATMENT

The identification and treatment of the underlying cause of the hypopigmentation are imperative in preventing further dyschromia in PIH patients. As long as the inflammation persists, repigmentation is difficult. Once this process is controlled, the stimulation of melanogenesis can be attempted. The treatment modalities for PIH include topical corticosteroids, topical immunomodulators such as tacrolimus and pimecrolimus, cosmetic cover-up products, and phototherapy with topical or oral PUVA or NB-UVB light. For topical PUVA, 8-methoxypsoralen is applied to the hypopigmented skin at concentrations of 0.1% or lower. The patient is exposed to the UVA light at a starting dose of 0.5 J/cm² approximately 30 minutes after application. The dose is then increased by 0.5 J/cm² at every treatment. Oral PUVA is used when the lesions are more generalized. Oral 8-methoxsalen (MOP) is given at a dose of 0.3 mg/kg, and treatments are administered twice weekly. The initial dose of UVA is usually 0.5 to 1.0 J/cm². NB-UVB phototherapy is administered twice weekly; with starting doses varying from 75 to 100 mJ/cm². The dose is then increased by 10% to 20% with each treatment. For all of the previously described treatments, the dose of phototherapy is gradually increased until minimal asymptomatic erythema occurs. Another treatment option is skin grafting, although the efficacy of this treatment is variable.[45]

PIEBALDISM

CLINICAL FEATURES

Piebaldism is a rare autosomal dominant disorder that affects 1 in 20,000 people worldwide. Although the exact prevalence is unknown, individuals of all races and genders are affected. The most characteristic manifestation of piebaldism is the white forelock, which is present at birth and may be the only sign in most patients;[46] approximately 80% to 90% of affected individuals have this manifestation. All of the hair strands in the forelock, along with the underlying skin, are depigmented. Located on the anterior midline scalp, the forelock is symmetrical and may have a triangular or diamond shape [**Figure 48-11A**]. In severe cases of piebaldism, the medial third of the eyebrows and eyelashes may also be depigmented.[47]

Another characteristic manifestation of piebaldism is nonprogressive leukoderma, distributed on the central forehead, central anterior trunk, and anterior mid-extremities [**Figure 48-11B**]. It is irregularly shaped and presents as well-circumscribed, milk-white patches, with hyperpigmented macules and patches. These are located within the depigmented skin and also on the adjacent normal skin. This leukoderma may extend from the abdomen to the flanks, but it usually does not appear on the mid-back. The hands and feet are also often spared, unlike in vitiligo; therefore, this is the main differential diagnosis.

Most patients are otherwise healthy and have no systemic symptoms, but piebaldism may rarely be associated with other disorders such as heterochromia iridis, Hirschsprung disease, neurofibromatosis type 1, Grover disease, and deafness.[48-51] Also, because the depigmentation of

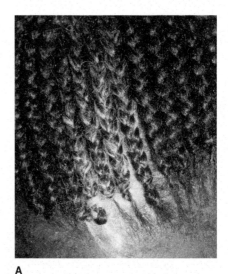

A

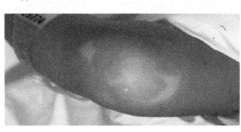

B

FIGURE 48-11. (A) Piebaldism on the forelock of a woman with darker skin of color. The white forelock, which is present at birth and may be the only sign in many patients, is the most characteristic manifestation of piebaldism. Note that both the hair strands in the forelock, and the underlying skin, are depigmented. **(B)** Another characteristic manifestation of piebaldism is nonprogressive leukoderma; here it presents as irregularly shaped, well-circumscribed, milk-white patches on the arm of a patient with skin of color.

piebaldism is striking in those with dark skin of color, there is a significant emotional burden on these patients.

DIAGNOSIS AND DIFFERENTIAL DIAGNOSIS

Diagnosis can be made based on an autosomal dominant inheritance pattern and a congenital presence of characteristic skin findings. The differential diagnosis of piebaldism consists of any condition that presents with a depigmented lesion or white forelock. This includes vitiligo, Vogt-Koyanagi-Harada syndrome, PIH, Alezzandrini syndrome, alopecia areata, tuberous sclerosis, and importantly, Waardenburg syndrome. The differential diagnosis should be further explored via ocular and auditory examinations. Less common syndromes that should also be considered are Ziprkowski-Margolis syndrome (also known as albinism-deafness syndrome or Woolf syndrome).

PATHOGENESIS

The clinical features of piebaldism can be explained by mutations in the *c-kit* proto-oncogene,[52] which is found in 75% of patients with this condition.[53] *c-kit* encodes the tyrosine kinase transmembrane receptors for the stem cell factor on the surface of melanoblasts in the neural crest.[54,55] These melanoblasts fail to proliferate, differentiate, and migrate to their residence in the skin.[56] There are numerous different mutation sites in *c-kit* that result in piebaldism of varying severity. Interestingly, a Val620Ala mutation results in a progression of the depigmented patches,[57] unlike classic piebaldism. Patients without the *c-kit* mutation have been reported to have a mutation in the *SLUG* gene, which is a zinc-finger neural crest transcription factor.[58]

HISTOLOGY

A histologic examination of piebaldism reveals an absence of melanocytes in the amelanotic skin.[59] The hyperpigmented macules within the depigmented skin and the normal adjacent skin are characterized by an abundance of melanosomes in the melanocytes and keratinocytes.[47]

TREATMENT

Piebaldism is unresponsive to the agents that are typically used for vitiligo, such as topical corticosteroids and phototherapy (PUVA or NB-UVB). The surgical techniques for treating piebaldism include autografts of the patient's normal skin into amelanotic areas, split-thickness grafts, and transplantation of autologous cultured melanocytes. These may require multiple procedures, with variable success.[60,61] More recently, Guerra et al[62] reported permanent repigmentation of piebaldism via the destruction of the amelanotic epidermis with the erbium-doped yttrium aluminium garnet (Er:YAG) laser, followed by a transplantation of autologous cultured epidermal grafts. The mean percentage of repigmentation for patients whose skin and hair had successfully repigmented was 95.45%.[16,62] In all patients, liberal sunscreen use and protection against sunburn are necessary. Also, patients with piebaldism can use cosmetic cover-up products as a means of camouflage.

PROGRESSIVE MACULAR HYPOMELANOSIS

CLINICAL FEATURES

PMH is a common skin disorder that is observed more frequently in young women with dark skin of color who originate from tropical climates. It can be seen in all individuals, but may be more noticeable in those with a dark skin color. PMH is characterized by the ill-defined hypopigmented macules that are located symmetrically on the trunk [**Figure 48-12**]. PMH rarely extends to the patient's extremities and face, neck, or proximal extremities.

In patients with PMH, there is usually no preceding pruritus, pain, or inflammation. In the majority of patients, the large hypopigmented patches (5 to 20 cm) on the front and back of the trunk originate from the central confluence of macules.[63,64] Solitary round macules are present on the lateral trunk. Under a Wood lamp, there is an accentuation of the macules, with red follicular fluorescent areas visible within the hypopigmented skin. This is absent in the adjacent normal skin and is therefore a key diagnostic sign of PMH.[64] It is thought that *Propionibacterium acnes* within the hair follicles may produce a porphyrin that causes this red follicular fluorescence.[65] Although *P. acnes* also causes acne vulgaris, preliminary analysis has shown that different subtypes of the species are related to each disease.[64]

The natural history of PMH, although not known with certainty, shows that it is a stable disease, sometimes with very slow progression

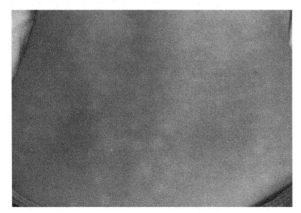

FIGURE 48-12. A Latina woman with progressive macular hypomelanosis. (Used with permission from Marcia Ramos-e-Silva, School of Medicine and University Hospital, Federal University of Rio De Janeiro, Brazil.)

over decades and spontaneous disappearance after mid-life.[64] This is supported by the observation that PMH has never been reported in the elderly.

PATHOGENESIS

The pathogenesis of PMH is unknown, although a melanopenic process is proposed. Relyveld et al[64] and Westerhof et al[65] hypothesized that a factor produced by strains of *P. acnes* interferes with the melanogenesis and subsequently causes hypopigmentation. These hypopigmented macules are located on parts of the skin that provide favorable growth conditions for *P. acnes*.[64,65]

HISTOLOGY

Histologic sections show decreased melanin content in the epidermis of lesional skin compared with the adjacent normal skin. The number of melanocytes is unchanged, and the dermis is normal.[65] Electron microscopy of patients with Fitzpatrick skin types V and VI shows a shift from large, stage IV, single melanosomes in keratinocytes from normal skin to small, stage I to III, aggregated, membrane-bound melanosomes in hypopigmented skin.[64,66,67]

DIAGNOSIS AND DIFFERENTIAL DIAGNOSIS

The diagnosis for PMH rests on a careful clinical examination and the performance of a KOH test on skin scrapings to exclude the major differential diagnosis of TV.[68] In addition, a Wood light examination for red follicular fluorescence in involved areas can be a helpful diagnostic finding.

The differential diagnosis consists of other disorders with acquired hypopigmentation, particularly on the trunk of the patient. This includes TV, seborrheic dermatitis, hypopigmented mycosis fungoides, tuberculoid or borderline tuberculoid leprosy, and PIH. Historically, extensive PA was considered in the differential for PMH, but more recently some authors have proposed that they are, indeed, the same disease.[69] However, there are some electron microscopic differences between extensive PA and PMH.[70]

TREATMENT

Several treatment modalities have been attempted, including topical and systemic antifungal agents and topical corticosteroids, all yielding poor results.[71] Relyveld et al[70] observed the successful treatment of PMH with PUVA therapy; however, after the cessation of this therapy, a recurrence of the hypopigmented lesions in the same distribution was immediately seen.[71] This can probably be explained by the temporary inhibition of *P. acnes* by PUVA, while melanogenesis was stimulated.[63] The hypothesis that *P. acnes* is the pathogenic factor in PMH was supported by a study conducted by Relyveld et al.[63] Their study showed that when both antimicrobial (benzoyl peroxide 5% hydrogel and clindamycin 1% lotion) and anti-inflammatory (fluticasone 0.05% cream) treatments were combined with UVA irradiation, the antibacterial treatment was significantly superior.[63]

The authors' recommended treatment regimen includes daily 5% benzoyl peroxide hydrogel and daily 1% clindamycin, in combination with UVB irradiation (both broadband and NB-UVB). The UVB should start at 20 J/m² twice a week for 12 weeks. Response rates vary, and maintenance treatments are recommended for patients who experience multiple recurrences over 1 year or recurrence within 3 months after the cessation of therapy.[63]

CONCLUSION

Hypopigmentation and depigmentation disorders affect individuals with all Fitzpatrick skin types. However, these conditions are often more apparent, and can be particularly distressing, for patients with darker skin of color. Hypopigmentation and depigmentation disorders include TV, IGH, PA, PIH, piebaldism, and PMH.

TV is caused by the fungus *P. ovale*. The most common treatment for TV is the application of 2.5% selenium sulfide lotion or 2% ketoconazole shampoo. Patients are to use the lotion or shampoo daily for a week and then once per week for a month. Thereafter, a once-a-month maintenance application is usually successful.

IGH is a very common acquired leukoderma and is often found in individuals over the age of 70 years. No consistently effective treatment is yet available, but the options include cryotherapy, intralesional corticosteroids, topical calcineurin inhibitors, topical and oral PUVA, skin grafts, and localized superficial dermabrasion.

PA mostly affects young children and adolescents and is more common in children with Fitzpatrick skin types IV to VI. PA treatment involves emollients such as petrolatum or 12% ammonium lactate lotion. Other reportedly effective modalities include tar emulsions, topical steroids, and topical or oral PUVA.

PIH is a common product of cutaneous inflammation and is much more noticeable in individuals with darker skin of color. It is essential that the underlying cause of the hypopigmentation is identified and treated before stimulation of melanogenesis can be attempted. The treatment modalities for PIH include topical corticosteroids, topical immunomodulators, and phototherapy.

Piebaldism is a rare autosomal dominant disorder and its most characteristic manifestation is the white forelock. This disorder is unresponsive to topical corticosteroids and phototherapy. However, physicians should note that a recent treatment that involves the destruction of the amelanotic epidermis with an Er:YAG laser, followed by transplantation of autologous cultured epidermal grafts has been successful.

PMH is more frequently found in young women with dark skin of color who originate from tropical climates. The recommended treatment for PMH includes 5% benzoyl peroxide hydrogel and 1% clindamycin, in combination with UVB irradiation.

The majority of the hypopigmentation and depigmentation disorders described in this chapter can be treated successfully; however, dermatologists should keep in mind the psychological and social effects these disorders can have on patients with darker skin of color.

REFERENCES

1. Halder RM, Nootheti PK. Ethnic skin disorders overview. *J Am Acad Dermatol.* 2003;48:S143-S148.
2. Halder RM, Nandedkar MA, Neal KW. Pigmentary disorders in ethnic skin. *Dermatol Clin.* 2003;21:617-628.
3. Nazzaro-Porro M, Passi S. Identification of tyrosinase inhibitor in culture of Pityrosporum. *J Invest Dermatol.* 1978;71:205-208.
4. Odom RB, James WD, Berger TG. Disorders resulting from fungi and yeast. In: *Andrews' Diseases of the Skin.* 9th ed. Philadelphia, PA: Saunders; 2000:388.
5. Charles CR, Sire DJ, Johnson BL, et al. Hypopigmentation in tinea versicolor: a histochemical and electron microscopic study. *Int J Dermatol.* 1973;12:48-58.
6. Karaoui R, Bou-Resli M, Al-Zaid NS, et al. Tinea versicolor: ultrastructural studies on hypopigmented and hyperpigmented skin. *Dermatologica.* 1981;162:69-85.
7. Borgers M, Cauwenbergh G, Van de Ven M, et al. Pityriasis versicolor and Pityrosporum ovale: morphogenetic and ultrastructural considerations. *Int J Dermatol.* 1987;26:586-589.
8. Galadari I, el Komy M, Mousa A, et al. Tinea versicolor: histologic and ultrastructural investigation of pigmentary changes. *Int J Dermatol.* 1992;31:253-256.
9. Falabella R. Idiopathic guttate hypomelanosis. *Dermatol Clin.* 1988;6:241-247.
10. Falabella R, Escobar C, Giraldo N, et al. On the pathogenesis of idiopathic guttate hypomelanosis. *J Am Acad Dermatol.* 1987;16:35-44.
11. Ortonne JP, Perrot H. Idiopathic guttate hypomelanosis. Ultrastructural study. *Arch Dermatol.* 1980;116:664-668.
12. Cummings KI, Cottel WI. Idiopathic guttate hypomelanosis. *Arch Dermatol.* 1966;93:184-186.
13. Bolognia JL, Pawelek JM. Biology of hypopigmentation. *J Am Acad Dermatol.* 1988;19:217-255.
14. Savall R, Ferrandiz C, Ferrer I, et al. Idiopathic guttate hypomelanosis. *Br J Dermatol.* 1980;103:635-642.
15. Wilson PD, Lavker RM, Kligman AM. On the nature of idiopathic guttate hypomelanosis. *Acta Derm Venereol.* 1982;62:301-306.
16. Kaya TI, Yazici AC, Tursen U, et al. Idiopathic guttate hypomelanosis: idiopathic or ultraviolet induced? *Photodermatol Photoimmunol Photomed.* 2005;21:270-271.
17. Wallace ML, Grichnik JM, Prieto VG, et al. Numbers and differentiation status of melanocytes in idiopathic guttate hypomelanosis. *J Cutan Pathol.* 1998;25:375-379.
18. Gilhar A, Pillar T, Eidelman S, et al. Vitiligo and idiopathic guttate hypomelanosis. Repigmentation of skin following engraftment onto nude mice. *Arch Dermatol.* 1989;125:1363-1366.
19. Ploysangam T, Dee-Ananlap S, Suvanprakorn P. Treatment of idiopathic guttate hypomelanosis with liquid nitrogen: light and electron microscopic studies. *J Am Acad Dermatol.* 1990;23:681-684.
20. Hexsel DM. Treatment of idiopathic guttate hypomelanosis by localized superficial dermabrasion. *Dermatol Surg.* 1999;25:917-918.
21. Kumarasinghe SP. 3–5 second cryotherapy is effective in idiopathic guttate hypomelanosis. *J Dermatol.* 2004;31:437-439.
22. Fox H. Partial depigmentation, chiefly on the face, in Negro children. *Arch Dermatol Syphilol.* 1923;7:268-269.
23. O'Farrell NM. Pityriasis alba. *AMA Arch Derm.* 1956;73:376-377.
24. Halder RM, Nandedkar MA, Neal KW. Pigmentary disorders in pigmented skins. In: Halder RM, ed. *Dermatology and Dermatological Therapy of Pigmented Skins.* Boca Raton, FL: CRC Press; 2005:114-143.
25. Watkins DB. Pityriasis alba: a form of atopic dermatitis. A preliminary report. *Arch Dermatol.* 1961;83:915-919.
26. Diepgen TL, Fartasch M, Hornstein OP. Evaluation and relevance of atopic basic and minor features in patients with atopic dermatitis and in the general population. *Acta Derm Venereol Suppl (Stockh).* 1989;144:50-54.
27. Blessmann Weber M, Sponchiado de Avila LG, Albaneze R, et al. Pityriasis alba: a study of pathogenic factors. *J Eur Acad Dermatol Venereol.* 2002;16:463-468.
28. Zaynoun ST, Jaber LA, Kurban AK. Oral methoxsalen photochemotherapy of extensive pityriasis alba. Preliminary report. *J Am Acad Dermatol.* 1986;15:61-65.
29. Dhar S, Kanwar AJ, Dawn G. Pigmenting pityriasis alba. *Pediatr Dermatol.* 1995;12:197-198.
30. Bassaly M, Miale A Jr, Prasad AS. Studies on pityriasis alba. A common facial skin lesion in Egyptian children. *Arch Dermatol.* 1963;88:272-275.
31. Martin RF, Lugo-Somolinos A, Sánchez JL. Clinicopathologic study on pityriasis alba. *Bol Asoc Med PR.* 1990;82:463-465.
32. Zaynoun ST, Aftimos BG, Tenekjian KK, et al. Extensive pityriasis alba: a histological histochemical and ultrastructural study. *Br J Dermatol.* 1983;108:83-90.
33. Urano-Suehisa S, Tagami H. Functional and morphological analysis of the horny layer of pityriasis alba. *Acta Derm Venereol.* 1985;65:164-167.
34. Wells BT, Whyte HJ, Kierland RR. Pityriasis alba: a ten-year survey and review of the literature. *Arch Dermatol.* 1960;82:183-189.
35. Galan EB, Janniger CK. Pityriasis alba. *Cutis.* 1998;61:11-13.
36. Galadari E, Helmy M, Ahmed M. Trace elements in serum of pityriasis alba patients. *Int J Dermatol.* 1992;31:525-526.
37. Shah AS, Supapannachart N, Nordlund JJ. Acquired hypomelanotic disorders. In: Levine N, ed. *Pigmentation and Pigmentary Disorders.* Boca Raton, FL: CRC Press; 1993:352-353.
38. Lin A. Topical immunotherapy. In: Wolverton SE, ed. *Comprehensive Dermatological Therapy.* Philadelphia, PA: Saunders; 2001:617-619.
39. Morelli JG, Norris DA. Influence of inflammatory mediators and cytokines on human melanocyte function. *J Invest Dermatol.* 1993;100:191S-195S.
40. Ellis DA, Tan AK. How we do it: management of facial hyperpigmentation. *J Otolaryngol.* 1997;26:286-289.
41. Ortonne JP, Bahadoran P, Fitzpatrick TB, et al. Hypomelanoses and hypermelanosis. In: Freedberg IM, Eisen AZ, Wolff K, et al, eds. *Fitzpatrick's Dermatology in General Medicine.* 6th ed. New York, NY: McGraw-Hill; 2003:857.
42. Grover R, Morgan BD. Management of hypopigmentation following burn injury. *Burns.* 1996;22:627-630.
43. Verma S, Patterson JW, Derdeyn AS, et al. Hypopigmented macules in an Indian man. *Arch Dermatol.* 2006;142:1643-1648.
44. Yang CC, Lee JY, Wong TW. Depigmented extramammary Paget's disease. *Br J Dermatol.* 2004;151:1049-1053.

45. Johnston GA, Sviland L, McLelland J. Melasma of the arms associated with hormone replacement therapy. *Br J Dermatol.* 1998;139:932.

46. Ward KA, Moss C, Sanders DS. Human piebaldism: relationship between phenotype and site of kit gene mutation. *Br J Dermatol.* 1995;132: 929-935.

47. Thomas I, Kihiczak GG, Fox MD, et al. Piebaldism: an update. *Int J Dermatol.* 2004;43:716-719.

48. Mahakrishnan A, Srinivasan MS. Piebaldism with Hirschsprung's disease. *Arch Dermatol.* 1980;116:1102.

49. Angelo C, Cianchini G, Grosso MG, et al. Association of piebaldism and neurofibromatosis type 1 in a girl. *Pediatr Dermatol.* 2001;18:490-493.

50. Kiwan RA, Mutasim DF. Grover disease (transient acantholytic dermatosis) and piebaldism. *Cutis.* 2002;69:451-453.

51. Spritz RA, Beighton P. Piebaldism with deafness: molecular evidence for an expanded syndrome. *Am J Med Genet.* 1998;75:101-103.

52. Spritz RA. The molecular basis of human piebaldism. *Pigment Cell Res.* 1992;5:340-343.

53. Ezoe K, Holmes SA, Ho L, et al. Novel mutations and deletions of the KIT (steel factor receptor) gene in human piebaldism. *Am J Hum Genet.* 1995;56:58-66.

54. Giebel LB, Strunk KM, Holmes SA, et al. Organization and nucleotide sequence of the human KIT (mast/stem cell growth factor receptor) proto-oncogene. *Oncogene.* 1992;7:2207-2217.

55. Boissy RE, Nordlund JJ. Molecular basis of congenital hypopigmentary disorders in humans: a review. *Pigment Cell Res.* 1997;10:12-24.

56. Syrris P, Heathcote K, Carrozzo R, et al. Human piebaldism: six novel mutations of the proto-oncogene KIT. *Hum Mutat.* 2002;20:234.

57. Richards KA, Fukai K, Oiso N, et al. A novel KIT mutation results in piebaldism with progressive depigmentation. *J Am Acad Dermatol.* 2001;44:288-292.

58. Sánchez-Martin M, Pérez-Losada J, Rodriguez-Garcia A, et al. Deletion of the SLUG (SNAI2) gene results in human piebaldism. *Am J Med Genet A.* 2003;122A:125-132.

59. Jimbow K, Fitzpatrick TB, Szabo G, et al. Congenital circumscribed hypomelanosis: a characterization based on electron microscopic study of tuberous sclerosis, nevus depigmentosus, and piebaldism. *J Invest Dermatol.* 1975;64:50-62.

60. Falabella R, Barona M, Escobar C, et al. Surgical combination therapy for vitiligo and piebaldism. *Dermatol Surg.* 1995;21:852-857.

61. Njoo MD, Nieuweboer-Krobotova L, Westerhof W. Repigmentation of leucodermic defects in piebaldism by dermabrasion and thin split-thickness skin grafting in combination with minigrafting. *Br J Dermatol.* 1998;139:829-833.

62. Guerra L, Primavera G, Raskovic D, et al. Permanent repigmentation of piebaldism by erbium:YAG laser and autologous cultured epidermis. *Br J Dermatol.* 2004;150:715-721.

63. Relyveld GN, Kingswijk MM, Reitsma JB, et al. Benzoyl peroxide/clindamycin/UVA is more effective than fluticasone/UVA in progressive macular hypomelanosis: a randomized study. *J Am Acad Dermatol.* 2006;55:836-843.

64. Relyveld GN, Menke HE, Westerhof W. Progressive macular hypomelanosis: an overview. *Am J Clin Dermatol.* 2007;8:13-19.

65. Westerhof W, Relyveld GN, Kingswijk MM, et al. Propionibacterium acnes and the pathogenesis of progressive macular hypomelanosis. *Arch Dermatol.* 2004;140:210-214.

66. Guillet G, Helenon R, Gauthier Y, et al. Progressive macular hypomelanosis of the trunk: primary acquired hypopigmentation. *J Cutan Pathol.* 1988;15:286-289.

67. Guillet G, Helenon R, Guillet MH, et al. Progressive and confluent hypomelanosis of the melanodermic metis. *Ann Dermatol Venereol.* 1992;119:19-24.

68. Holden CA, Berth-Jones J. Eczema, lichenification, prurigo and erythroderma. In: Burns T, Breathnach S, Cox N, Griffiths C, eds. *Rook's Textbook of Dermatology.* Vol 1, 7th ed. Oxford, United Kingdom: Blackwell; 2004:17-55.

69. Di Lernia V, Ricci C. Progressive and extensive hypomelanosis and extensive pityriasis alba: same disease, different names? *J Eur Acad Dermatol Venereol.* 2005;19:370-372.

70. Relyveld G, Menke H, Westerhof W. Letter to the editor: progressive and extensive hypomelanosis and extensive pityriasis alba: same disease, different names? *J Eur Acad Dermatol Venereol.* 2006;20:1363-1364.

71. Menke HE, Ossekoppele R, Dekker SK, et al. Nummulaire en confluerende hypomelanosis van de romp. *Ned Tijdsch Dermatol Venereol.* 1997; 7:117-122.

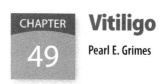

CHAPTER 49

Vitiligo

Pearl E. Grimes

KEY POINTS

- Vitiligo has an equal incidence in all types of skin color.

- Given the contrast between the depigmented patches and an individual's normal skin tones, this disease is most disfiguring for those with darker skin of color.

- Between 20% and 30% of patients report the disease in first- and second-degree relatives.

- In vitiligo, an absence of melanocytes is the predominant histologic change.

- The popular pathogenetic mechanisms for vitiligo include autoimmune, genetic, neural, biochemical, and autocytotoxic causes.

- Vitiligo patients have an increased frequency of other autoimmune disorders, including Hashimoto thyroiditis, Graves disease, pernicious anemia, and Addison disease.

- Baseline laboratory tests should include a comprehensive metabolic panel, and thyroid function, antinuclear antibody, and thyroid peroxidase antibody tests.

- The therapeutic objectives should include both the stabilization and repigmentation of the vitiliginous lesions.

- The therapies for limited areas of involvement include topical steroids, topical immunomodulators, calcipotriol, and targeted phototherapy.

- For patients with vitiligo affecting more than 15% to 20% of their body's surface area, optimal results can be achieved with narrow-band ultraviolet B phototherapy.

INTRODUCTION

Vitiligo is a relatively common acquired pigmentary disorder characterized by areas of depigmented skin resulting from the loss of epidermal melanocytes. Given the stark contrast between the depigmented patches and normal skin, this disease is most disfiguring in patients with darker skin of color [**Figure 49-1**]. Vitiligo is one of the most psychologically devastating skin diseases, and the psychological effects are influenced and exacerbated by societal perceptions of skin disfigurement and irregularities in skin color.[1,2] Patients with vitiligo often experience low self-esteem, isolation, job discrimination, stigmatization, depression, and embarrassment in social and sexual relationships.[3]

EPIDEMIOLOGY AND CLINICAL MANIFESTATIONS

The prevalence of vitiligo varies from 0.1% to 3% in various populations worldwide.[4] The onset may occur at any age; however, the peak incidence is during the second and third decades of life. One-fourth of patients with vitiligo are children. Although females are affected more often than males, the disease shows no racial or socioeconomic predilection. Vitiliginous lesions are typically asymptomatic, depigmented macules and patches that have no clinical signs of inflammation, although, at times, inflammatory vitiligo with erythematous borders has been reported. Hypopigmented and depigmented lesions may coexist in a vitiligo patient. Occasionally, the depigmented patches are pruritic. The macules or patches of vitiligo frequently begin on sun-exposed or periorificial facial skin and either remain localized or develop on other cutaneous sites. The areas of depigmentation vary in size from a few millimeters to many centimeters, and their borders are usually distinct.

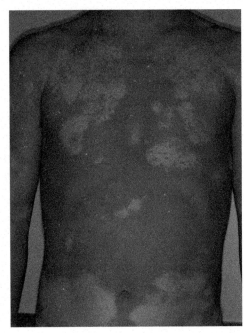

FIGURE 49-1. Generalized areas of depigmentation on the trunk and arms of a patient with darker skin of color.

Trichrome lesions are observed most often in individuals with darker skin of color. These lesions are characterized by zones of white, light-brown, and normal skin. Depigmented hair strands are often present in lesional skin and do not always preclude repigmentation of a lesion. In addition, there is a high incidence of premature graying of scalp hair in patients with vitiligo and in their families. The vitiliginous lesions can remain stable, or they can progress slowly for many years. Only in rare cases do patients undergo almost complete spontaneous depigmentation in a few years.

Vitiligo is classified into different subtypes based on the distribution of skin lesions. These subtypes include generalized (vulgaris), acral or acrofacial, localized, and segmental. The generalized pattern is characterized by symmetric depigmented macules or patches occurring in a random distribution. Acral or acrofacial vitiligo consists of depigmented macules confined to the extremities or the face and extremities, respectively. A subcategory of the acrofacial type is the lip-tip variety, in which lesions are confined to the lips and distal tips of the digits [**Figure 49-2**]. The generalized and acrofacial varieties are the most common. Segmental vitiligo occurs in a dermatomal or quasi-dermatomal distribution, most frequently along the distribution of the trigeminal nerve. The areas of depigmentation usually stabilize within a year and rarely spread beyond the affected dermatome. Segmental vitiligo is the least common subtype of vitiligo. In contrast to other types, it commonly begins in childhood.[5]

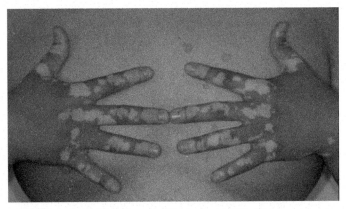

FIGURE 49-2. A patient with severe vitiligo involvement of the hands.

Melanocytes of the eye, ear, and leptomeninges may also be involved in vitiligo. In one study, depigmented areas of the retinal pigment epithelium and choroid were found in 39% of subjects.[6] These asymptomatic lesions did not interfere with visual acuity. However, another study reported a significantly lower incidence of ocular abnormalities.[7] Vitiligo is also a manifestation of Vogt-Koyanagi-Harada syndrome, which is characterized by chronic uveitis, poliosis, alopecia, dysacusia, vitiligo, and signs of meningeal irritation. This syndrome usually begins in the third decade of life and tends to be more severe among people with skin of color, especially Asians.

PATHOGENESIS

The predominant finding in the depigmented areas of vitiligo is an absence of epidermal melanocytes.[8] The precise cause of the loss of these epidermal melanocytes is unknown. Light microscopic and ultrastructural studies have revealed vacuolar degeneration of basal and parabasal keratinocytes and dermal lymphohistiocytic infiltrates.[9,10] Genetic, autoimmune, neural, biochemical, autocytotoxic, and melanocyte detachment mechanisms, as well as viral infections and oxidative stress, have been proposed to explain the pathogenesis of vitiligo. However, the autoimmune hypothesis remains the most well supported by current data.[8]

Genetic studies support a non-Mendelian inheritance pattern for vitiligo and suggest that vitiligo is a multifactorial, polygenic disorder.[11-13] Between 20% and 30% of vitiligo patients report the condition in their first- and second-degree relatives. The disease has been associated with specific genetic polymorphisms, such as human leukocyte antigen (HLA)-DR4, -Dw7, -DR7, -DR1, -B13, -Cw6, -DR53, and -A19; however, haplotypes may vary considerably within the populations studied.[11,12] Recently, a genome-wide linkage scan was performed in 71 Caucasian multiplex families with vitiligo.[13] The linkage was assessed using multipoint nonparametric linkage analysis. The autoimmunity susceptibility locus located on chromosome 1p31 showed a highly significant linkage, suggesting that it is a major susceptibility locus for individuals with Fitzpatrick skin types I to III. The additional signals on chromosomes 1, 7, 8, 11, 19, and 22 meet the genome criteria for a suggestive linkage. Genetic studies also vary between the populations being evaluated. Studies in Chinese families show linkage evidence to chromosome 4q13-q21, in contrast to data in Caucasian families.[14] These findings support significant genetic heterogeneity for vitiligo in different racial populations. Recently, the *NLRP1* gene (previously known as *NALP1*) on chromosome 17p13 was identified as the principal regulator of the innate immune system. The *NLRP1* gene encodes the NACHT (neuronal apoptosis inhibitor protein, major histocompatibility complex class 2 transcription activator, incompatibility locus protein from *Podospora anserina*, and telomerase-associated protein) domain leucine-rich repeat protein 1, which contributes to a group of epidemiologically associated autoimmune diseases, including vitiligo.[15] Other candidate genes reported to affect vitiligo susceptibility include *HLA, ACE, CAT, FOXD3, ESR1, COMT, PTPN22, PDGFRA, C12orf10, MITF, KIT, XBP1, FAS,* and *COX2* [**Table 49-1**].[8,11,12,16-18]

A 1996 study found that cytomegalovirus DNA was demonstrated in the involved and uninvolved skin of patients with vitiligo. No viral DNA was detected in the normal skin of matched control subjects.[19] A herpes simplex viral infection has been reported to trigger vitiligo in the Smyth line chicken animal model for vitiligo.[20] These findings suggest that in some cases vitiligo may be triggered by a viral infection.

The neural theory is supported by several clinical, biochemical, and ultrastructural observations.[21] These observations include the occurrence of segmental vitiligo; the demonstration of lesional autonomic dysfunction, such as increased sweating; and the demonstration of nerve ending-melanocyte contact. The last observation is rare in normal skin.

Abnormalities in the melanocortin system have been implicated in the pathogenesis of vitiligo. Defects in the melanocortin system reported in vitiligo include low α-melanocyte-stimulating hormone (α-MSH) plasma levels,[22] reduced α-MSH levels in melanocytes,[23,24] decreased prohormone convertases 1 and 2 (PC1 and PC2) expression

TABLE 49-1 Candidate genes reported to affect vitiligo susceptibility[8,11,12,16-18]

Gene symbol	Gene name	Gene symbol	Gene name
HLA	Human leukocyte antigen	PDGFRA	Platelet-derived growth factor receptor, α polypeptide
ACE	Angiotensin I converting enzyme	C12orf10	Chromosome 12 open reading frame 10
CAT	Catalase	MITF	Microphthalmia-associated transcription factor
FOXD3	Forkhead box D3	KIT	V-kit Hardy-Zuckerman 4 feline sarcoma viral oncogene homolog
ESR1	Estrogen receptor 1	XBP1	X-box binding protein 1
COMT	Catechol-O-methyl-transferase	FAS	Fas cell surface death receptor
PTPN22	Protein tyrosine phosphatase, non-receptor type 22 (lymphoid)	COX2	Cyclooxygenase 2
NLRP1	Nucleotide-binding oligomerization domain-like receptor family, pyrin domain containing 1		

in melanocytes,[23] increased melanocortin-1 receptor gene (*MC1R*) and *MC4R* messenger ribonucleic acid (mRNA) expression in nonlesional skin,[25] decreased pro-opiomelanocortin (POMC) mRNA expression in lesional skin,[25] and other defects.[26]

Several studies suggest that oxidative stress may be the initial event in the destruction of melanocytes.[27,28] A defective recycling of tetrahydrobiopterin, an increased production of hydrogen peroxide, and decreased catalase levels have been demonstrated in the affected skin of patients with vitiligo.[27,28] In addition, lesional catecholamine biosynthesis and release are increased. Peripheral blood studies of patients with vitiligo have shown low catalase and glutathione levels, whereas superoxide dismutase and xanthine oxidase are elevated.[29] Oxidative stress may contribute to melanocyte destruction in susceptible individuals, causing DNA damage as well as protein and lipid peroxidation. Recent studies suggest that oxidative stress may cause the aberrant immune responses observed in vitiligo. Reactive oxygen species can cause apoptosis and the release of neoantigens, which serve as autoantigens that initiate humoral and cell-mediated immune responses.[27,30]

The self-destruction hypothesis proposes that melanocytes may be destroyed by the phenolic compounds formed during the synthesis of melanin.[21] In vivo and in vitro studies have demonstrated the destruction of melanocytes by phenols and catechols. In addition, industrial workers who are exposed to catechols and phenols may develop depigmented patches. A number of environmentally ubiquitous compounds containing catechols, phenols, and sulfhydryls can induce hypopigmentation, depigmentation, or both. These compounds are encountered most often in industrial chemicals and cleaning agents. The possible mechanisms for altered pigment production by these compounds include melanocyte destruction via free radical formation, inhibition of tyrosinase activity, and interference with the production or transfer of melanosomes.[29]

There is a substantial amount of new data that further implicates immune mechanisms in the pathogenesis of vitiligo and suggests that vitiligo shares common linkages with other autoimmune diseases.[30,31] Historically, vitiligo has been reported in association with a number of autoimmune endocrinopathies and diseases. Thyroid disorders, in particular Hashimoto thyroiditis and Graves disease, are associated most commonly with vitiligo.[5] Other associated disorders include diabetes mellitus, alopecia areata, pernicious anemia, rheumatoid arthritis, autoimmune polyglandular syndrome, and psoriasis.[32-34] A survey of 2624 vitiligo probands in North America and the United Kingdom found that the prevalence of six autoimmune disorders was significantly increased in vitiligo probands and first-degree relatives.[5] These diseases included vitiligo, pernicious anemia, Addison disease, systemic lupus erythematosus, thyroid diseases (predominantly hypothyroidism), and inflammatory bowel disease.

Many humoral and cell-mediated immune aberrations have been reported in vitiligo patients. Numerous studies have documented an increased frequency of organ-specific autoantibodies in these patients.[35,36] Antithyroid (thyroglobulin, thyroid microsomal, and thyroid peroxidase), gastric parietal cell, and antinuclear antibodies are the most commonly associated autoantibodies that have been documented. Vitiligo patients who have organ-specific autoantibodies, unassociated with an overt autoimmune disease, have an increased risk of developing a subclinical or overt autoimmune disease.[35] The presence of antibodies to surface and cytoplasmic melanocyte antigens in the sera of vitiligo patients lends additional support for the autoimmune pathogenesis for this disease.[37-39] These antibodies can induce the destruction of melanocytes grown in the culture by complement-mediated lysis and antibody-dependent cellular cytotoxicity.[37,38] In addition, melanocyte antibodies, when passively administered to nude mice grafted with human skin, have a destructive effect on melanocytes within the skin graft.[40] Notably less common are antibodies targeting tyrosinase, tyrosinase-related proteins 1 and 2, melanocyte protein 17 (also known as glycoprotein 100 [gp100]), and melanin-concentrating hormone 1, which have been reported in vitiligo patients.[39] The transcription factors SOX9 and SOX10 have been identified as melanocytic autoantigens in autoimmune polyendocrine syndrome and idiopathic vitiligo.[41]

Recent studies provide additional insights into the role of cell-mediated immunity in the destruction of melanocytes, suggesting that cytotoxic T-lymphocytes may play a significant role in melanocyte destruction in vitiligo.[42,43] Numerous activated cytotoxic T-lymphocytes have been reported in the perilesional area of vitiliginous skin, often in apposition to disappearing melanocytes.[43] These infiltrating lymphocytes are predominantly cytotoxic cluster of differentiation 8-positive (CD8+) lymphocytes that express skin homing receptors (such as the cutaneous leukocyte-associated antigen receptor). Melanocyte-specific CD8 T-cells have been shown to mediate the destruction of melanocytes in human vitiligo skin.[44] In addition, other studies have demonstrated the presence of increased numbers of circulating CD8+ cytotoxic lymphocytes. These lymphocytes are reactive to the melanosomal proteins melan-A/melanoma antigen recognized by T-cells 1, gp100, and tyrosinase in HLA-A2-positive patients with vitiligo.[45-47]

In a recent study, patients with vitiligo had higher circulating T-cell counts compared to control subjects.[44] Compared with patients with stable vitiligo, the patients with active vitiligo had higher CD8+ T-cell counts and a significantly reduced CD4+:CD8+ ratio. Compared with control subjects, those with generalized vitiligo showed a significant decrease in their regulatory T-cell (Treg) percentage and counts, along with a significant reduction in FOXP3 expression. The Treg cell percentage and counts were significantly reduced in patients with active generalized vitiligo, compared with those whose disease was stable. These findings give further credence to aberrant T-cell formation in vitiligo.

Several investigations have also addressed the role of peripheral blood and lesional cytokine expression in the pathogenesis of vitiligo. Elevated levels of serum soluble interleukin (IL)-2 receptor, IL-6, and IL-8, and elevated lesional tissue levels of IL-2 have been reported in vitiligo patients.[48-50] These findings correlate with an increased level of T-cell activation. In biopsies of lesional, perilesional, and healthy skin, there were significantly lower levels of expression for the granulocyte colony-stimulating factor and stem cell factor reported in vitiliginous skin, but the expression of IL-6 and tumor necrosis factor-α (TNF-α) was increased in lesional skin.[51] Granulocyte colony-stimulating factor, basic fibroblast growth factor, and stem cell factor are paracrine cytokines secreted by keratinocytes. These paracrine cytokines stimulate melanogenesis and melanocyte proliferation, whereas IL-6 and TNF-α inhibit melanocyte proliferation and melanogenesis.[52] Together these findings suggest that keratinocyte function is also impaired in vitiliginous skin.

A subsequent report demonstrated an increased expression of TNF-α and interferon-γ in the lesional and adjacent healthy skin of patients with vitiligo, when compared with the skin of matched control subjects.[53] After 6 months of treatment with a twice-daily application of tacrolimus, a topical immunomodulator, there was a significant depression in the level of TNF-α expression in the lesional and adjacent healthy skin compared with baseline levels. This observation suggests that the suppression of TNF-α may be associated with the repigmentation of vitiliginous lesions.[53]

Whether these immunologic aberrations are primary or secondary events in the destruction of melanocytes in vitiligo remains controversial. However, regardless of which event is primary, many of the most effective therapies for vitiligo work via suppression or modulation of the immune response.

DIFFERENTIAL DIAGNOSIS

Other disorders characterized by depigmentation may occasionally clinically mimic vitiligo.[3] These include piebaldism, nevus depigmentosus, nevus anemicus, postinflammatory depigmentation or hypopigmentation, pityriasis alba, tinea versicolor, discoid lupus erythematosus, scleroderma, hypopigmented mycosis fungoides, and sarcoidosis. Therefore, in some instances, a skin biopsy may be necessary to substantiate a vitiligo diagnosis.

LABORATORY EVALUATION

In view of the association of vitiligo with a myriad of other autoimmune diseases, the routine baseline evaluation of a patient should include a thorough history and physical examination. Recommended laboratory tests include a complete blood count, erythrocyte sedimentation rate, comprehensive metabolic panel (including liver function tests), and autoantibody tests (such as antinuclear antibodies, thyroid peroxidase, and parietal cell antibodies).[26]

TREATMENT

The therapeutic objectives for vitiligo should include both the stabilization of the disease and the repigmentation of the patient's vitiliginous skin lesions. Repigmentation can be accomplished medically or, in patients with localized stable lesions, surgically. The choice of repigmentation therapies should be predicated on the age of the patient, the body surface area affected (severity), and the activity or progression of the disease. Many studies document enhanced repigmentation in patients with darker skin of color. The disease can be divided into four stages: limited (<10% involvement), moderate (10% to 25% involvement), moderately severe (26% to 50% involvement), and severe (>50% involvement).[3]

Commonly used medical therapies for vitiligo include topical and systemic steroids, topical calcineurin inhibitors, narrowband ultraviolet (UV) phototherapy, psoralen with ultraviolet A (PUVA), targeted phototherapy, nutritional vitamin supplementation, and calcipotriol[32-34,54] [**Table 49-2**].

■ STEROIDS

Mid- to high-potency topical corticosteroids are used as a first-line treatment in patients with limited forms of vitiligo.[3,5,26,32] Topical corticosteroids usually produce optimal results (75% repigmentation) on areas with greater sun exposure, such as the face and neck, on more recent lesions, and for patients with darker skin of color.[26] The response from topical corticosteroid use is poor in acral areas of the body. However, short-term use of steroids is safe and is an effective treatment in both children and adults.

A short course of oral prednisone for 1 to 2 weeks or a course of intramuscular triamcinolone acetonide injections (40 mg for 2 to 3 months) is often extremely helpful for stabilizing rapid progressive vitiligo.

TABLE 49-2	Therapeutic approaches for vitiligo	
Localized/Limited	Moderate/Severe	Recalcitrant
Topical steroids	Narrowband ultraviolet B	***Severe***
Topical PUVA	Oral PUVA	Depigmentation
PUVAsol	Systemic steroids	Monobenzene
Topical immunomodulators	Antioxidants/vitamins	***Localized***
Tacrolimus		Surgical
Pimecrolimus		Sheet grafts
Targeted phototherapy		Autologous punch grafts
Calcipotriol		Split-thickness grafts
Antioxidants/vitamins		Melanocyte transplants
		Cocultured epidermis

Abbreviations: PUVA, psoralen photochemotherapy with ultraviolet A; PUVAsol, psoralen and solar ultraviolet A.

However, prolonged use of systemic steroids is not advisable. Low-potency topical steroids are usually ineffective for patients with vitiligo. Topical mid- to high-potency steroids can be used safely for 2 to 3 months and then interrupted for 1 month, or tapered to low-potency preparations. Patients must be monitored closely for topical steroid side effects, which include skin atrophy, telangiectasias, hypertrichosis, acneiform eruptions, and striae.[55]

Lower potency and medium-potency (class III) classes of topical corticosteroids, such as mometasone furoate and methylprednisolone aceponate, have an increased benefit-to-risk ratio with fewer side effects.[26] Topical fluticasone propionate has a low potential for inducing local and systemically adverse effects.[56] Since the introduction of topical immunomodulators (such as tacrolimus and pimecrolimus), topical steroids are used less frequently in vitiligo patients.[57]

■ TOPICAL IMMUNOMODULATORS

Topical immunomodulatory agents such as tacrolimus and pimecrolimus offer several advantages in treating vitiligo. These agents are extremely well tolerated in children and adults, and they can be used for longer periods without evidence of atrophy or telangiectasias, which are common complications associated with long-term steroid use. This is a significant advantage in treating a chronic disease such as vitiligo. A comparison of the efficacy of topical immunomodulators and topical steroids in the treatment of vitiligo showed that the time frame from the start of treatment to the onset of repigmentation was significantly shorter in a group of 52 patients who were treated with topical immunomodulators, compared with 27 patients who were administered topical steroids.[57]

Tacrolimus is a topical immunomodulatory agent that affects T-cell and mast cell functions by binding to cytoplasmic immunophilins and by inactivating calcineurin.[58,59] Tacrolimus inhibits the synthesis and release of proinflammatory cytokines and vasoactive mediators from the basophils and mast cells.[59] Multiple studies have demonstrated its efficacy and safety for the treatment of atopic dermatitis[53,60,61] [**Figure 49-3**]. A 24-week study assessed the efficacy and safety of tacrolimus ointment in 23 patients with generalized vitiligo, with 19 patients completing the study.[53] At 24 weeks, 89% of the patients achieved varying levels of repigmentation, and there was a statistically significant decrease in their overall disease severity scores. Maximal repigmentation was observed on the face and neck areas (the areas with greater sun exposure), with 68% of patients achieving more than 75% repigmentation. Adverse events were minimal throughout the study.[53] Other studies have corroborated these results.[60-62] In a chart review of 101 patients diagnosed with vitiligo, topical tacrolimus was found to be more effective for the treatment of vitiligo in patients with skin of color.[63] Children and teenagers aged 2 to 15 years were treated with tacrolimus 0.03%, whereas individuals aged 16 years

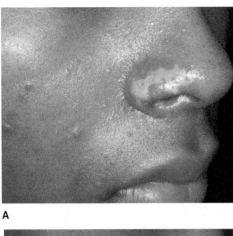

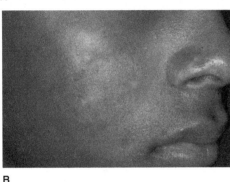

FIGURE 49-3. (A) Areas of facial depigmentation on a patient with skin of color. **(B)** The same area after 3 months of treatment with tacrolimus.

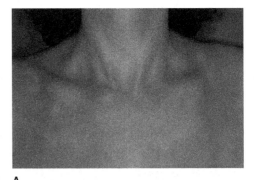

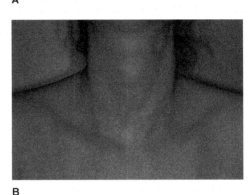

FIGURE 49-4. (A) A patient with depigmented patches of the neck and chest. **(B)** The same area after 30 narrowband ultraviolet B phototherapy treatments.

or older were treated with tacrolimus 0.1% ointment applied twice daily. The topical tacrolimus was efficacious in body lesions in patients of all skin tones, with superior efficacy observed in those with Fitzpatrick skin types III and IV.[63]

Pimecrolimus, which has a mechanism of action similar to tacrolimus, can also induce repigmentation of vitiliginous skin lesions.[62] The efficacy of pimecrolimus and clobetasol was compared in a right/left prospective study that focused on treating symmetric lesions; the two agents had comparable rates of repigmentation.[64] As with tacrolimus, pimecrolimus induces maximal repigmentation in the sun-exposed areas of a patient's body.

It is well recognized that there is an increased risk of skin cancer among transplant recipients who have been treated with cyclosporine[55] or systemically administered tacrolimus, given the immunosuppression induced by such agents.[65] The use of topical tacrolimus, however, has not been associated with systemic immunosuppression or an increased risk of skin and other malignancies in clinical studies.[66,67] However, in light of the reports documenting an increase in skin cancers and lymphomas in animal models, tacrolimus and pimecrolimus currently have 'black box' warning labels.[68] These animal studies should be interpreted with caution, given the massive dosages used in animal protocols. The labeling of these agents recommends that they should not be used in combination with UV light therapy, and that appropriate photoprotective precautions should be taken by patients.

▪ NARROWBAND ULTRAVIOLET B

Historically, topical and systemic PUVA was the "gold standard" for repigmenting vitiliginous skin lesions; however, PUVA-induced repigmentation rates vary considerably.[54,69] In addition, the adverse effects can be substantial, including phototoxicity and gastrointestinal irritation. Oral PUVA also requires the patient to use ocular protection for 12 to 24 hours following treatment.

Given the comparable efficacy of narrowband ultraviolet B (NB-UVB) phototherapy and its lack of systemic adverse effects, it has emerged as

the initial treatment of choice for patients with moderate to severe vitiligo [**Figure 49-4**]. NB-UVB involves the use of UV lamps with a peak emission of around 311 nm.[70] These shorter wavelengths provide higher energy fluences and induce less cutaneous erythema. NB-UVB induces local immunosuppression and apoptosis; stimulates the production of melanocyte-stimulating hormones, basic fibroblasts, growth factor, and endothelin-1; and increases melanocyte proliferation and melanogenesis. The first major study of NB-UVB in patients with vitiligo compared its efficacy with that of topical PUVA.[71] The study showed that significantly enhanced repigmentation was achieved in patients treated with NB-UVB compared with those treated with topical PUVA. The adverse effects were minimal in the group of patients treated with NB-UVB in contrast with the increased phototoxicity observed in the patients treated with topical PUVA. Subsequent studies have further confirmed the efficacy of NB-UVB and documented enhanced repigmentation rates when compared with PUVA phototherapy for vitiligo[72-76] [**Figure 49-5**].

The major advantages of NB-UVB include an established safety profile in both children and adults and a lack of systemic toxicity. NB-UVB does not require patients to use eye protection beyond the treatment exposure time. There have been no studies that have documented an increase in squamous cell carcinomas, basal cell cancers, or malignant melanomas in vitiligo patients treated with either PUVA or NB-UVB. This is in contrast with reports documenting an increase in squamous cell carcinomas and melanomas in psoriasis patients treated with PUVA.[77]

Lifetime prevalences of melanoma and nonmelanoma skin cancer (NMSC) in patients with nonsegmental vitiligo were compared with control subjects without vitiligo in a retrospective, comparative cohort survey.[78] Data from 1307 eligible survey questionnaires revealed that patients with vitiligo had a three-fold lower probability of developing melanoma and NMSC. The patients who were treated with NB-UVB and PUVA did not show dose-related trends of an increased age-adjusted lifetime prevalence of melanoma or NMSC.

A functional color yeast assay demonstrated overexpression of a functioning wild-type p53 protein in both the depigmented and healthy

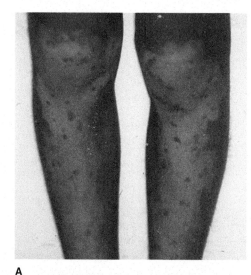

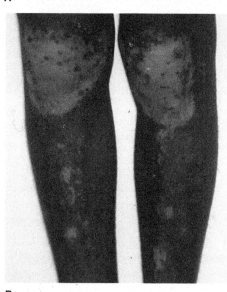

FIGURE 49-5. A patient with skin of color with depigmented lesions of the lower extremities. **(A)** before treatment with narrow-band ultraviolet B therapy and **(B)** after 26 treatments.

pigmented epidermis of patients with vitiligo compared with healthy control subjects.[79] This wild-type p53 overexpression may explain the possible low risk of skin cancers in patients with vitiligo. However, long-term follow-up studies are needed to fully assess the risks of NB-UVB.

The additive effect of tacrolimus ointment 0.1% applied once daily combined with NB-UVB in the treatment of vitiligo was recently evaluated in a randomized double-blind trial.[80] A total of 40 patients with stable symmetrical vitiligo were treated with tacrolimus ointment 0.1% on one side of their body and a placebo ointment on the other side. Whole-body NB-UVB was administered two or three times weekly for at least 3 months. In 27 patients, significant improvement was seen on the areas of vitiligo treated with tacrolimus. The results showed that combination therapy with NB-UVB and tacrolimus ointment 0.1% was more effective for patients than UVB treatment alone. This effect was dependent on the total dose of tacrolimus applied and was correlated with the number of topical tacrolimus applications, but not the number of UVB treatments.

TARGETED PHOTOTHERAPY

Targeted phototherapy systems have also demonstrated improved efficacy for the treatment of localized vitiligo.[81] These units deliver high-intensity light only to the patient's affected areas, while avoiding exposure of the healthy skin and lowering the cumulative UVB dose. In 1999, the effectiveness of UVB radiation microtherapy was first reported for repigmentation of segmental vitiligo in a small series of eight patients.[82] Five of these patients achieved more than 75% repigmentation.

Subsequent investigations have also documented the benefits of excimer laser systems and targeted phototherapy units.[83-86] The excimer laser produces monochromatic radiation at a wavelength of 308 nm. An open-label pilot investigation used the excimer laser to treat 29 affected areas of vitiligo in 18 patients.[83] In this study, lesions were treated three times per week for a maximum of 12 treatments; 23 vitiliginous areas on 12 patients received at least six treatments. Varying degrees of repigmentation were reported in 57% of the treated areas. Of the 11 affected areas that received all 12 treatments, 87% demonstrated some repigmentation.[83] A newly developed unit with a larger irradiation field was used recently on 37 patients.[87] Compared with other targeted units with small irradiation fields (<3 cm), this unit had an irradiation field of 36 × 14 cm, allowing the treatment of larger areas. Of the patients treated with this unit, 43% experienced 50% to 75% repigmentation of their lesions, and 49% of the patients had 76% to 100% repigmentation.

Targeted phototherapy systems can also work synergistically with topical therapies. Several studies have assessed the efficacy of combination treatment with an excimer laser and tacrolimus ointment or topical methoxsalen.[81,86] In a study of eight patients with vitiligo, the subjects were treated with an excimer laser and either topical tacrolimus or a placebo ointment.[86] In the study, 50% of the areas treated with the combination excimer laser and topical tacrolimus achieved 75% or greater repigmentation, compared with 20% for the placebo group.

Several studies show that maximal results are achieved with the excimer laser when patients are treated two or three times weekly. Optimal repigmentation is usually achieved on a patient's face, neck, and trunk areas.[88,89]

The therapeutic efficacy of targeted broadband UVB phototherapy in localized vitiligo is good but limited. In an evaluation of a high-dose targeted phototherapy system, 32 patients were treated twice or thrice weekly for a total of 20 to 60 sessions.[90] Visible repigmentation occurred in only four patients (12.5%), and improvement was observed only in facial lesions. Two patients achieved more than 75% repigmentation through the phototherapy system, whereas the other two patients experienced less than 25% repigmentation. Mild adverse events were reported in 3 of the 32 patients.[90]

VITAMINS

Preliminary open-label studies have documented stabilization and repigmentation in vitiligo patients who have been treated with high-dose vitamin supplementation, including daily doses of ascorbic acid (1000 mg), vitamin B$_{12}$ (1000 µg), and folic acid (1 to 5 mg).[91,92]

VITAMIN D ANALOGS

Calcipotriol is a synthetic analogue of vitamin D$_3$. Vitamin D$_3$ binds to vitamin D receptors in the skin, affecting melanocyte and keratinocyte growth and differentiation. It also inhibits T-cell activation.[93] Melanocytes are thought to express 1-α-dihydroxy vitamin D$_3$ receptors, which may have a role in stimulating melanogenesis. Several studies have assessed the efficacy of calcipotriol in combination with UV light therapy in patients with vitiligo.[93-98] Some have shown that when used in combination with UV light exposure, calcipotriol is a well-tolerated and efficacious treatment for both children and adults with vitiligo.[93,98,99] Recently, the efficacy of calcipotriol 0.05% ointment was reported in combination with clobetasol in a series of 12 patients with vitiligo.[96] Clobetasol was used in the morning, and calcipotriene was used in the evening. A total of 83% of patients responded to treatment with an average 95% repigmentation of their affected areas.

A further study showed that calcipotriene 0.005%/betamethasone dipropionate 0.05% ointment was effective and well tolerated in the treatment of 31 patients with vitiligo.[99] Patients received the combination of topical calcipotriol/betamethasone dipropionate twice daily for at least 12 weeks. The response was excellent in three patients (9.7%), moderate in six patients (19.4%), mild in eight patients (25.8%), and minimal in seven patients (22.6%), while seven patients (22.6%) experienced no repigmentation. The responsiveness was greater in patients at a progressive phase than in those at a stable phase.[99]

NOVEL AND EXPERIMENTAL VITILIGO THERAPIES

Afamelanotide, a potent and longer-lasting synthetic analogue of naturally occurring α-MSH, is a novel intervention for reduced α-MSH in patients with vitiligo.[23,100] Afamelanotide is delivered as a subcutaneous bioresorbable implant that promotes melanocyte proliferation and melanogenesis. The safety and efficacy of afamelanotide implants combined with NB-UVB were recently assessed in an observational study of four patients with generalized vitiligo.[100] The patients were treated three times weekly with NB-UVB, and then in the second month, they were administered a series of four monthly implants containing 16 mg of afamelanotide. Follicular and confluent areas of repigmentation were evident within 2 days to 4 weeks after the initial implant. Afamelanotide induced fast and deep repigmentation, as well as diffuse hyperpigmentation in all cases.[100] Afamelanotide is a potentially efficacious and accelerated treatment for vitiligo.

Prostaglandin E$_2$ (PGE$_2$) is a novel and potentially beneficial treatment for localized stable vitiligo. PGE$_2$ controls the proliferation of melanocytes through stimulant and immunomodulatory effects. In a consecutive series, repigmentation occurred in 40 of 56 patients with stable vitiligo treated with translucent PGE$_2$ 0.25 mg g^{-1}.[101] The patients applied the PGE$_2$ gel twice daily for 6 months. The mean onset of repigmentation was 2 months. The response was excellent in 22 of 40 patients, with complete repigmentation observed in 8 patients. The patients with a disease duration of 6 months showed the most significant response. Repigmentation occurred the earliest in the face and scalp.[101]

Bimatoprost, a topical prostaglandin, is associated with hyperpigmentation of periocular skin caused by increased melanogenesis. In a study by Narang,[102] 10 patients were treated with bimatoprost 0.03% ophthalmic solution twice daily for 4 months. Of the 10 patients, 3 had 100% repigmentation, 3 had 75% to 99% repigmentation, and 1 had 50% to 75% repigmentation. The best responses were observed on the face.[102]

It has been shown that the inducible heat shock protein 70 (HSP70i), a molecular link between stress and the resultant immune response, causes an inflammatory dendritic cell phenotype and is essential for depigmentation in vitiligo mouse models.[103] However, a mutant HSP70i (HSP70iQ435A) behaved differently by binding human dendritic cells and reducing their activation in a mouse model. Mice expressing a transgenic, melanocyte-reactive T-cell receptor treated with HSP70iQ435A-encoding DNA months before spontaneous depigmentation did not develop vitiligo. HSP70iQ435A used therapeutically in another rapid depigmentation model led to a 76% recovery of pigmentation and prevented the relevant T-cell populating of mouse skin. Ex vivo treatment of human skin with HSP70iQ435A prevented the shift from the quiescent to the effector T-cell phenotype associated with vitiligo.[103]

DEPIGMENTATION

Since the 1950s, monobenzylether of hydroquinone (MBEH), or monobenzene, has been used as a depigmenting agent for patients with extensive vitiligo. In general, MBEH causes permanent destruction of melanocytes and induces depigmentation locally and remotely from the sites of application. Hence the use of MBEH for other disorders of pigmentation is contraindicated.

Depigmentation is a viable therapeutic alternative in patients with over 50% cutaneous depigmentation who have demonstrated recalcitrance to repigmentation or in patients with extensive vitiligo who have no desire to undergo repigmentation therapies.[3] The major side effects of MBEH therapy are dermatitis and pruritus, which usually respond to topical and systemic steroids. Other side effects include severe xerosis,

alopecia, and premature graying. Additional depigmenting agents are 4-methoxyphenol and 88% phenol.[104] Alternatively, physical therapies may be used for depigmentation, such as Q-switched ruby and alexandrite lasers or cryotherapy. Second-line agents such as imatinib mesylate, imiquimod, and diphencyprone are also used.[104] Experimental agents currently under investigation include phenol derivatives, melanoma vaccines, interferon-γ, and busulfan.[104]

SURGICAL APPROACHES

Surgical therapies have been used for vitiligo for the past 25 years. Recently, substantial advances have been made in the techniques and protocols for harvesting and transplanting melanocytes. Surgical therapies remain viable options for patients with localized areas of depigmentation that have failed to respond to medical intervention.[72,105-107] The major advantage of transplantation procedures is the transfer of a reservoir of healthy melanocytes to the vitiliginous skin for proliferation and migration into areas of depigmentation. Transplantation procedures are contraindicated for patients with a history of hypertrophic scars or keloids.

Surgical therapies include autologous suction-blister grafts, minigrafts and punch grafts, split-thickness grafts, autologous melanocyte cultures, cultured epidermal suspensions, melanocyte-keratinocyte suspensions, and single-hair grafts [**Figure 49-6**].[108] A systematic review of autologous transplantation methods for vitiligo found that maximal repigmentation occurred in patients who were treated with split-thickness grafting and epidermal suction blister grafting.[72] Both of these treatment groups achieved success rates of 90% repigmentation. Other studies have reported the benefits of the transplantation of autologous melanocyte cultures and epidermal suspensions containing both melanocytes and keratinocytes.[105,106]

A study that included 117 patients assessed the influences of age, site of lesion, and type of disease on transplantation outcomes.[107] In this series, the best results were achieved for patients younger than 20 years of age and patients with segmental vitiligo. The grafting site did not significantly affect the outcome. In most instances, tattooing or

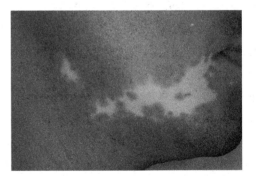

A

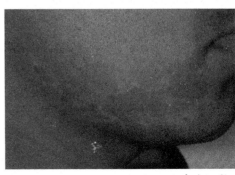

B

FIGURE 49-6. A young man with segmental vitiligo of the face (**A**) before grafting and (**B**) 3 months after autologous 1 mm punch grafting.

micropigmentation should be avoided given the risk of koebnerization and oxidation of the tattoo pigment causing further dyschromia.

CONCLUSION

Vitiligo is a pigmentary disorder with an equal incidence in all skin types. Due to the contrast between the affected areas and normal skin, this condition is most disfiguring in those with darker skin of color and can be psychologically devastating for this patient group.

The objectives for vitiligo treatment should include both the stabilization of the disease and the repigmentation of the vitiliginous skin lesions. Typically used medical therapies for vitiligo include topical and systemic steroids, topical calcineurin inhibitors, NB-UVB phototherapy, PUVA, targeted phototherapy, nutritional vitamin supplementation, and calcipotriol.

Topical immunomodulatory agents, such as tacrolimus and pimecrolimus, are a common first-line vitiligo treatment modality. These agents have proven to be very effective and can be used for long periods without substantial adverse effects. NB-UVB phototherapy is currently the initial treatment of choice for patients with moderate to severe vitiligo. This therapy has comparable efficacy to PUVA, and one of its major advantages is its established safety profile. Vitamin supplementation has been found to cause stabilization and repigmentation in vitiligo patients when administered in high doses. Calcipotriol (a synthetic analogue of vitamin D_3) in combination with UV light therapy is also a well-tolerated and effective treatment for cases of limited localized vitiligo.

Depigmentation and surgical therapies are viable treatment options for patients with severe or recalcitrant vitiligo. For the last 25 years, surgical therapies have been used as a form of vitiligo treatment, and recently, there has been significant progress in the area of harvesting and transplanting melanocytes. Studies have reported the benefits of split-thickness grafting and epidermal suction blister grafting, as well as the transplantation of autologous melanocyte cultures and epidermal suspensions containing both melanocytes and keratinocytes.

REFERENCES

1. Robins A. *Biological Perspectives on Human Pigmentation.* Cambridge, England: Cambridge University Press; 1991.
2. Grimes PE. Disorders of pigmentation. In: Dale DC, Federman DD, eds. *ACP Medicine.* New York, NY: WebMD Scientific American Medicine Inc.; 2003:526-534.
3. Porter J. The psychological effects of vitiligo: response to impaired appearance. In: Hann SK, Nordlund JJ, eds. *Vitiligo.* Oxford, United Kingdom: Blackwell Science; 2000:97-100.
4. Alkhateeb A, Fain PR, Thody A, et al. Epidemiology of vitiligo and associated autoimmune diseases in Caucasian probands and their families. *Pigment Cell Res.* 2003;16:208-214.
5. Grimes PE, Billips M. Childhood vitiligo: clinical spectrum and therapeutic approaches. In: Hann SK, Nordlund JJ, eds. *Vitiligo.* Oxford, England: Blackwell Science; 2000:61-70.
6. Albert DM, Wagoner MD, Pruett RC, et al. Vitiligo and disorders of the retinal pigment epithelium. *Br J Ophthalmol.* 1983;67:153-156.
7. Cowan CL Jr, Halder RM, Grimes PE, et al. Ocular disturbances in vitiligo. *J Am Acad Dermatol.* 1986;15:17-24.
8. Grimes PE. New insights and new therapies in vitiligo. *JAMA.* 2005;293:730-735.
9. Montes LF, Abulafia J, Wilborn WH, et al. Value of histopathology in vitiligo. *Int J Dermatol.* 2003;42:57-61.
10. Le Poole IC, Das PK. Microscopic changes in vitiligo. *Clin Dermatol.* 1997;15:863-873.
11. Majumder PP, Das SK, Li CC. A genetical model for vitiligo. *Am J Hum Genet.* 1988;43:119-125.
12. Nath SK, Majumder PP, Nordlund JJ. Genetic epidemiology of vitiligo: multilocus recessivity cross-validated. *Am J Hum Genet.* 1994;55:981-990.
13. Fain PR, Gowan K, LaBerge GS, et al. A genomewide screen for generalized vitiligo: confirmation of AIS1 on chromosome 1p31 and evidence for additional susceptibility loci. *Am J Hum Genet.* 2003;72:1560-1564.
14. Chen JJ, Huang W, Gui JP, et al. A novel linkage to generalized vitiligo on 4q13-q21 identified in a genomewide linkage analysis of Chinese families. *Am J Hum Genet.* 2005;76:1057-1065.
15. Jin Y, Mailloux CM, Gowan K, et al. NALP1 in vitiligo-associated multiple autoimmune disease. *N Engl J Med.* 2007;356:1216-1225.
16. Spritz RA. Recent progress in the genetics of generalized vitiligo. *J Genet Genomics.* 2011;38:271-278.
17. Zhang X. Genome-wide association study of skin complex diseases. *J Dermatol Sci.* 2012;66:89-97.
18. Al-Shobaili H. Update on the genetics characterization of vitiligo. *Int J Health Sci (Qassim).* 2011;5:167-179.
19. Grimes PE, Sevall J, Vojdani A. Cytomegalovirus DNA identified in skin biopsy specimens of patients with vitiligo. *J Am Acad Dermatol.* 1996;35:21-26.
20. Erf G, Bersi TK, Wang X, et al. Herpes virus connection in the expression of autoimmune vitiligo in Smyth line chickens. *Pigment Cell Res.* 2001;14:40-46.
21. Gauthier Y, Cario Andre M, Taïeb A. A critical appraisal of vitiligo etiologic theories: is melanocyte loss a melanocytorrhagy? *Pigment Cell Res.* 2003;16:322-332.
22. Pichler R, Sfetsos K, Badics B, et al. Vitiligo patients present lower plasma levels of alpha-melanotropin immunoreactivities. *Neuropeptides.* 2006;40:177-183.
23. Graham A, Westerhof W, Thody AJ. The expression of alpha-MSH by melanocytes is reduced in vitiligo. *Ann N Y Acad Sci.* 1999;885:470-473.
24. Spencer JD, Gibbons NC, Rokos H, et al. Oxidative stress via hydrogen peroxide affects proopiomelanocortin peptides directly in the epidermis of patients with vitiligo. *J Invest Dermatol.* 2007;127:411-420.
25. Kingo K, Aunin E, Karelson M, et al. Gene expression analysis of melanocortin system in vitiligo. *J Dermatol Sci.* 2007;48:113-122.
26. Taïeb A, Picardo M, VETF Members. The definition and assessment of vitiligo: a consensus report of the Vitiligo European Task Force. *Pigment Cell Res.* 2007;20:27-35.
27. Dell'Anna ML, Maresca V, Briganti S, et al. Mitochondrial impairment in peripheral blood mononuclear cells during the active phase of vitiligo. *J Invest Dermatol.* 2001;117:908-913.
28. Picardo M, Grammatico P, Roccella F, et al. Imbalance in the antioxidant pool in melanoma cells and normal melanocytes from patients with melanoma. *J Invest Dermatol.* 1996;107:322-326.
29. Dell'Anna ML, Picardo M. A review and a new hypothesis for non-immunological pathogenetic mechanisms in vitiligo. *Pigment Cell Res.* 2006;19:406-411.
30. Laddha NC, Dwivedi M, Mansuri MS, et al. Vitiligo: interplay between oxidative stress and immune system. *Exp Dermatol.* 2013;22:245-250.
31. Richmond JM, Frisoli ML, Harris JE. Innate immune mechanisms in vitiligo: danger from within. *Curr Opin Immunol.* 2013;25:676-682.
32. Njoo MD, Westerhof W. Vitiligo. Pathogenesis and treatment. *Am J Clin Dermatol.* 2001;2:167-181.
33. Kovacs S. Vitiligo *J Am Acad Dermatol.* 1998;38:6666.
34. Boissy R, Nordlund J. Molecular basis of congenital hypopigmentary disorders in humans: a review *Pigment Cell Res.* 1997;10:12-24.
35. Betterle C, Caretto A, De Zio AD, et al. Incidence and significance of organ-specific autoimmune disorders (clinical, latent, or only autoantibodies) in patients with vitiligo. *Dermatologica.* 1985;171:419-423.
36. Grimes PE, Halder RM, Jones C, et al. Autoantibodies and their clinical significance in a black vitiligo population. *Arch Dermatol.* 1983;119:300-303.
37. Naughton GK, Eisinger M, Bystryn JC. Detection of antibodies to melanocytes in vitiligo by specific immunoprecipitation. *J Invest Dermatol.* 1983;81:540-542.
38. Norris DA, Kissinger RM, Naughton GM, et al. Evidence for immunologic mechanisms in human vitiligo: patients' sera induce damage to human melanocytes in vitro by complement-mediated damage and antibody-dependent cellular cytotoxicity. *J Invest Dermatol.* 1988;90:783-789.
39. Ongenae K, Van Geel N, Naeyaert JM. Evidence for an autoimmune pathogenesis of vitiligo. *Pigment Cell Res.* 2003;16:90-100.
40. Gilhar A, Pillar T, Eidelman S, et al. Vitiligo and idiopathic guttate hypomelanosis. Repigmentation of skin following engraftment onto nude mice. *Arch Dermatol.* 1989;125:1363-1366.
41. Hedstrand H, Ekwall O, Olsson MJ, et al. The transcription factors SOX9 and SOX10 are vitiligo autoantigens in autoimmune polyendocrine syndrome type I. *J Biol Chem.* 2001;276:35390-35395.
42. Ghoneum M, Grimes PE, Gill G, et al. Natural cell-mediated cytotoxicity in vitiligo. *J Am Acad Dermatol.* 1987;17:600-605.

43. Ogg GS, Dunbar PR, Romero P, et al. High frequency of skin-homing melanocyte specific cytotoxic T-lymphocytes in autoimmune vitiligo. *J Exp Med.* 1998;188:1203-1208.

44. Harris JE, Harris TH, Weninger W, et al. A mouse model of vitiligo with focused epidermal depigmentation requires IFN-γ for autoreactive CD8+ z T-cell accumulation in the skin. *J Invest Dermatol.* 2012;132:1869-1876.

45. Lang KS, Caroli CC, Muhm A, et al. HLA-A2 restricted, melanocyte-specific CD8(+) T-lymphocytes detected in vitiligo patients are related to disease activity and are predominantly directed against melanA/MART1. *J Invest Dermatol.* 2001;116:891-897.

46. Palmero B, Campanelli R, Garbelli S, et al. Specific cytotoxic T-lymphocyte responses against melan-A/MART1, tyrosinase and gp100 in vitiligo by the use of major histocompatibility complex/peptide tetramers: the role of cellular immunity in the etiopathogenesis of vitiligo. *J Invest Dermatol.* 2001;117:326-332.

47. Mandelcorn-Monson RL, Shear NH, Yau E, et al. Cytotoxic T-lymphocyte reactivity to gp100, melanA/MART-1, and tyrosinase, in HLA-A2-positive vitiligo patients. *J Invest Dermatol.* 2003;121:550-556.

48. Yu HS, Chang KL, Yu CL, et al. Alterations in IL-6, IL-8, GM-CSF, TNF-alpha, and IFN-gamma release by peripheral mononuclear cells in patients with active vitiligo. *J Invest Dermatol.* 1997;108:527-529.

49. Honda Y, Okubo Y, Koga M. Relationship between levels of soluble interleukin-2 receptors and the types and activity of vitiligo. *J Dermatol.* 1997;24:561-563.

50. Caixa T, Hongwen F, Xiran L. Levels of soluble interleukin-2-receptor in the sera and skin tissue fluids of patients with vitiligo. *J Dermatol Sci.* 1999;21:59-62.

51. Moretti S, Spallanzani A, Amato L, et al. New insights into the pathogenesis of vitiligo: imbalance of epidermal cytokines at sites of lesions. *Pigment Cell Res.* 2002;15:87-92.

52. Imokawa G. Autocrine and paracrine regulation of melanocytes in human skin and in pigmentary disorders. *Pigment Cell Res.* 2004;17:96-110.

53. Grimes PE, Morris R, Avaniss-Aghajani E, et al. Topical tacrolimus therapy for vitiligo: therapeutic responses and skin messenger RNA expression of proinflammatory cytokines. *J Am Acad Dermatol.* 2004;51:52-61.

54. Grimes PE. Vitiligo. An overview of therapeutic approaches. *Dermatol Clin.* 1993;11:325-338.

55. Whitton ME, Pinart M, Batchelor J, et al. Interventions for vitiligo. *Cochrane Database Syst Rev.* 2010;1:CD003263.

56. Korting HC, Schöllmann C. Topical fluticasone propionate: intervention and maintenance treatment options of atopic dermatitis based on a high therapeutic index. *J Eur Acad Dermatol Venereol.* 2012;26:133-140.

57. Choi CW, Chang SE, Bak H, et al. Topical immunomodulators are effective for treatment of vitiligo. *J Dermatol.* 2008;35:503-507.

58. Tharp M. Calcineurin inhibitors. *Dermatol Ther.* 2002;15:325-332.

59. Kang S, Lucky AW, Pariser D, et al. Long-term safety and efficacy of tacrolimus ointment for the treatment of atopic dermatitis in children. *J Am Acad Dermatol.* 2001;44:S58-S64.

60. Tanghetti EA. Tacrolimus ointment 0.1% produces repigmentation in patients with vitiligo: results of a prospective patient series. *Cutis.* 2003;71:158-162.

61. Travis LB, Weinberg JM, Silverberg NB. Successful treatment of vitiligo with 0.1% tacrolimus ointment. *Arch Dermatol.* 2003;139:571-574.

62. Mayoral FA, Gonzalez C, Shah NS, et al. Repigmentation of vitiligo with pimecrolimus cream: a case report. *Dermatology.* 2003;207:322-323.

63. Silverberg JI, Silverberg NB. Topical tacrolimus is more effective for treatment of vitiligo in patients of skin of color. *J Drugs Dermatol.* 2011;10:507-510.

64. Coskun B, Saral Y, Turgut D. Topical 0.05% clobetasol propionate versus 1% pimecrolimus ointment in vitiligo. *Eur J Dermatol.* 2005;15:88-91.

65. Woodle ES, Thistlethwaite JR, Gordon JH, et al. A multicenter trial of FK506 (tacrolimus) therapy in refractory acute renal allograft rejection. A report of the Tacrolimus Kidney Transplantation Rescue Study Group. *Transplantation.* 1996;62:594-599.

66. Arellano FM, Wentworth CE, Arana A, et al. Risk of lymphoma following exposure to calcineurin inhibitors and topical steroids in patients with atopic dermatitis. *J Invest Dermatol.* 2007;127:808-816.

67. Thaci D, Salgo. R. The topical calcineurin inhibitor pimecrolimus in atopic dermatitis: a safety update. *Acta Dermatovenerol Alp Panonica Adriat.* 2007;16:60-62.

68. Ormerod AD. Topical tacrolimus and pimecrolimus and the risk of cancer: how much cause for concern? *Br J Dermatol.* 2005;153:701-705.

69. Grimes PE. Psoralen for photochemotherapy for vitiligo. *Clin Dermatol.* 1997;15:921-926.

70. Parrish JA, Jaenicke KF. Action spectrum for phototherapy of psoriasis. *J Invest Dermatol.* 1981;76:359-362.

71. Westerhof W, Nieuweboer-Krobotova L. Treatment of vitiligo with UV-B radiation vs topical psoralen plus UV-A. *Arch Dermatol.* 1997;133:1525-1528.

72. Njoo MD, Spuls PI, Bos JD, et al. Nonsurgical repigmentation therapies in vitiligo. Meta-analysis of the literature. *Arch Dermatol.* 1998;134:1532-1540.

73. Njoo M, Bos J, Westerhof W. Treatment of generalized vitiligo in children with narrow-band (TL-01) UVB radiation therapy. *J Am Acad Dermatol.* 2000;42:245-253.

74. Yones SS, Palmer RA, Garibaldinos TM, et al. Randomized double-blind trial of treatment of vitiligo: efficacy of psoralen-UV-A therapy vs narrow-band-UV-B therapy. *Arch Dermatol.* 2007;143:578-584.

75. Natta R, Somsak T, Wisuttida T, et al. Narrow-band ultraviolet B radiation therapy for recalcitrant vitiligo in Asians. *J Am Acad Dermatol.* 2003;49:473-476.

76. Bhatnagar A, Kanwar AJ, Parsad D, et al. Psoralen and ultraviolet A and narrow-band ultraviolet B in inducing stability in vitiligo, assessed by vitiligo disease activity score: an open prospective comparative study. *J Eur Acad Dermatol Venereol.* 2007;21:1381-1385.

77. Nijsten TE, Stern RS. The increased risk of skin cancer is persistent after discontinuation of psoralen + ultraviolet A: a cohort study. *J Invest Dermatol.* 2003;121:252-258.

78. Teulings HE, Overkamp M, Ceylan E, et al. Decreased risk of melanoma and nonmelanoma skin cancer in patients with vitiligo: a survey among 1307 patients and their partners. *Br J Dermatol.* 2013;168:162-171.

79. Schallreuter KU, Behrens-Williams S, Khaliq TP, et al. Increased epidermal functioning wild-type p53 expression in vitiligo. *Exp Dermatol.* 2003;12:268-277.

80. Nordal EJ, Guleng GE, Rönnevig JR. Treatment of vitiligo with narrow-band-UVB (TL01) combined with tacrolimus ointment (0.1%) vs. placebo ointment, a randomized right/left double-blind comparative study. *J Eur Acad Dermatol Venereol.* 2011;25:1440-1443.

81. Grimes PE. Advances in the treatment of vitiligo: targeted phototherapy. *Cosmet Dermatol.* 2003;16:18-22.

82. Lotti TM, Menchini G, Andreassi L. UV-B radiation microphototherapy. An elective treatment for segmental vitiligo. *J Eur Acad Dermatol Venereol.* 1999;13:102-108.

83. Spencer JM, Nossa R, Ajmeri J. Treatment of vitiligo with the 308 nm excimer laser: a pilot study. *J Am Acad Dermatol.* 2002;46:727-731.

84. Taneja A, Trehan M, Taylor C. 308-nm excimer laser for the treatment of localized vitiligo. *Int J Dermatol.* 2003;42:658-662.

85. Passeron T, Ostovari N, Zakaria W, et al. Topical tacrolimus and the 308 nm excimer laser: a synergistic combination for the treatment of vitiligo. *Arch Dermatol.* 2004;140:1065-1069.

86. Kawalek AZ, Spencer JM, Phelps RG. Combined excimer laser and topical tacrolimus for the treatment of vitiligo: a pilot study. *Dermatol Surg.* 2004;30:130-135.

87. Leone G, Iacovelli P, Paro Vidolin A, et al. Monochromatic excimer light 308 nm in the treatment of vitiligo: a pilot study. *J Eur Acad Dermatol Venereol.* 2003;17:531-537.

88. Hofer A, Hassan AS, Legat FJ, et al. Optimal weekly frequency of 308 nm excimer laser treatment in vitiligo patients. *Br J Dermatol.* 2005;152:981-985.

89. Hadi S, Tinio P, Al-Ghaithi K, et al. Treatment of vitiligo using the 308 nm excimer laser. *Photomed Laser Surg.* 2006;24:354-357.

90. Akar A, Tunca M, Koc E, et al. Broadband targeted UVB phototherapy for localized vitiligo: a retrospective study. *Photodermatol Photoimmunol Photomed.* 2009;25:161-163.

91. Montes LF, Diaz ML, Lajous J, et al. Folic acid and vitamin B12 in vitiligo: a nutritional approach. *Cutis.* 1992;50:39-42.

92. Bhattacharya SK, Dutta AK, Mandal SB, et al. Ascorbic acid in vitiligo. *Indian J Dermatol.* 1981;26:4-11.

93. Parsad D, Saini R, Verma N. Combination of PUVAsol and topical calcipotriol in vitiligo. *Dermatology.* 1998;197:167-170.

94. Ermis O, Alpsoy E, Cetin L, Yilmaz E. Is the efficacy of psoralen plus ultraviolet A therapy for vitiligo enhanced by concurrent topical calcipotriol? A placebo-controlled, double blind study. *Br J Dermatol.* 2001;145:472-475.

95. Baysal V, Yildirim M, Erel A, et al. Is the combination of calcipotriol and PUVA effective in vitiligo? *J Eur Acad Dermatol Venereol.* 2003;17:299-302.

96. Travis LB, Silverberg NB. Calcipotriene and corticosteroid combination therapy for vitiligo. *Pediatr Dermatol.* 2004;21:495-498.

97. Goktas EO, Aydin F, Senturk N, et al. Combination of narrow-band UVB and topical calcipotriol for the treatment of vitiligo. *J Eur Acad Dermatol Venereol.* 2006;20:553-557.

98. Kullavanijaya P, Lim HW. Topical calcipotriene and narrow-band ultraviolet B in the treatment of vitiligo. *Photodermatol Photoimmunol Photomed.* 2004;20:248-251.

99. Xing C, Xu A. The effect of combined calcipotriol and betamethasone dipropionate ointment in the treatment of vitiligo: an open, uncontrolled trial. *J Drugs Dermatol.* 2012;11:e52-e54.

100. Grimes PE, Hamzavi I, Lebwohl M, et al. The efficacy of afamelanotide and narrow-band UV-B phototherapy for repigmentation of vitiligo. *JAMA Dermatol.* 2013;149:68-73.

101. Kapoor R, Phiske MM, Jerajani HR. Evaluation of safety and efficacy of topical prostaglandin E2 in treatment of vitiligo. *Br J Dermatol.* 2009;160:861-863.

102. Narang G., Efficacy and safety of topical bimatoprost solution 0.03% in stable vitiligo: a preliminary study. World Congress of Dermatology, Seoul, Korea, June 2011.

103. Mosenson JA, Zloza A, Nieland JD, et al. Mutant HSP70 reverses autoimmune depigmentation in vitiligo. *Sci Transl Med.* 2013;5:174ra128

104. Gupta D, Kumari R, Thappa DM. Depigmentation therapies in vitiligo. *Indian J Dermatol Venereol Leprol.* 2012;78:49-58.

105. van Geel N, Ongenae K, De Mil M, et al. Double-blind placebo-controlled study of autologous transplanted epidermal cell suspensions for repigmenting vitiligo. *Arch Dermatol.* 2004;140:1203-1208.

106. Chen YF, Yang PY, Hu DN, et al. Treatment of vitiligo by transplantation of cultured pure melanocyte suspension: analysis of 120 cases. *J Am Acad Dermatol.* 2004;51:68-74.

107. Gupta S, Kumar B. Epidermal grafting in vitiligo: influence of age, site of lesion, and type of disease on outcome. *J Am Acad Dermatol.* 2003;49:99-104.

108. Falabella R, Barona MI. Update on skin repigmentation therapies in vitiligo. *Pigment Cell Melanoma Res.* 2009;22:42-65.

CHAPTER

50

Oculocutaneous Albinism

Pamela A. Morganroth
Thomas J. Hornyak

KEY POINTS

- Oculocutaneous albinism (OCA) is the most common congenital disorder that causes generalized hypopigmentation.

- The pigmentary dilution seen in OCA involves the skin, hair, and eyes.

- Each of the four types of OCA is defined by a specific gene mutation that results in impaired biosynthesis of melanin.

- Different OCA types can have distinctive pigmentation phenotypes.

- Patients with albinism should receive cutaneous evaluation and counseling to help prevent and treat photodamage and skin cancer as well as ophthalmologic management for the visual manifestations of OCA.

BACKGROUND

Oculocutaneous albinism (OCA) is the most common congenital disorder that causes generalized hypopigmentation. The pigmentary dilution seen in OCA involves the skin, hair, and eyes. There are four types of OCA (OCA1, OCA2, OCA3, and OCA4), each of which is defined by a specific gene mutation that results in impaired biosynthesis of melanin. **Table 50-1** summarizes the characteristic features of each OCA type.

This chapter describes the epidemiology, pathogenesis, and clinical features of each of the four types of OCA. Management of OCA, nitisinone as a possible OCA treatment, the historical anthropology of OCA, and the contemporary struggles of East Africans with OCA are also discussed.

EPIDEMIOLOGY

OCA has an estimated frequency of approximately 1 in 17,000 to 20,000 in the general population.[1-3] Although four types of OCA have been described, the vast majority of known OCA cases are OCA1 (40%) or

OCA2 (50%).[3] The frequencies of different forms of OCA have wide racial and geographic variation. OCA2 is more common in darker skin of color individuals; whereas the overall prevalence of OCA2 is only 1 in 36,000 in the United States, it is 1 in 10,000 in African Americans.[4] A much higher OCA2 prevalence of 1 in 1400 to 7000 is found in sub-Saharan Africa.[5,6] In contrast to OCA2, OCA1, which has a frequency of approximately 1 in 40,000 in most populations, is very uncommon among darker skin of color individuals.[2] Although OCA3 and OCA4 combined account for only 10% of worldwide OCA cases, they are seen at higher rates in select populations. OCA3 has an estimated prevalence of 1 in 8500 in South African blacks,[7] and OCA4 accounted for 27% of OCAs in a study of Japanese patients, making OCA4 the second most common type of OCA in this population (behind OCA1).[8]

PATHOGENESIS

The four well-characterized types of OCA all are inherited in an autosomal recessive pattern, and each type has been linked to a causative gene mutation.[3] Patients with OCA have a normal number of melanocytes, but gene mutations result in impaired biosynthesis of melanin. Melanin is synthesized and stored in melanosomes, which are specialized subcellular organelles specific to melanocytes and retinal pigmented epithelial cells. The melanosomes are transferred from melanocytes to keratinocytes through their dendritic processes.[9] There are two distinct types of melanin: eumelanin, which is brown-black and insoluble, and pheomelanin, which is red-yellow and soluble. The total amount and distribution of melanin within melanocytes and keratinocytes and the relative amount of eumelanin and pheomelanin present are both important in determining skin and hair color. Both eumelanin and pheomelanin are synthesized from the precursor tyrosine. Tyrosinase, which requires binding of copper for its catalytic activity, is the rate-limiting enzyme involved in the conversion of tyrosine to melanin and plays an important role in OCA.[10] **Figure 50-1** depicts the biosynthesis of melanin within the melanosome in conjunction with the localization of critical OCA-related proteins.

Because melanocytes are present in the epidermis, hair follicle, and eye, reduced melanin production in OCA leads not only to decreased pigmentation of the skin and hair but also to hypopigmentation of several ocular structures, including the iris and fundus.[11] Another characteristic ocular finding is misrouting of the optic nerve at the optic chiasm, resulting in nystagmus. Studies in mice have shown that tyrosinase likely plays an important role in the routing of these optic nerve fibers during ocular development.[3,12] Patients with OCA also have decreased visual acuity of variable severity, which is multifactorial and related to nystagmus, foveal hypoplasia, and refractive error.[11] Photophobia is another common problem in individuals with OCA.[2]

OCULOCUTANEOUS ALBINISM TYPE 1

OCA1 is caused by mutations in the tyrosinase gene (*TYR*) on chromosome 11q14.3.[13] Over 100 different mutations in *TYR* have been described.[7] Mutations causing complete loss of tyrosinase function result in OCA1A, whereas those that cause partial loss of tyrosinase activity lead to the milder phenotype of OCA1B.

OCA1A, the classic tyrosinase-negative OCA, presents with white skin, white hair, and translucent irides due to a complete lack of melanin synthesis [**Figure 50-2**]. Melanocytic nevi are amelanotic and appear pink. Denaturing of hair keratins may cause a mild yellow coloring of the hair over time, and the irides typically appear pink early in life and become blue-gray with age.[1,3] Otherwise, the phenotype does not change as the child ages, and the skin lacks the ability to tan. Due to the complete lack of melanin, OCA1A patients are extremely susceptible to skin cancer. OCA1 patients also have worse visual acuity than other OCA types, typically ranging from 20/100 to 20/400.[1,14]

At birth, OCA1B patients typically look similar to OCA1A patients, with minimal to no pigment in the skin, hair, and eyes. However, over

TABLE 50-1 Characteristics of oculocutaneous albinism (OCA), types 1A, 1B, 2, 3, and 4

	OCA1A	OCA1B	OCA2	OCA3	OCA4
Important subtypes		Temperature-sensitive OCA1B	Brown OCA	Rufous OCA	
Gene mutation	*TYR*	*TYR* (leaky mutation)	*OCA2 (P* gene)	*TYRP1*	*SLC45A2 (MATP, AIM1)*
Protein product	Tyrosinase	Tyrosinase	OCA2 (P protein)	Tyrosinase-related protein 1	Solute carrier family 45 member 2 (membrane-associated transporter protein, absent in melanoma 1 protein)
Chromosome	11q14.3	11q14.3	15q11.2-q12	9p23	5p13.3
Hair color	White	Minimal to no pigment at birth, yellow/blonde to brown with age	Yellow (may be blonde or red in Caucasians, light brown in brown OCA)	Ginger-red (rufous type), mild hypopigmentation (nonrufous)	Minimal to near-normal pigmentation
Skin color	White (with amelanotic pink melanocytic nevi)	Minimal to no pigment at birth, may darken with age	Creamy white (light brown in brown OCA)	Red-bronze (rufous type), mild hypopigmentation (nonrufous)	
Iris color	Pink or blue-gray		Blue-gray to brown	Blue-gray to brown	

the first 20 years of life, patients develop variable amounts of melanin, resulting in increased pigmentation of the skin and hair.[1,3] The hair color typically becomes a yellow or light blonde color and may turn dark blonde or brown as the years pass. Most OCA1B patients burn easily with sun exposure, but many do have the ability to tan. Those with some melanin synthesis in the skin and hair may develop pigmented melanocytic nevi, lentigines, and ephelides. The irides also can develop brown pigment, which may be restricted to the inner third of the iris, but some degree of iris translucency is typically retained throughout life

and can be seen with slit-lamp examination.[3] Visual acuity is commonly 20/100 to 20/200, although it may be as high as 20/60 in some patients.[14] Relative to their family members, patients may have prominent skin and hair hypopigmentation or subtle pigmentary change. Variants of OCA1B have been called yellow OCA, platinum OCA, and minimal pigment OCA.

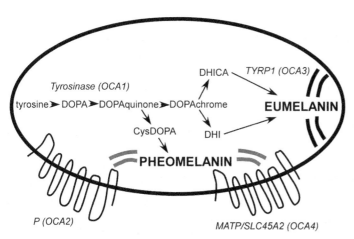

FIGURE 50-1. Roles of oculocutaneous albinism (OCA) proteins in melanosome structure and melanin biosynthesis. Depicted is a schematic structure of the melanosome, a subcellular organelle that is the intracellular site of melanin biosynthesis in the melanocyte. Melanin is synthesized via a cascade of enzymatic reactions starting with the amino acid tyrosine as a precursor. Tyrosinase, defective in OCA1, catalyzes the conversion of tyrosine to DOPAquinone through the intermediate dihydroxyphenylalanine (DOPA). Under conditions of eumelanin biosynthesis, DOPAquinone is rapidly converted to DOPAchrome. DOPAchrome is a precursor to two distinct metabolites: dihydroxyindolecarboxylic acid (DHICA), via the activity of DOPAchrome tautomerase (not depicted), and dihydroxyindole (DHI), via a slower, nonenzymatic conversion. Either can polymerize to form eumelanin, the brown-black form of melanin, which is deposited on intramelanosomal striations. TYRP1, defective in OCA3, may function as a DHICA oxidase[60] in addition to its role in stabilizing tyrosinase activity. Under conditions of pheomelanin (yellow-red melanin) biosynthesis, DOPAquinone is diverted via the intermediate cysteinylDOPA (CysDOPA) to form pheomelanin.[61] The proteins defective in OCA2 and OCA4 (the P protein and MATP/SLC45A2, respectively) do not have direct enzymatic roles in the formation of melanin. The P protein is a transmembrane protein important for melanosome acidification. MATP/SLC45A2 has the structure of a transporter transmembrane protein, but its precise role in melanosomal physiology is currently unknown.

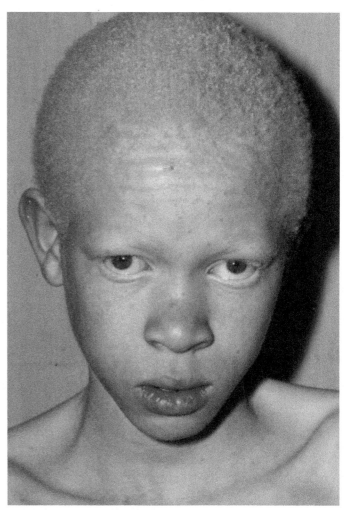

FIGURE 50-2. Note the white skin, blonde hair, and light eyes of this albino boy. (Used with permission from Barbara Leppard.)

One particularly interesting variant is temperature-sensitive OCA1B. These patients have a temperature-sensitive mutation in tyrosinase that causes the enzyme to become inactive at temperatures above 35°C.[15] This results in melanin synthesis limited to the cooler areas of the body. These patients are born with white hair. At puberty, they develop pigmented hairs on the extremities, but the hairs on the warmer scalp and axillary areas remain white.[1,3] Siamese cats also have a temperature-sensitive tyrosinase, which explains their typical fur pattern.[16] The kittens are white at birth but develop dark fur on the cooler face, ears, tail, and extremities as they age.

OCULOCUTANEOUS ALBINISM TYPE 2

OCA2 is caused by mutations in the *OCA2* gene (also known as the *P* gene) located on chromosome 15q11.2-q12.[2,17] The OCA2 protein is a melanosomal transmembrane protein with 12 domains that appears to play a role in regulation of melanosome pH.[18,19] Studies of mice with a deficiency in the OCA2 protein demonstrate a loss of the normal acidity of melanosomes.[20] The acidic environment in melanosomes may facilitate tyrosinase activity or other processes involved in melanin biosynthesis, such as melanosome biogenesis or the processing and transport of melanosomal proteins.[18] Many different *OCA2* mutations have been found to cause the OCA2 phenotype, but a single 2.7-kb deletion *OCA2* allele accounts for approximately 75% of mutations in sub-Saharan African OCA2 patients[21] and up to 50% of mutations in African American OCA2 patients.[22] Other distinct *OCA2* mutations are found commonly in different populations with a high frequency of OCA2.[3]

Africans and African Americans are much more commonly afflicted by OCA2 than Caucasians. Darker skin of color individuals with OCA2 have creamy white skin and yellow hair [**Figure 50-3**].[3] Hair may become darker with age, or alternatively, hair may become lighter, likely secondary to the normal phenomenon of hair graying. Iris color is variable, ranging from blue-gray to brown. Although these patients are unable to tan, they can develop pigmented melanocytic nevi, ephelides, and lentigines. Caucasian patients with OCA2 have a similar phenotype, with

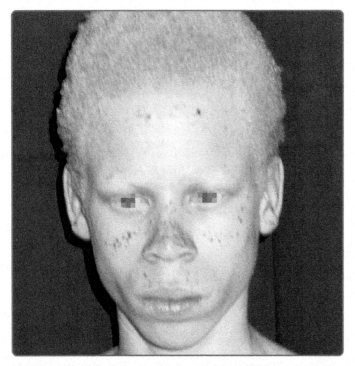

FIGURE 50-3. Yellow hair, creamy white skin, and pigmented ephelides in an African boy with OCA2. (Reproduced with permission from Goldsmith LA, et al. *Fitzpatrick's Dermatology in General Medicine.* 8th ed. New York, NY: McGraw-Hill; 2012.)

creamy white skin that does not tan coupled with the ability to develop pigmented skin lesions over time. Hair color in Caucasians with OCA2 is more variable, ranging from yellow to blonde to red, and Caucasians may experience darkening of hair with age. As with Caucasians with OCA1, the pigmentary dilution in Caucasians with OCA2 may be subtle, and patients may present with only ocular symptoms such as nystagmus. Visual acuity in OCA2 is usually 20/60 to 20/100, although acuity may be as high as 20/25.[23]

Brown OCA is an OCA2 variant with a mild phenotype that has been reported in Africans and African Americans. The phenotype is characterized by light brown hair and skin and blue-gray to brown irides at birth, with little pigmentary change as the child ages.[24] As with other OCA2 patients, nystagmus and decreased visual acuity are features. The brown pigmentation in the skin helps protect against actinic damage and skin cancer.[24]

OCA2 has an interesting association with Prader-Willi syndrome (PWS) and Angelman syndrome (AS), two genetic developmental disorders caused most frequently by a deletion on the paternal (PWS) or maternal (AS) chromosome 15q in the region containing the *OCA2* gene.[25,26] The genes responsible for PWS and AS are imprinted, which means that they are expressed only on the maternal or the paternal chromosome. Absence of the maternally derived chromosome 15q11-q13 region results in AS, whereas absence of the same area of the paternally derived chromosome results in PWS. Although deletions are the most common cause of PWS and AS, these diseases can also be caused by uniparental disomy and defects in the imprinting center region.[27,28] Some patients with PWS and AS have generalized hypopigmentation of the hair and skin, but these patients lack the characteristic ocular features of OCA.[23,25,26] In PWS, having a chromosome 15q deletion that includes the *OCA2* gene has been shown to correlate with the presence of hypopigmentation.[25] It is unclear why patients with PWS and AS develop this hypopigmentation when they have one normal *OCA2* gene on the allele without the 15q deletion, whereas individuals in OCA2 families who are heterozygotes for the *OCA2* mutation have normal pigmentation. However, abnormal extension of the imprinted region into the distal *OCA2* locus, which is normally not imprinted, could explain this phenomenon.[27] PWS and AS patients who manifest both the cutaneous and ocular features of OCA have also been reported, but these patients have an independent *OCA2* mutation on the chromosome 15 not affected by the PWS or AS 15q deletion.[23,28-30]

OCULOCUTANEOUS ALBINISM TYPE 3

OCA3 is caused by a mutation in the *TYRP1* gene on chromosome 9p23.[31] The protein product of *TYRP1*, tyrosinase-related protein 1 (TYRP1), belongs to the same protein family as tyrosinase and has a similar structure.[32] TYRP1 increases the tyrosine hydroxylase and dihydroxyphenylalanine (DOPA) oxidase activities of tyrosinase, which are crucial for melanin synthesis. Like other members of the tyrosinase-related protein family, TYRP1 also affects melanocyte proliferation and apoptosis.[33]

OCA3 is seen most frequently in South African patients, where the prevalence is approximately 1 in 8500.[34] These patients present with red-bronze skin, ginger-red hair, and blue-gray or brown irides.[35] This phenotype is known as rufous (red) OCA. In contrast to the other OCA types, rufous OCA patients typically have limited ocular disease with mild or no nystagmus.[34] Two specific *TYRP1* mutations are common in South African rufous OCA patients. One is a deletion mutation at codon 368 of exon 6 (resulting in a stop codon downstream at codon 384), and the other is a base substitution at codon 166 of exon 3 (leading to a stop codon in place of a serine).[34] Although OCA3 was initially considered to be exclusive to darker skin of color individuals, case reports have recently documented OCA3 in Caucasian and Asian patients from Pakistan, Germany, India, China, and Japan.[32,36-39] These patients have been reported to have a mild phenotype relative to other OCA types.

OCULOCUTANEOUS ALBINISM TYPE 4

OCA4 is a more recently described subset of OCA that is caused by *SLC45A2* (previously called *MATP* and *AIM1*) on chromosome 5p13.2.[40] This gene encodes solute carrier family 45 member 2 (SLC45A2), a protein with homology to plant sucrose proton symporters.[40] SLC45A2 is also expressed in a high percentage of melanoma cell lines.[41] The precise role of SLC45A2 in melanin synthesis is unknown, but tyrosinase is mislocalized in mouse melanocytes with homozygous *SLC45A2* mutations.[42] Although OCA4 is a rare variant in most countries, it is the second most common type of OCA in Japan (behind OCA1).[8]

The OCA4 phenotype is characterized by variable hypopigmentation of the skin, hair, and irides, ranging from minimal pigment to near-normal pigment.[8,40,43] Some patients may experience an increase in pigmentation during the first decade of life.[8] Nystagmus is noted in some but not all patients.[43] Visual acuity is typically between 20/100 and 20/200, but it can range from 20/30 to 20/400.[40] Clinically the phenotype cannot be distinguished from OCA2.[2]

SYNDROMES WITH GENERALIZED HYPOPIGMENTATION

There are several rare albinism syndromes that should be included in the differential diagnosis of OCA. These syndromes—Chédiak-Higashi syndrome, Hermansky-Pudlak syndrome, and Griscelli syndrome—present with a variable degree of generalized hypopigmentation, in addition to multiple systemic manifestations. In contrast to OCA, which is caused by impaired melanin biosynthesis, these albinism syndromes are caused by gene mutations that impair intracellular vesicle trafficking or transfer, which are important processes not only in melanocytes but also in a variety of other cell types. The key features of these rare syndromes are summarized in **Table 50-2**.[1,44,45]

GENETIC TESTING FOR OCULOCUTANEOUS ALBINISM

The diagnosis of OCA is typically made based on clinical findings. However, molecular genetic testing is needed to establish the OCA subtype due to substantial clinical overlap among the subtypes. Identification of the mutation responsible for OCA in a given patient enables carrier detection in family members when this is desired.[2]

MANAGEMENT OF OCULOCUTANEOUS ALBINISM

Patients with albinism are at increased risk for sunburns and skin cancer because they lack the protection from ultraviolet radiation traditionally provided by melanin. Therefore, these patients should engage in photoprotective behaviors from an early age, including avoidance of sun exposure (especially during the peak hours of 10 AM to 2 PM) and regular use of broad-spectrum sunscreens and photoprotective clothing. Education regarding photoprotection may be particularly important for parents with darker skin types who do not have problems with sun sensitivity themselves. Patients with albinism should have regular follow-up with a dermatologist. Basal cell and squamous cell carcinomas are the most common skin cancers seen in OCA patients, but both amelanotic and pigmented melanomas may also occur.[46,47]

Management of the multiple vision problems in OCA patients may include glasses (possibly bifocals) to aid in visual acuity, darkly tinted lenses to manage photophobia, and contact lenses or extraocular muscle surgery for nystagmus.[2] Eye patching may be needed for children with strabismus.[2] Patients may need special equipment at school to help them overcome their visual disabilities and succeed in the classroom.

The National Organization for Albinism and Hypopigmentation (NOAH), a U.S. support group for the albinism community, has a website that may be helpful for patients with albinism: http://www.albinism.org/. NOAH publishes a variety of informational bulletins discussing issues such as the social aspect of albinism, the impact of albinism on driving, and visual aids that can be helpful for people with albinism. In addition, for patients who might benefit from talking with or meeting others with albinism, NOAH has online forums as well as biennial national conferences.

FUTURE TREATMENT

Currently there are no effective medical treatments available for the hypopigmentation of the hair, skin, and eyes of patients with OCA. However, nitisinone, a U.S. Food and Drug Administration-approved drug for the treatment of hereditary tyrosinemia type 1, may be a future treatment option for OCA1B. Nitisinone [Orfadin; 2(-2-nitro-4 trifluoromethylbenzoyl)-1,3 cyclohexanedione] is a competitive inhibitor of 4-hydroxyphenylpyruvate dioxygenase, an enzyme involved in the tyrosine catabolic pathway.[48] Patients with hereditary tyrosinemia type 1 treated with nitisinone have a reduction in hepatotoxic and nephrotoxic intermediates. However, they also develop elevated plasma tyrosine levels as a side effect of nitisinone treatment, so it was hypothesized that this might be a useful medication for OCA.[48] In a recent study using a mouse model of OCA1B, treatment with nitisinone resulted not only in increased tyrosine but also improved stability and enzymatic function of tyrosinase.[48] The OCA1B mouse model treated with nitisinone had an increased number of pigmented melanosomes in both the retinal pigmented epithelium and the iridial and choroidal melanocytes, as well as visibly darker coat and iris pigmentation. Interestingly, prenatal nitisinone treatment (the mother mouse received nitisinone during her pregnancy) also resulted in improved skin and fur pigmentation in the baby OCA1B mouse model. An OCA1A mouse model was also

TABLE 50-2	Albinism syndromes with systemic manifestations		
	Griscelli (subtypes GS1-3)*	Hermansky-Pudlak (subtypes HPS1-7)	Chédiak-Higashi
Gene mutation	*MYO5A* (in GS1), *RAB27A* (in GS2), *melanophilin* (*MLPH*) (in GS3)	*HPS1*, *ADTB3A* (in HPS2), *HPS3*, *HPS4*, *HPS5*, *HPS6*, *DTNBP1* (in HPS7)	*LYST*
Pigmentary features	Pigmentary dilution of the skin, silvery-gray hair	Similar to tyrosinase-positive OCA (including ocular pathology)	Pigmentary dilution of skin and eyes, silvery hair
Systemic manifestations	Recurrent infections (GS2), hemophagocytic syndrome (GS2), neurologic problems (GS1)	Platelet dysfunction, pulmonary fibrosis, granulomatous colitis, kidney disease	Bleeding diathesis, recurrent infections, neurologic problems, accelerated phase (lymphoproliferation involving major organs)
Other key features	Large, irregularly distributed clumps of pigment in hair shafts; accumulation of melanosomes in melanocytes	Most common in Puerto Rico, lysosomal ceroid storage defects	Small, regularly distributed clumps of pigment in hair shafts; giant granules in neutrophils; giant melanosomes in melanocytes

Abbreviations: GS, Griscelli syndrome; HPS, Hermansky-Pudlak syndrome; OCA, oculocutaneous albinism.

*Elejalde syndrome (neuroectodermal melanolysosomal disease), which manifests with the hypopigmentation of Griscelli syndrome and severe neurologic disease is likely a variant of GS1.

treated with nitisinone, but the OCA1 mouse model did not experience increased ocular and cutaneous pigmentation.

Nitisinone holds promise as a potential treatment for OCA1B patients, both for increasing pigmentation of the skin, hair, and irides and also possibly for improving visual function. It is unclear whether nitisinone treatment in humans with OCA1B would improve visual defects, especially if it is not administered prenatally. Nitisinone in doses of 1 to 2 mg/kg/d orally have been well tolerated in humans,[49] and clinical studies are currently in development to examine whether nitisinone is a beneficial treatment for OCA.[48]

HISTORICAL ANTHROPOLOGY OF ALBINISM

Reports of albinos in Native American subpopulations in North and South America have been described for centuries. These subpopulations related to their albinos in markedly different ways. For example, in the Cuna Indian population of Panama, albinos were selected against culturally, with marriage discrimination and infanticide limiting the frequency of the trait in the population. In contrast, both the Hopi and Zuni tribes of the now Southwest United States actively protected their albino members, allowed them to marry nonalbinos, and integrated them fully into cultural activities. Historical estimates of the incidence of albinism in these various Native American populations have been used to calculate Darwinian fitness values of the individual albinism genotypes.[50]

The "Brandywine isolate," a small, triracial population in Brandywine, Maryland, is an example of a select small population studied intensively for its genetic attributes, which include a very high frequency of albinism. In this highly inbred population of mixed Caucasian, African, and Native American ancestry, the prevalence of OCA2 is estimated at 1 in 85 individuals (1.2% of the population of 5128).[50,51] The Brandywine isolate is believed to have originated with illegal interracial unions between Native Americans, Caucasian, and African Americans in the late seventeenth and eighteenth centuries.[52] The high prevalence of OCA2 in the inbred Brandywine isolate has been attributed to the founder effect (decrease in genetic variation that occurs when a small number of individuals create a new population) and decreased selection against albinism within the inbred population.[50]

CONTEMPORARY STRUGGLES OF EAST AFRICANS WITH ALBINISM

Many myths about albinism abound in Africa, and these myths have resulted in widespread brutal attacks on adults and children with albinism in Burundi, Tanzania, and other East African countries. The following commonly held beliefs provide motivation for murders and rapes of Africans with albinism: (1) albino body parts worn as amulets bring good luck, fortune, and health; (2) albino body parts are a necessary ingredient for witch doctor potions; and (3) sexual intercourse with an albino woman will cure human immunodeficiency virus infection.[53] During the past 10 years, over 100 Africans with albinism have been murdered so that their body parts could be sold for thousands of dollars in underground markets.[54] In addition, deceased individuals with albinism are frequently buried indoors in graves sealed with cement to prevent grave robbers from stealing albino body parts. Children with albinism are subjected to verbal and physical abuse at school and may also be shunned by family members.[53] Other social obstacles are created by beliefs that albinism can be spread by touching, albinos have low intelligence, albinos are fathered by Caucasian men, and albinos are possessed by ghosts of European colonists.[53]

Multiple nonprofit organizations are engaged in advocacy to combat the violence against Africans with albinism. Asante Mariamu is a group that was created to specifically address the threats faced by East Africans with albinism.[55] The group was named after Mariamu Stanford, a Tanzanian woman with albinism who was 5 months pregnant when she lost both of her arms and her unborn child during an attack by men who wanted her body parts for the black market. NOAH has also been very involved in efforts to stop the violence against Africans with albinism.[56] With the help of such organizations and recent international media attention, there have been multiple positive political developments. Jakaya Kikwete, Tanzania's president, has publically condemned the violence against people with albinism and, in 2008, appointed Al-Shymaa Kway-Geer, a woman with albinism, to Parliament as a symbol of his support of the albino community.[54] In 2010, the U.S. House of Representatives passed legislation (H.R. 1088) denouncing the brutal attacks on Africans with albinism and urging the U.S. and East African governments to take action to prevent further violence against people with albinism and bring the perpetrators to justice.[57]

Individuals with albinism in Africa also suffer from a high morbidity and mortality caused by skin cancers in sun-exposed areas. Africans with albinism often have difficulty succeeding in school and finding desirable indoor jobs for multiple reasons, including the visual disturbances associated with albinism and the prevalence of negative myths about people with albinism, including the belief that albinos have inferior intelligence.[53] Thus, Africans with albinism are often employed in menial outdoor jobs, which greatly increases their risk of developing skin cancers, especially when poverty prevents them from buying sunscreen.[53,58] Multiple studies have found a very high rate of skin cancers in Africans with albinism at a young age, especially squamous cell carcinoma (SCC) of the head and neck. Largely because of poverty, Africans with albinism often fail to seek treatment for skin cancer for several years after symptom onset and present with large tumors.[58] Furthermore, they are frequently prevented from finishing treatment due to lack of money.[58] Although specific incidence rates of SCC in Africans with albinism are lacking and are likely to vary as a function of distance from the equator, a survey of 305 Tanzanians with albinism performed in the early 1980s provides a glimpse at the extent of SCC within this population. Of 52 albinos between the ages of 11 and 20 followed for the 2-year period of the natural history study, 54% (n = 28) developed a skin malignancy.[59]

CONCLUSION

OCA has been reported in skin of color populations and in Africans and African Americans in particular. The four types of OCA cause generalized hypopigmentation of the skin and hair as well as ocular disorders. Different OCA types can have distinctive pigmentation phenotypes. Evaluation and counseling of patients with OCA are important to prevent and treat photodamage and skin cancer. Additionally, ophthalmologic management for visual manifestations of OCA is important.

REFERENCES

1. Ortonne J, Passeron T. Vitiligo and other disorders of hypopigmentation. In: Bolognia JL, Schaffer JV, eds. *Dermatology*. 3rd ed. New York, NY: Elsevier Limited; 2012.
2. Gronskov K, Ek J, Brondum-Nielsen K. Oculocutaneous albinism. *Orphanet J Rare Dis*. 2007;2:43.
3. Hornyak TJ. Albinism and other genetic disorders of pigmentation. In: Fitzpatrick TB, Wolff K, eds. *Fitzpatrick's Dermatology in General Medicine*. 7th ed. New York, NY: McGraw-Hill Medical; 2008.
4. Oetting WS, King RA. Molecular basis of albinism: mutations and polymorphisms of pigmentation genes associated with albinism. *Hum Mutat*. 1999;13:99-115.
5. Kromberg JG, Jenkins T. Prevalence of albinism in the South African negro. *S Afr Med J*. 1982;61:383-386.
6. Spritz RA, Fukai K, Holmes SA, Luande J. Frequent intragenic deletion of the P gene in Tanzanian patients with type II oculocutaneous albinism (OCA2). *Am J Hum Genet*. 1995;56:1320-1323.
7. Oetting WS, Fryer JP, Shriram S, King RA. Oculocutaneous albinism type 1: the last 100 years. *Pigment Cell Res*. 2003;16:307-311.
8. Suzuki T, Tomita Y. Recent advances in genetic analyses of oculocutaneous albinism types 2 and 4. *J Dermatol Sci*. 2008;51:1-9.

9. Park H-Y, Yaar M. Biology of melanocytes. In: Fitzpatrick TB, Wolff K, eds. *Fitzpatrick's Dermatology in General Medicine.* 7th ed. New York, NY: McGraw-Hill Medical; 2008.

10. Hearing VJ. Determination of melanin synthetic pathways. *J Invest Dermatol.* 2011;131:E8-E11.

11. Russell-Eggitt I. Albinism. *Ophthalmol Clin North Am.* 2001;14:533-546.

12. Lavado A, Jeffery G, Tovar V, de la Villa P, Montoliu L. Ectopic expression of tyrosine hydroxylase in the pigmented epithelium rescues the retinal abnormalities and visual function common in albinos in the absence of melanin. *J Neurochem.* 2006;96:1201-1211.

13. Tomita Y, Takeda A, Okinaga S, Tagami H, Shibahara S. Human oculocutaneous albinism caused by single base insertion in the tyrosinase gene. *Biochem Biophys Res Commun.* 1989;164:990-996.

14. King RA. Oculocutaneous albinism type 1. In: Pagon RA, Bird TD, Dolan CR, Stephens K, Adam MP, eds. *GeneReviews.* Seattle, WA: University of Washington; 1993.

15. King RA, Townsend D, Oetting W, et al. Temperature-sensitive tyrosinase associated with peripheral pigmentation in oculocutaneous albinism. *J Clin Invest.* 1991;87:1046-1053.

16. Imes DL, Geary LA, Grahn RA, Lyons LA. Albinism in the domestic cat (*Felis catus*) is associated with a tyrosinase (TYR) mutation. *Anim Genet.* 2006;37:175-178.

17. Rinchik EM, Bultman SJ, Horsthemke B, et al. A gene for the mouse pink-eyed dilution locus and for human type II oculocutaneous albinism. *Nature.* 1993;361(6407):72-76.

18. Brilliant M, Gardner J. Melanosomal pH, pink locus protein and their roles in melanogenesis. *J Invest Dermatol.* 2001;117:386-387.

19. Sitaram A, Piccirillo R, Palmisano I, et al. Localization to mature melanosomes by virtue of cytoplasmic dileucine motifs is required for human OCA2 function. *Mol Biol Cell.* 2009;20:1464-1477.

20. Puri N, Gardner JM, Brilliant MH. Aberrant pH of melanosomes in pink-eyed dilution (p) mutant melanocytes. *J Invest Dermatol.* 2000;115:607-613.

21. Kerr R, Stevens G, Manga P, et al. Identification of P gene mutations in individuals with oculocutaneous albinism in sub-Saharan Africa. *Hum Mutat.* 2000;15:166-172.

22. Durham-Pierre D, King RA, Naber JM, Laken S, Brilliant MH. Estimation of carrier frequency of a 2.7 kb deletion allele of the P gene associated with OCA2 in African-Americans. *Hum Mutat.* 1996;7:370-373.

23. Lewis RA. Oculocutaneous albinism type 2. In: Pagon RA, Bird TD, Dolan CR, Stephens K, Adam MP, eds. *GeneReviews.* Seattle, WA: University of Washington; 1993.

24. King RA, Creel D, Cervenka J, Okoro AN, Witkop CJ. Albinism in Nigeria with delineation of new recessive oculocutaneous type. *Clin Genet.* 1980;17:259-270.

25. Spritz RA, Bailin T, Nicholls RD, et al. Hypopigmentation in the Prader-Willi syndrome correlates with P gene deletion but not with haplotype of the hemizygous P allele. *Am J Med Genet.* 1997;71:57-62.

26. Smith A, Wiles C, Haan E, et al. Clinical features in 27 patients with Angelman syndrome resulting from DNA deletion. *J Med Genet.* 1996;33:107-112.

27. Cassidy SB, Schwartz S, Miller JL, Driscoll DJ. Prader-Willi syndrome. *Genet Med.* 2012;14:10-26.

28. Buiting K. Prader-Willi syndrome and Angelman syndrome. *Am J Med Genet C Semin Med Genet.* 2010;154C:365-376.

29. Fridman C, Hosomi N, Varela MC, Souza AH, Fukai K, Koiffmann CP. Angelman syndrome associated with oculocutaneous albinism due to an intragenic deletion of the P gene. *Am J Med Genet A.* 2003;119A:180-183.

30. Lee ST, Nicholls RD, Bundey S, Laxova R, Musarella M, Spritz RA. Mutations of the P gene in oculocutaneous albinism, ocular albinism, and Prader-Willi syndrome plus albinism. *N Engl J Med.* 1994;330:529-534.

31. Murty VV, Bouchard B, Mathew S, Vijayasaradhi S, Houghton AN. Assignment of the human TYRP (brown) locus to chromosome region 9p23 by nonradioactive in situ hybridization. *Genomics.* 1992;13:227-229.

32. Zhang KH, Li Z, Lei J, et al. Oculocutaneous albinism type 3 (OCA3): analysis of two novel mutations in TYRP1 gene in two Chinese patients. *Cell Biochem Biophys.* 2011;61:523-529.

33. Boissy RE, Zhao H, Oetting WS, et al. Mutation in and lack of expression of tyrosinase-related protein-1 (TRP-1) in melanocytes from an individual with brown oculocutaneous albinism: a new subtype of albinism classified as "OCA3." *Am J Hum Genet.* 1996;58:1145-1156.

34. Manga P, Kromberg JG, Box NF, Sturm RA, Jenkins T, Ramsay M. Rufous oculocutaneous albinism in southern African Blacks is caused by mutations in the TYRP1 gene. *Am J Hum Genet.* 1997;61:1095-1101.

35. Kromberg JG, Castle DJ, Zwane EM, et al. Red or rufous albinism in southern Africa. *Ophthalmic Paediatr Genet.* 1990;11:229-235.

36. Rooryck C, Roudaut C, Robine E, Musebeck J, Arveiler B. Oculocutaneous albinism with TYRP1 gene mutations in a Caucasian patient. *Pigment Cell Res.* 2006;19:239-242.

37. Yamada M, Sakai K, Hayashi M, et al. Oculocutaneous albinism type 3: a Japanese girl with novel mutations in TYRP1 gene. *J Dermatol Sci.* 2011;64:217-222.

38. Forshew T, Khaliq S, Tee L, et al. Identification of novel TYR and TYRP1 mutations in oculocutaneous albinism. *Clin Genet.* 2005;68:182-184.

39. Chiang PW, Spector E, Scheuerle A. A case of Asian Indian OCA3 patient. *Am J Med Genet A.* 2009;149A:1578-1580.

40. Suzuki T, Hayashi M. Oculocutaneous albinism type 4. In: Pagon RA, Bird TD, Dolan CR, Stephens K, Adam MP, eds. *GeneReviews.* Seattle, WA: University of Washington; 1993.

41. Harada M, Li YF, El-Gamil M, Rosenberg SA, Robbins PF. Use of an in vitro immunoselected tumor line to identify shared melanoma antigens recognized by HLA-A*0201-restricted T-cells. *Cancer Res.* 2001;61:1089-1094.

42. Costin GE, Valencia JC, Vieira WD, Lamoreux ML, Hearing VJ. Tyrosinase processing and intracellular trafficking is disrupted in mouse primary melanocytes carrying the underwhite (uw) mutation. A model for oculocutaneous albinism (OCA) type 4. *J Cell Sci.* 2003;116:3203-3212.

43. Inagaki K, Suzuki T, Shimizu H, et al. Oculocutaneous albinism type 4 is one of the most common types of albinism in Japan. *Am J Hum Genet.* 2004;74:466-471.

44. Scheinfeld NS. Syndromic albinism: a review of genetics and phenotypes. *Dermatol Online J.* 2003;9:5.

45. Schaffer JV, Paller AS. Primary immunodeficiencies. In: Bolognia JL, Schaffer JV, eds. *Dermatology.* 3rd ed. New York, NY: Elsevier Limited; 2012.

46. Perry PK, Silverberg NB. Cutaneous malignancy in albinism. *Cutis.* 2001;67:427-430.

47. Schulze KE, Rapini RP, Duvic M. Malignant melanoma in oculocutaneous albinism. *Arch Dermatol.* 1989;125:1583-1586.

48. Onojafe IF, Adams DR, Simeonov DR, et al. Nitisinone improves eye and skin pigmentation defects in a mouse model of oculocutaneous albinism. *J Clin Invest.* 2011;121:3914-3923.

49. Holme E, Lindstedt S. Nontransplant treatment of tyrosinemia. *Clin Liver Dis.* 2000;4:805-814.

50. Woolf CM. Albinism (OCA2) in Amerindians. *Am J Phys Anthropol.* 2005;(Suppl 41):118-140.

51. Witkop CJ Jr, Niswander JD, Bergsma DR, Workman PL, White JG. Tyrosinase positive oculocutaneous albinism among the Zuni and the Brandywine triracial isolate: biochemical and clinical characteristics and fertility. *Am J Phys Anthropol.* 1972;36:397-405.

52. Harte TJ. Social origins of the Brandywine population. *Phylon.* 1963;24:369-378.

53. Cruz-Inigo AE, Ladizinski B, Sethi A. Albinism in Africa: stigma, slaughter and awareness campaigns. *Dermatol Clin.* 2011;29:79-87.

54. Ladizinski B, Cruz-Inigo AE, Sethi A. The genocide of individuals with albinism in Africa. *Arch Dermatol.* 2012;148:1151.

55. Asante Mariamu. http://www.asante-mariamu.org/. Accessed December 7, 2012.

56. NOAH: The National Organization for Albinism and Hypopigmentation. http://www.albinism.org/. Accessed December 7, 2012.

57. Congress TLo. H.RES.1088 Library of Congress: Recognizing the plight of people with albinism in East Africa and condemning their murder and mutilation. http://thomas.loc.gov/cgi-bin/bdquery/z?d111:H.Res1088:. Accessed December 7, 2012.

58. Opara KO, Jiburum BC. Skin cancers in albinos in a teaching Hospital in eastern Nigeria - presentation and challenges of care. *World J Surg Oncol.* 2010;8:73.

59. Luande J, Henschke CI, Mohammed N. The Tanzanian human albino skin. Natural history. *Cancer.* 1985;55:1823-1828.

60. Kobayashi T, Urabe K, Winder A, et al. Tyrosinase related protein 1 (TRP1) functions as a DHICA oxidase in melanin biosynthesis. *EMBO J.* 1994;13:5818-5825.

61. Sturm RA, Teasdale RD, Box NF. Human pigmentation genes: identification, structure and consequences of polymorphic variation. *Gene.* 2001;277:49-62.

CHAPTER

51

Melasma

Amit G. Pandya
Shelly Rivas

KEY POINTS

- Melasma is an acquired, relapsing condition of bilateral facial hypermelanosis.

- Melasma predominantly affects women with skin of color.

- An association exists with exposure to ultraviolet radiation, hormonal influences, and genetic predisposition, although the exact cause remains unknown.

- Melasma negatively affects quality of life and can be socially stigmatizing.

- First-line therapy entails sun protection and sun avoidance in conjunction with topical depigmenting agents.

- The use of chemical peels, laser and light therapies should be reserved for refractory cases and used with caution in patients with skin of color to reduce the risk of postinflammatory hyperpigmentation.

Melasma is an acquired, relapsing disorder of the skin characterized by bilateral, hyperpigmented, irregularly shaped macules and patches on sun-exposed areas of the face [**Figure 51-1**]. The terms chloasma and 'mask of pregnancy' are synonymous with melasma. Melasma is a common cause of hyperpigmentation worldwide, particularly in women of childbearing age with skin of color. Although several therapies have been developed for this often recalcitrant condition, effective long-term treatment for melasma remains a challenge, resulting in psychological distress and social stigmatization.

EPIDEMIOLOGY AND PATHOGENESIS

Melasma affects more than 5 million people in the United States alone and serves as a significant source of psychological distress with a negative impact on the quality of life reported by those who seek treatment for it.[1,2] It predominantly affects women of Latino, African, Native American, and Asian descent.[3] Fitzpatrick skin types III and IV are most commonly affected, as evidenced by a recent multicenter survey of women from nine countries.[4] A population-based study of melasma in Hispanic women in the United States showed that 8.8% currently had melasma and 4% reported having had it in the past [**Figure 51-2**].[5] Other studies, including surveys of patients presenting to dermatology clinics, have shown rates as high as 40%.[6] The mean age of diagnosis is 34 years old, often years after the last pregnancy.[4] Melasma tends to be much less common after menopause.

The exact etiology of melasma has yet to be elucidated. There appears to be a strong association with hormones, ultraviolet (UV) light, and genetics. Recent data indicate that visible light may also play a role in the pathogenesis.

HORMONAL INFLUENCES

Melasma has long been associated with hormonal changes, with patients noticing initiation or exacerbation of the condition during pregnancy, after oral contraceptive use, and occasionally during hormone replacement therapy.[7,8] In a study conducted by Resnik,[7] 29% of women developed melasma after initiating oral contraceptives, whereas Ortonne et al[4] recently found that 25% of women using hormonal contraception claimed that their melasma appeared for the first time after its use in a multicountry study. While there is evidence for the proliferative effect of estrogen on melanocytes, levels of estrogen, progesterone, or melanocyte-stimulating hormone have not been found to be elevated in patients with melasma.[9,10] Unfortunately, melasma often persists for years after

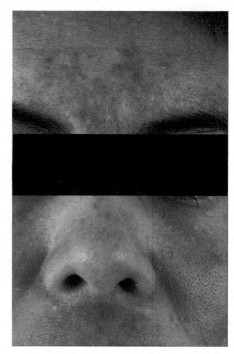

FIGURE 51-1. Melasma involving the cheeks symmetrically with prominent glabella, nasal, and upper lip involvement.

pregnancy or with discontinuation of oral contraceptives. Patients who develop melasma while taking oral contraceptives should discontinue the medication and avoid future use. Recent studies have also found increased vascularization and greater expression of vascular endothelial growth factor in keratinocytes in melasma lesions as compared to perilesional normal skin, although an association with hormone levels has not been observed.[11,12] In a study that sought to investigate the histopathologic characteristics of melasma in men compared with those of women, clinicians found that chronic UV radiation associated with paracrine cytokine signaling played an important role in the mechanism associated with hyperpigmentation in men [**Figure 51-3**].

ULTRAVIOLET RADIATION

Exposure to sunlight is perhaps the most important risk factor for melasma, evidenced by the worsening of melasma in patients with sun exposure. UV exposure causes upregulation of cytokines, leading to melanogenesis and melanocyte proliferation. In addition, melasma is more common in countries closer to the equator, and it tends to fade during the winter season.

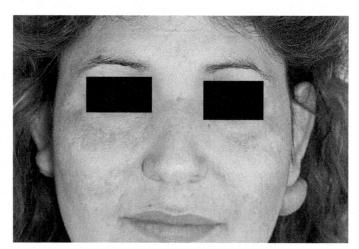

FIGURE 51-2. Melasma in a Hispanic woman involving the cheeks symmetrically.

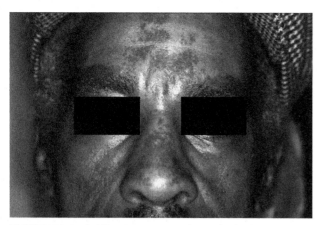

FIGURE 51-3. An African American man with centrofacial melasma. Clinicians postulate that chronic ultraviolet radiation plays an important role in the occurrence of melasma in men.

GENETIC PREDISPOSITION

In a recent study of 324 melasma patients surveyed globally, 48% reported a family history of melasma, predominantly in first-degree relatives, suggesting that genetic factors play a role in the etiology of melasma.[4] It was also found that African Americans were more likely to have a positive family history of melasma.[4] Additionally, a survey of pregnant women with melasma in Iran reported a 54.7% incidence of melasma in a family member.[13]

CLINICAL FEATURES

Melasma is diagnosed clinically with light tan to grayish-brown macules, visible on the malar areas, forehead, upper lip, and mandible. Symmetric, irregular lesions on the cheeks are the most common presentation and can be used to differentiate melasma from other disorders of facial hyperpigmentation. There are two major clinical patterns of melasma: centrofacial and malar. Mandibular melasma, or lower jawbone melasma, is a rarer clinical pattern, and it has been conjectured that without histopathologic evidence, the diagnosis of mandibular melasma should not be made because of its rarity.[14]

The centrofacial pattern is the most common and is characterized by lesions on the cheeks, nose, forehead, and chin [**Figure 51-4**]. The malar pattern presents with lesions localized to the cheeks and nose

[**Figure 51-5**], whereas the mandibular pattern predominantly presents with lesions along the jawline.[15] Wood lamp skin examinations are used to distinguish between melasma caused by epidermal versus dermal hyperpigmentation, with epidermal involvement showing enhancement of lesions under the light; however, a recent study showed that dermal melanin in patients with Wood lamp-enhanced melasma.[16] In comparing lesional skin to normal skin in melasma patients with Fitzpatrick skin types IV through VI, Grimes et al[16] showed that a Wood lamp examination indicated epidermal melasma in some patients; however, melanin was seen in the epidermis and dermis on light microscopy in all patients. These findings indicate that dermal melasma may be underrecognized using a Wood lamp examination.

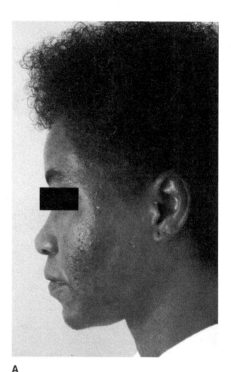

A

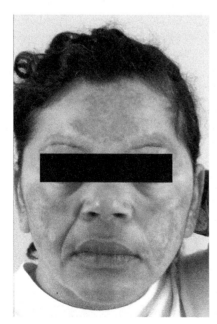

FIGURE 51-4. Centrofacial melasma in a skin of color patient. Note the characteristic lesions on the cheeks, nose, and forehead.

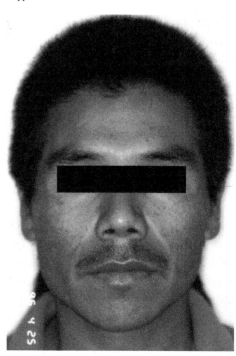

B

FIGURE 51-5. Malar melasma in an **(A)** African American patient and **(B)** Latin American patient. Note the localization of the lesions to the cheeks and nose.

TABLE 51-1 Differential diagnosis of melasma

Differential diagnosis	Notes
Postinflammatory hyperpigmentation	This usually occurs in the setting of previous trauma or inflammation to the affected area
Ephelides (freckles)	These can be distinguished by their smaller size and their earlier appearance in life, usually before puberty
Solar lentigines	These present with a more diffuse and asymmetrical pattern of distribution on the face, with evidence of solar damage to other parts of the face and body
Facial acanthosis nigricans	This should be considered if the lesion is velvety in texture and there are indications of insulin resistance in the patient (such as obesity) and similar lesions in flexural areas of the body
Medication-induced pigmentation	This is usually present in several areas of the body and it is uncommon for the pigmentation to be located exclusively on the face; a history of recent drug intake would be consistent with the diagnosis
Bilateral acquired nevus of Ota	This would present with darker gray pigmentation, and it is usually a congenital disorder

HISTOPATHOLOGY OF MELASMA

Histopathologically, melasma can present with the following patterns: epidermal, dermal, or compound (mixed). This classification is based on a study carried out by Sanchez et al[15] using lesional skin biopsies of melasma patients with Fitzpatrick skin types I to IV. In the epidermal type, melanin was found in the basal and suprabasal layers and in the presence of highly pigmented and highly dendritic melanocytes. In the dermal type, melanophages and melanosomes were seen in perivascular locations in the dermis with limited pigmentation in the epidermis.[15] Melanocytes in lesional skin are larger and with more prominent dendrites compared to normal skin.[17]

DIFFERENTIAL DIAGNOSIS

The differential diagnosis of melasma includes a variety of disorders of hyperpigmentation, which are listed in **Table 51-1**.

TREATMENT

Although no cure exists for melasma, it can be effectively managed [**Table 51-2**]. Among the first-line therapies are topical agents aimed at skin lightening, sun protection, and camouflage. Second-line therapies include chemical peels, light-based therapies, and lasers. Caution should be observed in patients with skin of color, because these latter therapies can worsen or enhance pigmentation of the skin. Although there have been recent developments in light and laser therapies, they tend to work better on patients with lighter skin types, and their effectiveness for those with darker skin types remains unclear. No single *panacea* exists

TABLE 51-2 Management therapies for melasma

First-line	Triple combination therapy containing hydroquinone, a retinoid, and a fluorinated steroid nightly, with use of daily sunscreen at SPF 30 or above and physical sunblock
	Hydroquinone 4% twice daily for up to 6 months, with daily use of sunscreen at SPF 30 or above and physical sunblock
Second-line	Glycolic acid peels every 4–6 weeks starting at 30% and increasing in concentration as tolerated, with daily use of sunscreen at SPF 30 or above and physical block
Third-line	Fractional laser therapy, intense pulsed light therapy, with daily use of sunscreen at SPF 30 or above and physical block

Abbreviation: SPF, sun protection factor.

Adapted with permission from Sheth VM, Pandya AG. Melasma: a comprehensive update part II. *J Am Acad Dermatol.* 2011;65:699-714.[31]

for melasma, and the most effective treatment involves a combination of therapies.

MINIMIZING ULTRAVIOLET EXPOSURE

The most important preventive measure for melasma is minimizing sun exposure through sun avoidance and frequent sunblock use. Frequent daily use of broad-spectrum sunscreen with a minimum sun protection factor of 30 as well as physical sunblocks such as zinc oxide and titanium dioxide is recommended. In addition, photosensitizing medications should be avoided. The use of clothing and hats and sun avoidance add further protection. Sunscreens help prevent melasma and also enhance the effectiveness of other topical treatments for melasma.[18,19] Because UV and visible light can cause an increase in melanin in all skin types,[20] the use of sunscreen is of utmost importance. This intervention is particularly important for women with darker skin types, given the widespread misconception of inherent protection from UV radiation.

CAMOUFLAGE

The use of camouflage makeup has been found to be useful in many patients with melasma. Several brands offer cosmetic coverage for a wide range of skin tones.

TOPICAL AGENTS

Topical treatment is aimed at preventing the development of pigment involved in the pathogenesis of melasma. This is achieved by various mechanisms, predominantly through the inhibition of tyrosinase, the rate-limiting enzyme in the melanin production pathway.[21] Hydroquinone, which is believed to act as a tyrosinase inhibitor, is considered the gold standard in melasma treatment either as a monotherapy or combination therapy. In a study by Ennes et al[22] comparing 4% hydroquinone to a placebo for the treatment of melasma, 38% of patients treated with hydroquinone had a complete clinical response versus only 8% in the placebo-treated group. Controversy regarding the safety of hydroquinone has existed for decades due to concerns that it can cause exogenous ochronosis and occupational vitiligo.[23] However, numerous studies have shown no adverse effects when hydroquinone was compared to controls, supporting its safe use.[24]

Tretinoin has also been found to be effective in the treatment of melasma as a monotherapy or in combination therapy. It is believed to work by stimulating keratinocyte turnover, decreasing melanosome transfer, and enhancing the absorption of depigmenting agents.[25] In a study conducted by Griffiths et al,[26] 68% of melasma subjects treated with 0.1% tretinoin showed clinical improvement versus 5% of vehicle-treated subjects over a period of 40 weeks. Similar results were reported in skin of color patients who used tretinoin 0.1% for 40 weeks.[27] In both studies, irritation was found to be the most common side effect. The long duration until improvement limits its use a monotherapy. Adapalene, a synthetic retinoid that causes less irritation than tretinoin, can be used as an alternative and has been shown to be as effective as tretinoin for the treatment of melasma.[28] The Kligman-Willis formula containing 5% hydroquinone, 0.1% tretinoin, and 0.1% dexamethasone was one of the first combination therapies found to be effective for the treatment of melasma.[29] In a more recent study using a formula containing 4% hydroquinone, 0.05% retinoic acid, and 0.01% fluocinolone acetonide, Taylor et al[30] found that 77% of patients using the formula showed complete or near-complete clearance of their melasma after 8 weeks when compared to a maximum of 46.8% of patients on dual combination therapy containing hydroquinone, tretinoin, or fluocinolone.

Other topical agents used for the treatment of melasma include azelaic acid, kojic acid, ascorbic acid, arbutin/deoxyarbutin, licorice extract, and soy.[31] These agents have varying degrees of effectiveness and have not been generally found to be superior to hydroquinone; however, they are useful alternatives when hydroquinone is not tolerated or unavailable. Studies examining the efficacy of azelaic acid have yielded promising results. In a recent Iranian study, patients who used 20% azelaic acid showed greater improvement in their melasma when compared to patients using 4% hydroquinone.[32] Another study in Filipino patients conducted by Verallo-Rowell et al[33] found a greater reduction of melasma using 20% azelaic acid versus 2% hydroquinone, and in patients with skin types IV to VI, Lowe et al[34] showed there was a significant improvement in melasma patients who used 20% azelaic acid versus its vehicle.

Tranexamic acid, a plasmin inhibitor, is another compound that has been targeted as a possible new treatment for melasma when used topically, orally, and intradermally. In a study of 100 Asian women with melasma, weekly injections of tranexamic acid were shown to produce a significant decrease in their Melasma Area and Severity Index (MASI) scores from a baseline of 13.22 to 7.57 after 12 weeks.[35] In another study, 25 patients used both oral and topical tranexamic acid concomitantly for 8 weeks resulting in a significant decrease in the melanin index in lesional skin, which also showed reduced vascularity and epidermal pigmentation on histologic examination.[36] Conversely, 23 melasma patients studied by Kanechorn et al[37] in a randomized, double-blind, split-face trial showed no significant difference in the depigmenting effect of 5% tranexamic versus its vehicle.

CHEMICAL PEELS

Chemical peels have shown modest benefit in the treatment of melasma and are considered a second-line therapy when used as an adjunct treatment. A study conducted by Sarkar et al[38] in which 40 patients with melasma underwent glycolic acid peels in addition to topical therapy with a modified Kligman-Willis formula (5% hydroquinone, 0.05% tretinoin, 1% hydrocortisone acetate) showed an 80% decrease in MASI scores. However, in a split-face study by Hurley et al[39] comparing the effect of 4% hydroquinone alone versus 4% hydroquinone plus glycolic acid peels, no difference was found in depigmenting effect. In a study measuring the effectiveness of salicylic acid peels, Grimes[40] reported improvement of melasma in six patients treated with a series of salicylic acid peels and 4% hydroquinone; however, a more recent controlled, split-face study showed no improvement with four salicylic acid peels.[41]

There are limited data available on the use of other chemical peeling agents, such as lactic acid, Jessner solution, and trichloroacetic acid. Given that the long-term efficacy of chemical peels as a monotherapy has not been established, their use should be limited to recalcitrant cases and as an adjunct therapy. Because irritation from chemical peels can result in postinflammatory hyperpigmentation, these peels should be used cautiously, particularly in patients with darker skin types.

LASERS

Laser and light treatment is considered a second- or third-line therapy for melasma and should only be considered in the most resistant cases. The risk of postinflammatory hyperpigmentation is greatest in darker-skinned individuals; these modalities should be used with extreme caution in these patients. A spot test is advised before laser treatment to determine the individual's response to treatment.

Studies with Q-switched, erbium-doped yttrium aluminium garnet, and ultrapulse carbon dioxide lasers have shown worsening of melasma and development of postinflammatory hyperpigmentation after treatment[42-44]; therefore, such therapies should be used judiciously in treating melasma or avoided altogether. The use of fractional laser therapy has shown promising results and is currently the only U.S. Food and Drug Administration-approved laser treatment for melasma. In a study of 10 patients with melasma with Fitzpatrick skin types III to V exposed to fractional laser therapy, 6 out of 10 patients had 75% to 100% clearance of their lesions.[45] Use of the fractional laser at a lower fluence and in conjunction with hydroquinone appears to yield the best results. The use of intense pulsed light (IPL), a nonlaser light source, has also produced optimistic results. In a study of 89 Asian females with melasma treated with IPL, mean MASI scores were shown to significantly decrease after four sessions.[46] A study of Taiwanese women with Fitzpatrick skin types III to VI treated with IPL in combination with hydroquinone for the treatment of melasma showed marked improvement compared to hydroquinone alone after 16 weeks of therapy.[47] Figueiredo and

Trancoso[48] compared patients with refractory melasma who were treated with a single session of IPL and triple combination therapy (hydroquinone 4%, tretinoin 0.05%, and fluocinolone acetonide 0.01%) to patients treated with triple therapy alone and found there was a better response in the IPL group, with the MASI score showing a 49.4% reduction after 6 months and 44.9% reduction after 12 months.

Copper bromide lasers, which can produce two beams of light, one for treating pigmented lesions and a second for treating vascular lesions, have shown promising outcomes recently. In a study of 10 Korean women treated with copper bromide laser, modest improvement of melasma was shown after only 8 weeks.[49] Furthermore, biopsies of lesional skin before and after treatment showed a decrease in epidermal melanin and melanosomes as well as a decrease in dermal vascularity,[49] pointing to a possibly new target, cutaneous vessels, in the treatment of melasma.

CONCLUSION

The exact etiology of melasma remains unknown, thus making treatment more challenging. While camouflage and avoidance of sun exposure can contribute to melasma control, topical agents, chemical peels, and lasers have also been proven effective in some studies; however, their use needs to be tailored to patients' Fitzpatrick skin types and history of treatment. The future of melasma treatment includes the targeting of cutaneous blood vessels, although further studies are needed to determine the efficacy of such an approach.

REFERENCES

1. Grimes PE. Melasma: etiologic and therapeutic considerations. *Arch Dermatol.* 1995;131:1453-1457.
2. Taylor A, Pawaskar M, Taylor SL, et al. Prevalence of pigmentary disorders and their impact on quality of life: a prospective cohort study. *J Cosmet Dermatol.* 2008;7:164-168.
3. Taylor SC. Epidemiology of skin diseases in ethnic populations. *Dermatol Clin.* 2003;21:601-607.
4. Ortonne JP, Arellano I, Berneburg M, et al. A global survey of the role of ultraviolet radiation and hormonal influences in the development of melasma. *J Eur Acad Dermatol Venereol.* 2009;23:1254-1262.
5. Werlinger KD, Guevara IL, Gonzalez CM, et al. Prevalence of self-diagnosed melasma among pre-menopausal Latino women in Dallas and Fort Worth, Tex. *Arch Dermatol.* 2007;143:424-425.
6. Sivayathorn A. Melasma in Orientals. *Clin Drug Invest.* 1995;10:34-40.
7. Resnik S. Melasma induced by oral contraceptive drugs. *J Am Med Assoc.* 1967;199:601-605.
8. Ponzio HA, Favaretto AL, Rivitti EA. Proposal of a quantitative method to describe melasma distribution in women. *J Cosmet Dermatol.* 2007;20:103-111.
9. Jee SH, Lee SY, Chiu HC, et al. Effects of estrogen and estrogen receptors in normal human melanocytes. *Biochem Biophys Res.* 1994;199:1407-1412.
10. Perez M, Sanchez JL, Aguilo F. Endocrinologic profile of patients with idiopathic melasma. *J Invest Dermatol.* 1983;81:543-545.
11. Kim EH, Kim YC, Lee E-S, et al. The vascular characteristics of melasma. *J Derm Sci.* 2007;46:111-116.
12. Jang YH, Sim JH, Hee YK, et al. The histopathologic characteristics of male melasma: comparison to female melasma and lentigo. *J Am Acad Dermatol.* 2012;66:642-649.
13. Moin A, Jabery Z, Fallah N. Prevalence and awareness of melasma during pregnancy. *Int J Dermatol.* 2006;45:285-288.
14. Panda S. Melasma study: methodological problems. *Indian J Dermatol.* 2011;56:772-773.
15. Sanchez NP, Pathak MA, Sato S. Melasma: a clinical, light microscopic, ultrastructural, and immunofluorescence study. *J Am Acad Dermatol.* 1981;4:698-709.
16. Grimes PE, Yamada N, Bhawan J. Light microscopic, immuno-histochemical and ultrastructural alterations in patients with melasma. *Am J Dermatopathol.* 2005;27:96-101.
17. Kang WH, Yoon KH, Lee ES, et al. Melasma: histopathological characteristics in 56 Korean patients. *Br J Dermatol.* 2002;146:228-237.
18. Pathak MA, Fitzpatrick TB, Kraus EW. Usefulness of retinoic acid in the treatment of melasma. *J Am Acad Dermatol.* 1986;15:894-899.

19. Grimes PE. A microsponge formulation of hydroquinone 4% and retinol 0.15% in the treatment of melasma and postinflammatory hyperpigmentation. *Cutis.* 2004;74:362-368.

20. Pathak MA, Riley FC, Fitzpatrick TB. Melanogenesis in human skin following exposure to long-wave ultraviolet and visible light. *J Invest Dermatol.* 1962;39:435-443.

21. Jimbow K, Obata H, Pathak M, et al. Mechanism of depigmentation by hydroquinone. *J Invest Dermatol.* 1974;62:436-449.

22. Ennes SB, Paschoalick RC, Mota de Avelar Alchorne M. A double-blind, comparative, placebo-controlled study of the efficacy and tolerability of 4% hydroquinone as a depigmenting agent in melasma. *J Dermatol Treat.* 2000;11:173-179.

23. Westerhof W, Kooyers TJ. Hydroquinone and its analogues in dermatology—a potential health risk. *J Cosmet Dermatol.* 2005;4:55-59.

24. Nordlund JJ, Grimes PE, Ortonne JP. The safety of hydroquinone. *J Eur Acad Dermatol Venereol.* 2006;20:781-787.

25. Ortonne JP. Retinoid therapy of pigmented disorders. *Dermatol Ther.* 2006;19:280-288.

26. Griffiths CE, Finkel LJ, Ditre CM, et al. Topical tretinoin (retinoic acid) improves melasma. A vehicle-controlled, clinical trial. *Br J Dermatol.* 1993;129:415-421.

27. Kimbrough-Green CK, Griffiths CEM, Finkel LJ, et al. Topical retinoic acid (tretinoin) for melasma in black patients. *Arch Dermatol.* 1994;130:727-733.

28. Dogra S, Kanwar AJ, Parsad D. Adapalene in the treatment of melasma: a preliminary report. *J Dermatol.* 2002;29:539-540.

29. Kligman AM, Willis I. A new formula for depigmenting human skin. *Arch Dermatol.* 1975;111:40-48.

30. Taylor SC, Torok H, Jones T, et al. Efficacy and safety of a new triple-combination agent for the treatment of facial melasma. *Cutis.* 2003;72:67-72.

31. Sheth VM, Pandya AG. Melasma: a comprehensive update part II. *J Am Acad Dermatol.* 2011;65:699-714.

32. Farshi S. Comparative study of therapeutic effects of 20% azelaic acid and hydroquinone 4% in the treatment of melasma. *J Cosmet Derm.* 2011;10:282-287.

33. Verallo-Rowell VM, Verallo V, Graupe K, et al. Double-blind comparison of azelaic acid and hydroquinone in the treatment of melasma. *Acta Derm Venereol Suppl (Stockh).* 1989;143:58-61.

34. Lowe NJ, Rizk D, Grimes P, et al. Azelaic acid 20% cream in the treatment of facial hyperpigmentation in darker-skinned patients. *Clin Ther.* 1998;20:945-959.

35. Lee JH, Park JG, Lim SH, et al. Localized intradermal microinjection of tranexamic acid for treatment of melasma in Asian patients: a preliminary clinical trial. *Dermatol Surg.* 2006;32:626-631.

36. Na JI, Choi SY, Yang SH, et al. Effect of tranexamic acid on melasma: a clinical trial with histological evaluation. *J Eur Acad Dermatol Venereol.* 2013;27:1035-1039.

37. Kanechorn NA, Niumphradit N, Manosroi A, et al. Topical 5% tranexamic acid for the treatment of melasma in Asians: a double-blind randomized controlled clinical trial. *J Cosmet Laser Ther.* 2012;14:150-154.

38. Sarkar R, Kaur C, Bhalla M, et al. The combination of glycolic acid peels with a topical regimen in the treatment of melasma in dark-skinned patients: a comparative study. *Dermatol Surg.* 2002;28:828-832.

39. Hurley ME, Guevara IL, Gonzales RM, et al. Efficacy of glycolic acid peels in the treatment of melasma. *Arch Dermatol.* 2002;138:1578-1582.

40. Grimes PE. The safety and efficacy of salicylic acid chemical peels in darker racial-ethnic groups. *Dermatol Surg.* 1999;25:18-22.

41. Kodali S, Guevara IL, Carrigan CR, et al. A prospective, randomized, split-face, controlled trial of salicylic acid peels in the treatment of melasma in Latin American women. *J Am Acad Dermatol.* 2010;63:1030-1035.

42. Taylor CR, Anderson RR. Ineffective treatment of refractory melasma and postinflammatory hyperpigmentation by Q-switched ruby laser. *J Dermatol Surg Oncol.* 1994;20:592-597.

43. Tse Y, Levine VJ, McClain SA, et al. The removal of cutaneous pigmented lesions with the Q-switched ruby laser and the Q-switched neodymium: yttrium-aluminum-garnet laser. A comparative study. *J Dermatol Surg Oncol.* 1994;20:795-800.

44. Angsuwarangsee SA, Polnikorn N. Combined ultrapulse CO_2 laser and Q-switched alexandrite laser compared with Q-switched alexandrite laser alone for refractory melasma: split-face design. *Dermatol Surg.* 2003;29:59-64.

45. Rokhsar CK, Fitzpatrick RE. The treatment of melasma with fractional photothermolysis: a pilot study. *Dermatol Surg.* 2005;31:1645-1650.

46. Li YH, Chen JZS, Wei HC, et al. Efficacy and safety of intense pulsed light in treatment of melasma in Chinese patients. *Dermatol Surg.* 2008;34:693-701.

47. Wang CC, Hui CY, Sue YM, et al. Intense pulsed light for the treatment of refractory melasma in Asian persons. *Dermatol Surg.* 2004;30:1196-200.

48. Figueiredo SL, Trancoso SS. Single-session intense pulsed light combined with stable fixed-dose triple combination therapy for the treatment of refractory melasma. *Dermatol Ther.* 2012;25:477-480.

49. Lee HI, Lim YY, Kim BJ, et al. Clinicopathologic efficacy of copper bromide plus/yellow laser (578 nm with 511 nm) for treatment of melasma in Asian patients. *Dermatol Surg.* 2010;36:885-893.

CHAPTER 52

Postinflammatory Hyperpigmentation/ Periorbital Hyperpigmentation

Candrice R. Heath
Raechele Cochran Gathers
Susan C. Taylor

KEY POINTS

- Hyperpigmentation is a common disorder affecting individuals with skin of color.

- Postinflammatory hyperpigmentation (PIH) may be secondary to inflammatory disease, infection, allergic contact or irritant reactions, injury from prior procedures or trauma, sites of papulosquamous or vesiculobullous disease, and medication reactions.

- Periorbital hyperpigmentation may be secondary to excessive epidermal or dermal melanin deposition, excessive or superficial vasculature or skin laxity, or periorbital fat pseudoherniation.

- Treatment, which should be directed toward the primary etiology, includes photoprotection, topical bleaching agents, chemical peels, lasers, dermal fillers, and surgical intervention.

- Although PIH and periorbital hyperpigmentation are not life threatening, they negatively affect quality of life.

Postinflammatory hyperpigmentation (PIH) is a common disorder that occurs in just about all individuals with skin of color [**Figure 52-1**]. This acquired hyperpigmentation may involve areas of prior inflammatory disease, infection, allergic contact or irritant reactions, injury from prior procedures or trauma, sites of papulosquamous or vesiculobullous disease, and medication reactions [**Figure 52-2, A to C**].[1-3] PIH commonly appears on the skin as brown to gray macules or patches.[4] Periorbital hyperpigmentation, often colloquially referred to as *dark circles,* is defined as bilateral, homogeneous, hyperchromic macules and patches primarily involving the upper and lower eyelids, but also sometimes extending toward the eyebrows, malar regions, and lateral nasal root.[5,6] Many causal factors have been implicated in the development of periorbital hyperpigmentation [**Table 52-1**]. Periorbital hyperpigmentation can be much more noticeable in skin of color populations[3] and is often a significant cosmetic concern because it can portend a fatigued, sad, or aged appearance.[7-9]

Both PIH and periorbital hyperpigmentation can be emotionally distressing for patients, affecting all aspects of their personal and professional lives.[4]

EPIDEMIOLOGY, ETIOLOGY, AND PATHOGENESIS

PIH affects women and men with equal incidence and may occur at any age. Although PIH may be more apparent in Fitzpatrick skin types III to VI, all skin types have the potential to develop PIH lesions [Figures 52-1 and 52-2]. The PIH in Fitzpatrick skin types III to VI patients may last longer and sometimes never completely fades.[1,2,10,11] Some authors have concluded that people with skin of color are more likely to develop

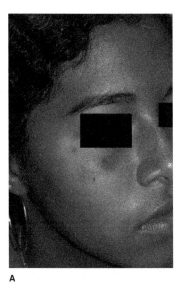 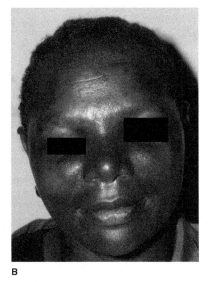 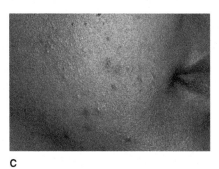

A   B   C

FIGURE 52-1. Hyperpigmentation on the face. **(A)** Postinflammatory hyperpigmentation from acne in a woman with skin type V. **(B)** Hyperpigmentation on the face of a woman with skin type VI. (Used with permission of Dr. Barbara J. Leppard.) **(C)** Hyperpigmentation on the cheek of a Hispanic woman with skin type IV.

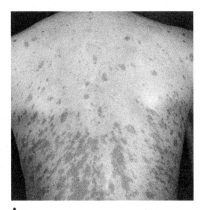

A

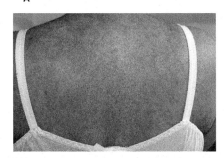

B

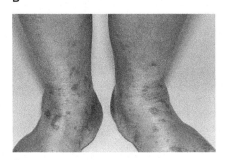

C

FIGURE 52-2. Postinflammatory hyperpigmentation may occur after drug eruption, lichen planus, psoriasis, tinea versicolor, or eczema. **(A)** Postinflammatory hyperpigmentation on the back of an East Indian woman with skin type IV. Reproduced with permission from Goldsmith LA, et al. *Fitzpatrick's Dermatology in General Medicine.* 8th ed. New York, NY: McGraw-Hill; 2012. **(B)** Postinflammatory hyperpigmentation on the back of an African American woman with skin type V. **(C)** Postinflammatory hyperpigmentation from lichen planus on the ankles and feet of a woman with skin type V.

PIH due to the large amount of melanin contained in melanosomes within the epidermis.[1,2] Other investigators have theorized that a person's tendency to develop PIH is related to the specific type of melanocyte present: weak, strong, or normal. After an inflammatory event or skin trauma, weak melanocytes result in hypopigmentation due to the decreased production of melanin, whereas strong melanocytes produce excess pigment, leading to hyperpigmentation.[2] Although melanin production may be increased in PIH, the number of melanocytes is normal.[1] Normal melanocytes continually produce appropriate quantities of melanin, resulting in normochromia.[2]

A myriad of stimuli may result in PIH [**Table 52-2**]. The hyperpigmented macules and patches seen in PIH result from mechanisms occurring in both the epidermal and the dermal layers of the skin. Inflammatory cells release mediators and cytokines that play a role in PIH.[3] In response to inflammation, arachidonic acid mediators such as prostaglandins and leukotrienes stimulate increased melanin synthesis and transport to keratinocytes.[10,12] Oleic acid and stem cell factor also have been implicated in the pathogenesis of PIH.[13,14] Inflammation may

TABLE 52-1	Etiology of periorbital hyperpigmentation

Most likely
- Fatigue/stress
- Hereditary factors
- Aging/photodamage
- Lifestyle factors (alcohol, smoking, caffeine)

Consider
- Postinflammatory
- Atopy
- Eye strain
- Hormonal
- Medications (oral contraceptives, antipsychotics, chemotherapeutics, etc.)

Always rule out
- Hepatic/renal disease
- Thyroid disease
- Addison disease
- Carcinoma
- Ecchymoses
- Vitamin K deficiency
- Hereditary blood disorder

TABLE 52-2	Stimuli producing postinflammatory hyperpigmentation
Dermatologic diseases	
Acneiform	
Papulosquamous	
Lichenoid	
Psoriasiform	
Vesiculobullous	
Infections	
Dermatologic therapy	
Topical agents	
Drug eruptions	
Cosmetic procedures	
Chemical peels	
Microdermabrasion	
Cryosurgery	
Laser therapy	
Intense pulse light therapy	
Fillers	
Trauma	

cause the disruption of melanocytes and the release of pigment into the dermis, a phenomenon called *pigment incontinence.*[2,10]

Periorbital hyperpigmentation has a distinct etiology, pathogenesis, and perceived epidemiology. Despite the perceived prevalence of periorbital hyperpigmentation, there are few comprehensive epidemiologic data. Although not rare in males, females may be affected more frequently due to hormonal factors.[8,9]

Many causal factors have been implicated in the development of periorbital hyperpigmentation [Table 52-2]. Genetics,[6,15,16] fatigue, stress and emotional lability, exhaustion of the periorbital muscles, and aging all may play a significant role. Lifestyle factors associated with periorbital hyperpigmentation may include alcohol overuse, smoking, and excessive intake of caffeinated beverages.[8] Various systemic etiologies also have been associated with periorbital hyperpigmentation, including cachexia, biliary disease, hyperthyroidism,[17] vitamin K deficiency, Addison disease, heart and kidney disease, and other circulatory conditions that may cause excessive fluid retention.[8] Periorbital hyperpigmentation also may be seen in ectodermal dysplasia,[18] erythema dyschromicum perstans,[19] and acanthosis nigricans. A rare autosomally dominant pattern of periorbital hyperpigmentation also may be seen.[15,16]

Patients with atopic dermatitis, contact dermatitis, or any airborne or food allergy may experience periorbital itching and irritation with ensuing periorbital hyperpigmentation.[8] Atopic individuals also may develop inferior lid discoloration (allergic shiners) resulting from mucosal edema and venous stasis of the paranasal sinuses.[19,20] Periorbital ecchymoses (raccoon eyes) resulting from anterior fossa fracture may lead to periorbital hyperpigmentation. Additionally, neoplasms must be considered. Eyelid melanoma and, in children, neuroblastoma metastatic to the orbits may lead to periorbital hyperpigmentation.[19] The dermal melanocytosis of nevus of Ota may present as isolated periorbital hyperpigmentation, often with a blue-green to dark gray hue. Finally, chronic use of some drugs, including oral contraceptives, hormone replacement therapy, antipsychotics, iron-containing compounds, gold, and chemotherapeutic agents, can lead to periorbital hyperpigmentation.[19] When assessing the patient with periorbital hyperpigmentation, a comprehensive history and directed review of systems should be performed. A complete medical evaluation may be necessary in cases of sudden onset, rapid progression, or unexplained symptomatology.

CLINICAL FINDINGS

◼ HISTORY

The chief complaint of patients with PIH may include dark marks, dark spots, uneven skin tone, discolorations, and blemishes. Patients

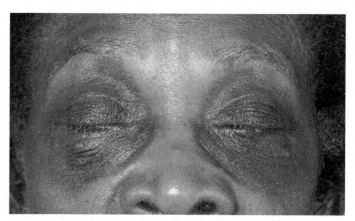

FIGURE 52-3. Woman with periorbital hyperpigmentation.

presenting with periorbital hyperpigmentation may complain of dark circles and appearing fatigued despite being well-rested.

◼ PHYSICAL FINDINGS

The morphology of the macules and patches of PIH is variable, but the borders are often hazy and are distributed in areas of prior inflammation. When melanin is deposited in the epidermis, the lesions tend to be brown, but melanin in the dermis causes lesions to have a dark gray or gray-blue hue.[1,2]

The clinical presentation of periorbital hyperpigmentation is related to its pathogenesis. Periorbital hyperpigmentation secondary to excessive epidermal melanin may appear brown in color [**Figure 52-3**]. Pigmentation secondary to excessive dermal melanin may appear blue-gray in color.[21]

Periorbital hyperpigmentation related to hypervascularity often has a violaceous or bluish color due to visibility of the dermal capillary network.[22] Applying pressure or stretching the affected skin often will lessen the appearance of the pigmentation. Periorbital hyperpigmentation due to periorbital edema is often characterized by variability and a purplish hue, and is often worse in the morning or after a salty meal.[5]

Pseudoherniation of the periorbital fat and skin laxity can result in the creation of dark shadows. Facial movements may cause repositioning of the muscles and skin, thus altering the pattern of light on the face and emphasizing the appearance of hyperpigmentation.[8]

◼ LABORATORY AND OTHER TESTS

While history and physical examination are usually sufficient to determine the primary cause of PIH and periorbital hyperpigmentation, confirmation by histologic examination may rarely be necessary. Evidence of PIH may be found in the epidermis, dermis, or both. Histologic characteristics of periorbital hyperpigmentation suggest that it may be caused by a number of pathogenetic factors, including epidermal and dermal hypermelanosis, excessive or superficial vasculature and periorbital edema, and shadowing of the skin secondary to anatomic factors such as skin laxity and pseudoherniation of periorbital fat.[5,8]

Under the Wood's light, lesions with increased epidermal pigment appear darker,[23] but this may not be useful in darker skin types.[21] Also, Wood's light exams do not always correlate histologically with the level of melanin in the skin—epidermal, dermal, or mixed.

Confocal in vivo reflectance microscopy is now being utilized as a noninvasive method of evaluating the level of melanin (epidermal vs. mixed) and to highlight the heterogeneous nature of hyperpigmentation within lesions. With continued development, confocal in vivo reflectance microscopy may become a future staple in hyperpigmentation research and patient clinical evaluation.[24–27]

DIFFERENTIAL DIAGNOSIS

The differential diagnosis of periorbital hyperpigmentation and PIH are detailed in **Table 52-3**; clinical manifestations are shown in **Figures 52-4 to 52-6**.

TABLE 52-3	Differential diagnosis of periorbital hyperpigmentation and postinflammatory hyperpigmentation	
Periorbital hyperpigmentation	**Postinflammatory hyperpigmentation**
Most likely	**Most likely**
• Postinflammatory hyperpigmentation • Irritant/allergic contact dermatitis	• Secondary to melasma, acne vulgaris, atopic dermatitis, trauma
Consider	**Consider**
• Nevus of Ota • Acanthosis nigricans • Erythema dyschromicum perstans • Fixed drug eruption	• Exogenous ochronosis • Amyloidosis (lichenoid/macular) • Tinea versicolor • Lichen planus • Acanthosis nigricans • Erythema dyschromicum perstans (ashy dermatosis) • Morphea
Always rule out	**Always rule out**
• Ecchymoses • Melanoma	• Addison disease • Systemic lupus erythematosus

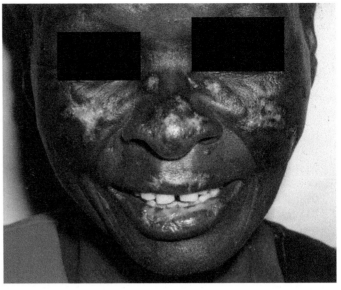

FIGURE 52-6. Hyperpigmentation secondary to discoid lupus on the face of a woman with skin type VI.

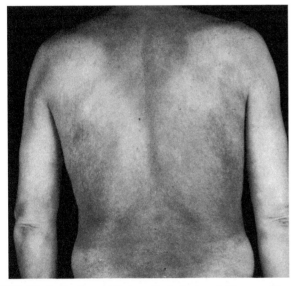

FIGURE 52-4. Macular amyloidosis on the back of an Arabian man. (Reproduced with permission from Wolff K. *Fitzpatrick's Color Atlas of Dermatology*, 5th ed. New York, NY: McGraw-Hill; 2005.)

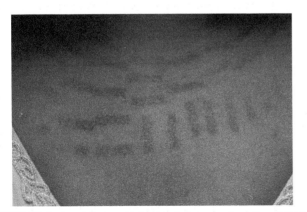

FIGURE 52-5. Laser hair removal-induced postinflammatory hyperpigmentation in an African American woman with skin type V.

COMPLICATIONS

PIH and periorbital hyperpigmentation may indicate other underlying diseases, but in and of themselves are benign physical findings. Nevertheless, many patients may be considerably frustrated by their cosmetic appearance. Further, the injudicious use of medicated and cosmetic creams may result in many side effects, including acne, dermatitis, skin fragility, and worsening hyperpigmentation.[9]

PROGNOSIS/CLINICAL COURSE

Epidermal pigment may take 6 to 12 months to fade, whereas dermal pigment may be present for years.[16] Underlying conditions, if left untreated, could result in new areas of PIH[28] and persistence or worsening of periorbital hyperpigmentation. Treating PIH is challenging, and some periorbital hyperpigmentation can be fairly resistant to treatment. However, many viable treatment options are available, particularly for epidermal hyperpigmentation. In patients with skin of color, conservative management and setting realistic patient expectations are key.

PREVENTION

The cornerstone of preventing or reducing PIH is to treat the underlying inflammatory condition. In addition, photoprotection with the use of a broad-spectrum sunscreen with a sun protection factor (SPF) of at least 30, coupled with protective clothing, hats, and sunglasses, is essential.[1,29] With that said, the location of the pigment plays a role in how helpful photoprotection may be. It is less likely to be helpful when the pigment is in the dermis, in which case the hyperpigmentation has a slate blue to brown color.[29]

Although diligent practice of photoprotection, proper nutritional and lifestyle choices, and avoidance of environmental triggers may help to decrease the incidence of periorbital hyperpigmentation, genetics and the normal aging process make it unlikely that periorbital hyperpigmentation can be avoided in all patients.

TREATMENT

The treatment of periorbital hyperpigmentation and PIH should be directed toward the primary cause of the hyperpigmentation [**Table 52-4**]. Often, several treatment modalities will need to be used

TABLE 52-4 **Etiology and treatment of periorbital hyperpigmentation**

Etiology	Treatment
Epidermal/dermal melanin	Sun protection
	Topical bleaching agents
	Chemical peels
	Laser
Superficial or excessive vasculature	Topical vitamin K preparations
	Laser
Skin laxity/fat pseudoherniation	Dermal fillers
	Botox
	Surgical intervention (blepharoplasty)

for optimal response. The goals of treatment are centered on inhibiting melanogenesis and increasing keratinocyte turnover.[30] Because of the lengthy treatment course, patients should be actively involved in the planning of any therapeutic regimen. Treatment options for both periorbital hyperpigmentation and PIH include photoprotection, various lightening agents, chemical peels, and laser therapy [**Table 52-5**].

Periorbital hyperpigmentation treatment may also include botulinum toxin, soft tissue fillers, and surgical intervention. Over-the-counter cosmetics may play a valuable role in camouflage. However, PIH resolution may be spontaneous, obviating the need for therapy.

■ SUNSCREEN

One of the cornerstones of treatment is often the use of a broad-spectrum (ultraviolet A [UVA]/ultraviolet B [UVB]) sunscreen. UVA, UVB, and visible light may stimulate melanogenesis and worsen the hyperpigmentation.[30] In addition, all-weather ultraviolet-coated sunglasses that block 99% to 100% of UVA/UVB are recommended.[8]

Topical skin-lightening agents and physical modalities such as chemical peels, microdermabrasion, and laser treatments also may be used to treat PIH.[1] However, the irritation and inflammation of these treatments may induce hyperpigmentation.[1]

■ SKIN-LIGHTENING AGENTS

A wide range of phenolic and nonphenolic lightening agents exist. Topical hydroquinone, a phenolic lightening agent, has been the "gold standard" for treating hyperpigmentation for more than a half century.[31]

TABLE 52-5 **Topical modalities for the treatment of hyperpigmentation**

Treatment	Clinical research studies demonstrating efficacy for the treatment of hyperpigmentation disorders
Hydroquinone 4%	Amer M, Metwalli M. Topical hydroquinone in the treatment of some hyperpigmentary disorders. *Int J Dermatol.* 1998;37:449-450.
	Haddad AL, Matos LF, Brunstein F, Ferreira LM, Silva A, Costa D Jr. A clinical trial, prospective, randomized, double-blind trial comparing skin whitening complex with hydroquinone vs placebo in the treatment of melasma. *Int. J Dermatol.* 2003;42:153-156.
Retinoids (eg tretinoin, tazarotene)	Griffiths CE, Finkel LJ, Ditre CM, Hamilton TA, Ellis CN, Voorhees JJ. Topical tretinoin (retinoic acid) improves melasma: a vehicle-controlled, clinical trial. *Br J Dermatol.* 1993;129:415-421.
	Kimbrough-Green CK, Griffiths CE, Finkel LJ, et al. Topical retinoic acid (tretinoin) for melasma in black patients: a vehicle-controlled clinical trial. *Arch Dermatol.* 1994;130:727-733.
	Grimes P, Callender V. Tazarotene cream for postinflammatory hyperpigmentation and acne vulgaris in darker skin: a double-blind, randomized, vehicle-controlled study. *Cutis.* 2006;77:45-50.
Corticosteroids (eg betamethasone 17-valerate 0.2%)	Neering H. Treatment of melasma (cholasma) by local application of a steroid cream. *Dermatologica.* 1975;151:349-353.
Hydroquinone 4% + tretinoin 0.05% + flucinolone acetonide	Taylor SC, Torok H, Jones T, et al. Efficacy and safety of a new triple-combination agent for the treatment of facial melasma. *Cutis.* 2003;72:67-72.
Hydroquinone 4% + retinol 0.15% + antioxidants	Cook-Bolden FE, Hamilton SE. An open-label study of the efficacy and tolerability of microencapsulated hydroquinone 4% and retinol 0.15% with antioxidants for the treatment of hyperpigmentation. *Cutis.* 2008;81:365-371.
Hydroquinone 4% + rentinol 0.15%	Grimes PE. A microsponge formulation of hydroquinone 4% and retinol in the treatment of melasma and postinflammatory hyperpigmentation. *Cutis.* 2004;74:362-368.
Azelaic acid	Lowe NJ, Rizk D, Grimes P, Billips M, Pincus S. Azelaic acid 20% cream in the treatment of facial hyperpigmentation in darker-skinned patients. *Clin Ther.* 1998;20:945-959.
	Verallo-Rowell VM, Verallo V, Graupe K, Lopez-Villafuerte L, Garcia-Lopez M. Double-blind comparison of azelaic acid and hydroquinone in the treatment of melasma. *Acta Derm Venereol Suppl (Stockh).* 1989;143:58-61.
	Balina LM, Graupe K. The treatment of melasma: 20% azelaic acid versus 4% hydroquinone cream. *Int J Dermatol.* 1991;30:893-895.
	Kakita LS, Lowe NJ. Azelaic acid and glycolic acid combination therapy for facial hyperpigmentation in darker-skinned patients: a clinical comparison with hydroquinone. *Clin Ther.* 1998;20:960-970.
Kojic acid	Lim JT. Treatment of melasma using kojic acid in a gel containing hydroquinone and glycolic acid. *Dermatol. Surg.* 1999;25:282-284.
	Garcia A, Fulton JE Jr. The combination of glycolic acid and hydroquinone or kojic acid for the treatment of melasma and related conditions. *Dermatol Surg.* 1996;22:443-447.
Glycolic acid	Hurley MD, Guevara IL, Gonzalez RM, Pandya AG. Efficacy of glycolic acid peels in the treatment of melasma. *Arch Dermatol.* 2002;138:1578-1582.
	Sarkar R, Kaur C, Bhalla M, Kanwar AJ. The combination of glycolic acid peels with a topical regimen in the treatment of melasma in dark-skinned patients: a comparative study. *Dermatol Surg.* 2002;28:828-832.
	Javaheri SM, Handa S, Kaur I, Kumar B. Safety and efficacy of glycolic acid facial peel in Indian women with melasma. *Int J Dermatol.* 2001;40:354-357.
	Lim JT, Tham SN. Glycolic acid peels in the treatment of melasma among Asian women. *Dermatol Surg.* 1997;23:177-179.
Salicylic acid	Grimes PE. The safety and efficacy of salicylic acid chemical peels in darker racial-ethnic groups. *Dermatol Surg.* 1999;25:18-22.
Trichloroacetic acid	Chun EY, Lee JB, Lee KH. Focal trichloroacetic acid peel method for benign pigmented lessions in dark-skinned patients. *Dermatol Surg.* 2004;30:512-516.

Hydroquinone prevents the conversion of tyrosine to dopa, in turn inhibiting the synthesis of melanin.[32] Hydroquinone is also thought to cause injury to existing melanocytes.[33] Commonly available in 3% and 4% prescription strengths, hydroquinones are most effective in the treatment of epidermal hyperpigmentation. Adverse events from hydroquinone use have been reported. Hydroquinone may induce irritation, erythema, and scaling.[1] In patients using hydroquinone as a spot treatment, halo hypopigmentation may occur around the treated hyperpigmented patch.[1] Additionally, exogenous ochronosis may occur after long-term hydroquinone use, often involving high hydroquinone concentrations.[31,34,35] Often, antioxidants such as vitamin C, retinoids, and α-hydroxyacids may be added to improve the efficacy of hydroquinone. Other agents include N-acetyl-4-cysteaminylphenol (NCAP), another phenolic agent not yet available in North America. As with hydroquinone, NCAP inhibits tyrosinase activity but also stimulates the production of pheomelanin rather than eumelanin.[36] NCAP may be more stable and less irritating than hydroquinone.

Retinoic acid inhibits melanin production.[37] Retinoids may induce skin lightening due to the epidermal melanin redistribution or dispersion.[39] Retinoids may be used to treat various types of hyperpigmentation, including PIH and periorbital hyperpigmentation.[38–40] Tretinoin, a vitamin A derivative, has been used in the treatment of hyperpigmentation, particularly epidermal melanin.[41] Tretinoin 0.1%, adapalene 0.1% gel, and tazarotene 0.1% cream all have demonstrated efficacy in improving PIH induced by acne vulgaris after 12 to 40 weeks of therapy. Topical steroids and hydroquinone may be added to tretinoin to improve its efficacy. Tazarotene and adapalene have been found to be comparable in efficacy to tretinoin for the treatment of hyperpigmentation, but with the added benefit of greater tolerability for adapalene.[42]

Topical azelaic acid, a naturally occurring nonphenolic dicarboxylic acid, has been used for its selective effect on abnormal melanocytes. Kojic acid, a naturally occurring hydrophilic fungal derivative, popular in Asia, is similar to hydroquinone in its mechanism of action but may cause contact dermatitis and erythema. The tyrosinase inhibitors azelaic acid and kojic acid also have been used in the treatment of PIH with varied efficacy and tolerability. They are generally considered second-line therapy and are used in situations where hydroquinone and/or retinoids cannot be used.[43,44] Azelaic acid is a weak competitive inhibitor of tyrosinase and specifically inhibits proliferation of abnormally hyperactive melanocytes. This selective antiproliferative action against abnormal melanocytes prevents the halo effect since normal melanocytes remain undisturbed.[30] Arbutin, another agent popular in Asia, is an extract of the bearberry plant. It is effective in higher concentrations but also may cause paradoxical hyperpigmentation. Finally, glycyrrhetinic acid, an extract from licorice (Glycyrrhiza glabra), may inhibit both inflammation and pigmentation.

CHEMICAL PEELS

Chemical peels may be useful in the treatment of hyperpigmentation.[32,33,45] Superficial salicylic acid peels have proven efficacy in darker skin types.[45] Glycolic acid peels also have been found to be effective. Despite the benefits of chemical peels, a risk of skin trauma and further hyperpigmentation still remains.[33] Trichloroacetic acid peels may be used with extreme caution because high concentrations of this deeply penetrating peel may cause postinflammatory hyperpigmentation.[46] Although tretinoin has been used as a topical leave on medication for decades, it is now also being used as a peeling agent with success.[47] Phenol peels, not commonly used in darker skin types, along with transconjunctival blepharoplasty, have been reported as therapeutic in skin type V.[48] Nonetheless, with this method, significant pigment irregularity is a possible adverse event. Despite their possible risks, when performed by a properly trained provider skilled in the treatment of skin of color, chemical peels are a useful therapeutic adjunct.[7] It should be noted that when periorbital hyperpigmentation is caused primarily by hypervascularity, chemical peels are contraindicated because they may worsen the clinical appearance.[8] Microdermabrasion alone or in addition with chemical peels and dermabrasion has been effective in treating PIH.[49,50]

Cryotherapy is not used for the treatment of PIH due to the unpredictability of results.

LASERS

Lasers that target pigment and vascularity are now a viable treatment option for darker skin types. Longer wavelengths and cooling devices have made laser therapy a valuable therapeutic alternative for skin of color patients. Various lasers, including the Q-switched ruby laser and the pulsed dye laser, have been used, although the potential adverse events may outweigh the benefit of the therapy.[51,52] The Q-switched ruby laser has been described in the treatment of periorbital hyperpigmentation.[53] Emitting a red light, it causes the selective destruction of melanized melanosomes.[54] With the Q-switched ruby laser, dyspigmentation may occur because a deeply pigmented epidermis may prevent the laser light from reaching the dermis.[46] This in turn leads to unintentional injury to the epidermis and results in dyspigmentation.[46] Considering the potential adverse side effects in patients with skin of color (especially those with darker skin), the safest laser to treat hyperpigmentation is the Q-switched Nd:YAG.[46] Both long-pulsed and low-fluence Q-switched Nd:YAG lasers have been used to treat periorbital hyperpigmentation in Fitzpatrick type III and IV Asian patients.[55,56] There have also been some recent successes combining certain laser modalities, like the low-fluence Q-switched Nd:YAG, with microdermabrasion and hydroquinone to synergistically improve pigmentation.[57,58] When using lasers, physicians must be aware that darker skin types may require more frequent visits and necessitate longer therapeutic time requirements, and as with other modalities, the pigment may not be completely cleared.

BOTULINUM TOXIN AND SOFT TISSUE FILLERS

Botulinum toxin type A may help to lessen the appearance of periorbital hyperpigmentation in cases where active musculature alters the pattern of light on the face and emphasizes dark shadows.[8] Restylane (hyaluronic acid) is the most popular filler for ethnic skin[7] and may be used to fill periorbital hollows and to restore volume, thus decreasing shadowing. Other fillers, including Sculptra (poly-L-lactic acid), which acts to stimulate collagen fiber production, are gaining popularity. Some researchers have even tried autologous fat transfer for Korean (Fitzpatrick skin types II and III) patients with thin, translucent skin of the lower eyelid.[59]

SURGERY

Blepharoplasty, either alone or in conjunction with other procedures, may be useful in eliminating periorbital hyperpigmentation caused by shadows cast by fat deposits and skin laxity.[8] Transconjunctival blepharoplasty, coupled with phenol peels, has been reported to be effective in darker skin types.[48]

COSMECEUTICALS

Cosmeceuticals have also gained popularity as treatments for hyperpigmentation.[30,46,60,61] Although response may be modest, over-the-counter cosmetics can improve the appearance of periorbital hyperpigmentation temporarily by helping to restore moisture and tone. A topical product containing growth factors obtained from cultured human foreskin fibroblasts, TNS (Skin Medica Co.), may help to diminish periorbital pigmentation.[7] Topical preparations containing vitamin K may be of some benefit because of their effect on the clotting mechanism. There are also many highly effective cosmetic concealers that can more than adequately mask the appearance of periorbital hyperpigmentation.

CONCLUSION

Hyperpigmentation is one of the most common cutaneous disorders occurring in individuals with skin of color. Although PIH and periorbital hyperpigmentation are often viewed as cosmetic problems, they can cause a significant impact on patients' self-esteem.[62] As more treatment modalities are proven efficacious and underlying etiologies are better elucidated, each patient should receive a tailored approach to improving postinflammatory and periorbital hyperpigmentation.

REFERENCES

1. Taylor SC, Burgess C, Callendar V, et al. Postinflammatory hyperpigmentation: evolving combination treatment strategies. *Cutis.* 2006;78:1-25.
2. Ruiz-Maldonado R, de la Luz Orozco-Covarrubias M. Postinflammatory hypo-pigmentation and hyperpigmentation. *Semin Cutan Med Surg.* 1996;16:36-43.
3. Halder R, Nootheti P. Ethnic skin disorders overview. *J Am Acad Dermatol.* 2003;48:S143-S148.
4. Chadurvedi SK, Singh G, Gupta N. Stigma experience in skin disorders: an Indian perspective. *Dermatol Clin.* 2005;23:635-642.
5. Freitag FM, Cestari TF. What causes dark circles under the eyes. *J Cosmet Dermatol.* 2007;6:211-215.
6. Maruri CA, Diaz LA. Dark circles around the eyes. *Cutis.* 1969;5:979-982.
7. Downie JB. Esthetic considerations for ethnic skin. *Semin Cutan Med Surg.* 2006;25:158-162.
8. Gendler EC. Treatment of periorbital hyperpigmentation. *Aesthet Surg J.* 2005;25:618-624.
9. Mashhood AA. Treatment of hyperpigmentation disorders. *J Pakistan Assoc Dermatol.* 2006;16:65-68.
10. Bose SK, Ortonne JP. Pigmentation: dyschromia. In: Baran R, Maibach HI, eds. *Cosmetic Dermatology.* London, United Kingdom: Martin Dunitz; 1994:277-298.
11. Stulberg DL, Clark N, Tovey D. Common hyperpigmentation disorders in adults: II. Melanoma, seborrheic keratoses, acanthosis nigricans, melasma, diabetic dermopathy, tinea versicolor, and postinflammatory hyperpigmentation. *Am Fam Physician.* 2003;68:1963-1968.
12. Tomita Y, Maeda K, Tagami H. Melanocyte-stimulating properties of arachidonic acid metabolites: possible role in postinflammatory pigmentation. *Pigment Cell Res.* 1992;5:357-361.
13. Kitawaki A, Tanaka Y, Takada K. New findings on the mechanism of postinflammatory pigmentation. *Pigment Cell Res.* 2003;16:603-615.
14. Maurer M, Galli SJ. Lack of significant skin inflammation during elimination by apoptosis of large numbers of mouse cutaneous mast cells after cessation of treatment with stem cell factor. *Lab Invest.* 2004;84:1593-1602.
15. Goodman RM, Belcher RW. Periorbital hyperpigmentation. *Arch Dermatol.* 1969;100:169-174.
16. Haddock N, Wilkin JK. Periorbital hyperpigmentation. *JAMA.* 1981;246:835.
17. Jeghers H. Pigmentation of the skin. *N Engl J Med.* 1944;23:122.
18. Lelis J. Autosomal recessive ectodermal dysplasia. *Cutis.* 1992;50:435-437.
19. Ing EB, Buncic JR, Weiser BA, et al. Periorbital hyperpigmentation and erythema dyschromicum perstans. *Can J Ophthalmol.* 1992;27:353-355.
20. Carlson R, Hering P. Allergic shiners. *JAMA.* 1981;246:835.
21. Gilchrest BA, Fitzpatrick TB, Anderson RR, et al. Localization of melanin pigmentation in the skin with Wood's lamp. *Br J Dermatol.* 1977;96:245-248.
22. Manuskiatti W, Fitzpatrick RE, Goldman MP. Treatment of facial skin using combinations of CO2, Q-switched alexandrite, flashlamp-pumped pulsed dye and Er:YAG lasers in the same treatment session. *Dermatol Surg.* 2000;26:114-120.
23. Paraskevas PR, Halpern AC, Marghoob AA. Utility of the Wood's light: five cases from a pigmented lesion clinic. *Br J Dermatol.* 2005;152:1039-1044.
24. Grimes PE, Yamada N, Bhawan J. Light microscopic, immunohistochemical, and ultrastructural alterations in patients with melasma. *Am J Dermatopathol.* 2005;27:96-101.
25. Ardigo M, Cameli N, Berardesca E, et al. Characterization and evaluation of pigment distribution and response to therapy in melasma using in vivo reflectance confocal microscopy: a preliminary study. *J Eur Acad Dermatol Venereol.* 2010;24:1296-1303.
26. Kang HY, Bahadoran P. Application of in vivo reflectance confocal microscopy in melasma classification. *J Am Acad Dermatol.* 2012;67:157.
27. Sheth VM, Pandya AG. Reply. *J Am Acad Dermatol.* 2012;67:157-158.
28. Lacz N, Vafaie J, Kihiczak N, et al. Postinflammatory hyperpigmentation: a common but not troubling condition. *Int J Dermatol.* 2004;43:362-365.
29. Epstein J. Postinflammatory hyperpigmentation. *Clin Dermatol.* 1989;7:55-65.
30. Reszko AE, Berson D, Lupo MP. Cosmeceuticals: practical applications. *Dermatol Clin.* 2009;27:401-416.
31. Halder RM, Richards GM. Topical agents used in the management of hyperpigmentation. *Skin Therapy Lett.* 2004;9:1-3.
32. Lawrence N, Bligard CA, Reed R, et al. Exogenous ochronosis in the United Stated. *J Am Acad Dermatol.* 1988;18:1207-1211.
33. Burns RL, Prevost-Blank PL, Lawry MA, et al. Glycolic acid peels for postinflammatory hyperpigmentation in black patients: a comparative study. *Dermatol Surg.* 1997;23:171-174.
34. Roberts W. Chemical peeling in ethnic/dark Skin. *Dermatol Ther.* 2004;17:196-205.
35. Levin CY, Maibach H. Exogenous ochronosis: an update on clinical features, causative agents and treatment options. *Am J Clin Dermatol.* 2001;2:213-217.
36. Olumide Y, Akinkugbe A, Altraide D, et al. Complications of chronic use of skin lightening cosmetics. *Int J Dermatol.* 2008;47:344-353.
37. Alena F, Dixon W, Thomas P, et al. Glutathione plays a key role in the depigmenting and melanocytotoxic action of N-acetyl-4-cysteaminylphenol in black and yellow hair follicles. *J Invest Dermatol.* 1995;104:792-797.
38. Romero C, Aberdam E, Larnier C, et al. Retinoic acid as modulator of UVB-induced melanocyte differentiation. *J Cell Sci.* 1994;107:1095-1103.
39. Bulengo-Ransby SM, Griffiths CEM, Kimbrough-Green CK. Topical tretinoin (retinoic acid) therapy for hyperpigmented lesions caused by inflammation of the skin in black patients. *N Eng J Med.* 1993;328:1438-1443.
40. Jacyk WK, Mpofu P. Adapalene gel 0.1% for topical treatment of acne vulgaris in African patients. *Cutis.* 2001;68:48S-54S.
41. Grimes P, Callender V. Tazarotene cream for postinflammatory hyperpigmentation and acne vulgaris in darker skin: a double-blind, randomized, vehicle-controlled study. *Cutis.* 2006;77:45-50.
42. Kimbrough-Green CK, Griffiths CEM, Finkel LJ, et al. Topical retinoic acid (tretinoin) for melasma in black patients: a vehicle-controlled clinical trial. *Arch Dermatol.* 1994;130:727-733.
43. Dogra S, Kanwar AJ, Parsad D. Adapalene in the treatment of melasma: a preliminary report. *J Dermatol.* 2002;29:539-540.
44. Lowe NJ, Rizk D, Grimes P, et al. Azelaic acid 20% cream in the treatment of facial hyperpigmentation in darker-skinned patients. *Clin Ther.* 1998;20:945-959.
45. Nakagawa M, Kawai K, Kawai K. Contact allergy to kojic acid in skin care products. *Contact Dermatitis.* 1995;32:9-13.
46. Grimes PE. The safety and efficacy of salicylic acid chemical peels in darker racial-ethnic groups. *Dermatol Surg.* 1999;25:18-22.
47. Konda S, Feria AN, Halder RM. New horizons in treating disorders of hyperpigmentation in skin of color. *Semin Cutan Med Surg.* 2012;31:133-139.
48. Faghihi G, Shahingohar A, Siadat AH. Comparison between 1% tretinoin peeling versus 70% glycolic acid peeling in the treatment of female patients with melasma. *J Drugs Dermatol.* 2011;10:1439-1442.
49. Epstein JS. Management of infraorbital dark circles: a significant concern. *Arch Facial Plast Surg.* 1999;1:303-307.
50. Cotellessa C, Peris K, Fargnoli MC, et al. Microabrasion versus microabrasion followed by 15% trichloracetic acid for treatment of cutaneous hyperpigmentation in adult females. *Dermatol Surg.* 2003;23:352-356.
51. Kunachak S, Leelaudomlipi P, Wongwaisayawan S. Dermabrasion: a curative treatment for melasma. *Aesthet Plast Surg.* 2001;25:114-117.
52. Taylor CR, Anderson RR. Ineffective treatment of refractory melasma and postinflammatory hyperpigmentation by Q-switched ruby laser. *J Dermatol Surg Oncol.* 1994;20:592-597.
53. Dierickx C, Goldman MP, Fitzpatrick RE. Laser treatment of erythematous/hypertrophic and pigmented scars in 26 patients. *Plast Reconstr Surg.* 1955;95:84-90.
54. Watanabe S, Nakai K, Ohnishi T. Condition known as dark rings under the eyes in the Japanese population is a kind of dermal melanocytosis which can be successfully treated by Q-switched ruby laser. *Dermatol Surg.* 2006;32:785-789.
55. Halder RM, Nootheti PK. Ethnic skin disorders overview. *J Am Acad Dermatol.* 2003;48:S143-S148.
56. Ma G, Lin XX, Hu XJ, et al. Treatment of venous infraorbital dark circles using a long-pulsed 1,064-nm neodymium-doped yttrium aluminum garnet laser. *Dermatol Surg* 2012;38:1277-1282.
57. Xu TH, Yang ZH, Li YH, et al. Treatment of infraorbital dark circles using a low-fluence Q-switched 1,064-nm Laser. *Dermatol Surg.* 2011;37:797-803.
58. Kauvar ANB. The evolution of melasma therapy: targeting melanosomes using low-fluence Q-switched neodymium-doped yttrium aluminum garnet lasers. *Semin Cutan Med Surg.* 2012;31:126-132.
59. Cho SB, Park SJ, Kim JS, et al. Treatment of post-inflammatory hyperpigmentation using 1064-nm Q-switched Nd:YAG laser with low fluence: report of three cases. *J Eur Acad Dermatol Venerol.* 2009;23:1206-1207.
60. Roh MR, Kim TK, Chung KY. Treatment of infraorbital dark circles by autologous fat transplantation: a pilot study. *Br J Dermatol.* 2009;160:1022-1025.

61. Woolery-Lloyd H, Kammer JN. Treatment of hyperpigmentation. *Semin Cutan Med Surg.* 2011;30:171-175.
62. Ladizinski B, Mistry N, Kundu R. Widespread use of toxic skin lightening compounds: Medical and psychosocial aspects. *Dermatol Clin.* 2011;29:111-123.
63. Ho SGY, Yeung CK, Chan NPY, et al. A retrospective analysis of the management of acne post-inflammatory hyperpigmentation using topical treatment, laser treatment, or combination topical and laser treatments in Oriental patients. *Lasers Surg Med.* 2011;43:1-7.

CHAPTER
53

Solar Lentigines

Dóris Hexsel
Manoela Porto

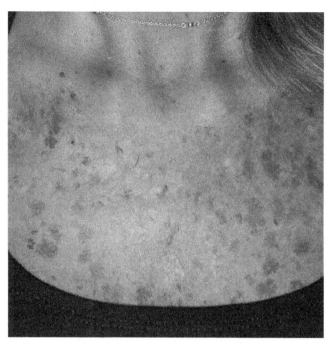

FIGURE 53-1. Solar lentigines on the chest of a patient who had early and intense sun exposure.

KEY POINTS

- Solar lentigines are hyperpigmented macules that are round or oval in shape with slightly irregular edges.
- They are common in skin of color populations except among South Asians with skin of color.
- Ultraviolet light exposure and genetic predisposition are the most important factors in the development of solar lentigines.
- Treatment may include physical modalities and depigmenting agents.
- Sun avoidance, protective clothing, sunscreen, and blocking agents are indicated to prevent solar lentigines.

INTRODUCTION

Solar lentigines (SLs) are benign, hyperpigmented macules that occur on sun-exposed areas of the skin.[1-4] They are induced by natural or artificial sources of ultraviolet (UV) radiation and are also called sun-induced freckles, sunburn freckles, freckles in adulthood, age spots, actinic lentigines, and senile lentigines.[5,6]

EPIDEMIOLOGY, ETIOLOGY, PATHOGENESIS, AND HISTOPATHOLOGY

This benign pigmentary disorder is prevalent among fair-skinned patients with Fitzpatrick skin types I or II (those who always burn and who tan a little or not at all).[5,7] The incidence increases with age, affecting more than 90% of those with Fitzpatrick skin type I to III older than 50 years.[2-4,8] SLs are also a clinical features of photoaging in East and Southeast Asian populations. In this skin of color population, discrete pigmentary changes, including SLs and mottled hyperpigmentation, are seen frequently.[9] In a study by Chung et al[10] of Koreans aged 30 to 92 years, hyperpigmented macules were the major pigmentary lesions associated with photoaging in women. The number of hyperpigmented macules increased with each decade of age in Fitzpatrick skin types I to III.[10]

Bastiaens et al[6] demonstrated that SLs have a positive association with cumulative lifetime sun exposure and early sun exposure [**Figure 53-1**]. There is also a possible genetic susceptibility to the development of SLs in response to acute or chronic UV exposure.[5] Aoki et al[11] demonstrated that SLs are induced by the mutagenic effect of repeated UV exposure in the past, leading to the characteristic enhancement of melanin production together with decreased proliferation and differentiation of lesional keratinocytes against a background of chronic inflammation.

SLs may appear after chronic photochemotherapy (6 to 8 months). However, individual susceptibility factors such as race, age, and tanning and burning responses to sunlight are important to determine the prevalence and density of SLs.[5] Recently, a study observed that, in addition to age and constitutive host factors, current intake of oral contraceptives or progestogen treatments may be associated with SLs.[12]

The histopathology of SLs shows a linear increase in melanocytes along the dermal-epidermal junction.[13] There is more melanin than normal in the adjacent epidermis and stratum corneum, but no atypicality or pigment incontinence is seen.[2,4,5,14] Moreover, melanocytes display increased activity, as manifested by marked dopa reactivity, elongated dendrites, numerous normal-appearing melanosomes, enlarged perikarya with developed rough endoplasmic reticula, numerous mitochondria, and hypertrophic Golgi complexes.[5]

One study observed two different histologic patterns of SLs among 40 Japanese women: one pattern demonstrated a flattened epidermis with basal melanosis, and the other pattern showed epidermal hyperplasia with elongated rete ridges composed of deeply pigmented basaloid cells. The flattened epidermis group showed a significantly thinner epidermis, more severe solar elastosis, and fewer Langerhans cells.[15] The presence of Langerhans cells in the epidermis of SLs might play a role in the remission of postinflammatory pigmentation due to aesthetic treatment.[15]

CLINICAL FINDINGS

SLs are macular hyperpigmented lesions that range in color from pale yellow to dark brown and vary in size from a few millimeters to 2 cm. Lesions are round or oval with slightly irregular, sharply defined edges.[1,2,7] They are more common in fair-skinned patients, such as those with Fitzpatrick skin phototypes I to III, and are less frequent in dark-skinned subjects.[2,3] A previous history of acute sunburn followed by the sudden appearance of large numbers of macular lesions is often found.[14] Usually similar lesions appear in the same area, such as the face, arms, hands [**Figure 53-2**], chest, and back.[1-4,7] SLs are diagnosed by clinical examination.[12] Other methods, such as dermoscopy and confocal microscopy (CM), also may be used in the diagnosis of SLs and for differential diagnoses [**Figure 53-3**].[9,16-21] CM obtains images from deep inside the skin without interference from scattered light.[19] Langley et al[20] evaluated SLs using CM and demonstrated an absence of atypical melanocytes. Yamashita et al[21] diagnosed SLs using CM and showed numerous aggregated melanosomes.

DIFFERENTIAL DIAGNOSIS

SLs can be distinguished from ephelides, lentigo simplex, pigmented actinic keratosis, flat seborrheic keratosis, melanocytic nevi, and malignant melanomas by their clinical appearance. Other lesions that may be misdiagnosed are 'flat' varieties of junctional melanocytic nevi,

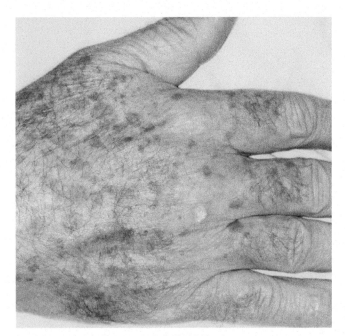

FIGURE 53-2. Solar lentigines on the back of the hand.

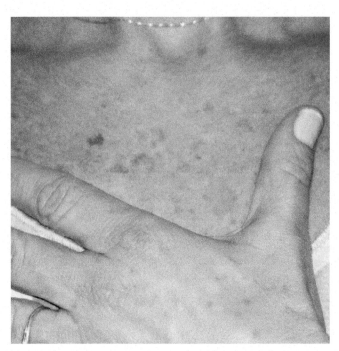

FIGURE 53-4. A 40-year-old patient showing solar lentigines on the chest and back of the hand. Lesions are more numerous in areas exposed to intermittent but repeated sun exposure (chest) than in areas chronically exposed to the sun (dorsal hand).

pigmented actinic keratoses, large cell acanthomas, and benign pigmented keratoses.[5,22]

Dalton et al[22] studied 147 patients with facial lentigo maligna (LM). In 30% of patients, SLs were present in the biopsy specimen. The presence of an associated SL can make the diagnosis of LM more difficult, leading to misdiagnosis.[22] Dermoscopy is helpful in the differential diagnoses of a number of skin lesions, such as seborrheic keratosis, lentigo simplex, melanoma in situ, lichen planus-like keratosis, and pigmented actinic keratosis.[9,17,18]

SLs may enlarge, darken, and become more irregular and 'fixed' over time, similar to the progression of LM.[5] It is possible that SLs will evolve into varieties of intraepidermal melanocytic dysplasia, which is similar to LM, in some individuals.[5] Recurrence after treatment also may occur.[23]

PROGNOSIS/CLINICAL COURSE

SLs may appear at any time in life, but most of the cases occur in people older than 50 years [**Figure 53-4**].[2] Once formed, it is possible that SLs may fade slightly or persist indefinitely. During the clinical course,

PREVENTION

Sun avoidance, protective clothing, and sunscreens are recommended for the prevention of SLs. These protective measures must be initiated in childhood and continued throughout life.[5]

TREATMENT

There are a number of treatment options for SLs, and they can be divided into two categories: physical modalities and topical therapies.[24] Physical modalities includes cryotherapy, chemical peels, lasers, pulsed light, and dermabrasion, whereas topical therapies involve the use of hypopigmenting agents such as hydroquinone, tretinoin, tazarotene, adapalene, and some combinations of these agents. These treatments are categorized according to the quality and level of evidence from clinical studies published in the literature in **Tables 53-1** and **53-2**.

CONCLUSION

SLs are commonly found among patients with Fitzpatrick skin phototypes I to III and are most common in people older than 50 years of age. These lesions are induced by natural or artificial sources of UV radiation. Therefore, protective measures must be initiated in childhood to prevent their appearance later in life.

A number of physical and topical therapies, either alone or in various combinations, have been demonstrated to be efficacious and safe. However, the results are often not permanent; recurrence is frequent, making management a challenge for dermatologists. Finally, additional double-blind studies are needed in order to identify better treatments for SLs.

FIGURE 53-3. Dermoscopy of solar lentigines, at 50× magnification.

TABLE 53-1 Summary of studies on physical modalities for the treatment of solar lentigines

Study/source (year of study)	Quality of evidence*	Level of evidence**	Number of subjects	Outcome and follow-up
Cryotherapy				
Raziee et al[26] (2008)	I	A	25	Cryotherapy was more likely to produce substantial lightening of SLs than 33% TCA ($P = 0.025$).
Lugo-Janer et al[27] (2003)	I	A	25	LN was more likely to produce significant lightening of SLs than 30% TCA solution ($P < 0.05$).
Chemical peels				
Chun et al[28] (2004)	IIa	B	49	Of the subjects, 86% showed a good clinical response with 10%–65% TCA, and the clinical results were maintained for 12 months after treatment.
Cook and Cook[29] (2000)	IIa	A	3100	There was a significant decrease with 40% TCA + 70% glycolic peel in irregular pigmentation of nonfacial skin, including SLs.
Laser therapy				
Rashid et al[30] (2002)	IIa	C	6	All patients showed improvement of 50% with 532 nm Nd:YAG laser, and no recurrence was reported after a 24-month follow-up.
Kopera et al[31] (1997)	IIa	A	8	A single course of Q-switched Ruby laser treatment resulted in fading of the lesions without scarring and no recurrence within a 6- to 8-week follow-up period.
Rosenbach et al[32] (2002)	IIa	B	11	There was a significant improvement with Alexandrite laser therapy among the treated lentigines: 2 lesions were graded as "good," 14 as "excellent," and 5 as "clear" compared with untreated areas at 4 weeks ($P < 0.001$).
Negishi et al[33] (2013)	I	A	193	Aggressive irradiation using Q-switched lasers resulted in a high PIH incidence, while having no advantage in efficacy.
IPL				
Kawada et al[34] (2002)	III	B	45	There was more than a 50% improvement in SLs in 40% of the patients after 4 treatments.
Kawana et al[35] (2007)	IIc	C	18	IPL was considered effective in 12 of 18 patients (66.6% improvement).
Kligman and Zhen[36] (2004)	IIc	C	23	There was a decrease in SLs after 3 treatments with IPL.
Sadighha et al[37] (2008)	IIa	A	91	Complete clearance was achieved in all patients and PIH occurred in 16.6% of patients with Fitzpatrick skin type IV.
Sasaya et al[38] (2011)	IIa	A	31	Out of the patients, 66% had more than 50% improvement after 5 treatments of IPL.
Microdermabrasion				
Cotellessa et al[39] (2003)	III	D	40	The combination of microdermabrasion with 15% TCA resulted in complete remission in 50% of patients.
Lasers + cryotherapy				
Stern et al[40] (1994)	IIa	C	13	Good results were reported in 61%, 62%, and 75% of patients treated with carbon dioxide laser, argon laser, and cryotherapy, respectively.
Todd et al[1] (2000)	IIa	B	27	After 12 weeks, the frequency-doubled Q-switched Nd:YAG laser provided significant lightening compared with the krypton laser ($P = 0.001$), the 532 nm diode-pumped vanadate laser ($P = 0.001$), and LN ($P = 0.001$).
Laser therapy + chemical peels				
Li and Yang[41] (1999)	IIa	A	20	The frequency-doubled Q-switched Nd:YAG laser proved to be significantly more effective than 35% TCA ($P = 0.0004$).
Dermabrasion + cryotherapy				
Hexsel et al[2] (2000)	IIa	B	10	Localized dermabrasion is an efficacious and effective technique comparable with LN. Moreover, dermabrasion was associated with fewer side-effects, such as hypochromia, than LN.
Chemical peels + cryotherapy				
Raziee et al[42] (2008)	I	B	25	Cryotherapy was more likely to produce substantial lightening of the SLs than 33% TCA solution.

Abbreviations: IPL, intense pulsed light therapy; LN, liquid nitrogen; Nd:YAG, neodymium-doped yttrium aluminium garnet; PIH, postinflammatory hyperpigmentation; SLs, solar lentigines; TCA, trichloroacetic acid

*The quality of evidence was graded according to a 6-point scale as follows: I = Evidence obtained from at least one properly designed randomized, controlled trial; IIa = Evidence obtained from well-designed controlled trials without randomization; IIb = Evidence obtained from well-designed cohort or case-control analytic studies, preferably from more than one center or research group; IIc = Evidence obtained from multiple time series with or without the intervention (dramatic results in uncontrolled experiments also could be regarded as this type of evidence); III = Opinions of respected authorities based on clinical experience, descriptive studies, or reports from expert committees; IV = Inadequate evidence due to problems of methodology (eg, sample size, length or comprehensiveness of follow-up, or conflicts with the evidence).[25]

**The level of evidence was classified on a 5-point scale as follows: A = There is good evidence to support the use of the procedure; B = There is fair evidence to support the use of the procedure; C = There is poor evidence to support the use of the procedure; D = There is fair evidence to support the rejection of the use of the procedure; E = There is good evidence to support the rejection of the use of the procedure.[25]

TABLE 53-2 Summary of studies on topical therapies for the treatment of solar lentigines

Study/source (year of study)	Quality of evidence*	Level of evidence**	Number of subjects	Outcome
Hydroquinone				
Petit and Piérard[43] (2003)	I	A	30	Reflectance spectrophotometric measurements showed a significant decrease in the differential melanin index by 3.5% and 8.7% after 1 and 2 months, respectively (P <0.05). Video image analysis showed a 17% decrease in the areas with SLs at 2 months (P <0.01). Melanin density in the stratum corneum was reduced by 4.9% (P <0.01) and 18.6% (P <0.001) after 1 and 2 months, respectively.
Tretinoin				
Weiss et al[44] (2006)	I	B	45	Tretinoin microsphere 0.1% gel was superior to a placebo in improving photodamage, including SLs, after 6 months (P = 0.0054).
Kang et al[45] (2005)	I	B	204	Tretinoin 0.05% cream resulted in significantly greater improvement to clinical signs of photodamage, including SLs, compared with a placebo (P <0.05).
Weinstein et al[46] (1991)	I	B	251	Overall improvement of photodamaged skin, including SLs, was reported in 79% of patients at a 0.05% dose compared with improvement in 57% of patients at a 0.01% dose and 48% of patients with the vehicle.
Rafal et al[47] (1992)	I	B	58	After 10 months, 83% of patients with facial lesions treated with tretinoin had lightening of these lesions compared with 29% of the patients treated with a placebo.
Tazarotene				
Kang et al[48] (2005)	I	B	568	Tazarotene cream was significantly more effective than a vehicle in reducing SLs (59% versus 28%, P <0.001) at week 24.
Phillips et al[49] (2002)	I	B	563	The application of 0.1% tazarotene produced clinical improvement in SLs compared with a placebo (55% versus 15%; P <0.001).
Adapalene				
Kang et al[50] (2003)	I	B	90	At 9 months, 57% and 59% of patients had lighter lesions in the 0.1% and 0.3% adapalene gel groups, respectively, compared with 36% in the control group (P <0.05).
Hydroquinone + tretinoin				
Yoshimura et al[51] (2000)	IIc	B	90	At 8 weeks, successful lightening of lesions was achieved in 82.2% of patients (excellent or good benefits).
Mequinol (4HA) + tretinoin				
Jarratt[52] (2004)	I	A	216	Combined 2% mequinol and 0.01% tretinoin solution was a highly effective and well-tolerated treatment for SLs and related hyperpigmented lesions, superior to 3% hydroquinone.
Fleischer et al[53] (2000)	I	A	1175	Combined 2% mequinol and 0.01% tretinoin demonstrated significant superiority over 4HA and vehicle (P = 0.0001).
Draelos[54] (2006)	IIc	C	259	Over 80% of all subjects responded to 2% 4HA 2% plus 0.01% tretinoin therapy and maintained clinical benefit at 4 weeks posttreatment.
Ortonne et al[55] (2004)	IIc	C	378	Of the target lesions of the arm and face treated with 4HA-RA, 80% and 88%, respectively, treated with 4HA-RA were clear or almost clear after 4 weeks of follow-up.
Undecylenoyl phenylalanine				
Katoulis et al[56] (2010)	I	B	30	Of the studied patients, 63.3% had moderate improvement and 36.6% had marked improvement with the active treatment.
L-ascorbic acid + phytic acid serum				
Khemis et al[57] (2011)	I	B	30	The pigmentation index for product-treated SLs was reduced, whereas that for vehicle-treated lesions remained. This reduction was statistically significant.

Abbreviations: 4HA, 4-hydroxyanisole; RA, retinoic acid; SLs, solar lentigines.

*The quality of evidence was graded according to a 6-point scale as follows: I = Evidence obtained from at least one properly designed randomized, controlled trial; IIa = Evidence obtained from well-designed controlled trials without randomization; IIb = Evidence obtained from well-designed cohort or case-control analytic studies, preferably from more than one center or research group; IIc = Evidence obtained from multiple time series with or without the intervention (dramatic results in uncontrolled experiments also could be regarded as this type of evidence); III = Opinions of respected authorities based on clinical experience, descriptive studies, or reports from expert committees; IV = Inadequate evidence due to problems of methodology (eg, sample size, length or comprehensiveness of follow-up, or conflicts with the evidence).[25]

**The level of evidence was classified on a 5-point scale as follows: A = There is good evidence to support the use of the procedure; B = There is fair evidence to support the use of the procedure; C = There is poor evidence to support the use of the procedure; D = There is fair evidence to support the rejection of the use of the procedure; E = There is good evidence to support the rejection of the use of the procedure.[25]

REFERENCES

1. Todd MM, Rallis TM, Gerwels JW, et al. A comparison of three lasers and liquid nitrogen in the treatment of solar lentigines: a randomized, controlled comparative trial. *Arch Dermatol.* 2000;136:841-846.

2. Hexsel DM, Mazzuco R, Bohn I, et al. Clinical comparative study between cryotherapy and local dermabrasion for the treatment of solar lentigo on the back of the hands. *Dermatol Surg.* 2000;26:457-462.

3. Grimes PE. Cosmetic issues of concern for potential surgical patients. In: Soriano T, Hexsel DM, Kim J, eds. *Aesthetic and Cosmetic Surgery for Darker Skin Types.* Philadelphia, PA: Lippincott Williams & Wilkins; 2008:49.

4. Baumann L. Disorders of pigmentation. In: Weisberg E, ed. *Cosmetic Dermatology: Principles and Practice.* New York, NY: McGraw-Hill; 2002:67.

5. Freedberg IM, Eisen AZ, Wolff K, et al, eds. *Fitzpatrick's Dermatology in General Medicine.* New York, NY: McGraw-Hill; 1999:1047.

6. Bastiaens M, Hoefnagel J, Westendorp R, et al. Solar lentigines are strongly related to sun exposure in contrast to ephelides. *Pigment Cell Res.* 2004;17:225.

7. Baran R, Maibach HI. Pigmentation: dyschromia. In: Baran R, Maibach HI, eds. *Cosmetic Dermatology.* London, United Kingdom: Martin Dunitz; 1994:282.

8. Sampaio SAP. Discromia. In: Sampaio SAP, Rivitti, EA, eds. *Dermatologia.* São Paulo, Brazil: Artes Medicas; 1998:277.

9. Goh SH. The treatment of visible signs of senescence: the Asian experience. *Br J Dermatol.* 1990;122:S105-S109.

10. Chung JH, Lee SH, Youn CS, et al. Cutaneous photodamage in Koreans. *Arch Dermatol.* 2001;137:1043-1051.

11. Aoki H, Moro O, Tagami H, et al. Gene expression profiling analysis of solar lentigo in relation to immunohistochemical characteristics. *Br J Dermatol.* 2007;156:1214-1223.

12. Ezzedine K, Mauger E, Latreille J, et al. Freckles and solar lentigines have different risk factors in Caucasian women. *J Eur Acad Dermatol Venereol.* 2013;27:e345-e356.

13. Champion RH, Burton JL, Burns DA, et al, eds. *Rook's Textbook of Dermatology.* Vol 2. Oxford, England: Blackwell Science; 2004:1719.

14. Baran R, Maibach HI. Pigmentation: dyschromia. In: Baran R, Maibbach HI, eds. *Textbook of Cosmetic Dermatology.* 3rd ed. London, United Kingdom: Taylor & Francis; 2005:396.

15. Yonei N, Kaminaka C, Kimura A, et al. Two patterns of solar lentigines: a histopathological analysis of 40 Japanese women. *J Dermatol.* 2012;39:829-832.

16. Rassner G, Steinert U, eds. *Dermatologia: Tratado e Atlas.* São Paulo, Brazil: Livraria Editora Santos; 1994:203.

17. Wang SQ, Katz B, Rabinovitz H, et al. Lessons on dermoscopy 11: solar lentigo. *Dermatol Surg.* 2000;26:1173.

18. Braun RP, Rabinovitz HS, Oliviero M, et al. Dermoscopy of pigmented skin lesions. *J Am Acad Dermatol.* 2005;52:109-121.

19. Nicholas A, Egerton IB, Lim AC, et al. Imaging the skin. *Australas J Dermatol.* 2003;44:19-27.

20. Langley RG, Burton E, Walsh N, et al. In vivo confocal scanning laser microscopy of benign lentigines: comparison to conventional histology and in vivo characteristics of lentigo maligna. *J Am Acad Dermatol.* 2006;55:88-97.

21. Yamashita T, Negishi K, Hariya T, et al. Intense pulsed light therapy for superficial pigmented lesions evaluated by reflectance-mode confocal microscopy and optical coherence tomography. *J Invest Dermatol.* 2006;126:2281.

22. Dalton SR, Gardner TL, Libow LF, et al. Contiguous lesions in lentigo maligna. *J Am Acad Dermatol.* 2005;52:859-862.

23. Kede MPV, Sabatovich O, eds. *Dermatologia Estética.* São Paulo, Brazil: Editora Atheneu; 2003:656.

24. Ortonne JP, Pandya AG, Hexsel DM, et al. Treatment of solar lentigines. *J Am Acad Dermatol.* 2006;54:262-271.

25. Williams HC. Healthcare needs assessment, second series. In: Stevens A, Raftery J, eds. *Dermatology.* Oxford, England: Radcliffe Medical Press; 1997:340.

26. Raziee M, Balighi K, Shabanzadeh-Dehkordi H, et al. Efficacy and safety of cryotherapy vs trichloroacetic acid in the treatment of solar lentigo. *J Eur Acad Dermatol Venereol.* 2008;22:316-319.

27. Lugo-Janer A, Lugo-Somolinos A, Sanchez JL. Comparison of trichloroacetic acid solution and cryosurgery in the treatment of solar lentigines. *Int J Dermatol.* 2003;42:829-831.

28. Chun EY, Lee JB, Lee KH. Focal trichloroacetic acid peel method for benign pigmented lesions in dark-skinned patients. *Dermatol Surg.* 2004;30:512-516.

29. Cook KK, Cook WR Jr. Chemical peel of nonfacial skin using glycolic acid gel augmented with TCA and neutralized based on visual staging. *Dermatol Surg.* 2000;26:994-999.

30. Rashid T, Hussain I, Haider M, et al. Laser therapy of freckles and lentigines with quasi-continuous, frequency-doubled, Nd:YAG (532 nm) laser in Fitzpatrick skin type IV: a 24-month follow-up. *J Cosmet Laser Ther.* 2002;4:81-85.

31. Kopera D, Hohenleutner U, Landthaler M. Quality-switched ruby laser treatment of solar lentigines and Becker's nevus: a histopathological and immunohistochemical study. *Dermatology.* 1997;194:338-343.

32. Rosenbach A, Lee SJ, John RH. Treatment of medium-brown solar lentigines using an alexandrite laser designed for hair reduction. *Arch Dermatol.* 2002;138:547-548.

33. Negishi K, Akita H, Tanaka S, et al. Comparative study of treatment efficacy and the incidence of post-inflammatory hyperpigmentation with different degrees of irradiation using two different quality-switched lasers for removing solar lentigines on Asian skin. *J Eur Acad Dermatol Venereol* 2013;27:307-312.

34. Kawada A, Shiraishi H, Asai M. Clinical improvement of solar lentigines and ephelides with an intense pulsed light source. *Dermatol Surg.* 2002;28:504-508.

35. Kawana S, Ochiai H, Tachihara R. Objective evaluation of the effect of intense pulsed light on rosacea and solar lentigines by spectrophotometric analysis of skin color. *Dermatol Surg.* 2007;33:449-454.

36. Kligman DE, Zhen Y. Intense pulsed light treatment of photoaged facial skin. *Dermatol Surg.* 2004;30:1085.

37. Sadighha A, Saatee S, Muhaghegh-Zahed G. Efficacy and adverse effects of Q-switched ruby laser on solar lentigines: a prospective study of 91 patients with Fitzpatrick skin type II, III, and IV. *Dermatol Surg.* 2008;34:1465-1468.

38. Sasaya H, Kawada A, Wada T, et al. Clinical effectiveness of intense pulsed light therapy for solar lentigines of the hands. *Dermatol Ther.* 2011;24:584-586.

39. Cotellessa C, Peris K, Fargnoli MC. Microabrasion versus microabrasion followed by 15% trichloroacetic acid for treatment of cutaneous hyperpigmentations in adult females. *Dermatol Surg.* 2003;29:352-356.

40. Stern RS, Dover JS, Levin JA, et al. Laser therapy versus cryotherapy of lentigines: a comparative trial. *J Am Acad Dermatol.* 1994;30:985.

41. Li YT, Yang KC. Comparison of the frequency-doubled Q-switched Nd:YAG laser and 35% trichloroacetic acid for the treatment of face lentigines. *Dermatol Surg.* 1999;25:202-204.

42. Raziee M, Balighi K, Shabanzadeh-Dehkordi H, et al. Efficacy and safety of cryotherapy vs. trichloroacetic acid in the treatment of solar lentigo. *J Eur Acad Dermatol Venereol* 2008;22:316-319.

43. Petit L, Piérard GE. Analytic quantification of solar lentigines lightening by a 2% hydroquinone-cyclodextrin formulation. *J Eur Acad Dermatol Venereol.* 2003;17:546-549.

44. Weiss JS, Shavin JS, Nighland M. Tretinoin microsphere gel 0.1% for photodamaged facial skin: a placebo-controlled trial. *Cutis.* 2006;78:426.

45. Kang S, Bergfeld W, Gottlieb AB. Long-term efficacy and safety of tretinoin emollient cream 0.05% in the treatment of photodamaged facial skin: a two-year randomized, placebo-controlled trial. *Am J Clin Dermatol.* 2005;6:245-253.

46. Weinstein GD, Nigra TP, Pochi PE. Topical tretinoin for treatment of photodamaged skin: a multicenter study. *Arch Dermatol.* 1991;127:659-665.

47. Rafal ES, Griffiths CE, Ditre CM, et al. Topical tretinoin (retinoic acid) treatment for liver spots associated with photodamage. *N Engl J Med.* 1992;326:368-374.

48. Kang S, Krueger GG, Tanghetti EA, et al. A multicenter, randomized, double-blind trial of tazarotene 0.1% cream in the treatment of photodamage. *J Am Acad Dermatol.* 2005;52:268-274.

49. Phillips TJ, Gottlieb AB, Leyden JJ, et al. Efficacy of 0.1% tazarotene cream for the treatment of photodamage: a 12-month multicenter, randomized trial. *Arch Dermatol* 2002;138:1486-1493.

50. Kang S, Goldfarb MT, Weiss JS, et al. Assessment of adapalene gel for the treatment of actinic keratoses and lentigines: a randomized trial. *J Am Acad Dermatol.* 2003;49:83-90.

51. Yoshimura K, Harii K, Aoyama T, et al. Experience with a strong bleaching treatment for skin hyperpigmentation in Orientals. *Plast Reconstr Surg.* 2000;105:1097-1108.

52. Jarratt M. Mequinol 2%/tretinoin 0.01% solution: an effective and safe alternative to hydroquinone 3% in the treatment of solar lentigines. *Cutis.* 2004;74:319-322.

53. Fleischer AB, Schwartzel EH, Colby SI, et al. The combination of 2% 4-hydroxyanisole (Mequinol) and 0.01% tretinoin is effective in improving the appearance of solar lentigines and related hyperpigmented lesions in two double-blind multicenter clinical studies. *J Am Acad Dermatol.* 2000;42:459.

54. Draelos ZD. The combination of 2% 4-hydroxyanisole (Mequinol) and 0.01% tretinoin effectively improves the appearance of solar lentigines in ethnic groups. *J Cosmet Dermatol.* 2006;5:239-244.

55. Ortonne JP, Camacho F, Wainwright N, et al. Safety and efficacy of combined use of 4-hydroxyanisole (Mequinol) 2%/tretinoin 0.01% solution and sunscreen in solar lentigines. *Cutis.* 2004;74:261-264.
56. Katoulis AC, Alevizou A, Bozi E et al. A randomized, double-blind, vehicle-controlled study of a preparation containing undecylenoyl phenylalanine 2% in the treatment of solar lentigines. *Clin Exp Dermatol.* 2010;35:473-476.
57. Khemis A, Cabou J, Dubois J, et al. A randomized controlled study to evaluate the depigmenting activity of L-ascorbic acid plus phytic acid-serum vs. placebo on solar lentigines. *Cosmet Dermatol.* 2011;10:266-272.

CHAPTER 54

Nevus of Ito/Ota

Marvi Iqbal
Zhong Lu

KEY POINTS

- Nevus of Ota is a dermal melanocytic hamartoma that is unilaterally distributed along the first and second branches of the trigeminal nerve. It presents clinically as a bluish gray hyperpigmentation of the skin.

- Nevus of Ito is a similar melanocytic condition, but the distribution is along the shoulder.

- It is felt that these melanocytic disorders represent melanocytes that did not migrate completely from the neural crest to the epidermis during the embryonic period.

- Nevi of Ito and Ota occur more frequently in skin of color populations from Asia and are rare in Caucasians.

INTRODUCTION

Oculodermal melanosis was first described by Hulke in 1861.[1] The entity nevus of Ota became known after it was described by Ota in 1939 as a bluish gray hyperpigmentation along the first and second divisions of the trigeminal nerve with occasional mucosal involvement[2] [**Figures 54-1** and **54-2**]. Nevus of Ito, described by Ito in 1954, is a similar melanocytic condition, but the distribution is along the shoulder[3] [**Figure 54-3**].

The etiology of nevi of Ota and Ito is unknown. It is possible that these melanocytic disorders represent melanocytes that did not migrate completely from the neural crest to the epidermis during the embryonic period.[4,5] It is also possible that hormones play a role in the development of a nevus of Ota because the two peaks of onset are at infancy and puberty, which account for 61.35% and 21.99% of patients, respectively. Other factors, such as ultraviolet light, infection, and trauma, also may play a role.[6,7]

Nevi of Ota and Ito occur more frequently in skin of color populations of Asian descent and are rare in Caucasians. Some studies have shown the incidence to be from 0.014% to 1.1%.[8,9] Nevus of Ota is more prevalent in women, with the male-to-female ratio being 1:4.8 to 5.68;[6] the ratio for nevus of Ito is unknown. Most patients with nevi of Ota or Ito do not have a family history of this condition.

CLINICAL AND HISTOLOGIC MANIFESTATIONS

Nevus of Ota is considered to be a dermal melanocytic hamartoma that is unilaterally distributed along the first and second branches of the trigeminal nerve. It appears as a blue-black or slate-gray macule. It may be classified according to the distribution of cutaneous involvement,[9] histologically based on the depth of melanocytic dermal involvement, and according to laser response.

Histologically, lesion of the nevus of Ota has a normal epidermis; the dendritic melanocytes are distributed in the papillary and midreticular dermis, surrounded by fibrous sheaths and parallel to the skin surface [**Figure 54-4**]. Transmission electron microscopy reveals that dendritic

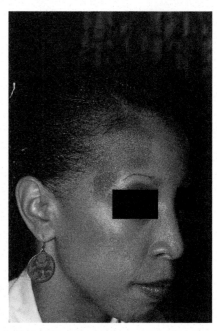

FIGURE 54-1. Nevus of Ota on the right forehead of an African American woman with Fitzpatrick type V skin.

melanocytes [**Figure 54-5**] contain more and larger melanosomes than normal melanocytes in the epidermis[10] [**Figure 54-6**]. Based on their location, there are five histologic groups: superficial (S), superficial dominant (SD), diffuse (Di), deep dominant (DD), and deep (D). S lesions tend to be in the cheek area, whereas D lesions are found more in the periorbital areas, temple, and forehead[3] [**Table 54-1**]. The ratio of S:SD:Di:DD:D is 3:2:3:1:1.[11]

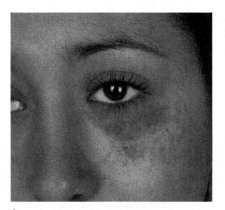

A

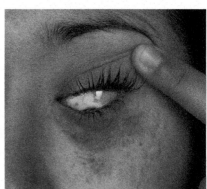

B

FIGURE 54-2. Nevus of Oto with (**A**) infraorbital hyperpigmentation and (**B**) scleral hyperpigmentation.

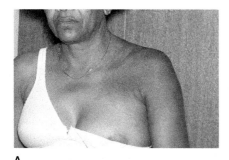

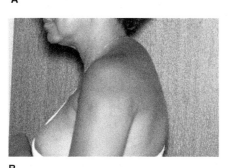

FIGURE 54-3. Nevus of Ito with hyperpigmentation along (**A**) the left shoulder and (**B**) the upper back.

Classification of nevi of Ota based on laser response is a novel approach, it is most likely developed since punch biopsy is rarely performed to diagnose this condition. The classification is as follows[12]:

1. Nevus of Ota without periorbital involvement, other birthmarks, and extracutaneous involvement

2. Nevus of Ota with periorbital involvement but without other birthmarks and extracutaneous involvement

3. Nevus of Ota with another birthmark but without extracutaneous involvement

4. Nevus of Ota with extracutaneous involvement

A similar classification for nevi of Ito does not exist, but histologically, nevi of Ito and Ota are described in the same way.

ASSOCIATED DISORDERS

Nevus of Ota at times may be associated with extracutaneous involvement. One type is known as *phakomatosis pigmentovascularis,* which is a congenital generalized hemangioma associated with nevus of Ota. This may present with systemic involvement such as ocular and neurologic disorders (eg, Sturge-Weber and Klippel-Trenaunay syndromes) and intracranial arteriovenous malformations.[13-16] Nevus of Ota also may be associated with ocular complications such as increased ocular pressure

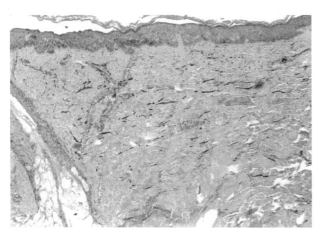

FIGURE 54-4. Melanocytes can be found within the dermis of nevi of Ota.

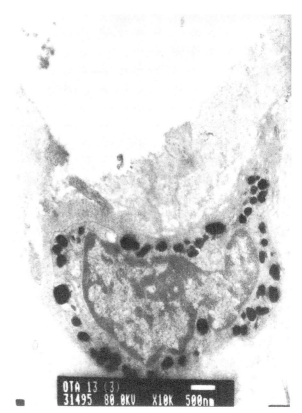

FIGURE 54-5. Dendritic melanocyte in nevus of Ota.

with or without glaucoma (10.3%), asymmetric cupping of the optic nerve head not associated with glaucoma (9.8%), uveitis (2.6%), cataracts (1%), and orbital melanoma (0.5%).[1] Although it is rare, nevus of Ota has been reported to be associated with malignant melanoma; most cases are orbital melanomas, but involvement of the skin and meninges has also been reported. In most of the reported cases, the patients were Caucasian, but other groups have been reported as well.[1] Only one case

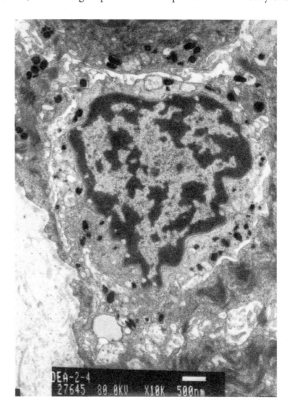

FIGURE 54-6. Normal melanocyte in epidermis.

TABLE 54-1	Comparison of nevi of Ota and Ito	
Nevi of Ota	**Nevi of Ito**	
Oculodermal melanosis	Shoulder melanosis	
Peaks of onset during infancy and puberty	Peaks of onset during infancy and puberty	
More frequent in Asians	More frequent in Asians	
Higher prevalence in woman	Unknown male-to-female ratio	
Deep (periorbital area and temple)		
Superficial (cheeks)		

TABLE 54-2	Laser therapy
Q-switched ruby laser	
Q-switched 1069-nm neodymium-doped yttrium aluminium garnet	
Q-switched alexandrite	
Recurrence of 0.6%–1.2% after complete clearance	

of melanoma has been reported with nevus of Ito.[16a] In terms of extracutaneous manifestations, although rare, nevus of Ito has been reported to occur simultaneously with nevus of Ota. Nevus of Ito also can be associated with sensory changes in the involved skin.[3]

TREATMENT

With the introduction of laser surgery based on the theory of selective photothermolysis, the treatment of nevus of Ota has improved significantly. Before laser theraph, treatment was limited to cryotherapy, dermabrasion, and surgical excision, all of which had significant risk of scarring and/or were unreliable. A study of 114 nevus of Ota patients treated with the Q-switched ruby laser found that most patients had an excellent response with four to five treatments, and no patient in the study had atrophic or hypertophic scarring.[17] The Q-switched ruby laser (694.3 nm, 6 J/cm², 30-nanosecond pulse) has been shown to interact selectively with cells that contain pigment, such as dermal melanocytes.[17] The Q-switched alexandrite and Q-switched 1064-nm neodymium-doped yttrium aluminium garnet (Nd:YAG) lasers also have been shown to be effective in the treatment of nevus of Ota.[18-22] According to a study on 522 Chinese patients with nevi of Ota treated with the Q-switched alexandrite laser, 278 patients achieved more than 75% clearance after two to six treatments.[18] Zygomatic, buccal, and forehead areas showed better response than ocular and temporal areas. Treatment session, interval, and fluence were significant factors that affected the treatment outcome.[18] The melanosomes degenerated by the laser irradiation and the dendritic melanocyte debri were gradually scavenged primarily by macrophages[19] [**Figure 54-7**]. It is recommended that the interval between the two laser sessions be 5 to 6 months long. According to several studies, the Nd:YAG laser was shown to be more effective than the Q-switched alexandrite laser in lightening the nevus of Ota, although the Q-switched alexandrite laser was better tolerated.[20,21] Nd:YAG laser is safe for skin types IV and V, and it is possible to achieve near total or marked improvement in 30% of patients after multiple treatments.[22] More recently, nonablative fractionated laser has been used to treat nevus of Ota, and there has been a report of successful treatment with a fractionated 1440-nm Nd:YAG laser.[23] It is important to keep in mind that there is a risk of recurrence of 0.6% to 1.2% after complete clearing with laser treatment [**Table 54-2**].[23] This is a special consideration in children when weighing the risks and benefits of multiple laser surgery treatments.

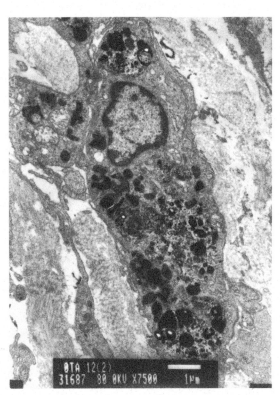

FIGURE 54-7. Degenerated melanosomes scavenged by macrophage.

REFERENCES

1. Chan HH, Kono T. Nevus of Ota: clinical aspects and management. *Skinmed.* 2003;59:200-210.
2. Bhattacharya SK, Girgla HS, Singh G. Naevus of Ota. *Int J Dermatol.* 1973; 12:344-347.
3. Lui H, Zhou Y. Nevi of Ota and Ito. www.e-medicine.com. Accessed February 15, 2015.
4. Kopf AW, Weidman AI. Naevus of Ota. *Arch Dermatol.* 1962;85:195-208.
5. Mishima Y, Mevorah B. Nevus of Ota and nevus of Ito in American Negroes. *J Invest Dermatol.* 1961;36:133-154.
6. Hidano A, Kajama H, Ikeda S, et al. Natural history of naevus of Ota. *Arch Dermatol.* 1967;95:187-195.
7. Stuart C. Naevus of Ota. *Br J Dermatol.* 1955;67:317.
8. Gonder JR, Ezell PC, Sheilds JA, et al. Ocular melanocytosis: a study to determine the prevalence rate of ocular melanocytosis. *Ophthalmology.* 1982; 89:950-952.
9. Tanino H. Uber eine in Japan haufig vorkommende Navusform: "Naevus fusco-caeruleus opthalmo-maxillaris Ota": I. Mitteilung:beobachtunguber lokalisation, verfarbung, anordnung and histologische veranderung. *Jpn J Dermatol.* 1939;46:435-451.
10. Lu Z, Chen J, Wang X, Fang L, et al. Effect of Q-switched Alexandrite laser irradiation on epidermal melanocytes in treatment of nevus of Ota. *Ch Med J.* 2003;116:597-601.
11. Hirayama T, and Suzuki T. A new classification of Nevus of Ota based on histopathological features. *Dermatologica.* 1991;183:169-172.
12. Chan HH, Lam LK, Wong DS, et al. Nevus of Ota: a new classification based upon the response to laser treatment. *Lasers Surg Med.* 2001;28:267-272.
13. Hasegawa Y, Yasuhara M. Phakomatosis pigmentovascularis type IVa. *Arch Dermatol.* 1985;121:651-655.
14. Massey EW, Brannon WL, Moreland M. Nevus of Ota and intracranial arteriovenous malformation. *Neurology.* 1979;29:1626-1627.
15. Ota M, Kawamura T, Ito N. Phakomatosis pigmentovascularis. *Jpn J Dermatol.* 1947;52:1-3.
16. Kumar A, Singh J. Naevus of Ota with primary retinitis pigmentosa: a syndrome. *Can J Ophthalmol.* 1985;20:261-263.
16a. Wise SR, Capra G, Martin P, et al. Malignant melanoma transformation within a nevus of Ito. *J Am Acad Dermatol.* 2010;62:869-874.
17. Watanabe S, Takahashi H. Treatment of nevus of Ota with the Q-switched ruby laser. *N Engl J Med.* 1994;331:1745-1750.
18. Lu Z, Fang L, Jiao S, et al. Treatment of 522 patients with nevus of Ota with Q-switched alexandrite laser. *Ch Med J.* 2003;116:226-230.
19. Lu Z, Chen J, Wang X, et al. Effect of Q-switched alexandrite laser irradiation on dermal melanocytes of nevus of Ota. *Ch Med J.* 2000;113:49-52.
20. Chan HH, King WWK, Chan ESY, et al. In vivo trial comparing patients' tolerance of Q-switched alexandrite and Q-switched neodymium:yttrium-aluminum-garnet lasers in the treatment of nevus of Ota. *Lasers Surg Med.* 1999;24:24-28.
21. Chan HH, Ying SY, Ho WS, et al. An in vivo trial comparing the clinical efficacy and complications of Q-switched 755-nm alexandrite and Q-switched 1064-nm (Nd-YAG) lasers in the treatment of nevus of Ota. *Dermatol Surg.* 2000;26:919-922.

22. Kar HK, Gupta L. 1064 nm Q switched Nd: YAG laser treatment of nevus of Ota: an Indian open label prospective study of 50 patients. *Indian J Dermatol Venereol Leprol.* 2011;77:565-570.
23. Polder KD, Landau JM, Vergilis-Kalner IJ, et al. Laser eradication of pigmented lesions: a review. *Dermatol Surg.* 2011;37:572-595.

Management of Hyperpigmentation

CHAPTER 55

So Yeon Paek
David Ozog
Henry W. Lim

KEY POINTS

- Acquired disorders of hyperpigmentation are commonly seen in patients with skin of color but are particularly challenging to treat in this population.
- Photoprotection is a safe and effective method of management.
- Topical agents, including hydroquinone, combination, and azelaic acid creams, are first-line treatments for hyperpigmentation.
- Glycolic acid and salicylic acid peels, and microdermabrasion have also demonstrated efficacy.
- Q-switched (QS) neodymium-doped yttrium aluminium garnet laser, intense pulsed light, and nonablative fractional photothermolysis are promising therapies.
- The erbium-doped yttrium aluminium garnet resurfacing laser, and lasers with shorter wavelengths (including the QS ruby and QS alexandrite laser) are not recommended for the treatment of acquired pigmentary disorders in patients with skin of color.

INTRODUCTION

Acquired disorders of hyperpigmentation, such as melasma [**Figures 55-1** and **55-2**] and postinflammatory hyperpigmentation (PIH), are among the most common conditions seen by dermatologists in patients with skin of color.[1] They are often refractory to standard methods of lightening, and patients with darker skin types are at greater risk for developing undesired hypo- or hyperpigmentation from depigmenting agents or procedures.[2] In this chapter, the treatment of hyperpigmentation with topical agents, peeling agents, and laser and light therapies is reviewed.

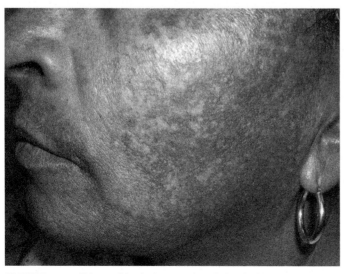

FIGURE 55-1. Melasma of the cheek in a patient with skin of color.

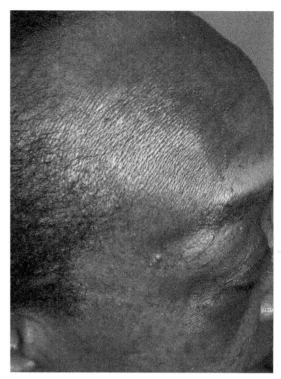

FIGURE 55-2. Melasma of the forehead in a patient with skin of color.

Key principles of management include prevention of dyspigmentation with photoprotection, disruption of melanogenesis through tyrosinase inhibition, and melanin removal.

TOPICAL AGENTS

SUNSCREENS

In addition to ultraviolet (UV) A (290 to 320 nm) and ultraviolet UV B (320 to 400 nm) radiation, long-wave visible light (400 to 760 nm) has also been shown to induce melanin formation and pigmentation.[3,4] Thus, photoprotection is a safe and effective first-line approach to depigmentation. Patients of all skin types should be advised to apply an oil-free, broad-spectrum UVA and UVB sunscreen with a sun protection factor (SPF) of at least 30.[5] In June 2011, the U.S. Food and Drug Administration (FDA) released its final rule on sunscreens, clearly stating the testing and labeling requirements for "broad-spectrum" statements.[6] As of December 2012, all major sunscreen manufacturers were mandated to accurately describe broad-spectrum coverage in accordance with these regulations. Seeking shade during the hours of 10:00 AM and 2:00 PM when UV rays are strongest, using photoprotective clothing and wide-brimmed hats, wearing sunglasses, and applying broad-spectrum sunscreens are essential approaches to avoid hyperpigmentation.[7]

HYDROQUINONE

The most commonly used topical depigmenting agent is hydroquinone cream. Available in 2% over-the-counter formulations or higher concentrations by prescription, hydroquinone is a hydroxyphenol that acts on the tyrosinase enzyme to inhibit conversion of dihydroxyphenylalanine (dopa) to melanin.[2] Hydroquinone is widely used in the United States and throughout the world. Its main side effects include ochronosis (due to accumulation of homogentisic acid in the dermis), nail discoloration, irritant and allergic contact dermatitis, and hypopigmentation of the surrounding normal skin (termed the 'halo effect').[8,9] Exogenous ochronosis [**Figure 55-3**] occurs primarily in patients with darker Fitzpatrick skin types after long-term application; it is not limited to use at higher concentrations, as there are reports of ochronosis occurring from 2% hydroquinone in the United States.[10] Early studies suggesting DNA

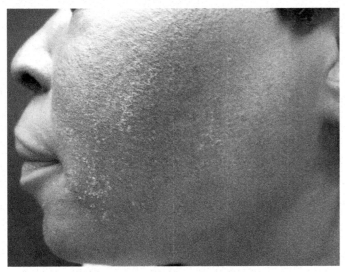

FIGURE 55-3. Exogenous ochronosis in a patient with darker skin of color.

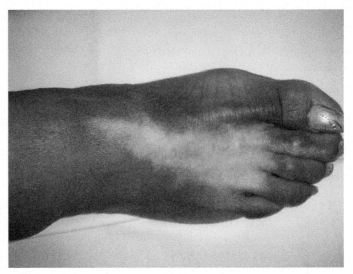

FIGURE 55-4. Steroid-induced hypopigmentation of the foot.

damage in rodents from hydroquinone have not yet been replicated in humans.[11] Therefore, although there is a proposed ruling by the U.S. FDA to remove hydroquinone from over-the-counter products due to concerns of exogenous ochronosis and carcinogenesis, it is still widely available and commonly used.

A derivative of hydroquinone, known as monobenzyl ether of hydroquinone, is applied as a 20% or 40% cream twice daily for 3 to 12 months for depigmentation therapy in advanced vitiligo. Skin irritation and allergic contact dermatitis are potential side effects.[12] Because monobenzyl ether of hydroquinone causes permanent depigmentation via melanocyte apoptosis, it is not recommended as a lightening agent for acquired disorders of hyperpigmentation.

COMBINATION CREAMS

The original Kligman-Willis formula, first reported in 1975, combined hydroquinone 5%, tretinoin 0.1%, and dexamethasone 0.1% in hydrophilic ointment.[13] Tretinoin increases epidermal penetration of hydroquinone and decreases potential steroid atrophy, while topical steroids reduce irritation and inhibit the synthesis of melanin. A triple combination cream containing fluocinolone acetonide 0.01%, hydroquinone 4%, and tretinoin 0.05% is a modern adaptation of the Kligman-Willis formula and has been shown to be effective in the treatment of melasma.[14-18]

AZELAIC ACID

Azelaic acid, a dicarboxylic acid found naturally in *Malassezia furfur*, the yeast responsible for pityriasis versicolor, is a depigmenting agent that functions as a tyrosinase inhibitor.[19] Studies comparing azelaic acid cream with hydroquinone demonstrated equal to improved efficacy of azelaic acid in the treatment of melasma and PIH.[20-23] Advantages of azelaic acid include a favorable safety profile and concomitant treatment of acne vulgaris; limiting factors include the long duration of treatment (it can be potentially months before improvement is seen) and development of allergic sensitization.[24,25]

KOJIC ACID

Kojic acid is a fungal metabolic product and antioxidant that also functions as a tyrosinase inhibitor to lighten skin. It is available in 1% to 4% cream or gel formulations, alone or in combination with hydroquinone and glycolic acid.[19,26] Clinical studies of kojic acid have shown marginal efficacy, with mostly equivocal results when compared with hydroquinone.[27,28] Allergic contact dermatitis is a well-known side effect, and many patients experience irritation from this agent, restricting the frequency of use.[29,30]

OTHER AGENTS

Other topical depigmenting agents with limited clinical investigations include soy, mulberry, licorice, arbutin, resveratrol, niacinamide, and *N*-acetyl glucosamine.[31,32] Topical corticosteroids are also known to induce hypopigmentation [**Figure 55-4**]. Although they have been used by some patients for depigmentation, topical corticosteroids are not recommended for this purpose because of their recognized side effects.

PEELING AGENTS

Alone or in combination with topical bleaching agents, chemical peels can be effective in treating pigmentary disorders. Glycolic acid and salicylic acid peels have been studied extensively and are reviewed below. The risks of deep chemical peels, such as phenol peels, outweigh the benefits and are not recommended in patients with skin of color. All peeling agents may produce undesirable side effects, including PIH, atrophy, erythema, telangiectasias, and infections.[33] Prior to their use, the provider should obtain a detailed history, including history of herpes simplex virus infection, adverse reaction to other cosmetic procedures, pregnancy, and presence of other concomitant skin conditions, such as psoriasis, which may be aggravated by the irritant effect of peeling agents. Patients must practice rigorous photoprotection after the procedure.

GLYCOLIC ACID PEELS

Composed of α-hydroxy acids from sugarcane juice, glycolic acid peels have been used effectively for melasma and PIH.[34] This superficial peel functions to remove the stratum corneum and increase penetration of topical agents. Glycolic acid peels have been used alone or in conjunction with hydroquinone, tretinoin, azelaic acid, adapalene, hydrocortisone creams, and lasers.[35-39] A study of 40 Indian women treated with a modified Kligman-Willis formula (2% hydroquinone, 0.05% tretinoin, and 1% hydrocortisone in a cream base) and glycolic acid peel (starting at 30% and increased to 40%) demonstrated greater improvement of melasma than with the topical agent alone.[36] Another trial evaluated the use of 20% azelaic acid cream and 0.1% adapalene gel with or without serial glycolic acid peels of increasing concentration (20% to 70%) for recalcitrant melasma and found increased improvement in the peel group.[37] Based on available data, improvement of pigmentation may be observed with multiple serial peels, starting at 30% glycolic acid and increasing as tolerated, in addition to application of topical agents.

SALICYLIC ACID PEELS

Salicylic acid is a β-hydroxy acid obtained from willow tree bark.[33] Salicylic acid peels have shown mixed results in the treatment of melasma and PIH in dark skin.[40,41] A study of six patients with melasma, along with 19 patients with acne, oily skin, and PIH, treated with 4% hydroquinone prior to 20% to 30% salicylic acid peels every 2 weeks for five sessions demonstrated moderate to significant improvement in two-thirds of patients, but also reported associated erythema, crusting, and dryness.[40] In a split-face trial, 10 subjects receiving two 20% salicylic acid peels and three 30% salicylic acid peels exhibited no statistically significant improvement of PIH.[41] Finally, a study of 24 Korean patients with PIH who received 30% salicylic acid peels biweekly for 3 months revealed significant colorimetric lightening after the first peel.[42] Although this depigmenting effect was not statistically significant, the authors concluded that salicylic acid peels may be used to lighten skin and reduce erythema in Asians.[42]

MICRODERMABRASION

Using crystals for physical exfoliation, microdermabrasion is a non-surgical, office-based procedure for rejuvenating the skin. It is used to treat photoaging and melasma in patients with skin of color.[43,44] The procedure is relatively safe, although patients have reported minor erythema and pain.[45] However, an open randomized trial of 10 patients who underwent either weekly microdermabrasion primed with 0.1% adapalene gel for 6 weeks or weekly microdermabrasion alone noted only marginal improvement for melasma in both groups.[46] Microdermabrasion may be useful as an adjunctive treatment to other modalities. Kauvar[47] demonstrated increased overall improvement in melasma treated with Q-switched (QS) neodymium-doped yttrium aluminium garnet (Nd:YAG) combined with microdermabrasion compared with QS Nd:YAG alone.[47]

LASER AND LIGHT THERAPY

Laser and light therapies are emerging treatment modalities for acquired disorders of pigmentation. Published evidence to support their use is limited to small clinical trials. Treatment with lasers is based on the concept of selective photothermolysis proposed by Anderson and Parrish.[48] Targets of laser energy (chomophores) have specific peak absorptions by various wavelengths. Chromophores dissipate this delivered heat at different rates depending on their shape and size. The thermal relaxation time (TRT) is the amount of time for 50% of the heat to dissipate from the chromophore after treatment. Anderson and Parrish[48] stated that as long as the laser energy is delivered to the chromophore in a shorter period of time than the TRT, the energy is restricted to the target, and collateral damage to surrounding tissue is minimized. For pigmentation, the main chromophore is melanin, which has a broad absorption between 630 and 1100 nm. The TRT of a melanosome is quite rapid (250 to 1000 nanoseconds [ns]), as this is a relatively small structure. Therefore, many of the lasers studied for melasma and PIH have been QS with pulse durations shorter than 250 ns and wavelengths between 694 and 1064 nm. The wavelength of these lasers affects not only the target and competing targets (primarily hemoglobin), but depth of penetration as well. In these visible and near-infrared ranges, higher wavelengths correlate with greater depth of penetration. However, higher energies must be used.

Lasers with shorter wavelengths, such as the QS ruby (694 nm) and QS alexandrite (755 nm) lasers, have limited penetration and may result in undesired hyperpigmentation due to absorption by endogenous melanin in patients with skin of color, whereas those with longer wavelengths, such as the QS Nd:YAG at 1064 nm, have reduced risk of inducing adverse discoloration.[49] Additional lasers used to treat pigmentary disorders include both ablative and nonablative devices. These lasers improve discoloration by allowing a shuttling of pigment (through microscopic exudative necrotic debris [MEND]) or direct ablation of superficial pigment. Intense pulsed light (IPL) is effective for epidermal melasma but less so with deep or mixed variants. The latter can be targeted with higher fluences, but increasing risk of PIH exists with darker

skin.[50] Laser and light therapy with any device should begin at low doses after test spots have been performed to minimize adverse events.[51,52]

Q-SWITCHED RUBY LASER

Emitting red light at 694 nm that reaches a skin depth of 2 to 3 mm, the QS ruby laser has been shown to induce PIH and worsen melasma in patients with darker skin types.[53,54] However, a study of 15 Korean women treated with a novel fractional QS ruby laser for six bimonthly sessions at low-energy settings did indicate a 30% improvement of melasma,[55] suggesting a possible role for a fractional QS ruby laser in this subset population. At this time, given the high incidence of PIH and conflicting results of studies, general use of the QS ruby laser is not recommended for the treatment of dyschromias in individuals with skin of color. However, the QS ruby laser is a mainstay of therapy for patients with a nevus of Ota/Ito, as suggested by studies demonstrating effective lightening in these lesions.[56]

Q-SWITCHED ALEXANDRITE LASER

The QS alexandrite laser (755 nm), which allows deeper skin penetration than the QS ruby (694 nm) because of its longer wavelength, is also standard therapy for the treatment of a nevus of Ota/Ito.[57-60] Two studies suggested improvement of refractory melasma when the QS alexandrite laser was combined with the pulsed carbon dioxide (CO_2) laser.[60,61] However, the development of severe PIH in treated patients limits its use.

Q-SWITCHED ND:YAG LASER

The QS neodymium-doped yttrium aluminum garnet Nd:YAG laser emits at 1064 nm and has been shown to successfully treat dermal melasma and PIH. It is the most commonly used laser to treat melasma. Two case reports of patients treated with 10 weekly QS Nd:YAG laser treatments, along with topical 7% α-arbutin and broad-spectrum sunscreen of SPF 50, revealed considerable reduction of hyperpigmentation.[62] A study of 27 female patients treated with low-fluence QS Nd:YAG laser and microdermabrasion every 4 weeks, along with hydroquinone 4% cream twice daily, tretinoin 0.05% cream nightly, and broad-spectrum sunscreen with a minimum SPF of 40 daily, demonstrated partial clearance of melasma, which was observed even after only one treatment.[47] Several other reports of pigmentary improvement in Korean women treated with the QS Nd:YAG laser support its use for melasma and PIH.[63-65] The longer wavelength of this laser makes it a safer option for treating dyschromias in darker skin types.

ER:YAG RESURFACING LASER

The erbium-doped yttrium aluminium garnet (Er:YAG) resurfacing laser, which emits at 2940 nm and targets water molecules, has been demonstrated to induce initial (within the first 10 days) postprocedure improvement of refractory melasma.[66,67] However, the development of persistent erythema, PIH requiring further treatment with topical and peeling agents for months, and higher incidence of pain with type IV to V skin constrain its use.[66,67]

INTENSE PULSED LIGHT

IPL therapy uses high-intensity visible light (range: 515 to 1200 nm) and was initially used to target vascular lesions.[68] A trial of 89 Chinese females with refractory epidermal or mixed melasma who received four treatments of IPL over 12 weeks demonstrated moderate to significant improvement.[69] A comparison of treatment with topical 4% hydroquinone cream and broad-spectrum sunscreen alone versus topical therapy with four IPL sessions in Asian women with skin types III and IV found significant reduction in refractory melasma.[70] Zoccali et al[71] found that IPL was more effective in treating epidermal melasma over three to five sessions in individuals with skin types III and IV than topical 4% hydroquinone cream and broad-spectrum sunscreen of SPF 15 alone. A study of 62 patients with refractory melasma treated with single-session IPL plus triple combination topical therapy cream (hydroquinone 4%, treti-noin 0.05%, and fluocinolone acetonide 0.01%) and broad-spectrum sunscreen versus topical agents alone demonstrated statistically signifi-cant improvement ($P <0.001$) in the IPL group with a 44.9% reduction after 12 months.[72] The authors noted that patients without forehead involvement had the greatest improvement. Best results with IPL were obtained when patients were pretreated with triple combination topical therapy and sunscreen.[72] Disadvantages of IPL treatment include des-quamation, erythema, edema, and PIH, usually limited to patients with deeper or mixed-type melasma and often responsive to topical hydro-quinone cream.

■ FRACTIONAL PHOTOTHERMOLYSIS

As the latest advancement in laser therapy, fractional laser resurfacing damages microscopic zones of lesional skin using thermal radiation while protecting healthy skin.[73] The original nonablative fractional pho-tothermolysis (NAFP) device was developed as a means to offset the side effects encountered with traditional ablative and nonablative lasers. First reported by Manstein et al[74] in 2004, the NAFP device uses an erbium-doped 1550-nm laser and allows for rapid healing, shorter recovery time, and reduction of undesired pigmentation, scarring, and infection, while maintaining efficacy of treatment. The mechanism by which NAFP induces pigmentary change involves the elimination of pigment via thermal damage, in a process known as the melanin shuttle.[75] Mela-nin is released from damaged skin and transported through MEND, and new keratinocytes and melanocytes repopulate the previously damaged area.[76] Histologic evaluation of tissue treated with NAFP demonstrates a decrease in melanin granule content and number of melanocytes.

NAFP with the 1550 nm erbium-doped laser is an FDA-approved procedure for the treatment of melasma, pigmented lesions, perior-bital rhytides, and scars from acne or surgeries.[77] Of these indica-tions, melasma is the most difficult to treat.[78] In a study of melasma patients with Fitzpatrick skin types III to V treated with a nonabla-tive fractional resurfacing laser, Rokhsar and Fitzpatrick[79] found that 6 of 10 patients showed significant improvement of pigmentation. Naito[80] found similar results in three of six Chinese patients with skin types III to IV and resistant melasma treated with NAFP. However, use of the erbium-doped NAFP in 25 Korean patients with melasma was only minimally effective.[81] A split-face study from the Netherlands comparing NAFP to triple combination topical therapy (hydroquinone 5%, tretinoin 0.05%, and triamcinolone acetonide 0.1% cream) for melasma in patients with skin types II to V showed inferiority of fractional photothermolysis, whereas another randomized controlled study by the same group demon-strated no difference in efficacy and comparable recurrence rates between laser and triple combination topical therapy.[82,83] Finally, a split-face study of melasma in 14 patients with skin types II to IV who received NAFP revealed improvement in only half of patients, with recurrence at weeks 26 to 28 and PIH in 2 of 12 patients.[84] All studies noted an increased incidence of PIH in patients with darker skin types, and pre- and post-treatment bleaching agents (hydroquinone and retinoids) and use of a broad-spectrum sunscreen of at least SPF 30 daily are recommended for patients with skin of color.[78] In addition, clinicians may consider lowering the treatment level (treatment settings 4 to 6 for light Asian skin and 2 to 3 for dark Asian skin) to reduce the risk of PIH in this population.[85]

The first use of novel ablative fractional photothermolysis CO_2 (10,600 nm) and Er:YAG (2940 nm) lasers was reported by Hantash et al[86] in 2007. Both lasers were shown to have superior efficacy in the treatment of scarring and photoaging previously only seen with tradi-tional ablative lasers.[86] However, they have not been studied specifically for melasma.

CONCLUSION

Management of acquired disorders of hyperpigmentation in patients with skin of color can be challenging [**Table 55-1**]. First-line therapies for depigmentation include prevention of hyperpigmentation with

TABLE 55-1	Depigmenting management strategies in patients with skin of color	
Treatment type	Therapy	Clinical recommendations
First line	Photoprotection	• Oil-free, broad-spectrum, UVA/UVB sunscreen with minimum SPF of 30 • Shade, photoprotective clothing, wide-brimmed hat, sunglasses
	HQ 4% cream	• Switch to non-HQ agent after long-term use to avoid exogenous ochronosis
	Combination creams	• May be used daily for prolonged treatment • Triple combination cream: fluocinolone aceton-ide 0.01%, HQ 4%, and tretinoin 0.05%
Second line	Azelaic acid cream	• Use in cases of HQ intolerance • Concomitant treatment of acne vulgaris
	Glycolic acid peels with 2% HQ cream before treatment	• Start with 30% glycolic acid and increase as tolerated • May repeat monthly
	Salicylic acid peels	• May be used for PIH but not effective for melasma • Greater efficacy in Asian skin than for darker skin types
	Microdermabrasion	• Minimal reported improvement but relatively safe
Third line[a]		
	QS Nd:YAG laser	• Safe for melasma and PIH, alone or in combi-nation with microdermabrasion or topical agents
	NAFP	• Adjunct therapy after failure of above • May become first- or second-line treatment once larger clinical trials are available
	IPL	• Effective for superficial melasma
Not recommended		
	Kojic acid cream or gel	• Equivocal outcomes • Allergic contact dermatitis is well known
	QS ruby laser	• Worsens melasma and induces PIH • Treatment of a nevus of Ota/Ito
	QS alexandrite laser	• Induces severe PIH • Treatment of a nevus of Ota/Ito
	Er:YAG resurfacing laser	• High incidence of pain and PIH in darker skin types

Abbreviations: Er:YAG, erbium-doped yttrium aluminium garnet; HQ, hydroquinone; IPL, intense pulsed light; NAFP, nonablative fractional photothermolysis; Nd:YAG, neodymium-doped yttrium aluminium garnet; PIH, postinflammatory hyperpigmentation; QS, Q-switched; SPF, sun protection factor; UV, ultraviolet.

[a]Pretreat all laser/light therapies with broad-spectrum sunscreen of at least SPF 30 and triple combina-tion cream (hydroquinone 4%, tretinoin 0.05%, and fluocinolone acetonide 0.01%).

photoprotection and inhibition of tyrosinase through topical creams, such as hydroquinone and a triple combination cream (fluocinolone acetonide 0.01%, hydroquinone 4%, and tretinoin 0.05%). Second-line agents include azelaic acid creams, glycolic acid peels with 4% hydro-quinone pretreatment, salicylic acid peels, and microdermabrasion. Finally, QS Nd:YAG lasers, NAFP, and IPL therapies may be used as third-line treatment modalities. Patients with darker skin types should be pretreated with a triple combination cream (fluocinolone acetonide 0.01%, hydroquinone 4%, and tretinoin 0.05%) and advised to apply broad-spectrum sunscreens of at least SPF 30 daily before and after any laser or light treatments. The following are not recommended for patients with skin of color: kojic acid creams or gels (because of the lack of documented efficacy), and QS ruby, QS alexandrite, and Er:YAG resurfacing lasers (because of their potential side effects).

REFERENCES

1. Alexis AF, Sergay AB, Taylor SC. Common dermatologic disorders in skin of color: a comparative practice survey. *Cutis.* 2007;80:387-394.

2. Grimes PE. Management of hyperpigmentation in darker racial ethnic groups. *Semin Cutan Med Surg.* 2009;28:77-85.

3. Mahmoud BH, Hexsel CL, Hamzavi IH, et al. Effects of visible light on the skin. *Photochem Photobiol.* 2008;84:450-462.

4. Mahmoud BH. Photobiologic effects of long wavelength UVA and visible light on melanocompetent skin. *J Invest Dermatol.* 2009;129:125.

5. Downie JB. Esthetic considerations for ethnic skin. *Semin Cutan Med Surg.* 2006;25:158-162.

6. Wang SQ, Lim HW. Current status of the sunscreen regulation in the United States: 2011 Food and Drug Administration's final rule on labeling and effectiveness testing. *J Am Acad Dermatol.* 2011;65:863-869.

7. Maier T, Korting HC. Sunscreens: which and what for? *Skin Pharmacol Physiol.* 2005;18:253-262.

8. Levin CY, Maibach H. Exogenous ochronosis. An update on clinical features, causative agents and treatment options. *Am J Clin Dermatol.* 2001;2:213-217.

9. Nordlund JJ, Grimes PE, Ortonne JP. The safety of hydroquinone. *J Eur Acad Dermatol Venereol.* 2006;20:781-787.

10. Hoshaw RA, Zimmerman KG, Menter A. Ochronosislike pigmentation from hydroquinone bleaching creams in American blacks. *Arch Dermatol.* 1985; 121:105-108.

11. Draelos ZD. Skin lightening preparations and the hydroquinone controversy. *Dermatol Ther.* 2007;20:308-313.

12. Lyon CC, Beck MH. Contact hypersensitivity to monobenzyl ether of hydroquinone used to treat vitiligo. *Contact Dermatitis.* 1998;39:132-133.

13. Kligman AM, Willis I. A new formula for depigmenting human skin. *Arch Dermatol.* 1975;111:40-48.

14. Taylor SC, Torok H, Jones T, et al. Efficacy and safety of a new triple-combination agent for the treatment of facial melasma. *Cutis.* 2003;72:67-72.

15. Torok HM, Jones T, Rich P, et al. Hydroquinone 4%, tretinoin 0.05%, fluocinolone acetonide 0.01%: a safe and efficacious 12-month treatment for melasma. *Cutis.* 2005;75:57-62.

16. Grimes P, Kelly AP, Torok H, et al. Community-based trial of a triple-combination agent for the treatment of facial melasma. *Cutis.* 2006;77:177-184.

17. Chan R, Park KC, Lee MH, et al. A randomized controlled trial of the efficacy and safety of a fixed triple combination (fluocinolone acetonide 0.01%, hydroquinone 4%, tretinoin 0.05%) compared with hydroquinone 4% cream in Asian patients with moderate to severe melasma. *Br J Dermatol.* 2008;159:697-703.

18. Ferreira Cestari T, Hassun K, Sittart A, et al. A comparison of triple combination cream and hydroquinone 4% cream for the treatment of moderate to severe facial melasma. *J Cosmet Dermatol.* 2007;6:36-39.

19. Halder RM, Richards GM. Topical agents used in the management of hyperpigmentation. *Skin Therapy Lett.* 2004;9:1-3.

20. Verallo-Rowell VM, Verallo V, Graupe K, et al. Double-blind comparison of azelaic acid and hydroquinone in the treatment of melasma. *Acta Derm Venereol Suppl (Stockh).* 1989;143:58-61.

21. Sarkar R, Bhalla M, Kanwar AJ. A comparative study of 20% azelaic acid cream monotherapy versus a sequential therapy in the treatment of melasma in dark-skinned patients. *Dermatology.* 2002;205:249-254.

22. Baliña LM, Graupe K. The treatment of melasma: 20% azelaic acid versus 4% hydroquinone cream. *Int J Dermatol.* 1991;30:893-895.

23. Lowe NJ, Rizk D, Grimes P, et al. Azelaic acid 20% cream in the treatment of facial hyperpigmentation in darker-skinned patients. *Clin Ther.* 1998; 20:945-959.

24. Del Rosso JQ. The use of topical azelaic acid for common skin disorders other than inflammatory rosacea. *Cutis.* 2006;77:22-24.

25. Graupe K, Cunliffe WJ, Gollnick HP, et al. Efficacy and safety of topical azelaic acid (20 percent cream): an overview of results from European clinical trials and experimental reports. *Cutis.* 1996;57:20-35.

26. Parvez S, Kang M, Chung HS, et al. Survey and mechanism of skin depigmenting and lightening agents. *Phytother Res.* 2006;20:921-934.

27. Garcia A, Fulton JE Jr. The combination of glycolic acid and hydroquinone or kojic acid for the treatment of melasma and related conditions. *Dermatol Surg.* 1996;22:443-447.

28. Lim JT. Treatment of melasma using kojic acid in a gel containing hydroquinone and glycolic acid. *Dermatol Surg.* 1999;25:282-284.

29. Mata TL, Sanchez JP, De La Cuadra Oyanguren J. Allergic contact dermatitis due to kojic acid. *Dermatitis.* 2005;16:55-86.

30. Serra-Baldrich E, Tribó MJ, Camarasa JG. Allergic contact dermatitis from kojic acid. *Contact Dermatitis.* 1998;39:86-87.

31. Konda S, Geria AN, Halder RM. New horizons in treating disorders of hyperpigmentation in skin of color. *Semin Cutan Med Surg.* 2012;31:133-139.

32. Davis EC, Callender VD. Postinflammatory hyperpigmentation: a review of the epidemiology, clinical features, and treatment options in skin of color. *J Clin Aesthet Dermatol.* 2010;3:20-31.

33. Roberts WE. Chemical peeling in ethnic/dark skin. *Dermatol Ther.* 2004;17:196-205.

34. Song JY, Kang HA, Kim MY, et al. Damage and recovery of skin barrier function after glycolic acid chemical peeling and crystal microdermabrasion. *Dermatol Surg.* 2004;30:390-394.

35. Gupta RR, Mahajan BB, Garg G. Chemical peeling—evaluation of glycolic acid in varying concentrations and time intervals. *Indian J Dermatol Venereol Leprol.* 2001;67:28-29.

36. Sarkar R, Kaur C, Bhalla M, et al. The combination of glycolic acid peels with a topical regimen in the treatment of melasma in dark-skinned patients: a comparative study. *Dermatol Surg.* 2002;28:828-832.

37. Erbil H, Sezer E, Tastan B, et al. Efficacy and safety of serial glycolic acid peels and a topical regimen in the treatment of recalcitrant melasma. *J Dermatol.* 2007;34:25-30.

38. Burns RL, Prevost-Blank PL, Lawry MA, et al. Glycolic acid peels for postinflammatory hyperpigmentation in black patients. A comparative study. *Dermatol Surg.* 1997;23:171-174.

39. Park KY, Kim DH, Kim HK, et al. A randomized, observer-blinded, comparison of combined 1064-nm Q-switched neodymium-doped yttrium-aluminium-garnet laser plus 30% glycolic acid peel vs. laser monotherapy to treat melasma. *Clin Exp Dermatol.* 2011;36:864-870.

40. Grimes PE. The safety and efficacy of salicylic acid chemical peels in darker racial-ethnic groups. *Dermatol Surg.* 1999;25:18-22.

41. Joshi SS, Boone SL, Alam M, et al. Effectiveness, safety, and effect on quality of life of topical salicylic acid peels for treatment of postinflammatory hyperpigmentation in dark skin. *Dermatol Surg.* 2009;35:638-644.

42. Ahn HH, Kim IH. Whitening effect of salicylic acid peels in Asian patients. *Dermatol Surg.* 2006;32:372-375.

43. Davis EC, Callender VD. Aesthetic dermatology for aging ethnic skin. *Dermatol Surg.* 2011;37:901-917.

44. Shim EK, Barnette D, Hughes K, et al. Microdermabrasion: a clinical and histopathologic study. *Dermatol Surg.* 2001;27:524-530.

45. Karimipour DJ, Karimipour G, Orringer JS. Microdermabrasion: an evidence-based review. *Plast Reconstr Surg.* 2010;125:372-377.

46. Bhalla M, Thami GP. Microdermabrasion: reappraisal and brief review of literature. *Dermatol Surg.* 2006;32:809-814.

47. Kauvar AN. Successful treatment of melasma using a combination of microdermabrasion and Q-switched Nd:YAG lasers. *Lasers Surg Med.* 2012; 44:117-124.

48. Anderson RR, Parrish JA. Selective photothermolysis: precise microsurgery by selective absorption of pulsed radiation. *Science.* 1983;220:524-527.

49. Battle EF Jr, Hobbs LM. Laser therapy on darker ethnic skin. *Dermatol Clin.* 2003;21:713-723.

50. Arora P, Sarkar R, Garg VK, et al. Lasers for treatment of melasma and postinflammatory hyperpigmentation. *J Cutan Aesthet Surg.* 2012;5:93-103.

51. Bhatt N, Alster TS. Laser surgery in dark skin. *Dermatol Surg.* 2008;34:184-194.

52. Alster TS, Tanzi EL. Laser surgery in dark skin. *Skinmed.* 2003;2:80-85.

53. Tse Y, Levine VJ, McClain SA, et al. The removal of cutaneous pigmented lesions with the Q-switched ruby laser and the Q-switched neodymium:yttrium-aluminum-garnet laser. A comparative study. *J Dermatol Surg Oncol.* 1994;20:795-800.

54. Taylor CR, Anderson RR. Ineffective treatment of refractory melasma and postinflammatory hyperpigmentation by Q-switched ruby laser. *J Dermatol Surg Oncol.* 1994;20:592-597.

55. Jang WS, Lee CK, Kim BJ, et al. Efficacy of 694-nm Q-switched ruby fractional laser treatment of melasma in female Korean patients. *Dermatol Surg.* 2011;37:1133-1140.

56. Watanabe S. Basics of laser application to dermatology. *Arch Dermatol Res.* 2008;300:S21-S30.

57. Kagami S, Asahina A, Watanabe R, et al. Treatment of 153 Japanese patients with Q-switched alexandrite laser. *Lasers Med Sci.* 2007;22:159-163.

58. Wang HW, Liu YH, Zhang GK, et al. Analysis of 602 Chinese cases of nevus of Ota and the treatment results treated by Q-switched alexandrite laser. *Dermatol Surg.* 2007;33:455-460.

59. Kang W, Lee E, Choi GS. Treatment of Ota's nevus by Q-switched alexandrite laser: therapeutic outcome in relation to clinical and histopathological findings. *Eur J Dermatol.* 1999;9:639-643.

60. Angsuwarangsee S, Polnikorn N. Combined ultrapulse CO2 laser and Q-switched alexandrite laser compared with Q-switched alexandrite laser

alone for refractory melasma: split-face design. *Dermatol Surg.* 2003; 29:59-64.

61. Nouri K, Bowes L, Chartier T, et al. Combination treatment of melasma with pulsed CO2 laser followed by Q-switched alexandrite laser: a pilot study. *Dermatol Surg.* 1999;25:494-497.

62. Polnikorn N. Treatment of refractory dermal melasma with the MedLite C6 Q-switched Nd:YAG laser: two case reports. *J Cosmet Laser Ther.* 2008;10:167-173.

63. Cho SB, Kim JS, Kim MJ. Melasma treatment in Korean women using a 1064-nm Q-switched Nd:YAG laser with low pulse energy. *Clin Exp Dermatol.* 2009;34:e847-e850.

64. Choi M, Choi JW, Lee SY, et al. Low-dose 1064-nm Q-switched Nd:YAG laser for the treatment of melasma. *J Dermatolog Treat.* 2010;21:224-228.

65. Cho SB, Park SJ, Kim JS, et al. Treatment of post-inflammatory hyperpigmentation using 1064-nm Q-switched Nd:YAG laser with low fluence: report of three cases. *J Eur Acad Dermatol Venereol.* 2009;23:1206-1207.

66. Manaloto RM, Alster T. Erbium:YAG laser resurfacing for refractory melasma. *Dermatol Surg.* 1999;25:121-123.

67. Ko NY, Ahn HH, Kim SN, et al. Analysis of erythema after Er:YAG laser skin resurfacing. *Dermatol Surg.* 2007;33:1322-1327.

68. Pathak MA, Riley FC, Fitzpatrick TB. Melanogenesis in human skin following exposure to long-wave ultraviolet and visible light. *J Invest Dermatol.* 1962; 39:435-443.

69. Li YH, Chen JZ, Wei HC, et al. Efficacy and safety of intense pulsed light in treatment of melasma in Chinese patients. *Dermatol Surg.* 2008;34:693-700.

70. Wang CC, Hui CY, Sue YM, et al. Intense pulsed light for the treatment of refractory melasma in Asian persons. *Dermatol Surg.* 2004;30:1196-1200.

71. Zoccali G, Piccolo D, Allegra P, et al. Melasma treated with intense pulsed light. *Aesthetic Plast Surg.* 2010;34:486-493.

72. Figueiredo Souza L, Trancoso Souza S. Single-session intense pulsed light combined with stable fixed-dose triple combination topical therapy for the treatment of refractory melasma. *Dermatol Ther.* 2012;25:477-480.

73. Tierney EP, Hanke CW. Review of the literature: treatment of dyspigmentation with fractionated resurfacing. *Dermatol Surg.* 2010;36:1499-1508.

74. Manstein D, Herron GS, Sink RK, et al. Fractional photothermolysis: a new concept for cutaneous remodeling using microscopic patterns of thermal injury. *Lasers Surg Med.* 2004;34:426-438.

75. Rahman Z, Alam M, Dover JS. Fractional Laser treatment for pigmentation and texture improvement. *Skin Therapy Lett.* 2006;11:7-11.

76. Goldberg DJ, Berlin AL, Phelps R. Histologic and ultrastructural analysis of melasma after fractional resurfacing. *Lasers Surgery Med.* 2008;40:134-138.

77. Katz TM, Goldberg LH, Firoz BF, et al. Fractional photothermolysis for the treatment of postinflammatory hyperpigmentation. *Dermatol Surg.* 2009;35:1844-1848.

78. Sherling M, Friedman PM, Adrian R, et al. Consensus recommendations on the use of an erbium-doped 1,550-nm fractionated laser and its applications in dermatologic laser surgery. *Dermatol Surg.* 2010;36:461-469.

79. Rokhsar CK, Fitzpatrick RE. The treatment of melasma with fractional photothermolysis: a pilot study. *Dermatol Surg.* 2005;31:1645-1650.

80. Naito SK. Fractional photothermolysis treatment for resistant melasma in Chinese females. *J Cosmet Laser Ther.* 2007;9:161-163.

81. Lee HS, Won CH, Lee DH, et al. Treatment of melasma in Asian skin using a fractional 1,550-nm laser: an open clinical study. *Dermatol Surg.* 2009;35:1499-1504.

82. Kroon MW, Wind BS, Beek JF, et al. Nonablative 1550-nm fractional laser therapy versus triple topical therapy for the treatment of melasma: a randomized controlled pilot study. *J Am Acad Dermatol.* 2011;64:516-523.

83. Wind BS, Kroon MW, Meesters AA, et al. Non-ablative 1,550 nm fractional laser therapy versus triple topical therapy for the treatment of melasma: a randomized controlled split-face study. *Lasers Surgery Med.* 2010;42:607-612.

84. Barysch MJ, Rümmelein B, Kolm I, et al. Split-face study of melasma patients treated with non-ablative fractionated photothermolysis (1540 nm). *J Eur Acad Dermatol Venereol.* 2012;26:423-430.

85. Chan HH, Manstein D, Yu CS, et al. The prevalence and risk factors of post-inflammatory hyperpigmentation after fractional resurfacing in Asians. *Lasers Surg Med.* 2007;39:381-385.

86. Hantash BM, Bedi VP, Kapadia B, et al. In vivo histological evaluation of a novel ablative fractional resurfacing device. *Lasers Surg Med.* 2007;39:96-107.

CHAPTER 56

Anatomy and Diseases of the Oral Mucosa

Diana V. Messadi
Anh D. Le
Ginat W. Mirowski
Heddie Sedano

KEY POINTS

- Leukoedema is the most common benign oral condition related to individuals with skin of color.
- No treatment is necessary for leukoedema.
- Oral cancer incidence rate is similar among African Americans and Caucasians, but the mortality rate is higher in African Americans due to late diagnosis and lack of access to medical care.
- Screening and early detection of oral cancer are important to decrease the high mortality and morbidity rates in African Americans.
- Physiologic oral pigmentation is due to greater melanocytic activity rather than higher number of melanocytes.
- Some oral conditions are seen more commonly in Native Americans.
- In contrast to cutaneous melanoma, oral melanoma is as equally prevalent in African Americans as in Caucasians.

INTRODUCTION

Evaluation of the patient with oral complaints requires an organized approach that consists of obtaining a complete medical, dental, dermatologic, family, and social and medication history. Also important are the use of medications, herbs, and vitamins, as well as a history of all possible allergic reactions, a physical examination, and evaluation of any available laboratory studies.

The physical examination includes evaluation of the musculoskeletal and soft tissues of the head and neck including lymph nodes, thyroid and salivary gland palpation, and a complete mucocutaneous examination including conjunctiva and nasal mucosa. Intraoral examination requires proper visualization with an intraoral dental mirror and a bimanual palpation of the soft and hard tissues of the head and neck including the lips, gingiva, temporomandibular joint, neck, and tongue. A complete evaluation requires the use of gauze to dry the mucosa and to facilitate visual inspection and palpation of the lips and tongue. Evaluation of the teeth and periodontal status is necessary as well.

Laboratory studies, including scrapings, cytology, serum studies, cultures, and biopsies, should be performed when indicated. This chapter will focus on the oral diseases that are commonly present in African Americans and other individuals with skin of color.

INTRAORAL EXAMINATION

The external margin of the lips (ie, the transition zone between skin and mucous membrane) is known as the *vermilion*. It is pink to brown in color, hairless, and covered by a thin dry epithelium; at the junction

of the vermilion and the lips, the *vermilion border* is slightly palpable except in advanced age or with chronic sun exposure [**Figure 56-1**].

Intraorally, the oral cavity is divided into the vestibule and the oral cavity proper. The vestibule is limited by the gingiva and the teeth medially and by the labial and buccal mucosa laterally. The superior and the inferior of the vestibule are called *vestibular sulci*. Anterior and lateral frena traverse the vestibular sulci from the lip and buccal mucosa to the gingival mucosa. The lateral frena are seen bilaterally at the maxillary and mandibular premolars.

The labial and buccal mucosa is normally pale pink in color, shiny, and kept moist by an extensive number of minor salivary glands that secret myxoid saliva directly onto the mucosa.

On the buccal mucosa, a horizontal line called the *linea alba*, of varying prominence, may be seen bilaterally reflecting the occlusal plane of the teeth. Stensen papilla, a papule that protects the opening of the Stensen duct (main excretory duct of the parotid gland), can be seen above the linea alba. Clear aqueous saliva is easily expressed from the Stensen duct by gently applying manual pressure over the parotid gland. Both labial and buccal mucosa contain numerous minor salivary glands that occasionally may produce a pebbly appearance. Fordyce granules appear as yellow to white, 1- to 2-mm, ectopic sebaceous glands that are present in the buccal mucosa in approximately 85% of the general population. These granules may also be seen on the vermilion and labial mucosa.

The mucosa of the hard palate is firmly attached to the underlying bone, rendering it slightly paler than the rest of the oral mucosa. The hard palate mucosa is covered by a thick layer of keratin. The incisive papilla is located in the anterior portion of the hard palate immediately behind the two central maxillary incisors. Adjacent and posterior to the incisive papilla, ridges called *palatal rugae* radiate laterally. The distribution and shape of these rugae are particular to each individual. The palatine raphe is a slightly elevated ridge that runs, in the palatal midline, from the incisive papilla to the soft palate.

Some individuals present a bony exostosis in the center of the hard palate of variable degree and shape, known as *torus palatinus*. This bony exostosis is inherited as an autosomal dominant trait, and generally it makes itself evident around puberty.

Minor, mostly mucous, salivary glands are also found bilaterally and off the midline in the posterior one-third of the hard palate. The excretory ducts of these glands appear as small, 1-mm, erythematous umbilicated papules.

Separating the hard from the soft palate is a vibrating line that is visible when saying "Ahh." The soft palate is rich in blood vessels and, hence, is redder than the hard palate, and it extends toward the fauces or folds. The palatoglossal folds are seen laterally and represent the fusion of the soft palate with the pharyngeal wall. The uvula is an extension of soft tissue located in the midline of the free border of the soft palate. Minor salivary glands are also found in the soft palatal mucosa.

The anterior two-thirds of the dorsal surface of the tongue is derived from the ectoderm and is the functional or tasting portion of the tongue. The posterior third is derived from the endoderm and is the lymphatic portion because it contains the lingual tonsils. This posterior portion is characterized by the laterally irregular nodular surface with cryptic openings, called *foliate papillae*. The division of these two tongues areas is established by the lingual "V," which actually is formed by 10 to 12, round and flat, vallate or circumvallate papillae converging at the midline of the tongue and at the apex of the "V" at the site of the foramen

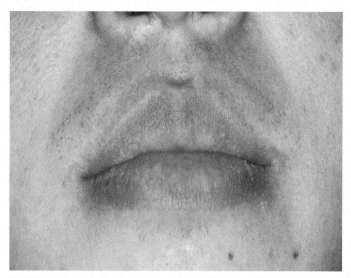

FIGURE 56-1. Lips showing the vermilion border, the junction between skin and oral mucosa, in an Asian man.

cecum, which represents the embryonal site of origin of parts of the thyroid gland.

The anterior two-thirds of the lingual dorsum is covered by papillae, giving this area a rough, white appearance. The filiform papillae are elongated and white in color due to keratinization of their end portions. In the vicinity of the lingual "V," they also have a "V" arrangement, but closer to the lingual tip, they acquire a horizontal arrangement. The fungiform papillae are small and red and are evenly distributed throughout the anterior dorsal tongue surface. Brown or black accumulation of melanin pigmentation can be seen in the fungiform papillae in African Americans and other people with skin of color in general. In some patients, the posterior lateral borders of the tongue present small lymphoid aggregates. The center of the lingual dorsum is occupied by a fissure of variable depth. Horizontal fissures can be seen in 5% of the population (fissure, scrotal tongue). The ventral surface of the tongue is shiny, smooth, and reddish and characteristically shows the ranine veins, which become varicose with age. The ventral surface is continuous with the oral floor. The lingual frenulum is located in the midline of the oral floor, extending from the mandibular gingiva to the ventral surface of the tongue.

The floor of the mouth is a continuation of the ventral lingual mucosa on the one side, and on the other side, it is reflected onto the gingiva. The openings of the submandibular and sublingual glands are seen as elevated, crater-like structures (sublingual caruncles) at each side of the lingual frenum. The sublingual folds are elevations seen at each side of the midline produced by the sublingual glands.

The gingiva is divided into free marginal gingiva and attached gingiva by the free marginal groove. The free marginal gingiva has an undulating or scalloped contour, and from its upper border emerge the interdental papillae with their characteristic triangular shape occupying the spaces between the teeth. The marginal end of the gingiva bends over the tooth surface and attaches itself to the tooth below the gingival border. The gingival sulcus, or crevice, is the space found between tooth and gingiva. The depth of the sulcus varies from 0.1 to 0.3 cm. The attached gingiva extends from the free gingival groove to the beginning of the alveolar crest and is continuous with the alveolar mucosa. Vestibular and lingual gingivae are essentially identical in clinical appearance, presenting a whiter color due to surface keratinization that is absent in the alveolar mucosa. An undulating band of melanin pigmentation of variable width and intensity of color can be seen in the gingiva of individuals of African descent and people with skin of color (discussed further later).

The geniohyoid processes are located bilaterally at each side of the mandibular midline on the lingual attached gingiva.

WHITE LESIONS

◼ LEUKOEDEMA

Leukoedema is an asymptomatic, symmetric, gray-white diffuse film on the oral mucosa that most commonly occurs bilaterally on the buccal mucosa, but it may also be noted on the floor of the mouth and palatopharyngeal tissues [**Figure 56-2, A and B**]. It is a common oral condition of unknown etiology. There may be an association between the development of leukoedema, poor oral hygiene, and abnormal biting patterns. Leukoedema has a greater prevalence in dark-skinned individuals, especially African Americans and Hispanics. It has been reported to be present in 70% to 90% of African American adults.[1] Because of this high prevalence, it has been speculated to be a variant of normal versus a pathologic process. However, some reports have shown that leukoedema is more severe in smokers and lessens with cessation. Diagnosis is made by stretching of the oral mucosa. The white opaque character of the lesion diminishes or disappears with the stretching and eversion of the oral mucosa. Any diffuse white lesions of the oral mucosa should always be stretched out to rule out any other underlying lesions. Histologically, oral lesions show parakeratosis and an increase in thickness of the oral mucosa epithelium with intracellular edema of the spinous layer. The cells of the spinous layer are large with pyknotic nuclei. Rete ridges may be elongated. No dysplasia or hypergranulosis is noted. No treatment is necessary for this benign condition. Leukoedema has no malignant potential.[2]

◼ SUBMUCOUS FIBROSIS

Oral submucous fibrosis (OSF) is a unique premalignant condition. It presents as a generalized white discoloration of the oral mucosa of individuals in India and Southeast Asia who chew betel quid, a blend of tobacco, slaked lime, areca nut (and its main constituent arecoline), and betel leaves. OSF is diagnosed based on clinical criteria including oral ulceration, paleness of the oral mucosa and burning sensation, hardening of the tissue, and presence of characteristic fibrous bands. The fibrosis involves the lamina propria and the submucosa and may often extend into the underlying musculature, resulting in the deposition of dense fibrous bands giving rise to the limited mouth opening that is a hallmark of this disorder.[3] Reports have shown that chemicals such as arecoline

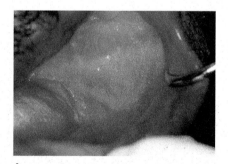

A

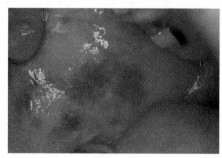

B

FIGURE 56-2. (A) Leukoedema of the buccal mucosa of an African American man. Lesions appear opalescent, whitish gray, and are usually bilateral. Lesions disappear when mucosa is stretched. **(B)** Some leukoedema lesions are accompanied by physiologic pigmentations.

appear to interfere with the molecular processes of deposition and/or degradation of extracellular matrix molecules such as collagen, causing imbalance in the normal process.[4] The most likely events that take place with regard to the above imbalance may be reduced phagocytosis of collagen by fibroblasts and up- or downregulation of key enzymes such as lysyl oxidase, matrix metalloproteinases, and tissue inhibitors of matrix metalloproteinases. The process may also be influenced by increased secretion of inflammatory cytokines and growth factors and decreased production of antifibrotic cytokines.[5] Reports have shown that the prevalence of OSF in India and Southeast Asia ranges from 0.04% to 24.4%. The highest rate of 24.4% was reported from a study of an aboriginal community of southern Taiwan, with a 69.5% areca quid-chewing prevalence rate. The malignant transformation rate of OSF is reported as 2.3% to 7.6%. Other possible etiologic factors include capsaicin in chilies and micronutrient deficiencies of iron, zinc, and essential vitamins. In addition, a possible autoimmune basis to the disease with demonstration of various autoantibodies and an association with specific human leukocyte antigens (HLAs) has been proposed. This raises the possibility of a genetic predisposition of some individuals to develop OSF. However, from the available scientific literature, it is clear that the regular use of areca nut is the major etiologic factor.[6]

Clinically, OSF presents as a chronic progressive disease leading to marked limitation of mouth opening and is characterized by the oral mucosa becoming stiff due to fibroelastic transformation of the juxta-epithelial and deeper connective tissue; ultimately, trismus, masticatory difficulty, dysphagia, and severe xerostomia predominate. Progressive fibrosis results in the development of painful mucosal atrophy and restrictive fibrotic bands [**Figure 56-3, A and B**]. Histologically, it is characterized by submucosal deposition of dense avascular connective tissue fibers with a number of inflammatory cell infiltrates [**Figure 56-4, A and B**]. The epithelium is hyperkeratotic with some epithelial atrophy seen in elderly patients. It is an irreversible condition with no effective treatment. Frequent monitoring for malignant transformation is essential, and surgical interventions may be necessary in more advanced cases to release fibrotic bands and improve trismus.[7]

SQUAMOUS CELL CARCINOMA

The incidence of oral cancer worldwide is approximately 500,000 new cases every year, accounting for approximately 3% of all malignancies, thus constituting a significant worldwide health problem.[8] The American Cancer Society estimated 40,250 new cases of these cancers in 2012 in the United States alone.[9] Between 2003 and 2007, the incidence rate among African American men in the United States was 16 per 100,000, which was similar to the rate among Caucasians, which was 15.5 per 100,000. The 5-year survival rate is 62% for Caucasian men and 38%

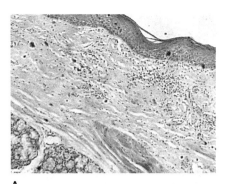

A

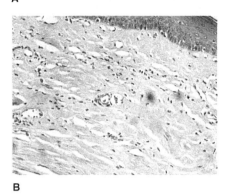

B

FIGURE 56-4. (A) This biopsy from the lip of the patient shown in Figure 56-3 shows marked fibrosis of the collagenic connective tissue with a moderate, mostly lymphocytic inflammatory infiltrate. The epithelium is atrophic and is covered by a thin layer of parakeratin. These are typical findings in submucous fibrosis. (Original magnification: ×100.) **(B)** This higher magnification of another field of the same biopsy shows similar findings. (Original magnification: ×200.)

for African American men. The annual mortality rate among African American males was 1.5 times higher than Caucasian males (3.9 vs 2.4 deaths per 100,000). The average age of diagnosis of oral and pharyngeal cancer for African American males is approximately 10 years younger than that for Caucasians. Among these diagnosed cancer lesions, only 19% are at the early stage as compared to 38% in Caucasian males.[10] This discrepancy in the morbidity and mortality rates has been attributed mainly to the more advanced or later stage at which the cancer was diagnosed in African American male patients. Oral cancer occurs mostly on the lips, tongue, floor of the mouth, palate, gingiva, alveolar and buccal mucosa, and oropharynx.[11]

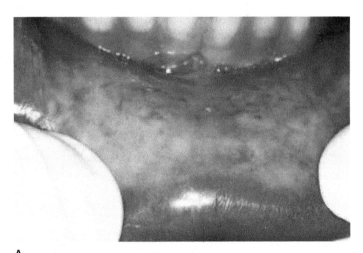

A

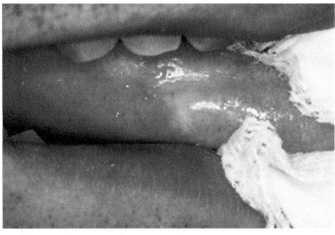

B

FIGURE 56-3. (A) Submucous fibrosis: mucosal atrophy. Lower lip mucosa of a Pakistani man who practiced the habit of chewing betel nut mixed with tobacco. Note the white, marble-like appearance of the mucosa. The patient had limited mouth opening and complained of mouth dryness. **(B)** Local fibrosis of the lateral tongue border of the same patient showing similar clinical findings.

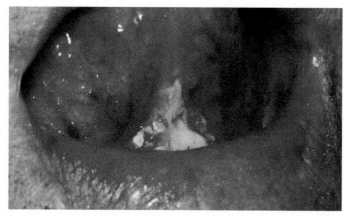

FIGURE 56-5. Squamous cell carcinoma of the floor of the mouth and ventral surface of the tongue.

The major risk factors are smoking and alcohol consumption. A number of oncogenic viruses may be associated with the development of squamous cell carcinoma (SCC), especially human papillomavirus (HPV) type 16; the tumor suppressor gene *p53* has also been implicated in the pathogenesis of SCC. Other major risk factors include age, ultraviolet exposure, immunosuppression, nutritional deficiency, and intraoral infection with syphilis, candidiasis (chronic), or HPV.[12]

Clinically, oral SCC may present as leukoplakia, erythroplakia, erythroleukoplakia, irregular endophytic masses with ulceration [**Figure 56-5**], or exophytic nodules [**Figure 56-6**]. High-risk anatomic sites for development of SCC are the ventrolateral tongue, floor of the mouth, and vermilion border of the lip. Gingival lesions are more common in women. Any persistent oral lesion should be biopsied. High-risk lesions including persistent ulcer in high-risk sites (eg, floor of mouth, site of previous SCC, site of previous radiation) have a high probability of being malignant. A second primary lesion of the aerodigestive tract is found in up to one-fourth of patients with oral SCCs. Oral SCCs in general have a high rate of metastasis, but the incidence depends on the site of involvement, duration of the lesion, and histologic grade. Overall, more posterior SCCs demonstrate higher rates of metastasis to regional lymph nodes. Distant metastases do occur and typically involve the lungs, liver, and bone. Ultimately, prognosis is best determined by clinical staging. Tobacco-cessation measures should be initiated.[13]

Histologically, oral SCC encompasses a wide range from well-differentiated (low-grade) lesions, in which the tumors resemble normal epithelium, to poorly differentiated or anaplastic (high-grade) lesions, where the tumor cells lose their resemblance to the epithelial tissues.

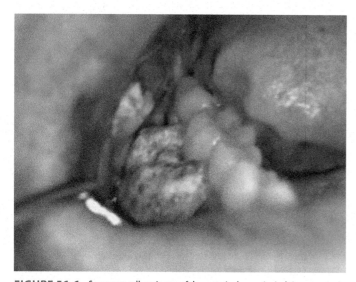

FIGURE 56-6. Squamous cell carcinoma of the posterior lower gingival tissues.

The treatment of choice is aggressive surgical intervention, and patients with lymph node involvement typically require surgery followed by external-beam radiation. Adjuvant therapy with chemotherapeutic agents or epidermal growth factor receptor inhibitors may be used in recurrent or metastatic cases. Additionally, systemic retinoids and antioxidants may serve a chemopreventive role in high-risk patients.[14]

HEREDITARY BENIGN INTRAEPITHELIAL DYSKERATOSIS

Hereditary benign intraepithelial dyskeratosis (HBID), also known as Witkop-von Sallman syndrome, was originally described by Witkop et al[15] in a triracial isolate of North Carolina (Haliwa-Saponi Indian tribe, inhabitants of Halifax County, hence the name), but a recent publication[16] reported a patient from Brazil with the syndrome. HBID is inherited as an autosomal dominant trait, and the gene has been mapped to the telomeric region of chromosome 4 (4q35).[17] The characteristic clinical findings include gelatinous plaques in the cornea of the eyes, both in the inner and outer surfaces. These foamy plaques may be present since early childhood and have a tendency to shed either during the fall or the summer. The cornea is markedly vascular and erythematous and eventually may be fully affected by the dyskeratotic lesions. Blindness may result from the repeated shedding and revascularization. Other ocular findings are photophobia and itchiness.[18-20]

The oral manifestations of HBID consist of a marked whitening of different degrees of both buccal mucosae. This thickening is formed by soft plaques and folds that are similar in appearance to the lesions of white sponge nevus. These lesions tend to increase in severity during the first 15 years of life, and there is no tendency to malignant transformation.[15,20,21]

Histologically, both ocular and oral lesions present acanthosis and vacuolization of the spinous cell layer of the epithelium and dyskeratosis with a typical "cell within a cell" appearance. Markedly eosinophilic cells called "tobacco cells" are also seen.[20,22]

The histology of the HBID lesions should be differentiated from that of Darier-White disease and that of oral desquamated cells seen in patients on methotrexate therapy.[22]

ACTINIC PRURIGO

Actinic prurigo (AP) is an idiopathic photodermatosis mainly affecting Native Americans and Mestizos, mostly from Latin America. AP also has been reported in the Inuit and occasionally in Caucasians and individuals of African or Asian descent. AP starts early in life with a slight predilection for women and children younger than 10 years of age.[23-29]

The pathogenetic mechanisms of AP are unknown, although an association with several HLA alleles has been reported.[30] It has been shown that there is a strong association between AP and the HLA allele DR4, specifically with the DRB1*0407 allele, which has been reported to be present in over 60% of patients with AP.[31-34] This finding has been confirmed in different populations and is most likely an important pathogenetic factor.[35]

AP affects the sun-exposed areas of the skin, manifesting as erythematous papules and lichenoid plaques that follow the initial presentation of a severe and persistent chronic pruritus. Occasionally, areas not exposed to the sun also can be affected. Cheilitis is found in over 80% of patients with skin lesions and is characterized by severe pruritus, pain, and tingling mostly of the vermilion border of the lips, especially the lower lip, which is known to have a higher rate of sun exposure compared to the upper lip [**Figure 56-7**]. AP cheilitis also has been reported as an isolated example in patients free of the dermatologic manifestations.[28] The appearance of the lips is disfiguring due to areas of ulceration eventuating in crust formation.[27]

The histopathologic findings mostly consist of acanthosis, spongiosis, basal cell vacuolation, and edema of the lamina propria. The surface is generally ulcerated and covered by a serohematic crust.[28] The underlying connective tissue presents a profuse lymphocytic inflammatory infiltrate and the typical presence of well-defined lymphoid follicles. Additionally, Langerhans cells, melanophages, and eosinophils can be identified.[27,28,36]

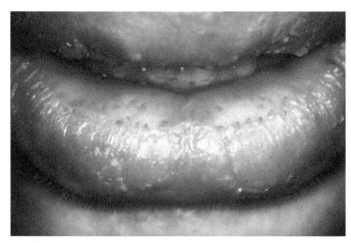

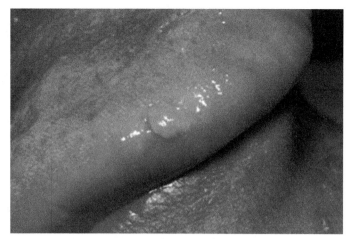

FIGURE 56-7. In actinic prurigo, the lower lip shows marked denudation of the superficial epithelial layers as well as pinpoint areas of ulceration. Also note the crust formation, especially on the upper lip.

FIGURE 56-8. Note the small nodules on the lateral border of the tongue on a Native American child with multifocal papillomavirus epithelial hyperplasia.

AP cheilitis is best treated with a combination of protection from the sun by means of hats and sunscreens, topical corticosteroids, and oral thalidomide.[25,26]

HEREDITARY POLYMORPHIC LIGHT ERUPTION

Hereditary polymorphic light eruption (HPLE) is prevalent in South, Central, and North American natives.[37,38] This is now considered to be a variant of AP; the main distinguishing feature is the fact that over 75% of affected individuals have other family members similarly affected. HPLE is inherited as an autosomal dominant condition. Fusaro and Johnson[37] have reported that 28% of their Caucasian patients and 53% of their African American patients with HPLE had a definite family history of Native American heritage. Patients with HPLE also develop cheilitis that persists into adulthood and that presents the same clinical findings, that is, pruritus, papular eruption, and excoriation of the lips.

MULTIFOCAL PAPILLOMAVIRUS EPITHELIAL HYPERPLASIA

Carlos and Sedano[39] proposed the name *multifocal papillomavirus epithelial hyperplasia* (MPVEH) based on the viral nature and clinical multifocality typical of this disease. MPVEH is a benign, proliferative, wartlike disease of the oral mucosa, sometimes affecting the anal/genital mucosa with a rare skin involvement. It shows an unusual racial and geographic distribution frequently seen in Inuit and native peoples from North, Central, and South America, Eskimos, and Africans.[40,41] Most authors report a female-to-male ratio of 2:1, and over 90% of cases are observed in patients in the first and second decades of life.[39,42,43] The first reports in the North American literature were those of Archard and colleagues,[40,44] who independently proposed the name *focal epithelial hyperplasia* and the eponym *Heck disease*. Praetorius-Clausen[45] demonstrated evidence of viral infection in biopsies of this lesion, and Pfister et al[46] identified the presence of HPV-13. Beaudenon et al[47] isolated another virus from lesions of this disease, which they named *HPV-32*.

Immunohistochemical studies and in situ hybridization have shown that the majority of cases of MPVEH demonstrate the presence of HPV (ie, HPV-13 or HPV-32). Even if HPV-13 and HPV-32 are considered the causative agents, other factors such as genetic predisposition, malnutrition, hygiene, and living conditions of affected individuals should be considered of etiologic importance.[48-52]

Clinically, MPVEH is characterized by multiple papulonodular eruptions located mostly on the buccal and lower lip mucosa, followed by the lateral border of the tongue. Rarely, lesions will be found in the palatal mucosa and on the ventral surface of the tongue. These lesions mostly have a smooth surface that can have the normal mucosal color, but in some patients, they can be corrugated and have a whitish color [**Figure 56-8**]. A small number of patients will present with additional lesions having a definite papilloma-like or papillated appearance[39] [**Figure 56-9**]. Familial incidence has been noted by several authors, and it can be explained by the viral contagious nature of the disease and a possible genetic predisposition.[53] The possibility that MPVEH can be transmitted through saliva has been recently suggested.[54] MPVEH has been reported almost exclusively in children and youngsters who live in extreme poverty.[42] Some cases have been documented in human immunodeficiency virus (HIV)-positive and acquired immunodeficiency syndrome (AIDS) patients.[55]

Histologically, biopsies of MPVEH present acanthosis of the superficial epithelium, and deeper epithelial layers present swollen cells, ballooning cellular degeneration, and individual cell keratinization. The epithelium at the connective tissue interface shows anastomosing rete ridges. The epithelial cellular appearance produced by nuclear abnormalities, which have been classically described as "mitosoid," or cell within a cell, is the typical distinguishing histologic feature of MPVEH[39,42,45,53] [**Figure 56-10**].

Surgical or laser ablation can be used to treat large lesions that interfere with mastication or that bleed when bitten. Most lesions disappear with time. Cimetidine, used as immune stimulant, has been tried,

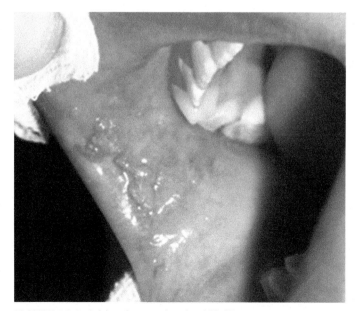

FIGURE 56-9. Left buccal mucosa of another child of Native American ancestry showing multiple hyperplastic nodes with a smooth surface typical of multifocal papillomavirus epithelial hyperplasia.

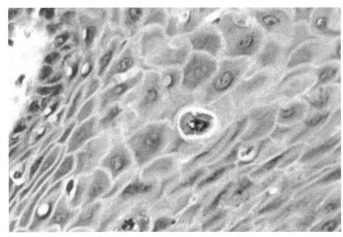

FIGURE 56-10. Microscopy of a lip lesion of multifocal papillomavirus epithelial hyperplasia showing the characteristic cell-within-a-cell or mitosoid appearance of some epithelial cells as well as cytoplasmic vacuolization.

especially in HIV-positive patients, with mixed results. Interferon-β has been used to treat some patients with positive results.[56]

ORAL PIGMENTED LESIONS

Oral pigmented lesions are frequently noted on physical examination and must be differentiated from signs of a malignant process or of a systemic condition.

◼ PHYSIOLOGIC (RACIAL) PIGMENTATION

The color of clinically normal gingiva is usually described as pale or coral pink; the color is also dependent on the gingiva's vascularity, keratinization, and the presence or absence of inflammation. There is, in fact, considerable variation in the color of normal gingiva, which results from differences in the amount of melanin pigment. The color of the gingiva varies depending on the complexion of the individual; pigmentation is prominent in the normal gingiva of Africans, Asians, Indians, South Americans, and Mediterraneans.[57] Physiologic pigmentation, which is due to greater melanocytic activity rather than a greater number of melanocytes, develops during the first two decades of life but may not come to the patient's attention until later. The color ranges from light to dark brown. The attached gingiva is the most common intraoral site of such pigmentation, where it appears as a bilateral, well-demarcated, ribbon-like, dark brown band that usually spares the marginal gingival.[58] People worldwide have various degrees of physiologic pigmentation, and the color varies from brown to black. The involvement may be in isolated patches or a diffuse speckling [**Figure 56-11, A and B**]. Pigmentation of the buccal mucosa, hard palate, and lips may also be seen as brown patches with less well-defined borders. The fungiform papillae on the dorsal surface of the tongue can show pigmentations. The pigmentation is asymptomatic, and no treatment is required.[58]

◼ LENTIGINES

Lentigines are common oral melanocytic lesions that appear as brown macules on the palate, gingiva, or lips. Microscopically melanocytic hyperplasia with elongation of the rete ridges is observed. Labial melanotic macules (focal melanosis) present as asymptomatic, well-circumscribed, 2- to 5-mm blue, black, or brown macules on the vermillion, with no malignant potential. The lower lip is more commonly affected, with less frequent involvement noted in the buccal mucosa, gingiva, palate, and tongue. The presence of pigmentation may be of cosmetic concern. Surgical excision is the most common treatment, but scarring may result. Cryosurgery has been reported to be effective but is not uniformly successful.[59] Histologically increased basal layer melanin without rete

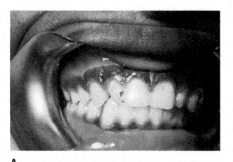

A

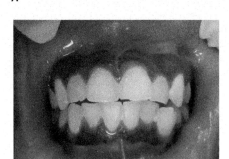

B

FIGURE 56-11. A and B. Well-delineated marginal gingival pigmentation in two African American men.

ridge elongation is observed with focal increase in melanin in the basal cell layer, lamina propria, or both.

Both lentigines and melanotic macules tend to be solitary and are more common in women. Solitary lesions may resemble an early malignant melanoma but are HMB-45 negative. When multiple labial macules are observed, one must consider a number of conditions including Peutz-Jeghers syndrome, Carney complex (NAME [nevi, atrial myxoma, myxoid neurofibromas, and ephelides] syndrome, LAMB [lentigines, atrial myxomas, and blue nevi] syndrome; LEOPARD [electrocardiographic conduction abnormalities, ocular hypertelorism, pulmonary stenosis, abnormalities of genitalia, retardation of growth, and deafness] syndrome), Laugier-Hunziker syndrome, and Addison disease.

◼ LAUGIER-HUNZIKER SYNDROME

Laugier-Hunziker (L-H) syndrome is a benign syndrome of unknown etiology characterized by macular hyperpigmentation on the oral and genital mucosa, conjunctiva, fingers, and toes and longitudinal melanonychia. L-H syndrome is seen commonly in middle-age Caucasian women, not infrequently in Chinese individuals, and rarely in African Americans or in men. Patients present with a variable number of gray to brown pigmented macules on the lips, buccal mucosa, hard palate, fingertips, labial commissures, gingiva, and floor of mouth [**Figure 56-12**]. In contrast to Peutz-Jeghers syndrome or Addison disease, there are no associated systemic or internal manifestations.[60,61] Dermoscopic findings show a parallel furrow pattern (PFP) with multiple dots on the lip and vulva, PFP on the palms and soles, and regular, homogeneous, brownish bands with indistinct borders on the toenails.[62] Others describe the pigmentation as regular brown reticular pattern with linear and curvilinear vasculature on oral mucosa, longitudinal homogeneous pigmentation on toenails, and parallel furrow on palms and soles.[63] Histology is consistent with mucosal melanosis (ie, pigmented basal keratinocytes with melanophages but no increase in melanocytes).[64]

The pigmented macules are effectively treated without scarring with the Q-switched neodymium:yttrium-aluminum-garnet (Nd:YAG) laser or the Q-switched alexandrite laser. In a study of 22 subjects, one session resulted in clearing of the lips in 18 patients (81.8%); 3 patients (13.6%) required three laser treatments, and 1 patient's pigmentation resolved in six sessions.[65]

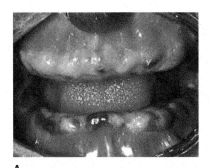

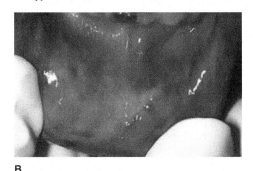

FIGURE 56-12. Laugier-Hunziker syndrome is characterized by mucosal pigmented macules, as seen here on the gingiva of an edentulous African American man **(A)** and involving the labial mucosa of the same individual **(B)**.

PEUTZ-JEGHERS SYNDROME

Peutz-Jeghers syndrome (PJS) is an autosomal dominant condition characterized by mucocutaneous hyperpigmentation, gastrointestinal hamartomas and polyposis, and multiple visceral malignant tumors.[66,67]

Mutations in the serine/threonine kinase *STK11/LKB1* tumor suppressor gene on chromosome 19p13.3 have been described.[68] Patients present in infancy and early childhood with mucocutaneous oral and anal pigmentation [**Figure 56-13, A and B**]. With time, mucosal pigmentation, particularly on the lips (95%) and the buccal mucosa (85%), will persist while the cutaneous pigmentation fades and decreases in diameter, particularly on the face in the periorbital region.[69]

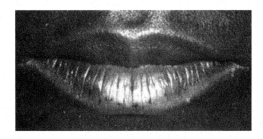

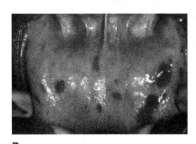

FIGURE 56-13. (A) Peutz-Jeghers syndrome is characterized by pigmented macules on the vermilion of this African American woman. **(B)** Note that the intraoral macules are significantly larger in diameter.

Polyps may occur in any part of the gastrointestinal tract, but jejunal hamartomatous polyps are a consistent feature. Intussusception, bowel obstruction, abdominal pain, and GI or rectal bleeding may be early signs. Malignant degeneration of the small intestinal polyps is rare but does occur in the colon. Intussusceptions and gastrointestinal bleeding are well described. An increase in colorectal, breast, small bowel, gastric, and pancreatic cancer has been documented, as have benign ovarian and testicular tumors. Extragastrointestinal polyps, namely, ureteral, bladder, renal pelvis, bronchial, and nasal polyps, also have been noted. Gynecomastia with testis tumors also may be seen. Surgical resection of polyps and medical surveillance are necessary for these patients.[70,71]

POSTINFLAMMATORY HYPERPIGMENTATION

Postinflammatory hyperpigmentation (PIH) can occur following any type of inflammation or trauma and is the most common complications of laser surgery among dark-skinned patients. This undesirable adverse effect is a major reason why laser resurfacing is much less popular among patients with darker skin. It has been postulated that inflammation may lead to hyperpigmentation via direct stimulation of melanocytes and release of endocrine inducers of pigmentation such as α-melanocyte–stimulating hormone. The resulted melanin secretion provides protection against future insult, via both ultraviolet absorption and reactive oxygen species-scavenging activities.[72]

Dermatologic diseases, including lichenoid dermatoses such as lichen planus, are known to be associated with PIH of any skin type, but patients with darker skin have more prominent PIH. In lichenoid dermatoses, the inflammatory zone between the epidermal and dermal junction contributes to the pigmentary incontinence that could lead to a great degree of PIH.

Traditionally, the gold standard topical agent for skin lightening is hydroquinone (HQ) 4%. However, it is not effective for dermal hyperpigmentation. Recently, new non–HQ-containing skin brightener formulations that contain SMA-432, a prostaglandin E_2 inhibitor have been reported as effective and equally well tolerated as the gold standard, 4% HQ.[73] Furthermore, new methods in facial rejuvenation using fractional laser resurfacing with modified density and energy have been reported to decrease the risk of PIH in individual patients.

MELANOACANTHOMA

Intraoral melanoacanthomas appear as darkly pigmented, well-demarcated irregular plaques that may ulcerate. Melanoacanthomas arise in response to a traumatic stimulus, usually on the buccal mucosa. They are most often reported in darker skinned women in the third decade of life but have been reported in children rarely. These reactive lesions may reach several centimeters in diameter in just a few weeks. A biopsy must be performed to exclude malignant melanoma. Dendritic melanocytes are seen throughout the mucosal epithelium, accompanied by acanthosis and spongiosis. Importantly, no pleomorphism or mitoses are observed. Often, a melanoacanthoma will regress spontaneously after removal of any ongoing trauma. Melanocytic nevi are composed of aggregates of nondendritic nevus cells, whereas amalgam tattoos will have finely granulated radiopaque particles.[74,75]

SMOKER'S MELANOSIS

This benign pigmentation develops in the anterior mandibular region, with less prominent pigmentation on the palate and buccal mucosa. Its prevalence varies from 15% to 31% of smokers, and it may reverse over months to years when smoking stops. Pipe smoking contributes to this even more than cigarettes. It is hypothesized that a component in tobacco stimulates melanocytes, although estrogen (eg, birth control pills) also may play a role. The intensity of the pigmentation is directly related to the duration and dose [**Figures 56-14 and 56-15**]. Histologically an increase in melanin production is noted. Although pigmentation is most pronounced in individuals with skin of color, Caucasians such as the Swedish population can also develop smoker's melanosis.

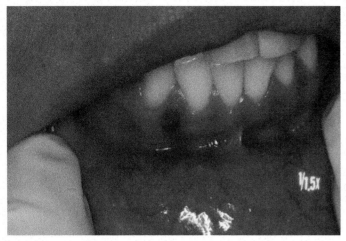

FIGURE 56-14. Well-circumscribed pigmented lesion of the lower gingiva in a heavy smoker.

ORAL MELANOMA

Oral mucosal malignant melanoma (OMM) is a rare tumor that may evolve within or at mucocutaneous junction. Contrary to popular belief, mucosal melanomas are often amelanotic. In contrast to cutaneous melanoma, oral melanoma is equally prevalent in African Americans and Caucasians. Primary OMM represents 0.2% to 8% of all melanomas diagnosed in Europe and represents 0.26% of all oral cavity cancers. A higher incidence has been reported in Japan and India. Due to the low incidence of OMM, the published data on the epidemiology, tumor behavior, treatment, patient survival rates, and prognostic information on primary OMMs are sparse and are mainly based on single case reports or small series.[76] Intraoral melanoma presents as an irregular pigmented macule, patch, or papule on the hard palate or maxillary gingiva in patients over the age of 50. Most oral melanomas arise de novo, from apparently normal mucosa. A definite precursor lesion has not yet been identified. Satellite lesions are frequently present surrounding the initial tumor.[77] Although often asymptomatic, advanced lesions may ulcerate or bleed. The clinical differential includes lymphoma or angiosarcoma. The histology reveals nested and single atypical melanocytes with microinvasions and multicentric metastatic disease noted early on. Oral melanoma is positive for S-100, HMB-45, Melan-A, and Mart 1.[78] The growth pattern resembles a nodular pattern. The prognosis is poor if greater than 2 mm. Clinical staging is based on local disease, regional lymph node disease, or disseminated disease at the time of diagnosis. Clinical workup should include a total-body skin examination, baseline computed tomography or magnetic resonance imaging, and a basic metabolic workup. The median survival time is 19 months, and the 5-year overall survival rate is 0% to 20%[79] [**Figure 56-16**].

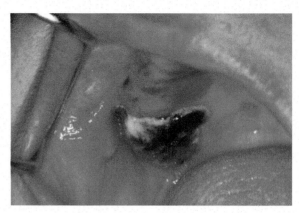

FIGURE 56-16. Oral melanoma of the palate in a 53-year-old Hispanic woman.

ORAL INFECTIOUS DISEASES

SYPHILIS

Infective syphilis is caused by the anaerobic filamentous spirochete *Treponema pallidum*. In the past decade, there has been a significant rise in the prevalence of infective syphilis in developed countries, including Eastern Europe and, to a lesser extent, Western Europe and the United States. In Eastern Europe, the increased frequency of syphilis has been predominantly in heterosexuals, whereas in the United Kingdom and United States, the outbreaks are among heterosexuals and homosexuals.[80,81]

From 2000 to 2004, the incidence of primary and secondary syphilis in the United States increased from 2.2 cases to 2.7 cases per 100,000 population.[82] Among the U.S. metropolitan centers, San Francisco has experienced a striking increase from an estimate of 5 cases in 1998 to 320 cases in 2004. Additionally, the rates of primary and secondary syphilis among African American were estimated to be 5.1 times higher in 2003 and 5.6 times higher in 2004, in comparison to those in Caucasians.[83]

The clinical presentation of syphilis varies depending on the disease stage.[84,85] The first stage, known as primary syphilis, is clinically evident 2 to 3 weeks after the initial inoculation, followed by the second stage, or secondary (disseminated) syphilis. Infected patients are highly contagious during the first two stages. Oral syphilitic lesions are rare but may occur at any stage. Primary syphilis is manifested orally as chancre at the site of inoculation, on the lips [**Figure 56-17**], tongue, palate, gingiva, and tonsils. The oral lesions usually present as a deep ulceration, with a red, purple, or brown base and an irregular, raised border, accompanied by regional lymphadenopathy. The ulceration of primary syphilis may be sometimes confused with other solitary ulcerative disorders, most notably traumatic ulceration. The diagnosis of primary syphilis may be

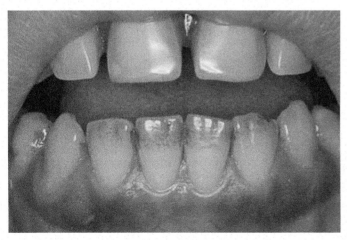

FIGURE 56-15. Diffuse pigmented lesion on the lower gingiva due to heavy smoking.

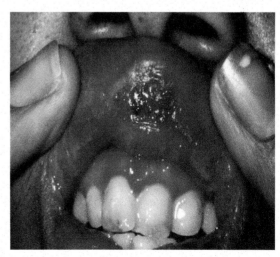

FIGURE 56-17. Chancre on upper lip of an African American patient.

difficult and relies on detailed history of the sexual and/or social lifestyles of the patient and the involved sexual partner. In the early disease stage, infected patients may not show a positive nonspecific reaginic test (ie, rapid plasma reagin [RPR] or Venereal Disease Research Laboratory [VDRL] tests), and this should be supplemented with specific tests for immunoglobulin G antibodies to *T. pallidum*. Definitive diagnosis of early syphilis is made through visualization of *T. pallidum* spirochetes on dark-field microscopy, with direct fluorescent antibody tests, or with polymerase chain reaction; however, these tests are usually impractical and time consuming.[86]

The oral manifestations of secondary syphilis vary and can be more extensive than those of the primary disease. Oral lesions usually arise in at least 30% of patients with secondary syphilis, manifested primarily as mucous patches and maculopapular lesions, and to a lesser extent, nodular lesions. *Macular syphilides* are macular lesions that arise on the hard palate and manifest as flat to slightly raised, firm, red lesions. *Papular syphilides* are rare and present as red, raised, firm round nodules with a gray, ulcerated center. These papules usually arise on the buccal mucosa or commissures. *Mucous patches* are oval to crescentic erosions or shallow ulcers covered by a gray mucoid exudate with an erythematous border. These patches usually arise bilaterally on the mobile surfaces of the oral cavity. Another rarer form, the ulceronodular disease, also known as lues maligna, is an explosive generalized form of secondary syphilis characterized by fever, headache, and myalgia, followed by a papulopustular eruption that rapidly transforms into necrotic, sharply demarcated ulcers bordered by hemorrhagic brown crusts. Lues maligna can arise on the gingivae, palate or buccal mucosa, tongue, and lower lip. Lesions may occur on the vermillion, mimicking SCC or keratoacanthoma.

After the second stage, patients may enter a period free of lesions or symptoms, known as latent syphilis, or may further progress to tertiary syphilis. In addition to serious complications involving the vascular system and central nervous system, less significant but more characteristic oral presentations are the foci of granulomatous inflammation, known as gumma, frequently seen on the palate or tongue. Diffuse atrophy of the dorsal tongue papillae can give rise to a condition known as luetic glossitis. Pregnant women may transmit the infection to the fetus during any stage of the disease, with the greatest developmental effect at the fourth month of gestation. The clinical changes secondary to fetal infection are known as congenital syphilis. Congenital syphilis was initially defined to comprise three pathognomonic diagnostic features, known as the Hutchinson triad—Hutchinson teeth, interstitial keratitis, and eighth nerve deafness. However, few patients exhibit all three features.

Concurrent HIV infection and syphilis is not uncommon, particularly in young adults and homosexuals. The recent increase in incidence of primary and secondary syphilis among hetero- and homosexuals has been correlated with high rates of HIV co-infection, high-risk sexual behavior, Internet partner recruitment, and drug use.[87] There have been some reports of prolonged primary disease and secondary disease in patients co-infected with HIV as compared to those not infected.[88] The guideline by the Centers for Disease Control and Prevention on sexually transmitted diseases in 2010[89] recommended cerebral spinal fluid (CSF) evaluation in any suspected, high-risk patient (HIV positive or negative) at any stage of disease, who has clinical evidence of neurologic involvement with syphilis (eg, cognitive dysfunction, motor or sensory deficits, cranial nerve palsies, ophthalmic or auditory symptoms, or signs of meningitis) and/or uveitis or other ocular manifestation associated with syphilis (iritis, neuroretinitis, or optic neuritis).

Treatment of syphilis-infected patients and their sexual contacts remains an important public health challenge. Standard therapy as recommended by the Centers for Disease Control and Prevention for treating syphilis is intramuscular injection of benzathine penicillin G or oral doxycycline in penicillin-allergic patients. Other alternatives include oral single-dose azithromycin, which has proven to be as effective in the treatment of syphilis in developing countries in which intramuscular administration of penicillin may be more problematic.[90] In the last decade, azithromycin treatment failure has been documented and is associated with mutations in certain *T. pallidum* strains. The prevalence of strains harboring these mutations varies throughout the United States and the world. In these regions where prevalence of the mutations is high, macrolides should not be considered for treatment of syphilis.[91]

SARCOIDOSIS

Sarcoidosis is a systematic granulomatous disorder of unknown etiology, affecting multiple organs, especially the lungs, lymph nodes, skin, and eyes. Most of the cases have been reported in patients of Caucasian (52%), African (29%), North African (11%), Hispanic (5%), and Asian (4%) origin.[92] In the head and neck region, the salivary glands are frequently affected and manifested clinically as parotid swelling and xerostomia. Oral lesions are relatively uncommon and, if present, usually occur in patients with chronic multisystemic sarcoidosis. Clinically, oral sarcoidosis appears as nontender swelling or firm, nodular lesions affecting the tongue, lips, oral mucosa, palate, and gingiva.[92] In the buccal mucosa, the lesions appear as nontender, well-circumscribed, brownish red or purplish swelling; as papules; or as submucosal nodules that occasionally ulcerate. Gingival manifestation may resemble gingival hypertrophy, gingivitis, and periodontitis leading to tooth mobility.[93,94] These lesions are most often asymptomatic and solitary, but may be multiple in a small percentage of cases.

The diagnosis of sarcoidosis is established based on clinical examination and radiologic and histopathologic features associated with the exclusion of other known causes of granuloma including foreign body granuloma, infectious etiologies (eg, tuberculosis, syphilis, leprosy, cat-scratch disease, mycosis), and other causes (eg, Crohn disease, Wegener disease). Treatment of oral sarcoidosis remains controversial. Not all cases require treatment because the symptoms may resolve spontaneously within 2 years in some patients.[95] Different treatments have been reported ranging from observation in asymptomatic patients to pharmacologic or surgical excision. Cases manifested as gingival hyperplasia and gingivitis may be controlled by scaling and strict oral hygiene. Oral corticosteroids remain the mainstay of treatment in painful and progressive lesions, either as single therapy or in conjunction with hydroxychloroquine, doxycycline, or immunosuppressive drugs such as methotrexate.[92]

PARACOCCIDIOIDOMYCOSIS (BLASTOMYCOSIS)

Paracoccidioidomycosis (PCM), also known as Lutz disease,[96] is a subacute or chronic systemic mycosis that is endemic to certain regions in South and Central America,[97] and is thus also known as *South American blastomycosis*. Brazil accounts for about 80% of the reported cases.[98] The causative agent is *Paracoccidioides brasiliensis*, a thermal dimorphic fungus. The primary mode of infection is respiratory, but all organs and mucous membranes can be affected by lymphatic dissemination. Oropharyngeal lesions were the most common sign on physical examination, followed by lymphadenopathy, dysphonia, and skin lesions. The most frequent sites for intraoral lesions of PCM are the oral mucosa, gingiva, and lip mucosa.[96] Frequently, the oral lesions constitute the first sign and site of confirmation of diagnosis.[99] The diagnosis can be carried out by biopsy or wet mounts of sputum, bronchoalveolar lavage products, or mucous membrane samples that are positive for *P. brasiliensis*. Antifungal agents such as the sulfamethoxazole-trimethoprim combination, amphotericin B, and especially azole derivatives are used in the therapeutic management of patients.[97,100] Antigen detection assay for the gp43 and gp70 molecules of *P. brasiliensis* is useful in early diagnosis and follow-up of patients with PCM.[101] Without treatment, the natural evolution of the disease is typically death. In patients with immunosuppression, such as AIDS patients, the infection can progress to full-blown disseminated disease.[102]

REFERENCES

1. Martin JL. Leukoedema: an epidemiological study in white and African-Americans. *J Tenn Dental Assoc*. 1997;77:18-21.

2. Neville BD, Damm DD, Allen CM, Bouquot JE. Developmental defects of the oral and maxillofacial region. In: *Oral and Maxillofacial Pathology.* Philadelphia, PA: Saunders; 2002:7-8.

3. Rajalalitha P, Vali S. Molecular pathogenesis of oral submucous fibrosis-collagen metabolic disorder. *J Oral Pathol Med.* 2005;34:321-328.

4. Jeng JH, Chang MC, Hahn LJ. Role of areca nut in betel quid-associated chemical carcinogenesis: current awareness and future perspectives. *Oral Oncol.* 2002;37:477.

5. Rajendran R. Oral submucous fibrosis: etiology, pathogenesis, and future research. *Bull WHO.* 1994;72:985.

6. Tilakaratne WM, Klinikowski MF, Takashi S, et al. Oral submucous fibrosis: review on etiology and pathogenesis. *Oral Oncol.* 2006;42:561-568.

7. Pei-Shan Ho, Yi-Hsin Yang A, Shieh T-Y, et al. Consumption of areca quid, cigarettes, and alcohol related to the comorbidity of oral submucous fibrosis and oral cancer. *Oral Surg Oral Med Oral Pathol Oral Radiol Endod.* 2007;104:647-652.

8. Johnson NW, Warnakulasuriya S, Gupta PC, et al. Global oral health inequalities in incidence and outcomes for oral cancer: causes and solutions. *Adv Dent Res.* 2011;23:237-246.

9. Siegel R, Naishadham D, Jemal, A. Cancer statistics. *CA Cancer J Clin.* 2012;62:10-29.

10. National Cancer Institute Surveillance, Epidemiology, and End Results Program. SEER Stat Fact Sheets: oral cavity and pharynx. http://seer.cancer.gov /statfacts/html/oralcav.htm. Accessed February 7, 2011.

11. Dodd VJ, Watson JM, Choi Y, Tomar SL, Logan HL. Oral cancer in African Americans: addressing health disparities. *Am J Health Behav.* 2008;32:684-692.

12. Rhodus NL. Oral cancer: leukoplakia and squamous cell carcinoma. *Dent Clin North Am.* 2005;49:143.

13. Noonan VL, Kabani S. Diagnosis and management of suspicious lesions of the oral cavity. *Otolaryngol Clin North Am.* 2005;38:21.

14. Sciubba JJ. Oral cancer: the importance of early diagnosis and treatment. *Am J Clin Dermatol.* 2001;2:239-251.

15. Witkop CJ Jr, Shankle CH, Graham JB, et al. Hereditary benign intraepithelial dyskeratosis. II. Oral manifestations and hereditary transmission. *Arch Pathol.* 1960;70:696-711.

16. Baroni A, Palla M, Aiello FS, et al. Hereditary benign intraepithelial dyskeratosis: case report. *Int J Dermatol.* 2009;48:627-629.

17. Allingham RR, Seo B, Rampersaud E, et al. A duplication in chromosome 4q35 is associated with hereditary benign intraepithelial dyskeratosis. *Am J Hum Genet.* 2001;68:491-494.

18. Shields CL, Shields JA, Eagle RC Jr. Hereditary benign intraepithelial dyskeratosis. *Arch Ophthalmol.* 1987;105:422-423.

19. Von Sallmann L Paton D. Hereditary benign intraepithelial dyskeratosis. I. Ocular manifestations. *Arch Ophthalmol.* 1960;63:421-429.

20. Haisley-Royster CA, Allingham RR, Klintworth GK, Prose NS. Hereditary benign intraepithelial dyskeratosis: report of two cases with prominent oral lesions. *J Am Acad Dermatol.* 2001;45:634-636.

21. Sadeghi EM, Witkop CJ Jr. Ultrastructural study of hereditary benign intraepithelial dyskeratosis. *Oral Surg.* 1977;44:567-577.

22. Cummings TJ, Dodd LG, Eedes CR, Klintworth GK. Hereditary benign intraepithelial dyskeratosis: an evaluation of diagnostic cytology. *Arch Pathol Lab Med.* 2008;132:1325-1328.

23. Cornelison RL Jr. Cutaneous diseases in Native Americans. *Dermatol Clin.* 2003;21:699-702.

24. Gómez A, Umana A, Trespalacios AA. Immune responses to isolated human skin antigens in actinic prurigo. *Med Sci Monit.* 2006;12:BR106-BR113.

25. Magaña M, Cervantes M. Histopathology of sun prurigo. *Rev Invest Clin.* 2000;52:391-396.

26. Chen M, Doherty SD, Hsu S. Innovative uses of thalidomide. *Dermatol Clin.* 2010;28:577-586.

27. Mounsdon T, Kratochvil F, Auclair P, et al. Actinic prurigo of the lower lip: review of the literature and report of five cases. *Oral Surg Oral Med Oral Pathol.* 1988;65:327-332.

28. Vega-Memije ME, Mosqueda-Taylor A, Irigoyen-Camacho ME, et al. Actinic prurigo cheilitis: clinicopathologic analysis and therapeutic results in 116 cases. *Oral Surg Oral Med Oral Pathol Oral Radiol Endod.* 2002;94:83-91.

29. Worret WI, Vocks E, Frias G, Burgdorf WH, Lane P. Actinic prurigo. An assessment of current status. *Hautarzt.* 2000;51:474-478.

30. Hojyo-Tomoka MT, Vega-Memije ME, Cortes-Franco R, et al. Diagnosis and treatment of actinic prurigo. *Dermatol Ther.* 2003;16:40-44.

31. Grabczynska SA, Hawk JL. What is actinic prurigo in Britain? *Photodermatol Photoimmunol Photomed.* 1997;13:85-86.

32. Grabczynska SA, McGregor JM, Kondeatis E, et al. Actinic prurigo and polymorphic light eruption: common pathogenesis and the importance of HLA-DR4/DRB1*0407. *Br J Dermatol.* 1999;140:232-236.

33. Millard TP, Kondeatis E, Cox A, et al. A candidate gene analysis of three related photosensitivity disorders: cutaneous lupus erythematosus, polymorphic light eruption and actinic prurigo. *Br J Dermatol.* 2001;145:229-236.

34. Zuloaga-Salcedo S, Castillo-Vazquez M, Vega-Memije E, et al. Class I and class II major histocompatibility complex genes in Mexican patients with actinic prurigo. *Br J Dermatol.* 2007;156:1074-1075.

35. Herrera-Geopfert R, Magaña M. Follicular cheilitis: a distinctive histopathologic finding in actinic prurigo. *Am J Dermatopathol.* 1995;17:357-361.

36. Calderón-Amador J, Flores-Langarica A, Silva-Sánchez A, et al. Epidermal Langerhans cells in actinic prurigo: a comparison between lesional and non-lesional skin. *J Eur Acad Dermatol Venereol.* 2009;23:438-440.

37. Fusaro RM, Johnson JA. Hereditary polymorphic light eruption of American Indians: occurrence in non-Indians with polymorphic light eruption. *J Am Acad Dermatol.* 1996;34:612-617.

38. Birt AR, Hogg GR. The actinic cheilitis of hereditary polymorphic light eruption. *Arch Dermatol.* 1979;115:699-702.

39. Carlos BR, Sedano HO. Multifocal papillomavirus epithelial hyperplasia. *Oral Surg Oral Med Oral Pathol.* 1994;77:631-635.

40. Archard HO, Heck JW, Stanley JR. Focal epithelial hyperplasia: an unusual oral mucosal lesion found in Indian children. *Oral Surg Oral Med Oral Pathol.* 1965;20:201-212.

41. Praetorius-Clausen F. Geographical aspects of oral focal epithelial hyperplasia. *Pathol Microbiol.* 1973;39:204-213.

42. Gonzalez LV, Gaviria AM, Sanclemente G, et al. Clinical, histopathological and virological findings in patients with focal epithelial hyperplasia from Colombia. *Int J Dermatol.* 2005;44:274-279.

43. Harris AMP, van Wyk CW. Heck's disease (focal epithelial hyperplasia): a longitudinal study. *Commun Dent Oral Epidemiol.* 1993;21:82-85.

44. Witkop CJ, Niswander JD. Focal epithelial hyperplasia in Central and South American Indians and Latinos. *Oral Surg Oral Med Oral Pathol.* 1965;20:213-217.

45. Praetorius-Clausen F. Histopathology of focal epithelial hyperplasia: evidence of viral infection. *Tandlaegebladet.* 1969;73:1013-1022.

46. Pfister H, Heltich J, Runne U, Chilf GN. Characterization of human papillomavirus type 13 from focal epithelial Heck lesions. *J Virol.* 1983;47:363-366.

47. Beaudenon S, Praetorius F, Kremsdorf D, et al. A new type of human papillomavirus associated with oral focal epithelial hyperplasia. *J Invest Dermatol.* 1987;88:130-135.

48. Garlick JA, Calderon S, Buchner A, Mitrani-Rosenbaum S. Detection of human papillomavirus (HPV) DNA in focal epithelial hyperplasia. *J Oral Pathol Med.* 1989;18:172-177.

49. Henke RP, Guèrin-Reverchon I, Milde-Langosch K, et al. In situ detection of human papillomavirus types 13 and 32 in focal epithelial hyperplasia of the oral mucosa. *J Oral Pathol Med.* 1989;18:419-421.

50. Padayachee A, van Wyk CW. Human papillomavirus (HPV) DNA in focal epithelial hyperplasia by in situ hybridization. *J Oral Pathol Med.* 1991;20:210-214.

51. Gültekin SE, Tokman Yildirim B, Sarisoy S. Oral focal epithelial hyperplasia: report of 3 cases with human papillomavirus DNA sequencing analysis. *Pediatr Dent.* 2011;33:522-524.

52. Garlick JA, Taichman LB. Human papillomavirus infection of the oral mucosa. *Am J Dermatopathol.* 1991;13:386-395.

53. Ledesma-Montes C, Garces-Ortiz M, Hernandez-Guerrero JC. Clinicopathological and immunocytochemical study of multifocal epithelial hyperplasia. *J Oral Maxillofac Surg.* 2007;65:2211-2217.

54. Lopez-Villanueva ME, Conde-Ferráez L, Ayora-Talavera G, Cerón-Espinosa JD, González-Losa Mdel R. Human papillomavirus 13 in a Mexican Mayan community with multifocal epithelial hyperplasia: could saliva be involved in household transmission? *Eur J Dermatol.* 2011;21:396-400.

55. Moerman M, Danielides VG, Nousia CS, et al. Recurrent focal epithelial hyperplasia due to HPV-13 in an HIV-positive patient. *Dermatology.* 2001;203:339-341.

56. Steinhoff M, Metze D, Stockfleth E, Luger TA. Successful topical treatment of focal epithelial hyperplasia (Heck's disease) with interferon-β. *Br J Dermatol.* 2001;144:1067-1069.

57. Kauzman A, Pavone M, Blanas P, Bradley G. Pigmented lesions of the oral cavity: review, differential diagnosis, and case presentations. *J Can Dent Assoc.* 2004;70:682-683.

58. Eisen D. Disorders of pigmentation in the oral cavity. *Clin Dermatol.* 2000;18:579-587.

59. Yeh C-J. Simple cryosurgical treatment of the oral melanotic macule. *Oral Surg Oral Med Oral Pathol Oral Radiol Endod.* 2000;90:12-13.

60. Gaeta GM, Satriano RA, Baroni A. Oral pigmented lesions. *Clin Dermatol.* 2002;20:286-288.

61. Lampe AK, Hampton PJ, Woodford-Richens K, et al. Hunziker syndrome: an important differential diagnosis for Peutz-Jeghers syndrome. *J Med Genet.* 2003;40:e77.

62. Gencoglan G, Gerceker-Turk B, Kilinc-Karaarslan I, et al. Dermoscopic findings in Laugier-Hunziker syndrome. *Arch Dermatol.* 2007;143:631-633.

63. Shih YC, Chiu CS, Chuang YH, Ko JH. Dermoscopic features in Laugier-Hunziker syndrome. *J Dermatol.* 2011;38:87-90.

64. Bouaziz J-D, Le Pelletier F. Additional conjunctival and penile pigmentation in Laugier-Hunziker syndrome: a report of two cases. *Int J Dermatol.* 2000;43:571-574.

65. Zuo YG, Ma DL, Jin HZ, et al. Treatment of Laugier-Hunziker syndrome with the Q-switched alexandrite laser in 22 Chinese patients. *Arch Dermatol Res.* 2010;302:125-130.

66. Peutz JLA. Very remarkable case of familial polyposis of mucous membrane of intestinal tract and nasopharynx accompanied by peculiar pigmentations of skin and mucous membrane. *Nederl Maandschr Geneesk.* 1921;10:134-146.

67. Jeghers H, McKusick VA, Katz KH. Generalized intestinal polyposis and melanin spots of the oral mucosa, lips and digits. *N Engl J Med.* 1949;241:993-1005, 1031-1036.

68. Hezel AF, Bardeesy N. LKB1; linking cell structure and tumor suppression. *Oncogene.* 2008;27:6908-69019.

69. OMIM. Peutz-Jeghers syndrome. http://omim.org/entry/175200. Accessed February 13, 2015.

70. Higham P, Alawi F, Stoopler ET. Medical management update: Peutz-Jeghers syndrome. *Oral Med Oral Pathol Oral Radiol Endod.* 2010;109:5-11.

71. vanLier MGF, Wagner A, Mathus-Vliegen EMH, Kuipers EJ, Steyerberg EW. High cancer risk in Peutz-Jeghers syndrome: a systematic review and Surveillance Recommendations. *Am J Gastroenterol.* 2010;105:1258-1264.

72. Chan HH, Manstein D, Yu CS, et al. The prevalence and risk factors of postinflammatory hyperpigmentation after fractional resurfacing in Asians. *Lasers Surg Med.* 2007;39:381-385.

73. Makino ET, Herndon JH, Sigler ML, Gotz V, Garruto J, Mehta RC. Clinical efficacy and safety of a multimodality skin brightener composition compared with 4% hydroquinone. *Drugs Dermatol.* 2012;11:1478-1482.

74. Fornatora ML, Reich RF, Haber S, Solomon F, Freedman PD. Oral melanoacanthoma: a report of 10 cases, review of the literature, and immunohistochemical analysis for HMB-45 reactivity. *Am J Dermatopathol.* 2003; 25:12-15.

75. Brooks JK, Sindler AJ, Scheper MA. Oral melanoacanthoma in an adolescent. *Pediatr Dermatol.* 2010;27:384-387.

76. Wang X, Wu HM, Ren GX, Tang J, Guo W. Primary oral mucosal melanoma: advocate a wait-and-see policy in the clinically N0 patient. *J Oral Maxillofac Surg.* 2012;70:1192-1198.

77. Speight PM. Mucosal malignant melanoma in tumours of the oral cavity and oropharynx. In: Barnes L, Eveson JW, Reichart D, Sidransky D, eds. *Head and Neck Tumours.* Lyon, France: IARC Press; 2005:206-207.

78. Tanaka N, Mimura M, Ichinose S, Odajima T. Malignant melanoma in the oral region: ultrastructural and immunohistochemical studies. *Med Electron Microsc.* 2001;34:198-205.

79. Sortino-Rachou AM, Cancela Mde C, Voti L, Curado MP. Primary oral melanoma: population-based incidence. *Oral Oncol.* 2009;45:254-258.

80. Ashton M, Sopwith W, Clark P, et al. An outbreak no longer: factors contributing to the return of syphilis in Greater Manchester. *Sex Transm Infect.* 2003;79:291-293.

81. Hughes G, Paine T, Thomas D. Surveillance of sexually transmitted infections in England and Wales. *Eur Surveill.* 2001;6:71-80.

82. Centers for Disease Control and Prevention. Primary and secondary syphilis—United States, 2002. *MMWR.* 2003;52:1117-1120.

83. Centers for Disease Control and Prevention (CDC). Primary and secondary syphilis: United States, 2003-2004. *MMWR Morb Mortal Wkly Rep.* 2006;55:269-273.

84. Centers for Disease Control and Prevention. *Sexually Transmitted Disease Surveillance, 2003.* Atlanta, GA: US Department of Health and Human Services; 2004.

85. Leão JC, Gueiros LA, Porter SR. Oral manifestations of syphilis. *Clin Dermatol.* 2006;61:161-166.

86. Augenbraun M, Rolfs R, Johnson R, et al. Treponemal-specific tests for the serodiagnosis of syphilis. Syphilis and HIV Study Group. *Sex Transm Dis.* 1998;25:549-552.

87. Wong W, Chaw JK, Kent CK, Klausner JD. Risk factors for early syphilis among gay and bisexual men seen in an STD clinic: San Francisco, 2002-2003. *Sex Transm Dis.* 2005;32:458-463.

88. Kumar B, Muralidhar S. Malignant syphilis: a review. *AIDS Patient Care STDs.* 2001;12:921-925.

89. Workowski KA, Berman SM. Sexually transmitted diseases treatment guidelines, 2010. *MMWR* 2010;59:1-109.

90. Riedner G, Rusizoka M, Todd J, et al. Single-dose azithromycin versus penicillin G benzathine for the treatment of early syphilis. *N Engl J Med.* 2005;353:1236-1244.

91. Grimes M, Sahi SK, Godornes BC, et al. Two mutations associated with macrolide resistance in Treponema pallidum: increasing prevalence and correlation with molecular strain type in Seattle, Washington. *Sex Transm Dis.* 2012;39:954-958.

92. Bouaziz A, Le Scanff J, Chapelon-Abric C, et al. Oral involvement in sarcoidosis: report of 12 cases. *Q J Med.* 2012;105:755-767.

93. Clayman L, MacLennan M, Dolan RL. Nonpainful swelling of the palate and loosening of the maxillary incisors. *J Oral Maxillofac Surg.* 1998;56:1327-1335.

94. Armstrong C, Napier S, Linden GJ. Sarcoidosis with gingival involvement: a case report. *J Periodontol.* 2004;75:608-612.

95. Kasamatsu A, Kanazawa H, Watanabe T, Matsuzaki O. Oral sarcoidosis: report of a case and review of literature. *J Oral Maxillofac Surg.* 2007;65:1256-1259.

96. Azenha MR, Caliento R, Brentegani LG, Lacerda SA. A retrospective study of oral manifestations in patients with paracoccidioidomycosis. *Braz Dent J.* 2012;23:753-757.

97. Marques SA. Paracoccidioidomycosis. *Clin Dermatol.* 2012;30:610-615

98. Severo CB, Dallo Bello AG, Oliviera FM, et al. Pleural effusion an unusual feature of paracoccidioidomycosis: report of two new cases with a systematic review of the literature. *Mycopathologia.* 2013;175:323-330.

99. de Abreu E Silva MA, Salum FG, Figueiredo MA, Cherubini K. Important aspects of oral paracoccidioidomycosis-a literature review. *Mycoses.* 2013; 56:189-199.

100. Queiroz-Telles F, Goldani LZ, Schlamm HT, et al. An open-label comparative pilot study of oral voriconazole and itraconazole for long-term treatment of paracoccidioidomycosis. *Clin Infect Dis.* 2007;45:1462-1469.

101. Marques-da-Silva SH, Colombo AL, Blotta MH, et al. Diagnosis of paracoccidioidomycosis by detection of antigen and antibody in bronchoalveolar lavage fluids. *Clin Vaccine Immunol.* 2006;13:1363-1366.

102. Blotta MH, Mamoni RL, Oliveira SJ, et al. Endemic regions of paracoccidioidomycosis in Brazil: a clinical and epidemiologic study of 584 cases in the southeast region. *Am J Trop Med Hyg.* 1999;61:390-394.

CHAPTER 57

Common Diseases of the Oral Mucosa

Anabella Pascucci

Nasim Fazel

KEY POINTS

- Examination of the oral mucosa should be a part of the complete skin examination.

- Familiarity with variations in normal oral anatomy is essential in distinguishing benign findings from conditions requiring treatment intervention.

- Recognition of common oral mucosal diseases and their characteristic signs and symptoms is important in initiating prompt and effective therapy.

BENIGN ORAL FINDINGS

GEOGRAPHIC TONGUE

Geographic tongue, also known as benign migratory glossitis, is an idiopathic inflammatory condition that is caused by a loss of filiform papillae on the dorsal tongue. It has a prevalence of 1% to 2.5% and

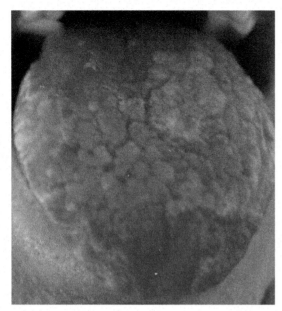

FIGURE 57-1. Geographic tongue: pink patches with white borders on the dorsal tongue.

is more common in children with diminishing frequency with age.[1] In some instances it can be associated with an underlying condition such as psoriasis, hormonal disturbances, diabetes, atopy, psychological stress, Reiter syndrome, Down syndrome, nutritional deficiencies, and fissured tongue. There are also rare reports of a genetic predisposition to the disorder. It has been found to be inversely associated with tobacco smoking.[2,3]

Geographic tongue is characterized by asymptomatic erythematous patches with a slightly raised border and a centrally denuded area. It typically involves the anterior two-thirds of the dorsal tongue. Patches have well-demarcated and irregular, serpiginous, raised, yellow to white

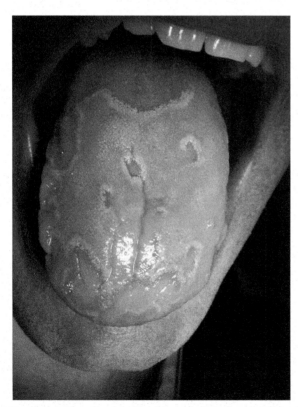

FIGURE 57-2. Geographic tongue. Note prominence of white borders. (Used with permission from Henry W. Lim, MD, Henry Ford Hospital, Detroit, MI.)

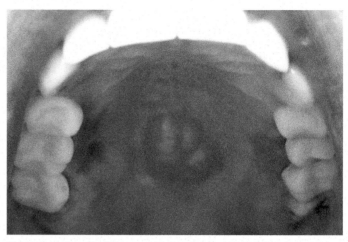

FIGURE 57-3. Palatal torus: prominent bony exostosis of the hard palate at the midline.

borders [**Figures 57-1 and 57-2**]. They are migratory, meaning that they change in shape and location over time, and may change within minutes or hours. The migratory pattern and irregular appearance of the lesions can be distressing to the patient. Although most often asymptomatic, some patients may complain of tongue sensitivity, burning, a foreign body sensation, or pain.[1,2] Most often, simply reassuring the patient is all that is necessary. However, in symptomatic patients, topical steroids, topical antifungals, topical antihistamines, topical anesthetics, and topical tacrolimus can be used.[2,4]

PALATAL AND LINGUAL TORI

The prevalence of oral tori is 12% to 15%.[5,6] Some studies have shown an association between oral tori and bruxism (grinding).[7] Genetic and environmental factors likely play a role in the development of tori. However, the etiology of tori is unknown.[8,9]

Tori present as asymptomatic bony sessile protuberances that develop during puberty. Torus palatinus occurs at the midline on the hard palate [**Figure 57-3**]. Torus mandibularis occurs on the lingual aspect of the mandible [**Figure 57-4**]. Oral tori are generally benign exostoses that do not require treatment. Tori may be surgically excised if they cause trauma or interfere with mastication or speech.[6,8,9]

BLACK HAIRY TONGUE

Black hairy tongue, also known as lingua villosa nigra, presents as a painless black plaque on the tongue anterior to the circumvallate papillae. It usually does not affect the anterior one-third of the tongue. It may

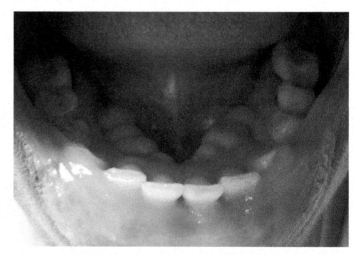

FIGURE 57-4. Lingual tori: multiple bony exostoses along the lingual aspect of the mandible.

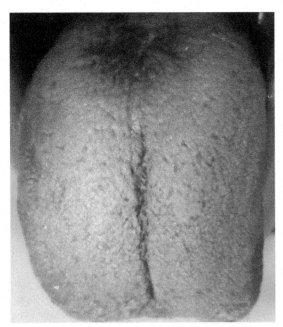

FIGURE 57-5. Black hairy tongue: elongated lingual papillae with dark discoloration on the dorsum of the tongue.

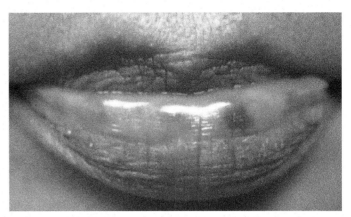

FIGURE 57-6. Labial melanotic macule: solitary, brown-colored, evenly pigmented macule on the lower lip proper.

cause alteration in taste and nausea or can be asymptomatic. The prevalence of black hairy tongue is variable and ranges from 0% to 53.8%.[10,11]

Black hairy tongue is a benign condition caused by elongation and hypertrophy of the filiform papillae with accumulation of keratin in patients with poor oral hygiene [**Figure 57-5**]. It is associated with smoking, alcohol abuse, coffee/tea drinking, xerostomia, trigeminal neuralgia, oral infections, immunosuppression, history of stem cell transplant, and history of radiation, and in some instances, it may be drug-induced. Implicated drugs include tetracycline, penicillin, erythromycin, lansoprazole, linezolid, olanzapine, and bismuth.[10-13]

Treatment includes improved oral hygiene, mechanical removal of the plaque with a hard toothbrush, and avoidance of predisposing factors. Retinoids, urea, and other keratolytic agents can also improve appearance.[10-13]

PIGMENTED LESIONS

LABIAL MELANOTIC MACULE

Labial melanotic macule is most common in women over the age of 30. The mean age is 47.3 years, with a female-to-male ratio of 2:1. Labial melanotic macule presents as an asymptomatic brown, blue, or black macule less than 10 mm in diameter. Lesions are usually solitary and most commonly present on the lower lip or gingiva [**Figure 57-6**]. Less commonly, they occur as multiple lesions and present on the upper lip or mucous membranes.[14-17]

It is unclear if they constitute a physiologic or reactive process. Labial melanotic macules are benign lesions that do not require treatment other than for cosmetic reasons. However, if there is any doubt in the diagnosis, then a biopsy should be performed to rule out a malignant process.[14-17]

ORAL MELANOCYTIC NEVI

The exact incidence of oral melanocytic nevi is unknown, but they are thought to be uncommon.

Oral melanocytic nevi may be congenital or acquired. Oral melanocytic nevi present as asymptomatic, solitary, small, well-circumscribed, brown, gray, blue, or black macules or papules. In rare instances, they may be nonpigmented. They are most commonly present on the palate, but also occur in decreasing order of frequency on the buccal mucosa,

vermillion border, and gingiva. They are very rare on the tongue or floor of the mouth. Histopathology varies depending on the type of nevus. Intramucosal nevi are the most common type, followed by compound nevi and blue nevi. Junctional nevi are rare. The malignant potential of oral nevi is unclear. Excision is usually recommended to rule out oral melanoma.[18-21]

AMALGAM TATTOOS

Amalgam tattoos generally present as an asymptomatic gray, black, or blue macule on the oral mucosa in the vicinity of a tooth restored with amalgam. Tattoos are most common on the gingival surface. They also occur on the alveolar and buccal mucosa and less commonly on the floor of the mouth[22-24] [**Figure 57-7**].

The prevalence of amalgam tattoos is unknown, but they are considered a common finding.

Amalgam tattoos are caused by the iatrogenic implantation of amalgam into soft tissues. Mercury and other metals such as silver, copper, zinc, and tin found in amalgam may also diffuse into surrounding tissues. Amalgam restorations are being used less frequently with the advent of composite fillings and tooth-colored dental materials that can withstand the forces of mastication.

Amalgam tattoos are sometimes biopsied to rule out a malignant process. Histopathology shows dark brown or black pigment granules in the superficial dermis, but that can also be found in the subcutaneous tissues. Granules are often arranged linearly among the collagen fibers and surrounding blood vessels. There is usually no associated inflammatory

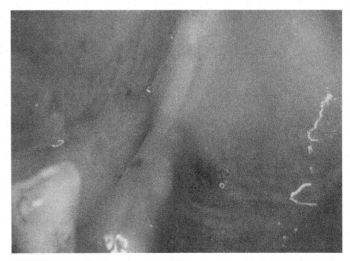

FIGURE 57-7. Amalgam tattoos: grayish blue-colored macules on the mandibular ridge and left buccal mucosa.

response. In the rare cases with an inflammatory response, it is usually consistent with a granulomatous reaction.

Amalgam tattoo is a benign lesion, and no treatment is necessary. However, if a patient has a metal allergy, treatment may be helpful. Tattoos can also be treated for cosmetic reasons. Treatment options include surgical excision, Q-switched ruby laser, and Q-switched alexandrite laser.[22-26]

INFECTIOUS ORAL DISEASES

HERPES LABIALIS AND PRIMARY HERPETIC GINGIVOSTOMATITIS

Herpes labialis and primary herpetic gingivostomatitis are caused by herpes simplex virus types 1 and 2, although both entities are more frequently caused by herpes simplex virus 1 (HSV-1). Primary infection may be asymptomatic or cause gingivostomatitis. Subsequent to primary infection, the herpes virus remains latent in the sensory ganglia with reactivation of the virus causing herpes labialis. Known triggers for reactivation include emotional stress, exposure to ultraviolet light, fever, or menstruation.[27-29]

The prevalence of HSV-1 increases during childhood, reaching 80% to 90% in adults. The peak incidence of primary herpetic gingivostomatitis within the pediatric population is between the ages of 6 months and 5 years due to the protective role of maternal antibodies during the first 6 months of life. A second peak occurs in the early 20s.[29,30]

Primary herpetic gingivostomatitis occurs as a result of initial exposure to the herpes virus through direct contact with a lesion or infected body fluids such as saliva. Characteristically, it presents with oral and extraoral vesicles, edematous hemorrhagic gums, and lymphadenopathy. Patients may experience prodromal symptoms of burning, itching, or tingling prior to the onset of clinically evident lesions. In some cases, patients may also complain of constitutional symptoms such as fever, malaise, and headache. Mucosal vesicles may occur on the tongue, gingiva, hard and soft palate, and lips. Vesicles quickly rupture to form painful ulcerations that heal without scarring. The ulcerated lesions may have a characteristic "punched out" appearance. Herpes labialis typically presents with a prodrome of tingling, burning, and/or itching prior to the development of a clinically evident lesion. The prodrome is followed by the development of erythematous grouped vesicles on the vermilion border and cutaneous lip [**Figures 57-8 and 57-9**]. Early recognition of prodromal symptoms is important, given that prompt initiation of antiviral therapy may abort or alleviate the severity of a flare.[28,29]

Primary herpetic gingivostomatitis is a self-limited condition that does not cause systemic complications in an immunocompetent individual; therefore, it does not require treatment. Palliation with topical

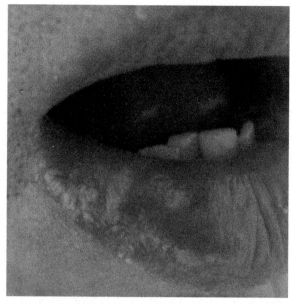

FIGURE 57-9. Herpes labialis: cluster of vesicles on an erythematous base involving the lower lip.

anesthetics such as benzocaine gel can facilitate oral intake. Immunocompromised individuals or children under 6 years of age with gingivostomatitis may benefit from systemic antiviral therapy to prevent complications such as eye infections (ocular herpes or herpetic keratoconjunctivitis) and herpetic whitlow of the digits. Antiviral agents include acyclovir, valacyclovir, and famciclovir. Herpes labialis is also self-limited, but recurrent disease may be uncomfortable and create a social stigma. Systemic antiviral therapy can reduce the duration and severity of symptoms. Treatment is most effective when it is started during the prodromal stage and within the first 72 hours of a clinically evident lesion. Prophylactic systemic antiviral therapy is indicated in patients with frequent outbreaks, which can decrease the frequency and severity of flares.[27,31-33]

ORAL CANDIDIASIS/THRUSH

Candida albicans is a commensal organism that is normally present in the gastrointestinal tract as well as oral and vaginal mucosa. *C. albicans* can cause infections of the oral, esophageal, and vaginal mucosa in susceptible individuals.[34] Approximately 50% of the population are commensal carriers of *C. albicans*, and it is isolated from 80% of patients diagnosed with oral candidiasis.[34]

The clinical presentation of oral candidiasis is variable. Pseudomembranous candidiasis, or thrush, presents as white plaques overlying an erythematous base that may also affect the oropharynx and esophagus in immunocompromised patients [**Figure 57-10**]. Lesions may be asymptomatic or associated with burning and pain. Pseudomembranous candidiasis is the type of candidiasis that is most frequently found in immunocompromised individuals and infants. Unlike other white lesions such as leukoplakia, oral candidiasis characteristically "wipes off" with the application of gauze. This clinical finding can help distinguish oral candidiasis from other white lesions.[35,36]

Erythematous candidiasis is the most common form of candidiasis in the general population and may occur in immunocompetent individuals. It has varying presentations, including angular cheilitis, acute atrophic candidiasis, chronic atrophic candidiasis, median rhomboid glossitis, and chronic multifocal candidiasis. Angular cheilitis presents with erythema and painful fissuring involving the labial commissures [**Figure 57-11**]. Most cases are caused by a combination of *C. albicans* and *Staphylococcus aureus*. Acute atrophic candidiasis presents as erythema of the tongue with atrophy of the lingual papillae, associated with a burning sensation. It is most often associated with the use of

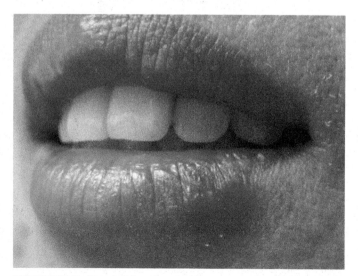

FIGURE 57-8. Herpes labialis, early stage: erythematous papule at the vermilion border of the lower lip.

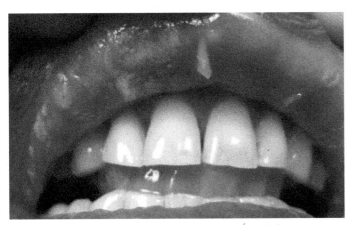

FIGURE 57-10. Pseudomembranous candidiasis: fluffy white plaques involving the upper labial mucosa.

TABLE 57-1	Systemic therapies for oral candidiasis	
Medication	Dosing regimen	Main adverse effects
Nystatin oral suspension 100,000 U/mL	5 mL qid, swish and swallow	Nausea, vomiting, diarrhea, and abdominal pain
Ketoconazole	200 mg/d	Hepatotoxicity, nausea, abdominal pain, diarrhea, and headache
Fluconazole	100 mg/d	Hepatotoxicity, leukopenia, nausea, abdominal pain, diarrhea, and headache
Itraconazole	100–200 mg/d	Hepatotoxicity, leukopenia, nausea, abdominal pain, diarrhea, and headache

Abbreviation: qid, four times a day.

broad-spectrum antibiotics. Chronic atrophic candidiasis presents with asymptomatic erythema and petechiae of the mucosa in denture wearers. Median rhomboid glossitis presents with a well-demarcated area of atrophy of the lingual papillae and characteristically affects the dorsal tongue anterior to the circumvallate papillae and at the midline. Chronic multifocal candidiasis occurs when erythematous candidiasis is present in more than one location. Hyperplastic candidiasis is the least common form of candidiasis and presents with a well-demarcated white plaque on the buccal mucosa, palate, or lateral tongue that cannot be wiped off. It may be indistinguishable from leukoplakia and is frequently biopsied to rule out squamous cell carcinoma.[35-37]

Topical antifungal agents are usually sufficient treatment for mild disease. Commonly used therapy includes topical polyene and azole antifungals, nystatin suspension, gentian violet, and amphotericin suspensions. Systemic antifungals may be necessary in refractory cases and in immunocompromised individuals. Systemic therapies include ketoconazole, fluconazole, miconazole, itraconazole, and amphotericin for azole-resistant strains[35,36] [**Table 57-1**].

ULCERATIVE ORAL DISEASES

▨ RECURRENT APHTHOUS STOMATITIS

Recurrent aphthous stomatitis (RAS) is the most common oral ulcerative condition in the United States. The age of onset is between 10 and 19 years of age with a wide range of reported prevalence up to 60%. There is a higher prevalence in women and those of higher socioeconomic status.[38,39] The etiology and pathogenesis of RAS remain unclear. Patients with a family history of RAS are more likely to have an earlier age of onset and a more severe course of the disease. Predisposing factors associated with RAS include incidental oral trauma or trauma secondary to dental procedures, nutritional deficiencies (including vitamin B_6 and B_{12}, folate, and zinc), iron deficiency anemia, immunologic factors, psychological stress, and some systemic disorders. Associated systemic diseases include human immunodeficiency virus (HIV), celiac disease, hematinic deficiencies, PFAPA syndrome (*periodic fever, aphthosis, pharyngitis, and adenitis*) [**Figure 57-12**], MAGIC syndrome (*mouth and genital ulcerations with inflamed cartilage*), and inflammatory bowel disease (including Crohn disease and ulcerative colitis).[38-41]

Aphthous ulcers present as recurrent, well-defined, shallow, round to oval ulcerations on the oral mucosa that have a necrotic center with a yellow-gray pseudomembrane and a surrounding halo of erythema. Lesions are painful and may cause difficulty with eating, swallowing, and speaking. The first episode usually occurs in adolescence, and most often there is a decreasing frequency and severity of episodes with age.[38-41]

RAS is divided into three clinical subtypes based on the morphology of the lesions: minor, major, and herpetiform. Minor aphthous stomatitis is the most common subtype, occurring in 70% to 80% of patients. Ulcerations are small (<10 mm) and shallow. Lesions typically involve the nonkeratinized mucosal surfaces including the buccal mucosa, labial mucosa, ventral tongue, soft palate, posterior oral pharynx, and floor of

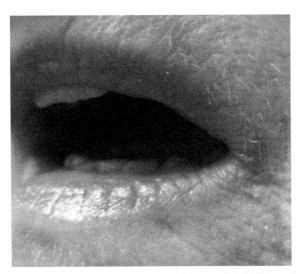

FIGURE 57-11. Angular cheilitis: erythema and fissuring at the left labial commissure.

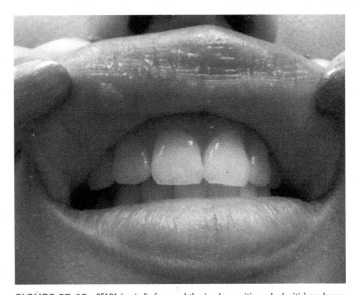

FIGURE 57-12. PFAPA (*periodic fever, aphthosis, pharyngitis, and adenitis*) syndrome: discrete ulceration with fibromembranous exudate involving the upper labial mucosa in the setting of pharyngitis, periodic fever, and adenitis.

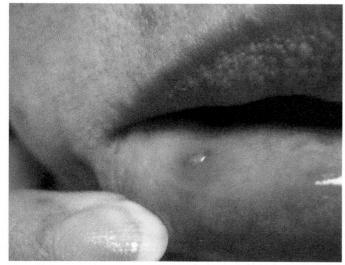

A

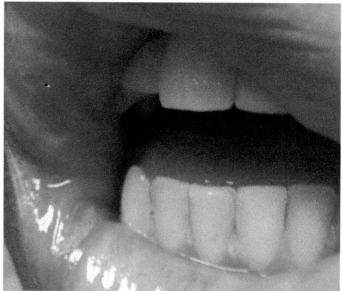

FIGURE 57-14. Major aphthous stomatitis: large well-circumscribed ulcerations on the upper and lower labial mucosa.

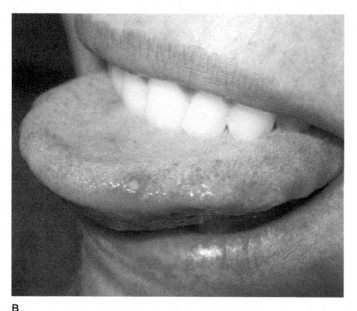

B

FIGURE 57-13. Minor aphthous stomatitis. **(A)** Well-circumscribed ulceration on an erythematous base involving the lower labial mucosa. **(B)** Well-circumscribed ulceration on an erythematous base involving the dorsal tongue.

classification system, which is based on the severity of the disease, can be helpful in determining the necessity for systemic therapy.[42]

The main goals of therapy in RAS are symptomatic relief, decreased healing time, and decreased recurrence. Topical treatment includes topical steroids, intralesional steroids, topical antibiotics, topical calcineurin inhibitors, and topical retinoids. Topical steroids are the mainstay of therapy. The more commonly used topical steroids include clobetasol gel, fluocinonide gel, and triamcinolone compounded in Orabase two to four times daily. Topical therapies, in general, are limited in their contact time due to the effects of normal salivary flow. Chlorhexidine gluconate 0.12% (Peridex) mouthrinse twice daily has been shown to reduce the number of ulcer days and increase disease-free intervals. Side effects include dysgeusia (abnormalities in taste perception) and yellow discoloration of the teeth, which resolves with routine in-office cleanings.[38-41,43,44]

Patients with frequent painful episodes most often require systemic therapy. The more commonly used systemic immunomodulatory

the mouth [**Figure 57-13**]. This is in sharp contrast to herpes simplex, which typically affects the keratinized mucosal surfaces of the gingiva, hard palate, and lip proper. Minor aphthous ulcers typically heal within 10 to 14 days without residual scarring. Major aphthous stomatitis is a rare severe presentation of RAS. Ulcerations are large (>10 mm) and occur on the soft palate, posterior oral pharynx, tongue, buccal and labial mucosa, soft palate, and faucial pillars [**Figure 57-14**]. Ulcers are painful, slow to heal, and often multiple, and may take up to 6 weeks to resolve. Deeper lesions tend to heal with residual scarring, which can lead to significant mucosal distortion. Herpetiform ulcers are the least common presentation. Patients have clusters of small painful ulcers that may coalesce to form larger ulcerations [**Figure 57-15**]. This subtype of aphthous stomatitis is seen more frequently in middle-aged women.[38-41]

The second classification system for RAS is based on the severity of the disease: simple versus complex aphthosis. Patients with simple aphthosis have fewer lesions, less frequent flaring, and minimal pain. Typically, lesions heal in 1 to 2 weeks without scarring. However, patients with complex aphthosis have more severe, continuous flaring, multiple lesions, marked pain, and frequent genital involvement. This

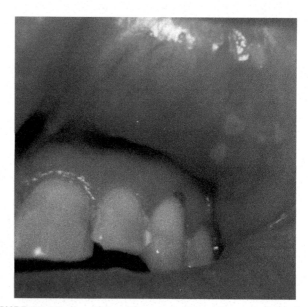

FIGURE 57-15. Herpetiform aphthous ulcers: cluster of discrete small ulcerations on the upper labial mucosa.

TABLE 57-2	Systemic therapies for recurrent aphthous stomatitis	
Medication	Dosing regimen	Main adverse effects
Colchicine	0.6 mg bid 0.6 mg tid 0.6 mg q am, 1.2 mg q pm	Myelosuppression, hepatotoxicity, diarrhea, nausea, vomiting, and headaches
Pentoxifylline	400 mg tid	Gastrointestinal disturbances, nausea, dizziness, and headaches
Dapsone	50–100 mg daily	Hemolytic anemia, methemoglobin-emia, and peripheral neuropathy
Thalidomide	50–100 mg daily	Sedation, neuropathy, neutropenia, constipation, and teratogenicity
Azathioprine	50–100 mg daily	Gastrointestinal disturbances, hepato-toxicity, and myelotoxicity

Abbreviations: bid, twice a day; tid, three times a day; q, every.

agents include colchicine, prednisone, pentoxifylline, thalidomide, dapsone, azathioprine, methotrexate, cyclosporine, interferon-α, and tumor necrosis factor (TNF) antagonists [**Table 57-2**]. Prednisone therapy can be very helpful in providing fairly immediate relief in cases of severe flaring when systemic therapies are indicated. It can be dosed in short courses at 40 to 80 mg daily with gradual taper. Long-term dosing is generally not recommended because of side effects such as weight gain and risk of osteoporosis. Although prednisone therapy can be very helpful in controlling a severe flare, it generally does not provide a sustained remission in patients with severe disease. Therefore, systemic therapy with other agents such as pentoxifylline, colchicine, or dapsone is required in these instances. Pentoxifylline is an orally active methylxanthine derivative that inhibits T- and B-cell activation and neutrophil adhesions. Dapsone can be used in combination with other agents such as colchicine.[38-41,43,44]

There is less information regarding the use of thalidomide, azathioprine, methotrexate, cyclosporine, interferon-α, and TNF antagonists.[38-41,43,44] Palliative agents can be used in conjunction with topical and systemic therapies to alleviate pain and facilitate oral intake during a flare. These include benzyl alcohol gel (Zilactin), amlexanox oral paste, sucralfate (1 g/10 mL) suspension, benzocaine gel (Orajel), viscous lidocaine 2% solution, and diphenhydramine elixir (12.5 mg/5 mL).[38-41,43,44]

■ BEHÇET DISEASE

The prevalence of Behçet disease (BD) is highest in countries bordering the Silk Road including China, Korea, Japan, Iran, and Turkey, with an estimated prevalence between 1 in 1000 and 1 in 10,000. It is more commonly seen in males, who are at higher risker of developing multiorgan system involvement and more severe presentations of the disease.[45-50]

The etiology of BD is unknown. It is thought to be an autoimmune process that is triggered by infectious or environmental factors in a genetically predisposed individual. Although HLA-B51 is the most strongly associated known genetic factor for BD, it only accounts for approximately 20% of the genetic risk. This suggests that other undiscovered genetic factors may exist. BD most commonly presents around the third decade with a male gender predilection. It is a chronic, relapsing systemic vasculitis that can affect multiple organ systems including the musculoskeletal, vascular, gastrointestinal, and neurologic systems. The severity of the disease and mortality risk are greatest in men and in the younger patient population. In 1990, the International Study Group (ISG) developed a set of criteria for the diagnosis of BD [**Table 57-3**]. The ISG criteria are based on the presence of recurrent oral ulcerations in all patients, plus two or more of the following: recurrent genital ulceration, eye lesions, skin lesions, and cutaneous pathergy. Recurrent oral ulcerations are defined as at least three episodes over a 12-month period presenting as any of the three morphologic patterns (ie, herpetiform or minor or major aphthous ulcers). The ISG criteria are the most uniformly accepted diagnostic criteria, with a sensitivity of 91% and a specificity of 96%.[45-53]

TABLE 57-3	International classification criteria of Behçet disease

Recurrent oral ulceration observed by physician or patient, at least three episodes in a 12-month period.
Plus two of the following:
    Recurrent genital ulceration
    Eye lesions: anterior uveitis, posterior uveitis, cells in the vitreous, or retinal vasculitis
    Skin lesions: erythema nodosum, pseudofolliculitis, papulopustular or acneiform nodules in postadolescent patients not on corticosteroids
    Pathergy ready by a physician at 24–48 hours

Most often, BD presents with oral ulcers, genital ulcers, and ocular disease. Recurrent oral ulcerations are the most common initial presentation of the disease and may precede other manifestations of the disease. They present as single or multiple ulcers with an erythematous border covered by a gray-white pseudomembrane that overlies a yellow fibrinous base [**Figure 57-16**]. Ulcers most commonly involve the buccal mucosa, pharynx, tongue, and lips and typically heal without scarring. Genital ulcers present similarly to oral ulcers, but can be larger and deeper with a greater likelihood of scarring. Genital ulcers in men are found most commonly on the scrotum, but may also occur on the penis or urethra. In women, they most commonly involve the labia minora and majora followed by the vulva and vagina [**Figure 57-17**].

In cases of gastrointestinal involvement ulcerations may be found in the esophagus, stomach, small and large intestine, and/or perianal area. The skin manifestations of BD include erythema nodosum, pseudofolliculitis, and papulopustular or acneiform nodules [**Figure 57-18, A and B**]. Ocular disease is commonly found in patients with BD and can cause visual impairment with risk of blindness. Ocular findings may include anterior and posterior uveitis, retinal vasculitis, cataracts, glaucoma, vitritis, retinitis, retinal edema, macular degeneration, thrombosis, disc edema, and retinal detachment [**Figure 57-19, A and B**]. Anterior uveitis generally has a good prognosis. However, posterior segment involvement of the eye can cause irreversible damage with loss of vision.[45-53]

Since BD is considered a systemic vasculitis, patients may develop vascular manifestations. These include superficial thrombophlebitis and deep vein thrombosis. Arterial thrombosis is less common but can involve the pulmonary arteries, aorta, renal arteries, coronary arteries, and peripheral arteries. Like many other systemic inflammatory disorders, BD can affect the joints. Arthralgias and arthritis are relatively common, occurring in up to half of cases, and may be the presenting sign. Neurologic manifestations usually occur later in the disease course.

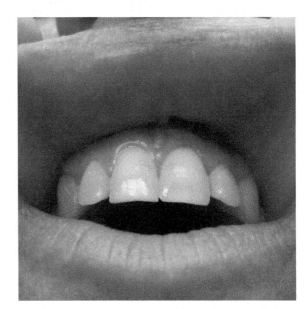

FIGURE 57-16. Behçet disease: multiple small discrete ulcerations on the labial mucosa of the upper lip.

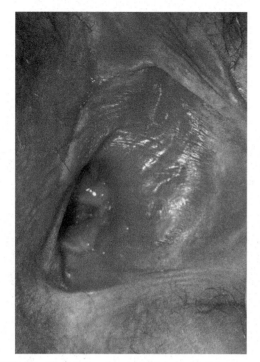

FIGURE 57-17. Behçet disease: ulcerations at the vulvar introitus.

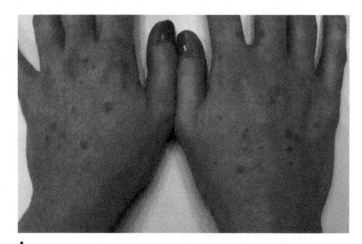

A

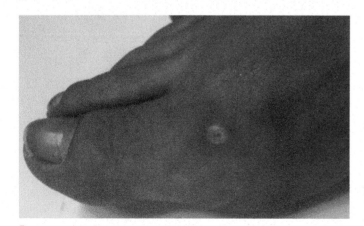

B

FIGURE 57-18. (A and B) Behçet disease: papulopustular lesions on the hands and feet.

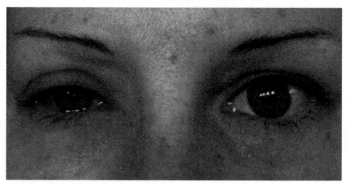

A

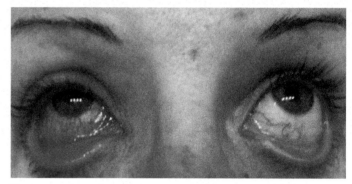

B

FIGURE 57-19. (A and B) Behçet disease: anterior uveitis and diffuse panscleritis with prominent conjunctival injection.

Symptoms include headache, seizures, meningitis, meningoencephalitis, cranial nerve palsies, and hemiplegia.[45-50,54]

The goals of treatment for BD are symptomatic relief, prevention of tissue damage, and reduction of the severity and frequency of attacks. However, younger patients and males have more severe disease and often require aggressive treatment.[55] Systemic therapies include corticosteroids, colchicine, dapsone, thalidomide, methotrexate, azathioprine, cyclophosphamide, cyclosporine, mycophenolate mofetil, interferon-α, and anti-TNF agents. The choice of therapy is dependent on the severity of symptoms and organ systems involved[47-50,55-60] [**Table 57-4**].

Systemic corticosteroids are used alone or in combination with other systemic medications to treat mucocutaneous lesions, acute uveitis, and neurologic disease. Corticosteroids are typically dosed at 1 mg/kg/d. Dapsone also inhibits the chemotactic activity of neutrophils and can be used in combination with colchicine. Thalidomide inhibits TNF

TABLE 57-4	**Systemic therapies for Behçet disease**	
Medication	Dosing regimen	Main adverse effects
Colchicine	0.6–1.2 mg every day	Myelosuppression, hepatotoxicity, diarrhea, nausea, vomiting, and headaches
Corticosteroids	1–1.5 mg/kg/d	Osteoporosis, hypertension, hyperglycemia, weight gain, and cataracts
Cyclosporine	5 mg/kg/d	Hypertension, headache, gingival hyperplasia, hyperlipidemia, hyperkalemia, hyperuricemia, and hypomagnesemia
Mycophenolate mofetil	1.5–3 g/d	Weakness, fatigue, headache, nausea, diarrhea, anorexia, and dysuria
Methotrexate	7.5–20 mg/wk	Hepatotoxicity, pancytopenia, teratogenicity, nausea, and anorexia
Azathioprine	2.5 mg/kg/d	Gastrointestinal disturbances, hepatotoxicity, and myelotoxicity

synthesis and is used to treat oral and genital ulcerations. Methotrexate is used to treat mucocutaneous lesions, ocular disease, and neurologic disease. Azathioprine suppresses both the cellular and humoral immune response and has been used to treat genital and oral ulcerations and arthritis and to prevent the development of eye disease. Cyclophospha-mide is an alkylating agent that has been proven useful for ocular disease and systemic vasculitis. It is reserved for severe cases not responding to other therapies due its severe toxicity. Cyclosporine is an immunosup-pressant that inhibits T-lymphocytes. It is used to treat mucocutaneous lesions and ocular disease. However, the use of cyclosporine should be limited to refractory cases due its systemic side effects and increased Behçet's-related neurologic manifestations in patients on cyclosporine therapy. Mycophenolate mofetil inhibits B and T-cells, thereby inhibiting both the humoral and cellular immune response. It has been used for the treatment of ocular manifestations. Interferon-α has been used for mucocutaneous disease, ocular disease, and arthritis. Anti-TNF agents such as etanercept, infliximab, and adalimumab have been useful for the treatment of all manifestations of BD including mucocutaneous lesions, ocular disease, arthritis, and vasculitis.[47-50,55-60]

ORAL LICHEN PLANUS

The prevalence of oral lichen planus (LP) has been reported in the range of 0.5% to 2.2%, with a gender predilection in women. It is most common in adults aged between 40 and 70, but can rarely occur in children. Children represent less than 5% of those affected. About half of patients with cutaneous LP go on to develop oral LP, and about a quarter of patients present with oral LP without skin manifestations.[61-70]

The pathogenesis of LP remains unclear. However, it is now established that LP is an immune reaction initiated by an unknown antigen in genetically predisposed individuals.[62,64,67,71-74] Hepatitis C virus has also been implicated in the pathogenesis of LP. Epidemiologic studies have shown a significant association between hepatitis C and LP.[75-77] An association has also been shown between human papilloma virus (HPV), especially HPV-16, and oral LP. The prevalence of HPV may be a factor in the malignant transformation of LP into squamous cell carcinoma.[78-81] Although the significance of the association of LP with hepatitis C and HPV remains unclear, it is important to screen patients for these viruses.

LP is a chronic inflammatory disorder that affects the skin, cutaneous appendages, and mucous membranes. Oral LP has a more chronic course and often causes long-term morbidity. Oral LP can present anywhere in the oral mucosa but most commonly involves the buccal mucosa, tongue, and gingiva. It is divided into six clinical subtypes, which include reticular, papular, plaque, atrophic, erosive, and bullous LP. Reticular oral LP is the most common presentation. It presents as fine white striae on the buccal mucosa and is usually asymptomatic. It may also be found on the lateral tongue and gingiva [**Figure 57-20, A and B**]. Papular oral LP presents as asymptomatic white papules and is thought to be underdiagnosed. Plaque-like oral LP presents with asymptomatic white plaques that can resemble leukoplakia most often present on the dorsal tongue and buccal mucosa [**Figure 57-21**]. It is more common in tobacco smokers. Atrophic oral LP presents as diffuse red plaques with surrounding white striae. Erosive oral LP is the second most common type of oral LP. It presents with irregular painful erosions covered with a pseudomembrane and has surrounding white striae [**Figure 57-22, A and B**]. It frequently causes a burning sensation, especially when exposed to certain foods. Patients often complain of an intolerance to spicy foods, hot beverages, and citrus fruits and juices to the extent that they may restrict these foods from their diet entirely. Bullous oral LP presents with bullae that rupture easily and cause painful erosions that range in size from millimeters to centimeters. It is the rarest form of oral LP.[62-64,67,70,82-84]

Oral LP poses a risk for malignant transformation, possibly due to chronic inflammation, although the underlying mechanism continues to be unclear. The risk of malignant transformation is highest with the erosive and atrophic patterns of oral LP.[62,67,78-82,84] The increased risk of malignant transformation of oral LP is not necessarily linked to other risk factors for squamous cell carcinoma such as tobacco and alcohol

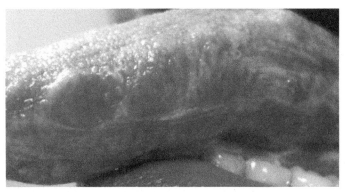

A

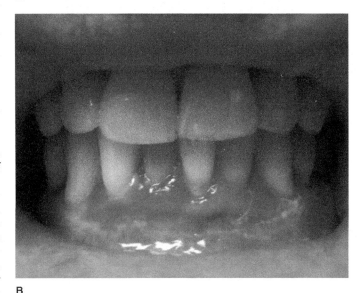

B

FIGURE 57-20. (A and B) Reticulated oral lichen planus: prominent white striations on the ventral tongue and gingivae.

use. It is also thought that immunosuppressive therapy and HPV exposure may have a synergistic role in the oral cancer morbidity of oral LP patients. The use of immunosuppressive drugs such as topical and systemic steroids may be associated with enhanced viral replication, which can theoretically affect the risk of malignant transformation.

LP can also affect other mucosal sites besides the oral mucosa, such as the esophagus, larynx, ocular mucosa, and genital mucosa. Esophageal LP is a rare manifestation of the disease that is thought to be under-reported and underrecognized. Esophageal symptoms may precede,

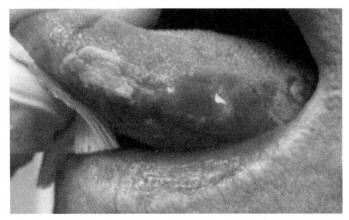

FIGURE 57-21. Plaque-like oral lichen planus: white-colored plaques on the lateral tongue.

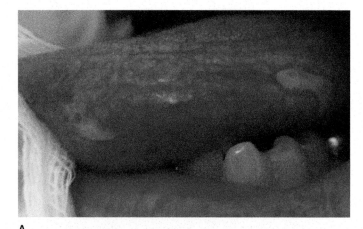

A

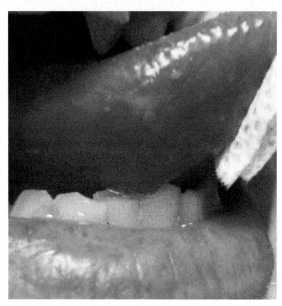

B

FIGURE 57-22. (A and B) Erosive oral lichen planus: ulcerations on the ventral tongue with surrounding reticulated white striations.

present simultaneously with, or develop after other manifestations of the disease. Esophageal LP is most common in middle-age women. The most commonly associated symptoms are dysphagia, odynophagia (pain with swallowing), and weight loss. Associated heartburn-like symptoms can lead to a misdiagnosis of gastroesophageal reflux disease. There have been rare cases of squamous cell carcinoma developing in association with esophageal LP; thus endoscopy should be performed in any LP patients with dysphagia or odynophagia.[63,85,86] Timely recognition and prompt initiation of therapy for esophageal involvement are important, given the associated sequelae of esophageal strictures, webs, and erosions.

Ocular LP can present with blepharitis or conjunctivitis. Patients with chronic keratoconjunctivitis can develop fibrosis, dryness, entropion, and corneal opacifications resulting in visual loss. Any patient with eye complaints should be evaluated by an ophthalmologist.[63,83,87-91] LP involving the genital mucosa is more common in perimenopausal and postmenopausal women. It has various presentations, including asymptomatic white reticular patches, erosive lesions, papulosquamous lesions, and hypertrophic lesions. Erosive genital LP is the most common subtype, and like oral erosive disease, it can cause significant pain and scarring with dyspareunia and impairment in sexual function. In women, scarring can lead to resorption of the labia minora and clitoral hood, as well as stenosis of the vaginal introitus. The long-term sequelae of the disease can cause disruption of sexual function and detrimentally

affect the patient's overall quality of life. Other associated symptoms are pruritus and burning.[61,63,83,84]

Whenever the diagnosis of LP is considered, a drug history should be completed to rule out a lichenoid drug reaction. Lichenoid drug reactions usually present in a photodistribution and do not have oral or other mucosal involvement. The most common implicated drugs are thiazide diuretics, β-blockers, angiotensin-converting enzyme inhibitors, spironolactone, and furosemide. Other rare diagnoses that may mimic LP are lichenoid contact reactions and lichenoid mycosis fungoides.[62,67,92-94]

The treatment of oral LP should be guided by the type of oral LP the patient exhibits. Reticular, papular, and plaque-type oral LP are usually asymptomatic and may not require treatment. However, atrophic, erosive, and bullous forms of the disease can cause pain and difficulty with eating, necessitating prompt initiation of therapy. Erosive and atrophic oral LP have been shown to rarely display malignant transformation, further necessitating aggressive treatment. It is important to recognize that oral LP is a chronic disease and requires long-term treatment and follow-up. First-line treatment of symptomatic oral LP is topical corticosteroids. Several small randomized controlled trials have shown significant improvement of symptoms in patients using potent topical corticosteroids versus placebo. Oral corticosteroids are used when patients do not respond to topical formulations or in patients with severe symptoms. Topical and oral retinoids have been used as a second-line treatment with varying results, although oral retinoids such as acitretin have been shown in randomized controlled trials to cause significant improvement in symptoms and disease. Topical retinoids have been used with some improvement in symptoms, but were less effective than topical corticosteroids in a head-to-head comparison. Topical calcineurin inhibitors have likewise been used as second-line treatment and have been shown to cause improvement in symptoms and the severity of disease when compared to placebo and were comparable to topical corticosteroids in a head-to-head trial. However, improvement was not sustained once therapy was discontinued. Topical cyclosporine has also been used with improvement in symptoms in oral LP. Randomized controlled trials comparing topical cyclosporine to high- and mid-potency corticosteroids showed no difference in efficacy.[62,67,82,95-124]

REFERENCES

1. Shulman JD, Carpenter WM. Prevalence and risk factors associated with geographic tongue among US adults. *Oral Dis.* 2006;12:381-386.
2. Assimakopoulos D, Patrikakos G, Fotika C, Elisaf M. Benign migratory glossitis or geographic tongue: an enigmatic oral lesion. *Am J Med.* 2002; 113:751-755.
3. van der Wal N, van der Kwast WA, van Dijk E, van der Waal I. Geographic stomatitis and psoriasis. *Int J Oral Maxillofac Surg.* 1988;17:106-109.
4. Ishibashi M, Tojo G, Watanabe M, Tamabuchi T, Masu T, Aiba S. Geographic tongue treated with topical tacrolimus. *J Dermatol Case Rep.* 2010; 4:57-59.
5. Jainkittivong A, Apinhasmit W, Swasdison S. Prevalence and clinical characterisics of oral tori in 1,520 Chulalongkorn University Dental School patients. *Surg Radiol Anat.* 2007;29:125-131.
6. Jainkittivong A, Langlais RP. Buccal and palatal exostoses: prevalence and concurrence with tori. *Oral Surg Oral Med Oral Pathol Oral Radiol Endod.* 2000;90:48-53.
7. Morrison MD, Tamimi F. Oral tori are associated with local mechanical and systemic factors: a case-control study. *J Oral Maxillofac Surg.* 2013;71:14-22.
8. Garcia-Garcia AS, Martinez-Gonzalez JM, Gomez-Font R, Soto-Rivadeneira A, Oviedo-Roldan L. Current status of the torus palatinus and torus mandibularis. *Med Oral Patol Oral Cir Bucal.* 2010;15:e353-e360.
9. Seah YH. Torus palatinus and torus mandibularis: a review of the literature. *Aust Dental J.* 1995;40:318-321.
10. Nisa L, Giger R. Black hairy tongue. *Am J Med.* 2011;124:816-817.
11. Vano-Galvan S, Jaen P. Black hairy tongue. *Cleve Clin J Med.* 2008;75:847-848.
12. Akay BN, Sanli H, Topcuoglu P, Zincircioglu G, Gurgan C, Heper AO. Black hairy tongue after allogeneic stem cell transplantation: an unrecognized cutaneous presentation of graft-versus-host disease. *Transplant Proc.* 2010;42:4603-4607.

13. Thompson DF, Kessler TL. Drug-induced black hairy tongue. *Pharmacotherapy.* 2010;30:585-593.

14. Ho KK, Dervan P, O'Loughlin S, Powell FC. Labial melanotic macule: a clinical, histopathologic, and ultrastructural study. *J Am Acad Dermatol.* 1993;28:33-39.

15. Kaugars GE, Heise AP, Riley WT, Abbey LM, Svirsky JA. Oral melanotic macules. A review of 353 cases. *Oral Surg Oral Med Oral Pathol.* 1993;76:59-61.

16. Page LR, Corio RL, Crawford BE, Giansanti JS, Weathers DR. The oral melanotic macule. *Oral Surg Oral Med Oral Pathol.* 1977;44:219-226.

17. Shen ZY, Liu W, Bao ZX, Zhou ZT, Wang LZ. Oral melanotic macule and primary oral malignant melanoma: epidemiology, location involved, and clinical implications. *Oral Surg Oral Med Oral Pathol Oral Radiol Endod.* 2011;112(1):e21-e25.

18. Buchner A, Hansen LS. Pigmented nevi of the oral mucosa: a clinicopathologic study of 32 new cases and review of 75 cases from the literature. Part II. Analysis of 107 cases. *Oral Surg Oral Med Oral Pathol.* 1980;49:55-62.

19. Buchner A, Leider AS, Merrell PW, Carpenter WM. Melanocytic nevi of the oral mucosa: a clinicopathologic study of 130 cases from northern California. *J Oral Pathol.* 1990;19:197-201.

20. Buchner A, Merrell PW, Carpenter WM. Relative frequency of solitary melanocytic lesions of the oral mucosa. *J Oral Pathol Med.* 2004;33:550-557.

21. Meleti M, Vescovi P, Mooi WJ, van der Waal I. Pigmented lesions of the oral mucosa and perioral tissues: a flow-chart for the diagnosis and some recommendations for the management. *Oral Surg Oral Med Oral Pathol Oral Radiol Endod.* 2008;105:606-616.

22. Buchner A, Hansen LS. Amalgam pigmentation (amalgam tattoo) of the oral mucosa. A clinicopathologic study of 268 cases. *Oral Surg Oral Med Oral Pathol.* 1980;49:139-147.

23. Pigatto PD, Brambilla L, Guzzi G. Amalgam tattoo: a close-up view. *J Eur Acad Dermatol Venereol.* 2006;20:1352-1353.

24. Tran HT, Anandasabapathy N, Soldano AC. Amalgam tattoo. *Dermatol Online J.* 2008;14:19.

25. Amano H, Tamura A, Yasuda M, et al. Amalgam tattoo of the oral mucosa mimics malignant melanoma. *J Dermatol.* 2011;38:101-103.

26. Shah G, Alster TS. Treatment of an amalgam tattoo with a Q-switched alexandrite (755 nm) laser. *Dermatol Surg.* 2002;28:1180-1181.

27. Arduino PG, Porter SR. Oral and perioral herpes simplex virus type 1 (HSV-1) infection: review of its management. *Oral Dis.* 2006;12:254-270.

28. Arduino PG, Porter SR. Herpes simplex virus type 1 infection: overview on relevant clinico-pathological features. *J Oral Pathol Med.* 2008;37:107-121.

29. Whitley RJ, Roizman B. Herpes simplex virus infections. *Lancet.* 2001;357:1513-1518.

30. Whitley RJ. Changing epidemiology of herpes simplex virus infections. *Clin Infect Dis.* 2013;56:352-353.

31. Cunningham A, Griffiths P, Leone P, et al. Current management and recommendations for access to antiviral therapy of herpes labialis. *J Clin Virol.* 2012;53:6-11.

32. Nasser M, Fedorowicz Z, Khoshnevisan MH, Shahiri Tabarestani M. Acyclovir for treating primary herpetic gingivostomatitis. *Cochrane Database Syst Rev.* 2008;4:CD006700.

33. Porter SR. Little clinical benefit of early systemic aciclovir for treatment of primary herpetic stomatitis. *Evid Based Dent.* 2008;9:117.

34. Kim J, Sudbery P. *Candida albicans*, a major human fungal pathogen. *J Microbiol.* 2011;49:171-177.

35. Farah CS, Lynch N, McCullough MJ. Oral fungal infections: an update for the general practitioner. *Aust Dent J.* 2010;55(Suppl 1):48-54.

36. Giannini PJ, Shetty KV. Diagnosis and management of oral candidiasis. *Otolaryngol Clin North Am.* 2011;44:231-240.

37. Rautemaa R, Ramage G. Oral candidosis: clinical challenges of a biofilm disease. *Crit Rev Microbiol.* 2011;37:328-336.

38. Chattopadhyay A, Shetty KV. Recurrent aphthous stomatitis. *Otolaryngol Clin North Am.* 2011;44:79-88.

39. Chavan M, Jain H, Diwan N, Khedkar S, Shete A, Durkar S. Recurrent aphthous stomatitis: a review. *J Oral Pathol Med.* 2012;41:577-583.

40. Femiano F, Lanza A, Buonaiuto C, et al. Guidelines for diagnosis and management of aphthous stomatitis. *Pediatr Infect Dis J.* 2007;26:728-732.

41. Liang MW, Neoh CY. Oral aphthosis: management gaps and recent advances. *Ann Acad Med Singapore.* 2012;41:463-470.

42. Baccaglini L, Lalla RV, Bruce AJ, et al. Urban legends: recurrent aphthous stomatitis. *Oral Dis.* 2011;17:755-770.

43. Altenburg A, Abdel-Naser MB, Seeber H, Abdallah M, Zouboulis CC. Practical aspects of management of recurrent aphthous stomatitis. *J Eur Acad Dermatol Venereol.* 2007;21:1019-1026.

44. Brocklehurst P, Tickle M, Glenny AM, et al. Systemic interventions for recurrent aphthous stomatitis (mouth ulcers). *Cochrane Database Syst Rev.* 2012;9:CD005411.

45. Dalvi SR, Yildirim R, Yazici Y. Behcet's syndrome. *Drugs.* 2012;72:2223-2241.

46. Davatchi F. Diagnosis/classification criteria for Behcet's disease. *Pathol Res Int.* 2012;2012:607921.

47. Hatemi G, Seyahi E, Fresko I, Hamuryudan V. Behcet's syndrome: a critical digest of the recent literature. *Clin Exp Rheumatol.* 2012;30(3 Suppl 72):S80-S89.

48. Mendes D, Correia M, Barbedo M, et al. Behcet's disease—a contemporary review. *J Autoimmun.* 2009;32:178-188.

49. Saadoun D, Wechsler B. Behcet's disease. *Orphan J Rare Dis.* 2012;7:20.

50. Yurdakul S, Yazici H. Behcet's syndrome. *Best Pract Res Clin Rheumatol.* 2008;22:793-809.

51. Criteria for diagnosis of Behcet's disease. International Study Group for Behcet's Disease. *Lancet.* 1990;335:1078-1080.

52. Mendoza-Pinto C, Garcia-Carrasco M, Jimenez-Hernandez M, et al. Etiopathogenesis of Behcet's disease. *Autoimmun Rev.* 2010;9:241-245.

53. Pineton de Chambrun M, Wechsler B, Geri G, Cacoub P, Saadoun D. New insights into the pathogenesis of Behcet's disease. *Autoimmun Rev.* 2012;11:687-698.

54. Malik AA, Halabi AM, Jamil G, Qureshi A. Rare manifestation of Behcet's syndrome: insight from multimodality cardiovascular imaging. BMJ Case Reports 2012;10.1136/bcr-2012-007148.

55. Hatemi G, Silman A, Bang D, et al. EULAR recommendations for the management of Behcet disease. *Ann Rheum Dis.* 2008;67:1656-1662.

56. Alexoudi I, Kapsimali V, Vaiopoulos A, Kanakis M, Vaiopoulos G. Evaluation of current therapeutic strategies in Behcet's disease. *Clin Rheumatol.* 2011;30:157-163.

57. Alpsoy E, Akman A. Behcet's disease: an algorithmic approach to its treatment. *Arch Dermatol Res.* 2009;301:693-702.

58. Ambrose NL, Haskard DO. Differential diagnosis and management of Behcet syndrome. *Nat Rev Rheumatol.* 2013;9:79-89.

59. Benitah NR, Sobrin L, Papaliodis GN. The use of biologic agents in the treatment of ocular manifestations of Behcet's disease. *Semin Ophthalmol.* 2011;26:295-303.

60. Evereklioglu C. Ocular Behcet disease: current therapeutic approaches. *Curr Opin Ophthalmol.* 2011;22:508-516.

61. Belfiore P, Di Fede O, Cabibi D, et al. Prevalence of vulval lichen planus in a cohort of women with oral lichen planus: an interdisciplinary study. *Br J Dermatol.* 2006;155:994-948.

62. Bricker SL. Oral lichen planus: a review. *Semin Dermatol.* 1994;13:87-90.

63. Eisen D. The evaluation of cutaneous, genital, scalp, nail, esophageal, and ocular involvement in patients with oral lichen planus. *Oral Surg Oral Med Oral Pathol Oral Radiol Endod.* 1999;88:431-436.

64. Eisen D. The clinical features, malignant potential, and systemic associations of oral lichen planus: a study of 723 patients. *J Am Acad Dermatol.* 2002;46:207-214.

65. Kanwar AJ, De D. Lichen planus in childhood: report of 100 cases. *Clin Exp Dermatol.* 2010;35:257-262.

66. McCartan BE, Healy CM. The reported prevalence of oral lichen planus: a review and critique. *J Oral Pathol Med.* 2008;37:447-453.

67. Mollaoglu N. Oral lichen planus: a review. *Br J Oral Maxillofac Surg.* 2000;38:370-377.

68. Sharma R, Maheshwari V. Childhood lichen planus: a report of fifty cases. *Pediatr Dermatol.* 1999;16:345-348.

69. Silverman S Jr, Gorsky M, Lozada-Nur F. A prospective follow-up study of 570 patients with oral lichen planus: persistence, remission, and malignant association. *Oral Surg Oral Med Oral Pathol.* 1985;60:30-34.

70. Sousa FA, Rosa LE. Oral lichen planus: clinical and histopathological considerations. *Braz J Otorhinolaryngol.* 2008;74:284-292.

71. Brant JM, Vasconcelos AC, Rodrigues LV. Role of apoptosis in erosive and reticular oral lichen planus exhibiting variable epithelial thickness. *Braz Den J.* 2008;19:179-185.

72. Ichimura M, Hiratsuka K, Ogura N, et al. Expression profile of chemokines and chemokine receptors in epithelial cell layers of oral lichen planus. *J Oral Pathol Med.* 2006;35:167-174.

73. Santoro A, Majorana A, Bardellini E, et al. Cytotoxic molecule expression and epithelial cell apoptosis in oral and cutaneous lichen planus. *Am J Clin Pathol.* 2004;121:758-764.

74. Spandau U, Toksoy A, Goebeler M, Brocker EB, Gillitzer R. MIG is a dominant lymphocyte-attractant chemokine in lichen planus lesions. *J Invest Dermatol.* 1998;111:1003-1009.

75. Lodi G, Giuliani M, Majorana A, et al. Lichen planus and hepatitis C virus: a multicentre study of patients with oral lesions and a systematic review. *Br J Dermatol.* 2004;151:1172-1181.

76. Lodi G, Pellicano R, Carrozzo M. Hepatitis C virus infection and lichen planus: a systematic review with meta-analysis. *Oral Dis.* 2010;16:601-612.

77. Shengyuan L, Songpo Y, Wen W, Wenjing T, Haitao Z, Binyou W. Hepatitis C virus and lichen planus: a reciprocal association determined by a meta-analysis. *Arch Dermatol.* 2009;145:1040-1047.

78. Bombeccari GP, Guzzi G, Tettamanti M, et al. Oral lichen planus and malignant transformation: a longitudinal cohort study. *Oral Surg Oral Med Oral Pathol Oral Radiol Endod.* 2011;112:328-334.

79. Gorsky M, Epstein JB. Oral lichen planus: malignant transformation and human papilloma virus: a review of potential clinical implications. *Oral Surg Oral Med Oral Pathol Oral Radiol Endod.* 2011;111:461-464.

80. Lo Muzio L, Mignogna MD, Favia G, Procaccini M, Testa NF, Bucci E. The possible association between oral lichen planus and oral squamous cell carcinoma: a clinical evaluation on 14 cases and a review of the literature. *Oral Oncol.* 1998;34:239-246.

81. Syrjanen S, Lodi G, von Bultzingslowen I, et al. Human papillomaviruses in oral carcinoma and oral potentially malignant disorders: a systematic review. *Oral Dis.* 2011;17(Suppl 1):58-72.

82. Eisen D. The clinical manifestations and treatment of oral lichen planus. *Dermatol Clin.* 2003;21:79-89.

83. Shaikh ZI, Arfan ul B, Mashhood AA, Qayyum A, Latif ur R. Mucosal lichen planus simultaneously involving oral mucosa, conjunctiva and larynx. *J Coll Physicians Surg Pak.* 2010;20:478-479.

84. Shklar G. Erosive and bullous oral lesions of lichen planus: histologic studies. *Arch Dermatol.* 1968;97:411-416.

85. Fox LP, Lightdale CJ, Grossman ME. Lichen planus of the esophagus: what dermatologists need to know. *J Am Acad Dermatol.* 2011;65:175-183.

86. Izol B, Karabulut AA, Biyikoglu I, Gonultas M, Eksioglu M. Investigation of upper gastrointestinal tract involvement and *H. pylori* presence in lichen planus: a case-controlled study with endoscopic and histopathological findings. *Int J Dermatol.* 2010;49:1121-1126.

87. Brewer JD, Ekdawi NS, Torgerson RR, et al. Lichen planus and cicatricial conjunctivitis: disease course and response to therapy of 11 patients. *J Eur Acad Dermatol Venereol.* 2011;25:100-104.

88. Crosby MB, Crosby CV, Wojno TH, Grossniklaus HE. Conjunctival lichen planus in a patient with herpes simplex virus keratitis. *Cornea.* 2009;28:936-937.

89. Pakravan M, Klesert TR, Akpek EK. Isolated lichen planus of the conjunctiva. *Br J Ophthalmol.* 2006;90:1325-1326.

90. Ramos-Esteban JC, Schoenfield L, Singh AD. Conjunctival lichen planus simulating ocular surface squamous neoplasia. *Cornea.* 2009;28:1181-1183.

91. Rozas Munoz E, Martinez-Escala ME, Juanpere N, Armentia J, Pujol RM, Herrero-Gonzalez JE. Isolated conjunctival lichen planus: a diagnostic challenge. *Arch Dermatol.* 2011;147:465-467.

92. Athavale PN, Shum KW, Yeoman CM, Gawkrodger DJ. Oral lichenoid lesions and contact allergy to dental mercury and gold. *Contact Derm.* 2003;49:264-265.

93. Rogers RS 3rd, Bruce AJ. Lichenoid contact stomatitis: is inorganic mercury the culprit? *Arch Dermatol.* 2004;140:1524-1525.

94. Schlosser BJ. Lichen planus and lichenoid reactions of the oral mucosa. *Dermatol Ther.* 2010;23:251-267.

95. Buajeeb W, Kraivaphan P, Pobrurksa C. Efficacy of topical retinoic acid compared with topical fluocinolone acetonide in the treatment of oral lichen planus. *Oral Surg Oral Med Oral Pathol Oral Radiol Endod.* 1997;83:21-25.

96. Buajeeb W, Pobrurksa C, Kraivaphan P. Efficacy of fluocinolone acetonide gel in the treatment of oral lichen planus. *Oral Surg Oral Med Oral Pathol Oral Radiol Endod.* 2000;89:42-45.

97. Carbone M, Arduino PG, Carrozzo M, et al. Topical clobetasol in the treatment of atrophic-erosive oral lichen planus: a randomized controlled trial to compare two preparations with different concentrations. *J Oral Pathol Med.* 2009;38:227-233.

98. Cawson RA. Treatment of oral lichen planus with betamethasone. *Br Med J.* 1968;13:86-89.

99. Conrotto D, Carbone M, Carrozzo M, et al. Ciclosporin vs. clobetasol in the topical management of atrophic and erosive oral lichen planus: a double-blind, randomized controlled trial. *Br J Dermatol.* 2006;154:139-145.

100. Corrocher G, Di Lorenzo G, Martinelli N, et al. Comparative effect of tacrolimus 0.1% ointment and clobetasol 0.05% ointment in patients with oral lichen planus. *J Clin Periodontol.* 2008;35:244-249.

101. Eisen D, Ellis CN, Duell EA, Griffiths CE, Voorhees JJ. Effect of topical cyclosporine rinse on oral lichen planus. A double-blind analysis. *N Engl J Med.* 1990;323:290-294.

102. Giustina TA, Stewart JC, Ellis CN, et al. Topical application of isotretinoin gel improves oral lichen planus. A double-blind study. *Arch Dermatol.* 1986;122:534-536.

103. Gonzalez-Moles MA, Morales P, Rodriguez-Archilla A. The treatment of oral aphthous ulceration or erosive lichen planus with topical clobetasol propionate in three preparations. A clinical study on 54 patients. *J Oral Pathol Med.* 2002;31:284-285.

104. Gorouhi F, Solhpour A, Beitollahi JM, et al. Randomized trial of pimecrolimus cream versus triamcinolone acetonide paste in the treatment of oral lichen planus. *J Am Acad Dermatol.* 2007;57:806-813.

105. Holmstrup P, Schiotz AW, Westergaard J. Effect of dental plaque control on gingival lichen planus. *Oral Surg Oral Med Oral Pathol.* 1990;69:585-590.

106. Iraji F, Faghihi G, Asilian A, Siadat AH, Larijani FT, Akbari M. Comparison of the narrow band UVB versus systemic corticosteroids in the treatment of lichen planus: a randomized clinical trial. *J Res Med Sci.* 2011;16:1578-1582.

107. Kellett JK, Ead RD. Treatment of lichen planus with a short course of oral prednisolone. *Br J Dermatol.* 1990;123:550-551.

108. Laeijendecker R, Tank B, Dekker SK, Neumann HA. A comparison of treatment of oral lichen planus with topical tacrolimus and triamcinolone acetonide ointment. *Acta Derm Venereol.* 2006;86:227-229.

109. Laurberg G, Geiger JM, Hjorth N, et al. Treatment of lichen planus with acitretin. A double-blind, placebo-controlled study in 65 patients. *J Am Acad Dermatol.* 1991;24:434-437.

110. Le Cleach L, Chosidow O. Clinical practice. Lichen planus. *N Engl J Med.* 2012;366:723-732.

111. McCaughey C, Machan M, Bennett R, Zone JJ, Hull CM. Pimecrolimus 1% cream for oral erosive lichen planus: a 6-week randomized, double-blind, vehicle-controlled study with a 6-week open-label extension to assess efficacy and safety. *J Eur Acad Dermatol Venereol.* 2011;25:1061-1067.

112. Ormerod AD, Campalani E, Goodfield MJ, BAD Clinical Standards Unit. British Association of Dermatologists guidelines on the efficacy and use of acitretin in dermatology. *Br J Dermatol.* 2010;162:952-963.

113. Passeron T, Lacour JP, Fontas E, Ortonne JP. Treatment of oral erosive lichen planus with 1% pimecrolimus cream: a double-blind, randomized, prospective trial with measurement of pimecrolimus levels in the blood. *Arch Dermatol.* 2007;143:472-476.

114. Radfar L, Wild RC, Suresh L. A comparative treatment study of topical tacrolimus and clobetasol in oral lichen planus. *Oral Surg Oral Med Oral Pathol Oral Radiol Endod.* 2008;105:187-193.

115. Scardina GA, Messina P, Carini F, Maresi E. A randomized trial assessing the effectiveness of different concentrations of isotretinoin in the management of lichen planus. *Int J Oral Maxillofac Surg.* 2006;35:67-71.

116. Sieg P, Von Domarus H, Von Zitzewitz V, Iven H, Farber L. Topical cyclosporin in oral lichen planus: a controlled, randomized, prospective trial. *Br J Dermatol.* 1995;132:790-794.

117. Sonthalia S, Singal A. Comparative efficacy of tacrolimus 0.1% ointment and clobetasol propionate 0.05% ointment in oral lichen planus: a randomized double-blind trial. *Int J Dermatol.* 2012;51:1371-1378.

118. Swift JC, Rees TD, Plemons JM, Hallmon WW, Wright JC. The effectiveness of 1% pimecrolimus cream in the treatment of oral erosive lichen planus. *J Periodontol.* 2005;76:627-635.

119. Thongprasom K, Chaimusig M, Korkij W, Sererat T, Luangjarmekorn L, Rojwattanasirivej S. A randomized-controlled trial to compare topical cyclosporin with triamcinolone acetonide for the treatment of oral lichen planus. *J Oral Pathol Med.* 2007;36:142-146.

120. Thorn JJ, Holmstrup P, Rindum J, Pindborg JJ. Course of various clinical forms of oral lichen planus. A prospective follow-up study of 611 patients. *J Oral Pathol.* 1988;17:213-218.

121. Volz T, Caroli U, Ludtke H, et al. Pimecrolimus cream 1% in erosive oral lichen planus—a prospective randomized double-blind vehicle-controlled study. *Br J Dermatol.* 2008;159:936-941.

122. Voute AB, Schulten EA, Langendijk PN, Kostense PJ, van der Waal I. Fluocinonide in an adhesive base for treatment of oral lichen planus. A double-blind, placebo-controlled clinical study. *Oral Surg Oral Med Oral Pathol.* 1993;75:181-185.

123. Yoke PC, Tin GB, Kim MJ, et al. A randomized controlled trial to compare steroid with cyclosporine for the topical treatment of oral lichen planus. *Oral Surg Oral Med Oral Pathol Oral Radiol Endod.* 2006;102:47-55.

124. Zegarelli DJ. The treatment of oral lichen planus. *Ann Dent.* 1993;52:3-8.

CHAPTER 58

Genital Lesions in Men

Theodore Rosen
Sean D. Doherty

KEY POINTS

- Genital lesions may have a unique appearance in patients with skin of color, and both the frequency and the appearance may vary between men and women.

- Some African Americans and Hispanics have higher rates of primary and secondary syphilis in comparison to other racial groups.

- In the United States, reported cases of chancroid generally occur in urban epidemics and are most common in men with darker skin of color.

- In tinea cruris, patients with darker skin of color may present with striking hyperpigmentation rather than erythema, and genital skin may not have scales.

- Psoriasis occurs less commonly in Americans with darker skin of color (0.1%) than in Caucasian Americans (1%), and lesions in individuals with darker skin of color may possess an atypical morphology and thus may require biopsy confirmation.

- A high mortality rate from genital squamous cell carcinoma has been reported in the past among those with darker skin of color, both in the United States and in Africa.

- Genital dermatoses may occur only on the genitalia or may occur anywhere on the body, and lesions may have a different appearance when found on genital skin compared with other anatomic sites.

INTRODUCTION

Genital lesions may have a unique appearance in individuals with skin of color. There also may be variation in both statistical frequency and clinical characteristics of selected lesions between men and women. Genital dermatoses include a wide variety of diagnoses, and lesions may occur only on the genitalia or also may occur elsewhere on the body. When lesions appear on genital skin, they may have a unique morphology. The thin, moist skin typically found in the genital region is at least partially responsible for the different characteristics of lesions in this region.[1] For example, the dry scale that may be a prominent manifestation of lesions elsewhere may not be present in the genital region. Furthermore, genital lesions and the concern over the possibility of a sexually transmitted infection (STI) may cause significant anxiety for the patient. Genital lesions may result from a variety of etiologies, including non-STI infectious agents, inflammatory cutaneous disorders, multisystem diseases, benign and malignant neoplasms, and exogenous factors.

It is often difficult to distinguish between one genital disorder and similar entities based solely on morphology. In various published studies, physicians have had an accuracy of only 33% to 80% in diagnosing genital lesions based solely on appearance.[2] The physician should not hesitate to perform additional diagnostic testing, including serologic studies, bacterial and viral cultures, cytologic studies, colposcopic examinations, incisional and excisional biopsies, and other appropriate studies. Additionally, a full-body skin check and a detailed review of systems may be necessary when evaluating a patient with genital lesions.

INFECTIOUS DISEASES

▥ SEXUALLY TRANSMITTED INFECTIONS

Syphilis

Epidemiology, Etiology, and Pathogenesis Syphilis is caused by the spirochete *Treponema pallidum*, with an incubation period of 9 to 90 days. The organism is transferred between individuals by direct sexual contact. Infection is most likely to occur through microbreaks in normal skin occurring during sexual activity but may occur though intact mucous membranes.[3]

In 2000, the rate of primary and secondary syphilis in the United States was the lowest since reporting began in 1941.[4] From 2001 to 2004, the rate increased 30% to 2.7 cases per 100,000 population.[4] The increased rate was primarily due to increases in cases of men who have had sex with men. Cumulative data from the Centers for Disease Control and Prevention also showed that rates of primary and secondary syphilis were higher in African Americans and Hispanics than in other groups.[4]

There is a notable association between syphilis and human immunodeficiency virus (HIV) infection. The diseases affect similar patient groups, and co-infection is common.[5] Additionally, syphilis increases sexual transmission of HIV by six- to seven-fold, likely secondary to the increased incidence of genital ulcers.[6]

Clinical Findings Syphilis presents initially with a solitary, painless, indurated ulceration (chancre) about 3 weeks (range: 9 to 90 days) after contact with an infected partner [**Figure 58-1**]. In men, the primary lesion is most commonly located on the distal penis and usually is accompanied by unilateral lymphadenopathy. This lesion of primary syphilis remits spontaneously and is followed in 1 to 2 months by secondary syphilis, a papulosquamous eruption that may involve the palms and soles, trunk, face, and genitalia. Secondary syphilis may be associated with exudative anogenital plaques (condylomata lata), which appear to be more common in individuals with skin of color[7] [**Figure 58-2**]. Atypical presentations of primary and secondary syphilis may occur in individuals who are co-infected with HIV or in individuals who have been infected with syphilis previously.[6]

Serologic testing is the most commonly used diagnostic technique. Nontreponemal antigen tests, including the rapid plasma reagin (RPR) and the Venereal Disease Research Laboratory (VDRL) tests, are used for screening, and treponema-specific tests, including the *T. pallidum* particle agglutination assay and fluorescent treponemal antibody absorption tests, are used to confirm the diagnosis. *T. pallidum* cannot be cultured, but it can be demonstrated directly by dark-field microscopy. The organism also can be detected in biopsy specimens using specific treponemal fluorescent antibody stains or silver stains such as the Warthin-Starry stain.[6] However, the latter stain also reacts with melanin, which may make diagnosis difficult in skin of color.[7] All individuals testing positive for syphilis also should be counseled and evaluated for HIV infection.

Complications The complications of syphilis occur years after primary infection in the tertiary stage. These include cardiovascular syphilis, gummatous disease, and late manifestations of neurosyphilis, including tabes dorsalis and general paresis. Late complications are seen in approximately one-third of untreated patients between 3 and 15 years

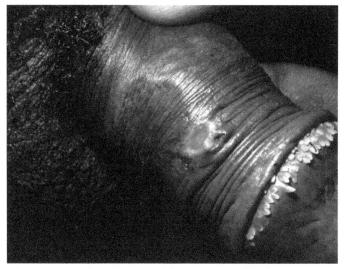

FIGURE 58-1. A patient with syphilis. Note the midshaft reepithelializing chancre and the incidental pearly penile papules on the corona.

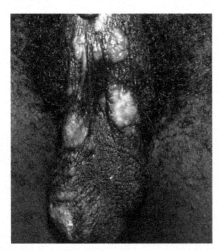

FIGURE 58-2. A patient with syphilis. The exophytic nodules typify condylomata lata.

after the initial infection. Neurosyphilis is exceedingly rare among patients who undergo the appropriate penicillin treatment; however, this form of the disease may result in meningitis, cranial neuritis, ocular involvement, and meningovascular disease.[6]

Prognosis/Clinical Course Untreated syphilis passes through four stages: primary, secondary, latent, and tertiary. Treatment of primary syphilis results in rapid disappearance of the chancre. Secondary syphilis occurs only in untreated or inadequately treated individuals. Since the primary chancre will resolve spontaneously without treatment within a month or two, the RPR titer should be followed in patients to confirm adequate treatment.

Chancroid

Epidemiology, Etiology, and Pathogenesis Chancroid is an STI caused by the Gram-negative coccobacillus *Haemophilus ducreyi*. The bacterium initiates an infective process within genital skin after epidermal microabrasions occur during sexual intercourse.[7] Like syphilis, chancroid is a genital ulceration associated with both increased occurrence and transmission rates of HIV.

H. ducreyi is the most common pathogen isolated in genital ulcer disease in Africa. In the United States, reported cases generally occur in urban epidemics and are most common in darker skin of color men.[8] The increased incidence in males is due to spread from infected commercial sex workers and the more rapid resolution of the infection in females.[8]

Clinical Findings After a 3- to 14-day incubation period, a pustule develops at the site of inoculation that rapidly evolves into a shallow, ragged, painful erosion. In men, the ulcers are found (in decreasing order of frequency) on the prepuce, coronal sulcus, glans, frenulum, and penile shaft. Autoinoculation frequently leads to the presentation of multiple ulcers [**Figure 58-3**]. Painful inguinal lymphadenopathy occurs in up to 50% of patients and is more common in men.[7] Percutaneous rupture with purulent drainage (bubo formation) is frequent [**Figure 58-4**].

Diagnosis of clinically suspicious lesions typically is confirmed by cultures on enriched and vancomycin-impregnated gonococcal and Mueller-Hinton agars under conditions of high humidity and high carbon dioxide tension.[9] Gram-stained ulcer material should not be used to diagnose chancroid due to the low specificity and sensitivity of this test.[7] The most sensitive and specific modality for diagnosis is mutiplex polymerase chain reaction (PCR), which has a resolved sensitivity and specificity for *H. ducreyi* of 98.4% and 99.6%, respectively.[8] Infected patients should be tested for HIV infection.

Complications Patients with chancroid are at a higher risk of HIV infection. Complications that occur in conjunction with chancroid include phimosis and additional destructive ulceration due to secondary bacterial infection.

Prognosis/Clinical Course If untreated, ulcers will persist for roughly 2 to 3 months before healing spontaneously with significant scar formation. Adequately treated chancroid resolves in approximately 10 days.[3]

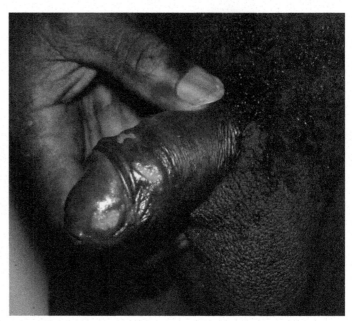

FIGURE 58-3. Multiple ulcers of chancroid on the genital skin of a male patient with skin of color.

Granuloma Inguinale

Epidemiology, Etiology, and Pathogenesis Granuloma inguinale, also called donovanosis, is caused by *Klebsiella granulomatis (once known as Calymmatobacterium granulomatis)* an intracellular Gram-negative encapsulated bacillus. Although sexual contact is the likely method of spread, there is some controversy regarding the mode of transmission.[10]

Endemic foci of granuloma inguinale are seen in New Guinea, Africa, Australia, and parts of India and China. Worldwide, the disease is more common in males than in females and is more common in men who have sex with men than others. There were fewer than 10 cases per year in the United States until 1989.[10] There was a higher incidence among individuals with darker skin of color in these cases. As with other genital ulcerative diseases, granuloma inguinale can increase the transmission rate of HIV infection.

Clinical Findings After an incubation period of 8 to 90 days (usually 2 to 3 weeks), a papule or nodule appears on the anogenital region. Erosion through the skin occurs rapidly, yielding a clean-based remarkably

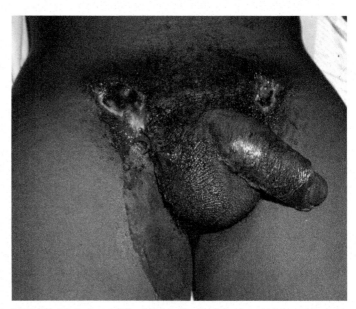

FIGURE 58-4. Ruptured inguinal lymph nodes (bubo formation) in a patient with untreated chancroid.

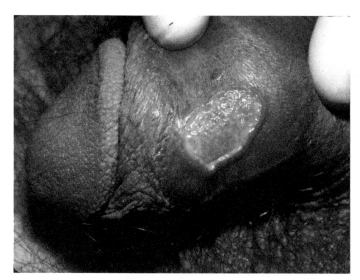

FIGURE 58-5. Rolled border and friable base typical of granuloma inguinale in a Hispanic patient from the Caribbean.

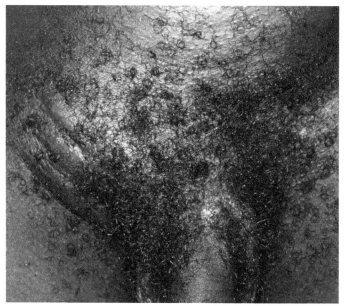

FIGURE 58-6. Pathognomonic pattern of inguinal adenopathy in lymphogranuloma venereum.

painless ulceration that bleeds readily to the touch and demonstrates a rolled border[11] [**Figure 58-5**]. The most common locations of lesions in men are the coronal sulcus, the subpreputial region, and the anus.[12] True adenopathy is rare, but involvement of nearby tissue may produce a periadenitis that may be mistaken for a lymph node, giving rise to the term pseudobubo.[13]

Diagnosis of granuloma inguinale may be made clinically in endemic areas with some confidence. In nonendemic areas, such as the United States, laboratory diagnosis requires a crush specimen from a punch biopsy stained with Wright or Giemsa stains. The biopsy specimen should be taken before cleaning the lesion or removing any necrotic tissue. Diagnosis is made by the visualization of Donovan bodies, deeply staining rods in the cytoplasm of macrophages. Ultrathin histologic sections may be necessary for good visualization of the causative organism.[13]

Complications The disease process can lead to fibrosis and keloid formation, causing genital deformation, paraphimosis, and lymphatic obstruction with localized elephantiasis. The lesions also may become infected secondarily. Extensive ulceration of the soft tissues can lead to fistula formation and genital mutilation. Additionally, there is an increased incidence of squamous cell carcinoma (SCC) occurring in long-standing lesions.[13]

Prognosis/Clinical Course If left untreated, granuloma inguinale will not remit spontaneously, although lesions may be stable for long periods of time. Hematogenous and lymphatic spread, along with autoinoculation, can lead to lesions in extragenital locations.[13] Proper treatment will halt lesion progression, but prolonged therapy may be required to allow complete healing.[14]

Lymphogranuloma Venereum

Epidemiology, Etiology, and Pathogenesis Lymphogranuloma venereum (LGV) is an STI caused by *Chlamydia trachomatis* (serotypes L1, L2a, L2b, and L3), a Gram-negative intracellular parasite. LGV is most common in tropical regions but does occur with a low incidence in the Western world. Very few cases are reported annually in the United States, and the disease is more commonly reported among men than women; however, this may be because early manifestations of the STI are more apparent in men.[14a] Recent outbreaks of LGV proctitis (due to serotype L2b) have been associated with groups of men who have sex with men.[14a]

Clinical Findings After a 1- to 2-week incubation period, LGV begins with a painless papule or shallow ulcer. The most common locations for the primary lesion in men are the coronal sulcus and the glans penis. The primary lesion lasts only 2 to 3 days and goes unnoticed in approximately 75% of patients. After 1 to 3 weeks, tender unilateral adenopathy develops. The lymphadenopathy involves the inguinal nodes more frequently than the femoral nodes but may involve both, giving rise to the groove sign of Greenblatt (corresponding to the inguinal ligament) [**Figure 58-6**]. Unfortunately, this nearly pathognomonic sign appears in only about 20% of LGV patients.[15] The lymph nodes become tender and fluctuant and are referred to as buboes. The nodes may develop multiple fistulas that drain purulent material. Systemic symptoms, including fever, malaise, headaches, and arthralgia, are common.[3] Diagnosis is made by culturing pus aspirated from the enlarged nodes. A Giemsa stain also may be performed on a smear to look for intracellular corpuscles of Gamma-Miyagawa.[13]

Complications Late complications include fibrosis and tissue destruction. Fibrosis may lead to elephantiasis of the penis and scrotum.[13]

Prognosis/Clinical Course If left untreated, LGV will persist for years and may result in the complications listed earlier. Treatment prevents these sequelae.

Genital Herpes

Epidemiology, Etiology, and Pathogenesis Genital herpes is a very prevalent disease, with at least 50 million people in the United States infected and an estimated 500,000 to 700,000 new cases occurring each year.[16] Genital herpes generally is caused by herpes simplex virus (HSV)-2, although a minority of these lesions may be caused by HSV-1, the usual etiologic agent of herpes labialis.[17] Darker skin of color individuals have a lower prevalence of HSV-1–induced lesions (1.3%) than the general population.[18] HSV is a double-stranded DNA virus that enters the body via direct skin-to-skin or mucosal contact, or contact with infected secretions. The virus multiplies in the epidermis before ascending the sensory nerve roots to the dorsal root ganglion, where it becomes latent. When the virus reactivates, it travels back down the sensory root, leading to a mucocutaneous outbreak.

Clinical Findings Primary lesions appear in an individual approximately 6 days after infection. The primary lesion consists of painful, grouped vesicles on an erythematous base that may rupture, leading to erosion or ulcer formation [**Figure 58-7**]. The lesion is found most commonly on the shaft or glans of the penis in men but may be located in the perianal area, thighs, or buttocks. Perianal lesions, including persistent large ulcerations, may be seen in homosexual men practicing receptive anal intercourse [**Figure 58-8**]. During the initial event, the patient may complain of fever, headaches, or malaise. Recurrent HSV outbreaks are usually less severe than the initial episode and typically are preceded by a prodrome of local pain or tingling.[16] The diagnosis of genital herpes

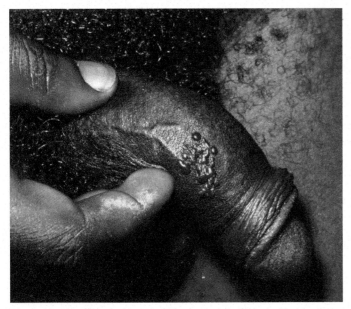

FIGURE 58-7. Genital herpes. The grouped vesicles are characteristic of herpes progenitalis.

usually can be made based on clinical appearance. If the diagnosis is in question, a Tzanck smear (showing viral acantholytic giant cells), viral culture, skin biopsy, or PCR test for HSV DNA may be performed.

Complications Rarely, men may develop urinary retention symptoms from urethral lesions. Perianal infection with proctitis is common in men who have sex with men.[16]

Prognosis/Clinical Course There is no cure for genital herpes. The recurrence rate for untreated genital herpes is variable, with a median of four episodes per year. HSV-1 recurs less frequently than HSV-2, and men tend to have more recurrences than women. Recurrences are most often spontaneous and unpredictable, but emotional stress, hormonal changes, or other factors may trigger them. Over time, recurrent episodes become less frequent. It should be noted that asymptomatic viral shedding may occur at any time, and it is estimated that some 70% of genital herpes is acquired when an uninfected individual has genital contact with an infected person who is shedding virus unknowingly. Male-to-female transmission is more efficient than the converse.

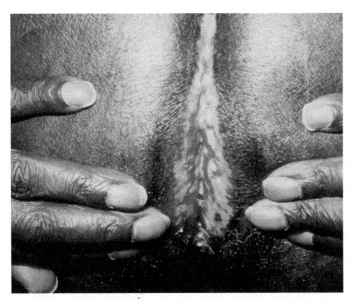

FIGURE 58-8. Genital herpes. This patient underwent persistent ulceration due to human immunodeficiency virus co-infection with the herpes simplex virus.

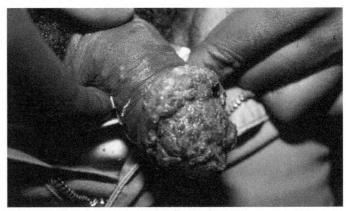

FIGURE 58-9. Neglected genital warts forming a large verrucous mass.

Genital Warts

Epidemiology, Etiology, and Pathogenesis Genital warts, or condylomata acuminata, are STIs caused by human papillomavirus (HPV) infection. HPV is a DNA virus with more than 100 different types. Types 6 and 11 are most commonly associated with genital warts (90%).[19] It is likely that more than half of sexually active adults in the United States have been infected with at least one type of genital HPV, but only about 1% of them have clinically apparent warts.[20]

Clinical Findings Visible lesions develop after an average interval of 2 to 3 months following sexual exposure to HPV.[21] Lesions occur most commonly on the penile shaft and glans in men. Genital warts can have variable appearances, but the most common appearance is that of mildly elevated, flat-topped papules. The classic wart (true condylomata acuminatum) is a filiform papilloma that is 3 to 10 mm high and 2 to 3 mm in diameter with a brush-like terminal end [**Figure 58-9**]. Genital warts usually can be diagnosed clinically, although a biopsy rarely may be required to differentiate genital warts from neoplastic growths.[22] Viral typing is not routine.[23]

Complications The HPV types 6 and 11 that cause genital warts are not oncogenic and do not carry a high risk of malignancy, like some other types of HPV. Rarely, long-standing genital warts theoretically have caused invasive SCC.[24] However, in this situation, the initial lesion may well have been an unrecognized malignant neoplasm from inception.

Prognosis/Clinical Course The course of HPV infections is variable, with lesions regressing spontaneously, persisting, resolving with therapy, or appearing after prolonged latency.[21] Most clinical manifestations of HPV infections are transient and become clinically undetectable within several years.[19]

Molluscum Contagiosum

Epidemiology, Etiology, and Pathogenesis Molluscum contagiosum is caused by the poxvirus molluscum contagiosum virus. This DNA virus is spread through sexual contact in adults. The virus occurs most commonly in underdeveloped areas and tropical climates.[24] The worldwide prevalence of molluscum contagiosum is 2% to 8%.[25]

Clinical Findings After an incubation period of 2 to 7 weeks or more, a papular eruption of multiple umbilicated lesions develops. The lesions are dome-shaped and opalescent in color [**Figure 58-10**]. The central umbilication is present 25% of the time and, if present, is pathognomonic for the disease. The papules may become inflamed, leading to an atypical appearance. In men, the lesions are found most commonly on the penile shaft but may be located anywhere in the groin, thighs, or lower abdomen when the infection is acquired sexually.[26] The diagnosis of molluscum contagiosum usually can be made from clinical appearance. If there is any uncertainty, a biopsy can be performed that will reveal intracytoplasmic inclusion bodies known as molluscum bodies or Henderson-Paterson bodies.

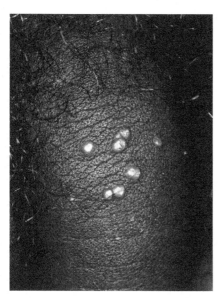

FIGURE 58-10. Many small, dome-shaped papules typical of molluscum contagiosum.

Complications If lesions become inflamed or are picked, they can lead to scarring. Immunocompromised individuals can develop generalized cutaneous infection.

Prognosis/Clinical Course In immunocompetent patients, the infection follows a self-limited course marked by spontaneous clearing within a few months. In patients with HIV infection or atopic dermatitis, or those undergoing immunosuppressive therapy, lesions can be atypical, widespread, or resistant to clearing even with therapy.[24]

Sclerosing Lymphangitis

Epidemiology, Etiology, and Pathogenesis Sclerosing lymphangitis occurs in men following vigorous sexual activity. It has an unknown etiology but may be related to trauma. The disease usually occurs in 20- to 40-year-old men without racial predilection.[27]

Clinical Findings Sclerosing lymphangitis is characterized by the acute onset of a flesh-colored, firm, cord-like lesion of the coronal sulcus [**Figure 58-11**] that may extend onto the penile shaft.[28] The lesion is normally painless but may be associated with some discomfort, especially with erection. The diagnosis can be made clinically. STIs, particularly gonococcal and nongonococcal urethritis, frequently occur in association with this condition. Patients thus should have a full workup for STIs.[28]

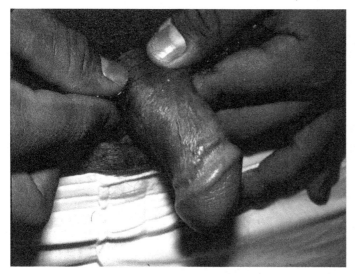

FIGURE 58-11. Cordlike induration seen in a patient with sclerosing lymphangitis.

Complications In rare instances, tenderness may persist for a long period of time.

Prognosis/Clinical Course The lesions usually resolve spontaneously within 1 to 2 months.[28]

▪ NONSEXUALLY TRANSMITTED INFECTIONS

Tinea Cruris

Epidemiology, Etiology, and Pathogenesis Tinea cruris is a common dermatophyte infection of the genital skin that occurs most commonly in postpubertal men of any racial group. The most common etiologic agent is *Trichophyton rubrum,* and the cutaneous infection is frequently secondary to concomitant toenail onychomycosis.

Clinical Findings Tinea cruris is classically characterized as erythematous, scaly, sharply demarcated plaques over the inner thighs to the crural crease, but patients with darker skin of color may present with striking hyperpigmentation rather than erythema, and genital skin may not have scale [**Figure 58-12**]. The eruption is typically annular and pruritic. Individuals with coarse hair may have papules within the leading edge of the eruption. In men, the infection usually spares the scrotum and shaft of the penis. The diagnosis of tinea cruris generally can be made clinically, especially if the individual has other dermatophyte fungal infections such as tinea pedis or onychomycosis. If the diagnosis of tinea cruris is unclear, a potassium hydroxide examination or culture of the peripheral scale may be performed.

Complications The condition may become extensive or may involve follicles.

Prognosis/Clinical Course Tinea cruris generally can be eradicated with therapy, although recurrences are not uncommon, and patients may require intermittent treatment. Some susceptible patients may require chronic suppressive therapy.

Leishmaniasis

Epidemiology, Etiology, and Pathogenesis Cutaneous leishmaniasis is a parasitic disease caused by various species of the *Leishmania* protozoan. The disease affects 1 to 2 million people each year, mainly in tropical and subtropical areas. Genital manifestations of leishmaniasis are quite rare because the cutaneous manifestations usually occur on exposed skin. Genital lesions have been described in farmers, miners, nude sunbathers, and individuals who normally sleep naked.[29] The disease is spread by the bite of the sandfly of genus *Lutzomyia* in the new world and *Phlebotomus* in the old world. The parasite is able to survive within macrophages in the host.[30] Clinical lesions develop secondary to continued release of cytokines as part of the host immune response.[31]

Clinical Findings After a 2- to 8-week or longer incubation, an erythematous papule develops at the site of the sandfly bite. The papule enlarges into a nodule that promptly ulcerates [**Figure 58-13**]. The

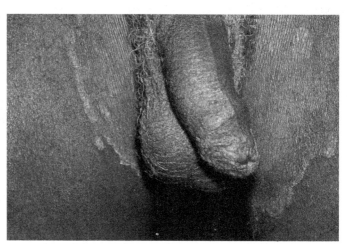

FIGURE 58-12. Tinea cruris characterized by annular scaling and erythema in the groin.

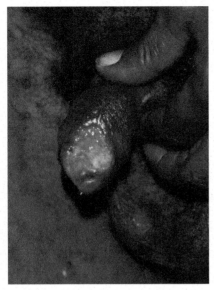

FIGURE 58-13. *Persistent painless ulcer of genital leishmaniasis.*

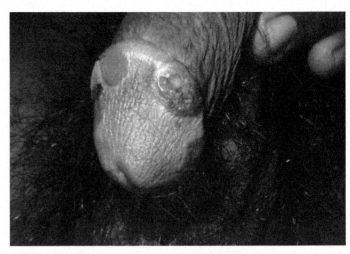

FIGURE 58-14. Plaques of psoriasis, both with and without scale.

ulcer is usually painless unless secondarily infected. When the disease occurs on the genitalia of men, the ulcers usually occur on the glans or scrotum.[29] The most common test to diagnose cutaneous leishmaniasis is a scraping from the center of the lesion following cleaning. Giemsa staining should reveal Leishman-Donovan bodies (amastigotes within monocytes). A biopsy of the lesion also can be performed to identify amastigotes. Newer tests, including culture on selective media and PCR assay, may enhance detection.[31]

Complications Cutaneous lesions can become disseminated, especially in immunosuppressed patients. The lesions also can become secondarily infected with bacteria and fungi. Untreated lesions may result in genital deformity.

Prognosis/Clinical Course Old world leishmaniasis tends to heal spontaneously in months, whereas new world lesions may take years to do so. Scarring usually results after involution.

INFLAMMATORY DISEASES

▉ PAPULOSQUAMOUS

Psoriasis

Epidemiology, Etiology, and Pathogenesis Psoriasis is a T-cell–mediated autoimmune disorder wherein keratinocyte proliferation follows aberrant cytokine elaboration and secretion.[32] Psoriasis occurs less commonly in Americans with darker skin of color (0.1%) than in Caucasian Americans (1%); however, in East Africa, psoriasis occurs in 1.4% of the darker skin of color population.[33] Psoriasis has a genetic basis, with 30% of affected individuals having an affected first-degree relative, but environmental factors also may play a role in the disease process.

Clinical Findings The typical lesions of psoriasis consist of erythematous plaques with an overlying silvery scale [**Figure 58-14**]. However, in skin of color, psoriasis may present as bluish-black, minimally scaly, flattened plaques. Psoriatic lesions occur most frequently over the scalp, elbows, and knees, although genital involvement does occur with some regularity. The lesions commonly occur over the elbows and knees because of the Koebner phenomenon, in which lesions occur at sites of injury or irritation. This phenomenon may have an effect on genital lesions as well because heat and friction produce mild irritation. When psoriasis occurs on genital skin, it may appear less thickened and with less scale due to the occluded, damp nature of genital skin. Psoriasis is common in the inguinal crease, upper inner thighs, perineum, scrotum, and penile shaft and glans. Although the diagnosis of psoriasis usually can be made based on clinical appearance, lesions in darker skin of color individuals may possess an atypical morphology and thus may require biopsy confirmation. Additionally, darker skin of color individuals are

less likely to have associated psoriatic features such as nail dystrophy that could assist in the diagnosis.[33] Genital psoriasis may be identical in clinical morphology to Reiter syndrome, although the latter is uncommon in African Americans.

Complications Psoriasis is associated with many comorbidities, including emotional distress, cardiovascular disease, renal insufficiency, arthritis, and an increased risk of lymphoma and nonmelanoma skin cancer. The local maceration that can occur in psoriasis, along with the use of topical corticosteroids, can increase the risk of infection with *Candida* or dermatophytes.

Prognosis/Clinical Course Psoriasis is a chronic disease with a waxing and waning clinical course. There is no cure for psoriasis, and treatments are aimed at managing the disease.

Lichen Planus

Epidemiology, Etiology, and Pathogenesis Lichen planus, like psoriasis, is probably related to errant T-cell autoimmunity.[34] Approximately 25% of men demonstrate genital involvement, usually of the glans.[2]

Clinical Findings Although the lesions of lichen planus typically appear as polygonal papules with a violaceous hue [**Figure 58-15**], variations are very common in skin of color. Lesions are usually deeper in color, and annular lesions are more common.[35] Erosive lichen planus can occur on the penis but is much more common in females; this is discussed in Chapter 59, Genital Lesions in Women. Although classic lichen planus is diagnosed clinically, genital lesions may require a biopsy for diagnosis.[34]

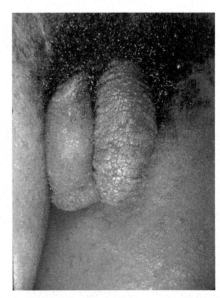

FIGURE 58-15. Numerous flat-topped violaceous papules of lichen planus.

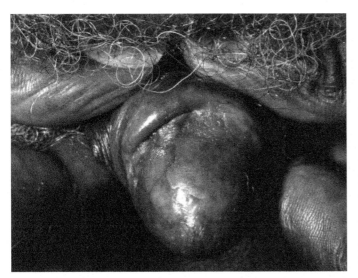

FIGURE 58-16. Shallow asymptomatic erosion of Zoon balanitis.

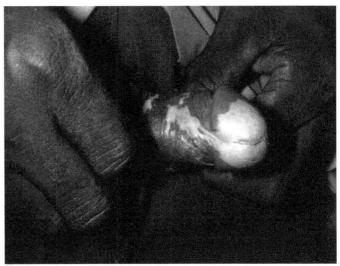

FIGURE 58-17. Depigmentation of vitiligo.

Complications Lichen planus is associated with systemic illnesses such as myasthenia gravis, ulcerative colitis, primary biliary cirrhosis, and chronic active hepatitis C. Chronic ulcerative lichen planus may degenerate into SCC. Phimosis may develop in uncircumcised men.[36] Lichen planus therapy is immunosuppressive, thereby increasing the risk of superimposed *Candida* and dermatophyte infections.

Prognosis/Clinical Course The course of lichen planus is variable. Some lesions remit spontaneously, whereas others persist. Nonerosive lesions, typical in men, are usually well controlled with therapy.

Zoon Balanitis

Epidemiology, Etiology, and Pathogenesis Zoon balanitis, or plasma cell balanitis, has an unknown etiology but generally occurs in older uncircumcised men of any racial group. It is thought that inflammation may be an inciting event in the disease process.[37]

Clinical Findings Zoon balanitis presents as a sharply demarcated, shiny, erythematous and geographic shallow erosion affecting the glans penis and/or the inner surface of the prepuce [**Figure 58-16**]. The lesion is usually asymptomatic. The diagnosis is established by biopsy, which must be performed to rule out SCC in situ.[38]

Complications Zoon balanitis does not usually lead to any complications.

Prognosis/Clinical Course Zoon balanitis may be well controlled or even eradicated with treatment. It is unclear if untreated disease resolves, persists indefinitely, or evolves into a more recognizable disease such as lichen planus. Rare cases of SCC have been reported to develop within this otherwise benign lesion.[39]

NONPAPULOSQUAMOUS

Vitiligo

Epidemiology, Etiology, and Pathogenesis Vitiligo is an autoimmune disease of uncertain etiology that results in the destruction of melanocytes; there are predisposing genetic loci explaining a familial predilection.[40] While there is no racial predilection, the disease is so obvious (and cosmetically distressing) in patients with skin of color that more patients who fall into this category may seek medical attention. Most vitiligo patients relate an onset before the age of 40; men and women are at equal risk.

Clinical Findings Areas of absolute depigmentation are apparent [**Figure 58-17**]. The periorificial regions of the face and the dorsum of the hands and feet are frequent sites of initial involvement. The glans penis is another favored area. Vitiligo must be differentiated from lichen sclerosus, which it may resemble.

Complications Vitiligo itself poses no other medical complications. However, thyroid dysfunction, pernicious anemia, and diabetes mellitus should be sought as potential comorbid conditions.[41]

Prognosis/Clinical Course The disease may unpredictably resolve, persist, or expand.

MULTISYSTEM DISEASES

NON-MALIGNANT

Behçet Syndrome

Epidemiology, Etiology, and Pathogenesis Behçet syndrome is a relatively uncommon disease that consists of a triad of oral ulcers, genital ulcers, and ocular inflammation. Anogenital ulcerations are found in roughly 90% of patients with Behçet syndrome and may be the presenting manifestation. Although common in the Middle East and Japan, this disorder is rare in both Africans and Americans with dark skin of color.[42]

Clinical Findings In men, the genital lesions of Behçet syndrome present as extremely painful, small, 'punched out' ulcers over the scrotum [**Figure 58-18**] and, less commonly, the penile shaft.[43] The diagnosis of Behçet syndrome is made clinically. The diagnostic criteria include the presence of oral aphthae plus any two of the following: genital ulceration, eye disease, other skin lesions, or skin pathergy (the formation of a pustule at the site of intracutaneously injected saline).

Complications Behçet syndrome may be associated with gastrointestinal symptoms, arthritis, thrombophlebitis, psychiatric problems, or neurologic defects. Patients also may manifest other cutaneous problems, including erythema nodosum and erythema multiforme. Ocular disease may be severe enough to lead to blindness.

Prognosis/Clinical Course The genital lesions follow a variable course. Some lesions will heal while other lesions will form. The systemic manifestations of the disease are more progressive.

MALIGNANT

Squamous Cell Carcinoma

Epidemiology, Etiology, and Pathogenesis SCC is the most common tumor of the penis, accounting for more than 95% of malignant genital neoplasms. In the Western world, penile carcinoma accounts for less than 1% of adult male cancers, but in some developing areas in Africa, Asia, and South America, the disease can constitute up to 17% of malignancies in men.[43a] The disease is seen most commonly in 50- to 70-year-old individuals. In the United States, African American men tend to present with genital SCC at a younger age and at a more advanced state than Caucasians.[44] A high mortality from genital SCC

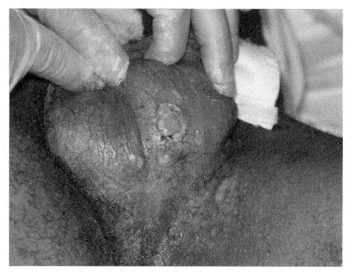

FIGURE 58-18. Multiple painful scrotal ulcers of Behçet syndrome.

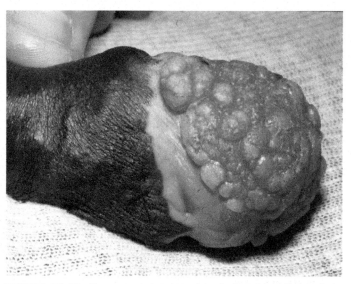

FIGURE 58-20. Verrucous, nonulcerating squamous cell carcinoma that required a partial penectomy.

also has been reported in the past among darker skin of color patients, both in the United States and in Africa.[45] Risk factors for the disease include not being circumcised as a child, HPV infection (subtypes 16, 18, 31, 33, 35, 51, and 52), tobacco use, ionizing radiation, chemical agents, and immunosuppression. SCC in situ is a precursor of invasive SCC, but only 10% of these lesions will transform.[46] Carcinoma in situ is often referred to as erythroplasia of Queyrat when it occurs on the glans and Bowen disease when it occurs on the shaft.

Clinical Findings In situ SCC presents as velvety papules and plaques or shallow nonhealing erosions on the glans or shaft of the penis [**Figure 58-19**]. Invasive SCC can occur on the penis or scrotum. The lesions may have variable clinical morphology but typically appear as friable and/or ulcerated nodules and plaques. They also may appear as red or brown flat-topped papules or plaques that are identical in appearance to in situ lesions. Alternatively, they may appear as a rock-hard, verrucous or hyperkeratotic nodules without evidence of ulceration [**Figure 58-20**]. The diagnosis of SCC is established with a biopsy.

Complications Invasive lesions that have persisted for many years can lead to significant destruction of tissue [**Figure 58-21**]. Destructive ulceration, also known as 'rodent ulcers,' can lead to autoamputation of the distal penis. Fatal metastases may be associated with invasive SCC.

Prognosis/Clinical Course Untreated invasive penile SCC will metastasize to the local lymph nodes and result in death, usually within a few years.

Kaposi Sarcoma

Epidemiology, Etiology, and Pathogenesis Kaposi sarcoma (KS) is a multicentric malignant tumor of lymphatic origin that can be one of four types: classic, endemic African, acquired immune deficiency syndrome–related, or transplant-related. The etiologic agent of all types of KS is human herpesvirus type 8.[47] The incidence of KS in the United States has decreased dramatically with the advent of highly active antiretroviral therapy for HIV infection.[48] There is no sex predilection in the United States. In Africa, KS is very common, accounting for up to 10% of all malignancies in some regions; men are affected 20 to 30 times more frequently than women in these areas.[49]

Clinical Findings Lesions that involve the genitalia can be either primary lesions or part of generalized disease. The lesional morphology is similar in all forms of KS, starting as soft, spongy macules and plaques that enlarge into hard, violaceous nodules and tumors [**Figure 58-22**]. In primary penile KS, lesions usually present as a violaceous nodule on the glans but may involve the foreskin, coronal sulcus, meatus, or rarely, the shaft. The lesions may be associated with significant edema.[50] The diagnosis of KS is confirmed with biopsy. Primary penile lesions are

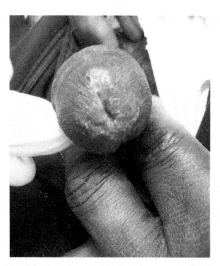

FIGURE 58-19. Velvety, erythematous erosion of squamous cell carcinoma in situ.

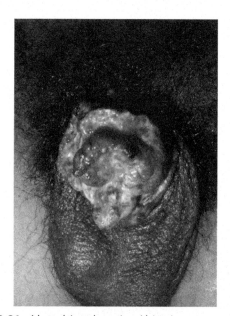

FIGURE 58-21. Advanced tissue destruction with invasive squamous cell carcinoma in a Hispanic patient from Panama.

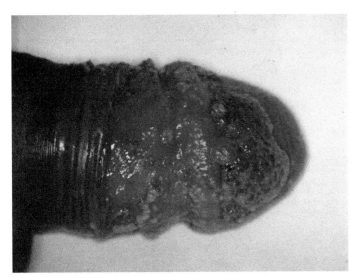

FIGURE 58-22. Purple-colored papules and nodules of Kaposi sarcoma.

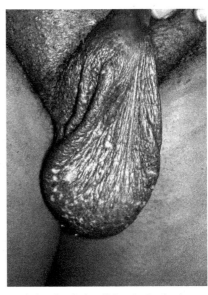

FIGURE 58-23. Thickened, scaly skin of lichen simplex chronicus.

most commonly associated with HIV infection, and all patients should be tested for HIV.[51]

Complications KS can metastasize to the lymph nodes, the gastrointestinal tract, the pulmonary system, or the oral cavity.[51]

Prognosis/Clinical Course In most classic and African endemic cases, progression of the disease is slow. Individuals with HIV-associated KS and some individuals with other forms of KS have a rapidly progressive course with rapid dissemination. Complete cure is attained rarely in individuals with disseminated disease. In transplant-associated KS, diminution of immunosuppression may lead to lesional involution.[51]

EXOGENOUS DISEASES

■ LICHEN SIMPLEX CHRONICUS

Epidemiology, Etiology, and Pathogenesis Lichen simplex chronicus (LSC) is an eczematous disease characterized by unremitting itching and scratching. Primary LSC arises de novo on normal-appearing tissue and has been called "the itch that rashes." Secondary LSC develops in the presence of a preexisting dermatologic disease. The triggers of primary LSC are psychological and environmental factors, and primary LSC often occurs in the presence of atopy, whereas the trigger of secondary LSC is the underlying dermatologic condition. The itch-scratch cycle is responsible for the condition in all types.[52] Darker skin of color individuals are more prone to developing and resistant to clearing lichenification than Caucasians.

Clinical Findings LSC presents as thickened, hyperpigmented plaque with accentuated skin markings and overlying scale that may be associated with discrete hyperkeratotic nodules (prurigo nodularis) [**Figure 58-23**]. In men, the scrotum is the most commonly involved site, but lesions also can occur on the proximal penis or the upper, inner thighs. In genital skin, the lesions may appear white and wrinkled instead of thickened and scaly secondary to the high moisture content of the area.[52] A variant of lichen simplex common in older men with darker skin of color exists in which thickening and hypo- and hyperpigmentation of the scrotum coexist. The diagnosis of LSC is made clinically with a compatible history of excessive itching that may be subconscious or occur at night. Biopsy findings are nonspecific.

Complications Scratching of the area may be so vigorous that genital distortion, fibrosis, and scarring may occur. The condition may mask other premalignant and malignant conditions (e.g., lichen sclerosus or SCC in situ). In individuals with dark skin, postinflammatory hyper- and hypopigmentation can occur even after the condition is well controlled.[52]

Prognosis/Clinical Course LSC is a chronic disease that will persist indefinitely without treatment, although severity will wax and wane. Recurrences are common.

Contact Dermatitis

Epidemiology, Etiology, and Pathogenesis Contact dermatitis is a common inflammatory skin reaction to external agents. Allergic contact dermatitis (ACD) is a delayed-type hypersensitivity reaction and requires a prior antigen sensitization, but irritant contact dermatitis (ICD) is a nonimmunologic skin response to direct damage from a skin irritant. In both cases, the offending agent may be transferred to the genitalia by the hand or by the mucosa of sexual partners. To date, many offending agents have been described for both ACD and ICD, but most cases of genital ACD result from topical cosmetic products, medications, latex condoms, or local anesthetic agents used to delay ejaculation by dulling sensation.[12,53-57]

Clinical Findings ACD of the genitalia presents as pruritic erythema and edema [**Figure 58-24**] that may have associated vesicles or bullae. The lesion may be painful as well. More chronic irritation shows scaly skin with accentuated skin markings. The high moisture content and friction of genital skin may spread the offending substance, making a geometric distribution less obvious than in other skin areas. The diagnosis of both ICD and ACD generally is made with a careful history because the clinical appearance and even biopsy may be nonspecific. Biopsy can be performed to rule out other possible diagnoses. Patch testing may be useful in some patients if the clinical findings suggest ACD but no offending agent can be determined by the history.[12]

Complications Severely irritating chemicals may cause erosions of the penis. Additionally, severe inflammation may damage melanocytes, leading to permanent dyschromia.

Prognosis/Clinical Course Patients allergic to one substance generally have a good prognosis once the offending agent is removed and anti-inflammatory treatment is initiated. Patients with more chronic symptoms and no obvious single etiology generally have a prolonged course with chronic management requirements.

Genital Bite Wounds

Epidemiology, Etiology, and Pathogenesis Human genital bites usually result from sexual activity and are reported infrequently due to embarrassment. Bites may be deliberate or accidental, and penile bites may cause serious damage that leads to disfigurement and sexual dysfunction. Genital bites may transmit many possible communicable infectious diseases, especially if the person inflicting the bite is at high

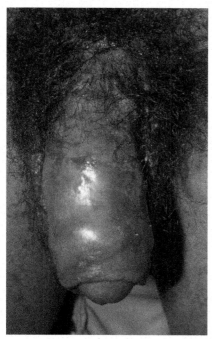

FIGURE 58-24. Allergic contact dermatitis, with marked pruritic erythema and edema, resulting from contact allergy to vaginal lubricant in a Hispanic male from Guatemala.

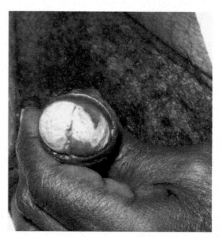

FIGURE 58-25. Necrotic ulceration characterizing a genital bite wound.

risk of contracting or carrying infectious diseases, such as prostitutes, men who have sex with men, intravenous drug abusers, or anyone receiving multiple blood transfusions prior to 1985. Rapidly progressive, necrotic genital infections following a bite generally are caused by oral flora such as *Eikenella corrodens,* a Gram-negative facultative anaerobe.[56,57]

Clinical Findings Genital bite wounds can present as lacerations, ulcers, cellulitis, or balanoposthitis. Diagnosis is made based on a careful history, which must include the health status of the biter, time elapsed since the injury, and the victim's medical condition, including his immune status. A wound culture for aerobic and anaerobic organisms always should be performed on these lesions. Baseline and follow-up tests for syphilis, hepatitis, and HIV should be obtained.

Complications Localized infection secondary to microorganisms carried in the saliva can be a very serious complication. Infections can lead to erosion and ulceration [**Figure 58-25**], cellulitis, abscess formation, lymphadenitis or lymphangitis, and infrequently, seeding of prosthetic joints or artificial heart valves. Rarely, sepsis may occur.[57]

Prognosis/Clinical Course If the bite did not cause anatomic damage to the penis and the wound does not become infected, the prognosis is good. Infections caught early and treated appropriately also have a good prognosis.

DIFFERENTIAL DIAGNOSES AND TREATMENTS

The various differential diagnoses and treatment options that should be considered for each form of genital lesion in men covered in this chapter are detailed in **Table 58-1**.

TABLE 58-1 Differential diagnoses and treatments for genital lesions in men[a]		
Lesion/disease	Differential diagnoses	Treatments
Syphilis	• Chancroid • Condylomata acuminata (external genital warts) • Fixed drug eruption • Genital aphthosis, including Behçet syndrome • Granuloma inguinale • Herpes progenitalis • Lymphogranuloma venereum • Papulosquamous diseases (eg, psoriasis, seborrhea) • Traumatic ulceration (eg, bite wounds, vacuum erection device)	Therapy of choice for a syphilis infection of less than 1 year in duration (primary, secondary, or early latent infections) consists of 2.4 MU of benzathine G penicillin intramuscularly. Tetracycline drugs are second-line agents. RPR titers should be followed to confirm successful treatment. Individuals with a clear-cut diagnosis of syphilis who fail to respond should be retested for HIV infection and treated with weekly benzathine G penicillin 2.4 MU intramuscularly for 3 weeks [**e-Table 58-1**].
Chancroid	• Aphthous ulcers and Behçet syndrome • Factitious ulceration • Granuloma inguinale • Herpes progenitalis • Lymphogranuloma venereum • Metastatic (extraintestinal) Crohn disease • SCC • Syphilis • Traumatic ulceration	Currently accepted treatments of equal efficacy include erythromycin, azithromycin, and ceftriaxone. Large, fluctuant nodes should be aspirated for symptomatic relief and to avoid rupture. Incision and drainage with subsequent wound packing also may be performed [**e-Table 58-2**].

(Continued)

TABLE 58-1   Differential diagnoses and treatments for genital lesions in men[a] (Continued)

Lesion/disease	Differential diagnoses	Treatments
Granuloma inguinale	• Cutaneous amebiasis • Behçet syndrome • Chancroid • Condylomata acuminata • Condylomata lata • Deep mycosis (in endemic areas) • Herpes progenitalis (severe) • Leishmaniasis (in endemic areas) • Scrofuloderma • SCC • Syphilis (primary) • Tuberculosis (cutaneous)	Several antimicrobial regimens are effective to treat granuloma inguinale. Few controlled trials have been published, and recommended regimens vary between the CDC and the WHO. The CDC recommends doxycycline and trimethoprim-sulfamethoxazole as first-line therapy, whereas the WHO guidelines recommend azithromycin.[12-14] All therapies should be continued for at least 3 weeks or until all lesions are healed. If improvement does not occur during the first few days of therapy, an intravenously administered aminoglycoside such as gentamicin may need to be added to the treatment regimen[14] [**e-Table 58-3**].
Lymphogranuloma venereum	• Chancroid • Genital herpes • Hodgkin disease • Syphilis • Ganglionic tuberculosis	Multiple antibiotics successfully treat lymphogranuloma venereum. Additionally, fluctuant nodes should be aspirated as often as necessary. Nodes should not be incised because fistulas may develop[3] [**e-Table 58-4**].
Genital herpes	• Aphthous ulcers • Behçet syndrome • Chancroid • Granuloma inguinale • Lymphogranuloma venereum • Pemphigus vulgaris • Syphilis • Traumatic ulceration	Because there is no cure for genital herpes, treatment is aimed at decreasing the duration and frequency of outbreaks, and the number of asymptomatic shedding episodes.[58] Oral antiviral medications, including acyclovir, valacyclovir, and famciclovir, are used for initial infections, recurrences, and suppressive therapy. All are effective if they are taken during the prodrome or at the first sign of recurrence. Topical therapies are not recommended. Alternative and complementary remedies have little scientific validation [**e-Table 58-5**].
Genital warts	• Condylomata lata (secondary syphilis) • Enlarged sebaceous glands (variation of normal) • Fibroepitheliomas (skin tags) • Lichen planus • Molluscum contagiosum • Pearly penile papules • SCC in situ (Bowen disease)	Treatment of genital warts includes patient- and physician-applied treatments and procedures. An important aspect of treatment is patient counseling because genital warts can cause significant patient distress, including concern about future malignancy. Most patients prefer treatments that they can perform at home without coming into the office. Immunomodulation (imiquimod) has been associated with the lowest recurrence rate of all modalities, but it is more effective in women (~75% clearance rate) than in men (~33% clearance rate).[63] One potential drawback to the use of imiquimod on skin of color is its capacity to induce local vitiligo-like depigmentation[60] [**e-Table 58-6**].
Molluscum contagiosum	• Condylomata acuminata • Cutaneous *Cryptococcus* (in HIV-positive patients) • Epidermal inclusion cyst (or milium) • Herpes simplex or herpes zoster • Lichen planus • Papular granuloma annulare • Sebaceous glands (variation of normal)	Although the lesions usually will resolve on their own, treatment will reduce the duration and infectivity of lesions. Therapy consists of mechanical treatments that remove the molluscum core or topical or systemic treatments. The value of the latter is questionable [**e-Table 58-7**].
Sclerosing lymphangitis	• Essentially pathognomonic • No substantial differential	Cessation or reduction in sexual activity is recommended while the lesion resolves. Very rarely, persistently tender lesions may require surgical removal of the indurated tissue [**e-Table 58-8**].
Tinea cruris	• Candidiasis • Contact dermatitis • Erythrasma • Neurodermatitis • Psoriasis • Tinea versicolor (rarely affects genital skin)	Multiple topical antifungals may be used to effectively clear tinea cruris. The two main classes are allylamines, including terbinafine and naftifine, and azoles, including clotrimazole, econazole, ketoconazole, miconazole, oxiconazole, sertaconazole, and sulconazole; alternative topical therapies include topical butenafine and ciclopirox creams.[61] It is very important to treat onychomycosis, if present, with appropriate systemic therapy. Patients also may require systemic therapy for extensive or refractory tinea cruris or for suppression [**e-Table 58-9**].
Leishmaniasis	• Amebiasis • Chancroid • Granuloma inguinale • Primary syphilis (chancre) • SCC	The treatment of choice for cutaneous leishmaniasis is pentavalent antimony. The antimonial agent used in the United States, sodium stibogluconate, must be obtained from the CDC, which can counsel the physician in its use. Antimonials have a high incidence of reversible side effects. Other treatments for leishmaniasis have been reported.[62] Azole antifungals may prove particularly useful for leishmaniasis acquired in the Middle East by contractors and service personnel serving in war zones [**e-Table 58-10**].

(Continued)

TABLE 58-1 Differential diagnoses and treatments for genital lesions in men[a] (Continued)

Lesion/disease	Differential diagnoses	Treatments
Psoriasis	• Bowen disease • Candidiasis • Contact dermatitis • Drug eruption • Eczema, including lichenified eczema • Lichen planus • Paget disease (extramammary) • Reiter syndrome • Seborrheic dermatitis • Tinea cruris • Zoon balanitis plasmacellularis	The first-line treatment for psoriasis, topical corticosteroid therapy, is more effective on the genitalia than elsewhere because the skin is thin and occluded by clothing. High-potency topical steroids should be avoided on the genitalia. Topical vitamin D derivatives may be used alone or in conjunction with corticosteroids. Topical calcineurin inhibitors appear promising, especially for treatment of anogenital psoriasis.[63] Other topical treatments, such as coal tar, anthralin, and topical retinoids, may be associated with prohibitive irritation when applied to genital skin. UV light is logistically difficult. The systemic agents used for severe psoriasis generally are not required for genital lesions [e-Table 58-11].
Lichen planus	• Bowen disease and bowenoid papulosis • Candidiasis • Condylomata acuminata (external genital warts) • Erythema multiforme • Fixed drug reaction • Granuloma annulare • Lichen simplex chronicus • Psoriasis • Scabies • Syphilis (secondary)	The papular disease that occurs on the genitalia of men is much easier to treat than the erosive variant, which is more common in women. First-line therapy consists of topical steroids or topical calcineurin inhibitors.[64] Systemic therapy should be considered only after failure of these topical modalities and, even then, only for as short a time as possible [e-Table 58-12].
Zoon balanitis	• SCC in situ • SCC (invasive) • *Candida* and *Pseudomonas* balanitis • Contact dermatitis • Psoriasis • Lichen planus	The treatment of choice for Zoon balanitis is circumcision, which may result in cure. Other less well-documented treatments include topical corticosteroids, topical retinoids, and topical tacrolimus. Although laser ablation (eg, carbon dioxide, Er:YAG) has been suggested as a therapeutic option,[65,66] the risk of permanent dyschromia in skin of color militates against this maneuver [e-Table 58-13].
Vitiligo	• Discoid lupus erythematosus • Hansen disease (tuberculoid) • Lichen sclerosus et atrophicus (most important) • Postinflammatory dyschromia • Seborrhea • Tinea versicolor (rare on genital skin)	A number of therapeutic modalities have been touted to induce repigmentation, but none are assured to succeed.[67] The likelihood of success is always better in recent-onset, limited disease occurring in younger patients compared with widespread vitiligo of long duration in older individuals. Genital skin is particularly difficult to approach surgically (eg, epidermal grafts and laser therapy) due to the risk of scar induction.[68] Genital skin is also a suboptimal area for phototherapy due to the difficulty in delivering the appropriate dose of phototherapy to the site. Standard therapy for genital vitiligo consists of application of topical steroids and/or topical calcineurin inhibitors.[67,69] Vitiliginous genital skin has been restored following transfer of noncultured keratinocyte-melanocyte cell suspensions.[70] When therapy is unsuccessful, careful camouflage, such as therapeutic tattoo, may be considered [e-Table 58-14].
Behçet syndrome	• Chancroid • Crohn disease (extraintestinal) • Granuloma inguinale • Herpes progenitalis • Syphilis • Traumatic ulceration	Traditional systemic treatment for Behçet syndrome consists of steroids (with or without various cytotoxic agents), dapsone, and colchicine.[71] Thalidomide has proven beneficial in a handful of cases. Recent reports suggest the utility of anti–tumor necrosis factor-α biologic drugs[72-74] [e-Table 58-15].
Squamous cell carcinoma	• Condylomata acuminata • Condylomata lata • Extramammary Paget disease • Lichen planus (SCC in situ) • Psoriasis (SCC in situ) • Seborrhea (SCC in situ) • Zoon balanitis (SCC in situ)	Treatment of invasive SCC involves resection of the tumor or ablation of the tumor if it is small. Mohs micrographic surgery is an increasingly used tissue-sparing alternative to traditional surgery. Laser ablation and radiation therapy also have been used. Patients with lymph node metastasis must undergo a lymphadenectomy. Courses of topical 5-fluorouracil or imiquimod may be attempted for in situ lesions before surgical extirpation or laser ablation is entertained[75] [e-Table 58-16].
Kaposi sarcoma	• Acral angiodermatitis • Angiokeratoma • Atypical acid-fast bacilli infection • Deep fungal infection • Lichen planus • Metastatic tumor from visceral malignancy • Soft tissue sarcoma	For penile lesions, surgical excision is recommended for small solitary lesions, whereas conservative radiation therapy may be useful for larger lesions. Intralesional chemotherapy may be used for isolated lesions. Adjuvant α or β interferon is used in some patients, but systemic chemotherapy is reserved for patients with visceral involvement or generalized lesions[50] [e-Table 58-17].

(Continued)

TABLE 58-1	Differential diagnoses and treatments for genital lesions in men (Continued)	
Lesion/disease	Differential diagnoses	Treatments
Lichen simplex chronicus	• Atopic dermatitis • Bowen disease • Candidiasis • Contact dermatitis (chronic) • Psoriasis • Pubic lice • Scabies • Tinea cruris	The treatment of lichen simplex chronicus involves identification of underlying disease, repair of barrier layer function, reduction of inflammation, and disruption of the itch-scratch cycle[52] [**e-Table 58-18**].
Contact dermatitis	• Bowen disease • Candidiasis • Extramammary Paget disease • Lichen simplex chronicus • Psoriasis • Seborrheic dermatitis	Treatment involves removal of the offending agents and topical anti-inflammatory treatment. Oral steroids are reserved for patients with severe disease. Patients with significant pruritus or pain may be helped by sedating antihistamines at night [**e-Table 58-19**].
Genital bite wounds	• Chancroid • Granuloma inguinale • Herpes progenitalis (severe) • Primary syphilis	Prompt treatment of human bite wounds should be initiated at presentation to avoid complications. The wound should be irrigated with a bactericidal and virucidal solution. Tetanus boosters need to be given if immunizations are not current. Broad-spectrum antibiotic treatment should be instituted empirically before culture results return because copious amounts of subcutaneous tissue in the genital area allow bacterial spread. The genital area carries a high risk for infection, so bite wounds are not closed[56,57] [**e-Table 58-20**].

Abbreviations: CDC, Centers for Disease Control and Prevention; Er:YAG, erbium-doped yttrium aluminium garnet; HIV, human immunodeficiency virus; RPR, rapid plasma reagin; SCC, squamous cell carcinoma; UV, ultraviolet; WHO, World Health Organization.[a]

CONCLUSION

Genital lesions in men may result from a variety of etiologies such as infectious diseases, including sexually transmitted infections, inflammatory diseases, multisystem benign and malignant neoplasms, and exogenous factors.

Genital dermatoses may occur only on the genitalia or elsewhere on the body, requiring the need for full-body checks because lesions may have a different appearance when found on genital skin compared with other anatomic sites. An example of this is psoriasis, which occurs less commonly in darker skin of color Americans than in Caucasian Americans and may possess an atypical morphology and require diagnosis by biopsy.

The most common STI in Africa, chancroid, is also prevalent in the United States and occurs in urban epidemics, most commonly in darker skin of color men. In the United States and Africa, there has also been a high mortality rate reported in darker skin of color patients from genital SCC.

REFERENCES

1. Goldman BD. Common dermatoses of the male genitalia. *Postgrad Med.* 2000;108:89-91.
2. Rosen T. Update on genital lesions. *JAMA.* 2003;290:1001-1005.
3. Lynch PJ, Edwards L. Infectious primary ulcers. In: Lynch PJ, Edwards L, eds. *Genital Dermatology.* New York, NY: Churchill-Livingstone;1994:205-212.
4. Centers for Disease Control and Prevention (CDC). Primary and secondary syphilis—United States, 2003-2004. *MMWR.* 2005;58:269-273.
5. Lynn WA, Lightman S. Syphilis and HIV: a dangerous combination. *Lancet Infect Dis.* 2004;4:456-466.
6. Zeltser R, Kurban AK. Syphilis. *Clin Dermatol.* 2004;22:461-468.
7. Lewis DA. Chancroid: clinical manifestations, diagnosis, and management. *Sex Transm Infect.* 2003;79:68-71.
8. Bong CTH, Bauer ME, Spinola SM. Haemophilus ducreyi: clinical features, epidemiology, and prospects for disease control. *Microbes Infect.* 2002;4:1141-1148.
9. Jones CC, Rosen T. Cultural diagnosis of chancroid. *Arch Dermatol.* 1991;127:1823-1827.
10. Rosen T, Tschen JA, Ramsdell W, et al. Granuloma inguinale. *J Am Acad Dermatol.* 1984;11:433-437.
11. Rosen T. Tropical infections: granuloma inguinale. In: *Clinical Dermatology in Black Patients.* Bari, Italy: PiGreco Press; 1995:169-170.
12. O'Farrell N. Donovanosis. *Sex Transm Infect.* 2002;78:452-457.
13. Lupi O, Madkan V, Tyring SK. Tropical dermatology: bacterial tropical diseases. *J Am Acad Dermatol.* 2006;54:589-578.
14. Centers for Disease Control and Prevention. Sexually transmitted diseases treatment guidelines 2002. *MMWR.* 2002;51:1-78.
14a. Ceovic R, Gulin SJ. Lymphogranuloma venereum: diagnostic and treatment challenges. *Infect Drug Resist.* 2015;8:39-47.
15. Rosen T, Brown TJ. Genital ulcers: evaluation and treatment. *Dermatol Clin.* 1998;16:673-685.
16. Beauman JG. Genital herpes: a review. *Am Fam Physician.* 2005;72:1527-1534.
17. Lynch PJ, Edwards L. Vesicular disease. In: Lynch PJ, Edwards L, eds. *Genital Dermatology.* New York, NY: Churchill-Livingstone; 1994:181-186.
18. Solomon J, Cannon MJ, Reyes M, et al. Epidemiology of recurrent genital herpes simplex virus types 1 and 2. *Sex Transm Infect.* 2003;79:456-459.
19. Dupin N. Genital warts. *Clin Dermatol.* 2004;22:481-486.
20. Koutsky L. Epidemiology of genital human papillomavirus infection. *Am J Med.* 1997;102:3-8.
21. Handsfield HH. Clinical presentation and natural course of anogenital warts. *Am J Med.* 1997;102:16-20.
22. Tyring S. Introduction: perspectives on human papillomavirus infection. *Am J Med.* 1997;102:1-2.
23. Kodner CM, Nasraty S. Management of genital warts. *Am Fam Physician.* 2004;70:2335-2342.
24. Smith KJ, Skelton H. Molluscum contagiosum: recent advances in pathogenic mechanisms, and new therapies. *Am J Clin Dermatol.* 2002;3:535-545.
25. Hanson D, Diven DG. Molluscum contagiosum. *Dermatol Online J.* 2003;9:2.
26. Lynch PJ, Edwards L. Skin-colored nodules. In: Lynch PJ, Edwards L, eds. *Genital Dermatology.* New York, NY: Churchill-Livingstone; 1994:137-148.
27. Kumar B, Narang T, Radotra BD, et al. Mondor's disease of the penis: a forgotten disease. *Sex Transm Infect.* 2005;81:480-482.
28. Rosen T, Hwong H. Sclerosing lymphangitis of the penis. *J Am Acad Dermatol.* 2003;49:916-918.
29. Grunwald MH, Amichai B, Trau H. Cutaneous leishmaniasis on an unusual site: the glans penis. *Br J Urol.* 1998;82:928.
30. Markle WH, Makhoul K. Cutaneous leishmaniasis: recognition and treatment. *Am Fam Physician.* 2004;69:458-460.

31. Richens J. Genital manifestations of tropical diseases. *Sex Transm Infect.* 2004;80:12-17.

32. Krueger G, Ellis CN. Psoriasis: recent advances in understanding its pathogenesis and treatment. *J Am Acad Dermatol.* 2005;53:S94-S100.

33. Rosen T. Diseases with unusual features: psoriasis. In: *Clinical Dermatology in Black Patients.* Bari, Italy: PiGreco Press; 1995:51-54.

34. Moyal-Barracco M, Edwards L. Diagnosis and therapy of anogenital lichen planus. *Dermatol Ther.* 2004;17:38-46.

35. Rosen T. Diseases with unusual features: lichen planus. In: *Clinical Dermatology in Black Patients.* Bari, Italy: PiGreco Press; 1995:36-40.

36. Farber EM, Nall L. Genital psoriasis. *Cutis.* 1992;50:263-266.

37. Moreno-Arias GA, Camos-Fresneda A, Llaberia C, et al. Plasma cell balanitis treated with tacrolimus 0.1%. *Br J Dermatol.* 2005;153:1204-1206.

38. Stern JK, Rosen T. Balanitis plasmacellularis circumscripta (Zoon's balanitis plasmacellularis). *Cutis.* 1980;25:57-60.

39. Davis-Daneshfar A, Trueb RM. Bowen's disease of the glans penis (erythroplasia of Queyrat) in plasma cell balanitis. *Cutis.* 2000;65:95-98.

40. Passeron T, Ortonne JP. Pathophysiology and genetics of vitiligo. *J Autoimmun Dis.* 2005;25:63S-68S.

41. Handa S, Kaur I. Vitiligo: clinical findings in 1436 patients. *J Dermatol.* 1999;26:653-657.

42. Jacyk WK. Behçet's disease in South African blacks: report of five cases. *J Am Acad Dermatol.* 1994;30:869-873.

43. Fisher BK, Margesson LJ. Inflammatory lesions of the penis. In: *Genital Skin Disorders: Diagnosis and Treatment.* St. Louis, MO: Mosby; 1998:40-64.

43a. Barnholtz-Sloan JS, Maldonado JL, Pow-sang J, et al. Incidence trends in primary malignant penile cancer. *Urol Oncol.* 2007;25:361-367.

44. Rippentrop JM, Joslyn SA, Konety BR. Squamous cell carcinoma of the penis: evaluation of data from the surveillance, epidemiology, and end results program. *Cancer.* 2004;101:1357-1363.

45. Hubbell CR, Rabin VR, Mora RG. Cancer of the skin in blacks: V. A review of 175 black patients with squamous cell carcinoma of the penis. *J Am Acad Dermatol.* 1988;18:292-298.

46. Kroon BK, Horenblas S, Nieweg OE. Contemporary management of penile squamous cell carcinoma. *J Surg Oncol.* 2005;89:43-50.

47. Pantanowitz L, Dezube BJ. Advances in the pathobiology and treatment of Kaposi sarcoma. *Curr Opin Oncol.* 2004;16:443-449.

48. Noy A. Update in Kaposi sarcoma. *Curr Opin Oncol.* 2003;15:379-381.

49. Rosen T. Diseases more often seen in blacks: Kaposi's sarcoma. In: *Clinical Dermatology in Black Patients.* Bari, Italy: PiGreco Press; 1995:90-92.

50. Micali G, Nasca MR, Pasquale RD, et al. Primary classic Kaposi's sarcoma of the penis: report of a case and review. *J Eur Acad Dermatol Venereol.* 2003;17:320-323.

51. Rosen T, Hoffman J, Jones A. Penile Kaposi's sarcoma. *J Eur Acad Dermatol Venereol.* 1999;13:71-73.

52. Lynch PJ. Lichen simplex chronicus (atopic/neurodermatitis) of the anogenital region. *Dermatol Ther.* 2004;17:8-19.

53. Bircher AJ, Hirsbrunner P, Langauer S. Allergic contact dermatitis of the genitals from rubber additives in condoms. *Contact Dermatitis.* 1993;28:125-126.

54. Foti C, Bonamonte D, Antelmi A, et al. Allergic contact dermatitis to condoms: description of a clinical case and analytical review of current literature. *Immunopharmacol Immunotoxicol.* 2004;26:481-485.

55. Kugler K, Brinkmeier T, Frosch PJ, et al. Anogenital dermatoses: allergic and irritative causative factors. Analysis of IVDK data and review of the literature. *J Dtsch Dermatol Ges.* 2005;3:979-986.

56. Rosen T, Conrad N. Genital ulcer caused by human bite to the penis. *Sex Transm Dis.* 1999;26:527-530.

57. Rosen T. Penile ulcer from traumatic orogenital contact. *Dermatol Online J.* 2005;11:18.

58. Gupta R, Wald A. Genital herpes: antiviral therapy for symptom relief and prevention of transmission. *Expert Opin Pharmacother.* 2006;7:665-675.

59. Scheinfeld N, Lehman DS. An evidence-based review of medical and surgical treatments of genital warts. *Dermatol Online J.* 2006;12:5.

60. Brown T, Zirvi M, Cotsarelis G, et al. Vitiligo-like hypopigmentation associated with imiquimod treatment of genital warts. *J Am Acad Dermatol.* 2005;52:715-716.

61. Gupta AK, Ryder JE, Chow M, et al. Dermatophytosis: the management of fungal infections. *Skinmed.* 2005;4:305-310.

62. Lee SA, Hasbun R. Therapy of cutaneous leishmaniasis. *Int J Infect Dis.* 2003;7:86-93.

63. Martin Ezquerra G, Sanchez Regana M, Herrera Acosta E, et al. Topical tacrolimus for the treatment of psoriasis on the face, genitalia, intertriginous areas and corporal plaques. *J Drugs Dermatol.* 2006;5:334-336.

64. Lonsdale-Eccles AA, Velangi S. Topical pimecrolimus in the treatment of genital lichen planus: a prospective case series. *Br J Dermatol.* 2005;153:390-394.

65. Retamar RA, Kien MC, Chouela EN. Zoon's balanitis: presentation of 15 patients, five treated with a carbon dioxide laser. *Int J Dermatol.* 2003;42:305-307.

66. Albertini JG, Holck DE, Farley MF. Zoon's balanitis treated with erbium: YAG laser ablation. *Lasers Surg Med.* 2002;30:123-126.

67. Grimes PE. New insights and new therapies for vitiligo. *JAMA.* 2005;293:730-735.

68. Falabella R. Surgical approaches for stable vitiligo. *Dermatol Surg.* 2005;31:1277-1284.

69. Kostovic K, Pasic A. New treatment modalities for vitiligo: focus on topical immunomodulators. *Drugs.* 2005;65:447-459.

70. Mulekar SV, Al Issa A, AL Eisa A, et al. Genital vitiligo treated by autologous, noncultured melanocyte-keratinocyte cell transplantation. *Dermatol Surg.* 2005;31:1737-1739.

71. Barnes CG. Treatment of Behçet's syndrome. *Rheumatology (Oxf).* 2006;45:245-247.

72. Atenzi F, Sarzi-Puttini P, Capsoni F, et al. Successful treatment of resistant Behçet's disease with etanercept. *Clin Exp Rheumatol.* 2005;23:729.

73. Connolly M, Armstrong JS, Buckley DS. Infliximab treatment for severe orogenital ulceration in Behçet's disease. *Br J Dermatol.* 2005;153:1073-1075.

74. Haugeberg G, Velken M, Johnsen V. Successful treatment of genital ulcers with infliximab in Behçet's disease. *Ann Rheum Dis.* 2004;63:744-745.

75. Orengo I, Rosen T, Guill CK. Treatment of squamous cell carcinoma in situ of the penis with 5% imiquimod cream: a case report. *J Am Acad Dermatol.* 2002;47:S225-S228.

CHAPTER
59

Genital Lesions in Women

Theodore Rosen
Christy B. Doherty

KEY POINTS

- Genital lesions may have a unique appearance in skin of color, and the appearance may vary between men and women.

- Genital lesions are difficult to diagnose based solely on morphology.

- Genital dermatoses may occur only on the genitals or may occur anywhere on the body, and lesions may have a different appearance when found on genital skin than when seen elsewhere on the body.

- Most recently, overall rates of primary and secondary syphilis were higher among darker skin of color Americans and Hispanics than among Caucasian Americans, although rates decreased among darker skin of color American females.

- Most women are unaware of the primary chancre. Cervical, anal, and oral lesions are possible, although extragenital chancres are apparently less common in darker skin of color individuals.

- Darker skin of color American patients, especially women, are reportedly more likely to develop condylomata lata in secondary syphilis than Caucasian Americans.

- The annular syphilid (round facial lesions located near orifices) is nearly unique to darker skin of color individuals.

- Vulvar contact dermatitis may present with edema, vesicles or bullae, erythema, and weeping. Patients with darker skin of color may show hyperpigmentation instead of erythema.

- The physician may need to perform additional studies, including biopsies, when evaluating genital lesions.

INTRODUCTION

Similar to those seen in men, genital lesions seen in women may have a unique appearance in skin of color individuals (see Chapter 58, Genital Lesions in Men). There may also be variation in both the statistical frequency and clinical characteristics of selected lesions between men and women.

INFECTIOUS DISEASES

◼ SEXUALLY TRANSMITTED INFECTIONS

Syphilis

Epidemiology, Etiology, and Pathogenesis Syphilis primarily affects young adults of both sexes. After rates of syphilis dropped to the lowest reported rate of 2.1 cases per 100,000 population in 2000, the primary and secondary syphilis rate increased to 2.7 between 2001 and 2004.[1] From 2000 to 2004, overall rates of primary and secondary syphilis were higher among darker skin of color Americans than among Caucasian Americans, although rates decreased among darker skin of color American females.[1] Syphilis is caused by the bacterial spirochete *Treponema pallidum* and is transmitted via sexual contact, likely by inoculation into tiny abrasions from sexual trauma.[2] After spreading to the regional lymph nodes, treponemes spread via a hematogenous route to other parts of the body.

Clinical Findings The primary lesion of syphilis is a solitary, painless ulcer (chancre) that develops in the genital area approximately 9 to 90 days after sexual contact with an infected individual [**Figure 59-1**].[3] The labia major and the perineal skin just adjacent to the vaginal orifice are the most frequent sites affected. Most women are unaware of the primary chancre.[4] Cervical, anal, and oral lesions are possible, although extragenital chancres are apparently less common in darker skin of color individuals.[3] Between 1 to 2 months after the chancre disappears, secondary syphilis presents with a generalized papulosquamous rash involving the palms, soles, trunk, face, and genitalia with or without concomitant lymphadenopathy, patchy alopecia, condylomata lata (exudative anogenital plaques), and/or mucous patches in the form of grayish-white round papules and thin plaques in the mouth and on the vulvar and perineal area. Darker skin of color individuals, especially women, are reportedly more likely to develop condylomata lata in secondary syphilis than Caucasian Americans.[3] The annular syphilid (round facial lesions located near orifices) is nearly unique to darker skin of color patients[3] [**Figure 59-2**].

Diagnosis may be made by identification of treponemes using dark-field microscopy of samples from primary chancre, condylomata lata,

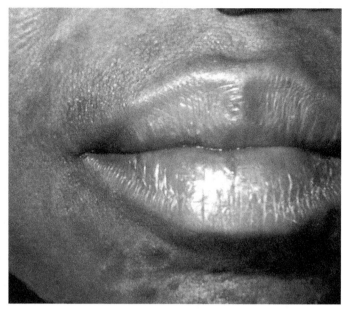

FIGURE 59-2. Secondary clues of perioral annular syphilis in an individual with darker skin of color.

genital mucosal lesions, skin papules, or lymph node aspirate.[2] Using specific treponemal fluorescent antibody stains or silver stains (ie, the Warthin-Starry stain), organisms may be detectable in biopsy specimens. However, silver also stains melanin, complicating the interpretation of biopsies from patients with darker skin of color.[3] Serologic tests available for confirmation are nontreponemal cardiolipin-based, such as the rapid plasma reagin (RPR) and the Venereal Disease Research Laboratory (VDRL) tests, or treponemal antigen-based, such as the *T. pallidum* particle agglutination (TPPA) or hemagglutination (TPHA) and fluorescent antibody absorption (FTA-abs) tests. A new diagnosis of syphilis mandates investigation for concomitant human immunodeficiency virus (HIV) infection.

Complications Tertiary syphilis is characterized by destructive gummas, manifesting dermatologically as heavily crusted granulomatous lesions of the skin. Neurologic and cardiovascular structures are vulnerable to gummatous syphilis as well.

Prognosis/Clinical Course Failure to receive adequate treatment at any stage of syphilis may result in the development of subsequent stages of the disease. However, adequate treatment of primary, secondary, or early latent infectious syphilis should result in disappearance of the clinical manifestations of active disease, although residual postinflammatory hyperpigmentation is possible in dark skin. The titer of RPR or VDRL and the clinical symptoms must be followed after treatment to verify therapeutic efficacy.

Granuloma Inguinale

Epidemiology, Etiology, and Pathogenesis Granuloma inguinale, also known as donovanosis, is caused by infection with an encapsulated Gram-negative rod called *Calymmatobacterium granulomatis*. Transmission is most likely due to sexual contact,[5] and infection is seen predominantly in sexually active individuals aged between 18 and 40 with a 3:1 male predominance.[6] This infection is endemic in New Guinea, Africa, Australia, and areas of India, China, and the Caribbean basin but rare in the United States.[6] Due to the natural geographic distribution of donovanosis, it is more likely to be encountered among those with skin of color.

Clinical Findings After a variable incubation period ranging from 2 weeks to 6 months, granuloma inguinale begins as a single or multiple nodules that erode to become well-defined, painless, friable ulcerations with a rolled border.[5] As lesions extend to involve normal surrounding skin, the ulcer base develops a beefy red color that resembles granulation tissue.[7] Despite ulceration, the lesions tend to be painless, and regional adenopathy is not a feature of this disorder. The most

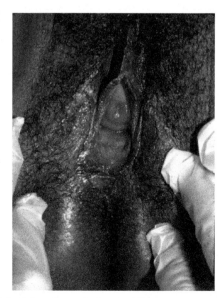

FIGURE 59-1. Solitary chancre of primary syphilis.

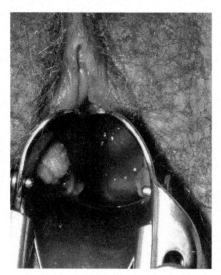

FIGURE 59-3. Granuloma inguinale with cervical lesions.

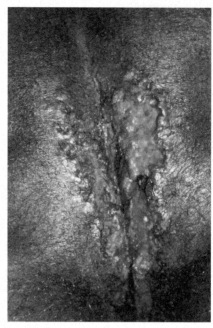

FIGURE 59-4. Perianal herpes simplex virus type 2–related erosions acquired via receptive anal intercourse.

commonly affected sites in females are the *labia minora* and perigenital area, although infection also may involve the cervix, uterus, and adnexa [**Figure 59-3**]. Diagnosis is based on the demonstration of Donovan bodies (intracellular bipolar-staining bacteria within histiocytes) with Giemsa, Wright, or silver stains performed on tissue crush preparations or biopsy specimens obtained from the leading edge of the ulcer. The use of cultures is impractical.

Complications With extensive and deep ulceration and necrosis of soft tissues, fistulas may form.[5] Mutilating genital destruction may eventuate in untreated disease. There is a small but real increased incidence of squamous cell carcinoma (SCC) of affected genital skin.

Prognosis/Clinical Course Lesions may stabilize but will not remit independent of treatment. Prolonged therapy may be necessary to allow for complete healing.[6]

Genital Herpes

Epidemiology, Etiology, and Pathogenesis Herpes simplex virus (HSV) is a sexually transmitted infection that enters the body through the skin or mucous membranes via direct sexual contact with the secretions or mucosal surfaces of an infected individual.[8] After multiplying initially in the epithelial layer, the virus travels in the sensory nerve roots to the dorsal root ganglion, where it becomes latent. Mucocutaneous outbreaks of HSV are triggered by the reactivation of the latent virus, which subsequently travels back down the nerve root. HSV type 2 (HSV-2) is more commonly causative in cases of genital herpes, as opposed to HSV type 1 (HSV-1), which is more closely associated with herpes labialis.

Genital herpes is a prevalent infection, with approximately 50 million Americans infected and 500,000 to 700,000 new infections per year.[8] HSV-2 seropositivity appears to be higher among darker-skinned individuals in the United States than among fairer-skinned individuals and more prevalent among women than among men, reflecting the greater ease of transmission from men to their female partners.[9,10]

Clinical Findings After an incubation period of 2 to 20 days (average: 7 days), primary lesions develop, consisting of painful, grouped vesicles that ultimately rupture to become painful ulcers[4] [**Figure 59-4**]. In women, ulcers may appear on the introitus, urethral meatus, labia, and perineum.[8] Women typically are afflicted with more severe disease, systemic symptoms, and complications than men. Cervical ulcerative lesions are possible, particularly with the initial outbreak. Additionally, women may complain of dysuria and urinary retention secondary to urethral lesions. Recurrent HSV outbreaks typically are milder than the initial outbreak, and women reportedly have fewer recurrences than men.

Although the diagnosis of genital herpes is largely clinical, it may be confirmed using viral culture, a Tzanck smear (showing viral

acantholytic giant cells), a polymerase chain reaction test for HSV DNA, or characteristic histopathology.

Complications Women are more susceptible to systemic complications, such as aseptic meningitis.[8] Perhaps the most dreaded complication is transmission to a neonate due to viral shedding in the genital tract during normal vaginal delivery. The risk of neonatal herpes is greatest (approximately 50%) when a woman has acquired the disease during gestation and has active lesions at the time of delivery. Conversely, the risk is lowest (approximately 0.04%) when the disease is long-standing and there are no active lesions at the time of delivery.

Prognosis/Clinical Course There is no cure for herpes, and recurrence of lesions is expected, with an average of four outbreaks per year. Individuals who experience more severe primary infections appear to have recurrent episodes more frequently.

Genital Warts (Condylomata Acuminata)

Epidemiology, Etiology, and Pathogenesis Genital warts, or condylomata acuminata, are caused by human papillomavirus (HPV), most commonly, types 6 and 11.[11] Transmission of the virus in most adults is primarily sexual. Seroprevalence suggests that 1% of sexually active American adults have visible genital warts, whereas at least 15% have subclinical infection.[12] Sexually active women under the age of 25 years have the highest rates of genital HPV infection.

Clinical Findings Lesions typically develop 2 to 3 months after exposure and begin as small papules that may develop into skin-colored to reddish, filiform, asymptomatic papules [**Figure 59-5**]. The skin around the vaginal introitus and perianal area is affected most commonly, but the cervix also may have lesions[11]. Although genital warts are chiefly a clinical diagnosis, confirmation may be achieved through biopsy.

Complications Invasive SCC arising from long-standing genital warts is possible but rare.[13]

Prognosis/Clinical Course HPV infections tend to have a fluctuating clinical course of visible lesions, latency, and recurrence.[14] However, most clinically apparent lesions eventually resolve in several months to years.

■ NONSEXUALLY TRANSMITTED INFECTIONS

Tinea Cruris

Epidemiology, Etiology, and Pathogenesis Tinea cruris (ringworm of the groin) is caused most commonly by *Trichophyton rubrum*, the

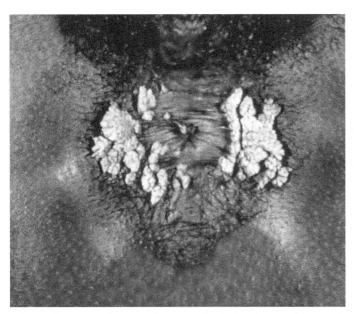

FIGURE 59-5. Aggregate cauliflower-shaped masses typical of anogenital warts.

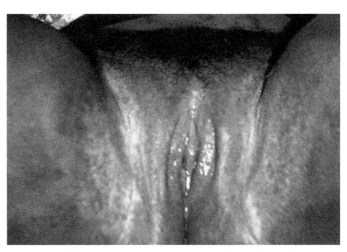

FIGURE 59-7. Erythema and edema extending from the vulva to the inner thigh due to a severe *Candida* infection.

same organism responsible for most cases of tinea corporis.[15] This condition is less common in women than in men and typically affects young adults.[4] Infection can be spread via sexual contact with infected skin or through autoinoculation from tinea pedis by shaving upward toward the bikini line.

Clinical Findings A pruritic, erythematous, scaling rash develops over weeks that involves any area from the proximal inner thigh area to the crural crease. In women, the rash has a propensity to involve the hair-bearing portion of the vulva. Patients with darker skin of color may present with striking hyperpigmentation instead of erythema [**Figure 59-6**]. A peripheral border with overlying scale lends to an annular appearance, but it is not always present. Feet also should be examined because concurrent onychomycosis is often present.

Tinea cruris may be diagnosed clinically, but the diagnosis can be confirmed by potassium hydroxide (KOH) examination or fungal culture of the peripheral scale. Care should be taken to distinguish tinea from candidiasis. Whereas tinea cruris tends to have annular lesions with central clearing and no satellite lesions, candidiasis presents with confluent erythema and satellite pustules.

Complications Follicular or extensive involvement makes the infection more difficult to clear.

Prognosis/Clinical Course Affected individuals are at elevated risk for recurrence, although infections may be eradicated temporarily with therapy. Ongoing intermittent therapy with topical antifungals may be indicated to prevent return of the infection.[16]

Candidiasis

Epidemiology, Etiology, and Pathogenesis Candidiasis is a muco-cutaneous yeast infection found commonly in women, particularly immunocompromised individuals. Most infections are due to *Candida albicans,* an organism found in the vagina and gastrointestinal tract of healthy women that becomes pathogenic under the influence of factors such as medication (eg, antibiotics, corticosteroids, or chemotherapy), disease (eg, diabetes or immunodeficiency), and hormones (eg, due to pregnancy or birth control pills). The source of the infection may be a sexual partner.

Clinical Finding Women may develop candidal vaginitis, vulvitis, or vulvovaginitis, with presenting symptoms being moderate to severe itching or burning and a varying amount of curd-like vaginal discharge. Inflammation with satellite pustules may be seen within the vestibule, in the interlabial crease and over the labia minora and majora. If infection is more severe, inflammation may be found in the crural fold and on the upper inner thigh [**Figure 59-7**]. Vulvar edema, at times severe, may be present. Diagnosis is clinical, with confirmation via culture and/or KOH wet mount.

Complications In patients with persistent infection, constant scratching may lead to secondary lichenification, excoriation, and chronic swelling that resembles lichen simplex chronicus or chronic contact dermatitis.[4] In severe infections, particularly those seen in immunocompromised patients, erosions may complicate the disease course.

Prognosis/Clinical Course In most cases, treatment is necessary to clear the infection. Women with vulvovaginitis are susceptible to recurrence because *Candida* is a normal inhabitant of the gastrointestinal tract and vagina. Frequently recurrent or chronic vaginal candidiasis is a common problem, and there is no simple remedy.[17] It is important that women with recurrent symptoms be evaluated for bacterial vaginosis, *Trichomonas* infection, and infection with a non-*albicans Candida* species, because these conditions will not respond well to conventional treatment.

INFLAMMATORY DISEASES

▨ PAPULOSQUAMOUS

Lichen Planus

Epidemiology, Etiology, and Pathogenesis Lichen planus (LP) is a papulosquamous skin condition thought to be related to T-cell autoimmunity.[18] Vulvovaginal LP most commonly affects women aged between 30 and 60 years. Once thought to be an uncommon occurrence, genital LP is being diagnosed more frequently, especially in women, because

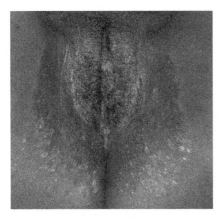

FIGURE 59-6. Hyperpigmented, scaly patch of tinea cruris in a woman with skin of color.

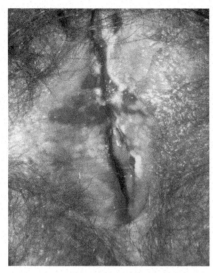

FIGURE 59-8. Erosive lichen planus resembling genital herpes. (Used with permission from Libby Edwards, MD.)

more physicians are familiar with the entity and its wide morphologic range. Approximately 1% of the general population has oral LP; of women with oral LP, 20% to 25% also have genital disease.[19]

Clinical Findings Individuals with genital LP may complain of severe pruritus and, if there is scarring, dyspareunia. Vulvar LP, particularly the erosive variant, typically is associated with inflammatory vaginitis, and patients may bleed during sexual intercourse or gynecologic examination and complain of purulent, irritating vaginal discharge.[18]

Genital LP lesions vary widely in morphology, but the most common and most difficult to treat is the erosive variant [**Figure 59-8**]. Erosive LP occurs more often in women than in men and occurs on the moist skin of the vulva and within the vagina. The most common site to be affected by erosive lesions is the posterior vulvar vestibule, from which lesions extend to involve the labia minora. Individuals also may exhibit superficial gingival erosions, termed vulvovaginal-gingival syndrome.

Vulvar LP, when associated with generalized LP, resembles the more classic violaceous, polygonal, papular or plaque morphology seen on extragenital skin and involves the labia or mons pubis.[20] In individuals with darker skin of color, classic lesions are typically deeper in color due to the larger amount of melanin displaced from the epidermis.[19]

The least common form of vulvar LP is the hypertrophic variant, which presents with extensive white scarring of the periclitoral area that extends along the interlabial sulcus to the introitus. White hyperkeratotic papules may have classic-appearing reticulate surface markings.

Diagnosis is achieved through biopsy of a noneroded red or white macule or papule.[18] The edge of the erosion should be taken when sampling such a lesion. Direct and indirect immunofluorescence can exclude an autoimmune blistering disorder.

Complications With chronic erosive disease, inflamed and eroded surfaces may adhere and result in adhesions and disappearance of the normal external architecture, including loss of the labia minora, agglutination of the clitoral prepuce with covering of the clitoris by scar tissue, and narrowing of the introitus.[20] Although uncommon, erosive LP of the mouth or vulva eventually may develop into SCC.[18] It should be suspected in a chronic, indurated or granulated ulcer or in a white hyperkeratotic, poorly demarcated papule or plaque.

Prognosis/Clinical Course Nonerosive LP lesions may be well controlled with topical corticosteroids, and the disease may remit spontaneously. Erosive disease tends to be chronic, recalcitrant, and scarring. The course of erosive LP is one of exacerbations with slow healing, recurrent secondary infections, and slow response to therapy.

◼ NONPAPULOSQUAMOUS

Lichen Sclerosus et Atrophicus

Epidemiology, Etiology, and Pathogenesis Lichen sclerosus is a chronic inflammatory skin condition that most commonly affects middle-aged women.[21] Various studies give a female-to-male ratio that ranges from 6:1 to 10:1.[21] Although the etiology is largely unknown, there appears to be a genetic susceptibility and a connection with autoimmune mechanisms. Lichen sclerosus is thought to exhibit the Koebner phenomenon such that trauma and injury may trigger symptoms in vulnerable individuals.

Clinical Findings Genital lesions may appear as a complete or incomplete 'figure of eight' pattern of hypopigmentation around the vulva and anus, with patients complaining of intractable pruritus and soreness of the affected areas. Dysuria, dyspareunia, and pain with defecation are not uncommon. Skin changes include the development of areas of pallor ranging from small polygonal patches to large plaques, as well as atrophic, fragile skin with telangiectasias, purpura, erosions, and tender fissures. Biopsy is used to confirm the diagnosis of lichen sclerosus and to rule out malignant degeneration.

Complications Scarring may disrupt the normal architecture of the genitalia.[21] The labia minora may fuse or be entirely resorbed, the clitoris may become buried, and the introitus may narrow. Additionally, approximately 3% to 5% of vulvar lichen sclerosus lesions progress to SCC.[21]

Prognosis/Clinical Course Individuals treated properly do well, often with cessation of symptoms and no further scarring. However, there is no reversal of existing scarring, and the disease does not remit permanently. Therefore, ongoing topical therapy generally is indicated to maintain control of disease. Surgery may be required to lyse scars that interfere with normal functioning. High potency topical corticosteroids and topical calcineurin inhibitors seem to be particularly effective in the management of lichen sclerosus et atrophicus in women.[22-24]

Vitiligo

Epidemiology, Etiology, and Pathogenesis Vitiligo is a chronic condition characterized by skin depigmentation due to an autoimmune response which destroys the melanocytes; while the etiology is uncertain, a familial predilection is noted.[25] The disease is very apparent in skin of color, and often extremely psychologically distressing for the patient; this may explain why more patients with skin of color seek treatment in comparison to patients of other populations who are equally affected. The vast majority of cases exhibit onset of the disease before the age of 40 years and there is no gender predilection.

Clinical Findings White/depigmented patches on the skin are the major clinical finding of vitiligo. Frequent sites of involvement tend to be sun-exposed areas, such as the dorsa of the hands and feet and periorificial regions of the face. Other general areas include the armpits, genitals, and navel. In women, involvement of the vulva in common [**Figure 59-9**].

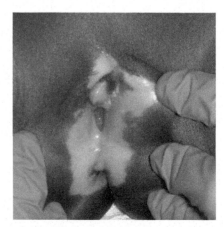

FIGURE 59-9. Genital vitiligo often begins at an early age, as in this patient. (Used with permission from Noah Scheinfeld, MD.)

Complication The presence of the disease itself does not result in any other medical complications. However, potential comorbid conditions include thyroid dysfunction, pernicious anemia, and diabetes mellitus.[26]

Prognosis/Clinical Course Vitiligo is highly unpredictable and it is not possible to calculate if depigmented patches will resolve, spread progressively, or remain stable and persist indefinitely. The speed of the spread of depigmentation also varies.

MULTISYSTEM DISEASES

▨ CROHN DISEASE

Epidemiology, Etiology, and Pathogenesis Crohn disease (CD) is a chronic granulomatous disorder that may involve any portion of the gastrointestinal tract.[27] The disease typically begins between the ages of 20 and 30 years but can persist into the geriatric years. Cutaneous manifestations occur in 22% to 44% of patients with CD.[27a] The skin can be involved by direct extension from the gastrointestinal tract or via involvement away from the gastrointestinal tract, so-called metastatic CD. Genital involvement in CD is less frequent in men than in women. About 2% of women with CD have vulvar involvement.[27] The etiology of CD is unknown, but proposed causes include an unrecognized infectious agent or a disturbed immunologic reaction to an intestinal organism in genetically vulnerable individuals.

Among those with inflammatory bowel disease seen in the United States, Caucasians and African Americans are equally likely to manifest CD, whereas those of Hispanic origin more often have ulcerative colitis.[28]

Clinical Findings There are three patterns of anogenital CD involvement. Contiguous disease represents direct extension from the involved intestine with the formation of sinuses/fistulas involving the skin. Metastatic disease, albeit rare, consists of ulcers and swelling in the vulvar area. There are also nonspecific mucocutaneous lesions, including aphthous ulcers and pyoderma gangrenosum. Female patients with metastatic CD classically present with painful swelling and ulceration of the vulvar or perianal area. The classic ulcerations are deemed 'knife cut' linear fissures and are located along the labiocrural fold [**Figure 59-10**]. Ulcers also may be solitary, deep, and necrotic. The diagnosis of cutaneous CD is based on a biopsy showing the typical granulomatous change.

Complications Patients may present with complications directly related to the underlying inflammatory bowel disease, such as enteric fistulas, granulomatous salpingitis and oophoritis, vulvar abscesses, destructive perineal disease, and vulvar granulomas.[27] Complications unrelated to

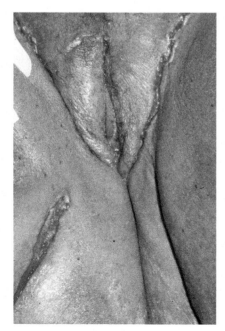

FIGURE 59-10. Cut-like perigenital erosions characteristic of Crohn disease. (Used with permission from Libby Edwards, MD.)

bowel involvement include anemia, dysmenorrhea, Bowen disease of the vulva or vagina, and pyoderma gangrenosum (at any body site).

Prognosis/Clinical Course Anogenital lesions are chronic but should improve if the gastrointestinal manifestations of the disease are controlled.[29]

TUMORS

▨ NON-MALIGNANT

Benign Cysts

Epidemiology, Etiology, and Pathogenesis Benign genital cysts are very common, with an estimated prevalence of 1 in 200 women affected; this is thought to be an underestimation because most cysts are not reported.[30] Cyst formation appears to increase with age but has no racial predilection.

Epidermal inclusion cysts are the most common genital cyst in women.[31] They develop from buried epithelial fragments, most commonly following an episiotomy or other surgical procedure, or from a blockage in the pilosebaceous duct. Bartholin duct cysts are due to ductal obstruction within one of the two major vulvar vestibular glands, typically from a previous infection or inspissated mucus. Vestibular mucous cysts are simple cysts of the vulvar vestibule composed of mucus-secreting epithelium. Skene duct cysts (uncommon paraurethral duct cysts) are caused by obstruction of the Skene ducts, most commonly secondary to gonorrheal infection.[32]

Clinical Findings Vaginal cysts are most commonly found incidentally on examination, but patients may complain of mild discomfort, vaginal pressure, or urinary incontinence or retention.

Epidermal inclusion cysts are classically round, firm, smooth, and mobile; overlying skin may have a yellowish color. Bartholin duct cysts present as round or ovoid cystic lesions at the 5 or 7 o'clock positions on the hymenal ring. Cysts are usually 1 to 4 cm in diameter, but lesions may cause enough swelling to block the entire introital area. Vestibular mucous cysts range from 0.5 to 1.5 cm in diameter. These are typically located around the introitus and are mobile, nontender, and yellowish or bluish. Skene duct cysts are located near the edge of the urethral meatus, are mobile, and are skin-colored or translucent. Diagnosis of cysts is clinical, but a biopsy may confirm the diagnosis.

Complications If cystic lesions continue to grow, they may obstruct the urethral meatus or the vaginal introitus. Cysts may become infected and subsequently tender.

Prognosis/Clinical Course Asymptomatic, small cysts need not be treated and likely will not become problematic. However, cysts causing pain or urinary symptoms should not be expected to remit spontaneously and should be treated by excision.

▨ MALIGNANT

Squamous Cell Carcinoma

Epidemiology, Etiology, and Pathogenesis SCC accounts for 85% to 90% of malignant tumors of the vulva, and neoplasms may be classified as either intraepithelial or invasive.[33a] Intraepithelial SCC may be referred to as squamous cell carcinoma *in situ*, vulvar intraepithelial neoplasia, or squamous intraepithelial lesion. SCC in situ has been associated with HPV types 16, 18, 31, 33, 35, 51, and 52. Advanced age, immunosuppression, and smoking appear to contribute to the development of SCC in situ.[31,33] Multifocal intraepithelial neoplasia affects women aged between 20 and 50 years, whereas women over the age of 60 are more likely to be afflicted by solitary intraepithelial neoplasia. The risk of developing invasive vulvar cancer increases with age. Studies have shown that among darker skin of color women, rates of in situ squamous cell tumors have increased by 7.9% per year from 1973 through 1998.[34] Whether this increased incidence is simply related to the enhanced use of biopsies to investigate suspicious vulvar lesions or represents a true population dynamic is not known.

Clinical Findings Multifocal intraepithelial neoplasia, also called bowenoid papulosis, is characterized by papules and plaques of variable color with clearly defined borders that appear scattered on the

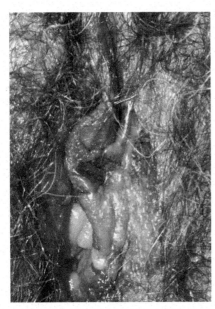

FIGURE 59-11. Multifocal plaques of variable color typify in situ squamous cell carcinoma in a Hispanic woman.

vestibule, outer labia minora, and labia majora [**Figure 59-11**]. Women tend to have larger lesions than men, reaching 2 to 3 cm in diameter.[31] Additionally, women may have significantly more lesions than men. Solitary intraepithelial neoplasia, also termed Bowen disease, typically presents as a single pink or erythematous, sharply bordered patch or plaque. Plaques may have a velvety appearance. Approximately half of the affected women complain of pruritus with solitary lesions. Invasive vulvar cancer typically presents as erythematous or white, unifocal lesions that may ulcerate or become nodular morphologically. Lesions appear on the posterior *fourchette*, labia minora, or interlabial sulcus.[31,33]

Vulvar cancer typically is suspected clinically and confirmed via biopsy. Gross examination of the vulva should be followed by a colposcopic examination of the vulva, vagina, and cervix. Potential areas of active HPV infection can be identified by the use of topically applied diluted acetic acid, with biopsies taken from the acetowhite regions.

Complications Large lesions (>2 cm), invasive SCC, and SCC of the mucous membranes are associated with a high risk of recurrence and metastasis.[35] Additionally, SCC arising in injured or chronically diseased skin is associated with an approximate risk of metastasis of 40%.[35]

Prognosis/Clinical Course In the absence of metastatic disease, most patients with primary SCC have an excellent prognosis.

Contact Dermatitis

Epidemiology, Etiology, and Pathogenesis Contact dermatitis is an inflammatory reaction to external material. Possible triggers for genital contact dermatitis include seminal fluid, spermicides, latex condoms, lubricant jelly, perfumes (eg, feminine hygiene sprays, scented soaps, or scented tampons), self-adhesive feminine napkins, topical antibiotics (eg, neomycin), and moisturizers (eg, lanolin).[36] Irritant contact dermatitis (ICD) is caused by prolonged or repeated exposure to irritating substances, whereas allergic contact dermatitis (ACD) is a true allergy to a low dose of a chemical substance. ACD involves a delayed-type hypersensitivity reaction, whereas ICD does not require prior sensitization.

Clinical Findings Vulvar contact dermatitis may present with edema, vesicles or bullae, erythema, and weeping. Patients with darker skin of color may show hyperpigmentation instead of erythema. Secondary lichenification or excoriation may be present. Compared with more generalized contact dermatitis, chronic contact dermatitis in the genital area may have a decreased amount of visible scale due to the high-moisture environment. Contact dermatitis is a diagnosis based largely on history because clinical appearance and even a biopsy may be nonspecific. However, a biopsy can be performed to rule out other possible diagnoses, and patch testing may be useful to confirm ACD.

Complications Hyper- or hypopigmentation may occur due to melanocyte damage from severe inflammation.

Prognosis/Clinical Course If patients are able to avoid the offending substance and receive anti-inflammatory therapy, they have a good prognosis. Patients with chronic symptoms and no obvious etiology generally have a prolonged course with long-term management.

DIFFERENTIAL DIAGNOSES AND TREATMENT OPTIONS

The differential diagnoses and treatment options for each form of genital lesion in women covered in this chapter are detailed in **Table 59-1**.

TABLE 59-1	Differential diagnoses and treatments for genital lesions in women[a]	
Lesion/disease	**Differential diagnosis**	**Treatment**
Syphilis	• Behçet syndrome • Chancroid • Condylomata acuminata (external genital warts) • Fixed drug eruption (secondary syphilis) • Granuloma inguinale • Herpes progenitalis (genital herpes) • Lichen planus (secondary syphilis) • Lymphogranuloma venereum • Psoriasis (secondary syphilis) • Traumatic ulcer	First-line therapy for systemic syphilis consists of 2.4 MU of benzathine G penicillin G intramuscularly. Doxycycline, tetracycline and erythromycin are second-line agents that can be used in the case of a penicillin allergy. Treatments are outlined in detail in **e-Table 59-1**.
Granuloma inguinale	• Behçet syndrome • Chancroid • Condylomata acuminatum (external genital warts) • Condylomata lata • Deep mycosis • Herpes progenitalis • Leishmaniasis (rare on the genitalia) • Lymphogranuloma venereum • Squamous cell carcinoma • Syphilis • Tuberculosis of the skin	Lesions will not resolve without treatment and prolonged therapy may be necessary. Doxycycline, trimethoprim-sulfamethoxazole, or azithromycin are first-line treatments for systemic granuloma inguinale. Ciprofloxacin is a second-line option and erythromycin should be used for pregnant patients [e-**Table 59-2**].

(Continued)

TABLE 59-1   Differential diagnoses and treatments for genital lesions in women[a] (Continued)

Lesion/disease	Differential diagnosis	Treatment
Herpes	• Aphthous ulcers • Behçet syndrome • Chancroid • Granuloma inguinale • Lymphogranuloma venereum • Pemphigus vulgaris or vegetans • Syphilis • Trauma	There is no cure for herpes. Treatments for systemic genital herpes are outlined in **e-Table 59-3**. Antiviral medications (acyclovir, valacyclovir, famciclovir) have been specifically developed for the treatment of genital herpes.
Genital warts (condylomata acuminata)	• Molluscum contagiosum • Lichen planus • Enlarged sebaceous glands • Condylomata lata • Vulvar intraepithelial neoplasia	Imiquimod, a prescription medication that acts as an immune response modifier, is used to treat genital warts. Podofilox is a second-line option. Both patient- and physician-applied treatments are available [**e-Table 59-4**]. Cryotherapy, laser ablation, surgical excision, and electro-desiccation may also be utilized.
Tinea cruris	• Candidiasis • Contact dermatitis • Erythrasma • Neurodermatitis • Psoriasis • Tinea versicolor (rarely affects genital skin)	Both topical and oral systemic options exist for the treatment of tinea cruris. Terbinafine and naftifine are the first line of treatment. **e-Table 59-5** outlines these in more detail, as well as potential second-line treatment options.
Candidiasis	• Contact dermatitis • Darier disease • Eczema • Hailey-Hailey disease • Lichen simplex chronicus • Psoriasis • Seborrheic dermatitis • Tinea cruris • Vulvar vestibulitis	Several different treatment strategies have been used, such as continuous or intermittent suppressive therapy with oral or topical antifungals. However, long-term studies evaluating such protocols are not available. **e-Table 59-6** outlines the treatment options, including both topical (clotrimazole, miconazole, nystatin, kentoconazole and ciclopirox) and oral (itraconazole and fluconazole) first-line treatments. Pregnant patients should receive oral therapy only.
Lichen planus	• Erosive disease • Candidiasis • Cicatricial pemphigoid • Lichen sclerosus • Lupus erythematosus • Pemphigus vulgaris • Papulosquamous form • Bowen disease • Condylomata acuminata (genital warts) • Erythema multiforme • Fixed drug reaction • Lichen sclerosus • Lichen simplex chronicus • Psoriasis • Scabies • Secondary syphilis	**e-Table 59-7** lists treatment options, including erosive, nonerosive, vaginal, and second-line options.
Lichen sclerosus et atrophicus	• Lichen planus (chronic) • Morphea • Postinflammatory dyschromia • Squamous cell carcinoma in situ/vulvar intraepithelial neoplasia • Vitiligo	Triamcinolone 0.01% or clobetasol 0.05% are first-line treatments for lichen sclerosus. Second-line options also exist (tacrolimus and pimecrolimus). Treatment regimens are available in **e-Table 59-8**.
Vitiligo	• Discoid lupus erythematosus • Hansen disease (tuberculoid) • Lichen sclerosus et atrophicus (most important) • Postinflammatory dyschromia • Seborrhea • Tinea versicolor (rare on genital skin)	Cosmetic coverup products or a therapeutic tattoo are camouflage options. Repigmentation therapeutic modalities are available (eg, keratinocyte-melanocyte transfers, epidermal grafts, or excimer laser treatment), although these are not guaranteed (see Table 58-1, Chapter 58, Genital Lesions in Men). Corticosteroids are a potential first-line therapy.

(Continued)

TABLE 59-1   Differential diagnoses and treatments for genital lesions in women[a] (Continued)

Lesion/disease	Differential diagnosis	Treatment
Crohn disease	• Actinomycosis • Angioedema • Behçet syndrome • Chancroid • Extramammary Paget disease • Factitious dermatitis • Filariasis • Fixed drug eruption • Granuloma inguinale • Hidradenitis suppurativa	There is no cure for Crohn disease. Treatment is designed to control the disease, suppress symptoms, and decrease the frequency and duration of symptomatic episodes. While surgery is not curative, it can conserve portions of the gastrointestinal tract and improve quality of life. The majority of patients will require surgery at some point during their lives.
Benign cysts	• Fibroma • Furuncle (tender, hot, and red at inception) • Hidradenitis suppurativa (purulent discharge) • Lipoma • Neuroma • Nevus • Xanthoma	**e-Table 59-9** lists treatment options.
Squamous cell carcinoma	• Acrochorda (skin tags) • Bartholin duct obstruction • Condylomata acuminata (genital warts) • Epidermal inclusion cyst • Hemangioma • Hidradenomas • Lentigo • Lichen sclerosus • Mucous cysts • Seborrheic keratoses • Varicosities • Verrucae	Invasive squamous cell carcinoma treatment usually involves resection or ablation (if the tumor is small). Alternatives to traditional surgery include Mohs micrographic surgery, laser ablation, and radiation therapy. Topical imiquimod may be prescribed for *in situ* lesions. More information on treatment can be found in Chapter 45, Squamous Cell Carcinoma, and Chapter 58, Genital Lesions in Men.
Contact dermatitis	• Atopic dermatitis • Bowen disease (squamous cell carcinoma in situ) • Candidiasis • Intertrigo (nonspecific) • Lichen simplex chronicus • Paget disease • Psoriasis • Tinea	Both topical and systemic treatment options are outlined in **e-Table 59-9**, including triamcinolone, hydroxyzine, and prednisone.

[a]All e-tables appear online and are available at mhprofessional.com/DermatologySkinofColor.

CONCLUSION

It is important for dermatologists to bear in mind that additional diagnostic testing may be necessary for patients with skin of color presenting with genital lesions, because morphology alone may not be enough to distinguish between a genital disorder and similar entities. Full-body skin checks may also be necessary. This is the case for both male and female skin of color patients with skin of color, in whom there is also variation in both the statistical frequency and clinical characteristics of the genital lesions.

Female patients with sexually transmitted syphilis infections may be unaware of the primary chancre and extragenital chancres that are less common in darker skin of color patients. Darker skin of color American patients, especially women, are reportedly more likely to develop condylomata lata in secondary syphilis than Caucasian Americans. The rates of both primary and secondary syphilis are higher among darker skin of color Americans and Hispanics than among Caucasian Americans, although rates are decreasing among darker skin of color American females.

REFERENCES

1. Centers for Disease Control and Prevention (CDC). Primary and secondary syphilis—United States, 2003–2004. *MMWR.* 2005;55:269-273.
2. Goh BT. Syphilis in adults. *Sex Transm Inf.* 2005;81:448-452.
3. Rosen T. Diseases with unusual features: syphilis. In: *Clinical Dermatology in Black Patients.* Bari, Italy: PiGreco Press; 1995:59-63.
4. Fisher BK, Margesson LJ. Infectious diseases of the vulva. In: *Genital Skin Disorders: Diagnosis and Treatment.* St. Louis, MO: Mosby; 1998:128-149.
5. Lupi O, Madkan V, Tyring SK. Tropical dermatology: bacterial tropical diseases. *J Am Acad Dermatol.* 2006;54:559-578.
6. Centers for Disease Control and Prevention. Sexually transmitted diseases treatment guidelines 2002. *MMWR Recomm Rep.* 2002;51:1-78.
7. Rosen T. Tropical infections: granuloma inguinale. In: *Clinical Dermatology in Black Patients.* Bari, Italy: PiGreco Press; 1995:169-170.
8. Beauman JG. Genital herpes: a review. *Am Fam Physician.* 2005;72:1527-1534.
9. Solomon J, Cannon MJ, Reyes M, et al. Epidemiology of recurrent genital herpes simplex virus types 1 and 2. *Sex Transm Inf.* 2003;79:456-459.
10. Fleming DT, Leone P, Esposito D, et al. Herpes virus type 2 infection and genital symptoms in primary care patients. *Sex Transm Dis.* 2006;33:416-421.
11. Dupin N. Genital warts. *Clin Dermatol.* 2004;22:481-486.
12. Koutsky L. Epidemiology of genital human papillomavirus infection. *Am J Med.* 1997;102:3-8.
13. Kodner CM, Nasraty S. Management of genital warts. *Am Fam Physician.* 2004; 70:2335-2342.
14. Handsfield HH. Clinical presentation and natural course of anogenital warts. *Am J Med.* 1997;102:16-20.
15. Nadalo D, Montoya C. What is the best way to treat tinea cruris? *J Fam Pract.* 2006;55:256-258.
16. Huang DB, Ostrosky-Zeichner L, Wu JJ, et al. Therapy of common superficial fungal infections. *Dermatol Ther.* 2004;17:517-522.

17. Hay RJ. The management of superficial candidiasis. *J Am Acad Dermatol.* 1999;40:S35-S42.

18. Moyal-Barracco M, Edwards L. Diagnosis and therapy of anogenital lichen planus. *Dermatol Ther.* 2004;17:38-46.

19. Rosen T. Diseases with unusual features: lichen planus. In: *Clinical Dermatology in Black Patients.* Bari, Italy: PiGreco Press; 1995:36-40.

20. Fisher BK, Margesson LJ. Inflammatory diseases of the vulva. In: *Genital Skin Disorders: Diagnosis and Treatment.* St. Louis, MO: Mosby; 1998:154-176.

21. Powell JJ, Wojnarowska F. Lichen sclerosus. *Lancet.* 1999;353:1777-1783.

22. Ginarte M, Toribio J. Vulvar lichen sclerosus successfully treated with topical tacrolimus. *Eur J Obstet Gynecol Reprod Biol.* 2005;123:123-124.

23. Luesley DM, Downey GP. Topical tacrolimus in the management of lichen sclerosus. *Br J Obstet Gynaecol.* 2006;113:832-834.

24. Goldstein AT, Marinoff SC, Christopher K. Pimecrolimus for the treatment of vulvar lichen sclerosus: a report of 4 cases. *J Reprod Med.* 2004;49:778-780.

25. Passeron T, Ortonne JP. Pathophysiology and genetics of vitiligo. *J Autoimmun.* 2005;25:63S-68S.

26. Handa S, Kaur I. Vitiligo: clinical findings in 1436 patients. *J Dermatol.* 1999;26:653-657.

27. Feller ER, Ribaudo S, Jackson ND. Gynecologic aspects of Crohn's disease. *Am Fam Physician.* 2001;64:1725-1728.

27a. Burgdorf W. Cutaneous manifestations of Crohn's disease. *J Am Acad Dermatol.* 1981;5:689-695.

28. Basu D, Lopez I, Kulkarni A, Sellin JH. Impact of race and ethnicity on inflammatory bowel disease. *Am J Gastroenterol.* 2005;100:2254-2261.

29. Lynch PJ, Edwards L. Noninfectious primary ulcers. In: Lynch PJ, Edwards L, eds. *Genital Dermatology.* New York, NY: Churchill-Livingstone; 1994:213-221.

30. Eilber KS, Raz S. Benign cystic lesions of the vagina: a literature review. *J Urol.* 2003;170:717-722.

31. Fisher BK, Margesson LJ. Tumors and cysts of the vulva. In: *Genital Skin Disorders: Diagnosis and Treatment.* St. Louis, MO: Mosby; 1998:154-176.

32. Rosen T. Unusual presentation of gonorrhea. *J Am Acad Dermatol.* 1982;6:369-372.

33. Tyring SK. Vulvar squamous cell carcinoma: guidelines for early detection and treatment. *Am J Obstet Gynecol.* 2003;189:S17-S23.

33a. Cancer Network. Practice Guidelines: Vulvar Cancer. www.cancernetwork.com/articles/practice-guidelines-vulvar-cancer. Accessed July 17, 2015.

34. Howe HL, Wingo PA, Thun MJ, et al. Annual report to the nation on the status of cancer (1973-1998), featuring cancers with recent increasing trends. *J Natl Cancer Inst.* 2001;93:824-842.

35. Alam M, Ratner D. Cutaneous squamous cell carcinoma. *N Engl J Med.* 2001;344:975-983.

36. Sonnex C. Genital allergy. *Sex Transm Inf.* 2004;80:4-7.

Dermatologic Infections

Cutaneous Manifestations of Human Immunodeficiency Virus

Miguel R. Sanchez

KEY POINTS

- Human immunodeficiency virus (HIV) infection is associated with a wide range of dermatologic conditions.

- Mucocutaneous findings, such as thrush, sebopsoriasis, and herpes zoster, may manifest as the initial clinical presentation of HIV infection.

- Some HIV-associated skin conditions first appear with deteriorating immunity, especially when CD4 counts fall less than 200 cells/μL. The appearance of the skin disease can reflect the patient's immune status.

- Antiretroviral therapy dramatically reduces morbidity and mortality for HIV-infected patients and has a profound effect on the appearance and course of many skin conditions, ie, Kaposi sarcoma (KS). However, skin problems may continue to affect individuals living with HIV.

INTRODUCTION

Approximately 37 million people worldwide were living with human immunodeficiency virus (HIV) in 2014; alarmingly, more than 19 million were unaware of their infection.[1] Although there is no racial predominance, individuals with skin of color bear the brunt of the infection globally, with 70% of HIV cases residing in sub-Saharan Africa with the predominant mode of transmission being heterosexual sexual activity. It is estimated that there are 5 million HIV-infected people in Asia and the Pacific and 1.7 million in Latin America.[1] In the United States, the main form of transmission continues to be male-to-male sexual activity.[1] According to statistics from the Centers for Disease Control and Prevention (CDC), African Americans—predominantly men who have sex with men (MSM)—account for 47% of new cases of HIV infection in the United States; African American women constitute 30% of cases.[2] Hispanics are also disproportionally affected, accounting for 21% of new HIV cases.[1] HIV depletes cluster of differentiation (CD) 4 cells, leading to profound immunodeficiency that results in infectious, inflammatory, neoplastic autoimmune, and metabolic disease.

Some infections or atypical presentations of skin diseases are highly suggestive of HIV infection and warrant evaluation for the virus.[3] While combination antiretroviral treatment (ARVT) revolutionized the treatment of HIV infection and effectively reduced the frequency and severity of opportunistic skin infections and malignancies, only 30% of those living with HIV control their infection.[4] Some skin diseases (such as warts [**Figure 60-1**], psoriasis, photodermatitis, molluscum, contagiosum, prurigo nodularis, and pruritic disorders) remain common concerns in individuals with low CD4 counts. Patients adequately treated with ARVT may still develop xerosis, eczema, drug reactions, lipodystrophy, immune reconstitution inflammatory syndrome-related diseases, and even Kaposi sarcoma (KS).[3]

NONVIRAL AND NONBACTERIAL DISEASES

EXANTHEM OF ACUTE RETROVIRAL SYNDROME

Acute retroviral syndrome (ARS) has been reported in 25% to 75% of new HIV infections; it may present within 2 to 4 weeks and up to 3 months after initial exposure to the virus.[5] In most cases, the symptoms resolve within 5 days but can persist for several weeks. Patients often present with fever, malaise, myalgia, pharyngitis, and lymphadenopathy. Skin findings have been described in 30% to 50% of cases and consist of a measles-like eruption or scattered, pink round to oval, 10- to 15-mm macules/patches on the chest, trunk [**Figure 60-2**], upper extremities, and face.[5] Major aphthous ulcers on the oral and/or anogenital mucosa occur in 3.1% of HIV cases.[6] It is important to note that HIV antibody tests do not become positive for 10 to 24 weeks after HIV exposure; therefore, the diagnosis of HIV infection in ARS cases requires DNA or ribonucleic acid testing.[5,7,8]

SEBORRHEIC DERMATITIS

Seborrheic dermatitis used to be the most common manifestation of HIV infection, affecting as many as 70% of cases.[9,10] In Mali, where seborrheic dermatitis is uncommon, the disease has been used as a marker of HIV infection.[9] Patients with fair immune function have typical erythema with greasy yellowish white scales in the nasolabial folds, ears, eyebrows, scalp, and/or beard areas; however, with progression to acquired immune deficiency syndrome (AIDS), the skin changes become more severe, widespread, and recalcitrant to treatment [**Figure 60-3**].[9] The face, chest, axillae, and groin may also be affected and the lesions become thicker and more sharply defined. In the lower part of the face, petaloid patches may appear or the changes may be symmetrically spread in a "butterfly" fashion along the malar area.[10] These features are similar to inverse psoriasis or sebopsoriasis and there may be no distinguishing feature to differentiate between the two diseases. In addition to yellow scaling, exudative crusts may cover the lesions on the scalp, perinasal and retroauricular areas and inverse folds. In skin of color, lesions often develop or heal with hyper- or hypopigmentation.[10] Antifungals (eg, imidazole) and low-potency topical corticosteroids are effective; however, higher potency corticosteroids or calcineurin inhibitors may be required in some cases.[9]

PSORIASIS

Psoriasis is uncommon in HIV-infected African Americans, mirroring the overall lower prevalence of the condition in this population.[11] While the prevalence of psoriasis in HIV-infected individuals is similar to that of the general population, psoriasis may be more severe and recalcitrant, and psoriasis arthritis may be more prevalent in AIDS patients.[12] Prior to ARVT, the development of HIV-associated psoriasis was a predictor of profound immunosuppression and indicated a poor prognosis.[13] Most HIV-infected psoriasis cases have typical lesions. A distinguishing feature is the presence of more than one type of psoriasis (inverse, classic plaque, annular or polycyclic, and pustular) in the same patient. In immunosuppressed persons, psoriasis spreads aggressively, does not respond well to treatment, and is more often associated with arthritis.[12] In South Africa, erythrodermic psoriasis was reported to be the most common form of the disease.[14] Patients with reactive arthritis-like psoriasis syndrome (RAPS) have Reiter syndrome-like findings

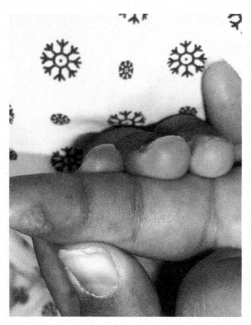

FIGURE 60-1. Multiple exophytic verruca vulgaris (warts) on a human immunodeficiency virus–infected man. (Used with permission from the Ronald O. Perelman Department of Dermatology, NYU School of Medicine, NYU Langone Medical Center, NY.)

such as palmoplantar psoriasiform plaques that may develop pustules and crusting. AVRT is indicated for moderate-to-severe psoriasis with significant improvement seen as viral loads decline. Mild limited disease usually responds to topical corticosteroids and more extensive disease to phototherapy, such as narrow-band ultraviolet (UV)-B therapy or psoralen plus UVA (PUVA).[15] Acitretin is particularly effective for pustular psoriasis and RAPS. Systemic immunosuppressants such as methotrexate and cyclosporine are the last options to be considered because of the increased risk of opportunistic infections.[15] However, methotrexate has been used effectively and without complications in some cases.[16] Cyclosporine may be needed in recalcitrant cases of pustular or erythrodermic

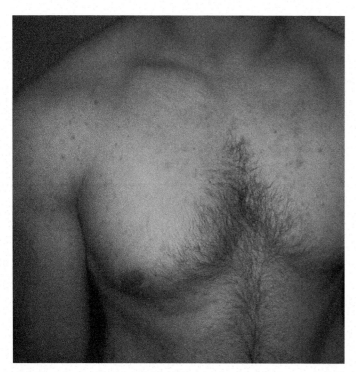

FIGURE 60-2. Poorly defined pink macules on the trunk of a man with acute retroviral syndrome. (Used with permission from the Ronald O. Perelman Department of Dermatology, NYU School of Medicine, NYU Langone Medical Center, NY.)

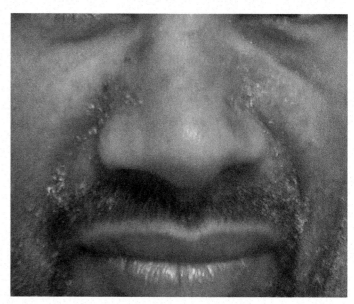

FIGURE 60-3. Severe seborrheic dermatitis with hypopigmented borders on the nasolabial folds of a Hispanic man. (Used with permission from the Ronald O. Perelman Department of Dermatology, NYU School of Medicine, NYU Langone Medical Center, NY.)

psoriasis, and tumor necrosis factor-alpha (Tnf-α) inhibitors and other biologics may be necessary in therapeutically resistant cases without hepatitis C coinfection.[15] Oral tacrolimus should be avoided in immunosuppressed patients or those taking medicines used to treat HIV infection; however, recent research indicates adjusted doses may be safe.[17]

■ XEROSIS

Dry skin, especially along the anterior lower legs, is a common complaint among those living with HIV. This worsens both with progressive immunosuppression and the duration of time on ARVT[10]; transepidermal water loss is greater in African American skin than Caucasian skin, which may predispose the former group to xerosis.[18] In severe cases, small, fine irregular, polygonal darker scales characteristic of acquired ichthyosis may develop.[10] Alpha hydroxy acid preparations, such as lactic acid or urea, are the treatment of choice, in addition to moisturizers and the avoidance of exacerbating factors, such as frequent or prolonged bathing. Dry skin may also become more pronounced and pruritic in the winter months.

■ ECZEMA

Dry skin is prone to the development of eczema because the skin barrier is damaged and irritating substances can more readily penetrate the stratum corneum. The changes lead to intense itching, excoriations, and even prurigo nodularis. Although HIV mainly impairs cell-mediated immunity, immunoglobulin E levels are often elevated and some patients develop atopic dermatitis.[19,20] Treatment should be administered promptly to avoid the occurrence of eczema-related postinflammatory pigmentation, a disfiguring and long lasting side effect which often develops in individuals with skin of color. In addition to emollients, the treatment of choice is medium- to high-potency topical corticosteroids. Barrier repair creams may also improve lesions. Tacrolimus ointment has a warning to avoid in patients with immunosuppression but experience indicates it is safe if used in limited steroid atrophic areas or in patients with pan-steroid tropical agent allergy. Considering the link between atopic dermatitis and *Staphylococcus aureus* colonization, skin decontamination may be beneficial.[21] Numerous therapies are available for the treatment of atopic dermatitis, including narrow-band UVB phototherapy and immunosuppressants such as cyclosporine and mycophenolic acid. Dupilumab (a monoclonal antibody) may be an effective alternative to therapeutically recalcitrant cases of atopic dermatitis.[22]

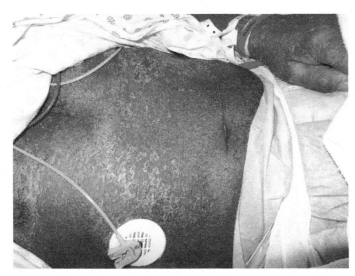

FIGURE 60-4. Toxic epidermal necrolysis due to vancomycin in a patient with human immunodeficiency virus. (Used with permission from the Ronald O. Perelman Department of Dermatology, NYU School of Medicine, NYU Langone Medical Center, NY.)

DRUG ERUPTIONS

The risk of drug eruptions in HIV-infected individuals can be up to10-fold higher than that of the general population.[23] Reaction rates to certain drugs (eg, combined sulfamethoxazole and trimethoprim) are even higher and independent of glutathione deficiency, slow acetylation, or active non-HIV viral infections.[24] Exanthematous morbilliform eruptions from sulfamethoxazole/trimethoprim have reached rates of 47% when higher than usual doses were used to treat *Pneumocystis jiroveci* pneumonia.[25] Penicillins and other antibiotics are also frequent causes of drug reactions. Antiretrovirals produce a wide spectrum of cutaneous adverse effects. Indinavir can cause ingrown toe nails and alopecia, and saquinavir may cause oral ulcerations.[26] Morbilliform eruptions have been reported in 2% to 8% of patients treated with some protease inhibitors, including darunavir, lopinavir/ritonavir, fosamprenavir, atazanavir, and tipranavir/ritonavir.[26] Pruritus and maculopapular, urticarial, vesiculobullous, or pustular eruptions develop in 5% to 7% of cases treated with tenofovir.[26] In the majority of cases, the eruption resolves spontaneously even if the drug responsible is not discontinued. However, progression to hypersensitivy syndrome, Stevens-Johnson syndrome (SJS), or toxic epidermal necrolysis (TEN) [**Figure 60-4**] is always a risk for HIV patients.[27,28] The antiretroviral agents, abacavir and nevirapine, have very high incidences of acute hypersensitivity. Abacavir is one of the most frequent causes of systemic hypersensitivity reactions, which usually occur within the first 6 weeks of treatment.[29] In an international collaborative study, nevirapine was responsible for 83% of 18 cases of SJS/TEN;[30] however this may not have been precipitated by HIV because rates were similar among HIV-seronegative individuals taking nevirapine for prophylaxis.[31] In a prospective study in Kenya, cutaneous hypersensitivity eruptions, most caused by thiacetazone, were seen in 20% of HIV-seropositive but only 1% of HIV-seronegative cases within the initial 16 weeks of tuberculosis treatment.[32] Screening for human leukocyte antigen B*5701 allele, which is associated with a higher likelihood of developing a hypersensitivity reaction, may detect persons who are at increased risk of potentially lethal drug effects from abacavir.[33]

LIPODYSTROPHY

Lipodystrophy is seen predominantly in those undergoing long-term ARVT which includes certain protease inhibitors and nucleoside reverse-transcriptase inhibitors (particularly stavudine). Some protease inhibitors (eg, nelfinavir) and nucleoside reverse-transcriptase inhibitors (abacavir and tenofovir) do not produce these changes.[34] Patients

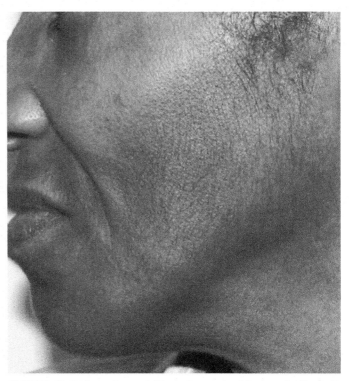

FIGURE 60-5. Human immunodeficiency virus-associated lipodystrophy. (Used with permission from the Ronald O. Perelman Department of Dermatology, NYU School of Medicine, NYU Langone Medical Center, NY.)

undergo loss of adipose tissue in the face, limbs, and buttocks together with accumulation of fat in the dorso-cervical area, abdomen, and breasts [**Figure 60-5**]. These changes are associated with a metabolic syndrome consisting of hyperinsulinemia due to insulin resistance, hyperglycemia, and hyperlipidemia.[34]

IMMUNE RECONSTITUTION INFLAMMATORY SYNDROME

Paradoxically, with the recovery of immunity following ARVT, a subset of patients develop clinical deterioration in areas of previous or current infectious (eg, cytomegalovirus, hepatitis B or C, tuberculosis, and *Cryptococcus*), neoplastic (KS) and autoimmune involvement. Dermatologic manifestations of immune reconstitution inflammatory syndrome (IRIS) include the onset or rapid worsening of molluscum or warts, development of epidermodysplasia verruciformis-like human papillomavirus (HPV) lesions, reactivation of herpes zoster and ulcerative oral or anogenital herpes, ulcerations from *Mycobacterium avium*, upgrading of leprosy to the lepromatous spectrum, rapid progression of leishmaniasis, and flare-ups of acne and pruritic papular eruptions (PPEs).[35,36] The etiology involves an exaggerated immune response to antimicrobial or other antigens.[35] Systemic corticosteroids may be required in some cases to prevent disabling, destructive, or lethal organ damage.[36]

PRURITUS, PRURIGO NODULARIS, PRURITIC PAPULAR ERUPTION, AND EOSINOPHILIC FOLLICULITIS

Individuals living with HIV often complain of itching, which may be primary (HIV-associated pruritus) or secondary to cutaneous diseases such as eczema, scabies, drug reactions, PPEs, or eosinophilic folliculitis (EF). Chronic abrasion of the skin results in thick, pigmented hyperkeratotic plaques and nodules (prurigo nodularis).[10] The prevalence of PPE in Africans and Haitians with HIV varies from 12% to 46%.[37] In some developing countries, PPE is the most frequent HIV-related skin manifestation and often the first marker of HIV infection.[37,38] The typical eruption consists of multiple, scattered,

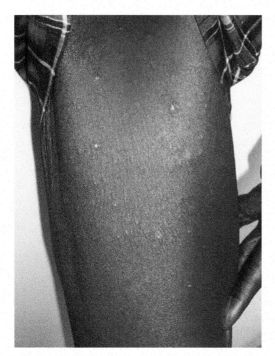

FIGURE 60-6. Discrete excoriated papules in a patient with pruritic papular eruption of human immunodeficiency virus. (Used with permission from the Ronald O. Perelman Department of Dermatology, NYU School of Medicine, NYU Langone Medical Center, NY.)

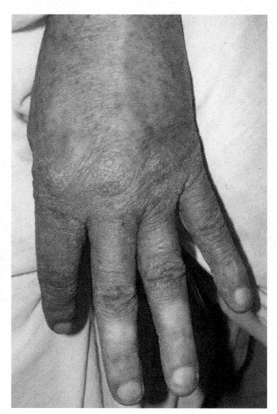

FIGURE 60-7. Hyperkeratotic crusted plaques in a man with crusted (Norwegian) scabies. Similar lesions were present on the trunk, feet, face, and ears. (Used with permission from the Ronald O. Perelman Department of Dermatology, NYU School of Medicine, NYU Langone Medical Center, NY.)

discrete, lichenified papules on the extremities [**Figure 60-6**], neck, and upper back. In most cases, the cause is arthropod bites or stings or hypersensitivity to the assault, as in papular urticaria.[39] In contrast to PPE, HIV-related EF is characterized histologically by the presence of aneosinophil-rich perivascular infiltrate that is concentrated near the follicular isthmus and sebaceous ducts and by spongiosis in the follicular epithelium.[40] Usually, the agent responsible is a human follicle-inhabiting arthropod, such as mites of the *Demodex* species.[41] In EF, crops of discrete, intensely pruritic, pink or pigmented papules and sterile papulopustules erupt on the face, chest, neck, back, and lateral extensor surfaces of the upper extremities.[40] The lesions become excoriated, eroded, and lichenified.[10] The eruption waxes and wanes over time even without treatment; however, the pruritus usually prompts patients to seek urgent medical attention.[41] The pigmentary changes associated with both EF and PPE may be very disconcerting to patients with skin of color.[10] Medium- to super-high-potency corticosteroids are usually required. Systemic corticosteroids rapidly halt pruritus and the development of new lesions. Phototherapy is considered by many to be the treatment of choice for EF.[10] Acitretin, cyclosporine, and indomethacin have proven beneficial in cases of recalcitrant EF.[41]

PHOTODERMATITIS AND PIGMENTARY CHANGES

Photosensitivity to UV-B and, to a lesser extent, UV-A has been reported in HIV-infected patients; of these patients, many had CD4 counts less than 200 cells/μL and most had concomitant EF and/or were on sulfamethoxazole-trimethoprim prophylaxis.[42] The study also suggested that HIV-infected Native Americans may be predisposed to photosensitivity.[42] Chronic actinic dermatitis usually affects African Americans and may be the initial manifestation of HIV infection although most of these patients are markedly immunosuppressed.[43] The proclivity to photodermatitis can impact on the use of phototherapy as a treatment of skin disease.[10,43] Mucocutaneous pigmentary changes are common in those with skin of color living with HIV, mainly as a result of postinflammatory pigmentation and drug-induced effects. Zidovudine often causes dose-dependent hyperpigmentation of the skin and oral mucosa as well as longitudinal melanonychia. Emtricitabine causes hyperpigmentation

of the palms, soles, nails, and oral mucosa, almost exclusively in patients with skin of color.[10]

NONINFECTIOUS HAIR/NAIL DISEASES

Alopecia areata, diffuse alopecia (potentially inflammatory), telogen effluvium, and strikingly elongated eyelashes have been reported in individuals living with AIDS.[44] Beau lines and thin brittle nails are common in patients with malnutrition and those with chronic illnesses.[45]

SCABIES

Scabies in HIV infection is a devastating problem in some economically developing countries. With advanced HIV infection, *Sarcoptes scabiei* infestation presents as the hyperkeratotic crusted scabies type with a widespread distribution of plaques over the head, dorsa [**Figure 60-7**], palms, and soles. Diagnosis may be hindered by the absence of typical burrows and pruritus; however, a skin scraping will show numerous mites. Oral ivermectin is usually required as well as repeated applications of permethrin.[46]

VIRAL MANIFESTATIONS

HERPES SIMPLEX VIRUS

In the general population, the herpes simplex virus (HSV) disproportionately afflicts African Americans of both genders.[47] As many as 70% of all HIV-infected individuals are infected with HSV.[48] In most HIV cases, the oral and anogenital herpetic lesions are identical to those of the general population and typically consist of small ulcers in the mucosal surfaces or discrete vesicles that tend to be grouped and rest on an erythematous base [**Figure 60-8**].[10] Clinical herpes infections in immunocompromised patients tend to be prolonged, severe, painful, and

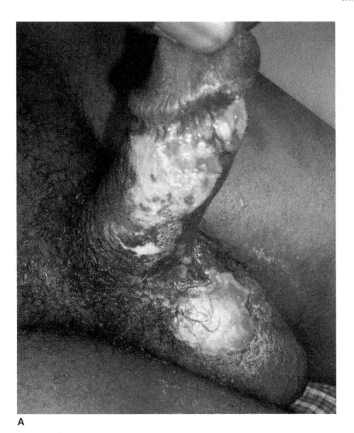

A

B

FIGURE 60-8. **(A)** Multiple, large, horizontally expanding, weeping genital ulcers with bright red bases and irregular edges secondary to acyclovir-resistant herpse simplex virus (HSV)-2. **(B)** Chronic, slowly expanding, tumor-like nodule with ulcerated surface caused by HSV-2. (Used with permission from the Ronald O. Perelman Department of Dermatology, NYU School of Medicine, NYU Langone Medical Center, NY.)

atypical.[49] Patients with CD4 counts less than 100 cells/μL may develop gradually enlarging ulcers that do not heal and are often resistant to thymidine kinase inhibitors at normal doses. Rare variants include hypertrophic, verrucous, and vegetative types and discrete subcutaneous painful nodules.[10] Mucocutaneous contact with active lesions carries a high risk of HIV transmission—particularly to sexual partners—and the risk remains high even after the lesions have healed.[10,49] Nucleic acid amplification is a very sensitive diagnostic test for HSV and obviates the need for biopsies, viral cultures, and Tzanck smears.[49] Thymidine kinase inhibitors—such as acyclovir, famciclovir, and valacyclovir—remain the therapeutic gold standard. In some cases, higher and more prolonged doses than usually recommended may be needed.[49] Foscarnet is indicated for acyclovir-resistant strains that fail to respond to imiquimod and/or compounded cidofovir gel.[49] Suppressive therapy prevents the development of lesions in HIV-infected individuals but does not decrease the risk of HIV or HSV-2 transmission to susceptible sexual partners.[49] HSV may disseminate in profoundly immunocompromised HIV-infected individuals.

VARICELLA ZOSTER VIRUS

Approximately 20% of HIV-infected persons develop herpes zoster, the incidence of which is 15-fold higher than that of the general adult population.[48] Up to 75% of HIV-associated zoster patients are African American.[50] Varicella zoster virus (VZV) is more likely to reactivate when CD4 counts fall less than 200 cells/μL; at this degree of immunosuppression, there is also a rare risk of dissemination. Administration of ARVT eventually reduces zoster rates; however, VZV reactivation induced by IRIS elevates the risk of developing herpes zoster by two- to four-fold between 4 and 16 weeks after initiation of the antiretroviral agents.[49] Characteristic findings include a dermatomal band-like patch or plaque of painful erythema studded with grouped vesicles and occasional bullae [**Figure 60-9**]. In HIV-immunosuppressed cases, the eruption extends aggressively, vesicles coalesce, and response to therapy is slow. Acute retinal necrosis may be a complication even in cases without trigeminal distribution.[51] Live attenuated varicella vaccines have been shown to be safe and are recommended for HIV patients with CD4 counts more than 200 cells/μL without a history of the vaccination or evidence of VZV immunity.[52] Treatment with thymidine kinase inhibitors at the recommended doses should be initiated within the first week as soon as the lesions develop and continued for 7 to 10 days or even longer if the lesions resolve slowly. Intravenous acyclovir is reserved for extensive skin lesions and dissemination. Varicella zoster immunoglobulin should be given to susceptible or exposed HIV-infected adolescents and adults.

HUMAN PAPILLOMAVIRUS

Human papilloma virus (HPV) infection rates are very high in HIV-positive patients.[53] Warts (condyloma acuminata) grow and spread more rapidly, require more aggressive therapy and are more prone to recur [**Figure 60-10**]. While 80% to 90% of HPV cases are cleared from the body in 2 years without treatment, HPV can also lie dormant for years with the sudden appearance of clinical lesions.[47] In HIV-immunocompromised individuals, elevations of viral loads and CD4 counts following ARVT may not influence the course of HPV.[54] Some cases of devastatingly aggressive warts have occurred as a result of ARVT-induced immune reconstitution. Infection with oncogenic HPV types accounts for most vulvar, vaginal, penile, anal, and oropharyngeal cancers.[55] Treatment of warts consists of destructive and immunomodulating therapies that can be used alone or in combination with the following: cryotherapy, chemical ablation with trichloroaceticacid, podophyllin/podophyllotoxin or cantharidin, laser or electrocautery, surgical resection, chemoimmunotherapy with imiquimod or sinecatechins, and topical chemotherapy with fluorouracil.[10,47] Therapeutically recalcitrant warts should be biopsied to exclude squamous cell carcinoma (SCC). Cervical cytologic

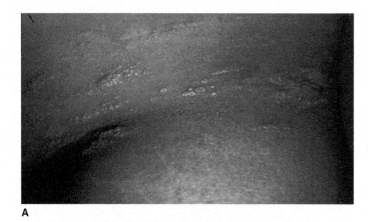

A

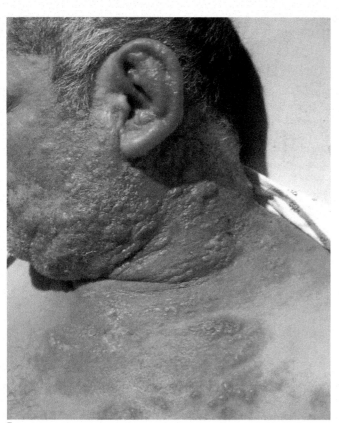

B

FIGURE 60-9. (A) Herpes zoster in the classic dermatomal distribution. **(B)** Severe herpes zoster in a Hispanic man. (**[B]** Used with permission from the Ronald O. Perelman Department of Dermatology, NYU School of Medicine, NYU Langone Medical Center, NY.)

screening is recommended 12 months after any sexual activity and then 6 months later.[49]

OTHER VIRAL INFECTIONS

Molluscum contagiosum presents as 1- to 3-mm flesh-colored or white, umbilicated, hemispheric, exophytic, highly transmissible papules on the face [**Figure 60-11**], arms, and trunk of healthy children. Healthy adults who contract the infection through sexual contact usually have papules on the anogenital area, pubis, groin, and upper thighs. In patients with CD4 counts less than 200 cells/μL, the lesions grow rapidly to 10 mm or larger, spread more aggressively, tend to coalesce, persist indefinitely, and respond poorly to therapy. In this patient group, lesions erupt on the face, arm, and upper trunk, rather than the anogenital area. The treatment is the same as for warts; curettage following ethyl chloride

is also a popular procedure. However, without improvement in immune function, it is very difficult to contain the infection.

The Epstein-Barr virus causes oral hairy leukoplakia presenting as white plaques with shaggy, corrugated surfaces, mainly along the sides of the mouth. The lesions spontaneously resolve with ART-induced enhancement of immune function.[10] Polyomaviridae have been implicated as the cause of Merkel cell tumors, which may be more common in HIV-infected persons,[56] as well as trichodysplasia spinulosa, a folliculocentric papular eruption consisting of central spiny excrescences on the face which has been reported in several immunodeficiency conditions.[54]

BACTERIAL DISEASES

Certain community-acquired pathogens, such as *Staphylococcus aureus*, methicillin-resistant *S. aureus* (MRSA), and *Pseudomonas aeruginosa*, have a higher frequency in HIV-infected individuals than among the healthy population.[46] The presence of *S. aureus* colonization predisposes patients to skin and soft tissue infections such as folliculitis, abscesses [**Figure 60-12**], furuncles, carbuncles, ecthyma, and cellulitis as well as less common types of infection, such as pyomyositis, fasciitis, and botryomycosis.[46] Whenever possible, the choice of antibiotics should be guided by cultures and sensitivities.[57] Limited superficial folliculitis usually responds to topical clindamycin, mupirocin, retapamulin, sodium fusidate, and benzoyl peroxide. Incision and drainage is the treatment of choice for abscesses but antibiotics are recommended for patients with significant immunosuppression.[57] Sulfamethoxazole-trimethoprim, clindamycin, and doxycycline can be used to treat community-acquired MRSA while oral tedizolid and linezolid are reserved for more serious infections. Vancomycin remains the gold standard of *S. aureus* antibiotic. Strategies to eradicate colonization include combination regimens of chlorhexidine cleanser solution, benzoyl peroxide, dilute bleach baths, and intranasal and topical (in the body folds) mupirocin.[57]

Pseudomonas can cause cellulitis in immunosuppressed individuals and commonly colonizes or infects skin wounds. Bacillary angiomatosis, seen infrequently in markedly immunodeficient patients, and is caused by either *Bartonella henselae* or *Bartonella quintana*.[58] Clinical findings consist of red, hemispheric, exophytic papules ranging in size from 2 to 20 mm; these papules may occur singly or in the hundreds. Less often, painful, dusky, subcutaneous nodules are observed instead.[58] The recommended treatment is erythromycin or doxycycline administration for 2 weeks to 2 months. Lifelong treatment may be required. *M. avium*-intracellulare complex may present as deep pustules and indurated crusted plaques.

SYPHILIS

The prevalence of syphilis is increased among HIV-infected individuals.[59] In the United States, African Americans and Hispanics had disproportionately higher rates of infectious syphilis than the general population in 2013, with African American and Hispanic men accounting for rates of 27.9 and 11.6, respectively, compared to a rate of 5.4 for Caucasian men.[59] MSM accounted for 83.9% of primary and secondary syphilis cases among men in 2012.[59] Most cases of primary syphilis present with the typical chancre. Secondary syphilis typically presents with papulosquamous eruptions [**Figure 60-13**]. Other presentations of syphilis (multiple chancres or psoriasiform or noduloulcerative eruptions) occur infrequently regardless of HIV status.[60]

Serologic tests are reliable but higher than expected post-treatment titers and delayed reactivity resulting in false-negative tests may occur.[47] Long-acting benzathine G penicillin remains the best treatment. As in immunocompetent patients, one injection is given for early syphilis (primary, secondary, or latent syphilis of less than a year's duration) and three injections a week are given for latent syphilis (more than 1 year's or of unknown duration). Additional doses do not decrease treatment failure rates or progression to symptomatic neurosyphilis, which develops

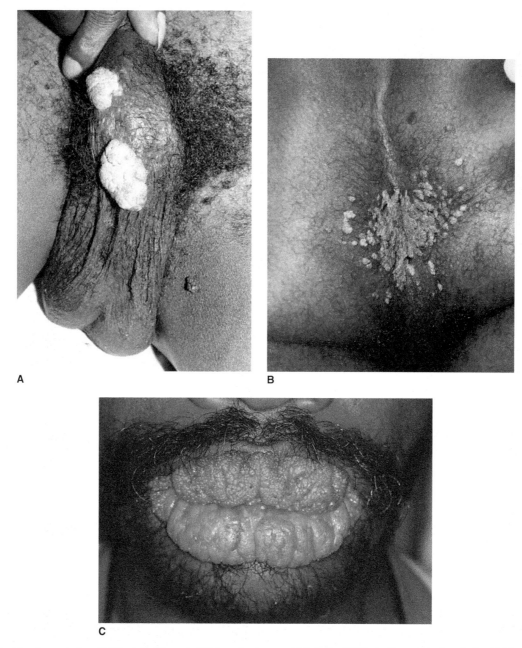

FIGURE 60-10. Condylomata acuminata on (**A**) the shaft of the penis, (**B**) the perianal area, and (**C**) the lips. ([**B**] Used with permission from the Ronald O. Perelman Department of Dermatology, NYU School of Medicine, NYU Langone Medical Center, NY.)

in 0.5% of cases despite adequate treatment.[61] Doxycycline is a possible alternative for penicillin in allergic individuals but azithromycin is not recommended for patients with HIV.[48] It is essential that patients are aware of potential symptoms of neurosyphilis. These should be evaluated clinically and serologically every 3 months for a year and then every 6 to 12 months following treatment of early syphilis and every 6 months following treatment of late latent syphilis.[48]

◼ SUPERFICIAL FUNGAL INFECTIONS

Oropharyngeal candidiasis (thrush) presents with painless, creamy white exudate that scrapes off easily and is located on the mouth and pharynx [**Figure 60-14**].[46] It is typically seen among patients with CD4 counts of less than 200 cells/μL.[46] Other presentations include angular cheilitis and erythematous patches on the anterior or posterior upper palate or diffusely on the tongue. Effective treatments include mucoadhesive buccal tablets of miconazole, itraconazole or posaconazole, oral suspensions, and oral fluconazole.[48]

HIV-infected individuals are prone to rapidly spreading and extensive dermatophytic fungal infections, including tinea pedis, corporis [**Figure 60-15**], manuum, or capitis, and onychomycosis.[62] White subungual onychomycosis is a marker of advanced immunodeficiency.[63] Topical antifungals may suffice for localized fungal infections but systemic antifungals are needed for widespread infection, tinea capitis, and most cases of onychomycosis.

Opportunistic Deep Fungal Infections Following the introduction of ARVT, the incidence of opportunistic deep fungal infections among patients with CD4 counts of 50 to 150 cells/μL decreased in developed countries, but it still remains a critical problem in other populations with limited health resources.[48] Opportunistic deep fungal infections are a group of systemic infections considered to be AIDS-defining and associated with dissemination and high mortality. The presence of skin lesions expedites diagnosis. In disseminated cases, many morphologies may be seen, including acneiform papules or pustules; ulcers; warty, vegetating, infiltrative, or granulomatous plaques; nodules; masses; bullae;

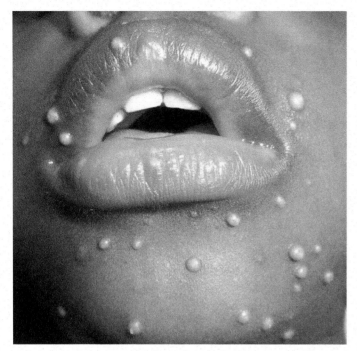

FIGURE 60-11. Disseminated molluscum contagiosum on the face of a child. (Used with permission from the Ronald O. Perelman Department of Dermatology, NYU School of Medicine, NYU Langone Medical Center, NY.)

sinusitis; subcutaneous swellings; and vasculitis-like lesions. However, characteristic lesions for these fungal infections have been described in most HIV-infected cases.[10,46]

Histoplasmosis involves the skin in approximately 5% of disseminated cases in the United States in comparison to 66% of cases in Brazil, usually from dissemination or reactivation of a previous infection.[64] Most disseminated cases have reddish papules and pustules that become necrotic [**Figure 60-16**].[65] Oral ulcers are common. The skin is affected in approximately 10% to 15% of cryptococcosis cases; disseminated cutaneous *Cryptococcus* infections are noted in 6% of HIV-infected patients.[66] Skin lesions may appear days to weeks before the diagnosis of systemic disease, especially meninigitis.[67] Typically, the pink, dimpled, exophytic papules become centrally ulcerated.[67] Penicilliosis, caused by *Penicillium marneffei*, nearly exclusively occurs in South or Southeast Asia.[68] An eruption consisting of small, flesh colored, molluscum-resembling papules with centers that become necrotic and ulcerated is present in 70% of disseminated cases.[68]

MALIGNANCIES

▪ EPIDEMIC KAPOSI SARCOMA

HIV potentiates oncogenesis; epidemic KS together with non-Hodgkin lymphomas and invasive cervical carcinomas are the three AIDS-defining malignancies.[69] Once the AIDS manifestation most dreaded by patients, KS now predominantly affects Caucasians.[70] Since the availability of ARVT, rates have decreased over eight-fold, mortality has decreased by 90% and tumors are more indolent and tend to regress spontaneously.[69] Human herpesvirus-8, the virus that causes KS, transforms endothelial cells into spindle-like cells which HIV induces to proliferate and form slit-like vascular channels.[69] KS is characterized by violaceous (or reddish brown in skin of color), smooth, papules, plaques, and/or nodules ranging from a few millimeter to several centimeter in size and which are often symmetrical and follow the Langer lines on the trunk, extremities, face/neck [**Figure 60-17**], and oral-anogenital mucosa. Enlarging and coalescent lesions, especially in the lower extremities, may ulcerate or become lymphedematous. The upper gastrointestinal tract is asymptomatically affected in up to 80% of KS cases, but lung involvement generally indicates an ominous prognosis.[69]

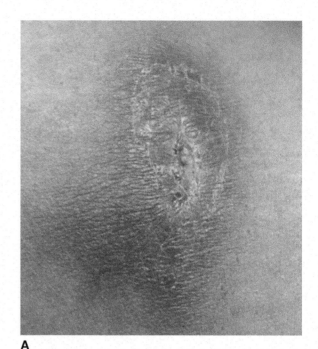

A

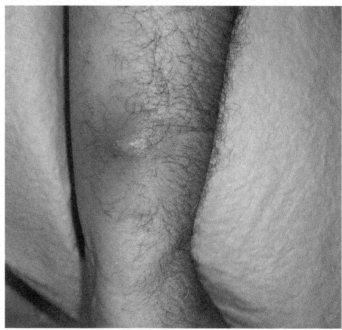

B

FIGURE 60-12. (A) Drained methicillin-resistant *Staphylococcus aureus* (MRSA) abscess. **(B)** Abscess with surrounding cellulitis caused by MRSA on the forearm of a Hispanic man. (**[B]** Used with permission from the Ronald O. Perelman Department of Dermatology, NYU School of Medicine, NYU Langone Medical Center, NY.)

ARVT represents the first-line treatment for slowly progressive disease while ARVT and chemotherapy are indicated for visceral and/or rapidly progressive disease. Chemotherapy is added for visceral and/or rapidly progressive disease.[69] Local treatments for small discrete neoplasms include cryotherapy, intralesional vinblastine, alitretinoin gel, and possibly imiquimod. KS is very radiosensitive but this modality is rarely used due to concern regarding its long-term side effects.

▪ SKIN CANCER

Although factors such as aging influence rates of cancer in the general population, HIV infection significantly increases the risk of cervical, anal, oral, and vulvar SCC related to oncogenic strains of HPV.[71] In

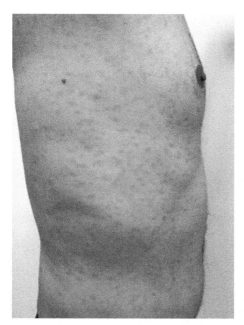

FIGURE 60-13. Typical eruption of secondary syphilis consisting of erythematous, round to oval, barely raised papules following the Langer lines on the trunk of a man. (Used with permission from the Ronald O. Perelman Department of Dermatology, NYU School of Medicine, NYU Langone Medical Center, NY.)

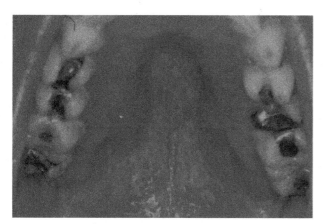

FIGURE 60-14. Oral candidiasis.

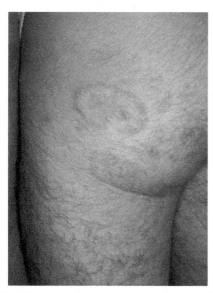

FIGURE 60-15. Widespread tinea corporis on the buttocks of a man infected with human immunodeficiency virus. (Used with permission from the Ronald O. Perelman Department of Dermatology, NYU School of Medicine, NYU Langone Medical Center, NY.)

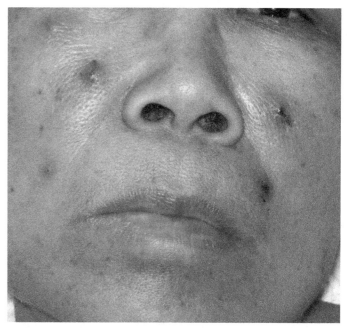

FIGURE 60-16. Case of disseminated histoplasmosis with erythematous pustules that became necrotic and hemorrhagic. (Used with permission from the Ronald O. Perelman Department of Dermatology, NYU School of Medicine, NYU Langone Medical Center, NY.)

comparison to those without the infection, HIV-infected individuals are diagnosed with basal cell carcinoma twice as often and with SCC three times as often.[71] Rapidly growing and metastatic SCC and Bowen disease have been reported in association with HIV.[72] Anal cancer rates are elevated in MSM and markedly increased in HIV-infected MSM, although there seems to be an independent association with HIV infection.[73] Some state health departments have recommended anal cytological examinations every 1 to 3 years in HIV-infected MSM, depending on immunologic status.[74] Basal cell carcinoma can be more aggressive and, in rare cases, eruptive; however, most neoplasms are of the superficial spreading type.[75] ARVT may give patients a lower risk of developing nonmelanoma skin cancers.[76] Malignant melanomas appear to behave more aggressively in HIV-immunosuppressed individuals.[77]

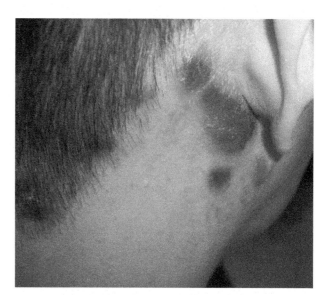

FIGURE 60-17. Violaceous nodular plaques characteristic of epidemic Kaposi sarcoma involving the head and neck. (Used with permission from the Ronald O. Perelman Department of Dermatology, NYU School of Medicine, NYU Langone Medical Center, NY.)

CONCLUSION

Over the past decade, the number of individuals living with HIV has increased, in part due to ARVT which has reduced the frequency and severity of opportunistic skin infections and malignancies. However, the number of new infections per year remains very high—particularly among certain populations. Although there is no racial predominance; individuals with skin of color (particularly African Americans and Hispanics) may be disproportionately affected by HIV. Additionally, MSM are at increased risk of infection as the primary form of transmission is male-to-male sexual activity. The course of the virus suppresses the normal function of the immune system and leads to a state of profound immunodeficiency. Some cutaneous conditions are indicators of HIV infection and the appearance of the skin can reflect the patient's immune status. Skin diseases remain a common concern for HIV-infected individuals; even with adequate treatment, patients may still suffer from a wide range of dermatologic conditions.

REFERENCES

1. UNAIDS. Fact sheet: 2014 statistics. http://www.unaids.org/en/resources/campaigns/HowAIDSchangedeverything/factsheet. Accessed August 23, 2015.
2. Centers for Disease Control and Prevention (CDC). Disparities in diagnoses of HIV infection between blacks/African Americans and other racial/ethnic populations: 37 states, 2005-2008. *MMWR Morb Mortal Wkly Rep*. 2011;60(4):93–98.
3. Maurer TA. Dermatologic manifestations of HIV infection. *Top HIV Med*. 2005;12:149–154.
4. Bradley H, Hall HI, Wolitski RJ, et al. Vital signs: HIV diagnosis, care, and treatment among persons living with HIV—United States, 2011. *MMWR Morb Mortal Wkly Rep*. 2014;63:1113–1117.
5. Khambaty MM, Hsu SS. Dermatology of the patient with HIV. *Emerg Med Clin North Am*. 2010;28:355–368.
6. Muzyka BC, Glick M. Major aphthous ulcers in patients with HIV disease. *Oral Surg Oral Med Oral Pathol*. 1994;77:116–120.
7. Hulsebosch HJ, Claessen FA, vanGinkel CJ, et al. Human immunodeficiency virus exanthem. *J Am Acad Dermatol*. 1990;23:483–486.
8. Abrams DI. Clinical manifestations of HIV infection, including persistent generalized lymphadenopathy and AIDS-related complex. *J Am Acad Dermatol*. 1990;22:1217–1222.
9. Chatzikokkinou P, Satiropoulos K, Katoulis A, et al. Seborrheic dermatitis: an early and common skin manifestation in HIV patients. *Acta Dermatovenerol Croat*. 2008;16:226–230.
10. Sanchez M, Friedman-Kien AE. Skin manifestations of HIV infection. In: Wormser G, ed. *AIDS and Other Manifestations of HIV Infection*. 4th ed. Waltham, MA: Academic Press; 2004:655–688.
11. Gelfand JM, Stern RS, Nijsttten T, et al. The prevalence of psoriasis in African Americans: results from a population-based study. *J Am Acad Dermatol*. 2005;52:23–26.
12. Cedeno-Laurent F, Gómez-Flores M, Mendez N, et al. New insights into HIV-1-primary skin disorders. *J Int AIDS Soc*. 2011;14:5.
13. Morar N, Willis-Owen SA, Maurer T, et al. HIV-associated psoriasis: pathogenesis, clinical features, and management. *Lancet Infect Dis*. 2010;10:470–478.
14. Okoduwa C, Lambert WC, Schwartz RA, et al. Erythroderma: review of a potentially life-threatening dermatosis. *Indian J Dermatol*. 2009;54:1–6.
15. Menon K, Van Voorhees AS, Bebo BF Jr, et al. Psoriasis in patients with HIV infection: from the medical board of the National Psoriasis Foundation. *J Am Acad Dermatol*. 2010;62:291–299.
16. Haustein UF, Rytter M. Methotrexate in psoriasis: 26 years' experience with low-dose long-term treatment. *J Eur Acad Dermatol Venereol*. 2000;14:382–388.
17. Bickel M, Anadol E, Vogel M, et al. Daily dosing of tacrolimus in patients treated with HIV-1 therapy containing a ritonavir-boosted protease inhibitor or raltegravir. *J Antimicrob Chemother*. 2010;65:999–1004.
18. Wesley NO, Maibach HI. Racial (ethnic) differences in skin properties: the objective data. *Am J Clin Dermatol*. 2003;4:843–860.
19. Horváth A. Total and specific IgE in sera of HIV positive and HIV negative homosexual male (regulation of IgE synthesis in HIV infection). *Acta Biomed Ateneo Parmense*. 1992;63:133–145.
20. Rudikoff D. The relationship between HIV infection and atopic dermatitis. *Curr Allergy Asthma Rep*. 2002;2:275–281.
21. Gong JQ, Lin L, Lin T, et al. Skin colonization by Staphylococcus aureus in patients with eczema and atopic dermatitis and relevant combined topical therapy: a double-blind multicentre randomized controlled trial. *Br J Dermatol*. 2006;155:680–687.
22. Beck LA, Thaçi D, Hamilton JD, et al. Dupilumab treatment in adults with moderate-to-severe atopic dermatitis. *N Engl J Med*. 2014;371:130–139.
23. Coopman SA, Johnson RA, Platt R, et al. Cutaneous disease and drug reactions in HIV infection. *N Engl J Med*. 1993;328:1670–1674.
24. Eliaszewicz M, Flahault A, Roujeau JC, et al. Prospective evaluation of risk factors of cutaneous drug reactions to sulfonamides in patients with AIDS. *J Am Acad Dermatol*. 2002;47:40–46.
25. Caumes E, Roudier C, Rogeaux O, et al. Effect of corticosteroids on the incidence of adverse cutaneous reactions to trimethoprim-sulfamethoxazole during treatment of AIDS-associated *Pneumocystis carinii pneumonia*. *Clin Infect Dis*. 1994;18:319–323.
26. Borrás-Blasco J, Navarro-Ruiz A, Borrás C, et al. Adverse cutaneous reactions associated with the newest antiretroviral drugs in patients with human immunodeficiency virus infection. *J Antimicrob Chemother*. 2008;62:879–888.
27. Todd G. Adverse cutaneous drug eruptions and HIV: a clinician's global perspective. *Dermatol Clin*. 2006;24:459–472.
28. Harr T, French LE. Toxic epidermal necrolysis and Stevens-Johnson syndrome. *ChemImmunol Allergy*. 2012;97:149–166.
29. Chaponda M, Pirmohamed M. Hypersensitivity reactions to HIV therapy. *Br J Clin Pharmacol*. 2011;71:659–671.
30. Fagot JP, Mockenhaupt M, Bouwes-Bavinck JN, et al. Nevirapine and the risk of Stevens-Johnson syndrome or toxic epidermal necrolysis. *AIDS*. 2001;15:1843–1848.
31. Centers for Disease Control and Prevention (CDC). Serious adverse events attributed to nevirapine regimens for postexposure prophylaxis after HIV exposures—worldwide, 1997-2000. *MMWR Morb Mortal Wkly Rep*. 2001;49:1153–1156.
32. Nunn P, Gicheha C, Hayes R, et al. Cross-sectional survey of HIV infection among patients with tuberculosis in Nairobi, Kenya. *Tuber Lung Dis*. 1992;73:45–51.
33. Ma JD, Lee KC, Kuo GM. HLA-B*5701 testing to predict abacavir hypersensitivity. *PLoS Curr*. 2010;2:RRN1203.
34. Finkelstein JL, Gala P, Rochford R, et al. HIV/AIDS and lipodystrophy: implications for clinical management in resource-limited settings. *J Intern AIDS Soc*. 2015;18:19033.
35. Walker NF, Scriven J, Meintjes G, et al. Immune reconstitution inflammatory syndrome in HIV-infected patients. *HIV AIDS (Auckl)*. 2015;7:49–64.
36. Novak RM, Richardson JT, Buchacz K, et al. HIV Outpatient Study (HOPS) Investigators. Immune reconstitution inflammatory syndrome: incidence and implications for mortality. *AIDS*. 2012;26:721–730.
37. Resneck JS Jr, Van Beek M, Furmanski L, et al. Etiology of pruritic papular eruption with HIV infection in Uganda. *JAMA*. 2004;292:2614–2621.
38. Liautaud B, Pape JW, DeHovitz JA, et al. Pruritic skin lesions: a common initial presentation of acquired immunodeficiency syndrome. *Arch Dermatol*. 1989;125:629–632.
39. Resnick JS Jr, Van Beek M, Furmanski L, et al. Etiology of pruritic papular eruption with HIV infection in Uganda. *JAMA*. 2004;292:2614–2621.
40. Afonso JP, Tomimori J, Michalany NS, et al. Pruritic papular eruption and eosinophilic folliculitis associated with human immunodeficiency virus (HIV) infection: a histopathological and immunohistochemical comparative study. *J Am Acad Dermatol*. 2012;67:269–275.
41. Ellis E, Scheinfeld N. Eosinophilic pustular folliculitis: a comprehensive review of treatment options. *Am J Clin Dermatol*. 2004;5:189–197.
42. Vin-Christian K, Epstein JH, Maurer TA, et al. Photosensitivity in HIV-infected individuals. *J Dermatol*. 2000;27:361–369.
43. James WD, Berger T, Elston D. *Andrews' Diseases of the Skin: Clinical Dermatology*. 12th ed. Philadelphia, PA: Elsevier;2015:35.
44. Jordaan HF. Common skin and mucosal disorders in HIV/AIDS. *S Afr Fam Pract*. 2008;50:14–23.
45. Singh G. Nails in systemic disease. *Indian J Dermatol Venereol Leprol*. 2011;77:646–651.
46. Hogan MT. Cutaneous infections associated with HIV/AIDS. *Dermatol Clin*. 2006;24:473–495.
47. Centers for Disease Control and Prevention. 2012 Sexually Transmitted Diseases Surveillance. www.cdc.gov/std/stats12/figures/49.htm. Accessed August 23, 2015.
48. Panel on Opportunistic Infections in HIV-Infected Adults and Adolescents. Guidelines for Prevention and Treatment of Opportunistic Infections in HIV-Infected Adults and Adolescents: recommendations from the Centers for Disease Control and Prevention, the National Institutes of Health, and the HIV Medicine Association of the Infectious Diseases Society of America. http://aidsinfo.nih.gov/contentfiles/lvguidelines/adult_oi.pdf. Accessed April 20, 2015.
49. Workowski KA, Bolan GA; Centers for Disease Control and Prevention. Sexually transmitted diseases treatment guidelines, 2015. *MMWR Recomm Rep*. 2015;64:1–137.

50. Blank LJ, Polydefkis MJ, Moore RD, et al. Herpes zoster among persons living with HIV in the current antiretroviral therapy era. *J Acquir Immune Defic Syndr.* 2012;61:203–207.

51. Gnann JW Jr, Whitley RJ. Clinical practice: herpes zoster. *N Engl J Med.* 2002;347:340–346.

52. Koenig HC, Garland JM, Weissman D, et al. Vaccinating HIV patients: focus on human papillomavirus and herpes zoster vaccines. *AIDS Rev.* 2013;15:77–86.

53. Palefsky J. Human papillomavirus-related disease in people with HIV. *Curr Opin HIV AIDS.* 2009;4:52–56.

54. Altman K, Vanness E, Westergaard RP. Cutaneous manifestations of human immunodeficiency virus: a clinical update. *Curr Infect Dis Rep.* 2015;17:464.

55. Forman D, de Martel C, Lacey CJ, et al. Global burden of human papillomavirus and related diseases. *Vaccine* 2012;30:F12–F23.

56. Wieland U, Silling S, Scola N, et al. Merkel cell polyomavirus infection in HIV-positive men. *Arch Dermatol.* 2011;147:401–406.

57. Liu C, Bayer A, Cosgrove SE, et al. Clinical practice guidelines by the Infectious Diseases Society of America for the treatment of methicillin-resistant *Staphylococcus aureus* infections in adults and children. *Clin Infect Dis.* 2011;59:e18–e55.

58. Stevens DL, Bisno AL, Chambers HF, et al. Practice guidelines for the diagnosis and management of skin and soft tissue infections: 2014 update by the Infectious Diseases Society of America. *Clin Infect Dis.* 2014;59:147–159.

59. Patton ME, Su JR, Nelson R, et al. Primary and secondary syphilis: United States, 2005-2013. *MMWR Morb Mortal Wkly Rep.* 2014;63:402–406.

60. Gregory N, Sanchez M, Buchness MR. The spectrum of syphilis in patients with human immunodeficiency virus infection. *J Am Acad Dermatol.* 1990;22:1061–1067.

61. Centers for Disease Control and Prevention (CDC). Symptomatic early neurosyphilis among HIV-positive men who have sex with men: four cities, United States, January 2002-June 2004. *MMWR Morb Mortal Wkly Rep.* 2007;56:625–628.

62. Aly R, Berger T. Common superficial fungal infections in patients with AIDS. *Clin Infect Dis.* 1996;22:S128–S132.

63. Elewski BE. Onychomycosis: pathogenesis, diagnosis, and management. *Clin Microbiol Rev.* 1998;11:415–429.

64. Karimi K, Wheat LJ, Connolly P, et al. Differences in histoplasmosis in patients with acquired immunodeficiency syndrome in the United States and Brazil. *J Infect Dis.* 2002;186:1655–1660.

65. Cohen PR, Bank DE, Silvers DN, et al. Cutaneous lesions of disseminated histoplasmosis in human immunodeficiency virus-infected patients. *J Am Acad Dermatol.* 1990;23:422–428.

66. Moskowitz DG. Cutaneous Cryptococcus Clinical Presentation. http://emedicine.medscape.com/article/1093087-clinical. Accessed August 22, 2015.

67. Murakawa GJ, Kerschmann R, Berger T. Cutaneous Cryptococcus infection and AIDS: report of 12 cases and review of the literature. *Arch Dermatol.* 1996;132:545–548.

68. Ranjana KH, Priyokumar K, Singh TJ, et al. Disseminated *Penicillium marneffei* infection among HIV-infected patients in Manipur state, India. *J Infect.* 2002;45:268–271.

69. Sanchez M. Kaposi's sarcoma. In: Rigel DS, Robinson JK, Ross MI, et al, eds. *Cancer of the Skin.* 2nd ed. Baltimore, MD: Saunders; 2011:168–178.

70. Hiatt KM, Nelson AM, Lichy JH, et al. Classic Kaposi sarcoma in the United States over the last two decades: a clinicopathologic and molecular study of 438 non-HIV-related Kaposi sarcoma patients with comparison to HIV-related Kaposi sarcoma. *Mod Pathol.* 2008;21:572–582.

71. Silverberg MJ, Leyden W, Warton EM, et al. HIV infection status, immunodeficiency, and the incidence of non-melanoma skin cancer. *J Natl Cancer Inst.* 2013;105:350–360.

72. Berthelot C, Cockerell CJ. Cutaneous neoplastic manifestations of HIV disease. In: Cockerell CJ, Calame A, eds. *Cutaneous Manifestations of HIV Disease.* London, UK: CRC Press; 2012.

73. Sigel K, Dubrow R, Silverberg M, et al. Cancer screening in patients infected with HIV. *Curr HIV/AIDS Rep.* 2011;8:142–152.

74. Palefsky JM. Anal cancer prevention in HIV-positive men and women. *Curr Opin Oncol.* 2009;21:433–438.

75. Gordon Spratt EA, Fischer M, Kamino H. Eruptive basal-cell carcinomas in the setting of human immunodeficiency virus infection. *Dermatol Online J.* 2012;18:1.

76. Zhao H, Shu G, Wang S. The risk of non-melanoma skin cancer in HIV-infected patients: new data and meta-analysis. *Int J STD AIDS.* 2015;pii:0956462415586316.

77. Kubica AW, Brewer JD. Melanoma in immunosuppressed patients. *Mayo Clin Proc.* 2012;87:991–1003.

Mucocutaneous Viral Infections

Andrew J. Thompson
Ashley E. Ojeaga
Marigdalia K. Ramirez-Fort
Harrison P. Nguyen
Farhan Khan
Stephen K. Tyring

KEY POINTS

- Varicella-zoster virus (shingles) often presents with a prodrome of dermatomal pain, pruritus, and dysesthesia prior to the onset of a rash, which is localized to a unilateral dermatome.

- People with skin of color are less likely than fairer skinned individuals to develop shingles.

- Genital herpes presents with chronic, recurrent episodes of painful vesicles and subsequent ulceration and requires diagnostic testing with viral culture, polymerase chain reaction analysis, or serology to establish the correct diagnosis.

- Kaposi sarcoma, caused by human herpesvirus type 8, most commonly presents as violaceous lesions on the skin of the lower extremities, mucocutaneous surfaces, lymph nodes, or viscera.

- Anogenital warts are caused by human papillomavirus types 6 and 11 in the majority of cases.

- Common warts are most often observed in children, and they usually present with cauliflower-like papules on the dorsa of the hands or fingers.

- Molluscum contagiosum infection causes pearly white or skin-colored papules with central umbilication.

INTRODUCTION

Despite the U.S. population becoming increasingly multiracial and multi ethnic, there is limited evidence-based data regarding skin of color. It is crucial for our understanding of skin of color to improve so that we can advance treatment of diseases including viral infections. The goal of this chapter is to discuss important epidemiologic factors of common viral infections that have cutaneous manifestations. We will also highlight the pathogenesis, clinical manifestations, diagnosis, and treatment options of these viral infections.

VARICELLA-ZOSTER VIRUS

Varicella-zoster virus (VZV) is a human neurotropic virus that causes varicella (chickenpox) and zoster (shingles). Primary infection causes varicella, a mild and self-limited disease of childhood. The virus subsequently establishes latency. VZV reactivates and causes herpes zoster when individuals have a decline in cell-mediated immunity. In a population-based cohort investigation, the effect of race on the risk of acquiring herpes zoster was examined in individuals older than 65 years of age.[1] There were significantly fewer cases among darker skin of color subjects compared to fairer skinned subjects. In another study that included 3206 subjects older than 64 years of age, African Americans were one-fourth as likely as Caucasian patients to experience zoster infection.[2]

■ PATHOGENESIS

Up to 90% of nonimmune household contacts develop primary varicella infection after exposure to an infected individual.[3] VZV is transmitted by respiratory secretions from the nasopharynx or by direct contact with infected skin lesions. Individuals are infectious from 2 days prior to the onset of the rash until all of the vesicles have crusted.

During primary varicella infection, the virus establishes latency in cranial nerve ganglia, dorsal root ganglia, and autonomic ganglia. A decline in T-cell proliferation in response to VZV antigens is thought to be involved in the process of reactivation. This reactivation occurs more commonly in the elderly, individuals infected with human immunodeficiency virus (HIV), organ transplantation recipients, and those treated with chemotherapy, radiotherapy, and long-term corticosteroids.[3] Reactivation of VZV typically occurs once in a lifetime; recurrent reactivation of VZV or "recurrent shingles" is a rare phenomenon among the immunocompetent.[4-6]

CLINICAL MANIFESTATIONS

Primary varicella is usually a mild self-limited disease in children. Infected adults may have prodromal symptoms including fever, chills, headache, and myalgias prior to onset of the rash, but in children, the rash is frequently the first sign of varicella infection.[7] The pruritic skin lesions appear as crops of red macules on the head and spread inferiorly to the trunk and extremities. The skin lesions become papular and develop into clear superficial vesicles on an erythematous base [**Figure 61-1**], which later become pustular followed by crust formation and resolution. The most common complication of varicella is bacterial superinfection, most frequently caused by *Staphylococcus aureus* or *Streptococcus pyogenes*.[8] The superinfection may cause cellulitis, impetigo, or furuncles. Varicella pneumonia is a complication that presents within 1 to 6 days after onset of the rash. The mortality rate of varicella pneumonia is 10% in immunocompetent individuals and 30% in immunocompromised individuals.[3] A prodrome of dermatomal pain, pruritus, and dysesthesia precedes the appearance of the herpes zoster rash in most patients.[3] The pain may be either constant or intermittent and may mimic the pain of acute appendicitis, biliary or renal colic, cholecystitis, peptic ulcer, myocardial infarction, pleurisy, or a prolapsed intervertebral disk. This pain is most severe in the elderly and immunocompromised patients. Rarely, individuals with dermatomal pain do not develop a skin lesion; this is known as *zoster sine herpete*. The rash of zoster is usually localized to a unilateral dermatome, most frequently involving the ophthalmic division of the trigeminal nerve (V_1) and the thoracic nerves [**Figure 61-2**]. The eruption initially presents with erythematous macules and papules, which evolve into vesicles on an erythematous base. After 3 to 4 days, pustules form and gradually crust. This is usually

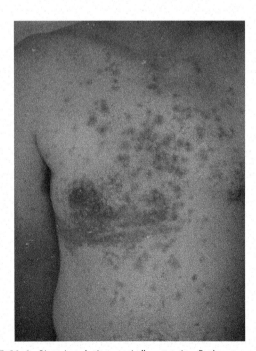

FIGURE 61-1. Disseminated primary varicella-zoster virus. Erythematous macules and papules on the trunk.

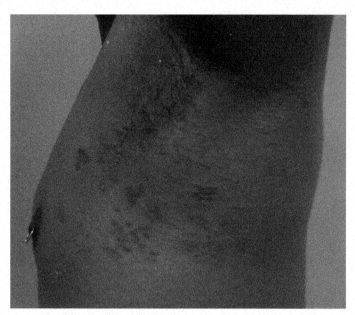

FIGURE 61-2. Herpes zoster. Erythematous papules and vesicles on an erythematous base in a thoracic spinal nerve 4 (T4) distribution.

followed by complete healing, but hyperpigmentation commonly occurs in individuals with darker skin tones.[3]

During the reactivation of VZV, the virus travels down peripheral sensory nerves to the skin. By unknown mechanisms, the involved nerves are irritated resulting in postherpetic neuralgia (PHN). There are several risk factors for PHN, including herpes zoster infection at an older age, more severe acute pain, more severe rash, and the presence of a painful prodrome.[9-11] PHN affects more than one-third of individuals over 60 years old and presents as pain that may be accompanied by pruritus, paresthesia, dysesthesia, or anesthesia.[3] The pain of PHN usually decreases significantly within 3 to 6 months following acute zoster infection. However, some individuals may experience postherpetic pain for more than 5 years.[12] When cranial nerve V_1 is involved in zoster infection, multiple ocular complications, including blindness, may occur.[3] Disseminated herpes zoster is a complication primarily in immunocompromised patients and has a mortality rate of 40%.[13]

DIAGNOSIS

Varicella and zoster are diagnosed clinically. However, herpes simplex virus (HSV) may cause a dermatomal rash that is morphologically indistinguishable from herpes zoster. Although the vesicular fluid can be examined with the Tzanck smear, it does not distinguish varicella zoster from HSV; both infections result in multinucleated giant cells and epithelial cells containing intranuclear inclusions. Viral culture, serology, direct immunofluorescence, dot-blot hybridization, and real-time polymerase chain reaction (PCR) may be used to differentiate VZV from HSV. Real-time PCR has higher sensitivity compared to viral culture.[14] Patient history may also aid in differentiation. Recurrent herpes zoster is rare in immunocompetent patients, whereas infection by HSV may recur anywhere from 1 to 10 times per year. An immunocompetent patient presenting with a recurrent dermatomal vesicular eruption should prompt suspicion for infection by HSV.

TREATMENT

Children with varicella infection should receive symptomatic treatment for fever and pruritus. Treatment with acyclovir is most beneficial when initiated within 24 hours of the onset of the rash[3] [**Table 61-1**]. Acyclovir is approved for the treatment of varicella in individuals older than 2 years of age. Early treatment results in decreased pruritus and fewer lesions after 28 days.[15] Varicella zoster immune globulin is recommended for pregnant, varicella-seronegative women who are exposed to

TABLE 61-1   Varicella treatment

Healthy children: oral acyclovir (20 mg/kg) 4 times a day for 5 days.

Children who weigh more than 40 kg and immunocompetent adults: oral acyclovir 800 mg 4 times a day for 5 days; valacyclovir 1 g 3 times a day and famciclovir 500 mg 3 times a day for 7 days are also frequently used but not approved by the U.S. Food and Drug Administration for treatment of primary varicella in adults.

Immunocompromised individuals: intravenous acyclovir (10 mg/kg) every 8 hours for 7–10 days.

Symptoms	Treatment
Fever	Antipyretics (acetaminophen): children should not be given aspirin because of its association with Reye syndrome.
Pruritus	Oral antihistamines including diphenhydramine and loratadine, calamine lotion, or tepid baths with baking soda. Fingernails should be clipped to minimize scratching.

VZV. The live attenuated varicella-zoster vaccine has a 96% seroconversion rate in healthy children.[3] The vaccine is close to 100% protective from severe chickenpox and 90% protective from all disease.[16]

There are several antiviral medications available for the treatment of herpes zoster, and these medications are most beneficial when initiated within 72 hours of the onset of the rash[17] [**Table 61-2**]. Acyclovir accelerates healing of the eruption, decreases acute pain, and reduces both the incidence and duration of PHN.[18] Intravenous acyclovir is indicated for immunocompromised individuals, for immunocompetent patients with significant complications, and for those unable to take oral medications. Adverse effects of acyclovir include headache, nausea, diarrhea, nephrotoxicity, and neurotoxicity. Compared to acyclovir, valacyclovir decreases the median duration of pain caused by zoster.[3] Valacyclovir has similar side effects as acyclovir, but it is not associated with neurotoxicity or nephrotoxicity. Famciclovir is also indicated for the treatment of zoster and has the same efficacy as valacyclovir in the treatment of zoster.[15]

There are multiple treatment options to reduce the pain associated with PHN. The duration and severity of PHN are reduced with early initiation of antiviral medications. Additional treatment options include tricyclic antidepressants, anticonvulsants, and topical medications. Tricyclic antidepressants reduce the pain associated with PHN. However, they have significant anticholinergic side effects, including dry mouth, blurred vision, and urinary retention. Gabapentin reduces the pain and sleep disturbances associated with PHN. Capsaicin cream is

TABLE 61-2   Zoster treatment

Immunocompetent individuals: oral acyclovir 800 mg 5 times daily for 7–10 days; oral valacyclovir 1 g 3 times daily for 7 days, oral famciclovir 500 mg 3 times daily for 7 days

Immunocompromised individuals: intravenous acyclovir 10 mg/kg every 8 hours for 7 days

Symptoms	Treatment
Pain	Analgesics
Pruritus	Oral antihistamines, calamine lotion

also effective in decreasing the pain associated with PHN but causes a burning sensation.[3] The burning may be alleviated by pretreatment with topical lidocaine patch.

HUMAN HERPESVIRUSES

Human herpesviruses (HHVs) are a diverse group of double-stranded, enveloped DNA viruses that belong to the family Herpesviridae. These viruses are ubiquitous and highly adapted to their human hosts. All of the HHVs establish both productive and latent infections for the lifetime of the host, with severe symptoms and complications of infection typically limited to young or immunocompromised individuals. In most HHV infections, reactivation of latent virus results in recurrent disease.

HERPES SIMPLEX VIRUSES

When infection with HSV type 1 (HSV-1) or type 2 (HSV-2) occurs from the umbilicus to the knees, the disease is entitled genital herpes. Genital herpes is a common sexually transmitted disease that presents with chronic, recurrent episodes of painful vesiculation with subsequent ulceration. Genital herpes is most frequently caused by HSV-2, but recently an increasing number of cases have been found to be a result of HSV-1 infection.[19] Asymptomatic shedding is the most common cause of transmission to sexual partners.[20] The strongest risk factor is the number of lifetime sexual partners. Individuals with genital herpes have a two- to four-fold increased risk of HIV infection.[21-23] Antiviral medications treat acute episodes and are effective in reduction of viral shedding and the total number of recurrences.

The National Health and Nutrition Examination Survey (NHANES) assessed 40,000 subjects from 1988 to 1994 for antibodies to HSV-2. The seroprevalence of HSV-2 in subjects 12 years of age and older was 21.9%.[24] The seroprevalence was 25.6% among women and 17.8% among men.[24] The seroprevalence was 17.6% among Caucasians, 45.9% among African Americans, and 22.3% among Mexican Americans.[24]

PATHOGENESIS

Primary HSV transmission occurs through direct contact with infected individuals who are shedding HSV from either skin or genital secretions.[25] Approximately 70% of genital HSV-2 is transmitted during periods of asymptomatic shedding.[19] During primary infection, HSV enters the body through mucocutaneous surfaces and replicates in the epithelial cells. HSV subsequently establishes latency in the sacral dorsal root ganglia. During reactivation, HSV travels from dorsal root ganglia down the nerve roots to the mucocutaneous surfaces. Several precipitating factors are associated with HSV reactivation; however, most recurrences have no identifiable cause.[25] HSV reactivation may result in asymptomatic viral shedding or clinical signs and symptoms of infection.

CLINICAL MANIFESTATIONS

Primary HSV-1 or HSV-2 genital infection may result in asymptomatic infection or prodromal symptoms of localized pain, burning, and pruritus or may have constitutional symptoms. The lesions initially present as ill-defined erythema with subsequent papulovesicular formation [**Figure 61-3**]. The vesicular fluid eventually becomes purulent; the pustule then resolves, leaving a shallow erosion. Lesions most commonly occur on the external genitalia, perianal area, upper thighs, and buttocks. Primary lesions last between 2 and 6 weeks. Episodes may be associated with tender inguinal or femoral lymphadenopathy. Cervical lesions may cause intermittent vaginal bleeding or discharge. The clinical presentations of HSV-1 and HSV-2 infections are morphologically indistinguishable.[26] The recurrence rate of HSV-1 infection is significantly lower compared to HSV-2 infection.[27] Without antiviral medications, the recurrence rate of HSV-1 infection is approximately one time per year, whereas the median HSV-2 recurrence rate is four times

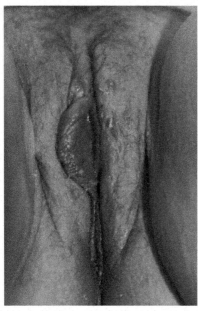

FIGURE 61-3. Herpes simplex virus type 1. Erythematous papulovesicles on female external genitalia.

per year.[25] The recurrence rates of both HSV-1 and HSV-2 infections decrease over time. Individuals with severe primary infections have more frequent recurrences.[28] Recurrences usually present with prodromal symptoms of localized pain, tingling, and pruritus. The skin lesions are often unilateral, and there are fewer lesions compared to the initial episode. The lesions usually last for 1 week. Systemic symptoms are rare during recurrent episodes.[29]

Eczema herpeticum is the manifestation of reactivated latent HSV-1 or HSV-2 in unusual locations (eg, face, neck, chest, arms, hands, ankles) or a presentation of disseminated primary infection by HSV-1 or HSV-2. Eczema herpeticum is morphologically identical to lesions of HSV primary infection and reactivation [**Figure 61-4**]. Any anatomic region may be involved, but it is most often seen on the face and neck.

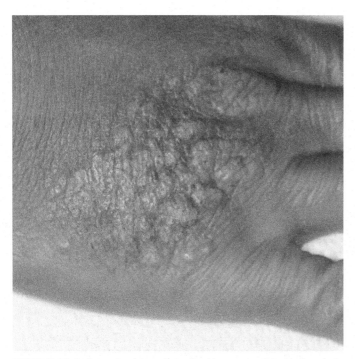

FIGURE 61-4. Eczema herpeticum. Grouped vesicles on an erythematous base on the dorsal hand.

TABLE 61-3	Genital herpes treatment

Antiviral agent:

Acyclovir

Initial infection: 200 mg 5 times daily or 400 mg 3 times daily for 7–10 days

Recurrences: 200 mg 5 times daily or 400 mg 3 times daily for 5 days

Suppressive therapy: 400 mg twice daily

Valacyclovir

Initial infection: 1 g twice daily for 7–10 days

Recurrences: 500 mg twice daily for 3–5 days

Suppressive therapy: 1 g daily in patients with more than 9 episodes per year; 500 mg daily in patients with fewer outbreaks

Famciclovir

Initial infection: 250 mg 3 times daily for 7–10 days

Recurrences: 125 mg twice daily for 5 days

Suppressive therapy: 250 mg twice daily

DIAGNOSIS

Clinical diagnosis of genital herpes has low sensitivity and specificity. Thus, diagnostic testing is essential to establish a correct diagnosis. A swab of the genital lesion can be assessed with viral culture or PCR analysis. Viral culture allows identification of HSV in the majority of primary infections but in fewer than 50% of recurrent episodes. PCR has a higher sensitivity compared to viral culture.[30] Serology may be used as indirect evidence of HSV infection and is only useful when the test distinguishes HSV-1 from HSV-2 infection. Serology is important in individuals with subclinical infections. It is also used to diagnose recurrent episodes because viral culture has a low sensitivity.[26]

TREATMENT

Oral nucleoside analogues, including acyclovir, valacyclovir, and famciclovir, are used to improve symptoms of genital herpes [**Table 61-3**]. They may be used for either episodic treatment or long-term suppressive therapy. Side effects of these antiviral medications are infrequent and include nausea, vomiting, diarrhea, and headache. Intravenous acyclovir is indicated for disseminated disease. Helicase-primase inhibitors are novel potent inhibitors of HSV replication and are currently undergoing clinical trials to evaluate efficacy in episodic and suppressive treatment of genital herpes.[31,32]

The selection of episodic or suppressive therapy should be based on the number of recurrences. Episodic therapy is generally indicated for individuals with mild and infrequent recurrences. Prophylactic therapy is used for patients with frequent and severe outbreaks and/or who are intimate with HSV seronegative partners. Individuals with more than six recurrences per year should be considered for suppressive therapy.[33] For both episodic and suppressive therapy, treatment may be with acyclovir, valacyclovir, or famciclovir.

HUMAN HERPESVIRUS TYPE 8

Human herpesvirus type 8 (HHV-8), or Kaposi sarcoma-associated herpesvirus (KSHV), is a member of the *Rhadinovirus* genus of Gammaherpesviruses subfamily. HHV-8 is the etiologic agent of almost all types of Kaposi sarcoma (KS), a multicentric malignant neoplasm characterized by spindle-shaped tumors of the lymphatic endothelium. There are four clinical variants of KS: classic KS, endemic African KS, acquired immunodeficiency syndrome (AIDS)-associated KS, and iatrogenic KS. HHV-8 is also thought to contribute to the development of primary effusion lymphoma (PEL) and multicentric Castleman disease (MCD).

Unlike the majority of HHVs, HHV-8 infection is not ubiquitous, and a racial predilection is geographically observed.[34-37] In North America, northern Europe, and Asia, HHV-8 seroprevalence rates are relatively low (0% to 5%).[34] Intermediate rates (5% to 20%) are observed in the

Middle East, Mediterranean, and Caribbean, whereas high rates (>50%) have been detected in central and southern Africa.[34] HHV-8 prevalence also varies among population groups within geographical regions. In South America, increased rates of HHV-8 prevalence have been observed in Brazilian and Ecuadorian Amerindians compared to other groups.[36] Likewise, increased prevalence among some groups in China has also been reported.[37]

■ PATHOGENESIS

HHV-8 transmission occurs primarily through saliva.[35] Sexual transmission is common in developed countries, especially among homosexuals.[38,39] HHV-8 can also be transmitted through childbirth,[38] intravenous drug use, organ transplantation, and blood transfusion.[35] HHV-8 infects endothelial cells, triggering morphologic changes resulting in spindle cell morphology.[40] The infection persists for the life of the host, although the infection predominates in a latent state in the majority of cells.[40,41]

■ CLINICAL MANIFESTATIONS

KS most commonly presents as violaceous lesions on the skin of the lower extremities[39] that are often associated with edema [**Figure 61-5**]. There are several morphologic variants of KS; however, lesions are typically classified in three clinical stages: patchy, plaque, and nodular.[42] Initially, lesions present as small, violaceous flat macules that characterize the patchy stage. These lesions may then coalesce to form plaques. Once the disease progresses to the nodular stage, brown elevated nodules or tumors are observed.[43] The tumors may ulcerate or infiltrate subsequent tissues.

The four variants of KS differ in their clinical manifestations. Classic KS commonly affects older men of Mediterranean, Jewish, or Eastern European decent and is characterized by violaceous lesions presenting on the lower extremities.[38,41] Endemic African KS is most prevalent in sub-Saharan Africa and presents as localized plaques and nodules in

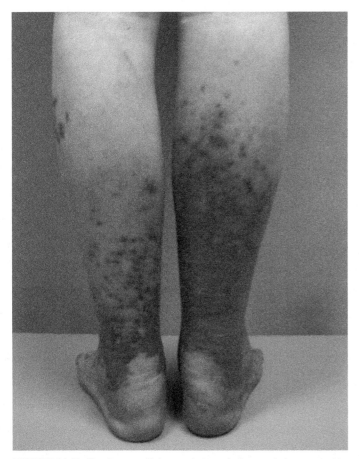

FIGURE 61-5. Kaposi sarcoma. Violaceous plaques and edema on the lower extremities bilaterally.

one of four clinical subvariants: nodular, florid, infiltrative, and lymphadenopathic.[41] The lymphadenopathic form is aggressive, and visceral involvement is common. AIDS-associated KS typically presents in homosexual males as bulky lesions associated with lymphatic obstruction and edema. Lesions spread to oral and perioral locations in over 50% cases and can cause speech and eating difficulties.[44] Gastrointestinal involvement is also common, occurring in 80% of patients.[44] Iatrogenic KS is associated with immunosuppression and organ transplantation; disease involves lymph nodes, mucosa, and visceral organs in 50% of cases.[38]

■ DIAGNOSIS

KS is diagnosed through histologic and immunohistochemistry tests.[42] Histologically, HHV-8 infection is characterized by dilated, abnormally shaped blood vessels with extravasated erythrocytes, hemosiderin, and fibrosis.[38] The three progressive stages of KS are histologically different, and lesions can be microscopically identified at each stage of development. The patch stage is characterized by minimal perivascular lymphoplasmacytic infiltrate and subtle proliferation of slit-like vascular spaces within the reticular dermis.[43,44] The proliferation of spindle-shaped cells with slit-like vascular spaces is observed as the disease progresses into the plaque stage.[42-44] At this stage, hemosiderin and hyaline bodies are apparent as the disease advances into the superficial subcutaneous tissue.[44] During the nodular stage, well-defined intradermal nodules of spindle cells arranged in fascicles with slit-like vascular spaces are predominantly observed.[43,44] Cytologic atypia, erythrocytes, and plasma cells are often observed.[43]

■ TREATMENT

KS is incurable but can be electively palliated through various treatments. Treatment of KS varies with the type and level of progression of the disease. Localized KS is often treated with surgical excision, cryotherapy, and radiation therapy.[38,39] In extensive or recurrent KS, treatment is systemic and can include chemotherapy, intralesional injections of vinblastine, surgery, immunotherapy, and radiation.[38] The progression of AIDS-associated KS is most successfully decelerated with highly active antiretroviral therapy (HAART). In iatrogenic KS, the disease typically regresses following a reduction in immunosuppressive therapy.

PARVOVIRUS B19

Parvovirus B19 is a small DNA virus that causes erythema infectiosum, which presents with a slapped-cheek rash on malar eminences and a pink reticular eruption on the trunk and extensor surfaces. A study of 800 stored serum samples demonstrated that there were no racial differences in B19 seropositive rates.[45]

■ PATHOGENESIS

Transmission occurs via aerosol droplets through the respiratory route.[46] Individuals are usually not infectious once the rash appears. During infection, B19 lyses erythroid precursor cells. The rash subsequently occurs due to immune complex deposition.[47]

■ CLINICAL MANIFESTATIONS

In children, erythema infectiosum (fifth disease) is the most common clinical presentation of B19 infection. Seven to 11 days after exposure, individuals may experience prodromal symptoms of low-grade fever, headache, coryza, and nausea. Nine to 13 days after exposure, patients present with "slapped cheek" erythematous edematous plaques on malar eminences. Associated symptoms include malaise, myalgias, pharyngitis, and conjunctivitis. Pink macules and papules present on the trunk and extensor surfaces. This eruption may involve the palms and soles. The rash often has a lacy, reticular pattern due to central clearing [**Figure 61-6**]. Over the next several weeks, the rash may recur with emotional stress, temperature change, sunlight, exercise, and bathing.[47]

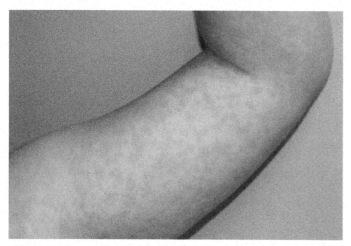

FIGURE 61-6. Parvovirus B19. Pink macules with a lacy, reticular pattern on the arm.

Subsequently, the rash resolves spontaneously with no permanent sequelae.

In adults, B19 infection is more frequently asymptomatic, does not present with erythema infectiosum, but causes arthralgias, fever, and lymphadenopathy.[48] Parvovirus B19 is associated with papular purpuric gloves and socks syndrome. This syndrome is most common in young adults. Prodromal symptoms may include low-grade fever, fatigue, and arthralgias. Individuals experience rapidly progressive painful and pruritic symmetrical swelling and erythema of the distal hands and feet. This progresses to papular-purpuric lesions of the distal extremities with sharp demarcation ending at the wrists and ankles.[47] Symptoms usually resolve within 1 to 3 weeks with no known sequelae.

DIAGNOSIS

Laboratory findings are unremarkable in most patients with erythema infectiosum.[49] Diagnosis is based on clinical presentation of a slapped-cheek rash on malar eminences and a lacy rash on the trunk, neck, and extensor surfaces.

When the clinical presentation is unclear, B19 immunoglobulin (Ig) M is used for diagnosis. IgM is detectable within a few days after onset of illness and for up to 6 months.[50] It has 89% sensitivity and 99% specificity.[51] B19 IgG is found 7 days after onset of infection and for up to several years and is clinically used to confirm prior infection.

TREATMENT

Usually, erythema infectiosum does not require specific treatment. If necessary, supportive treatment is the only indicated therapy [**Table 61-4**].

HUMAN PAPILLOMAVIRUS

Human papillomaviruses (HPVs) are small, nonenveloped, double-stranded DNA viruses classified as members of the Papillomaviridae family. HPV specifically invades and replicates in cells of the basal layer of the stratified epithelium and mucous membranes, stimulating proliferation in the skin.[52] The virus has an incubation period between 3 weeks and 8 months[53] and may be latent for several months to years.

TABLE 61-4	Parvovirus B19 treatment
Symptoms	Treatment
Arthralgias	Nonsteroidal anti-inflammatory medications
Pruritus	Oral antihistamines, starch baths
Fever	Antipyretics
Malaise	Bed rest

There are over 100 identified types of HPV. Some of the most common nononcogenic or low-risk types include HPV-2, -3, -6, -10, and -11. HPV-6 and HPV-11 are sexually transmitted from one person to another. The viruses penetrate skin and mucosal microabrasions in the anogenital area, causing genital warts.[54] Transmission can also occur from mother to infant at childbirth.[55] HPV-2, -3, and -10 are associated with cutaneous warts and transmitted via contact with an HPV-induced lesion from an infected individual. They are also associated with the development of epidermodysplasia verruciformis (EV).[53] Oncogenic HPVs such as HPV-16, -18, -31, and -45 are associated with over 95% of all cervical cancers and over 50% of all penile, vulvar, and vaginal cancers.[56] Worldwide, cervical cancer is the second most common cancer in women.[57] HPV-16 is responsible for 60% to 70% of HPV-positive cervical cancers, whereas HPV-18, the second most common HPV associated with cervical cancer, is responsible for 10% to 20% of cases.[53]

Racial differences occur in the prevalence of various types of HPV infection. Therefore, a clear pattern of racial difference in overall HPV infection is not yet established. The frequencies of cutaneous[56] and genital warts[58] have been reported to be higher in Caucasians than those with skin of color. On the other hand, increased incidence rates of cervical cancer are observed among Hispanics, African Americans, and American Indian/Alaska Natives compared to non-Hispanic Caucasians.[59]

HUMAN PAPILLOMAVIRUS TYPES 6 AND 11

HPV-6 and HPV-11 are low-risk mucosal types of HPV that cause 90% of all cases of anogenital warts. HPV-6 and HPV-11 are also the causative agents in cervical intraepithelial neoplasia and recurrent respiratory papillomatosis. In addition, HPV-6 causes vulvar intraepithelial neoplasia, whereas HPV-11 causes pharyngeal, nasal, and conjunctival papillomas.

Clinical Manifestations Genital warts clinically manifest as visible, painless papules associated with pruritus and discharge that develop within 3 months of primary infection.[54] The penis, vulva, vagina, cervix, perineum, and perianal areas are most commonly affected. Papules vary in color and can be pearly, filiform, or plaque-like. Urethral, vaginal, and coital bleeding may occur. Lesions may regress, remain inactive, or progress spontaneously. Recurrence is common, typically occurring in 67% of cases.[53]

Diagnosis The diagnosis of genital warts normally occurs through direct physical examination with bright light and magnification.[54] Colposcopy with acetic acid is often used to aid in visualization of infected cervical or vaginal tissue.[60] Histologic examination of genital warts reveals acanthosis, parakeratosis, hyperkeratosis, and the morphologic atypical koilocytosis. Clinically suspicious lesions demonstrating induration, ulceration, and pigmentation should be biopsied to evaluate for malignant transformation.[60]

Treatment of Genital Warts There is no cure for genital warts, and treatment is to ameliorate symptoms and remove symptomatic warts.[61] Surgical treatments include cryotherapy, electrosurgery, surgical excision, and laser surgery.[61] Nonsurgical therapies include podophyllotoxin, imiquimod, 5-fluorouracil, sinecatechins, and the antiviral cidofovir.[54,61]

HUMAN PAPILLOMAVIRUS TYPE 2

HPV-2 is a low-risk mucosal type that induces verruca vulgaris. Common warts occur most frequently in children. Lesions are typically harmless and resolve on their own. HPV-2 also causes the majority of verruca plantaris, or mosaic plantar warts, which are often mistaken for corns or callous.

Clinical Manifestations Common warts typically present as cauliflower-like papules on the dorsa of the hands or fingers, but may be palmar, periungal, or plantar.[62,63] Lesions infrequently present on the face, neck, lips, or oral mucosa. They may be flat or dome-shaped and can occur singly or in clusters. Lesions are characterized as filiform, endophytic, digitate, or multidigitate.[64] Although most warts have an irregular, hyperkeratotic, asymmetric, brownish-gray surface, the size and shape of individual warts vary.[62]

Mosaic plantar warts are horny, granular, and irregular patches located on the soles of the feet.[60] Each patch consists of many small individual cores clustered together in a mosaic pattern, with small capillaries extending perpendicular to the plane of the surface.[65] Generalized verrucosis is a rare clinical presentation of a disseminated HPV infection associated with severe immunodeficiency status.[66]

Diagnosis The diagnosis of palmar/plantar warts is clinical. In HPV-2-induced warts, histologic findings include hyperkeratosis with focal parakeratotic columns, hypergranulosis, dilated capillaries in dermal papillae,[63] acanthosis, and papillomatosis.[57,63,64] Koilocytosis features include vacuolization of granular cells with unusual, pyknotic nuclei enclosed by a perinuclear halo and prominent condensed keratohyaline granules of different sizes, shapes, and stainability.[63,64]

HUMAN PAPILLOMAVIRUS TYPES 3 AND 10

HPV-3 and HPV-10 cause verruca plana, or plane (flat) warts. They additionally cause HPV-associated EV, a lifelong disease characterized by widespread, large, and irregular plane wart-like lesions. EV also clinically manifests as red-brown macules and plaques and pityriasis versicolor-like lesions.

Clinical Manifestations Plane warts are slightly raised, small, skin-colored, flat-topped papules that commonly appear on the palmar and dorsal hands.[64] Flatter and pigmented lesions may appear on the cheeks, chin, and forehead.[63] Lesions are often multiple and irregularly disseminated and can be grouped, confluent, or linearly distributed.[63,64]

HPV-3/-10–induced EV clinically manifests as disseminated, flat, plane wart-like lesions on the extremities, back, face, and dorsal hands.[67,68] Lesions may be confluent with uneven polycyclic borders.[67,68] EV also manifests as erythematous, slightly scaly, pityriasis versicolor-like macules on the face, neck, trunk, and arms.[67,68] EV lesions become malignant in one-third of cases, typically manifesting as actinic keratosis,[68] Bowen disease, invasive squamous cell carcinoma, and basal cell carcinoma.[67]

Diagnosis Diagnosis of plane warts and HPV-3/-10–induced EV is based on histologic findings. Histologic findings can be subtle and include a loose stratum corneum without areas of parakeratosis, slight papillomatosis, and minimal koilocytosis in the upper spinous and granular layers.[63] In HPV-3–associated warts, koilocytosis is characterized by perinuclear vacuolization with strongly basophilic nuclei, resembling bird eyes, located in the center of cells.[63] Hyperkeratosis, papillomatosis, and parakeratosis are more pronounced in HPV-10–associated warts.[63,64]

Treatment of Cutaneous Warts The treatment of cutaneous warts is dependent on the symptoms, the extent and duration of lesions, and the patient's immunologic status.[63] When warts are located in cosmetically essential areas, topical treatments such as tretinoin cream, 5-fluorouracil, cantharidin, imiquimod and salicylic acid are preferred. However, topical treatment is often gradual and may be required for weeks or months. Destructive therapies help achieve quick results and include curettage, electrodessication, and cryosurgery with liquid nitrogen.[63] Additional therapies include intralesional bleomycin, intralesional recombinant interferon-α, cidofovir, and induction with dinitrochlorobenzene.[63]

There is no specific treatment for EV. Patients with EV must undergo regular full-body skin examinations and protect themselves against ultraviolet (UV) exposure with UVA and UVB sunscreens with a sun protection factor (SPF) of 50 or higher.[64] EV skin lesions rarely regress spontaneously, and tumors are often removed via surgery, cryotherapy, or laser.[68] Benign lesions can be successfully treated with 0.05% to 0.1% retinoic acid with 5% 5-fluorouracil ointment.[68] When EV occurs on the face, skin grafts are typically performed on the forehead as a preventative therapy. Treatment with retinoids and interferon-α has demonstrated synergetic antiproliferative and antiangiogenic effects.[68]

Rare cases of generalized verrucosis are managed by treating the underlying immunodeficiency. In cases with severe disfigurement, a combination of surgical debridement and antiviral therapy is indicated.[66]

HAND, FOOT, AND MOUTH DISEASE

Hand, foot, and mouth disease (HFMD) is a viral illness caused by enteroviruses, most commonly coxsackievirus (CV) A16.[69] HFMD is usually a mild week-long illness that affects children between the ages of 2 and 10 years. There is no racial predilection for HFMD.[70]

PATHOGENESIS

CVA16, A6, A9, A10, B1, B3, and B5 and enterovirus 71 are all causal agents of HFMD.[71] Although CVA16 is the most common cause of HFMD, CVA6 outbreaks have recently been increasing. In 2008, there was an outbreak of HFMD in Finland due to CVA6. This same strain of CVA6 caused an outbreak in Japan that resulted in three children developing encephalitis or encephalopathy.[72,73] Enteroviruses are transmitted most often through the fecal–oral route. There may also be respiratory and oral–oral transmission. Minor viremia is generally dependent on patient age; children less than 2 years old have a longer period of viremia compared to older children and adults. Major viremia occurs during replication of the virus at the secondary infection sites, including skin, mucous membranes, central nervous system, heart, and other organs.

CLINICAL MANIFESTATIONS

Typically, HFMD starts with a 1- to 2-day prodrome of malaise, fatigue, low-grade fever, sore throat, and anorexia. The majority of patients develop small vesicles on the tongue or oral mucosa, which rapidly rupture to form shallow erosions.[71,74] Up to 70% of individuals develop an eruption on the dorsum of the hands, feet, palms, and soles [**Figure 61-7**]. The eruption evolves from papules to papulovesicles to vesicles.[74,75] Vesicles are asymptomatic or tender. There is crusting of the vesicles with residual red or pink spots and eventual desquamation before the illness resolves [**Figure 61-8**]. Associated symptoms may include diarrhea, joint pain, and lymphadenopathy.[74] Individuals frequently have both oral and cutaneous manifestations but do not need both for the diagnosis of HFMD.

DIAGNOSIS

Serologic assay by complement fixation for coxsackievirus B (CVB) (1 to 6) and CVA (2, 4, 7, 9, 10, and 16) antibodies is frequently used for detection of the more common coxsackievirus strains. CVA6 and EV71 are not readily detected with standard serologic assays and grow poorly in culture. Thus, real-time reverse transcription PCR is favored for detection of enterovirus infection.[76] The virus can be detected during the early acute phases of infection, but secretion of virus in saliva and skin occurs for a much shorter time than fecal shedding.

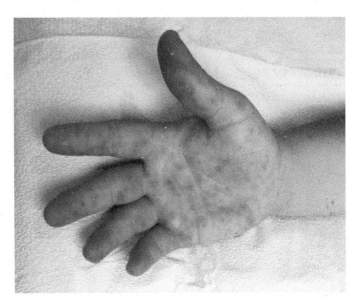

FIGURE 61-7. Hand, foot, and mouth disease. Erythematous papulovesicles on the hands bilaterally.

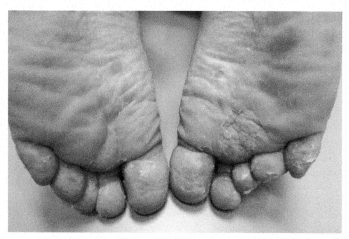

FIGURE 61-8. Hand, foot, and mouth disease. Desquamation of the toes bilaterally.

TREATMENT

There is no specific treatment for HFMD. Symptomatic treatment is outlined in **Table 61-5**.

MOLLUSCUM CONTAGIOSUM

Molluscum contagiosum (MC) is a cutaneous viral infection that is commonly observed in both healthy and immunocompromised school-age children. The infection is caused by a member of the Poxviridae family, the molluscum contagiosum virus (MCV).

There were an estimated 280,000 patient visits per year for MC in the United States alone during the 1990s.[77] MC is ubiquitously observed, and several epidemiologic studies conducted on specific racial populations in the United States have similarly concluded that skin color does not appear to impact the prevalence of MCV infection.[78-80] Instead, other comorbidities, such as atopic dermatitis, eczema, and immunosuppressive conditions, significantly increase the frequency and severity of molluscum disease.

PATHOGENESIS

MCV likely enters the skin through small abrasions and replicates in the lower layers of the epidermis.[81] The estimated incubation period varies from 14 days to 6 months. When active infection commences, the epidermis hypertrophies, extending into the underlying dermis, and characteristic molluscum bodies (also known as Henderson-Paterson bodies) within cells of the stratum spinosum form. As infection progresses, the molluscum bodies enlarge while hyperplasia of the basal cell layer replaces the spinosa layer. The hypertrophied spinosa cells then project toward the stratum corneum, forming the characteristic umbilicated lesions.[82]

CLINICAL MANIFESTATION

MC presents as single or multiple small, pearly white or flesh-colored papules that typically have a central umbilication [**Figure 61-9**]. The lesions vary in size, from 1 mm to 1 cm in diameter, and are generally asymptomatic.[83] However, in immunosuppressed patients, MC can

TABLE 61-5	Hand, foot, and mouth disease treatment
Symptoms	Treatment
Fever	Antipyretics: children should not be given aspirin due its association with Reye syndrome.
Anorexia	Drink water and avoid intake of fruit juices and sodas because they can irritate oral lesions.
Sore throat	Saline water rinses and gargles 2 or 3 times daily. Prepare with ½ teaspoon of salt and 1 glass of warm water.

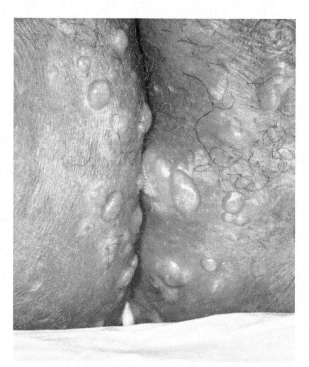

FIGURE 61-9. Molluscum contagiosum. Multiple white and skin-colored papules with central umbilication on the buttocks.

be a severe infection with hundreds of lesions developing throughout the body. MCV is transmitted through close physical contact with an infected individual or with a fomite.[84] MC usually begins in a localized area of the skin, although the lesions can be transmitted to other areas of the body, such as genital, perineal, pubic, and surrounding skin, through autoinoculation. Rarely, MC can also spread to the oral region as well as to the conjunctiva and cornea.[85,86] In atopic patients, eczema can develop around the papules approximately a month after their onset. The eczema, which has also been observed in nonatopic children, occurs in upward of 30% of patients and, importantly, increases the risk of autoinoculation.[87]

DIAGNOSIS

The diagnosis of MC is clinical. For challenging cases, the use of a magnifying lens or a dermatoscope to visualize the characteristic central umbilication often aids in diagnosis. Histopathology yields the final diagnosis in clinically unequivocal cases. Histopathology typically demonstrates epidermal hyperplasia producing a crater filled with molluscum bodies. Molluscum bodies, which are large (up to 35 μm), discrete, ovoid intracytoplasmic inclusion bodies, appear as large acidophilic granular masses, pushing the nucleus and numerous keratohyaline granules aside.

CLINICAL MANAGEMENT

MC in immunocompetent patients is self-limited; lesions typically resolve without intervention within 6 to 9 months. One study reported spontaneous resolution in 94.5% of patients within 6.5 months after initial infection; moreover, the same study reported that 23% of study participants were cured within 1 month after the first consultation with a dermatologist.[88] Current therapeutic intervention in the treatment of MC is intended merely to accelerate the eradication process.

To date, there is insufficient evidence to support that any treatment is definitively effective.[84] Nevertheless, curettage, cryotherapy, and cantharidin are considered to be first-line treatment strategies used in clinical practice. Cantharidin—the most popular method of treatment among American dermatologists—is a topical blistering agent that is applied directly to the lesions, usually with the blunt end of a cotton swab.[84] To prevent further autoinoculation or transmission, the site of treatment should then be covered with a bandage and should be washed with soap and water 2 to 6 hours after application. Treatments can be repeated every 2 to 4 weeks and are contraindicated for lesions located on the face, genitalia, or perianal regions.

Immunocompromised patients can develop severe, persistent disease and are at risk for developing concomitant infections by opportunistic pathogens. Surgical management, such as curettage, should be avoided because wounds increase the risk of additional infection. Instead, imiquimod applied three nights per week is recommended.[89] Clearance of recalcitrant, refractory lesions in HIV-positive patients has also been achieved through the use of intravenous or topical cidofovir, a nucleotide analog of deoxycytidine monophosphate.[90] Systemic cidofovir can be toxic on the kidneys, so topical cidofovir is favored. The authors achieved complete resolution of a severe case of MC on the face of an HIV patient in 2 months of treatment with the use of topical cidofovir compounded into a 2% ointment. Patients with atopic dermatitis are at risk for increased scar formation, so curettage is not advisable.

CONCLUSION

Individuals with skin of color are a diverse group and include multiple racial and ethnic groups. Ideally, the epidemiology of cutaneous viral infections should include information concerning the incidence, prevalence, mortality, and utilization of healthcare services. However, this information is limited for the majority of viral infections. With improvements in evidence-based data regarding skin of color, we will be better able to effectively diagnose viral infections and manage these conditions in this population.

REFERENCES

1. Schmader K, George LK, Burchett BM, et al. Racial and psychosocial risk factors for herpes zoster in the elderly. *J Infect Dis.* 1998;178:67-70.
2. Schmader K, George LK, Burchett BM, et al. Racial differences in the occurrence of herpes zoster. *J Infect Dis.* 1995;171:701-704.
3. Creed R, Satyaprakash D, Tyring SK. Varicella-zoster virus. In: Tyring SK, ed. *Mucocutaneous Manifestations of Viral Diseases.* 2nd ed. London: Informa Healthcare; 2010:98-122.
4. Epstein E. Recurrences in herpes zoster. *Cutis.* 1980;26:378-379.
5. Hope-Simpson RE. The nature of herpes zoster: a long-term study and a new hypothesis. *Proc R Soc Med.* 1965;58:9-20.
6. Helgason S, Sigurdsson JA, Gudmundsson S. The clinical course of herpes zoster: a prospective study in primary care. *Eur J Gen Pract.* 1996;2:1.
7. Dennehy PH. Varicella-zoster virus infections. In: Elzouki AY, Harfi HA, Stapleton FB, eds. *Textbook of Clinical Pediatrics.* Berlin: Springer-Verlag Berlin Heidelberg; 2012:1185-1189.
8. Aebi C, Ahmed A, Ramilo O. Bacterial complications of primary varicella in children. *Clin Infect Dis.* 1996;23:698-705.
9. Jung BF, Johnson RW, Griffin DR, et al. Risk factors for postherpetic neuralgia in patients with herpes zoster. *Neurology.* 2004;62:1545-1551.
10. Whitley RJ, Shukla S, Crooks RJ. The identification of risk factors associated with persistent pain following herpes zoster. *J Infect Dis.* 1998;189:S71-S75.
11. Whitley RJ, Weiss HL, Soong SJ, et al. Herpes zoster: risk categories for persistent pain. *J Infect Dis.* 1999;179:9-15.
12. Watson P. Clinical evidence handbook: postherpetic neuralgia. *Am Fam Physician.* 2011;84:690-692.
13. Weaver BA. Herpes zoster overview: natural history and incidence. *J Am Osteopath Assoc.* 2009;109:S2-S6.
14. Stranska R, Schuurman R, de Vos M, et al. Routine use of a highly automated and internally controlled real-time PCR assay for the diagnosis of herpes simplex and varicella-zoster virus infections. *J Clin Virol.* 2003;30:39-44.
15. Tyring SK, Beutner KR, Tucker BA, et al. Antiviral therapy for herpes zoster: randomized, controlled clinical trial of valacyclovir and famciclovir therapy in immunocompetent patients 50 years and older. *Arch Fam Med.* 2000;9:863-869.
16. Gershon AA. Viral vaccines of the future. *Pediatr Clin North Am.* 1990;37:689-707.
17. Stankus SJ, Dlugopolski M, Packer D. Management of herpes zoster (shingles) and postherpetic neuralgia. *Am Fam Physician.* 2000;61:2437-2444.
18. Crooks RJ, Jones DA, Fiddian AP. Zoster-associated chronic pain: an overview of clinical trials with acyclovir. *Scand J Infect Dis Suppl.* 1991;80:62-68.
19. Azwa A, Barton SE. Aspects of herpes simplex virus: a clinical review. *J Fam Plann Reprod HealthCare.* 2009;35:237-242.
20. Mertz GJ. Asymptomatic shedding of herpes simplex virus 1 and 2: implications for prevention of transmission. *J Infect Dis.* 2008;198:1098-1100.
21. Freeman EE, Weiss HA, Glynn JR. Herpes simplex virus 2 infection increases HIV acquisition in men and women: systematic review and meta-analysis of longitudinal studies. *AIDS.* 2006;20:73-83.
22. Barnabas RV, Celum C. Infectious co-factors in HIV-1 transmission herpes simplex virus type-2 and HIV-1: new insights and interventions. *Curr HIV Res.* 2012;10:228-237.
23. Corey L, Wald A, Celum CL, et al. The effects of herpes simplex virus-2 on HIV-1 acquisition and transmission: a review of two overlapping epidemics. *J AIDS.* 2004;35:435-445.
24. Fleming DT, McQuillan GM, Johnson RE, et al. Herpes simplex virus type 2 in the United States, 1976 to 1994. *N Engl J Med.* 1997;337:1105-1111.
25. Gupta R, Warren T, Wald A. Genital herpes. *Lancet.* 2007;370:2127-2137.
26. Beauman JG. Genital herpes: a review. *Am Fam Physician.* 2005;72:1527-1534.
27. Lafferty WE, Coombs RW, Benedetti C, et al. Recurrences after oral and genital herpes simplex virus infection: influence of anatomic site and viral type. *N Engl J Med.* 1987;316:1444-1449.
28. Benedetti J, Corey L, Ashley R. Recurrence rates in genital herpes after symptomatic first-episode infection. *Ann Intern Med.* 1994;121:847-854.
29. Corey L, Adams HG, Brown ZA, et al. Genital herpes simplex virus infections: clinical manifestations, course, and complications. *Ann Intern Med.* 1983;98:958-972.
30. Ramaswamy M, McDonald C, Smith M, et al. Diagnosis of genital herpes by real time PCR in routine clinical practice. *Sex Transm Infect.* 2004;80:406-410.
31. Tyring S, Wald A, Zadeikis N, et al. ASP2151 for the treatment of genital herpes: a randomized, double-blind, placebo- and valacyclovir-controlled, dose-finding study. *J Infect Dis.* 2012;205:1100-1110.
32. Field HJ, Mickleburgh I. The helicase-primase complex as a target for effective herpesvirus antivirals. *Adv Exp Med Biol.* 2013;767:145-159.
33. Patel R, Tyring S, Strand A, et al. Impact of suppressive antiviral therapy on the health related quality of life of patients with recurrent genital herpes infection. *Sex Transm Infect.* 1999;75:398-402.
34. Moore P. The emergence of Kaposi's sarcoma-associated herpesvirus (human herpesvirus 8). *N Engl J Med.* 2000;343:1411-1413.
35. Uldrick TS, Whitby D. Update on KSHV epidemiology, Kaposi sarcoma pathogenesis, and treatment of Kaposi sarcoma. *Cancer Lett.* 2011;305:150-162.
36. Mohanna S, Maco V, Bravo F, Gotuzzo E. Epidemiology and clinical characteristics of classic Kaposi's sarcoma, seroprevalence, and variants of human herpesvirus 8 in South America: a critical review of an old disease. *Int J Infect Dis.* 2005;9:239-250.
37. Zhang T, Shao X, Chen Y, et al. Human herpesvirus 8 seroprevalence, China. *Emerg Infect Dis.* 2012;18:150-152.
38. Antman K, Chang Y. Kaposi's sarcoma. *N Engl J Med.* 2000;342:1027-1038.
39. Schwartz RA, Micali G, Nasca MR, Scuderi L. Kaposi sarcoma: a continuing conundrum. *J Am Acad Dermatol.* 2008;59:179-206.
40. Ballon G, Cesarman E. Castleman's disease. In: Paul JP, Volberding A, eds. *Viral and Immunological Malignancies.* Hamilton, Ontario, Canada: BC Decker Inc; 2006:108-121.
41. Geraminejad P, Memar O, Aronson I, Rady PL, Hengge U, Tyring SK. Kaposi's sarcoma and other manifestations of human herpesvirus 8. *J Am Acad Dermatol.* 2002;47:641-655.
42. Fukumoto H, Kanno T, Hasegawa H, Katano H. Pathology of Kaposi's sarcoma-associated herpesvirus infection. *Front Microbiol.* 2011;2:175.
43. Ackerman AB, Gottlieb GJ. Atlas of the gross and microscopic features. In: Gottlieb GJ, Ackerman AB, eds. *Kaposi's Sarcoma: A Text and Atlas.* Philadelphia, PA: Lea & Febiger; 1988:29-110.
44. Hudnall SD, Yen-Moore A, Tyring SK. Human herpesvirus 8. In: Tyring SK, Yen Moore A, Lupi O, eds. *Mucocutaneous Manifestations of Viral Diseases.* 2nd ed. London: Informa Healthcare; 2010:184-197.
45. Ooi SL, Hooi PS, Chua BH, et al. Seroprevalence of human parvovirus B19 infection in an urban population in Malaysia. *Med J Malaysia.* 2002;57:97-103.
46. Anderson MJ, Higgins PG, Davis LR, et al. Experimental parvoviral infection in humans. *J Infect Dis.* 1985;152:257-265.
47. Gripp AC, Fontenelle E, Wiss K. Parvovirus B19. In: Tyring SK, Yen Moore A, Lupi O, eds. *Mucocutaneous Manifestations of Viral Diseases.* 2nd ed. London: Informa Healthcare; 2010:253-262.
48. Feder HM, Anderson I. Fifth disease. A brief review of infections in childhood, in adulthood, and in pregnancy. *Arch Intern Med.* 1989;149:2176-2178.

49. Condon FJ. Erythema infectiosum-report of an area-wide outbreak. *Am J Public Health.* 1949;49:528-535.

50. Cohen BJ, Mortimer PP, Pereira MS. Diagnostic assays with monoclonal antibodies for the human serum parvovirus-like virus (SPLV). *J Hyg.* 1983;91:113-130.

51. Doyle S, Kerr S, O'Keeffe G, et al. Detection of parvovirus B19 IgM by antibody capture enzyme immunoassay: receiver operating characteristic analysis. *J Virol Methods.* 2009;90:143-152.

52. Satyaprakash A, Mansur C. Human papillomaviruses. In: Tyring SK, Yen Moore A, Lupi O, eds. *Mucocutaneous Manifestations of Viral Diseases.* 2nd ed. London: Informa Healthcare; 2010:207-252.

53. Sterling JC. Introduction. In: Sterling JC, Tyring SK, eds. *Human Papillomaviruses: Clinical and Scientific Advances.* London, United Kingdom: Arnold; 2001:1-7.

54. Dupin N. Genital warts. *Clin Dermatol.* 2004;22:481-486.

55. Doorbar J, Sterling JC. The biology of human papillomaviruses. In: Sterling JC, Tyring SK, eds. *Human Papillomaviruses: Clinical and Scientific Advances.* London, United Kingdom: Arnold; 2001:10-23.

56. Schachner L, Ling NS, Press S. A statistical analysis of a pediatric dermatology clinic. *Pediatr Dermatol.* 1983;1:157-164.

57. Parkin DM, Pisani P, Ferlay J. Estimates of the worldwide frequency of eighteen major cancers in 1985. *Int J Cancer.* 1993;54:594-606.

58. Oriel JD. Natural history of genital warts. *Br J Vener Dis.* 1971;47:1-13.

59. U.S. Cancer Statistics Working Group. *United States Cancer Statistics: 1999–2009 Incidence and Mortality Web-based Report.* Atlanta, GA: U.S. Department of Health and Human Services, Centers for Disease Control and Prevention and National Cancer Institute; 2013.

60. Chin-Hong PV, Palefsky JM. External genital warts. In: Klausner JD, Hook III EW, eds. *Current Diagnosis & Treatment of Sexually Transmitted Diseases.* New York, NY: McGraw Hill; 2007.

61. Shykhon M, Kuo M, Pearman K. Recurrent respiratory papillomatosis. *Clin Otolaryngol Allied Sci.* 2002;27:237-243.

62. Moore AY, Tyring SK. Cutanous warts. In: Sterling JC, Tyring SK, eds. *Human Papillomaviruses: Clinical and Scientific Advances.* London, United Kingdom: Arnold; 2001:52-59.

63. Gruβendorf-Conen EI. Papillomavirus-induces tumors of the skin: cutaneous warts and epidermodysplasia verruciform. In: Syrjänen KJ, Gissmann L, Koss LG, eds. *Papillomaviruses and Human Disease.* Heidelberg, Germany: Springer-Verlag; 1987:159-181.

64. Montgomery AH, Montgomery RM. Mosaic type of plantar wart: its characteristics and treatment. *Arch Derm Syphiol.* 1948;57:397-399.

65. Alisjahbana B, Dinata R, Sutedja E, et al. Disfiguring generalized verrucosis in an Indonesian man with idiopathic CD4 lymphopenia. *Arch Dermatol.* 2010; 146:69-73.

66. Cobb MW. Human papillomavirus infection. *J Am Acad Dermatol.* 1990;22: 547-566.

67. Jablonska S, Majewski S. Epidermodysplasia verruciformis: immunological and clinical aspects. In: zur Hausen H, ed. *Human Pathogenic Papillomaviruses.* Heidelberg, Germany: Springer-Verlag; 1994:157-175.

68. Majewski S, Jablonska S. Epidermodysplasia verruciformis. In: Sterling JC, Tyring SK, eds. *Human Papillomaviruses: Clinical and Scientific Advances.* London, United Kingdom: Arnold; 2001:90-101.

69. Xu W, Liu C, Yan L, et al. Distribution of enteroviruses in hospitalized children with hand, foot and mouth disease and relationship between pathogens and nervous system complications. *Virol J.* 2012;9:8.

70. Ghosh SK, Bandyopadhyay D, Ghosh A, et al. Mucocutaneous features of hand, foot and mouth disease: a reappraisal from an outbreak in the city of Kolkata. *Indian J Dermatol Venereol Leprol.* 2010;76:564-566.

71. Yang F, Zhang T, Hu Y, et al. Survey of enterovirus infections from hand, foot and mouth disease outbreak in China, 2009. *Virol J.* 2011;8:508.

72. Fujimoto T, Iizuka S, Enomoto M, et al. Hand, foot and mouth disease caused by coxsackievirus A6, Japan, 2011. *Emerg Infect Dis.* 2012;18:337-339.

73. Aizaki K, Tsuru T, Okumura K, et al. Three pediatric cases of group A coxsackievirus-associated encephalitis/encephalopathy. *No To Hattatsu.* 2012; 44:397-400.

74. Conner KB, Tyring SK. Enteroviruses. In: Tyring SK, Yen Moore A, Lupi O, eds. *Mucocutaneous Manifestations of Viral Diseases.* 2nd ed. London, United Kingdom: Informa Healthcare; 2010:407-418.

75. Lynch DP. Oral manifestations of viral diseases. In: Tyring SK, ed. *Mucosal Immunology and Virology.* London, United Kingdom: Springer-Verlag; 2006: 99-156.

76. Oberste MS, Pallansch MA. Enterovirus molecular detection and typing. *Red Med Microbiol.* 2005;16:163-171.

77. Molino AC, Fleischer AB, Feldman SR. Patient demographics and utilization of healthcare services for molluscum contagiosum. *Pediatr Dermatol.* 2004;21:628-632.

78. Becker TM, Blount JH, Douglas J, et al. Trends in molluscum contagiosum in the United States, 1966-1973. *Sex Transm Dis.* 1986;13:88-92.

79. Braue A, Ross G, Varigos G, et al. Epidemiology and impact of childhood molluscum contagiosum: a case series and critical review of the literature. *Pediatr Dermatol.* 2005;22:287-294.

80. Reynolds MG, Holman RC, Yorita Christensen KL, et al. The incidence of molluscum contagiosum among American Indians and Alaskan Natives. *PLoS One.* 2009;4:e5255.

81. Pierard-Franchimont C, Legrain A, Pierard GE. Growth and regression of molluscum contagiosum. *J Am Acad Dermatol.* 1983;9:669-672.

82. Shelley WB, Burmeister V. Demonstration of a unique viral structure: the molluscum viral colony sac. *Br J Dermatol.* 1986;115:557-562.

83. Rogers M, Barnetson RSC. Diseases of the skin. In: McIntosh N, Helms P, Smyth R, et al, eds. *Forfar and Arneil's Textbook of Pediatrics.* 5th ed. New York, NY: Churchill Livingstone; 2008.

84. Van der Wouden JC, van der Sande R, van Suijlekom-Smit LWA, et al. Interventions for cutaneous molluscum contagiosum. *Cochrane Database Syst Rev.* 2009;4:CD004767.

85. Whitaker SB. Intraoral molluscum contagiosum. *Oral Surg Oral Med Oral Pathol.* 1991;72:334-336.

86. Rao VA, Baskaran RK, Krishnan MM. Unusual cases of molluscum contagiosum of eye. *Indian J Opthalmol.* 1985;33:263-265.

87. Silverberg NB, Sidbury R, Mancini AJ. Childhood molluscum contagiosum: experience with cantharidin therapy in 300 patients. *J Am Acad Dermatol.* 2000;43:503-507.

88. Takemura T, Ohkuma K, Nagai H, et al. The natural history of molluscum contagiosum. *Ex Treat Dermatol Dis.* 1983;5:667-670.

89. Liota E, Smith KJ, Buckley R, et al. Imiquimod therapy for molluscum contagiosum. *J Cutan Med Surg.* 2000;4:76.

90. Meadows KP, Tyring SK, Pavia AT, et al. Resolution of recalcitrant molluscum contagiosum virus lesions in human immunodeficiency virus-infected patients treated with cidofovir. *Arch Dermatol.* 1997;133:987-990.

CHAPTER	**Bacterial Infections**
62	Lauren S. Meshkov Rajiv I. Nijhawan Jeffrey M. Weinberg

KEY POINTS

- Individuals with skin of color may develop a wide range of cutaneous infections involving either Gram-positive or Gram-negative organisms.

- In most cases, these infections do not differ significantly from those that occur in the general population.

- *Staphylococcus aureus* and *Streptococcus pyogenes* are the two major Gram-positive organisms that are most often implicated in common skin and soft tissue infections.

- Gram-negative infections of the skin occur more commonly in children, patients with diabetes, and immunocompromised patients.

- Although empirical antibiotic treatment is an important first step in treating bacterial infections, once the diagnosis is established, treatment should then be dictated by the antibiotic sensitivities of the cultured organism.

BACTERIAL BIOFILMS AND THE SKIN

The human body plays host to a diverse world of bacteria, both as single-celled planktonic organisms and in sessile groups. Microbial flora of the skin largely exists within biofilms, sessile bacterial communities encased in an extracellular matrix, with the ability to communicate and regulate its own growth and metabolism.[1] Biofilms exist in both healthy and pathologic skin and may be protective or destructive, influencing host inflammatory cells and host metabolism and conferring antibiotic resistance. Therapeutic approaches to dermatologic disease have shifted recently, as biofilms may require more than traditional culture-based treatment.[2]

Biofilm studies are revealing new information about the skin's bacterial environment. These studies help explain why noninfectious diseases like acne vulgaris, miliaria, and atopic dermatitis respond to antibiotics and why certain lesions have anatomic predilections.[2] More alarming however, are in vitro studies of biofilms that are 50 to 500 times more resistant to antibiotics than their planktonic counterparts.[3,4] This is due to several mechanisms: a physical barrier that prevents antibiotic diffusion,[5] slowed growth and metabolism of centrally located organisms that escape peripheral antibiotic activity, regulatory genes that change bacterial phenotype in response to environmental stress, spore-like forms that shut down antibiotic targets,[6] and frequent gene transfer through genomic islands of horizontally acquired DNA segments.[7] The complex interaction between biofilms and antibiotic therapy demands attention from the dermatologist, as inappropriate usage with sub-minimum inhibitory concentrations may enhance biofilm formation and confer further resistance.[8,9]

ANTIBIOTIC RESISTANCE

The widespread use of antibiotics for bacterial skin infections contributes to the emergence of resistant organisms and poses a serious threat to public health. Dermatologists wrote approximately 9.5 million prescriptions for oral antibiotics in 2009 alone,[10] and antibiotic resistance is growing among normal skin flora. The first penicillin-resistant *Staphylococcus aureus* was discovered in 1941, shortly after the drug's introduction. Up to 78% of all staphylococcal skin infections are now due to methicillin-resistant *S. aureus* (MRSA).[11] MRSA continues to display resistance to a range of drugs, including mupirocin, erythromycin, clindamycin, tetracycline, sulfonamides, chloramphenicol, cephalosporins, and quinolones.[12]

Propionibacterium acnes, the bacteria involved in acne formation, is just one organism that has shown resistance to oral tetracyclines and topical clindamycin,[13] the most common systemic and topical medications prescribed by dermatologists in 2009.[10] As a result, the recommended treatment now includes topical clindamycin with a benzoyl peroxide agent, retinoids, or clindamycin in a combination product rather than as monotherapy.[14,15] Systemic antibiotics for acne should be limited to the shortest duration possible in order to reduce antibiotic resistance.[16]

Antibiotic resistance is not only the result of overuse, but is also caused by infection prophylaxis with topical antibiotics. Seventy-two percent of dermatologists encourage topical antibiotic use after dermatologic procedures, despite the low incidence of postoperative infections[17] and despite allergic contact dermatitis to bacitracin and neomycin.[18] MRSA resistance to mupirocin has grown from 1.6% between 1995 and 1999 to 7% between 2000 and 2004.[19] This is problematic because mupirocin is the cornerstone of treatment for MRSA impetigo infections and nasal carriage.[11]

Clinicians should be aware of local resistance patterns and choose antibiotics based on the target organism, patient profile, and necessity of treatment. Extended courses of antibiotics are not recommended, although in the case of true infections, strict adherence to dosage and duration is imperative.

GRAM-POSITIVE INFECTIONS [TABLE 62-1]

S. aureus and *Streptococcus pyogenes* are the two major Gram-positive organisms most often implicated in common skin and soft tissue infections. Infections usually begin and remain contained at the site of a minor wound or skin abrasion, but once the skin is penetrated, the risk increases for systemic conditions such as sepsis, local necrosis, and endocarditis.

TABLE 62-1 Common Gram-positive bacterial infections

Erythrasma
Impetigo, ecthyma
Infectious folliculitis
Abscess, furuncle, carbuncle
Paronychia
Cellulitis, erysipelas
Blistering distal dactylitis
Cutaneous anthrax
Staphylococcal scalded skin syndrome
Toxic shock syndrome
Scarlet fever

The following infections are typically diagnosed clinically and treated empirically. Gram-positive organisms are treated with an antibiotic, such as a penicillinase-resistant penicillin, a cephalosporin, a macrolide, or a flouroquinolone.[20] Although empiric antibiotic therapy is often important, treatment should be tailored to culture results and antibiotic sensitivities of the offending organisms.

CUTANEOUS MRSA INFECTION

The cost of treating a MRSA infection exceeds that of a methicillin-sensitive *S. aureus* (MSSA) infection by almost $19,000.[21] As the incidence of MRSA increases worldwide, dermatologists must distinguish between community-acquired MRSA (CA-MRSA) and hospital-acquired MRSA (HA-MRSA) strains to best determine treatment.

CA-MRSA most often affects individuals with close infected contacts and those who are exposed to crowded conditions, such as members of athletic teams, prisoners, and military personnel. In identifying those with CA-MRSA, a social history may prove important and should include the following information: intravenous drug use, tobacco use, a recent tattoo, men who have sex with other men, pregnant women, children, newborns, and those with low socioeconomic status. Medical risk factors include recent antibiotic use, chronic skin disease, human immunodeficiency virus, nasal colonization, and history of endocarditis.[22] CA-MRSA carries the *SCCmec* type IV or V gene, which leads to increased interleukin-8, skin necrosis, and leukocytoclasis, but not multidrug resistance. HA-MRSA carries the *mecA* gene, which encodes penicillin-binding protein 2a, protects cell wall synthesis, and induces multidrug resistance.[23] HA-MRSA develops in susceptible patients who are hospitalized for over 48 hours. Transmission occurs through skin-to-skin contact, disruption of the skin barrier, or contaminated equipment.[22]

Clinical Description Cutaneous MRSA infections often begin as papules and pustules on the lower extremities that may progress to abscesses with or without necrotic centers. Of those with MRSA skin infections, 58.8% have abscesses, 38.5% have cellulitis, 9.1% have folliculitis/furunculosis, and 2.3% have impetigo.[23] Rare MRSA presentations include acute paronychia, ulcers, necrotizing fasciitis, pyomyositis, bullous erysipelas, staphylococcal scalded skin syndrome, staphylococcal toxic shock syndrome, and purpura fulminans.[23,24]

Treatment Bacterial culture is required to diagnose cutaneous MRSA and to determine appropriate treatment. MRSA colonization is established via a swab and culture of the anterior nasal vestibule. Incision and drainage are required for MRSA abscesses. If an MRSA-confirmed patient suffers systemic symptoms, the Infectious Diseases Society of America recommends blood culture and antibiotic susceptibility testing.[25] Severe MRSA infections warrant an infectious disease consultation and parenteral antibiotics for at least 7 to 10 days.[11] CA-MRSA may be treated with trimethoprim-sulfamethoxazole, doxycycline or minocycline, clindamycin, or rifampin. HA-MRSA may be treated with vancomycin, quinupristin/dalfopristin, or tigecycline. β-Lactam antibiotics cannot be used in either CA-MRSA or HA-MRSA, although it is acceptable to treat a presumed MSSA infection with β-lactam drugs if the patient lacks risk factors for MRSA and there is low MRSA incidence in the geographic region.[22] A thorough epidemiologic history will help distinguish between CA-MRSA and HA-MRSA.

NASAL CARRIAGE AND COLONIZATION OF *S. AUREUS*

The nasal mucosa is a natural habitat for *S. aureus*. Colonization is usually transient, but in those with diabetes, chronic eczema, or atopic diathesis, there is a higher risk of skin disease and wound infection.[11] Between 70% and 90% of atopic patients have *S. aureus* colonization due to an impaired epidermal barrier function and better bacterial adhesion in sites of T-helper 2 cell-mediated inflammation.[26] Reduced antimicrobial sphingosine lipids[27] and less dermcidin in the sweat[28] also contribute to colonization.

Treatment Colonized atopic patients may be treated with antiseptics, disinfectant baths, silver-threaded clothing or silver-containing therapies, anti-inflammatory topicals such as tacrolimus or pimecrolimus, or corticosteroids preventatively for previously infected areas.[29] Nasal eradication of laboratory-confirmed MRSA may be accomplished with mupirocin and chlorhexidine soap, but intranasal mupirocin prophylaxis and regular decolonization are not recommended due to increased antibiotic resistance.[11] Frequent hand washing will help prevent spread.

ERYTHRASMA

Erythrasma is a chronic bacterial infection caused by *Corynebacterium minutissimum* that affects the intertriginous areas of the axillae, groin, and toes. Because of these typical locations, it can often mimic a fungal infection.

Clinical Description The skin lesions [**Figure 62-1**] are typically sharply marginated, reddish-brown macules, sometimes with hyperkeratotic white maceration, erosion, or fissures, especially in the webbing of the toes. The condition may be pruritic with resultant secondary excoriation and lichenification.

Treatment As prophylactic measures, looser fitting clothing and the use of an absorbing powder such as Zeasorb AF powder may be useful.[20] The treatment of choice includes a 14-day course of erythromycin 250 mg every other day. Second-line treatments include tetracycline and chloramphenicol. Clarithromycin may also prove to be effective. In interdigital areas, or if erythromycin treatment fails, a combination of topical clindamycin, Whitefield's ointment, sodium fusidate ointment, or antibacterial soaps may be necessary for both treatment and prophylaxis. Whitefield's ointment has shown to have greater efficacy than erythromycin for interdigital areas.[30]

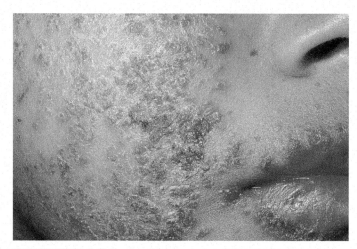

FIGURE 62-2. Nonbullous impetigo.

IMPETIGO/ECTHYMA

Impetigo may be bullous or nonbullous in nature, with *S. aureus* being the primary causative agent for bullous impetigo. In industrialized countries, nonbullous impetigo is also primarily caused by staphylococci, whereas in developing nations, nonbullous impetigo can also be caused by *S. pyogenes*, a group A β-hemolytic *Streptococcus*, or both organisms. When both bacteria are found, it is thought to be due to primary infection with *Streptococcus* and secondary infection with *Staphylococcus*. The bacteria initially infect the superficial layer of the epidermis. Although some lesions will resolve spontaneously, others will extend into the dermis, thus causing ecthyma.

Clinical Description Nonbullous impetigo, which accounts for more than 70% of impetigo cases, presents with small superficial pustules that quickly rupture and evolve into a crusted plaque, often of a honey color that appears "stuck on" [**Figure 62-2**]. Surrounding erythema may be present. Patients lack constitutional symptoms. The most common location for these lesions is the face, but any area may be involved. The lesions are often scattered and discrete, but without treatment will likely coalesce. Autoinoculation may lead to infection at distant sites. Nonbullous impetigo characteristically heals without scarring.

Bullous impetigo is characterized by vesicles containing cloudy-to-yellow fluid arising from skin of normal color, without surrounding erythema [**Figure 62-3**]. Bullous impetigo occurs when staphylococci produce toxins (namely, exfoliative toxins A and B), which causes

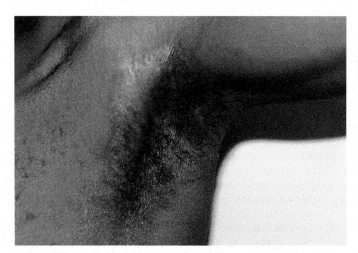

FIGURE 62-1. Skin lesions of erythrasma typically appear in intertriginous areas such as the axillae.

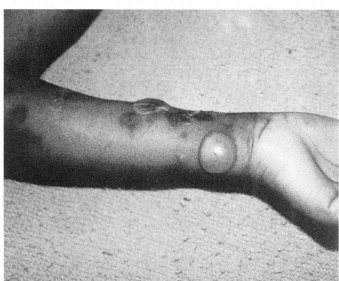

FIGURE 62-3. Bullous impetigo.

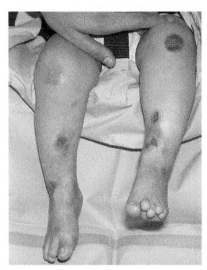

FIGURE 62-4. Ecthyma.

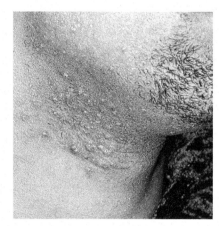

FIGURE 62-5. Infectious folliculitis.

splitting of the epidermis. Both types of impetigo are most common in, but not limited to, intertriginous areas.

Ecthyma, a deeper form of streptococcal impetigo, presents with punched out ulcerations of the epidermis with a surrounding thick adherent crust [**Figure 62-4**]. Surrounding areas of erythema may occur. Lymphangitis or lymphadenopathy may be associated with ecthyma. Unlike nonbullous impetigo, ecthymas are more commonly found on the extremities and may heal with scarring.

Treatment Pathogen identification in superficial impetigo is unnecessary, because 70% of impetigo infections are caused by *S. aureus*.[31] Topical treatment includes mupirocin applied three times daily to the involved skin and nares, as approximately 25% of people are carriers of *S. aureus*. Although treatment helps reduce autoinoculation and communicable spread, treatment also contributes to the growing resistance of *S. aureus* against mupirocin.[32] Because mupirocin is a cornerstone of MRSA treatment, many authors recommend it be reserved for MRSA carriers with recurrent infections only.[11,23] Although a 1- or 2-week course of mupirocin may not be enough time for the emergence of resistant strains, prolonged treatment with mupirocin is not advised for chronic conditions.[33]

Retapamulin 1% ointment applied twice daily for 5 days is an effective alternative to mupirocin, offering broader coverage of *S. pyogenes* and MSSA.[23] Retapamulin shows no evidence of bacterial resistance due to a three-fold mechanism that interferes with the 50s subunit of the bacterial ribosome, blocks p-site interactions, and inhibits peptidyl transfer.[34] A recent study showed that retapamulin inhibited 99% of *S. aureus* isolates in vitro with 4, 16, and 32 times more activity against MSSA, MRSA, and *Streptococcus*, respectively,[31] but there are limited studies on its use in impetigo. Sodium hypochlorite bleach baths and fusidic acid are alternatives.[32]

To eliminate staphylococcal carriage in impetigo patients, rifampin and dicloxacillin are often used, as well as the topical antiseptics polyhexanide, polyvidone, octenidine, and chlorhexidine. For severe infections or impetigo caused by β-hemolytic group A *Streptococcus*, first-line treatment has shifted toward oral cephalexin, dicloxacillin, and amoxicillin/clavulanic acid due to erythromycin and penicillin resistance.[11] Penicillin-allergic patients may take erythromycin. CA-MRSA in impetigo is increasingly common in the pediatric population, and treatment includes clindamycin, trimethoprim-sulfamethoxazole, tetracycline, and flouroquinolones.[12]

INFECTIOUS FOLLICULITIS

Infectious folliculitis affects the upper portion of the hair follicle. When the infection extends to the entire length of the follicle, it is called sycosis. The etiology may include bacterial, fungal, or viral infections.

Bacteria include *S. aureus* (seen in both superficial and deep folliculitis), *Pseudomonas aeruginosa* (associated with hot tub folliculitis), and Gram-negative folliculitis (associated with acne vulgaris and those who have been treated with oral antibiotics).[35]

Clinical Description Skin lesions typically show a papule or pustule that is confined to the hair follicle but may exhibit surrounding erythema [**Figure 62-5**]. Pustules may rupture, leading to erosions with crusts that can be scattered or more frequently clustered. The superficial infection can progress to an abscess, especially when the causative agent is *S. aureus*.

Although the superficial infection typically heals without scarring, in darkly pigmented people, there can be considerable postinflammatory hypo- and/or hyperpigmentation. Also of note in more darkly pigmented skin is pseudofolliculitis barbae (PFB). PFB is an inflammatory disorder characterized by the formation of papules, pustules, and hyperpigmentation from ingrown hairs often complicated by an *S. aureus* superinfection. Men with skin of color are especially prone to PFB due to the curly nature of their hair, which is more prone to becoming ingrown and sometimes infected. It is estimated that PFB affects 45% to 83% of men with darker skin of color who shave regularly. In a recent published study, it was found that twice-daily applications of benzoyl peroxide 5%/clindamycin 1% gel showed reductions in papule and pustule counts ranging from 38.2% at week 2 to 63.9% at week 10.[36] Another type of folliculitis that affects skin of color is keloidal folliculitis. This condition occurs at the nape of the neck with chronically occurring papules and pustules that often lead to extensive hypertrophic scarring and keloid formation. Resulting hair loss may occur in the area. Keloidal folliculitis may also become complicated by bacterial superinfection.

Treatment Affected areas should be cleansed with antibacterial soap or a benzoyl peroxide preparation. Antiseptic or antimicrobial therapy is indicated for widespread folliculitis or immune deregulation. Treatment may include the antiseptics polyhexinide, polyvidone, octenidine, and chlorhexidine, or the oral antibiotics ampicillin or trimethoprim-sulfamthoxazole.[11] Gram-negative folliculitis in acne and rosacea patients is best treated with isotretinoin (0.5 to 1 mg/kg daily for 4 to 5 months).[20] For treatment of pseudomonal folliculitis, please see the section on Gram-negative infections.

ABSCESS, FURUNCLE, AND CARBUNCLE

Abscesses, furuncles, and carbuncles represent a progression in severity of a process usually caused by a *Staphylococcus* infection.[20] An abscess is a well-circumscribed collection of pus associated with tissue destruction and localized inflammation. A furuncle is acute and deeper than an abscess, is tender and erythematous, and develops around a hair follicle. A carbuncle is a deeper and more extensive lesion and is made up of a confluence of abscesses. The most common cause is *S. aureus*, and these infections occur mostly in individuals who are nasal carriers of this organism.

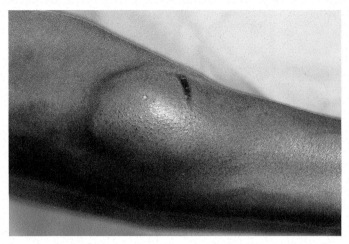

FIGURE 62-6. Abscess.

Clinical Description Cutaneous abscesses present initially as warm, tender, red nodules [**Figure 62-6**] that can occur anywhere on the skin, but typically occur in areas of trauma, burns, or IV catheter insertion. Abscesses will typically enlarge without treatment and form a pus-filled cavity. Furuncles are firmer, tender nodules, larger than abscesses, that occur on hair-bearing skin, such as the beard, neck, scalp, axillae, and buttocks [**Figure 62-7**]. Furuncles may be very painful, develop a surrounding area of cellulitis, and have associated constitutional symptoms. After several days, the nodules will rupture and expel pus and necrotic tissue. Multiple coalescing furuncles comprise a carbuncle, which is typically found on the nape of the neck, back, or thighs. Constitutional symptoms are often present. The involved area is erythematous and indurated and develops a yellow central crater. Carbuncles often resolve with a permanent scar that is very apparent.

Treatment It is advisable for patients susceptible to staphylococcal infections to cleanse daily with an antibacterial soap or a benzoyl peroxide wash. Additionally, mupirocin ointment applied daily to the nares or other known carrier sites is recommended. Application of heat to the lesion can promote consolidation and may even aid in spontaneous drainage if done early in the course of the disease. However, patients must be instructed not to manipulate lesions, particularly on the face, to avoid sinus vein thrombosis.[11] Usually, incision and drainage provide adequate treatment, particularly in otherwise healthy individuals. However, oral antibiotics can hasten resolution and are an absolute requirement for immunosuppressed individuals. Effective oral antibiotics include dicloxacillin, cephalexin, and erythromycin, with clindamycin recommended for penicillin-allergic patients.[11] Intravenous vancomycin is recommended for the most severe cases.

PARONYCHIA

Whereas the chronic form of paronychia is caused by the yeast *Candida albicans*, the acute form is typically caused by *S. aureus* and is seen in people with hand trauma or those chronically exposed to hand washing or moisture.

Clinical Description In acute paronychia, the proximal and/or lateral nail fold is erythematous, hot, and tender and, if not treated, may evolve into an abscess.

Treatment Treatment includes incision and drainage of an abscess, topical disinfectants, and oral or topical antibiotics.[37] Cephalexin or clindamycin is recommended.[11]

PITTED KERATOLYSIS

Pitted keratolysis, caused by *Micrococcus sedentarius*, is a condition that affects only the feet, specifically the toe web spaces and the soles, with lesions being most notable on areas of pressure such as the ball or heel of the foot.[38] Predisposing factors include occlusive footwear and hyperhidrosis.

Clinical Description Cutaneous findings show pitting of varying depth within the thickly keratinized skin of one or both soles. The pits range from 1 to 8 mm in diameter and can become confluent.

Treatment Decreasing or minimizing moisture through the selection of less occlusive footwear and the use of an absorbent powder is often a successful treatment modality. Additional treatment may include washing affected areas with a benzoyl peroxide preparation and the daily application of either a topical benzoyl peroxide or an erythromycin gel.

CELLULITIS AND ERYSIPELAS

Cellulitis Cellulitis, although a general term for several types of infections, is, in general, an acute, edematous suppurative inflammation of the dermis and subcutaneous tissues.[39] *S. aureus* and group A *Streptococcus* (GAS) are most commonly identified, but other bacteria may include group B *Streptococcus* in the newborn, pneumococcus, and Gram-negative bacilli. It is often associated with systemic symptoms such as fever, malaise, and chills.

Clinical Description Lesions are macular and firm, poorly demarcated from uninvolved skin, and painful upon palpation [**Figure 62-8**]. Necrosis of the overlying epidermis may occur with resulting epidermal sloughing. In some cases, the infection may lead to both dermal and subcutaneous

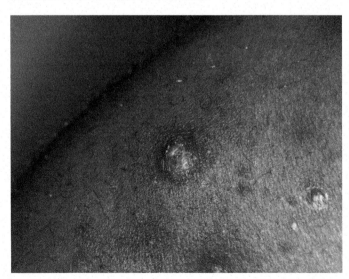

FIGURE 62-7. Furuncle.

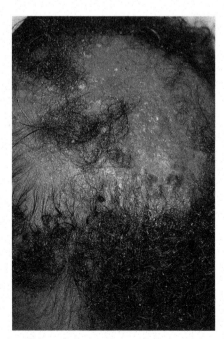

FIGURE 62-8. Cellulitis.

abscess formation and necrotizing fasciitis. Cellulitis is typically found on the extremities and is usually associated with lymphangitis.

Erysipelas Erysipelas is an acute infection of the dermal and subcutaneous tissues that is typically red, hot, and tender. It is most frequently caused by GAS and rarely by *S. aureus*. *Streptococcus* infection is associated with a high morbidity rate. Risk factors for erysipelas include venous insufficiency, toe web intertrigo, lymphedema, and obesity.[40]

Clinical Description Erysipelas differs from cellulitis in that it is a painful, raised, indurated plaque with borders that are markedly distinguishable from the surrounding noninvolved skin. In severe cases, bullous, pustular, or necrotic areas may develop. Patients typically report a prodrome of headache, malaise, and fever. The legs have become the most common areas of infection, with fewer cases affecting the face.[41]

Gangrenous Cellulitis A more severe form of cellulitis is gangrenous cellulitis, or necrotizing fasciitis. In general, gangrenous cellulitis is characterized by the rapid progression of infection with necrosis of both subcutaneous tissue and the overlying skin. The clinical picture, as well as the name of the disease, differs depending on the bacterial organism involved, as well as comorbid conditions and anatomic location of the infection. In general, there is local erythema, heat, and pain in the involved area. Constitutional symptoms are typically present and increase over time. Often there are visible gangrenous changes characterized by a dusky blue hue of the affected area. Vesicles may develop with subsequent rupture of bullae, which is commonly associated with numbness and a black necrotic eschar formation, similar in appearance to a third-degree burn. In some cases, the appearance of the skin may not adequately reflect subcutaneous destruction of small blood vessels and nerve destruction that can produce an anesthetic area.

Treatment is closely aligned with the diagnosis and severity of disease and ranges from incision and drainage to the antibiotics clindamycin and linezolid,[11] and/or surgical debridement of necrotic tissue to life-saving amputations. Of particular concern is necrotizing fasciitis, typically occurring on the leg of an elderly adult with an underlying chronic illness and generally caused by group A β-hemolytic *Streptococcus*. This infection is associated with a high fatality rate and may present with symptoms similar to toxic shock syndrome (discussed later).

Treatment Treatment of cellulitis may be divided into local care, including elevation, immobilization, and the application of cool saline dressings, to systemic antimicrobial therapy that addresses the most frequent isolates, streptococci (groups A, G, and B) and *S. aureus*.[41]

Comorbidities such as diabetes or immunosuppression should also be considered in treatment decisions. The gold standard used to determine the involved organism is a culture obtained from the portal of entry. Often the responsible organism remains elusive and is identified in only about 5% of cases through positive cultures.[41] Empiric treatment for mild cellulitis or erysipelas consists of oral dicloxacillin, which covers both staphylococci and streptococci. Empiric antimicrobial treatment for moderate or severe cellulitis consists of an intravenous cephalosporin (cefazolin or ceftriaxone) or nafcillin (vancomycin in patients with an allergy to penicillin), followed by dicloxacillin or an oral cephalosporin for 7 to 14 days. In patients with recurrent leg cellulitis, identification of interdigital fissures caused by dermatophytes and treatment with topical antifungal agents will likely prevent further recurrences. Daily prophylaxis with oral penicillin G (or amoxicillin) has been suggested for patients who have had more than two episodes of cellulitis at the same site.[41]

BLISTERING DISTAL DACTYLITIS

Blistering distal dactylitis is most often due to GAS, but group B *Streptococcus* may also be a causative agent. Cases of staphylococcal dactylitis have also been reported with an identical clinical picture. Blisters typically occur in children and adolescents.

Clinical Description Blistering distal dactylitis is characterized by a large, purulent, fluid-filled blister on the distal finger or toe pad that often extends distally to the nails. There is often a surrounding erythematous base.

Treatment Blistering distal dactylitis readily responds to incision and drainage, compresses, and oral antibiotics such as penicillin or erythromycin.[42]

CUTANEOUS ANTHRAX

Humans acquire anthrax infections from contact with infected animals or contaminated animal products, such as hides, wool, hair, and ivory tusks. More than 95% of naturally occurring anthrax is the cutaneous form.[43] Cutaneous anthrax is caused by *Bacillus anthracis*.

Clinical Description The primary lesion of anthrax is a painless, pruritic papule occurring at the site of inoculation that appears 1 to 7 days after exposure. One to 2 days after the appearance of the primary lesion, small vesicles surround the papule, or alternatively, a clear or serosanguineous fluid-containing vesicle develops. As the vesicle enlarges, satellite vesicles may develop. A nonpitting, gelatinous edema surrounds the lesion and may become massive, particularly when the primary lesion involves the neck or face. Low-grade fever and malaise are frequent. Necrosis of the vesicle results in the formation of an ulcer covered by a black eschar. The eschar resolves with minimal scarring. Regional lymphadenopathy is present initially. Secondary infection with streptococci or *S. aureus* is uncommon, but fever with lymphangitis, local pain, and purulent drainage is indicative of secondary infection. Bacteremia is a rare complication.[43]

Treatment Without antibiotic treatment, mortality may approach 20%. Incision or debridement of an early-stage lesion should be avoided because it may increase the possibility of bacteremia. For mild cases of cutaneous anthrax in adults, oral treatment with ciprofloxacin 500 mg every 12 hours is recommended. If the strain is susceptible, oral doxycycline at 100 mg every 12 hours or amoxicillin 500 mg every 8 hours is a suitable alternative. Treatment should be continued for 7 to 10 days, unless bioterrorism is suspected, which would necessitate treatment for 60 days. Severe cutaneous anthrax is treated with the same drugs and dosages as inhalation anthrax. The recommended initial therapy for adults with clinically evident inhalation anthrax is 400 mg of ciprofloxacin given intravenously every 12 hours.[43]

STAPHYLOCOCCAL SCALDED SKIN SYNDROME

Staphylococcal scalded skin syndrome (SSSS) is an epidermolytic disease that is caused by two distinct toxins released by a strain of *S. aureus* of phage group II, primarily type 71. The toxins cause erythema with associated detachment of the superficial layers of the epidermis. SSSS occurs in newborns and infants younger than 2 years of age and in immunocompromised adults. There are several different forms of SSSS that range in severity. At one end of the spectrum is the completely localized form, called *bullous impetigo*, and at the other end are more generalized and extensive forms.[44]

Clinical Description The localized form of SSSS is characterized by clusters of intact purulent bullae that rupture and produce erythematous and crusted erosive lesions. The most common sites are the intertriginous areas of the axillae, groin, and neck, as well as periorificial area on the face. The erythema typically deepens in color, and the skin becomes very tender. Lesions become more widespread with time, and there may be accompanying fever. The erythematous eruption can rapidly progress to flaccid bullae that exfoliate, producing a denuded epidermis and a resultant tender and oozing erythematous base.

Treatment Therapy includes baths and compresses for debridement and the use of nonstick dressings.[11] Topical antiseptics include chlorhexidine or polyhexanide solutions and topical antimicrobial agents such as mupirocin, bacitracin, fusidic acid, and sulfadiazine ointment. Successful systemic antimicrobial therapy includes oral cephalexin, clindamycin, or doxycycline for local disease and intravenous nafcillin or cefazolin for generalized disease.[11,13] In known carriers of MRSA, intravenous vancomycin or linezolid is recommended.[11] In severe disease, fluid and electrolyte loss must be replaced.

TOXIC SHOCK SYNDROME

Toxic shock syndrome (TSS) is an acute toxin-mediated febrile illness that is caused by the production and release of exotoxins by *S. aureus*. Systemic symptoms include acute onset of fever, hypotension, generalized skin and mucosal erythema, and multisystem failure. TSS occurs more commonly but not exclusively in women who are using vaginal tampons of high absorbency for extended lengths of time. Nonmenstrual cases, associated with localized infections, surgery, or insect bites, have increased and now account for approximately one-third of all cases. Patients with nonmenstrual TSS have a higher mortality rate than those with menstrual TSS.[45]

Clinical Description The classic cutaneous findings of TSS include a generalized scarlatiniform erythroderma with accompanying fever and hypotension. There is often extensive, generalized, nonpitting, nondependent edema and edema of the feet. One to 2 weeks following resolution of the erythema, there is desquamation of the palms and soles. Intense erythema of the bulbar conjunctivae, mouth, tongue, pharynx, vagina, and tympanic membranes may occur. Often these areas display ulceration. Strawberry tongue and subconjunctival hemorrhages are also typical. Nonspecific gastrointestinal symptoms may also be a manifestation of disease.

Treatment The treatment of TSS is generally supportive.[46] Admission to the intensive care unit for management of fluid replacement for shock, careful organ system monitoring, and intravenous antibiotic therapy for staphylococcal colonization or infection may occur. Commonly prescribed antibiotics include flucloxacillin or cefazolin in combination with clindamycin.[11] In severe cases, methylprednisolone has been given, but benefit is uncertain. In vitro studies have shown that immune globulins may have a future role in the treatment of TTS.

SCARLET FEVER

Scarlet fever is an acute infection of the tonsils and/or skin by an exotoxin-producing strain of GAS. It typically occurs in children.[47]

Clinical Description The initial site of infection is typically the tonsils or pharynx, with resultant pharyngitis or tonsillitis, although a skin lesion or infected wound may be the initiator. The first sign of scarlet fever is finely punctuate erythema on the upper trunk, which may be accentuated in skin folds. The palms and soles are typically spared. The face is flushed with perioral pallor. The initial punctuate lesions become confluent and scarlatiniform. Scattered petechiae and distant lesions may occur [**Figure 62-9**]. The exanthem fades within 4 to 5 days and is followed by truncal and extremity desquamation and exfoliation of the palms and soles. The tongue is characteristically white with scattered hyperkeratotic red papillae (white strawberry tongue). The hyperkeratotic membrane is sloughed and gives way to a strawberry tongue on day 4 or 5. Punctuate erythema and petechiae can also occur in the palate.

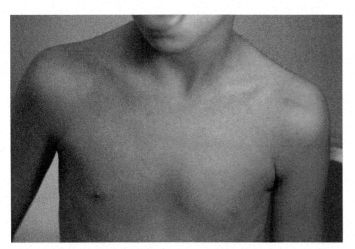

FIGURE 62-9. Scarlet fever exanthem.

The patient often appears acutely ill, and there is often appreciable anterior cervical lymphadenitis.

Treatment Treatment includes acetaminophen for fever or discomfort. Penicillin is the drug of choice because of its efficacy in preventing rheumatic fever. Clindamycin can also be used for treatment. Human immune globulin contains toxin-neutralizing antibodies and, if given at an early stage of invasive disease, may have a beneficial effect.[47]

GRAM-NEGATIVE INFECTIONS [TABLE 62-2]

Gram-negative infections of the skin are more common in three groups: children, patients with diabetes, and immunocompromised patients. These infections are typically treated with a second- or third-generation cephalosporin.[20]

CAT SCRATCH DISEASE

Cat scratch disease is usually caused by the Gram-negative bacillus *Bartonella henselae*.[48] It is a relatively benign, self-limited disease that typically occurs after being scratched by a cat, but can occur even after contact with a cat without a history of a scratch, bite, or lick.

Clinical Description Following a cat scratch, the area of inoculation develops a small, firm papule or pustule that may be tender. Lesions typically occur on exposed skin. Associated regional lymphadenitis and large tender lymph nodes occur. Alternatively, the site of inoculation of *B. henselae* may be a mucous membrane. In that case, a light yellow granulation on the palpebral conjunctivae, with associated preauricular or cervical lymphadenopathy, occurs. Most patients are afebrile.

Treatment The literature does not definitely report effective antibiotic therapy for cat scratch disease primarily due to that fact that it is a disease in which most patients are not seriously ill and spontaneous resolution is common.[49] The disease is typically self-limiting with a maximum duration of 2 months, although longer disease duration has been reported. Antimicrobial therapy has not been proven to alter the course of the disease. However, ciprofloxacin, doxycycline, and erythromycin are therapeutic suggestions.[50] A small, prospective, comparative study demonstrated that azithromycin may shorten the duration of lymphadenopathy.[51] In a minority of patients (about 15%) with typical cat scratch disease, the affected lymph node undergoes suppuration and becomes exquisitely tender. Drainage with a large-bore needle usually results in the almost immediate relief of pain. However, incision and drainage are seldom necessary and may result in the development of a chronic sinus tract.

TULAREMIA

Tularemia is cause by *Francisella tularensis*, a Gram-negative coccobacillus, which is transmitted through direct contact with the flesh of infected animals, typically rabbits and squirrels. Routes of transmission include a puncture or abrasion in the skin, autoinoculation, ingestion, or inhalation. Although accidental exposure can occur through arthropod bites, handling infected animals, or breathing in aerosols, cases are usually isolated and contained. It is important to note that transmission via inhalation is very serious in contrast to cutaneous transmission. The high infectivity of tularemia makes it a major concern to public health officials as a possible biological weapon.[52]

Clinical Description Tularemia has six potential presentations: ulceroglandular, glandular, oculoglandular, oropharyngeal, typhoidal, and pneumonic forms. The ulceroglandular form is the most common and the one that typically presents with skin lesions. If there is an identifiable

TABLE 62-2 Gram-negative infections
Cat scratch disease
Tularemia
Cutaneous *Pseudomonas aeruginosa* infections

inoculation site, it is typically an erythematous, tender papule that enlarges with raised, well-demarcated crusted borders surrounded by an area of cellulitis. There is a depressed center that is covered by a black eschar, evidence of rapid necrosis. Mucous membranes involved include the conjunctivae, and typically a purulent, painful, edematous conjunctivitis occurs, with small yellow nodules visible on the conjunctivae. A high fever, chills, headache, and malaise typically accompany the rash, and as bacteremia ensues, painful regional lymphadenopathy develops.

Treatment Management focuses on prevention with complete protective gear when handling wild rabbits. For treatment, streptomycin 1 to 2 g/d until the patient has been afebrile for 7 to 10 days is effective. Gentamicin, tetracycline, and quinolones are also effective.[53]

CUTANEOUS *PSEUDOMONAS AERUGINOSA* INFECTIONS

Pseudomonas aeruginosa produces a host of bacterial infections and is of concern because of its propensity for infecting hospitalized and compromised patients.[54] *Pseudomonas* rarely infects healthy people but instead infects hosts with disruption of the normal flora, with disruption of a normal cutaneous barrier by introduction of a foreign object, or following an injury or trauma. Once local invasion occurs, ecthyma gangrenosum, a necrotizing soft tissue infection, ensues and is associated with blood vessel invasion, sepsis, vascular occlusion, and infarction of tissue throughout the body.

Clinical Description *Pseudomonas* has the potential to colonize many areas on the body and, therefore, can present in a number of manners. *Pseudomonas* colonizes the undersurface of nails in patients with onychomycosis, the hair follicles of healthy individuals exposed to infected hot tubs, and in macerated intertriginous spaces. Outbreaks of *Pseudomonas* may occur in people using hot tubs and whirlpools. Follicular erythematous papules and pustules occur on submerged areas of skin and typically last from 7 to 10 days. *Pseudomonas* hot foot syndrome manifests with tender nodules on the soles of children's feet after using a wading pool.

Treatment Treatment for mild cutaneous cases is usually supportive, with antipruritic agents administered orally or topically. Acetic acid 5% compresses applied for 20 minutes twice daily can also be used for symptomatic relief, as well as sodium hypochlorite solution applied twice daily or topical tobramycin otic or ophthalmic drops under the nail plate.[55] Adequate chlorination and control of the pH level in hot tubs can prevent hot-tub folliculitis.[51] A course of oral ciprofloxacin 500 mg twice daily for 7 days may be warranted if systemic manifestations, including fever, chills, and lymphadenopathy, are present. In patients with immunodeficiencies, granulocytopenia must first be corrected with a colony-stimulating factor. Thereafter, sensitivity-appropriate antimicrobial therapy can be instituted. Antimicrobial therapy for bacteremia is also tailored according to the specific sensitivity of the encountered strain. Antibiotics are given as monotherapy or in combination, as *P. aeruginosa* infections have particularly high mortality rates and the strongest multidrug resistance among all bacteria.[55] Effective agents include aminoglycosides, ciprofloxacin, colistin, and a limited number of β-lactams such as piperacillin, ticarcillin, ureidopenicillins, ceftazidime, carbapenems, aztreonam, and cefepime, which retains the broadest spectrum of activity against *P. aeruginosa*.[55] To prevent further damage to skin and underlying organs, areas of infarction should be surgically debrided once the infection is controlled.[54] For burn victims, topical antimicrobials, such as silver compounds and mafenide acetate, may decrease invasive burn wound sepsis.[55]

In summary, individuals with skin of color may develop a wide range of cutaneous infections involving either Gram-positive or Gram-negative organisms. In general, most infections do not differ significantly from those that occur in the general population. As expected, *S. aureus* and *S. pyogenes* are Gram-positive organisms that are most often implicated in common skin and soft tissue infections. In contrast, Gram-negative infections occur more commonly in children, patients with diabetes, and immunocompromised patients. In most cases, treatment is dictated by the antibiotic sensitivities of the cultured organism.

REFERENCES

1. Donlan RM, Costerton JW. Biofilms: survival mechanisms of clinically relevant microorganisms. *Clin Microbiol Rev.* 2002;15:167-193.
2. Vlassova N, Han A, Zenilman JM, James G, Lazarus GS. New horizons for cutaneous microbiology: the role of biofilms in dermatological disease. *Br J Dermatol.* 2011;165:751-759.
3. Prosser BL, Taylor D, Dix BA, Cleeland R. Method of evaluating effects of antibiotics on bacterial biofilm. *Antimicrob Agents Chemother.* 1987;31:1502-1506.
4. Mah TF, O'Toole GA. Mechanisms of biofilm resistance to antimicrobial agents. *Trends Microbiol.* 2001;9:34-39.
5. Anderson GG, O'Toole GA. Innate and induced resistance mechanisms of bacterial biofilms. *Curr Top Microbiol Immunol.* 2008;322:85-105.
6. Lewis K. Persister cells and the riddle of biofilm survival. *Biochemistry (Mosc).* 2005;70:267-274.
7. Driffield K, Miller K, Bostock JM, et al. Increased mutability of *Pseudomonas aeruginosa* in biofilms. *J Antimicrob Chemother.* 2008;61:1053-1056.
8. Dunne WM. Effects of subinhibitory concentrations of vancomycin or cefamandole on biofilm production by coagulase-negative staphylococci. *Antimicrob Agents Chemother.* 1990;34:390-393.
9. Linares JF, Gustafsson I, Baquero F, Martinez JL. Antibiotics as intermicrobial signaling agents instead of weapons. *Proc Natl Acad Sci USA.* 2006; 103:19484-19489.
10. Leyden JJ, Del Rosso JQ, Webster GF. Clinical considerations in the treatment of acne vulgaris and other inflammatory disorders: Focus on antibiotic resistance. *Cutis.* 2007;79(6 Suppl):9-25.
11. Schofer H, Bruns R, Effendy I, et al. Diagnosis and treatment of *Staphylococcus aureus* infections of the skin and mucous membranes. *J Dtsch Dermatol Ges.* 2011;9:953-967.
12. Silverberg N, Block S. Uncomplicated skin and skin structure infections in children: diagnosis and current treatment options in the United States. *Clin Pediatr.* 2008;47:211-219.
13. Del Rosso JQ, Leyden JJ. Status report on antibiotic resistance: implications for the dermatologist. *Dermatol Clin.* 2007;25:127-132.
14. Rosen T. Antibiotic resistance: an editorial review with recommendations. *J Drugs Dermatol.* 2011;10:724-733.
15. Leyden JJ, Del Rosso JQ, Webster GF. Clinical considerations in the treatment of acne vulgaris and other inflammatory disorders: a status report. *Dermatol Clin.* 2009;27:1-15.
16. Toossi P, Farshehian M, Malekzad F, et al. Subantimicrobial-dose doxycycline in the treatment of facial acne. *J Drugs Dermatol.* 2008;7:1149-1152.
17. Neville JA, Housman TS, Letsinger JA, Fleischer AB Jr, Feldman SR, Williford PM. Increase in procedures performed at dermatology office visits from 1995 to 2001. *Dermatol Surg.* 2005;31:160-162.
18. Drucker CR. Update on topical antibiotics in dermatology. *Dermatol Ther.* 2012;25:6-11.
19. Simor AE, Stuart TL, Louie L, et al. Mupirocin-resistant, methicillin-resistant *Staphylococcus aureus* strains in Canadian hospitals. *Antimicrob Agents Chemother.* 2007;51:3880-3886.
20. Stulberg DL, Penrod MA, Blatny RA. Common bacterial skin infections. *Am Fam Physician.* 2002;66:119-124.
21. Filice G, Nyman J, Lexau C, et al. Excess costs and utilization associated with methicillin resistance for patients with *Staphylococcus aureus* infection. *Infect Control Hosp Epidemiol.* 2010;31:365-373.
22. Hansra NK, Shinkai K. Cutaneous community-acquired and hospital-acquired methicillin resistant *Staphylococcus aureus*. *Dermatol Ther.* 2011;24:263-272.
23. Kil E, Heymann W, Weinberg JM. Methicillin-resistant *Staphylococcus aureus*: an update for the dermatologist. Part 2: pathogenesis and cutaneous manifestations. *Cutis.* 2008;81:247-254.
24. Elston D. Community acquired methicillin resistant *Staphylococcus aureus*. *J Am Acad Dermatol.* 2007;56:1-16.
25. Stevens D, Bisno A, Chambers H, et al. Practice guidelines for the diagnosis and management of skin and soft tissue infections. *Clin Infect Dis.* 2005;41:1373-1406.
26. Cho SH, Strickland I, Tomkinson A, et al. Preferential binding of *Staphylococcus aureus* to skin sites of Th2-mediated inflammation in a murine model. *J Invest Dermatol.* 2001;116:658-663.
27. Arikawa J, Ishibashi M, Kawashima M, et al. Decreased levels of sphingosine, a natural antimicrobial agent, may be associated with vulnerability of the stratum corneum from patients with atopic dermatitis to colonization by Staphylococcus aureus. *J Invest Dermatol.* 2002;119:433-439.
28. Rieg S, Steffen H, Seeber S, et al. Deficiency of dermcidin derived antimicrobial peptides in sweat of patients with atopic dermatitis correlates with an impaired innate defense of human skin in vivo. *J Immunol.* 2005;174:8003-8010.

29. Hung SH, Lin YT, Chu CY, et al. *Staphylococcus* colonization in atopic dermatitis treated with fluticasone or tacrolimus with or without antibiotics. *Ann Allergy Asthma Immunol.* 2007;98:51-56.

30. Holdiness MR. Management of cutaneous erythrasma. *Drugs.* 2002;62:1131-1141.

31. Yang LP, Keam SJ. Retapamulin: a review of its use in the management of impetigo and other uncomplicated superficial skin infections. *Drugs.* 2008;68:855-873.

32. Bangert S, Levy M, Hebert AA. Bacterial resistance and impetigo treatment trends: a review. *Pediatr Dermatol.* 2012;29:243-248.

33. Axelsson I. Treatment of impetigo: save mupirocin. *BMJ.* 2004;329:979.

34. Yan K, Madden L, Choudhry AE, et al. Biochemical characterization of the interactions of the novel pleuromutilin derivative retapamulin with bacterial ribosomes. *Antimicrob Agents Chemother.* 2006;50:3875-3881.

35. Boni R, Nehrhoff B. Treatment of gram-negative folliculitis in patients with acne. *Am J Clin Dermatol.* 2003;4:273-276.

36. Cook-Bolden FE, Barba A, Halder R, et al. Twice-daily applications of benzoyl peroxide 5%/clindamycin 1% gel versus vehicle in the treatment of pseudofolliculitis barbae. *Cutis.* 2004;73(6 Suppl):18-24.

37. Scott PM. Drainage for an acute paronychia. *JAAPA.* 2002;15:57-58.

38. Takama H, Tamada Y, Yano K, et al. Pitted keratolysis: clinical manifestations in 53 cases. *Br J Dermatol.* 1997;137:282-285.

39. Hedrick J. Acute bacterial skin infections in pediatric medicine: current issues in presentation and treatment. *Paediatr Drugs.* 2003;5(Suppl 1):35-46.

40. Bonnetblanc JM, Bedane C. Erysipelas: recognition and management. *Am J Clin Dermatol.* 2003;4:157-163.

41. Swartz MN. Clinical practice. Cellulitis. *N Engl J Med.* 2004;350:904-912.

42. McCray MK, Esterly NB. Blistering distal dactylitis. *J Am Acad Dermatol.* 1981;5:592-594.

43. Carucci JA, McGovern TW, Norton SA, et al. Cutaneous anthrax management algorithm. *J Am Acad Dermatol.* 2002;47:766-769.

44. Schenfeld LA. Images in clinical medicine. Staphylococcal scalded skin syndrome. *N Engl J Med.* 2000;342:1178.

45. Manders SM. Infectious disease update. *Dermatol Clin.* 2001;19:749-756.

46. Manders SM. Toxin-mediated streptococcal and staphylococcal disease. *J Am Acad Dermatol.* 1998;39:383-398.

47. Bialecki C, Feder HM Jr, Grant-Kels JM. The six classic childhood exanthems: a review and update. *J Am Acad Dermatol.* 1989;21:891-903.

48. Lamps LW, Scott MA. Cat-scratch disease: historic, clinical, and pathologic perspectives. *Am J Clin Pathol.* 2004;121(Suppl):S71-S80.

49. Adal KA, Cockerell CJ, Petri WA Jr. Cat scratch disease, bacillary angiomatosis, and other infections due to *Rochalimaea. N Engl J Med.* 1994;330:1509-1515.

50. Margileth AM. Cat scratch disease. *Adv Pediatr Infect Dis.* 1993;8:1-21.

51. Bass JW, Freitas BC, Freitas AD, et al. Prospective randomized double blind placebo-controlled evaluation of azithromycin for treatment of cat-scratch disease. *Pediatr Infect Dis J.* 1998;17:447-452.

52. Gallagher-Smith M, Kim J, Al-Bawardy R, et al. Francisella tularensis: possible agent in bioterrorism. *Clin Lab Sci.* 2004;17:35-39.

53. Senol M, Ozcan A, Karincaoglu Y, et al. Tularemia: a case transmitted from a sheep. *Cutis.* 1999;63:49-51.

54. Werlinger KD, Moore AY. Therapy of other bacterial infections. *Dermatol Ther.* 2004;17:505-512.

55. Wu DC, Chan WW, Metelitsa AI, et al. *Pseudomonas* skin infection: clinical features, epidemiology, and management. *Am J Clin Dermatol.* 2011;12:157-169.

CHAPTER **63**

Fungal and Yeast Infections

Johnathan J. Ledet
Boni E. Elewski
Aditya K. Gupta

KEY POINTS

- Fungal infections affect people of all races.
- Susceptibility to fungal infection is influenced by a variety of factors including socioeconomic status, geographic location, and cultural or religious practices.
- Dermatophytes cause most superficial fungal infections.
- In the immunocompromised host, nondermatophyte molds and yeasts are also cutaneous pathogens.

INTRODUCTION

Fungi are ubiquitous worldwide, and cutaneous fungal infections are common among most races.[1] Keratinized tissues including stratum corneum, nails, and hair are an adaptive substrate for the superficial mycoses, such as dermatophytes, which are the primary causative agent of fungal infections. The immune system generally provides adequate defense against fungal invasion; consequently, nondermatophyte molds and yeasts are more common in those with primary or secondary immunodeficiency.

The presence of cutaneous mycoses does not appear to be a reflection of differences in the biologic characteristics of skin color. However, underlying immunologic diseases such as human immunodeficiency virus (HIV) infection and acquired immunodeficiency syndrome (AIDS) are of epidemic proportions in Africa, and studies in this region have identified higher incidences of associated fungal infections.[2] Climatic differences affect the ability of fungi to grow; high ambient temperature and humidity provide an ideal setting for fungal proliferation. Additional factors such as occlusive clothing and footwear worn in cooler settings may provide suitable microclimates for mycotic activity. Cultural or religious customs, such as communal bathing, may create opportunities for the transmission of fungi. Variation in hygienic practices also may explain increased susceptibility to fungal invasion.

This chapter provides an overview of superficial fungal infections that are common to most skin types, including individuals with skin of color. Tinea capitis and seborrheic dermatitis, which are covered in detail in Chapters 84 and 23, are fungal infections found more frequently in people with skin of color.

MYCOLOGIC EXAMINATION

Accurate diagnosis of a fungal infection is necessary before selecting an appropriate treatment regimen. Mycologic methods are similar for most mycoses, the goal being confirmation of the presence of fungi and identification of the pathogenic species. Light microscopy and fungal culture are used to determine whether fungal organisms are present in the specimen evaluated. Direct examination is performed using 10% to 20% potassium hydroxide (KOH) to dissolve the surrounding keratin. In addition, calcofluor white or periodic acid–Schiff (PAS) stain may be added to the KOH preparation to enhance visibility of the fungal organism.[3,4] The KOH test can indicate the presence or absence of a fungal element but does not give information as to the type of fungal element detected. Due to sampling error and nonproliferating fungi that may not be visible on microscopic examination, a negative microscopic result is not necessarily indicative of fungus-free tissue. A KOH result revealing septate hyphae in the setting of clinical suspicion of fungal infection may be sufficient to initiate treatment. Biopsy is generally not required. Because antifungal agents have different spectra of activity, organism identification is an integral part of disease management.[3,4] If the diagnosis cannot be made by light microscopy, samples must be obtained for culture. Dermatophyte test medium is a simple method of verification of dermatophyte presence or absence. Cultures containing cycloheximide and chloramphenicol are used to deter the growth of nonpathogenic molds and bacteria that may mask proliferation of the dermatophytes.[3] The use of both microscopy and culture as diagnostic tools reduces the rate of false-negative results and aids in accurate diagnosis.[3,4]

THERAPY

Topical antifungals are first-line therapy for dermatophyte infections in those with uncomplicated, localized infections because they are widely regarded as safe and effective. Irritant and contact dermatitis represent potential adverse reactions due to various vehicle components. The main drug classes of topical antifungal agents include imidazoles, triazoles, allylamines, benzylamines, and polyenes. Azoles inhibit 14-α-demethylase, preventing synthesis of ergosterol, which is required for fungal cell membrane integrity. Per U.S. Food and Drug Administration (FDA) guidelines, ketoconazole (oral tablets) should not be used as first-line treatment for any fungal infections, and it has been withdrawn from European national markets secondary to risk of severe liver injury and drug interactions.

Most azoles are fungistatic, but some can be fungicidal at high concentrations. Allylamines and benzylamine inhibit squalene epoxidase, which results in fungicidal levels of intracellular squalene. Polyene antifungal agents, along with ciclopirox olamine, bind to the fungi cell membrane and increase permeability; they can be both fungistatic and fungicidal. Other topical agents used for therapy include flucytosine, selenium sulfide, undecylenic acid, and iodoquinol.

Systemic antifungal therapy is required for some dermatophyte infections such as onychomycosis, tinea unguium, tinea manuum, tinea capitis, and widespread dermatophytosis. Commonly used systemic antifungals include azoles, echinocandins, and griseofulvin. Echinocandins interfere with cell wall synthesis and alter permeability by inhibiting synthesis of β-(1,3)-D-glucan. Griseofulvin inhibits mitosis in dermatophytes by interacting with microtubules. Therapeutic regimens for different infections can be found in Tables 63-1 to 63-4.

PITYRIASIS VERSICOLOR (TINEA VERSICOLOR)

DEFINITION

Pityriasis (tinea) versicolor (PV) is a noncontagious chronic benign disorder characterized by scaly hypo- or hyperpigmented superficial patches on the trunk and proximal upper extremities.[5,6] With the exception of children, it seldom occurs on the face and is rare on the lower extremities.

EPIDEMIOLOGY

PV occurs when the round yeast form transforms to the mycelial form. PV is distributed worldwide geographically; however, it is more common in tropical climates. The disease affects mainly young adults of both sexes, although in tropical zones it is also common in infancy and even in neonates.[5] PV is generally rare before puberty and in old age, possibly due to alterations in sebum production. Without treatment, PV is commonly a chronic disease. After treatment, recurrence of PV is common, affecting 60% of patients 1 year after treatment and 80% 2 years after treatment.[7]

A study done by the University of Wake Forest that analyzed National Ambulatory Medical Care data between 1990 and 1999 found that visit rates to physicians for PV were highest among African American patients and American Indians/Eskimos.[8] An epidemiologic report showed that PV in the United States occurs in 2.2% of the dark skin of color population.[9] In southeast London, England, between January and March 1996, a diagnosis of PV was seen in 3.8% of patients.[10] Furthermore, in Rwanda on the continent of Africa, PV was one of the most commonly reported cutaneous diseases.[11]

ETIOLOGY

The lipophilic yeast *Malassezia* species are the etiologic agents of PV. *Malassezia globosa*[12,13] and *Malassezia sympodialis*[14] may be the most common etiologic agents, whereas *Malassezia furfur* has been isolated in some lesions.[15] *Malassezia* yeasts are a part of normal skin flora (predominantly *Malassezia sympodialis*); however, in individuals who develop PV, the organisms transform from saprophytic, round-celled, or the yeast phase to the mycelial phase. Tropical climates provide the right environment for this conversion due to their high temperature and humidity. Factors such as immunodeficiency, poor nutrition, hyperhidrosis, pregnancy, and use of oral contraceptives and corticosteroids have been implicated in nontropical climates.[14] Genetic susceptibility is also likely.[16] Due to the lipophilic nature of the yeast, the frequent use of palm oil, other natural oils, or cocoa butter on the skin may promote growth of the yeast. These substances contain high concentrations of complex lipids (eg, glycol stearate, squalene, lanolin, mineral oil, and spermaceti), some of which have been proven to enhance growth of *M. furfur* in culture media.[17] In addition, these substances may act to occlude the skin, resulting in an increased carbon dioxide concentration, altered microflora, and altered pH range, leading to a subsequent overgrowth of fungi.[18] Frequent application of these products may occur in some cultures but should be avoided in at-risk populations.

HISTOPATHOLOGY

Lesional skin samples show that *Malassezia* is present in all layers of the stratum corneum but least often in the lower part of the horny layer. The normal horizontal direction of the skin cells may be disrupted in the superficial and middle layers of the stratum corneum when the organism enters the keratinocytes.[19,20] The skin cells may swell and split, expelling the cell matrix and organelles, resulting in a "clear zone" around the invading yeast cells. Alternatively, the keratin within the invaded cells may be replaced by lipid-dense material.[21]

Hyperpigmented lesions of PV contain more spores and hyphae than either normal or hypopigmented skin. Merkel cells that contain melanosomes and secretory granules may have increased activity, and melanocytes may appear larger, singly distributed, and hypertrophic. Melanin production may be inhibited by azelaic acid or lipoxygenase produced by *Malassezia*, which contribute to the hypopigmentation.[22] Perivascular inflammation and lymphocyte infiltration have been reported in both hypopigmented and hyperpigmented skin.[23] In hypopigmented lesions, there may be a decrease in melanosomes in the stratum spinosum, and the horny layer may be hyperkeratotic.[23,24]

DIAGNOSIS AND CLINICAL APPEARANCE

In individuals with skin of color, PV lesions present as flaky, round or oval maculae with a fine scale that are either hypo- or hyperpigmented. Some patients experience mild pruritus, but for most, PV is asymptomatic and mainly a cosmetic concern. A stretching or scratching of the skin is used to visualize the scale. Areas of involvement usually have confluent lesions and typically include the upper trunk and shoulders. The face is frequently involved in children. When flexural areas are involved, this is referred to as "inverse" PV.

The diagnosis of PV is confirmed by KOH preparations of skin scrapings that demonstrate pseudohyphae and yeast cells. Wood light examination is a useful diagnostic tool for cases of PV in which *M. furfur* is the etiologic agent.[25] The lesions appear bright yellow or gold in color. Culturing the yeast is not necessary for diagnosis, because the organism is part of normal flora. The differential diagnosis includes pityriasis alba, vitiligo, chloasma, tinea corporis, pityriasis rotunda, pityriasis rosea, secondary syphilis, pinta, and seborrheic dermatitis. The distinguishing feature of PV is a characteristic "spaghetti and meatballs" appearance under microscopy that results from the transformation of the yeast to a mycelial form.

TREATMENT

Both topical and oral medications have demonstrated efficacy in the treatment of PV. Nonspecific agents, such as 1% to 2.5% selenium sulfide and 30% to 50% propylene glycol, can physically or chemically remove infected stratum corneum. Ketoconazole has the best minimum inhibitory concentration against all species of *Malassezia*, but the other topical azoles are also effective. The allylamines are less effective topically and are ineffective orally. A variety of shampoos contain pyrithione zinc and are also effective against *Malassezia*.

Patients who suffer from severe or widespread involvement of the skin with PV may benefit from oral therapy [**Table 63-1**]. Treatment

TABLE 63-1	Treatment regimens for pityriasis versicolor	
Drug	**Dose**	**Duration**
Fluconazole[a]	400 mg once	Repeat in 7 days
Itraconazole[a]	200 mg daily	5–7 days

[a]Regimen not approved by the U.S. Food and Drug Administration for this indication.

selection requires a number of considerations: extent and location of lesions, risks and benefits of treatment modality, age of patient, likelihood of compliance, and cost. Relapse commonly occurs, and there is interest in the development of prophylactic treatment.

TINEA NIGRA

Tinea nigra is a superficial mycosis that presents as an infection of the stratum corneum affecting the palms, soles, neck, and trunk.[26,27] It is a misnomer since it is not caused by a dermatophyte but has the name tinea. This infection occurs most commonly in tropical and subtropical climates, but does occur in the United States, particularly in the southern coastal areas.[27] The causative agent, *Hortaea werneckii* (formerly *Exophiala wernickii*), resides in sewage, soil, decaying vegetation, wood, and humid environments.[27,28] Clinical lesions commonly present as slightly scaly, brown to greenish black velvety macules. Lesions may develop as one or several spots and spread centrifugally, darkening at the border.[26,27,29] Heavily pigmented macules may resemble acral melanocytic nevi or even melanoma. Tinea nigra is generally darker and lacks the furrows seen in dermoscopy of acral nevi. Skin biopsy shows hyperkeratosis without dermal inflammation. KOH preparation of scrapings shows dematiaceous hyphae in the upper layers of the stratum corneum that are brownish or olive-colored with branching septate.[28,29] Diagnosis can be made readily by examination of a KOH preparation and can be confirmed by culture; a skin biopsy will also confirm the diagnosis. The therapy of choice for tinea nigra is topical imidazoles; other reported successful therapies include keratinolytic agents like urea, salicylic acid, and Whitfield ointment.[27,29,30] Oral griseofulvin and terbinafine are ineffective.

PIEDRA

Piedra is a superficial asymptomatic infection of the hair shaft. Two varieties of piedra exist: black piedra and white piedra.[31,32] Piedras are distinguished by both clinical appearance and microscopic examination. White piedra is found in the temperate regions of South America, Europe, Asia, and the southern United States. *Trichosporon beigelii* is the cause of white piedra, which commonly infects the beard, mustache, or pubic hair. The infection causes weakening and breaking of the hair by growing through the hair shaft.[31,33,34] KOH examination of white piedra shows nondematiaceous hyphae with blastoconidia and arthoconidia. Clinically, it has loosely adherent nodules that are softer and vary in color from light brown to white. These nodules lack the organized appearance of black piedra.[31,32,34,35] *T. beigelii* can also cause a systemic infection in immunocompromised patients known as trichosporonosis.

Black piedra is caused by *Piedraia hortae* and frequently infects scalp, facial hair, and only rarely pubic hair. Black piedra is common in tropical regions of South America, the Far East, and the Pacific Islands and is less frequent in Africa and Asia.[34,35] KOH preparation of black piedra reveals hard, brown-black nodules on the hair shaft that are cemented together and resemble organized tissue. Nodules vary in size and are gritty to touch. Microscopic examination distinguishes piedra from nits, hair casts, developmental hair defects, and trichomycosis axillaris. Oral terbinafine has been reported to be an effective therapy for black piedra. Treatment for white piedra includes imidazoles, ciclopirox olamine, 2% selenium sulfide, 6% precipitated sulfur in petrolatum, chlorhexidine solutions, and zinc pyrithione.[33,35] Clipping of infected hairs would be a solution to both black and white piedra.

TINEA CORPORIS/CRURIS (RING WORM, JOCK ITCH)

■ DEFINITION

Tinea corporis (ringworm) includes all superficial dermatophyte infections of the glabrous skin, not including the scalp, beard, face, hands, feet, and groin.[33] Tinea cruris (jock itch) includes infections of the genitalia, pubic area, perineal and perianal skin,[33] and often the upper thigh.[4]

■ ETIOLOGY AND EPIDEMIOLOGY

A number of dermatophytes may cause tinea corporis; however, *Trichophyton tonsurans*, *Trichophyton rubrum*, *Trichophyton mentagrophytes*, and *Microsporum canis* are usually the causative organisms.[34] They are also common in individuals who have primary or secondary immunodeficiencies. Tinea corporis is common in children, especially wrestlers and those with family pets with *M. canis*. Tinea cruris is usually caused by *T. rubrum*, *T. mentagrophytes*, or *Epidermophyton floccosum*.[34] A common predisposing factor for these dermatophyte infections in adults is excessive perspiration.[34] Other factors that predispose individuals include occlusive clothing, contact with contaminated clothing or furniture, immunosuppression, and external exposure sites (eg, locker rooms, gymnasiums, wrestlers, outdoor occupations).[34] There is a high incidence of tinea corporis/cruris in hot, humid areas of the world, with males being affected by tinea cruris more often than females.[34]

■ PATHOGENESIS

The responsible dermatophytes generally reside in the stratum corneum and do not penetrate below the epidermis.[36] The skin responds to the superficial infection by increasing proliferation, and this results in scale and epidermal thickening.[36]

■ CLINICAL MANIFESTATIONS

Tinea corporis may take several clinical forms and may be mild to severe. In individuals with skin of color, the lesions may not be erythematous but rather brown or gray in color. Lesions are typically annular with a central clearing but may assume other patterns such as circinate, oval, or arcuate. Likewise, with tinea cruris, the characteristic red scaling plaques may in fact be tan, brown, or gray in color and extend down the sides of the inner thighs, waist area, and buttocks.[37]

■ HISTOPATHOLOGY

Histopathologically, fungal organisms can be seen in the stratum corneum. If compact orthokeratosis is found in a section, there should be a search for fungal hyphae facilitated by staining with PAS.[34]

■ DIAGNOSIS AND LABORATORY FINDINGS

Diagnosis can be established through review of the patient history and physical examination. However, there is greater diagnostic accuracy if the clinical diagnosis is verified by KOH and/or culture.[36] The affected area should be disinfected with alcohol or cleansed with water, and a 15-blade scalpel should be used to obtain a specimen from the active border of the infection.[38]

■ TREATMENT

Noninflammatory, less severe cases of tinea corporis and cruris infections can be treated with topical antifungals such as econazole, clotrimazole, or ciclopirox. Systemic treatment (eg, terbinafine, itraconazole, fluconazole) should be considered when the infection is inflammatory or involves a large surface area of skin, when host immunity is reduced or abnormal, or when there is chronic or recurrent infection with a poor response to topical therapy[28] [**Table 63-2**]. Other factors that determine the choice of therapy include the overall health of the patient, the causative organism, site and extent of the infection, patient preference (oral vs topical treatment), and the cost-effectiveness of therapy.[38]

TABLE 63-2   Systemic treatment for tinea corporis/cruris

Drug	Dose	Duration
Terbinafine	250 mg/d	2–4 weeks
Itraconazole	200 mg/d	2 weeks
Fluconazole	150 mg once weekly	2 weeks
Griseofulvin	250 mg every 12 hours	Until infection clears

TINEA PEDIS (ATHLETE'S FOOT)

EPIDEMIOLOGY

Tinea pedis (athlete's foot) is one of the most common superficial fungal infections, affecting at least 10% of the world population at any given time.[39] Prevalence rates for Europe and Asia are similar, ranging from 3% to 27%[40,41] and 4% to 20%,[42,43] respectively. In the Middle East, approximately 10% of the population is affected.[44] In general, race does not appear to affect the distribution of this disease. Tinea pedis is more common in men and the elderly.[40] Predisposing factors include diabetes, obesity, trauma, immunosuppression, and certain occupations and hobbies.

ETIOLOGY

The dermatophytes *T. rubrum, T. mentagrophytes*, and *E. floccosum* are the most common causal organisms of tinea pedis.[45,46] Nondermatophyte pathogens such as *Scytalidium dimidiatum* and *Scytalidium hyalinum* are also associated with this disease.[45] Nondermatophyte pathogens are typically recalcitrant to conventional therapy and perhaps best treated with keratolytics.

CLINICAL MANIFESTATIONS

Tinea pedis has three clinical types: interdigital, hyperkeratotic (moccasin), and vesicobullous.[45,47] Interdigital (dermatophytosis simplex), the most prevalent and often chronic form, usually affects the toe web space between the fourth and fifth toes, followed by the toe web space between the third and fourth toes. The skin may appear white and macerated with red erosions.[47] The formation of diffuse hyperkeratosis and desquamative erythema on the sole and toes in a chronic and nonseasonal manner is characteristic of hyperkeratotic tinea pedis. This form is often accompanied by tinea unguium and generally is caused by *T. rubrum*.[48] The vesicobullous form, frequently caused by *T. mentagrophytes*, is characterized by inflammatory vesicles or bullous lesions.[39] It is sometimes associated with a secondary infection (dermatophytosis complex), itching, and maceration.[47] Severe cases are difficult to diagnose because secondary bacterial infections causing inflammation can mask the primary condition.[47]

TREATMENT

Patients should be examined for other fungal infections, especially onychomycosis, because the nails can acts as a reservoir of infection.[39,47] Prophylactic measures include wearing nonocclussive footwear and changing socks and shoes regularly.[39] Regular applications of antifungal foot powders may be helpful.[49] Public baths and pools are major sources of infection by dermatophytes,[50] and using these facilities without footwear should be avoided. Washing the feet with soap and thoroughly drying them also have been found to reduce the presence of dermatophytes.[50] Topical antifungal agents can be used to treat tinea pedis in most cases. Application of a topical antifungal (eg, azoles, allylamines, or ciclopirox) for 1 month is generally curative. Oral griseofulvin, fluconazole, ketoconazole, itraconazole, and terbinafine have been used but are not all FDA approved for therapy of tinea pedis [**Table 63-3**].

TABLE 63-3	Systemic treatment for tinea pedis	
Drug	Dose	Duration
Terbinafine	250 mg daily	2–4 weeks
Itraconazole	200 mg daily	2 weeks
Itraconazole	200 mg twice daily	1 week (1 pulse)
Fluconazole	200 mg once weekly	4–6 weeks
Microsize griseofulvin	500 mg every 12 hours	4–8 weeks
Ultramicrosize griseofulvin	250–375 mg every 12 hours	4–8 weeks

[a]For recalcitrant fungal infections, the prescribing limit is 1 g/d.

ONYCHOMYCOSIS (TINEA UNGUIUM)

DEFINITION

Onychomycosis is a fungal infection involving the nail unit.

ETIOLOGY

Approximately 90% of infections are caused by dermatophytes, with *T. rubrum* being the most commonly isolated etiologic agent.[51,52] Other dermatophyte pathogens include *T. mentagrophytes* and *E. floccosum*.[53] Nondermatophyte molds such as *Scopulariopsis brevicaulis, Acremonium* species, *Aspergillus* species, *Scytalidium* species, *Onychocola canadensis, Alternaria* species, and *Fusarium* species are responsible for 2.1% to 12.5% of onychomycotic infections depending on geographic location.[54] *Candida albicans* causes disease in immunocompromised individuals but can also cause primary onycholysis, paronychia, and occasionally nail plate involvement in healthy patients.[54]

EPIDEMIOLOGY

Onychomycosis accounts for nearly 50% of all nail disorders.[53,55] North American epidemiologic studies suggest prevalence rates between 8% and 13.8%.[51,53] Slightly higher prevalence rates were reported for Europe (23% to 26%) and East Asia (22%).[56] The distribution of onychomycosis does not appear to be directly affected by race,[53] although cultural and socioeconomic factors may play a role. Dermatophytes were isolated from communal bathing areas in several Muslim mosques in a South African study; the incidence of infection reported in males regularly attending these mosques was higher than in non-Muslim males from the same community.[57]

Toenails generally are affected more often than fingernails.[51] Predisposing factors include diabetes mellitus, peripheral arterial disease, compromised immune system, smoking, increasing age, and male gender.[58]

PATHOGENESIS

There are four main routes of entry into the nail unit, each with a corresponding clinical presentation.[59,60] Total dystrophic onychomycosis results from the progression of one or more of the four main presentations or from simultaneous invasion of all nail tissues as a result of immunosuppression.[59]

HISTOPATHOLOGY

Histologic examination reveals fungal elements (spores or hyphae) in the stratum corneum, deep portion of the nail plate, or hyponychium depending on the clinical type.[61]

DIAGNOSIS

The differential diagnosis of onychomycosis includes psoriasis, chronic onycholysis, lichen planus, yellow nail syndrome, and trauma.[55] Clinical suspicion of onychomycosis calls for mycologic examination of the affected nail. Samples should be collected from different sites of the nail unit, including proximal nail clippings, curetted subungual debris, and nail plate shavings from the diseased portion of the nail, in order to maximize positive results.[62]

TREATMENT

Oral antifungal agents are the most effective treatments currently available for onychomycosis [**Table 63-4**]. The mechanism of action of azole (itraconazole) and allylamine (terbinafine) antifungal agents involves the inhibition of ergosterol biosynthesis, an essential component of the fungal cell membrane. These drugs penetrate the nail unit via the nail bed. Modern topical antifungal nail lacquers and solutions, such as ciclopirox 8%, amorolfine 5%, and efinaconazole 10%, exploit the use of a concentration gradient that promotes penetration of the active

TABLE 63-4	Systemic treatment for onychomycosis	
Drug	Dose	Duration
Terbinafine	250 mg daily	Fingernails—6 weeks
Terbinafine	250 mg daily	Toenails—12 weeks
Itraconazole pulse	200 mg twice daily	Fingernails—1 week/month for 2 months
Itraconazole pulse	200 mg twice daily	Toenails—1 week/month for 3 months
Itraconazole continuous	200 mg daily	Fingernails—6 weeks
Itraconazole continuous	200 mg daily	Toenails—12 weeks
Fluconazole	200–400 mg once weekly	Fingernails/toenails—until clear

compound to the affected portion of the nail. Topical nail lacquers may provide a safe alternative for patients with onychomycosis of mild to moderate disease severity. Removal of the affected portion of the nail by chemical or mechanical means may be used as an adjunct to antifungal therapy to reduce the fungal burden. Nail avulsion or debridement without concomitant antifungal therapy has a high potential for relapse.[63]

CUTANEOUS CANDIDIASIS

Candida species are part of the normal human cutaneous microflora but may become pathogenic when host factors such as immune status are altered. Lesions may affect several body sites, including nails [see "Onychomycosis (Tinea Unguium)" above], with warm, moist intertriginous areas being affected most frequently. *C. albicans* is the main etiologic agent.

▓ CLINICAL MANIFESTATIONS

Cutaneous candidiasis occurs in moist, macerated folds of skin. It presents as pruritic, erythematous, macerated areas.[64]

▓ LABORATORY FINDINGS/HISTOPATHOLOGY

For superficial candidal infections, examination of skin scrapings shows typical budding yeasts with hyphae or pseudohyphae in the stratum corneum. Culture results in whitish, mucoid colonies within 2 to 5 days.[65]

▓ TREATMENT

Anticandidal topical therapy includes clotrimazole, econazole, ketoconazole, miconazole, ciclopirox, and nystatin. Oral itraconazole or fluconazole may be considered if oral therapy is warranted.[66]

CONCLUSION

Fungi are ubiquitous, and individuals of all races may be affected. Susceptibility to fungal infection is influenced by a variety of factors including socioeconomic status, geographic location, and cultural or religious practices. Topical antifungals are first-line therapy for dermatophyte infections in those with uncomplicated, localized infections.

Systemic antifungal therapy is required for some dermatophyte infections such as onychomycosis, tinea unguium, tinea manuum, tinea capitis, and widespread dermatophytosis.

REFERENCES

1. Taylor SC. Epidemiology of skin diseases in ethnic populations. *Dermatol Clin.* 2003;21:601-607.
2. Hartshorne ST. Dermatological disorders in Johannesburg, South Africa. *Clin Exp Dermatol.* 2003;28:661-665.
3. Weinberg JM, Koestenblatt EK, Tutrone WD, et al. Comparison of diagnostic methods in the evaluation of onychomycosis. *J Am Acad Dermatol.* 2003;49:193-197.
4. Elewski BE, Leyden J, Rinaldi MG, Atillasoy E. Office practice-based confirmation of onychomycosis: a US nationwide prospective survey. *Arch Intern Med.* 2002;162:2133-2138.
5. Crespo E, Delgado F. *Malassezia* species in skin diseases. *Curr Opin Infect Dis.* 2002;15:133.
6. Vander Straten MR, Hossain MA, Ghannoum MA. Cutaneous infections, dermatophytosis, onychomycosis, and tinea versicolor. *Infect Dis Clin North Am.* 2003;17:87-112.
7. Faergemann J. *Pityrosporum* species as a cause of allergy and infection. *Allergy.* 1999;54:413.
8. Mellen LA, Vallee J, Feldman SR, et al. Treatment of pityriasis versicolor in the United States. *J Dermatolog Treat.* 2004;15:18-92.
9. Halder RM, Nootheti PK. Ethnic skin disorders overview. *J Am Acad Dermatol.* 2003;48:S143.
10. Child FJ, Fuller LC, Higgins EM, et al. A study of the spectrum of skin disease occurring in a black population in southeast London. *Br J Dermatol.* 1999;141:512-517.
11. Van Hecke E, Bugingo G. Prevalence of skin disease in Rwanda. *Int J Dermatol.* 1980;19:526-529.
12. Gupta AK, Kohli Y, Summerbell RC, et al. Quantitative culture of *Malassezia* species from different body sites of individuals with or without dermatoses. *Med Mycol* 2001;39:243-251.
13. Nakabayashi A, Sei Y, Guillot J. Identification of *Malassezia* species isolated from patients with seborrheic dermatitis, atopic dermatitis, pityriasis versicolor and normal subjects. *Med Mycol.* 2000;38:337.
14. Bolognia JL, Jorizzo JL, Schaffer JV, eds. *Dermatology.* 3rd ed. Philadelphia, PA: Saunders, Elsevier; 2012:1252-1258.
15. Mayser P, Gross A. IgE antibodies to *Malassezia furfur, M. sympodialis* and *Pityrosporum orbiculare* in patients with atopic dermatitis, seborrheic eczema or pityriasis versicolor, and identification of respective allergens. *Acta Dermatol Venereol.* 2000;80:357-361.
16. Gueho E, Boekhout T, Ashbee HR, et al. The role of *Malassezia* species in the ecology of human skin and as pathogens. *Med Mycol.* 1998;36:220S.
17. Porro MN, Passi S, Caprilli F, et al. Induction of hyphae in cultures of *Pityrosporum* by cholesterol and cholesterol esters. *J Invest Dermatol.* 1977;69:531-534.
18. King RD, Cunico RL, Maibach HI, et al. The effect of occlusion on carbon dioxide emission from human skin. *Acta Dermatol Venereol.* 1978;58:135-138.
19. Gupta AK, Bluhm R, Summerbell R. Pityriasis versicolor. *J Eur Acad Dermatol Venereol.* 2002;16:19-33.
20. Borgers M, Cauwenbergh G, Van de Ven MA, et al. Pityriasis versicolor and *Pityrosporum ovale*: morphogenetic and ultrastructural considerations. *Int J Dermatol.* 1987;26:586.
21. Gupta AK, Bluhm R, Summerbell R. Pityriasis versicolor. *J Eur Acad Dermatol Venereol.* 2002;16:19-33.
22. Nazzaro-Porro M, Passi S. Identification of tyrosinase inhibitors in cultures of *Pityrosporum. J Invest Dermatol.* 1978;71:205-208.
23. Galadari I, el Komy M, Mousa A, et al. Tinea versicolor: histologic and ultrastructural investigation of pigmentary changes. *Int J Dermatol.* 1992; 31:253-256.
24. Crespo-Erchiga V, Martos AO, Casano AV, et al. Mycology of pityriasis versicolor. *J Mycol Med.* 1999;9:143.
25. Savin R. Diagnosis and treatment of tinea versicolor. *J Fam Pract.* 1996; 43:127-132.
26. Knox J, Mullins F, Spiller W. Tinea nigra. *J Invest Dermatol.* 1956;27:187-192.
27. Abliz P, Fukushima K, Takizawa K, Miyaji M, Nishimura K. Specific oligonucleotide primers for identification of *Hortaea werneckii*, a causative agent of tinea nigra. *Diagn Microbiol Infect Dis.* 2003;46:89-93.
28. Mok WY. Nature and identification of *Exophiala werneckii. J Clin Microbiol.* 1982;16:976-978.
29. McKinlay JR, Barrett TL, Ross EV. Picture of the month: tinea nigra. *Arch Pediatr Adolesc Med.* 1999;153:305-306.
30. Burke WA. Tinea nigra: treatment with topical ketoconazole. *Cutis.* 1993; 52:209-211.
31. Figueras MJ, Guarro J, Zaror L. New findings in black piedra infection. *Br J Dermatol.* 1996;135:157-158.
32. Smith JD, Murtishaw WA, McBride ME. White piedra (trichosporosis). *Arch Dermatol.* 1973;107:439-442.
33. Gupta AK, Chaudhry M, Elewski B. Tinea corporis, tinea cruris, tinea nigra, and piedra. *Dermatol Clin.* 2003;21:395-400.
34. James W, Berger T, Elston D. Diseases resulting from fungi and yeasts. In: *Andrew's Diseases of the Skin: Clinical Dermatology.* 11th ed. Philadelphia, PA: Saunders, Elsevier; 2011:642-657.
35. Assaf RR, Weil ML. The superficial mycoses. *Dermatol Clin.* 1996;14:57-67.

36. Drake LA, Dinehart SM, Farmer ER, et al. Guidelines of care for superficial mycotic infections of the skin: tinea corporis, tinea cruris, tinea faciei, tinea manuum, and tinea pedis. Guidelines/Outcomes Committee, American Academy of Dermatology. *J Am Acad Dermatol.* 1996;34:282.

37. Weinstein A, Berman B. Topical treatment of common superficial tinea infections. *Am Fam Physician.* 2002;65:2095-2102.

38. Gupta AK, Einarson TR, Summerbell RC, et al. An overview of topical antifungal therapy in dermatomycoses: a North American perspective. *Drugs.* 1998;55:645-674.

39. Gupta AK, Chow M, Daniel CR, et al. Treatments of tinea pedis. *Dermatol Clin.* 2003;21:431-462.

40. Perea S, Ramos MJ, Garau M, et al. Prevalence and risk factors of tinea unguium and tinea pedis in the general population in Spain. *J Clin Microbiol.* 2000;38:3226-3230.

41. Lupa S, Seneczko F, Jeske J, et al. Epidemiology of dermatomycoses of humans in central Poland: III. Tinea pedis. *Mycoses.* 1999;42:563-565.

42. Ungpakorn R, Lohaprathan S, Reangchainam S. Prevalence of foot diseases in outpatients attending the Institute of Dermatology, Bangkok, Thailand. *Clin Exp Dermatol.* 2004;29:87-90.

43. Cheng S, Chong L. A prospective epidemiological study on tinea pedis and onychomycosis in Hong Kong. *Chin Med J (Engl).* 2002;115:860-865.

44. Falahati M, Akhlaghi L, Lari AR, et al. Epidemiology of dermatophytoses in an area south of Tehran, Iran. *Mycopathologia.* 2003;156:279.

45. Lopes JO, Alves SH, Mari CR, et al. A ten-year survey of tinea pedis in the central region of the Rio Grande do Sul, Brazil. *Rev Inst Med Trop Sao Paulo.* 1999;41:75-77.

46. Vella ZL, Gatt P, Boffa MJ, et al. Characteristics of superficial mycoses in Malta. *Int J Dermatol.* 2003;42:265-271.

47. Masri-Fridling GD. Dermatophytosis of the feet. *Dermatol Clin.* 1996;14:33-40.

48. Tanuma H. Pathogenesis and treatment of hyperkeratotic tinea pedis in Japan. *Mycoses.* 1999;42:21-28.

49. Pierard G, Wallace R, De Doncker P. Biometrological assessment of the preventive effect of a miconazole spray powder on athlete's foot. *Clin Exp Dermatol.* 1996;21:344.

50. Watanabe K, Taniguchi H, Katoh T. Adhesion of dermatophytes to healthy feet and its simple treatment. *Mycoses.* 2000;43:45-50.

51. Gupta AK, Jain HC, Lynde CW, et al. Prevalence and epidemiology of onychomycosis in patients visiting physicians' offices: a multicenter Canadian survey of 15,000 patients. *J Am Acad Dermatol.* 2000;43:244-248.

52. Foster KW, Ghannoum MA, Elewski BE. Epidemiologic surveillance of cutaneous fungal infection in the United States from 1999 to 2002. *J Am Acad Dermatol.* 2004;50:748-752.

53. Ghannoum MA, Hajjeh RA, Scher R, et al. A large-scale North American study of fungal isolates from nails: the frequency of onychomycosis, fungal distribution, and antifungal susceptibility patterns. *J Am Acad Dermatol.* 2000;43:641-648.

54. Tosti A, Piraccini BM, Lorenzi S, et al. Treatment of nondermatophyte mold and *Candida* onychomycosis. *Dermatol Clin.* 2003;21:491-497.

55. Lynde C. Nail disorders that mimic onychomycosis: what to consider. *Cutis.* 2001;68:8-12.

56. Haneke E, Roseeuw D. The scope of onychomycosis: epidemiology and clinical features. *Int J Dermatol.* 1999;38:7S.

57. Raboobee N, Aboobaker J, Peer AK. Tinea pedis et unguium in the Muslim community of Durban, South Africa. *Int J Dermatol.* 1998;37:759-765.

58. Gupta AK, Konnikov N, Lynde CW, et al. Onychomycosis: predisposed populations and some predictors of suboptimal response to oral antifungal agents. *Eur J Dermatol.* 1999;9:633-638.

59. Baran R, Hay RJ, Tosti A, et al. A new classification of onychomycosis. *Br J Dermatol.* 1998;139:567-571.

60. Tosti A, Baran R, Piraccini BM, et al. "Endonyx" onychomycosis: a new modality of nail invasion by dermatophytes. *Acta Dermatol Venereol.* 1999;79:52-53.

61. Jerasutus S. Histology and histopathology. In: Scher RK, Daniel CR III, eds. *Nails: Therapy, Diagnosis, Surgery.* 2nd ed. Philadelphia, PA: Saunders; 1997:55-98.

62. Hull PR, Gupta AK, Summerbell RC. Onychomycosis: an evaluation of three sampling methods. *J Am Acad Dermatol.* 1998;39:1015-1017.

63. Hettinger DF, Valinsky MS. Treatment of onychomycosis with nail avulsion and topical ketoconazole. *J Am Podiatr Med Assoc.* 1991;81:28-32.

64. Darmstadt GL, Dinulos JG, Miller Z. Congenital cutaneous candidiasis: Clinical presentation, pathogenesis, and management guidelines. *Pediatrics.* 2000;105:438-444.

65. Hay RJ. The management of superficial candidiasis. *J Am Acad Dermatol.* 1999;40:35S.

66. Blatchford NR. Treatment of oral candidiasis with itraconazole: a review. *J Am Acad Dermatol.* 1990;23:565-567.

CHAPTER 64

Parasitic Infections

Shobita Rajagopalan

KEY POINTS

- Parasitic infestations and infections are encountered commonly in developing countries, where the environment is ideal for them to thrive. International travel to tropical destinations plays an important part in the acquisition of parasitic diseases.

- Factors such as geography, environment, and low socioeconomic status causing overcrowding and pollution, poor hygiene, food and water contamination, malnutrition, delayed access to medical care, and the presence of appropriate vectors play an important role in transmission of parasitic diseases.

- Skin diseases associated with parasitic infection or infestations, including scabies and cutaneous larva migrans, are encountered in skin of color patients.

INTRODUCTION

Parasites are ubiquitous in nature and associated with a variety of diseases in many different hosts. They are more common in regions of the world where various environmental factors, including climate, population dynamics, food and water sources, and the presence of appropriate vectors, enable them to thrive. In addition, host factors such as nutritional status and immune function play a key role in the transmission and acquisition of parasitic diseases and determine disease severity. Genetic susceptibility to specific parasites may also play a role. Susceptible individuals who travel to destinations where parasites are endemic are at increased risk for acquiring parasitic illnesses.

Racial differences in skin properties, such as including epidermal melanin content, melanosome dispersion, hair structure, and fibroblast and mast cell size and structure may explain differences in disease prevalence and presentation among different groups.[1-4]

Various skin disorders, including those caused by or associated with parasitic infection or infestation, are commonly encountered in people with skin of color, that is, African Americans, Asians, Hispanics/Latinos, and Native Americans. Complex interactions between the host factors, such as genetic makeup, nutritional status, and immune function, and environmental factors, such as geography and climate, play a key role in disease acquisition. Socioeconomic indicators such as poverty, overcrowding, and decreased access to medical care may also contribute to parasitic disease acquisition.[3,4]

This chapter will review some common and important parasitic illnesses that are known to cause significant skin disease in humans and focus on possible race-related variations in disease presentation. Skin manifestations of specific parasitic diseases that will be covered include the ectoparasitic infestation scabies and the cutaneous migratory endoparasitic phenomenon known as cutaneous larva migrans.

SCABIES

BACKGROUND

Scabies is a common and highly contagious ectoparasitic infestation of global and public health significance caused by the arthropod *Sarcoptes scabiei* var. *hominis*. Scabies affects all individuals regardless of age, gender, race/ethnicity, or socioeconomic status. Worldwide, an estimated 300 million cases occur annually.[5] Prevalence rates in developing countries are higher than those in developed nations. Overcrowding, poor hygiene, delayed diagnosis and treatment, and lack of public education are some of the factors that contribute to the prevalence of scabies in both industrial and nonindustrial nations. In developed countries, scabies epidemics occur primarily in institutional settings, such as prisons, long-term care facilities such as nursing homes, and hospitals. Prevalence rates are observed to be higher in children and sexually active individuals than in other persons. The more severe and crusted variant of scabies, known as *Norwegian scabies* (so named because of its initial description in Norway in the mid-1800s), is common in patients with poor sensory perception due to entities such as leprosy and in immunocompromised persons (after organ or tissue transplantation or with human immunodeficiency virus [HIV] infection) and the aged.[6] These populations typically present with clinically atypical lesions and are frequently misdiagnosed, thus delaying treatment and enhancing the risk of local epidemics. Although scabies is a readily treatable infestation, it remains relatively common primarily because of diagnostic difficulty, inadequate treatment of patients and their contacts, and improper environmental control measures.

PATHOPHYSIOLOGY

The scabies mite is an obligate parasite and completes its entire life cycle on humans.[7] Animal scabies mites may cause mild and transient symptoms in humans that generally do not persist. Prolonged direct contact with infested individuals facilitates transmission. Mites can live up to 3 days away from human skin; thus fomites such as infested bedding or clothing may be an additional rare source of transmission. The life cycle of the scabies mite is approximately 30 days and is spent within the human epidermis. After copulation, the male mite dies, and the female mite burrows into the superficial skin layers and lays a total of 60 to 90 eggs. The eggs incubate and hatch after 3 to 8 days. About 90% of the hatched mites die, but those that survive go through various stages of molting and reach maturity after approximately 2 weeks. The female adults, who never leave their burrows, die after 1 to 2 months. In classic scabies, 5 to 15 mites (range, 3 to 50) may live on the host skin.

During the initial month of scabies infestation, infested individuals remain relatively asymptomatic. However, approximately 4 weeks into and with subsequent infestation, a delayed-type hypersensitivity reaction develops to the mites, eggs, and scybala (packet of feces). With reinfestation, the sensitized individual may develop a rapid reaction (often within hours). The resulting skin eruption and its associated intense pruritus are the hallmark of classic scabies.

Norwegian Scabies In immunocompromised hosts, frail elderly persons, and physically and/or mentally handicapped persons and in individuals with sensory nerve impairment, the fulminant distinctive and highly contagious hyperinfestation due to the crusted or Norwegian form of scabies is relatively common. In this variant of scabies, numerous mites infest the host. Rare cases have been described in immunocompetent patients. Extensive, widespread crusted lesions appear with thick, hyperkeratotic scales over the elbows, knees, palms, and soles. The number of mites in a patient with crusted scabies can exceed 1 million. In these cases, the mite can survive off the host for up to 7 days, feeding on the sloughed skin in the local environment, such as bed sheets, clothing, and chair covers. Failure to implement environmental control measures in this situation may result in relapse and reinfestation after successful treatment of the host. Serum immunoglobulin E (IgE) and immunoglobulin G (IgG) levels are extremely high in these patients, yet the immune reaction does not seem to be protective. Cell-mediated immune responses in classic scabies demonstrate a predominantly CD4 T-cell infiltrate in the skin, whereas one study suggests CD8 T-cell predominance in crusted scabies. Atypical infestations also can occur in infants and young children.

CLINICAL MANIFESTATIONS

The historical aspects of scabies infestations are quite reliable in suggesting the diagnosis.[8] The incubation period prior to onset of symptoms depends on whether the infestation is an initial exposure or a relapse/reinfestation. Previously sensitized individuals can develop

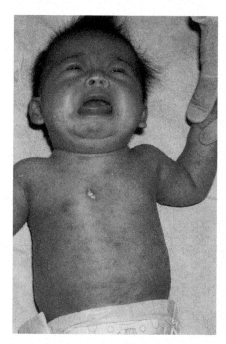

FIGURE 64-1. A Hispanic infant with generalized scabies.

symptoms within hours of reexposure. The hypersensitivity reaction is responsible for the intense pruritus that is the clinical hallmark of the disease.

Lesion distribution, intractable pruritus that is worse at night, and similar symptoms in close contacts immediately should raise a high index of suspicion for scabies. Lesion distribution differs in adults and children. Adults manifest lesions primarily on the flexor aspects of the wrists, the interdigital web spaces of the hands, the dorsal feet, axillae, elbows, waist, buttocks, and genitalia.[9] Secondary lesions may occur as a result of rubbing and scratching, and they may be the only clinical manifestation of the disease. Pruritic papules and vesicles on the scrotum and penis in men and the areolae in women are highly characteristic. Infants and small children develop lesions predominantly on the face, scalp, neck, palms, and soles, although any site may be involved [**Figure 64-1**]. Widespread pruritic eczematous eruptions in any skin site are common in immunocompromised and elderly patients.

Burrows are a pathognomonic sign of classic scabies and represent the intraepidermal tunnel created by the moving female mite. They appear as inapparent, serpiginous, grayish, threadlike elevations ranging from 2 to 10 mm long [**Figure 64-2**]. Common locations for burrows include the webbed spaces of the fingers; the flexor surfaces of the wrists, elbows, and axillae; the belt line; the feet; the scrotum in men; and the areolae in women. In infants, burrows are commonly located on the palms and soles. The actual mites are not visible with the naked eye and can be visualized only with microscopy.

Complications of scabies are rare and generally result from vigorous rubbing and scratching. Disruption of the skin barrier puts the patient at risk for secondary bacterial invasion, primarily by *Streptococcus pyogenes* and *Staphylococcus aureus*. Superinfection with *S. pyogenes* can precipitate acute poststreptococcal glomerulonephritis and even rheumatic fever. More common pyodermas include impetigo and cellulitis, which rarely may result in sepsis. Scabies infestations can exacerbate underlying eczema, psoriasis, and other preexisting dermatoses. Even with appropriate treatment, scabies can leave in its wake residual eczematous dermatitis and/or postscabietic pruritus, which can be debilitating and recalcitrant. Crusted or Norwegian scabies can result in extensive involvement of the skin and carries an increased mortality rate because of the frequency of secondary bacterial infections resulting in sepsis [**Figure 64-3**].

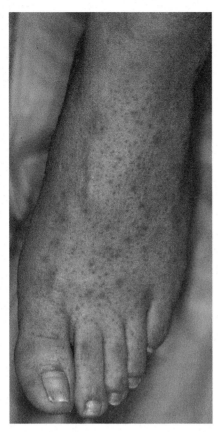

FIGURE 64-2. Classic scabies eruption showing burrows.

LABORATORY DIAGNOSIS

Light Microcopy The diagnosis is confirmed by light microscopic identification of mites, larvae, ova, or scybala in skin scrapings[10,11]. In rare cases, mites are identified in biopsy specimens obtained to rule out other dermatoses. Characteristic histopathology common to a variety of arthropod reactions in the absence of actual mites also may suggest the diagnosis. Excision of a burrow may reveal mites, larvae, ova, and feces within the stratum corneum. A superficial and deep dermal infiltrate composed of lymphocytes, histiocytes, mast cells, and eosinophils is characteristic. Spongiosis and vesicle formation with exocytosis of eosinophils and occasional neutrophils is present. Biopsy of older lesions may be nondiagnostic and reveal fibrosis and scale crusts. Crusted scabies demonstrates massive hyperkeratosis of the stratum corneum with numerous mites in all stages of development. Psoriasiform hyperplasia

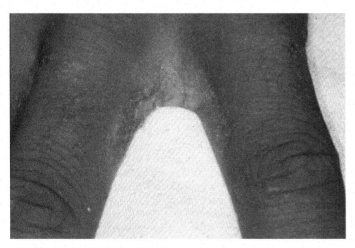

FIGURE 64-3. Scabies infestation of the finger and web spaces.

of the underlying epidermis with spongiotic foci and occasional epidermal microabscesses is present. The dermis shows a superficial and deep chronic inflammatory infiltrate with interstitial eosinophils. Nodular variants of scabies reveal a dense, mixed, superficial, and deep dermal inflammatory cell infiltrate. Lymphoid follicles may be present, and the infiltrate occasionally extends into the subcutaneous fat.

Other Tests Elevated IgE titers and eosinophilia may be found in some patients with scabies. Clinically inapparent infection can be detected by amplification of *Sarcoptes* DNA in epidermal scale by polymerase chain reaction.[12] Immunosuppression, either via medication or disease related, may be associated with crusted scabies.

TREATMENT

The mainstay of scabies treatment is the application of topical scabicidal agents and/or systemic pharmacologic (oral) drug treatment.[13,14]

The following medications are approved by the U.S. Food and Drug Administration (FDA) for the treatment of scabies.

Permethrin Cream 5% (Brand Name: Elimite) Permethrin is FDA approved for the treatment of scabies in persons aged over 2 months old. Permethrin is a synthetic pyrethroid that kills the scabies mite and eggs and is the drug of choice for the treatment of scabies. Two (or more) applications, each about a week apart, may be necessary to eliminate all mites, particularly when treating severe crusted (Norwegian) scabies.

Crotamiton Lotion 10% and Crotamiton Cream 10% (Brand Names: Eurax; Crotan) Crotamiton is FDA approved for the treatment of scabies in adults only. Frequent treatment failures have been reported with crotamiton.

Lindane Lotion 1% Lindane is FDA approved organochloride for the treatment of scabies. Lindane is not recommended as a first-line therapy. Overuse, misuse, or accidentally swallowing lindane can be toxic to the brain and other parts of the nervous system; its use should be restricted to patients who have failed treatment with, or cannot tolerate other medications that pose less risk. Because of reported neurotoxicity, lindane should not be used to treat premature infants, persons with a seizure disorder, women who are pregnant or breast-feeding, or infants and children, frail elderly, and persons who weigh less than 110 pounds who have compromised epidermal skin barrier function (marked irritation, erosions, ulcerations).

Ivermectin (Brand Name: Stromectol) Ivermectin is a synthetic macrocyclic lactone belonging to the avermectin group of antibiotics. It is active against a number of human and animal endoparasites and ectoparasites. Ivermectin, although not FDA approved for scabies treatment, is effective in most cases of typical scabies at a dose of 200 to 250 µg/kg given at diagnosis and repeated in 7 to 14 days. Crusted scabies may require three or more doses given at 1- to 2-week intervals. Ivermectin is an ideal agent in patients in whom topical therapy is difficult or impractical, such as in widespread institutional infestations and bedridden patients.[15,16] Ivermectin is contraindicated in patients with allergic sensitization or nervous system disorders and in women who are pregnant or breast-feeding. Children younger than 5 years or weighing less than 15 kg should not be treated with ivermectin.

Patients may experience pruritus for up to 2 weeks after successful treatment. If itching persists beyond this time, the patient must be reevaluated to ensure the correct diagnosis, adequate treatment, and simultaneous treatment of contacts and environment. A second treatment course may be indicated. Rarely, individuals with a history of atopy may require a tapered dose of prednisone for the treatment of severe pruritus. Intranodular injection of dilute corticosteroids may be necessary in patients with nodular scabies. Because of the heavy mite burden, patients with crusted scabies may require repeated applications of topical scabicides or simultaneous treatment with topical permethrin and oral ivermectin.

Symptomatic treatment may require oral antihistamines and topical antipruritics/anesthetics such as menthol (Sarna) and pramoxine (Prax). More severe symptoms may require a short course of topical or oral steroids. Secondary infections may require antibiotics, which should be prescribed based on culture and sensitivity.

Detailed verbal and written instructions are critical for compliance and complete eradication and prevention of spread to contacts and are as follows:

- Family members and close contacts must be evaluated and treated, even if they do not have symptoms. Pets do not require treatment. All carpets and upholstered furniture should be vacuumed and the vacuum bags immediately discarded.

- Patients must be instructed to launder clothing, bed linens, and towels used within the last week in hot water the day after treatment is initiated and again in 1 week. Items that cannot be washed may be professionally dry cleaned or sealed in plastic bags for 1 week.

- Patients with crusted scabies or their caregivers should be instructed to remove excess scale to allow penetration of the topical scabicidal agent and decrease the burden of infestation. This can be achieved with warm-water soaks followed by application of a keratolytic agent such as 5% salicylic acid in petrolatum or Lac-Hydrin cream. (Salicylic acid should be avoided if large body surface areas are involved because of the potential risk of salicylate poisoning.) The scales then are debrided mechanically with a tongue depressor or similar non-sharp device.

COMPLICATIONS

Treatment failures are uncommon if guidelines are followed. Residual pruritus may require antihistamines or a short course of topical or oral corticosteroids. Secondary bacterial infection usually as a result of *Streptococcus* or *Staphylococcus* species requires administration of an empirical course of antibiotics; although antibiotic susceptibility is usually predictable, culture and sensitivity data should be followed to appropriately tailor the regimen. Scabietic nodules may require intranodular corticosteroid injection for complete resolution. Flaring or reactivation of preexisting eczema or atopic dermatitis requires the use of standard eczema treatments.

PROGNOSIS

Prognosis is usually excellent with proper diagnosis and treatment in otherwise healthy individuals, as well as in immunocompromised or institutionalized hosts.

CUTANEOUS LARVA MIGRANS

BACKGROUND

Cutaneous larva migrans (CLM) is a common dermatology condition caused by the migratory larvae of animal hookworms characteristically encountered in travelers returning from tropical and subtropical destinations.[17] Cases also have been reported from the southwestern United States. CLM is characterized by an erythematous, serpiginous, pruritic cutaneous eruption caused by accidental percutaneous penetration and subsequent migration of larvae of various nematode parasites. The animal hookworm, *Ancylostoma braziliense*, is the species found most frequently in humans.[18,19] These hookworms generally live in the intestines of domestic pets such as dogs and cats and shed their eggs via feces to soil (usually moist soil and sandy areas of beaches or under houses). Humans are incidental hosts and are infected by contact with contaminated soil found in endemic areas of tropical and subtropical regions. The hookworm larvae burrow through intact skin and stay confined to the upper dermis. Migration of larvae through the skin results in an intensely pruritic, linear, or serpiginous track known as a *creeping eruption* [**Figure 64-4**]. Creeping eruptions are not unique to CLM and occur in many other human skin diseases.

In the United States, among helminthic infestations, CLM is rated second to pinworm. The condition is benign and self-limited but can cause a disturbing pruritus. There is neither a specific racial nor gender

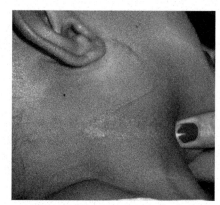

FIGURE 64-4. Cutaneous larva migrans.

predilection for CLM; exposure to animal nematode larvae plays the key role in disease acquisition. In addition, CLM can affect persons of all ages, but it tends to be seen more commonly in children than in adults.

ETIOLOGY AND PATHOGENESIS

Common causes include the following:

- *Ancylostoma braziliense* (hookworm of wild and domestic dogs and cats) is the most common cause. It can be found in the central and southern United States, Central America, South America, and the Caribbean.

- *Ancylostoma caninum* (dog hookworm) is found in Australia.

- *Uncinaria stenocephala* (dog hookworm) is found in Europe.

- *Bunostomum phlebotomum* (cattle hookworm)

    Rare causes include the following:

- *Ancylostoma ceylonicum*

- *Ancylostoma tubaeforme* (cat hookworm)

- *Necator americanus* (human hookworm)

- *Strongyloides papillosus* (parasite of sheep, goats, and cattle)

- *Strongyloides westeri* (parasite of horses)

- *Ancylostoma duodenale*

    The life cycle of the parasites begins when eggs are passed from animal feces into warm, moist soil, where the larvae hatch. The larvae initially feed on soil bacteria and molt twice before the infective third stage. By using their proteases, larvae penetrate through follicles, fissures, or intact skin of the new host. After penetrating the stratum corneum, the larvae shed their natural cuticle and begin migration within a few days. In their natural animal hosts, the larvae are able to penetrate into the dermis and are transported via the lymphatic and venous systems to the lungs. They break through into the alveoli and migrate to the trachea, where they are swallowed. In the intestine, they mature sexually, and the cycle begins again as their eggs are excreted. Humans are accidental hosts, and the larvae are believed to lack the collagenase enzymes required to penetrate the basement membrane to invade the dermis. Therefore, the disease remains limited to the skin when humans are infected.

CLINICAL FEATURES

Patients complain of tingling/prickling at the site of exposure within 30 minutes of penetration of larvae, intense pruritus, and erythematous, often linear lesions that advance and are associated with a history of sunbathing, walking barefoot on the beach, or similar activity in a tropical location.[20,21] Predispositions include hobbies and occupations that involve contact with warm, moist sandy soil and tropical/subtropical travel. Persons at risk include those who walk barefoot or sunbathe on the beach, children in sandboxes, carpenters, electricians, plumbers, farmers, gardener, and pest exterminators.

Cutaneous signs include pruritic, erythematous, edematous papules and/or vesicles; serpiginous, slightly elevated, erythematous tunnels that are 2- to 3-mm wide and track 3 to 4 cm from the penetration site; nonspecific dermatitis; vesicles with serous fluid; secondary impetiginization; and tract advancement of 1 to 2 cm/d. Systemic signs include peripheral eosinophilia (Löffler syndrome), migratory pulmonary infiltrates, and increased IgE levels but are rarely seen. Lesions typically are distributed on the distal lower extremities, including the dorsal surfaces of the feet and the interdigital spaces of the toes, but also can occur in the anogenital region, the buttocks, the hands, and the knees.

Differential diagnosis includes allergic contact dermatitis, epidermal dermatophytosis, erythema chronicum migrans, migratory myiasis, photoallergic dermatitis, and larva currens caused by *Strongyloides stercoralis*.

LABORATORY DIAGNOSIS

Diagnosis is based mostly on the classic clinical appearance of the eruption. Some patients may demonstrate peripheral eosinophilia on a complete blood count and increased IgE levels on total serum immunoglobulin determinations.

Skin biopsy samples from the advancing edge of a tract may show a larva (periodic acid–Schiff positive) in a suprabasalar burrow, basal layer tracts, spongiosis with intraepidermal vesicles, necrotic keratinocytes, and an epidermal and upper dermal chronic inflammatory infiltrate with many eosinophils.

TREATMENT

Even though the condition is self-limited, the intense pruritus and risk for infection mandate treatment.[22] Topical modalities such as ethyl chloride spray, liquid nitrogen, phenol, piperazine citrate, electrocautery, and radiation therapy were used unsuccessfully because their effectiveness is limited for multiple lesions and hookworm folliculitis and may need daily applications for several days. Topical application of a 10% to 15% thiabendazole solution/ointment/cream to the affected area has been shown to be effective.[20-24]

Systemic treatment with thiabendazole is currently considered the treatment of choice. Other effective alternative treatments include albendazole, mebendazole, and ivermectin. The treatment course results in decreased pruritus within 24 to 48 hours, and lesions/tracts resolve in 1 week.

Thiabendazole Thiabendazole is the drug with which there has been the most experience in the oral treatment of CLM.[24-27] Thiabendazole is minimally effective when given as a single dose. The best results have been observed with 50 mg/kg/week of oral thiabendazole for four weeks.[28a] However, thiabendazole is less well tolerated than either albendazole or ivermectin. Reported adverse effects include nausea, vomiting, dizziness, and headache.[28]

Albendazole Albendazole is a third-generation heterocyclic antihelminthic drug used in the treatment of intestinal helminth infection, for example, ascariasis, enterobiasis, ancylostomiasis, trichuriasis, and strongyloidiasis. Albendazole treatment of CLM with a single dose of 400 mg, the same dose for 3 and 5 consecutive days, and with an 800-mg daily dose for 3 consecutive days has been shown to yield successful results.[29-32] However, other studies suggest that for tourists with CLM treated with albendazole, the regimen should be 400 to 800 mg/d for 3 to 5 days.[33] Albendazole is generally well tolerated when use for the treatment of CLM. However, the rare side effect of gastrointestinal pain and diarrhea after receiving albendazole 800 mg by mouth on 3 consecutive days has been reported.[34,35]

Ivermectin Ivermectin, briefly described in the section on scabies, is also active against *Onchocerca volvulus* and other nematodes, including gastrointestinal helminths. Its mechanism of action is poorly understood.[36,37] A single 12-mg dose of ivermectin resulted in 100% cure rates among patients with CLM.

COMPLICATIONS

Complications such as secondary bacterial infection, usually with *S. pyogenes*, may lead to cellulitis and impetigo and prolonged pruritus, and local or general allergic reactions may occur.

PROGNOSIS

The prognosis of CLM is excellent. This is a self-limiting disease. Humans are accidental, dead-end hosts, with the larva dying and the lesions resolving within 4 to 8 weeks or as long as a year in rare cases.

PREVENTION

Persons who travel to tropical regions and pet owners should be made aware of CLM. Because tourists are usually infected by walking or lying on tropical sandy beaches contaminated by dog feces, the best way to prevent CLM is to wear shoes when walking in sandy areas. It also may be prudent to lie on sand washed by the tide or to use a mattress; avoid lying on dry sand, even on a towel.

CONCLUSION

Parasitic infestations and infections are encountered in both developing and developed countries. Although they occur in people with skin of color, there does not appear to be a specific predisposition. Other factors such as travel, geography, environment, and socioeconomic and immune status seemingly play important roles in acquiring these disorders.

REFERENCES

1. Bari AU, Khan MB. Pattern of skin diseases in black Africans of Sierra Leone, West Africa. *J Clin Diagn Res*. 2007;1:361-368.
2. Shriver MD. Ethnic variation as a key to the biology of human disease. *Ann Intern Med*. 1997;127:401-403.
3. Fitzpatrick TB. The validity and practicality of sun reactive skin type I through VI. *Arch Dermatol*. 1988;124:869-871.
4. Maibach HI. Racial (ethnic) differences in skin properties: the objective data. *Am J Clin Dermatol*. 2003;4:843-860.
5. Burkhart CG, Burkhart CN, Burkhart KM. An epidemiologic and therapeutic reassessment of scabies. *Cutis*. 2000;65:233-240.
6. Guldbakke KK, Khachemoune A. Crusted scabies: a clinical review. *J Drugs Dermatol*. 2006;5:221-227.
7. Burgess I. Sarcoptes scabiei and scabies. *Adv Parasitol*. 1994;33:235-292.
8. Elgart ML. Scabies. *Dermatol Clin*. 1990;8:253-263.
9. Fitzpatrick TB, Johnson RA, Wolff K. Insect bites and infestations. In: Fitzpatrick TJ, Johnson RA, Wolff K, Polano MK, Suurmond R, eds. *Color Atlas and Synopsis of Clinical Dermatology*. 3rd ed. New York, NY: McGraw-Hill; 1997:836-861.
10. Brodell RT, Helms SE. Bedside testing: the diagnostic cornerstone of dermatology. *Compr Ther*. 1997;23:211-217.
11. Johnston G, Sladden M. Scabies: diagnosis and treatment. *Br Med J*. 2005;331:619-622.
12. Bezold G, Lange M, Schiener R, et al. Hidden scabies: diagnosis by polymerase chain reaction. *Br J Dermatol*. 2001;144:614-618.
13. Centers for Disease Control and Prevention. Scabies treatment. http://www.cdc.gov/parasites/scabies/health_professionals/meds.html. Accessed February 19, 2015.
14. Elgart GW, Meinking TL. Ivermectin. *Dermatol Clin*. 2003;21:277-282.
15. Huffam SE, Currie BJ. Ivermectin for *Sarcoptes scabiei* hyperinfestation. *Int J Infect Dis*. 1998;2:152-154.
16. Aubin F, Humbert P. Ivermectin for crusted (Norwegian) scabies. *N Engl J Med*. 1995;332:612.
17. Caumes E, Carrière J, Guermonprez G, et al. Dermatoses associated with travel to tropical countries: a prospective study of the diagnosis and management of 269 patients presenting to a tropical disease unit. *Clin Infect Dis*. 1995;20:542-548.
18. Beaver PC. Larva migrans: a review. *Exp Parasitol*. 1956;5:587-621.
19. Chaudhry AZ, Lonworth DL. Cutaneous manifestations of intestinal helminthic infections. *Dermatol Clin*. 1989;7:275-290.
20. Davies HD, Sakuls P, Keystone JS. Creeping eruption: a review of clinical presentation and management of 60 cases presenting to a tropical disease unit. *Arch Dermatol*. 1993;129:588-591.
21. Jelineck T, Maiwald H, Northdurft HD, Loscher T. Cutaneous larva migrans in travelers: synopsis of histories, symptoms and treatment of 98 patients. *Clin Infect Dis*. 1994;19:1062-1066.

22. Caumes E. Treatment of cutaneous larva migrans. *Clin Infect Dis.* 2000; 30:811-814.

23. Davis CM, Israel RM. Treatment of creeping eruption with topical thiabendazole. *Arch Dermatol.* 1968;97:325-326.

24. Katz R, Hood WR. Topical thiabendazole for creeping eruption. *Arch Dermatol.* 1966;94:643-645.

25. Katz R, Ziegler J, Blank H. The natural course of creeping eruption and treatment with thiabendazole. *Arch Dermatol.* 1965;91:420-424.

26. Jacksonville Dermatology Society. Creeping eruption treated with thiabendazole. *Arch Dermatol.* 1965;91:425-426.

27. Stone OJ, Mullins JF. Thiabendazole effectiveness in creeping eruption. *Arch Dermatol.* 1965;91:427-429.

28a. Caumes E. Treatment of cutaneous larva migrans. *Clin Infect Dis.* 2000; 30:811-814.

28. Thomas J, Lugagne J, Rosso AM, et al. Traitement de la dermatite vermineuse rampante par le ÿhiabendazole (à propos de 50 cas). *Marseille Med.* 1969;9:718-721.

29. Vakil BJ, Bandisode MS, Gaitonde BB, et al. Clinical trials with a new antihelminthic, thiabendazole. *J Trop Med Hyg.* 1955;58:287-295.

30. Coulaud JP, Binet D, Voyer C, et al. Traitement du syndrome de larva migrans cutanée "larbish" par l'albendazole: à propos de 18 observations. *Bull Soc Pathol Exot Filiales.* 1982;75:534-537.

31. Wlliams HC, Monk B. Creeping eruption stopped in its tracks by albendazole. *Clin Exp Dermatol.* 1989;14:355-356.

32. Orihuela AR, Torres JR. Single dose of albendazole in the treatment of cutaneous larva migrans. *Arch Dermatol.* 1990;126:398-399.

33. Jones SK, Reynolds NJ, Oliwiecki S, Harman RRM. Oral albendazole for the treatment of cutaneous larva migrans. *Br J Dermatol.* 1990;122:99-101.

34. Sanguigni S, Marangi M, Teggi A, De Rosa F. Albendazole in the therapy of cutaneous larva migrans. *Trans R Soc Trop Med Hyg.* 1990;84:831.

35. Pungpak S, Bunnag D, Chindanond D, Radmoyos B. Albendazole in the treatment of strongyloidiasis. *Southeast Asian J Trop Public Health.* 1987;18: 202-207.

36. Caumes E, Carrière J, Datry A, et al. A randomized trial of ivermectin versus albendazole for the treatment of cutaneous larva migrans. *Am J Trop Med Hyg.* 1993;49:641-644.

37. Goa KL, McTavish D, Clissold SD. Ivermectin: a review of its antifilarial activity, pharmacokinetic properties and clinical efficacy in onchocerciasis. *Drugs.* 1991;42:640-658.

CHAPTER

Onchocerciasis

65

Chinwe Laura Onyekonwu
Gladys Angela Ozoh
Uche Rowland Ojinmah

KEY POINTS

- Onchocerciasis is a chronic, disabling vector-borne disease caused by infestation with the filarial nematode worm *Onchocerca volvulus* that not only leads to physical and psychosocial sequelae, but also causes profound socioeconomic problems.

- An estimated 37 million people are afflicted, especially in sub-Saharan Africa, with Nigeria accounting for about one-third of the world's cases.

- Clinical presentation reflects variations in a host's immune response to the parasite.

- The classic lesion is the onchocercoma, a firm, painless nodule that occurs in the subcutaneous tissue.

- Most of the burden of the skin disease occurs as a result of severe, intolerable pruritus.

- Mass treatment with ivermectin in affected communities has been highly successful in reducing the disease burden.

- There remains a need for sustainability of control measures to maintain the gains in management of the disease.

Onchocerciasis (river blindness) is a vector-borne parasitic disease caused by the filarial nematode worm, *Onchocerca volvulus*. Infection is acquired through the bite of the insect vector, blackflies of the genus *Simulium*, which breed in fast-flowing streams and rivers. Members of the *Simulium damnosum* complex are the major vectors in Africa, whereas numerous other species are vectors of the disease in Latin America.[1] People residing in rural areas near fast-flowing rivers and streams have the highest risk of acquiring onchocerciasis. Although the disease occurs in Yemen and in six countries in Central and South America, 99% of the disease occurs in 27 sub-Saharan African countries stretching between 15°N and 14°S, from Senegal in the west to Ethiopia in the east, where it causes blindness and skin disease.[2]

Onchocerciasis is a chronic, disabling disease that is a major public health problem and an even more profound socioeconomic problem that extends beyond the infected individual, affecting families, communities, and countries as a whole.[1] It results in significant morbidity, psychosocial problems, and reduction in quality of life of those affected. Impaired social interaction, low morale, stigmatization, and the socioeconomic impact of the disease must be emphasized. The manifestations of the disease have resulted in abandonment of vast areas of fertile land and a poor attitude with regard to work. The disease has led to the collapse and desertion of families and vast communities and is one of the top five causes of blindness in the world, ranking second to trachoma as a cause of infectious blindness.[3,4]

Estimates indicate that 37 million individuals, mostly in tropical Africa, are infected.[5,6] Nigeria accounts for about one-third of the world's cases of onchocerciasis, and 60% of the cases occur in West Africa, with 18 to 20 million persons at risk of infection, 7.9 million affected, and 200,000 blind from the disease.[7] O'Neill first reported the presence of filariae in cases of "craw-craw," as onchocerciasis is called in West Africa, in 1875. The term *Onchocerca* is derived from the Greek word *ogkos*, meaning "swelling or mass," and *kerkos*, meaning "tail."[8]

Clinical presentations of onchocerciasis reflect variations in the host's immune response to the parasite, and these range from endemic normal individuals (putatively immune) who are disease free and have a good cellular immune response to the parasite, to individuals with low cellular immunity (with or without generalized onchodermatitis) and significant immune tolerance to millions of microfilariae with tissue damage progressing over many years. Individuals with a strong antibody response and hyperreactive onchodermatitis and human immunodeficiency virus (HIV)-positive patients with a weakened antibody response make up the other groups of susceptible individuals. Geographic variation in the clinical picture of individuals with onchocerciasis also occurs and may be related to vector biting habits. Most of the burden of onchocercal skin disease is due to severe intolerable pruritus. The cutaneous manifestations of onchocerciasis are discussed in this chapter.

EPIDEMIOLOGY

The epidemiology of onchocerciasis is determined by several factors including the host's response, parasite and vector competence, the geographic environment (proximity of the home or dwelling to fly breeding sites), and social and demographic influences; even in the same geographic area, onchocerciasis has distinctly variable endemic rates.

Genetic variations in populations exist among the different foci of onchocerciasis worldwide and affect the biology of the parasites.[1] The parasite and the blackfly vector have reciprocal effects on each other's survival at various stages of the parasite's life cycle.[9] The strains of the parasite evidently differ in their pathogenicity and distribution in the human body.[10]

In West African savannah (nonforest) areas, ocular involvement is common and affects the anterior segment of the eye, leading to severe blindness, although the posterior eye segment may also be involved.[11] Conversely, onchocercal skin disease occurs in the African forest areas where ocular disease is infrequent and, when it occurs, usually involves the posterior eye segment. Lymphatic involvement and skin manifestations (eg, pruritus, chronic papular dermatitis, nodules, depigmentation) are more common in the rainforest than in the savannah. In fact, concentrations of dermal microfilariae have been shown to be 50% higher in the savannah than in the forest, but the number of palpable nodules in the forest communities was 50% higher than in the savannah.[12]

ETIOLOGY AND PATHOGENESIS

O. volvulus is a parasitic filarial nematode worm belonging to the family Filarioidea whose five-stage life cycle occurs in two different hosts: blackflies (the obligate intermediate host) and humans (the only natural vertebrate host). However, infection of nonhuman primates such as the chimpanzee is likely. The life cycle of *O. volvulus* is depicted in **Figure 65-1**.

Blackflies of the genus *Simulium*, which are tiny ferocious biters, are the only vectors of *O. volvulus*. At least 15 different species of blackflies can transmit onchocerciasis, and they vary by terrain and continent (eg, *S. damnosum* in Africa). Their eggs require fast-running rivers for breeding grounds. *Simulium* bites by day and can make long wind-assisted flights covering several kilometers. Infection occurs when a blackfly introduces an *O. volvulus* stage 3 larva (L_3) into the host during a blood meal (Figure 65-1). These immature larval forms of the parasite create nodules in subcutaneous tissues where they molt to the L_4 and juvenile adult stages within 1 to 2 months, whereas mature adult worms capable of producing microfilariae develop within 10 to 15 months of infection. Development to the adult stage occurs in humans. The adult worms pair and mate in the human host, and unlike most nematodes that produce eggs, the female *Onchocerca* gives birth daily to thousands of microscopic larvae known as *microfilariae*. These larvae mature into adult worms in about 1 year.

The life span of microfilariae is 6 to 30 months, in contrast to the adult female worm life span, which is 2 to 15 years.[13,14] The microfilariae move throughout the body, and when they die, they cause a variety of symptoms and signs, including a dermatitis, nodular lesions, pigmentary alterations, edema, and severe itching. The inflammatory response against dying microfilariae over years of repeated infection causes

gradual and eventually blinding sclerosal opacification of the anterior eye by local inflammation and of the posterior eye by an autoimmune mechanisms.[15] Apart from blindness, a high microfilaria load has been identified as a factor reducing the life span of infected individuals.[16]

A rickettsial bacterium, *Wolbachia* was discovered in the late 1990s to exist in a symbiotic relationship with *O. volvulus*, inhabiting the endodermis of female *O. volvulus* worms and various stages of its intrauterine embryos, and appears to have coevolved with *Onchocerca*.[17] The basis of the symbiosis is thought to be metabolic, although a possible role for *Wolbachia* in immune evasion has received little attention.[18] *Wolbachia* also contributes to the clinical presentation of filarial infections since bacterial products released from both living and dead worms activate the mammalian innate immune system, triggering the release of pro-inflammatory mediators.[18]

CLINICAL FINDINGS

Onchocerciasis is characterized by dermal, lymphatic, and ocular manifestations. The classic lesion of onchocerciasis is the onchocercoma, a subdermal nodule most often seen over bony prominences on the head, scapular girdle, ribs, pelvic girdle, trochanters, knees, and ankles that contains encapsulated adult worms, usually two or three with daughter microfilariae. Nodules may vary in size from as small as 0.2 cm in diameter to as large as 6.0 cm and occasionally even larger. Removal of these nodules historically formed the core strategy of control programs in Mexico and Guatemala.[19] However, some studies have suggested that considerable numbers of female worms are hidden in deep-lying, non-visible nodules, which may be sufficient to maintain a large population of microfilariae in the skin and eyes.[20,21]

Onchocercomas are often found over the bony prominences of the torso and hips in Africans, whereas in South Americans, where it is sometimes called *Robles disease*,[22] the predominant strains characteristically produce nodules on the head and shoulders.[23] Cases of onchocercoma presenting as a breast mass[24] or as deep nodules in the pelvis[25] have been described. An angiogenic protein produced by the adult female is

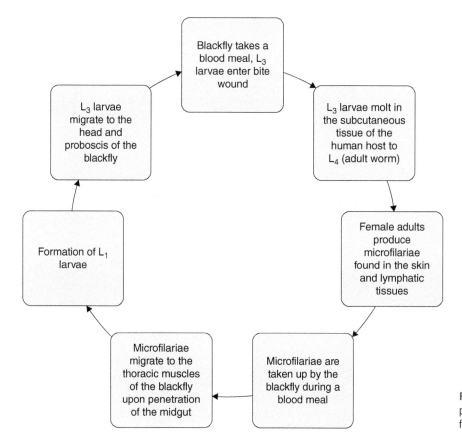

FIGURE 65-1. Life cycle of *Onchocerca volvulus*. (Used with permission from the World Health Organization/African Programme for Onchocerciasis.)

believed to play a role in the formation of the nodules. Each adult worm is estimated to produce 1600 microfilariae per day.[26] The presence of onchocercomata does not correlate with microfilarial load.[25] A risk factor for onchocerciasis infection in children in endemic areas, apart from exposure to infected blackflies, may be maternal onchocercal infection during the gestational period.[27]

The most common skin presentation of onchocerciasis is a diffuse papular dermatitis, often with intense pruritus with geographic variation in the exact clinical presentation. These variations occur due to such factors as variability in host response, parasite strain, and biting habits of different *Simulium* vector species. Onchocercal dermatitis is usually associated with the presence of microfilariae in the skin and is typically generalized and symmetrical.[1] Recently infected patients often demonstrate a strong T-helper 1 (T_H1)-type immune response, whereas in those with chronic disease, the cutaneous manifestations can be differentiated across a spectrum, from pruritic lichenification on one end to asymptomatic depigmentation (the "leopard skin" pattern) on the other.[28]

Systemic manifestations of onchocerciasis may also occur and can present as weight loss, musculoskeletal pain, and inguinal hernias.

CLASSIFICATION

Broadly, cutaneous manifestations of onchocerciasis may be classified into early and late lesions [**Table 65-1**]. Several other classifications for onchocercal dermatitis are in existence, but Murdoch et al[29] developed

TABLE 65-1   Clinical features of cutaneous onchocerciasis
Symptoms
Pruritus
• Severe pruritus, the most distressing clinical manifestation, interferes with the ability to sleep, work, farm, or interact socially.
• The itching may be so severe that patients scratch with twigs, stones, and knives, resulting in bleeding wounds, sores, and pain.[7]
Emotional disturbance
• Agitation, emotional disturbances, and stigmatization may drive the victim to suicide.[8]
Signs
• Itching may be mild and intermittent or severe and continuous, leading to superficial excoriation, crusts, secondary infection, and ulceration.
• **Early skin lesions (onchodermatitis)**
• Urticaria
• Macules
• Papules
• Pustules
• Subcutaneous edema including swelling of limbs or groin area
• Scaling
• Lichenification
• Lymphadenopathy (particularly in the inguinal and femoral region)
• Cellulitis, lymphangitis, and lymphadenitis
• Excoriations
• Nodules (onchocercomata) found over bony prominences
• Sowda (intensely itchy localized papules, pustules, pachydermia, and darkening of the skin seen in chronic hyperreactive onchodermatitis)
• **Late skin lesions**
• Atrophy (shiny, fragile skin described as "lizard skin")
• Dermal scarring and loss of elasticity
• Loose and hanging skin (face: leonine facies; axilla and groin: hanging groin)
• Spotty depigmentation over the shin (leopard skin; see Figure 65-5)
• Genital elephantiasis
• Elephantiasis of the limbs (associated with sowda)

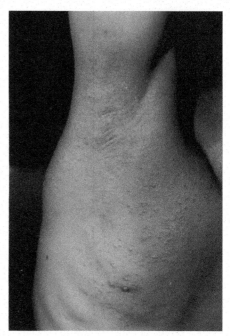

A

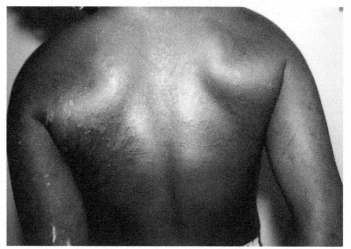

B

FIGURE 65-2. (A) Acute papular onchodermatitis in a young African boy. **(B)** Acute papular onchodermatitis on the back.

a classification scheme for standardization and comparison of surveys conducted from different parts of the world. This classification describes five main categories of onchocercal dermatitis: (1) acute papular onchodermatitis [**Figure 65-2, A and B**], (2) chronic papular onchodermatitis [**Figure 65-3**], (3) lichenified onchodermatitis/sowda [**Figure 65-4**], (4) atrophy, and (5) depigmentation [**Figure 65-5**], with activity, severity (presence of itching or excoriation), and distribution grading as appropriate. Other associated features include lymphadenopathy, lymphedema, onchocercoma [**Figure 65-6**], and hanging groin.

It has been found that patients with onchocerciasis have a higher possibility of converting to HIV positivity than do those without onchocerciasis when exposed to the HIV virus, and treatment of onchocerciasis in HIV-infected patients may reduce viral replication.[30]

DIFFERENTIAL DIAGNOSIS

The differential diagnosis of cutaneous onchocerciasis varies by the clinical manifestations of the disease. **Table 65-2** outlines differential diagnoses by manifestation.

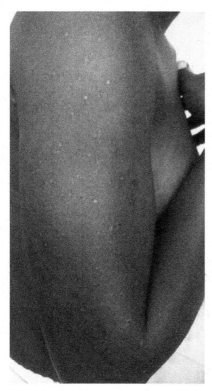

FIGURE 65-3. Chronic papular onchodermatitis on the upper limb.

LABORATORY DIAGNOSIS

Diagnostic tests include skin snip microscopy for microfilariae, which lacks sensitivity, and the diethylcarbamazine (DEC) patch test.[30] Newer biochemical methods include skin-snip polymerase chain reaction, enzyme-linked immunosorbent assays, enzyme immunoassays, and antigen surveys. Recent developments include antibody-based rapid diagnostic tests.[31] Microfilariae may be seen on slit-lamp examination of the cornea and anterior chamber of the eye.

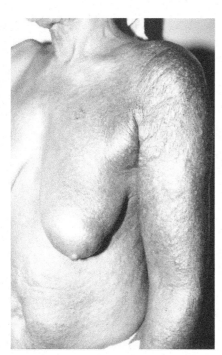

FIGURE 65-4. Lichenified onchodermatitis.

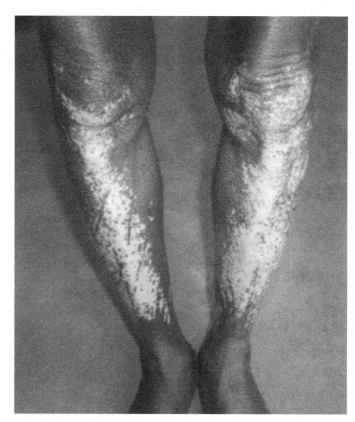

FIGURE 65-5. Bilateral onchocercal depigmentation (leopard skin).

COMPLICATIONS

Complications include secondary bacterial infection, cellulitis, lymphangitis or recurrent lymphangitis, and blindness in the eruptive phase.

TREATMENT

The African Programme for Onchocerciasis (APOC) was launched by the World Health Organization (WHO) for distribution of ivermectin (Mectizan) following the discovery and approval of the microfilaricidal drug. APOC currently covers 19 endemic countries in Africa. Ivermectin is given at a dose of 100 to 150 μg/kg every 3 months, every 6 months, or yearly, depending on symptoms, until the adult worms die (about 10 to 15 years).

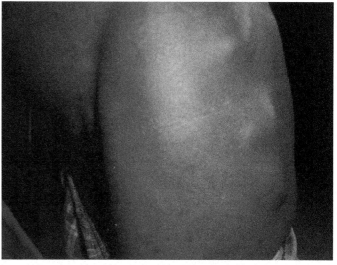

FIGURE 65-6. Multiple onchocercal nodules on the greater trochanter area.

TABLE 65-2 Differential diagnosis of cutaneous onchocerciasis
Manifestation:
Localized nodules
• Epidermoid cyst
• Juxta-articular nodules
• Fibroma
• Lipoma
• Podoconiosis
Generalized eruptive rash
• Pyoderma
• Dermatitis herpetiformis
• Pityriasis lichenoides chronic
• Urticaria
• Lichen planus
• Tinea incognito
• Drug eruption
• Scabies
• Secondary syphilis
• Lichen simplex chronicus
• Chronic idiopathic urticaria

DEC, given at a dose of 25 to 50 mg three times a day and increased weekly by 25 mg up to 100 mg, is no longer recommended due to the severe reactions (Mazzotti reaction) that arise as a result of destruction of microfilariae. Suramin, a drug that targets adult worms, is given at a dose of 4 g over 6 weeks for adults over 60 kg, starting with a test dose of 0.2 g, but it is toxic and is rarely used now.

Amocarzine has been investigated as an oral onchocercacidal drug. Targeting endosymbiotic *Wolbachia* species with doxycycline therapy (100 to 200 mg/d for 6 weeks) has shown promising results.[32] An antiparasitic drug, moxidectin is currently being studied by the WHO for use in onchocerciasis.[33] Nodulectomy, with or without ivermectin, may be undertaken for cosmetic purposes.

CONTROL AND PREVENTION

Great progress has been made in the last 30 years in the control of onchocerciasis both in Africa and in the Americas, largely due to international public and private partnerships, sustained funding of regional programs, and new tools and technology. Until the advent of ivermectin, larvicidal campaigns against the insect vector were the only practical approach for onchocerciasis control. The insecticides used were effective against the vectors but safe for the remainder of the environment because they were biodegradable. They included the organophosphates temephos, chlorphoxin, and pyracolos. Although dichlorodiphenyltrichloroethane (DDT) was relatively cheap, it later fell out of favor because of its persistence in the environment and fears of toxicity. Newer larvicides in use include biocides such as *Bacillus thuringiensis* sp. *isrealensis*[34] (serotype BT H14). This bacterium infects and kills mosquitos and blackfly larvae. Vector reinvasion was a problem, but expanding the zones of application of larvicidal agents, supplemented by mass ivermectin chemotherapy, has been a successful strategy. With the phasing out of the Onchocercal Control Programme (OCP) and the mass distribution of ivermectin, the Mectizan Expert Committee and the Mectizan Donation Program were able to organize and promote distribution of the drug.

A unique global partnership was launched in 1995 by the APOC (among 19 endemic African countries), WHO, the World Bank, and afflicted communities with the following objective: "To establish, within a period of 12 years, effective and self-sustainable, community-directed treatment with ivermectin throughout the remaining endemic areas in Africa and to eliminate the disease by vector control in selected foci."[35,36]

However, over the years, constraints to the sustainability of ivermectin distribution[37] have been identified as a threat to the gains achieved in the prevention and treatment of the disease.

REFERENCES

1. Rodriguez-Perez MA, Unnasch TR, Real-Najarro O. Assessment and monitoring of onchocerciasis. *Adv Parasitol.* 2011;77:175-226.
2. World Health Organization: Onchocerciasis and its control. Report of a WHO Expert Committee on Onchocerciasis Control. *World Health Organ Tech Rep Ser.* 1995;852:1-104.
3. Etyáale D. Onchocerciasis and trachoma control: what has changed in the past two decades? *Community Eye Health.* 2008;21:43-45.
4. Hotez PJ, Bottazzi ME, Franco-Parades C, et al. The neglected tropical diseases of Latin America and the Caribbean: a review of disease burden and distribution and a roadmap for control and elimination. *PLoS Negl Trop Dis.* 2008;2:e300.
5. African Programme for Onchocerciasis Control, APOC. Final Communiqué of the 11th Session of the Joint Action Forum of APOC, Paris, France. Ouagadougou, Burkina Faso: APOC; 2005.
6. Basánez MG, Pion SD, Churcher TS, et al. River blindness: a success story under threat? *PLoS Med.* 2006;3:e371.
7. Edungbola L. The status of human onchocerciasis in Kainji reservoir basin areas 20 years after the impoundment of the lake. *Trop Geogr Med.* 1986;38:263-270.
8. Brown L, Huges AM, Sykes J, et al, eds. *The New Shorter Oxford English Dictionary on Historical Principles.* Oxford, England: Oxford University Press; 1993.
9. Basánez MG, Churcher TS, Grillet ME. *Onchocerca-Simulium* interactions and the population and evolutionary biology of *Onchocerca volvulus. Adv Parasitol.* 2009;68:263-313.
10. Duke BO, Lewis DJ, Moore PJ. *Onchocerca Simulium* complexes. I Transmission of forest and Sudan-savannah strains of *Onchocerca volvulus*, from Cameroon, by *Simulium damnosum* from various West African bioclimatic zones. *Ann Trop Med Parasitol.* 1966;60:318-326.
11. Remme J, Dadzie KY, Rolland A, et al. Ocular onchocerciasis and intensity of infection in the community. I. West African Savannah. *Trop Med Parasitol.* 1989;40:340.
12. Anderson J, Fuglsang H, Hamilton PJ, et al. Studies on onchocerciasis in the United Cameroon Republic I. Comparison of populations with and without *Onchocerca volvulus. Trans R Soc Trop Med Hyg.* 1974;68:190-208.
13. Somorin AO. Onchocerciasis. *Int J Dermatol.* 1983;22:182-188.
14. Karam M, Schulz-Key H, Remme J. Population dynamics of *Onchocerca volvulus* after 7 to 8 years of vector control in West Africa. *Acta Trop.* 1987;44:445-457.
15. Hall LR, Pearlman E. Pathogenesis of onchocercal keratitis (river blindness). *Clin Microbiol Rev.* 1999;12:445-453.
16. Little MP, Breitling LP, Basanez MG, et al. Association between microfilarial load and excess mortality in onchocerciasis: an epidemiological study. *Lancet.* 2004;363:1514-1521.
17. Brattig NW. Pathogenesis and host responses in human onchocerciasis: impact of *Onchocerca* filariae and *Wolbachia* endobacteria. *Microbes Infect.* 2004;6:113-128.
18. Hansen RDE, Trees AJ, Bah GS, et al. A worm's best friend :recruitment of neutrophils by *Wolbachia* confounds eosinophil degranulation against the filarial nematode *Onchocerca ochengi. Proc R Soc B.* 2011;278:2293-2302.
19. Rodriguez-Perez MA, Rivas-Alcala AR. Problems in the investigation of the control of *Onchocerca volvulus* in Mexico. *Salud Publica Mex.* 1991;33:493-503.
20. Schulz-Key H. Observations on the reproductive biology of *Onchocerca volvulus. Acta Leiden.* 1990;59:27-44.
21. Duke BO. Human onchocerciasis: an overview of the disease. *Acta Leiden.* 1990;59:9-24.
22. World Health Organization. Onchocerciasis (river blindness). Report from the Tenth InterAmerican Conference on Onchocerciasis, Guayaquil, Ecuador. *Wkly Epidemiol Rec.* 2001;76:205-212.
23. Wolf R, Orion E, Matz H. Onchocerciasis (river blindness). *Isr Med Assoc J.* 2003;5:522-523.
24. Zavieh K, McCarthur C, Eswaran SL, et al. *Onchocerca volvulus* breast mass: case report from Cameroon and literature review. *Mo Med.* 2004;101:608-610.
25. Okulicz JF, Stibich AS, Elston DM, et al. Cutaneous onchocercoma. *Int J Dermatol.* 2004;43:170-172.

26. Mawson AR, WaKabongo M. Onchocerciasis-associated morbidity: hypothesis. *Trans R Soc Trop Med Hyg.* 2002;96:541-542.

27. Kirch AK, Duerr HP, Boatin B, et al. Impact of parental onchocerciasis and intensity of transmission on development and persistence of *Onchocerca volvulus* infection in offspring: an 18 year follow-up study. *Parasitology.* 2003;127:327-335.

28. Timmann C, Abraha RS, Hamelmann C, et al. Cutaneous pathology in onchocerciasis associated with pronounced systemic T-helper 2-type responses to *Onchocerca volvulus. Br J Dermatol.* 2003;149:782-787.

29. Murdoch ME, Hay RJ, Mackenzie CD, et al. A clinical classification and grading system of the cutaneous changes in onchocerciasis. *Br J Dermatol.* 1993;129:260-269.

30. Ozoh G, Boussinesq M, Bissek AZ, et al. Evaluation of the diethylcarbamazine patch to evaluate onchocerciasis endemicity in Central Africa. *Trop Med Int Health.* 2007;12:123-129.

31. Udall DN. Recent updates on onchocerciasis: diagnosis and treatment. *Clin Infect Dis.* 2007;44:53-60.

32. Hoerauf A, Mand S, Volkmann L, et al. Doxycycline in the treatment of human onchocerciasis: kinetics of *Wolbachia* endobacteria reduction and of inhibition of embryogenesis in female Onchocerca worms. *Microbes Infect.* 2003;5:261-273.

33. TDR for Research on Diseases of Poverty. A new drug for onchocerciasis. http://www.who.int/tdr/research/ntd/onchocerciasis/moxidectin/en/index.html. Accessed January 15, 2013.

34. Hougard JM, Back C. Perspectives on the bacterial control of vectors in the tropics. *Paristol Today.* 1992;8:364-368.

35. APOC/WHO Website. Country profiles. http://www.who.int/apoc/countries/en/. Accessed January 15, 2013.

36. Seketeli A, Adeoye G, Eyamba A, et al. The achievements and challenges of the African Programme for Onchocerciasis Control (APOC). *Ann Trop Med Parasitol.* 2002;96:S15-S28.

37. Abiose A, Homeida M, Lisse B, et al. Onchocerciasis control strategies. *Lancet.* 2000;356:1523.

CHAPTER

66

Leprosy

Rie Roselyne Yotsu
Norihisa Ishii
Shobita Rajagopalan

KEY POINTS

- Leprosy is a mycobacterial infection that affects the skin and the peripheral nerves.

- There are over 200,000 new cases of leprosy diagnosed every year around the world.

- Various skin symptoms are associated with the disease depending on the immune reaction of the host (patient), including hypopigmentation, erythema, and nodules.

- Multidrug therapy, which is a combination of dapsone, rifampicin, and clofazimine, effectively cures the disease and is recommended as the first-line therapy by the World Health Organization.

- Deformities as a consequence of the disease lead to social discrimination and stigma and, hence, the need for early detection and treatment.

Leprosy is a chronic bacterial infection caused by the intracellular microorganism *Mycobacterium leprae*. The bacteria have affinity for the peripheral nerves and skin, resulting in neuropathy and skin symptoms, which are cardinal manifestations of the disease. The diagnosis of this disease may be a challenge due to a wide variety of manifestations that are determined by the interplay between the bacilli and host immune responses, which eventually determine the clinical spectrum of the disease. If not treated early, the progressive nature of this chronic infectious disease may cause deformities of the face and limbs, loss of eyesight, and other long-term complications.

EPIDEMIOLOGY

Leprosy is seen most commonly in people with skin of color predominantly in developing countries in tropical and subtropical regions including India, Brazil, and Indonesia.[1] Socioeconomic factors, including poverty, overcrowding, and poor sanitation, are known to play a significant role in the increased disease prevalence in these regions.

Sporadic cases encountered in developed nations often occur among immigrants from countries where the disease is endemic.

ETIOLOGY AND PATHOGENESIS

M. leprae, the lepra bacillus, an acid-fast organism, was first discovered by G.H. Armauer Hansen in the year 1873. The organism is approximately 0.2 μm in width and 8 μm in length [**Figure 66-1**]. It grows best at a temperature around 31°C; thus, it thrives in cooler areas of the body such as the earlobes, nose, and testicles, and areas where the peripheral nerves are close to the skin. It is a slow-growing organism that needs 11 to 13 days to multiply. Otherwise, many of the characteristics of the bacilli are still unknown because the organism cannot be cultured in any laboratory media. In animal models, limited multiplication can be observed in the nude mouse foot pads.[2]

Nonetheless, recent advances in genome sequencing have contributed to the better knowledge of the disease. The first genome sequence of *M. leprae*, completed in 2001, revealed that only half of the small genome contains protein-coding genes, whereas the remainder consists of pseudogenes and noncoding regions.[3] The number of pseudogenes is much larger in the *M. leprae* genome compared to other mycobacteria.[4] Despite this genetic damage, a specialized intracellular environment free from evolutionary competition with other pathogens has allowed the organism to survive.[3,5,6]

The incubation period of leprosy typically ranges from 1 to 5 years, although this continues to be debated. Some experts argue that the incubation period can vary from several months to 30 years.[7,8] The mode of transmission is not yet clear, but it is commonly known to occur via nasal and oral droplets from the bacilliferous patients, or less commonly, through breaks in the skin.[9,10] Close and repeated contact with these patients is a source of transmission. Upon multidrug therapy treatment, however, infectivity is quickly eliminated.

Once *M. leprae* bacilli gain entry into the host, they have an affinity for neural tissue, especially the Schwann cells, as well as skin. The subsequent manifestations of leprosy that ensue depend on host immune responses, which will be discussed in the following section.

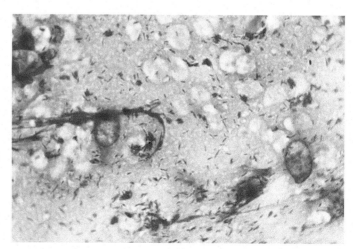

FIGURE 66-1. *Mycobacterium leprae* (skin slit smear, Ziehl-Neelsen stain, ×1000).

TABLE 66-1	Classification of leprosy
Ridley-Jopling classification	
TT = tuberculoid leprosy	
LL = lepromatous leprosy	
BT = borderline tuberculoid leprosy	
BL = borderline lepromatous leprosy	
BB = mid-borderline leprosy	
I = indeterminate leprosy	
World Health Organization classification	
PB = paucibacillary	
MB = multibacillary	

CLASSIFICATION OF LEPROSY

A range of clinical, bacteriologic, and histologic findings are found in leprosy depending on the immune response of a patient to *M. leprae*. In 1966, Ridley and Jopling[11] focused on this characteristic and classified leprosy into six types [**Tables 66-1 and 66-2**]. Infection with *M. leprae* may produce a localized disease in a partially resistant patient, namely, the *tuberculoid type* (TT), and a disseminated generalized disease in a highly susceptible patient with little or no immunity, namely, the *lepromatous leprosy type* (LL). A disease spectrum between these two polar varieties is referred to as the *borderline forms*, which consist of borderline tuberculoid (BT), mid-borderline (BB), and borderline lepromatous (BL). Classification of borderline forms is based on the different degrees in which the patient resembles the characteristics of the polar varieties (TT and LL). The polar varieties are immunologically stable, whereas the borderline forms are immunologically unstable and progress to either a gradual decline toward the lepromatous pole or improvement toward the tuberculoid pole. An *indeterminate* form (I), which consists of the development of an early lesion before the disease becomes active, can be self-healed or may develop to any of the other forms of leprosy.

Another classification for leprosy, which is more practical to use at field level and to facilitate treatment, has been developed by the World Health Organization (WHO) and consists of just two categories [Tables 66-1 and 66-2]. It classifies patients by the number of lesions; those with

five or fewer skin lesions are classified as having the paucibacillary (PB) form, and those with six or more lesions are classified as having the multibacillary (MB) form. As for the correlation between the two classification systems, I, TT, and part of BT are generally equivalent to PB, and part of BT, BB, BL, and LL are equivalent to MB.

Very rarely, patients present with disease that solely involves the nerves, without any skin lesions, and this form is known as *pure neuritic leprosy* (PNL).

The different manifestations of infection due to the same bacilli depend on the immunity of the host against *M. leprae*. Furthermore, there is a strong relationship between clinical manifestations and cytokine profiles within the skin lesions. T-helper (T_H) 1 cytokines secreted by the T_H cells, such as interleukin (IL)-2, interferon-γ, and tumor necrosis factor, play important roles in cellular immune responses in PB/TT. These cytokines stimulate the number and activity of macrophages and maintain inflammation. On the other hand, T_H2 cytokines, including IL-4, IL-5, and IL-10, augment humoral immune responses that suppress macrophage activity and allow the bacilli to proliferate. This immune response predominates in MB/LL. Thus, there is an inverse correlation in the cytokine profiles that create the basis of PB/TT and MB/LL leprosy.

INDICATION OF LEPROSY

When leprosy is suspected, it is essential to determine the presence of the eight characteristics listed below. Once leprosy is confirmed, these characteristics may assist in determining the correct classification.

1. Number of skin lesions
2. Distribution and symmetry of skin lesions
3. Definition and clarity of skin lesions
4. Hypoesthesia and anesthesia
5. Loss of sweating and reduced hair growth
6. Distribution, extent, and nature of peripheral nerve involvement
7. Mucosal and systemic involvement
8. Number of *M. leprae* bacilli

▣ TUBERCULOID LEPROSY (TT/PB)

TT affects skin and peripheral nerves [**Figure 66-2**]. Skin lesions are single with sharp borders. They may be macules or plaques. The lesions are hypoesthetic or definitely anesthetic, where the skin sensory innervation compensates for the damage. Autonomic nerve damage within the lesions is often severe; the skin texture is rough and dry. By usual methods of examination, no *M. leprae* can be found in TT.

In histopathology, a dermal granulomatous infiltrate is seen that may have a linear pattern as it follows the course of a nerve. Epithelioid cells and Langhans giant cells are surrounded by lymphocytes. The cutaneous nerves are edematous, and there is an absence of the bacilli.

TABLE 66-2	Summary of classification and characteristics of leprosy	
WHO Classification	**Paucibacillary (PB)**	**Multibacillary (MB)**
Ridley-Jopling classification	(I) TT	(B) LL ⋀ BT BB BL
Cellular immunity against *M. leprae*	Good	Poor/No
Dominant T cells and cytokines	T_H1, IL-2, IFN-γ, IL-12	T_H2, IL-4, IL-5, IL-10
Slit skin smear	Negative	Positive
Skin lesions		
Number	Few	Many
Size	Variable	Small
Surface	Dry	Shiny
Sensation	Absent	Slightly diminished
Hair	Absent	Not affected initially
Histology	Epithelioid cells Nerve destruction Sarcoid-like granuloma	Foam cells Xanthoma-like Acid-fast bacilli
Infectious	No	Yes

Abbreviations: B, Borderline; BT, Borderline tuberculoid leprosy; BB, Borderline Borderline leprosy; BL, Borderline lepromatous leprosy; I, indeterminate leprosy; IFN-γ, interferon-γ; IL, interleukin; LL, lepromatous leprosy; T_H, T helper; TT, tuberculoid leprosy; WHO, World Health Organization.

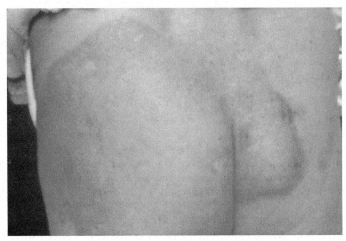

FIGURE 66-2. Tuberculoid leprosy. Single anesthetic plaque on the buttocks.

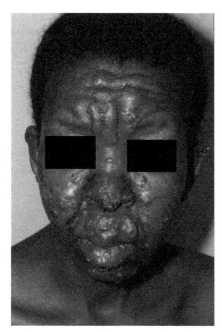

FIGURE 66-3. Lepromatous leprosy. Extensive papules, nodules, and plaques. Note loss of eyebrows. (Used with permission from Barbara Leppard.)

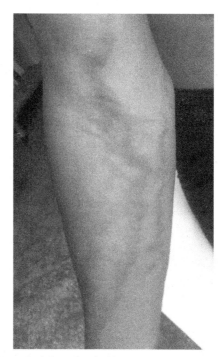

FIGURE 66-4. Borderline tuberculoid leprosy. Anesthetic annular erythema with satellite lesions on the arm.

LEPROMATOUS LEPROSY (LL/MB)

The early lesions of LL usually consist of macules or nodules that are widely and symmetrically distributed [**Figure 66-3**]. The surface may be shiny and moist. Touch and pin-prick sensation are usually unimpaired in early lepromatous macules, but sweating may be diminished. Hair, eyelashes, and eyebrows may be lost.

Histopathologic examination reveals a diffuse infiltrate of foamy histiocytes (macrophages) along with plasma cells and lymphocytes in the dermis. A band of normal-appearing dermis, called an Unna band or Grenz zone, separates the epidermis from the infiltrate. Bacilli can be observed anywhere in the dermis, but often, they are seen inside the histiocytes. When the patient is undergoing successful treatment, fragmented bacilli can be observed.

BORDERLINE TYPES

Skin manifestations and histopathologic findings in the borderline types contain both characteristics of TT/PB and LL/MB. When it more closely resembles TT/PB, it is diagnosed as borderline tuberculoid leprosy (BT) [**Figure 66-4**]; and when it more closely resembles LL/MB, it is diagnosed as borderline lepromatous leprosy (BL) [**Figure 66-5**]. In between conditions are diagnosed as mid-borderline leprosy (BB).

INDETERMINATE LEPROSY (I)

Indeterminate leprosy is an early and transitory stage of leprosy found in patients (usually children) whose immunologic status has yet to be determined. There is scattered nonspecific histiocytic and lymphocytic infiltration, histopathologically resembling leprosy.

PURE NEURITIC LEPROSY (PNL)

In the purely neural form of leprosy, there may be involvement and enlargement of one or more peripheral nerves without skin involvement. This form usually presents with signs and symptoms of nerve deficit, such as gradual weakness in the hand or a sudden foot drop or anesthesia in the extremity. The diagnosis usually can be made based on the presence of anesthetic skin and definite nerve enlargement.

DIAGNOSIS

There are three cardinal signs of leprosy: (1) loss or impairment of skin sensations, (2) thickening of the nerves, and (3) the presence of

M. leprae bacilli in slit skin smears from skin or biopsy materials. The sites where peripheral nerves are potentially palpable are shown in **Figure 66-6**.[12] The presence of one of the three signs is sufficient to establish a diagnosis.

Clinical diagnosis is confirmed by obtaining slit skin smears from affected areas of the body. Slit skin smears are the most important laboratory test used in the diagnosis and prognosis of leprosy. The epidermis is slit open to a depth of 2 to 3 mm using a very sharp sterile scalpel [**Figure 66-7**]. Care should be taken not to go deep and draw blood. The smear can be stained for acid-fast bacilli [Figure 66-1].

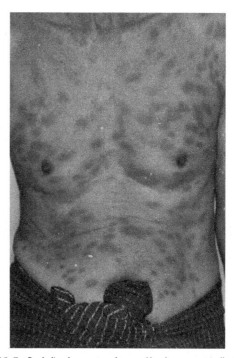

FIGURE 66-5. Borderline lepromatous leprosy. Macules symmetrically distributed on the trunk.

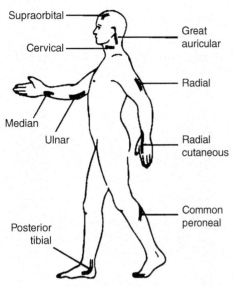

FIGURE 66-6. Sites to examine for peripheral nerve enlargement as described by Hastings RC and Opromolla DVA (*Leprosy*. 2nd ed. New York, NY: Churchill-Livingstone; 1994). (Used with permission from Marisol LLC, Muscat, Sultanate of Oman.)

Biopsy samples are subjected to acid-fast staining in addition to conventional histopathologic stains in order to demonstrate the presence of *M. leprae*; however, bacilli are not usually detected in PB patients. The presence of neural inflammation is a histologic characteristic of leprosy that can differentiate it from other granulomatous disorders. Polymerase chain reaction (PCR) is a sensitive method for the detection of *M. leprae* DNA that is widely used for diagnosis in advanced countries.[8,13,14]

▨ BACTERIOLOGIC INDEX

The evaluation of smears from each site is made according to grades 0 to 6. The average grade arrived at after examining the smears from the four sites is calculated to find the bacteriologic index (BI). The BI continues to be a valuable test to assess a patient's progress.

TREATMENT

▨ CHEMOTHERAPY

A common regimen for the treatment of both PB and MB leprosy is desirable. The WHO Technical Advisory Group recommends that all leprosy patients, both PB and MB, should be treated with a multidrug therapy (MDT) regimen for a period of 6 to 12 months.

MDT treatment may vary based on the age of the patient and the type of leprosy and is determined by bacilloscopy for number of lesions. **Table 66-3** outlines treatment for PB and MB leprosy recommended by the WHO. The treatment for PB patients includes daily doses of dapsone 100 mg and a monthly dose of rifampicin 600 mg over a 6-month

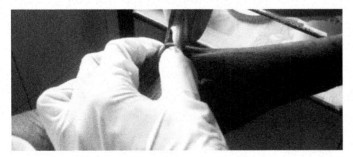

FIGURE 66-7. Slit skin smear.

TABLE 66-3	Treatment of leprosy with multidrug therapy (MDT)		
Multibacillary (MB) leprosy			
	Rifampicin	Dapsone	Clofazimine
Adult, 50–70 kg	600 mg/month*	100 mg/d	50 mg/d and 300 mg/month*
Child, 10–14 years	450 mg/month*	50 mg/d	50 mg/d and 150 mg/month*
Younger than 10	300 mg/month*	25 mg/d	50 mg twice a week and 100 mg/month*
Paucibacillary (PB) leprosy			
	Rifampicin	Dapsone	
Adult, 50–70 kg	600 mg/month*	100 mg/d	
Child 10–14 years	450 mg/month*	50 mg/d	
Younger than 10	300 mg/month*	25 mg/d	

*: Administered once monthly as a single dose.

period. MB patients are administered dapsone 100 mg and clofazimine 50 mg once a day in addition to monthly administration of rifampicin 600 mg and clofazimine 300 mg for 12 months. The WHO has designed two easy-to-use blister pack medication kits for PB and MB patients in developing countries. The kits contain enough medication for 28 days and are supplied at no cost to registered patients. Treatment is automatically terminated at the end of the prescribed regimen because, in public health terms, it is reasonable to conclude that transmission is unlikely after initiation of MDT. Many countries, however, prefer longer treatments, especially in MB cases.

Rifampicin is an effective bactericidal agent against *M. leprae* within a few days of administering a single 600-mg dose. Dapsone is bacteriostatic or weakly bactericidal against *M. leprae* and was the mainstay of leprosy treatment for many years until widespread resistant strains appeared. Clofazimine binds preferentially to mycobacterial DNA and exerts a slow bactericidal effect on *M. leprae* by inhibiting mycobacterial growth. Skin discoloration, ranging from red to black, is one of the most troublesome side effects of clofazimine, although the pigmentation fades slowly in most cases after withdrawal. A characteristic ichthyosis is also sometimes evident. Other effective chemotherapeutic agents against *M. leprae* include ofloxacin, minocycline, levofloxacin, sparfloxacin, moxifloxacin, and clarithromycin.[15]

▨ COMPLICATIONS AND LEPRA REACTIONS

There are two main types of complications: (1) those due to massive invasion of tissue by *M. leprae* and (2) those due to lepra reactions.

Lepra reactions are acute inflammatory complications that occur in treated or untreated leprosy and often present as medical emergencies in these patients. There are two major clinical types of lepra reactions that affect 30% to 50% of all leprosy patients.[16-18] Severe inflammation associated with these reactions results in nerve injury accompanied by subsequent loss of sensation, paralysis, and deformity. The different types of reactions appear to have different underlying immunologic mechanisms; however, the factors that initiate them are unknown. Reversal reactions (type 1 reactions) manifest as erythema and edema of dermal lesions and tender peripheral nerves with rapid loss of nerve function [**Figures 66-8 and 66-9**]. They generally occur during the first several months of treatment and occasionally after treatment.[19,20]

Erythema nodosum leprosum (ENL, or type 2 reactions) occurs in LL and BL patients with higher bacterial loads in their lesions.[21] ENL can begin during the first or second year of treatment, but also before or after treatment. Patients are febrile with skin nodules accompanied by iritis, neuritis, lymphadenitis, orchitis, bone pain, dactylitis, arthritis, and proteinuria, which are difficult to treat [**Figure 66-10**].[22]

BT, BB, and BL patients tend to develop type 1 reversal reaction. LL patients tend to develop ENL type 2 reaction. Both conditions are managed with prednisolone, an anti-inflammatory treatment. When patients with ENL type 2 reactions are not responding to prednisolone,

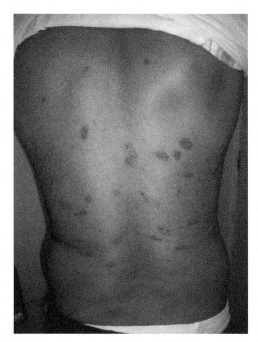

FIGURE 66-8. Type 1 leprosy reaction: swelling of old lesions.

thalidomide is used as the second-line treatment. Thalidomide needs to be administered with caution because it has serious adverse effects, particularly teratogenicity.[23]

PREVENTION AND CONTROL

Early case detection and timely and appropriate initiation of MDT are critical to minimize leprosy-related impairments and deformities [**Figure 66-11**]. It is especially important to identify patients before they develop reactions, because most complications caused by leprosy are consequences of reactions. Prevention of disabilities is one of the major

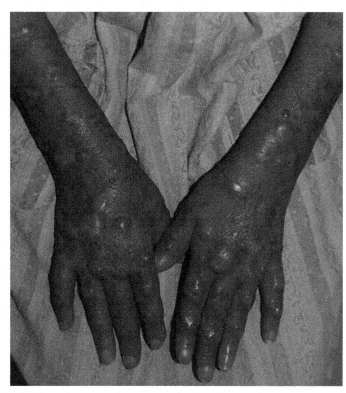

FIGURE 66-10. Type 2 leprosy reaction: erythema nodosum leprosum.

strategies practiced in endemic countries among people affected with leprosy. Rehabilitation is an important need in this population.

CONCLUSION

Early diagnosis and early treatment of leprosy are critically important to reduce peripheral nerve damage including loss of sensory, motor, and autonomic nerve function, with subsequent deformity from repeated trauma of the skin. Recognition and management of leprosy reactions lead to fewer consequences of nerve damage and have an impact on the quality of life for those affected by the disease and the stigma it generates. The disease and its associated deformities have been responsible for social stigmatization and discrimination against patients and their families in many societies. Thus, prevention of nerve damage and management and rehabilitation of impairments are important components of a leprosy control program.

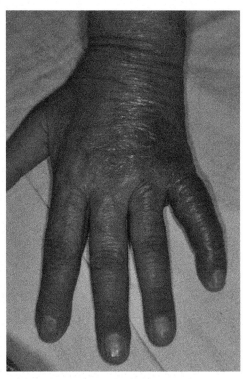

FIGURE 66-9. Type 1 leprosy reaction: swelling of hand.

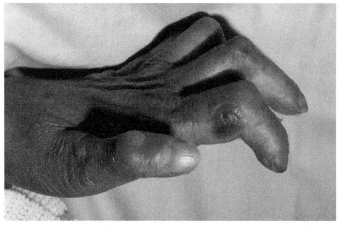

FIGURE 66-11. Claw and ape hand owing to ulnar and median nerve palsy. (Used with permission from Barbara Leppard.)

REFERENCES

1. World Health Organization. Global leprosy situation, 2011. *Wkly Epidemiol Rec.* 2012;87:317-328.
2. Shepard CC. Temperature optimum of *Mycobacterium leprae* in mice. *J Bacteriol.* 1965;90:1271-1275.
3. Cole ST, Eiglmeier K, Parkhill J, et al. Massive gene decay in the leprosy bacillus. *Nature.* 2001;409:1007-1011.
4. Brosch R, Gordon SV, Eiglmeier K, et al. Comparative genomics of the leprosy and tubercle bacilli. *Res Microbiol.* 2000;151:135-142.
5. Lawrence JG, Hendrix RW, Casjens S. Where are the pseudogenes in bacterial genomes? *Trends Microbiol.* 2001;9:535-540.
6. Vissa V, Brennan P. The genome of *Mycobacterium leprae*: a minimal mycobacterial gene set. *Genome Biol.* 2001;2:1023.
7. Britton W. *Leprosy.* London, United Kingdom: Mosby; 1999.
8. Suzuki K, Udono T, Fujisawa M, et al. Infection during infancy and long incubation period of leprosy suggested in a case of a chimpanzee used for medical research. *J Clin Microbiol.* 2010;48:3432-3434.
9. Davey TF, Rees RJ. The nasal dicharge in leprosy: clinical and bacteriological aspects. *Leprosy Rev.* 1974;45:121-134.
10. McDougall AC, Rees RJ, Weddell AG, et al. The histopathology of lepromatous leprosy in the nose. *J Pathol.* 1975;115:215-226.
11. Ridley DS, Jopling WH. Classification of leprosy according to immunity. *Int J Leprosy.* 1966;34:255-273.
12. Pfaltzgraff R, Ramu G. *Leprosy.* 2nd ed. New York, NY: Churchill Livingstone; 1994.
13. Nakamura K, Akama T, Bang PD, et al. Detection of RNA expression from pseudogenes and non-coding genomic regions of *Mycobacterium leprae*. *Microb Pathog.* 2009;47:183-187.
14. Suzuki K, Takigawa W, Tanigawa K, et al. Detection of *Mycobacterium leprae* DNA from archaeological skeletal remains in Japan using whole genome amplification and polymerase chain reaction. *PloS One.* 2010;5:e12422.
15. Ishii N, Sugita Y, Sato I, et al. Sparfloxacin in the treatment of leprosy patients. *Int J Dermatol.* 1997;36:619-621.
16. Kumar B, Dogra S, Kaur I. Epidemiological characteristics of leprosy reactions: 15 years experience from north India. *Int J Lepr Other Mycobact Dis.* 2004;72:125-133.
17. Becx-Bleumink M, Berhe D. Occurrence of reactions, their diagnosis and management in leprosy patients treated with multidrug therapy; experience in the leprosy control program of the All Africa Leprosy and Rehabilitation Training Center (ALERT) in Ethiopia. *Int J Lepr Other Mycobact Dis.* 1992;60:173-184.
18. Scollard DM, Smith T, Bhoopat L, et al. Epidemiologic characteristics of leprosy reactions. *I Int J Lepr Other Mycobact Dis.* 1994;62:559-567.
19. Britton W. The management of leprosy reversal reactions. *Leprosy Rev.* 1998;69:225-234.
20. Croft RP, Nicholls PG, Richardus JH, et al. Incidence rates of acute nerve function impairment in leprosy: a prospective cohort analysis after 24 months (The Bangladesh Acute Nerve Damage Study). *Lepr Review.* Mar 2000;71(1):18-33.
21. Manandhar R, LeMaster JW, Roche PW. Risk factors for erythema nodosum leprosum. *Int J Lepr Other Mycobact Dis.* 1999;67:270-278.
22. Lockwood DN. The management of erythema nodosum leprosum: current and future options. *Lepr Rev.* 1996;67:253-259.
23. Zeldis JB, Williams BA, Thomas SD, et al. S.T.E.P.S.: a comprehensive program for controlling and monitoring access to thalidomide. *Clin Ther.* 1999;21:319-330.

CHAPTER 67

Leishmaniasis

Emmanuel Olaniyi Onayemi

KEY POINTS

- Leishmaniasis is a chronic protozoan infection, described independently in 1903 by Leishman and Donovan.

- There are at least 20 species of the protozoa that cause leishmaniasis in humans.

- Certain species of leishmaniasis cause visceral leishmaniasis (eg, *Leishmania infantum* and *Leishmania donovani*), and others cause cutaneous disease (eg, *Leishmania major* and *Leishmania tropica*).

- Emerging research has demonstrated that these species-specific presentations may not be absolute because some species can cause both types of infections.

- The transmission of infection is primarily through the bite of sandflies of the genus *Phlebotomus* (Old World) or *Lutzomyia* (New World). Rarely, transmission can occur through shared syringes, by blood transfusion, or congenitally from mother to infant.

- The sandfly usually bites at night and outdoors, although they have rarely been reported to bite during the day and indoors.

- Leishmaniasis presents with lesions of the skin, mucous membranes, or internal organs, and the presentation is dependent on a number of factors including the infecting species of *Leishmania*, its virulence, number of parasites inoculated, site of bite, and the nutritional status and immune response of the host.

- Diagnosis can be made clinically, particularly in endemic areas, or via microscopic examination of Giemsa-stained smear, leishmanin skin test, histologic examination of biopsy specimen, or serologic techniques including polymerase chain reaction technology.

- Treatment modalities include topical or systemic chemotherapy, physical methods, and surgical intervention.

- Recovery from infection confers lifelong immunity.

- Prevention is always superior to treatment and cure.

INTRODUCTION

Leishmaniasis is a chronic parasitic infection caused by inoculation of the *Leishmania* protozoan during the bite of an infected sandfly of the genus *Phlebotomus* in the Old World or *Lutzomyia* in the New World. The insect becomes infected when it bites infected humans or mammals such as rodents that harbor the *Leishmania* parasites.[1] The sandfly usually bites at night and outdoors, but when disturbed in its habitat, it can bite during the day and indoors. However, on rare occasions, transmission can occur by shared syringes among intravenous drug users, by transfusion of infected blood, and congenitally from an infected mother to her infant.[2]

Four clinical forms of leishmaniasis exist: cutaneous, diffuse cutaneous, mucocutaneous, and visceral types. Clinical variants depend on the causative species of the *Leishmania*. There are at least 20 species of the protozoa that cause infections in humans, and some species cause visceral leishmaniasis (eg, *Leishmania infantum* and *Leishmania donovani*), whereas other species cause cutaneous disease (eg, *Leishmania major* and *Leishmania tropica*). Emerging research has shown that these species-specific presentations may not be absolute because some species can cause both types of infections. The virulence of the protozoan also determines the clinical outcome in the host. Additional determinants of clinical outcome include the number of parasites inoculated, the site of the bite, the nutritional status of the host, and integrity of the host immunity.

The diagnosis of leishmaniasis may be clinical, particularly in endemic areas. However, supportive laboratory diagnosis involves microscopic examination of Giemsa-stained smear, leishmanin skin test (Montenegro test), histologic examination of biopsy specimen, and serologic techniques including polymerase chain reaction (PCR) technology. Various treatment modalities are available for the management of leishmaniasis, and these can be used singly or in combination. Treatments include topical or systemic chemotherapy, physical methods, and surgical intervention. Recovery from infection confers lifelong immunity from reinfection by the same species of *Leishmania*.[3] Control measures involve early diagnosis and prompt treatment with effective chemotherapy, as well as vector and reservoir host control to eliminate transmission. The role of health education cannot be overemphasized, because prevention still remains a better option than treatment and cure.

ETIOLOGY

Leishmaniasis occurs in four continents and is endemic in 88 countries, most of which are developing countries. Cutaneous leishmaniasis of the Old World is caused by *L. major*, *L. tropica*, *Leishmania aethiopica*, *L. donovani*, and *L. infantum*, whereas that of the New World is due to *Leishmania braziliensis*, *Leishmania guyanensis*, *Leishmania panamensis*, *Leishmania peruviana*, *Leishmania mexicana*, *Leishmania amazonensis*, and *Leishmania venezuelensis*. Old World visceral leishmaniasis is caused by parasites of *L. donovani* and *L. infantum*. A few cases of Old World visceral leishmaniasis caused by *L. tropica* have been reported. The etiologic agent for New World visceral leishmaniasis is *L. infantum*, and the disease is similar to that seen in the Old World.[2]

EPIDEMIOLOGY

Leishmaniasis is endemic in 88 countries with an estimated 10 million people suffering from the disease. The population at risk is more than 350 million people, whereas estimated incidence is 2 million new cases per year, with the ratio of cutaneous leishmaniasis to visceral leishmaniasis being 3:1. At least one person gets infected with cutaneous leishmaniasis every 20 seconds.[2]

Leishmaniasis occurs in a focal distribution and in remote locations.[4] Cutaneous leishmaniasis is endemic in the northern Mediterranean littoral west of Greece and in North Africa,[5,6] Asia, Central and South America, Brazil, and the Middle East.[7]

PATHOGENESIS

The host immunity plays a leading role in the expression of the disease. Promastigotes inoculated into the skin by the bite of a sandfly are engulfed by histiocytes and monocytes, in which they multiply. *Leishmania* protozoa then invade human macrophages and replicate intracellularly. A raised, erythematous papule or plaque develops at the site of the bite within weeks or months [**Figure 67-1**]. Good protective immune response of the host results in localized cutaneous leishmaniasis. Mucocutaneous leishmaniasis occurs in humans with an intense inflammatory response, whereas disseminated cutaneous leishmaniasis occurs in situations where there is extensive proliferation of the promastigotes but with minimal inflammatory response and no tendency for visceral involvement. When there is little immune response by the host or in the case of immunosuppression, visceral leishmaniasis results.

CLINICAL FEATURES

CUTANEOUS LEISHMANIASIS

Synonyms include Aleppo boil, Baghdad boil, chiclero ulcer, Delhi boil, uta, Lahore sore, Oriental sore, and leishmaniasis tropica.

Cutaneous leishmaniasis is the most common form of leishmaniasis. It affects the skin and sometimes the mucous membranes and presents as sores, which usually begin at the site of the bite of the sandfly. Lesions occur primarily on exposed parts of the body. In a few patients, sores develop on mucous membranes of the mouth, tongue, gums, lips, and nose. The lesion then ulcerates and may become secondarily infected with bacteria. In many species (eg, *L. major*), the lesion frequently heals spontaneously with atrophic scarring [**Figure 67-2**]. Lesions may heal and reappear as satellite lesions around the site of the original lesion. They may also reappear along the route of lymphatic drainage [**Figure 67-3**].

MUCOCUTANEOUS LEISHMANIASIS

Mucocutaneous leishmaniasis is caused primarily by *L. braziliensis* and *L. panamensis* and is seen mostly in Bolivia, Brazil, and Peru. These species of the *Leishmania* protozoa cause spread of the infection to the mouth and upper respiratory tract through lymphatic or hematologic dissemination. In conditions of depressed immunity, other species can behave in a similar fashion.[2] In a few patients, sores may develop on mucous membranes of the mouth, tongue, gums, lips, and nose. Mucous membrane lesions are most often caused by *L. braziliensis*, but cases caused by *L. aethiopica* have also been rarely described.

Mucocutaneous leishmaniasis can occur as late as 20 years after a cutaneous lesion. It is the most feared form of cutaneous leishmaniasis because it produces destructive and disfiguring lesions of the face. Known risk factors include malnutrition, site of primary lesion above the waist, multiple or large lesions, and delayed healing of primary cutaneous leishmaniasis. Clinically, nodules on the nose [**Figure 67-4**], with thickened skin of the nose, and obstruction of the nostrils due to infiltration of the anterior nasal septum occur. Eventually, there may be collapse and broadening of the nose.[2] Mucocutaneous leishmaniasis rarely heals spontaneously, and death often occurs from secondary bacterial infections with intercurrent pneumonia.

VISCERAL LEISHMANIASIS

Synonyms include kala-azar, death fever, and dum-dum fever.

Visceral leishmaniasis is caused by parasites of the *L. donovani–L. infantum* complex. *L. tropica* has been associated with a few cases.[2] Infection is usually asymptomatic, and those who subsequently develop clinical infection may have underlying malnutrition and/or immunosuppression. Visceral leishmaniasis manifests in different clinical forms

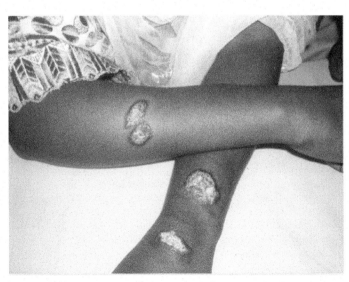

FIGURE 67-1. Crusted plaques of cutaneous leishmaniasis on the arms and left wrist.

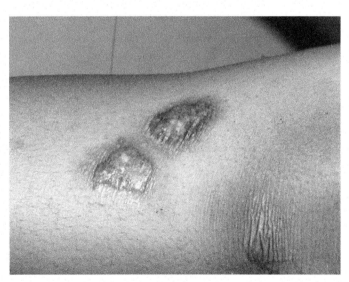

FIGURE 67-2. Spontaneously healing cutaneous leishmaniasis with atrophic scars.

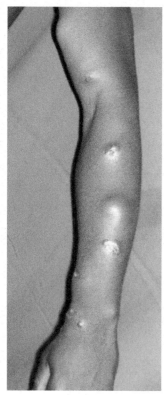

FIGURE 67-3. Cutaneous leishmaniasis with sporotrichoid spread along lymphatic drainage.

depending on whether or not it is endemic, sporadic, or epidemic in nature, and there may be accompanying cutaneous manifestations like those of cutaneous leishmaniasis.[8]

In endemic areas, the infection is usually chronic, and children are particularly predisposed to acquiring it. In sporadic cases, any age group may be affected, and nonindigenous people entering an endemic zone are most often affected. The epidemic form of visceral leishmaniasis can be fatal, and all age groups are susceptible except those who have developed immunity from a previous epidemic.[2] After an incubation period that ranges from 10 days to over 1 year, fever develops, either insidiously or abruptly. Noticeable symptoms include fatigue, discomfort from the presence of the enlarged spleen, cough, diarrhea, and epistaxis. Gross splenomegaly, hepatomegaly, and lymphadenopathy may be

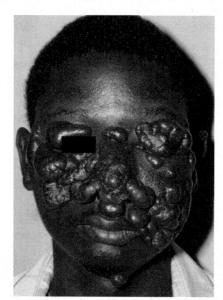

FIGURE 67-4. Mucocutaneous leishmaniasis with multiple nodules clustered on the face, destroying the nasal cartilage.

demonstrated in some endemic zones.[8] There may be clinical evidence of malnutrition with hyperpigmentation of the skin. Intercurrent infections are common. Comorbidity with human immunodeficiency virus has modified the classical presentation of visceral and other forms of leishmaniasis.[2]

POST–KALA-AZAR DERMAL LEISHMANIASIS

In East Africa and on the Indian subcontinent, between 5% and 20% of patients develop a rash after the visceral disease has healed, either spontaneously or following treatment. The rash erupts after 6 months to a year of apparent cure of visceral leishmaniasis. However, a small number of patients with post–kala-azar dermal leishmaniasis have no previous history of visceral disease. In Sudan, it may occur concurrently with visceral leishmaniasis.[2] The rash may initially be hypopigmented macules, which later become papular or nodular and infiltrative, and may be seen on the cheeks, chin, ears, and extensor aspects of forearms, buttocks, and lower legs.[2,8] The rash heals spontaneously over a few months in Africans but rarely in Indian patients.[2]

DIAGNOSIS OF LEISHMANIASIS

Diagnosis is based on clinical suspicion, especially in endemic areas, and appropriate laboratory investigations with correct interpretation of results.[8-11] Differential diagnoses are presented in **Table 67-1**.

Appropriate investigations include the following procedures.

CUTANEOUS SCRAPING

This simple and commonly used test is 70% to 75% sensitive and is performed under local anesthesia. The procedure is as follows:

- Remove crust on the skin's surface.
- Clean and dry the site with sterile gauze.
- Scrape the margin and central area of the ulcer.
- Make multiple slides (five or more slides).
- Fix the slides with methanol.
- Stain with Giemsa, and examine under oil immersion. Amastigotes are seen in monocytes or extracellularly.
- Observe the nucleus and the rod-shaped kinetoplast, a mitochondrial structure containing extranuclear DNA. The kinetoplast differentiates *Leishmania* from other small organisms such as *Histoplasma*.

NEEDLE ASPIRATION

This test is useful for nodular and papular lesions. The procedure is as follows:

- Inject 0.1 mL of normal saline into the border of the rash through the intact skin.
- Aspirate fluid while moving the needle back and forth under the skin; the fluid is useful for culture (blood agar Nicolle-Novy-MacNeal media).

PUNCH BIOPSY

- Take a punch 2 to 3 mm along the active lesional border.
- Make tissue-impression smears from a biopsy sample by rolling the cut portion on a slide after blotting excess blood.

TABLE 67-1	Differential diagnoses of cutaneous leishmaniasis
• Bacterial skin infections	• Blastomycosis
• Cutaneous anthrax	• Eczema
• Fungal skin infections	• Leprosy
• *Mycobacterium marinum*	• Myiasis
• Sarcoidosis	• Skin cancer
• Sporotrichosis	• Syphilis
• Tuberculosis	• Yaws
• Verrucous lesions	

MOLECULAR TECHNIQUE USING PCR

This is the gold standard for diagnosis. The PCR test is highly sensitive and specific. Antibodies are detected most consistently.

LEISHMANIN SKIN TEST (MONTENEGRO TEST)

Isoenzyme Analysis Isoenzyme analysis is important for species identification and consists of enzyme electrophoresis of cultured amastigotes.

Monoclonal Antibodies These are directed against *Leishmania* antigen. This test has very high sensitivity and specificity. However, it is not readily available for routine use.

SEROLOGY

This is generally not useful due to low sensitivity and specificity. Antibody is present in low titer and cross-reacts with leprosy, malaria, and trypanosomal infections.

XENODIAGNOSIS

This involves the laboratory inoculation of domestic animal when parasite load is low.

TREATMENT AND PREVENTION [TABLES 67-2 AND 67-3]¹²⁻¹⁶

Indications for treating leishmaniasis include cosmetically disfiguring lesions, multiple lesions, nodular lymphangitis, large or chronic lesions, mucocutaneous disease, lesions in immunosuppressed patients, lesions over joints, and worsening lesions.

TABLE 67-2	Leishmaniasis treatments

Intralesional injections
- The WHO recommendation for treatment of CL is intralesional antimonials (eg, sodium stibogluconate and meglumine antimoniate).
- WHO recommends infiltration with 1–3 mL under the edge of the lesion and the entire lesion until the surface has blanched.
- The infiltration could be administered every 5–7 days for a total of 2–5 treatments.
- Cure rate for intralesional antimonials is 72%–97% in various series.
- Intralesional antimonials are more effective for *Leishmania major* than *Leishmania tropica*.

Other intralesional therapies
- Local injections of hypertonic sodium chloride solution or zinc sulphate have been reported to be as effective as local sodium stibogluconate in a few Iraqi patients.

Topical treatments
- Paromomycin ointments
- Imiquimod: although not very effective alone, it is used in combination with meglumine antimoniate
- Topical amphotericin B
- Cryotherapy
- Localized controlled heat
- Carbon dioxide laser

Oral therapies
- Azoles
- Azithromycin
- Miltefosine
- Zinc sulphate

Intramuscular and intravenous drugs
- Systemic antimonials
- Drugs combinations with antimonials
- Pentamidine
- Amphotericin B

New promising agents
- Bisphosphonates
- Quinolones

Abbreviations: CL, cutaneous leishmaniasis; WHO, World Health Organization.

TABLE 67-3	Methods of leishmaniasis prevention

- Avoidance of sandflies, although this may be difficult in endemic areas.
- Prevention of sandfly bites:
  - Use of insect repellent, especially by travelers
  - Wearing protective clothing
  - Proper netting of windows
- Use of pyrethroid-impregnated bed nets (used in Burkina Faso, Sudan, and Columbia).
- House and space spraying with insecticides
- Destruction of rodent reservoirs.
- Vaccine development, which is underway
- The combination of killed promastigotes plus bacillus Calmette-Guérin (BCG) vaccine (which is being tested in Iran, Sudan, and Ecuador)

Each case needs to be individualized based on parasite species, extent of disease, host immune and nutritional status, geographic region, and cost and availability of therapeutic agents. Patients should be monitored until the lesion is completely healed. Follow-up at 6 months is then appropriate.

CONCLUSION

Leishmaniasis, which is a significant public health concern throughout the developing world, presents with lesions of the skin, mucous membrane, or internal organs. Caused by a number of different species of *Leishmania*, it is transmitted primarily through the bite of sandflies. The institution of various methods of prevention is superior to treatment and cure.

REFERENCES

1. World Health Organization. Neglected tropical diseases. http://www.who.int/neglected_diseases/diseases/en/. Accessed February 19, 2015.
2. World Health Organization. Control of the leishmaniasis. *World Health Organ Tech Rep Ser*. 2010;949:186.
3. Fitzpatrick TB, Johnson RA, Wolff K, Suurmond D. Cutaneous and mucocutaneous leishmaniasis. In: *Color Atlas & Synopsis of Clinical Dermatology*. 4th ed. New York, NY: McGraw-Hill Companies; 2001.
4. Bern C, Maguire JH, Alvar J. Complexities of assessing the disease burden attributable to leishmaniasis. *PLoS Negl Trop Dis*. 2008;2:e313.
5. Bellazoug S, Ammar-Khodja A, Belkoid M, et al. La leishmaniose cutanée du Nord d'Algerie. *Bull Soc Pathol Exot Filiales*. 1985;75:615-622.
6. Briffa CV. Cutaneous leishmaniasis in the Maltese Islands. *Br J Dermatol*. 1985;113:370-371.
7. World Health Organization (WHO). Leishmaniasis. In: *Thirteenth Programme Report. Special Programme for Research and Training in Tropical Diseases (TDR)*. Geneva, Switzerland: WHO Publications; 1997:100-111.
8. Vega-Lopez R, Hay RJ. Parasitic worms and protozoa. In: Burns T, Breathnach S, Cox N, Griffiths C, eds. *Rook's Textbook of Dermatology*. 7th ed. New York, NY: Wiley; 2004:1-48.
9. James WD, Berger TG, Elston D. *Andrews' Diseases of the Skin: Clinical Dermatology*. New York, NY: Saunders Elsevier; 2006.
10. Reithinger R, Dujardin J-C. Molecular diagnosis of leishmaniasis: current status and future applications. *J Clin Microbiol*. 2007;45:21-25.
11. Sharifi I, FeKri AR, Aflatonian MR, et al. Randomised vaccine trial of single dose of killed *Leishmania major* plus BCG against anthroponotic cutaneous leishmaniasis in Bam, Iran. *Lancet*. 1998;351:1540-1543.
12. Murray HW, Berman JD, Davies CR, Saravia NG. Advances in leishmaniasis. *Lancet*. 2005;366:1561-1577.
13. Minodiera P, Parolab P. Cutaneous leishmaniasis treatment. A review. *Trav Med Infect Dis*. 2007;5:150-158.
14. Markle WH, Makhoul K. Leishmaniasis. *Am Fam Physician*. 2004;69:1455-1460.
15. Machado PRL, Lessa H, Lessa M, et al. Oral pentoxifylline combined with pentavalent antimony: a randomized trial for mucosal leishmaniasis. *Clin Infect Dis*. 2007;44:788-793.
16. Lrajhi AA, Ibrahim EA, De Vol EB, et al. Fluconazole for the treatment of cutaneous leishmaniasis caused by *Leishmania major*. *N Engl J Med*. 2002;346:891-895.

Cutaneous Manifestations of Systemic Diseases

Diabetes Mellitus

Lynn McKinley-Grant
Sridhar Dronavalli
Sanna Ronkainen

KEY POINTS

- Common dermatoses such as intertrigo, tinea corporis, hair loss, and pruritus can be signs of diabetes.

- A recognition of the early cutaneous manifestations of diabetes can direct the healthcare provider to test for this condition or to refer the patient to a specialist for diabetes treatment. This may result in decreased morbidity and mortality in diabetic patients.

- Diabetes rates are higher among obese patients, and in many regions of the world, obesity is occurring with an increased prevalence.

- Genetics can affect an individual's likelihood of developing diabetes.

- Diabetes affects every organ of the body, but the highest morbidity is in the heart and kidneys. If patients are treated early and make the appropriate lifestyle changes, the symptoms of diabetes can usually be well managed.

- Some common cutaneous conditions induced by diabetes include skin infections, granuloma annulare, diabetic dermopathy, necrobiosis lipoidica diabeticorum, diabetic bullae, leg and foot ulcers, scleredema, and acanthosis nigricans.

INTRODUCTION

Cutaneous manifestations of diabetes are seen daily in the practice of all medical specialties. An estimated 25.8 million Americans have diabetes, and approximately one-quarter are unaware of their condition.[1] A further 79 million individuals have elevated blood sugar levels consistent with prediabetes.[1] In the United States, type 2 diabetes is currently most prevalent among Native Americans and African Americans, whereas the lowest prevalence is found among Asian Americans [Table 68-1].[2-4] However, it is important to note that the patient population seen by healthcare providers is changing, and this is likely to impact diabetes statistics in the United States. The U.S. Census Bureau projects that by the year 2060, the U.S. population will shift from 63% to 43% Caucasian, whereas the Latino/Hispanic population will increase to 31%, the African American population to 14.7%, the Asian American population to 8.2%, and the Native American population to 1.5%.[5]

EPIDEMIOLOGY

Diabetes is classified by type. Type 1 diabetes is a disease characterized by an autoimmune destruction of the pancreas β-cells, and this leads to a complete lack of insulin secretion. Type 1 diabetes is typically seen at a younger age and is more common in patients with a family history of other autoimmune diseases.

Type 2 diabetes is a disease of impaired insulin secretion and/or insulin resistance; these often occur simultaneously. The patient's pancreas is capable of secreting insulin; however, there is a dysregulation of the cellular response to insulin. Type 2 diabetes has a significant genetic component; therefore, a patient's family history must be considered in the diagnosis. The primary contributing factor to the increase in type 2 diabetes is obesity. This is the most common form of this condition and accounts for up to 95% of cases. Individuals with type 2 diabetes are almost always overweight or obese.[6] Although type 2 diabetes most commonly develops in adulthood, pediatric type 2 diabetes is becoming increasingly common as obesity becomes a growing problem among children and adolescents.[2-4]

In the United States, diabetes is observed nationwide. However, there is a striking preponderance of diabetes cases in the American South, in a distribution of contiguous states and counties known as the "diabetes belt."[7]

ETIOLOGY AND GENETICS

In addition to lifestyle, development of type 2 diabetes is also 30% to 70% attributable to genetic factors.[8] It appears that most of the genetic components associated with type 2 diabetes are associated with β-cell dysfunction.[9] One gene that has been shown to contribute to type 2 diabetes is the *TCF7L2* gene.[10] For people with one or two copies of this gene, there is an increased risk of 1.5 to 2.4 times, respectively. This gene is associated with impaired insulin secretion and increased gluconeogenesis.[10]

African Americans and Native Americans have a higher prevalence of type 2 diabetes than other racial groups.[2,3] The increased genetic predisposition of diabetes in these populations is thought to be polygenetic. In a genome-wide association study of African Americans, one single-nucleotide polymorphism (SNP) (rs7560163 located between the *RND3* and *RBM43* genes) reached statistical significance, with several other SNPs showing potential associations.[11] In the Pima Indian population, it has been shown that SNPs in the *SIRT1* gene are correlated with insulin resistance.[12] However, the Pima Indians consist of two separate populations with vastly different rates of diabetes. One group is in rural Mexico and live on a subsistence diet, whereas the other is in Arizona, living on a Western diet.[13] The rates of diabetes in Mexico and Arizona are 6.9% and 38%, respectively, suggesting a significant environmental component to the development of type 2 diabetes.[13] In 2010, the age-adjusted prevalence was 12.6 per 100 persons in African Americans and 16.1 per 100 persons in Native Americans. In comparison, the prevalence was 11.8 per 100 in Hispanic Americans and 7.1 per 100 in Caucasian Americans.[14]

TREATMENT

Type 1 diabetes is typically managed with insulin injections. In extenuating circumstances, type 1 diabetics may undergo whole-organ pancreatic or kidney-pancreatic transplants. This occurs in patients who have extreme difficulty in managing their blood glucose levels or who have end-stage renal disease requiring a kidney transplant. Islet cell-specific transplants have been performed in clinical trials.[15] Of those receiving kidney-pancreas or pancreas transplants in 2012, 22% and 11%, respectively, were African American.[16] From 2003 to 2004, 53.2% of African Americans and 57.4% of Caucasian Americans who had been on the transplant list for more than 2 years received their required transplants.[2]

TABLE 68-1	The prevalence of type 2 diabetes in correlation with obesity in Caucasians, Hispanics, African Americans, Native Americans, and Asian Americans[2-4]				
	Non-Hispanic Caucasians (%)	Hispanics (%)	Non-Hispanic African Americans (%)	Native Americans (%)	Asian Americans (%)
Obesity	26.1	31.9	36.8	39.4	11.6
Type 2 diabetes	7.1	11.8	12.6	17.5	9.1

CLINICAL FINDINGS

Cutaneous manifestations of diabetes mellitus have been reported in 30% and more than 80% of patients.[9,17] These signs and symptoms can be noted on a physical examination and include central obesity, acanthosis nigricans (AN), bacterial and fungal skin infections, pruritus, hair loss, onychomycosis, necrobiosis lipoidica, bulla, scleredema, foot and leg ulcers, and granuloma annulare (GA). Diabetic patients may also present with xerosis, ichthyosis, brittle nails, loss of leg hair, diabetic thick skin, and hyperpigmentation.[18a] Some of these symptoms or conditions are very early cutaneous signs of diabetes and provide useful indications in the diagnostic workup.

Elevated glucose levels cause direct changes in the skin and can specifically induce skin thickening.[18] Painless, thick, waxy changes can occur on the dorsal hands and are localized over the joints. This often limits a patient's ability to straighten their small joints, which is a condition called cheiroarthropathy, or limited joint mobility syndrome.[19,20] While the waxy changes can have a yellow hue, the skin is typically tight and shiny, which is most notable on the palmar surfaces. Patients can be identified by the 'prayer sign': when asked to press their hands together as if in prayer, they are unable to straighten their fingers. This will be most prominent in their fourth and fifth digits. Cheiroarthropathy is seen in 8% to 36% of diabetics and occurs more frequently in patients with a longer duration of diabetes and insulin dependence. One study in a Nigerian population showed that insulin-dependent patients were twice as likely as non-insulin-dependent diabetics to have cheiroarthropathy, despite the fact that all patients in both groups had the same blood glucose controls.[21] In severe cases of limited joint mobility syndrome, the tightness and waxiness extend to the dorsal aspect of the hand, and sclerosis of the tendon sheaths can occur.[20] Diabetic cheiroarthropathy can be a major factor in limiting the motion of an individual's small joints. The treatment for thickened skin is typically physical therapy to preserve the patient's range of motion.

CUTANEOUS INFECTIONS

Infections of the skin can be the presenting sign of diabetes mellitus. *Streptococcus*, *Staphylococcus*, and methicillin-resistant *Staphylococcus aureus* cellulitis and folliculitis are more common in patients with diabetes.[22] Uncontrolled diabetes can increase the risk of cutaneous infections for a multitude of reasons. It has been shown that insulin-dependent diabetics have a higher carrier rate of *S. aureus*.[23] On the cellular level, both the T-cell and neutrophil functions are impaired, particularly in a ketotic state.[24] Tight glucose management has been shown to improve the intracellular bactericidal action of neutrophils.[25]

Neuropathic patients who develop foot ulcers are at risk for polymicrobial infections of those wounds, which can be further complicated by fasciitis and/or osteomyelitis. These wounds require debridement or, in severe cases, an amputation of the affected limb. Necrotizing fasciitis is the most concerning infection that is encountered in diabetic patients because it has a 62% mortality rate for patients older than 60 years of age.[26] It presents classically with pain that spreads rapidly beyond the erythematous and edematous borders [**Figure 68-1**]. The treatment for this infection must be a combination of aggressive debridement and broad-spectrum antibiotics.

Malignant otitis externa is an infection of the external auditory canal and the surrounding skull, which is most commonly caused by *Pseudomonas aeruginosa*. It presents with pain, otorrhea, and hearing loss without a fever.[22] If it is left untreated, cranial osteomyelitis and central nervous system (CNS) involvement can occur. The treatment includes aggressive debridement of the area and antipseudomonal antibiotics, such as ciprofloxacin.

An uncommon infection with high morbidity, rhinocerebral mucormycosis, is more frequently seen in diabetic patients, particularly those with diabetic ketoacidosis. The causative agent is typically *Rhizopus* or *Mucor* fungi. Approximately 50% of all patients presenting with mucormycosis have diabetes.[27] In vitro studies have shown that the ketoacidotic state impairs the inhibition of this fungi, allowing an invasion into the tissue, bone, and even the CNS. The typical presentation is an elderly patient with a rapid onset of facial cellulitis, periorbital edema, and fever. Less commonly, mucormycosis can also occur outside the sinuses, for instance on the chest and extremities. [**Figure 68-2**]. This results in a necrotizing fasciitis-like clinical picture.[28] The diagnosis can be confirmed with a biopsy that shows broad, nonseptate hyphae branching at 90-degree angles within a vessel wall, alongside obliterative thrombosis of the vessel. Prompt treatment is needed, including the correction of blood glucose levels, administration of amphotericin B, and debridement of the infected region.

Superficial fungal infections with tinea corporis, caused by *Trichophyton rubrum* [**Figure 68-3**] and *Candida albicans*, are also commonly seen in diabetic patients. These include intertrigo [**Figure 68-4**], thrush, vaginitis, and balanitis.

GRANULOMA ANNULARE (GA)

GA is a common dermatosis in children, with a peak incidence at 4 years of age [**Figure 68-5**].[29] This condition may be associated with diabetes; however, its correlation is controversial, and a 2002 case-control study showed no association.[30] GA is twice as common in females compared with males.

The etiology of GA is unknown; clinically, it appears as an annular cluster of papules. These are typically found on the hands and feet, although they can occur anywhere on the body. In patients with skin of color, the papules vary from skin-colored to erythematous, ranging

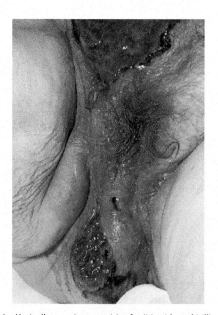

FIGURE 68-1. Vaginally occurring necrotizing fasciitis with methicillin-resistant *Staphylococcus aureus*. Due to its high mortality rate, this is one of the most serious infections that can develop in diabetic patients. (Used with permission from the Department of Dermatology, Washington Hospital Center, Washington, DC.)

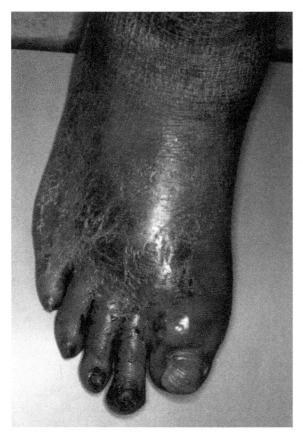

FIGURE 68-2. A dark skin of color patient with mucormycosis of the foot. This condition may occur on the chest or the extremities of individuals with diabetes. (Used with permission from the Department of Dermatology, Washington Hospital Center, Washington, DC.)

from pink to purple to brown. Histologically, palisading granulomas with increased central mucin are seen in the dermis. GA is typically painless and self-limited; therefore, it is managed conservatively. However, it can result in postinflammatory hyperpigmentation, particularly in patients with skin of color.

Differential Diagnosis The differential diagnosis of GA includes necrobiosis lipoidica diabeticorum (NLD) and sarcoidosis.

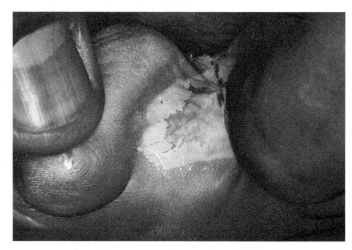

FIGURE 68-4. A case of intertrigo in a patient with dark skin of color. Superficial fungal infections, including intertrigo, often occur in patients with diabetes. (Used with permission from the Department of Dermatology, Washington Hospital Center, Washington, DC.)

NECROBIOSIS LIPOIDICA DIABETICORUM (NLD)

NLD is a rare condition that is seen in fewer than 0.5% of diabetic patients, the majority of whom are women.[31] NLD typically develops in individuals who are 30 to 40 years of age and may predate the onset of diabetes.[6] Both immune and antibody mediation have been suggested as a potential cause for this condition.[15] An element of microangiopathy has been noted, and these lesions reportedly have lower oxygen tension than normal skin.[32]

The painful lesions of NLD are most often seen on the anterior tibial surfaces of both lower legs [**Figure 68-6A**]. In patients with dark skin of color, they begin as small, yellow/brown-bluish/purple patches (depending on the background pigment), with a reddish border and a yellow/brown center [**Figure 68-6B**]. As the lesions grow, the central area will atrophy and turn waxy, whereas the outer border will darken. In about one-third of cases, particularly those subject to trauma, ulceration of the lesions will also occur.[6,15]

Histologically, the lesions are marked by a collagen degeneration, as well as palisading granulomatous inflammation of the dermis and the subcutaneous tissues. This occurs with a significant presence of plasma cells and lipid

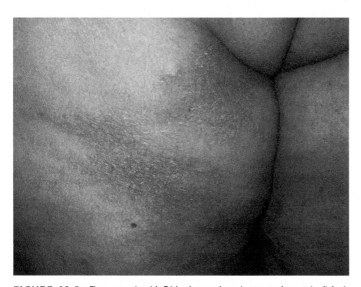

FIGURE 68-3. Tinea corporis with *Trichophyton rubrum* is commonly seen in diabetic patients. (Used with permission from the Department of Dermatology, Washington Hospital Center, Washington, DC.)

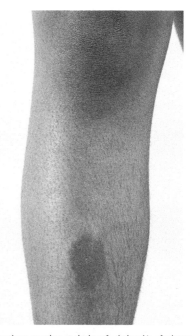

FIGURE 68-5. Granuloma annulare on the leg of a darker skin of color patient. This condition is common in children, although its association with diabetes is controversial. (Used with permission from the Department of Dermatology, Washington Hospital Center, Washington, DC.)

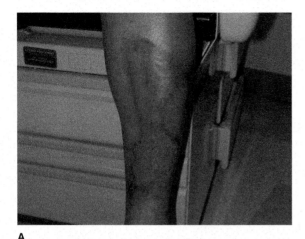

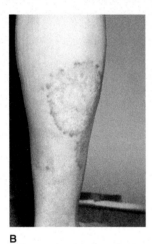

FIGURE 68-6. **(A)** Necrobiosis lipoidica diabeticorum on a patient's anterior tibia. **(B)** A red-brown/yellowish shiny plaque with a dark brown-red serpiginous border, alongside a few punctuate lesions with scales and a loss of hair follicles. (Used with permission from the Department of Dermatology, Washington Hospital Center, Washington, DC.)

droplets. The inflammation of blood vessels, capillary basement membrane thickening, and the obliteration of vessel lumina are also observed.[6]

Treatment Sometimes the lesions will disappear when glycemic control is achieved. However, intralesional and topical steroids, compression stockings, ultraviolet-B and -A1 phototherapy, hyperbaric oxygen therapy, and tumor necrosis factor-α inhibitors are also useful in treating NLD.[33]

Differential Diagnosis The differential diagnosis for NLD includes sarcoidosis, pretibial myxedema, GA, and stasis dermatitis.

■ DIABETIC BULLAE

Diabetic bullae are considered a diagnostic indication of diabetes [**Figure 68-7**]. Bullae occur equally in men and women. The cause is unknown, and the onset is often sudden.[6] Although this condition is most often seen in patients with long-standing diabetes, it is sometimes already present when diabetes is first diagnosed. Spontaneous tense serous bullae occur primarily on the lower extremities, particularly on the acral areas.[34] Bullae usually appear on a pigmented base as round pale-yellow blisters containing clear fluid. If the bullae have ruptured, there will be a gray or yellowish flaccid piece of skin overlying a pink base. They will generally be surrounded by normal skin with no inflammation. Bullae are painless and heal without scarring. The histology shows they are subepidermal.

Treatment If they are causing the patient discomfort, large bullae should be aspirated. Otherwise, the treatment should focus on preventing infectious complications.

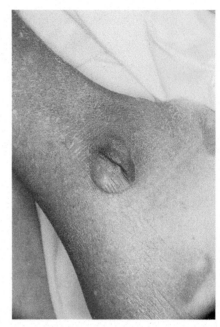

FIGURE 68-7. Diabetic bullae, as pictured here, are a hallmark of diabetes. They are seen most often as a blister on the lower extremities. (Used with permission from the Department of Dermatology, Washington Hospital Center, Washington, DC.)

Differential Diagnosis The differential diagnosis includes fixed drug eruption, porphyria cutanea tarda, bullous pemphigoid, and other autoimmune bullous diseases.

■ LEG AND FOOT ULCERS

Leg and foot ulcers commonly occur in patients who have poorly controlled diabetes, with a recent study noting a lifetime risk of up to 25% in diabetics [**Figure 68-8**].[35] These ulcers often pose significant health risks and can result in chronic infections, gangrene, and lower limb amputations.

Diabetic foot ulcers are usually due to peripheral neuropathy (60%), ischemic arterial disease (15%), or a combination of both factors (15%). A structural foot deformity may lead to areas of higher pressure, and when this is coupled with decreased sensation, it can result in the formation of an ulcer. In addition, poor glucose control contributes to poor wound healing. Recent evidence supports this, showing that higher serum values of hemoglobin A1C are correlated with slower wound healing.[36]

Clinically, ulcers typically form at sites of high pressure or friction. There is often a thickened callus covering the ulcer or a hyperkeratotic rim around it. These ulcers are usually painless as they occur in patients with peripheral neuropathy. When ischemic disease is contributing to the ulcer formation, there is often shiny taut skin and a loss of hair on the distal lower extremities. Foot deformities and evidence of prior ulcers often coexist. The histopathology reveals necrotic tissue and is usually not helpful in the diagnosis of the ulcer.

Treatment The treatment of diabetic foot ulcers is difficult and requires a multidisciplinary approach. Aggressive debridement is needed to remove the necrotic tissue, whereas pressure offloading is often necessary to allow the affected areas to heal.[37] A bacterial colonization of the ulcers is common, so judicious use of antibiotics is warranted. If there is concomitant soft tissue or bone infection, longer courses of antibiotics are necessary. If arterial ischemia is contributing to the ulcer formation or difficulties in wound healing, a revascularization procedure may be necessary. Bioengineered skin grafts can also be used in combination with the aforementioned treatment strategies. If revascularization is not possible or the infection cannot be controlled, then limb amputation may be necessary. It is important to prevent diabetic patients from developing ulcers through the use of regular foot inspections and pressure-offloading shoes that inhibit callus formations.

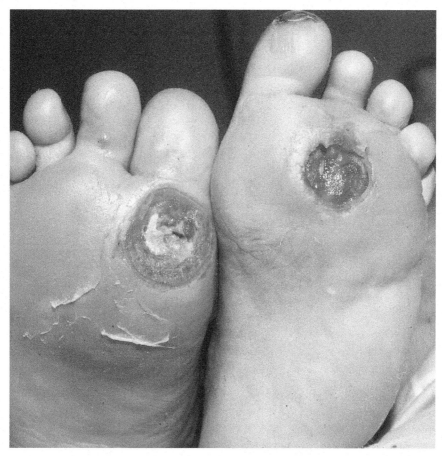

FIGURE 68-8. A case of diabetic ulcers located on the soles of a patient's feet. This condition occurs in individuals with poorly controlled diabetes and can result in serious complications. (Used with permission from the Department of Dermatology, Washington Hospital Center, Washington, DC.)

ACANTHOSIS NIGRICANS (AN)

AN is a common skin condition associated with insulin resistance and obesity, particularly in patients with metabolic syndrome. It can also be seen in those with other endocrinologic disorders (such as acromegaly, Cushing syndrome, and leprechaunism) or an internal malignancy (such as gastric cancer). AN occurs more commonly in African American, Hispanic, and Southeast Asian patients. Hyperinsulinemia has been associated with AN and may result in the activation of the insulin growth factor receptors on keratinocytes. This can lead to epidermal proliferation.

AN consists of thick velvety hyperpigmented plaques, most commonly seen on the neck and axillae [**Figure 68-9**]. It can also occur on the lips, umbilicus, areolae, submammary region, elbows, and hands. The form of AN associated with endocrine disorders is often insidious at onset, whereas paraneoplastic AN usually presents acutely. In African American skin, the plaques are dark brown to black; in Asian or Hispanic skin, they are light brown to dark brown. The histology shows papillomatosis, hyperkeratosis, and acanthosis in patients with AN.

Treatment The primary treatment for this condition involves tight glycemic control and weight loss. Patients with AN are likely to require much higher insulin doses to achieve a glycemic control, due to their often coexistent insulin resistance. Retinoic acid, α-hydroxy acids, calcipotriol, hydroquinones, neodymium-doped yttrium aluminum garnet (Nd:YAG) laser therapy, and systemic retinoids have also been used to treat AN with varying rates of success.[38]

SCLEREDEMA (SCLEREDEMA ADULTORUM OF BUSCHKE)

Scleredema is a rare skin disease that is commonly associated with diabetes. It is usually seen in obese patients with poor glycemic control. It

is 10 times more common in men than in women, and it has an increased incidence in older age groups.[39] The exact pathogenesis is unknown, but it is thought to be related to the dermal deposition of glycosaminoglycans and collagen. The stimulation of fibroblasts by insulin promotes the fibroblast production of collagen and mucin.

Clinically, scleredema is characterized by indurated erythematous skin of the upper back, shoulders, and posterior neck [**Figure 68-10**].

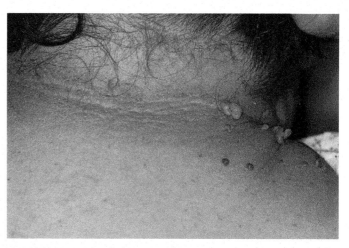

FIGURE 68-9. A skin of color patient with hyperpigmented plaques of acanthosis nigricans occurring on the neck. These skin changes are not seen exclusively in diabetic patients but are an indicator of insulin resistance. (Used with permission from the Department of Dermatology, Washington Hospital Center, Washington, DC.)

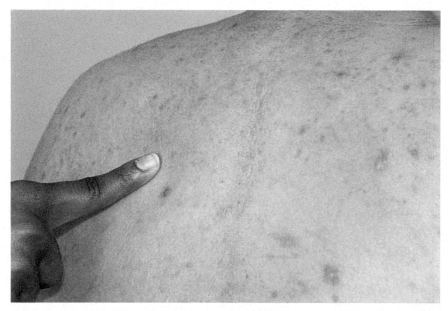

FIGURE 68-10. Scleroderma on the back of a male patient. This condition is most often seen in men with poor glycemic control. (Used with permission from the Department of Dermatology, Washington Hospital Center, Washington, DC.)

The infiltration of the dermis often results in a *peau d'orange* appearance of the skin. Scleredema is slowly progressive and can lead to a restricted range of motion. However, patients do not typically have increased rates of morbidity or mortality. The histopathology reveals a thickened dermis with large bungles of collagen and clear spaces representing mucin.

Treatment   The form of scleredema associated with diabetes has been found to respond poorly to treatment. Tight diabetic control does not result in an improvement of this skin disease either. Treatments include intralesional and topical steroids, extracorporeal photopheresis, intravenous immunoglobulin, UVA1 phototherapy, and psoralen plus ultraviolet A therapy.[40]

■ DIABETIC DERMOPATHY

Diabetic dermopathy is a common rash, usually located on the shins of diabetic patients [**Figure 68-11**]. These lesions are seen in at least 50%

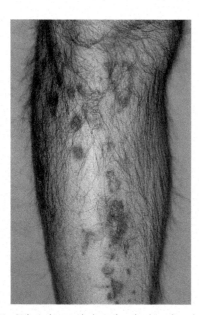

FIGURE 68-11. Diabetic dermopathy located on the shins of a male patient. This is the most common cutaneous manifestation of diabetes but can be hard to identify in individuals with darker skin of color. (Used with permission from the Department of Dermatology, Washington Hospital Center, Washington, DC.)

of diabetics, making them the most common skin marker of diabetes.[41] The frequency of these lesions increase with a patient's age and the duration of the disease. It is seen more commonly in those with type 1 diabetes and in males. The development of these lesions is likely related to trauma, as the darker color is associated with blood extravasation and breakdown.

Diabetic dermopathy presents with well-circumscribed hyper- and hypopigmented macules and patches on the lower extremities. They are most commonly seen on patients' anterior shins. These lesions can be difficult to identify in those with darker skin of color. They often heal with atrophy and hyperpigmentation. The histology shows a thickening of the capillaries in the dermis, a perivascular lymphocytic infiltrate, and scattered hemosiderin.

Treatment   The treatment for diabetic dermopathy is not usually efficacious, and tight glycemic control does not lead to an improvement of the lesions.[42] Although these lesions are not specific to diabetes, they often occur with other vascular complications of diabetes.

CONCLUSION

The spectrum of cutaneous manifestations in diabetes is broad. Patients may present with GA, NLD, diabetic bullae, leg and foot ulcers, and scleredema. However, the most common skin findings are usually diabetic dermopathy, cutaneous infections, and AN.

Infections of the skin include polymicrobial infections, malignant otitis externa, rhinocerebral mucormycosis, and superficial fungal infections. These are generally treated with antibiotics, aggressive debridement, and/or correction of blood glucose levels. However, in severe cases, amputation of the affected limb may be required.

Diabetic dermopathy is the most common cutaneous manifestation of diabetes. Unfortunately, controlling the patient's glycemic levels does not affect the severity of these lesions. Therefore, the treatment options for this condition are limited.

AN is commonly associated with insulin resistance and obesity. As a result, AN is treated through tight glycemic control and weight loss. Other treatment options include retinoic acid, α-hydroxy acids, calcipotriol, hydroquinones, Nd:YAG laser therapy, and systemic retinoids.

In addition to the aforementioned conditions, diabetic patients may also present with several other nonspecific findings, including xerosis, ichthyosis, brittle nails, the loss of leg hair, diabetic thick skin, and hyperpigmentation. It is important for dermatologists to recognize the increased incidence of these skin changes in diabetic patients and, if necessary, alter their treatment plan accordingly.

REFERENCES

1. American Diabetes Association. Diabetes basics. http://www.diabetes.org/diabetes-basics/diabetes-statistics/. Accessed January 9, 2013.

2. Centers for Disease Control and Prevention. Summary health statistics for U.S. adults: National Health Interview Survey, 2010. http://www.cdc.gov/nchs/data/series/sr_10/sr10_252.pdf. Accessed January 30, 2013.

3. Barnes PM, Adams PF, Powell-Grimes E. Health characteristics of the American Indian or Alaska Native adult population: United States, 2004–2008. http://www.cdc.gov/nchs/data/nhsr/nhsr020.pdf. Accessed January 30, 2013.

4. Flegal KM, Carroll MD, Kit BK, et al. Prevalence of obesity and trends in the distribution of body mass index among US adults, 1999-2010. *JAMA*. 2012;307:491-497.

5. American Census Bureau. Population by race and Hispanic origin: 2012 and 2060. http://www.census.gov/newsroom/releases/img/racehispanic_graph.jpg. Accessed January 1, 2013.

6. Ahmed I, Goldstein B. Diabetes mellitus. *Clin Dermatol*. 2006;24:237-246.

7. Pinhas-Hamiel O, Zeitler P. The global spread of type 2 diabetes mellitus in children and adolescents. *J Pediatr*. 2005;146:693-700.

8. Centers for Disease Control and Prevention. Prevalence of diabetes, 2007. http://www.cdc.gov/diabetes/statistics/prev/national/menuage.htm. Accessed January 12, 2013.

9. Wahid Z, Kanjee A. Cutaneous manifestations of diabetes mellitus. *J Pak Med Assoc*. 1998;48:304-305.

10. Genetic Services Policy Project. Type 2 diabetes and genetic technology: a policy brief. http://depts.washington.edu/genpol/docs/PolicyBriefT2D.pdf. Accessed November 20, 2008.

11. Palmer ND, McDonough CW, Hicks PJ, et al. A genome-wide association search for type 2 diabetes genes in African Americans. *PLoS One*. 2012;7:e29202.

12. Dong Y, Guo T, Traurig M, et al. SIRT1 is associated with a decrease in acute insulin secretion and a sex specific increase in risk for type 2 diabetes in Pima Indians. *Mol Genet Metab*. 2011;104:661-665.

13. Schulz LO, Bennett PH, Ravussin E, et al. Effects of traditional and Western environments on prevalence of type 2 diabetes in Pima Indians in Mexico and the U.S. *Diabetes Care*. 2006;29:1866-1871.

14. American Diabetes Association. Diagnosis and classification of diabetes mellitus. *Diabetes Care*. 2007;30:S42-S47.

15. Ngo BT, Hayes KD, DiMiao DJ, et al. Manifestations of cutaneous diabetic microangiopathy. *Am J Clin Dermatol*. 2005;6:225-237.

16. Litonjua P, Piñero-Piloña A, Aviles-Santa L, et al. Prevalence of acanthosis nigricans in newly-diagnosed type 2 diabetes. *Endocr Pract*. 2004;10:101-106.

17. Schmults CA. Scleroderma. *Dermatol Online J*. 2003;9:11.

18a. Sehgal VN, Srivastava G, Aggarwal AK, et al. Noninsulin-dependent, type II diabetes mellitus-related dermatoses: part II. *Skinmed*. 2011;9:302-308.

18. Collier A, Matthews DM, Kellett HA, et al. Change in skin thickness associated with cheiroarthropathy in insulin dependent diabetes mellitus. *Br Med J (Clin Res Ed)*. 1986;292:936.

19. Lyons TJ, Kennedy L. Non-enzymatic glycosylation of skin collagen in patients with type 1 (insulin-dependent) diabetes mellitus and limited joint mobility. *Diabetologia*. 1985;28:2-5.

20. Nashel J, Steen V. Scleroderma mimics. *Curr Rheumatol Rep*. 2012;14:39-46.

21. Akanji AO, Bella AF, Osotimehin BO. Cheiroarthropathy and long term diabetic complications in Nigerians. *Ann Rheum Dis*. 1990;49:28-30.

22. Muller LM, Gorter KJ, Hak E, et al. Increased risk of common infections in patients with type 1 and type 2 diabetes mellitus. *Clin Infect Dis*. 2005;41:281-288.

23. Tuazon CU. Skin and skin structure infections in the patient at risk: carrier state of *Staphylococcus aureus*. *Am J Med*. 1984;76:166-171.

24. Calvet HM, Yoshikawa TT. Infections in diabetes. *Infect Dis Clin North Am*. 2001;15:407-421.

25. Gallacher SJ, Thomson G, Fraser WD, et al. Neutrophil bactericidal function in diabetes mellitus: evidence for association with blood glucose control. *Diabet Med*. 1995;12:916-920.

26. Hoeffel JC, Hoeffel F. Necrotizing fasciitis and purpura fulminans. *Plast Reconstr Surg*. 2002;109:2165.

27. Joshi N, Caputo GM, Weitekamp MR, et al. Infections in patients with diabetes mellitus. *N Engl J Med*. 1999;341:1906-1912.

28. Muthukumarassamy R, Sumit KR, Vikram K, et al. Necrotising soft tissue infection of fungal origin in two diabetic patients. *Mycoses*. 2006;10:1111.

29. Felner EI, Steinberg JB, Weinberg AG. Subcutaneous granuloma annulare: a review of 47 cases. *Pediatrics*. 1997;100:965-967.

30. Nebesio CL, Lewis C, Chuang TY. Lack of an association between granuloma annulare and type 2 diabetes mellitus. *Br J Dermatol*. 2002;146:122-124.

31. Muller SA, Winkelmann RK. Necrobiosis lipoidica diabeticorum. A clinical and pathological investigation of 171 cases. *Arch Dermatol*. 1966;93:272-281.

32. Boateng B, Hiller D, Albrecht HP, et al. Cutaneous microcirculation in pretibial necrobiosis lipoidica. Comparative laser Doppler flowmetry and oxygen partial pressure determinations in patients and healthy probands. *Hautarzt*. 1993;44:581-586.

33. Erfurt-Berge C, Seitz AT, Rehse C, et al. Update on clinical and laboratory features in necrobiosis lipoidica: a retrospective multicentre study of 52 patients. *Eur J Dermatol*. 2012;22:770-775.

34. Lipsky BA, Baker PD, Ahroni JH. Diabetic bullae: 12 cases of a purportedly rare cutaneous disorder. *Int J Dermatol*. 2000;39:196-200.

35. Namazi, MR, Yosipovitch, G. Diabetes mellitus. In: Callen JP, Jorizzo JL, eds. *Dermatological Signs of Internal Disease*. 4th ed. Philadelphia, PA: Saunders; 2009:189-198.

36. Christman AL, Selvin E, Margolis DJ, et al. Hemoglobin A1c predicts healing rate in diabetic wounds. *J Invest Dermatol*. 2011;131:2121-2127.

37. Gordon KA, Lebrun EA, Tomic-Canic M, et al. The role of surgical debridement in healing of diabetic foot ulcers. *Skinmed*. 2012;10:24-26.

38. Kapoor S. Diagnosis and treatment of acanthosis nigricans. *Skinmed*. 2010;8:161-164.

39. Martín C, Requena L, Manrique K, et al. Scleredema diabeticorum in a patient with type 2 diabetes mellitus. *Case Rep Endocrinol*. 2011;2011:560273.

40. Aichelburg MC, Loewe R, Schicher N, et al. Successful treatment of poststreptococcal scleredema adultorum Buschke with intravenous immunoglobulins. *Arch Dermatol*. 2012;148:1126-1128.

41. Ragunatha S, Anitha B, Inamadar AC, et al. Cutaneous disorders in 500 diabetic patients attending diabetic clinic. *Indian J Dermatol*. 2011;56:160-164.

42. Levy L, Zeichner JA. Dermatologic manifestation of diabetes. *J Diabetes*. 2012;4:68-76.

CHAPTER 69

Hepatic Disease

Lynn McKinley-Grant
Nasir Aziz
Daniel Callaghan

KEY POINTS

- Early cutaneous signs of hepatic disease can depend on the etiology of the disease, particularly whether the disease is viral, resulting from nonalcoholic fatty liver disease, or autoimmune.

- There is a higher incidence of hepatic diseases in people with skin of color. In Caucasians, there is a higher incidence of primary biliary cirrhosis.

- The skin findings in end-stage hepatic failure include jaundice, spider angiomas, pruritus, and many others.

- Mixed cryoglobulinemia is the most common extrahepatic manifestation of hepatitis C, but only a small proportion of patients with cryoglobulins have a clinically evident form of hepatitis C.

- Lichen planus and hepatitis C have a strong clinical correlation.

INTRODUCTION

The epidemiology of liver disease shows that it is more prevalent in individuals with skin of color. In general, the skin gives the first clues to the signs and symptoms of liver disease. According to the Centers for Disease Control and Prevention, chronic liver disease/cirrhosis was the fifth most common cause of death among Native Americans and Alaskan Natives in 2009 and was the sixth most common cause of death among the Hispanic/Latino populations.[1] The liver can be affected by a wide variety of disease processes, many of which show no predilection for skin color or gender and others which occur more widely in those with darkly pigmented skin. The causes of these diseases range from viral infections and metabolic disorders to drugs and alcohol, but the end result shared by all forms of liver disease is that, when left unchecked, the liver eventually becomes fibrotic and cirrhotic.

NONALCOHOLIC FATTY LIVER DISEASE

■ EPIDEMIOLOGY

Worldwide, nonalcoholic fatty liver disease (NAFLD) is the most common cause of chronic liver disease.[2] NAFLD is a metabolic disorder that results from the accumulation of triglycerides in the hepatocytes and, as such, is strongly associated with obesity, insulin resistance, and the metabolic syndrome. Certain cultural or racial groups are known to be at greater risk of developing this disease, with the prevalence being highest in Hispanics, followed by Asians and Caucasians.[3] The lowest prevalence is in African Americans.[3] Patients with psoriasis have also been found to have a greater risk of developing NAFLD, which has been attributed to the higher prevalence of diabetes, obesity, and hypertension among psoriasis patients.[4,5]

■ PATHOGENESIS

The pathogenesis of NAFLD is not yet fully understood. Hispanics suffer from the highest rates of NAFLD, and it was initially speculated that this was a result of the high prevalence of obesity and insulin resistance within that population. However, the fact that African Americans suffer from higher rates of obesity and insulin resistance, yet have a lower prevalence of NAFLD, suggests that other factors are associated with the disease's pathogenesis.[6,7]

This discrepancy could be due to variations in the enzyme adiponutrin, which hydrolyzes triacylglycerol in adipocytes. One allele in *PNPLA3*, the gene that encodes adiponutrin, has been associated with increased hepatic inflammation and fat levels and has been found to be most common in Hispanics.[8] Conversely, another allele of *PNPLA3* has been associated with lower hepatic fat levels and has been found more commonly in African Americans.[8]

■ CLINICAL FEATURES

The majority of patients with NAFLD are asymptomatic. Patients occasionally have nonspecific symptoms including fatigue, malaise or vague right upper quadrant abdominal discomfort, and spider angiomas [**Figure 69-1**].[9] However, given the association of NAFLD with insulin resistance, obesity, and the metabolic syndrome, the signs and symptoms more specific to these diseases should prompt clinicians to test

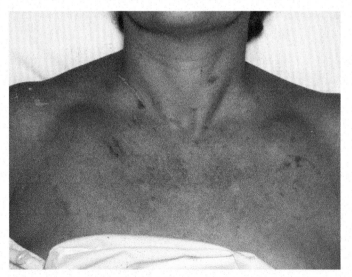

FIGURE 69-1. Spider angiomas on the chest and back are commonly seen in nonalcoholic fatty liver disease and other forms of hepatic failure. (Used with permission from the Department of Dermatology, Washington Center, Washington DC.)

for NAFLD as well. For example, acanthosis nigricans, which is often seen in the setting of insulin resistance, has been connected to NAFLD. Although one study based out of the United States found that only 14% of adults with nonalcoholic steatohepatitis (NASH) had acanthosis nigricans,[10] another study in Sri Lanka found that 80% of adults with NAFLD also had acanthosis nigricans.[11]

■ TREATMENT

Unfortunately, no definitive treatment for NAFLD or NASH is available as yet, except for diet and lifestyle modifications.[12]

LICHEN PLANUS

■ EPIDEMIOLOGY

The reported prevalence of lichen planus (LP) in the general population varies widely; however, it has been estimated to be 0.9% to 1.2%.[13] For more information, see Chapter 26. It is a disease that mostly affects the middle-aged and has also been found to affect women more than men by a ratio of roughly 2:1.[13] In most cases, the disease shows no preference for any specific racial group.[14] However, there has been a report highlighting an increased incidence of oral involvement among villagers in India, especially among those using chewing tobacco.[15]

Although LP has long been associated with the hepatitis C virus (HCV), this relationship has remained controversial given the fact that several studies have shown no association between the two.[16] For example, although studies out of Taiwan,[17] Japan,[18] Egypt,[19] and Thailand[20] have all found statistically significant relationships between HCV and LP, similar studies out of Turkey,[21] China,[22] and Nepal[23] have not. Interestingly, although a study out of Nigeria did find a relationship between HCV and LP, it found an association between HCV and cutaneous LP as opposed to oral LP, with which HCV is traditionally associated.[24] Furthermore, the HCV-positive patients from Nigeria more frequently had hypertrophic LP rather than the atrophic-erosive LP found in numerous other studies throughout the world.[24] Based on these inconsistencies, which may be a result of the small sample sizes within individual studies, the association between LP and HCV has remained controversial.

With that in mind, several recent meta-analyses have confirmed the association between HCV and LP. One study demonstrated a five-fold increased risk of LP among HCV patients as well as a five-fold increased risk of HCV seropositivity among LP patients.[25] An earlier study found an overall 2.5-fold increased prevalence of LP in HCV patients.[14] However, both studies showed geographical variability in this association due to the varied prevalence of HCV infection. A higher prevalence of HCV infections was found in patients with LP in Japan, the Mediterranean regions, and the United States.[14,25] Interestingly, similar geographical variability has been demonstrated for other dermatologic disorders associated with HCV, including porphyria cutanea tarda (PCT) and mixed cryoglobulinemia (MC).[14,25]

■ PATHOGENESIS

The histology of LP is characterized by the degeneration of the basal keratinocytes, a dense band-like subepithelial lymphohistiocytic infiltrate, and increased numbers of intraepithelial lymphocytes. The exact pathogenesis leading to these changes is still unclear, and research has largely focused on oral LP lesions. LP is believed to be an autoimmune disease, with cluster of differentiation 8 (CD8)-positive cytotoxic T-cells having been found to accumulate in these lesions. These T-cells are thought to lead to the destruction of antigen-specific basal keratinocytes.[26] Several cytokines, including interferon-γ, tumor necrosis factor-α, interleukin (IL)-6, and IL-8, are also believed to be involved.[16] Although experimental data suggest that HCV is associated with the pathogenesis of oral LP due to common epitopes shared with these basal keratinocytes, several studies were unable to find similar epitopes shared between them.[27,28] As a result of this lack of data, it is now thought that HCV contributes to the pathogenesis of LP as a result of the CD8+ T-cells targeting epithelial cells expressing HCV antigens.[27,28]

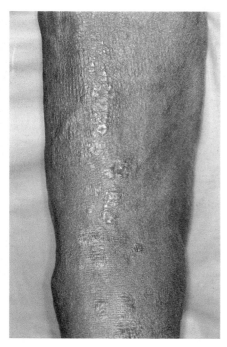

FIGURE 69-2. A patient with lichen planus on the forearm. Lichen planus is believed to be caused by the T-cell-mediated destruction of antigen-specific basal keratinocytes. (Used with permission from the Department of Dermatology, Washington Center, Washington DC.)

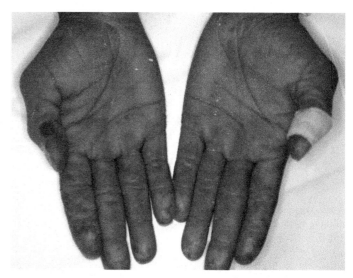

FIGURE 69-3. Mixed cryoglobulinemia of the hands. (Used with permission from the Department of Dermatology, Washington Center, Washington DC.)

CLINICAL FEATURES

The skin lesions of LP are characterized by pruritic, violaceous, shiny polygonal papules and plaques with overlying delicate white lines, referred to as Wickham striae [**Figure 69-2**].[29] Wickham striae are pathognomonic for LP and are especially found in lesions on flexor surfaces.[16,30] Notably they can result in long-term residual hyperpigmentation, which is more common in darkly pigmented individuals.[31] Conversely, oral LP is characterized by symmetrical, reticular lesions in addition to papules, plaques, erythematous lesions, and erosions. Rather than being pruritic, the erosive lesions are actually quite painful.[31] Oral lesions are also commonly associated with HCV.[29,32] Anogenital LP shares characteristics with both the skin and oral manifestations of the disease.[31] Ungual LP is characterized by nail plate thinning with longitudinal ridging and fissuring, with or without pterygium.[33]

TREATMENT

Skin LP lesions will typically resolve spontaneously within 1 to 2 years.[34] Skin lesions are initially treated with high-potency topical steroids.[29] If initial therapy fails, topical calcineurin inhibitors, intralesional corticosteroids, systemic corticosteroids, retinoids, narrowband ultraviolet B therapy, psoralen plus ultraviolet A treatment, and hydroxychloroquine have all been found to be effective.[29,35] LP lesions in the mucous membranes are generally more resistant to treatment, and even when treated, recurrence is common.[34] For oral LP, high-potency topical steroids are the first line of treatment. If these should fail, topical retinoids, topical calcineurin inhibitors, and intralesional corticosteroids, among other treatments, can be used.[29,36,37]

MIXED CRYOGLOBULINEMIA (MC)

EPIDEMIOLOGY

MC is recognized as the most common extrahepatic manifestation of HCV [**Figures 69-3 and 69-4**].[38] Cryoglobulins are seen in 19% to 54% of HCV patients, whereas only 10% to 30% of patients with cryoglobulins have a clinically evident form of the disease.[39,40] Conversely, 40% to 90% of individuals with MC have HCV, whereas 5% to 10% of

MC patients are HCV-negative. HCV-negative MC may be associated with such diseases as multiple myeloma, chronic lymphocytic leukemia, systemic lupus erythematosus, Sjögren syndrome, and other viral infections.[38,41] The prevalence of MC has been found to vary based on geographic location, with a greater prevalence in southern Europe when compared to both northern Europe and North America.[42]

PATHOGENESIS

The pathogenesis of MC is ultimately a result of the cryoglobulins, which are immune complexes made up of HCV proteins, polyclonal anti-HCV immunoglobulin G (IgG) antibodies, and monoclonal immunoglobulin M (IgM) rheumatoid factor (RF) antibodies that are deposited in the vascular endothelium. IgM RF binds the anti-HCV IgG, and upon being deposited in the vessel wall, the complement system is activated, leading to the vasculitis that results in MC's clinical manifestations.[29,32,42] Cryoglobulins can also precipitate intravascularly at temperatures below 37°C (98.6°F).[43]

CLINICAL FEATURES

The most common clinical manifestations of MC are palpable purpura (80% to 90%), urticarial vasculitis (10%), and livedo reticularis of the legs.[41] Other cutaneous manifestations can include edema or Raynaud

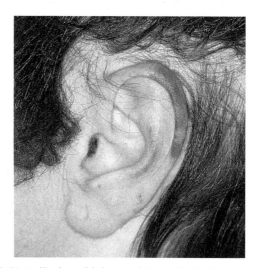

FIGURE 69-4. Mixed cryoglobulinemia of the ear. (Used with permission from the Department of Dermatology, Washington Hospital Center, Washington DC.)

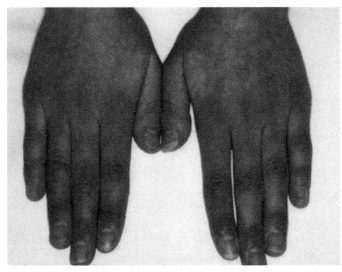

FIGURE 69-5. Porphyria cutanea tarda presenting with postinflammatory hypopigmentation and hyperpigmentation. (Used with permission from the Department of Dermatology, Washington Hospital Center, Washington DC.)

phenomenon [**Figure 69-5**].[38] In more severe MC, cutaneous manifestations can include ulcers, which are commonly found in the supramalleolar region; these may become necrotic and progress to gangrene.[42] Notably, patients with HCV who develop MC generally present with cutaneous lesions more frequently than those with noncutaneous manifestations.[41]

PATHOLOGY

MC is a vasculitis that affects both small- and medium-sized vessels. The histopathology reveals a leukocytoclastic vasculitis with a deposition of immune complexes made up of IgM RF and IgG along with complement component 3 and neutrophils into the vessel wall.[42] Whether the cryoglobulinemia is designated as type I, II, or III depends on whether or not the immunoglobulins are monoclonal, polyclonal, or mixed, respectively.[41] Additionally, MC can also manifest as necrotizing vasculitis with fibrinoid necrosis of the vessel wall.[42]

TREATMENT

Given the wide variety of clinical manifestations of MC, it is challenging to develop broad treatment recommendations. Any treatment regimen should accomplish three goals: (1) eradicate the HCV; (2) limit or prevent B-cell proliferation; and (3) contain and symptomatically treat the associated vasculitis along with limiting the damage caused by the circulating cryoglobulins. For this reason, the first line of treatment should be pegylated interferon along with ribavirin to treat the underlying HCV. Rituximab can be considered in patients who suffer from severe MC; if this fails, colchicine is occasionally used, despite the limited data concerning its efficacy. Although high-dose pulse glucocorticoids can also be used for severe MC, the long-term use of steroids is discouraged, even at low doses.[44-47]

NECROLYTIC ACRAL ERYTHEMA

EPIDEMIOLOGY

Necrolytic acral erythema (NAE) is an uncommon dermatosis that may be an early cutaneous marker for HCV infection. The age of onset is broad, between 11 and 60 years, but it most commonly occurs between the ages of 35 and 55 years. There is no gender predilection.[48] It has been found that 87% of patients diagnosed with NAE are unaware of their underlying HCV infection, which presents a rare opportunity to suspect and diagnose HCV based solely on the skin findings.[49]

The majority of cases have been reported from Egypt.[50] There are several possible explanations for this. Egyptian patients may be more susceptible to this cutaneous association with HCV. Alternately, this could simply reflect a higher prevalence of HCV in Egypt, which ranges from 15% to 20% compared to approximately 3% worldwide.[50] Finally, it could simply reflect greater awareness of this entity among Egyptian physicians. A recent study from the United States found a low prevalence (1.7%) of NAE among a cohort of 300 chronic HCV-infected patients.[50] The vast majority of patients were of African origin (92%). The authors speculated that the lower incidence could be attributed to the difference in HCV genotypes seen in the United States compared with Egypt.[50]

CLINICAL FEATURES

NAE typically presents as psoriasiform, erythematous to violaceous, and hyperpigmented papules and plaques with sharp borders; scales and erosion are also seen.[51-53] Acute lesions can appear vesiculobullous with erythematous borders, whereas chronic lesions can appear erythematous to violaceous with a more pronounced scale and hyperpigmented borders. Lesions typically occur on acral areas, especially the lower extremities. Less common areas of involvement include the trunk and upper extremities.[49,54,55] Although these lesions can simulate psoriasis, the palmoplantar areas are usually spared in NAE, which can help to differentiate the two diagnoses.[56]

PATHOLOGY

Histology shows psoriasiform changes with epidermal necrosis.[46,47,54] A histologic review of 30 cases found that early NAE is characterized by acanthosis, epidermal spongiosis, and superficial perivascular inflammation.[54] In its fully developed state, psoriasiform hyperplasia with parakeratosis, subcorneal pustules, epidermal pallor, and necrotic keratinocytes can be seen. Although the clinical and histologic overlap can make it difficult to distinguish NAE from psoriasis, discerning features include the foci of epidermal necrosis and the pallor.[49]

PATHOGENESIS

The pathogenesis of NAE remains unclear, although it is widely believed to have a multifactorial etiology. Given its association with nearly every case of NAE, it is possible that HCV plays a direct role in the pathogenesis either through the HCV ribonucleic acid, peptides, or other mechanisms. However, there have been no successful attempts in isolating hepatitis C viral particles within the involved lesions, giving rise to the hypothesis that NAE may be due to an autoimmune response to the viral or host antigens.[51-53] Although a direct correlation exists between the severity of the cutaneous disease and the degree of hepatic damage, the fact that it has not been reported in other cirrhotic conditions excludes chronic liver damage as the chief cause.[57]

Furthermore, the pathogenesis of NAE is believed to have a metabolic component as well. This hypothesis is a result of the observation that amino acid or zinc supplementation can clear the skin lesions of NAE. Specifically, hypoaminoacidemia may deplete the protein stores, in turn causing the keratinocyte necrolysis seen in NAE. On the other hand, zinc deficiency leads to an impairment of nutrient delivery to the tissues, possibly resulting in dysfunctional epidermal proliferation and differentiation.[57]

TREATMENT

Once diagnosed, patients who have their HCV treated with a combination of interferon-α and ribavirin will often experience the complete resolution of their NAE lesions within several months.[58] There have also been reports of the skin lesions clearing up after patients undergo a liver transplantation.[50] Additionally, zinc supplementation has been found to resolve the lesions;[49] although it is not always successful, zinc supplements should be taken by all NAE patients regardless of their serum zinc levels because the probable benefit greatly outweighs any risks. Notably, these lesions have repeatedly been found to be unresponsive to topical steroid treatments in the majority of patients.[49,53,57]

PORPHYRIA CUTANEA TARDA

PATHOGENESIS

PCT is the most common type of cutaneous porphyria, which is a group of disorders that result in a build-up of porphyrins in the body. PCT is due to the decreased activity of uroporphyrinogen III decarboxylase (UROD) in the liver.[59,60] Most patients have the sporadic form of the disease (type I). Approximately 20% to 30% of patients have gene mutations affecting the UROD enzyme, which result in the familial form (type II).[59-61] This form of PCT results in 50% reduced enzyme activity, both in the liver and erythrocytes. Finally, although type III is characterized by a family history of the disease, the defective URO-D is only in the liver, similar to that seen in type I PCT. Although most patients with the sporadic form experience symptoms in their 20s and 30s, the familial subtype has an earlier onset. Inheritance is autosomal dominant with low penetrance.[61]

There are multiple precipitating factors, all of which are associated with the inhibition of hepatic UROD activity. These include iron overload, alcohol ingestion, estrogen, HCV, and HIV infections. Data from different countries differ widely with regard to the significance of various factors contributing to the pathogenesis of PCT. Concomitant HCV infection occurs in 56% to 85% of patients with PCT in southern Europe, Japan, and the United States, whereas rates are much lower in northern France, Germany, and New Zealand (0% to 23%).[59]

CLINICAL FEATURES

The accumulation of porphyrins in the liver causes liver damage, and their circulation in the plasma results in cutaneous phototoxicity. Patients present with skin fragility, noninflammatory vesicles, and bullae in a photodistribution [**Figures 69-5 and 69-6**].[60] Crusts and erosions are often present, and the lesions leave milia and scars after they have healed.[60,62] The dorsal hands and forearms are common locations. Other symptoms include periorbital hypertrichosis, mottled dyspigmentation, and sclerodermoid changes that can affect both the sun-exposed and sun-protected areas of the skin.[61]

TREATMENT

The standard treatment for acquired PCT is a phlebotomy, which reduces hepatic iron and therefore decreases iron's inhibition of UROD oxidation.[63] Low dose hydroxychloroquine (200 mg once or twice weekly) has also been used with success.

PRIMARY BILIARY CIRRHOSIS

EPIDEMIOLOGY

The incidence and prevalence of primary biliary cirrhosis (PBC) appear to vary based on geographic location, with an annual incidence ranging between 0.7 and 49 cases per 1,000,000 people and a prevalence ranging between 6.7 and 402 cases per 1,000,000.[64-66] However, little is known about how PBC varies between different races or distinct cultural groups given that most studies originate from European countries. Additionally, the leading study conducted in the United States was performed in a predominantly Caucasian community.[66] Given the fact that it is an autoimmune disease, it should come as no surprise that PBC predominantly affects females, with only approximately 7% to 11% of patients being male.[67] It predominantly affects individuals in their fifth decade of life and is generally not seen in patients under 25 years old.[68]

CLINICAL MANIFESTATIONS

Although fatigue is the most common symptom of PBC, affecting up to 78% of patients, local or diffuse pruritus is a more specific symptom. Although pruritus was once found in 20% to 70% of patients with PBC, the prevalence of pruritus in PBC has been decreasing given the trend toward diagnosing PBC in patients before they are symptomatic.[68] When pruritus does manifest, it is either local or diffuse and is usually worse at night. Uncommon cutaneous manifestations of PBC include

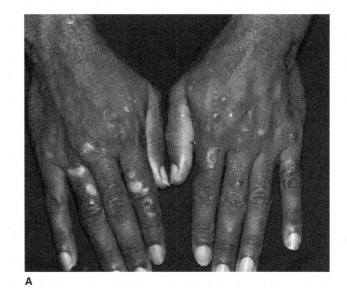
A

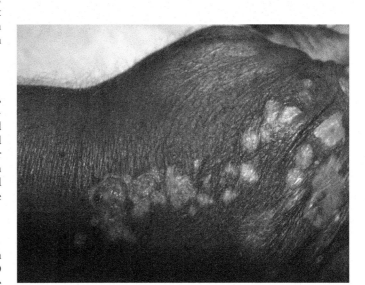
B

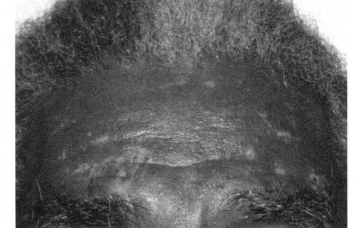
C

FIGURE 69-6. (A) Porphyria cutanea tarda (PCT) presenting with postinflammatory hypopigmentation and milia on the hands. **(B)** Acute PCT with impetiginized bullae in a patient. **(C)** A patient with PCT in a sun-exposed area, the forehead, with postinflammatory hypopigmentation. ([A] Image appears with permission from VisualDx. (B&C) Used with permission from the Department of Dermatology, Washington Center, Washington DC.)

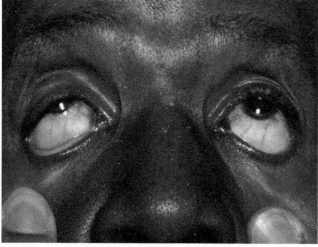

A

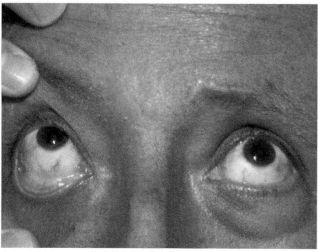

B

FIGURE 69-7. The brown pigment in the sclera of the eye in patients with darker skin types (**A**) is often difficult to distinguish from jaundice (**B**). As seen in these images, the natural brown is not diffuse through the sclera like that of the yellow discoloration of jaundice. (Used with permission from the Department of Dermatology, Washington Center, Washington DC.)

Raynaud phenomenon and calcinosis cutis. Cutaneous manifestations can also present secondary to PBC's role in subsequent diseases such as the xanthelasmas and xanthomas seen with hyperlipidemia, the spider angiomas seen with portal hypertension, and the jaundice seen with advanced liver disease [**Figure 69-7**].[69]

▓ PATHOLOGY

PBC has four histologic stages that may exist simultaneously in any given PBC patient. Stage 1 is characterized by inflammation localized to the portal triads. In stage 2, this inflammation spreads to the surrounding parenchyma. Stage 3 demonstrates fibrous septa that connect the portal triads. Finally, stage 4 PBC is defined by the regenerative nodules characteristic of cirrhosis.[70]

▓ PATHOGENESIS

The exact pathogenesis of PBC is currently unclear; however, it is known to be an autoimmune disorder. Roughly 90% of PBC patients have antimitochondrial antibodies (AMAs).[68] These AMAs develop when something triggers an individual to lose tolerance to the pyruvate dehydrogenase complexes (pyruvate dehydrogenase complex E2 component) found on the mitochondria.[71] This is hypothesized to be a multifactorial process, with genetics, epigenetics, and environmental factors all contributing to the pathogenesis.[72]

▓ TREATMENT

The only drug approved by the U.S. Food and Drug Administration for PBC is ursodeoxycholic acid (UDCA), which is optimally dosed at 13 to 15 mg/kg/d. Such a regimen may decrease the need for a liver transplantation. However, UDCA does not treat underlying symptoms such as pruritus, which needs to be treated separately. Given the role of liver-produced substances, which contribute to the pruritus, it can be treated with bile acid sequestrants such as cholestyramine. Alternative drugs that can be used for pruritus cases that prove refractory to this therapy include rifampicin, naltrexone, and sertraline.[69]

CONCLUSION

Every type of liver disease will have a skin manifestation associated with it. Therefore, because dermatologists are often the first physicians to be consulted regarding these cutaneous indications, it is imperative that they become very familiar with the manifestation of liver diseases and the systemic disorders indicated by their presence. Additionally, patients may present with end-stage hepatic disease with skin manifestations, and these manifestations should help the practitioner make the appropriate diagnosis and referral.

REFERENCES

1. Barnes PM, Adams PF, Powell-Griner E. Health characteristics of the American Indian or Alaska Native adult population: United States, 2004–2008. www.cdc.gov/nchs/data/nhsr/nhsr020.pdf. Accessed July 30, 2013.
2. Ong JP, Younossi ZM. Epidemiology and natural history of NAFLD and NASH. *Clin Liver Dis.* 2007;11:1-16.
3. Weston SR, Leyden W, Murphy R, et al. Racial and ethnic distribution of nonalcoholic fatty liver in persons with newly diagnosed chronic liver disease. *Hepatology.* 2005;41:372-379.
4. Madanagobalane S, Anandan S. The increased prevalence of non-alcoholic fatty liver disease in psoriatic patients: a study from South India. *Australas J Dermatol.* 2012;53:190-197.
5. Gisondi P, Targher G, Zoppini G, et al. Non-alcoholic fatty liver disease in patients with chronic plaque psoriasis. *J Hepatol.* 2009;51:758-764.
6. Pagadala MR, McCullough AJ. Non-alcoholic fatty liver disease and obesity: not all about body mass index. *Am J Gastroenterol.* 2012;107:1859-1861.
7. Mohanty SR, Troy TN, Huo D, et al. Influence of ethnicity on histological differences in non-alcoholic fatty liver disease. *J Hepatol.* 2009;50:797-804.
8. Romeo S, Kozlitina J, Xing C, et al. Genetic variation in PNPLA3 confers susceptibility to nonalcoholic fatty liver disease. *Nat Genet.* 2008;40:1461-1465.
9. McCullough AJ. The clinical features, diagnosis and natural history of nonalcoholic fatty liver disease. *Clin Liver Dis.* 2004;8:521-533.
10. Uwaifo GI, Tjahjana M, Freedman RJ, et al. Acanthosis nigricans in patients with nonalcoholic steatohepatitis: an uncommon finding. *Endocr Pract.* 2006;12:371-379.
11. Dassanayake AS, Kasturiratne A, Rajindrajith S, et al. Prevalence and risk factors for non-alcoholic fatty liver disease among adults in an urban Sri Lankan population. *J Gastroenterol Hepatol.* 2009;24:1284-1288.
12. Sourianarayanane A, Pagadala MR, Kirwan JP. Management of non-alcoholic fatty liver disease. *Minerva Gastroenterol Dietol.* 2013;59:69-87.
13. Lozada-Nur F, Miranda C. Oral lichen planus: epidemiology, clinical characteristics, and associated diseases. *Semin Cutan Med Surg.* 1997;16:273-277.
14. Liu S, Yao SP, Wei W, et al. Hepatitis C virus and lichen planus: a reciprocal association determined by a meta-analysis. www.scholar.qsensei.com/content/169k06. Accessed July 31, 2013.
15. Ahmed SM, Ahmed MN, Rather AR. Squamous cell carcinoma arising from lichen planus. *JK Science.* 2003;5:174-175.
16. Rübsam K, Schroll A, Weisenseel P, et al. Lichen planus and hepatitis virus infections: causal association? *J Dtsch Dermatol Ges.* 2011;9:464-468.
17. Lin LH, Lu SY, Lu SN. Seroprevalence of anti-HCV among patients with oral lichen planus in Southern Taiwan. *Oral Surg Oral Med Oral Pathol Oral Radiol Endod.* 2010;109:408-414.
18. Nagao Y, Sata M. A retrospective case-control study of hepatitis C virus infection and oral lichen planus in Japan: association study with mutations in the core and NS5A region of hepatitis C virus. *BMC Gastroenterol.* 2012;12:31.
19. Zyada MM, Fikry HE. Immunohistochemical study of syndecan-1 down-regulation and the expression of P35 protein in oral lichen planus: a

clinicopathologic correlation with hepatitis C infection in the Egyptian population. *Ann Diagn Pathol.* 2010;14:153-161.

20. Klanrit P, Thongprasom K, Rojanawatsirivej S, et al. Hepatitis C virus infection in Thai patients with oral lichen planus. *Oral Dis.* 2003;9:292-297.

21. Dervis E, Serez K. The prevalence of dermatologic manifestations related to chronic hepatitis C virus infection in a study from a single center in Turkey. *Acta Dermatovenerol Alp Panonica Adriat.* 2005;14:93-98.

22. Zhou Y, Jiang L, Liu J, et al. The prevalence of hepatitis C virus infection in oral lichen planus in an ethnic Chinese cohort of 232 patients. *Int J Oral Sci.* 2010;2:90-97.

23. Garg VK, Karki BM, Agrawal S, et al. A study from Nepal showing no correlation between lichen planus and hepatitis B and C viruses. *J Dermatol.* 2002;29:411-413.

24. Daramola OO, Ogunbiyi AO, George AO. Evaluation of clinical types of cutaneous lichen planus in anti-hepatitis C virus seronegative and seropositive Nigerian patients. *Int J Dermatol.* 2003;42:933-935.

25. Lodi G, Pellicano R, Carrozzo M. Hepatitis C virus infection and lichen planus: a systematic review with meta-analysis. *Oral Dis.* 2010;16:601-612.

26. Sugerman PB, Savage NW, Walsh LJ, et al. The pathogenesis of oral lichen planus. *Crit Rev Oral Biol Med.* 2002;13:350-365.

27. Farhi D, Dupin N. Pathophysiology, etiologic factors, and clinical management of oral lichen planus, part I: facts and controversies. *Clin Dermatol.* 2010;28:100-108.

28. Mahboobi N, Agha-Hosseini F, Lankarani KB. Hepatitis C virus and lichen planus: the real association. *Hepat Mon.* 2010;10:161-164.

29. Chung CM, Nunley JR. Overview of hepatitis C and skin. *Dermatol Nurs.* 2006;18:425-430.

30. Soylu S, Gül U, Kiliç A. Cutaneous manifestations in patients positive for anti-hepatitis C virus antibodies. *Acta Derm Venereol.* 2007;87:49-53.

31. Le Cleach L, Chosidow O. Clinical practice: lichen planus. *N Engl J Med.* 2012;366:723-732.

32. Jackson JM. Hepatitis C and the skin. *Dermatol Clin.* 2002;20:449-458.

33. Goettmann S, Zaraa I, Moulonguet I. Nail lichen planus: epidemiological, clinical, pathological, therapeutic and prognosis study of 67 cases. *J Eur Acad Dermatol Venereol.* 2012;26:1304-1309.

34. Usatine RP, Tinitigan M. Diagnosis and treatment of lichen planus. *Am Fam Physician.* 2011;84:53-60.

35. Byrd JA, Davis MD, Rogers RS 3rd. Recalcitrant symptomatic vulvar lichen planus: response to topical tacrolimus. *Arch Dermatol.* 2004;140:715-720.

36. Byrd JA, Davis MD, Bruce AJ, et al. Response of oral lichen planus to topical tacrolimus in 37 patients. *Arch Dermatol.* 2004;140:1508-1512.

37. Torti DC, Jorizzo JL, McCarty MA. Oral lichen planus: a case series with emphasis on therapy. *Arch Dermatol.* 2007;143:511-515.

38. Lauletta G, Russi S, Conteduca V, et al. Hepatitis C virus infection and mixed cryoglobulinemia. *Clin Dev Immunol.* 2012;2012:502156.

39. Houghton M, Weiner A, Han J, et al. Molecular biology of the hepatitis C viruses: implications for diagnosis, development and control of viral disease. *Hepatology.* 1991;14:381-388.

40. Zignego AL, Ferri C, Pileri SA, et al. Extrahepatic manifestations of hepatitis C virus infection: a general overview and guidelines for a clinical approach. *Dig Liver Dis.* 2007;39:2-17.

41. Rebora A. Skin diseases associated with hepatitis C virus: facts and controversies. *Clin Dermatol.* 2010;28:489-496.

42. Charles ED, Dustin LB. Hepatitis C virus-induced cryoglobulinemia. *Kidney Int.* 2009;76:818-824.

43. LoSpalluto J, Dorward B, Miller W Jr, et al. Cryoglobulinemia based on interaction between a gamma macroglobulin and 7S gamma globulin. *Am J Med.* 1962;32:142-147.

44. Pietrogrande M, De Vita S, Zignego AL, et al. Recommendations for the management of mixed cryoglobulinemia syndrome in hepatitis C virus-infected patients. *Autoimmun Rev.* 2011;10:444-454.

45. Misiani R, Bellavita P, Fenili D, et al. Interferon alfa-2a therapy in cryoglobulinemia associated with hepatitis C virus. *N Engl J Med.* 1994;330:751-756.

46. Ferri C, Marzo E, Longombardo G, et al. Interferon-alpha in mixed cryoglobulinemia patients: a randomized, crossover-controlled trial. *Blood.* 1993;81:1132-1136.

47. Sansonno D, De Re V, Lauletta G, et al. Monoclonal antibody treatment of mixed cryoglobulinemia resistant to interferon alpha with an anti-CD20. *Blood.* 2003;101:3818-3826.

48. Hayat W, Zahra K, Malik LM, et al. Necrolytic acral erythema: an unusual cutaneous presentation of hepatitis C virus infection. *J Pak Assoc Dermatol.* 2012;22:66-69.

49. Abdallah MA, Hull C, Horn TD. Necrolytic acral erythema: a patient from the United States successfully treated with oral zinc. *Arch Dermatol.* 2005;141:85-87.

50. Raphael BA, Dorey-Stein ZL, Lott J, et al. Low prevalence of necrolytic erythema in patients with chronic hepatitis C virus infection. *J Am Acad Dermatol.* 2012;67:962-968.

51. El-Ghandour TM, Sakr MA, El-Sebai H, et al. Necrolytic acral erythema in Egyptian patients with hepatitis C virus infection. *J Gastroenterol Hepatol.* 2006;21:1200-1206.

52. Patel U, Loyd A, Patel R, et al. Necrolytic acral erythema. *Dermatol Online J.* 2010;16:15.

53. Tabibian JH, Gerstenblith MR, Tedford RJ, et al. Necrolytic acral erythema as a cutaneous marker of hepatitis C: report of two cases and review. *Dig Dis Sci.* 2010;55:2735-2743.

54. Abdallah MA, Ghozzi MY, Monib HA, et al. Necrolytic acral erythema: a cutaneous sign of hepatitis C virus infection. *J Am Acad Dermatol.* 2005;53:247-251.

55. Hivnor CM, Yan AC, Junkins-Hopkins JM, et al. Necrolytic acral erythema: response to combination therapy with interferon and ribavirin. *J Am Acad Dermatol.* 2004;50:S121-S124.

56. Bentley D, Andea A, Holzer A, et al. Lack of classic histology should not prevent diagnosis of necrolytic acral erythema. *J Am Acad Dermatol.* 2009;60:504-507.

57. Fielder LM, Harvey VM, Kishor SI. Necrolytic acral erythema: case report and review of the literature. *Cutis.* 2008;81:355-360.

58. Halpern AV, Peikin SR, Ferzli P, et al. Necrolytic acral erythema: an expanding spectrum. *Cutis.* 2009;84:301-304.

59. Rossmann-Ringdahl I, Olsson R. Porphyria cutanea tarda in a Swedish population: risk factors and complications. *Acta Derm Venereol.* 2005;85:337-341.

60. Robinson-Bostom L, DiGiovanna JJ. Cutaneous manifestations of end-stage renal disease. *J Am Acad Dermatol.* 2000;43:975-986.

61. Chantorn R, Lim HW, Shwayder TA. Photosensitivity disorders in children: part I. *J Am Acad Dermatol.* 2012;67:1093.

62. Shieh S, Cohen JL, Lim HW. Management of porphyria cutanea tarda in the setting of chronic renal failure: a case report and review. *J Am Acad Dermatol.* 2000;42:645-652.

63. Ramsay CA, Magnus IA, Turnbull A, et al. The treatment of porphyria cutanea tarda by venesection. *Q J Med.* 1974;43:1-24.

64. Kantartzis K, Gastaldelli A, Magkos F, et al. Diabetes and nonalcoholic fatty liver disease. *Exp Diabetes Res.* 2012;2012:404632.

65. Lazaridis KN, Talwalkar JA. Clinical epidemiology of primary biliary cirrhosis: incidence, prevalence, and impact of therapy. *J Clin Gastroenterol.* 2007;41:494-500.

66. Kim WR, Lindor KD, Locke GR 3rd, et al. Epidemiology and natural history of primary biliary cirrhosis in a US community. *Gastroenterology.* 2000;119:1631-1636.

67. Smyk DS, Rigopoulou EI, Pares A, et al. Sex differences associated with primary biliary cirrhosis. *Clin Dev Immunol.* 2012;2012:610504.

68. Nguyen DL, Juran BD, Lazaridis KN. Primary biliary cirrhosis. *Best Pract Res Clin Gastroenterol.* 2010;24:647-654.

69. Lindor KD, Gershwin ME, Poupon R, et al. Primary biliary cirrhosis. *Hepatology.* 2009;50:291-308.

70. Kaplan MM, Gershwin ME. Primary biliary cirrhosis. *N Engl J Med.* 2005;353:1261-1273.

71. Gershwin ME, Rowley M, Davis PA, et al. Molecular biology of the 2-oxo-acid dehydrogenase complexes and anti-mitochondrial antibodies. *Prog Liver Dis.* 1992;10:47-61.

72. Selmi C, Mayo MJ, Bach N, et al. Primary biliary cirrhosis in monozygotic and dizygotic twins: genetics, epigenetics, and environment. *Gastroenterology.* 2004;127:485-492.

CHAPTER 70

Internal Malignancy

Jewell Gaulding
Cindy E. Owen
Jeffrey P. Callen

Internal malignancies can result in cutaneous paraneoplastic syndromes that may precede the diagnosis of the malignancy or herald a relapse. Awareness of these paraneoplastic syndromes can result in earlier diagnosis of internal malignancy. As discussed in this chapter, people with skin of color present later to the healthcare system with internal malignancies and therefore have a poorer prognosis.[1] Based on data in the United States, this chapter will cover the epidemiology of malignancy by race and ethnicity, as well as characteristics of paraneoplastic dermatoses.

EPIDEMIOLOGY

AFRICAN AMERICANS

In the United States, African Americans have the highest death rates and the shortest survivals for the majority of cancers. Research is still ongoing to determine if these health disparities are due to discrepancies in access to healthcare or other factors.[1] Cancer is the second leading cause of death in African Americans. From 2005 to 2009, the death rate for all cancers combined was 33% higher among African American men and 17% higher among African American women when compared to their Caucasian counterparts.[1] The most common types of cancer among African American women are breast (33%), lung (13%), and colorectal (11%) cancers.[1] The most common types of cancer among African American men are prostate (37%), lung (14%), and colorectal (10%) cancers.[1]

Cancer deaths among African Americans are primarily due to lung cancer, followed by prostate and colorectal cancers in men, and breast and colorectal cancers in women. Racial discrepancies in cancer death rates are mainly due to breast and colorectal cancers in women and prostate, lung, and colorectal cancers in men. The discrepancies are due to higher incidence among African Americans and shorter survival due to diagnosis at a later stage coupled with decreased access to treatment.

HISPANICS/LATINOS

Cancer was the leading cause of death in the Hispanic/Latino population in 2009; however, the incidence and death rates for all cancers combined are lower in Hispanics when compared to non-Hispanic whites.[2] Malignancies that have higher incidence and mortality in this population include stomach, liver, cervix, and gallbladder cancer.

The most common malignancies among Hispanic men are prostate (29%), colorectal (11%), lung (9%), kidney (6%), and liver (6%) cancers, with lung cancer causing the most cancer deaths, followed by colorectal, liver, and prostate cancers.[2] Among Hispanic women, the most common malignancies are breast (29%), colorectal (8%), thyroid (8%), and lung (7%) cancers, with breast cancer accounting for the most cancer deaths, followed by lung and colorectal cancers.[2] Although Hispanics/Latinos have lower incidence and death rates, they are more likely to present with more advanced disease than non-Hispanic whites.

ASIAN AMERICANS AND PACIFIC ISLANDERS

Asian Americans and Pacific Islanders have a lower incidence rate than the non-Hispanic white population for the most common cancers. This population has a higher incidence of cancers associated with infection, including hepatocellular and stomach cancers. Asians and Pacific Islanders have the highest incidence of and mortality from liver cancer when compared to all racial and ethnic groups in both men and women.

NATIVE AMERICANS AND ALASKAN NATIVES

Data for Native Americans and Alaskan Natives are limited, but the Cancer Registry and Indian Health Service are currently working together to resolve this problem. It is known that this population has a higher incidence of renal carcinoma than any other racial or ethnic population, which may be attributable to a high prevalence of smoking and obesity.

TREND IN INCIDENCE

Data from 2005 to 2009 show the following trends in incidence of cancer for all sites:

- *Men:* African American > Caucasian American > American Indian/Alaskan Native > Hispanic/Latino > Asian American/Pacific Islander
- *Women:* Caucasian American > African American > American Indian/Alaskan Native > Hispanic/Latino > Asian American/Pacific Islander

BREAST CANCER

Among African American women, breast cancer is the most common malignancy and second most common cause of cancer death. Among women under age 45, the incidence rate is higher in African American women than in Caucasian women.[1]

Breast cancer survival rates are lower among African American women than Caucasian women for two reasons: later stage of detection and worse stage-specific survival. Caucasian women are more likely to be diagnosed with breast cancer at a local stage and tend to participate more in early detection and treatment strategies.[1] There is some evidence that the biologic behavior of breast cancer may be more aggressive in African Americans than in Caucasians.[3,4]

Breast cancer is the most common malignancy and the primary cause of cancer death among Hispanic women. Breast cancer incidence is roughly 40% lower among Hispanic women than among non-Hispanic white women. This may be due in part to a reduced use of hormone-replacement therapy among Hispanic women, protective reproductive patterns such as younger age at first birth and multiparity, and underdiagnosis secondary to fewer Hispanic women undergoing mammography.[2,5] Hispanic women are approximately 20% more likely to die from breast cancer than Caucasian women at a similar age and stage of diagnosis.[6] Caucasian women are more likely to be diagnosed with breast cancer at an earlier stage and with a smaller-sized tumor.[7]

COLORECTAL CANCER

Colorectal cancer is the third most common malignancy and third most common cause of cancer death among African American men and women.[1] Incidence rates are higher and survival rates are lower among African Americans than among Caucasians.[1] A reason for the former has not been elucidated, whereas the latter is secondary to decreased access to care, reduced delivery of treatment, and a possible difference in tumor biology.[8]

Among Hispanics/Latinos, colorectal cancer is the second most common malignancy, and incidence rates are 12% to 16% lower than in non-Hispanic whites.[2] Hispanics are more likely to be diagnosed at an advanced stage and are less likely to survive after diagnosis.[6] This may be due to lower screening rates and decreased access to healthcare compared to non-Hispanic whites.[2] Malignancies of the colon and rectum are the second most common cause of cancer death among Hispanic men and the third most common cause of cancer death among Hispanic women.[2]

LUNG CANCER

Malignancies of the lung and bronchus are the second most common type of cancer and the number one cause of cancer death among African Americans.[1] Incidence rates are about 11% lower for African American women compared to Caucasian women but are almost 20% higher among African American men compared to Caucasian men.[1] Survival rates are slightly lower among African Americans.[1] One study demonstrated that African Americans diagnosed with early-stage lung cancer were less likely to receive surgical intervention, which is the only treatment that results in a cure.[9]

Lung cancer is the third most common malignancy among Hispanic/Latino males and the fourth most common malignancy among Hispanic/Latino females.[2] Incidence rates are approximately 50% lower in the Hispanic/Latino population than in the non-Hispanic white population.[2] This can be attributed to lower rates of cigarette use among Hispanics/Latinos.[10] Lung cancer accounts for the most cancer-related deaths among Hispanic men, but this malignancy is second to breast cancer for number of deaths among Hispanic women.[2]

PROSTATE CANCER

Among African American and Hispanic men, prostate cancer is the most common malignancy.[1,2] Prostate cancer is the second most common cause of cancer death in African American men.[1] Prostate cancer is the fourth most common cause of cancer death in Hispanic men.[2]

The annual incidence rate is approximately 63% higher among African American men than among Caucasian men, the reason for which is not well understood.[1] Among Hispanic men, prostate cancer rates are about 10% lower than in non-Hispanic whites.[2] The death rate is 2.4 times higher among African American men, and prostate cancer is more likely to be diagnosed at an earlier stage in Caucasian men.[1]

INTERNAL MALIGNANCY AND SKIN MANIFESTATIONS

Internal malignancies can result in manifestations on the skin. These signs can be malignant or nonmalignant. This can be due to cells from an internal malignancy penetrating the skin representing metastasis or local/regional spread [**Figure 70-1, A and B**] or a nonmalignant skin disorder that occurs in association with a malignancy known as a paraneoplastic dermatosis. In instances when paraneoplastic dermatoses arise prior to the identification of a neoplasm, recognition of the cutaneous manifestation can aid in diagnosis of the malignancy. Helen Curth suggested several criteria for assessing the relationship between an internal malignancy and a possible cutaneous finding; these have become known as Curth's postulates [**Table 70-1**].[11]

Paraneoplastic dermatoses can present with signs due to metabolic products of malignancy, or as proliferative, inflammatory, bullous, and

TABLE 70-1	Curth's postulates[a]
Postulates	**Definitions**
1. Concurrent onset	The dermatosis and malignancy occur concurrently.
2. Parallel course	If the malignancy is treated successfully or recurs, the dermatosis follows a similar course.
3. Uniformity	A specific malignancy is consistently associated with a specific dermatosis.
4. Statistical significance	There is a statistically significant association between the malignancy and the dermatosis based on case-control studies.
5. Genetic basis	There is a genetic association between the malignancy and dermatosis.

[a]Curth's postulates are criteria used to help establish a relationship between an internal malignancy and a cutaneous disorder. All criteria do not have to be met.

other skin disorders. Skin signs can also signify heritable conditions that are associated with malignancy (genodermatoses with associated malignancy are not discussed in this chapter).

PARANEOPLASTIC DERMATOSES DUE TO METABOLIC PRODUCTS OF MALIGNANCY

HYPERPIGMENTATION DUE TO ECTOPIC ADRENOCORTICOTROPHIC HORMONE PRODUCTION

Cushing syndrome as a result of ectopic adrenocorticotrophic hormone (ACTH) production from an internal malignancy is the most common paraneoplastic syndrome induced by hormones. The classical findings of Cushing syndrome include glucose intolerance or diabetes, hypokalemic metabolic alkalosis, hypertension, muscle wasting, proximal muscle weakness, and, of particular interest, severe hyperpigmentation.[12] The hyperpigmentation associated with Cushing syndrome is believed to be due to α-melanocyte-stimulating hormone (α-MSH), which is a proopiomelanocortin (POMC)-derived peptide.[13] This hormone is located in the pituitary as well as the skin, and there is evidence that ACTH, a precursor of α-MSH, activates the same receptor as α-MSH, which is expressed by melanocytes.[13] Therefore, with increased ACTH from an ectopic site, there is increased synthesis of melanin leading to hyperpigmentation.[13] The most common internal malignancy causing ectopic Cushing syndrome is small-cell lung carcinoma. Ectopic Cushing syndrome is also associated with carcinoid tumors, thymomas, and pheochromocytomas.

NECROLYTIC MIGRATORY ERYTHEMA

Necrolytic migratory erythema (NME) is present in approximately 70% of patients with pancreatic α-islet cell tumors that secrete glucagon known as glucagonomas. NME is a transitory, weeping eczematous or psoriasiform eruption that normally occurs in skin flexures and acral sites and most commonly affects the genital and anal area. Additional features may include weight loss, diabetes, anemia, abdominal pain, thromboembolic phenomena, diarrhea, alopecia, and stomatitis.[14] NME has been described as pathognomonic for glucagonoma; however, there have been reports that this eruption may also occur in patients without a glucagon-producing tumor, and this has been referred to as pseudo-glucagonoma syndrome.[15]

AMYLOIDOSIS

Amyloidosis results from improperly folded proteins and polypeptides that interact to form insoluble protein aggregates. Amyloidosis occurs when these insoluble protein aggregates deposit into various organs and tissues. In primary (AL) amyloidosis, monoclonal light chains are deposited in various tissues including the kidney and the skin. Clinical mucocutaneous findings include petechiae, purpura, and ecchymosis,

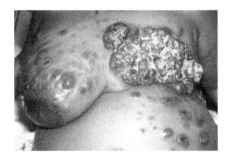

A

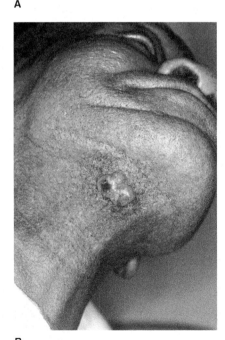

B

FIGURE 70-1. (A) Metastatic breast disease in an African American woman after a mastectomy with multiple dome-shaped nodules in both breasts and the skin of the chest and abdomen. Both nodules and plaques have necrosis. **(B)** Metastatic lung disease in an elderly African American man with multilobule nodule on the chin with unshaven surrounding area. (Used with permission from the Department of Dermatology, Washington Hospital Center, Washington DC.)

which occur after minor trauma. Bullous lesions, dermal thickening, waxy papules and plaques, and enlarged shoulder pads may also occur. AL amyloidosis can be isolated or occur in association with multiple myeloma or, less commonly, Waldenström macroglobulinemia.[16]

PARANEOPLASTIC PROLIFERATIVE DISORDERS

◼ ACANTHOSIS NIGRICANS

Acanthosis nigricans normally presents as hyperpigmented plaques with a velvety texture located in intertriginous areas. Although commonly associated with obesity and insulin resistance, acanthosis nigricans can also be one of the first signs of malignancy. Acanthosis nigricans is more common in people with darker skin, with a prevalence of 34% in American Indians, 13.3% in African Americans, 5.5% in Latinos, and less than 1% in Caucasians.[17,18] The association of acanthosis nigricans with internal malignancy is rare. Cancer should be considered in patients who are older than 35, are cachectic or complaining of weight loss, or have a rapid onset or unusual distribution.[19] The most common malignancy associated with this disease is gastric cancer; however, other cancers, including hepatocellular carcinoma and adenocarcinomas of the lung, ovary, endometrium, kidney, pancreas, bladder, and breast, have also been reported.[20-24] Acanthosis nigricans in association with malignancy usually has a different clinical presentation than acanthosis nigricans in association with obesity or insulin resistance [**Figure 70-2, A and B**].

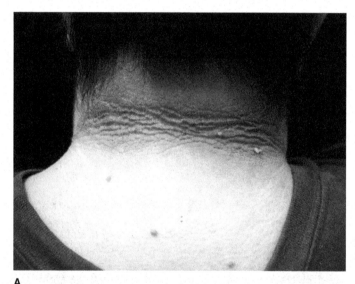

A

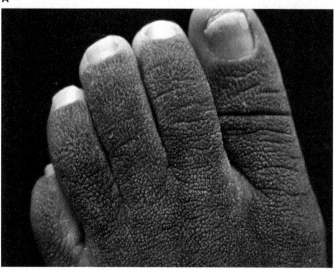

B

FIGURE 70-2. (A) Acanthosis nigricans. Hyperpigmented, velvety plaques on the neck. **(B)** Diffuse acanthosis nigricans with involvement of the dorsal foot.

In the former, these velvety, hyperpigmented plaques can arise in unusual locations (such as mucosal sites), in combination with multiple skin tags, with the sudden onset of seborrheic keratoses known as the sign of Leser-Trélat, or with tripe palms.[25] Acanthosis nigricans that is progressing at a rapid rate, that is prominent on the soles and palms, or that involves mucous membranes should increase suspicion for malignancy.

◼ SIGN OF LESER-TRÉLAT

Multiple pruritic seborrheic keratoses, often with an inflammatory base, erupting suddenly due to a malignancy is known as the sign of Leser-Trélat.[26] The location of this sudden eruption can occur anywhere on the body but most commonly occurs on the back and chest. Other locations include the extremities, face, abdomen, neck, axilla, and groin.[27] There does not seem to be a significant difference in incidence among males or females, and racial predilection has not been reported.[27] The most common malignancies associated with the sign of Leser-Trélat are gastrointestinal adenocarcinoma, breast and lung cancers, or lymphoproliferative disorders.[28] It is likely that the neoplasm produces cytokines and other growth factors that lead to the rapid appearance of the seborrheic keratoses.

◼ TRIPE PALM

Tripe palm is a condition where the palms, and on occasion the soles, appear velvety and thickened, with an appearance resembling the stomach lining of ruminants ("tripe").[28] This condition is accompanied by acanthosis nigricans approximately 75% of the time.[28] The cancers predominantly associated with this condition are gastric or bronchogenic carcinomas; however, tripe palm has been described in conjunction with a number of other malignancies.[29] Tripe palm was the initial presenting feature in undiagnosed malignancy in 40% of cases, and one review reported that 94% of cases of tripe palm occurred in conjunction with malignancy.[30] Due to the strong connection of this paraneoplastic dermatosis with malignancy, a full cancer screening should be done in adults who are diagnosed with this condition.

◼ BAZEX SYNDROME

Bazex syndrome presents with psoriasiform lesions located on acral areas, most commonly the helix of the ear and the nose.[31] Other areas that are less commonly affected include the nails, hands, feet, elbows, and knees.[28] In dark-skinned individuals, macular hyperpigmentation may be located in the same distribution, and bullae on the hands and feet are also possible.[28,32] Swelling, erythema, and dystrophy of the nails are characteristic. On a biopsy of the lesion, the most common findings are hyperkeratosis, acanthosis, parakeratosis, dyskeratotic keratinocytes, and infiltration of perivascular lymphocytes.[28] The most common malignancies associated with Bazex syndrome are squamous cell carcinomas in the oral cavity/pharynx/larynx, lung, and esophagus.[33]

◼ HYPERTROPHIC OSTEOARTHROPATHY

Hypertrophic osteoarthropathy is also known as pachydermoperiostosis, and the triad of this condition includes thickening of the skin in prominent folds and creases such as the scalp and forehead, clubbing of the fingers, and new periosteum formation in the radius, tibia, and phalanges. Secondary hypertrophic osteoarthropathy is usually associated with non–small-cell lung cancer and other intrathoracic diseases such as cystic fibrosis, infections, and cyanotic cardiac shunts.[34]

PARANEOPLASTIC INFLAMMATORY DISORDERS

◼ SWEET SYNDROME

Sweet syndrome is also known as acute febrile neutrophilic dermatosis and presents with a set of symptoms and findings that include fever, peripheral neutrophilia, and dermal nonvasculitic infiltration by neutrophils.[35] The lesions consist of tender, red to purple papules, plaques, or nodules that are well demarcated and most commonly located on the upper extremities, face, and neck, but can occur anywhere [**Figure 70-3**].[35]

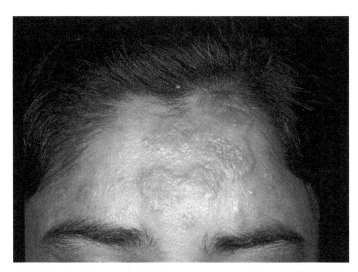

FIGURE 70-3. Sweet syndrome. Erythematous to violaceous plaques on the forehead.

Furthermore, the lesions can be pustular, and the plaques and nodules can become ulcerated.[36] Up to half of patients with Sweet syndrome have an underlying disease, and approximately 10% of patients have this cutaneous eruption in association with a premalignant illness or malignancy. Malignancy-associated Sweet syndrome occurs most commonly with

acute myeloblastic leukemia; however, it has also been seen in conjunction with solid malignancies and premalignant syndromes such as myelodysplastic syndrome.[36] There is not a racial predilection for Sweet syndrome.[37]

DERMATOMYOSITIS

Dermatomyositis is characterized by cutaneous findings along with progressive, symmetrical, proximal muscle weakness. A violaceous rash involving the periorbital region, known as a heliotrope rash, and scaly purple papules and plaques over bony prominences, commonly the hands, known as Gottron papules, are considered pathognomonic cutaneous findings for this inflammatory myopathy. In African Americans, the only finding of the heliotrope rash may be periorbital edema.[38] Other cutaneous findings of this condition are poikiloderma in sun-exposed areas [**Figure 70-4, A to C**], malar erythema (usually involving nasolabial folds), telangiectasias around nails with ragged cuticles [**Figure 70-4D**], and photosensitivity. Malignancies associated with dermatomyositis frequently include ovarian (most common), breast, uterine, lung, gastric, colorectal, and pancreatic; however, a wide range of tumors have been reported.[39] Dermatomyositis associated with malignancy is less common in African American women compared to Caucasian women.[38] In patients of Chinese descent with dermatomyositis, nasopharyngeal carcinoma composes 40% to 80% of the associated malignancies.[40] The malignancies that are associated with dermatomyositis are frequently diagnosed within 3 years of the diagnosis of dermatomyositis, with most being detected within a year.[41]

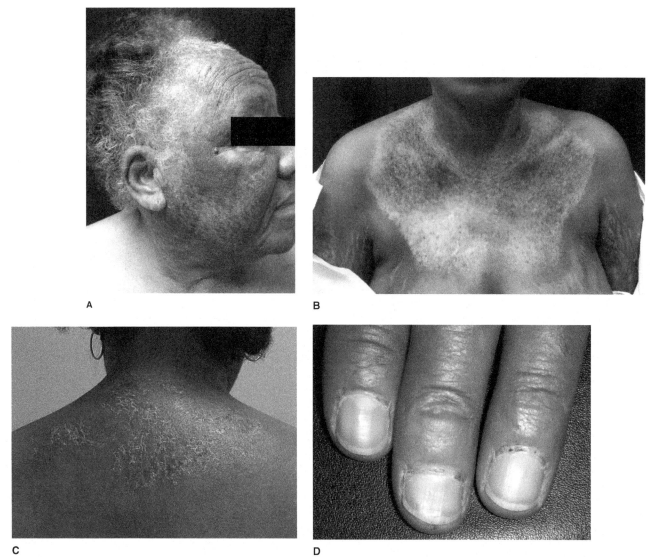

A   B

C   D

FIGURE 70-4. Dermatomyositis. (**A–C**) Poikiloderma of sun-exposed areas including the face, chest, and back (the so-called "shawl sign"). (**D**) Ragged cuticles and dilated capillary loops of the nail fold.

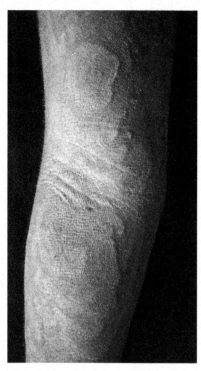

FIGURE 70-5. Erythema gyratum repens. Concentric annular plaques resembling wood grain seen in a patient who also has diffuse acanthosis nigricans.

PITYRIASIS ROTUNDA

Pityriasis rotunda presents with circular, sharply demarcated hyperpigmented or hypopigmented patches. There are usually multiple lesions typically located on the truck that may become confluent. Pityriasis rotunda has been described in Japanese, West Indians, South African blacks, and African Americans.[42] Malignancies that are associated with this disorder include hepatocellular carcinoma; carcinoma of the esophagus, palate, prostate, and stomach; and multiple myeloma and chronic lymphocytic leukemia.[42]

ERYTHEMA GYRATUM REPENS

Erythema gyratum repens is a reactive erythema that presents as scaly macular, papular, or bullous serpiginous bands that are arranged in parallel configuration with a wood-grain appearance [**Figure 70-5**]. The lesions migrate rapidly and normally involve the trunk and proximal extremities with sparing of the palmar and plantar surfaces, but can occur anywhere on the body. This condition is typically pruritic and is one of the most specific skin signs of internal malignancy. Greater than 80% of patients with this condition have an underlying malignancy. Lung cancer is the most common associated malignancy, followed by esophageal and breast cancers.[43] Therefore, patients with this condition should undergo a workup for an underlying malignancy. Most reports of erythema gyratum repens have been in Caucasians; however, reporting bias may exist.[29]

PARANEOPLASTIC BULLOUS DISORDERS

PARANEOPLASTIC PEMPHIGUS (ALSO KNOWN AS PARANEOPLASTIC AUTOIMMUNE MULTIORGAN SYNDROME)

Paraneoplastic pemphigus presents with painful stomatitis. Cutaneous lesions can resemble erythema multiforme or lichen planus and can include tense bullae. This disorder is typically associated with malignancies such as chronic lymphocytic leukemia and non-Hodgkin lymphoma or lymphoproliferative disorders such as Castleman disease and Waldenström macroglobulinemia.[44] There is no known racial predilection for

paraneoplastic pemphigus. Detecting anti-plakin antibodies on indirect immunofluorescence testing using the patient's serum, along with clinical and histopathologic findings that are consistent, makes the diagnosis. Computed tomography of the chest, abdomen, and pelvis should be obtained in patients who are suspected of having paraneoplastic pemphigus but have not been diagnosed with a malignancy. The syndrome can affect multiple organ systems, with death occurring most commonly due to bronchiolitis obliterans.

ANTI-EPILIGRIN CICATRICIAL PEMPHIGOID

Anti-epiligrin (also known as anti-laminin 5 or anti-laminin 332) cicatricial pemphigoid (AECP) is an autoimmune blistering disease characterized by painful lesions of the oral mucosa and skin that may be vesiculobullous and/or erosive with an erythematous base. In a series of 35 patients of various racial and ethnic origins (Caucasian, Japanese, Hispanic, African American, Chinese, and Korean), all of the patients had oral mucosal involvement and more than half had ocular involvement (66%).[45] Other mucosal surfaces involved include laryngeal (51%), nasal (46%), pharyngeal (46%), esophageal (20%), genital (31%), and anal (11%).[45] Severe gingival destruction, loss of teeth, restriction in mobility of the tongue or pharynx, blindness, dysphonia, airway compromise requiring tracheostomy, and aspiration are potential complications. Thirty patients in the series had mild to moderate skin lesions.[45]

The diagnosis for AECP requires the following: erosive and/or blistering lesions of mucous membranes, in situ deposits of immunoglobulin (Ig) G autoantibodies in epidermal basement membranes or IgG autoantibodies in circulation that bind on the dermal side of 1-M NaCl split human skin, and circulating IgG that immunoprecipitates laminin 5 on extracts or conditioned media of radiolabeled human keratinocytes.[45] Malignancies associated with this condition are lung, stomach, colon, and endometrial adenocarcinomas.[46] The time between onset of blisters and cancer diagnosis ranged from 14 months before to 14 months after the diagnosis of AECP.[45]

OTHER PARANEOPLASTIC DISORDERS

POEMS SYNDROME

POEMS syndrome, also known as Crow-Fukase syndrome, is a rare condition that is due to an underlying plasma cell dyscrasia, such as osteosclerotic myeloma or solitary plasmacytoma. The largest initial reports of this disease were from Japan; however, reports have shown that this syndrome also occurs in Caucasians, African Americans, and Hispanics.[47] The acronym POEMS refers to several features of the syndrome: polyneuropathy, organomegaly, endocrinopathy, monoclonal plasma cell disorder, and skin changes.[48] The most common skin changes seen are hyperpigmentation and angiomas [**Figure 70-6A**], although other skin changes such as sclerodermatous thickening, acquired facial lipoatrophy, plethora, acrocyanosis, hypertrichosis, hyperhidrosis, infiltrated livedo lesions, and clubbing have been reported.[49] Glomeruloid hemangiomas [**Figure 70-6B**] have been proposed to be a specific cutaneous marker of POEMS syndrome when present.[50] The pathogenesis of POEMS syndrome is not completely understood; however, an imbalance of proinflammatory cytokines coupled with a derangement in production of vascular endothelial growth factor (VEGF) has been proposed.[51] If this syndrome is suspected, serum and urine electrophoresis with immunofixation should be performed and serum VEGF levels obtained. In cases without serum and urine electrophoresis findings, a bone marrow biopsy may need to be performed if there is high clinical suspicion. In addition, all patients should have a bone survey to look for osteosclerotic lesions.

EXTRAMAMMARY PAGET DISEASE

Extramammary Paget disease (EMPD) is a rare cutaneous neoplastic condition that accounts for approximately 1% of vulvar cancers.[52] EMPD presents as a nonhealing dermatitis in areas that contain

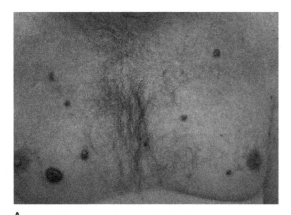

A

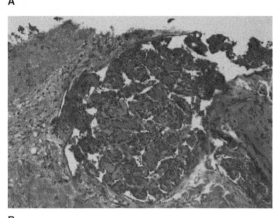

B

FIGURE 70-6. POEMS syndrome. **(A)** Numerous hemangiomas of the trunk in a patient with POEMS. **(B)** Histopathology of a glomeruloid hemangioma with intravascular capillary growth resembling renal glomeruli, a finding thought to be relatively specific to POEMS.

apocrine glands with a well-demarcated pruritic and erythematous plaque [**Figure 70-7**]. The vulva is the most common location for the lesion, followed by perineal, perianal, scrotal, and penile skin. Burning, irritation, swelling, pain, or bleeding may also be present. This disease more commonly affects women and Caucasians, although there seems to be a male predominance in Asians.[53,54] To make the diagnosis of

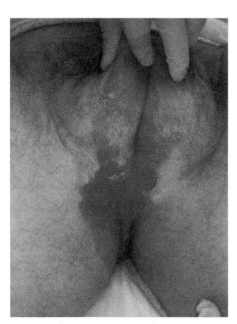

FIGURE 70-7. Extramammary Paget's disease—erythematous, well-demarcated, partially eroded plaque of the genital area.

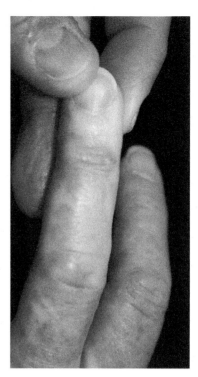

FIGURE 70-8. Multicentric histiocytosis—lightly erythematous papules of the fingers.

EMPD, intraepidermal, infiltrating Paget cells are identified by histopathology. Immunohistochemistry is used to differentiate EMPD from other conditions that have pagetoid spread on histology, such as Bowen disease and superficial spreading melanoma, as well as to identify the cell of origin when EMPD is associated with an underlying malignancy.[53] Approximately 25% of patients with EMPD also have an underlying in situ or invasive neoplasm. Perianal EMPD has a higher frequency of associated cancer than vulvar EMPD.[53] Vulvar EMPD is not usually associated with an internal malignancy; however, associations have been reported with endocervical, vaginal, urethral, bladder, and endometrial cancer. When EMPD of the male genitalia arises, it is more commonly associated with urethral, bladder, prostate, or testicular cancer. Perianal EMPD, on the other hand, has a strong association with anal, rectal, or colon cancer.[53]

MULTICENTRIC RETICULOHISTIOCYTOSIS

Multicentric reticulohistiocytosis (MRH) presents with severe erosive arthritis and widespread flesh-colored to yellow-brown papulonodular lesions typically on the face, hands, forearms, and ears [**Figure 70-8**]. Lesions on the fingernails have a "coral bead" appearance. In one-third of patients, xanthelasma has been noted. Other symptoms such as weight loss, fever, and weakness may also occur. This condition has been reported in many nations, such as Argentina, Malaysia, India, and China, and has been seen in different ethnic groups.[55] MRH has been associated with a number of malignancies with breast, hematologic, and gastric cancers being the most common.[56] Therefore, in every patient diagnosed with MRH, it is important to complete a thorough internal malignancy workup.

REFERENCES

1. Desantis C, Naishadham D, Jemal A. Cancer statistics for African Americans, 2013. *CA Cancer J Clin.* 2013;63:151-166.
2. Siegel R, Naishadham D, Jemal A. Cancer statistics for Hispanics/Latinos, 2012. *CA Cancer J Clin.* 2012;62:283-298.
3. Carey LA, Perou CM, Livasy CA, et al. Race, breast cancer subtypes, and survival in the Carolina Breast Cancer Study. *JAMA.* 2006;295:2492-2502.

4. Dunn BK, Agurs-Collins T, Browne D, Lubet R, Johnson KA. Health disparities in breast cancer: biology meets socioeconomic status. *Breast Cancer Res Treat.* 2010;11:281-292.

5. Sweeney C, Baumgartner KB, Byers T, et al. Reproductive history in relation to breast cancer risk among Hispanic and non-Hispanic white women. *Cancer Causes Control.* 2008;19:391-401.

6. Jemal A, Clegg LX, Ward E, et al. Annual report to the nation on the status of cancer, 1975-2001, with a special feature regarding survival. *Cancer.* 2004;101:3-27.

7. Miller BA, Hankey BF, Thomas TL. Impact of sociodemographic factors, hormone receptor status, and tumor grade on ethnic differences in tumor stage and size for breast cancer in women. *Am J Epidemiol.* 2002;155:534-545.

8. Polite BN, Dignam JJ, Olopade OI. Colorectal cancer model of health disparities: understanding mortality differences in minority populations. *J Clin Oncol.* 2006;24:2179-2187.

9. Bach PB, Cramer LD, Warren JL, Begg CB. Racial differences in the treatment of early-stage lung cancer. *N Engl J Med.* 1999;341:1198-1205.

10. Cokkinides VE, Bandi P, Siegel RL, Jemal A. Cancer-related risk factors and preventive measures in US Hispanics/Latinos. *CA Cancer J Clin.* 2012;62:353-363.

11. Curth HO. Skin lesions and internal carcinoma. In: Andrade R, Gumport SL, Popkin GL, et al, eds. *Cancer of the Skin.* Philadelphia, PA: WB Saunders; 1976:1308-1309.

12. Pivonello R, De Martino MC, De Leo M, Lombardi G, Colao A. Cushing's syndrome. *Endocrinol Metab Clin North Am.* 2008;37:135-149.

13. Wakamatsu K, Graham A, Cook D, Thody AJ. Characterisation of ACTH peptides in human skin and their activation of the melanocortin-1 receptor. *Pigment Cell Res.* 1997;10:288-297.

14. Thiers BH, Sahn RE, Callen JP. Cutaneous manifestations of internal malignancy. *CA Cancer J Clin.* 2009;59:73-98.

15. Marinkovich MP, Botella R, Datloff J, Sangueza OP. Necrolytic migratory erythema without glucagonoma in patients with liver disease. *J Am Acad Dermatol.* 1995;32:604-609.

16. Kyle RA, Durie BG, Rajkumar SV, et al. Monoclonal gammopathy of undetermined significance (MGUS) and smoldering (asymptomatic) multiple myeloma: IMWG consensus perspectives risk factors for progression and guidelines for monitoring and management. *Leukemia.* 2010;24:1121-1127.

17. Stoddart ML, Blevins KS, Lee ET, Wang W, Blackett PR; Cherokee Diabetes Study. Association of acanthosis nigricans with hyperinsulinemia compared with other selected risk factors for type 2 diabetes in Cherokee Indians: the Cherokee Diabetes Study. *Diabetes Care.* 2002;25:1009-1014.

18. Gilkison C, Stuart CA. Assessment of patients with acanthosis nigricans skin lesion for hyperinsulinemia, insulin resistance and diabetes risk. *Nurse Pract.* 1992;17:26, 28, 37.

19. Stuart CA, Gilkison CR, Keenan BS, Nagamani M. Hyperinsulinemia and acanthosis nigricans in African Americans. *J Natl Med Assoc.* 1997;89:523-527.

20. Krawczyk M, Mykała-Cieśla J, Kołodziej-Jaskuła A. Acanthosis nigricans as a paraneoplastic syndrome. Case reports and review of literature. *Pol Arch Med Wewn.* 2009;119:180-183.

21. Kamińska-Winciorek G, Brzezińska-Wcisło L, Lis-Swiety A, Krauze E. Paraneoplastic type of acanthosis nigricans in patient with hepatocellular carcinoma. *Adv Med Sci.* 2007;52:254-256.

22. Serap D, Ozlem S, Melike Y, et al. Acanthosis nigricans in a patient with lung cancer: a case report. *Case Rep Med.* 2010;2010.

23. Oh CW, Yoon J, Kim CY. Malignant acanthosis nigricans associated with ovarian cancer. *Case Rep Dermatol.* 2010;2:103-109.

24. Longshore SJ, Taylor JS, Kennedy A, Nurko S. Malignant acanthosis nigricans and endometrioid adenocarcinoma of the perimetrium: the search for malignancy. *J Am Acad Dermatol.* 2003;49:541-543.

25. Yeh JS, Munn SE, Plunkett TA, Harper PG, Hopster DJ, du Vivier AW. Coexistence of acanthosis nigricans and the sign of Leser-Trélat in a patient with gastric adenocarcinoma: a case report and literature review. *J Am Acad Dermatol.* 2000;42:357-362.

26. Schwartz RA. Sign of Leser-Trélat. *J Am Acad Dermatol.* 1996;35:88-95.

27. Moore RL, Devere TS. Epidermal manifestations of internal malignancy. *Dermatol Clin.* 2008;26:17-29.

28. Kurzrock R, Cohen PR. Cutaneous paraneoplastic syndromes in solid tumors. *Am J Med.* 1995;99:662-671.

29. Chung VQ, Moschella SL, Zembowicz A, Liu V. Clinical and pathologic findings of paraneoplastic dermatoses. *J Am Acad Dermatol.* 2006;54:745-762.

30. Cohen PR, Grossman ME, Almeida L, Kurzrock R. Tripe palms and malignancy. *J Clin Oncol.* 1989;7:669-678.

31. Poligone B, Christensen SR, Lazova R, Heald PW. Bazex syndrome (acrokeratosis paraneoplastica). *Lancet.* 2007;369:530.

32. Abreu Velez AM, Howard MS. Diagnosis and treatment of cutaneous paraneoplastic disorders. *Dermatol Ther.* 2010;23:662-675.

33. Sarkar B, Knecht R, Sarkar C, Weidauer H. Bazex syndrome (acrokeratosis paraneoplastica). *Eur Arch Otorhinolaryngol.* 1998;255:205-210.

34. Azar L, Khasnis A. Paraneoplastic rheumatologic syndromes. *Curr Opin Rheumatol.* 2013;25:44-49.

35. Cohen PR. Sweet's syndrome revisited: a review of disease concepts. *Int J Dermatol.* 2003;42:761-778.

36. Buck T, González LM, Lambert WC, Schwartz RA. Sweet's syndrome with hematologic disorders: a review and reappraisal. *Int J Dermatol.* 2008;47:775-782.

37. Cohen PR. Sweet's syndrome—a comprehensive review of an acute febrile neutrophilic dermatosis. *Orphanet J Rare Dis.* 2007;2:34.

38. Kovacs SO, Kovacs SC. Dermatomyositis. *J Am Acad Dermatol.* 1998;39:899-920.

39. Hill CL, Zhang Y, Sigurgeirsson B, et al. Frequency of specific cancer types in dermatomyositis and polymyositis: a population-based study. *Lancet.* 2001;357:96-100.

40. Ee HL, Ng PP, Tan SH. Exacerbation of amyopathic dermatomyositis in Orientals: a high alert for nasopharyngeal carcinoma. *Australas J Dermatol.* 2004;45:77-78.

41. Wakata N, Kurihara T, Saito E, Kinoshita M. Polymyositis and dermatomyositis associated with malignancy: a 30-year retrospective study. *Int J Dermatol.* 2002;41:729-734.

42. Grimalt R, Gelmetti C, Brusasco A, Tadini G, Caputo R. Pityriasis rotunda: report of a familial occurrence and review of the literature. *J Am Acad Dermatol.* 1994;31:866-871.

43. Boyd AS, Neldner KH, Menter A. Erythema gyratum repens: a paraneoplastic eruption. *J Am Acad Dermatol.* 1992;26:757-762.

44. Mahajan VK, Sharma V, Chauhan PS, et al. Paraneoplastic pemphigus: a paraneoplastic autoimmune multiorgan syndrome or autoimmune multiorganopathy? *Case Rep Dermatol Med.* 2012;2012:207126.

45. Egan CA, Lazarova Z, Darling TN, Yee C, Yancey KB. Anti-epiligrin cicatricial pemphigoid: clinical findings, immunopathogenesis, and significant associations. *Medicine (Baltimore).* 2003;82:177-186.

46. Egan CA, Lazarova Z, Darling TN, Yee C, Coté T, Yancey KB. Anti-epiligrin cicatricial pemphigoid and relative risk for cancer. *Lancet.* 2001;357:1850-1851.

47. Dispenzieri A, Kyle RA, Lacy MQ, et al. POEMS syndrome: definitions and long-term outcome. *Blood.* 2003;101:2496-2506.

48. Nakanishi T, Sobue I, Toyokura Y, et al. The Crow-Fukase syndrome: a study of 102 cases in Japan. *Neurology.* 1984;34:712-720.

49. Barete S, Mouawad R, Choquet S, et al. Skin manifestations and vascular endothelial growth factor levels in POEMS syndrome: impact of autologous hematopoietic stem cell transplantation. *Arch Dermatol.* 2010;146:615-623.

50. Tsai CY, Lai CH, Chan HL, Kuo TT. Glomeruloid hemangioma—a specific cutaneous marker of POEMS syndrome. *Int J Dermatol.* 2001;40:403-406.

51. Soubrier M, Dubost JJ, Serre AF, et al. Growth factors in POEMS syndrome: evidence for a marked increase in circulating vascular endothelial growth factor. *Arthritis Rheum.* 1997;40:786-787.

52. Curtin JP, Rubin SC, Jones WB, Hoskins WJ, Lewis JL Jr. Paget's disease of the vulva. *Gynecol Oncol.* 1990;39:374-377.

53. Shepherd V, Davidson EJ, Davies-Humphreys J. Extramammary Paget's disease. *BJOG.* 2005;112:273-279.

54. Lam C, Funaro D. Extramammary Paget's disease: summary of current knowledge. *Dermatol Clin.* 2010;28:807-826.

55. Islam AD, Naguwa SM, Cheema GS, Hunter JC, Gershwin ME. Multicentric reticulohistiocytosis: a rare yet challenging disease. *Clin Rev Allergy Immunol.* 2013;45:281-289.

56. Snow JL, Muller SA. Malignancy-associated multicentric reticulohistiocytosis: a clinical, histological and immunophenotypic study. *Br J Dermatol.* 1995;133:71-76.

Neurofibromatosis

Yuichi Yoshida

KEY POINTS

- Neurofibromatosis type 1 (NF1) is a neurocutaneous genetic disorder caused by mutation of the *NF1* gene on chromosome 17q11.2, whereas neurofibromatosis type 2 (NF2) is a genetically distinct disorder caused by mutation of the gene on chromosome 22q12.2 encoding merlin.

- The worldwide prevalence of NF1 is approximately 1 in 3000 individuals with no relation to race.

- NF1 is characterized by café-au-lait spots, freckling, neurofibromas, Lisch nodules, cerebral tumors, and osseous abnormalities.

- Clinical manifestations of NF1 are variable in each individual, and the overall degree of severity and complications are not predictable.

- Patients with NF1 have increased risk of malignancies.

- Age-specific annual monitoring and treatment of complications by appropriate specialists are important for management of NF1.

INTRODUCTION

Neurofibromatosis type 1 (NF1; Online Mendelian Inheritance in Man [OMIM] #162200), also known as von Recklinghausen disease, is one of the most common neurocutaneous genetic disorders.[1] NF1 is characterized by café-au-lait spots, freckling, neurofibromas, Lisch nodules, cerebral tumors, and osseous abnormalities. Clinical manifestations are variable even within the same family members. However, it has been estimated that two-thirds of patients with NF1 have a relatively mild phenotype without life-threatening complications.

Neurofibromatosis type 2 (NF2; OMIM #101000) is a genetically distinct disorder caused by mutation of the gene on chromosome 22q12.2 encoding merlin.[2] NF2 is much less common than NF1 with an incidence of 1 in 25,000 live births (prevalence of 1 in 100,000 individuals).[3] NF2 is characterized by tumors of the central nervous system (vestibular schwannomas, meningioma, and glioma), schwannoma of the peripheral nervous system, and juvenile posterior subcapsular lenticular opacities/juvenile cortical cataract.[4] Cutaneous tumors are seen in 59% to 68% of patients and are usually schwannomas (not neurofibromas). Although pigmented spots are seen in 33% to 48% of patients, they are often singular and are not typical features of NF2. Therefore, pigmented spots are not included in the diagnostic criteria for NF2.

The primary emphasis of this chapter is the more common NF1.

Epidemiology

The worldwide prevalence of NF1 is approximately 1 in 3000 individuals with nearly 100% penetrance.[5] The birth incidence of NF1 is similar to its prevalence. No racial predilection has been reported for NF1. About half of NF1 cases are nonfamilial sporadic cases. Mosaic NF1 (segmental neurofibromatosis) is characterized by a regionally limited distribution of the features of NF1. The estimated incidence of mosaic NF1 is approximately 1 in 36,000 to 40,000 individuals (0.003%) in the general population.[6]

The overall risk of malignancies in patients with NF1 is 36% by the age of 70 years, being 2.7 times higher than that in the general population in the United Kingdom.[7] The most common associated malignancies in NF1 are malignant peripheral nerve sheath tumor (MPNST) (14% risk; standardized incidence ratio [SIR], 122) and brain tumors (7.9% risk; SIR, 22.6). In addition, women with NF1 (<50 years old) are at higher risk for breast cancer than the general population with no relation to race (SIR, 4.41).[8] It has been reported that children with NF1 also have an increased risk of cancers (6.45 times higher risk than the general population) in Japan.[9] Disease-associated malignancies have also been reported in patients with mosaic NF1.[10] The average age at death in patients with NF1 is about 15 years earlier than healthy individuals. It is important for physicians to be aware of the increased risk of malignancies in patients with NF1.

ETIOLOGY/GENETICS

The *NF1* gene was cloned on chromosome 17q11.2 in 1990.[11,12] Hotspots of the mutation have not been found in NF1 because of the large size of the gene. The *NF1*-encoded protein product, neurofibromin, contains a guanosine triphosphatase–activating protein (GAP)-related domain and functions as a negative regulator of rat sarcoma viral oncogene homolog (RAS)-mediated signaling (tumor suppressor activity). Therefore, mutation of the *NF1* gene increases signaling through the intracellular Ras/mitogen-activated protein kinase (MAPK) and phosphatidylinositol 3-kinase (PI3K)/AKT/mammalian target of the rapamycin (mTOR) pathway.[13]

Although the pathogenesis of NF1-associated features has not been fully elucidated, loss of heterozygosity or biallelic mutation of the *NF1* gene in different cell lineages is related to several complications. Biallelic *NF1* inactivation in melanocytes has been shown in café-au-lait spots.[14] In addition, *NF1* haploinsufficiency plays an important role in the tumor microenvironments. Interaction between $NF1^{-/-}$ Schwann cells and $NF1^{+/-}$ mast cells is essential for the development of neurofibromas.[15] Because plexiform neurofibroma (PNF) arises during early childhood, the timing of biallelic *NF1* loss in an embryonic Schwann cell lineage is critical for the formation of PNF.[16] It has been suggested that abnormally differentiated Remak bundles (nonmyelinated axon–Schwann cell unit) are the cells of origin for PNF.[17] In contrast, it has been proposed that skin-derived precursors are the cells of origin for cutaneous neurofibroma.[18] Loss of both *NF1* alleles has been shown in pilocytic astrocytomas[19] and in the lesion of osseous dysplasia.[20] In addition to loss of *NF1* function, other gene mutations, such as mutations in *TP53* and *CDKN2A*, are related to the development of MPNST from PNF.[21]

Mosaic NF1 is caused by a postzygotic somatic mutation of the *NF1* gene in the affected region.[22] Patients with mosaic NF1 are at risk of having a child with generalized NF1 because the parental gametes as well as the regional skin may be affected.[23]

CLINICAL FINDINGS

NF1 is usually diagnosed based on clinical criteria of the National Institutes of Health (NIH) [**Table 71-1**].[24] Since many of the features in NF1 are age-dependent,[25,26] it is necessary to follow suspected cases for several years before a diagnosis can be made. Although café-au-lait spots and PNF are usually seen at birth, it is difficult for infant patients without a family history to fulfill the criteria. The overall degree of severity and complications in each individual are not predictable. Genotype-phenotype correlations have not been established in NF1 except for

TABLE 71-1	**The diagnostic criteria for Neurofibromatosis Type 1 (NF1) (National Institutes of Health)**

1. Six or more café-au-lait macules (>5 mm in prepubertal individuals and >15 mm in postpubertal individuals)
2. Two or more neurofibromas of any type or one plexiform neurofibroma
3. Freckling in the axillary or inguinal regions
4. Optic glioma
5. Two or more Lisch nodules (iris hamartomas)
6. A distinctive osseous lesion (sphenoid dysplasia or thinning of long bone cortex, with or without pseudarthrosis)
7. A first-degree relative with NF1 by the above criteria

Note: Fulfillment of two or more diagnostic criteria is required for the diagnosis of NF1.

Source: Data from Neurofibromatosis. Conference statement. National institutes of health consensus development conference. *Arch Neurol.* 1988;45(5):575-578.

whole-gene deletion (severe phenotype)[27] and a specific three-base-pair deletion in exon 17 of the *NF1* gene (mild phenotype).[28] Therefore, molecular testing for NF1 has recently become available in some countries (with preimplantation genetic diagnosis also being possible), but its routine application for patients is not recommended.

MAJOR CLINICAL FINDINGS INCLUDED IN THE DIAGNOSTIC CRITERIA OF NF1

Café-au-lait spots are well-circumscribed, light to dark brown macules with smooth borders [**Figure 71-1**]. They can be present at birth or become apparent in early childhood and grow proportionately to body growth. They are sometimes seen with Mongolian spots in Asian patients [**Figure 71-2**]. A giant café-au-lait spot has irregular borders compared with an ordinary café-au-lait spot [**Figure 71-3**], and PNF often develops in an overlying hyperpigmented region.

Freckling consists of a small brown macule, 1 to 3 mm in diameter, typically seen on the axillae and groin beginning at 3 years of age [**Figure 71-4**]. Freckling is sometimes seen on the face or the trunk.

Neurofibroma can be classified into cutaneous neurofibroma and PNF (nodular PNF and diffuse PNF). Cutaneous neurofibromas are soft, dome-shaped, flesh-colored nodules, 1 to 2 cm in diameter [**Figure 71-5**]. They are detectable in most patients at puberty and increase in number and size with age or pregnancy. Blue-red and pseudoatrophic macules, unusual variants of cutaneous neurofibromas, can arise before puberty[29] [**Figure 71-6**]. Cutaneous neurofibromas are usually asymptomatic but sometimes cause itching. On the other hand, PNF is thought to be a congenital tumor and is seen in about 30% of patients. Nodular PNF develops in and along multiple branches of nerve plexuses [**Figure 71-7**] and can also be seen within diffuse PNF. Diffuse PNF enlarges gradually during one's lifetime, resulting in disfigurement and impaired quality of life (QOL) [**Figure 71-8**]. Cutaneous neurofibromas are always benign, whereas PNF has a potential for malignant transformation (MPNST). When a patient complains of pain caused by rapid growth of the tumor,

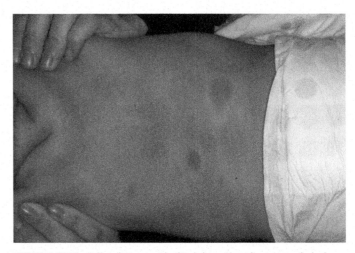

FIGURE 71-2. Café-au-lait spots with white halos on Mongolian spots on the back.

fluorine-18-fluorodeoxyglucose–positron emission tomography/computed tomography (CT) is a useful noninvasive method to identify malignant change in preexisting PNF.[30]

CT or magnetic resonance imaging is useful for the diagnosis of optic glioma (typically low-grade pilocytic astrocytoma) if there are visual and neurologic problems [**Figure 71-9**]. The incidence of optic glioma is less than 1% in Asian populations.[26] Glioma also occurs in the brain in up to 3% of patients [**Figure 71-10**].

Lisch nodules are small pigmented nodules in the iris detectable from 3 years of age and are found in most adult patients [**Figure 71-11**]. Slit-lamp examination by an ophthalmologist may aid in the diagnosis. Treatment for Lisch nodules is not required.

The most frequent osseous abnormalities associated with NF1 include sphenoid wing dysplasia, long bone dysplasia (tibial pseudarthrosis), and scoliosis.[31] Sphenoid wing dysplasia is rarely seen (<1%) with or

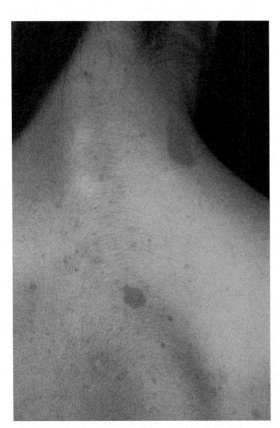

FIGURE 71-1. Multiple brown macules (café-au-lait spots) on the back.

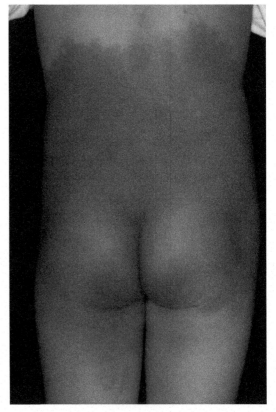

FIGURE 71-3. A giant café-au-lait spot on the buttocks.

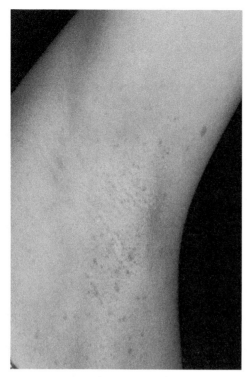

FIGURE 71-4. Multiple small pigmented macules (freckling) on the axilla.

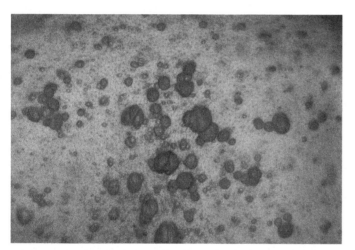

FIGURE 71-5. Multiple soft brown-pink nodules (cutaneous neurofibromas) on the trunk.

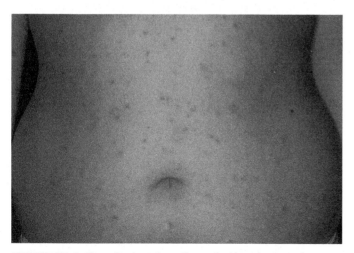

FIGURE 71-6. Blue-red and pseudoatrophic macules (unusual variants of cutaneous neurofibromas) on the abdomen.

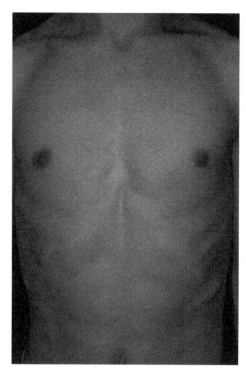

FIGURE 71-7. Nodular plexiform neurofibroma on the abdomen.

without PNF in the orbit and can result in a pulsating exophthalmos or brain herniation in some cases [**Figure 71-12**]. Sphenoid wing dysplasia and long bone dysplasia (approximately 2%) are usually identified in infancy. Scoliosis is apparent until puberty in up to 10% of NF1 patients [**Figure 71-13**].

ADDITIONAL CLINICAL FINDINGS

Hairy fuscoceruleus spots are blue-brown macules with or without coarse hairs seen in 20% of Asian patients with NF1[32] [**Figure 71-14**]. A glomus tumor is a small, bluish, painful tumor that arises in the

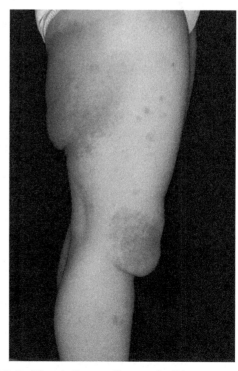

FIGURE 71-8. Diffuse plexiform neurofibroma on the thigh.

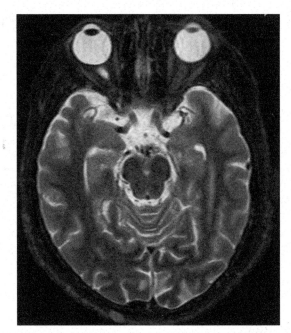

FIGURE 71-9. Optic glioma in the right optic nerve (magnetic resonance imaging).

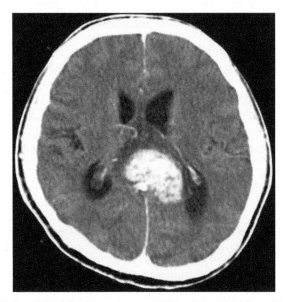

FIGURE 71-10. Pilocytic astrocytoma with hemorrhage in the brain (computed tomography).

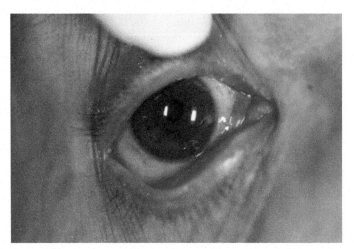

FIGURE 71-11. Lisch nodules in the iris.

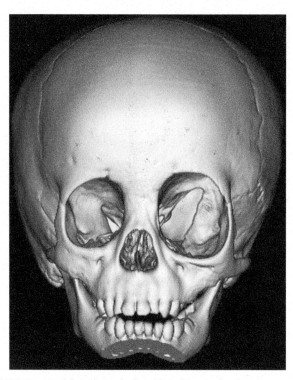

FIGURE 71-12. Sphenoid wing dysplasia (three-dimensional computed tomography).

subungual regions of the fingers and toes in up to 5% of NF1 patients[33] [**Figure 71-15**]. Surgical excision is the only effective treatment for a glomus tumor. Learning disabilities occur in about half of the patients. Cardiovascular abnormalities such as hypertension caused by renal artery stenosis (2%) or pheochromocytoma (2%) rarely occur in association

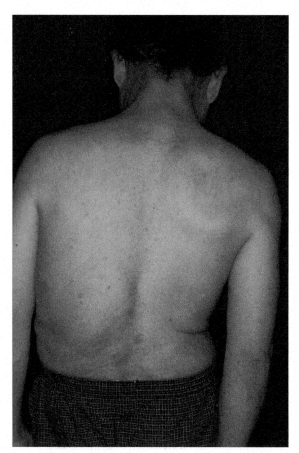

FIGURE 71-13. Scoliosis.

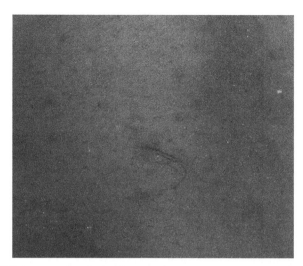

FIGURE 71-14. Hairy fuscoceruleus spot.

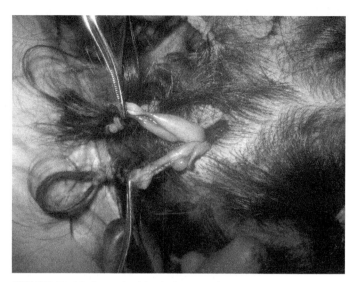

FIGURE 71-16. Resected nodular plexiform neurofibroma on the scalp.

with NF1. NF1 patients have an increased risk of developing gastrointestinal stromal tumors.[34]

DIFFERENTIAL DIAGNOSIS

In 2007, Legius syndrome (NF1-like syndrome) resembling NF1 was identified. Legius syndrome (OMIM #611431) is caused by mutations in the *SPRED1* gene on chromosome 15q13.2, resulting in overactivation of the RAS/MAPK pathway.[35] Patients with Legius syndrome have multiple café-au-lait spots and macrocephaly with or without freckling but lack other typical features of NF1 (eg, neurofibromas, Lisch nodules, optic glioma, and bone abnormalities). It has been estimated that about 2% of individuals with a clinical diagnosis of NF1 according to the NIH criteria in fact had Legius syndrome.[36] Several clinical syndromes, such as Noonan syndrome, Costello syndrome, cardiofaciocutaneous syndrome, and LEOPARD syndrome, with mutations in genes encoding proteins of the RAS signaling pathways have characteristic features overlapping with those of NF1 (RASopathies).[37]

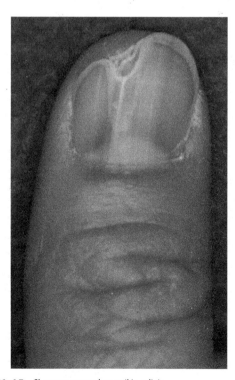

FIGURE 71-15. Glomus tumor under a nail in a digit.

TREATMENT

Age-specific annual monitoring and patient education are important for the management of NF1. Café-au-lait spots and freckling can be treated with a variety of lasers or intense pulsed radiofrequency.[38] However, the results are not always satisfactory because repigmentation or postinflammatory hyperpigmentation may be seen after treatment in some cases. Cosmetic advice on skin camouflaging can be given.

Cutaneous neurofibromas are most commonly removed by surgical excision to improve cosmetic appearance or address social problems or QOL issues in patients with the disease. Carbon dioxide laser is useful for the removal of small regions.

PNF has a risk of malignant transformation. In addition, diffuse PNF sometimes causes life-threatening massive intratumor hemorrhage after minor trauma. Therefore, it is preferable to treat diffuse PNF by surgery or embolization.[39] However, large PNF is a therapeutic challenge, especially if the tumor is located in the head or neck region. Symptomatic nodular PNF can also be surgically treated [**Figure 71-16**], but removal may result in a neurologic deficit. The standard care for MPNST is wide surgical excision and postoperative radiotherapy with or without chemotherapy. However, MPNST is frequently resistant to those therapies and has a poor overall prognosis.[40]

Optic glioma is often asymptomatic, and treatment is not always required. However, chemotherapy with vincristine and cisplatin is performed in symptomatic cases for management of optic glioma. There are concerns about an increased risk of further malignancies and the development of moyamoya syndrome after radiation therapy for optic glioma in patients with NF1.[41,42]

If osseous abnormalities are found, early referral to an orthopedist or neurosurgeon is desirable because management is often difficult.

CONCLUSION

Although we focused on cutaneous manifestations in this chapter, it is important for dermatologists to refer patients with NF1 to appropriate specialists for management of extracutaneous complications such as psychiatric disorders (learning disabilities and attention deficit hyperactivity disorder), cardiovascular abnormalities, and gastrointestinal stromal tumors.

Recent targeted strategies have revealed several interesting molecular therapies for NF1. Various drugs blocking the RAS-MAPK or mTOR pathways are under investigation for treatment of NF1.[43] For example, a tyrosine kinase inhibitor, imatinib mesylate, can inhibit c-kit in addition to blocking c-abl and platelet-derived growth factor. A phase II clinical trial of imatinib mesylate showed that the size of PNF was reduced in some cases.[44]

Clinical trials involving pharmacologic inhibition of mTOR are ongoing, but no published results are available. In the future, these novel medical therapies may be useful for treatment of complications related to NF1.

REFERENCES

1. Boyd KP, Korf BR, Theos A. Neurofibromatosis type 1. *J Am Acad Dermatol.* 2009;61:1-14.
2. Rouleau GA, Merel P, Lutchman M, et al. Alteration in a new gene encoding a putative membrane-organizing protein causes neurofibromatosis type 2. *Nature.* 1993;363:515-521.
3. Asthagiri AR, Parry DM, Butman JA, et al. Neurofibromatosis type 2. *Lancet.* 2009;373:1974-1986.
4. Gutmann DH, Aylsworth A, Carey JC, et al. The diagnostic evaluation and multidisciplinary management of neurofibromatosis 1 and neurofibromatosis 2. *JAMA.* 1997;278:51-57.
5. Lammert M, Friedman JM, Kluwe L, et al. Prevalence of neurofibromatosis 1 in German children at elementary school enrollment. *Arch Dermatol.* 2005; 141:71-74.
6. Ruggieri M, Huson SM. The clinical and diagnostic implications of mosaicism in the neurofibromatoses. *Neurology.* 2001;56:1433-1443.
7. Walker L, Thompson D, Easton D, et al. A prospective study of neurofibromatosis type 1 cancer incidence in the UK. *Br J Cancer.* 2006;95:233-238.
8. Madanikia SA, Bergner A, Ye X, et al. Increased risk of breast cancer in women with NF1. *Am J Med Genet A.* 2012;158A:3056-3060.
9. Matsui I, Tanimura M, Kobayashi N, et al. Neurofibromatosis type 1 and childhood cancer. *Cancer.* 1993;72:2746-2754.
10. Dang JD, Cohen PR. Segmental neurofibromatosis and malignancy. *Skinmed.* 2010;8:156-159.
11. Cawthon RM, Weiss R, Xu GF, et al. A major segment of the neurofibromatosis type 1 gene: cDNA sequence, genomic structure, and point mutations. *Cell.* 1990;62:193-201.
12. Wallace MR, Marchuk DA, Andersen LB, et al. Type 1 neurofibromatosis gene: identification of a large transcript disrupted in three NF1 patients. *Science.* 1990;249:181-186.
13. Gottfried ON, Viskochil DH, Couldwell WT. Neurofibromatosis type 1 and tumorigenesis: molecular mechanisms and therapeutic implications. *Neurosurg Focus.* 2010;28:E8
14. De Schepper S, Maertens O, Callens T, et al. Somatic mutation analysis in NF1 café au lait spots reveals two NF1 hits in the melanocytes. *J Invest Dermatol.* 2008;128:1050-1053.
15. Zhu Y, Ghosh P, Charnay P, et al. Neurofibromas in NF1: Schwann cell origin and role of tumor environment. *Science.* 2002;296:920-922.
16. Wu J, Williams JP, Rizvi TA, et al. Plexiform and dermal neurofibromas and pigmentation are caused by NF1 loss in in desert hedgehog-expressing cells. *Cancer Cell.* 2008;13:105-116.
17. Zheng H, Chang L, Patel N, et al. Induction of abnormal proliferation by nonmyelinating Schwann cells triggers neurofibroma formation. *Cancer Cell.* 2008;13:117-128.
18. Le LQ, Shipman T, Burns DK, et al. Cell of origin and microenvironment contribution for NF1-associated dermal neurofibromas. *Cell Stem Cell.* 2009;8: 453-463.
19. Gutmann DH, Donahoe J, Brown T, et al. Loss of neurofibromatosis 1 (NF1) gene expression in NF1-associated pilocytic astrocytomas. *Neuropathol Appl Neurobiol.* 2000;26:361-367.
20. Stevenson DA, Zhou H, Ashrafi S, et al. Double inactivation of NF1 in tibial pseudarthrosis. *Am J Hum Genet.* 2006;79:143-148.
21. Brems H, Beert E, de Ravel T, et al. Mechanisms in the pathogenesis of malignant tumors in neurofibromatosis type 1. *Lancet Oncol.* 2009;10:508-515.
22. Tinschert S, Naumann I, Stegmann E, et al. Segmental neurofibromatosis is caused by somatic mutation of the neurofibromatosis type 1 (*NF1*) gene. *Eur J Hum Genet.* 2000;8:455-459.
23. Consoli C, Moss C, Green S, et al. Gonasomal mosaicism for a nonsense mutation (R1947X) in the *NF1* gene in segmental neurofibromatosis type 1. *J Invest Dermatol.* 2005;125:463-466.
24. Neurofibromatosis. Conference statement. National Institutes of Health consensus development conference. *Arch Neurol.* 1988;45:575-578.
25. Ferner RE, Huson SM, Thomas N, et al. Guidelines for the diagnosis and management of individuals with neurofibromatosis 1. *J Med Genet.* 2007;44:81-88.
26. Niimura M. Neurofibromatosis in Japan. In: Ishibashi Y, Hori Y, eds. *Tuberous Sclerosis and Neurofibromatosis: Epidemiology, Pathophysiology, Biology and Management.* Amsterdam, the Netherlands: Elsevier Science Publishers; 1990:23.
27. Lepping KA, Kaplan P, Viskochil D, et al. Familial neurofibromatosis 1 microdeletions: cosegregation with distinct facial phenotype and early onset of cutaneous neurofibromata. *Am J Med Genet.* 1997;73:197-204.
28. Upadhyaya M, Huson SM, Davies M, et al. An absence of cutaneous neurofibromas associated with a 3-bp inframe deletion in exon 17 of the NF1 gene (c.2970-2972 delAAT): evidence of a clinically significant NF1 genotype-phenotype correlation. *Am J Hum Genet.* 2007;80:140-151.
29. Westerhof W, Konrad K. Blue-red macules and pseudoatrophic macules: additional cutaneous signs in neurofibromatosis. *Arch Dermatol.* 1982;118:577-581.
30. Treglia G, Taralli S, Bertagna F, et al. Usefulness of whole-body fluorine-18-fluorodeoxyglucose positron emission tomography in patients with neurofibromatosis type 1: a systematic review. *Radiol Res Pract.* 2012;2012:431029.
31. Alwan S, Tredwell SJ, Friedman JM. Is osseous dysplasia a primary features of neurofibromatosis 1 (NF1)? *Clin Genet.* 2005;67:378-390.
32. Niimura M. Aspects in neurofibromatosis from the viewpoint of dermatology. *J Dermatol.* 1992;19:868-872.
33. Stewart DR, Sloan JL, Yao L, et al. Diagnosis, management, complications of glomus tumors of the digits in neurofibromatosis type 1. *J Med Genet.* 2010;47:525-532.
34. Mussi C, Schildhaus HU, Gronchi A, et al. Therapeutic consequences from molecular biology for gastrointestinal stromal tumor patients affected by neurofibromatosis type 1. *Clin Cancer Res.* 2008;14:4550-4555.
35. Brems H, Chmara M, Sahbatou M, et al. Germline loss-of-function mutations in SPRED1 cause a neurofibromatosis 1-like phenotype. *Nat Genet.* 2007;39:1120-1126.
36. Messiaen L, Yao S, Brems H, et al. Clinical and mutational spectrum of neurofibromatosis type 1-like syndrome. *JAMA.* 2009;302:2111-2118.
37. Tidyman WE, Rauen KA. The RASopathies: developmental syndromes of Ras/MAPK pathway dysregulation. *Curr Opin Genet Dev.* 2009;19:230-236.
38. Yoshida Y, Sato N, Furumura M, et al. Treatment of pigmented lesions of neurofibromatosis 1 with intense pulsed-radio frequency in combination with topical application of vitamin D3 ointment. *J Dermatol.* 2007;34:227-230.
39. Yoshida Y, Yamamoto O. Ultrasonic dissection for diffuse plexiform neurofibroma. *Dermatol Surg.* 2010;36:1773-1774.
40. Widemann BC. Current status of sporadic and neurofibromatosis type 1-associated malignant peripheral nerve sheath tumor. *Curr Oncol Rep.* 2009;11:322-328.
41. Sharif S, Ferner R, Birch JM, et al. Second primary tumors in neurofibromatosis 1 patients treated for optic glioma: substantial risks after radiotherapy. *J Clin Oncol.* 2006;24:2570-2575.
42. Ullrich NJ, Robertson R, Kinnamon DD, et al. Moyamoya following cranial irradiation for primary brain tumors in children. *Neurology.* 2007;68:932-938.
43. ClinicalTrials.gov. A service of the U.S. National Institutes of Health. http://www.clinicaltrials.gov. Accessed February 28, 2015.
44. Robertson KA, Nalepa G, Yang FC, et al. Imatinib mesylate for plexiform neurofibroma in patients with neurofibromatosis type 1: phase 2 trial. *Lancet Oncol.* 2012;13:1218-1224.

CHAPTER 72

Tuberous Sclerosis Complex

Mari Wataya-Kaneda

KEY POINTS

- Tuberous sclerosis complex (TSC) is an autosomal dominant disease characterized by generalized hamartoma formation in nearly every organ, with various manifestations occurring throughout the individual's lifetime.

- Skin manifestations of TSC include angiofibromas, forehead plaques, hypomelanotic macules, shagreen patches, and ungual fibromas.

- Hypomelanotic macules are observed in more than 90% of patients with TSC and are evident at birth or during early infancy. More than three hypomelanotic macules are useful for the diagnosis of TSC in infant.

- Hypomelanotic macules are off-white in color and usually oval, polygonal, or ash leaf shaped, but sometimes appear as scattered numerous small white macules. Hypomelanotic macules present on the scalp, eyelashes, and eyebrows cause poliosis.

- The hypomelanotic macules in TSC have a normal number of melanocytes but decreased number and size of melanosomes.

TUBEROUS SCLEROSIS COMPLEX

Tuberous sclerosis complex (TSC) is an autosomal dominant inherited genetic disorder that can affect any organ in the body, with the most common findings observed in the skin, brain, kidneys, lungs, retina, and heart.[1]

The first description of TSC was provided in the early1800s by Ryer. TSC was initially described approximately 150 years ago by von Recklinghausen. Bourneville provided a detailed description of the neurologic symptoms and gross pathology in the central nervous system in 1880. Kirpicznik first recognized TSC to be a genetic disease in 1910, and Berg described the dominant inheritance of TSC in 1913. In 1993,[2] the *TSC2* gene was identified on chromosome 16p13, and in 1997, the *TSC1* gene was cloned on chromosome 9q34.[3] In 2002, the complex consisting of hamartin and tuberin, which are encoded by tumor suppressor genes *TSC1* and *TSC2*, respectively, was reported to regulate the mammalian target of rapamycin (mTOR).[4]

EPIDEMIOLOGY

Prior to the 1980s, the incidence of TSC ranged between 1/100,000 and 1/200,000 individuals.[5] Recent studies have estimated a frequency of 1/6000 to 1/10,000 live births. TSC occurs in all races and ethnic groups, and in both genders.[6]

GENETICS AND PATHOGENESIS

TSC is an autosomal dominant disease characterized by hamartoma formation. It was recognized to be a genetic disease over 100 years ago (by Kirpicznik in 1910). Two genes, *TSC1*[3] and *TSC2*,[2] which encode hamartin and tuberin, respectively, have been shown to be responsible for TSC. Hamartin and tuberin associate physically in vivo and function in the same complex. The hamartin–tuberin complex inhibits the mTOR pathway.[7] Therefore, mutations of *TSC1* or *TSC2*, which cause abnormalities in hamartin and tuberin, respectively, result in defects of the inhibition of mTOR signaling. mTOR is a protein kinase with many functions in the regulation of protein synthesis, metabolism, differentiation, growth, and migration. Constitutive activation of mTOR is associated with abnormal cellular proliferation, which occurs in the hamartomatous lesions of TSC.

CLINICAL FINDINGS

TSC affects nearly every organ, with a variety of manifestations occurring at various times throughout the individual's lifetime. The two most commonly affected organs are the brain and skin; other commonly affected organs include the heart, kidneys, lungs, and eyes.

DERMATOLOGIC MANIFESTATIONS

Skin lesions are the most frequently observed manifestations of TSC.[8-10] The skin manifestations of TSC include angiofibromas, forehead plaques, hypomelanotic macules, shagreen patches, and ungual fibromas.

Facial Angiofibromas and Forehead Plaques Facial angiofibromas are the most emblematic lesions of TSC. Angiofibromas generally appear at approximately 2 to 5 years of age as small papules or telangiectasia [**Figure 72-1**]. Angiofibromas tend to grow during puberty[9] and continue until adulthood [**Figure 72-2**]. They predominate on the central areas of the face, particularly the nasolabial folds and nose, and extend symmetrically onto the cheeks and chin [**Figure 72-3**]. Approximately 75% to 90% of TSC patients[1,8,9,11-13] are affected by facial angiofibromas.

Forehead plaques are irregular, rubbery to firm connective tissue nevi. They are commonly located unilaterally on the forehead [**Figure 72-4**]. However, they may also be found on the scalp [**Figure 72-5**], jaw, and lower cheek extending to the neck [**Figure 72-6**].

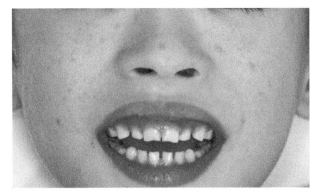

FIGURE 72-1. Angiofibromas in a Japanese boy with tuberous sclerosis complex. Red papules on the face are observed.

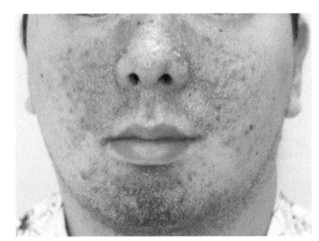

FIGURE 72-2. Facial angiofibroma on adolescent.

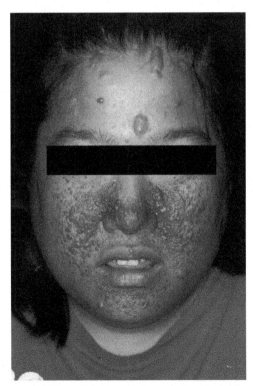

FIGURE 72-3. Angiofibromas and forehead plaques in a Japanese female with tuberous sclerosis complex. Dark red to skin-colored papules, some of which are fused to create plaques in the middle of the face, are observed.

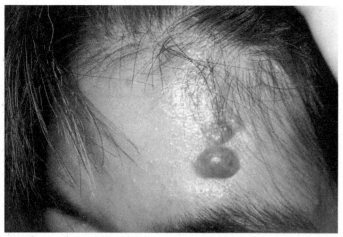

FIGURE 72-4. Forehead plaques on the left forehead of a Japanese female with tuberous sclerosis complex.

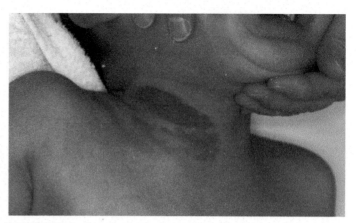

FIGURE 72-6. Connective tissue nevi presenting as plaques on the neck.

Differential Diagnosis The differential diagnosis of angiofibromas includes common skin lesions such as acne, warts, and syringomas. Acne vulgaris and acne rosacea are transient inflammatory diseases, and lesions are accompanied by comedones or pustules. Syringomas are multiple, small, skin-colored papules that usually appear on the lower eyelids after middle age.

Hypomelanotic Macules Hypomelanotic macules are observed in more than 90% of patients with TSC[1,8,9,11-16] and are evident at birth or during early infancy.[9,17,18] Hypomelanotic macules are off-white in color and usually oval, polygonal, or ash leaf shaped and are called "ash leaf spots" [**Figure 72-7**]. When present on the scalp, eyelashes, and eyebrows, hypomelanotic macules cause poliosis. The hypomelanotic macules observed in patients with TSC contain a normal number of melanocytes but with poorly developed dendritic processes as well as melanosomes, which are decreased in number and size.[19]

Differential Diagnosis

- Nevus anemicus is a disorder caused by vascular abnormalities, not pigmentation.

- Piebaldism is characterized by areas of complete depigmentation (white patches) devoid of melanocytes histologically on the ventral trunk and central forehead that usually contain small pigmented patches within their border.

- Vitiligo is an acquired disorder with areas of complete depigmentation (white patches) that lack melanocytes histologically.

- Idiopathic guttate hypomelanosis appears in adulthood rather than infancy.

- Postinflammatory,[9] postinfectious, and posttraumatic hypopigmentation may be differentiated by antecedent history of inflammation, infection, or trauma, respectively.

Shagreen Patches The reported prevalence of shagreen patches in TSC patients ranges from 20% to 57%.[8,9,10-12,20] Typical shagreen patches are firm or rubbery irregular plaques ranging in size from 1 to 10 cm; the color may be skin-colored or slightly pink or brown. They are commonly distributed asymmetrically on the lower back [**Figure 72-8**]. They can be single or multiple and can be misdiagnosed as verrucae [**Figure 72-9**]. Histologically, shagreen patches exhibit sclerotic collagen bundles with reduced elastic fibers. Atypical shagreen patches appear similar to large collagen hamartomas.[8,9,12,21]

Differential Diagnosis

- Buschke-Ollendorff syndrome lesions, although similar to shagreen patches, can occur anywhere on the body and histologically contain increased elastic fibers.

- Multiple endocrine neoplasia type 1 (MEN1), Birt-Hogg-Dube syndrome, and Cowden syndrome exhibit connective tissue nevi with increased collagen, termed collagenomas.

- The collagenomas observed in MEN1 and Birt-Hogg-Dube syndrome appear as multiple, whitish, skin-colored papules or nodules on the trunk and proximal extremities without a propensity for the lower back.[22,23]

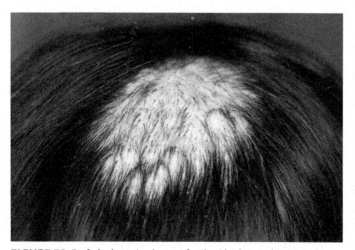

FIGURE 72-5. Scalp plaques in a Japanese female with tuberous sclerosis complex.

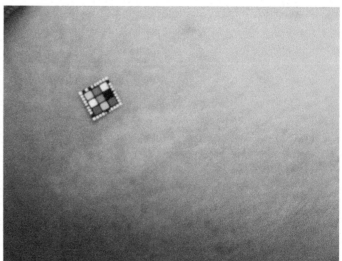

FIGURE 72-7. Hypomelanotic macules on the buttock in a Japanese female with tuberous sclerosis complex.

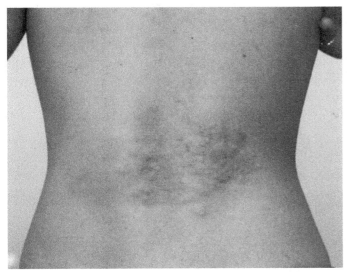

FIGURE 72-8. Shagreen patches with lumpy surfaces and a leathery appearance on the lower back in a Japanese female with tuberous sclerosis complex.

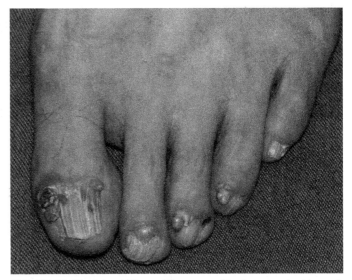

FIGURE 72-10. Periungual fibromas (Koenen tumors) in a Japanese male with normal-colored fibrotic plaques and dystrophic nails.

- The collagenomas observed in Cowden syndrome are histologically distinctive, having prominent clefts between collagen bundles, and are well circumscribed.[24]
- Eruptive collagenoma and familial cutaneous collagenoma are typically oval in shape and distributed on the trunk or extremities.[25]

Ungual Fibromas Ungual fibromas usually appear later than other TSC-associated skin lesions. The reported prevalence in TSC patients varies from 15% to 80%[8,9,12,26]; they eventually affect up to 88% of adults with TSC.[9,12] Ungual fibromas are usually multiple, are common on the toes, and may occur under the nail plate (subungual fibromas) or around the nail plate (periungual fibromas). They exert pressure on the nail matrix, creating longitudinal grooves in the nail [**Figure 72-10**]. Sometimes, nail grooves without evident tumors are found [**Figure 72-11**].

Differential Diagnosis

- Acquired traumatic periungual fibromas are usually solitary and occur on the fifth toe.[27]

Other Skin Lesions

- Molluscum fibrosum pendulum involves skin-colored or hyperpigmented skin tags [**Figure 72-12**].
- Dental enamel pitting is present in 90% of patients with TSC [**Figure 72-13**].

TREATMENT OF DERMATOLOGIC MANIFESTATION

Because most dermatologic manifestations of TSC are not life threatening, treatment is usually aimed at improving the cosmetic appearance of the skin, which is a vital component of a patient's self-esteem and impacts their quality of life.

Facial angiofibromas are treated with numerous methods, including[1,2]:

- Cryosurgery
- Laser therapy
  - Flat and red lesions can be treated with a vascular laser, such as YAG, Alexandria, pulsed dye, or intense pulsed light.
  - Raised and normal-colored lesions are treated with a carbon dioxide (CO_2) laser.
  - Raised and red lesions require the use of both CO_2 and vascular lasers.
- Dermabrasion (helpful when a large surface area of the face is involved[3])
- Excision (only appropriate for a small number of lesions[3])
- Skin graft surgery

Surgical treatment appears to be an effective approach; however, it is not without limitations.

- Anesthesia or sedation is usually required for surgical treatment because patients are often young children or have severe mental retardation. In certain circumstances, surgical treatments may need to be performed under general anesthesia.

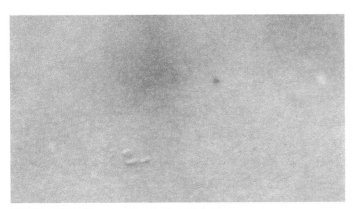

FIGURE 72-9. Shagreen patches that look like warts.

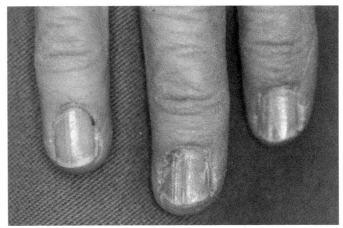

FIGURE 72-11. Periungual fibromas with nail grooves without an evident tumor in a Japanese female with tuberous sclerosis complex.

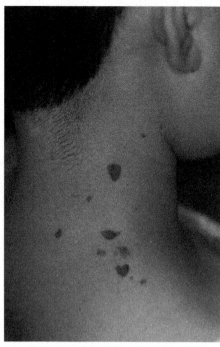

FIGURE 72-12. Molluscum fibrosum pendulum on the right lateral neck in a Japanese female with tuberous sclerosis complex.

- Affected patients have a high incidence of preexisting medical problems that may preclude surgical treatment, such as respiratory compromise, deteriorated kidney function, refractory epilepsy, and symptomatic rhabdomyoma.
- Undergoing tumor resection followed by skin grafting under general anesthesia is difficult, and postoperative care is necessary.

These observations raise the possibility of a new therapy for TSC using inhibitors of mTOR, such as rapamycin (sirolimus). Although the oral administration of rapamycin reduces the incidence of tumors,[28,29] it is associated with significant side effects. As a result, the topical administration of rapamycin is recommended for skin lesions. Several reports of topical rapamycin treatment have been published.[29-31]

SYSTEMIC MANIFESTATIONS OF TUBEROUS SCLEROSIS COMPLEX

Neurologic Manifestations

- Cortical and subcortical tubers.
- Subependymal nodules and subependymal giant cell astrocytomas.
- Epilepsy, reported in 75% to 95% of patients with TSC, begins during the first year of life in 70% of TSC patients.[32-37] Sixty-two percent of these patients develop refractory epilepsy.[38]

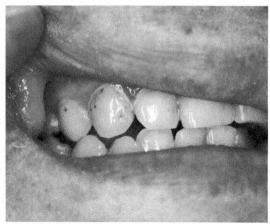

FIGURE 72-13. Dental enamel pitting.

- Cognitive impairment of some degree occurs in approximately 50% of individuals with TSC.
- Autism/autism spectrum disorders commonly occur in TSC patients, affecting 25% to 50% of children with TSC.[32,39-42]

Renal Manifestations

- Angiomyolipoma, renal cysts, and renal cell carcinoma

Pulmonary Manifestations

- Lymphangioleiomyomatosis and multinodular multifocal pneumocyte hyperplasia

Cardiac Manifestations

- Cardiac rhabdomyoma occurs at a high frequency and is an important cause of death in infancy; however, it regresses with age.

DIAGNOSIS

Numerous clinical manifestation appear in patients with TSC. However, many are age-related and not pathognomonic. Therefore, a diagnosis is usually made according to established diagnostic criteria.[43]

DIFFERENTIAL DIAGNOSIS OF TUBEROUS SCLEROSIS COMPLEX

Among adult patients, it is important to distinguish TSC without neurologic symptoms from Birt-Hogg-Dube syndrome (BHD), which is in the differential diagnosis.[44] As with TSC, the symptoms of BHD include facial tumors and renal tumors; however, the facial tumors associated with BHD are fibrofolliculomas or trichodiscomas, not angiofibromas. In addition, the renal tumors associated with BHD are chromophobe/oncocytic renal cell carcinomas or oncocytomas, not angiomyolipomas.

Distinguishing between TSC and MEN1, which is also in the differential diagnosis, is important.[45] MEN1 is associated with angiofibroma and collagenoma, as is TSC[46]; however, the diagnosis of MEN1 requires more than two endocrine tumors.

CONCLUSION

TSC is an autosomal dominant disorder characterized by the formation of hamartomas in a wide range of human tissues. Mutation in either the *TSC1* or *TSC2* tumor suppressor gene is responsible for the disorder. TSC occurs in all races and ethnic groups and in both genders. There are numerous characteristic cutaneous and neurologic manifestations of the disorder.

REFERENCES

1. Schwartz RA, Fernandez G, Kotulska K, Jozwiak S. Tuberous sclerosis complex: advances in diagnosis, genetics, and management. *J Am Acad Dermatol.* 2007;57:189-202.
2. European Chromosome 16 Tuberous Sclerosis Consortium. Identification and characterization of the tuberous sclerosis gene on chromosome 16. *Cell.* 1993;75:1305-1315.
3. van Slegtenhorst M, de Hoogt R, Hermans C, et al. Identification of the tuberous sclerosis gene TSC1 on chromosome 9q34. *Science.* 1997;277:805-808.
4. Inoki K, Li Y, Zhu T, Wu J, Guan KL. TSC2 is phosphorylated and inhibited by Akt and suppresses mTOR signalling. *Nat Cell Biol.* 2002;4:648-657.
5. Nevin NC, Pearce WG. Diagnostic and genetical aspects of tuberous sclerosis. *J Med Genet.* 1986;5:273-280.
6. National Institute of Neurological Disorders and Stroke. Tuberous sclerosis. http://www.ninds.nih.gov/disorders/tuberous_sclerosis/tuberous_sclerosis.htm. Accessed February 28, 2015.
7. Inoki K, Li Y, Xu T, Guan KL. Rheb GTPase is a direct target of TSC2 GAP activity and regulates mTOR signaling. *Genes Dev.* 2003;17:1829-1834.
8. Jozwiak J, Galus R. Molecular implications of skin lesions in tuberous sclerosis. *Am J Dermatopathol.* 2008;30:256-261.
9. Jozwiak S, Schwartz RA, Janniger CK, Michalowicz R, Chmielik J. Skin lesions in children with tuberous sclerosis complex: their prevalence, natural course, and diagnostic significance. *Int J Dermatol.* 1998;37:911-917.

10. Hake S. Cutaneous manifestations of tuberous sclerosis. *Ochsner J.* 2010;10: 200-204.

11. Hallett L, Foster T, Liu Z, Blieden M, Valentim J. Burden of disease and unmet needs in tuberous sclerosis complex with neurological manifestations: systematic review. *Curr Med Res Opin.* 2011;27:1571-1583.

12. Webb DW, Clarke A, Fryer A, Osborne JP. The cutaneous features of tuberous sclerosis: a population study. *Br J Dermatol.* 1996;135:1-5.

13. Dabora SL, Jozwiak S, Franz DN, et al. Mutational analysis in a cohort of 224 tuberous sclerosis patients indicates increased severity of TSC2, compared with TSC1, disease in multiple organs. *Am J Hum Genet.* 2001;68:64-80.

14. Au KS, Williams AT, Roach ES, et al. Genotype/phenotype correlation in 325 individuals referred for a diagnosis of tuberous sclerosis complex in the United States. *Genet Med.* 2007;9:88-100.

15. Yates JR, Maclean C, Higgins JN, et al. The Tuberous Sclerosis 2000 Study: presentation, initial assessments and implications for diagnosis and management. *Arch Dis Child.* 2011;96:1020-1025.

16. Staley BA, Vail EA, Thiele EA. Tuberous sclerosis complex: diagnostic challenges, presenting symptoms, and commonly missed signs. *Pediatrics.* 2011;127:e117-125.

17. Fitzpatrick TB, Szabo G, Hori Y, et al. White leaf-shaped macules. Earliest visible sign of tuberous sclerosis. *Arch Dermatol.* 1968;98:1-6.

18. Fitzpatrick TB. History and significance of white macules, earliest visible sign of tuberous sclerosis. *Ann N Y Acad Sci.* 1991;615:26-35.

19. Jimbow K. Tuberous sclerosis and guttate leukodermas. *Semin Cutan Med Surg.* 1997;16:30-35.

20. Sogut A, Ozmen M, Sencer S, et al. Clinical features of tuberous sclerosis cases. *Turk J Pediatr.* 2002;44:98-101.

21. Torrelo A, Hadj-Rabia S, Colmenero I, et al. Folliculocystic and collagen hamartoma of tuberous sclerosis complex. *J Am Acad Dermatol.* 2012;66:617-621.

22. Darling TN, Skarulis MC, Steinberg SM, et al. Multiple facial angiofibromas and collagenomas in patients with multiple endocrine neoplasia type 1. *Arch Dermatol.* 1997;133:853-857.

23. Asgharian B, Turner ML, Gibril F, et al. Cutaneous tumors in patients with multiple endocrine neoplasm type 1 (MEN1) and gastrinomas: prospective study of frequency and development of criteria with high sensitivity and specificity for MEN1. *J Clin Endocrinol Metab.* 2004;89:5328-5336.

24. Requena L, Gutierrez J, Sanchez Yus E. Multiple sclerotic fibromas of the skin. A cutaneous marker of Cowden's disease. *J Cutan Pathol.* 1992;19:346-351.

25. Uitto J, Santa Cruz DJ, Eisen AZ. Connective tissue nevi of the skin. Clinical, genetic, and histopathologic classification of hamartomas of the collagen, elastin, and proteoglycan type. *J Am Acad Dermatol.* 1980;3:441-461.

26. Aldrich CS, Hong CH, Groves L, et al. Acral lesions in tuberous sclerosis complex: insights into pathogenesis. *J Am Acad Dermatol.* 2010;63:244-251.

27. Carlson RM, Lloyd KM, Campbell TE. Acquired periungual fibrokeratoma: a case report. *Cutis.* 2007;80:137-140.

28. Hofbauer GF, Marcollo-Pini A, Corsenca A, et al. The mTOR inhibitor rapamycin significantly improves facial angiofibroma lesions in a patient with tuberous sclerosis. *Br J Dermatol.* 2008;159:473-475.

29. Haemel AK, O'Brian AL, Teng JM. Topical rapamycin: a novel approach to facial angiofibromas in tuberous sclerosis. *Arch Dermatol.* 2010;146:715-718.

30. Rauktys A, Lee N, Lee L, Dabora SL. Topical rapamycin inhibits tuberous sclerosis tumor growth in a nude mouse model. *BMC Dermatol.* 2008;8:1.

31. Kaufman McNamara E, Curtis AR, Fleischer AB Jr. Successful treatment of angiofibromata of tuberous sclerosis complex with rapamycin. *J Dermatolog Treat.* 2012;23:46-48.

32. Curatolo P, Napolioni V, Moavero R. Autism spectrum disorders in tuberous sclerosis: pathogenetic pathways and implications for treatment. *J Child Neurol.* 2010;25:873-880.

33. Franz DN, Bissler JJ, McCormack FX. Tuberous sclerosis complex: neurological, renal and pulmonary manifestations. *Neuropediatrics.* 2010;41:199-208.

34. Curatolo P, Brinchi V. Antenatal diagnosis of tuberous sclerosis. *Lancet.* 1993; 341:176-177.

35. Thiele EA. Managing epilepsy in tuberous sclerosis complex. *J Child Neurol.* 2004;19:680-686.

36. Devlin LA, Shepherd CH, Crawford H, Morrison PJ. Tuberous sclerosis complex: clinical features, diagnosis, and prevalence within Northern Ireland. *Dev Med Child Neurol.* 2006;48:495-499.

37. Holmes GL, Stafstrom CE. Tuberous sclerosis complex and epilepsy: recent developments and future challenges. *Epilepsia.* 2007;48:617-630.

38. Chu-Shore CJ, Major P, Camposano S, Muzykewicz D, Thiele EA. The natural history of epilepsy in tuberous sclerosis complex. *Epilepsia.* 2010;51: 1236-1241.

39. Curatolo P, Porfirio MC, Manzi B, Seri S. Autism in tuberous sclerosis. *Eur J Paediatr Neurol.* 2004;8:327-332.

40. de Vries PJ, Hunt A, Bolton PF. The psychopathologies of children and adolescents with tuberous sclerosis complex (TSC): a postal survey of UK families. *Eur Child Adolesc Psychiatry.* 2007;16:16-24.

41. Hunt A, Shepherd C. A prevalence study of autism in tuberous sclerosis. *J Autism Dev Disord.* 1993;23:323-339.

42. Smalley SL, Tanguay PE, Smith M, Gutierrez G. Autism and tuberous sclerosis. *J Autism Dev Disord.* 1992;22:339-355.

43. Roach ES, Gomez MR, Northrup H. Tuberous sclerosis complex consensus conference: revised clinical diagnostic criteria. *J Child Neurol.* 1998;13: 624-628.

44. Menko FH, van Steensel MA, Giraud S, et al. Birt-Hogg-Dube syndrome: diagnosis and management. *Lancet Oncol.* 2009;10:1199-1206.

45. Piecha G, Chudek J, Wiecek A. Multiple endocrine neoplasia type 1. *Eur J Intern Med.* 2008;19:99-103.

46. Vidal A, Iglesias MJ, Fernandez B, Fonseca E, Cordido F. Cutaneous lesions associated to multiple endocrine neoplasia syndrome type 1. *J Eur Acad Dermatol Venereol.* 2008;22:835-838.

CHAPTER 73

Renal Disease

Lynn McKinley-Grant
Jon Klinton Peebles

KEY POINTS

- All adults and children with renal disease can develop skin complications—these may arise from the uremic state or be due to the medical treatment received for the condition, for instance dialysis or kidney transplantation.

- More than 20 million people aged 20 years or older in the United States alone have chronic kidney disease, which is fatal if not treated with dialysis or kidney transplantation.

- The most important causes of chronic renal disease are diabetes and hypertension. Racial factors may play a role in the susceptibility to chronic renal failure because there is a strong association of hypertensive end-stage renal disease in African American families.

- Cutaneous manifestations are to be expected in any patient who undergoes dialysis treatment. Many of the skin changes that occur in patients with chronic renal failure are also found in patients undergoing dialysis.

- In contrast to dialysis treatment, cutaneous signs of renal failure may actually resolve if renal transplantation is successful.

- However, posttransplant patients are at risk of developing primary cutaneous malignancies as well as cutaneous and mucosal lesions. It is particularly important to recognize the latter in pediatric patients with skin of color, as they are more common in African American and Hispanic children.

INTRODUCTION

All adults and children with renal disease can develop cutaneous manifestations. These may arise from the uremic state as well as due to the medical treatments used to address the renal disease, for example, dialysis or kidney transplantation. Many of the systemic diseases that affect people with skin of color are diseases that result in the end-organ involvement of the kidney as part of the disease's natural progression.

The major etiologies of renal disease in patients with skin of color are diabetes and hypertension. Other diseases linked to renal insufficiency include connective tissue diseases, systemic lupus erythematosus (SLE), scleroderma, gout, and sickle cell anemia. Advances in medicine have helped increase the life expectancy of people suffering from renal diseases, but treatment, which can include medications, dialysis, and renal transplantation, may encourage the development of associated dermatologic conditions.[1]

RENAL DISEASE

CHRONIC KIDNEY DISEASE AND FAILURE

Chronic kidney disease (CKD) is a long-term condition defined by the gradual loss of kidney function. It is the precursor to end-stage renal disease (ESRD), which is fatal if not treated with dialysis or transplantation.

Epidemiology More than 20 million people aged 20 years or older in the United States alone suffer from CKD.[2] It is more common among women than men and is found in more than 35% of patients with diabetes and in over 20% of patients with hypertension. According to statistics from the Centers for Disease Control and Prevention, almost 110,000 patients in the United States began treatment for ESRD in 2007.[2] In the United States, 7 out of 10 new cases of ESRD in 2006 recorded either diabetes or hypertension as the primary cause.[2] Other etiologies are less common, including glomerulonephritis, hereditary kidney disease, and myelomas.

Genetic Predisposition African Americans were nearly four times more likely to develop ESRD than Caucasians in 2007,[2] with the incidence of renal failure being 998 per 1 million. Diabetes mellitus is currently the number one cause of renal failure in African Americans, who are twice as likely to have diabetes as Caucasian Americans of a similar age.[3]

According to the 2007–2009 National Health Interview Survey data, 7.1% of non-Hispanic Caucasians, 8.4% of Asian Americans, and 11.8% of Hispanics were diagnosed with diabetes. Compared to non-Hispanic Caucasian adults, the risk of diagnosed diabetes was 18% higher among Asian Americans and 69% higher among Hispanics.[3] Overall, Hispanics have 1.5 times the rate of kidney failure of non-Hispanic Caucasians.[2]

ACUTE RENAL FAILURE

Acute renal failure is the result of a rapid and often reversible deterioration in renal function. In general, it takes place over a period of hours to days, with the underlying etiology often being due to a disorder termed acute tubular necrosis. Many commonly used medications can result in acute renal failure secondary to acute tubular necrosis, and a large number of these, including aminoglycoside antimicrobials and antineoplastic agents, have concurrent cutaneous manifestations. In addition to intrinsic renal causes, acute renal failure can be the result of prerenal damage and postrenal obstruction.[3,4]

CHRONIC RENAL FAILURE

Chronic renal failure is a slow and progressive decrease in renal function that typically occurs over a period of months to years. It is generally irreversible and, without intervention, progresses to ESRD in a fairly predictable pattern through four stages that often overlap.[5,6]

Epidemiology Chronic renal failure can have many causes, the most important of which are diabetes mellitus and hypertension.[7] However, other causes that are commonly seen include glomerulonephritis, rheumatologic disease (the most common of which is SLE), interstitial nephritis, neoplasms, cholesterol emboli, infiltrative disorders (eg, systemic amyloidosis), and infection with a streptococcal species, human immunodeficiency virus (HIV), or hepatitis C or B. Additionally, it is important to consider congenital etiologies and genetic predisposition. As CKD has been found to cluster in families, there are clearly genetic and familial factors at play. Racial factors may play a role in this susceptibility because there is a strong association of renal disease in African American families with hypertensive ESRD. In addition, there is evidence that the rate of progression is faster among African American males.[4-6]

Pathology The pathology of renal disease affects one or more of the four basic components of the kidney: the blood vessels, interstitium, tubules, and glomeruli.[7] The pathologic mechanisms vary depending on which component is targeted. For example, glomerular injuries are often caused by immunologic conditions, including autoimmune diseases such as SLE and scleroderma, whereas tubular injuries are often caused by medications and drug toxicity.[4-6]

Genetic Predisposition Chronic renal disease can also be due to a number of congenital anomalies. Almost 10% of all individuals are born with potentially significant malformations of the urinary system. Renal dysplasias and hypoplasias account for 20% of chronic renal failure cases in children. Autosomal dominant polycystic kidney disease is responsible for approximately 10% of chronic renal failure cases in adults.[7] Genetic predispositions to renal maldevelopment, such as those associated with the *Wilms tumor 1* gene, cause genitourinary anomalies. In addition, several metabolic defects, such as cystinuria and the various types of renal tubular acidosis, can predispose patients to be more susceptible to kidney damage and subsequent renal failure.[7]

Other Predisposing Conditions of Chronic Renal Failure The vasculitides, a group of disorders that feature blood vessel inflammation, are important causes of renal failure with concurrent cutaneous manifestations, especially in childhood. In particular, Henoch-Schönlein purpura (HSP) is the most common systemic vasculitis of childhood and has a higher prevalence in Asian children than in African American children.[8,9] HSP is a variant of leukocytoclastic vasculitis characterized by the deposition of immunoglobulin A (IgA)-containing immune complexes in small vessels, most commonly in the skin, kidney, and gastrointestinal tract.[8] There is a strong association with streptococcal and viral infections, but the exact precipitating factor is not known. Classically, there are four manifestations: palpable purpura, colicky abdominal pain, renal involvement, and arthralgia/arthritis.[8-10] The other common vasculitides that can cause renal failure in adults include polyarteritis nodosa and Wegener granulomatosis.

Other rare, yet important, predisposing conditions to renal failure include lysosomal storage disorders (LSDs), such as Fabry disease, the second most common LSD after Gaucher disease, resulting from a deficiency of α-galactosidase A.[11] Renal insufficiency is a key clinical feature of the disease, along with angiokeratomas, pain, hearing loss, neuropathy, and hypohidrosis. Importantly, dermatologists have discovered many new probands for Fabry disease and these can therefore be said to play a key role in diagnosing the disease.[12,13] The dermatologic hallmark of Fabry disease is angiokeratoma corporis diffusum, which consists of small vascular lesions most commonly found in a bathing suit distribution. One study reported that 1.2% of males receiving dialysis in Japan were affected by Fabry disease.[14] A study from Spain on 18.5% of all patients receiving hemodialysis diagnosed 34 new patients with Fabry disease, indicating that the prevalence and incidence of this condition may be underestimated.[15]

Alport syndrome is an example of a genetic disorder caused by mutations in the *COL4A* gene family, which encode type IV collagen α-chain isoforms, resulting in renal disease without skin findings. However, it can be diagnosed by skin biopsy.[16-18] Several cases of Alport syndrome occurring in African American and Chinese patients have been documented in the literature; the disease is characterized by a family history of hematuria, sensorineural deafness, ocular abnormalities, and progressive renal failure.[16,18,19]

UREMIA

Pathogenesis Uremia is a syndrome associated with the deterioration of renal function. A symptomatic patient will demonstrate biochemical aberrations, often beginning with azotemia, characterized by abnormally high levels of nitrogen-containing compounds in the blood. There are numerous skin manifestations associated with the development and persistence of uremia, and the precise causes of the skin findings remain unclear. Some authors suggest that these cutaneous disorders do not have as much to do with the uremic syndrome itself but are instead tied to the underlying pathologic process that induced the primary renal disease.[20] Others, however, report that the skin findings and evidence from biopsy results are more likely related to the duration and severity of the renal failure process and not to the underlying etiology.[20]

CUTANEOUS MANIFESTATIONS OF RENAL DISEASE

GENERALIZED XEROSIS

Xerosis is defined as dry or roughened skin. Although it is most commonly seen in patients on dialysis, it is found in uremic patients as well. Features include complaints of pruritus and dry, fissured skin with scaling. It is often most pronounced over the extensor surfaces of the extremities and can be complicated by fissures, ulcers, lichen simplex chronicus, cellulitis, and irritant or contact dermatitis. Although the pathogenesis is largely unknown, the prevailing theory is one of decreased integrity of the stratum corneum with abnormal transepidermal water loss, possibly as a result of uremic toxins or deposition. Additionally, compromised eccrine gland secretion may lead to epithelial dehydration, although several authors have reported no correlation between xerotic skin and stratum corneum water content.[21]

ACQUIRED ICHTHYOSIS

Acquired ichthyosis is identified by the appearance of 'fish scales' in a generalized distribution. Acquired ichthyosis is known to be associated with numerous conditions, all of which should be kept in mind for the differential diagnosis. Acquired ichthyosis is a known entity that can result from uremia, with clinical features overlapping with those of xerosis and pruritus.

Treatment Treatment options for xerosis and acquired ichthyosis include the avoidance of irritants, the use of either mild soap or none at all in cleansing the skin, and the frequent use of emollients (see also the section on pruritus).[22]

UREMIC PRURITUS

Pruritus has been described by patients as a deep itching sensation, as well as akin to an insect bite when combined with very dry skin. It is one of the most common cutaneous manifestations of chronic renal failure and can be related to many different causes of renal disease. Pruritus can occur with the onset of dialysis treatment and can be significantly exacerbated by a change in the dialysate. Notably, pruritus is not commonly associated with acute renal failure but is linked to longstanding uremia and ESRD. Pruritus has been shown to affect 15% to 49% of patients with chronic renal failure and up to 50% to 90% of the dialysis population.[22] A recent case-controlled study in Egyptian hemodialysis patients demonstrated that pruritus was more common in diabetic uremics than in nondiabetic uremics.[23]

The clinical features of uremic pruritus can be generalized or localized and are typically not associated with a rash. Excoriations can be prominent, and an escalation to lichen simplex chronicus lesions and prurigo nodularis may be seen [**Figure 73-1**]. Pathophysiologically,

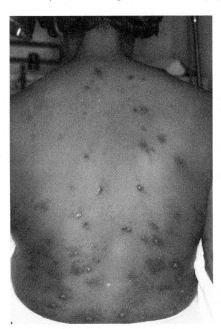

FIGURE 73-1. Prurigo nodularis on the back of a female patient with chronic renal disease. This condition is characterized by pruritic nodules which are discrete, symmetrically distributed and hyperpigmented. They are greater than 0.5 cm in both width and depth. Note the sparing of the relatively unreachable area of mid- and upper back. (Used with permission from the Department of Dermatology, Washington Hospital Center, Washington, DC.)

numerous etiologies have been proposed, including skin changes related to xerosis, deposition of urochrome and/or uremic toxins, calcium and phosphate dysregulation from secondary hyperparathyroidism of renal failure, hyperthyroidism, mast-cell proliferation, immune dysfunction, elevated pro-inflammatory cytokines, and/or hypovitaminosis D.[24] Higher contents of calcium, phosphorus, and magnesium have been found in the skin of patients with uremic pruritus in comparison to controls.[25] Histamine is one of the few mediators definitively linked to clinical pruritus, and it is thought that mast-cell proliferation in the setting of renal failure may lead to increased amounts of histamine.[22,23]

The differential diagnosis of pruritus is extensive; however, in cases of suspected renal failure, particular considerations would include hepatobiliary disease, atopic reactions, and malignancies, such as lymphoma, leukemia, and myeloma.

Treatment The treatment for uremic pruritus can be difficult. Current approaches have been largely empirical, and there is a lack of firm, evidence-based treatment regimens.[26] While renal transplantation is often the best option in severe renal disease, pruritus can be managed in the following ways:

- Moisturizers and proper hydration.

- Keratolytics.

- Antihistamines.

- Phototherapy. Both narrowband and broadband ultraviolet B (UVB) therapy have been shown to be beneficial, although there are recent studies that suggest that the effectiveness of this treatment is not clear and that further investigation is warranted.[27]

- Topical tacrolimus. This is an additional option but should be used with caution in patients with renal failure, given its immunosuppressive properties. Attention should also be paid to routine skin cancer screening.

- Cholestyramine. This should especially be considered for patients with concurrent biliary diseases.

- Ondansetron. This is more commonly used to prevent nausea and vomiting, which can be a significant comorbidity in this patient population.[28]

- Omega-3 fatty acids. These were found to be more effective than placebos in long-term treatment.[29]

- Gabapentin. This drug has had moderate success in the treatment of uremic pruritus, although a recent study found that desloratadine may be a superior choice because it provides significant relief and is better tolerated than gabapentin.[30,31]

- Cromolyn sodium. A topical cromolyn sodium 4% cream was found to be effective in a randomized double-blind study, whereas a study in Japan has led to the approval of nalfurafine hydrochloride for the treatment of uremic pruritus.[31-35]

- Baby oil and zinc sulfate supplementation. These have been suggested as inexpensive, safe, and simple options for managing pruritic symptoms and improving the quality of life of patients with ESRD.[36,37]

PIGMENTARY CHANGES

Pallor A variety of pigmentary skin alterations have been linked to chronic renal failure and uremia. Although most of these pigmentary changes are more closely associated with dialysis treatment, uremia and renal failure itself can result in skin pallor. In addition, the skin may have a yellowish tinge in a generalized distribution, which can be difficult to appreciate in patients with skin of color. The underlying pathogenesis is thought to be due to a combination of both anemia and the urochrome deposition. Specifically, the yellowish tinge can be attributed to the accumulation of carotenoids and nitrogenous pigments. Although often subtle in individuals with skin of color, it can be seen in every patient population and is well documented in East Asian patients as well as patients from the Indian subcontinent and Egypt.[23,38] The differential diagnosis should include all possible causes of anemia and chronic disease, from the most common etiologies—such as iron and other vitamin and mineral deficiencies—to rarer, more serious causes—such as neoplasia and sources of jaundice.

Hyperpigmentation Uremia may also result in a photodistributed or generalized brown hyperpigmentation, thought to be due to the increased amounts of melanin present in the epidermal basal layer and papillary dermis. Uremic patients are thought to have decreased metabolism of β-melanocyte-stimulating hormone (β-MSH) by the compromised kidneys.[39] This leads to elevated serum levels of β-MSH with subsequent melanin production stimulated by the melanocytes.

Bruising In addition to pallor and hyperpigmentation, easy bruising is common in the uremic patient. The distribution is largely at sites of trauma and is due to hemostatic abnormalities, including platelet dysfunction.

■ NAILS

Nail findings can be valuable clues in the examination of the skin of a patient with renal failure. The nails may display a spectrum of disease findings, from alopecia areata and psoriasis to renal and hepatic insufficiency. Two types of nail findings are commonly described in renal failure: Mees lines and half-and-half nails. Mees lines are lines of discoloration across the nails and are characterized by partial leukonychia of the nail plate. Clinically, half-and-half nails show a whitish or normal proximal portion and an abnormally brown distal portion that does not fade with pressure. This latter, or more distal, portion of the nail represents more than one-third of the nail plate. As with many other findings in renal failure, half-and-half nails are not always seen and are more prominent in dialysis patients. Although some patients will display no nail findings, leukonychia is actually more common than half-and-half nails, although this entity is not specific to the setting of renal disease.[40,41]

As with the hyperpigmentation of renal failure, the pathogenesis of these nail findings has been attributed to increased levels of plasma β-MSH. Histologically, increased melanin pigment is seen within the nail plate.[40-42]

■ UREMIC FROST

Although a rare condition today, uremic frost was once described as a classic manifestation of chronic renal failure. This condition manifests itself as a discoloration of the face. White deposits are noted about the face, nostrils, and neck; these are believed to be due to the eccrine deposition of crystallized urea from sweat after evaporation. Although uncommon, it is a manifestation of profound untreated azotemia. Usually, blood urea levels are greater than 200 mg/dL. The skin exhibits a gray, almost metallic, hue with underlying hyperpigmentation, pallor, and sometimes fine scale. However, the appearance may not be classic in patients with skin of color. A high index of suspicion is warranted in patients with cutaneous abnormalities and a history of longstanding, untreated renal failure.[43] Another variant, erythema papulatum uremicum, is a condition in which large papules and nodules on an erythematous base appear on the palms, soles, forearms, and face. Within weeks, the lesions can desquamate and develop fissures.[38] As with uremia in general, dialysis treatments have fortunately rendered this condition quite rare.

Drug reactions, although quite common in the general population, occur more commonly in patients with chronic renal failure due to the routine administration of many drugs and the delayed clearance rate imposed by uremia. The most common offenders in this population are penicillins, sulfonamides, and cephalosporins.

CUTANEOUS MANIFESTATIONS OF DIALYSIS

Cutaneous manifestations are to be expected in any patient who undergoes dialysis treatments for any extended period of time. Many of the skin changes that occur in patients with chronic renal failure are also found in patients undergoing dialysis. It is important to keep in mind that dialysis has increased the life expectancy of patients with ESRD and has thereby provided the time and opportunity for these

TABLE 73-1	Iatrogenic skin manifestations of hemodialysis
Manifestation	**Details**
Pruritus	This is a frequent complaint. It may be severe and worsen with dialysis.[31,32] Severe, intractable symptoms may be a manifestation of another underlying disorder. It is associated with Ekbom syndrome (also known as delusional parasitosis), which is a rare, false belief that one is infested with parasites—this belief is due to the itching sensation of pruritus.[47]
Xerosis	
Cutaneous pigmentation	
Acquired ichthyosis	
Half-and-half nails	
Perforating dermatoses, bullous dermatoses, and calcifying disorders	
Arteriovenous shunt dermatitis	This may occur in up to 8% of patients undergoing long-term dialysis.[46]
Other graft site complications	Eczema may be seen at sites of arteriovenous fistula or catheter insertion. Pseudo-Kaposi sarcoma may also be seen at fistula sites, with purple nodules or papules that slowly become scaly, violaceous, crusted patches.[48-50] Vigilance is needed to prevent infectious complications at cannula sites, for instance overwhelming sepsis.
Gynecomastia	Protein-energy malnutrition can occur with chronic renal failure. Pituitary gonadotropic and testicular functions may remain suppressed following treatment. With an increase in daily protein intake, a subtle hormone surge can lead to transient gynecomastia.
Nephrogenic systemic fibrosis	This condition is rare, although recent studies suggest that the disorder is seen in over one-tenth of hemodialysis patients.[83-85]

cutaneous changes to appear. Although many of these changes overlap with those of uremia and ESRD in general, there are several dermatologic conditions that are specific to dialysis. In light of this intersection, dialysis-associated cutaneous changes can be grouped into two broad categories: (1) cutaneous manifestations in patients with ESRD/chronic renal failure on hemodialysis and (2) iatrogenic skin manifestations of hemodialysis. The first category demonstrates overlap with uremic skin manifestations as described in the previous section, whereas the second category will be discussed in detail here [**Table 73-1**].[44-47]

The iatrogenic manifestations associated with dialysis include arteriovenous shunt dermatitis and other graft site complications, gynecomastia, and, rarely, nephrogenic systemic fibrosis, which will be discussed later. Arteriovenous shunt dermatitis may occur in up to 8% of patients on long-term hemodialysis treatment.[46] Some authors report patients developing eczema both at the site of the arteriovenous fistula as well as at the site of catheter insertion. Interestingly, cases of pseudo-Kaposi sarcoma have been documented at the fistula site, which appears as purple nodules or papules that slowly become scaly, violaceous, crusted patches.[48-50] Constant vigilance must be exercised by caregivers to prevent infectious complications at the cannula site because it is not uncommon for patients to develop overwhelming sepsis from catheter-related infections.[44]

Other conditions reported to be associated to varying degrees with dialysis treatment include dermatosis papulosa nigra, acrochorda, prurigo nodularis, idiopathic guttate hypomelanosis, insulin-induced lipoatrophy, vitiligo,[44] papular urticaria, onychoschizia (splitting of the distal nail plate into layers at the free edge), and Schamberg disease. A number of hair abnormalities have also been reported in the setting of dialysis treatment, mostly consisting of sparse body hair and diffuse alopecia with very dry hair.[44] The pathogenesis of this process is thought to be due to the decreased secretion of sebum secondary to uremia in association with the intermittent frequency of dialysis treatments.[44,48]

Additionally, acquired perforating dermatoses and a spectrum of bullous dermatoses, especially pseudoporphyria, can develop in association with hemodialysis. Both of these groups of disorders are discussed separately below.

◼ BULLOUS DERMATOSES: PORPHYRIA CUTANEA TARDA AND PSEUDOPORPHYRIA CUTANEA TARDA

The bullous dermatoses represent a spectrum of blistering disorders that are associated with hemodialysis. Broadly, patients can develop two types of bullous dermatosis in the setting of chronic renal failure.[49,50] One is a true porphyria, such as the well-known porphyria cutanea tarda (PCT), and the other is pseudoporphyria, also known as dialysis porphyria.

PCT is a disorder of heme biosynthesis due to a deficiency in uroporphyrinogen decarboxylase, resulting in a photodistributed vesicobullous eruption of the skin. The disorder can be categorized as acquired or inherited, with important distinctions between the two. In the acquired form, the enzymatic deficiency is localized to the liver, whereas the inherited form affects all tissues, including erythrocytes, in an autosomal dominant fashion. PCT is a known adverse effect of dialysis treatment, with a reported incidence of 1.2% to 18% of hemodialysis patients.[51] Pseudoporphyria in the setting of chronic renal disease was first described in 1975 and has since been well documented in the literature.[52] Interestingly, pseudoporphyria of chronic renal failure in the absence of dialysis has also been reported.

Clinical Features Clinical features of PCT and pseudoporphyria consist of skin fragility, tense subepidermal vesicles and bullae in a photodistribution, preferentially affecting the dorsal hands [**Figure 73-2**] and forearms.[20,52] The face and feet are often involved. Crusts and erosions are typically present, and lesions heal with significant scarring and milia formation.[20,52] Facial hypertrichosis and hyperpigmentation can occur. In the true porphyrias, sclerodermoid plaques can sometimes be seen on any skin surface, regardless of sun exposure.[46] However, hypertrichosis and sclerodermoid plaques are not typical features of pseudoporphyria.[53]

Pathogenesis and Etiology The pathogenesis of the inherited porphyrias is due to enzyme deficiencies in the biosynthetic pathway of heme synthesis. In PCT, a deficiency of uroporphyrinogen decarboxylase results in the accumulation of porphyrins in the liver, plasma, and skin. Once deposited in the skin, oxidative free radicals are generated, which cause photosensitivity, blisters, and scarring once exposed to ultraviolet light.

The cause of pseudoporphyria, on the other hand, is largely unknown. Although most patients with pseudoporphyria do not have elevated levels of porphyrins, there are some whose plasma porphyrin levels are slightly above the normal range. Photoactive drugs have also been implicated in triggering the onset of pseudoporphyria.[54-57] Hepatitis C or HIV infection, iron overload, alcohol, and various medications (including valproate, sulfonamides, hydroxychloroquine, estrogens, and diaminodiphenyl sulfone) are all exacerbating factors in the development of these bullous disorders in patients with chronic renal failure.[58,59]

Differential Diagnosis These disorders may have the following differential diagnoses: blistering disorders, including bullous pemphigoid, pemphigus vulgaris, bullous SLE, epidermolysis bullosa acquisita, and linear IgA dermatosis.[52-55] Plasma porphyrin profiles often distinguish between pseudoporphyria and PCT. However, patients with pseudoporphyria can have elevated porphyrin levels, albeit not as elevated as those seen in PCT.[39]

Treatment The standard treatment for acquired PCT is phlebotomy, which reduces the hepatic iron load and therefore decreases the inhibitory effect of iron on uroporphyrinogen decarboxylase oxidation. Because many of these patients are anemic, small volume phlebotomy (100-200 mL per weekly session) should be used. Additional therapies

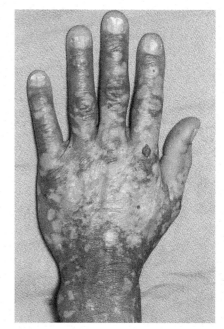

A

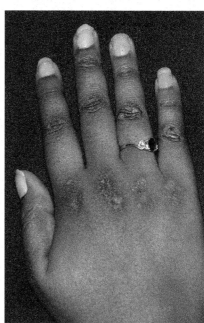

B

FIGURE 73-2. Cases of porphyria cutanea tarda on the back of the hand of a male (**A**) and female patient (**B**). (Used with permission from the Department of Dermatology, Washington Hospital Center, Washington, DC.)

that have proved successful in several cases include erythropoietin and deferasirox.[40,46,59-63]

◼ CALCINOSIS CUTIS AND CALCIPHYLAXIS

Clinical Features and Differential Diagnosis Calcinosis cutis is the term used to indicate the deposition of calcium salts in the skin and soft tissues [**Figure 73-3 A**]. Associated with altered calcium and phosphate metabolism, this is a form of metastatic calcification in the setting of ESRD and is a benign nodular process.

Clinically, calcinosis cutis presents as firm papules, plaques, or nodules near joints or on the fingertips. While most of these lesions are painless, periarticular deposits leading to joint dysfunction can be painful. Some of the lesions of calcinosis cutis can emit a white chalky discharge.[46,64,65]

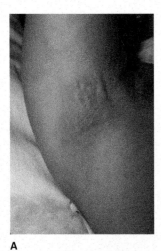

A

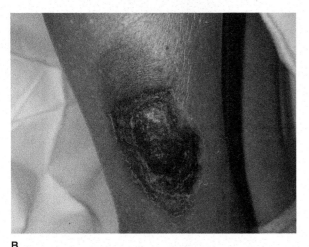

B

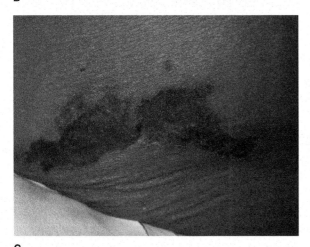

C

FIGURE 73-3. **(A)** A case of calcinosis cutis axilla in a Hispanic female patient. **(B)** Calciphylaxis with necrotic plaque on an edematous erythematous base appearing on the lower extremity of an African American patient on dialysis. **(C)** Calciphylaxis can be seen on the proximal lower extremity of a patient on dialysis; the acute onset of this condition manifested with painful burgundy, necrotic, depressed plaques. (Used with permission from the Department of Dermatology, Washington Hospital Center, Washington, DC.)

Another disorder of calcium deposition is calciphylaxis [**Figure 73-3, B and C**]. It is much more severe than calcinosis cutis and is never benign and frequently lethal.[40] It occurs when calcium is deposited not only in the dermis and subcutis but also intravascularly. Calciphylaxis is usually accompanied by intimal fibroplasia, vascular occlusion, and soft tissue necrosis.

Easily distinguishable from the benign calcinosis cutis, calciphylaxis presents with the acute onset of intense, debilitating cutaneous pain.

Initially, the site may be only mildly erythematous or demonstrate retiform purpura, but the condition rapidly progresses to stellate ulcerations with central necrosis or eschar formation.

The differential diagnosis of calciphylaxis composes a spectrum of disorders that must be definitively ruled out, including connective tissue disease, several forms of vasculitis (eg, cryoglobulinemia), deep fungal infections, systemic oxalosis, and hypercoagulable states and embolic events.

Treatment and Prognosis Treatment for calcinosis cutis is usually only required if the deposits are unusually large. However, many patients benefit from a low-phosphate diet. The lesions will typically resolve once serum calcium and phosphorus levels are normalized.

However, the prognosis for those suffering from calciphylaxis is poor as mortality rates approach 60% to 80%, with sepsis as the leading cause of death.[66a] Appropriate prevention should be emphasized regarding the risk factors previously discussed. Bisphosphonates, cinacalcet, phosphate binders, sodium thiosulfate, and low calcium dialysates have all been used with varying treatment success.[64-71]

PRURITUS AND ACQUIRED PERFORATING DERMATOSIS

Several perforating diseases are associated with chronic renal failure. These are often grouped under the umbrella term acquired perforating dermatosis (APD). This term includes, but is not limited to, Kyrle disease [**Figure 73-4**], reactive perforating collagenosis, perforating disorder of uremia, elastosis perforans serpiginosa, and perforating folliculitis. Most commonly associated with diabetes mellitus and renal disease, these disorders represent a disturbance in the dermal-epidermal barrier and a disruption in the transepidermal elimination of dermal substances.[72,73] Normal transepidermal elimination is a process in which altered connective tissue components within the dermis, in the form of collagen or elastic fibers, are eliminated through the epidermis with little damage to the surrounding structures.[22,74] There is a predilection for these disorders in African American patients. It is important to note that these disorders have also been documented in renal failure patients who were not receiving dialysis treatment.[46,74,75]

Clinical Features The clinical features of these disorders consist of grouped dome-shaped papules or nodules that are usually 1 to 10 mm in diameter. These keratotic papules and nodules are often found initially on the trunk and lower extremities and gradually come to involve the upper extremities and other areas. Verrucous follicular-based papules are prominent in Kyrle disease. On darker skin, brown or hyperpigmented papules are often observed. In Kyrle disease, the scalp and face tend to become involved only after the trunk and extremities, while the lesions of elastosis perforans serpiginosa are most commonly found on

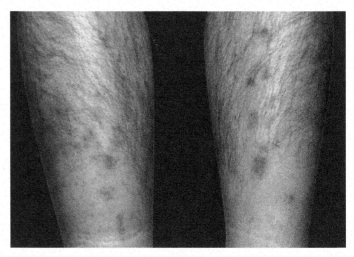

FIGURE 73-4. Kyrle disease is a perforating skin condition characterized by the presence of large keratotic papules distributed widely throughout the body, as seen on this patient. (Used with permission from the Department of Dermatology, Washington Hospital Center, Washington, DC.)

the face and neck. Importantly, the spontaneous resolution of developed individual lesions can occur simultaneously with the continued development of newer lesions. Pruritus, when it occurs, can contribute to the Koebnerization of the lesions.[74-80]

Etiology Although the exact pathogenesis of APD remains unknown, defective transepidermal elimination is thought to be at the root of these disorders.[72-74] Interestingly, both ESRD and diabetes mellitus have been shown to be associated with elevated serum fibronectin. An ongoing theory suggests that, given the role of fibronectin in the chemotaxis of neutrophils and its ability to incite epithelial migration and proliferation, fibronectin deposition in the dermal matrix could be responsible for the disease process. Additional hypotheses include defects in vitamin A and/or vitamin D metabolism.[73,74]

Histologically, the features of each of the APD disorders overlap because they all share defective transepidermal elimination. The elimination canal and/or extruded material are typically the factors that best determine the correct diagnosis. As such, there is often a need to analyze focal, serial sections in the histology examination. Generally, the epidermis surrounds a plug of necrotic material composed of collagen, elastin, nuclear debris, and leukocytes extruded through the epithelium. In Kyrle disease, abnormal clones of keratinocytes perforate through the epidermis down to the dermis. In reactive perforating collagenosis, abnormal collagen is thought to be extruded from the dermis through the epidermis. Thickened elastic fibers are typically seen in elastosis perforans serpiginosa. Finally, perforating folliculitis is characterized by follicular plugs and curled-up hairs that perforate through the follicle into the dermis.[65,73-78]

Differential Diagnosis Dermatoses ranging from Sweet syndrome to the genodermatoses can be a differential diagnosis for pruritus and APD. Additionally, elastosis perforans serpiginosa can be associated with Ehlers-Danlos syndrome, Marfan syndrome, osteogenesis imperfecta, and Down syndrome, and an effect of D-penicillamine administration.[75,76] Additionally, APD may be a manifestation of internal malignancy. It has been reported in a patient with stage IV colon cancer with hepatic metastases as well as in a patient with a periampullary villous adenoma initially presenting with jaundice.[75-78]

Treatment Treatment has been largely ineffective and generally focuses on the symptomatic relief of pruritus. Options include antihistamines, keratolytics, UVB phototherapy, a combination of psoralen and ultraviolet A therapy, allopurinol, cryosurgery, corticosteroids, and topical and systemic retinoids.[74,75,79-81] However, treatment with narrowband UVB radiation has been reported to be effective in some patients, and there are also case reports documenting success with photodynamic therapy.[80,81] The spontaneous resolution of established lesions does occur, as described earlier, as part of the natural history of the disease process. However, complete resolution with no further recurrences is not typical.[79-82]

◼ NEPHROGENIC SYSTEMIC FIBROSIS

Nephrogenic systemic fibrosis (NSF) was first described in 1997 as nephrogenic fibrosing dermopathy and represents a thickening of the skin and multiorgan fibrosis in patients with renal failure or renal insufficiency [**Figure 73-5**].

Epidemiology Recent studies suggest that NSF is seen in over one-tenth of hemodialysis patients. To date, no racial or gender predilections have been observed nor has a genetic predisposition been identified. However, there is a higher percentage of people with skin of color on hemodialysis than Caucasians.[83-85]

Pathogenesis Although the exact pathogenesis remains unknown, gadolinium exposure has been proposed as a precipitating factor, as has erythropoietin exposure.[83-88] Histologically, there is a proliferation of dermal fibroblasts and dendritic cells.[83-89]

Clinical Features This condition presents with indurated papules and plaques ranging in color from dark brown to purple that coalesce to

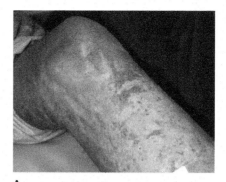

A

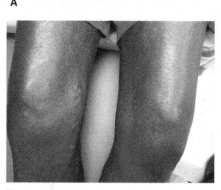

B

FIGURE 73-5. **(A)** Nephrogenic systemic fibrosis following anasarca in a 23-year-old African American male patient requiring hemodialysis after a kidney transplant rejection. Clinical findings included a sclerotic band on the medial aspects of the legs and thighs. **(B)** Nephrogenic systemic fibrosis of the bilateral knees after magnetic resonance imaging in an African American male patient on hemodialysis. (Used with permission from the Department of Dermatology, Washington Hospital Center, Washington, DC.)

cause a diffuse hardening of the skin, with a wood-like texture, *peau d'orange* plaques, and subcutaneous nodules. These typically begin in the lower extremities and move upward and proximally to involve the trunk and upper extremities. The disease can progress to involve the joints, causing contractures and sclerodactyly. Although the clinical features of NSF do not often include pain, joint involvement can be painful depending on the severity. Affected areas can become pruritic; if the disease is protracted, painful and burning sensations may occur. The systemic involvement of various organ systems has been reported, including the heart, lungs, kidneys, eyes (yellow scleral plaques), and muscles.[84,90-98]

Differential Diagnosis The differential diagnosis can be wide when considering NSF, although the clinical picture and setting of renal failure are typically helpful. In the earlier stages of disease, the condition may resemble nonspecific drug reactions, cellulitis, or panniculitis.[84,85] The diagnosis of NSF is based primarily on the clinical picture and skin biopsy.[84,90-98]

Treatment Treatment of NSF is often disappointing because the disease tends to be refractory to many treatments. Although renal transplantation can be effective, symptoms can persist even with improvement of the underlying renal failure or even in the face of dialysis treatment and transplantation.[93,99]

CUTANEOUS MANIFESTATIONS OF RENAL TRANSPLANTATION

Patients with ESRD undergoing successful renal transplantation often have an improved quality of life as well as increased survival compared to patients receiving long-term dialysis treatment. Cutaneous signs of renal failure may actually resolve if renal transplantation is successful, which is in contrast to treatment with dialysis. However, there are numerous dermatologic considerations in the posttransplant population because these patients are at risk of developing a number of cutaneous and mucosal lesions. It is important to recognize cutaneous manifestations and skin changes in the posttransplant setting, especially with regard to pediatric patients with skin of color, because these effects are more common in African American and Hispanic children.[100,101]

The potential side effects of immunosuppressive medications in the posttransplant setting are staggering, and awareness of these issues is crucial.[22,102,103] Infectious complications can occur in the cases of chronic renal failure, independent of transplantation status.[104-106] Infection with *Staphylococcus aureus* is more common in transplant recipients on chronic immunosuppressants, because the bacterial activation of the Toll-like receptors and subsequent immunologic attack on the virus is impaired.[105,106] Additionally, renal transplantation patients commonly suffer from the following infectious agents: herpes simplex, herpes zoster, varicella zoster, cytomegalovirus, *Candida* paronychia, *Candida* intertrigo, tinea cruris, diffuse folliculitis, and molluscum contagiosum.[106,107] Warts caused by the human papilloma virus and tinea versicolor are common in this population, and the onset of infection is usually late.[108,109] Other bacterial etiologies include *Bartonella henselae*, *Mycobacterium tuberculosis*, and atypical mycobacteria.[109,110]

Malignancies are common after any organ transplantation. Most of these are primary cutaneous malignancies, particularly squamous cell carcinoma and premalignant keratoses, for which immunosuppression is a known risk factor. Additionally, lymphomas are an important consideration in the renal transplant population, as are Merkel cell carcinomas and dermatofibrosarcoma protuberans.[99,111-116]

In addition to the infectious, iatrogenic, and neoplastic consequences of renal transplantation, several miscellaneous benign skin lesions can also occur, including acrochordons and seborrheic keratoses. Xerosis is also highly associated with this procedure.[112,116,117]

CONCLUSION

All patients with renal disease can develop cutaneous manifestations, either in the adult or pediatric setting, and these can range from benign conditions to life-threatening complications. There is a high prevalence of cutaneous conditions in patients with renal disease, with most patients showing at least one dermatologic manifestation. These skin complications may arise from the uremic state itself or occur as a result of the treatment received, most notably dialysis or kidney transplantation. The most common conditions are xerosis and pruritus. Additionally, a variety of pigmentary skin alterations linked to chronic renal failure and uremia have been seen in every patient population; it is therefore important to examine patients carefully for any skin changes, as these may be subtle in individuals with skin of color. Depending on the condition, treatment options may target the condition itself or provide symptomatic relief. Kidney transplantation can alleviate or completely resolve certain skin symptoms; however, this should only be considered in severe cases. Even relatively benign skin disorders can negatively affect the mental and physical health of the patient. The early recognition and treatment of cutaneous complications by a dermatologist can therefore immeasurably relieve patient suffering, increase quality of life, and decrease morbidity in patients with renal disease.

REFERENCES

1. McKinley-Grant L, Warnick M, Singh S. Cutaneous manifestations of systemic diseases. In: Kelly AP, Taylor SC, eds. *Dermatology for Skin of Color.* New York, NY: McGraw-Hill Professional; 2009:486.
2. Centers for Disease Control and Prevention. 2013 National Chronic Kidney Disease Fact Sheet. www.cdc.gov/diabetes/pubs/pdf/kidney_factsheet.pdf. Accessed March 29, 2013.
3. Centers for Disease Control and Prevention. National Diabetes Fact Sheet, 2011. www.cdc.gov/diabetes/pubs/pdf/ndfs_2011.pdf. Accessed March 29, 2013.
4. Mitch WE. Acute renal failure. In: Goldman L, Ausiello D, eds. *Cecil Textbook of Medicine.* 22nd ed. Philadelphia, PA: Saunders Co.; 2004:703-708.
5. Luke RG. Chronic renal failure. In: Goldman L, Ausiello D, eds. *Cecil Textbook of Medicine.* 22nd ed. Philadelphia, PA: Saunders Co.; 2004:708-716.
6. Meguid El Nahas A, Bello AK. Chronic kidney disease: the global challenge. *Lancet.* 2005;365:331-340.
7. Kumar V, Abbas AK, Fausto N, et al. *Robbins and Cotran: Pathologic Basis of Disease.* 8th ed. Philadelphia, PA: Saunders Co.; 2009:Chapter 20.
8. González LM, Janniger CK, Schwartz RA. Pediatric Henoch-Schönlein purpura. *Int J Dermatol.* 2009;48:1157-1165.
9. Gardner-Medwin JM, Dolezalova P, Cummins C, et al. Incidence of Henoch-Schönlein purpura, Kawasaki disease, and rare vasculitides in children of different ethnic origins. *Lancet.* 2002;360:1197-1202.
10. Tizard EJ, Hamilton-Ayres MJ. Henoch Schonlein purpura. *Arch Dis Child Educ Pract Ed.* 2008;93:1-8.
11. Linthorst GE, Hollak CE, Korevaar JC, et al. alpha-Galactosidase A deficiency in Dutch patients on dialysis: a critical appraisal of screening for Fabry disease. *Nephrol Dial Transplant.* 2003;18:1581-1584.
12. Tse KC, Chan KW, Tin VP, et al. Clinical features and genetic analysis of a Chinese kindred with Fabry's disease. *Nephrol Dial Transplant.* 2003;18:182-186.
13. Chen CH, Shyu PW, Wu SJ, et al. Identification of a novel point mutation (S65T) in α-galactosidase A gene in Chinese patients with Fabry disease: mutations in brief no. 169 online. *Hum Mutat.* 1998;11:328-330.
14. Tanaka M, Ohashi T, Kobayashi M, et al. Identification of Fabry's disease by the screening of alpha-galactosidase A activity in male and female hemodialysis patients. *Clin Nephrol.* 2005;64:281-287.
15. Herrera J, Miranda CS. Prevalence of Fabry's disease within hemodialysis patients in Spain. *Clin Nephrol.* 2014;81:112-120.
16. Bekheirnia MR, Reed B, Gregory MC, et al. Genotype-phenotype correlation in X-linked Alport syndrome. *J Am Soc Nephrol.* 2010;21:876-883.
17. Cook C, Friedrich CA, Baliga R. Novel COL4A3 mutations in African American siblings with autosomal recessive Alport syndrome. *Am J Kidney Dis.* 2008;51:e25-28.
18. Mukerji N, Dodson K. X-linked Alport syndrome: a case report. *Internet J Nephrol.* 2002;1:13399.
19. Zhang Y, Wang F, Ding J, et al. Genotype-phenotype correlations in 17 Chinese patients with autosomal recessive Alport syndrome. *Am J Med Genet A.* 2012;158A:2188-2193.
20. Robinson-Bostom L, DiGiovanna JJ. Cutaneous manifestations of end-stage renal disease. *J Am Acad Dermatol.* 2000;43:975-986.
21. Ponticelli C, Bencini PL. Uremic pruritus: a review. *Nephron.* 1992;60:1-5.
22. Abdelbaqi-Salhab M, Shalhub S, Morgan MB. A current review of the cutaneous manifestations of renal disease. *J Cutan Pathol.* 2003;30:527-538.
23. Attia EA, Hassan SI, Youssef NM. Cutaneous disorders in uremic patients on hemodialysis: an Egyptian case-controlled study. *Int J Dermatol.* 2010;49:1024-1030.
24. Mettang M, Weisshaar E. Pruritus: control of itch in patients undergoing dialysis. *Skin Therapy Lett.* 2010;15:1-5.
25. Navarro-González JF, Mora-Fernández C, García-Pérez J. Clinical implications of disordered magnesium homeostasis in chronic renal failure and dialysis. *Semin Dial.* 2009;22:37-44.
26. Kfoury LW, Jurdi MA. Uremic pruritus. *J Nephrol.* 2012;25:644-652.
27. Ko MJ, Yang JY, Wu HY, et al. Narrowband ultraviolet B phototherapy for patients with refractory uraemic pruritus: a randomized controlled trial. *Br J Dermatol.* 2011;165:633-639.
28. To TH, Clark K, Lam L, et al. The role of ondansetron in the management of cholestatic or uremic pruritus: a systematic review. *J Pain Symptom Manage.* 2012;44:725-730.
29. Ghanei E, Zeinali J, Borghei M, et al. Efficacy of omega-3 fatty acids supplementation in treatment of uremic pruritus in hemodialysis patients: a double-blind randomized controlled trial. *Iran Red Crescent Med J.* 2012;14:515-522.
30. O'Connor NR, Corcoran AM. End-stage renal disease: symptom management and advance care planning. *Am Fam Physician.* 2012;85:705-710.
31. Greaves MW. Itch in systemic disease: therapeutic options. *Dermatol Ther.* 2005;18:323-327.
32. Marquez D, Ramonda C, Lauxmann JE, et al. Uremic pruritus in hemodialysis patients: treatment with desloratadine versus gabapentin. *J Bras Nefrol.* 2012;34:148-152.
33. Inui S. Nalfurafine hydrochloride for the treatment of pruritus. *Expert Opin Pharmacother.* 2012;13:1507-1513.
34. Feily A, Dormanesh B, Ghorbani AR, et al. Efficacy of topical cromolyn sodium 4% on pruritus in uremic nephrogenic patients: a randomized double-blind study in 60 patients. *Int J Clin Pharmacol Ther.* 2012;50:510-513.
35. Kumagai H, Ebata T, Takamori K, et al. Efficacy and safety of a novel κ-agonist for managing intractable pruritus in dialysis patients. *Am J Nephrol.* 2012;36:175-183.
36. Lin TC, Lai YH, Guo SE, et al. Baby oil therapy for uremic pruritus in haemodialysis patients. *J Clin Nurs.* 2012;21:139-148.

37. Najafabadi MM, Faghihi G, Emami A, et al. Zinc sulfate for relief of pruritus in patients on maintenance hemodialysis. *Ther Apher Dial.* 2012;16:142-145.

38. Leena JA, Islam MMSU, Ahmed AS, et al. Cutaneous manifestations of chronic kidney disease: an observational study in 100 cases. *Faridpur Med Coll J.* 2012;7:33-36.

39. Gilkes JJ, Eady RA, Rees LH, et al. Plasma immunoreactive melanotrophic hormones in patients on maintenance haemodialysis. *Br Med J.* 1975;1: 656-657.

40. Markova A, Lester J, Wang J, et al. Diagnosis of common dermopathies in dialysis patients: a review and update. *Semin Dial.* 2012;25:408-418.

41. Salem A, Al Mokadem S, Attwa E, et al. Nail changes in chronic renal failure patients under haemodialysis. *J Eur Acad Dermatol Venereol.* 2008;22:1326-1331.

42. Martinez MA, Gregório CL, Santos VP, et al. Nail disorders in patients with chronic renal failure undergoing haemodialysis. *An Bras Dermatol.* 2010;85: 318-323.

43. Walsh SR, Parada NA. Images in clinical medicine: uremic frost. *N Engl J Med.* 2005;352:e13.

44. Udayakumar P, Balasubramanian S, Ramalingam KS, et al. Cutaneous manifestations in patients with chronic renal failure on hemodialysis. *Indian J Dermatol Venereol Leprol.* 2006;72:119-125.

45. Fuchs E, Lynfield Y. Dialysis acne. *J Am Acad Dermatol.* 1990;23:125.

46. Cordova KB, Oberg TJ, Malik M, et al. Dermatologic conditions seen in end-stage renal disease. *Semin Dial.* 2009;22:45-55.

47. Trigka K, Dousdampanis P, Fourtounas C. Delusional parasitosis: a rare cause of pruritus in hemodialysis patients. *Int J Artif Organs.* 2012;35:400-403.

48. Morton CA, Lafferty M, Hau C, et al. Pruritus and skin hydration during dialysis. *Nephrol Dial Transplant.* 1996;11:2031-2036.

49. Labidi J. Porphyria cutanea tarda in a chronic hemodialysis patient. *Saudi J Kidney Dis Transpl.* 2010;21:919-922.

50. Korting GW. Porphyria cutanea tarda-like aspects in two prolonged hemodialysis patients (author's transl). *Dermatologica.* 1975;150:58-61.

51. Frank J, Poblete-Gutierrez R. Porphyria. In: Bolognia JL, Jorizzo JL, Rapini RP, eds. *Dermatology.* 2nd ed. New York, NY: Elsevier; 2008:641-652.

52. Gafter U, Mamet R, Korzets A, et al. Bullous dermatosis of end-stage renal disease: a possible association between abnormal porphyrin metabolism and aluminum. *Nephrol Dial Transplant.* 1996;11:1787-1791.

53. Green JJ, Manders SM. Pseudoporphyria. *J Am Acad Dermatol.* 2001;44: 100-108.

54. Day RS, Eales L. Porphyrins in chronic renal failure. *Nephron.* 1980;26:90-95.

55. Glynne P, Deacon A, Goldsmith D, et al. Bullous dermatoses in end-stage renal failure: porphyria or pseudoporphyria? *Am J Kidney Dis.* 1999;34:155-160.

56. Goldsmith DJ, Black MM. Skin disorders in the setting of renal failure: invited editorial. *J Eur Acad Dermatol Venereol.* 2001;15:392-398.

57. Poh-Fitzpatrick MB, Masullo AS, Grossman ME. Porphyria cutanea tarda associated with chronic renal disease and hemodialysis. *Arch Dermatol.* 1980; 116:191-195.

58. Ramsay CA, Magnus IA, Turnbull A, et al. The treatment of porphyria cutanea tarda by venesection. *Q J Med.* 1974;43:1-24.

59. Anderson KE. The porphyrias. In: Goldman L, Ausiello D, eds. *Cecil Textbook of Medicine.* 22nd ed. Philadelphia, PA: Saunders Co.; 2004:1292-1300.

60. Peces R, Enríquez de Salamanca R, Fontanellas A, et al. Successful treatment of haemodialysis-related porphyria cutanea tarda with erythropoietin. *Nephrol Dial Transplant.* 1994;9:433-435.

61. Pandya AG, Nezafati KA, Ashe-Randolph M, et al. Deferasirox for porphyria cutanea tarda: a pilot study. *Arch Dermatol.* 2012;148:898-901.

62. Schanbacher CF, Vanness ER, Daoud MS, et al. Pseudoporphyria: a clinical and biochemical study of 20 patients. *Mayo Clin Proc.* 2001;76:488-492.

63. Callen JP. Dermatologic manifestations in patients with systemic disease. In: Bolognia JL, Jorizzo JL, Rapini RP, eds. *Dermatology.* 2nd ed. New York, NY: Elsevier; 2008:675-692.

64. Rivet J, Lebbé C, Urena P, et al. Cutaneous calcification in patients with end-stage renal disease: a regulated process associated with in situ osteopontin expression. *Arch Dermatol.* 2006;142:900-906.

65. Enelow TJ, Huang W, Williams CM. Perforating papules in chronic renal failure: metastatic calcinosis cutis with transepidermal elimination. *Arch Dermatol.* 1998;134:98-99, 101-102.

66. Tan O, Atik B, Kizilkaya A, et al. Extensive skin calcifications in an infant with chronic renal failure: metastatic calcinosis cutis. *Pediatr Dermatol.* 2006; 23:235-238.

66a. Magro CM, Simman R, Jackson S. Calciphylaxis: a review. *J Am Col Certif Wound Spec.* 2011;2:66-72.

67. Hayden MR, Tyagi SC, Kolb L, et al. Vascular ossification-calcification in metabolic syndrome, type 2 diabetes mellitus, chronic kidney disease, and calciphylaxis-calcific uremic arteriolopathy: the emerging role of sodium thiosulfate. *Cardiovasc Diabetol.* 2005;4:4.

68. Guldbakke KK, Khachemoune A. Calciphylaxis. *Int J Dermatol.* 2007;46: 231-238.

69. Hafner J, Keusch G, Wahl C, et al. Calciphylaxis: a syndrome of skin necrosis and acral gangrene in chronic renal failure. *Vasa.* 1998;27:137-143.

70. Ackermann F, Levy A, Daugas E, et al. Sodium thiosulfate as first-line treatment for calciphylaxis. *Arch Dermatol.* 2007;143:1336-1337.

71. Edwards RB, Jaffe W, Arrowsmith J, et al. Calciphylaxis: a rare limb and life threatening cause of ischaemic skin necrosis and ulceration. *Br J Plast Surg.* 2000;53:253-255.

72. Rapini RP. Perforating diseases. In: Bolognia JL, Jorizzo JL, Rapini RP, eds. *Dermatology.* 2nd ed. New York, NY: Elsevier; 2008:1461-1467.

73. Saray Y, Seçkin D, Bilezikçi B. Acquired perforating dermatosis: clinicopathological features in twenty-two cases. *J Eur Acad Dermatol Venereol.* 2006;20:679-688.

74. Patterson JW. The perforating disorders. *J Am Acad Dermatol.* 1984;10: 561-581.

75. Schreml S, Hafner C, Eder F, et al. Kyrle disease and acquired perforating collagenosis secondary to chronic renal failure and diabetes mellitus. *Case Rep Dermatol.* 2011;3:209-211.

76. Pereira AC, Baeta IG, Costa Júnior SR, et al. Elastosis perforans serpiginosa in a patient with Down's syndrome. *An Bras Dermatol.* 2010;85:691-694.

77. Jeon H, Sarantopoulos GP, Gharavi NM, et al. Acquired perforating dermatosis associated with metastatic colon cancer. *Dermatol Online J.* 2011;17:7.

78. Korula A, Thomas M, Noronha J. Acquired perforating dermatosis: an innocuous lesion with possibly ominous implications. *Cutis.* 2010;86:242-244.

79. Tsai TF, Yeh TY. Allopurinol in dermatology. *Am J Clin Dermatol.* 2010;11: 225-232.

80. Sezer E, Erkek E. Acquired perforating dermatosis successfully treated with photodynamic therapy. *Photodermatol Photoimmunol Photomed.* 2012; 28:50-52.

81. Ohe S, Danno K, Sasaki H, et al. Treatment of acquired perforating dermatosis with narrowband ultraviolet B. *J Am Acad Dermatol.* 2004;50:892-894.

82. Headley CM, Wall B. ESRD-associated cutaneous manifestations in a hemodialysis population. *Nephrol Nurs J.* 2002;29:525-527, 531-529.

83. Basak P, Jesmajian S. Nephrogenic systemic fibrosis: current concepts. *Indian J Dermatol.* 2011;56:59-64.

84. Mendoza FA, Artlett CM, Sandorfi N, et al. Description of 12 cases of nephrogenic fibrosing dermopathy and review of the literature. *Semin Arthritis Rheum.* 2006;35:238-249.

85. Todd DJ. Nephrogenic systemic fibrosis: what nephrologists need to know. www.cardiologyrounds.org/crus/nephus_0607_07.pdf. Accessed May 20, 2014.

86. High WA, Ayers RA, Chandler J, et al. Gadolinium is detectable within the tissue of patients with nephrogenic systemic fibrosis. *J Am Acad Dermatol.* 2007;56:21-26.

87. Boyd AS, Zic JA, Abraham JL. Gadolinium deposition in nephrogenic fibrosing dermopathy. *J Am Acad Dermatol.* 2007;56:27-30.

88. Peak AS, Sheller A. Risk factors for developing gadolinium-induced nephrogenic systemic fibrosis. *Ann Pharmacother.* 2007;41:1481-1485.

89. Nazarian RM, Mandal RV, Kagan A, et al. Quantitative assessment of dermal cellularity in nephrogenic systemic fibrosis: a diagnostic aid. *J Am Acad Dermatol.* 2011;64:741-747.

90. U.S. Food and Drug Administration. Public Health Advisory: update on magnetic resonance imaging (MRI) contrast agents containing gadolinium and nephrogenic fibrosing dermopathy. www.fda.gov/Drugs/DrugSafety/PostmarketDrugSafetyInformationforPatientsandProviders/ucm124344. htm. Accessed March 29, 2013.

91. Daram SR, Cortese CM, Bastani B. Nephrogenic fibrosing dermopathy/nephrogenic systemic fibrosis: report of a new case with literature review. *Am J Kidney Dis.* 2005;46:754-759.

92. Galan A, Cowper SE, Bucala R. Nephrogenic systemic fibrosis (nephrogenic fibrosing dermopathy). *Curr Opin Rheumatol.* 2006;18:614-617.

93. Introcaso CE, Hivnor C, Cowper S, et al. Nephrogenic fibrosing dermopathy/nephrogenic systemic fibrosis: a case series of nine patients and review of the literature. *Int J Dermatol.* 2007;46:447-452.

94. Mackay-Wiggan JM, Cohen DJ, Hardy MA, et al. Nephrogenic fibrosing dermopathy (scleromyxedema-like illness of renal disease). *J Am Acad Dermatol.* 2003;48:55-60.

95. Cowper SE. Nephrogenic fibrosing dermopathy: the first 6 years. *Curr Opin Rheumatol.* 2003;15:785-790.

96. Swartz RD, Crofford LJ, Phan SH, et al. Nephrogenic fibrosing dermopathy: a novel cutaneous fibrosing disorder in patients with renal failure. *Am J Med.* 2003;114:563-572.

97. Streams BN, Liu V, Liégeois N, et al. Clinical and pathologic features of nephrogenic fibrosing dermopathy: a report of two cases. *J Am Acad Dermatol.* 2003;48:42-47.

98. Piera-Velázquez S, Sandorfi N, Jiménez SA. Nephrogenic systemic fibrosis/nephrogenic fibrosing dermopathy: clinical aspects. *Skinmed.* 2007;6:24-27.

99. Tremblay F, Fernandes M, Habbab F, et al. Malignancy after renal transplantation: incidence and role of type of immunosuppression. *Ann Surg Oncol.* 2002;9:785-788.

100. Khosravi M, Golchai J, Mokhtari G. Muco-cutaneous manifestations in 178 renal transplant recipients. *Clin Transplant.* 2011;25:395-400.

101. Ulrich C, Hackethal M, Meyer T, et al. Skin infections in organ transplant recipients. *J Dtsch Dermatol Ges.* 2008;6:98-105.

102. Sandhu K, Gupta S, Kumar B, et al. The pattern of mucocutaneous infections and infestations in renal transplant recipients. *J Dermatol.* 2003;30:590-595.

103. Moloney FJ, Keane S, O'Kelly P, et al. The impact of skin disease following renal transplantation on quality of life. *Br J Dermatol.* 2005;153:574-578.

104. Formicone F, Fargnoli MC, Pisani F, et al. Cutaneous manifestations in Italian kidney transplant recipients. *Transplant Proc.* 2005;37:2527-2528.

105. Nunley JR. Dermatologic manifestations of renal disease. www.emedicine.medscape.com/article/1094846-overview. Accessed May 20, 2014.

106. Seçkin D, Güleç TO, Demirağ A, et al. Renal transplantation and skin diseases. *Transplant Proc.* 1998;30:802-804.

107. Silkensen JR. Long-term complications in renal transplantation. *J Am Soc Nephrol.* 2000;11:582-588.

108. Rüdlinger R, Smith IW, Bunney MH, et al. Human papillomavirus infections in a group of renal transplant recipients. *Br J Dermatol.* 1986;115:681-692.

109. Itin PH, Battegay M. Skin problems in immunodeficient patients. *Curr Probl Dermatol.* 2012;43:9-17.

110. Menni S, Beretta D, Piccinno R, et al. Cutaneous and oral lesions in 32 children after renal transplantation. *Pediatr Dermatol.* 1991;8:194-198.

111. Avermaete A, Altmeyer P, Bacharach-Buhles M. Non-malignant skin changes in transplant patients. *Nephrol Dial Transplant.* 2002;17:1380-1383.

112. Kobayashi TT, David-Bajar KM. Cutaneous manifestations of renal disease. In: Fitzpatrick JE, Morelli JG, eds. *Dermatology Secrets Plus.* 4th ed. Philadelphia, PA: Elsevier Mosby; 2011:274-279.

113. Euvrard S, Kanitakis J, Claudy A. Skin cancers after organ transplantation. *N Eng J Med.* 2003;348:1681-1691.

114. Dreno B. Skin cancers after transplantation. *Nephrol Dial Transplant.* 2003;18:1052-1058.

115. Kasiske BL, Vazquez MA, Harmon WE, et al. Recommendations for the outpatient surveillance of renal transplant recipients: American Society of Transplantation. *J Am Soc Nephrol.* 2000;11:S1-86.

116. Moloney FJ, Keane S, O'Kelly P, et al. The impact of skin disease following renal transplantation on quality of life. *Br J Dermatol.* 2005;153:574-578.

117. Silverberg NB, Singh A, Echt AF, et al. Lingual fungiform papillae hypertrophy with cyclosporin A. *Lancet.* 1996;348:967.

CHAPTER 74

Sarcoidosis

Jennifer David
Candrice R. Heath
Susan C. Taylor
Lynn McKinley-Grant

KEY POINTS

- Sarcoidosis is a granulomatous disease that can affect any organ system.

- In the United States, sarcoidosis has a higher prevalence in African Americans and Caucasians of Scandinavian descent.

- Sarcoidal lesions manifest with multiple morphologic features and can be mimickers of other inflammatory skin disease. Early detection of skin disease requires a systemic workup for pulmonary and other organ involvement.

- There is a connection between genetic and environmental exposure factors in patients with sarcoidosis.

INTRODUCTION

Sarcoidosis is a multisystem, granulomatous disease that can affect any organ system. The skin is the most common extrathoracic location.[1,2] Even though the first documented case of cutaneous sarcoidosis dates back to 1869, its etiology remains an enigma.[2-5] Evidence suggests that sarcoidosis develops when a genetically susceptible individual comes in contact with an unknown antigen (eg, bacterial, viral, or environmental) and their body elicits an immunologic cascade that produces noncaseating granulomas most commonly found in the lung, skin, heart, and liver [**Figure 74-1**]. Cutaneous sarcoid lesions have the unique capability of mimicking both rare and common skin disorders, often making diagnosis a challenge. Sarcoidosis is found more commonly in skin of color groups. Not only is sarcoidosis more common in patients with skin of color, but these patients also present with more advanced disease and have a poorer prognosis. There are numerous well-known historical and modern figures who had or have sarcoidosis. Such celebrities include Floyd Mayweather, Sr. (former boxer/trainer), Mahalia Jackson (gospel singer), Bernie Mac (comedian), Reggie White (American football player), Daisy Fuentes (actress/model), Manning Marable (author), Ludwig van Beethoven (musician), and Tisha Campbell Martin (actress/model), to name a few.

EPIDEMIOLOGY

Sarcoidosis affects all races and ethnicities.[4,5] In the United Sates, there is a higher prevalence in African Americans (35.5 to 64 cases/100,000) and other groups with skin of color compared to Caucasians (10.9 to 14 cases/100,000).[6] Scandinavia has the world's highest prevalence of reported cases (50 to 60 cases/100,000).[2-4,7]

A worldwide review of sarcoidosis that included 3676 patients of Japanese, Caucasian, darker skin of color American, Puerto Rican, and Mexican descent reported no gender predilection, and most patients were diagnosed before the age of 40.[8] A study in Singapore highlighted 25 patients and found that although Indian patients represented only 7.7% of the general population, they made up 52% of sarcoidosis patients in the study.[9]

Research data also show that, in the United States, morbidity and mortality rates are higher in African Americans than in Caucasians.[4,5] African Americans are also more likely to have cutaneous sarcoidosis.[4] Sarcoidosis may also occur in the liver, bone, and lymph nodes.[10] A study of 165 African Americans with sarcoidosis in Georgia found that 90% had comorbidities, the most frequent being hypertension, diabetes mellitus, anemia, gastroesophageal reflux disease, and heart failure.[11] This study also found that females had an increased frequency and clustering of chronic illness.[11]

PROGNOSIS

Most patients will experience spontaneous resolution of cutaneous lesions; however, the long-term prognosis depends primarily on the extent of systemic disease.[12,13] Conversely, the degree of cutaneous involvement does not necessarily reflect the severity of systemic disease, and the prognostic value of cutaneous lesions alone remains unclear.[10,12-15] Early recognition of skin lesions hastens systemic evaluation, allowing prompt treatment.

Race is a factor in a patient's clinical course and prognosis.[16] Darker skin of color individuals, including those of West Indian descent, have a higher rate of extrapulmonary involvement, chronic uveitis, lupus pernio, cystic bone lesions, and chronic progressive disease; poorer long-term prognosis; and higher rate of relapse compared with Caucasians.[15-18] Erythema nodosum is more common in Caucasians, and reports have shown that 80% of patients with erythema nodosum and acute inflammatory manifestations of sarcoidosis have spontaneous remission.[13] Death from sarcoidosis is mostly due to the failure of vital organs such as the heart and lungs.[13]

ETIOLOGY, GENETICS, AND EPIGENETICS

Although sarcoidosis has been studied extensively through the years, the exact etiology is unknown. Evidence suggests that exposure to an unknown antigen (unidentified bacterial, viral, or environmental

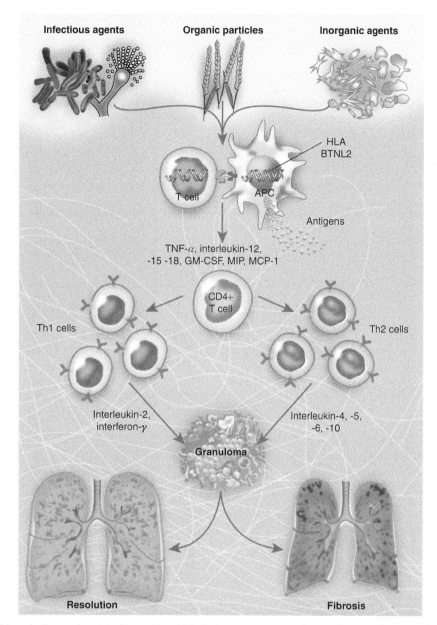

FIGURE 74-1. Illustration of the molecular cascade suspected in sarcoidosis. Molecular mimicry seems to be the most important factor for the heterogeneous clinical presentation and the immunopathogenesis of sarcoidosis. APC, antigen-presenting cell; GM-CSF, granulocyte-macrophage colony-stimulating factor; HLA, human leukocyte antigen; MCP-1, monocyte chemoattractant protein-1; MIP, macrophage inflammatory protein; Th, T helper; TNF-α, tumor necrosis factor-α.

antigen) elicits a noncaseating granulomatous reaction in genetically susceptible individuals.[2,5,7,13,19] Extensive research evaluating the major histocompatibility complex[19] genes and their role in sarcoidosis susceptibility has uncovered human leukocyte antigen (HLA)-DRB1 as a sarcoidosis susceptibility gene in Asians and Caucasians.[11] In those with skin of color, the HLA-DQB1 locus was identified as a susceptibility gene for sarcoidosis. In the United States, African Americans or individuals with darker skin of color have been shown to have greater HLA type II diversity compared to those of European descent. The genetic variances in HLA haplotypes are thought to explain some of the racial differences in prevalence, manifestations, and course.[11,14]

A recent genome-wide association study in a German population and two subsequent studies in European populations found that a nonsynonymous single-nucleotide polymorphism, rs1049550, within the *annexin A11* (*ANXA11*) gene was associated with susceptibility to sarcoidosis.[20] Regions of *ANXA11* were genotyped for 1689 sarcoidosis cases and 1252 controls. Sarcoidosis associations in the United States were identified only in African Americans (95% confidence interval 0.40 to 0.97).[20]

Fine mapping in African American women confirmed the importance of the 10p12 locus (where the *ANXA11* gene is located) to sarcoidosis.[20]

Further genetic testing found that in African American nuclear families that included two or more siblings with sarcoidosis, the strongest signal was at marker D5S407 on chromosome 5q11.2 based on full- and half-sibling pairs.[21] The results suggest a sarcoidosis susceptibility gene in African Americans on chromosome 5q11.2 and a gene that protects this population from sarcoidosis on 5p15.2.[21]

Socioeconomic factors such as income, education level, and health insurance coverage are thought to play a role in disease variation between ethnic and racial groups. The Case Controlled Etiologic Study of Sarcoidosis, sponsored by the National Heart, Lung, and Blood Institute, identified associations between disease severity and ethnic and racial groups as well as with socioeconomic factors.[22] The study revealed that African Americans, particularly those with lung-only sarcoidosis, were more likely to have been exposed to burning wood, whereas Caucasians were more likely to have a history of agricultural dust exposure.[22] Siblings of patients with sarcoidosis had a five times higher risk of sarcoidosis than the general population.[21,22] Additionally, at the end of the 2-year study, lower income African American patients were more likely to experience disease progression and new organ involvement without resolution.[22]

Certain environmental and occupational exposures have been associated with increased risk of disease.[23] Farming, raising birds, and teaching middle or high school are occupations that have been associated with higher incidences of sarcoidosis. Exposures to insecticides, pesticides, and damp environments are the attributed factors that place these professions at higher risk.[24]

Several case reports have revealed a relationship between hepatitis C virus (HCV) and sarcoidosis. Some authors link the emergence of sarcoidosis to interferon-α treatment for HCV, whereas others suggest that HCV itself can cause sarcoidosis.[25] Even though there is no strong evidence to suggest a direct causality, it may be beneficial to screen newly diagnosed sarcoid patients for hepatitis C.

CLINICAL FINDINGS

Of patients with systemic sarcoidosis, 25% have cutaneous involvement.[10,26,27] Cutaneous lesions vary in morphology and can occur in conjunction with or independent of systemic disease.[8,10] Lesions can be specific (showing noncaseating granulomatous histology) or nonspecific.[8,26,27] On physical examination, lesions can appear as indurated, violaceous plaques and nodules on the face (lupus pernio); firm red to brown papules on the face and neck that have an 'apple jelly' appearance on diascopy; hypopigmented macules; scars; ulcers; and nonspecific lesions of septal panniculitis (erythema nodosum).

◾ NONSPECIFIC SKIN LESIONS

Erythema Nodosum   Erythema nodosum is the most common nonspecific skin lesion and is the hallmark of acute sarcoidosis [**Figure 74-2**]. It is seen most commonly in those of European, Puerto Rican, and Mexican descent and is less common in patients of African or Asian descent.[8,9,28] Other less common nonspecific lesions of sarcoidosis include calcifications, erythema multiforme, prurigo, and clubbing of the nails.[28]

Löfgren Syndrome   Löfgren syndrome is a type of acute sarcoidosis characterized by erythema nodosum and associated with bilateral hilar adenopathy, symmetric arthralgias/arthritis, fever, and anterior uveitis. It affects mostly young women of African, Scandinavian, or Puerto

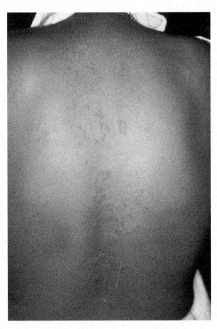

FIGURE 74-3.   Sarcoidosis in an African American woman with discrete brown annular papules and plaques on the back. (Used with permission from the Department of Dermatology, Washington Hospital Center, Washington, DC.)

Rican descent and is associated with a good prognosis, with >90% of patients experiencing spontaneous resolution within 2 years.[29]

◾ SPECIFIC SKIN LESIONS (CONTAINING NONCASEATING GRANULOMAS)

Distinctive Forms of Specific Lesions

Papules and Plaques   Papules are the most common cutaneous finding in sarcoidosis [**Figure 74-3**]. They can be localized or general and are typically firm, red-brown to violaceous, and <1 mm in size. On diascopy, lesions can demonstrate an 'apple jelly' color. Sarcoid papules occur.[28-39] Plaques, on the other hand, have more pronounced erythema, are greater than 5 mm, and tend to infiltrate more deeply. Patients with plaques also tend to have chronic disease and more scarring.[8,30]

Lupus Pernio   Lupus pernio is most common in women with skin of color and is the hallmark of fibrotic disease. The lesions present as indolent, indurated, red-brown to purple, swollen, shiny skin changes on the nose, lips, cheeks, and ears [**Figure 74-4**]. These lesions can be quite disfiguring and, when the nose is involved, granulomatous infiltration of the mucosa and bone can occur.[28-30]

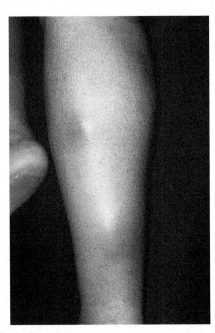

FIGURE 74-2.   African American woman with erythema nodosum with multiple tender erythematous nodules on the posterior tibia. (Used with permission from the Department of Dermatology, Washington Hospital Center, Washington, DC.)

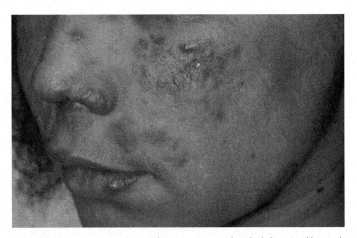

FIGURE 74-4.   Lupus pernio sarcoidosis in a woman with multiple brown and burgundy papules on the cheek, rim of the nares, and lip. (Used with permission from the Department of Dermatology, Washington Hospital Center, Washington, DC.)

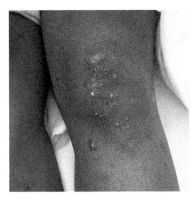

FIGURE 74-5. Sarcoidosis in an African American woman with multiples scars on the knee specked with purple-brown hyperkeratotic papules in the scars and surrounding areas. (Used with permission from the Department of Dermatology, Washington Hospital Center, Washington, DC.)

Scar Sarcoidosis Inactive scars can become infiltrated with sarcoidal lesions and assume an erythematous or violaceous hue [**Figure 74-5**]. Lesions within scars can remain asymptomatic and represent benign disease or, as some authors suggest, disease exacerbation.[31]

Minor Forms of Specific Lesions

Psoriasiform Psoriasiform sarcoidosis is a rare cutaneous presentation of the disease and often resembles psoriasis. The lesions present as erythematous plaques with a scale. Some authors theorize that some cases may represent sarcoidosis developing as a Koebner reaction within existing psoriasis.[29,30]

Subcutaneous Nodules Subcutaneous nodular sarcoidosis is also called Darier-Roussy sarcoidosis. Subcutaneous nodules are a rare form of sarcoidosis that occur more frequently in Caucasians than persons with skin of color. Lesions are characterized as firm, mobile, painless nodules ranging in size from 0.5 to 2 cm[30,32] [**Figure 74-6**].

Ulcerative Ulceration of sarcoidal lesions is rare and can occur *de novo* or develop within existing lesions [**Figure 74-7**]. Histopathology reveals noncaseating granulomas within ulcerations and the surrounding tissue. Darker skin of color individuals and women have a two-fold increased incidence of ulcerative lesions, which occur most commonly on the lower extremities.[33]

Hypopigmented Macules Hypopigmented sarcoidosis most commonly presents as macular lesions [**Figure 74-8**]; however, on palpation, they may have substance and are better characterized as lightly colored papules or nodules.[34,35] These lesions are more easily appreciated in patients with dark skin, and the presence of disease is confirmed via skin biopsy. The list of differential diagnoses for hypopigmented macules is exhaustive; thus, biopsy of indurated lesions or those with a contiguous papule yield higher diagnostic probability.[35]

Ichthyosiform Ichthyosiform sarcoidosis [**Figure 74-9**] presents as large rhomboidal hyperpigmented scaling plaques that are usually asymptomatic and involve the lower extremities. Clinically these lesions closely resemble ichthyosis vulgaris; however, histology will reveal compact orthokeratosis with a diminished or absent granular layer and multiple noncaseating granulomas within the dermis.[36-38] One study reviewed 19 cases of ichthyosiform sarcoidosis in non-Caucasian people and found 76% of the patients' lesions preceded or coincided with their diagnosis of systemic sarcoidosis.[36] Ultimately, 95% developed systemic disease in addition to their cutaneous lesions.[36]

Erythrodermic Erythroderma is an extremely rare variant of cutaneous sarcoidosis. To date, there are no cases of erythrodermic sarcoidosis in skin of color patients presented in the English literature. These lesions are described as erythematous patches that increase in number and size and eventually coalesce into an all-encompassing rash.[39] Histology reveals multiple small granulomas within the dermis with perivascular and periappendageal inflammatory infiltrates.[40] Sézary syndrome has

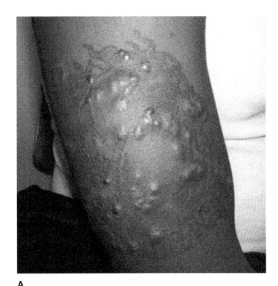

A

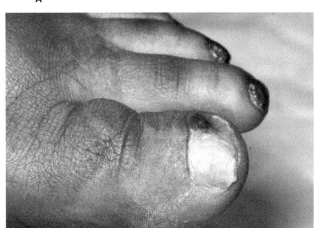

B

FIGURE 74-6. (**A**) Darier-Roussy sarcoidosis: multiple red nodules and papules in the markings of a tattoo on the upper extremity. (**B**) Sarcoidosis lesion occurring on the toe. (Used with permission from the Department of Dermatology, Washington Hospital Center, Washington, DC.)

been reported to have epithelioid granulomas that resemble sarcoidosis; thus, it is important to exclude this as a diagnosis.[41]

Scalp and Nails Sarcoidosis of the scalp is most common among darker skin of color women and typically presents as a scarring alopecia

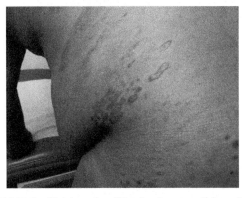

FIGURE 74-7. Sarcoidosis in an obese African American man with brown linear plaques, some ulcerated, on the abdomen. (Used with permission from the Department of Dermatology, Washington Hospital Center, Washington, DC.)

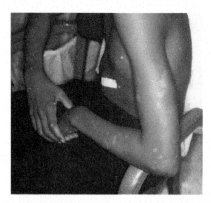

FIGURE 74-8. Sarcoidosis in an African American patient with hypopigmented macules and patches that, on palpation, have some induration. (Used with permission from the Department of Dermatology, Washington Hospital Center, Washington, DC.)

that can be localized or diffuse [**Figure 74-10**].[42] Scalp involvement is highly associated with systemic disease and does not respond well to treatment.[42]

Nail involvement is rare in sarcoidosis and can present as dystrophy, discoloration, clubbing, subungual hyperkeratosis, longitudinal ridging, or splinter hemorrhages. It is usually a marker of chronic disease.[43-45]

OTHER

Extremely rare clinical presentations of cutaneous sarcoidosis have been reported. Those not discussed in the previous sections include lichen nitidus papules [**Figure 74-11**],[46] verrucous lesions,[28] morpheaform plaques,[47] pustular lesions,[28] and lower extremity swelling.[48] Mucosal involvement is rare; however, lupus pernio lesions of the nose can infiltrate through to the nasal mucous membrane. Additionally, granulomatous lesions of sarcoidosis have been reported to affect the oral [**Figure 74-12**] and anogenital mucosa.[49]

DIAGNOSIS

Sarcoidosis is a great mimicker of many diseases, and the clinical presentation varies widely, making diagnosis a challenge. A comprehensive evaluation is imperative when sarcoidosis is suspected and should

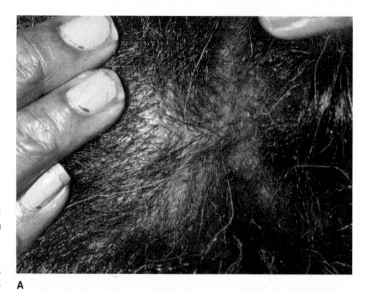

A

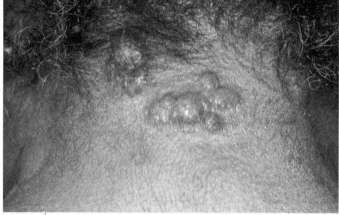

B

FIGURE 74-10. Systemic sarcoidosis in an African American woman after liver transplant with annular plaques on (**A**) the scalp and (**B**) posterior neck. (Used with permission from the Department of Dermatology, Washington Hospital Center, Washington, DC.)

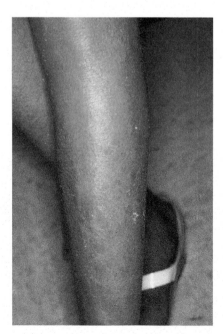

FIGURE 74-9. Sarcoidosis ichthyosis in an African American woman with ichthyotic erythematous-brown scale on the lower extremities. (Used with permission from the Department of Dermatology, Washington Hospital Center, Washington, DC.)

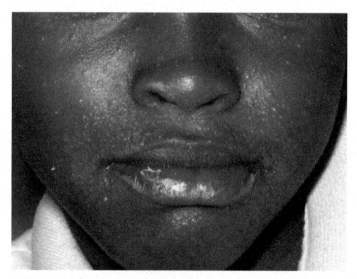

FIGURE 74-11. Lichen nitidus in a young child is an extremely rare clinical presentation of cutaneous sarcoidosis. (Used with permission from the Department of Dermatology, Washington Hospital Center, Washington, DC.)

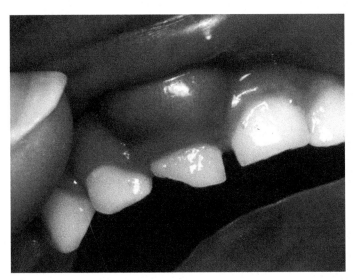

FIGURE 74-12. Lupus pernio lesion infiltrating into the mucosal membrane. (Used with permission from the Department of Dermatology, Washington Hospital Center, Washington, DC.)

include clinical, radiologic, and histopathologic evaluations.[22,50] Approximately 30% to 50% of patients are asymptomatic and are diagnosed on routine chest radiographs. One-third of patients have nonspecific symptoms of fever, fatigue, weight loss, and malaise.[50a] This presentation is more common in people with skin of color, including Asian Indians.[50]

Initial tests such as a biopsy, radiograph, or laboratory studies can be performed by dermatologists; however, it might be necessary to coordinate care with other specialists (rheumatologist, pulmonologist, or ophthalmologist). Initial evaluation for suspected cases of sarcoidosis include complete blood count, blood urea nitrogen, creatinine, liver enzymes, serum calcium, antinuclear antibodies, anti–double-stranded DNA, chest X-ray, pulmonary function, skin biopsy, and angiotensin-converting enzyme tests.[49,50]

The diagnosis of sarcoidosis is confirmed by the presence of noncaseating granulomas on biopsy. Also, although no longer commonly used, a positive Kveim-Siltzbach reaction can be elicited.[51]

TREATMENT

There is no cure for sarcoidosis, and treating cutaneous sarcoid lesions can be difficult. Therapies often focus on symptomatic relief and controlling the disease activity. Treatment regimens in the past were based primarily on anecdotal evidence and case reports. As more double-blind randomized controlled studies are published, it has been possible to incorporate evidence-based medicine into clinical decision-making[52,53] [**Table 74-1**].

Topical and intralesional corticosteroids are first-line agents for the treatment of cutaneous sarcoid lesions. The anti-inflammatory properties of corticosteroids inhibit granuloma formation. For mild disease limited to the skin, twice-daily application of potent topicals such as halobetasol and clobetasol may be all that is required for successful treatment.[53-55] Papular and plaque sarcoidosis lesions are best treated with intralesional injections of triamcinolone, 3 to 20 mg/mL, repeated every 4 weeks until lesions flatten.[53,54] Systemic corticosteroids are indicated for lesions that are refractory to local treatment, widespread, or indicate a potential for scarring. Dosing of prednisone ranges from 40 to 80 mg/d and is tapered over a course of weeks to months depending on clinical response. Topical and intralesional corticosteroids carry the risk of causing cutaneous atrophy and hypopigmentation. Hypopigmentation is more obvious in patients with skin of color and can lead to increased emotional stress. Common adverse effects of systemic corticosteroids include osteoporosis, peptic ulcers, impaired wound healing, acne, hyperglycemia, Cushing syndrome, and adrenal insufficiency.[53] Although corticosteroids are an

TABLE 74-1	Selected treatments for sarcoidosis and their respective scientific level of evidence			
Treatment	**Dosing**	**Adverse effects**	**Evidence level**	**Reference**
Topical corticosteroid (clobetasol, halobetasol)	0.05% ointment twice a day for 3–4 weeks or under occlusive dressing; applied once a week for 3–5 weeks	Hypopigmentation, skin atrophy	2a	Khatri et al[30] Volden[54] Veien and Brodthagen[69]
Intralesional corticosteroid (triamcinolone)	10 mg/mL every 4 weeks	Hypopigmentation, skin atrophy	4	Bersani and Nichols[55] Veien and Brodthagen[69]
Oral corticosteroids (prednisone)	Initially 0.5–1 mg/kg/d for 3–4 weeks then gradually tapered to maintenance dose of 10 mg/d	*Short term:* Gastrointestinal irritation, mood disturbances *Long term:* Osteoporosis, hypertension, acne, hyperglycemia, Cushing syndrome	4	Veien and Brodthagen[69] Saxe et al[70]
Hydroxychloroquine	200–400 mg/d (maximum of 6.5 mg/kg/d)	Corneal opacity (less likely than chloroquine), anorexia, dizziness, hepatotoxicity, renal damage	2a	Siltzbach and Teirstein[63] Brodthagen and Gilg[64] Jones and Callen[65]
Chloroquine	250–750 mg/d for a maximum of 3.5 mg/kg/d	Corneal opacity, anorexia, dizziness, hepatotoxicity, renal damage	2a	Morse et al[66] Hirsch[67]
Methotrexate	7.5–25 mg/wk orally, subcutaneously, or intramuscularly	Hepatic and renal toxicity, pneumonitis, gastrointestinal disturbances, neutropenia	2b	Lacher[68] Veien and Brodthagen[69] Lower and Baughman[71]
Doxycycline/minocycline/ cyclosporine	Doxycycline or minocycline 200 mg/d	Photosensitivity, vulvovaginitis, dizziness, teeth discoloration	2b	Schmitt et al[72] Pia et al[73] Marshall and Marshall[74]
Thalidomide	50–400 mg/d	Teratogenicity, nausea, renal toxicity, neuropathy	2b	Baughman and Lowe[62]
Infliximab	3–7 mg/kg intravenously at 0, 2, and 6 weeks (3–10 mg/kg) and then every 6 weeks	Tuberculosis reactivation, infections, lymphoma	2b	Doty et al[75] Saleh et al[76]
Adalimumab	40 mg every 2 weeks	Tuberculosis reactivation, infections, lymphoma	2b	Heffernan and Smith[77] Philips et al[19]

Source: Data from Heath C, David J, Taylor S. Sarcoidosis: Are there differences in your skin of color patients? *J Amer Acad Dermatol.* 2012 Jan;66(1):121.e1-14.

effective and accepted treatment modality for cutaneous sarcoidosis, there are few controlled clinical trials published to date that standardize dosing and length of treatment intervals.

Chloroquine and hydroxychloroquine are antimalarial agents used commonly to treat cutaneous sarcoidosis. They suppress the body's inflammatory response by inhibiting antigen presentation thus preventing granuloma formation.[56] Antimalarials can be used alone or in conjunction with corticosteroid therapy. Like corticosteroids, they are a standard treatment option even though controlled clinical trials are lacking. Adverse effects include corneal opacity, anorexia, dizziness, hepatotoxicity, hair bleaching, and renal damage.[56-58] Patients are advised to follow up regularly with an ophthalmologist to monitor for corneal deposits. It is also imperative for patients of Mediterranean, African, or Southeast Asian descent to be screened for glucose-6-phosphate dehydrogenase deficiency before being prescribed antimalarials to avoid precipitating an episode of hemolytic anemia.

Methotrexate is a second-line agent and used for recalcitrant sarcoidosis or when corticosteroid therapy is no longer an option. Weekly dosing of 10 to 15 mg is an effective therapeutic range. Potential adverse effects include hepatic toxicity, gastrointestinal disturbances, and hypersensitivity pneumonitis.[59-61]

Alternative agents for treating cutaneous sarcoidosis include tetracycline antibiotics, allopurinol, isotretinoin, thalidomide, infliximab, cyclosporine, and laser therapy. While published case reports and small trials of the aforementioned therapies have demonstrated promising results, randomized, double-blind, controlled trials with longitudinal follow-up are still needed to establish evidence-based justification.[53,62]

REFERENCES

1. James WD, Berger TG, Elston DM, eds. *Andrews' Diseases of the Skin: Clinical Dermatology.* 10th ed. Toronto, Ontario, Canada: Saunders Elsevier; 2006.
2. Haimovic A, Sanchez M, Judson M, et al. Sarcoidosis: a comprehensive review and update for the dermatologist: part I. Cutaneous disease. *J Am Acad Dermatol.* 2012;66:699.e1-699.e18.
3. Hosoda Y, Sasagawa S, Yasuda N. Epidemiology of sarcoidosis: new frontiers to explore. *Curr Opin Pulm Med.* 2002;8:424-428.
4. Rybicki BA, Major M, Popovich J Jr, et al. Racial differences in sarcoidosis incidence: a 5-year study in a health maintenance organization. *Am J Epidemiol.* 1997;145:234-241.
5. Iannuzzi MC, Rybicki BA, Teirstein AS. Sarcoidosis. *N Engl J Med.* 2007;357:2153-2165.
6. Labow TA, Atwood WG, Nelson CT. Sarcoidosis in the American Negro. *Arch Dermatol.* 1964;89:682-689.
7. Rybicki BA, Maliarik MJ, Major M, et al. Epidemiology, demographics, and genetics of sarcoidosis. *Semin Respir Infect.* 1998;13:166-173.
8. James DG, Neville E, Siltzbach LE. Worldwide review of sarcoidosis. *Ann N Y Acad Sci.* 1976;322:334.
9. Chong WS, Tan HH, Tan SH. Cutaneous sarcoidosis in Asians: a report of 25 patients from Singapore. *Clin Exp Dermatol.* 2005;30:120-124.
10. Mana J, Marcoval J, Graells J, et al. Cutaneous Involvement in sarcoidosis: relationship to systemic disease. *Arch Dermatol.* 1997;133:882-888.
11. Rybicki BA, Maliarik MJ, Poisson LM, et al. Sarcoidosis and granuloma genes: a family-based study in African Americans. *Eur Respir J.* 2004;24:251-257.
12. Olive KE, Kartaria YP. Cutaneous manifestations of sarcoidosis to other organ system involvement, abnormal laboratory measurements, and disease course. *Arch Intern Med.* 1985;145:1811-1814.
13. English JC, Patel PJ, Greer KE. Sarcoidosis. *J Am Acad Dermatol.* 2001;44:725-746.
14. Cox C, David-Allen A, Judson M. Sarcoidosis. *Med Clin North Am.* 2005;89:817-828.
15. Minus HR, Grimes PE. Cutaneous manifestations of sarcoidosis in Blacks. *Cutis.* 1983;32:361-364.
16. Isreal HL, Karlin P, Menduke H, et al. Factor affecting outcome of sarcoidosis. Influence of race, extrathoracic involvement, and initial radiologic lung lesions. *Ann N Y Acad Sci.* 1986;465:609-618.
17. Honeybourne D. Ethnic differences in the clinical features of sarcoidosis in South-East London. *Br J Dis Chest.* 1980;74:63-69.
18. Evans M, Sharma O, LaBree L, et al. Differences in clinical findings between Caucasians and African Americans with biopsy-proven sarcoidosis. *Ophthalmology.* 2007;114:325-333.
19. Philips MA, Lynch J, Azmi FH. Ulcerative cutaneous sarcoidosis responding to adalimumab. *J Am Acad Dermatol.* 2005;53:917.
20. Levin AM, Iannuzzi MC, Montgomery CG, et al. Association of ANXA11 genetic variation with sarcoidosis in African Americans and European Americans. *Genes Immun.* 2013;14:13-18.
21. Ianuzzi MC. Genetics of sarcoidosis. *Sem Respir Crit Care Med.* 2007;28:15-21.
22. Judson MA, Baughman RP, Thompson BW, et al. Two year prognosis of sarcoidosis: the ACCESS experience. *Sarcoidosis Vasc Diffuse Lung Dis.* 2003;20:204-211.
23. Kreider ME, Christie JD, Thompson B, et al. Relationship of environmental exposures to the clinical phenotype of sarcoidosis. *Chest.* 2005;128:207-215.
24. Newman L. A case control etiologic study of sarcoidosis: environmental and occupational risk factors. *Am J Respir Crit Care Med.* 2004;165:1324-1330.
25. Brjalin V, Salupere R, Tefanova V, et al. Sarcoidosis and chronic hepatitis C: a case report. *World J Gastroenterol.* 2012;18:5816-5820.
26. Samtsov AV. Cutaneous sarcoidosis. *Int J Dermatol.* 1992;31:385-391.
27. Hanno R, Callen JP. Sarcoidosis: a disorder with prominent cutaneous features and their interrelationship with systemic disease. *Med Clin North Am.* 1980;64:847-866.
28. Elgart ML. Cutaneous sarcoidosis: definitions and types of lesions. *Clin Dermatol.* 1986;4:35-45.
29. Mañá J, Marcoval J. Skin manifestations of sarcoidosis. *Presse Med.* 2012;41:6.
30. Khatri KA, Chotzen VA, Burrall BA. Lupus pernio: successful treatment with a potent topical corticosteroid. *Arch Dermatol.* 1995;131:617-618.
31. Chudomirova K, Velichkva L, Anavi B. Recurrent sarcoidosis in skin scars accompanying systemic sarcoidosis. *J Eur Acad Dermatol Venerol.* 2003;17:360-361.
32. Vainsencher D, Winkelmann RK. Subcutaneous sarcoidosis. *Arch Dermatol.* 1984;120:1028-1031.
33. Albertini JG, Tyler W, Miller OF III. Ulcerative sarcoidosis: case report and review of literature. *Arch Dermatol.* 1997;133:215-219.
34. Mashek H, Kalb R. Hypopigmentation of the extremities. *Arch Dermatol.* 1998;134:744-747.
35. Hall RSH, Floro JF, Kin LE. Hypopigmented lesions in sarcoidosis. *J Am Acad Dermatol.* 1984;11:1163-1164.
36. Cather JC, Cohen PR. Ichthyosiform sarcoidosis. *J Am Acad Dermatol.* 1999;40:862-865.
37. Banse-Kupin L, Pelachyk JM. Ichthyosiform sarcoidosis: Report of two cases and a review of the literature. *J Am Acad Dermatol.* 1987;17:616-620.
38. Rosenberg B. Ichthyosiform sarcoidosis. *Dermatol Online J.* 2005;11:15.
39. Yoon CH, Lee CW. Case 6: Erythrodermic form of cutaneous sarcoidosis. *Clin Exp Dermatol.* 2003;28:575-576.
40. Greer KE, Harman LE, Kayne AL. Unusual cutaneous manifestations of sarcoidosis. *Southern Med J.* 1977;65:666-668.
41. Gregg PJ, Kantor GR, Telang GH, et al. Sarcoidal tissue reaction in Sézary syndrome. *J Am Acad Dermatol.* 2000;43:372-376.
42. House NS, Welsh JP, English JC 3rd. Sarcoidosis-induced alopecia. *Dermatol Online J.* 2012;18:4.
43. Momen S, Al-Niaimi F. Sarcoid and the nail: review of the literature. *Clin Exp Dermatol* 2013;38:119-125.
44. Patel KB, Sharma OP. Nails in sarcoidosis: response to treatment. *Arch Dermatol.* 1983;119:277-278.
45. Losada-Campa A, de la Torre-Fraga C, Gomez de Liano A, et al. Histopathology of nail sarcoidosis. *Acta Derm Venerol.* 1995;75:404-405.
46. Okamoto H, Horio T, Izumi T. Micropapular sarcoidosis simulating lichen nitidus. *Dermatological.* 1985;165:253-255.
47. Burov EA, Kantor GR, Isaac M. Morpheaform sarcoidosis: report of three cases. *J Am Acad Dermatol.* 1998;39:345-348.
48. Ramanan AV, Denning DW, Baildam EM. Cutaneous childhood sarcoidosis—a rare disease refractory to treatment. *Rheumatology.* 2003;42:1565-1571.
49. Fernandez-Faith E, McDonnell J. Cutaneous sarcoidosis: differential diagnosis. *Clin Dermatol.* 2007;25:276-287.
50a. Aladesanmi OA. Sarcoidosis: an update for the primary care physician. *MedGenMed.* 2004;6:7.
50. Hunninghake GW, Costabel U, Ando M, et al. ATS/ERS/WASOG statement on sarcoidosis. *Am J Resp Crit Care Med.* 1999;160:736-755.
51. Kirsner RS, Kerdel FA. Sarcoidosis. In: Arnt KA, Leoit PE, Robinson JK, et al., eds. *Cutaneous Medicine and Surgery: An Integrated Program in Dermatology,* Vol. 1. London, United Kingdom: Saunders; 1996:433-437.
52. Heath C, David J, Taylor S. Sarcoidosis: are there differences in your skin of color patients? *J Am Acad Dermatol.* 2012;66:121.e1–14.
53. Doherty C. Evidence-based therapy for cutaneous sarcoidosis. *Drugs.* 2008;68:1361-1383.
54. Volden G. Successful treatment of chronic skin diseases with clobetasol propionate and a hydrocolloid occlusive dressing. *Acta Dermato Venereologica.* 1992;72:69-71.

55. Bersani T, Nichols C. Intralesional triamcinolone for cutaneous palpebral sarcoidosis. *Am J Ophthalmol*. 1985;99:561-562.

56. Fox RI, Kang HI. Mechanism of action of antimalarial drugs: inhibition of antigen processing and presentation. *Lupus*. 1993;1:S9-S12.

57. Veien NK. Cutaneous sarcoidosis: prognosis and treatment. *Clin Dermatol*. 1986;4:75-87.

58. Zic JA, Horowitz DH, Arzubiaga C, et al. Treatment of cutaneous sarcoidosis with chloroquine: review of the literature. *Arch Dermatol*. 1991;127:1034-1040.

59. Lower E, Baughman R. Prolonged use of methotrexate for sarcoidosis. *Arch Intern Med*. 1995;155:846.

60. Henderson C, Ilchyshyn A, Curry A. Laryngeal and cutaneous sarcoidosis treated with methotrexate. *J R Soc Med*. 1994;87:632-633.

61. Rajendran R, Theertham M, Salgia R, et al. Methotrexate in the treatment of cutaneous sarcoidosis. *Sarcoidosis*. 1994;11:S335-S338.

62. Baughman R, Lowe E. Newer therapies for cutaneous sarcoidosis: the role of thalidomide and other agents. *Am J Clin Dermatol*. 2004;5:385-394.

63. Siltzbach L, Teirstein A. Chloroquine therapy in 43 patients with intrathoracic and cutaneous sarcoidosis. *Acta Medica Scand Suppl*. 1964;425:302-308.

64. Brodthagen H, Gilg I. Hydroxychloroquine in the treatment of sarcoidosis. In: Turiaf J, Chabot J, eds. *La Sarcoidose: Rapports de la IV Conference International*. Paris, France: Mason and Co.; 1967:764-767.

65. Jones E, Callen JP. Hydroxychloroquine is effective therapy for control of cutaneous sarcoidal granulomas. *J Am Acad Dermatol*. 1990;23:487-489.

66. Morse S, Cohn Z, Hirsch J, et al. The treatment of sarcoidosis with chloroquine. *Am J Med*. 1961;30:779-784.

67. Hirsch J. Experimental treatment with chloroquine. *Am Rev Respir Dis*. 1961;84:52-58.

68. Lacher M. Spontaneous remission or response to methotrexate in sarcoidosis. *Ann Intern Med*. 1968;69:1247.

69. Veien N, Brodthagen H. Cutaneous sarcoidosis treated with methotrexate. *Br J Dermatol*. 1977;97:213-216.

70. Saxe N, Benatar SR, Bok L, et al. Sarcoidosis with leg ulcers and annular facial lesions. *Arch Dermatol*. 1984;120:93-96.

71. Lower E, Baughman R. Prolonged use of methotrexate for sarcoidosis. *Arch Intern Med*. 1995;155:846.

72. Schmitt C, Fabi S, Kukreja T, et al. Hypopigmented cutaneous sarcoidosis responsive to minocycline. *J Drugs Dermatol*. 2012;11:385-389.

73. Pia G, Pascalis L, Aresu G, et al. Evaluation of the efficacy and toxicity of the cyclosporine A-flucortolone-methotrexate combination in the treatment of sarcoidosis. *Sarcoidosis Vasc Diffuse Lung Dis*. 1996;13:146-152.

74. Marshall TG, Marshall FE. Sarcoidosis succumbs to antibiotics—implications for autoimmune disease. *Autoimmun Rev*. 2004;3:295-300.

75. Doty JD, Mazur JE, Judson MA. Treatment of sarcoidosis with infliximab. *Chest*. 2005;127:1064-1071.

76. Saleh S, Ghodsian S, Yakimova V, et al. Effectiveness of infliximab in treating selected patients with sarcoidosis. *Respir Med*. 2006;100:2053-2059.

77. Heffernan MP, Smith DI. Adalimumab for treatment of cutaneous sarcoidosis. *Arch Dermatol*. 2006;142:17-19.

CHAPTER

75

Sickle Cell Disease

Salam Al-Kindi
Lynn McKinley-Grant
Titilola Sode

KEY POINTS

- Sickle cell disease (SCD) is prevalent in sub-Saharan Africa, the Middle East, India, and most tropical climates where malaria is present.

- The SCD group of disorders can include all genotypes (eg, HbSS, HbSC, and HbSβ-thalassemia), unlike sickle cell anemia which occurs only with the HbSS genotype. SCD is characterized by recurrent vaso-occlusive crises, anemia, and a predisposition for infections.

- Patients with SCD commonly present with jaundice and/or pallor.

- A physical examination of the patient should include nonpathognomonic skin findings, stroke, pectus excavatum, body habitus, and an

enlarged spleen, as well as the cutaneous symptoms of renal failure (see Chapter 73, Renal Disease).

- Leg ulcers are a common cutaneous manifestation of SCD.

- In children, hand-foot syndrome (dactylitis) is typically the first cutaneous marker of this condition.

INTRODUCTION

Although it likely occurred for many years before it was first identified, sickle cell disease (SCD) was initially described by Dr. James Herrik in 1910.[1] Dr. Herrik was a cardiologist in Chicago who came across SCD while evaluating a West Indian patient, Walter Noel. His intern described Noel's blood smear as having "many pear-shaped and elongated forms - some small."[1] SCD has a unique set of cutaneous manifestations with which dermatologists should be familiar. These symptoms include leg ulcers and skin infections; however, the first manifestation of SCD is often hand-foot syndrome. This syndrome usually presents in early childhood.

ETIOLOGY AND GENETICS

SCD is a commonly inherited hemoglobinopathy. It is caused by a mutation in the gene that encodes for the β chain of hemoglobin (hemoglobin S) on chromosome 11. This mutation replaces a hydrophilic amino acid (glutamic acid) with a hydrophobic amino acid (valine). Consequently, noncovalent polymerization of hemoglobin occurs and distorts the red blood cells. The result is an abnormally rigid and sickle-shaped erythrocyte, especially when the oxygen tension is low. Problems occur because the sickle-shaped erythrocytes cannot easily navigate through small capillaries. This leads to vaso-occlusion, ischemia, hemolysis, and anemia. As a result, patients can suffer from a number of complications including strokes, infections, dactylitis, leg ulcerations and, most notably, pain crises.[2] Sickle cell anemia refers to the condition caused by a homozygous mutation (HbSS), whereas SCD characterizes all of the genotypes. This includes carriers of the trait (HbAS) and other abnormal forms of hemoglobin in combination with hemoglobin S (ie, C, D, E, and β-thalassemia).[3]

EPIDEMIOLOGY

SCD is widespread in tropical regions, including sub-Saharan Africa, India, and the southern coast of the Arabian Peninsula. Studies show that the sickle cell trait is a protective factor against malaria, and therefore, it presents with high frequency in endemic regions due to genetic selection. However, migration has increased the prevalence of this disease across Europe and the Americas.[2,4,5]

■ AFRICA

Africa has by far the highest prevalence of SCD. Epidemiologic analysis estimates that 85% of all sickle cell disorders and more than 70% of all affected births occur in Africa.[5] Central, eastern, and western Africa appear to share a higher prevalence of the disease (with the sickle cell trait ranging from 5% to 40%) compared to northern and southern regions of the continent, where the trait ranges from 1% to 2%.[6] For example, in the West African country of Nigeria, which is the most populated country in Africa with 162 million inhabitants, 24% of the population are carriers and SCD occurs in around 2% of all births.[4] Therefore, in Nigeria alone, more than 150,000 children are born annually with SCD.[4] Furthermore, certain tribes also have increased frequencies of the sickle cell trait. For example, among the Baamba tribe located in west Uganda, 45% of the population are carriers.[4] Estimates from a global epidemiology study of sickle hemoglobin in neonates show that approximately 64% and 75% of neonates who are born annually with the sickle cell trait and sickle cell anemia, respectively, come from sub-Saharan Africa.[7] In fact, 50% of all neonates with either the trait or

SCD come exclusively from three countries, two of which are located in Africa (Nigeria and the Democratic Republic of Congo).[7]

Several different haplotypes of the β-globin gene have been identified. In Africa, there are four major haplotypes that have been characterized by their region: Senegal, Benin, Bantu, and Cameroon.[6] Each haplotype differs in its clinical severity. The Senegal haplotype results in the most benign form of SCD, whereas the Benin, Cameroon, and Bantu haplotypes are typically more severe due to their lower levels of hemoglobin F.[6]

MIDDLE EAST AND INDIA

The Middle East encompasses portions of western Asia as well as portions of North Africa. The first case of SCD in the Middle Eastern region was recorded in Egypt in 1951.[8] However, it is likely that the disease existed in this area for much longer. In fact, it was recently proposed by a German team, from Hamburg's Bernhard Noct Institute for Tropical Medicine, that King Tutankhamen had SCD. Their theory is that he was so weakened by the SCD that a case of malaria was enough to cause his early death. Therefore, his crippling condition may not have been a hunting injury as earlier proposed, but sickle cell leg ulcers.[9,10]

SCD has now been recognized in nearly every country in the Middle Eastern region. The frequency of this disease varies between and within countries, with reported prevalence rates ranging from less than 1% in certain regions (Yemen, Palestine, Syria, and Lebanon) to much higher rates in other areas.[8] For example, in Egypt, the overall prevalence of SCD is low; however, within oases, the prevalence is between 9% and 22%.[11] Similar trends are seen in Sudan, where populations in western areas of the country have a higher rate of occurrence.[12] A Saudi-Indian haplotype has been identified in several countries in this region, which is mild in severity. However, African haplotypes, such as the Benin haplotype, have also been identified throughout the region.[8,13,14]

SCD is similarly prevalent in India. Throughout various regions of the country, the frequency of the sickle cell gene varies, ranging from 0.05 to 0.31; Madhya Pradesh has the highest prevalence of SCD, while Orissa has the lowest number of homozygous individuals.[15] The prevalence of SCD also varies among tribes. For example, in Nilgiris, most tribes, including the Irula, Paniya, and Mullukurumba, have a sickle cell trait frequency of more than 30%.[16] However, it appears that the prevalence of carriers is specifically higher in Paniya and Mullukurumba tribes living in the western region of Nilgiris.[16] It is estimated that 22.7% and 16.9% of neonates born annually with the sickle cell trait and SCD, respectively, are from the Saudi–Indian region.[7]

THE AMERICAS

SCD affects approximately 100,000 individuals in the United States and approximately 102,000 African American and 2600 Hispanic infants are born annually with sickle cell disorders.[17] This condition typically affects individuals who are of African, Asian, Caribbean, and Mediterranean descent. It is estimated that 1 in 365 African Americans and 1 in 16,305 Hispanics have SCD.[17]

SCD is also prevalent among certain regions of Latin America. For example, in Brazil, where there is a large African population as a result of the trans-Atlantic slave trade, it is estimated that 5% to 6% of the population has the sickle cell trait.[18] Consequently, there is an estimated incidence of 700 to 1000 affected infants born each year.[18] In Cuba, approximately 3% to 7% of the population is affected by SCD, and there are around 100 new cases reported annually.[19] SCD is also prevalent in other Latin American countries, such as Panama, Colombia, and Venezuela.

MODE OF DIAGNOSIS

Typically, patients with SCD present after the age of 6 months, when the adult level of hemoglobin is established. However, presentations earlier than that are also seen, and clinical examination may reveal pallor and jaundice. Laboratory findings include anemia and reticulocytosis in the full blood counts. Patients will have irreversibly sickled cells, polychromasia, and sometimes target cells on the peripheral smear. A sickle solubility test will indicate the presence of sickle hemoglobin, and it is

therefore often used as a screening test. However, the confirmatory tests include hemoglobin electrophoresis and high-performance liquid chromatography (HPLC). These are used to quantify the hemoglobin variants present (where normal adult hemoglobin is replaced by hemoglobin S or one of its variants). In addition, molecular confirmation is occasionally required, particularly in the presence of other hemoglobin disorders.

Universal neonatal screening is available in countries such as the United States and UK. The majority of screening programs in the United States use a combination of isoelectric focusing, hemoglobin electrophoresis, and HPLC. Antenatal testing can also be completed by a chorionic villus biopsy during the first trimester or by amniocentesis during the second trimester.[2,20]

Differential diagnoses include disorders affecting the joints, such as gout, septic arthritis, connective tissue disease, avascular necrosis, and Perthes disease. Diseases presenting with a painful abdomen should also be included, such as an acute abdomen, cholelithiasis, hepatic vein thrombosis, and pancreatitis. Osteomyelitis is another major differential diagnosis because the painful bone crisis is nearly identical in the presentation of both conditions. Pulmonary embolisms are also a part of the differential diagnosis because its presentation is similar to acute chest syndrome. Finally, trauma should additionally be considered, because pain is typically a major symptom upon presentation.[21]

CUTANEOUS MANIFESTATIONS

SKIN COLOR

Hemolysis and chronic anemia occur secondary to the abnormal shape and fragility of sickled erythrocytes. Therefore, pallor and jaundice are the predominant skin color features in SCD patients. In fact, jaundice in an infant can be one of the earliest signs of SCD.[20]

LEG ULCERS

Epidemiology The prevalence of leg ulcers affecting individuals with SCD in North America ranges from 2.5% to 10%.[22,23] In Africa, it is estimated to affect between 1.5% and 13.5% of patients with a sickle cell disorder.[23] A study done in Lagos, Nigeria, showed that 1.7% of patients (14 of 834) had leg ulcers, and those affected were predominantly male with a ratio of 6:1.[24] Leg ulcers are especially prevalent among Jamaican patients of West African origin, where up to 70% of those with SCD are affected.[25] A study from Saudi Arabia revealed no incidence of leg ulcers among patients with SCD.[26] It appears that leg ulcers predominantly affect individuals with sickle cell anemia, rather than those with SCD. Other risk factors include male gender, older than 20 years, low levels of hemoglobin F, use of hydroxyurea, environmental factors, personal hygiene, and low socioeconomic status.[27]

Etiology and Clinical Findings Patients with SCD, who are between the ages of 10 and 50 years, can develop deforming, sore, and indolent leg ulcers [**Figure 75-1**]. The exact etiology is unclear, but it appears to be related to the repeated injury of small vessels by sickled cells, a decreased oxygen delivery to the distal blood vessels, venous incompetence, and persistent inflammation.[20] There may also be an association between lupus anticoagulant and sickle cell patients with chronic leg ulcers.[28] Ulcers occur in areas of the leg with less subcutaneous fat and decreased blood flow. The skin overlaying the medial and lateral malleoli is the most frequent site of ulcer formation. However, they are also found on the dorsum of the foot and the region around the Achilles tendon. They can often appear in areas of trauma. Typically, the lesions present as round and punched-out ulcerations [**Figure 75-2**] with a raised border and a deep necrotic base [**Figure 75-3**]. Eventually, hyperpigmentation and hardening of the skin develop around the ulcer. Frequently, there is evidence of postinflammatory hyperpigmentation in areas of healed ulcers. There is often severe tenderness with palpation.[29,30] Unfortunately, these ulcers are slow to heal, resistant to treatment, and often recurrent.[31]

Treatment Several treatments have been proposed to manage leg ulcers in this population of patients. Interventions include systemic therapy, topical pharmaceuticals, reconstructive surgery, skin or cell

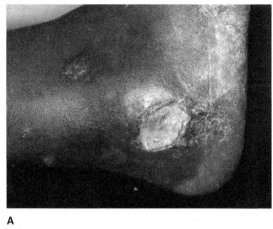

A

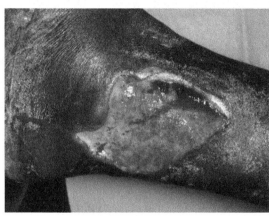

B

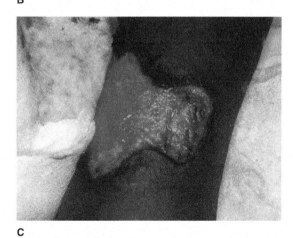

C

FIGURE 75-1. (A-C) Leg ulcers are painful and progress from small to large with a deep necrotic base. (Used with permission from Dr. Anisa Mosam, University of KwaZulu-Natal, Durban, South Africa.)

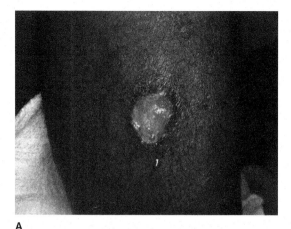

A

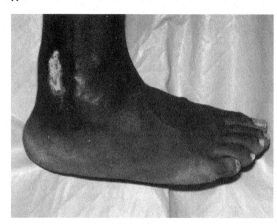

B

FIGURE 75-2. (A and B) Leg ulcers with a round, raised border and deep necrotic base. (Used with permission from Dr. Anisa Mosam, University of KwaZulu-Natal, Durban, South Africa.)

transplant, and laser treatments [**Table 75-1**].[32] Despite the variety of options available, a single effective modality of treatment has not yet emerged. Standard treatments typically include bed rest, hygienic maintenance, and dressings, such as Unna boots.[20] A review of several randomized control trials assessing the efficacy of systemic pharmaceutical therapy and topical pharmaceutical therapy was primarily inconclusive.[32] However, it showed that treatment with arginine-glycine-aspartic acid (RGD) peptide had some effectiveness in reducing the ulcer's size.[32]

PSEUDOXANTHOMA ELASTICUM

Pseudoxanthoma elasticum (PXE) is a rare hereditary systemic disorder that primarily impacts the cutaneous, ocular, and vascular structures. The cutaneous lesions are histologically characterized by fragmented elastic fibers and calcium deposits in the mid to deep dermis. The lesions are typically small, yellow papules, with areas of coalescence, especially in the antecubital fossa, popliteal fossa, axillae, and inguinal regions. These lesions have been described as having a 'plucked chicken' or 'gooseflesh' appearance. In patients with darker skin of color, the lesions are oval-shaped, hyperpigmented plaques along the skin line [**Figure 75-4**]. They are usually mildly pruritic. Over time, the involved areas may become increasingly lax and redundant.[33] Since the 1950s, an acquired form of PXE has been linked to SCD.[34] It is often reported as milder than the hereditary form of PXE. Also, unlike patients with hereditary PXE who present in childhood, patients with SCD typically present with PXE in their second decade of life. Although a genetic link between PXE and SCD does not exist, oxidative damage from chronic hemolysis and iron overload is most likely the mechanism that produces a PXE-like picture in SCD patients.[34,35] The treatment of PXE is usually focused on the ophthalmologic and cardiovascular aspects of this condition.

HAND-FOOT SYNDROME/DACTYLITIS
Epidemiology

Hand-foot syndrome is a form of dactylitis found in children who have SCD. Watson et al. reported that at least 52 cases of hand-foot syndrome were identified in the United States between 1941 and 1962.[36] Each case presented in young African American children with SCD. Most of these children were younger than 2 years; however, five of the patients were 6 years old.[36] A more recent cumulative study, conducted by the Cooperative Study of Sickle Cell Disease, showed that between the ages of 6 and 12 months, approximately 31% of infants with SCD experienced hand-foot syndrome.[37] However, it did not present in children over the age of 4 years. Furthermore, in this study, hand-foot syndrome

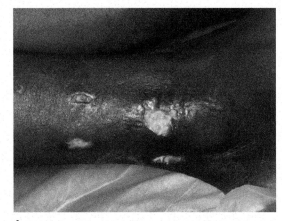

A

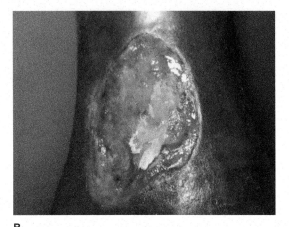

B

FIGURE 75-3. (A and B) Early presentation of leg ulcers can appear with multiple, punched-out ulcers that are generally resistant to treatment. (Used with permission from Dr. Anisa Mosam, University of KwaZulu-Natal, Durban, South Africa.)

predominantly affected those with the homozygous form of SCD, rather than other genotypes (ie, HbSC or HbSA).[37] A chart review in Saudi Arabia revealed that 3.5% of 143 subjects with homozygous SCD presented with hand-foot syndrome before the age of 12 months.[26]

This condition has also been identified in India. A study of 496 patients, performed in Nagpur, revealed that 35 individuals with SCD had experienced hand-foot syndrome. These subjects were young children all under 7 years of age.[38]

Clinical Findings Dactylitis appears as swelling of the hands and feet in infants and young children with SCD. As the amount of hemoglobin F decreases during the first few years of life, children become more susceptible to sickling. This is especially the case in regions more distal to the lungs where the levels of well-oxygenated blood are lower. Therefore, during a sickling crisis, children present with the swelling of any, or all four, extremities as a result of vaso-occlusion and ischemic infarction.[39]

The swelling is localized to the dorsum of the hands and feet and extends to the digits. The overlying skin appears to be tense and shiny, and there is an effacement of the skin folds. Palpation reveals that the swelling is nonpitting and nonfluctuant. Children typically have limited mobility in the affected regions. Initially, radiologic changes only show the soft tissue swelling. However, bone changes can usually be observed after 2 weeks. These changes typically include a mixture of radiolucent and hyperdense areas that give bones a moth-eaten appearance. X-rays can also reveal a periosteal elevation and opaque transverse lines in the areas of prior necrosis. Patients may also have an elevated temperature and leukocytosis. In most cases, symptoms typically resolve within 1 to 4 weeks without any long-term complications. For more severe cases, areas of necrosis may

TABLE 75-1	Medical interventions for sickle cell disease-induced leg ulcers
Class of intervention	**Examples**
Systemic pharmaceuticals	Isoxsuprine hydrochloride
	L-Carnitine
	Recombinant human erythropoietin
	Antithrombin III concentrate
	Bosentan
	Zinc sulphate
	Arginine butyrate
Topical pharmaceuticals	Antibiotics
	Collagen dressing
	Natural honey
	Granulocyte-macrophage colony-stimulating factor
	Arginine-glycine-aspartic acid (RGD) peptide matrix
	Solcoseryl
	Steroids
Surgical interventions	Free flap transfer
	Human skin equivalents graft
	Allogeneic keratinocytes application
Other	Laser therapy
	Hyperbaric oxygen therapy
	Acetic acid wet-to-dry dressings

result in the shortening of digits, leaving these children with a permanent deformity [**Figure 75-5**].[39]

Treatment Hand-foot syndrome is a self-limited phenomenon. Therefore, the care offered by physicians is usually largely supportive, including hydration, analgesics, antibiotics in the presence of fever and leukocytosis, and reassurance for the patient's parents and family.[20,39]

SYSTEMIC MANIFESTATIONS WITH NONPATHOGNOMONIC SKIN FINDINGS

Other complications of SCD can be divided into acute or chronic symptoms depending on their origin. Some of the acute complications are listed in **Table 75-2**. Chronic complications include a predisposition for the formation of gallstones, avascular necrosis, osteoporosis, pulmonary hypertension, renal abnormalities, and growth impediments.

Treatment The overall management is aimed at addressing the increased risk for infection, anemia, bone marrow aplasia, and painful crises. Individuals are typically given prophylactic penicillin until the

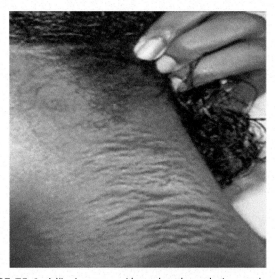

FIGURE 75-4. A Nigerian woman with pseudoxanthoma elasticum on the neck that waxed and waned with alteration in hydroxyurea dosing. (Used with permission from the Department of Dermatology, Washington Hospital Center, Washington, DC.)

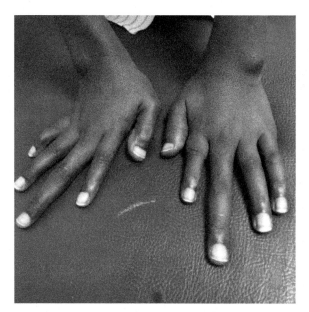

FIGURE 75-5. Hand-foot syndrome is a form of dactylitis found in children who have sickle cell disease. End stages of chronic dactylitis may result in shortening of the digits, leaving children with a permanent deformity, as above. (Used with permission from Dr. Frances O. Ajose, FRCP, Lagos State University Teaching Hospital, Nigeria.)

age of 5 years, as well as the appropriate vaccinations to prevent an infection from encapsulated organisms (such as the pneumococcal, *Haemophilus influenzae* type b, and meningococcal vaccines). Patients may require blood transfusions or exchange transfusions to treat symptomatic anemia or to support severe life-threatening complications, such as a stroke or acute chest syndrome.

Folic acid is often given as a daily regimen to reduce the risk of bone marrow aplasia in patients with chronic hemolysis. Effective pain management is extremely important for the quality of life of these individuals. Physicians usually prescribe a variety of analgesics and encourage patients to maintain an appropriate level of hydration.[20] Typically, patients also receive hydroxyurea as a disease-modifying drug. This is also used to increase their hemoglobin F levels. Bone marrow transplants offer the only curative therapy available for those with this disease.

CONCLUSION

SCD is one of the most common hemoglobin disorders experienced by individuals around the world. It is characterized by anemia, a predisposition to infection, and vaso-occlusive episodes that culminate in painful crises, acute chest syndromes, and strokes. It has a unique set of cutaneous manifestations, including leg ulcers, hand-foot syndrome, and an association with PXE. Because these manifestations are closely linked with disease pathologies, they often require different diagnostic and therapeutic approaches that demand an appropriate awareness by dermatologists.

TABLE 75-2 Acute complications of sickle cell disease

Complication	Comments
Acute painful episodes (vaso-occlusive crisis)	The most distressing complication experienced by >90% of all patients with sickle cell disease.
Acute chest syndrome	A life-threatening complication that mimics adult distress syndrome in its worst form.
Stroke	Potentially including thrombotic or hemorrhagic strokes or silent infarcts.
Sequestration	Red cells are sequestered in the spleen, liver, lungs, and potentially other organs.
Anemia	Perhaps due to hyperhemolytic or aplastic causes or an infection.
Infections	Usually due to splenic and immune dysfunction.
Priapism	Male patients may experience prolonged painful penile erections.

REFERENCES

1. Steensma DP, Kyle RA, Shampo MA. Walter Clement Noel—first patient described with sickle cell disease. *Mayo Clinic Proc.* 2010;85:e74-e75.
2. Rees DC, Williams TN, Gladwin MT. Sickle-cell disease. *Lancet.* 2010;376: 2018-2031.
3. Ashley-Koch A, Yang Q, Olney RS. Sickle hemoglobin (HbS) allele and sickle cell disease: a HuG Ereview. *Am J Epidemiol.* 2000;151:839-845.
4. World Health Organization. Fifty-Ninth World Health Assembly: Report by the secretariat. http://apps.who.int/gb/ebwha/pdf_files/WHA59-REC3/WHA59_REC3-en.pdf. Accessed April 12, 2013.
5. Modell B, Darlison M. Global epidemiology of haemoglobin disorders and derived service indicators. *Bull World Health Organ.* 2008;86:480-487.
6. Diallo D, Tchernia G. Sickle cell disease in Africa. *Curr Opin Hematol.* 2002;9: 111-116.
7. Piel FB, Patil AP, Howes RE, et al. Global epidemiology of sickle haemoglobin in neonates: a contemporary geostatistical model-based map and population estimates. *Lancet.* 2013;381:142-151.
8. El-Hazmi MA, Al-Hazmi AM, Warsy AS. Sickle cell disease in Middle East Arab countries. *Indian J Med Res.* 2011;134:597-610.
9. Hawass Z, Gad YZ, Ismail S, et al. Ancestry and pathology in King Tutankhamun's Family. *JAMA.* 2010;303:638-647.
10. Wuyts A. King Tut died from sickle-cell disease, not malaria. *The Independent,* June 25, 2010. www.independent.co.uk/life-style/history/king-tut-died-from-sicklecell-disease-not-malaria-2010531.html. Accessed April 12, 2013.
11. El-Beshlawy A, Youssry I. Prevention of hemoglobinopathies in Egypt. *Hemoglobin.* 2009;33:S14-S20.
12. Osman NOM, Afladni MHI. The prevalence of sickle cell anaemia in northern areas of Algadaref State, Sudan. http://www.sjph.net.sd/files/vol5i2/SJPH-vol5i1-p22-24.pdf. Accessed April 12, 2013.
13. Gelpi A. Sickle cell disease in Saudi Arabs. *Acta Haematol.* 1970;43:89-99.
14. Alkindi S, Al Zadjali S, Al Madhani A, et al. Forecasting hemoglobinopathy burden through neonatal screening in Omani neonates. *Hemoglobin.* 2010;34:135-144.
15. Kaur M, Das GP, Verma IC. Sickle cell trait and disease among tribal communities in Orissa, Madhya Pradesh and Kerala. *Indian J Med Res* 1997; 105: 111-116.
16. Ramasamy S, Balakrishnan K, Pitchappan RM. Prevalence of sickle cells in Irula, Kurumba, Paniya and Mullukurumba tribes of Nilgiris (Tamilnadu, India). *Indian J Med Res.* 1994;100:242-245.
17. Hassell KL. Population estimates of sickle cell disease in the US. *Am J Prev Med.* 2010;38:S512-S521.
18. Lyra IM, Gonçalves MS, Braga JA, et al. Clinical, hematological, and molecular characterization of sickle cell anemia pediatric patients from two different cities in Brazil. *Cad Saude Publica.* 2005;21:1287-1290.
19. Granda H, Gispert S, Dorticos A, et al. Cuban programme for prevention of sickle cell disease. *Lancet.* 1991;337:152-153.
20. National Heart, Lung, and Blood Institute. *The Management of Sickle Cell Disease.* Bethesda, MD: National Institutes of Health; 2002:15-18.
21. Driscoll MC. Sickle cell disease. *Pediatr Rev.* 2007;28:259-268.
22. Halabi-Tawil M, Lionnet F, Girot R, et al. Sickle cell leg ulcers: a frequently disabling complication and a marker of severity. *Br J Dermatol.* 2008;158: 339-344.
23. Minniti CP, Eckman J, Sebastiani P, et al. Leg ulcers in sickle cell disease. *Am J Hematol.* 2010;85:831-833.
24. Akinyanju O, Akinsete I. Leg ulceration in sickle cell disease in Nigeria. *Trop Geogr Med.* 1979;31:87-91.
25. Cumming V, King L, Fraser R, et al. Venous incompetence, poverty and lactate dehydrogenase in Jamaica are important predictors of leg ulceration in sickle cell anaemia. *Br J Haematol.* 2008;142:119-125.
26. Perrine RP, Pembrey ME, John P, et al. Natural history of sickle cell anemia in Saudi Arabs: a study of 270 subjects. *Ann Intern Med.* 1978;88:1-6.
27. Ladizinski B, Bazakas A, Mistry N, et al. Sickle cell disease and leg ulcers. *Adv Skin Wound Care.* 2012;25:420-428.
28. Olayemi EE, Bazuaye GN. Lupus anticoagulant and leg ulcers in sickle cell anemia. *Indian J Dermatol.* 2009;54:251-254

29. Serjeant GR, Serjeant BE, Mohan JS, et al. Leg ulceration in sickle cell disease: medieval medicine in a modern world. *Hematol Oncol Clin North Am.* 2005;19:943-956.

30. Serjeant GR. Leg ulceration in sickle cell anemia. *Arch Intern Med.* 1974;133: 690-694.

31. Serjeant GR, Galloway RE, Gueri MC. Oral zinc sulphate in sickle-cell ulcers. *Lancet.* 1970;2:891-893.

32. Martí-Carvajal AJ, Knight-Madden JM, Martinez-Zapata MJ. Interventions for treating leg ulcers in people with sickle cell disease. *Cochrane Database Syst Rev.* 2012;11:CD008394.

33. Laube S, Moss C. Pseudoxanthoma elasticum. *Arch Dis Child.* 2005;90:754-756.

34. Aessopos A, Farmakis D, Loukopolous D. Elastic tissue abnormalities resembling pseudoxanthoma elasticum in β-thalassemia and the sickling syndromes. *Blood.* 2002;99:30-35.

35. Hassan S, Kaya B. Pseudoxanthoma elasticum-like syndrome in a patient with sickle cell anaemia. *Br J Haematol.* 2010;148:342.

36. Watson RJ, Burko H, Megas H, et al. The hand-foot syndrome in sickle-cell disease in young children. *Pediatrics.* 1963;31:975-982.

37. Gill FM, Sleeper LA, Weiner SJ, et al. Clinical events in the first decade in a cohort of infants with sickle cell disease. Cooperative study of sickle cell disease. *Blood.* 1995;86:776-783.

38. Babhulkar S, Pande K, Babhulkar S. The hand-foot syndrome in sickle-cell haemoglobinopathy. *J Bone Joint Surg Br.* 1995;77:310-312.

39. Diggs L. Bone and joint lesions in sickle-cell disease. *Clin Orthop.* 1967;52: 119-144.

CHAPTER
76

Thyroid Disease

Lynn McKinley-Grant
Naurin Ahmad

KEY POINTS

- Dermatologists may be the first to see patients with thyroid-related conditions and should therefore be familiar with the cutaneous manifestations of thyroid dysfunction.

- The early recognition of hypo- and hyperthyroidism often lies with the dermatologist as both disorders can have a pronounced impact on the skin.

- The triggering factors of thyroid disease include iodine deficiency and autoimmune diseases such as diabetes, vitiligo, and alopecia.

- The incidence of thyroid disease is higher in Caucasian populations than in those with darker skin of color. Skin and hair manifestations of thyroid conditions will still present in patients with skin of color; however, they may appear in a more subtle form than in those with fairer skin.

- Graves disease is the most common hypothyroid disease associated with cutaneous manifestations. Patients with Graves disease may show clinical signs of acropachy or myxedema.

- The thyroid cancer syndromes include Sipple syndrome, Cowden syndrome, LAMB (lentigines, atrial myxomas, mucocutaneous myxomas, and blue nevi) syndrome, and NAME (nevi, atrial myxomas, myxoid neurofibromas, and ephelides) syndrome. Papillary carcinoma is the most common form of thyroid cancer in North America.

INTRODUCTION

Dermatologists may be among the first medical professionals to be consulted by individuals with hypo- and hyperthyroid disease. This is because the common dermatoses related to thyroid hormone dysfunction and/or thyroid-specific lesions (eg, cysts or malignancies) are often the first symptoms that patients become aware of. Therefore, dermatologists should be familiar with the broad and varied cutaneous

manifestations of an underlying systemic thyroid disease in order to make the correct diagnosis.

EPIDEMIOLOGY

Worldwide, the most common cause of primary thyroid disease is a dietary iodine deficiency; however, this is rarely seen in the Western world.[1] Several studies have found that, when compared with other patient groups, African Americans have a lower prevalence of thyroid disease.[2,3] Autoimmume thyroid disease is associated with other autoimmune diseases, including vitiligo, alopecia, and diabetes mellitus.[4-6] Hyperthyroidism tends to affect women more than men (at a ratio of 5:1) and has an overall prevalence of 1%.[7] Some studies suggest that there may be a lower incidence of hyperthyroidism in African American patients.[1] However, research on indigenous Africans in South Africa suggested that these patients presented more frequently with a complicated form of the disease, including cardiac failure, overt myopathy, and infiltrative ophthalmopathy.[8] The presentation is often late and severe, and this may reflect potential educational, socioeconomic, and cultural differences between the African and Caucasian populations in Africa, as well as delays in diagnoses.

A recent study demonstrated that the prevalence of subclinical hypothyroidism among pregnant women was fairly high among Indian patients.[9] They also had high rates of thyroid peroxidase (TPO) antibody positivity.[9] Therefore, screening for hypothyroidism is often included as a routine test to improve maternal and fetal outcomes.

Among Americans, there is a lower rate of thyroid cancer in patients with darker skin of color than in Caucasians. The highest prevalence is found in white non-Hispanics and Asians/Pacific Islanders between the ages of 14 and 45 years.[10,11] A 2011 study using the Surveillance, Epidemiology, and End Results (SEER) Program data demonstrated that papillary thyroid cancer rates among women were highest among Asian and lowest among African Americans; follicular cancer rates did not vary substantially by race/ethnicity; medullary cancer rates were highest among Hispanics and Caucasians; and anaplastic rates were highest among Hispanics.[12] The study showed that both papillary and follicular thyroid cancer rates among men were highest among the Caucasian group; medullary cancer rates were highest among Hispanics; and anaplastic rates were highest among Asians.[12]

An epidemiologic study documented the prevalence rates of thyroid cancer in the African continent.[13] The study found prevalence rates of 6.7% to 72.1% for papillary cancer, 4.9% to 68% for follicular cancer, 5% to 21.4% for anaplastic cancer, and 2.6% to 13.8% for medullary cancer. Interestingly, in the case of differentiated thyroid cancer, the authors noted that the more frequent occurrence of papillary cancer compared to follicular cancer may be attributable to the widespread iodization programs in Africa.[13]

PATHOPHYSIOLOGY OF CLINICAL MANIFESTATIONS

Thyroid hormones are mediated through the thyroid hormone receptor and have a wide array of effects on the skin, hair, and nails. The action of thyroid hormones on other organs and tissues may also have secondary manifestations on the skin. The clinical manifestations of thyroid hormone imbalances are often first seen in the skin, and the skin is an important clue in determining thyroid hormonal disruption.

The hypothalamic response to low levels of circulating thyroid hormones, triiodothyronine (T_3) and thyroxine (T_4), is to release thyrotropin-releasing hormone (TRH). TRH then stimulates the anterior pituitary gland to produce thyroid-stimulating hormone (TSH). Once TSH is released, it acts on the thyroid gland, leading to an increased production of T_3 and T_4. The primary thyroid hormone produced by the thyroid gland is T_4 and, to a lesser extent, T_3. T_4 is then converted to the active hormone T_3 by intracellular deiodinases. The presence of adequate amounts of thyroid hormone then sends negative feedback back to the brain to decrease the production of TSH and TRH.

Studies have identified thyroid hormone receptors in epidermal keratinocytes, skin fibroblasts, hair arrector pili muscle cells, vascular endothelial cells, Schwann cells, and cells relating to the hair follicle.[14] Thus the cutaneous manifestations of thyroid disease are vast and have a wide array of dermatologic symptoms.

HYPERTHYROIDISM

Hyperthyroidism is a condition of the thyroid gland in which there is an overproduction of thyroid hormone. The causes of hyperthyroidism are often the presence of a toxic multinodular goiter, Graves disease, solitary thyroid nodules, thyroiditis, and/or an unsuspected intake of thyroid hormone.

In hyperthyroidism, the texture of the skin often changes, becoming more warm, soft, and velvety. Patients also experience generalized hyperhidrosis, most prominently on their palms and soles [**Figure 76-1**]. These symptoms may be a result of the increased blood flow and peripheral vasodilation. Due to these vascular changes, facial flushing and palmar erythema have also been noted.[15] Nails often have a concave contour with distal onycholysis, also known as Plummer nail, or twenty-nail dystrophy may be present [**Figure 76-2**]. The hair tends to be soft and fine with occasional nonscarring alopecia. As the hair shafts of patients with darker skin of color may be coarser, the presence of dry and brittle hair may be more subtle on examination and, therefore, easy to miss.

Hyperpigmentation has also been noted in the creases of acral areas and the gingival and buccal mucosa.[16] In patients with skin of color, mucosal pigmentation and the darker pigmentation of acral skin may be present as a natural variant, making subtle changes in thyroid-related hyperpigmentation more difficult to evaluate.

GRAVES DISEASE

Epidemiology Graves disease is the hyperthyroid disorder most commonly associated with dermatologic manifestations. It is an autoimmune disorder in which B-lymphocytes produce thyroid-stimulating immunoglobulins. These activate the thyroid gland's TSH receptor to cause increased thyroid hormone production.[17,18] Some studies have demonstrated that the human leukocyte antigen DRB3*020/DQA1*0501 haplotype is associated with Graves disease in patients with darker skin of color.[19]

Cutaneous Manifestations Patients with Graves disease have a distinct subset of the clinical manifestations of thyroid disease, including

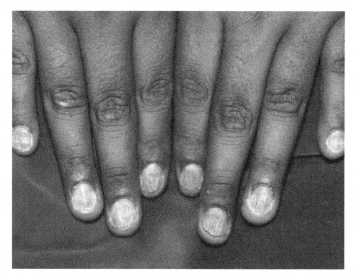

FIGURE 76-2. Twenty-nail dystrophy in a hypothyroid patient with darker skin of color. (Used with permission from the Department of Dermatology, Washington Hospital Center, Washington, DC.)

goiters, exophthalmos [**Figure 76-3**], infiltrative dermopathy (myxedema), and thyroid acropachy [**Figure 76-4**]. Many of these patients also have a smooth palpable midline goiter. A bruit is often heard with a stethoscope, signaling the increased vascularity of the gland. Approximately 25% of patients with Graves disease also develop significant ophthalmopathy secondary to the deposition of hyaluronic acid in the extraocular muscles and retro-orbital tissues.[20] This often results in lid lag and stare, as well as eyelid retraction.

Treatment When hyperthyroidism is suspected, a TSH test should be performed. If the TSH is low, and the free T_3 and T_4 levels are elevated, this confirms the diagnosis of hyperthyroidism. Thyroid-stimulating antibodies should also be monitored if Graves disease is a possibility. The TSH receptor antibodies test is more expensive, but it is a specific indicator for Graves disease. After the laboratory diagnosis is made, a 24-hour radioactive iodine uptake scan is typically performed to evaluate for Graves disease (high uptake, homogenous goiter), toxic nodule (high uptake, hot nodule), or thyroiditis (low uptake, cold scan).[21]

In Graves disease, treatment options include radioactive iodine, antithyroid medications (propylthiouracil/methimazole), or a thyroidectomy. Other less common therapies include lithium, cholestyramine,

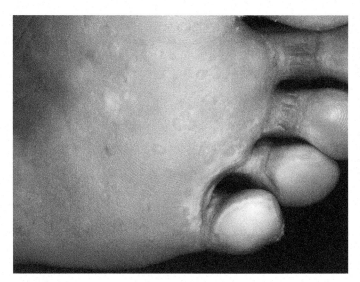

FIGURE 76-1. Plantar hyperhidrosis in a patient with hyperthyroidism. (Used with permission from the Department of Dermatology, Washington Hospital Center, Washington, DC.)

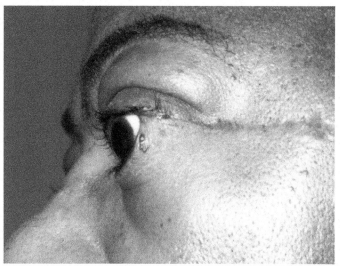

FIGURE 76-3. Exopthalmos in a patient with skin of color suffering from Graves disease. (Used with permission from the Department of Dermatology, Washington Hospital Center, Washington, DC.)

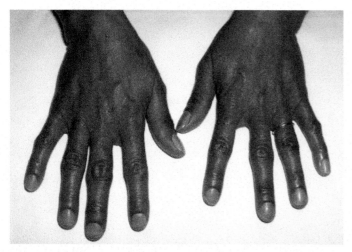

FIGURE 76-4. Thyroid acropachy in a patient with darker skin of color suffering from an autoimmune thyroid disease. (Used with permission from the Department of Dermatology, Washington Hospital Center, Washington, DC.)

and charcoal hemoperfusion. Treating the underlying hyperthyroid states does not usually result in an improvement of the ophthalmopathy.[19] Other treatment options include nonsteroidal anti-inflammatory drugs, oral steroids, radiation therapy, and surgical decompression.

◼ INFILTRATIVE DERMOPATHY (MYXEDEMA)

Epidemiology Infiltrative dermopathy (myxedema) occurs almost exclusively in Graves hyperthyroidism. It occurs only in up to 4% of patients and is secondary to glycosaminoglycan deposition in the dermis.[15,16,22,23]

Cutaneous Manifestations Myxedema presents as hyperpigmented or violaceous papules and plaques, nonpitting edema, and induration. It is frequently referred to as having a *peau d'orange* appearance.[24] This condition commonly occurs on the lower extremities, such as with pretibial myxedema [**Figure 76-5**], but can occur in other locations such as the upper back, neck, extremities, shoulders, and palms.[25] Typically

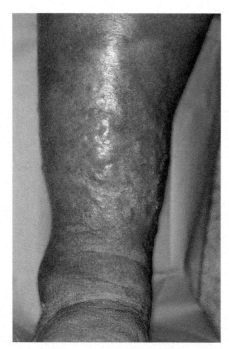

FIGURE 76-5. Pretibial myxedema in the lower extremity of a patient. (Used with permission from the Department of Dermatology, Washington Hospital Center, Washington, DC.)

this dermopathy is asymptomatic, but it can cause pruritus and, rarely, pain.[22] Myxedema can be seen in both hypo- and hyperthyroidism. In cutaneous myxedema, hyaluronic acid is the major glycosaminoglycan that accumulates in the dermis. This has a hygroscopic property and can therefore swell up to 1000 times its dry weight when hydrated, which leads to boggy edematous plaques.[26]

Treatment The treatment of pretibial myxedema is directed at both the pruritus and for cosmesis with topical steroids under occlusion.[24] Because there is a higher risk of postinflammatory hypopigmentation in skin of color, topical steroids should be used with caution. The use of compression stockings may also be helpful.

◼ ACROPACHY

Epidemiology Acropachy occurs in fewer than 1% of patients with Graves disease.[24,27] It usually occurs in conjunction with infiltrative dermopathy and ophthalmopathy.[24,27]

Cutaneous Manifestations Acropachy presents as clubbing and edema of the digits.[24,27] Patients may also have a periosteal reaction and experience pain around the distal bones.[24,27] The classic triad is that of digital clubbing, hand and foot edema, and a periosteal reaction in the long bones.

Treatment Therapy for acropachy is limited to the treatment of Graves disease, and the condition will often resolve when the thyroid disease has been more effectively controlled.[27] The treatment of hyperthyroidism is dependent on the etiology of the disorder. Symptom control can be achieved with β-blockers. In Graves disease, treatment options include radioactive iodine, antithyroid medications (propylthiouracil/methimazole), or a thyroidectomy. Other less common therapies include lithium, cholestyramine, and charcoal hemoperfusion.

HYPOTHYROIDISM

Hypothyroidism is a condition of the thyroid gland that results in an impaired production of the thyroid hormones T_3 and T_4.[15] Hypothyroidism can result from primary causes (such as a disease of the thyroid gland, an iodine deficiency, previous external radiation to the head or neck, a partial or total thyroidectomy, antithyroid drugs, and infiltrative diseases) or secondary causes (such as diseases of the pituitary gland and hypothalamic axis).[15] In the United States, the majority of primary thyroid disease cases are related to Hashimoto thyroiditis, which is an autoimmune disorder.[1,28] Patients with Hashimoto thyroiditis develop antibodies against the thyroglobulin protein and/or the peroxidase enzyme in the thyroid gland.[15] Autoimmune primary hypothyroidism is the most common type of hypothyroidism in the Western world, and it most frequently affects women between the ages of 30 and 50.[28] Some cases of this condition are drug-induced, with the offending drugs including lithium and iodine, interferon-α, and interleukin-2. Bexarotene has been shown to cause central hypothyroidism.[29]

◼ CUTANEOUS MANIFESTATIONS

The development of a thyroid goiter is the most common and visible manifestation of hypothyroidism related to an iodine deficiency. However, goiters can be seen in both hyper- and hypothyroid disease states and are not specific to a particular disease. Goiters are firm bulging masses that are located in the midpharyngeal region and can be uniform or nodular.[30] Goiters are often a significant cosmetic concern, but when significantly enlarged, they can also cause airway obstruction and compression.

The other cutaneous manifestations of hypothyroidism include skin thickening, diffuse nonscarring alopecia, and nail atrophy and brittleness [**Figure 76-6**]. Generalized xerosis involving the extensor surfaces and cool clammy skin are also often noted.[27] The skin's cool temperature and pale appearance is likely due to vasoconstriction and the decreased metabolic rate. However, dermatologists should note that pale skin may be more difficult to distinguish in patients with skin of color. Diffuse nonscarring alopecia has been noted in up to 50% of individuals with

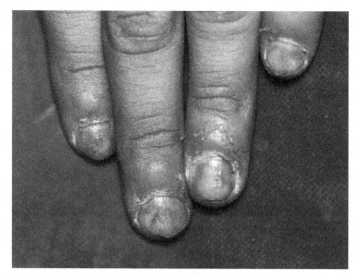

FIGURE 76-6. Dystrophic nails and xerosis on the digits of a patient with hypothyroidism. (Used with permission from the Department of Dermatology, Washington Hospital Center, Washington, DC.)

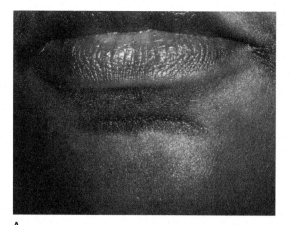

A

B

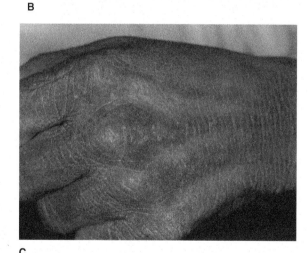

C

FIGURE 76-7. Acanthosis nigricans is a skin disorder that results in velvety markings with a light brown to black color. Hypothyroidism is one of the many potential causes for this condition. **(A)** Acanthosis nigricans of the mouth area. **(B)** Acanthosis nigricans of the neck. **(C)** Acanthosis nigricans of the hands. (Used with permission from the Department of Dermatology, Washington Hospital Center, Washington, DC.)

hypothyroidism.[31] There are also reports of a yellowing or pseudojaundice of the skin on the acral surfaces and nasolabial folds, secondary to decreased carotene metabolism.[18] Another potential manifestation is the nonscarring thinning, or loss, of the lateral eyebrows (madarosis). In addition, periorbital edema, facial puffiness, macroglossia, coarse facial features, and flat affect (lack of emotional reactivity) are often noted. Hypothyroid patients may also have decreased sebum production leading to the presence of less lipophilic flora and, instead, the presence of *Candida albicans*. These patients are at higher risk for *C. albicans*–caused folliculitis.[32]

Puri examined 50 Indian patients with a thyroid disease (72% with hypothyroidism and 28% with hyperthyroidism).[31] The majority of patients with hyperthyroidism displayed warm, moist skin and an elevated temperature. The other findings included diffuse nonscarring alopecia, pretibial myxedema, Plummer nails, facial flushing, and palmar and plantar hyperhidrosis. Interestingly, hyperpigmentation of the skin was noted in this population as well. The most common cutaneous feature of hypothyroidism in Indian patients included dry xerotic skin, pallor, nail changes, keratoderma, a loss of the lateral third of the eyebrow, and myxedematous facies.[31] Patients with hypothyroidism were also found to have associated autoimmune conditions such as vitiligo, alopecia areata, and dermatitis herpetiformis.[31]

Hashimoto thyroiditis can also be associated with other autoimmune diseases such as alopecia areata, vitiligo, and morphea.[33-35] It has also been described in association with acanthosis nigricans [**Figure 76-7**], granuloma annulare, keratosis pilaris, melasma, mucinosis, and lichen sclerosus et atrophicus.[36-40]

A case-control study of patients with vitiligo in India demonstrated that 14 of 50 patients (28%) had TPO antibody positivity.[41] Subclinical hypothyroidism was found in 14 of 50 patients (28%), mostly among those in the TPO antibody–positive group. Thyroid disease was prevalent in 20 of 50 patients (40%) when the TPO antibody–positive group was considered collectively alongside those with subclinical hypothyroidism.[41]

▪ TREATMENT

A lab diagnosis of a high TSH and low T$_4$ is often noted. In the case of central hypothyroidism, the TSH will be normal or low, and the free T$_4$ will also be low. In the case of an autoimmune thyroid disease, the most common antibodies detected are TPO (found in 95% of patients) and thyroglobulin antibodies (found in up to 60% of patients).[16] Thyroid hormone replacement (levothyroxine) is the mainstay of therapy

for autoimmune hypothyroidism. For the drug-induced form of this disease, the removal of the offending medications or toxins is essential.

THYROID CANCER

▪ EPIDEMIOLOGY

Thyroid cancer is the most common malignancy of the endocrine system.[42] Typically the presentation is that of a solitary nodule; however, in rare cases this cancer can present with metastatic disease. The incidence of thyroid cancer is increasing more rapidly in women than any other cancer, and it is the third most rapidly rising cancer in men.[15] In general, this form of cancer has a low mortality rate, depending on the subtype. It is seen most commonly in women aged 15 to 30 and >60 years.[16]

Although African Americans have a lower incidence of thyroid cancer, there is still an unfortunate social disparity in the survival outcomes for this group.[42] Americans with thyroid cancer have a significantly lower 5-year survival rate compared with Caucasians. A study using data from the SEER program demonstrated that African American patients were 2.3 times more likely to be diagnosed with an anaplastic disease.[42] They were also nearly 80% more likely to be diagnosed with a follicular disease. Compared with Caucasian patients, African Americans were nearly twice as likely to have large tumors (≥4 cm).[42]

Thyroid cancer is rarely fatal if detected early. Therefore, the familiarity with its cutaneous manifestations can aid in early detection, especially because there are several rare syndromes that have cutaneous manifestations and are associated with thyroid cancer. Papillary carcinoma is the most common form of thyroid cancer in North America.[43]

CUTANEOUS MANIFESTATIONS

Follicular carcinoma of the thyroid may have a greater propensity to metastasize to the skin. This is followed by papillary thyroid carcinoma, anaplastic carcinoma, and then medullary carcinoma. Some studies suggest that papillary may exceed follicular carcinoma in terms of metastases.[43]

However, there is medical agreement that the scalp is the most common site of skin metastases, which usually present as skin-colored papulonodules. These can be painful, pruritic, or ulcerative. Skin metastases are rarely the presenting sign of thyroid cancer; instead, this often presents as a sign of metastatic disease.[43,44]

DIAGNOSIS AND LABORATORY DATA

Testing for the presence of thyroid transcription factor 1 (TTF-1) antibodies is useful when suspecting thyroid metastatic lesions. Thyroglobulin expression can identify papillary and follicular cell carcinomas, but it is not seen in lung cancers. Medullary carcinomas have markers such as synaptophysin, chromogranin, and cluster of differentiation 56, as well as calcitonin.[43]

THYROID CANCER SYNDROMES

Although these syndromes are rare, the presence of any associated clinical findings should prompt the dermatologist to refer the patient. An investigation and diagnostic examination of an underlying thyroid malignancy will be required, as well as possible genetic testing.

Multiple Endocrine Neoplasia Type 2 Multiple endocrine neoplasia (MEN) type 2, or Sipple syndrome, is a rare familial disorder caused by mutations in the *RET* proto-oncogene. MEN type 2A is associated with medullary thyroid cancer, as well as pheochromocytoma and parathyroid adenoma.[45] MEN type 2B, also known as multiple mucosal neuroma syndrome, is associated with medullary thyroid carcinoma, pheochromocytoma, marfanoid habitus, and mucosal ganglioneuromas.[45] MEN types 2A and 2B are inherited in an autosomal dominant pattern and have very high, if not complete, penetrance.[14] Given the almost 100% penetrance of medullary thyroid carcinoma in these patients, and its tendency to occur at an early age, a prophylactic thyroidectomy is often performed.[46]

CARNEY COMPLEX

Carney complex is a rare autosomal dominant disease associated with thyroid follicular hyperplasia and thyroid carcinoma.[47] It is also known as LAMB syndrome (consisting of mucocutaneous lentigines, atrial myxomas, cardiomucocutaneous myxomas, and multiple blue nevi) or NAME syndrome (consisting of nevi, atrial myxomas, mucinosis of the skin, and endocrine overactivity). Carney complex is most commonly caused by mutations in the *PRKAR1A* gene on chromosome 17q23-q24,[47] which potentially functions as a tumor suppressor gene.[48]

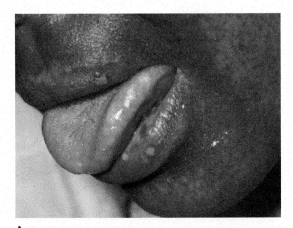

A

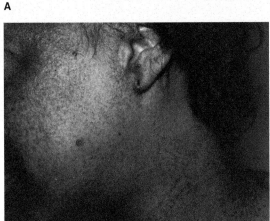

B

FIGURE 76-8. Symptoms of Cowden syndrome in a patient with darker skin of color. This syndrome is characterized by multiple noncancerous, tumor-like growths called hamartomas. These growths are most commonly found on the skin and mucous membranes, such as the lining of the mouth (**A**), nose, and eye (**B**). (Used with permission from the Department of Dermatology, Washington Hospital Center, Washington, DC.)

COWDEN SYNDROME

Cowden syndrome, or multiple hamartoma syndrome, is a rare autosomal dominant condition. It is thought to be the result of a loss-of-function mutation in the *phosphatase and tensin homolog* (*PTEN*) tumor suppressor gene.[49,50] It is characterized by multiple hamartomas and an increased risk of certain clinical features, including intestinal hamartomatous polyps, trichilemmomas, and a predisposition to breast carcinoma, follicular carcinoma of the thyroid, and endometrial carcinoma. Common cutaneous manifestations of Cowden syndrome are trichilemmomas on the face and papillomatous lesions that usually present on the face and/or mucous membranes, including the gums. A 'cobblestone' appearance of the tongue or gums may also present as a cutaneous indicator [**Figure 76-8**], as well as keratoses, which are hard growths on the skin. These often present on a patient's palms or the soles of their feet.

CONCLUSION

In conclusion, the manifestations of thyroid disease in the skin are vast and varied depending on the type of disease and its severity. Manifestations of thyroid conditions in the skin and hair will still present in patients with skin of color; however, they may appear in a more subtle form. There are many disparities in the outcomes of thyroid cancer and disease among patients with skin of color. These differences may mostly be related to the socioeconomic status of a patient, delays in diagnoses, and the patient's access to care in developing nations.

The role of the dermatologist is essential in recognizing the cutaneous manifestations of thyroid disease in the early stages. Increased awareness of the cutaneous symptoms of these conditions is likely to improve patient diagnoses and the initiation of treatment.

REFERENCES

1. Vanderpump MP. The epidemiology of thyroid disease. *Br Med Bull.* 2011;99:39-51.
2. Kanaya AM, Harris F, Volpato S, et al. Association between thyroid dysfunction and total cholesterol level in an older biracial population: the health, aging and body composition study. *Arch Intern Med.* 2002;162:773-779.
3. Sichieri R, Baima J, Marante T, et al. Low prevalence of hypothyroidism among black and Mulatto people in a population-based study of Brazilian women. *Clin Endocrinol.* 2007;66:803-807.
4. Daneshpazhooh M, Mostofizadeh GM, Behjati J, et al. Anti-thyroid peroxidase antibody and vitiligo: a controlled study. *BMC Dermatol.* 2006;6:3.
5. González GC, Capel I, Rodríguez-Espinosa J, et al. Thyroid autoimmunity at onset of type 1 diabetes as a predictor of thyroid dysfunction. *Diabetes Care.* 2007;30:1611-1612.
6. Seyrafi H, Akhiani M, Abbasi H, et al. Evaluation of the profile of alopecia areata and the prevalence of thyroid function test abnormalities and serum autoantibodies in Iranian patients. *BMC Dermatol.* 2005;5:11.
7. Hollowell JG, Staehling NW, Flanders WD, et al. Serum TSH, T4, and thyroid antibodies in the United States population (1988–1994): National Health and Nutrition Examination Study (NHANES III). *J Clin Endocrinol Metab.* 2002;87:489-499.
8. Kalk WJ. Atypical features of hyperthyroidism in blacks. *S Afr Med J.* 1980;57:707-710.
9. Gayathri R, Lavanya S, Raghavan K. Subclinical hypothyroidism and autoimmune thyroiditis in pregnancy: a study in south Indian subjects. *J Assoc Physicians India.* 2009;57:691-693.
10. Morris LGT, Sikora AG, Myssiorek DJ, et al. Racial patterns of thyroid cancer incidence in the United States. Presented at the American Academy of Otolaryngology Head and Neck Surgery (AAOHNS) Meeting, September 17, 2007. http://www.newswise.com/articles/lower-rate-of-thyroid-cancer-in-african-americans-may-be-caused-by-lax-detection-efforts. Accessed January 13, 2012.
11. Waguespack, S, Wells, S, Ross, J, et al. Thyroid cancer. In: Bleyer A, O'Leary M, Barr R, et al, eds. *Cancer Epidemiology in Older Adolescents and Young Adults 15 to 29 Years of Age, Including SEER Incidence and Survival: 1975-2000.* Bethesda, MD: National Cancer Institute; 2006:143-154.
12. Aschebrook-Kilfoy B, Ward MH, Sabra MM, et al. Thyroid cancer incidence patterns in the United States by histologic type, 1992–2006. *Thyroid.* 2011;21:125-134.
13. Ogbera AO, Kuku SF. Epidemiology of thyroid diseases in Africa. *Indian J Endocrinol Metab.* 2011;15:S82-S88.
14. Safer JD. Thyroid hormone action on skin. *Curr Opin Endocrinol Diabetes Obes.* 2012;19:388-393.
15. Doshi DN, Blyumin ML, Kimball AB. Cutaneous manifestations of thyroid disease. *Clin Dermatol.* 2008;26:283-287.
16. Diven DG, Gwinup G, Newton RC. The thyroid. *Dermatol Clin.* 1989;7:547-558.
17. Burman KD, McKinley-Grant L. Dermatologic aspects of thyroid disease. *Clin Dermatol* 2006;24:247-255.
18. Ai J, Leonhardt JM, Heymann WR. Autoimmune thyroid diseases: etiology, pathogenesis, and dermatologic manifestations. *J Am Acad Dermatol.* 2003;48:641-659.
19. Chen QY, Nadell D, Zhang XY, et al. The human leukocyte antigen HLA DRB3*020/DQA1*0501 haplotype is associated with Graves' disease in African Americans. *J Clin Endocrinol Metab.* 2000;85:1545-1549.
20. Daumerie C. Epidemiology. In: Wiersinga WM, Kahaly GJ, eds. *Graves' Orbitopathy: A Multidisciplinary Approach—Questions and Answers.* 2nd ed. Basel, Switzerland: Karger Publishers; 2010:33-39.
21. Tallstedt I, Lundell G, Tørring O, et al. Occurence of ophthalmopathy after treatment for Graves' hyperthyroidism. *N Engl J Med.* 1992;326:1733-1738.
22. Fatourechi V, Pajouhi M, Fransway AF. Dermopathy of Graves' disease (pretibial myxedema). Review of 150 cases. *Medicine (Baltimore).* 1994;73:1-7.
23. Fatourechi V. Pretibial myxedema: pathophysiology and treatment options. *Am J Clin Dermatol.* 2005;6:295-309.
24. Anderson CK, Miller OF 3rd. Triad of exophthalmos, pretibial myxedema, and acropachy in a patient with Graves' disease. *J Am Acad Dermatol.* 2003;48:970-972.
25. Georgala S, Katoulis AC, Georgala C, et al. Pretibial myxedema as the initial manifestation of Graves' disease. *J Eur Acad Dermatol Venereol.* 2002;16:380-383.
26. Parving HH, Hansen JM, Nielsen SL, et al. Mechanisms of edema formation in myxedema-increased protein extravasation and relatively slow lymphatic drainage. *N Engl J Med.* 1979;301:460-465.
27. Fatourechi V, Ahmed DD, Schwartz KM. Thyroid acropachy: report of 40 patients treated at a single institution in a 26-year period. *J Clin Endocrinol Metab.* 2002;87:5435-5441.
28. Slatosky J, Shipton B, Wahba H. Thyroiditis: differential diagnosis and management. *Am Fam Physician.* 2000;61:1047-1052.
29. Smit JW, Stokkel MP, Pereira AM, et al. Bexarotene-induced hypothyroidism: bexarotene stimulates the peripheral metabolism of thyroid hormones. *J Clin Endocrinol Metab.* 2007;92:2496-2499.
30. Heymann WR. Advances in cutaneous manifestations of thyroid disease. *Int J Dermatol.* 1997;36:641-645.
31. Puri N. A study on cutaneous manifestations of thyroid disease. *Indian J Dermatol.* 2012;57:247-248.
32. Dekio S, Imaoka C, Jidoi J. Candida folliculitis associated with hypothyroidism. *Br J Dermatol.* 1987;117:663-664.
33. Lyakhovitsky A, Shemer A, Amichai B. Increased prevalence of thyroid disorders in patients with new onset alopecia areata. *Australas J Dermatol.* 2015;56:103-106.
34. Kasumagic-Halilovic E, Prohic A, Begovic B, et al. Association between vitiligo and thyroid autoimmunity. *J Thyroid Res.* 2011;2011:938257.
35. Lee HJ, Kim MY, Ha SJ, et al. Two cases of morphea associated with Hashimoto's thyroiditis. *Acta Derm Venereol.* 2002;82:58-59.
36. Dix JH, Levy WJ, Fuenning C. Remission of acanthosis nigricans, hypertrichosis, and Hashimoto's thyroiditis with thyroxine replacement. *Pediatr Dermatol.* 1986;3:323-326.
37. De Paola M, Batsikosta A, Feci L, et al. Granuloma annulare, autoimmune thyroiditis, and lichen sclerosus in a woman: randomness or significant association? *Case Rep Dermatol Med.* 2013;2013:289084.
38. Lutfi RJ, Fridmanis M, Misiunas AL, et al. Association of melasma with thyroid autoimmunity and other thyroidal abnormalities and their relationship to the origin of the melasma. *J Clin Endocrinol Metab.* 1985;61:28-31.
39. Ertam I, Karaca N, Ceylan C, et al. Discrete papular dermal mucinosis with Hashimoto thyroiditis: a case report. *Cutis.* 2011;87:143-145.
40. Kreuter A, Kryvosheyeva Y, Terras S, et al. Association of autoimmune diseases with lichen sclerosus in 532 male and female patients. *Acta Derm Venereol.* 2013;93:238-241.
41. Kumar KV, Priya S, Sharma R, et al. Autoimmune thyroid disease in patients with vitiligo: prevalence study in India. *Endocr Pract.* 2012;18:194-199.
42. Hollenbeak CS, Wang L, Schneider P, et al. Outcomes of thyroid cancer in African Americans. *Ethn Dis.* 2011;21:210-215.
43. Alwaheeb S, Ghazarian D, Boerner SL, et al. Cutaneous manifestations of thyroid cancer: a report of four cases and review of the literature. *J Clin Pathol.* 2004;57:435-438.
44. Schwartz RA. Cutaneous metastatic disease. *J Am Acad Dermatol.* 1995;33:161-186.
46. Richards ML. Type 2 multiple endocrine neoplasia. http://misc.medscape.com/pi/iphone/medscapeapp/html/A123447-business.html. Accessed January 13, 2013.
45. Marquard J, Eng C. Multiple endocrine neoplasia type 2. In: Pagon RA, Adam MP, Ardinger HH, et al., Eds. GeneReviews®. Seattle, WA: University of Washington, 2015.
47. Online Mendelian Inheritance in Man. Carney Complex, Type 1; CNC1. http://omim.org/entry/160980. Accessed February 26, 2013.
48. Online Mendelian Inheritance in Man. Protein Kinase, cAMP-dependent, Regulatory, Type I, alpha; PRKAR1A. http://omim.org/entry/188830. Accessed February 26, 2013.
49. Online Mendelian Inheritance in Man. Phosphatase and Tensin Homolog; PTEN. http://www.omim.org/entry/601728. Accessed February 26, 2013.
50. Online Mendelian Inheritance in Man. Cowden Syndrome 1; CWS1. http://www.omim.org/entry/158350. Accessed February 26, 2013.

Cosmetic Dermatology

Photoaging

CHAPTER 77

Chee Leok Goh
Angeline Anning Yong

KEY POINTS

- Race, cultural behavior, nature of occupation, hobbies, and smoking habit can affect the photoaging process.
- The skin of people with skin of color varies considerably in its response to sun exposure and the process of photoaging in view of the wide range of skin phototypes.
- The melanin in darker skin type appears to confer protection against the photoaging effect of ultraviolet B and A radiation.
- Fairer-skinned individuals tend to develop earlier onset of photoaging and develop more prominent wrinkles and skin laxity than those with skin of color.
- People with skin of color tend to have less coarse wrinkles, skin sagging, telangiectasia, actinic keratoses, and skin cancers but tend to manifest with more pigmentary disorders (eg, lentigo and melasma) and uneven skin tones. In addition, as a result of the reduced extrinsic aging changes, signs of intrinsic aging, such as volume loss, can appear accentuated.

INTRODUCTION

Skin aging in all skin types can be divided into two basic processes: intrinsic aging and extrinsic aging (photoaging).[1] Intrinsic aging is a natural process that occurs with time and manifests as skin thinning, laxity, fine wrinkles, and xerosis.[2] Race, anatomic sites, and hormonal changes can influence the intrinsic aging process.[3] On the other hand, extrinsic aging results in premature skin aging on chronically photodamaged skin. Photoaging is characterized by deep wrinkles, senile purpura, pigmentary disorders (eg, solar lentigines and seborrheic keratoses), telangiectasis, skin sagging, actinic keratoses, and skin cancers.[2] Race, cultural behavior, nature of occupation, hobbies, and smoking habit can affect the photoaging process.[3] There are differences in photoaging changes between people with skin of color and Caucasians.

DEFINING SKIN OF COLOR

Most of the world's population are individuals with skin of color, including Asians, Hispanics, and Africans. Asians can be subdivided into East Asians (Chinese, Koreans, Japanese), Southeast Asians (Indonesians, Malaysians, Singaporeans, Thais, Cambodians, Vietnamese, Filipinos), and South Asians (Bangladeshis, Pakistanis, Sri Lankans, Indians). Both East Asians and Southeast Asians are of Mongoloid background. Those from East Asia have lighter skin color, whereas Southeast Asians have darker brownish skin color. South Asians, on the other hand, are of Caucasian origin but have brown to dark brown skin.[4]

Hispanics are a large group with varied skin color. A large number of Hispanics worldwide are brown-skinned, but European Hispanics who are of Caucasian origin are lighter in skin color. There are also Hispanics who are of mixed ancestry, with Caucasian and African American or Native American heritage. The geographic areas for brown-skinned Hispanics include North America, Mexico, Central and South America, and the Caribbean.[4]

Thus the term *skin of color* includes an extremely heterogeneous group of peoples. Patients with skin of color generally have Fitzpatrick skin phototypes III to VI. With this wide range of skin colors, the skin of people with skin of color varies considerably in its response to sun exposure and the process of photoaging.[4]

PHOTOAGING IN SKIN OF COLOR

Photoaging is observed in people of all racial groups.[5] However, people with skin of color have delayed or less pronounced photoaging changes and have different dominant manifestations. This is believed to be due to the increased epidermal melanin in pigmented skin, which confers a natural photoprotective effect.[6,7]

Ultraviolet (UV) radiation has been established as an important factor in promoting the development of cutaneous malignancies and photoaging. In a 1979 study, Kaidbey et al[8] compared the transmission of UV radiation on Caucasian and dark skin of color cadaver skin. They found that the mean protective factor for UVB in the epidermis of dark skin of color was 13.4 compared with 3.4 in the lighter-skinned epidermis, and the mean UVB transmission into the dermis was 5.7% in the epidermis of dark skin of color versus 29.4% in the epidermis of lighter-colored skin.[8] For UVA, the mean protective factor of dark skin of color epidermis was 5.7 compared to 1.8 in lighter-colored epidermis, and the mean UVA transmission into dark skin of color epidermis was 17.5% compared with 55.5% for lighter-colored epidermis.[8] Therefore, three to four times more UVA reaches the upper dermis of fairer-skinned individuals than that of people with dark skin of color. The main site of UV filtration in the former was the stratum corneum, whereas the malpighian layers removed twice as much UVB radiation as the overlying stratum corneum in the latter.[8]

Studies have also demonstrated differences in the damaging effects of chronic sun exposure in skin of color. Yamaguchi et al[9] reported that the incidence of UV-induced apoptosis was greater in darker skin compared to lighter skin, suggesting that photodamaged cells may be more efficiently removed in darker skin.[9] Del Bino et al[10] reported the relationship between skin color and response to UV exposure using ex vivo light and dark skin samples. A biologically efficient UV dose was determined for each sample by quantifying sunburn cells. The biologic markers include DNA damage, apoptosis, and p53 accumulation. A statistically significant correlation was reported between the biologically efficient dose and DNA damage. In light, intermediate, and tanned skin samples, DNA-damaged lesions were distributed throughout the epidermis and the uppermost dermal cells. In brown and dark skin samples, DNA-damaged lesions were confined to the suprabasal epidermal layers. These results demonstrate a progressive decrease in sensitivity to UV exposure with increasing skin pigmentation. This susceptibility was thought to be predictive of an individual's proneness to developing the damaging effects of chronic sun exposure, skin cancer, and photoaging, confirming that skin pigmentation can have a natural protective role against photodamage.[10]

RACIAL DIFFERENCES IN PHOTOAGING

Although all people are prone to photoaging, Caucasian or fairer-skinned individuals tend to develop earlier onset of photoaging and develop more prominent wrinkles and skin laxity than those with skin of color. People with skin of color tend to have less coarse wrinkles, skin sagging, telangiectasia, actinic keratosis, and skin cancers but tend to manifest with more pigmentary disorders and uneven skin tones.[11] As a result of the reduced extrinsic aging changes, signs of intrinsic aging, such as volume loss, can appear accentuated.

SPECIFIC PHOTOAGING CHANGES IN SKIN OF COLOR

■ PHOTOAGING IN DARK SKIN OF COLOR

Photoaging does occur in individuals with dark skin of color but is uncommon or mild because the epidermis and upper dermis are protected against photodamage by the increased number of melanosomes and melanin in the keratinocytes. Photoaging is seen more frequently in African Americans than in Africans or Afro-Caribbeans. This may be because African Americans consist of a heterogeneous mix of African, Caucasian, and Native American ancestry.[4] Published reports on photoaging in individuals with dark skin of color have been limited to African Americans.

Histologic preservation of epidermal and dermal components has been demonstrated in sun-exposed African American skin in contrast to sun-exposed Caucasian skin. Montagna and Carlisle[12] compared 19 dark-skinned women of African descent and 19 lighter-skinned women and found that long-term sun exposure resulted in only minor changes in the former compared to profound alterations in the latter. The majority of the lighter-skinned women aged between 45 and 50 years had wrinkles beside the lateral canthi of the eyes and at the corners of the mouth, whereas none of the dark skin of color women showed any obvious wrinkles. In their study, punch biopsies obtained from the malar eminences showed that in fair sun-exposed skin, the stratum lucidum was usually distorted, swollen, and distinctly cellular, whereas darker sun-exposed skin remained compact and rarely showed any evidence of alteration in the stratum lucidum regardless of age. A greater amount of solar elastosis was also found in fairer skin compared to darker skin.[12] This presence of elastotic material in fairer skin is an important factor in dermal photodamage.[13] Elastotic tissue is constantly resorbed and replaced with other elastotic tissue and large collagenous fiber bundles, resulting in shrinkage and reduction of dermal volume. This process occurs less precipitously in the facial skin of young and middle-aged women with dark skin of color.[12] Consequently, a naturally youthful appearance can be maintained well into later life, with photoaging appearing usually late in the fifth or sixth decades of life in this group.[14]

Clinical features of photoaging in African Americans include fine wrinkling and laxity with aging, particularly in the deeper muscular layers of the face, with sagging of malar fat pads toward the nasolabial fold.[15] Hyperpigmentation and uneven skin tone have also been reported to be a greater concern in African American skin compared to Caucasian skin.[16] Mottled pigmentation and dermatosis papulosa nigra (DPN) are other common manifestations of photoaging in individuals with dark skin of color [**Figure 77-1**]. Although the pathogenesis for the formation of DPN is not completely understood, Niang et al[17] proposed that UV radiation is a potential pathogenic factor because lesions were found to be limited to sun-exposed areas in the African population of Senegal.

■ PHOTOAGING IN HISPANICS

Sanchez[18] showed that photoaging was the third most common dermatologic diagnosis in 1000 Hispanic patients treated in a dermatology practice in the United States, accounting for 16.8% of visits. Because the Hispanic population comprises individuals of varying skin phototypes, the lighter-pigmented Hispanics tend to exhibit photoaging signs similar to Caucasians individuals, whereas the darker-skin Hispanics tend show

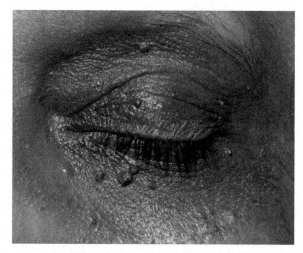

FIGURE 77-1. Clinical features of photoaging in individuals with dark skin of color include mottled pigmentation and dermatosis papulosa nigra, as seen in this patient. (Courtesy of National Skin Centre, Singapore.)

photoaging signs similar to African Americans and other populations of African descent.[19]

Photoaging in European and lighter-skin Hispanics occurs in the same frequency and degree as in Caucasians. As such, the clinical manifestation is primarily wrinkling rather than pigmentary alterations. Coarse wrinkling also appears at the same age at which it would appear in Caucasians. Darker-skin Hispanics who have skin phototypes IV and V and who live in sunny tropical climates such as Mexico, Central America, or South America tend to have clinical photoaging manifestations similar to those of South Asians and African Americans. These manifestations include fine wrinkling and mottled pigmentation. Melasma is a common pigmentary disorder [**Figure 77-2**] that occurs in the late fourth through sixth decades of life.[4] Hernández-Pérez and Ibiett[20] listed photoaging effects in Salvadorans, including fine wrinkles, dilated pores, thick skin, oily skin, telangiectasias, lentigines, and laxity of the skin, which responded well to intense pulsed light treatment.

■ PHOTOAGING IN ASIANS

Much attention has been directed toward the effects, prevention, and treatment of photoaging, in particular skin discoloration, in Asians in recent years. Many studies on photoaging have been carried out recently in East and Southeast Asians with skin of color. In East and South East Asia, photoaging is common because of the geographic proximity to the equator where sunlight exposure is continuous throughout the year. In

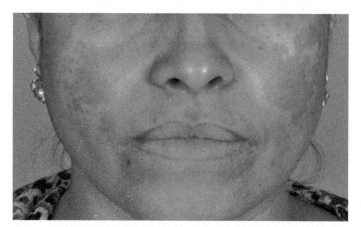

FIGURE 77-2. Darker-skinned Hispanics who have skin phototypes IV and V tend to have photoaging changes that are similar to South Asians and African Americans. This patient has melasma over her cheeks.

addition, the traditional desire of Asians to have fair and flawless facial skin, uniform in color and texture, has led to individuals seeking treatment of pigmentary disorders that are associated with photoaging in skin of color. Thus, the pigmentary changes associated with photoaging in Asians with skin of color are significant cosmetic problems for these patients.[21]

Characteristic features of photoaging in the Asian population with skin of color have been well described. The effects are attributed not only to inherent genetic differences in the biologic defenses of the skin, but may also be augmented by the different cultural practices related to sun exposure. Unlike Caucasians, Asians, such as Koreans, Japanese, and Chinese, traditionally avoid direct sunlight by wearing long-sleeved clothes, carrying umbrellas, or seeking shade. Asians have natural photoaging protection, including a thicker stratum corneum, and increased epidermal melanin. The primary difference between Caucasian and Asian skin, however, is attributed to melanocytic function. Because Asian skin is more pigmented, its acute and chronic cutaneous responses to UV radiation differ from Caucasian skin.[22]

In an evaluation of 1500 Asian patients with skin phototypes III and IV from Singapore, Indonesia, and Malaysia, Goh[23] reported that the main features of photoaging included hyperpigmentation, tactile roughness, and coarse and fine wrinkling. However, skin wrinkling was not readily apparent in these populations until about 50 years of age, and even then, the extent of wrinkling was less marked than in Caucasian skin.

In another study conducted on Chinese and Japanese patients by Griffiths et al,[24] pigmentary changes seemed to be a more important feature in photoaged skin than wrinkling. Histologic diagnoses of photoaging in this group include seborrheic keratoses, solar lentigines, and solar elastosis.[24]

A later study by Chung,[22] however, showed that rhytide formation could also be a major feature of photoaging in Koreans. This study showed that Asians have thicker, coarser, and deeper rhytides concentrated on the forehead as well as the periocular and perioral areas, whereas Caucasians have relatively fine wrinkles on their cheeks and the crow's feet area.[22] These differences in the pattern of skin wrinkling suggest the possibility that there may be wrinkle-associated genes or single-nucleotide polymorphisms in certain genes, such as those for collagen, elastin, or matrix metalloproteinase.[22] However, no scientific evidence has been established to date. In Koreans, patterns of pigmentary change related to aging have been shown to be dependent on gender. The most common pigmented lesions in sun-exposed skin include ephelides (freckling), melasma, lentigo, mottled pigmentation, and pigmented seborrheic keratoses. The appearance of solar lentigines increases with age and is more common in women, whereas the incidence of seborrheic keratosis also increases with age but is more common in men.[25]

Nonetheless, the primary clinical feature of photoaging in East and Southeast Asians is that of discrete pigmentary changes, which predominate over acquired rhytides. These include solar lentigines, pigmented seborrheic keratoses, and mottled hyperpigmentation [**Figure 77-3, A–C**], with very little manifestation of skin wrinkling. Sun-induced facial melasma is also more common in this group than in Caucasians and should be considered a form of actinic dyspigmentation and a contributor to photoaging in this instance.[4,21,26] It is not uncommon for photoaging in these individuals to present as a combination of multiple skin pigmentary disorders (eg, lentigines, melasma, acquired dermal melanocytosis) [**Figure 77-4**].

There are few studies describing photoaging changes in South Asians with skin of color. Sun-related hyperpigmentation, seborrheic keratoses, and DPN have been reported to be seen with increasing age, but fine wrinkling is not as apparent.[21]

Durai et al[2] reported 500 consecutive elderly individuals with skin phototypes IV and V attending the dermatology outpatient department in Puducherry, India, and found that the majority (83%) of the cases were found to have chronologic aging without photoaging, and only a minority (17%) of cases had photoaging along with chronologic aging.[2] Cutaneous changes suggestive of photoaging such as dyspigmentation (13%), freckles (4.8%), thick skin (3.2%), deep wrinkles (2.4%), melasma

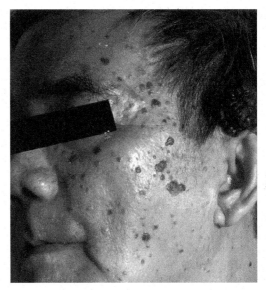

A

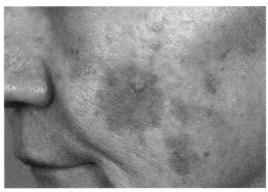

B

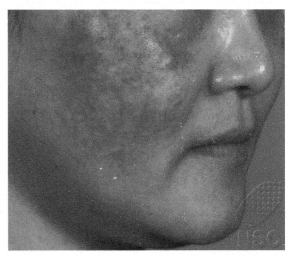

C

FIGURE 77-3. **(A–C)** Photoaging in Chinese is characterized by solar lentigines, flat pigmented seborrheic keratoses, mottled hyperpigmentation, and fine wrinkles. (Courtesy of National Skin Centre, Singapore.)

(2.4%), citrine skin (1%), senile purpura (1%), pseudostellate scars (0.4%), acrokeratoelastoidosis marginalis (0.4%), and lentigines (0.2%) were less frequently observed in this study than other reports. In contrast, Beauregard and Gilchrest[27] observed elastosis in 95.6%, lentigines in 70.6%, senile purpura in 11.9%, and stellate pseudoscars in 5.9% of his Caucasian patients in the United States.

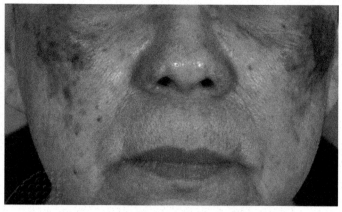

FIGURE 77-4. Typical photoaging changes in a Chinese woman include combination pigmentary disorders (eg, melasma, lentigines, acquired dermal melanocytosis) on sun-exposed areas with little fine wrinkling. Coarse wrinkling is generally absent. (Courtesy of National Skin Centre, Singapore.)

OTHER CONTRIBUTORY FACTORS TO PHOTOAGING IN SKIN OF COLOR

◼ SMOKING

Smoking has been associated with an increased risk of premature photoaging and rhytide formation. This has been found predominantly in fairer skin and less often in skin of color.[28] In Caucasians, premature wrinkling was found to increase with the number of smoking pack-years. Kadunce et al[29] found that individuals who smoked more than 50 pack-years were 2.3 to 4.7 times more likely to develop facial wrinkles than nonsmokers. When excessive sun exposure and smoking coexisted, their effects on wrinkling on skin were synergistic. In the brown skin of Koreans, the odds ratios of wrinkling associated with 30 and 50 pack-years of smoking were 2.8 and 5.5, respectively, after controlling for age, gender, and sun exposure.[25] The effects of sun exposure and smoking were synergistic and presented an 11-fold increased risk for wrinkling compared to nonsmokers in a less sun-exposed group.[25] Yin et al[30] also reported a 22-fold increase in more severe skin wrinkling in Japanese participants who smoked more than 30 pack-years and were exposed to the sun for more than 2 hours per day, compared to those of the same age who never smoked and had sun exposure levels of less than 2 hours per day.[30] These studies suggest that cigarette smoking is an independent risk factor for the development of rhytides in Asians, as in the Caucasians. Furthermore, cigarette smoking also acts synergistically with the effects of aging and sun exposure. These studies have not been performed in other skin of color populations.

◼ RECREATIONAL ACTIVITIES AND OUTDOOR OCCUPATIONS

Many individuals with skin of color live in sunny, tropical areas and are employed in outdoor occupations or engage in outdoor recreational activities that expose their skin to sunlight. Individuals with skin of color often do not believe or understand that they need photoprotection when involved in either recreational or occupational activities that result in sun exposure. It has been shown that many of these people do not protect themselves with sunscreen when exposed to the sun, and studies have shown that sunscreen use is less prevalent in the African American and Hispanic populations than among Caucasians.[31,32] This is changing now as public education concerning sun exposure and proper protection has become more widespread.[33]

CONCLUSION

Aging is a global problem, and the desire to halt, retard, or reverse this process is observed in all patient population. Although Caucasian skin is more prone to UV light injury while those with skin of color are more protected against its effect, the latter also exhibit their own characteristic photoaging changes.

The cutaneous manifestations of photoaging can differ significantly between Caucasians and those with skin of color. Pigmentation disorders are more commonly observed with photoaging in individuals with skin of color, whereas wrinkles and telangiectasia are more common in Caucasians. As in light-skinned individuals, adequate photoprotection is important in preventing the detrimental effects of UV radiation in individuals with skin of color

REFERENCES

1. Gilchrest BA. Skin aging and photoaging: an overview. *J Am Acad Dermatol.* 1989;21:610-613.
2. Durai PC, Thappa DM, Kumari R, et al. Aging in elderly: chronological versus photoaging. *Indian J Dermatol.* 2012;57:343-352.
3. Farage MA, Miller KW, Elsner P, et al. Intrinsic and extrinsic factors in skin aging: a review. *Int J Cosmet Sci.* 2008;30:87-95.
4. Halder RM, Richards GM. Photoaging in patients of skin of color. In: Rigel DS, Weiss RA, Lim HW, et al, eds. *Photoaging.* New York, NY: Marcel Dekker; 2004:55-63.
5. Griffiths CE, Goldfarb MT, Finkel LJ, et al. Topical tretinoin treatment of hyperpigmented lesions associated with photoaging in Chinese and Japanese patients: a vehicle-controlled trial. *J Am Acad Dermatol.* 1994;30:76-84.
6. Kligman AM. Solar elastosis in relation to pigmentation. In: Fitzpatrick TB, Pathak MA, Harber L, et al, eds. *Sunlight and Man.* Tokyo, Japan: University of Tokyo Press; 1974:157-163.
7. Pathak MA, Fitzpatrick TB. The role of natural photoprotective agents in human skin. In: Fitzpatrick TB, Pathak MA, Harber L, et al, eds. *Sunlight and Man.* Tokyo, Japan: University of Tokyo Press; 1974:725-750.
8. Kaidbey KH, Agin PP, Sayre RM, et al. Photoprotection by melanin: a comparison of black and Caucasian skin. *J Am Acad Dermatol.* 1979;1:249-260.
9. Yamaguchi Y, Takahashi K, Zmudzka BZ, et al. Human skin responses to UV radiation: pigment in the upper epidermis protects against DNA damage in the lower epidermis and facilitates apoptosis. *FASEB J.* 2006;20:1486-1488.
10. Del Bino S, Sok J, Bessac E, et al. Relationship between skin response to ultraviolet exposure and skin color type. *Pigment Cell Res.* 2006;19:606-614.
11. Rawlings AV. Ethnic skin types: are there differences in skin structure and function? *Int J Cosmet Sci.* 2006;28:79-93.
12. Montagna W, Carlisle K. The architecture of black and white facial skin. *J Am Acad Dermatol.* 1991;24(6 Pt 1):929-937.
13. Montagna W, Kirchner S, Carlisle K. Histology of sun-damaged human skin. *J Am Acad Dermatol.* 1989;21(5 Pt 1):907-918.
14. Halder RM. The role of retinoids in the management of cutaneous conditions in blacks. *J Am Acad Dermatol.* 1998;39(2 Pt 3):S98-S103.
15. Matory WE. Skin care. In: Matory WE, ed. *Ethnic Considerations in Facial Aesthetic Surgery.* Philadelphia, PA: Lippincott-Raven; 1998:100.
16. Grimes P, Edison BL, Green BA, et al. Evaluation of inherent differences between African American and white skin surface properties using subjective and objective measures. *Cutis.* 2004;73:392-396.
17. Niang SO, Kane A, Diallo M, et al. Dermatosis papulosa nigra in Dakar, Senegal. *Int J Dermatol.* 2007;46(suppl 1):45-47.
18. Sanchez MR. Cutaneous diseases in Latinos. *Dermatol Clin.* 2003;21:689-697.
19. Taylor SC. Skin of color: biology, structure, function and implications for dermatologic disease. *J Am Acad Dermatol.* 2002;46(suppl 2):S41-S62.
20. Hernández-Pérez E, Ibiett EV. Gross and microscopic findings in patients submitted to nonablative full-face resurfacing using intense pulsed light: a preliminary study. *Dermatol Surg.* 2002;28:651-655.
21. Munavalli GS, Weiss RA, Halder RM. Photoaging and nonablative photorejuvenation in ethnic skin. *Dermatol Surg.* 2005;31:1250-1261.
22. Chung JH. Photoaging in Asians. *Photodermatol Photoimmunol Photomed.* 2003;19:109-121.
23. Goh SH. The treatment of visible signs of senescence: the Asian experience. *Br J Dermatol.* 1990;122:105-109.
24. Griffiths CE, Goldfarb MT, Finkel LJ, et al. Topical tretinoin treatment of hyperpigmented lesions associated with photoaging in Chinese and Japanese patients: a vehicle-controlled trial. *J Am Acad Dermatol.* 1994;30:76-84.
25. Chung JH, Lee SH, Youn CS, et al. Cutaneous photodamage in Koreans: influence of sex, sun exposure, smoking, and skin color. *Arch Dermatol.* 2001; 137:1043-1051.
26. Alexis AF, Rossi A. Photoaging in skin of color. *Cosmet Dermatol.* 2011;24: 367-370.

27. Beauregard S, Gilchrest BA. A survey of skin problems and skin care regimens in the elderly. *Arch Dermatol.* 1987;123:1638-1643.

28. Allen HB, Johnson BL, Diamond SM. Smoker's wrinkles? *JAMA.* 1973;225:1067-1069.

29. Kadunce DP, Burr R, Gress R, et al. Cigarette smoking: risk factor for premature facial wrinkling. *Ann Intern Med.* 1991;114:840-844.

30. Yin L, Morita A, Tsuji T. Epidemiological and molecular study on the premature skin aging induced by environmental factors: ultraviolet exposure and tobacco smoking. *J Invest Dermatol.* 2000;114:803A.

31. Hall HI, Jones SE, Saraiya M. Prevalence and correlates of sunscreen use among US high school students. *J Sch Health.* 2001;71:453-457.

32. Dawn M. Holman, Zahava Berkowitz, Gery P. Guy Jr., Nikki A. Hawkins, Mona Saraiya, Meg Watson. Patterns of sunscreen use on the face and other exposed skin among US adults. *J Am Acad Dermatol.* epub May 19, 2015.

33. Agbai O, Buster K, Sanchez M, et al. Skin cancer and photoprotection in people of color: a review and recommendations for physicians and the public. *J Am Acad Dermatol.* 2014;70:748-762.

CHAPTER 78

Chemical Peels, Microdermabrasion, Hair Transplantation, and Sclerotherapy

Valerie D. Callender
Cherie M. Young
Chesahna Kindred

KEY POINTS

- With rising populations of skin of color, dermatologic surgeons must understand and recognize the particular issues and needs relevant to those with darker skin.

- Among all patients of color, the most frequently performed cosmetic procedures are soft tissue fillers, botulinum toxin injections, microdermabrasion, and chemical peels. Additionally, hair transplantation is becoming increasingly popular.

- Although the exact number of hair transplant procedures performed in persons of color is unknown, it is clear that as the awareness of alopecia in men and women grows, the numbers of hair transplantations in this group of patients will increase.

Cosmetic procedures are becoming increasingly more popular, and over the past 5 years, the number of cosmetic procedures performed has increased by approximately 2 million.[1] The most common nonsurgical procedures performed in 2012 were botulinum toxin injections, hyaluronic acid fillers, laser hair removal, microdermabrasion, and chemical peels.[1] Caucasian patients typically desire cosmetic procedures that diminish signs of photoaging: fine lines, rhytides, dyschromia, telangiectasias, and keratoses. In contrast, patients of color most often request cosmetic procedures for disorders of pigmentation, primarily postinflammatory hyperpigmentation (PIH).[2-5] Two of the most common nonsurgical cosmetic procedures being performed in the United States, which address disorders of pigmentation, are chemical peels and microdermabrasion,[1] and these procedures and techniques may require modifications and special considerations when performed in patients of color. Of note is the fact that sought after cosmetic procedures, such as sclerotherapy, may result in the complication of PIH.

Alopecia occurs commonly in skin of color populations, leading to demand for hair transplantation surgery. Racial differences in hair and hair follicle morphology may necessitate differences in surgical instrument selection and surgical technique.

With rising populations of skin of color come increasing demands on cosmetic dermatologic surgeons, who must understand and recognize the particular issues and needs relevant to those with darker skin. Because the bulk of published data on cosmetic procedures thus far has focused on the Caucasian population, performing aesthetic procedures on patients with skin of color remains a challenge. Clearly, the medical community must expand its knowledge of the cosmetic issues relevant to this growing patient population. In this chapter the safety and efficacy of the following procedures in skin of color will be reviewed: chemical peels, microdermabrasion, hair transplantation, and sclerotherapy.

CHEMICAL PEELS

Chemical peeling is the process of applying one or more chemical agents to the skin for the purpose of exfoliating the epidermis or dermis, thus creating a wound that subsequently reepithelializes. Chemical peels are performed using superficial, medium-depth, or deep peeling agents. Superficial peels, with agents such as glycolic acid (GA), salicylic acid (SA), lactic acid (LA), Jessner's solution, trichloracetic acid (TCA) in concentrations of 10% to 30%, and lipohydroxy acid (LHA) in concentrations of 5% to 10%, penetrate the stratum corneum to the papillary dermis. Medium-depth peels reach the upper reticular dermis and include TCA (35% to 50% concentration), Jessner's solution combined with TCA 35%, GA 70% combined with TCA 35%, and phenol 88%. Deep chemical peels using the Baker-Gordon phenol formula penetrate to the midreticular dermis. Superficial and medium-depth peels may be performed safely on Fitzpatrick skin types IV to VI [**Table 78-1**].

TYPES OF PEELING AGENTS

Many agents are available for use in chemical peeling. The choice of agent should depend in part on its established safety and efficacy profiles in individuals of color. Although few published studies have evaluated peeling in darker skin, we have experienced excellent results in the treatment of skin of color patients.

Glycolic Acid GA, the most readily available peeling agent, belongs to a family of naturally occurring α-hydroxy acids (AHAs).[6] AHA peels have been used to treat a host of skin conditions, including melasma, hyperpigmentation disorders, photodamage, and acne. Improvement of these skin conditions has been observed with the use of AHA peels by their ability to thin the stratum corneum, diminish intercellular bonding,[7] promote epidermolysis, disperse basal layer melanin, and increase collagen synthesis within the dermis.[8]

A skin test always should precede treatment with GA peels in skin of color patients. Most chemical peeling is performed with GA concentrations ranging from a low of 30% to a high of 70%. Peeling with a 70% gel formulation delivers a high concentration of GA to the skin with a reduced risk of scarring.[6] Both superficial and medium-depth peeling are possible with GA, with increased concentrations of GA and a lower pH producing deeper peels.

Asian skin in particular shows benefits with GA peels, which are used often to treat facial skin with PIH, ephelides, lentigines, and melasma.[9] Compared with other superficial peeling agents, GA may produce more benefit in darker skin that is dry and sensitive.[10]

Lactic Acid Lactic acid is also an AHA peeling agent, with properties similar to GA.[11] It has been found to be safe and effective in the treatment of melasma and acne scarring in darker skin types and is a relatively inexpensive treatment.

Phytic Acid This is a newer AHA agent with a low pH. The advantage of this agent in comparison with the traditional AHA agents is that it does not require neutralization, and therefore, excessive peeling is avoided. Side effects that are typically observed with traditional AHAs, such as burning, do not occur with these peels. The phytic acid peel solution is applied and left on the face overnight .These peels are applied once a week if necessary. Five to six sessions are usually required to achieve adequate lightening, and they have been found to be safe and effective in the treatment of melasma in darker skin types, although studies are needed for further evaluation.[11]

Pyruvic Acid This is considered an α-keto-peel that has keratolytic, antimicrobial, and sebostatic properties. It also has the ability to stimulate the formation of new collagen and elastin fibers.[11]

TABLE 78-1	Studies evaluating chemical peels in FST IV-VI patients					
Author, year	Population studied	Diagnosis	Topical therapy	Type of peel	Response	Adverse events
Burns et al,[25] 1997	19 skin type IV–VI African Americans	PIH	T 0.05% cream + 2% HQ/10% GA	GA 50% GA 68%	Decreased HASI by 50% in peel group vs 42% in controls	Erythema, superficial desquamation, and vesiculation
Lim and Tham,[33] 1997	10 Asian women	Melasma, fine wrinkles	20% HQ and 10% HQ	GA 20%–70%	NSS	20% redness burns and transient PIH
Wang et al,[34] 1997	40 Asians	Acne	15% GA	GA 35% GA 50%	Significant resolution in acne	5.6% PIH, HSV flare, and mild skin irritation
Grimes,[13] 1999	25 V–VI African American and Hispanic women and men	Acne, PIH, melasma, oily skin, enlarged pores, and rough texture	4% HQ	SA 20% SA 30%	88% moderate to significant improvement	15% temporary crusting hypopigmentation, dryness, and hyperpigmentation
Javaheri et al,[28] 2001	25 East Indian women and men	Melasma	Sunscreen SPF 15, 10% GA, and oral acyclovir	GA 50%	46.7% epidermal, 27.8% mixed, 0% dermal	Hyperpigmentation
Al-Waiz and Al-Sharqi,[23] 2002	15 Dark-skinned women and men	Acne scars	RA cream in 3 patients	Jessner's solution + TCA 35%	6.6% significant 53.3% moderate 26.6% mild 6.6% minimal 6.6% no response	73.4% transient PIH
Sarkar et al,[26] 2002	40 East Indian patients	Melasma	HQ 5% + T 0.05% + HC 1% cream	GA peel in 20 patients	Decreased MASI in all patients, faster in peel group	Erythema, superficial desquamation, HSV, vesiculation, and PIH
Lee and Kim,[35] 2003	35 Korean patients	Acne vulgaris	N/A	30% salicylic acid peels	Decrease in inflammatory and noninflammatory lesion counts	Tolerable
Khunger et al,[29] 2004	10 East Indian women	Melasma	N/A	Split-faced study: 1% tretinoin peel vs 70% GA	Significant decrease in MASI; no difference between right vs left sides	Minimal
Kadhim and Al-Waiz,[19] 2005	12 Dark-skinned women and men	Periorbital wrinkles (fine/medium-sized)	N/A	Jessner's solution + TCA 35%	33% marked 25% moderate 25% mild 8% minimal 8% no response	Mild

Abbreviations: GA, glycolic acid; HASI, hyperpigmentation area severity index; HC, hydrocortisone acetate; HSV, herpes simplex virus; HQ, hydroquinone; MASI, melasma area severity index; N/A, not applicable; NSS, not statistically significant; PIH, postinflammatory hyperpigmentation; RA, retinoic acid; SA, salicylic acid; SPF, sun protection factor; T, tretinoin; TCA, trichloroacetic acid.

Although beneficial in the treatment of pigmentary disorders, the intense burning associated with this type of peeling agent has limited its use. There are no published studies with its use in skin of color.

Salicylic Acid SA is one of the older peeling agents and is used frequently. It belongs to the β-hydroxy acid family that occurs naturally in willow tree bark.[6] In 3% to 5% concentrations, SA is an effective keratolytic agent that improves the penetration of other peeling agents. One study assessing the keratolytic effect of SA in guinea pig skin demonstrated a reduction in the intercellular cohesiveness of the horny cells.[12] SA has anti-inflammatory properties and therefore decreases the PIH that can result from peeling.[11]

SA also has been found to be an effective comedolytic agent and is also used in the treatment of acne. It has been formulated in a variety of vehicles. Ethanol solutions of SA produce excellent benefits for many conditions, including acne, melasma, and PIH, in dark-skinned patients.[13]

Lipohydroxy Acid This is a newer derivative of SA that has an additional fatty chain with increased lipophilicity.[11] It modifies the stratum corneum, making it thinner, flexible, and resistant to wrinkling and cracking.[14] It possesses antibacterial, anti-inflammatory, antifungal, and anticomedonic properties and has a more targeted mechanism of action and greater keratolytic effect than the traditional SA.[14,15] It has a similar pH to the normal skin and has been proven to be tolerable and safe in darker skin types.[14] LHA peels do not require neutralization and are used mostly in the treatment of acne.[14,16]

Salicylic Mandelic Acid Peel This is a newer class of chemical peels that involves a combination of an AHA (mandelic acid) with a β-hydroxy acid (SA). There are no data published in its use in skin of color, but its benefit is in the slow and uniform penetration of the AHA, making it ideal for sensitive skin, and the quick penetration of the SA, with its added benefit of decreasing PIH.[11,17] These peels have proven to be efficacious for the treatment of acne and PIH.[11]

Trichloroacetic Acid TCA is an inorganic compound found in crystalline form. TCA 10% to 30% solutions deliver a superficial peel; however, the risks of PIH and scarring increase with the use of higher concentrations in skin of color. TCA may be used alone or in combination with GA or SA. Used in combination with GA, it has been demonstrated to improve mottled facial pigmentation.[6] TCA is also an effective treatment for acne scarring in skin of color patients.

Obagi Blue Peel This is a type of TCA peel that is composed of a fixed concentration of TCA with the blue peel base, consisting of glycerine, saponins, and a nonionic blue color base. A reduction in the surface tension of TCA, water, and glycerin occurs, which ensures a slow and more uniform penetration of TCA.[18]

Jessner's Solution Jessner's solution has been in use as a superficial peeling agent for several decades and penetrates into the papillary dermis. It is a combination of resorcinol 14 g, SA 14 g, and lactic acid 14 g in ethanol 95%. These three keratolytic agents used together produce a synergistic effect.

Jessner's solution is well tolerated in Fitzpatrick skin types IV to VI individuals, and an advantage of this agent is that it contains the phenolic skin-lightening agent resorcinol. Medium-depth peels using a combination of Jessner's solution followed by a 35% concentration of TCA have been found to be safe and effective in treating acne scars in patients with dark skin.[19]

Amino Fruit Acid Peel This is a relatively new class of chemical peels. There have been no studies on skin of color patients, but these peels have been effective in antiaging and treating photopigmentation in lighter-skinned patients.[20]

PATIENT SELECTION

Primary indications for chemical peels in patients with Fitzpatrick skin types IV to VI are PIH and melasma unresponsive to topical bleaching agents.[10,21] Other indications in darker-skinned individuals are acne vulgaris, acne scarring, oily skin, rough skin texture, pseudofolliculitis barbae, solar lentigines, and periorbital rhytids.[6,19] Within skin types IV to VI, individuals vary widely in their responses to chemical peeling, and therefore, the type of peel must be selected carefully.

INDICATIONS FOR CHEMICAL PEELS

Postinflammatory Hyperpigmentation Chemical peels are often effective for the treatment of postinflammatory hyperpigmentation because the procedure removes excess pigment from the skin.

Performing test spots with the peeling agent at specific sites of hyperpigmentation is a technique sometimes used in darker skin to establish how the skin will react to a particular agent. Peels are performed at 1-month intervals. All patients should be reminded that treatment of PIH may require an extended period of time, ranging up to 6 months, and that progress is made in small increments.

Melasma Chemical peels can be an effective method of removing excess epidermal pigment in the epidermal and mixed types of melasma [**Figure 78-1**]. The mechanism of action of chemical peels for the treatment of melasma involves a controlled chemical burn to the skin.[22] Dermal melasma is extremely difficult to treat, and attempting to treat this condition with deep chemical peels may result in scarring.[9]

Acne Vulgaris Chemical peels improve acne as well as acne-associated PIH. Staged peels, in which the patient returns for repeated treatments using the same concentration and formulation of a mild superficial peeling agent, are often used for skin of color. Both GA and SA have excellent safety profiles in patients with Fitzpatrick skin types IV to VI.[6,13,21] The choice of peeling agent depends on the physician's preference and/or experience.

Newer chemicals, such as the polyhydroxy acids, have been found to be extremely effective peeling agents for acne and pigmentary disorders in Asian skin.[9] Additionally, these agents are well tolerated in patients with dry, sensitive skin. Because the molecules in these agents are larger, they penetrate the epidermis more slowly, eliminating burning and irritation that sometimes occurs with AHA-containing products.

Scars Chemical peels for the treatment of scars are often beneficial in patients with skin of color, but hypertrophic scars do not usually respond well to the procedure. Medium-depth peels, which penetrate into the upper reticular dermis, are more effective peeling agents in the treatment of atrophic or crater-like acne scars and pitted or ice-pick scars that have a dermal component.[23]

CONTRAINDICATIONS

There are several contraindications to chemical peeling in skin of color. These contraindications include:

- Active herpes simplex infection, or verrucae
- Atopic dermatitis
- Wounded, sunburned, or excessively sensitive skin
- Inflammatory rosacea
- Isotretinoin use within a year

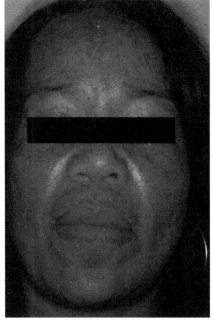

A

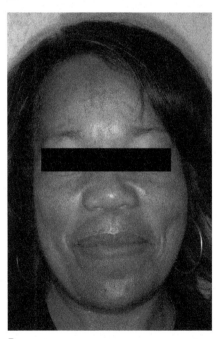

B

FIGURE 78-1. Before (**A**) and after (**B**) chemical peel for the treatment of melasma with improvement in the pigmentation on the cheek, upper lip and chin.

- Salicylate allergy (for SA peels)
- Pregnancy or active breast-feeding

TECHNIQUE

Prior to treating a patient with a chemical peel, a careful history should be obtained and a thorough skin examination performed. Patients should avoid the following procedures 1 week prior to chemical peeling: electrolysis, waxing, use of depilatory creams, and laser hair removal. Two to 5 days prior to the procedure, patients should discontinue use of topical retinoids and products that contain retinol, AHA, β-hydroxy acid, or benzoyl peroxide. Prophylactic antiviral therapy should be given to patients with a history of herpes simplex infection. Prior to applying chemical peeling agents to the skin, all makeup should be removed, the eyes should be protected with moistened cotton pads or eye shields, and petrolatum should be applied to sensitive areas, such as the corners of the nose and lips.

For the treatment of pigmentary disorders, pre- and posttreatment hyperpigmentation therapy is often essential and consists of treating the affected areas for 1 month prior to and after peeling with a combination skin-lightening agent containing hydroquinone, azelaic acid, or other cosmeceuticals with skin-lightening properties.[24] Peeling then can be performed using a 20% to 30% SA solution, 50% to 70% GA solution, Jessner's solution, or TCA 10% to 50%. The peel is applied with sponges or brushes for approximately 3 to 5 minutes, neutralized when appropriate, and then rinsed off.

SA peels are also used to treat active acne and oily skin. A 20% to 30% solution is applied to the skin with a sponge applicator and to individual papules and pustules with a cotton-tipped swab. Pustules and papules are often unroofed in the process. Typically, 4 to 5 minutes of a tingling or burning sensation occur before a white frost appears, signaling the end of the peel. This white frost of SA peels represents crystalline precipitation rather than protein agglutination associated with deep-peel frost. Patients are usually pleased with the results of this peel, and compliance remains high with the recommended three to six treatments. The number of peels performed is based on the severity of the acne, and patients usually tolerate the procedure well.

GA peels, available in many formulations and strengths, are also used for the treatment of acne. For skin of color, a partially buffered solution of 30% to 50% may be used.[6] The peeling agent contacts the skin for 2 to 4 minutes and then is rinsed off with cool water. Acne surgery performed with a comedone extractor on unroofed lesions often produces excellent results.

TCA peels in skin of color patients must be performed cautiously beginning with low concentrations. After a TCA peel, a white frost usually marks the end point [**Figure 78-2**]. It is important to note that in some skin types V to VI, this frost is not desired in skin types V to VI because it is associated with higher risks of adverse effects.

A combination of 70% GA gel and 25% TCA also has been used successfully for peeling,[6] with the gel formulation limiting the harshness of the TCA. First, GA gel is applied generously; then TCA is applied over it. The peel remains on the face for 2 to 4 minutes before removal. The procedure is usually repeated in 4 to 6 weeks, and if tolerated well, the peel may be left on 1 or 2 minutes longer with subsequent treatments.

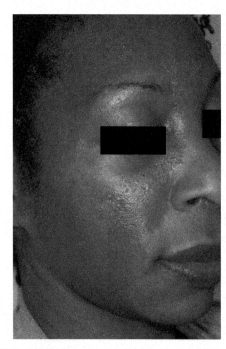

FIGURE 78-2. Patient undergoing a trichloracetic acid peel showing the white frost indicating the end point of the peel.

FOLLOW-UP AND PATIENT INSTRUCTIONS

Following the peel, patients are instructed to wash the skin with gentle cleansers, apply emollients twice daily, and use daily sun protection (SPF 30). When treating disorders of pigmentation, an effective interval between superficial peels is 3 to 6 weeks. Following the last peel of the series, the patient is maintained on daily ultraviolet (UV) protection sunscreen and often receives nightly application of a hydroquinone-based skin lightening agent for a 4- to 8-week period. Chronic melanocyte suppression can be accomplished by rotating the skin-lightening agents to avoid any of the adverse side effects of any one agent.[6] Topical retinoids, azelaic acid, or other cosmeceutical skin-lightening agents as maintenance therapy also can be used as an alternative to hydroquinone therapy.

OUTCOME

Several studies have looked at the efficacy and safety of a variety of chemical peels used to treat conditions common to skin of color [Table 78-1]. Many of the studies have found this procedure to be safe with very minimal side effects in this population.

Serial GA peels appear to enhance the efficacy of a topical regimen when treating PIH in patients with dark skin. In a study of 19 patients with Fitzpatrick skin types IV, V, and VI and facial PIH, a control group was treated with 2% hydroquinone–10% GA twice daily and tretinoin cream 0.05% at night.[25] The active peel group received the same topical regimen plus a series of six serial GA peels. Greater improvement was noted in the chemical peel group, although this difference was not statistically significant.

Several studies have assessed the efficacy of GA peels in the treatment of melasma in Indian patients. One study showed that serial GA peels with a topical regimen were an effective treatment for melasma in 40 dark-skinned East Indian women with Fitzpatrick skin types III to V.[26] The women were divided into two groups; one received serial GA peels combined with a topical regimen, which was a modified Kligman's formula (hydroquinone 5%, tretinoin 0.05%, and hydrocortisone acetate 1% in a cream base). The other group received only Kligman's formula. At 21 weeks, the group that received the GA peels showed a trend toward significantly improved results. Few side effects were noted in the peel group, and they included mild burning, erythema, and transient PIH.

Another study compared TCA (20% to 35%) to GA (10% to 20%) in the treatment of melasma in 40 East Indian women.[27] This study concluded that the GA peel had fewer side effects than the TCA peel, as well as the added advantage of skin rejuvenation. The GA group was pretreated with 12% GA cream, and the TCA group was pretreated with 0.1% tretinoin cream. The patients were treated with the lower doses of the respective peels (10% GA or 20% TCA) for the first two sessions and then the higher doses (20% GA or 35% TCA) for the second two sessions. The sessions were 2 weeks apart. In the GA group, 95% of patients reported mild burning and 15% had erythema, whereas in the TCA group, 75% reported moderate to severe burning and 15% had erythema.[27]

Other investigators evaluated the safety and efficacy of GA peels in 25 East Indian subjects with melasma.[28] Participants were asked to carry out a prepeel program of daily application of topical sunscreens and 10% GA lotion at night for 2 weeks. The women then were treated with a 50% GA facial peel once a month for 3 consecutive months. Results showed improvement in melasma in 91% of patients. Those with epidermal melasma had a better response than those with the mixed type. There were no significant side effects.

Another study compared the efficacy of GA peels versus tretinoin peels in the treatment of melasma in East Indian women.[29] The results show that there was no statistically significant difference between the two agents, and both resulted in a significant decrease in melasma area severity index (MASI).

A small study evaluating the treatment of superficial acne scarring with the use of 92% lactic acid was performed in seven East Indian patients.[30] These patients were treated with 92% lactic acid every 2 weeks for four sessions. This treatment was shown to be safe, and regarding efficacy, one patient had >75% clearance, three had 50% to 75% clearance, two had 26% to 50% clearance, and one had <25% clearance.[30]

Lactic acid peels have also been studied in the treatment of melasma in patients with Fitzpatrick skin type IV. A study that included 20 subjects with melasma were treated with pure lactic acid every 3 weeks until the desired response was achieved, to a maximum of six sessions. Sixty percent of the subjects completed the study, and they all showed marked improvement with no side effects.[31]

Another split-face study compared the use of 92% lactic acid with the Jessner's solution peel for the treatment of melasma. The majority of the patients included in this study had Fitzpatrick skin type IV and had sessions performed every 3 weeks until the desired response was achieved. All patients showed marked improvement with both treatments, with no side effects observed. Lactic acid was found to be as effective and safe as Jessner's solution for the treatment of melasma.[32]

Several studies have also assessed the efficacy and safety of chemical peels in treating Asian skin. Asians and Asian Americans have been found to respond well to staged GA peels.[33,34] A split-face study was performed that evaluated the safety and efficacy of GA peels in 10 Asian women with melasma and Fitzpatrick skin types IV and V.[33] Each woman underwent eight peels and at least one peel with 70% solution. At the end of 26 weeks, GA peels lightened the skin in all women compared with baseline. Up to 33% lightening of melasma occurred in six patients, and as much as 66% occurred in four patients. None of the patients experienced scarring or worsening of melasma. However, the results were not statistically significant as the sample was small.

Forty Asian patients with acne vulgaris were treated with a series of GA peels (35% to 70%) with significant improvement in acne lesions.[34] Side effects occured in 5.6% of the patients and included PIH, herpes simplex virus reactivation, and mild skin irritation.

The efficacy and safety of SA peels have been evaluated in skin of color. A study that assessed the efficacy and safety of 20% and 30% SA peels in 25 patients (9 with acne, 5 with PIH, 6 with melasma, and 5 with rough, oily skin and enlarged pores) with skin types V and VI, determined that they were safe and effective.[12] Side effects were mild or minimal and occurred in 16% of patients, with three experiencing transient hyperpigmentation that resolved in 7 to 14 days.

The efficacy and safety of SA peels in the treatment of acne vulgaris in Asian patients have been assessed.[35] Thirty-five Korean patients with acne vulgaris were treated with 30% SA peels biweekly for 12 weeks. There was a decrease in both inflammatory and noninflammatory acne lesion counts, and there was no change in stratum corneum hydration, skin surface lipid, skin pH, and transepidermal water loss from baseline levels.[35] Side effects were tolerable, further demonstrating the safety and efficacy of SA peels in skin of color patients.

While the risk of transient hyperpigmentation with medium-depth peeling is high, at least one group of investigators has found medium-depth chemical peels to be safe and effective in dark-skinned Iraqi patients.[23] Treatment was mainly for crater-like and ice-pick scars and consisted of three sessions held 1 month apart. Moderate improvement was seen in 53.3%, significant improvement in 6.6%, and a mild response in 26.1%. Peeling was performed with a combination of Jessner's solution followed by 35% TCA. Of note, transient PIH developed in 73.4% of patients, but all pigmentary changes resolved within 3 months.

A study also was performed on darker-skinned patients for the treatment of periorbital wrinkling (fine to medium) using medium-depth peels. Twelve patients underwent two to four peeling sessions with a combination of Jessner's solution followed by 35% TCA; each session was performed 1 month apart.[9] On completing the study, 33% of the subjects showed marked, 25% moderate, 25% mild, and 8% minimal improvement of periorbital wrinkling. Eight percent of the patients revealed no response to treatment. The treatment was tolerated well, with mild side effects occurring in 33% of patients.

Although most of the studies performed in skin of color using chemical peels have had small sample sizes, these studies reveal that, overall, chemical peels are safe to use in skin of color and are very efficacious.

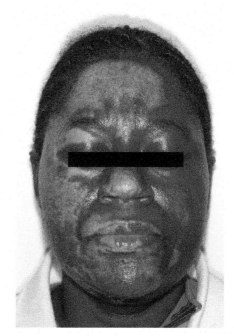

FIGURE 78-3. Patient with postinflammatory hypopigmentation from chemical peeling.

COMPLICATIONS

As with any cosmetic procedure, there is the risk of complications with the use of chemical peels in the skin of color population. However, the proper use of chemical peels in properly selected patients significantly diminishes this risk. Although superficial peeling agents, such as GA and SA, are generally well tolerated and safe in darker skin,[8,12] even superficial peeling may result in some scarring, hyperpigmentation, or hypopigmentation in susceptible individuals [**Figure 78-3**]. Other complications include persistent erythema, milia formation, and infection. For this reason, it is best to initiate peeling with agents at low concentrations and to perform skin testing prior to initiating a full procedure.

Time is an important variable when peeling with GA because this peel must be neutralized with water or 1% bicarbonate solution to discontinue keratolysis. Additionally, stronger solutions must be used cautiously because scarring has been reported following a 15-minute application of a 70% solution.[36,37]

Chemical peel is not recommended for removal of dermal pigment in Fitzpatrick skin types IV to VI.[8] Peeling to the depth needed to reach this pigmentation carries increased risks for scarring and permanent depigmentation.

Although Jessner's solution is usually well tolerated in Fitzpatrick skin types V and VI, caution must be used with this peel because resorcinol also may produce depigmentation in Fitzpatrick skin types V and VI.[9]

Deeper peels, such as the Baker phenol peel, as a rule are not used in darker skin because they are associated with complications such as hyperpigmentation, hypopigmentation, scarring, and keloid formation.[38] This peel is also associated with cardiac, renal, and hepatic toxicity.

MICRODERMABRASION

Microdermabrasion was first performed in Italy in 1985 by Marini and LoBrutto,[39] and since its introduction in the United States in 1996,[40] it has become one of the most popular cosmetic treatments among patients. Microdermabrasion is noninvasive, requires little or no recovery time, and may be performed safely on all Fitzpatrick skin types.[39]

PATIENT SELECTION

Microdermabrasion is an excellent option for the patient who is unable to tolerate peels or for whom extensive recovery time is not an option.

It is felt to be equivalent in efficacy to a superficial chemical peel and is less invasive than the carbon dioxide or Er:YAG laser.[39] Indications for microdermabrasion are similar to those for chemical peels and include acne, acne scarring, hyperpigmentation, photodamage, facial rejuvenation, enlarged pores, textural changes, and striae.[39,40]

■ CONTRAINDICATIONS

There are several relative contraindications to performing microdermabrasion:

- Active skin infections (eg, herpes simplex, verruca vulgaris, impetigo)
- Acute skin inflammation (eg, atopic dermatitis, rosacea, pustular acne)
- Koebnerizing skin conditions (eg, psoriasis, lichen planus, vitiligo)
- Isotretinoin use within 1 year

■ EQUIPMENT AND TECHNIQUE

Most microdermabrasion systems use aluminum oxide crystals, which are angular and create microtrauma from high crystal flow and numerous passes.[40,41] Other machines employ less abrasive sodium chloride and sodium bicarbonate crystals that also minimize the pulmonary risks associated with chronic aluminum exposure.[42] Other units that are available use a diamond wand and are crystal-free.

A typical microdermabrasion procedure, which does not require topical anesthesia, consists of superficially abrading the skin with either a diamond chip or fine crystals, which are simultaneously delivered to and vacuumed off the skin. The number of passes in a session varies with the patient's tolerance and desired effect, but most patients require two or three passes. Depth of ablation depends on the amount of force used to spray the crystals onto the skin, the flow rate of the crystals, the crystal size, and the angle at which the crystals are applied to the skin.[43]

Three levels of microdermabrasion may be used in the treatment of the skin[43]:

- Level one produces a superficial abrasion of the epidermis for gentle exfoliation.
- Level two is more aggressive, extends to the papillary dermis, and is used to treat superficial scars, striae, and fine wrinkles.
- Level three is most aggressive, extends to the level of the papillary and upper reticular dermis, and is used to treat striae.

It is important to note that levels two and three must be used with caution in skin of color due to an increased risk of hyperpigmentation.

■ FOLLOW-UP AND PATIENT INSTRUCTIONS

Following a treatment with microdermabrasion, patients are instructed to use mild cleansers, emollients, and sun protection (SPF 30). For maximal results, microdermabrasion is recommended 2 to 4 weeks apart for four to six treatments until desired results have been achieved.

■ OUTCOME

Histologically, significant epidermal changes have been demonstrated after microdermabrasion treatment. Hernandez-Perez and Ibiett[44] performed biopsies before and after microdermabrasion treatments. After five sessions, there was an increase in epidermal thickness ranging from 0.01 to 0.1 mm. Freedman et al[45] also revealed epidermal thickening in their study. After three passes of microdermabrasion, epidermal thickness, as well as papillary dermal thickness, increased significantly.

Changes in epidermal barrier function, such as transepidermal water loss, hydration, pH, and sebum production, may be responsible for the improved texture and overall appearance of the skin following microdermabrasion.[40,41] A study was performed in eight patients, three of whom were African American and two Hispanic. This was a split-face study where half the face was treated with aluminum oxide microdermabrasion and the other half with sodium chloride microdermabrasion. Each patient received three passes. Transepidermal water loss, stratum corneum hydration, skin pH, and sebum production were measured,

and it was revealed that microdermabrasion enhanced skin hydration and improved epidermal barrier function.[40]

An animal study was performed looking at enhanced penetration of hydrophilic and lipophilic substances following microdermabrasion.[46] It was found that after partially ablating and homogenizing the stratum corneum with microdermabrasion, there was increased penetration of hydrophilic substances into the skin.

Another study examined the changes in lipid levels in the stratum corneum following microdermabrasion. A statistically significant increase in the ceramide level was observed after two microdermabrasion treatments.[47] Following the third and fourth sessions, the ceramide level returned to baseline. This study provides the first evidence of changes in the lipid barrier following microdermabrasion treatments.

The benefits of microdermabrasion have been proven for the treatment of acne and acne scarring. Investigators demonstrated the efficacy of the procedure in 25 patients with grade II or III acne.[48] The patients received eight treatments at weekly intervals. Overall, 96% of the patients were pleased with their results and reportedly would recommend this procedure to others.

The efficacy of microdermabrasion was also accessed in 28 patients ranging in age from 40 to 75 with Fitzpatrick skin types I to IV by Shim et al.[39] Of those enrolled, there were 14 patients with photoaging, 11 with comedonal acne or milia, and 3 with severe acne scarring. Following 12 to 14 weeks of treatment, microdermabrasion produced statistically significant improvement in skin roughness, mottled pigmentation, and overall skin appearance, but not in rhytides. Some acne scarring improved, but most patients required deeper ablation. Adverse events, namely, PIH, did not occur.[39]

Microdermabrasion is also useful for other types of facial scarring. A study evaluated 41 Asian patients with scars (16 acne scars, 18 traumatic scars, 3 surgical scars, 2 chickenpox scars, 1 burn scar, and 1 other scar) that were treated with microdermabrasion over a 2-year period in a Taiwan hospital. All patients reported good to excellent clinical results.[49] Mean frequencies of treatment were 19 treatments for acne scars, 4 for traumatic scars, 4 for surgical scars, and 5.5 for chickenpox scars.

Of note, some investigators have found that dual therapy consisting of microdermabrasion and combination lightening agents has benefits in melasma, but additional research is needed.[50]

More recently, microdermabrasion has been used for other indications such as vitiligo. A study was performed demonstrating the efficacy of pimecrolimus 1% cream combined with microdermabrasion in the treatment of nonsegmental childhood vitiligo. This was a 3-month, randomized, placebo-controlled study in which three vitiliginous patches were treated in each subject.[51] One lesion was treated with pimecrolimus 1% cream alone, another lesion was treated with microdermabrasion on day 1 followed by the application of pimecrolimus 1% cream and the third lesion was treated with placebo. The treatment course was for 10 days, and microdermabrasion was performed on day 1 until erythema was observed on the skin. Pimecrolimus 1% cream was applied to the affected areas daily for the duration of the treatment course.[51]

Sixty-five children were enrolled and 60 completed the study. Significant clinical response was noted as greater than 50% repigmentation of the treated lesions.[51] A total of 60.4% of the patches treated with combination treatment showed a significant clinical response at the 3-month follow-up, compared with 32.1% and 1.7% of those treated with pimecrolimus alone and placebo, respectively. The only side effect noted was a mild burning sensation in 30% of the patients treated with microdermabrasion.[51]

Another study demonstrated the efficacy of vitiligo treated with microdermabrasion in combination with 5-fluorouracil cream. The response rate with this combination treatment was 73.3%.[52]

■ COMPLICATIONS

Very few complications have been observed with the use of microdermabrasion. Following treatment, patients may experience mild erythema. Other complications may include development of petechiae, purpura, or skin wounding if the vacuum suction power is increased, which, in turn, may result in PIH.[49]

Ocular complications from the crystals may occur; therefore, it is recommended that patients keep their eyes closed or apply disposable eye shields during the procedure. Patients with a history of herpes simplex also should be treated with antiviral prophylaxis prior to microdermabrasion because the procedure can cause reactivation of the virus.[53]

HAIR TRANSPLANTATION

Hair transplantation techniques have evolved and improved tremendously over the years. Follicular unit transplantation (FUT) was developed to provide a more naturally appearing cosmetic result in males with androgenetic alopecia.[54,55] Since then, hair transplantation has become more popular and has expanded to include women and other populations interested in correcting their hair loss. According to the International Society of Hair Restoration Surgery Practice Census, there were approximately 310,624 hair transplant procedures performed worldwide in 2012, and of these, the majority were performed in Asia.[56] Although the exact number of hair transplant procedures performed in persons of color is unknown, it is clear that as the awareness of alopecia in men and women grows, the numbers of hair transplantations in this group of patients will increase.[57] Thus, there are several racial differences in hair morphology, surgical instrumentation, and surgical technique in hair transplant surgery that will be discussed [**Table 78-2**].

FUT involves removing follicular groups or follicular units from the permanently hair-bearing rim hair (donor area) and inserting them into tiny incisions produced in the area of hair loss (recipient area). Racial variations in the hair characteristics of individuals is by far the most important difference in hair transplant surgery. Patients of African descent have extremely curly hair and a curved hair follicle [**Figure 78-4**] compared with the straight hair and straight hair follicle in Caucasian and Asian patients. Larger grafts typically are used in patients of color because of this distinct curl pattern within the dermis. There are major concerns that exist during donor harvesting and graft preparation, mainly transection of the hair follicle, which can affect graft survival.

Differences in hair densities between the races also exist. Patients of African descent exhibit lower densities when compared with other races,[55,58] and this lower density results in a lower number of donor grafts needed for a hair transplantation procedure.

▨ PATIENT SELECTION

The most common indication for hair transplantation is for the management of androgenetic alopecia in men with male-pattern baldness (MPB). Adjunctive medical therapy with topical minoxidil 5% or finasteride is recommended in younger patients to slow the progression of MPB before considering a hair transplantation procedure. The medical and surgical treatment of androgenetic alopecia in men with dark skin of color[59,60] is similar to that in other population groups, but those men who wear their hair closely shaved in a "fade" haircut will have difficulty in camouflaging the resulting donor scar produced by hair transplant surgery.

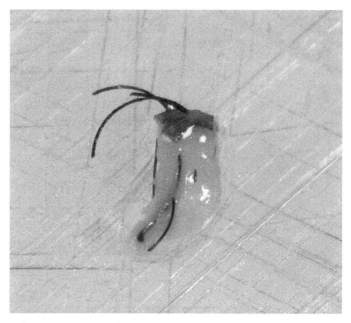

FIGURE 78-4. Hair follicles from an African American patient demonstrating the curly nature of African American hair.

Women also suffer from hair loss. The most common type of alopecia in women is female-pattern hair loss (FPHL), or androgenetic alopecia, affecting 13% of premenopausal women and 37% of postmenopausal women.[61] In women, hair loss is characterized by a diffuse thinning of the hair over the crown and frontal scalp with preservation of the anterior hairline. In all patients, topical minoxidil 2% is the mainstay of medical therapy for FPHL, but an increasingly popular option for women with FPHL is hair transplantation.[62]

Hair transplantation surgery is an effective treatment for traction alopecia, or traumatic alopecia marginalis, in African American women or those with dark skin of color[57,58,63,64] [**Figure 78-5**]. Surgical correction in these patients can take the form of either multi-follicular unit grafts, flap rotations, or FUT. Each method is effective and has advantages and disadvantages. The choice of surgical treatment is usually individualized

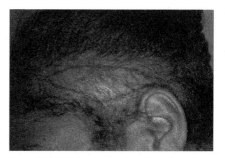

A

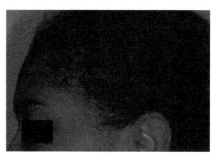

B

FIGURE 78-5. (A) Patient with traction alopecia prior to hair transplantation. (B) Twelve months after hair transplantation.

TABLE 78-2	Hair transplantation differences in persons with skin of color		
	Dark skin of color	Caucasians	Asians
Hair shape	Curly	Straight, wavy	Straight
Hair follicle	Curved	Straight	Straight
Hair density	0.6 FU/mm²	1 FU/mm²	1 FU/mm²
Hair groupings	Three	Two	Two
Indications	AGA, TA, CCCA	AGA	AGA
Recipient sites	>1.2 mm	<1.2 mm	<1.2 mm
Keloid risk	High	Low	Moderate

Abbreviations: AGA, androgenetic alopecia; CCCA, central centrifugal cicatricial alopecia; TA, traction alopecia.

to the patient depending on the severity of hair loss, the patient's desires, the flexibility of the scalp, and the shape of the hair. In many cases, a combination of techniques is the best choice.

Central centrifugal cicatricial alopecia (CCCA) is scarring alopecia, distributed in the midscalp and vertex, that primarily affects women with dark skin of color.[64,65] Although uncommon and often misdiagnosed as androgenetic alopecia, CCCA can occur in African American males.[66-68] Previous terminology includes *hot-comb alopecia,*[69] *chemically induced alopecia,*[70] and *follicular degeneration syndrome.*[71] CCCA develops in a roughly circular patch on the crown or vertex region of the scalp, with the area of inflammation and scarring increasing in circumference as the condition progresses.[53] Early changes consisting of only hair breakage and scalp pruritus/tenderness at the vertex have been documented histopathologically as CCCA.[72] Eventually, the scalp becomes smooth and shiny with loss of follicular ostia. The hair remaining in the scarred zone is short and brittle. The cause of CCCA is unknown, and treatment consists of aggressive anti-inflammatory treatments, such as corticosteroids and oral antibiotics, to address the symptoms and stop progression. Inflammation may be decreased with high-potency topical corticosteroids used daily, with special attention to the vehicle and the patient's hair grooming practices. Intralesional corticosteroid therapy performed monthly using triamcinolone acetonide at a concentration of 2.5 to 5.0 mg/mL suppresses dermal inflammation. Surgical correction with hair transplantation surgery is also an option after 9 months or more of medical therapy and a biopsy-proven noninflamed scalp.[57,64,73]

CONTRAINDICATIONS

The contraindications for hair transplantation are similar in all racial groups, but patients of color have a higher incidence of keloid and hypertrophic scarring.[57,73,74] A careful and detailed history of keloid formation along with a physical examination to check for other scars should be performed.

SURGICAL TECHNIQUE

Performing hair transplantation in patients with curly hair is challenging, and steps to avoid transection of the hair follicle within the grafts demand special attention and skill. The surgical equipment required to perform hair transplantation is listed in **Table 78-3**. Anesthesia is obtained by infiltrating 1% or 2% lidocaine with epinephrine for both donor and recipient areas. In addition, normal saline is injected into the donor area prior to excision of the donor strip to provide maximum skin turgor and to straighten the hair and hair follicles, thus allowing for less transection

TABLE 78-3	**Hair transplantation equipment**
1.	Aluminum rattail comb
2.	Hair densitometer
3.	Hibiclens solution
4.	Gauze
5.	Lidocaine with epinephrine
6.	Normal saline for skin turgor
7.	Scalpel with no. 15 blade
8.	Tissue clamps
9.	Hyfrecator and disposable sterile tips
10.	3-0 or 4-0 Prolene suture material
11.	Stereomicroscope or loupe magnification
12.	Cutting board with fiberoptic box lighting
13.	Persona blade (DermaBlade)
14.	Jeweler's forceps—straight, curved
15.	Petri dishes with saline
16.	Nokor needles—16 and 18 gauge
17.	Spearpoint blades—nos. 90 and 91
18.	Punches—2 to 4 mm
19.	Spray bottle with saline

while harvesting the donor strip. There are four steps in performing a hair transplantation procedure that will be discussed: donor harvesting, graft preparation, recipient-site creation, and graft placement.

Donor Harvesting This initial step involves excising a single strip of donor tissue from the occipital area of scalp in such a way that transection of hair follicles is limited and the resulting scar is undetectable. The length and width of the harvested tissue are determined by the hair density of the individual and the number of grafts needed to cover the area of hair loss. Follicular unit extraction (FUE)[75] is a newer technique available for hair transplantation. This method uses small punch excisions (1 mm) to extract the follicular units from the donor site.[75] Although this technique decreases the amount of scarring resulting from conventional harvesting, the complications include a higher transection rate and an increase in the amount of time to harvest the follicular units.[75,76] Trichophytic closure[77] is a technique currently used to minimize the scar by trimming the epidermis of one edge of the wound before suturing the wound margins together. Undermining the wound margins, which results in less tension, and limiting the width to less than 1 cm, also aid in minimizing the size of the donor scar.

Graft Preparation During this step, the donor strip is converted into individual grafts of different sizes. Caution must be taken with curly hair to avoid transection of the hair follicle, so a curved blade is often used to match the curvature of the hair. Flexible blades such as the DermaBlade are very useful in dissecting individual follicular units, particularly in patients with curved hair follicles.[78] These blades easily bend to match the curvature of the hair follicle [**Figure 78-6**]. The advantages of the use of flexible blades are a decrease in the transection rate of the hair follicle, a decrease in the need for multiple cuts because the flexible blade can cut closer along the entire length of the hair follicle, and the flexibility of the blade allows it to conform quickly and easily to the degree of curvature of the hair follicle.[78] The grafts that are created contain one to four hair follicular units and are placed in saline until they are ready to be inserted into the recipient sites.

Recipient-Site Creation and Graft Placement A number of surgical instruments can be used to create recipient sites in areas of hair loss. We select instrumentation based on the degree of curl of the hair—the greater the curl, the larger is the recipient site. Typically, the recipient site ranges from 1.2 to 2.0 mm in size in patients with a significant curl pattern.

COMPLICATIONS

Most African American patients have excellent cosmetic results from hair transplantation surgery and experience a low risk of keloidal scarring.

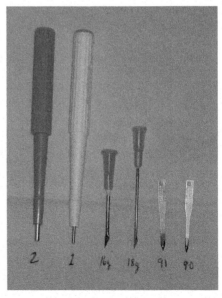

FIGURE 78-6. Hair transplantation: surgical instruments for recipient sites.

However, at least one case of a large keloidal scar following hair transplantation has been reported. This was a 60-year-old African American man with male-pattern alopecia and no previous history of keloidal scarring.[79] The scar developed over a large portion of the patient's scalp. This represents a significant potential complication, particularly in African American and Asian patients with a history of scarring. To avoid this complication, test grafting is recommended in some patients before a hair transplantation procedure.[80,81] If normal healing occurs in the donor area and recipient site after 3 months, the patient is a good candidate for a full transplantation procedure.

SCLEROTHERAPY

Varicose veins are a very common cosmetic complaint and are observed in a large majority of the population. In fact, 41% of women in the fifth decade of life have varicose veins, whereas 72% have varicosities in the seventh decade.[82] Sclerotherapy for varicose and spider veins is a common procedure performed in dermatologic practices and has been used by dermatologists since the 1980s.[83,84] It is a first-line therapy for treatment of small varicose veins.

PATIENT SELECTION

A detailed history and physical examination should be performed on all patients with varicose veins considering sclerotherapy. Based on an individual's history and physical examination, a noninvasive diagnostic test of the venous system may be necessary.[85] The "gold standard" of this testing is duplex ultrasound, which assesses for blood clots within the veins. After the patient has been deemed a good candidate, informed consent is obtained.

CONTRAINDICATIONS

- Reflux at the saphenofemoral junction
- Patients confined to bed
- Severely restricted arterial flow to legs
- History of deep venous thrombosis
- Allergy to sclerosing agents

- Obesity
- Pregnancy

TYPES OF SCLEROSING AGENTS

Numerous classes of sclerosing agents are available [**Table 78-4**]. The selection of an agent depends on factors such as the size and location of the vessel undergoing treatment. There are three major classes of sclerosing agents, and they include osmotic, detergent, and corrosive agents. Osmotic solutions are milder and less capable of initiating a cascade of inflammation, which could result in PIH, a common side effect of sclerotherapy in patients with skin of color.

Sclerosing agents are effective in treatment by causing endothelial damage of the vein, which induces fibrosis of the veins, followed by eventual resorption of the vessel.[86]

Hypertonic saline is used in different concentrations ranging from 10% to 30%. Although allergenicity is low with this solution, it may cause skin necrosis if extravasation occurs at the injection site. Ulcerations after injection of hypertonic saline are the leading cause of malpractice cases associated with sclerotherapy in the United States.[87] Pain associated with hypertonic saline injections is due to irritation of the nerves in the adventitia and muscular tissue.[88] Other potential side effects with the use of hypertonic saline are exacerbation of hypertension, necrosis of the cortex of the kidneys, hemolysis, hematuria, central nervous system disorders,[87] hypernatremia,[88] and membranous fat necrosis.[86]

The hypertonic saline and dextrose solution contains a mixture of dextrose, sodium chloride, propylene glycol, and phenethyl alcohol. It is predominantly marketed in Canada and used for treatment of smaller vessels. It is used off label in the United States for the treatment of telangiectasias.

Polidocanol is a detergent-based sclerosing agent that contains hydroxypolyethoxydodecane dissolved in distilled water with 5% ethanol. It was approved by the U.S. Food and Drug Administration (FDA) as a sclerosing agent in the United States in June 2010 for the treatment of lower extremity veins, with the 0.5% concentration being used for telangiectasias and the 1% concentration being used for small reticular veins.[86] The recommended volume of injection is less than 10 mL for patients weighing 50 kg or more or a dose of 2 mg/kg.[88] Injection with this agent is relatively painless, and it has a low incidence of cutaneous

TABLE 78-4	Comparison of commonly used sclerosing agents				
Sclerosing solution	Category	Advantages	Disadvantages	Vessels treated	Concentrations
Sodium tetradecyl sulfate (Sotradecol)	Detergent	FDA approved Painless unless injected extravascularly	May cause breakdown rarely found to be equivalent to polidocanol in clinical studies	All sizes	0.1%–0.2% telangiectasias 0.2%–0.5% reticular 0.5%–1.0% varicose 1.0%–3.0% axial varicose
Polidocanol	Detergent	Painless Low ulceration risk at low concentrations		Small to medium	0.25%–0.5% telangiectasias 0.5%–1.0% reticular 1.0%–3.0% varicose
Hypertonic saline	Hyperosmolar	Low risk of allergic reactions	Ulcerogenic Painful to inject	Small	23.4%–11.7% telangiectasias 23.4% reticular
Hypertonic saline + dextrose (Sclerodex)	Hyperosmolar	Low risk of allergic reaction Mild stinging Low ulcerogenic potential	Not FDA approved Relatively weak sclerosant	Small	Undiluted—telangiectasias Undiluted—reticular
Sodium morrhuate (Scleromate)	Detergent	FDA approved	Allergic reactions highest	Small	Undiluted—telangiectasias Undiluted—reticular
Chromated glycerin (glycerin with 6% chromium salt; Scleremo)	Chemical irritant	Low skin ulcer potential	Not FDA approved Very weak sclerosant	Smallest	Undiluted to one-half strength—telangiectasias
Glycerin—plain	Chemical irritant	Painless, low risk of allergic reaction, decreased risks of pigmentation and matting	FDA approved for reduction of cerebral edema	Smallest	50%–72%
Polyiodinated iodine (Varigloban)	Chemical irritant	Highly corrosive allows treatment of largest veins	Not FDA approved Avoid in iodine-allergic patients	Largest	1%–2% for up to 5-mm veins 2%–6% for the largest veins

Abbreviation: FDA, U.S. Food and Drug Administration.

necrosis. In a study of 285 Chinese patients, polidocanol 0.5%, 1%, and 3% (dose used was dependent on the type of varicose vein being treated) was found to be efficacious, with all response rates >85%, superior to placebo, and safe.[89]

Sodium tetradecyl sulfate is considered a detergent and is a very effective sclerosing agent. It is also FDA approved for the treatment of lower extremity veins. In high doses, this agent has been reported to cause an increased incidence of posttreatment pigmentation.

Sodium morrhuate consists of a 5% solution of salts of saturated and unsaturated fatty acids in cod liver oil. This agent has an increased potential for cutaneous necrosis and is used rarely for treatment of varicose veins due to its side effects. Fatalities due to anaphylaxis from this agent have been reported.[90]

Chromated glycerin is considered a chemical irritant and is not approved by the FDA. It is a weak sclerosing agent but does have the ability to destroy the endothelium.

Polyiodinated iodine is also a chemical irritant and a strong sclerosing agent. It has a very toxic effect on the endothelium and is not approved by the FDA.

TECHNIQUE

Sclerotherapy is performed beginning with treatment of the largest proximal varicosities and extending to the smaller distal vessels. Injection is performed using a 30-gauge needle that is inserted at a 10- to 30-degree angle with the bevel up. Initial treatment of telangiectatic webs begins with the lowest concentration of sclerosing agents. The agents used most commonly are 0.1% sodium tetradecyl sulfate or 0.2% polidocanol. Sclerosing usually occurs 1 to 6 months after the procedure is done, and if it is not successful, the concentration is increased during subsequent treatments.

Foam sclerotherapy is a technique that consists of a detergent sclerosing agent that is combined with air and is found to be more potent than liquid sclerosing agents.[91]

COMPLICATIONS

Hyperpigmentation following sclerotherapy [**Figure 78-7**] occurs at a rate of 0.3% to 10%, with rates as high as 30% in some studies.[92] The cause of this complication appears to be multifactorial and includes type and concentration of the sclerosing agent [**Table 78-5**], technique used, intravascular pressures, and postsclerotherapy care.[93] Initially, this pigmentation is due to deposition of hemosiderin, and eventually the hemosiderin is replaced by melanin. Within 6 months, the hyperpigmentation clears in 70% of patients.[93] For more persistent cases of hyperpigmentation, various treatments, including hypopigmenting agents, chemical peeling, and lasers,[94] which have demonstrated limited success, have been used.

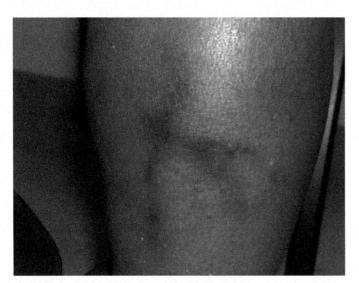

FIGURE 78-7. Hyperpigmentation following sclerotherapy.

TABLE 78-5	Sclerosing agents associated with hyperpigmentation
Chromated glycerin (glycerin with 6% chromium salt)	
Hypertonic saline	
Hypertonic saline + dextrose	
Polidocanol	
Polyiodinated iodine	
Sodium tetradecyl sulfate	

Other complications of sclerotherapy include erythema, edema, pruritus, pain, urticaria, localized hypertrichosis, telangiectatic matting, cutaneous necrosis and ulceration, superficial thrombophlebitis, and pulmonary embolism.

PATIENT INSTRUCTIONS AND FOLLOW-UP

Four to 8 weeks are usually allowed between subsequent treatments if needed. Patients are instructed to wear compression stockings for at least 2 weeks following treatment with sclerotherapy. Graduated 20 to 30 or 30 to 40 mm Hg support hose are recommended after treatment of larger veins, and over-the-counter 15 mm Hg compression stockings are recommended for smaller veins. In a study that evaluated postsclerotherapy compression with class II (30 to 40 mm Hg) stockings in 37 women who underwent sclerotherapy for leg telangiectasia, hyperpigmentation decreased from 40.5% to 28.5%.[95] Edema in the ankle and calf also was reduced.

CONCLUSION

This chapter reviews several cosmetic procedures performed in skin of color patients and some of the challenges providers must be aware of when performing these procedures. The cosmetic procedures reviewed are being performed more than ever in skin of color patients, and as noted, they are safe and effective in this population when performed with skill and caution.

REFERENCES

1. American Society for Aesthetic Plastic Surgery (ASAPS). 2012 Statistics on Cosmetic Surgery. www.surgery.org/press/statistics-2011.php. Accessed February 5, 2013.
2. Taylor SC. Cosmetic problems in skin of color. *Skin Pharmacol Appl Skin Physiol.* 1999;12:139-143.
3. Grimes PE. Skin and hair cosmetic issues in women of color. *Dermatol Clin.* 2000;18:659-665.
4. Grimes PE. Skin of color: disease and cosmetic issues of major concern. *Cosmet Dermatol.* 2003;16:1-4.
5. Callender VD. Cosmetic surgery in skin of color. *Cosmet Dermatol.* 2003;16: 53-56.
6. Roberts WE. Chemical peeling in ethnic/dark skin. *Dermatol Ther.* 2004;17: 196-205.
7. Van Scott EJ, Yu RJ. Hyperkeratinization, corneocyte cohesion, and alpha hydroxy acids. *J Am Acad Dermatol.* 1984;11:867-879.
8. Tung RC, Bergfeld WF, Vidimos AT, Remzi BK. Alfa-Hydroxy acid-based cosmetic procedures: guidelines for patient management. *Am J Clin Dermatol.* 2000;1:1-88.
9. Kakita LS. The use of chemical peels in Asian skin. In: Moy R, Luftman D, Kakita LS, eds. *Glycolic Acid Peels.* New York, NY: Marcel Dekker; 2002: 141-153.
10. Grimes PE. Glycolic acid peels in blacks. In: Moy R, Luftman D, Kakita LS, eds. *Glycolic Acid Peels.* New York, NY: Marcel Dekker; 2002:179-186.
11. Sarkar R, Bansal S, Garg VK. Chemical peels for melasma in dark-skinned patients. *J Cutan Aesthet Surg.* 2012;5:247-253.
12. Huber C, Christophers E. "Keratolytic" effect of salicylic acid. *Arch Dermatol Res.* 1977;257:293-297.
13. Grimes PE. The safety and efficacy of salicylic acid chemical peels in darker racial-ethnic groups. *Dermatol Surg.* 1999;25:18-22.
14. Rendon M, Berson DS, Cohen JL, et al. Evidence and considerations in the application of chemical peels in skin disorders and aesthetic resurfacing. *J Clin Aesthet Dermatol.* 2010;3:32-43.

15. Corcuff P, Fiat F, Minodo AM, et al. A comparative ultrastructural study of hydroxyacids induced desquamation. *Eur J Dermatol.* 2002;12:XXXIX-XLIII.
16. Uhoda E, Pierard-Franchimont C, Pierard GE. Comedolysis by a lipohydroxyacid formulation in acne-prone subjects. *Eur J Dermatol.* 2003;13:65-68.
17. Taylor MB. Summary of mandelic acid for the improvement of skin conditions. *Cosmet Dermatol.* 1999;12:26-28.
18. Obagi ZE, Obagi S, Alaiti S, et al. TCA-based bluepeel: a standardized procedure with depth control. *Dermatol Surg.* 1999;25:773-780.
19. Kadhim KA, Al-Waiz M. Treatment of periorbital wrinkles by repeated medium-depth chemical peels in dark-skinned individuals. *J Cosmet Dermatol.* 2005;4:18-22.
20. Klein M. Amino fruit acids: the new cosmeceutical. *Cosmet Dermatol.* 2000;13:25-28.
21. Grimes PE. Agents for ethnic skin peeling. *Dermatol Ther.* 2000;13:159-164.
22. Sheth VM, Pandya AG. Melasma: a comprehensive update: part II. *J Am Acad Dermatol.* 2011;65:699-714.
23. Al-Waiz M, Al-Sharqi AI. Medium-depth chemical peels in the treatment of acne scars in dark-skinned individuals. *Dermatol Surg.* 2002;28:383-387.
24. Kindred C, Okereke UR, Callender VD. Skin lightening agents: an overview of prescription, office-dispensed and OTC products. *Cosmet Dermatol.* 2012;5:18-26.
25. Burns RL, Prevost-Blank PL, Lawry MA, et al. Glycolic acid peels for postinflammatory hyperpigmentation in black patients: a comparative study. *Dermatol Surg.* 1997;23:171-175.
26. Sarkar R, Kaur C, Bhalla M, et al. The combination of glycolic acid peels with a topical regimen in the treatment of melasma in dark-skinned patients: a comparative study. *Dermatol Surg.* 2002;28:828-832.
27. Kumari R, Thappa DM. Comparative study of trichloroacetic acid versus glycolic acid chemical peels in the treatment of melasma. *Indian J Dermatol Venereol Leprol.* 2010;76:447.
28. Javaheri AM, Handa S, Kaur I, et al. Safety and efficacy of glycolic acid facial peel in Indian women with melasma. *Int J Dermatol.* 2001;40:354-357.
29. Khunger N, Sarkar R, Jain RK. Tretinoin peels versus glycolic peels in the treatment of melasma in dark-skinned patients. *Dermatol Surg.* 2004;30:756-760.
30. Sachdeva S. Lactic acid peeling in superficial acne scarring in Indian skin. *J Cosmet Dermatol.* 2010;9:246-248.
31. Sharquie KE, Al-Tikreety MM, Al-Mashhadani SA. Lactic acid as a new therapeutic peeling agent in melasma. *Dermatol Surg.* 2005;31:149-154.
32. Sharquie KE, Al-Tikreety, Al-Mashhadani SA. Lactic acid chemical peels as a new therapeutic modality in melasma in comparison to Jessner's solution chemical peels. *Dermatol Surg.* 2006;32:1429-1436.
33. Lim JT, Tham SN. Glycolic acid peels in the treatment of melasma among Asian women. *Dermatol Surg.* 1997;23:177-179.
34. Wang CM, Huang CL, Hu CT, et al. The effect of glycolic acid on the treatment of acne in Asian skin. *Dermatol Surg.* 1997;23:23-29.
35. Lee HS, Kim IH. Salicylic acid peels for the treatment of acne vulgaris in Asian patients. *Dermatol Surg.* 2003;29:1196-1199.
36. Brody H. *Chemical Peeling.* St Louis, MO: Mosby-Year Book; 1992.
37. Atzore L, Brundu MA, Orru A, et al. Gylcolic acid peeling in the treatment of acne. *J Eur Acad Dermatol Venereol.* 1999;12:119-122.
38. Camacho FM. Medium-depth and deep chemical peels. *J Cosmet Dermatol.* 2005;4:117-128.
39. Shim EK, Barnette D, Hughes K, et al. Microdermabrasion: a clinical and histopathologic study. *Dermatol Surg.* 2001;27:524-530.
40. Rajan P, Grimes PE. Skin barrier changes induced by aluminum oxide and sodium chloride microdermabrasion. *Dermatol Surg.* 2002;28:390-393.
41. Jackson BA. Cosmetic considerations and nonlaser cosmetic procedures in ethnic skin. *Dermatol Clin.* 2003;21:703-712.
42. Masalkhi A, Walton SP. Pulmonary fibrosis and occupational exposure to aluminum. *J Ky Med Assoc.* 1994;92:59-61.
43. Lim JT. Microdermabrasion. In: Grimes PE, ed. *Aesthetic and Cosmetic Surgery for Darker Skin Types.* Philadelphia, PA: Lippincott Williams & Wilkins; 2008:147-153.
44. Hernandez-Perez M, Ibiett V. Gross and microscopic findings in patients undergoing microdermabrasion for facial rejuvenation. *Dermatol Surg.* 2001;27:637-640.
45. Freedman BM, Rueda-Pedraza E, Waddell SP. The epidermal and dermal changes associated with microdermabrasion. *Dermatol Surg.* 2001;27:1031-1034.
46. Lee WR, Tsai RY, Fang CL, et al. Microdermabrasion as a novel tool to enhance drug delivery via the skin: an animal study. *Dermatol Surg.* 2006;32:1013-1022.
47. Lew BL, Cho Y, Lee MH. Effect of serial microdermabrasion on the ceramide level in the stratum corneum. *Dermatol Surg.* 2006;32:376-379.
48. Lloyd J. The use of micordermabrasion for acne: a pilot study. *Dermatol Surg.* 2001;27:329-331.
49. Tsai RY, Wang CN, Chan HL. Aluminum oxide crystal microdermabrasion: a new technique for treating facial scarring. *Dermatol Surg.* 1995;21:539-542.
50. Dual regimen for facial melasma. *Dermatol Times.* 2003;24:47.
51. Farajzadeh S, Daraei Z, Esfandiarpour I, et al. The efficacy of pimecrolimus 1% cream combined with microdermabrasion in the treatment of nonsegmental childhood vitiligo: a randomized placebo-controlled study. *Pediatr Dermatol.* 2009;26:286-291.
52. Sethi S, Mahajan BB, Guptta RR, et al. Comparative evaluation of the therapeutic efficacy of dermabrasion, dermabrasion combined with topical 5% 5-fluorouracil cream, and dermabrasion combined with topical placentrex gel in localized stable vitiligo. *Int J Dermatol.* 2007;46:875-879.
53. Warmuth IP, Bader R, Scarborough DA, et al. Herpes simplex infection after microdermabrasion. *Cosmet Dermatol.* 1999;12:13.
54. Bernstein RM, Rassman WR, Szaniawski W, et al. Follicular transplantation. *Int J Aesthet Rest Surg.* 1995;3:119-132.
55. Bernstein RM, Rassman WR. The aesthetics of follicular transplantation. *Dermatol Surg.* 1997;23:785-799.
56. International Society of Hair Restoration Surgery. 2013 Practice Census Results. www.ishrs.org. Accessed August 2013.
57. Callender VD. Hair transplantation for pigmented skins. In: Halder RM, ed. *Dermatology and Dermatological Therapy of Pigmented Skins.* London, United Kingdom: Taylor and Francis; 2006:245-257.
58. Sperling LC. Hair density in African-Americans. *Arch Dermatol.* 1990;135:656-658.
59. Pierce HE. The uniqueness of hair transplantation in black patients. *J Dermatol Surg Oncol.* 1997;3:533-535.
60. Earles RM. Hair transplantation, scalp reduction, and flap rotation in black men. *J Dermatol Surg Oncol.* 1986;12:87-91, 95-96.
61. Olsen EA. Female pattern hair loss. *J Am Acad Dermatol.* 2001;45:S70-S80.
62. Unger WP, Unger RH. Hair transplanting: an important but often forgotten treatment for female pattern hair loss. *J Am Acad Dermatol.* 2003;49:853-860.
63. Earles RM, Harland CC, Bull RH, et al. Surgical correction of traumatic alopecia marginalis or traction alopecia in black women. *J Dermatol Surg Oncol.* 1986;12:78-82.
64. Callender VD, McMichael AJ, Cohen GF. Medical and surgical therapies for alopecias in black women. *Dermatol Ther.* 2004;17:164-176.
65. Sperling LC. A new look at scarring alopecia. *Arch Dermatol.* 2000;136:235-242.
66. Sperling LC, Skelton HG, Smith KJ, et al. Follicular degeneration syndrome in men. *Arch Dermatol.* 1994;130:763-769.
67. Rondina A, Gathers RC. A case of central centrifugal cicatrical alopecia in an African-American man. *J Am Acad Dermatol.* 2009;60:AB102.
68. Davis EC, Reid SD, Callender VD, Sperling LC. Differentiating central centrifugal cicatricial alopecia and androgenetic alopecia in African-American men: report of 3 cases. *J Clin Aesthet Dermatol.* 2012;5:37-40.
69. Lopresti P, Papa CM, Kligman AM. Hot comb alopecia. *Arch Dermatol.* 1968;98:234.
70. Nicholson AG, Harland CC, Bull RH, et al. Chemically induced cosmetic alopecia. *Br J Dermatol.* 1993;128:537-541.
71. Sperling L, Sau P. The follicular degeneration syndrome in black patients: Hot comb alopecia, revisited and revised. *Arch Dermatol.* 1992;128:68-74.
72. Callender VD, Rucker-Wright D, Davis EC, Sperling LC. Hair breakage as a presenting sign of early or occult central centrifugal cicatricial alopecia: clinicopathologic findings in 9 patients. *Arch Dermatol.* 2012;148:1047-1052.
73. Callender VD, Young CM. Alopecias and hair restoration in women. In: Grimes PE, ed. *Aesthetic and Cosmetic Surgery for Darker Skin Types.* Philadelphia, PA: Lippincott Williams & Wilkins; 2008:287-295.
74. Shaffer J, Taylor S, Cook-Bolden F. Keloidal scars: a review with a critical look at therapeutic options. *J Am Acad Dermatol.* 2002;46:S41-S62.
75. Harris JA. Follicular unit extraction. *Facial Plast Surg Clin North Am.* 2013;21:375-384.
76. Callender V, Davis E. Hair transplantation. In: Alexis A, Barbosa VH, eds. *Skin of Color a Practical Guide to Dermatologic Diagnosis and Treatment.* New York, NY: Springer; 2013:351-370.
77. Marzola M. Trichophytic closure of the donor area. *Hair Transplant Forum Int.* 2005;15:113-116.
78. Callender VD, Davis EC. Hair transplantation technique: a flexible blade for preparing curly hair grafts. *Dermatol Surg.* 2011;37:1032-1034.
79. Brown MC, Johnson T, Swanson NA. Extensive keloids following hair transplantation. *J Dermatol Surg Oncol.* 1990;16:867-869.
80. Pierce HE. Hair replacement surgery in black patients. In: Pierce HE, ed. *Cosmetic Plastic Surgery in Non-White Patients.* New York, NY: Grune & Stratton; 1982:70-75.

81. Meyer M. Hair restoration in patients of African descent. In: Unger W, Shapiro R, eds. *Hair Transplantation*, 4th ed. New York, NY: Marcel Decker; 2004:595-602.

82. Engel A, Johnson ML, Haynes SG. Health effects of sunlight exposure in the Unites States: results from the first national health and nutrition examination survey 1971-1974. *Arch Dermatol*. 1988;124:72.

83. Weiss RA, Weiss MA. Sclerotherapeutic agents used for treatment of spider and varicose veins: update 2002. *J Drugs Dermatol*. 2002;1:53-59.

84. Duffy DM. Small vessel sclerotherapy: an overview. *Adv Dermatol*. 1988;3:221.

85. Weiss RA. Vascular studies of the legs for venous or arterial disease (review). *Dermatol Clin*. 1994;12:175.

86. Peterson JD, Goldman MP, Weiss RA, et al. Treatment of reticular and telangiectatic leg veins: double-blind, prospective comparative trial of polidocanol and hypertonic saline. *Dermatol Surg*. 2012;38:1322-1330.

87. Duffy DM. Sclerosants: a comparative review. *Dermatol Surg*. 2010;36:1010-1025.

88. Goldman MP, Guex JJ, Weiss RA. *Sclerotherapy: Treatment of Varicose and Telangiectatic Veins*, 5th ed. Philadelphia, PA: Saunders Elsevier; 2011.

89. Zhang J, Jing Z, Schliephake DE, et al. Efficacy and safety of Aethoxysklero (polidocanol) 0.5%, 1% and 3% in comparison with placebo solution for the treatment of varicose veins of the lower extremities in Chinese patients (ESA-China Study). *Phlebology*. 2012;27:184-190.

90. van Haarst EP, Liasis N, Van Ramshorst B, et al. The development of valvular incompetence after deep vein thrombosis: a 7-year follow-up study with duplex scanning. *Eur J Vasc Endovasc Surg*. 1996;12:295.

91. Rao J, Goldman MP. Stability of foam in sclerotherapy: differences between sodium tetradecyl sulfate and polidocanol and the type of connector used in the double system technique. *Dermatol Surg*. 2005;31:19-22.

92. Goldman MP. Sclerotherapy treatment for varicose and telangiectatic leg veins. In: Coleman WP, Hanke WK, Alt TH, Asken S, eds. *Cosmetic Surgery of the Skin*. Philadelphia, PA: BC Decker; 1991:197.

93. Weiss RA, Weiss MA. Resolution of pain associated with varicose and telangiectatic leg veins after compression sclerotherapy. *J Dermatol Surg Oncol*. 1990;16:333.

94. Tafazzoli A, Rostan E, Goldman MP. Q-switched ruby laser treatment for postsclerotherapy hyperpigmentation. *Dermatol Surg*. 2000;26:653-656.

95. Goldman MP. How to utilize compression after sclerotherapy. *Dermatol Surg*. 2002;28:860-862.

<table>
<tr><td>CHAPTER
79</td><td></td></tr>
</table>

Neuromodulators and Fillers

Valerie D. Callender
Cherie M. Young
Chesahna Kindred

KEY POINTS

- Individuals of racial minorities underwent 21% of the cosmetic procedures performed in the United States in 2012.

- Hispanics accounted for 8% of those cosmetic procedures; African Americans, 7%; Asians, 5%; and other non-Caucasians, 2%.

- Although photodamage is less of a concern in skin of color, all races experience brow furrows, frown lines, and crow's feet from repeated facial muscle contractions that are amenable to improvement with botulinum toxin.

- Soft tissue augmentation with dermal fillers is used in the treatment and correction of fine lines, nasolabial folds, marionette lines, tear trough deformities, lip augmentation, volume loss, and acne scars in skin of color patients.

Cosmetic procedures are more popular now than ever before. The American Society for Aesthetic Plastic Surgery (ASAPS) reports that in 2012 alone, surgeons performed over 10 million cosmetic surgical and nonsurgical procedures in the United States.[1] The most frequently performed surgical cosmetic procedure was breast augmentation, followed by liposuction, abdominoplasty, eyelid surgery, and rhinoplasty.[1] The most popular nonsurgical procedures were botulinum toxin injections, hyaluronic acid fillers, laser hair removal, microdermabrasion, and chemical peels. Over the past few years, the demand for such procedures has grown dramatically. Individuals are seeking cosmetic procedures that are less invasive, more affordable, and with minimal downtime.[2] According to the ASAPS, the overall number of procedures performed has increased 250% since 1997.[1] This trend is likely to continue as new advances in surgical techniques and materials unfold.

Not only are more people turning to cosmetic dermatology for answers to their cosmetic needs, but also the group of patients who seek cosmetic procedures has become more diverse. In 2012, individuals of racial minorities underwent 21% of the cosmetic procedures performed in the United States. Hispanics accounted for 8% of those procedures; African Americans, 7%; Asians, 5%; and other non-Caucasians, 2%; with the most common minimally invasive procedures being injectable fillers and botulinum toxin type A.[1]

Skin of color represent the majority of the world and approximately one-third of the U.S. population. The U.S. Census Bureau reported that in the year 2010, the resident population included 38.9 million African Americans, 50.5 million Hispanic Americans, and 15.2 million Asian Americans, Pacific Islanders, and Native Americans.[3] The non-Caucasian population in the United States is projected to grow even more in years to come, with the Hispanic population showing the most significant increases.

COSMETIC PROCEDURES

Because skin of color patients have unique cosmetic issues, they seek the procedures that best address their needs. Individuals with skin of color demonstrate less pronounced signs of extrinsic aging (photoaging) when compared with those with lighter-colored skin.[4] Additionally, when the signs of photoaging begin to manifest in darker-skinned individuals, it is at a later age. This is largely due to the photoprotective effects of eumelanin in more darkly pigmented skin.[5]

Intrinsic aging in patients with skin of color typically manifests in the midfacial region.[6] Clinically, the malar fat pads descend, leading to a tear trough deformity, infraorbital hollowing, mid-face volume loss, and deepening of the nasolabial folds. Perioral rhytides and lip atrophy are less common findings [**Figure 79-1**]. These classic signs of mid-face

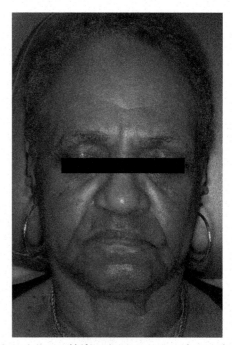

FIGURE 79-1. A 68-year-old African American woman with signs of aging including infraorbital hollowing, tear trough deformity, descent of the fat pads, and deepening of the nasolabial folds.

aging are a result of gravity-dependent sagging, volumetric loss, and soft tissue and skeletal alterations. Botulinum toxin type A and soft tissue fillers are used most often in skin of color patients to address these issues. When used with understanding and caution, most cosmetic procedures are safe and effective for use in patients with skin of color. In this chapter, the safety and efficacy of botulinum toxin injection and soft tissue filler augmentation will be reviewed.

BOTULINUM TOXIN

Although photodamage is less of a concern in skin of color, all races experience the brow furrows, frown lines, and crow's feet that repeated facial muscle contractions produce over time. Botulinum toxin A (BTX-A) is an effective treatment to reverse these effects by temporarily relaxing the muscles in the upper face, resulting in smoother skin and a more relaxed, youthful appearance.

Botulinum neurotoxins are derived from various strains of *Clostridium botulinum*. Currently, there are seven serotypes of botulinum toxin—A, B, Cα, D, E, F, and G[7]—of which serotypes A and B are available commercially. Botulinum toxin works by inhibiting the exocytosis of the neurotransmitter acetylcholine from the nerve into the synaptic space of the neuromuscular junction. Within the nerve cytoplasm exists the SNARE (soluble *N*-ethylmaleimide-sensitive factor attachment protein receptor) protein complex that is responsible for the exocytosis of acetylcholine [**Figure 79-2**]. The cleavage sites on the SNARE complex differ between the serotypes; BTX-A cleaves synaptosome-associated membrane protein 25 (SNAP-25), whereas botulinum toxin B cleaves vesicle-associated membrane protein (VAMP). This cleavage results in the inhibition of acetylcholine exocytosis and chemodenervation of the nerves that stimulate that muscle or eccrine sweat gland.

There are three U.S. Food and Drug Administration (FDA)-approved formulations of BTX-A available in the United States: onabotulinumtoxin A (Botox; Allergan, Irvine CA), abobotulinumtoxinA (Dysport; Medicis/Valeant, Phoenix, AZ), and incobotulinumtoxin A (Xeomin; Merz Aesthetics, Greensboro, NC).

INDICATIONS

- Glabellar brow furrow "frown lines" (FDA-approved indication)
- Horizontal frontalis forehead lines
- Periocular crow's feet
- Lateral brow lift
- Nasal bunny lines
- Perioral rhytides
- Marionette lines
- Dimpled chin
- Platysmal banding of the neck
- Axillary hyperhidrosis (FDA-approved indication)
- Palm and sole hyperhidrosis

TREATMENT

BTX-A is available in a crystallized form, which may be reconstituted with sterile preservative-free 0.9% saline before injection. It is injected intramuscularly in small amounts with a tuberculin syringe and a 30-gauge needle. Benefits first become noticeable within 3 to 5 days following treatment, with peak effects occurring at 1 to 3 weeks. These effects last an average of 3 to 6 months. For many patients, repeated injections maintain longer-lasting effects.

Glabellar Brow Furrow BTX-A injections are administered into the procerus muscle and corrugators with a 30-gauge needle and a tuberculin or diabetic syringe [**Figure 79-3**]. There are usually five separate injection points.[8] Based on the muscle mass, 20 to 30 Botox units (BU), 20 to 30 Xeomin units (XU), or 50 to 70 Dysport units (DU) are injected intramuscularly. Topical anesthesia is usually not required. Patients are

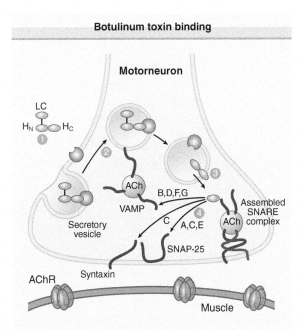

Botulinum toxin binding

Motorneuron

FIGURE 79-2. The heavy chain domain of the botulinum neurotoxin complex binds to the plasma membrane receptor (1) and the complex is internalized (2). The light chain fragment is then released into the cytoplasm (3), where it cleaves the SNARE (soluble *N*-ethylmaleimide-sensitive factor attachment protein receptor) protein complex at a site determined by the neurotoxin serotype (4). This disruption of the SNARE complex prevents exocytosis of acetylcholine (ACh) into the synaptic space of the neuromuscular junction. A through G, neurotoxin serotypes; AChR, acetylcholine receptor; LC, light chain; H$_C$, heavy chain C-terminus; H$_N$, heavy chain N-terminus; SNAP-25, synaptosome-associated protein of 25 kDa; VAMP, vesicle-associated membrane protein. (Reproduced with permission from Turton K, Chaddock JA, Acharya KR. Botulinum and tetanus neurotoxins: structure, function and therapeutic utility. *Trends Biochem Sci.* 2002 Nov;27(11):552-558.)

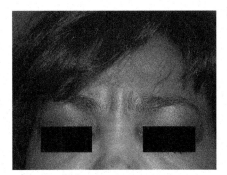

A

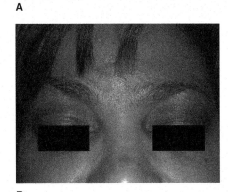

B

FIGURE 79-3. Before **(A)** and after **(B)** botulinum toxin A injections for glabellar brow furrows.

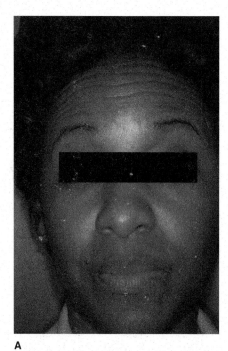

A

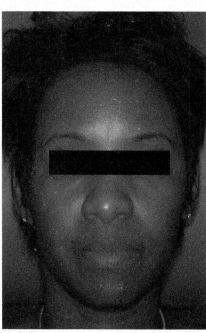

B

FIGURE 79-4. Before **(A)** and after **(B)** botulinum toxin A injections for horizontal forehead lines.

instructed not to massage or manipulate the area of injection and to remain upright for at least 2 to 4 hours.

Horizontal Forehead Lines The dose of BTX-A varies from 12 to 20 BU/XU or 20 to 50 DU based on muscle mass [**Figure 79-4**]. The lower third of the frontalis muscle is avoided in order not to produce brow ptosis. In a patient who has not been injected before, it is best to inject the glabellar brow area first and wait 2 weeks before injecting the forehead area.[9]

Crow's Feet The injection point for the crow's feet area (orbicularis oculi muscle) is approximately 1 cm lateral to the lateral canthus.[10] This injection is performed intradermally as a "wheal" in one to three injection points and then gently massaged laterally. The dose of BTX-A varies from 2 to 5 BU/XU or 10 DU per site and 10 to 18 BU/XU or 20 to 30 DU per side.

Hyperhidrosis BTX-A can be used to treat focal axillary hyperhidrosis.[11] Performing a Minor's starch-iodine test prior to the injections helps to demonstrate the area of axillary sweating. Topical anesthesia is recommended. Intradermal injections at doses between 2.5 and 4.0 units of BTX-A are placed into the skin 1 to 2 cm apart. A total of 50 units of BTX-A is used for each axilla. Results are expected in 2 to 4 days and can last up to 12 months.

Palmar hyperhidrosis also can be treated with BTX-A.[12] Anesthesia is obtained by the use of a topical anesthetic under occlusion; regional block of the median, ulnar, and radial nerves; ice; or high-intensity vibration. Each palm requires 100 units of BTX-A, and the technique consists of multiple intradermal injections of 2 to 3 units each spaced approximately 1 to 2 cm apart. Results may vary; a period of 6 to 12 months of anhydrosis is common.

OUTCOME

Multiple clinical studies have evaluated the safety and efficacy of botulinum toxin injections in skin of color patients. These populations include Asians, Latino/Hispanics, and African Americans.[13–22]

A 4-month randomized, double-masked dosing study for treatment of glabellar lines in women with skin types V and VI was performed to assess the efficacy of two dosing regimens of onabotulinumtoxin A (Botox): 20 units versus 30 units. Both dosing regimens were found to be well tolerated in the skin of color subjects.[22]

A 5-month study using abobotulinumtoxin A (Dysport), a purified BTX-A hemagglutin complex, was performed and demonstrated promising results in African American ptatients.[23] This was a phase III, randomized, double-blind, placebo-controlled study that involved 816 subjects, 160 of whom were African American. The dosages ranged from 50 to 70 units in women and 60 to 80 units in men. The African American patients displayed a higher response rate, as well as a slightly longer median duration of action with abobotulinumtoxin A (Dysport) treatment than those of other population groups. Treatment with abobotulinumtoxin A was found to be relatively safe in all treatment groups, although African Americans did exhibit a slightly increased incidence of ocular events (6% in African Americans vs 4% in other population groups) and a lower incidence of injection site reactions (3% in African Americans vs 5% in other population groups).

More recently, a post hoc analysis of six clinical trials compared the effectiveness and tolerability of abobotulinumtoxin A (Dysport) in the treatment of glabellar lines in skin of color patients, as compared to fairer-skinned patients.[24] Three of the trials compared the time to onset of response, response at day 30, durability of response, and safety and tolerability of a fixed 50-unit dose of abobotulinumtoxin A in skin of color and fairer-skinned patients, whereas one study assessed the same parameters of a dose of abobotulinumtoxin A adjusted to muscle mass in dark skin of color and fairer-skinned patients. It was found that the onset of response was similar in skin of color and fairer-skinned patients, but the response rate at 30 days after treatment was greater in skin of color patients. Adverse event rates were similar between the two populations.

To date, there have been no clinical trials assessing the effectiveness and side effect profile of incobotulinumtoxin A (Xeomin) in skin of color patients.

COMPLICATIONS

Local skin reactions can occur with BTX-A, such as swelling, erythema, and bruising. Most are mild and transient. Mild headache and flulike symptoms have been reported as well. A small percentage of patients experience transient ptosis that usually resolves within 2 to 4 weeks. Treatment with apraclonidine eye drops stimulates Muller muscles to lift the eyelids and correct the ptosis.[25] Injection of a minimally dilute solution approximately 1 cm or more above the brow, and postinjection counseling to emphasize the importance of remaining upright for 6 hours after the injection without massaging or manipulating the injected site will help to minimize the risk of ptosis.

SOFT TISSUE AUGMENTATION

Soft tissue augmentation with dermal filler is used in the treatment and correction of fine lines; nasolabial folds; marionette lines; tear trough deformities; lip, cheek, chin, and hand augmentation; volume loss; and acne scars. According to the ASAPS 2012 statistics, there were 1.62 million soft tissue filler injections, 1.423 million hyaluronic acid injections, 129,674 calcium hydroxylapatite injections, and 69,965 poly-L-lactic acid injections.[1] Hyaluronic acid fillers are used most often in soft tissue augmentation due to their longer duration of action and excellent safety profile compared with collagen fillers. Volumizing with an array of dermal fillers with different properties can improve aesthetic outcomes in skin of color patients. Collagen-based fillers (Zyderm, Zyplast, Cosmoderm, Cosmoplast, and Evolence) are no longer available and will not be discussed. Current available dermal fillers with skin of color data will be reviewed, and special considerations in patients with skin of color will be discussed [**Table 79-1**].

HYALURONIC ACID FILLERS

Hyaluronic acid (HA) fillers may be the agents of choice for soft tissue augmentation in patients with darker skin [**Figure 79-5**]. Compared with bovine collagen, these agents carry a significantly lower risk of allergic hypersensitivity reaction. As a result, preliminary skin testing is not required. HA is a glycosaminoglycan consisting of alternating units of D-glucuronic acid and N-acetyl-D-glucosamine disaccharides. It is found in the extracellular matrix of connective tissue in the skin, vitreous humor, synovial fluid, umbilical cord, and the capsules of certain microorganisms. Hypersensitivity secondary to trace amounts of proteins in the HA raw material or impurities of bacterial fermentation have occurred, but the introduction of more purified forms has reduced the incidence of this reaction. HA is a hydrophilic substance that attracts and holds water. Once injected into the skin, it attracts water and hydrates the skin. It is stabilized in the skin by cross-linking, which provides a longer duration than collagen fillers.

Restylane and Perlane Restylane and Perlane are derived from non-animal streptococcal bacteria. They both contain 20 mg/mL of HA and are cross-linked using butane-diol-diglycidyl ether (BDDE). They differ in the gel bead size—Restylane 250 μm, 100,000 units/mL, which is considered a small gel particle HA (SGP-HA), compared with Perlane 1000 μm, 10,000 units/mL, which is a large gel particle HA (LGP-HA). Both are FDA approved for the treatment of moderate to severe facial rhytides, and the duration of effect is 6 to 12 months.[25] Recently, SGP-HA has been approved for lip augmentation.[26]

Both Restylane and Perlane contain 0.3% preservative-free lidocaine, which helps to anesthetize the treated area within seconds. This allows for a more comfortable injection for the patient.

A multicenter, prospective, randomized (split-face), patient-blinded comparative study was performed to evaluate the safety and effectiveness

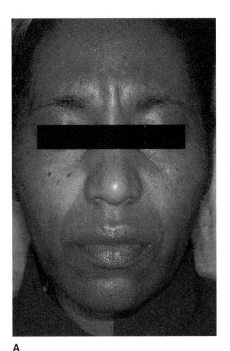

A

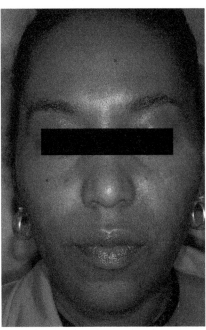

B

FIGURE 79-5. Before (**A**) and after (**B**) hyaluronic acid filler treatment for nasolabial folds and botulinum toxin A injections for glabellar brow furrows.

of SGP-HA (Restylane) and LGP-HA (Perlane) in the treatment of moderate to severe nasolabial folds in 150 subjects with skin types IV to VI.[27,28] Most of the patients were African American, and the Fitzpatrick skin types included 30% skin type IV, 45% skin type V, and 25% skin type VI. The results demonstrated duration of effect of at least 6 months with both SGP-HA (Restylane) (73%) and LGP-HA (Perlane) (70%), and postinflammatory hyperpigmentation occurred in 5% to 7% of injection sites. These adverse events were considered mild to moderate and resolved within 12 weeks. No keloidal or hypertrophic scarring related to the injection was seen during the study.

Another randomized, evaluator-blinded study was performed assessing the effectiveness and safety of SGP-HA (Restylane) for lip augmentation.[26] This 6-month study included Fitzpatrick skin types I to VI. One

TABLE 79-1	Dermal fillers in skin of color		
Filler	Dyschromia	HTS/Keloid	Study/Author
Restylane	9%	None	NLF, Taylor et al[27]
	None	None	Lips, Glogau et al[26]
Perlane	6%	None	NLF, Taylor et al[27]
Juvederm	7.5%	None	NLF, Grimes et al[29]
Belotero	N/A	N/A	N/A
Radiesse	None	None	NLF, Marmur et al[34]
Sculptra	N/A	N/A	N/A
ArteFill	N/A	N/A	N/A
Laviv	N/A	N/A	N/A

Abbreviations: HTS, hypertrophic scar; N/A, nonapplicable; NLF, nasolabial folds.

hundred eighty subjects were randomized, with 135 receiving treatment with SGP-HA and 45 receiving no treatment. Forty-one of the subjects (23%) had Fitzpatrick skin types IV, V, or VI. At week 8, 95% and 94% of the subjects who received SGP-HA for the upper and lower lips, respectively, were responders to treatment. Of those who did not receive treatment, the response rates were 36% for the upper lip and 38% for the lower lip. A subgroup analysis of patients with Fitzpatrick skin types IV, V, and VI found a similar response pattern. The most common adverse events reported in this study were pain, swelling, tenderness, bruising, and erythema, most of which were mild to moderate and lasted 5 to 10 days after the procedure.

Juvederm Ultra and Juvederm Ultra Plus Juvederm Ultra and Juvederm Ultra Plus are derived from nonanimal streptococcal bacteria. They are formulated with Hylacross technology to allow a higher concentration of cross-linked HA. This HA product also contains preservative-free lidocaine 0.3%, allowing for greater tolerability of the procedure by the patient.

A multicenter, double-blind, randomized, within-subject controlled study was performed to examine the efficacy and safety of HA-based fillers (Juvederm Ultra, Ultra Plus, and 30) versus cross-linked bovine collagen.[29] Subjects received nasolabial fold treatment of HA filler on one side and bovine treatment on the contralateral side. There were 423 subjects who completed the 24-week study, of whom 26% were non-Caucasian. Subject demographics included 12% Hispanics, 11% African Americans, and 2% Asians. All Fitzpatrick skin types (I to VI) were involved in the study, which included 20% type IV, 13% type V, and 3% type VI. The results demonstrated that the HA fillers resulted in longer-lasting clinical results than the bovine collagen, and the efficacy was similar for Caucasians and non-Caucasian subjects. In addition, there was no increased incidence of hyperpigmentation or hypertrophic scarring in the non-Caucasian subjects compared with the Caucasian subjects.

Belotero Balance Belotero is a recently FDA-approved monophasic HA-based dermal filler. It differs from the other approved HA fillers due to its cohesive polydensified matrix technology (CPM-HA). A recent study was conducted comparing its efficacy and safety profile with that of Restylane and Juvederm. Adverse events were unremarkable, and they all revealed equivalent efficacy.[30]

One split-face study compared the use of CPM-HA (Belotero) with bovine collagen. One hundred eighteen patients were randomized, with the majority being Caucasian (96.6%).[31] At the end of 24 weeks, twice the percentage of subjects maintained correction on the Belotero side as compared with the side treated with bovine collagen. The majority of the subjects reported one or more adverse events. They were mild to moderate events that were related to the injection process rather than the device and resolved in less than 7 days. Data in skin of color patients are not currently published, but clinical trials have been performed in this patient population.

Calcium Hydroxyapatite (CaHA, Radiesse) Radiesse is a semipermanent filler that, once injected into the deep dermis, forms a scaffold on which collagenesis occurs. It is used in the correction of nasolabial folds, marionette lines, jowls, cheeks, and chin. CaHA is not recommended for the lips, and the longevity varies from 3 to 12 months.[32]

To achieve pain reduction, Radiesse is mixed with 2% lidocaine prior to injection[33] [**Figure 79-6**]. This is done by drawing the lidocaine into a 3-mL syringe. This syringe is then attached to the syringe containing the Radiesse by using a luer lock connector. Approximately 10 mixing strokes are performed to adequately combine the two ingredients prior to injection.

A randomized split-face study was performed assessing the pain reduction and efficacy of premixing CaHA with 2% lidocaine for the treatment of nasolabial folds.[33] Subjects were randomized to receive CaHA alone in one nasolabial fold and CaHA mixed with lidocaine in the other nasolabial fold and completed pain assessments immediately after injection, 1 hour after injection, and 1 month after treatment. Subjects reported less

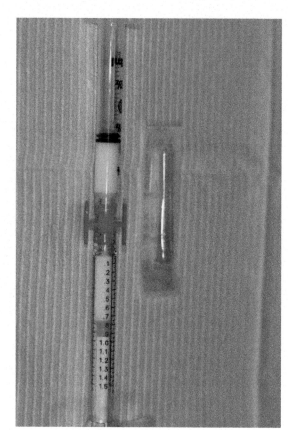

FIGURE 79-6. Calcium hydroxyapatite technique for mixing with 2% lidocaine prior to injection.

pain in the nasolabial fold treated with CaHA mixed with lidocaine, and aesthetic results were found to be equivalent for both treatments.

A postapproval open-label clinical study was initiated to assess adverse effects of Radiesse in persons of color.[34] One hundred subjects with Fitzpatrick skin types IV to VI whose nasolabial folds were treated with subdermal injections of Radiesse were followed for 6 months. Subject characteristics included 85 African Americans, 12 Hispanics, 2 Asians, and 1 other with Fitzpatrick skin types as follows: 24 with skin type IV, 35 with skin type V, and 41 with skin type VI. At the end of the study, results showed no reports of hypertrophic scarring, keloid formation, or dyspigmentation.

POLY-L-LACTIC ACID (SCULPTRA)

Poly-L-lactic acid (PLLA) was first FDA approved in 2004 to treat acquired lipodystrophy in patients with human immunodeficiency virus (HIV) infection[35,36] who were treated with highly active antiretroviral therapy (HAART). Since that time, Sculptra has been successfully used for the correction of nasolabial folds, mid- and lower face volume loss, and other signs of aging.[37] The injectable PLLA is biodegradable and biocompatible and produces a gradual and significant increase in skin thickness, improving the appearance of folds and sunken areas by fibroplasia.

PLLA is immunologically inert, so pretreatment skin testing is not required. Each vial contains a freeze-dried PLLA powder that is reconstituted with 6 to 7 mL of bacteriostatic sodium chloride 24 to 48 hours prior to treatment (off label). Prior to injecting, 2 mL of 1% lidocaine with or without epinephrine is added to the suspension and then shaken. Additional anesthesia can be used if necessary and includes topical agents, local infiltration, and nerve blocks.

Multiple treatment sessions are required at 4- to 6-week intervals, with the effects lasting up to 2 years. Results are not immediate, and touch-ups may be required. Vigorous massage of all injected areas is performed immediately after treatment and in some cases for 5 days after treatment. This step is extremely important to ensure proper distribution of the material and to decrease the possible formation of nodules.

Although studies have not been conducted in skin of color patients, clinicians have found that when treating these patients with PLLA, most require increased intervals between treatments.[38] With proper patient selection and administration technique, PLLA has been used effectively in patients with skin of color.

POLYMETHYLMETHACRYLATE (ARTEFILL)

ArteFill is a polymeric microsphere-based filler that was FDA approved in 2006 for the correction of nasolabial folds. It consists of polymethylmethacrylate (PMMA) microspheres suspended in 3.5% bovine collagen and 0.3% lidocaine and offers patients permanent, long-term correction of nasolabial folds. The bovine collagen is absorbed within 1 month of injection and is replaced by the patient's own connective tissue within 3 months.[39]

Previous studies have also assessed the effectiveness of ArteFill for the treatment of atrophic acne scars. In an open-label pilot study with 14 patients, some improvement in the correction of acne scars was observed in 96% of treated scars 8 months after treatment.[40] There were no adverse events noted. There are no published data for the use of Arte-Fill in skin of color patients, and therefore, further studies are needed.

AUTOLOGOUS COLLAGEN

There are two bioengineered forms of human collagen: allogenic and autologous. Allogenic collagen is provided from cadaver skin specimens and from discarded skin specimens obtained during plastic and reconstructive surgery.[41] Cosmoderm and Cosmoplast are derived from human collagen (foreskin). They have a low incidence of cross-reactivity, so skin testing is not required. All forms of these collagen-type fillers are no longer available.

Autologous collagen is prepared from the patient's own tissue. As a result, this type of collagen is not allergenic and does not transmit exogenous infection. Because it contains intact dermal collagen fibers, it may be more resistant to enzymatic degradation. Two examples of autologous collagen are Autologen and Isolagen.[42] Autologen is no longer available. Isolagen preliminary phase III data were introduced in 2005.

Recently, the FDA approved the use of autologous fibroblasts (Laviv) for the treatment of nasolabial folds in adults.[43] A phase III study was performed using autologous cultured fibroblast injection for the treatment of facial contour deformities such as nasolabial folds, acne scars, and glabellar lines.[44] One hundred fifty-one patients were treated, with 4.8% being Asian, 1.4% Hispanic, and 1.4.% African American. The fibroblast-treated patients had a much greater response than those treated with placebo, with the response lasting at least 12 months after treatment and a favorable safety profile.

SIDE EFFECTS OF FILLERS

Common side effects of HA fillers include bruising at injection site, erythema, edema, and slight pain. One side effect that clinicians should be aware of with the use of HAs is the Tyndall effect. This occurs when the filler is placed too superficially in the skin and a bluish hue appears.[45] The bluish color results from light reflection from particles contained in a clear material (filler). When the light is scattered from these particles, a bluish hue can result (Tyndall effect). This is most commonly seen in the treatment of the lower eyelid. If this effect occurs or the development of nodules occur, correction is done by injecting hyaluronidase. Hyaluronidase is an enzyme that dissolves HA quickly and efficiently. It should be noted that although effective for the treatment of certain side effects, hyaluronidase carries its own risks including allergic reactions.[46]

Since 2003, postapproval studies have been performed using HA and calcium hydroxylapatite fillers in patients with Fitzpatrick skin types IV to VI to assess the safety of dermal fillers in this population.[2,47] These studies were performed to assess the rates of keloid formation, dyschromias, hypertrophic scarring, and hypersensitivity reactions in skin of color.[2,40] There were no reports of keloid formation, and there was mild hypertrophic scarring with HA fillers in one study.[2,26,28]

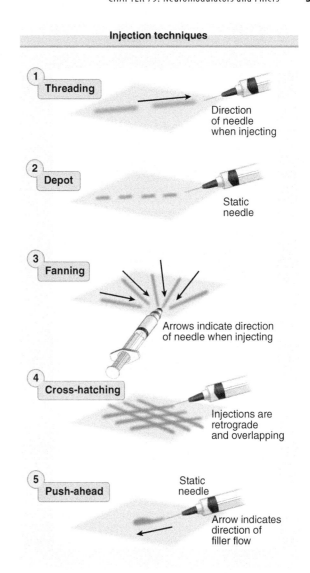

FIGURE 79-7. Injection techniques. (Reproduced with permission from Goldsmith LA, Katz SI, Blichrest BA, et al. *Fitzpatrick's Dermatology in General Medicine.* 8th ed. New York, NY: McGraw-Hill; 2012.)

The rate of dyschromia was similar between Caucasian and non-Caucasian patients, with no pigmentary changes being observed with patients treated with calcium hydroxylapatite.[2,26,28,32] The pigmentary changes observed in the use of HA fillers may be due to the superficial placement of these fillers as opposed to the subdermal placement of the calcium hydroxylapatite fillers.[2,34]

Minimizing the risks associated with injection of fillers should include decreasing the number of punctures to the skin, using the linear threading technique, avoiding serial punctures and fanning [**Figure 79-7**], mid-deep dermal placement, and postinjection topical application of a corticosteroid to decrease inflammation.[48]

CONCLUSION

Cosmetic procedures are desired by skin of color patients and continue to become more popular in this population. Noninvasive surgical procedures involving minimal downtime are the preferred method in achieving aesthetic results. It is important for the medical community to understand the needs of our patients and to be able to treat them in the appropriate manner. It has been proven that BTX-A and soft tissue fillers are relatively safe and effective in the treatment of cosmetic concerns in skin of color patients; however, more clinical studies are warranted.

REFERENCES

1. American Society for Aesthetic Plastic Surgery (ASAPS). 2012 statistics on cosmetic surgery. www.surgery.org/press/statistics-2011.php. Accessed May 5, 2013.

2. Davis EC, Callender VD. Aesthetic dermatology in aging ethnic skin. *Dermatol Surg.* 2011;37:1-17.

3. U.S. Census Bureau. www.census.gov. Accessed January 2013.

4. Halder RM, Richards GM. Photoaging in patients of skin of color. In: Rigel DS, Weiss RA, Lion HW, et al, eds. *Photoaging.* New York, NY: Marcel Dekker; 2004:55-63.

5. Kaidbey KH, Agin PP, Sayre RM, et al. Photoprotection by melanin: a comparison of black and Caucasian skin. *J Am Acad Dermatol.* 1979;1:249-260.

6. Harris MO. The aging face in patients of color: minimally invasive surgical facial rejuvenation—a targeted approach. *Dematol Ther.* 2004;17:206-211.

7. Aoki KR. Pharmacology and immunology of botulinum toxin serotypes. *J Neurol.* 2001;248:3S.

8. Carruthers JA, Lowe NJ, Menter MA, et al. A multicentre, double-blind, randomized, placebo-controlled study of efficacy and safety of botulinum toxin type A in the treatment of glabellar lines. *J Am Acad Dermatol.* 2002;46:840-849.

9. Carruthers A, Carruthers J. Clinical indications and injection technique for the cosmetic use of botulinum A exotoxin. *Dermatol Surg.* 1998;24:1189-1194.

10. Lowe NJ, Lask G, Yamauchi P, et al. Bilateral, double-blind, randomized, comparison of three doses of botulinum toxin type A and placebo in patients with crow's feet. *J Am Acad Dermatol.* 2002;47:834-840.

11. Lower NJ, Glaser DA, Eadie N, et al. Botulinum toxin type A in the treatment of primary axillary hyperhidrosis: a 52-week multicenter double-blind, randomized, placebo-controlled study of efficacy and safety. *J Am Acad Dermatol.* 2007;56:604-606.

12. Shelley WB, Talanin NY, Shelley ED. Botulinum toxin therapy for palmar hyperhidrosis. *J Am Acad Dermatol.* 1998;38(2 Pt 1):227-229.

13. Ahn KY, Park MY, Park DH, et al. Botulinum toxin A for the treatment of facial hyperkinetic wrinkle lines in Koreans. *Plast Reconstr Surg.* 2000;205:778-784.

14. Lew H, Yun YS, Lee SY, et al. Effect of botulinum toxin A on facial wrinkle lines in Koreans. *Ophthalmologica.* 2002;216:50-54.

15. Hexsel DM, De Almeida AT, Rutowitsch M, et al. Multicenter, double-blind study of the efficacy of injections with botulinum toxin type A reconstituted up to six consecutive weeks before application. *Dermatol Surg.* 2003;29:523-529.

16. Harii K, Kawashima M. A double-blind, randomized, placebo controlled, two-dose comparative study of botulinum toxin type a for treating glabellar lines in Japanese subjects. *Aesthet Plast Surg.* 2008;32:724-730.

17. Kawashima M, Harii K. An open-label, randomized, 64-week study repeating 10- and 20-U doses of botulinum toxin type A for treatment of glabellar lines in Japanese subjects. *Int J Dermatol.* 2009;48:768-776.

18. Farafvash MR, Arad S. Clostridium botulinum a type A toxin for the treatment of upper face animation lines: an Iranian experience. *J Cosmet Dermatol.* 2007;6:152-158.

19. Chang SP, Tsai HH, Chen WY, et al. The wrinkles soothing effect on the middle and lower face by intradermal injection of botulinum toxin type A. *Int J Dermatol.* 2008;47:1287-1294.

20. Kadunc BV, Trindade de Almeida AR, Vanti AA, Di Chiacchio N. Botulinum toxin A adjunctive use in manual chemabrasion: controlled long-term study for treatment of upper perioral vertical wrinkles. *Dermatol Surg.* 2007;33:1066-1072.

21. Grimes PE, Shabazz D. A four month randomized, double-blind evaluation of the efficacy of botulinum toxin type A for the treatment of glabellar lines in women with skin types V and VI. *Dermatol Surg.* 2009;35:429-436.

22. Kane M, Brandt F, Rohrich R, et al. Evaluation of variable-dose treatment with a new U.S. botulinum toxin type A (Dysport) for correction of moderate to severe glabellar lines: results from a phase III, randomized, double-blind, placebo-controlled study. *Plast Reconstr Surg.* 2009;124:1619-1629.

23. Taylor SC, Callender VD, Albright CD, et al. AbotulinumtoxinA for reduction of glabellar lines in patients with skin of color: post hoc analysis of pooled clinical trial data. *Dermatol Surg.* 2012;38:1804-1811.

24. Wollina U, Konrad H. Managing adverse events associated with botulinum toxin type A: a focus on cosmetic procedures. *Am J Clin Dermatol.* 2005;6:141-150.

25. Narins RS, Brandt F, Leyden J, et al. A randomized, double-blind, multicenter comparison of the efficacy and tolerability of Restylane versus Zyplast for the correction of nasolabial folds. *Dermatol Surg.* 2003;29:588-595.

26. Glogau RG, Bank D, Brandt F, et al. A randomized, evaluator-blinded, controlled study of the effectiveness and safety of small gel particle hyaluronic acid for lip augmentation. *Dermatol Surg.* 2012;38:1180-1192.

27. Taylor SC, Burgess CM, Callender VD. Safety of nonanimal stabilized hyaluronic acid dermal fillers in patients with skin of color: a randomized, evaluator-blinded comparative trial. *Dermatol Surg.* 2009;35:1653-1660.

28. Taylor SC, Burgess CM, Callender VD. Efficacy of variable-particle hyaluronic acid dermal fillers in patients with skin of color: a randomized, evaluator-blinded comparative trial. *Dermatol Surg.* 2010;36:741-749.

29. Grimes PE, Thomas JA, Murphy DK, et al. Safety and effectiveness of hyaluronic acid fillers in skin of color. *J Cosmet Dermatol.* 2009;8:162-168.

30. Prager W, Wissmueller E, Havermann I, et al. A prospective, split-face, randomized, comparative study of safety and 12-month longevity of three formulations of hyaluronic acid dermal filler for the treatment of nasolabial folds. *Dermatol Surg.* 2012;38:1143-1150.

31. Narins RS, Coleman III W, Donofrio L, et al. Nonanimal sourced hyaluronic acid-based dermal filler using a cohesive matrix technology is superior to bovine collagen in the correction of moderate to severe nasolabial folds: results from a 6-month, randomized, blinded, controlled, multicenter study. *Dermatol Surg.* 2010;36:730-740.

32. Sadick NS, Katz BE, Roy D. A multicenter, 47-month study of safety and efficacy of calcium hydroxylapatite for soft tissue augmentation of nasolabial folds and other areas of the face. *Dermatol Surg.* 2007;33:S122-S127.

33. Marmur E, Green L, Busso M. Controlled, randomized study of pain levels in subjects treated with calcium hydroxylapatite premixed with lidocaine for correction of nasolabial folds. *Dermatol Surg.* 2010;36:309-315.

34. Marmur ES, Taylor SC, Grimes PE, et al. Six-month safety results of calcium hydroxylapatite for treatment of nasolabial folds in Fitzpatrick skin types IV to VI. *Dermatol Surg.* 2009;35:1641-1645.

35. Valantin MA, Aubron-Olivier C, Ghosn J, et al. Polylactic acid implants (New-Fill) to correct facial lipoatrophy in HIV-infected patient: results of the open-label study VEGA. *AIDS.* 2003;17:2471-2477.

36. Burgess CM, Quiroga RM. Assessment of the safety and efficacy of poly-L-lactic acid for the treatment of HIV-associated facial lipoatrophy. *J Am Acad Dermatol.* 2005;52:233-239.

37. Narins RS, Baumann L, Brandt FS, et al. A randomized study of the efficacy and safety of injectable poly-L-lactic acid versus human-based collagen implant in the treatment of nasolabial fold wrinkles. *J Am Acad Dermatol.* 2010;62:448-462.

38. Hamilton TK, Burgess CM. Considerations for the use of injectable poly-L-lactic acid in people of color. *J Drugs Dermatol.* 2010;9:451-456.

39. Lemperle G, Knapp TR, Sadick NS, et al. ArteFill permanent injectable for soft tissue augmentation: I. Mechanism of action and injection techniques. *Aesthetic Plast Surg.* 2010;34:264-272.

40. Epstein RE, Spencer JM. Correction of atrophic scars with artefill: an open-label pilot study. *J Drugs Dermatol.* 2010;9:1062-1064.

41. Baumann L. Cosmoderm/Cosmoplast (human bioengineered) for the aging face. *Facial Plast Surg.* 2004;20:125-128.

42. West TB, Alster TS. Autologous human collagen and dermal fibroblasts for soft tissue augmentation. *Dermatol Surg.* 1998;24:510-512.

43. Zeng W, Zhang S, Liu D, et al. Preclinical safety studies on autologous cultured human skin fibroblast transplantation. *Cell Transplant.* 2014;23:39-49.

44. Weiss RA, Weiss MA, Beasley KL, et al. Autologous cultured fibroblast injection for facial contour deformities: a prospective, placebo-controlled, phase III clinical trial. *Dermatol Surg.* 2007;33:263-268.

45. Hirsch RJ, Narurkar V, Carruthers J. Management of injected hyaluronic acid induced Tyndall effects. *Lasers Surg Med.* 2006;38:202-204.

46. Van Dyke S, Hays GP, Caglia AE. Severe acute local reactions to a hyaluronic acid-derived dermal filler. *J Clin Aesthet Dermatol.* 2010;3:32-35.

47. Lim LM, Dang JM, Francis J, et al. Executive summary: dermal filler devices. Food and Drug Administration (online). http://www.fda.gov/ohrms/dockets/ac/08/briefing/2008-4391b1-01%20-%20FDA%20Executive%20Summary%20Dermal%20Fillers.pdf. Accessed May 30, 2013.

48. Callender VD, Narurkar VA, Davis EC. Cosmetic treatments for skin of color. In: Taylor S, Badreshia-Bansal S, Callender V, Gathers R, Rodriquez D, eds. *Treatments for Skin of Color.* 1st ed. Beijing, China: Saunders Elsevier; 2011:309-348.

<table>
<tr><td>CHAPTER</td><td rowspan="2"># Skin and Lip Typology</td></tr>
</table>

CHAPTER 80

Skin and Lip Typology

Diane Baras
Lawrence Caisey

KEY POINTS

- Diversity of skin color covers a large and continuous color space where different racial groups overlap each other.
- Racial or ethnic origins and cultural backgrounds play a major role in self-perception of skin tone, undoubtedly influencing makeup strategy.
- Four main makeup strategies have been identified.
- The lip color space is as large as the skin color space.

INTRODUCTION

The ideal makeup is a tailor-made product that respects a woman's individuality. Individual uniqueness can be characterized by biophysical as well as psychological features. A thorough understanding of a woman based on her own characteristics entails these two dimensions.

The diversity of women comes from the various types of skin tone, lips, and eyelashes, all of which could be enhanced, corrected, or transformed by makeup according to the user's expectations.

These expectations are linked to self-perception of the biophysical properties of the face. A woman's features and concerns about skin tone, lips, and lashes strongly depend on racial or ethnic origin, as well as on the cultural and geographic environment. There may be a discrepancy between self-perception and objective assessment.

Objective assessments are provided by instrumental measurements of physical and biophysical properties of the face. Several characteristics are recorded, such as color and unevenness of skin tone and morphologic and biomechanical hydration properties of the lips. Such measurements emphasize the diversity among different population groups as well as within each individual group.

This chapter expands on the main results of our dual approach, combining qualitative assessments and quantitative measurements in women with different skin of color and cultural background. It focuses on the two main cosmetic supports of the facial appearance: skin complexion and lips through their colorimetric features.

THE COLOR OF THE SKIN

For most women, applying a "colored" makeup to the skin is the first step, or foundation, of the makeup routine. A woman enhances her face by matching or changing the color of her skin.

A qualitative and quantitative study was conducted on a large panel of diverse women to better understand how individual women think about their makeup strategy and how it is influenced by skin color, race, ethnicity, and geographic location. The study consisted of (1) an examination of various skin colors or hues to define skin color worldwide, to highlight the differences between racial groups, and to observe the diversity within each group; (2) an exploration of how women self-perceive facial skin complexion, what their ideal skin tone is, how they managed to achieve it, specifically what they did, and how much they were satisfied with their makeup results; and (3) a colorimetric assessment of makeup results and comparison between that data and a woman's feelings.

Our investigations involved two studies, the first of which began in 1999 and now includes 3721 women living in nine countries, that determined the skin color of women. In 2003, colorimetric measurements were performed on 507 women from different racial groups before and after applying foundation. Measurements were followed by an in-depth interview to record the subject's self-description of her face as well as

her satisfaction level. Data were tabulated in a way to assess the needs of women.

SKIN TONES: A HIGH DIVERSITY

A number of studies have explored the differences in skin color among different population groups. However, they often do not provide adequate information about the diversity and intermixing of the involved populations. The scale of most of these studies was small, and the places where measurements were performed were too limited to reflect the large range of skin tones within each racial group or to reveal the overlapping of skin color range between groups.[1-7] In our study, which began in 1999, we measured skin tones and classified them independent of racial origin in order to emphasize their diversity and overlap.

Panel A total of 3721 female volunteers from six different racial origins living in nine different geographic locations have been included. They range in age from 18 to 65 years and include 1993 Asians, 160 Indians, 1120 Caucasians, 219 Hispanics, 127 French Africans, and 102 African Americans [**Table 80-1**]. None suffer from disease that might impair or change color or facial skin condition.

Methods Forehead and cheek color is measured using a spectroradiometer inside a Chromasphere. The Chromasphere, developed and patented by L'Oreal Research,[8] is a stable, reliable, and diffuse lighting system that faithfully mimics natural daylight (CIE illuminant D65). This device does not involve contact measurements that have the potential to alter blood flow when pressure is applied to the skin, thus altering skin color. The volunteer places her face into the Chromasphere, and standardized cameras are used to obtain pictures of the face.[9] The unevenness of skin color is then assessed through image analysis.

A spectroradiometer that measures the reflectance of forehead and cheek in the visible light range (400-700 nm) was used. The recorded spectrum is expressed in the CIE 1976 standard colorimetric space L^*C^*hD65/10°, where each color is described through three coordinates that reflect perception by human eye: h for hue angle (angular coordinate), C^* for chroma (radius coordinate), and L^* for lightness (z axis) [**Figure 80-1**]. The hue h is the approximate psychosensorial translation of the dominant wavelength. This is why the hue is that aspect of a color described with names such as *red* and *yellow*. The chroma C^*, or saturation, refers to the pureness or vividness. Highly colorful skin is vivid and intense, whereas less colorful skin appears more muted, even close to gray. The lightness L^*, or brightness coordinate, grades skin color (more or less light, more or less dark) using a gray scale.

Statistics Significant differences between racial groups were demonstrated using univariate analysis on L^*, C^*, and h data on both forehead and cheeks. The diversity of skin tones was described using principal component analysis (PCA) from L^*, C^*, and h data on forehead and cheeks of subjects. PCA allowed us to classify skin tones from different population groups on a hierarchical ascending classification.

Results From measurements performed on 3721 volunteers, a large color space has been defined [**Figure 80-2**]. The darkest skin tones were found in African American, French African, and Indian women. At the opposite end of the spectrum, Caucasians had the lightest complexions and the reddest cheeks. Asian and Indian women had the yellowest skin [**Figure 80-3**]. Interestingly, Caucasian, Asian, and Hispanic women

TABLE 80-1	Population and place of residence of the 3721 female volunteers involved in the study	
Population	Place of residence	Frequency
African American	United States	102
Asian	China, Japan, Korea, Thailand	1993
Caucasian	France, Russia, United States	1120
French African	France	127
Hispanic	Brazil, United States	219
Indian	India	160

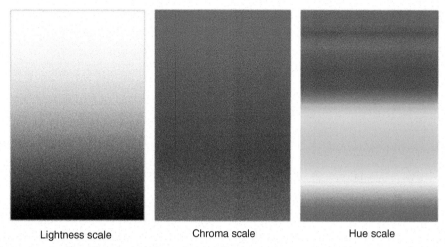

Lightness scale   Chroma scale   Hue scale

FIGURE 80-1. Scales of lightness, chroma, and hue. When the chroma/saturation is low, the color appears gray.

covered the same lightness range, Caucasian and Hispanic women the same chroma (saturation) range, and African American and Caucasian women the same hue range [Figure 80-3]. These are the first data that highlight this type of diversity between groups. However, such analyses do not evaluate the diversity within each population group, which motivated us to investigate differences within the skin color space.

Our classification emphasizes six groups of skin tones [Figure 80-2 and **Figure 80-4**].

Group 1 encompasses the darkest and the less saturated skin tones ($L^* = 42.0$; $C^* = 19.4$ on the forehead; Figure 80-3), including African American, French African, Brazilian, and Indian women.

Group 2 is composed of women with significantly lighter skin than group 1 but still significantly darker skin than in the other groups ($L^* = 54.4$ on forehead; Figure 80-3). It includes not only some African American, French African, and Indian women, but also some Asian (living in Thailand) and Hispanic (living in Brazil and the United States) women. Even among dark skin, there is a high level of diversity.

Group 3 has significantly lighter and the most saturated skin ($L^* = 61.2$ and $C^* = 26.5$ on the forehead; Figure 80-3). These skin tones could be termed *tanned skin*. This group is the meeting point where many racial or ethnic groups (eg, Caucasian, Asian, Hispanic, and French African) overlap one other.

Group 4, primarily composed of Caucasian women, but also some Asian and Hispanic women who also show such "pink" skin tones, displays significant redness ($h = 51.4$ and 46.3 on forehead and cheeks, respectively; Figure 80-3).

Group 5 has the lightest skin tones, with a good balance between red and yellow components and a low saturation level that reinforces the white visual appearance of the skin ($L^* = 66.2$, $C^* = 22.1$, and $h = 55.9$ on the forehead; Figure 80-3). With the exception of French Africans, African Americans, and Indians, all the racial or ethnic groups are found

in Group 5. Group 6, which includes not only Asian but also Caucasian and Hispanic women, has skin that is significantly yellow ($h = 59.9$ on forehead; Figure 80-3). Contrary to prejudgment, group 6 is not insignificant in proportion.

It is essential to note that these results show a tremendous diversity of skin color covering a large and continuous color space where different racial or ethnic groups overlap one another.

▣ SELF-PERCEPTION AND SATISFACTION LEVEL OF SKIN COLOR BEFORE AND AFTER APPLYING FOUNDATION MAKEUP

In 2006, we reported a study[10] on self-perception of facial skin by women from different population groups, showing how it was influenced by skin color, origin, and living place.

Panel The study involved 507 healthy women from distinct population groups using foundation on a daily basis and living in different geographic locations (112 French Caucasians in Paris, 107 American Caucasians in New York, 118 Japanese in Tokyo, and 75 African Americans and 95 Hispanic Americans in New York). The volunteers were 25 to 65 years old, including 170 women aged 25 to 35 years, 174 women aged 36 to 45 years, and 163 women aged 46 to 65 years.

Methods Fourteen women selected from each group were involved in semidirected, in-depth interviews based on a specific guideline to establish self-perception about their skin complexion. The interviewer belonged to the same specific population group in each case. The interviews were designed to explore self-perceptions and description of skin complexion and skin tone by the volunteers and their expectations from liquid foundation.

Results For the African American women, skin color was an important part of their identity. They described themselves as "people of color."

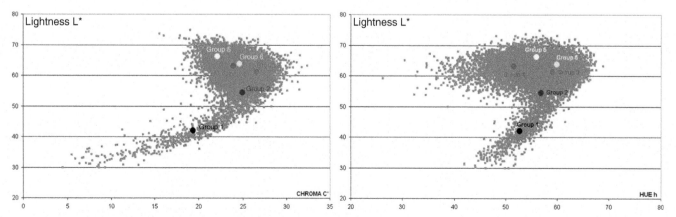

FIGURE 80-2. The worldwide skin color space depicted in two dimensions: **(A)** C^*, L^* and **(B)** h, L^*.

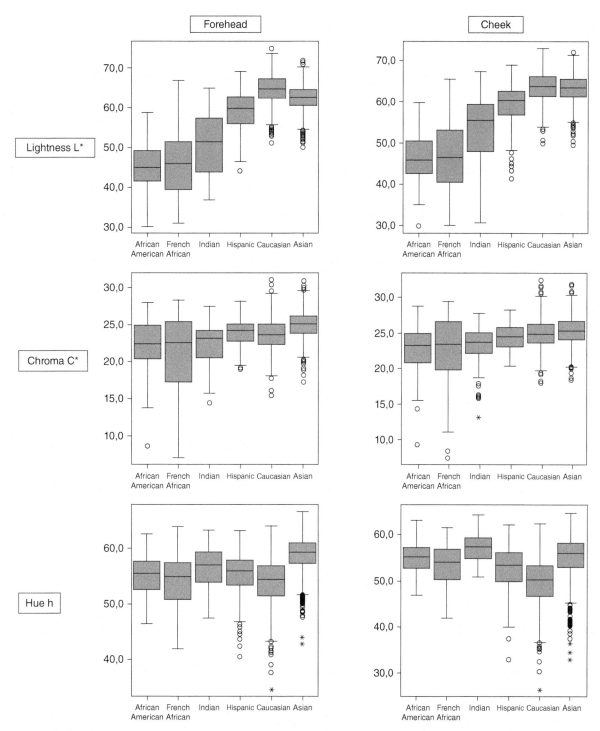

FIGURE 80-3. Boxplots bringing out the ranges of lightness, chroma, and hue of the different population groups on the forehead and cheek. It is interesting to note that Caucasian and Asian women practically cover the same lightness range, Caucasian and Hispanic women the same chroma range, and French African and African American women the same hue range.

In general, dark skin complexion was well regarded by the African American community. It was reflected in the use of positive expressions to describe their skin tone, such as "dark chocolate" and "mahogany" to depict dark skin and "toast" or "pecan" for lighter hues. None of the women used negative words about color itself. While women appeared to be fairly satisfied with their skin tone, they were concerned about color and texture unevenness. Subjects frequently complained about light/dark color variations, visible texture irregularities such as dark marks or scars, and skin blemishes such as pimples, wrinkles, rough skin, large pores, and facial hair.

The major issue addressed when applying foundation was to provide evenness by covering up blemishes. Makeup application resulted in shades darker than the natural skin tone. Women in this group chose shades at least as dark as their darkest skin area to even face color. They

also expected shades that brought glow and clarity from dullness. They used "vibrant" shades that were dark but not dull, such as "ebony," or with a slightly reddish undertone, such as "mahogany." A few individuals chose to lighten darker areas with a light foundation.

These interviews show that African American women have a positive self-perception of their own color. Although they declared themselves not satisfied with their usual foundation product because appropriate foundation shades were not available in stores, they managed to improve evenness by mixing several products.

Two independent groups of Caucasian women were also involved in the study; one included women in Paris, France, and the other one was made up of American women living in New York. We noticed a clear similarity between the results obtained from these two groups. The range of color used to depict skin included descriptors such as "beige," "medium beige,"

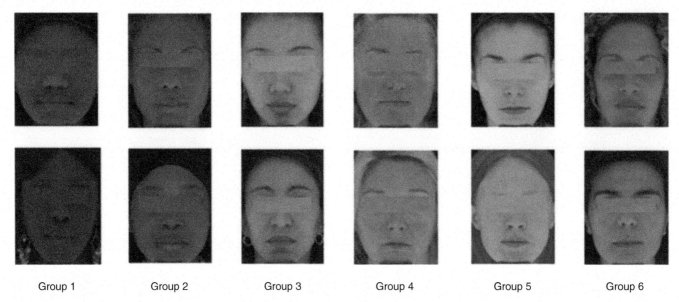

| Group 1 | Group 2 | Group 3 | Group 4 | Group 5 | Group 6 |

FIGURE 80-4. The six groups of skin tones reflecting the diversity in skin color.

and "bronze-like." Skin defects most commonly mentioned included pimples, acne, blackheads, and wrinkles. They were often described as "redness" by the French subjects and as "dark blotches" by the American group. However, as a general observation from the in-depth interviews, we noted that Caucasian women were the least concerned group about skin unevenness. Ideal facial skin complexion was depicted as a healthy look with even color and radiance. Most women chose a shade slightly darker than their skin tone, which they felt allowed them to look "healthy" ("*bonne mine*"), provided a better coverage by covering the darkest areas or skin imperfections, and thereby helped them obtain evenness of color. They selected colors that impart a "healthy" look, such as "tan" or "bronze-like" colors—"sun tan," "gold," "sand on the beach." Otherwise, they selected "rosy-orangy" (the French group) and "blush pink" (the American group) to enhance a glowing look.

In this study, Asian skin was represented by Japanese women. It is worth noting that Japanese women described their skin complexion using a skin tone scale: pink, ocher, and beige. Some of them described themselves as "yellow." Japanese women did not describe their yellow skin color as a source of dissatisfaction, but seemed to be more concerned by unevenness of their skin color because of the presence of pigment spots. Makeup strategies in this group consistently focused on improving skin evenness, irrespective of age or skin tone subgroup. Interestingly, the Japanese women were the only group that expected a "lightly tinted," "white," lucid, and bright skin color. They chose "white peach," "boiled egg," and "chinaware" shades or a color not different from the bare skin of the neck. To achieve this, they "played with color" by blending different foundation shades and by balancing powder and foundation shades.

Unlike the preceding groups, Hispanic Americans originated from a wide range of geographic areas that may have resulted in specific cultural characteristics. The Hispanic group included women from Puerto Rico, Dominica, Cuba, Venezuela, and Mexico, and many were recent immigrants. In contrast to the African American group, we found that some Hispanic American women tended not to enhance their own skin color by using descriptors such as "olive" and "dull." They complained about the "yellow tone" of their skin, which had a negative association with conditions such as jaundice and other types of sickness. Furthermore, they commented on uneven color, notably beneath the eyes, and reddish marks. The perception of skin color influenced makeup strategy. They expected color evenness with "one color all over the face" and a "healthy" skin color. This meant enhancing the yellow skin using shades that bring radiance, such as "golden bronze," "sun kissed," and "honey." Their approach to cosmetics undoubtedly also was influenced by the fact that the Hispanic American group included women from a wide range of cultural backgrounds, which likely contributed to a

certain discrepancy between skin makeup result and declared cosmetic approach. Even when subjects verbally described a consistent desire to seek darker skin tones with a view to achieve a "sun kissed" skin color and to resolve perceived unevenness, the result was either lightened or darkened or reddened skin.

To clarify our conclusions from the previous study, a new qualitative study was carried out more recently on self-perception and makeup expectations of women according to their native countries. The in-depth interviews took place in Los Angeles, Miami, and New York. Women involved in the study in Los Angeles originated from Mexico, Honduras, Guatemala, and Nicaragua, with an equal number of light, medium, and dark complexions according to their self-perceptions to get a wide range of skin tones. Women involved in Miami originated from Cuba, Colombia, Venezuela, and Argentina with the same distribution over the lightness scale. Women involved in New York were natives of Puerto Rico and the Dominican Republic, with an equal number of light, medium, and dark complexions too. The women were aged 25 to 65 years.

This study confirmed that the self-perception and approach of Hispanic Americans to cosmetics is undoubtedly influenced by lightness of skin complexion and native country. Those with the lightest skin were the least satisfied with skin complexion, except for women of Cuban and Mexican origin. A too light skin tone was referred to as "pale," "yellowish," "illness," and "sickly." A medium complexion was much more appreciated, especially in women from the Dominican Republic, Puerto Rico, and South America. Although not unsatisfied with medium complexions, Cuban and Mexican women expressed preference for lighter complexions. The darkest skin tones were very well appreciated, and women referred to tanned skin as robust to the sun and not sickly.

However, the level of satisfaction with skin tone depended on social background and native country. The darkest complexions were hard to come to terms with for Mexican and Central American women, whereas the lightest skin tones were reported to be "less discriminating," "more elegant," and "cleaner." Women from Puerto Rico and the Dominican Republic were much more satisfied with their dark complexions, particularly because they were living in New York, where the high level of mixing between people of different backgrounds and origins makes complexion less of a source of concern.

Cuban women living in Miami belonged to a large community, which could explain why they generally accepted dark complexions very well. They did, however, express appeal for "rosy" tones. Women from South America living in Miami often came from favored social backgrounds and so assumed a dark skin tone. All in all, the ideal color this group identified was a "tanned," "bronze" skin tone that brings radiance to the face. To achieve such a complexion, women with fair skin tones chose

TABLE 80-2 Percentage of each makeup strategy in different population groups

	Makeup strategies			
	"Golden look"	"Matching"	"Glow Look"	"Whitening"
French Caucasian	**54%**	20%	20%	6%
Russian Caucasian	**32%**	**54%**	14%	0%
American Caucasian	**33%**	**31%**	**28%**	8%
African American	**35%**	14%	**46%**	5%
French African	**36%**	20%	**38%**	6%
American Hispanic	**32%**	19%	**41%**	8%
Chinese	2%	14%	**48%**	**37%**
Japanese	6%	22%	**46%**	**26%**

Note: The percentages higher than 25% are highlighted in boldface.

darker shades, especially those native of the Dominican Republic. Those originating from Mexico and Cuba preferred to slightly lighten the skin with "rosy" or "bronze" shades that corrected the disliked "yellow" component. Most of those with medium complexions looked for a matching foundation. However, they preferred to slightly darken the face if they could not get the appropriate shade, except for Cuban, Mexican, and some Puerto Rican women, who sought to slightly lighten the skin. Those with the darkest skin tones liked to match their own skin tones, but because of uneven skin color, they finally decided to darken the face and achieve a homogeneous result.

Regarding the colorimetric overlap of the different groups, it is obvious that racial origin and cultural background play a major role in self-perception of skin tone and undoubtedly influence makeup strategy.

◼ THE COLOR OF THE SKIN AFTER APPLYING MAKEUP: MAIN STRATEGIES, SPECIFICITIES, AND COMMON STRATEGIES

The second stage of the 1999 study was to colorimetrically assess and classify women's makeup strategies. Women were asked to apply their usual and most preferred foundation with their own makeup routine. Measurements were done before (see the first part of the study) and

after making up. The difference was computed for each color coordinate L^*, C^*, and h on both forehead and cheek to evaluate makeup strategy.

Panel The trial involved 2047 women aged 18 to 65 years from five different origins who lived in five different geographic locations: 1319 Asians (living in China and Japan), 432 Caucasians (living in France, Russia, and the United States), 98 Hispanics living in the United States, 112 French Africans, and 86 African Americans.

Statistics Makeup strategies were investigated from the differences in L^*, C^*, and h coordinates (ΔL^*, ΔC^*, and Δh, respectively) on the forehead and cheek using PCA. PCA brought out the significant components on which a hierarchical ascending classification was carried out to classify the strategies.

Results There emerged four main strategies involving the three attributes: lightness L^*, saturation C^*, and hue h [**Table 80-2 and Figure 80-5**]. The first strategy made the skin darker, with most of the women making the skin more saturated and/or redder at the same time ($\Delta L^* = -1.6$, $\Delta C^* = +1.3$, $\Delta h = -2.1$ on forehead and $\Delta L^* = -1.9$, $\Delta C^* = -1.3$, $\Delta h = -1.6$ on cheek). We named it the "golden look." The second main strategy did not change the color, thus matching the skin tone. We named it "matching." The third main strategy made the skin redder and slightly less saturated

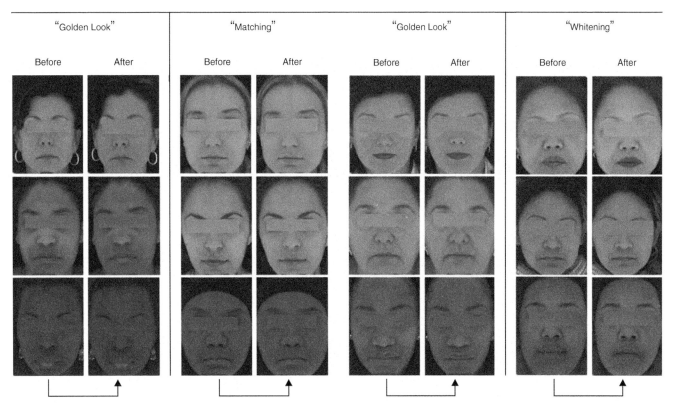

FIGURE 80-5. The four main strategies of women from different skin color groups.

($\Delta h = -2.0$, $\Delta C^* = -1.1$ on forehead; $\Delta h = -1.6$, $\Delta C^* = -1.0$ on cheek). We named it the "glow look." The last strategy made the skin highly less saturated to mute the color, with most of the women making the skin redder and lighter at the same time ($\Delta C^* = -3.0$, $\Delta h = -3.2$, $\Delta L^* = +1.4$ on forehead and $\Delta C^* = -2.7$, $\Delta h = -2.5$, $\Delta L^* = +1.3$ on cheek). We named it "whitening."

A sizeable portion of the African American women (35%; Table 80-2 and Figure 80-5) made their skin darker, which shows good consistency with the qualitative study. Many of the women explained that a darkening strategy was the easiest way to homogenize and/or the way to get a vibrant dark complexion. However, 46% preferred the "glow look," which does not alter the lightness, and 14% made up the skin without changing skin tone. We found that only 5% of African American women made the skin strongly less saturated and at the same time lighter and redder. This extreme strategy could be considered as a "whitening" strategy. The weak percentage confirms that most of the African American women are not willing to lighten their skin tone.

Most of the Chinese and Japanese women (85% and 72%, respectively) [Table 80-2 and Figure 80-5] made their skin less saturated. More detailed analysis showed that 37% and 26%, respectively, obtained a visible "white" appearance by strongly unsaturating the skin and making it lighter and redder. Only 14% of the Chinese and 22% of the Japanese women decided not to change their skin tone. It is worth noting that skin complexion in Asia strongly influences makeup strategy. Women who decide to strongly unsaturate skin have a bare skin tone significantly darker and more saturated, and women who decide to match their skin tone have significantly less saturated and redder skin, which means a pinkish complexion. Cross-correlating all data, we may suggest that the ideal Asian skin tone is a fair, not too saturated, and pink-ochre skin complexion.

In good agreement with their expectations, most Caucasian women made the skin darker (54% of French, 32% of Russian, and 33% of American Caucasians, respectively) [Table 80-2 and Figure 80-5]. Twenty percent and 31% of the French and American women, respectively, preferred to match their skin tone. The percentage increased to 54% in Russian Caucasians. Still consistent with the in-depth interview, 20% and 28% of the French and American women, respectively, brought a glow look to their faces. Few of these women decided to lighten their skin. Six percent of the French and 8% of the American women made the skin highly less saturated principally to mute a too vivid color.

As detailed in the qualitative study, the makeup strategies are much more varied in Hispanic women depending on native country and skin complexion. Nevertheless, 41% preferred to get a "glow look," and 32% darkened the skin to get a "tanned," "bronze" complexion [Table 80-2 and Figure 80-5], whereas 19% chose to match their skin tone. When looking deeper, only 8% strongly unsaturated the skin to get an apparent whitening/lightening effect.

There is a real diversity of makeup strategies. The matching strategy is transversal across different population groups. It is the way to enhance a well-appreciated skin color by hiding unevenness. The darkening strategy is either a way to homogenize the face or a way to make the skin more "tanned" and "radiant." The brightening strategy that goes through the unsaturation of color is either a way to mute a too vivid color or a cultural routine to get brightened fair skin.

CONCLUSION

A woman's uniqueness is striking with regard to the diversity of skin tones and various perceptions, expectations, and makeup strategies. Taking into account this diversity is of prime importance when formulating a makeup foundation range. It also means that proper advice should be provided to women to help them in selecting the most appropriate shades of makeup, which entails using their own words to meet their expectations.

THE LIPS

Lip makeup has a special place in the makeup routine. It could be the overall finish of the makeup routine or a way to enlighten skin tone. Unlike skin tone makeup, lip makeup is highly diversified in terms of color ranges and optical effects from matte to extreme shiny. Anatomically, lips are composed of the upper and lower vermilion borders and the perilabial skin that includes the area from the nose to the chin.

▉ LIP COLOR

Our approach consisted in defining the color space of the vermilion border, juxtaposing it to the skin color space, enlightening various contrasts, and determining the differences between different populations.

Panel The colorimetric study included 1940 subjects—166 French Caucasian, 169 Russian Caucasian, 292 Chinese, 315 Japanese, 409 American Caucasian, 416 African American, and 160 Indian women.

Methods Colorimetrical measurements were done inside the Chroma-sphere using a spectroradiometer as described earlier.

Statistics The significant differences between population groups were demonstrated using univariate analysis on L^*, C^*, and h data. The limit for significance was $P < 0.05$.

Results Surprisingly, the lip color space is as large as skin color space [**Figure 80-6**]. Some differences between groups were brought out.

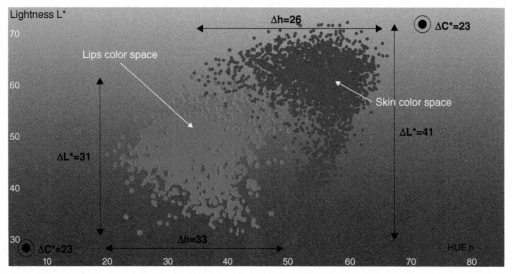

FIGURE 80-6. The lip and skin color spaces.

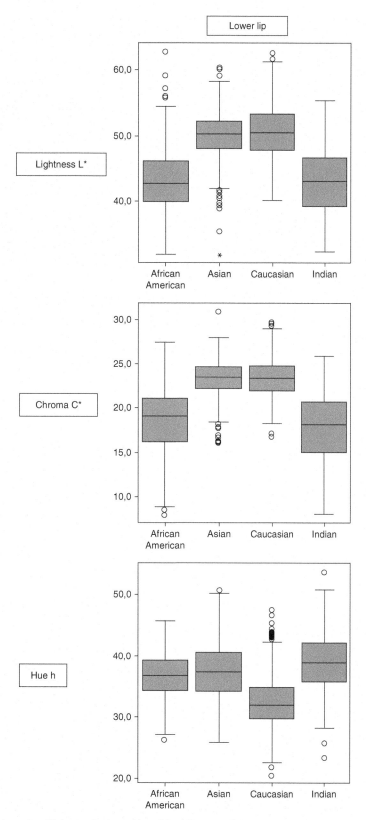

FIGURE 80-7. Boxplots bringing out the ranges of lightness, chroma, and hue of the different population groups on the lower lip. It is interesting to note that Caucasian and Asian women practically cover the same lightness and chroma ranges but are distinguished by the hue. African American and Indian women also have the same lightness and chroma ranges, but Indian lips are significantly more yellowish.

Indian and African American women have the darkest and least saturated lips ($L^* = 42.9$ and 43.1, $C^* = 17.7$ and 18.5, respectively) [**Figure 80-7**], whereas Asian and Caucasian women showed the lightest and most saturated lip complexions ($L^* = 50.0$ and 50.6, $C^* =$ 23.3 and 23.4, respectively) [Figure 80-7]. However, the hue distinguished Caucasian and Asian women. Caucasian women have redder lips than Asian women, and Indian women have the most yellowish lips ($h = 32.4$, 37.5, and 39.1, respectively) [Figure 80-7].

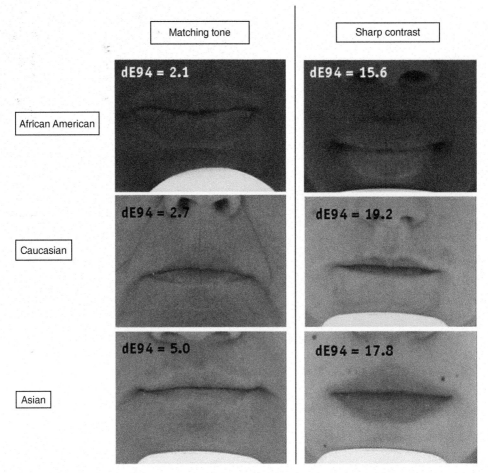

FIGURE 80-8. Various contrasts between the vermilion border and the perilabial skin expressed by the dE94 value.

◼ LIP COLOR CONTRAST

Comparison of the vermilion border and perilabial skin color refers to colorimetric contrasts. Indeed, lips can be likened to a colored object placed on a colored background (ie, the skin tone). The resulting contrast effect may change our visual perception of the color of the lips in relation to the color of skin tone. This issue was documented by the following study.

Panel A total of 914 women were involved in a colorimetric study using the same devices as described earlier to characterize the contrast between vermilion border and perilabial skin—238 African American, 238 American Caucasian, 225 French Caucasian, and 213 Japanese women equally distributed in the three age ranges of 18 to 35, 36 to 50, and 51 to 65 years.

Statistics A comparison between the vermilion border and the perilabial skin was carried out using the Student t test in cases of normal distribution, and the nonparametric Wilcoxon test was used if this was not the case. The difference was significant if $P < 0.05$.

Results Measurements show widely varying contrasts between the vermilion border and the perilabial skin from sharp differences to matching tones [**Figure 80-8**]. In all population groups except African American women, lips were made up to appear significantly darker than the perilabial skin [**Figure 80-9**]. In African American women, the vermilion border was lighter or darker, impacting the contrast [**Figure 80-10**]. Not surprisingly, the lips of women are significantly redder than the perilabial skin. However, some women show matching tones between lips and skin that decrease lip highlighting visually. In each group, there was no significant difference in saturation between the lips and perilabial skin. Consequently, lips could be either more saturated or less saturated than the skin.

CONCLUSION

The great number of contrasts between skin and lips offers a new perspective to enhance skin tone, lip color, or both. New studies should be conducted to explore the most appreciated contrasts for women. Other lip characteristics, such as morphologic, biomechanical, and hydration properties, could be investigated. Women express various concerns about these characteristics that also strongly depend on their racial origin, as well as on cultural and geographic environment.

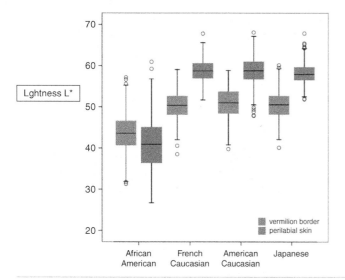

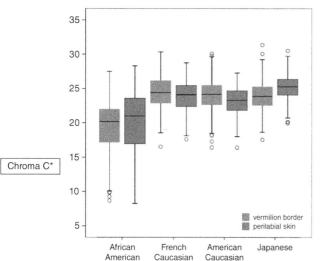

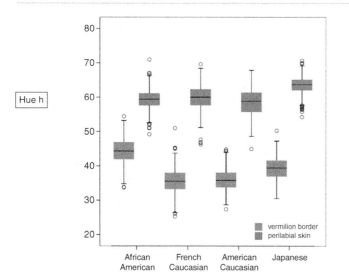

FIGURE 80-9. Boxplots bringing out the differences of lightness, chroma, and hue between the vermilion border and the perilabial skin.

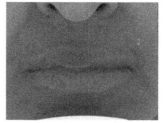

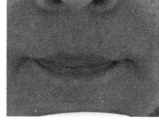

L*(perilabial skin) - L*(vermilion border) = −12.8   L*(perilabial skin) - L*(vermilion border) = +10.2

FIGURE 80-10. Two extreme contrasts.

REFERENCES

1. Sonoda I, Hirai Y, Okabe N, et al. On the preference of the color of makeup products related to the skin color in Japanese women. *J Soc Cosmet Chem.* 1987;21:219-224.
2. Lee KY, Shimagami K, Sato M, et al. Measurement of the color for bare skin and foundation-applied skin in women in their 20s: comparison of Japanese and Korean. *J Physiol Anthropol Appl Hum.* 2001;20:301.
3. Richards GM, Oresajo CO, Halder RM. Structure and function of ethnic skin and hair. *Dermatol Clin.* 2003;21:595-600.
4. Morizot F, Jdid R, Dheurle S, et al. Features related to skin pigmentation: differences between Japanese and French women. *Skin Res Technol.* 2005;11:76-77.
5. Minami J, Minami T. Designing the color of cosmetic foundations: Analysis on consumers' opinions about changing face color and measurement of colorimetric properties of foundation layers. *FRAGR J.* 1999;27:21-26.
6. Chardon A, Cretois I, Hourseau C. Skin colour typology and sun tanning pathways. *Int J Cosmet Sci.* 1991;13:191-208.
7. Liu W, Wang XM, Lai W. Skin color measurement in the Chinese female population: analysis of 407 cases from four cities of China. *Int J Dermatol.* 2007;46:835-839.
8. Giron F. Dispositif d'acquisition d'au moins une image d'au moins une partie du visage ou de la chevelure d'une personne. French patent 0111215. Paris, France: L'Oréal; 2001.
9. Caisey Bluteau L, Aubert J. Procédé et dispositif de mesure de la couleur. French patent 9606425. Paris, France, L'Oréal, 1996.
10. Caisey L, Grangeat F, Lemasson A, et al. Skin color and makeup strategies of women from different racial or ethnic groups. *Int J Cosmet Sci.* 2006;28:427-437.

CHAPTER
81

Laser Treatments

Lori M. Hobbs
Lisa R. Ginn
Zhong Lu

KEY POINTS

- The use of lasers in persons with skin of color requires an understanding of laser physics and laser tissue interactions. Epidermal melanin in skin of color acts as a competing chromophore; this not only decreases the effect of laser treatment, but is also likely to cause nonselective thermal injury to the epidermis.

- With the proper selection of device, wavelength, and parameters, cutaneous dermatologic lasers can be used safely on individuals with skin of color. To minimize unwanted side effects, the use of aggressive parameters is discouraged.

- With the ideal candidate and the proper clinical setting, intense pulsed light (IPL) often treats numerous dermatologic conditions. However, IPL must be used with caution in patients with skin phototypes IV and is not the desired treatment for those with phototypes V or VI.

- Fractional lasers show promise in the treatment of melasma, acne scarring, and skin rejuvenation in patients with darker phototypes.
- Test spots are highly encouraged when treating people with darker skin phototypes.
- Skin cooling and postoperative skin care are highly recommended for patients with skin of color.

INTRODUCTION

The demographics of the United States is changing, as racial minority populations are steadily growing. From 2000 to 2010, the African American population increased by 12%, and the Hispanic and Asian populations both increased by 43%.[1] As a result, dermatologists must embrace this growth by increasing their understanding of skin of color so as to deliver quality dermatologic care to patients of all skin phototypes.

In the subspecialty of dermatologic lasers, there are several factors to consider in order to optimize patient treatment. The choice of laser, appropriate parameters, an understanding of skin optics and tissue response, and the early treatment of untoward events are key to successfully treating patients with skin of color.

LASER–TISSUE INTERACTION FOR SKIN OF COLOR

A laser (light amplification by the stimulated emission of radiation) is made up of a pumping system, the lasing medium, and the optical cavity. The light that is emitted from the laser beam is monochromatic, coherent, collimated, and of high energy. Once the laser light reaches the skin, it can be reflected, scattered, transmitted, or absorbed. Laser light is absorbed by chromophores, which are 'light-loving' substances within the skin. There are three main endogenous chromophores in the skin: melanin, hemoglobin (oxyhemoglobin), and water [**Figure 81-1**]. Each chromophore has a specific peak absorption wavelength in the electromagnetic spectrum. Tattoo ink is considered an exogenous chromophore. Once absorbed, laser energy is transferred to other kinds of energy, for example heat, which may have various effects.

Laser light can be delivered onto the skin in either a continuous, quasi-continuous, or pulsed mode. Pulsed lasers emit a beam of light on the skin in pulses of (1) long duration, measured in milliseconds (ms); (2) short duration, measured in nanoseconds (ns); or (3) ultra-short duration, measured in picoseconds (ps).

MECHANISM OF LASER THERAPY

According to the Grotthuss-Draper law, light must be absorbed by the skin in order to have an effect. Successful laser therapy is based on the theory of selective photothermolysis, which allows the selective targeting of chromophores without damaging the surrounding tissue. Using the appropriate laser light, the selective heating of a target chromophore is achieved and heat is confined within the target chromophore. However, it is imperative that the pulse duration is equal to or shorter than the thermal relaxation time (TRT), which is the time necessary for the target tissue to cool down to half the temperature to which it was initially heated.[2] For example, by selecting a specific hemoglobin-targeting wavelength and using a brief pulse duration equal to or less than the TRT of blood vessels in the treatment of vascular lesions, there is selective thermal coagulation and damage of blood vessels with minimal damage to the surrounding tissues. When treating pigment lesions, Q-switched systems emit maximum energy output in pulses that are significantly shorter than the 100-ns TRT of melanosomes, creating a shock wave and/or cavitation damage to the melanosome. It is believed that the melanosome or target chromophore undergoes a photoacoustic (both light and sound) effect.

LASER TREATMENT ON SKIN OF COLOR

In skin of color, the large quantity of melanin within the epidermis creates the ultimate, fundamental challenge for laser surgeons. The wide absorption spectrum of melanin (250 to 1200 nm) is the target of all visible and near-infrared dermatologic lasers. Acting as a competing chromophore with the chromophore actually targeted for the absorption of laser energy, the epidermal melanin in skin of color not only decreases the effect of laser treatment, but is also likely to cause nonselective thermal injury to the epidermis. Blistering, crusting, scarring, and pigmentary discoloration can therefore ensue and can sometimes be permanent. Longer wavelengths, longer pulse durations, efficient cooling devices, and conservative fluence have been used in the attempt to at least partially solve this problem. Longer wavelengths are less easily absorbed by the melanin-rich epidermis, helping to spare heat within the epidermis and reaching the target chromophores. Efficient cooling, using either contact or noncontact cooling devices, is imperative so as to protect the epidermis from untoward events. Conservative fluences are crucial in treating darker skin tones, because high fluences cause too much heat within the epidermis and surrounding dermal tissues. In this

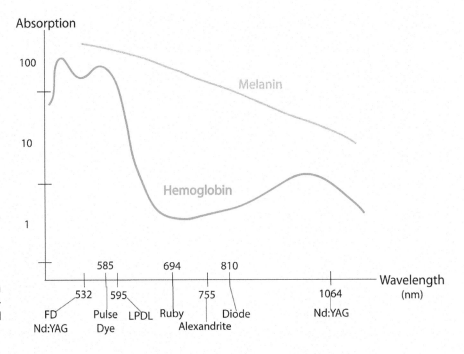

FIGURE 81-1. The absorption spectrum of hemoglobin and melanin with commonly used lasers. FD, frequency-doubled; LPDL, long-pulsed dye laser; Nd:YAG, neodymium-doped yttrium-aluminum-garnet.

respect, it is necessary for dermatologists to perform test spots on their patients, ensuring that the spot used for testing is in a representative and inconspicuous area.

Ablative resurfacing, known to improve photoaging and dyschromia, vaporizes the epidermis and a portion of the dermis, creating a controlled cutaneous thermal destruction with resulting re-epithelialization, neocollagenesis and new elastic fibrils. Traditional laser resurfacing with the carbon dioxide (CO_2) and erbium-doped yyttrium-aluminum-garnet (er:YAG) repeatedly produced impressive results, but are associated with a high risk of scarring, infection and pigmentary alteration. Phototypes I and II are ideal candidates for ablative resurfacing, but patients with skin phototypes IV -VI are at high risk for scarring and pigmentary changes. Nonablative fractional photothermolysis or fractional laser resurfacing bridged the gap between skin types and risks, while offering an effective therapeutic option for all skin types with a higher safety profile.

Nonablative lasers are used to treat a variety of skin disorders ranging from superficial rhytides, to acne scarring, to textural irregularities and pigmentary and vascular dermatologic disorders. Melasma, dyschromia from photoaging, minocycline-induced hyperpigmentation, nevus of Ota and striae alba have all been reportedly treated successfully with fractional laser resurfacing.

While numerous treatments are necessary, the down time and risk of significant side-effects are minimal compared to traditional laser resurfacing.

Radiofrequency technology continues to advance rapidly, offering skin rejuvenation treatment options for patients of all skin phototypes. Intense focused ultrasound therapy is the newest technology in the arena of noninvasive skin tightening devices. Clinical results vary and often are perceived as subtle for all of these nonablative devices, and not every patient can be treated successfully.

LASER AND LIGHT-BASED TREATMENTS FOR COMMON SKIN DISORDERS

VASCULAR DISORDERS

Port-Wine Stains Port-wine stains (PWS) affect 0.3% to 0.5% of newborns.[3,4] Occurring less often in African Americans, there is an equal frequency in males and females [**Figure 81-2**]. PWS are thought to be related to the varying depth of the ectatic vessels, which are typically 30 to 300 μm in diameter, in the papillary and reticular dermis. There is a deficiency of nerves in the papillary plexus of the affected skin. Interestingly, with PWS, the adjacent bone and soft tissue can become hyperplastic.

The most common location of a PWS is on the face, with only one-third of stains occurring on nonfacial areas.[5] In general, PWS get darker and worsen over time. Approximately two-thirds of all patients develop nodularity by the fifth decade of life.[5] Negative prognostic variables for laser treatment are lesions with a 'cobblestone' texture, patients over 50 years old, those with Fitzpatrick skin phototypes V and VI, and those with larger lesions or nonfacial PWS.[6,7]

The pulsed dye laser (PDL), with a wavelength of 585 or 595 nm, is traditionally the laser of choice in the treatment of PWS for all individuals. Specifically the variable PDL, with a 595-nm wavelength and equipped with cooling, is the ideal laser for treating PWS in skin phototypes IV to VI. The slightly longer wavelength of the 595-nm PDL allows for deeper penetration into the dermis and the ectatic vasculature of the PWS, and is thus a better choice for darker-skinned individuals.[8-10]

The TRT of different blood vessels is important in determining the appropriate pulse duration. For smaller vessels (of ≤20 μm in diameter), a pulse duration of 450 μs is adequate; vessels with a larger diameter (30 to 150 μm) should have a pulse duration of approximately 1 to 10 ms.[11] Longer pulse durations are generally indicated for darker skin types (V and VI), which require pulse durations of 10 ms or longer in most clinical situations.

It is crucial that test spots are performed on patients before they undergo laser treatment of the entire lesion. These test spots allow

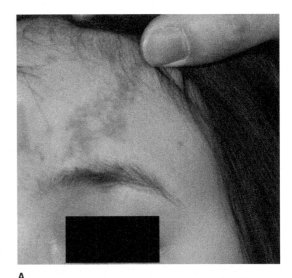

A

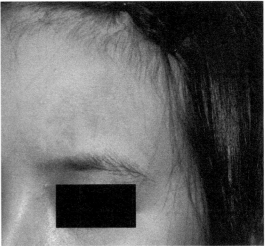

B

FIGURE 81-2. (A) Port-wine stain on the forehead of a young female patient before treatment. **(B)** Significant improvement was observed after three pulsed dye laser treatments at 595 nm. (Used with permission from Dr. Zhong Lu, Dermatology Department, Huashan Hospital, Fudan University, Shanghai, China.)

determination of the appropriate fluence and should be performed by delivering several juxtaposed pulses onto the PWS lesion. Varying fluences should be used to determine the best clinical outcome. Stacked or double pulsing is not recommended for patients with skin of color. The patient should return after 1 month so the dermatologist can check the clinical outcome of the test spot. The treatment should then be performed at a setting that provokes a clinical subpurpuric tissue response. With the PDL, transient violaceous discoloration of the treated area is normal. Limited exposure to sun, heat, and exercise is an important postlaser care measure to prevent the recanalization of the blood vessels.

Conventionally, 4-week treatment intervals are the most common. Decreasing the treatment intervals and initiating treatment early can result in better treatment outcomes and responses, as was seen in a study of 24 infants with PWS by Anolik et al.[12] The reason for this may be two-fold: infant skin is commonly subjected to less sun exposure and is also thinner than adult skin. In skin of color, intervals between treatments should allow sufficient time for the skin to heal.

As the PWS lightens with subsequent laser treatments, due to the decreasing number of chromophores, higher fluences are necessary. The exact number of treatments necessary to improve the color and texture of PWS in patients with skin of color is unknown.

The side effects of treating PWS with lasers are minimal, although transient hyperpigmentation has been reported in 44% to 46% of patients.[13] Transient hypopigmentation, permanent hypopigmentation, and scarring are rarely encountered.[14]

Unfortunately, the results of treating PWS with laser therapy remain disappointing. It is reported that only 10% to 20% of patients obtain a complete resolution of their PWS.[15,16] Hence, the majority of treated patients either experience lighter PWS or no change at all. For a patient with skin of color, the rate of any significant degree of improvement is thought to be significantly less than that of the general population.

There are new therapies that may help address difficult-to-treat PWS and thus may benefit darker-skinned individuals. Emerging light-based technology includes the use of longer wavelength devices—such as the 755-nm alexandrite laser, 810-nm diode laser, or the 1064-nm neodymium-doped yttrium-aluminum-garnet (Nd:YAG) laser—either simultaneously with PDL or alone.[17,18] Although there is deeper penetration with these adjunct lasers, there is decreased absorption by the hemoglobin, which thus requires the use of higher fluences for sufficient photocoagulation. This can result in the nonselective bulk-like heating of the surrounding tissue, thus increasing the risk of scarring.[17] Interestingly, the PDL/Nd:YAG dual laser is a system that works by first using the 595-nm PDL to cause a conversion of the oxyhemoglobin to methemoglobin, which has an absorption peak near 1064 nm. The subsequent synergistic use of the 1064-nm Nd:YAG then decreases the amount of fluence necessary for the photocoagulation of the blood vessels.[18] Unfortunately, there are no published reports of this laser on patients with skin of color, so it is not known if this combination is successful on their skin types.

Combining PDL with the prescription of posttreatment imiquimod has shown promise; this combination was seen to improve PWS in a recent small study.[19] The proposed mechanism of action of imiquimod is the inhibition of angiogenesis. However, more clinical trials are needed to establish its true efficacy and safety. Likewise, the immunosuppressant sirolimus, a macrolide antibiotic, has antiangiogenic properties that appear to help reduce PWS when used in combination with PDL therapy.[20]

Intense pulsed light (IPL) is a broadband light source that emits noncoherent light in wavelengths of between 500 and 1200 nm. IPL provides an option for the treatment of PWS in individuals with lighter complexions and has been used to treat patients with skin phototype IV. Ho et al were able to achieve a 25% to 50% clearance in a group of patients with skin phototype IV undergoing five to seven treatments every 3 to 4 weeks.[21] However, IPL is not recommended for the treatment of PWS in patients with darker phototypes. Patients with skin of color are more likely to experience hyperpigmentation, vesiculation, hypopigmentation, scarring, and permanent hair reduction.

Lastly, another vascular laser device used in the treatment of PWS is the frequency-doubled 532-nm Nd:YAG laser. It is best suited for patients with lighter skin types of phototype IV or fairer.

Hemangiomas Infantile hemangiomas occur in 10% of children.[22] There is a greater predilection in Caucasians compared with African Americans and in females compared with males [**Figure 81-3**].[22,23] Hemangiomas are benign vascular tumors of the skin. There is a rapid intermittent growth phase within the first year of life; the tumors usually reach their maximum size by the time the patient is 9 months old. It is during this proliferation phase that there is the highest risk of complications, which can include bleeding, ulceration, infection, or the obstruction of vital organs.[24,25] Regression is approximately 90% complete by the time the patient reaches the age of 9 years.[26] Generally, laser treatment for hemangiomas is not necessary because the majority involute or resolve spontaneously, and thus a 'wait and see' philosophy is commonly adopted. However, new ideologies are slowly emerging advocating the early intervention and treatment of hemangiomas, especially complicated ones.

Approximately 10% of hemangiomas will require active medical treatment to avoid the advent of life-threatening complications.[27] Treatment modalities range from topical and oral β-adrenergic blockers, such as propranolol, to topical corticosteroids, oral glucocorticoids, intralesional steroid injections, lasers, and surgical excision.[28]

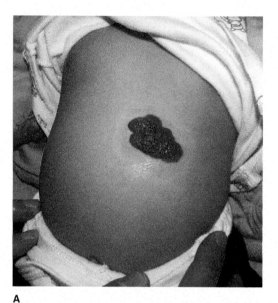

A

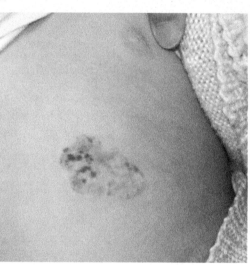

B

FIGURE 81-3. (A) Hemangioma on the stomach of an infant before treatment. **(B)** Significant improvement was observed after four long-pulsed neodymium-doped yttrium-aluminum-garnet laser treatment at 1064 nm. (Used with permission from Dr. Zhong Lu, Dermatology Department, Huashan Hospital, Fudan University, Shanghai, China.)

Treatments aim to halt any further growth of the hemangioma, accelerate regression, and prevent loss of function. When using lasers as an early adjunctive treatment modality for uncomplicated hemangiomas in darker-skinned patients, it is important that the benefits clearly outweigh the risks.

The laser of choice for the treatment of hemangiomas is PDL. The 595-nm PDL reaches a depth of 1.5 mm, and thus superficial hemangiomas respond better to PDL than others.[29-31] Propranolol can help to reduce the size of thicker hemangiomas. For patients receiving propranolol, laser treatments are sometimes performed during or just prior to the weaning of propranolol to counteract any potential rebound growth effects. With the 595-nm PDL, the number of treatments varies depending on the patient—therapy is usually continued until involution is achieved. Pre- and postcooling are beneficial. As with PWS lesions, initial treatments for hemangiomas should be performed at pulse durations that result in a clinical subpurpuric change in the skin. It is best to maintain a conservative fluence during the initial treatment. In subsequent visits, the parameters can be adjusted according to clinical outcome and tissue response. Some experts advocate treating patients more frequently, for example every 2 weeks instead of every 4 to 6 weeks. However, there should be enough time between treatments for the patient and/or doctor to notice any adverse cutaneous changes.

Similar to PWS therapies, adjunctive therapies seem promising for the treatment of hemangiomas in the future—particularly the use of imiquimod and sirolimus combined with PDL treatment and the single use of long-pulsed Nd:YAG lasers.

Leg Veins Sclerotherapy remains the gold standard for the treatment of leg veins. However, laser therapy may be considered for patients who have an allergy to the sclerosing agent, a fear of needles, small vessels that cannot be cannulated, postsclerotherapy matted telangiectasias, vessels in areas that are prone to ulceration, for instance the ankle, or superficial vasculature.

The following light sources are typically used to treat leg veins: 595-nm PDL; 800-, 810-, 940-, and 980-nm diode lasers; 1064-nm Nd:YAG; and 515- to 1200-nm IPL.[32] Wavelengths of between 700 and 1200 nm penetrate into the skin to a depth of approximately 3 mm, thereby targeting the superficial vessels. High fluences are required to achieve photocoagulation of the blood vessels. Pulse durations of 40 to 60 ms are adequate for leg veins measuring 0.2 to 0.8 mm in diameter, based on a TRT of 20 to 300 ms.[33] Clinically there is usually evidence of immediate vessel clearance, intravascular thrombosis, and rupture of the vessel resulting in purpura. With all factors taken into consideration, blue and larger vessels respond better to the 1064-nm Nd:YAG laser in comparison to the smaller red vessels. The fluence for larger vessels (1.5 to 3 mm in diameter) is generally lower and ranges from 100 to 200 J/cm^2 with longer pulse durations. For smaller vessels, the fluence is typically higher, in the range of 250 to 400 J/cm^2 with shorter pulse durations. Spot sizes of 2 to 3 mm are typical. With laser-assisted leg vein therapy, multiple treatments are necessary. Unlike sclerotherapy, compression stockings are not necessary.

It should be stated that treatment for patients with skin phototype V should be approached cautiously; cosmetic laser treatment of leg veins is not recommended for those with phototype VI. Moreover, IPL in particular is not the best treatment for patients with skin of color, especially those with phototypes IV to VI.

For optimal results, it is best that individuals undergoing laser leg vein treatment are not tanned. Additionally, it is prudent to first treat conditions like venous insufficiency, feeder vessels, and larger varicosities. Pre- and postlaser cooling are necessary to protect the skin from thermal damage and altered pigmentation. Postinflammatory hyperpigmentation is a common side effect, often lasting several months. However, cutaneous ulceration is rare.

HYPERTROPHIC SCARS AND KELOIDS

While both hypertrophic scars and keloids are forms of scarring, hypertrophic scars are confined to the borders of the skin injury, whereas keloids extend beyond this boundary. African Americans have the highest incidence of keloids, reported to be as high as 16%.[34]

PDL is effective in remodeling scar tissue and reducing the appearance of scars, although the mechanism of this effect is not yet fully understood. Young scars fare better with PDL. Nouri et al[35] found decreased formation of scar tissue when treating postsurgical scars with the 585-nm PDL on the day of suture removal. Additionally, adjunctive therapy with compression stockings was found to improve the height and erythema of burn scars.[36] The use of intralesional triamcinolone and the antimetabolite 5-fluorouracil immediately after PDL treatment showed more improvement than with PDL alone.[37]

The 595-nm PDL is a better choice in treating patients with skin of color.[38] It has been observed that purpuric pulse durations with conservative fluences improve erythematous hypertrophic scars and keloidal scars. For skin of color, longer pulse durations are recommended, and multiple treatments are necessary.

Fractional laser technology and the long-pulsed Nd:YAG are efficacious in reducing scars and pigmentary alterations. These are discussed in subsequent sections of this chapter.

PSORIASIS

Psoriasis is a chronic inflammatory skin disorder that is characterized by silvery scaly erythematous papules and plaques. It affects males and females equally and is estimated to occur in 2.6% of individuals in the United States.[39]

The PDL and excimer laser are used in the control of psoriasis vulgaris, with the latter being the most commonly used one. Hacker and Rasmussen[40] initially used PDL to treat psoriasis vulgaris in 1992. It is thought that the PDL targets the altered microvasculature in the psoriatic lesion. Generally, the parameters used for psoriasis vulgaris are mild to moderate fluence with a purpuric or short pulse duration on a spot size of 5 to 10 mm. PDL treatments can be used in conjunction with topical, oral, and injectable treatments. There was a 71% improvement, with a remission period of 10.7 months, seen in hand and feet psoriasis after treatment with PDL and either salicylic acid or calcipotriol.[41] There seems to be no difference between short PDL systems (0.450 ms) and long PDL systems (1.5 ms).[23]

For nail psoriasis, Oram et al[42] used the 595-nm PDL in five patients; although subungual hyperkeratosis and onycholysis responded well, nail pitting did not. Treewittayapoom et al[43] treated one hand (40 nails) with the 595-nm PDL on a 7-mm spot at 9 J/cm^2 for 6 ms, with 20 ms of cryogen and a 10-ms delay. The other hand (39 nails) was treated with the 595-nm PDL at 6 J/cm^2 for 0.45 ms, with 20 ms of cryogen and 10-ms delay, again on a 7-mm spot. The lateral and proximal nail folds were treated, including the lunula. Two passes were performed with a 10% overlap on a monthly basis for a total of 6 months. The fingernails on both hands improved from their baseline, independent of pulse duration.[43] Huang et al[44] used tazarotene 0.1% cream on all nails. A 7-mm spot on one hand was treated with the 595-nm PDL at 9 J/cm^2, for a pulse duration of 1.5 ms, with 30 ms of cryogen and a 30-ms delay. The treatment included one pass of pulses with a 10% overlap to the proximal and lateral nail folds. Investigators found a statistically significant decrease in the Nail Psoriasis Severity Index score in the PDL treatment group versus the non-PDL treatment group.[44]

The treatment of psoriasis in skin of color with the PDL has not shown consistent results. To enhance treatment with the PDL, it is best to remove scale prior to treatment. Conservative fluences and multiple treatments every 2 to 4 weeks are necessary. A more reliable and reproducible laser to help control psoriasis is the excimer laser. The 308-nm excimer laser has been approved by the U.S. Food and Drug Administration to treat mild, moderate, and severe psoriasis.[45] The xenon chloride laser produces a 308-nm monochromatic band of ultraviolet (UV) B radiation. Unlike traditional narrowband UVB (NB-UVB), the excimer laser only targets the affected psoriatic papules and plaques, sparing uninvolved skin. This allows for higher dosimetry to be used on the involved skin. The initial starting dose is dependent on the minimal erythema dose, which is then adjusted on subsequent treatments as per the clinical response. The mechanism of action is through T-cell cytotoxicity.

With their initial left-right comparison study of traditional NB-UVB versus the excimer laser, Bónis et al[45] demonstrated that there was less cumulative dosing, fewer treatments, and shorter treatment duration with the latter. Other studies have confirmed longer periods of remission with fewer treatments when using the excimer laser compared to traditional-phototherapy. Therefore, there is a lower cumulative dose of UV light with a lower risk for carcinogenicity. The side effects are localized to the treated site and include crusting, erythema, burning, and superficial erosion.

It appears that the excimer laser works best for truncal psoriasis. However, the excimer laser can be used in the treatment of scalp psoriasis and palmoplantar psoriasis. In addition, the excimer laser can be used in combination with other treatments, or as a monotherapy.

VERRUCA VULGARIS

Warts can prove very difficult to treat, and the PDL and CO_2 laser are the most common laser devices known to be effective. However, the CO_2 ablative laser is not recommended in skin of color. The PDL is a therapeutic option. In patients with skin of color, it is recommended for the initial treatment to either keep the pulse duration short while

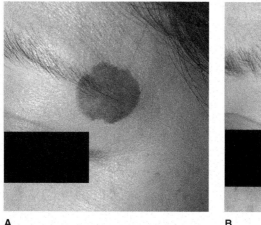
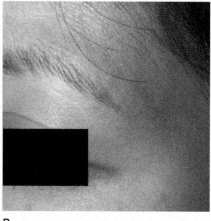

A   **B**

FIGURE 81-4. Lentigo near the eyebrow before **(A)** and after **(B)** treatment with the Q-switched ruby laser. (Used with permission from H. Lui, MD.)

decreasing the fluence or to keep the fluence moderate with a longer pulse duration. Subsequent treatments can be altered depending on the clinical response. During the pulse delivery onto the skin, the patient should not experience any graying, vesiculation, or extreme discomfort. The PDL can be used alone or in combination with other forms of treatment. Clearance rates are reportedly as high as 62.7% after an average of 3.4 treatments.[46,47]

PIGMENTED LESIONS

Q-switched lasers are well suited to treat patients with skin of color for a variety of pigmented dermatologic disorders. The three major Q-switched laser systems are the Q-switched ruby (694 nm), alexandrite (755 nm), and Nd:YAG (1,064 nm) lasers. The Q-switched ruby laser is best suited for patients with phototype IV or lighter, whereas the Q-switched alexandrite laser is best for phototype V or lighter. The Q-switched Nd:YAG laser can be used for all skin types. The frequency-doubled Nd:YAG (532 nm) is another Q-switched laser system, but is not used commonly for patients with darker phototypes.

Additionally, the fractional laser is used on all skin types and has gained acceptance for improving a variety of pigmentary disorders. IPL has gained popularity not only in medical offices, but medical spas. Nevertheless, it should be stated that although patients with skin phototype IV can use these treatments with caution, IPL is not suitable for patients with phototypes V or VI.

LENTIGINES

Often appearing as signs of aging and sun damage, lentigines are considered cosmetically undesirable by most patients. For fair-complexioned

individuals, the Q-switched ruby laser is efficacious. In addition, the frequency-doubled 532-nm Q-switched Nd:YAG laser is an alternative if it is used at the lowest possible fluence. Usually, only one or two treatment sessions are needed. Postinflammatory hyperpigmentation is common in patients with skin phototype IV and darker; it is more common with the use of lower-wavelength Q-switched lasers. Typically, frostlike whitening is observed as an after effect. It is important that the patient avoids excessive sun exposure when healing from the laser treatment [**Figures 81-4, and 81-5**].

The IPL system has been used to treat lentigines. Kawada et al[48] treated 66 Japanese patients with facial lentigines and ephelides using three to five IPL treatments. Approximately 48% of patients showed more than 50% improvement, with 20% of patients experiencing over 75% clearing of the lentigines. The expected mild crusting with pigmented lesions was experienced by over half of the patients, and one patient was burned. The authors postulated that this was due to the darker lesion and darker skin tone.[48] Wang et al[49] found a preference for the IPL for lentigines and the Q-switched alexandrite laser for ephelides, when comparing the two treatments in a group of Asian women.

DERMATOSIS PAPULOSA NIGRA

Dermatosis papulosa nigra (DPN) is a condition of benign pigmented lesions commonly associated with darker skin. However, only a few analyses of the effect of laser treatment on this condition have been reported.[50] A comparison of 532-nm potassium-titanyl-phosphate (KTP) laser treatment with electrodesiccation found the laser to be safe, effective, and well-tolerated alternative form of treatment for DPN in patients with darker skin. Additionally, KTP laser treatment has the

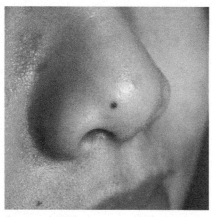
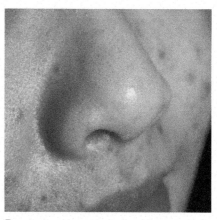

A   **B**

FIGURE 81-5. Blue nevus on the tip of the nose before **(A)** and after **(B)** one treatment with the Q-switched ruby laser. (Used with permission from H. Lui, MD.)

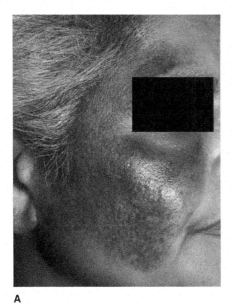
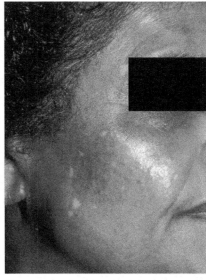

A   B

FIGURE 81-6. Nevus of Ota before **(A)** and after **(B)** several Q-switched ruby laser treatments. Note the mild transient hypopigmentation but excellent clearance. (Used with permission from H. Lui, MD.)

advantage of being less painful for the patient.[51] It is essential that the smallest spot size (1 to 2 mm) is used so as to limit treatment to the surface of the individual DPNs and avoid injury to the surrounding skin.

NEVI OF ITO AND OTA

These dermomelanocytic lesions are best treated with Q-switched laser systems. Multiple treatments are necessary to achieve a clinically acceptable outcome. On average, treatments range from four to eight sessions and can be performed every 1 to 2 months. It is believed that 2-month intervals between treatments may reduce the overall number of treatments required over time. Watanabe and Takahashi[52] found good results after three or more treatments with the Q-switched ruby laser on 114 Asian patients with a nevus of Ota. As previously stated, the choice of device should be based on the individual patient's phototype, with the Q-switched ruby laser most suitable for type IV, the Q-switched alexandrite laser for types IV and V, and the Q-switched Nd:YAG laser for all types.

In addition, depending on the clinical response and the depth of the dermal melanocytes, laser systems may need to be interchanged. The longer-wavelength lasers are better suited for the more deeply situated dermal melanocytic cells. Chan et al[53] found that the Q-switched Nd:YAG laser was clinically more effective than the Q-switched alexandrite laser after three or more treatments. The most common side effect was transient postinflammatory altered pigmentation [**Figure 81-6**].

MELASMA

Melasma is a common disorder of hyperpigmentation that is most commonly found in women with skin phototypes III through VI who live in areas of intense sunlight exposure. Other factors that are thought to play a role in the pathogenesis of melasma include hormonal factors, phototoxic drug effects, ovarian dysfunction, and underlying thyroid disease. However, recent studies have shown that melasma may also have a vascular component in its pathogenesis,[54] as well as a genetic predisposition.[55]

Although still not reported in the U.S. literature, there are reports of success abroad and the increased popularity of treating melasma with the Q-switched laser using a technique referred to as 'laser toning' or 'laser facial.' It is widely used in Asian countries for skin rejuvenation and melasma.[56] In Thailand, Wattanakrai et al[57] treated 22 Asian patients in a split-face study. The combination of the Q-switched laser and 2% hydroquinone topical therapy was compared to treatment with the 1064-nm Q-switched Nd:YAG on a 6-mm spot size, with a fluence of 3 to 3.8 J/cm[2] for five sessions at 1-week intervals. The monotherapy laser showed

improvement in relative lightness and in the melasma area and severity. However, mottled hypopigmentation developed in three patients. In addition, the improvement in hyperpigmentation proved temporary in four of the 22 patients; these patients developed rebound hyperpigmentation. All patients had recurrence of the melasma.[57] To avoid serious side effects, it is recommended that too many (eg, >6 to 10 sessions) or overly frequent (eg, every week) sessions with the Q-switched Nd:YAG laser be avoided. Hypopigmentation should be investigated after every session, and further treatments should be stopped if evidence of this side effect is found.[58] To summarize, the use of the Q-switched laser in the treatment of melasma needs greater study and analysis to determine its efficacy and safety.

Overall, the IPL system appears to modestly improve melasma when used as an adjunctive therapy in cases of melasma refractory to topical therapy alone.[59] In one study, 89 Asian females who were unresponsive to topical therapy and chemical peels were treated with IPL every 3 weeks for a total of four sessions.[60] Melanin and erythema measurements showed improvement. Interestingly, the IPL system has been reported in the literature to exacerbate subclinical melasma when aggressive fluences are used. Negishi et al[61] postulated that patients with latent melasma detected by UV photography should be treated with mild IPL parameters to avoid erythema. It is important to note that IPL-induced erythema should only last a few minutes and not hours. Nonablative lasers are helpful in improving melasma in patients with skin phototypes IV to VI. The nonablative long pulse 1064-nm laser has also been noted, in unpublished reports, to improve melasma as well as postinflammatory pigmentation changes. The exact mechanism of this improvement is unclear. However, there appears to be dermal remodeling with the release of cytokines, which enhances the quality of the skin. Multiple treatments every 3 to 6 weeks are necessary, but the treatment is a safe option for all phototypes with limited risk for patients with tanned skin. Adjunctive treatments with topical retinoids, sunscreens, and hydroquinone, as well as the use of chemical or mechanical peels, are helpful to improve the condition. The laser parameters with the long-pulsed 1064-nm laser should use a 5-mm spot size for 0.3 ms and 5 Hz, with a fluence range of 11 to 14 J/cm[2] depending on skin tone.

Another nonablative laser technique that is helpful in controlling melasma is fractional photothermolysis. After treatment with fractional laser resurfacing, patients with melasma showed a decrease in the number of melanocytes as well as the amount of melanin granules within the keratinocytes on light and electron microscopy.[62] Lee et al[63] studied 25 Asian patients with melasma who received four monthly treatments;

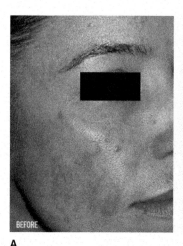 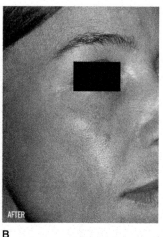

A   **B**

FIGURE 81-7. Melasma before (**A**) and after (**B**) four fractional laser treatments at 7 mJ/cm², treatment level 5, with 14% coverage. (Used with permission from Dr. Howard Conn, MD.)

early improvement was found overall, but a decline in improvement was noted at 24 weeks, and a loss of efficacy was seen at 6 months. No change in elasticity was noted in the group, and hyperpigmentation was observed in 13% of the patients.[63] When treating melasma in patients with skin of color, low density and low depth of penetration are recommended. The recommended density for the 1550-nm erbium-doped fractional nonablative laser is 11% to 14% (level 4 or 5) with an energy level of 6 to 8 mJ/cm². To avoid a rebound effect, it is best not to perform continued treatments in an effort to achieve 100% clearance. Strict sun avoidance and pre- and posttreatment hydroquinone are imperative [**Figure 81-7**].

Overall, the complex pathogenesis and the recurrent and refractory nature of melasma make it difficult to treat.

LASER AND LIGHT-BASED COSMETIC TREATMENTS

SKIN REJUVENATION

There is evidence that PDL has thermal effects on perivascular tissue to induce neocollagenesis. This concept is well established in the literature. The earliest studies were done by Zelickson et al[64] in patients with perioral and periorbital wrinkling; 10 patients were considered to have mild rhytides, and 10 patients had moderate rhytides. A 585-nm PDL was used, with a fluence of 3 to 6.5 J/cm² and pulse duration of 450 μs on spots of 7 to 10 mm in diameter. Approximately 14 months after the initial treatment, there was a 90% clinical improvement for those with mild rhytides and a 40% improvement for those with moderate rhytides. Histologically, there was increased staining of the elastin and collagen fibrils in the papillary dermis and increased mucin.[64] In a split-face study, Hsu et al[65] found a statistically significant improvement in periorbital rhytides following one to two sessions of the 585-nm PDL. Histologically, there was an increase in type III procollagen, type I collagen mRNA, and chondroitin sulfate.[65] Furthermore, after one PDL treatment to treat facial rhytides, an increase in dermal collagen was observed using ultrasonography.[66] These findings suggest that the PDL promotes new collagen production through the release of certain mediators within the skin. Neocollagenesis is seen after as little as one to two treatments with PDL. However, PDL skin rejuvenation is best used in patients with lighter phototypes.

The IPL system has been used to improve skin texture. In a cohort of 97 Asian patients with skin phototypes IV and V, Negishi et al[67] observed improvement in pigmentation, telangiectasias, and skin texture in 90%, 83%, and 65% of patients, respectively. Cut-off filters for shorter wavelengths were used, and the patients underwent multiple treatments. There were no reports of scarring or changes in pigmentation.[67] However, transient erythema and blistering have been noted with the use of IPL in Chinese patients.[68] Hernandez-Perez and Ibiett[69] treated five Hispanic

women using five IPL sessions. Moderate to very good improvements were noted in their patients' skin, including for conditions like mild rhytides and dilated pores. Histologically, there was a statistically significant difference in epidermal thickness, suggesting not only a dermal improvement but also an epidermal textural improvement.[69] However, it is the authors' opinion that the IPL should not under any circumstance be used on patients with skin phototypes V or VI.

Fractional laser therapy is now considered a fundamental device for treatment for skin rejuvenation. The remodeling of collagen within the treatment zones facilitates skin rejuvenation. In addition to long-pulse 1064 nm devices, new technology has led to the use of fractional, nonablative Q-switched 1064-nm Nd:YAG laser systems for treating acne scarring as well as performing skin rejuvenation.

TATTOO REMOVAL

It is estimated that 21% of adults in the United States have at least one tattoo.[70] Tattoos can be exogenous (eg, decorative or amateur) or traumatic (eg, asphalt, gravel). Laser-assisted tattoo removal is considered the gold-standard treatment. With laser-assisted tattoo removal, there is decreased risk of scarring and pigmentary alteration. Professional tattoos generally require more treatments than amateur tattoos. Traumatic tattoos can often be cleared after only a few treatments.

Depending on the absorption spectrum of the ink, a particular wavelength can be chosen. Red inks are best treated with a 532-nm laser, whereas green or teal inks are best treated with a 755-nm laser, and black ink can be treated with 694-, 755-, or 1064-nm lasers. However, the 1064-nm laser has been used most frequently to remove black tattoo ink and is the wavelength of choice when treating pigmented skin.[71]

There are few precautions and contraindications to be aware of concerning laser tattoo removal. The most severe reaction, and hence contraindication, is an allergy to the tattoo ink. In this case, the tattoo should either be surgically removed or vaporized with an ablative laser. Second, cosmetic tattoos that use flesh tones or white inks may undergo immediate pigment darkening with Q-switched lasers. This occurs when the ferric oxide in the ink is reduced to ferrous oxide by the laser. This pigment-darkening reaction cannot always be removed successfully.[72] Therefore, a test spot is highly recommended before treatment begins. Third, although not a contraindication, patients who are known to form keloids should be treated with caution. Although somewhat controversial, it is prudent to wait a minimum of 6 months after using isotretinoin, a medication primarily used for cystic acne, before most laser procedures to reduce the risk of scarring and keloid formation.[73,74] Tattoos resulting from combustible substances, for example gunpowder or fireworks, can cause ignition when treated with Q-switched lasers.[75] Lastly, those who are taking gold salts have been known to develop chrysiasis with the Q-switched lasers.[76]

The majority of tattoos are never completely removed. For the most part, faint to imperceptible remnants of color remain; this signifies an excellent outcome. Shorter-wavelength lasers often cause hypopigmentation, although this is transient in most cases and rarely permanent. Patients who 'do-over' or 'cover-up' their original tattoo with a second one are at risk for further side effects. Negative prognostic variables include smoking, older tattoos, short treatment intervals, brightly colored tattoos, tattoos with white ink, and tattoos located on the legs and feet; these were noted by Bencini et al[77] in their prospective study of 397 patients.

New on the market is the ultra-short Q-switched laser system. This technology provides a faster and more precise deposit of light energy to the target, causing the target to heat and expand more rapidly, resulting in the more precise and efficient dissolution of the ink or pigment. This means that there is less disruption of the surrounding tissue. The benefits of using ultra-short Q-switched devices (measured in ps) include lower fluences, faster clearance of the tattoo or pigment target, and fewer side effects.[78-80] In particular, the 1064-nm ultra-short Q-switched laser shows promise in pigmented skin, although studies are pending.

HAIR REMOVAL

Laser-assisted hair removal is used to ensure the permanent reduction of hair. Multiple treatments are necessary. Thick black hairs show

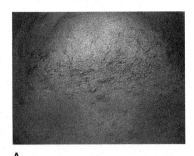

A

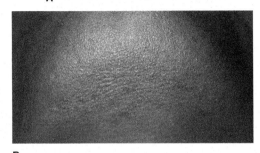

B

FIGURE 81-8. Before **(A)** and after **(B)** four treatments of laser-assisted hair removal. A 1064-nm long-pulsed laser was used on a 10-mm spot at 30 to 35 J/cm^2. (Used with permission from Dr. Samuel Lederman, MD.)

the best response to treatment, with gray, blonde, white, red, and light brown hairs showing either no or little response to laser-assisted hair removal. Side effects are rare; one uncommon side effect is the aberrant induction of hair growth, which mostly occurs in persons of Mediterranean descent. Anecdotally, it has been observed that those with fine to intermediate hairs located in the temple area or the lateral forehead are at greater risk. The increased hair growth is often difficult to treat and requires multiple treatments, sometimes with alternative laser-assisted hair removal devices [**Figure 81-8**].

NONINVASIVE BODY CONTOURING

Liposuction is one of the most common surgical cosmetic procedures in the United States. However, there is a need for a noninvasive treatment modality to rid unwanted adipose tissue. Although results are not as impressive as tumescent surgical liposuction, noninvasive devices for reducing adipose tissue have a high safety profile with little to no recovery time. Results typically can be seen as early as 30 to 90 days and as early as 2 weeks with some devices. Generally, multiple treatments are necessary to achieve noticeable results.

Three major categories exist for noninvasive non-light-based body contouring devices that decrease adipose tissue: radiofrequency, ultrasonography and cryolipolysis.

Radiofrequency devices cause skin tightening and produce volumetric heating of the fat causing cellular death of the adipocyte while sparing the overlying epidermal and dermal tissue.[81] However, patients with indwelling metal devices such as pacemakers or hip replacements are not candidates. High-intensity focused ultrasonography uses focused ultrasonic sound waves which cause thermocoagulation to disrupt the subcutaneous adipose tissue without affecting the overlying skin and surrounding structures. Pulsed (non-thermal) focused ultrasound mechanically destroys fat cells through cavitation. Newer ultrasound devices combine focused with nonfocused devices and high frequency and low frequency to achieve body contouring. Cryolipolysis involves the controlled application of cold temperatures to adipose tissue, thus selectively damaging the adipocyte without compromising the epidermis and dermis. The inflammatory response begins 72 hours after treatment, with clinical results seen between 30 to 90 days after treatment.[82] Side-effects are temporary bruising, erythema and altered sensation. More data are needed to determine its safety in persons with cold urticaria, cryoglobulinemia and the like.

CONCLUSION

Laser treatment of skin of color presents a great challenge for dermatologists and laser surgeons. However, skin of color is not a contraindication. A better understanding of laser-tissue interaction is very important when treating darker skin tones. Test spots, skin cooling, mild settings, and careful postoperative skin care are highly recommended to minimize untoward results.

REFERENCES

1. U.S. Census Bureau. Overview of Race and Hispanic Origin: 2010; 2010 Census Briefs. http://www.census.gov/prod/cen2010/briefs/c2010br-02.pdf Accessed February 10, 2012.
2. Anderson RR, Parrish JA. Selective thermolysis: precise microsurgery by selective absorption of pulsed radiation. *Science.* 1983;220:524-527.
3. Jacobs HA, Walton RG. The incidence of birth marks in the neonate. *Pediatrics.* 1976;58:218-222.
4. Alper JC, Holmes LB. The incidence and significance of birthmarks in a cohort of 4641 newborns. *Pediatr Dermatol.* 1983;1:58-68.
5. Geronemus R, Ashinoff R. The medical necessity of evaluation and treatment of port-wine stains. *J Dermatol Surg Oncol.* 1991;17:76-79.
6. Morelli JG, Weston WL, Huff JC, et al. Initial lesion size as a predictive factor in determining the response of port-wine stains in children treated with pulsed dye laser. *Arch Pediatr Adolesc Med.* 1995;149:1142-1144.
7. Ho WS, Chan HH, Ying SY, et al. Laser treatment of congenital facial port wine stains: long term efficacy and complication in Chinese patients. *Lasers Surg Med.* 2002;30:44-47.
8. Tong AK, Tan OT, Eng JB, et al. Ultrastructure: effects of melanin pigment on target specificity using a pulsed dye laser (577 nm). *J Invest Dermatol.* 1987;6:747-752.
9. Van Kampen EJ, Zijlstra WG. Determination of hemoglobin and its derivatives. In: Sobotka H, Stewart CP, eds. *Advances in Clinical Chemistry.* Vol 8. New York, NY: Academic Press; 1965:158-187.
10. Scherer K, Lorenz S, Wimmershoff M, et al. Both the flashlamp-pumped dye laser and the long pulsed tunable dye laser can improve results in port-wine stain therapy. *Br J Dermatol.* 2001;145:79-84.
11. Anderson RR. Laser-tissue interactions in dermatology. In: Arndt KA, Dover JS, Olbricht SM, eds. *Lasers in Cutaneous and Aesthetic Surgery.* Philadelphia, PA: Lippincott-Raven; 1977:25-51.
12. Anolik R, Newlove T, Weiss ET, et al. Investigation into optimal treatment intervals of facial port-wine stains using the pulsed dye laser. *J Am Acad Dermatol.* 2012;67:985-990.
13. Sommer S, Sheehan-Dare RA. Pulsed dye lser treatment of port-wine stains in pigmented skin. *J Am Acad Dermatol.* 2000;42:667-671.
14. Chang CJ, Kelly KM, van Gemert MJ, et al. Comparing the effectiveness of 585 nm vs 595 nm wavelength pulsed dye laser treatment of port wine stains in conjunction with cryogen spray cooling. *Lasers Surg Med.* 2002;31:352-358.
15. Huikeshoven M, Koster PH, de Borgie CA, et al. Redarkening of port-wine stains 10 years after pulsed-dye-laser treatment. *N Engl J Med.* 2007;356: 2745-2746.
16. Kelly KM, Choi B, Mc Farlane S, et al. Description and analysis of treatments for port-wine stain birthmarks. *Arch Facial Plast Surg.* 2005;7:287-294.
17. Chen JK, Ghasri P, Guillermo A, et al. An overview of clinical and experimental treatment modalities for port wine stains. *J Am Acad Dermatol.* 2012;67: 389-304.
18. Alster TS, Ranzi EL. Combined 595-nm and 1064-nm laser irradiation of recalcitrant and hypertrophic port-wine stains in children and adults. *Dermatol Surg.* 2009;35:914-919.
19. Tremaine AM, Armstrong JA, Yu-Chin H, et al. Enhanced port-wine stain lightening achieved with combined treatment of selective photothermolysis and imiquimod. *J Am Acad Dermatol.* 2011;66:634-641.
20. Jia W, Sun V, Tran N, et al. Long-term blood vessel removal with combined laser and topical rapamycin antiangiogenic therapy: implications for effective port-wine stain treatment. *Lasers Surg Med.* 2010;42:105-112.
21. Ho WS, Ying SY, Chan PK, et al. Treatment of port wine stains with intense pulsed light: a prospective study. *Dermatol Surg.* 2004;30:887-891.
22. Kilcline C, Frieden IJ. Infantile hemangiomas: how common are they? A systematic review of the medical literature. *Pediatr Dermatol.* 2008;25:168-173.
23. Kanada K, Reyes-Merin M, Munden A, et al. A prospective study of cutaneous findings in newborns in the United States: correlation with race, ethnicities, and gestational status using up dated classification and nomenclature. *J Pediatr* 2012;161:240-245.
24. Drolet BA, Esterly NB, Frieden IJ. Hemangioma in children. *N Engl J Med.* 1999;341:173-181.

25. Kim HJ, Colombo M, Frieden IJ. Ulcerated hemangiomas: clinical characteristics and response to therapy. *J Am Acad Dermatol.* 2001;44:962-972.

26. Bowers RE, Graham EA, Tomlinson KM. The natural history of the strawberry nevus. *Arch Dermatol.* 1960;82:667-680.

27. Li J, Chen X, Zhao S, et al. Demographic and clinical characteristics and risk factors for infantile hemangioma. *Arch Dermatol.* 2011;9:1049-1056.

28. Maguiness SM, Frieden IJ. Current management of infantile hemangiomas. *Semin Cutan Med Surg.* 2010;29:106-114.

29. Kono T, Hiroyuki S, William FG. Comparison study of traditional pulsed dye laser versus a long-pulsed dye laser in the treatment of early childhood hemangiomas. *Lasers Surg Med.* 2005;38:112-115.

30. Rizzo C, Brightman L, Chapas AM, et al. Outcomes of childhood hemangiomas treated with the pulsed-dye laser with dynamic cooling: a retrospective chart analysis. *Dermatol Surg.* 2009;35:1947-1954.

31. Hunzeker C, Geroneumus R. Treatment of superficial infantile hemangiomas of the eyelid using the 595-nm pulsed dye laser. *Dermatol Surg.* 2010; 36:590-597.

32. McCoppin HH, Hovenic WW, Wheeland RG. Laser treatment of superficial leg veins: a review. *Dermatol Surg.* 2011;37:729-741.

33. Parlette EC, Groff WF, Kinshella MJ, et al. Optimal pulse durations for the treatment of leg telangiectasias with a neodymium YAG laser. *Lasers Surg Med.* 2006;38:98-105.

34. Craft N. Keloids: current concepts in pathogenesis and treatment. *Cosmet Dermatol.* 2002;15:35-39.

35. Nouri K, Elsaie ML, Vejjabhinanta V, et al. Comparison of the effects of short-and-long-pulse durations when using a 585-nm pulsed dye laser in the treatment of new surgical scars. *Lasers Med Sci.* 2010;25:121-126.

36. Bailey JK, Burkes SA, Visscher MO, et al. Multimodal quantitative analysis of early pulsed-dye-laser treatment of scars at a pediatric burn hospital. *Dermatol Surg.* 2012;38:1490-1496.

37. Asilian A, Darougheh A, Shariati F. New combination of triamcinolone, 5-fluorouracil, and pulsed-dye laser for treatment of keloid and hypertrophic scars. *Dermatol Surg.* 2006;32:907-915.

38. Goldman MP, Fitzpatrick RE. Laser treatment of scars. *Dermatol Surg.* 1995; 21:685-687.

39. Koo J. Population-based epidemiologic study of psoriasis with emphasis on quality of life assessment. *Dermatol Clin.* 1996;14:485-496.

40. Hacker SM, Rasmussen JE. The effect of flash lamp-pulsed dye laser on psoriasis. *Arch Dermatol.* 1992;128:853-855.

41. de Leeuw J, Tank B, Bjerring P, et al. Concomitant treatment of psoriasis of the hands and feet with the pulsed dye laser and topical calcipotriol, salicylic acid, or both; a prospective open study in 41 patients. *J Am Acad Dermatol.* 2006;54:266-271.

42. Oram Y, Karincaoglu Y, Koyuncu E, et al. Pulsed dye laser in the treatment of nail psoriasis. *Dermatol Surg.* 2010;36:377-381.

43. Treewittayapoom C, Singvahanont P, Chanprapaph K, et al. The effect of different pulse durations in the treatment of nail psoriasis with the 595-nm pulsed dye laser: a randomized, double blind, intrapatient left-to-right study. *J Am Acad Dermatol.* 2012;66:807-812.

44. Huang YC, Chou CL, Chiang YY. Efficacy of pulsed dye laser plus topical tazarotene versus topical tazarotene alone in psoriatic nail disease: a single-blind, intrapatient left-to-right controlled study. *Lasers Surg Med.* 2013;45:102-107.

45. Bónis B, Kemény L, Dobozy A, et al. 308-nm excimer laser for psoriasis. *Lancet.* 1997;350:1522.

46. Kopera D. Verrucae vulgaris: flashlamp-pumped pulsed dye laser treatment of 120 patients. *Int J Dermatol.* 2003;42:904-908.

47. Lui A, Moy R, Ross EV, et al. Pulsed dye laser and pulsed dye laser-mediated photodynamic therapy in the treatment of dermatologic disorders. *Dermatol Surg.* 2012;38:351-366.

48. Kawada A, Shiraishi H, Mutsuyo A, et al. Clinical improvement of solar lentigines and ephelides with an intense pulsed light source. *Dermatol Surg.* 2002;28:504-508.

49. Wang CC, Sue YM, Yang CH, et al. A comparison of Q switched alexandrite laser and intense pulsed light for the treatment of freckles and lentigines in Asian persons: a randomized, physician-blinded, split face comparison trial. *J Am Acad Dermatol.* 2006;54:804-810.

50. Shah S, Alster T. Laser treatment of dark skin. *Am J Clin Dermatol.* 2010; 11:389-397.

51. Kundu RV, Joshi SS, Suh KY, et al. Comparison of electrodesiccation and potassium titanyl-phosphate laser for treatment of dermatosis papulosa nigra. *Dermatol Surg.* 2009;35:1079-1083.

52. Watanabe S, Takahashi H. Treatment of nevus of Ota with the Q-switched ruby laser. *N Engl J Med.* 1994;331:1745-1750.

53. Chan HH, Ying SY, Ho WS, et al. An in vivo trial comparing the clinical efficacy and complications of Q-switched 755-nm alexandrite and Q-switched 1064-nm (Nd-YAG) lasers in the treatment of nevus of Ota. *Dermatol Surg.* 2000;26:919-922.

54. Kim EH, Kim YC, Lee E-S, et al. The vascular characteristics of melasma. *J Derm Sci.* 2007;46:111-116.

55. Ortonne JP, Arellano I, Berneburg M, et al. A global survey of the role of ultraviolet radiation and hormonal influences in the development of melasma. *J Eur Acad Dermatol Vernereol.* 2009;23:1254-1262.

56. Arora P, Sarkar R, Garg WK, et al. Lasers for treatment of melasma and postinflammatory hyperpigmentation. *J Cutan Aesthet Surg.* 2012;5:93-103.

57. Wattanakrai P, Mornchan R, Eimpunth S. Low-fluence Q-switched neodymium-doped yttrium aluminum garnet (1,064 nm) laser for the treatment of facial melasma in Asians. *Dermatol Surg.* 2010;36:76-87.

58. Arora P, Sarkar R, Garg VK, et al. Lasers for treatment of melasma and postinflammatory hyperpigmentation. *J Cutan Aesthet Surg.* 2012;5:93-103.

59. Sheth VM, Panndya AG. Melasma: a comprehensive update: part II. *J Am Acad Dermatol.* 2011;65:699-714.

60. Li TH, Chen JZ, Wei HC, et al. Efficacy and safety of intense pulsed light in treatment of melasma in Chinese patients. *Dermatol Surg.* 2008;34:693-700.

61. Negishi K, Kushikata N, Tezuka Y, et al. Study of the incidence and nature of "very subtle epidermal melasma" in relation to intense pulsed light treatment. *Dermatol Surg.* 2004;30:881-886.

62. Goldberg DJ, Berlin AL, Phleps R. Histologic and ultrastructural analysis of melasma after fractional resurfacing. *Lasers Surg Med.* 2008;40:134-138.

63. Lee HS, Won CH, Lee DH, et al. Treatment of melasma in Asian skin using a fractional 1,550 nm: an open clinical study. *Dermatol Surg.* 2009;35: 1499-1504.

64. Zelickson BD, Kilmer SL, Bernstein E. Pulsed dye laser therapy for sun damage skin. *Lasers Surg Med.* 1999;25:229-236.

65. Hsu TS, Zelickson B, Dover JS, et al. Multicenter study of the safety and efficacy of a 585 nm pulsed-dye laser for the nonablative treatment of facial rhytides. *Dermatol Surg.* 2005;31:1-9.

66. Moody BR, McCarthy JE, Hruza GJ. Collagen remodeling after 585-nm pulsed dye laser irradiation: an ultrasonographic analysis. *Dermatol Surg.* 2003;29:997-999.

67. Negishi K, Tezuka Y, Kudshikata N, et al. Photorejuvenation for Asian skin by intense pulsed light. *Dermatol Surg.* 2001;27:627-632.

68. Chan HH, Chan E, Kono T, et al. The use of variable pulse width frequency doubled Nd:YAG 532 nm laser in the treatment of port-wine stain in Chinese patients. *Dermatol Surg.* 2000:26:657-661.

69. Hernandez-Perez E, Ibiett E. Gross and microscopic findings in patients submitted to nonablative full face resurfacing using intense pulsed light: a preliminary study. *Dermatol Surg.* 2001;27:627-632.

70. Braverman S. One in five U.S. adults now has a tattoo: yet over two in five without a tattoo say adult tattoos are less attractive. http://www. Harrisinterative.com/vault/harris%20poll%2022%20-tatoos_2.23.12.pdf. Accessed February 23, 2012.

71. Kilmer S. Laser treatment of tattoos. *Dermatol Clin.* 1997;15:409-417.

72. Anderson R, Geronemus R, Kilmer S, et al. Cosmetic tattoo ink darkening. A complication of Q-switched and pulsed-laser treatment. *Arch Dermatol.* 1993;129:1010-1014.

73. Bernstein L, Geronemus R. Keloid formation with the 585-nm pulsed dye laser during isotretinoin treatment. *Arch Dermatol.* 1997;133:111-112.

74. Alissa A. Concomitant Use of Laser and Isotretinoin, How Safe. Grapevine, TX: American Society for Laser Medicine and Surgery; 2011.

75. Taylor C. Laser ignition of traumatically embedded firework debris. *Lasers Surg Med.* 1998;22:157-158.

76. Almoallium H, Klinkhoff A, Arthur A, et al. Laser induced chrysiasis: disfiguring hyperpigmentation following Q-switched laser therapy in a woman previously treated with gold. *J Rheumatol.* 2006;33:620-621.

77. Bencini PL, Cazzaniga S, Tourlaki A, et al. Removal of tattoos by Q-switched laser. *Arch Dermatol.* 2012;148:1364-1369.

78. Ross V, Naseef G, Lin G, et al. Comparison of responses to tattoos to picosecond and nanosecond Q-switched neodymium: YAG lasers. *Arch Dermatol.* 1998;134:167-71.

79. Nazanin S, Metelista A, Petrell K, et al. Treatment of tattoos with a picosecond alexandrite laser. A prospective trial. *Arch Dermatol.* 2012;148:1360-1363.

80. Izikson L, Farinelli W, Sakamoto F, et al. Safety and effectiveness of black tattoo clearance in a pig model after a single treatment with a novel 758 nm 500 picosecond laser: a pilot study. *Lasers Surg Med.* 2010;42:640-646

81. Weiss RA. Noninvasive radio frequency for skin tightening and body contouring. *Semin Cutan Med Surg.* 2013;32:9-17.

82. Jewell ML, Solish NJ, Desilets CS. Noninvasive body sculpting technologies with an emphasis on high-intensity focused ultrasound. *Aesthetic Plast Surg.* 2011;35:901-912.

CHAPTER 82

Tissue-Tightening Treatments

Shoshana Marmon
Henry H.L. Chan

KEY POINTS

- Genetic and environmental factors impact the development, extent, and unique patterns of skin laxity in aging.

- The facelift is a longstanding treatment for correcting sagging skin, but recently patients are choosing less invasive approaches.

- Currently, patients can choose invasive or less invasive tissue laxity treatments including utilization of lasers and light sources, radiofrequency energy, focused ultrasound, laser-assisted lipolysis, or a combination of approaches.

- Nonablative lasers are a widespread therapy for skin laxity, noted for their relative safety in skin of color patients and for a shorter recovery period.

- Infrared light techniques are a less painful treatment option, whereas radiofrequency modalities are the mainstay of skin laxity therapy with long-proven results.

- Focused ultrasound and laser lipolysis are newer modalities that have demonstrated greater efficacy than lasers and light source treatments.

- Most patients require a combination of treatments and modalities to achieve desired results.

- Larger, controlled trials are necessary to achieve an objective comparison of various tissue-tightening treatments, especially with regard to the use of these modalities in people with skin of color.

INTRODUCTION

Tissue laxity is one of the most recognizable signs of aging. Both genetic and environmental factors contribute to the morphologic appearance of aged skin. Extrinsic aging, caused by external factors, results from a cumulative exposure to ultraviolet light and is manifested by signs of photodamage such as dyspigmentation, roughness, and keratosis.[1,2] Intrinsic aging, which is tied to internal factors, is linked with an individual's unique biological makeup and is largely genetically predetermined. Due to the photoprotective effect of epidermal melanin, aging in skin of color is considered to be more heavily influenced by intrinsic, rather than extrinsic, factors.[3] Therefore, both one's gender and genetic makeup have a defining impact on the progression, degree, and distinct pattern of skin laxity in aging.

The sagging of facial skin was compared between Japanese men and women in a study by Ezure et al.[4] Although both males and females were found to have similar age-related decreases in tissue elasticity in the mid-face, men, when compared with women, were noted to have an increased laxity in the lower eyelid area.[4]

The connection between pigmented and fair complexions and the rate and presentation of facial aging has been well studied. Thong et al[5] demonstrated that melanosomes in keratinocytes differ in both size and distribution among African Americans, Asians, and Caucasians. Using electron microscopy, they found that the melanosomes of lighter skin types are smaller and clustered, whereas the melanosomes in those with darker skin of color are larger and more widely dispersed.[5] The distribution and size of the melanosomes in darker skin of color, grossly noted as pigment, confer a protection against exposure to ultraviolet light, which would otherwise promote an aged look.

Although the presence or lack of epidermal melanin is central to the differential phenotype of aged skin, recent research has begun to uncover heretofore unrecognized histologic, molecular, and genetic factors that contribute to the pathogenesis of tissue laxity, both via their interplay with melanin and in its absence.[6] In a recent study by Fantasia et al,[7] the levels of elastin fibers and transforming growth factor-β (TGF-β) were compared between skin biopsies of African Americans and Caucasians. TGF-β is critical to the resilience of human skin through its ability to upregulate the expression of elastin and other extracellular matrix proteins.[7,8] Chronologic aging compromises the structural integrity of dermal connective tissue, and there is a loss of elasticity, which manifests as skin thinning, wrinkling, and sagging. Interestingly, both TGF-β and TGF-β receptor expression were found to be higher in African American skin compared with Caucasian skin.[7] This correlated with higher levels of the elastin messenger ribonucleic acid that were identified in dermal fibroblasts derived from African Americans.[7] Correspondingly, Caucasians often display earlier signs of wrinkling and tissue laxity than those with darker skin of color.[9,10]

In the past few decades, there has been a rapidly burgeoning interest in the field of tissue tightening. There are now a variety of choices in both devices and methodology to address sagging skin on the face and body.[11] Although facelift remains the gold standard and results in the most significant improvement in skin laxity, it is associated with a substantial recovery time, expense, and risk.[1,12] Thus, many of today's discerning cosmetic patients are demanding less invasive approaches and are willing to settle for, and at times prefer, a less dramatic outcome. Today's options include both invasive and noninvasive modalities including the utilization of lasers and light sources, radiofrequency (RF) energy, focused ultrasound (US), laser-assisted lipolysis, and combination approaches.[11]

A significant demand for these procedures is currently found in Asia. Facial skin laxity in the Asian patient presents as deepening of the nasolabial folds, drooping of the malar cheek, and the development of jowls [**Figure 82-1**].[13,14] Wrinkling in Asians is considered to present chronologically later than in Caucasians.[9,10] However, it has also been reported

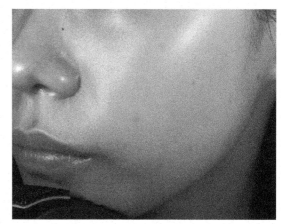

A

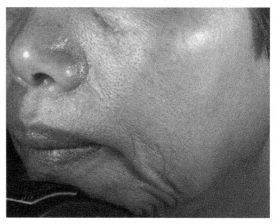

B

FIGURE 82-1. **(A)** Taut facial skin in a 24-year-old Asian woman. **(B)** Tissue laxity and the development of jowls in a 61-year-old Asian woman. (Used with permission from Dr. Henry Hin Lee Chan.)

that Asian individuals develop more severe rhytides on their forehead and around their mouth and eyes, when compared with their Caucasian counterparts.[15] Much of the latest cutting-edge research evaluating novel tissue-tightening devices in skin of color has been generated from studies investigating these techniques in Asian patients, classically Fitzpatrick skin types II to V. Unfortunately, there remains a relative paucity of data about these modalities being used in heavily pigmented skin, such as phototype VI. Patients should be warned that interventional approaches such as the face lift or ablative carbon dioxide (CO_2) resurfacing provides better results in comparison to noninvasive tissue tightening.[1] This chapter will discuss current tissue-tightening techniques and review the available data on their safety and efficacy in skin of color.

LASERS

This following section will review the current research and techniques particular to lasers and their use in skin tightening. For a discussion of the general principles and uses of lasers in skin of color, please refer to Chapter 81.

Lasers used in tissue tightening can be divided into two main categories: nonablative and ablative. Unlike ablative devices, nonablative lasers leave the epidermis intact while generating a large amount of heat in the dermis. The use of nonablative lasers for tissue tightening has become increasingly more widespread due to their relative safety in pigmented skin and the minimal associated down time. However, the degree of improvement with these techniques still lags behind that of traditional interventional or ablative approaches.[16,17] A fundamental impediment to the laser's efficacy is the result of the light scatter that occurs during the transmission of the laser energy through the tissue. This property makes it difficult to achieve significant depths of penetration without the use of sufficiently higher energy, which could damage the epidermis and result in postinflammatory hyperpigmentation (PIH) or scarring in those with darker skin of color.[18] One way to increase the amount of deliverable energy has been the adjunctive use of superficial cooling devices during treatment.[18] In this way, the epidermis is protected, and somewhat deeper penetration and heat can be generated while minimizing the pain and adverse effects. A well-studied and commonly used nonablative laser is the long-pulse 1064-nm neodymium-doped yttrium-aluminum-garnet (Nd:YAG) laser.[19] This laser has a long proven history of efficacy and safety in epilation in darker skin of color, including Fitzpatrick skin types IV through VI.[20] The advantage of using this laser in skin of color is a longer wavelength, allowing for penetration that bypasses the epidermal melanin.[20] A study by Key[21] compared skin tightening from a single treatment with the Nd:YAG laser to that achieved with a 1-cm^2 fast tip monopolar RF device in a split-face analysis. RF energy was administered to one side of the face using a repeat pulse pattern. Each patient received 450 pulses without pulse stacking. The other side of the face was treated with a laser at a fluence of 40 J/cm^2 for the cheek and 20 to 30 J/cm^2 for the forehead. The authors reported that under these conditions, a single treatment with the Nd:YAG laser resulted in a greater improvement than a single treatment with the RF device.[21] An important caveat to this study was that all of the patients were women with Fitzpatrick skin types I and II.[21]

A noteworthy obstacle to the use of the Nd:YAG laser, especially in sensitive areas, is the discomfort associated with this treatment.[22] At times, the pain can be so severe that it necessitates aborting the procedure. Kono et al[22] addressed this issue by comparing two different mechanisms to reduce the pain during treatment sessions: cryogen spray cooling (CSC) versus pneumatic skin flattening (PSF). In this split-face trial, Asian patients with skin phototypes III and IV who had facial skin laxity were subjected to Nd:YAG laser and CSC on one side of the face, while the other side was treated with Nd:YAG laser and PSF. The authors reported that the use of PSF with the Nd:YAG laser was associated with less pain than the use of CSC with the Nd:YAG laser. Neither of the adjunctive measures affected the efficacy of the procedure.[22]

Recently, Lee et al[23] reported that a single session of 1444-nm pulsed Nd:YAG laser therapy resulted in a mild to moderate improvement in both the cheek laxity and the nasolabial fold depth in a small study of 10 Korean patients. A histologic analysis of posttreatment biopsy specimens from five volunteers showed increases in skin thickness, collagen fibers, and the expression of Ki-67, a marker of cell proliferation.[23] Additionally, real-time reverse transcriptase polymerase chain reaction revealed a substantial increase in levels of TGF-β from the baseline, which persisted at the 3-month follow-up.[23] The 1444-nm pulsed Nd:YAG laser was initially introduced for use in laser-assisted lipolysis, as it has a greater affinity for water and a prior study showed that it is more lipolytic than the 1064-nm Nd:YAG laser.[24]

Ablative lasers, such as the high-energy pulsed CO_2 and erbium-doped yttrium-aluminium-garnet (Er:YAG) lasers, function by vaporizing the intact epidermis while simultaneously generating a large amount of thermal energy in the dermis. Although it has been demonstrated that this technique is extremely effective for tissue tightening and facial rejuvenation, it is also associated with a lengthy recovery period and an increased potential for infection. These adverse effects mean this treatment is often unappealing for today's patients. Importantly, the use of these lasers in much darker skin of color is relatively contraindicated, due to the significant risk of postinflammatory dyspigmentation and scarring. An alternative to the classic ablative laser is fractional laser resurfacing. In this technique, microscopic thermal zones are created with intervening areas of intact epidermis. This allows for a more rapid repair of the damaged tissue and a decreased propensity for infection.[25] This approach has nearly revolutionized the use of lasers in facial rejuvenation because it can cause a significant clinical improvement in photodamage while minimizing both risks and down time.[26] A recent report by Lee et al[27] used a fractionated 2940-nm short-pulse Er:YAG laser to address photodamage in a small study of 29 Korean patients. The authors reported that after treatment, all patients showed some degree of improvement in tissue laxity, while only half of the treatment group had a mild reduction in facial wrinkles.[27]

Another device that has been shown to induce tissue tightening is fractional delivery of the ablative 10,600-nm CO_2 laser [**Figure 82-2**].[28] However, although it is effective in facial rejuvenation and improvement of skin laxity, when used in Chinese patients with Fitzpatrick skin types III and IV, a significant risk of PIH was noted, especially at high fluences.[29] A retrospective study of Chinese patients similarly demonstrated an increased incidence of PIH after undergoing fractional resurfacing with the 1540-nm erbium glass laser.[30] Furthermore, the authors reported that the development of PIH appeared to correlate with an increased pulse density and inadequate epidermal cooling in patients with darker skin of color.[30] Kono et al[17] attempted to optimize the use of the 1550-nm laser for laser resurfacing in Asian skin by thoroughly testing a variety of treatment parameters.[17] The results revealed that an increased pulse density, rather than high fluences, was more closely associated with PIH, erythema, swelling, and decreased patient satisfaction.[17]

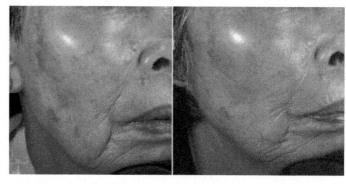

FIGURE 82-2. Before (**A**) and 7 months after (**B**) a single fractional carbon dioxide ablative laser treatment. (Used with the permission of Dr. Henry Hin Lee Chan.)

INFRARED LIGHT

Infrared light has also gained popularity in the armamentarium of nonablative tissue-tightening modalities. This technique delivers thermal energy to the tissues that promotes a wound-healing response with collagen contraction and dermal remodeling over time. An infrared light source has the ability to operate at fluences significantly lower than that of other nonablative RF devices. This potentially provides a less painful alternative for the treatment of facial sagging.[31] Chua et al[32] investigated the use of infrared light with epidermal cooling for facial skin laxity in Asian patients with Fitzpatrick skin types IV and V. In this study, patients were exposed to infrared light in three treatment sessions at 4-week intervals. Both physicians and patients performed a final analysis of the outcome at a 6-month follow-up. It was noted that in all subjects, there were varying degrees of mild to moderate improvement in their skin laxity after treatment.[32] Additionally, there was a high rate of patient satisfaction, with only minimal discomfort reported during the procedure. The most common side effect was blistering, which was transient and resolved without sequelae. A limitation of this study was the lack of an internal control, as the entire face or neck of each patient was treated in all cases.[32] A subsequent trial performed a split-face analysis for the treatment of skin laxity using the same device and similar treatment parameters. In this study, Chinese women with Fitzpatrick skin types III and IV were treated with an infrared device on one side of their face while the other side was left untouched.[12] The results revealed both a subjective and clinical mild to moderate improvement in the facial laxity on the treated side. These results were compiled both 1 and 3 months following the final treatment. As in the prior study, one patient experienced blistering, which had fully resolved by the follow-up appointment.[12] Thus, a nonablative infrared device with contact cooling appears to be a viable option for mild to moderate tissue tightening in skin of color.[31]

RADIOFREQUENCY

One of the earliest modalities developed to specifically target tissue laxity in a noninvasive manner was RF energy.[11] The electromagnetic spectrum of RF energy ranges from 300 MHz to 3 kHz.[11] Similar to a laser, heat is generated in the dermis through the delivery of RF energy to the skin. This results in an immediate tissue contraction and damage to the dermal collagen, with a subsequent wound-healing response that occurs over months. However, unlike lasers, RF energy creates an electric field that is transduced through the skin, independent of a chromophore presence.[11] The number of devices using RF energy has increased dramatically since the introduction of the first monopolar RF device in 2003.[11,33] Additionally, the modifications to existing devices, and the development of new protocols for their use, have further expanded the available options for the delivery of RF energy. RF devices are categorized as monopolar, bipolar, or tripolar, based on the arrangement of electrodes used in the treatment.[11,33]

Monopolar RF devices contain a single electrode that transmits current through to a grounding plate. When compared with a bipolar system, the delivery of electromagnetic energy via a monopolar device allows for an increased penetration depth but a less controlled current distribution.[11] Kushikata et al[34] used a monopolar RF device to evaluate skin tightening in Japanese females with skin phototypes III and IV who had lower facial laxity and wrinkles. At the 3- and 6-month assessment points, 30.5% and 25.6% of the patients reported a substantial improvement in their jowls, respectively.[34] A smaller number of patients admitted to a similarly positive outcome in the severity of their nasolabial folds and marionette lines over the same time frame. A physician assessment, largely based on before and after photography, revealed a slightly greater percentage of improvement after treatment. The patients experienced only minor complications such as edema, mild blistering, and PIH, all of which were transient.[34]

Although the monopolar RF is perhaps the best studied modality for facial laxity treatment, numerous small-scale studies with varying treatment parameters and grading systems have failed to show a significant and consistent degree of improvement.[35] A large-scale study by Dover et al[35] attempted to remedy this discrepancy and, in the process, develop a reproducible and effective protocol for this device. The authors compared a high-energy, single-pass treatment technique with a low-energy, multiple-pass technique using monopolar RF in 5700 patients.[35] The results revealed that the multiple-pass protocol was associated with less pain and a significantly better outcome in terms of immediate and long-term (6 months) tissue tightening. Importantly, the patient feedback on heat sensation was found to be crucial in determining the optimum energy parameters to be used during treatments.[35]

FOCUSED ULTRASOUND

Ultrasonography has been a mainstay of diagnostic clinical medicine for many years. High-intensity focused ultrasound (HIFU) differs from the traditional diagnostic US by the utilization of significantly higher energies and lower frequencies.[36] This technique has become an important therapeutic tool by virtue of its ability to visualize and treat benign and malignant solid tumors in a noninvasive manner. This, therefore, avoids postoperative morbidity and mortality.[36] In the past few years, the technology used in HIFU has been modified and approved by the Food and Drug Administration for the rejuvenation of lax skin on the face and neck. Focused US for tissue-tightening purposes delivers millisecond pulses of 0.5 to 10 J/cm² of energy, as opposed to the approximately 100 J/cm² used in HIFU.[11] The acoustic waves are transduced through the skin and converted into heat, causing a controlled injury to the dermis. This results in an immediate contractile response and long-term collagen remodeling, which eventuates in skin tightening [**Figure 82-3**].

A significant advantage of the focused US is its depth of penetration. It can penetrate up to 6 to 7.8 mm, as opposed to the 2- to 4-mm depth achieved by other deep tissue heating devices such as RF, laser, and infrared light sources.[37-39] Therefore, the heat generated can infiltrate into the mid-deep reticular dermis and approach the superficial musculoaponeurotic system.[37-39] Adjunctively, the visualization of subdermal target tissue is possible during the procedure, enabling an even more precise approach. In a study by Suh et al,[40] 22 Korean patients with Fitzpatrick skin types III to VI were exposed to one session of a focused US treatment for the treatment of facial skin laxity. All of the patients were noted to have some degree of objective (physician-graded) improvement, while more than 70% of the patients reported subjective improvement in the severity of their nasolabial folds and jaw line laxity 2 months after their treatment. A histologic analysis of the biopsy samples from a subset of patients revealed a more parallel arrangement of their elastic fibers and increased collagen in their dermis.[40]

Another report specifically investigated the safety and adverse effect profile of the focused US treatment in Chinese patients with skin phototypes III and IV.[37] In this study, volunteers underwent between one and three treatments at 4-week intervals with transcutaneous focused US technology. As per the protocol, a lower frequency transducer was used to deliver energy to regions of the face with an increased

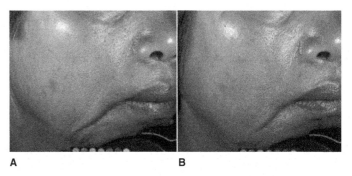

FIGURE 82-3. Baseline (**A**) and 5 months after (**B**) a single treatment with a focused ultrasound. (Used with the permission of Dr. Henry Hin Lee Chan.)

concentration of subcutaneous fat, such as the cheek and preauricular region. A higher frequency hand piece was used to treat thin-skinned areas such as the forehead and temple. Immediately after the treatment, erythema and edema were noted in 77.9% and 60.3% of the patients, respectively. However, this was transient and largely resolved within 1 week.[37] Focal bruising was experienced in 25% of cases but was no longer noticeable 1 month after the procedure.[37] Two patients developed minor, localized PIH on the forehead that slowly improved. Importantly, upon changing the transducer to one with a smaller diameter, no further cases of PIH occurred. Although no anesthetic agents were used in this study, it is suggested that more adequate pain control measures be pursued because severe pain was reported in more than half of the participants.[37] This study illustrates that although the focused US device is currently considered as the most effective nonablative modality for tissue tightening, even small modifications in treatment parameters can have a significant impact on potential adverse effects. While the absorption of ultrasonic energy is not affected by melanin, the thermal injury produced can still pose a risk of PIH in patients with darker skin of color, especially at high energies.[37]

LASER LIPOLYSIS

Laser lipolysis is a minimally invasive treatment for the removal of excess fatty tissue and the improvement of tissue laxity.[41] A purported advantage of this procedure over conventional liposuction is the potential for reduced scarring and shorter recovery times. The lipolytic effect is dependent on the degree of thermal energy that is transmitted via an optic fiber into the adipose tissue.[42] The heat generated melts the underlying fat and induces vessel coagulation and dermal remodeling. The tissue-tightening effect of the laser attempts to remedy the after effect of sagging or loose skin that is common after treatment with traditional liposuction. To date, there are only rare reports examining this approach in patients with skin of color. A single preliminary study by Sun et al[42] used the 1064-nm Nd:YAG laser to treat localized deposits of adiposity in 35 Asian subjects. The authors reported that there was a substantial improvement in the treated areas, with a significant reduction in fat. Also, the procedure was associated with significantly less bleeding, edema, and postoperative complications than with conventional liposuction. Importantly, other than transient ecchymosis in three patients, which quickly resolved, no other adverse effects were reported.[42]

COMBINATION APPROACHES

Treatment of the aging face, regardless of genetic makeup, often requires multiple modalities to achieve the desired cosmetic outcome. Yu et al[14] examined the safety and efficacy of a nonablative device that addressed tissue laxity in Asian skin through the combination of infrared light with bipolar RF energy. In this small prospective trial, 19 Chinese patients, with skin phototypes III to V, received three treatments at 3-week intervals with the aforementioned device.[14] At 3 months posttreatment, a variably mild to moderate degree of improvement was observed in the mid and lower face in 26.3% to 47.3% of the patients.[14] No significant long-term adverse effects were reported. However, mild superficial crusting was noted in patients following 7% of the treatment sessions.[14] This was similar to the complication reported in prior studies using infrared light for tissue tightening.[32] Because this was a small pilot study, additional testing in a larger number of patients is needed to confirm the reproducibility of these results and optimize the treatment parameters for this combination device.[14]

CONCLUSION

Over the years there has been substantial progress in the development of new devices and methodologies seeking to achieve tissue tightening. However, further research and testing are still required to establish a more complete body of knowledge in this area. Most laser and light sources have only been successful in improving skin laxity in small studies with stringent parameters in a select subset of patients. Serious head-to-head controlled trials are necessary to objectively compare the efficacy of the tissue-tightening techniques reviewed in this chapter. Nonablative lasers are often a more readily available and attractive option. However, they have yet to rival long-proven devices such as RF and newer modalities such as focused US devices in the improvement of wrinkles and skin laxity. Similarly, patients need to be cautioned that while the technology of noninvasive tissue tightening is advancing at a rapid pace, there is nothing that can deliver results comparable to those obtained by interventional approaches such as the face lift or ablative CO_2 resurfacing. As such, physicians must carefully tailor an appropriate treatment regimen for each individual's unique presentation and concerns. Finally, a thorough discussion of risks, benefits, and limitations of each procedure is of the utmost importance in managing patient expectations and ensuring a satisfactory outcome.

REFERENCES

1. Alexiades-Armenakas M, Rosenberg D, et al. Blinded, randomized, quantitative grading comparison of minimally invasive, fractional radiofrequency and surgical face-lift to treat skin laxity. *Arch Dermatol.* 2010;146:396-405.
2. Rabe JH, Mamelak AJ, McElgunn PJ, et al. Photoaging: mechanisms and repair. *J Am Acad Dermatol.* 2006;55:1-19.
3. Davis EC, Callender VD. Aesthetic dermatology for aging ethnic skin. *Dermatol Surg.* 2011;37:901-917.
4. Ezure T, Yagi E, Kunizawa N, et al. Comparison of sagging at the cheek and lower eyelid between male and female faces. *Skin Res Technol.* 2011;17:510-515.
5. Thong HY, Jee SH, Sun CC, et al. The patterns of melanosome distribution in keratinocytes of human skin as one determining factor of skin colour. *Br J Dermatol.* 2003;149:498-505.
6. Rawlings AV. Ethnic skin types: Are there differences in skin structure and function? *Int J Cosmetic Sci.* 2006;28:79-93.
7. Fantasia J, Lin CB, Wiwi C, et al. Differential levels of elastin fibers and TGF-beta signaling in the skin of Caucasians and African Americans. *J Dermatol Sci.* 2013;70:159-165.
8. Kahari VM, Olsen DR, Rhudy RW, et al. Transforming growth factor-beta up-regulates elastin gene expression in human skin fibroblasts. Evidence for post-transcriptional modulation. *Lab Invest.* 1992;66:580-588.
9. Vierkotter A, Krutmann J. Environmental influences on skin aging and ethnic-specific manifestations. *Dermatoendocrinol.* 2012;4:227-231.
10. Nouveau-Richard S, Yang Z, Mac-Mary S, et al. Skin ageing: A comparison between Chinese and European populations. A pilot study. *J Dermatol Sci.* 2005;40:187-193.
11. Bogle MA, Dover JS. Tissue tightening technologies. *Dermatol Clin.* 2009;27:491-499, vii.
12. Chan HH, Yu CS, Shek S, et al. A prospective, split face, single-blinded study looking at the use of an infrared device with contact cooling in the treatment of skin laxity in Asians. *Laser Surg Med.* 2008;40:146-152.
13. Chan HH. Effective and safe use of lasers, light sources, and radiofrequency devices in the clinical management of Asian patients with selected dermatoses. *Laser Surg Med.* 2005;37:179-185.
14. Yu CS, Yeung CK, Shek SY, et al. Combined infrared light and bipolar radiofrequency for skin tightening in Asians. *Laser Surg Med.* 2007;39:471-475.
15. Chung JH. Photoaging in Asians. *Photodermatol Photoimmunol Photomed.* 2003;19:109-121.
16. Chan HH, Lam LK, Wong DS, et al. Use of 1,320 nm Nd:YAG laser for wrinkle reduction and the treatment of atrophic acne scarring in Asians. *Laser Surg Med.* 2004;34:98-103.
17. Kono T, Chan HH, Groff WF, et al. Prospective direct comparison study of fractional resurfacing using different fluences and densities for skin rejuvenation in Asians. *Laser Surg Med.* 2007;39:311-314.
18. Chan HH, Lam LK, Wong DS, et al. Role of skin cooling in improving patient tolerability of Q-switched Alexandrite (QS Alex) laser in nevus of Ota treatment. *Laser Surg Med.* 2003;32:148-151.
19. Yeung CK, Shek SY, Chan HH. Hair removal with neodymium-doped yttrium aluminum garnet laser and pneumatic skin flattening in Asians. *Dermatol Surg.* 2010;36:1664-1670.
20. Alster TS, Bryan H, Williams CM. Long-pulsed Nd:YAG laser-assisted hair removal in pigmented skin: a clinical and histological evaluation. *Arch Dermatol.* 2001;137:885-889.

21. Key DJ. Single-treatment skin tightening by radiofrequency and long-pulsed, 1064-nm Nd: YAG laser compared. *Laser Surg Med.* 2007;39:169-175.

22. Kono T, Kikuchi Y, Groff WF, et al. Split-face comparison study of cryogen spray cooling versus pneumatic skin flattening in skin tightening treatments using a long-pulsed Nd:YAG laser. *J Cosmet Laser Ther.* 2010;12:87-91.

23. Lee SH, Roh MR, Jung JY, et al. Effect of subdermal 1,444-nm pulsed neodymium-doped yttrium aluminum garnet laser on the nasolabial folds and cheek laxity. *Dermatol Surg.* 2013;39:1067-1078.

24. Tark KC, Jung JE, Song SY. Superior lipolytic effect of the 1,444 nm Nd:YAG laser: comparison with the 1,064 nm Nd:YAG laser. *Laser Surg Med.* 2009;41:721-727.

25. Manstein D, Herron GS, Sink RK, et al. Fractional photothermolysis: a new concept for cutaneous remodeling using microscopic patterns of thermal injury. *Laser Surg Med.* 2004;34:426-438.

26. Jih MH, Kimyai-Asadi A. Fractional photothermolysis: a review and update. *Semin Cutan Med Surg.* 2008;27:63-71.

27. Lee HM, Haw S, Kim JE, et al. A fractional 2940 nm short-pulsed, erbium-doped yttrium aluminium garnet laser is effective and minimally invasive for the treatment of photodamaged skin in Asians. *J Cosmet Laser Ther.* 2012;14:253-259.

28. Rahman Z, MacFalls H, Jiang K, et al. Fractional deep dermal ablation induces tissue tightening. *Laser Surg Med.* 2009;41:78-86.

29. Chan NP, Ho SG, Yeung CK, et al. Fractional ablative carbon dioxide laser resurfacing for skin rejuvenation and acne scars in Asians. *Laser Surg Med.* 2010;42:615-623.

30. Chan HH, Manstein D, Yu CS, et al. The prevalence and risk factors of post-inflammatory hyperpigmentation after fractional resurfacing in Asians. *Laser Surg Med.* 2007;39:381-385.

31. Ruiz-Esparza J. Near [corrected] painless, nonablative, immediate skin contraction induced by low-fluence irradiation with new infrared device: a report of 25 patients. *Dermatol Surg.* 2006;32:601-610.

32. Chua SH, Ang P, Khoo LS, et al. Nonablative infrared skin tightening in type IV to V Asian skin: a prospective clinical study. *Dermatol Surg.* 2007;33:146-151.

33. Krueger N, Sadick NS. New-generation radiofrequency technology. *Cutis.* 2013;91:39-46.

34. Kushikata N, Negishi K, Tezuka Y, et al. Non-ablative skin tightening with radiofrequency in Asian skin. *Lase Surg Med.* 2005;36:92-97.

35. Dover JS, Zelickson B; 14-Physician Multispecialty Consensus Panel. Results of a survey of 5,700 patient monopolar radiofrequency facial skin tightening treatments: assessment of a low-energy multiple-pass technique leading to a clinical end point algorithm. *Dermatol Surg.* 2007;33:900-907.

36. Kennedy JE. High-intensity focused ultrasound in the treatment of solid tumours. *Cancer.* 2005;5:321-327.

37. Chan NP, Shek SY, Yu CS, et al. Safety study of transcutaneous focused ultrasound for non-invasive skin tightening in Asians. *Laser Surg Med.* 2011;43:366-375.

38. Gliklich RE, White WM, Slayton MH, et al. Clinical pilot study of intense ultrasound therapy to deep dermal facial skin and subcutaneous tissues. *Arch Facial Plast Surg.* 2007;9:88-95.

39. White WM, Makin IR, Barthe PG, et al. Selective creation of thermal injury zones in the superficial musculoaponeurotic system using intense ultrasound therapy: a new target for noninvasive facial rejuvenation. *Arch Facial Plast Surg.* 2007;9:22-29.

40. Suh DH, Oh YJ, Lee SJ, et al. An intense-focused ultrasound tightening for the treatment of infraorbital laxity. *J Cosmet Laser Ther.* 2012;14:290-295.

41. McBean JC, Katz BE. Laser lipolysis: an update. *J Clin Aesthet Dermatol.* 2011;4:25-34.

42. Sun Y, Wu SF, Yan S, et al. Laser lipolysis used to treat localized adiposis: a preliminary report on experience with Asian patients. *Aesthet Plastic Surg.* 2009;33:701-705.

Liposuction

Rajiv I. Nijhawan
Maritza I. Perez
Collette Ara-Honore

KEY POINTS

- Liposuction surgery, one of the most popular aesthetic procedures performed by cosmetic surgeons, is a sculpting technique that reduces cosmetically unwanted adipose tissue in localized areas to achieve a more desirable and slender silhouette.

- Non-Caucasians as a group represented 21% of patients on whom cosmetic surgery was performed in 2011 with the following breakdown: 8% Hispanics, 7% African Americans, 5% Asians, and 1% other non-Caucasians.

- Advances in liposuction, including the development of smaller cannulas, blunt-tipped cannulas, quieter and more efficient aspirators, power liposuction, and laser-assisted lipolysis, have optimized results and improved safety.

INTRODUCTION

Liposuction surgery is a sculpting technique developed to reduce cosmetically unwanted adipose tissue, in localized areas, to achieve a more desirable and slender silhouette. Advancements in instrumentation, anesthesia, technique, and training continue to ensure the utmost safety of patients as well as optimal outcomes. The American Society for Aesthetic Plastic Surgery ranks liposuction as the most frequently performed cosmetic procedure, with over 325,000 liposuctions being completed in the United States in 2011, representing an 84% increase since 1997.[1] Non-Caucasians represented 21% of patients on whom cosmetic surgery was performed in 2011: 8% Hispanics, 7% African Americans, 5% Asians, and 1% other non-Caucasians. Dermatologists perform approximately one-third of liposuction procedures in the United States.[2]

HISTORICAL PERSPECTIVE

The idea of fat removal has been around for almost a century. Charles Dujarrier, credited with the earliest attempt at localized fat removal, used a uterine curette to remove subcutaneous fat from the knees and calves of a dancer but accidentally injured a femoral artery that resulted in amputation of the affected leg in 1921.[3] In 1964, Schrudde tried to remove fat from the leg through incision and curettage, but the postoperative course was complicated by the development of hematomas and seromas.[4] Also in the 1960s, Pitanguy performed resection of skin and fat of the thigh, but incision scars made the outcome less than ideal.[5]

MODERN LIPOSUCTION

The era of modern liposuction began in 1976 when Arpad and Giorgio Fisher of Italy described the use of suction attached to blunt-tipped cannulas, which were inserted into 5-mm skin incisions, enabling suction of unwanted adipose tissue.[6] Later, Fournier in Paris developed the "dry technique" in which no fluids were infiltrated into the patient prior to liposuction[7]; Illouz, also in Paris, preferred the "wet technique" in which a solution of hypotonic saline and hyaluronidase infiltrated the adipose tissue prior to aspiration.[8] Both became leaders in the field, and American cosmetic surgeons traveled to Europe to learn their techniques. A task force from the American Society of Plastic and Reconstructive Surgeons attempted to monopolize this procedure by having Illouz sign a contract to only train plastic surgeons, but Fournier refused and continued to train physicians in different specialties.[8]

Julius Newman, an American otolaryngologist who coined the term *liposuction*, taught the first liposuction course in the United States and, in 1982, formed the American Society of Liposuction Surgery. Liposuction became part of the core surgical curriculum in dermatology in 1987, the same year that dermatologist Dr. Jeffrey Klein described tumescent anesthesia.[9] The tumescent technique revolutionized liposuction surgery and has been used subsequently in other dermatologic procedures such as hair transplants and dermabrasion.[10,11] Of note, the American Academy of Dermatology (AAD) became the first society to publish guidelines for liposuction in 1991,[12] and the American Society for Dermatologic Surgery (ASDS) published their guidelines in 2000.[13] Smaller cannulas (some with a diameter less than 0.6 mm) were developed, blunt-tipped cannulas became standard to decrease injury to blood vessels and minimize bleeding, aspirators became more efficient and quieter, and finally, before the turn of the century, power liposuction was introduced.[14-16]

In 1992, Apfelberg[17] first described the liquefying action of a laser on adipose tissue; however, it was Blugerman, Schavelzon, and Goldman who introduced the concept of the pulsed 1064-nm Nd:YAG laser to liquefy fat.[18] The laser energy is delivered by an optical fiber through tiny skin incisions and can be used in conjunction with suctioning. Not until October 2006 did the U.S. Food and Drug Administration approve the first laser lipolysis system called SmartLipo (Cynosure, Inc., Westford, MA) for the surgical incision, excision, vaporization, ablation, and coagulation of all soft tissues and for laser-assisted lipolysis.[18] With the advent of this more effective and minimally invasive surgical alternative to traditional liposuction, the surgeon can dissolve fat before it is removed and sculpt one's body as a result of the laser energy's accompanying collagen shrinkage and tissue tightening.

GOALS OF TREATMENT AND PATIENT SELECTION

The goal of liposuction is to remove localized areas of excess adipose tissue through tiny skin incisions using small, blunt cannulas. This procedure results in loss of inches and a more desirable body contour. The cannulas, which vary in size, length, and design, are introduced into the incision sites and crisscrossed over the area to produce a smooth, even result. While the removal of the subcutaneous fat shows immediate postoperative improvement, subsequent retraction of the skin may take up to 6 months after the procedure, resulting in continued short-term enhancement.

The ideal candidate is a nonoverweight, healthy adult with good skin elasticity who has isolated areas of fat that are unresponsive to diet and exercise. Bilateral full-skin-thickness "pinch tests" from proposed sites provide the surgeon and patient with an estimate of the amount of removable fat, quality of skin tone, and symmetry and an assessment of underlying muscle integrity. Areas with good skin elasticity and without excess amounts of skin are ideal as liposuction surgery only removes adipose tissue and not the overlying skin layers. Cutaneous abnormalities such as striae, hyperpigmentation, and cellulite should be pointed out to the patient. Hypertrophic scars and keloids, which are more common in skin of color populations, are relative contraindications. Surgical consent forms serve the important role of ensuring that patients understand the associated benefits, limitations, and risks.

Basic metabolic panels, complete blood counts, coagulation profiles, and human immunodeficiency virus (HIV) evaluations should be performed on all patients prior to the procedure. Electrocardiograms and chest X-rays are ordered on patients over 40 years of age. Abnormalities require clearance by the primary care physician.

EQUIPMENT

Basic equipment for liposuction includes an infiltration system for tumescent fluid infusion, an aspirator (and backup) with disposable containers, and blunt-tipped cannulas of varying lengths, diameters, and styles. A cardiac monitor (with pulse oximetry, blood pressure, pulse, and respiration readings) is advisable. For emergencies, a "crash cart" with oxygen/oxygen mask, intravenous (IV) kit, and medications such as atropine, diazepam, hydrocortisone sodium succinate, epinephrine, and lidocaine should be readily available.

TECHNIQUE

■ ANESTHESIA

First described by dermatologist Jeffery Klein,[9] tumescent (*tumesc*, "balloon up") anesthesia is a drug-delivery system designed to optimize the anesthetic effect of lidocaine at the target tissue site, minimize lidocaine absorption, and maximally expand the defined compartment. We use a dilute solution of lidocaine at a concentration of 0.1% with an epinephrine dilution of 1:1,000,000 by placing 50 mL of 1% lidocaine with epinephrine 1:100,000 into 500 mL of lactated Ringer's solution. Tissue expansion buffers the underlying tissue by preventing trauma and provides local hydrostatic pressure to decrease bleeding.[10,11,19] The use of tumescent anesthesia eliminates the need for general anesthesia and its associated risks and has revolutionized physicians' approach to liposuction by minimizing complications and maximizing patient outcomes. While some authors report safety with higher doses, a well-accepted safe maximum dose is 55 mg/kg for a patient within normal weight-to-height ratio; men may be more sensitive and require a 15% dosage reduction.[10,11,20] Of note, lidocaine is metabolized by the cytochrome P450 isozyme 3A4; therefore, other drugs metabolized by this isozyme should be used with caution in patients undergoing tumescent liposuction.[21]

While some specialties prefer to perform liposuction in a hospital-based setting, dermatologic surgeons have demonstrated the safety of tumescent anesthesia as an outpatient surgical procedure.[22] In a retrospective survey of 66,570 liposuction procedures, a serious adverse event rate was 0.68 per 1000 cases with no deaths being reported, while statistics indicate that hospital-based liposuction results in 3.5 times as many malpractice claims compared with outpatient liposuction.[22,23]

■ GENERAL

Prophylactic oral antibiotics and antimicrobial skin cleansers are started 24 hours before the procedure; the former is continued for 1 week after surgery. In addition, phytonadione (vitamin K) is initiated 1 week prior to liposuction surgery and continued for 1 week after. With the consent of the primary care physician, drugs that inhibit cytochrome P450-3A4 are discontinued in the perioperative period as well as over-the-counter medications and supplements that may thin the blood (eg, ibuprofen, vitamin E). Prior to infiltration of tumescent anesthesia, vital signs and measurements are recorded with the patient in an upright position, digital photographs are taken, and areas to be suctioned are marked and agreed upon by the patient. After sterile prepping and draping, incisions are strategically placed in less noticeable locations (eg, submental, umbilical, lateral thorax, groin) that provide the most direct subcutaneous tissue access. The lowest effective and safe concentrations and volumes of tumescent anesthesia are used. Tumescence is adequate when the tissue is firmly ballooned. Small cannulas (diameters <4 mm) are preferred. The cannula, parallel to the skin's surface with the apertures directed toward the fascia, is inserted into the deep layers of fat. The nondominant hand rests on the skin overlying the cannula and serves as a guide. During suctioning, the pinch test is performed frequently to ensure symmetry. On completion, incision sites are dressed and/or sutured, and compression garments are worn for 7 to 14 days depending on the area.[13,14]

Laser-assisted lipolysis has several advantages over traditional liposuction either as an adjunct or by itself. The skin-tightening effect, which can continue up to several months after procedure, is the most significant advantage. This effect is especially noticeable if done on a small body area (ie, submental area, calves, bilateral arms, male breasts, and ankles).[18] Additionally, there is less scarring due to the small cannula size that is required with the laser.[18] Because this procedure is minimally invasive, there is less trauma, which significantly decreases bleeding, bruising, and swelling, and thus minimizes recovery time (averaging 1.5 days to return to normal activity).[18]

POPULATION CONSIDERATIONS

The number of cosmetic procedures performed on non-Caucasians continues to increase. Therefore, it is imperative for the clinician to recognize subtle differences in body type among patients of other population groups so that optimum results may be achieved and dermatologists may better anticipate cultural and patient-specific preferences.[24] Regardless of race, the universal ideal proportion of the waist-to-hip ratio (WHR) is 0.7,[25] which should always be considered when discussing potential areas for liposuction. In our experience, the primary differences in regard to body habitus that have been observed are that African Americans tend to have larger buttocks,[26] Asians tend to have more lower than upper abdominal fat, and Hispanic women tend to have more prominent lateral thighs and hips.[26]

There are also differences in patients' desired outcomes. Researchers have established that African American beauty ideals are more accepting of a curvaceous body type as opposed to Caucasian women.[27] Hence, some African American women are seemingly content with a larger gluteal dimension, but do not like saddlebags and prefer a lumbar hyperlordosis. We have also noted population differences in the texture of the subcutaneous tissue, with the subcutaneous and truncal fat of African American men being more fibrous than that of other groups. The same area in East Indian men is less fibrous than in other groups. We are unaware of any studies comparing the morphology of subcutaneous fat in different groups, but there are data suggesting racial differences in visceral-to-subcutaneous fat ratios. African Americans, Hispanics, and Asians seem to have more subcutaneous fat than age-matched Caucasians.[28-32]

AREAS MOST FREQUENTLY TREATED WITH COSMETIC LIPOSUCTION

SUBMANDIBULAR/NECK [FIGURE 83-1, A–D]

Removal of small quantities of adipose tissue (35 to 100 mL) results in an immediately noticeable improvement in the patient's profile. Familiarity with cutaneous anatomic landmarks and experience in liposuction are prerequisites. A 3-mm horizontal submental crease incision provides cannula access from the angle of the mandibles laterally to the arch of the cricoid cartilage inferiorly. Suctioning is completed external to the platysma and medial to the sternocleidomastoid muscle using 1.5- to 3-mm-diameter nonaggressive standard cannulas. Unique to this area, the dermis is gently abraded, thereby enhancing skin contraction. Care should be taken to avoid the marginal branch of the mandibular nerve by lifting the skin away from the mandible and orienting the cannula medially and inferiorly. Postoperative compression garments are worn for 7 days.

BREASTS/CHEST [FIGURE 83-2, A–D]

Correctable causes of male gynecomastia/pseudogynecomastia should be excluded by history (drugs) and physical examination (symmetry and masses) preoperatively.[33,34] A 3- to 4-mm incision is made at the level of the serratus anterior in the anterior axillary line. Tissue debulking is completed simultaneously with mechanical tumescent solution infiltration (175 to 350 mL/breast). Aggressive grater and loop cannulas may be used, except under the areola and nipple. Suction is complete when the skin lies completely flat against the chest wall. Postoperative compression garments are worn for 3 weeks to ensure maximum skin contraction.

For women, a baseline mammogram is mandatory, and any abnormalities must be investigated prior to surgery. Because the process can be painful with a prolonged recuperation time, the procedure can be performed in a two-step process by first performing the suction mammoplasty on the non-dominant–sided breast. The amount of tumescent anesthesia can be calculated by observing how much fluid is displaced when a breast is immersed into a 1000-mL fluid-filled beaker. If 500 mL is displaced, then 500 mL of tumescent anesthesia should be used. The volume of fat extracted is typically half the tumescent anesthesia.

UPPER ARMS [FIGURE 83-3, A AND B]

The skin of the upper arms is subject to dimpling and should be suctioned gently with nonaggressive cannulas to prevent damage to internal neurovascular components. One 2- to 3-mm incision over the olecranon fossa is sufficient for tumescent infusion and suction of fat external to the triceps muscle. Nonaggressive, 22-cm long manual cannulas that are 3-mm or less in diameter and reciprocating power liposuction can be useful. The thin skin of the upper arm is subject to irregularities and may not contract well; therefore, err on the side of removing less. Proper positioning of the patient's arm when approaching the axilla avoids injury to the eighth cervical and first thoracic nerves of the brachial plexus. Compression garment should be worn for 2 weeks postoperatively.

ABDOMEN [FIGURE 83-4, A–D]

Anecdotally, clinical variations in fat distribution and abdomen texture are discernible among various population groups. African Americans and Latinos tend to accumulate fat in the upper and lower abdomen, while Asians and East Indians have greater fat accumulations in the lower abdomen.

For all patients, the abdomen, waist, and upper flanks should be treated simultaneously to maximize patient satisfaction. Suctioning of the lower abdomen can be completed successfully through incisions in the umbilicus (leaving no visible scar) and groin (midway between the femoral canal and the anterosuperior iliac spine). Treatment of the upper abdomen requires additional incisions. Placing incisions asymmetrically in moles or inframammary creases is favored. Tumescent fluid infusion volumes (1.5 to 4 L) should be titrated to patient comfort levels. Suctioning is performed in the deep fat planes using vertical to-and-fro strokes with moderately aggressive short (15 cm) followed by long manual and power cobra cannulas whose apertures are directed away from the skin surface. Power sculpting significantly decreases physician fatigue and is soothing to the patient. Frequent pinching of the skin ensures symmetry. The tunnels created in the subcutaneous tissue should be drained after the fat has been removed by suctioning of residual tumescent fluid in order to decrease postoperative drainage. Patients should be instructed to gently massage the skin toward the incision in lukewarm showers with each dressing change. Male patients should be informed of possible scrotal swelling; females may experience vulvar swelling. In both cases, resolution occurs in less than 7 days without sequelae. Compression garments should be worn for 2 weeks.

FLANKS [FIGURE 83-4, C AND D; FIGURE 83-5, A–F]

Liposuction of the male flank can be challenging. African American and Hispanic men, regardless of age, seem to have more dense flank tissue than their age-matched East Indian and Asian counterparts. Aggressive debulking and suctioning with pinto and candy cane cannulas can be effective. Powered cannulas may also be helpful; however, the thickness of the skin precludes their use exclusively.

One incision in the skin overlying the tubercle of the iliac crest is adequate for tumescence and suctioning small to medium flanks (350 mL or less). Larger flanks require an additional incision in the skin overlying the tenth rib in the midaxillary line. These sites also provide access to the lower back and waistline without visible scarring. Two weeks of postoperative compression are generally well tolerated. The skin of the flanks is forgiving, and contraction is excellent.

HIP/LATERAL THIGH/BUTTOCKS [FIGURE 83-6, A AND B]

Clinically, the quality of the subcutaneous tissue of the lateral thigh and hip is similar. Cosmetically, the contour of both can be disconcerting, even for otherwise slender women, and both areas may be suctioned in concert. Lower concentrations of Xylocaine in the tumescent solution are well tolerated (150 to 300 mL/hip or thigh). Most patients want to attain or maintain the soft downward slope from the waistline to the hip and the gentle curve of the lateral thigh, and less aggressive suctioning preserves this balanced silhouette. Contouring of the hip is achieved by nonaggressive suction with a two-port standard cannula through an

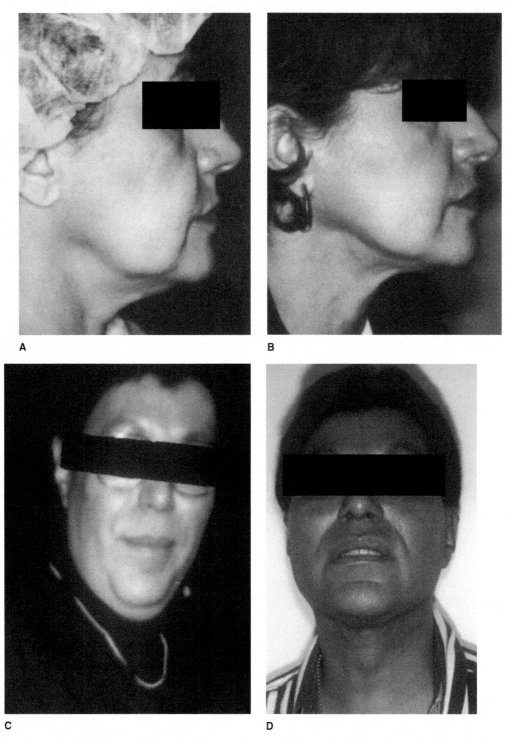

FIGURE 83-1. A Hispanic woman before (**A**) and after (**B**) liposuction of the neck and submandibular area. A Hispanic man before (**C**) and 6 months after (**D**) a similar procedure.

anterior gluteal incision. An infragluteal crease incision hides the scar of lateral thigh suctioning. A benefit of tumescent anesthesia is that patients can stand up during the procedure, allowing the surgeon to check for symmetry. Power sculpting works well in both areas. Hip and lateral and medial thigh compression for 10 days postoperatively helps to ensure good contraction.

▩ MEDIAL THIGH [FIGURE 83-7, A–D]

In contrast to the lateral thigh, the skin of the medial thigh extending from the labia majora to the inner knee is similar to the skin of the upper arm and is not forgiving. The skin is thin and more sensitive, and the fat is deep. Tumescence can be achieved with 75 to 150 mL of fluid infused

into the inferomedial border of the protuberance, and 2-mm standard reciprocating cannulas are a good choice for this area. Suctioning should be less aggressive and confined to the deeper plane to avoid the "doll" medial thigh appearance.

OUTCOMES FOR PEOPLE WITH SKIN OF COLOR

African Americans, Asians, Africans, East Indians, Hispanics, and other non-Caucasians comprise 21% of the patients undergoing cosmetic procedures. For procedures that disrupt the integrity of the skin of these individuals, adverse effects may include the development of keloids and/ or hyperpigmentation. At the earliest sign of persistent erythema or faint

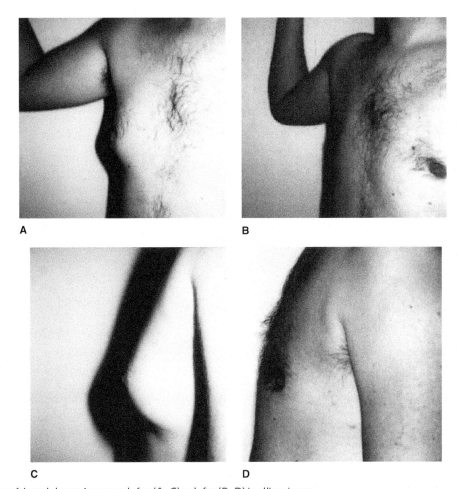

FIGURE 83-2. Liposuction of the male breast. Appearance before (**A, C**) and after (**B, D**) in a Hispanic man.

hyperpigmentation or in patients who develop hyperpigmentation in scars/incision sites, application of hydroquinone 4% cream twice a day is initiated. Often patients are told to mix the hydroquinone with a low- to mid-potency topical corticosteroid if notable inflammation is observed. The response to these self-compounded bleaching regimens has been excellent in the authors' opinion. Dyspigmentation of skin overlying the suctioned site has not been seen. With the exception of the neck, cannulas are kept away from the dermis.

Variations have been observed in tissue density. The density and fibrous component of the subcutaneous tissue seem greater in African Americans, Africans, and Hispanics compared with East Indians, Asians, and Caucasians. However, no difference has been noted in healing or outcome. Finally, and most importantly, body habitus, that is, contours and fat distribution, differs in various population groups. Beauty is culturally defined. The surgeon should respect these differences when performing liposuction surgery.

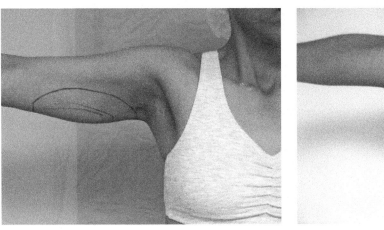
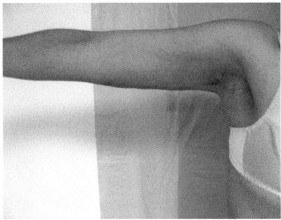

FIGURE 83-3. Liposuction of the upper arms. Appearance of arm before (**A**) and 2 weeks after (**B**) in a Hispanic female.

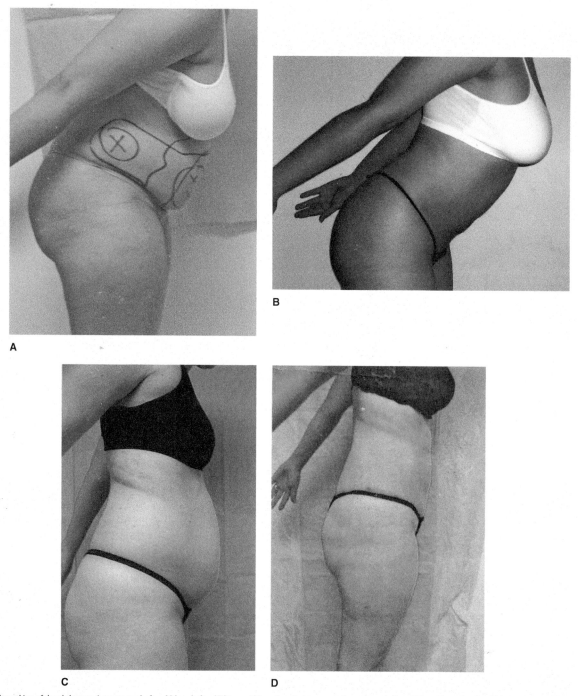

FIGURE 83-4. SmartLipo of the abdomen. Appearance before **(A)** and after **(B)** in an African American woman. Appearance before **(C)** and 2 weeks after **(D)** in another African American woman (with SmartLipo of the flanks as well).

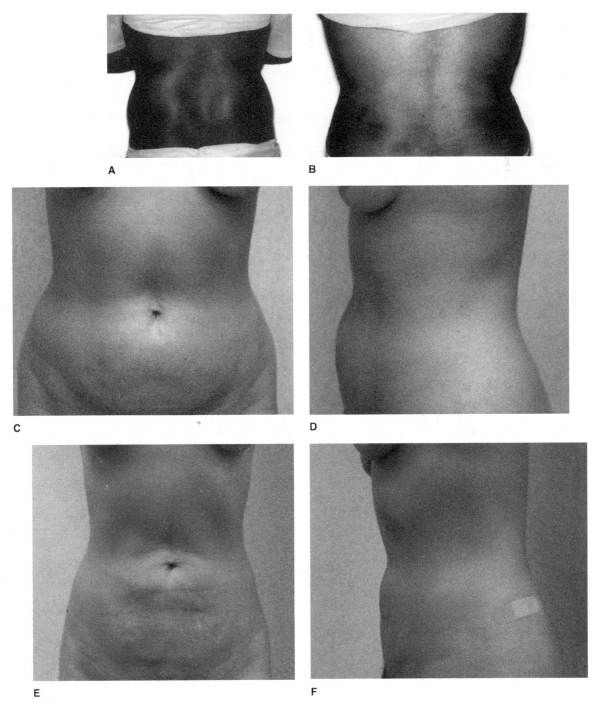

FIGURE 83-5. Liposuction of the flank and lower back. Appearance before (**A**) and after (**B**) in an East Indian man. Appearance before [(**C**) frontal view; (**D**) lateral view] and 6 weeks after [(**E**) frontal view; (**F**) lateral view] in a Hispanic woman.

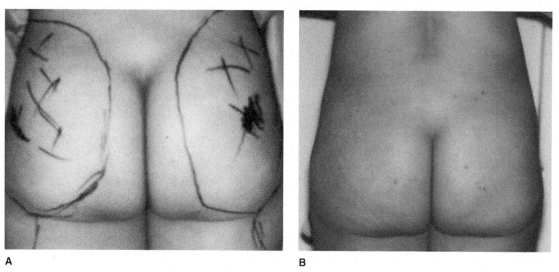

FIGURE 83-6. Liposuction of the hip, lateral thigh, and buttocks. Appearance before **(A)** and after **(B)** in a Hispanic woman.

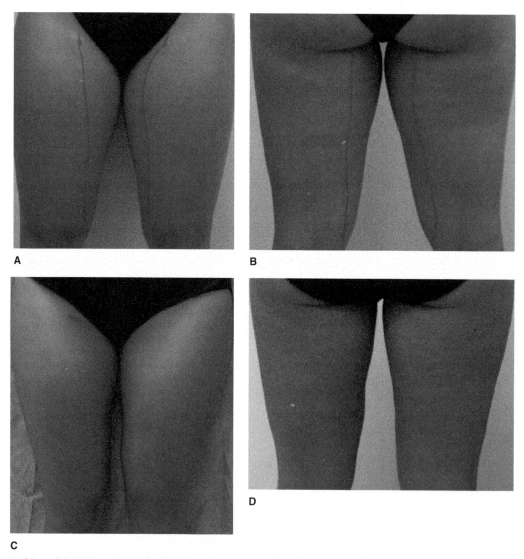

FIGURE 83-7. Liposuction of the medial thigh. Appearance before **(A, B)** and after **(C, D)** in a Hispanic woman.

COMPLICATIONS

Since liposuction is typically performed on an elective basis, the benefits as compared to the risks must be thoroughly considered. Potential complications from liposuction must be discussed with each patient preoperatively, and they include hypertrophic scarring, postinflammatory pigment alteration, skin ulceration or necrosis, seromas, infections, pulmonary emboli, pulmonary edema, hypotension, abdominal and thoracic wall perforations, hemorrhage, lidocaine toxicity, cardiac arrhythmias, hospitalization, and even death.[23] Of note, dermatologists performing liposuction have an excellent safety record, with serious adverse events occurring in less than 0.1% of cases.[2,22,23,35,36] The risk of complications is decreased by adhering to established guidelines, including adequate physician training, patient selection, proper technique, separating multiple procedures, limiting the amount and type of anesthesia, and meticulous pre-, intra-, and postoperative monitoring/care.

CONCLUSION

The surgeon with an artistic eye and proper technique will find that the results of liposuction are excellent. Patients are pleased with their new, improved contour and the positive effect it has on their lifestyles.[37] The most important considerations include patient selection and communication and individualizing the technique. Dermatologic surgeons have also pioneered liposuction for noncosmetic indications such as for axillary hyperhidrosis, lipomas, and lymphedema.[38-42]

REFERENCES

1. 15th Annual Cosmetic Surgery National Data Bank Statistics. The Authoritative Source for Current US Statistics on Cosmetic Surgery. New York: The American Society for Aesthetic Plastic Surgery; 2012.
2. Yu T, Perez M. Dermatologic liposuction: safety record and techniques. *Cosmet Dermatol.* 2004;17:209-212.
3. Dolsky RL, Newman J, Fetzek JR, et al. Liposuction. History, techniques, and complications. *Dermatol Clin.* 1987;5:313-333.
4. Schrudde J. Lipexheresis (liposuction) for body contouring. *Clin Plast Surg.* 1982;11:445-456.
5. Pitanguy I. Trochanteric lipodystrophy. *Plast Reconstr Surg.* 1964;34:280-286.
6. Fischer A, Fischer G. First surgical treatment for molding body's cellulite with three 5 mm incisions. *Bull Int Acad Cosmet Surg.* 1976;3:35.
7. Fournier PF. Reduction syringe liposculpturing. *Dermatol Clin.* 1990;8:539-551.
8. Flynn TC, Coleman WP II, Field LM, et al. History of liposuction. *Dermatol Surg.* 2000;26:515-520.
9. Klein J. The tumescent technique for liposuction surgery. *Am J Cosmetic Surg.* 1987;4:263-267.
10. Ostad A, Kageyama N, Moy RL. Tumescent anesthesia with a lidocaine dose of 55 mg/kg is safe for liposuction. *Dermatol Surg.* 1996;22:921-927.
11. Lillis PJ. Liposuction surgery under local anesthesia: limited blood loss and minimal lidocaine absorption. *J Dermatol Surg Oncol.* 1988;14:1145-1148.
12. Drake LA, Ceilley RI, Cornelison RL, et al. Guidelines of care for liposuction. Committee on Guidelines of Care. *J Am Acad Dermatol.* 1991;24:489-494.
13. Lawrence N, Clark RE, Flynn TC, et al. American Society for Dermatologic Surgery guidelines of care for liposuction. *Dermatol Surg.* 2000;26:265-269.
14. Weber PJ, Wulc AE, Jaworsky C, et al. Warning: traditional liposuction cannulas may be dangerous to your patient's health. *J Dermatol Surg Oncol.* 1988;14:1136-1138.
15. Collins PS. Selection and utilization of liposuction cannulas. *J Dermatol Surg Oncol.* 1988;14:1139-1143.
16. Coleman WP 3rd. Powered liposuction. *Dermatol Surg.* 2000;26:315-318.
17. Apfelberg D. Laser-assisted liposuction may benefit surgeons, patients. *Clin Laser Mon.* 1992;10:193-194.
18. McBean JC, Katz BE. Laser lipolysis: an update. *J Clin Aesthet Dermatol.* 2011;4:25-34.
19. Hagerty T, Klein P. Fat partitioning of lidocaine in tumescent liposuction. *Ann Plast Surg.* 1999;42:372-375.
20. Butterwick KJ, Goldman MP, Sriprachya-Anunt S. Lidocaine levels during the first two hours of infiltration of dilute anesthetic solution for tumescent liposuction: rapid versus slow delivery. *Dermatol Surg.* 1999;25:681-685.
21. Taro D. Cytochrome P450 enzyme drug interactions. *Drug Newsletter.* 1995;14:59-61.
22. Coleman WP, Hanke CW, Glogau RG. Does the specialty of the physician affect fatality rates in liposuction? A comparison of specialty specific data. *Dermatol Surg.* 2000;26:611-615.
23. Housman TS, Lawrence N, Mellen BG, et al. The safety of liposuction: results of a national survey. *Dermatol Surg.* 2002;28:971-978.
24. Prendergast TI, Ong'uti SK, Ortega G, et al. Differential trends in racial preferences for cosmetic surgery procedures. *Am Surg.* 2011;77:1081-1085.
25. Singh D. Universal allure of the hourglass figure: an evolutionary theory of female physical attractiveness. *Clin Plast Surg.* 2006;33:359-370.
26. Lee EI, Roberts TL, Bruner TW. Ethnic considerations in buttock aesthetics. *Semin Plast Surg.* 2009;23:232-243.
27. Dawson-Andoh NA, Gray JJ, Soto JA, et al. Body shape and size depictions of African American women in JET magazine, 1953-2006. *Body Image.* 2011;8:86-89.
28. Deurenberg P, Bhaskaran K, Lian PL. Singaporean Chinese adolescents have more subcutaneous adipose tissue than Dutch Caucasians of the same age and body mass index. *Asia Pac J Clin Nutr.* 2003;12:261-265.
29. Huang TT, Johnson MS, Figueroa-Colon R, et al. Growth of visceral fat, subcutaneous abdominal fat, and total body fat in children. *Obes Res.* 2001;9:283-289.
30. Okosun IS, Liao Y, Rotimi CN, et al. Impact of birth weight on ethnic variations in subcutaneous and central adiposity in American children aged 5-11 years. A study from the Third National Health and Nutrition Examination Survey. *Int J Obes Relat Metab Disord.* 2000;24:479-484.
31. Lovejoy JC, Smith SR, Rood JC. Comparison of regional fat distribution and health risk factors in middle-aged white and African American women: the Healthy Transitions Study. *Obes Res.* 2001;9:10-16.
32. Lovejoy JC, de la Bretonne JA, Klemperer M, et al. Abdominal fat distribution and metabolic risk factors: effects of race. *Metabolism.* 1996;45:1119-1124.
33. Braunstein GD, Glassman HA. Gynecomastia. *Curr Ther Endocrinol Metab.* 1997;6:401-404.
34. Thompson DF, Carter JR. Drug-induced gynecomastia. *Pharmacotherapy.* 1993;13:37-45.
35. Bernstein G, Hanke CW. Safety of liposuction: a review of 9478 cases performed by dermatologists. *J Dermatol Surg Oncol.* 1988;14:1112-1114.
36. Hanke CW, Bernstein G, Bullock S. Safety of tumescent liposuction in 15,336 patients. National survey results. *Dermatol Surg.* 1995;21:459-462.
37. Goyen MR. Lifestyle outcomes of tumescent liposuction surgery. *Dermatol Surg.* 2002;28:459-462.
38. Field LM. Liposuction surgery (suction-assisted lipectomy) for symmetric lipomatosis. *J Am Acad Dermatol.* 1988;18:1370.
39. Pinski KS, Roenigk HH Jr. Liposuction of lipomas. *Dermatol Clin.* 1990;8:483-492.
40. Payne CM, Doe PT. Liposuction for axillary hyperhidrosis. *Clin Exp Dermatol.* 1998;23:9-10.
41. Dolsky RL. Gynecomastia. Treatment by liposuction subcutaneous mastectomy. *Dermatol Clin.* 1990;8:469-478.
42. Brorson H, Svensson H. Complete reduction of lymphoedema of the arm by liposuction after breast cancer. *Scand J Plast Reconstr Surg Hand Surg.* 1997;31:137-143.

Pediatrics

Candrice R. Heath
Joni M. Mazza
Nanette B. Silverberg

KEY POINTS

- It is expected that children with skin of color will constitute about 15% of all dermatology visits by the year 2050.
- Children with skin of color are more susceptible to keloid and hypertrophic scar development, and many will develop a pigmentary alteration in response to inflammatory skin conditions.
- African American children are more susceptible to dry scalp, traction related hair loss, and tinea capitis.

INTRODUCTION

Children of color are often underserved in their needs, because the majority of dermatology textbooks have been written about Caucasian children and most prescription drugs have been tested primarily in Caucasian children. Currently there is only one atlas[1] in print that describes children of color. Children of color have several unique concerns that affect their development of illness and response to therapy.

Ten percent of visits to pediatricians are for skin issues, and 30% of all dermatology appointments are made for children.[2] By the year 2050, almost half of the U.S. population will be non-Caucasian.[3] Thus it is expected that children of color will constitute about 15% of all dermatology visits by the year 2050.[4]

Children of color have specific reactions to injury. They are more susceptible to keloid and hypertrophic scar development.[2] Most darkly pigmented children will develop a pigmentary alteration in response to inflammatory skin conditions, including atopic dermatitis, pityriasis rosea, and acne.[3] In fact, pigmentation, both hyperpigmentation and hypopigmentation, may be more noticeable and consequently more disturbing to children, especially adolescents of color. Furthermore lichenoid dermatologic responses are more common in children of color, resulting in cases of lichenoid atopic dermatitis, hypertrophic lichen planus, and lichenoid contact dermatitis.

Immunologic and metabolic reaction patterns in children of color are different as well. Higher rates of diabetes, poor vitamin D levels due to melanin-related sun protection, and alterations in enzymes such as low levels of glucose-6-phsophate dehydrogenase (G6PD) may all serve to contribute to skin disease development and ability to tolerate standard dermatologic therapeutics (eg, dapsone).

Other concerns include curved hair follicles and reduced flow of sebum on the hair shaft,[4] leaving the African American child more susceptible to dry scalp, traction-related hair loss, tinea capitis, and as an adult, central centrifugal cicatricial alopecia.

This chapter is meant to provide an overview of skin conditions seen in children of color and includes 10 sections: newborn skin conditions, dermatitis, papulosquamous disorders, acneiform skin conditions, autoimmune and collagen vascular diseases, vascular birthmarks, pigmentary diseases, traumatic, hair disorders, and infections. The sections will be limited to conditions not covered elsewhere in the text or will provide added information pertinent to pediatric patients supplemental to other chapters. Due to the complexity of the topic, only a limited number of conditions are covered in depth. The readers are encouraged to contribute to the literature regarding children of color, as it is limited in nature at this time.

SECTION I: NEWBORN SKIN CONDITIONS

NORMAL VARIATIONS

Pigmentation is quite variable in early childhood in children of color. At birth, pigmentation is often limited to the hair and genitalia, especially in children with dark skin of color. However, these children are often noted to have or develop pigmentation in the folds, periorificially, and over the genitalia. Asian children have distinctive patterns of pigmentary alteration, including 4% who have nevus depigmentosus and the more uncommon dermal melanocytosis known as nevus of Ito or Ota. Furthermore, it is typical for young children of color to have thin, straighter hair in infancy and toddler years as well as a reduced risk of keloid scarring compared to school-age children. Therefore, the risk of tinea capitis and keloids does not rise until age 3 years. Other normal variants of infancy in childhood include pigmentary mosaicism and greater tendency toward postinflammatory hypopigmentation.

MONGOLIAN SPOTS

Mongolian spots are birthmarks, typically located over the lower back and buttocks of children. Also known as dermal melanocytosis, these benign lesions represent entrapment of melanocytes within the dermis during migration from the neural crest. This deeper deposition of pigment gives the characteristic blue color due to the Tyndall effect. While these birthmarks can be found in all races they are significantly more common in children with skin of color. Lesions have been reported in 96% of African American and 46% of Hispanic children.[5] More recently, studies have demonstrated Mongolian spots in 62% of Chinese, 71% of Iranian, and 26% of Turkish children, but less than 10% of Caucasian infants.[2,6-8]

Lesions are typically seen at birth or within the first few weeks of life. They present as asymptomatic, hyperpigmented, blue to blue-gray macules and patches, typically located over the sacral, gluteal, or lumbar regions, though they can be found in any location. Most lesions occur as an isolated incident in an otherwise healthy child, but they have been seen in association with other anomalies, such as phakomatosis pigmentovascularis types 2 and 5, and inborn errors of metabolism, such as GM1 gangliosidosis and Hurler and Hunter disease.[9,10] Histopathology shows spindle-shaped dendritic melanocytes scattered throughout collagen in the dermis.

The differential diagnosis of Mongolian spots includes blue nevi, nevus of Ota, and nevus of Ito, given the characteristic blue-gray color that these lesions share. Mongolian spots can also be mistaken for bruises and have been implicated in misdiagnoses of child abuse.[11] For this reason, it is strongly recommended that clinicians document all melanocytic lesions, because their persistence, compared to quickly fading ecchymotic lesions, aids in making the proper diagnosis.

Most cases resolve with age, with complete clearance generally noted by age 6. These lesions have not been shown to have malignant potential, so treatment is observation. Medical makeup can be used to camouflage lesions for special occasion until spontaneous clearance occurs.[12,13]

TRANSIENT NEONATAL PUSTULAR MELANOSIS

Also known as transient neonatal pustulosis, transient neonatal pustular melanosis (TNPM) is a benign self-limited disease, seen primarily in newborns with skin of color. Lesions typically present as 1- to 3-mm flaccid, fragile blisters, small collarettes of scale, or even as hyperpigmented macules representing lesions that healed in utero. The vesicles and pustules rupture easily and generally heal within 48 hours. While this rash can appear anywhere on the body, it is most often seen on the face, neck, back, and buttocks.[14,15] TNPM is seven to eight times more common in African American newborns, being present in approximately 4.4% of African American as compared with 0.6% of Caucasian newborns,[16] although current data on overall incidence rates, as well as incidence in other groups with skin of color, have been sparse.

The etiology of this condition remains unknown. In a recent report looking at the correlation of skin findings in newborns with maternal factors, TNPM was seen predominantly in the children of women who had vaginal deliveries, while interestingly erythema toxicum neonatorum, a rash commonly in the differential of TNPM, was seen more frequently after cesarean section. On histopathology, subcorneal and intracorneal collections of neutrophils, and occasionally eosinophils, can be visualized. Although biopsy is usually unnecessary, Wright-stained smear of pustules demonstrates neutrophils, few or no eosinophils, and cellular debris.[11] The differential includes erythema neonatorum toxicum, acropustulosis of infancy, herpes simplex virus, milia, miliaria, and syphilis.

This condition is benign and self-limited; thus, the primary treatment is providing reassurance to the families. It is important to explain to parents that the hyperpigmentation may take weeks to months to resolve.

CLEAR CELL PAPULOSIS

Clear cell papulosis is a rare, benign condition, first described in 1987.[17] It tends to present in early childhood, typically between 4 months and 5 years of age. Lesions are described as asymptomatic groups of oval to round, hypopigmented macules or flat-topped papules, distributed over the lower abdomen or along the milk line in children. The majority of cases have been described in Asian children, and a genetic component has been suggested based on the fact that several reports have been in siblings. A 2007 case report described the condition in three Hispanic children in the United States.[18] The etiology remains unknown.

The findings on histopathology can be very subtle and may be misdiagnosed as normal skin if a clinical–histopathologic correlation is not made. Hematoxylin and eosin stains can show hyperkeratosis, mild to moderate acanthosis, and decreased pigment in the basal layer, with the characteristic feature of clear cells, larger than neighboring keratinocytes, with ample, pale cytoplasm. In a review of all reported cases (n = 38), with 28 cases reporting histopathology, the majority of lesions expressed positivity for mucin (24 of 27 cases), carcinoembryonic antigen (24 of 24), epithelial membrane antigen (20 of 20), cytokeratin (CK) AE1 and/or AE3 (28 of 28), gross cystic disease fluid protein 15 (9 of 10), cell adhesion molecule 5.2 (14 of 14), CK-7 (6 of 6), and colloidal iron (6 of 7). All were negative for S100.[19] Fontana-Masson staining shows decreased melanin staining.[20]

The differential includes postinflammatory hypopigmentation, vitiligo, tinea versicolor, nevus depigmentosus, verruca plana, hypopigmented mycosis fungoides, and pityriasis lichenoides chronica.

There is no known treatment for this condition. Spontaneous resolution tends to be seen by the end of childhood. A case series of 19 patients showed spontaneous regression in 85% of patients at a median follow-up of 11.5 years.[21] Early reports had expressed concern that these lesions could be a precursor of extramammary Paget disease, although this has not been supported in the literature.[14] For this reason, long-term surveillance seems judicious.

SECTION II: DERMATITIS

SEBORRHEIC DERMATITIS

Seborrheic dermatitis, also known as cradle cap, is a self-limited, erythematous to yellow, greasy, scaly, inflammatory eruption that is distributed on the scalp, face, postauricular, and intertriginous areas. Seborrheic dermatitis is common in the pediatric population, with a bimodal distribution most typically presenting in infants and adolescents.

The pathogenesis of seborrheic dermatitis is not entirely clear. The predilection for areas of increased sebaceous gland density and correlation with increased hormonal production in the first year of life and during adolescence suggest an etiologic role for sebum and sebaceous glands. The lipophilic yeast *Pityrosporum ovale* (*Malassezia ovalis*), has also been implicated. This normal constituent of skin flora may, in some individuals, be an inciting factor for the release of inflammatory cytokines and abnormal host response to yeast colonization.

In infants, seborrhea generally presents during the first few months of life with a peak incidence at 3 months.[22] Typically it occurs as erythema and scaling on the scalp or as greasy, scaly plaques on the face and/or intertriginous areas. Accompanying maceration can be noted, requiring therapy for *Candida* overgrowth in some settings. In adolescents, the scalp is the most commonly affected area, although eyebrows and nasolabial folds can also be affected. Petalloid (small, circinate or ovoid) lesions can be seen in both age groups. While the vast majority of lesions improve with time, pigmentary alteration remains a concern in patients with skin of color. Pruritus tends to be minimal in these patients, which often helps distinguish seborrhea from atopic dermatitis. In prepubertal children, seborrheic dermatitis may present as fine scale. All children in this age group warrant a fungal culture to rule out tinea capitis.[23] Diagnosis is based on clinical examination. Differential includes atopic dermatitis, psoriasis, pityriasis alba, pityriasis versicolor, dermatophytosis, Langerhans cell histiocytosis, nutritional deficiency, and immunodeficiency.

For infants, even without treatment, most cases of mild seborrhea will clear spontaneously by 8 to 12 months of age. Infantile scalp seborrhea can be managed by frequent shampooing with a gentle shampoo. Ketoconazole shampoo can also be used in harder to treat cases.[24] If thick or adherent scale is present, removal with mineral oil or baby oil and a soft brush or comb can also be used. If inflammation is present, the patient will benefit from topical corticosteroid solution or lotion. In infants with seborrhea on other areas of the body, low-strength topical steroids or antifungals can also be effective.[25]

The treatment for adolescents is essentially the same. Mild cases of scalp disease can be managed with shampoos containing selenium sulfide or zinc pyrithione. Thicker scale can be removed with mineral oil or the use of salicylic acid shampoo or P&S Liquid. Topical steroid lotions, gels, oils, or foams can be added as needed. Nonscalp sites can be treated with topical steroids or topical antifungals. Pimecrolimus 1% cream (not approved in the United States for children under the age of 2 years) has shown promising results in adult skin of color patients[26] and may be used in adolescents, although use in infants is currently not recommended. Additionally, a nonsteroidal cream has demonstrated similar efficacy to topical steroids in the treatment of seborrheic dermatitis,[27] but no studies have specifically looked at usage in pediatric patients with skin of color.

ATOPIC DERMATITIS

Atopic dermatitis (also called "eczema"), the cutaneous form of atopy, is an itchy, chronic skin condition that remits and relapses.[28] Patients with atopic dermatitis develop eczematous plaques in typical distribution, including facial and extensor surfaces in infancy, flexural areas in childhood, and hands/feet in adulthood.[28] African American children, children with dark skin of color, and Latino children are more likely to experience eczema flares that are lichenoid in nature,[29] whereas facial and nipple atopic dermatitis are sites more common in Asian children. In Latino children, nipple eczema seems to increase with age, whereas genital involvement decreases with age.[30] Triggers for atopic dermatitis include exposure to irritants such as fragrance, wool, or harsh cleansers or global immunologic triggers including viral infections and stress.[28]

One of the minor features of atopic dermatitis, the infraorbital crease, is more common in African America/African origin and Asian children.[31] Children of color often experience tremendous pigmentary alteration upon resolution of atopic dermatitis.

The incidence of eczema in the United States may be as high as 17.1%, with empirical diagnosis in 10.7%.[1] Atopic dermatitis appears to be more common in children who are of African origin than Caucasian children in developed countries such as England. In the United States, children who are African American and Asian/Pacific Islanders are more likely to seek care for atopic dermatitis.[33] Foreign-born children in the United States have a lower incidence of eczema, but the beneficial effect of foreign birth wanes over 10 years.[34] Thus many immigrants of color have lower risk of early childhood eczema presentation. African American children are more likely to have a positive prick test and wheezing than their Caucasian counterparts.[35] Other segments of children of color have specific issues related to atopic dermatitis including extensive postinflammatory changes in Hispanic and Asian children, extreme facial sensitivity, and greater confounding ichthyosis vulgaris.

Children of color have special needs when they have atopic dermatitis, including African American children who have greater transepidermal water loss and lower pH.[36,37] Most clinical trials in print addressed atopic dermatitis primarily in Caucasian children. A recent review article demonstrated that in atopic dermatitis trials where the patient's race was recorded, the mixture of patients was 62.1% Caucasian, 18.0% African American, 6.9% Asian, and 2.0% Hispanic.[38]

The differential diagnosis of atopic dermatitis includes seborrheic dermatitis in infancy and contact dermatitis.

Therapy of atopic dermatitis includes four steps: (1) moisturization and gentle skin care, (2) topical medicaments for flares and prevention of flares, (3) treatment of pruritus and sleep disturbance, and (4) control of infections and colonizations. Little to no data suggest that any differences are required in the therapeutics of patients with skin of color. The following paragraphs summarize the sparse data on these topics.

Skin care and moisturization are the core of long-term control of atopic dermatitis. Xerosis appears to be a more common issue in patients of African or Afro-Caribbean descent versus Caucasians, with 100%, 92%, and 16% of adult females of these races, respectively, using daily emollients.[39] Ichthyosis vulgaris may be noted in almost 10% of the Asian population, and this too requires extra emollient use.

Topical medications appear to be effective in all children with skin of color. Of the topical corticosteroids available, no data have been published reviewing differential response by race or skin of color groups. However, the presence of lichenoid changes in patients with dark skin of color, particularly lichen simplex chronicus, requires use of a higher potency agent. There is a single study that suggests that children with skin of color may require a higher potency of topical tacrolimus than their Caucasian counterparts, but pimecrolimus seems equally efficacious in all racial groups.[40] Asian patients across Korea and Japan seem to have a similar response to tacrolimus as patients in the United States.[41] Some ethnic preferences exist in prescribing. African origin and African American patients prefer and better tolerate petrolatum-based products. Middle Eastern patients may culturally prefer oil-based medicaments.

Pruritus and sleep disturbance seem to have no racial differences. The presence of a lower pH of the skin in those with dark skin of color or African American children would predict less superinfection with *Staphylococcus aureus*, due to superior enhancement of the acid mantle; however, no data exist to support this theory. The therapy of atopic dermatitis that resists topical agents is enhanced with narrowband ultraviolet B (NB-UVB), even in darkly pigmented patients. However, the prolonged dosage (time-wise) required in the darkest children prevents young patients from being able to tolerate therapy. Other caveats to phototherapy include rapid enhancement of tanning and hyperpigmentation in Asian and Hispanic patients and aggravated risk of melasma in menstruating females, especially those on oral contraceptives. Because patients with skin of color are less prone to skin cancer, they may have lower risk of the skin cancer with long-term phototherapy. However, this has not yet been fully proven. Therefore, counseling regarding potential skin cancer risk with phototherapy should be uniform through all population groups.

ALLERGIC CONTACT DERMATITIS

Allergic contact dermatitis is no more or less prevalent in children of color. However, early exposures may occur as a result of cultural practices, resulting in early onset of contact dermatitis. These include propensity to early piercing in African American and Hispanic children in the United States and usage of henna tattoos in South Asians, which expose patients to paraphenylenediamine. Because nickel contact is the most common form of allergic contact dermatitis worldwide, the differential presentation by race requires comment. Children with dark skin of color and Hispanic and African American children have greater lichenification and lichenoid contact dermatitis. Hence, widespread nickel contact and id reactions, also lichenoid in nature, can mimic lichen planus or juvenile dermatomyositis.

Furthermore, usage of nickel-laden jewelry is a hard habit to break and requires extensive counseling on avoidance techniques, including testing (dimethylglyoxime) and not purchasing new metal items with nickel content and avoiding contact with nonessential metals including grommets, piercings, and belt buckles.[42,43]

SECTION III: PAPULOSQUAMOUS DISORDERS

PSORIASIS

Psoriasis is a common skin condition affecting 3% of Caucasian Americans and 1.5% of African Americans [**Figure 84-1**]. Racial prevalence differences are highlighted by a study from California. The prevalence of psoriasis overall was 19 per 10,000, but the prevalence was 29 per 10,000 in non-Hispanic Caucasians, 20 per 10,000 in Asian/Pacific Islanders, 16 per 10,000 in Hispanic Caucasians, and 6 per 10,000 in African Americans.[44] Triggers in pediatric psoriasis include upper respiratory infections and stress.[45]

Psoriasis typically presents with erythematous plaques with overlying scale on the scalp and extensor surfaces in Caucasian patients. Associated pitting of the nails and guttate lesions on the body are other manifestations commonly noted in childhood.[45] Differences in clinical appearance of psoriasis of adulthood in those with dark skin of color and Caucasians have been highlighted by McMichael et al,[46] who surveyed 29 dermatologists who indicated that the illness manifested with greater hyperpigmentation and less erythema in dark skin of color individuals than in Caucasians. The differences in pediatric psoriasis have been reviewed by Silverberg,[47] highlighting less hyperkeratosis in scalp lesions (resulting in near absence of pityriasis amiantacea in dark skin of color, Hispanic, and Asian children with psoriasis) and, similar to adults, the presence of greater hyperpigmentation and thicker lesions,

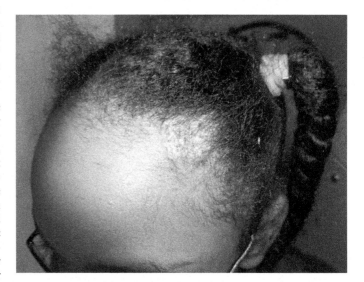

FIGURE 84-1. Psoriasis in a girl with traction alopecia. Note the extension of the plaque onto the forehead. A potassium hydroxide or fungal culture would be best to rule-out the possibility of tinea capitis in this child.

but less erythema and scale. Data suggest that pruritus and family history of pediatric psoriasis with arthritis are greater in Caucasian (Dutch) children than in Singaporean children.[48] The differences in incidence of psoriatic comorbidities such as obesity, hyperlipidemia, and arthritis by race in children have not been addressed in the literature.

Therapeutically, topical corticosteroids, topical calcipotriene and betamethasone,[49] phototherapy, and systemic therapies such as etanercept can be used successfully in individuals of color without major differences in safety or efficacy.[50] In the authors' experiences, calcipotriene can enhance postinflammatory hyperpigmentation in patients with Fitzpatrick types IV to VI. Other caveats for therapy are the damaging effects of harsh shampoos on hair in girls with dark skin of color and on sensitive facial skin in Asian children. Use of emolliating agents is often preferable in these groups as an alternative.

PITYRIASIS ROSEA

Pityriasis rosea is a self-limited papulosquamous inflammatory dermatosis of the skin. The etiology is presumed to be viral, and both human herpes virus (HHV)-6 and HHV-7 have been found in the skin and saliva, supporting the idea that pityriasis rosea is a viral exanthema with a prolonged course of disease beyond the initial stages of the infection. Disease usually begins with the herald patch followed by lesions along Langer lines that erupt centrally over 6 weeks and clear over another 6 weeks.[51]

As in Caucasian children with pityriasis rosea, children with skin of color experience pruritus and have a herald patch. However, the morphology and distribution of pityriasis rosea deviate from the typical description of pityriasis rosea in Caucasian children, which typically includes salmon-colored plaques limited to the central body and inner arms that heal without residual cutaneous alterations.

In a study of 50 African American children with pityriasis rosea, facial and scalp involvement was found more often than in their Caucasian counterparts. In contrast to the typical papulosquamous plaques seen in pityriasis rosea, children with skin of color often have papular lesions. Postinflammatory hyperpigmentation or hypopigmentation may be noted as papulosquamous lesions flatten and clear.[52,53] Amer et al[53] found that 48% of the African American children studied had residual hyperpigmentation. Some of the children studied had both hyperpigmentation and hypopigmentation.[52,53] Hypopigmentation was found most commonly following papular or papulovesicular lesions.[52] The erythema of lesions may not be apparent in those with darker skin tones, where violaceous to flesh-colored lesions can also be noted. However, hyperkeratosis at the border of the lesions may be prominent.[52] Pruritus may also be a prominent feature,[52,53] which can cause loss of sleep and discomfort.

The differential diagnosis includes secondary syphilis; therefore, a rapid plasma reagin test for syphilis should be performed in those who have reached sexual maturation, given that there is a surge of syphilis cases in 15 to 24 year olds.[54] Psoriasis would likely be more erythematous with greater overlying hyperkeratosis, the so-called *micaceous scale* noted in lesions over the knees, elbows, and scalp, which are sites not noted in pityriasis rosea. If guttate psoriasis is suspected, nail pitting may be suggestive of the diagnosis, and biopsy can be used as a clinical clue in favor of psoriasis. Papular eczema, tinea corporis, and pityriasis lichenoides may mimic papular pityriasis rosea, the herald patch, and generalized pityriasis rosea, respectively. Biopsy can distinguish most of these diagnoses.

Treatment is symptomatic for pruritus, with topical mid-potency corticosteroids and oral antihistamines being beneficial in some cases. NB-UVB can help with more extensive cases, but resolution without therapy is the norm. Postinflammatory pigmentary alteration can last months to a few years, with no described therapies available. Prevention is not possible, given that HHV-6 and HHV-7 are excreted asymptomatically in the saliva of individuals previously infected.

LICHEN PLANUS

Lichen planus is an uncommon dermatosis of childhood that is characterized by purple, polygonal, violaceous (especially in darkly pigmented patients), flat-topped papules and plaques that can affect the skin. The oral mucosa is a common site of lesions in adults, with about half of

cases having white plaques, but is a rare site in children, especially children of color. Disease can be triggered by hepatitis B infection, which is a bit more common in Asia, or by hepatitis B vaccine. Lesions are usually noted on the flexural surfaces of the wrists, but can be generalized and eruptive, a presentation seen in Hispanic children. Lesions in children of Hispanic and African origin/African American backgrounds may present as purple to violaceous, hyperpigmented, hypertrophic plaques overlying the shins [**Figure 84-2**]. Mosaicism is a bit more common in pediatric lichen planus, and linear lichen planus, which follows the lines of Blaschko, is often noted on the abdomen or legs, but may affect any region of the body.[55] Characteristically, intense residual hyperpigmentation remains as a sequela following resolution of lichen planus lesions. Although most literature does not report a racial predilection, a retrospective review of 36 cases of pediatric lichen planus in Wisconsin revealed a predominance in children with dark skin of color.[56]

Workup should include hepatitis B titers in children who were not vaccinated. Biopsy can demonstrate typical histology, namely interface dermatitis along the dermo-epidermal junction (DEJ), but will then vary based on stage of the lesion. As lesions evolve and progress, destruction of the basal layer can result in a "saw-tooth" pattern at the DEJ, with overlying epidermal hyperplasia and orthokeratosis. Civatte bodies, which represent necrotic keratinocytes within the epidermis, can also be seen in lichen planus. Hypertrophic lichen planus [**Figure 84-2**] can present histologically as pseudoepitheliomatous hyperplasia and may mimic hypertrophic or verrucous lupus. Dermoscopy will demonstrate Wickham striae, which are usually not visible with the naked eye, especially in hypertrophic lesions.

Therapy of lichen planus in childhood depends on the type of lesions and location. Topical corticosteroids remain the mainstay of therapy, but intralesional corticosteroids can aid in clearance of hypertrophic lesions. A case of linear lichen planus treated with some success using topical adapalene has been described. Oral corticosteroids and NB-UVB can be used to control eruptive and/or severe or generalized cases. Therapy becomes extremely important for many children with generalized disease due to severe pruritus. Antihistamines can be added adjunctively for sleep disturbance. The natural history in childhood is generally spontaneous resolution in 3 to 5 years, which suggests that more aggressive immunosuppression should be limited to the most extensive cases.[57]

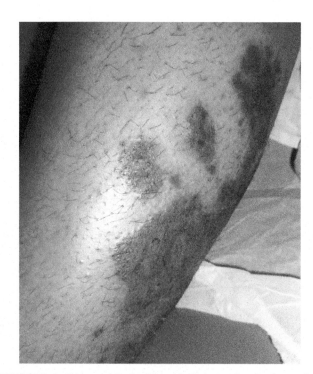

FIGURE 84-2. This teenage boy has lichen planus lesions on the calves that are slightly hypertrophic and quite violaceous. Note the erythematous border.

MYCOSIS FUNGOIDES

Mycosis fungoides (MF) is the most common form of cutaneous T-cell lymphoma (CTCL) composed primarily of memory T lymphocytes. Mycosis fungoides rarely occurs in children, adolescents, or young adults[58] and is therefore primarily considered an adult disease. It may, however, occasionally present during the first 10 years of life.[59] The hypopigmented variant of MF is more common in younger patients and in those with Fitzpatrick skin types IV to VI and often has delayed diagnosis compared to other variants of MF.[57] Childhood-onset hypopigmented MF usually does not progress to more severe disease stages and thus has an excellent prognosis.[56] The differential diagnosis include vitiligo, tinea versicolor, pityriasis lichenoides et varioliformis acuta (PLEVA) and pityriasis lichenoides chronicum (PLC). For cases in children of Caribbean origin, human T lymphotropic virus-1 testing may be needed. Therapies for MF include topical corticosteroids, NB-UVB, and psoralen with ultraviolet A (PUVA), with the latter two therapies to be used only in children capable of standing in a phototherapy booth and using appropriate eyewear, usually ages 6 and 12 or above, respectively.[60]

PITYRIASIS LICHENOIDES ET VARIOLIFORMIS ACUTA AND PITYRIASIS LICHENOIDES CHRONICUM

PLEVA and PLC represent the acute and chronic versions of a lymphocytic vasculitis, respectively. Clinically, PLEVA often presents as a sudden eruption of crops of erythematous macules, papules, or papulovesicles. Although lesions tend to occur on the chest and back, extension to extremities is not uncommon. This benign condition tends to be self-limited, with most patients achieving clearance of lesions in 1 to 3 years. PLC is considered the chronic form of PLEVA and therefore also commonly affects children and young adults. The pathophysiology of PLEVA and PLC is similar in all population groups. The lesions of PLEVA and PLC may leave behind patchy postinflammatory hypopigmentation[61] that can be particularly distressing in patients with skin of color. The hypopigmentation may be extensive and even involve the face. The differential diagnosis for PLEVA and PLC lesions includes pityriasis rosea and guttate psoriasis, but the residual hypopigmentation may raise concern for other skin disorders. Hypopigmented MF should also be considered in the differential diagnosis due to reports of patients with PLC coexisting with hypopigmented MF.[62] PLC has even rarely preceded lymphomatoid papulosis and MF.[63] Repetitive biopsies are needed to identify disease progression when lesional clearance or altered morphology occurs. Therapies for pityriasis lichenoides include topical corticosteroids, oral antibiotics, and phototherapy; however, the disease is usually resolves in 3 to 5 years.

SECTION IV: ACNEIFORM SKIN CONDITIONS

ACROPUSTULOSIS OF INFANCY

This condition occurs at birth or during infancy. Crops of intensely pruritic vesicles and pustules occur on the soles, palms, and dorsal surfaces of acral sites. The lesions will resolve within a few days, leaving a hyperpigmented macule that can be more difficult to discern in pigmented skin. New crops recur within a few weeks. The condition is rare but typically affects infants of color. A scabies prep must always be done prior to making the diagnosis, because the two conditions have very similar presentations and because 50% of cases have a preceding scabies infection as a trigger for the blistering process.[64] Therapeutic options include strong topical steroids, antihistamines, and in severe cases, dapsone orally, which should be given only in children who are not deficient in glucose-6-phosphate dehydrogenase enzyme. Therapy with dapsone requires careful blood count monitoring for dose-related hemolysis.[65]

ACNE

In a study of a pediatric dermatology clinic in Miami, acne was one of the leading diagnoses. Similarly, acne has been noted to be one of the most common diagnoses for patients with skin of color seeking pediatric dermatologic care worldwide. Acne can be seen in neonate, infant, toddler, childhood, preadolescent, and adolescent forms. Children aged 1 to 7 years should be referred for endocrine workup when acne is noted, because this is an uncommon time of life for acne and can reflect the presence of precocious puberty or an adrenal tumor.[66]

Hair oils and/or pomades have been identified as a contributory factor for forehead acne in adults of color. Hair care practices are traditionally passed on from one generation to the next. Due to the coiled and textural hair properties in patients of African descent (see Chapter 37), many children, young girls in particular, undergo time-consuming hair care cultural practices to make the hair more manageable.

Pomades, oils, and other greasy products may be used in skin of color populations during hair care routines. These substances are comedogenic, resulting in monomorphic, closed comedones localized to the forehead. Papules and pustules may also be present.[67] Using hair care products that are less comedogenic and avoiding hair scarves that occlude the forehead are all preventative measures.[68] Three hundred thirteen skin of color patients with acne were studied (239 were of African American or African Caribbean descent, 55 were Hispanic, and 19 were Asian or from other racial/ethnic groups, such as Indians and Pakistanis); 46.2% reported using hair oil or pomade, and 70.3% of the hair oil/pomade users had forehead acne.[69,70]

Acne in children of color usually begins on the forehead with open and closed comedones and small papules, progressing at times to papules and pustules [**Figure 84-3**]. Closed comedones will respond to topical retinoids, but amending hair care routines may prove very beneficial. Cysts are uncommon in African American patients with acne. When acne is noted primarily over the forehead with little or no lesions in the V_2 or V_3 region of the face, pomade exposure should be suspected as an aggravating factor.

Treatment of acne varies around the world, but generally follows the paradigm recently published by the American Acne and Rosacea Society. Mild disease, consisting of open and closed comedones or papules, will benefit from a topical retinoid and benzoyl peroxide product for antibacterial properties. Moderate disease often requires the inclusion of oral antibiotics and/or oral contraceptives in girls of child-bearing potential. Severe disease or scarring acne merits use of isotretinoin in some cases. A recent review of adolescent acne in children of color has identified some specific usage patterns that vary worldwide, including extensive use of adapalene in Asia, where it is available over the counter. Other therapeutic tips include the use of azelaic acid for reduction of lesions and hyperpigmentation, addition of mild chemical peels, and topical hydroquinones for hyperpigmentation.[71]

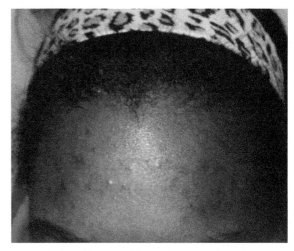

FIGURE 84-3. Forehead acne with postinflammatory hyperpigmentation in this preteen may have been exacerbated by pomade usage and *Pityrosporum* overgrowth.

▐ PERIORIFICIAL DERMATITIS

Periorificial dermatitis (also known as facial Afro-Caribbean eruption) consists of erythematous papules distributed in the perioral, perinasal, and periocular regions of the face. Often the papules are asymptomatic but may be pruritic or have a burning sensation. The vermillion border is generally spared. The granulomatous variant of periorificial dermatitis is more common in patients with skin of color. The distribution is the same, but the papules are typically flesh colored.[72] Involvement of the groin has been described in a cohort of Caucasian children with periorificial dermatitis, but we have never seen a case of genital involvement in the past 15 years in our skin of color center.[73]

Pediatric sarcoidosis may also affect the face with red-brown or violaceous flat-topped papules,[74,75] which may be mistaken for periorificial dermatitis. In the United States, pediatric sarcoidosis, though rare, is more common in children with dark skin of color[75-77] and thus should be considered in the differential diagnosis.

The exact etiology of periorificial dermatitis is unknown. Corticosteroid (topical/inhaled) use, contact irritants/allergens, and lip licking have been implicated, but many cases are deemed idiopathic.[76]

SECTION V: AUTOIMMUNE AND COLLAGEN VASCULAR DISEASES

▐ SARCOIDOSIS

Sarcoidosis is a chronic granulomatous disease that can affect any organ system of the body, including the skin, and is characterized histologically by noncaseating granulomas. In the United States, the incidence of this condition is significantly higher in African Americans compared with Caucasians (34 per 100,000 vs 11 per 100,000, respectively), and the prevalence in African Americans is 10 times that of Caucasian patients. The underlying cause remains unknown, although there is clearly a genetic component, because African Americans with an affected first-degree relative have a 2.5-fold increased risk of developing the disease.

Although this disease most commonly affects patients in the second to fourth decades of life, sarcoidosis can also occur in children. Two forms have been described. Patients with early-onset childhood sarcoidosis variant have rash and uveitis, and those under 5 years old may have arthritis.[78] Older children with sarcoidosis present with symptoms similar to adult-onset sarcoidosis. These symptoms include lymphadenopathy, pulmonary involvement, fever, malaise, and weight loss.[75,79]

▐ LUPUS

Lupus erythematosus is a multisystem autoimmune disorder caused by a variety of antibodies, primarily directed against nuclear antigens. Four major clinical variants are noted in childhood: neonatal lupus erythematosus, a vertically transmitted variant; systemic lupus erythematosus (SLE); subacute cutaneous lupus erythematosus; and discoid lupus erythematosus. Although discoid lupus and subacute cutaneous lupus resemble the adult types, unlike adult cases, the majority of cutaneous lupus cases will progress to systemic lupus, requiring frequent serologic follow-up.

Pediatric patients account for 10% to 20% of reported cases of SLE, and SLE more commonly affects African American, Afro-Caribbean, Asian, and Hispanic children.[80-82] Pediatric-onset SLE is more severe than adult-onset SLE. Pediatric patients with skin of color have more severe disease than fairer-skinned children with SLE.[81,82] Despite adequate treatment, many patients with pediatric SLE die before the age of 30 year.[81] The therapy of systemic lupus is beyond the scope of this article; however, cutaneous disease is often treated with topical and/or pulsed corticosteroids and/or hydroxychloroquine (in patients without G6PD deficiency, which is not uncommon in males of African descent).

Neonatal lupus is a distinct variant from SLE. Infants born with neonatal lupus have mothers with diagnosed or undiagnosed autoimmune disease. These mothers have a propensity for SLE, Sjögren syndrome, rheumatoid arthritis, or mixed connective tissue disease.[83,84] Despite the mother's autoimmune risk, only 1% of infants with circulating maternal

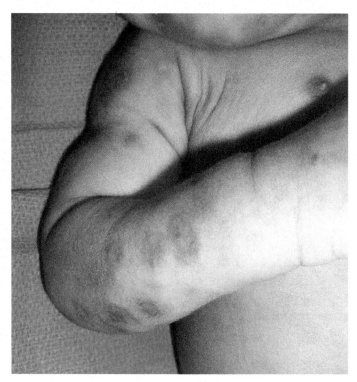

FIGURE 84-4. This 1-month-old African American female infant has a subacute cutaneous lupus-like lesions in the setting of neonatal lupus erythematosus. Her mother had undiagnosed Sjögren disease.

autoantibodies will develop neonatal lupus.[81,85] Infants born to mothers with these risk factors, if known, should be monitored closely. Of those with neonatal lupus, about 23% will have cutaneous symptoms at birth, and by 6 weeks of age, that number increases to 50%.[80]

Clinically, the lesions of neonatal lupus can be annular erythematous plaques [**Figure 84-4**],[86] periorbital erythema, or atrophic, scaly, telangiectatic discoid lesions.[80] The most common locations affected are the face and scalp,[84,86] but lesions may occur on other places like the trunk, extremities, and intertriginous areas. Even though the lesions may only be present for a few weeks or months, dyspigmentation and residual telangiectasias may remain for a year.[83,86] Neonatal lupus lesions often spontaneously resolve, but diligent sun protection and topical corticosteroids are necessary.[86]

The most serious complication of neonatal lupus is the risk of congenital heart block,[87] with complete heart block being the most common presentation.[85] It occurs in 1% to 2% of babies born to mothers with anti-Ro/SSA autoantibodies.[85] Pregnant women with positive anti-Ro/SSA or anti-La/SSB autoantibodies are at risk of having a child with congenital heart block.[85] In these women, the risk of congenital heart block in future pregnancies is about 10% to 20%.[88]

Neonatal lupus may or may not increase one's chance for developing SLE. Some reports suggest no increase beyond the risk conferred by family tendency.[84,89] Others report a general increased risk of autoimmunity.[86,88]

SECTION VI: VASCULAR BIRTHMARKS

▐ INFANTILE HEMANGIOMAS

Infantile hemangiomas are the most common benign tumors of childhood. Female and fairer-skinned newborns are most commonly affected, and the incidence of these lesions overall has been on the rise.[90] Recently, a study reviewing the National Hospital Discharge Survey (NHDS) newborn database from 1979 to 2006 confirmed that female, Caucasian patients remain the most commonly affected. Girls had a 1.43 times greater risk of infantile hemangioma than boys. Caucasians had a 1.5,

1.8, and 3.6 times greater risk than African Americans, Asians, and Native Americans, respectively. Interestingly, although the incidence is rising in Caucasians, the same is not true in skin of color newborns.[91] An important limitation to this study is that most hemangiomas will not develop or be detected prior to hospital discharge.

In 2002, a retrospective chart review of 327 patients demonstrated that Hispanic patients were more likely to have segmental lesions than Caucasians (30% vs 16%, respectively) and all other population groups combined (30% vs 15%, respectively). Additionally, Hispanics were found to have a much higher association with PHACE (posterior cranial fossa malformations, facial hemangiomas, arterial anomalies, aortic coarctaion and other cardiac defects, and eye abnormalities) syndrome and a significantly higher rate of complications. Hispanics also demonstrated slightly higher rates of mucosal involvement, and a larger number of patients needed to be treated with systemic medication.[92]

SECTION VII: PIGMENTARY DISEASES

VITILIGO

Vitiligo (formerly vitiligo vulgaris) is a chronic loss of pigmentation that is usually considered autoimmune in nature due to the association with personal and family history of autoimmune diseases in individuals with generalized variants of vitiligo. The incidence of vitiligo is 0.5% to 2% of the worldwide population.[93-96] Vitiligo can begin at any age, although about 50% of patients develop lesions before the age of 20 and 25% before the age of 8.[97,98] A Chinese population-based study of 17,345 individuals identified the incidence of vitiligo as 0.56% of the population, 0.71% in men and 0.45% women. Children in the first decade of life (0 to 9 years) had a prevalence of 0.1% and children in the second decade (10 to 19 years) had a prevalence of 0.36%; 64% of all cases occur prior to the age of 20 years in China. One of the lowest incidences reported to date was in an Egyptian cohort of 2194 children from the Sinai Desert, where only 0.18% of children developed vitiligo. Females were more likely to develop vitiligo. In 10 to 19 year olds, the incidence was 0.23% in males and 0.52% in females,[99] corroborating historic data indicating that vitiligo of childhood is more common in females.[100,101]

Many genetic and environmental factors contribute to vitiligo development, but no specific differences in genetic origin have been noted based on race although this may be discerned in the near future.[102-104] Vitiligo is a polygenic or multifactorial disease, with 23% twin concordance.[105-108] Pigmentation genes (eg, *TYR, OCA2* and its transcription downregulator *HERC2, MC1R*), major histocompatibility complex (MHC) genes (HLA-A*02:01),[109] and T-cell (autoreactive T-cell cytotoxicity)[110] and B-cell (autoantibody production and cellular adjuvants of T cells) genes have been linked to vitiligo development (*CTLA4, BACH2, CD44, IKZF4, LNK*).[111] Oxidative stress,[112] innate immunity (eg, *NLRP-1*, formerly *NALP-1*), genes that affect apoptosis (*CASP7*), polymorphisms in genes that regulate anti-inflammatory activity, including glutathione *S*-transferase[113] and the vitamin D receptor, and final promotion of melanocyte cell death via keratinocytes,[114,115] will cause melanocytorrhagy (poor cellular attachment of melanocytes, resulting in extreme susceptibility to the Koebner phenomenon),[116] promoting cellular apoptosis or other forms of cellular death of the melanocyte.[117] Vitiligo can also be exacerbated by chemical exposures, termed *chemical vitiligo* or *chemical leukoderma* chemical vitiligo is not uncommonly seen in teenagers who might use chemicals to cover up the vitiliginous areas.[118]

There are several variants of vitiligo: generalized, segmental, acrofacial, mucosal, and universal [**Figure 84-5**]. The diagnosis is usually made clinically, with Wood's lamp highlighting for confirmation; however, biopsy can be performed in atypical cases, confirming absence of melanocytes in the affected areas. Generalized disease or nonsegmental vitiligo appears in intertriginous areas, over bony prominences, or in the periorificial regions of the body. Localization to orifices, fingertips, toes, and genitalia is not uncommon. Trichrome vitiligo is a variant most commonly noted in children or young adults with skin types III

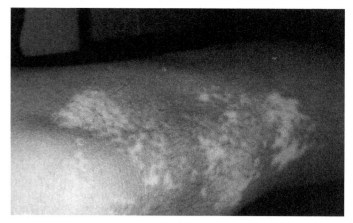

FIGURE 84-5. This Hispanic teenage male is experiencing good perifollicular repigmentation of his vitiligo with topical clobetasol.

to V, in whom a combination of partially and fully depigmented skin on a normally pigmented background is seen.[119] Commonly involved sites that are underreported include the oral mucosa and the palms and soles, leading to extension onto the face and dorsal extremities. Slow depigmentation will occur over a lifetime, some say due to friction, causing gradual extension in involved regions. Universal depigmentation can occur but is rare.[120]

Segmental vitiligo cases account for a third of childhood cases, and 87% of cases occur by age 20 years, appearing as depigmentation usually with poliosis and rapidly spreading across a broad Blaschkoid segment of the skin.[121] Worldwide, children with segmental vitiligo have not been reported to develop thyroid disease, whereas 10.7% to 26% of children with generalized vitiligo have thyroid abnormalities.[122-125] Occasional overlap exists, in which case children should be treated in a similar manner as those with nonsegmental disease. Halo nevi and poliosis can be clues to this conversion.[126,127] Thyroid disease, as measured by thyroid-stimulating hormone, triiodothyronine and/or thyroxine, and anti-TPO antibodies, was found to correlate with disease location on the upper extremities in one study, but this was not corroborated in a survey-based study of U.S. children. The upper extremities are an uncommon site of segmental disease, which is usually truncal, facial, or located on the hip/lower extremities, further supporting the idea that nonsegmental vitiligo, rather than segmental disease, is associated with thyroid autoimmunity.[128]

Particularly in patients with skin of color, the disease can be quite disfiguring, resulting in long-term psychosocial consequences.[129,130]

Psychological impairment affects 51.1% of children with vitiligo, with 13% of children and adolescents with disease experiencing severe impairments and even 10.7% of children with less than 25% body surface are a involvement having moderate to severe deficits in their quality-of-life scores on the Children's Dermatology Life Quality Index.[130]

It is especially important to consider that early therapy (before 5 years of disease duration) is most effective, using tacrolimus[131] and most other treatments. Many parents may wish to defer therapy because their child is not bothered by the lesions. However, a recent study demonstrated that although 45.6% of children aged 0 to 6 years and 50% of children aged 7 to 14 years are not bothered by their lesions, only 4.1% of teenagers (age 15 to 18 years) feel similarly. Therefore, it is reasonable to initiate therapy early in an effort to reduce self-consciousness at a later date. Because facial and leg lesions seem to be most associated with self-consciousness, these sites should be addressed early. These children are also at risk for bullying and teasing, especially when the face is involved.[127,129,132] Cosmetic camouflage can be quite important for some children.[133] Psychotherapy may help children cope with their disease.[134] Data that indicate whether children of color have more or less psychological distress with the disease are lacking.

A second autoimmune disease will strike 8.4% of children with vitiligo, especially thyroid disease, rheumatoid arthritis (1.1%), psoriasis (1.1%), and alopecia areata (0.8%).[135] Other reports outside the United States have associated childhood vitiligo with celiac disease, Addison disease, and pemphigus vulgaris.[136,137,138]

Therapies can work via rescue of damaged pigment cells, control of the autoimmune inflammatory process, free radical quenching and reduction of oxidative damage, and induction of repigmentation through melanocyte reservoirs (eg, hair bulbs). Vitiligo is an inflammatory disorder even if inflammation is not visible to the naked eye.[139]

Topical therapies include tacrolimus ointment, a calcineurin inhibitor. Tacrolimus can be used on genitalia and the face, especially the eyelids, because it does not cause atrophy or glaucoma that corticosteroids might. Results are often excellent for focal disease, especially on the head and neck.[140,141] Tacrolimus is more effective in patients with Fitzpatrick skin types III and IV.[142] In one study, children were nine times more likely to have a good response than adults with vitiligo, with a 76.92% response rate in segmental disease.[143]

Treatment with topical tacrolimus should be initiated as soon as possible, because use after 5 years of active disease reduces efficacy. This has been confirmed in both American mixed racial and Thai cohorts.[143]

Tacrolimus 0.1% ointment has been shown to be as effective as clobetasol propionate 0.05% for head and neck vitiligo lesions in children (age 2 to 16 years), but clobetasol is superior on the body.[144] Calcipotriene 0.005% ointment nightly can enhance corticosteroid results.[145,146] Limitation due to atrophy suggests that a class II topical corticosteroid may be safer than clobetasol for long-term use. Topical tacrolimus has a black box warning against use before 2 years of age because of a theoretical risk of malignancy.

Pimecrolimus 1% cream can also be used for facial lesions with some success. It is better accepted than tacrolimus ointment by many because of its cream base. A Turkish cohort randomized children with vitiligo to receive either mometasone 0.1% cream or pimecrolimus 1% cream. At 3 months, 65% and 42% of patients experienced repigmentation, respectively, but mometasone 0.1% cream (a class IV corticosteroid) worked best on the body.[147] Pimecrolimus 1% cream may be significantly more effective when paired with either microdermabrasion preceding the pimecrolimus application or excimer laser adjunctively.[148,149]

NB-UVB (311 to 313 nm) phototherapy, has shown varying degrees of success,[150,151] but no controlled studies have been conducted in children, and no current recommendations exist as to the duration of treatment and safe cumulative dose. Psoralen plus UVA is generally not used in children given the higher side effect profile; in adults, NB-UVB has been shown to be as effective as PUVA. Excimer laser (308 nm) can selectively treat patches of vitiligo while sparing the surrounding skin from UV exposure. A study of 17 patients under the age of 18 treated with an excimer laser for a duration of 2 months to 1.8 years demonstrated >50% repigmentation.[152,153] Combining this treatment with a calcineurin inhibitor may enhance its effect.[154] Surgical interventions are reserved for special cases of segmental or localized vitiligo that have been unresponsive to conventional treatments.

ACROPIGMENTATION OF DOHI

Acropigmentation of Dohi, also known as dyschromatosis symmetrica hereditaria and symmetrical dyschromatosis, is a rare genetic disorder with autosomal dominant inheritance[155,156] with high penetrance.[157] There have also been reports of recessive inheritance.[157-159] The gene identified in acropigmentation of Dohi is adenosine deaminase acting on RHA 1 (ADAR1).[158] Most cases of acropigmentation of Dohi in the literature detail patients from Japan, but patients from other places, like India, have also been reported.[155,156]

Characteristically, the depigmentation is mottled, patchy, and reticulated. The dyspigmentation is most commonly limited to the dorsal hands and dorsal feet. However, it may also appear on the arms and legs. The pigmentation begins before the age of 6 years. The pigmentation spreads to the extremities only in 50% of those affected. The other 50% also have involvement of the face. By adolescence, the total amount

of skin involvement is solidified, remains stable, and is permanent.[157,158] The differential diagnosis includes Dowling-Degos disease, reticulate pigmentation of Kitamura, dyschromatosis universalis hereditaria, and xeroderma pigmentosa.

In 1986, Taki et al[159] performed a thin split-skin graft procedure where a graft was harvested from their patient's abdomen and applied to recipient sites on the dorsal hands. At 13 months follow-up, there was no clinical evidence of the dyschromatosis symmetrica hereditaria reoccurring in the recipient sites.[159] This condition is genetic and not preventable. The skin involvement remains stable after adolescence, but there are reports of patients developing dystonia and mental deterioration.[157]

COLE SYNDROME

Cole syndrome, also known as dyskeratosis congenita of Zinsser-Cole-Engman, Zinsser-Cole-Engman syndrome, dyskeratosis congenita, Hoyeraal-Hreidarsson syndrome, or Revesz syndrome, results from defects in DKC1 (X-linked), which codes for dyskerin, TERC (autosomal dominant), which codes for mRNA for telomeres, TERT (autosomal dominant), which codes for telomerase enzyme, and NOP10 (autosomal recessive). These four genes only account for 40% of the people with Cole syndrome.[160] NHP2, TIN2, C16orf57, and TCAB1 genes may also cause Cole syndrome. Patients with Cole syndrome have short telomeres and difficulty properly maintaining the telomeres.[161]

Patients with Cole syndrome have dystrophic nails, oral leukoplakia, and reticulated hyperpigmentation of the face, neck, and shoulders. Other organ systems affected include the gastrointestinal, dental, genitourinary, neurologic, pulmonary, ophthalmic, and skeletal systems. The presenting findings are most commonly reticulated hyperpigmentation and nail dystrophy. The most life-threatening feature of this syndrome is bone marrow failure, which usually appears in early adulthood. Half of Cole syndrome patients develop aplastic anemia by the time they are 20 years old, and most patients will have bone marrow failure by age 30 years. Specific early childhood variants exist; these are called Hoyeraal-Hreidarsson syndrome and Revesz syndrome. Those with Hoyeraal-Hreidarsson syndrome demonstrate low T and B cells during childhood.[162]

The diagnosis can be made when the classic clinical findings are present, despite the patient having no hematologic abnormality. However, in a patient with hematologic abnormalities without the classic clinical findings, flow cytometry with fluorescence in situ hybridization can be used to evaluate the length of the telomeres in leukocytes. Unlike other acquired forms of aplastic anemia, the telomeres are short in all subsets of leukocytes in patients with Cole syndrome.[162]

The differential diagnosis includes graft-versus-host disease and Rothmund-Thomson syndrome. The treatment of choice is stem cell transplantation from a matched sibling. Alternative treatments for those with hematopoietic dysfunction that have shown varied success include androgens with or without granulocyte colony-stimulating factor.[160]

The prognosis is grim. While those with autosomal dominant inheritance have milder disease, whereas those with X-linked inherited disease have a severe course. Neuropsychiatry problems are more common in patients with dyskeratosis congenital.[162] Patients usually succumb to aplastic anemia, failed bone marrow transplant, or malignancies. There is a risk of head, neck, oropharyngeal, and gastrointestinal system cancers and squamous cell carcinomas.[160]

ERYTHEMA DYSCHROMICUM PERSTANS

Erythema dyschromicum perstans (EDP), also known as ashy dermatosis, or los cientos is uncommon.[163] EDP, a pigmentation disorder, most commonly affects the young adult population in patients of color.[163,164] However, pediatric cases have been reported. EDP was initially described in South Americans and most commonly affects Hispanics. It has also been reported in people of other racial groups including those of African descent, Caucasians, Asians, and East Indians.[164] Prepubertal cases are more common in Caucasians compared with Hispanics.[164,165] No sex predilection has been found in children, but in adults, the disease is more common in females.[164,166]

Some cases of EDP have followed exposure to pharmaceutical drugs, infections, ammonium nitrate, intestinal parasites, oral contrast media, cobalt, and chlorothalonil, among others, but the exact cause of EDP is unknown.[164,166] Genetic susceptibility also likely plays a role.[166]

In EDP, the clinical hue of the 0.5- to 3-cm macules and patches is slate gray to blue.[166] The slate gray oval macules, patches, and plaques begin on the trunk and spread centrifugally, also affecting the extremities.[164] The lesions may also be polycyclic or irregularly shaped.[166] When the lesions first appear, they are often surrounded by erythema, but the erythema resolves as lesions expand. Not only may the border of the lesion be erythematous, but it may also be elevated. Although the histologic pattern of EDP itself is nonspecific, skin biopsy can help distinguish EDP from other pigment disorders. The differential diagnosis includes extensive fixed drug eruption, lichen planus, lichen planus pigmentosus, lichen planus-like drug eruption, incontinentia pigmenti, pinta, Addison disease, contact dermatitis, hemochromatosis, and leprosy.[164-166]

EDP is difficult to treat and often lasts for many years in adults, whereas it often resolves after 2 to 3 years in children.[164,165] Treatments that have been tried for EDP include clofazimine, dapsone, antibiotics, corticosteroids, chemical peels, vitamins, tetracyclines, antihistamines, griseofulvin, isoniazid, chloroquine, and psychotherapy.[163] Photoprotection is essential in preventing further darkening of the lesions. The exact etiology of EDP is unknown.

EDP may pose a significant cosmetic problem for those affected. However, EDP does not lead to any systemic abnormalities.

MELANONYCHIA STRIATA

Melanonychia striata (childhood longitudinal melanonychia) is a longitudinal pigmentation of the nail plate emanating from the matrix through the full nail in a linear fashion. Although very common in Asian and African American adults (especially over the age of 50 years) as well as in Hispanic patients, this finding is not generally noted until patients are older and nail trauma becomes more prominent with sports-related activity and use of occlusive footwear. In a Chinese study, the appearance of melanonychia striata was not noted under the age of 20 years and was seen in 0.6% of patients aged 20 to 29 and 1.7% of patients aged 50 or older.[167] Therefore, adolescents may be more likely to suffer from this condition. The following are reasons to biopsy the matrix to rule out melanocytic neoplasm (including melanoma): solitary lesion, black or variegate coloration, 6 mm or greater in width, changing, and/or Hutchinson sign.[168] Lesions should be followed carefully in patients with skin of color to detect early malignancies, because acral melanomas are more common in patients with skin of color, especially those with dark skin of color. Clues that suggest the banality of a lesion are light tan color, multiple lesions, presence of family history, and bilaterality.[168] Dermoscopy of the nail plate generally shows fine striate color in regular bands; however, when pigmentation of the nail bed at the free margin of the nail is noted, melanocytic neoplasm is more likely.[169,170]

SECTION VIII: TRAUMATIC

CUPPING AND COINING (CAO GIO)

A child with erythematous annular patches or linear streaks will cause alarm in any provider unfamiliar with the cultural practice of cupping. Heated cups are placed on the skin.[171] As the air within the cup cools, suction occurs. The skin under the cup may become edematous, and then ecchymoses appear.[48,172] If medical providers are unsure if the lesions they observe are consistent with this cultural practice, a culturally competent pediatric dermatologist or child abuse team may be consulted for swift confirmation. Cao gio is a form of folk medicine

practiced by Southeast Asians. The healers are practicing traditional folk medicine when they rub a coin or a spoon heated in oil on an ill child's neck, spine, and ribs. The practice usually causes linear purpura or ecchymoses but can cause a burn or abrasion. Both of these practices can be mistaken for child abuse.[173]

SECTION IX: HAIR DISORDERS

TRICHORRHEXIS NODOSA

Trichorrhexis nodosa is a hair shaft anomaly in which broomstick deformity occurs in the hair shaft causing brittle hair and breakage at the site of the deformity. While trichorrhexis nodosa can be seen in several genodermatoses, the condition can also be acquired. Acquired proximal trichorrhexis nodosa has been described in skin of color patients as fragile, easily breakable hair that clinically resembles hair that has been cut very close to the scalp, without evidence of alopecia or hair loss. Large areas of the scalp can be involved, often the occiput or frontal scalp, but not the entire scalp. This condition is likely related to chemical, thermal, or mechanical hair treatments and can occur even after years of hair processing with no adverse effects. The hair breakage can also persist for years after the discontinuation of traumatic hair processing. An underlying genetic susceptibility has been suggested.[174] Diagnosis can be made via clipped hair mounts or through trichoscopy of hair in vivo for lighter skinned patients or via dermoscopy of clipped hairs against a white background.[175]

BUBBLE HAIRS

Bubble hair occurs in people of all races. In children of African descent, various techniques are used to help with hair manageability. Due to tightly coiled hair shafts, braids, chemical relaxers, and heat are often used to straighten the hair shafts for ease of hair styling in children and adults. Bubble hair, with air-filled spaces in the hair shaft, is caused by the application of thermal heat to the hair shaft. The bubbles in the hair shaft are filled with a gas. The heat may be delivered by an overheating blow dryer, curling iron, or flat iron. Blow dryers operating at ≥175°C may cause bubble hair.[176]

Clinical examination may reveal dry, wiry, coarse, lusterless hair or areas of alopecia due to hair breakage.[176,177] Trichorrhexis nodosa and trichoptilosis may also be present. Bubbles are visible on light microscopy, while electron microscopy demonstrates loss of cortical and medulla cells at the affected sites along the hair shaft.[178] The differential diagnosis includes trichorrhexis nodosa, trichoptilosis, and monilethrix.

Cutting off the damaged hair may be a quick fix. However, without proper prevention practices like limiting the amount or temperature of heat applied to the hair shaft, bubble hair may recur. Patients should be advised to avoid prolonged exposure to hot dryers and curling irons.[177] Detwiler et al[176] suggest that hair trapped in the coils of hair dryers contributes to overheating of the hair dryer. Hair dryer coils should be free of hair and free of any obstruction. Bubble hair is an acquired hair shaft abnormality. New hair, unexposed to the heat necessary to form bubble hair, inherently will not have the bubble hair abnormality.

HYPERTRICHOSIS

A child's genetic predisposition drives the amount of normal hair that is present. Some ethnic groups like Hispanics and those of Indian descent commonly have a higher density of body hair. A study performed on 422 Caucasian girls and 434 African American girls revealed that 8.9% and 48.8%, respectively, were observed to have upper lip hair. The limitation highlighted in the study concerned whether the authors found more hair on the upper lips of African American girls because it was just easier to see.[179]

Hypertrichosis, unlike nonidiopathic hirsutism, is not driven by androgens. In addition to genetic predisposition, hypertrichosis may be caused by medications.[180]

Newborns are often covered with soft, fine lanugo hair. As newborns mature, the lanugo hair is reduced and replaced with body

TABLE 84-1 Causes of hypertrichosis in childhood[225-231]

Excess hair
Localized acquired hypertrichosis (eg, following cast application, corticosteroid use)
Congenital
    Lanugo hypertrichosis
    Hypertrichosis lanuginosa
    Mucopolysaccharidosis
    Congenital hypothyroidism
    Vellus hypertrichosis
    Ambras syndrome
    Terminal hair hypertrichosis
    X-linked dominant hypertrichosis
Genetic defect
    Trisomy
    Turner syndrome
    Bloom syndrome
    Cornelia de Lange syndrome
    Hypertrichosis cubiti
    Coffin-Siris syndrome
    Rubinstein-Taybi syndrome
    Seckel syndrome
    Cerebro-oculofacioskeletal syndrome
        Gorlin syndrome
        Schinzel Giedion midface retraction syndrome
    Barber Say syndrome

site-dependent vellus and terminal hairs. The differential diagnosis is reviewed in **Table 84-1.**

After establishing an underlying diagnosis, some patients or parents may seek cosmetic improvement. On a patient-by-patient basis, hair removal methods may be explored. Lasers, including the long-pulse alexandrite (755 nm) with cooling, long-pulse Nd:YAG (1064 nm) with cooling, and long-pulse ruby (694 nm), have been used successfully in treating children.[181] Children are at risk for the well-known potential side effects of lasers including, burns, discomfort, postinflammatory pigment alteration, and damage to the eyes. The child's Fitzpatrick skin type should determine the specific laser chosen and settings. To increase pediatric patient comfort, topical anesthetics are often used. However, care must be taken to abide by dosage guidelines to avoid systemic side effects.[182]

Depilatories are commonly used among adults, but have also been used in children with hypertrichosis. Irritation is a potential side effect, and therefore, a test spot should be performed. Increasing the time between depilatory applications will also decrease irritation. Topical hydrocortisone may be applied following the depilatory treatment to reduce irritation.[183]

TRACTION ALOPECIA

Traction alopecia typically presents as thinning at the temporal and frontal regions of the scalp and represents years of prolonged tension on the hair, typically from tight hairstyles such as braiding. In early stages, the traction can also cause an associated folliculitis. This preventable condition, if recognized early, can be corrected by discontinuing the tight hairstyles and removing the tension and pull on the hair follicle. Full regrowth can be demonstrated within months. However, if these practices continue into adulthood, the perifollicular inflammation can lead to permanent scar formation. In these cases, treatment with intralesional steroid injections may be helpful to prevent further scarring.[174]

Alopecia areata, particularly the ophiasis pattern, is the main differential diagnosis of traction alopecia. These conditions can occasionally be distinguished by the presence of terminal hairs still present in the affected areas of patients with traction alopecia.[184] A hybrid variant termed football-shaped alopecia has been described as a localized ovoid (football-shaped) area of alopecia areata in the midline anterior crown. Often this hair loss is permanent. This is hypothesized to be due to follicular damage initiated by traction.[185] Dermoscopy may identify yellow bodies at the hair follicle in alopecia areata, discerning these two etiologies.[186]

SECTION X: INFECTIONS

TINEA CAPITIS

Tinea capitis (known as ringworm in the vernacular) is a dermatophyte infection of the hairs and scalp. Although tinea capitis can affect any age group, children between the ages of 3 and 11 years are the most likely to develop disease. Tinea capitis is more common in Hispanic children and those with dark skin of color, such as African American children, although Asian and Caucasian children may also develop disease if exposed.[187,188] Mothers and caretakers of small children with tinea capitis may also develop disease. In the United States, *Trichophyton tonsurans* is the most common dermatophyte to cause tinea capitis.[188] This dermatophyte was introduced in the United States from Puerto Rico and Latin America in the 1970s. Prior to the 1970s, most tinea capitis was caused by highly inflammatory zoonotic dermatophytes that fluoresced under Wood lamp. From 1974 to 1994, a rise in the number of *T. tonsurans* cases in San Francisco, California, was reported.[188] *T. tonsurans*, which causes an endothrix, does not fluoresce and is found only in humans. *T. tonsurans* is not severely inflammatory, in most cases, and now accounts for more than 90% of the cases in the United States.[187] It has also become the leading etiology in most developed nations.

There is a belief that many hairstyling cultural practices contribute to the increased rate of tinea capitis in African American and Hispanic children.[189] Application of oils, pomades, and grease to the scalp and infrequent washing are some of the practices that contributed to this belief. However, in multivariate analysis, the application of oil or grease and specific hairstyles such as braids, pony tails, or natural hairstyling did not increase the rate of tinea capitis infection in African Americans. In fact, use of conditioners was noted to be of potential benefit for prevention.[190] Hair oils are popular in Asian culture. Some of the oils used in Asian culture like amla oil, mustard oil, and coconut oil decrease dermatophyte infections.[191] Similarly, pomades with selenium sulfide may be of benefit for prevention of disease.

The presentations of tinea capitis caused by *T. tonsurans* are usually noninflammatory including seborrhea-like symptoms of hyperkeratosis. Noninflammatory changes include black dots from broken hairs and alopecia sometimes mimicking alopecia areata. Inflammatory findings such as kerions, pustules, erythema, and nuchal lymph nodes may also be noted.[192] In the African American community, the seborrheic dermatitis-like presentation may be "treated" with the applications of oil, pomade, or grease. This may lead to delayed presentation for care or obscure a clinician's recognition of the underlying tinea capitis during examination. Secondary findings may include id reactions, which consist of skin-colored fine papules and occipital lymphadenopathy.[193] Silent carriage can be noted and may account for transmission in households.

Occipital lymphadenopathy is an important diagnostic finding. In one study, 100 consecutive children (98 of whom were African American) who presented to a pediatric clinic with alopecia, scaling of the scalp, occipital lymphadenopathy, or pruritus underwent a scalp fungal culture. The scalp fungal cultures were positive in 68 of the children. Fifty-five children presented with alopecia and occipital lymphadenopathy. These 55 children were all found to have positive fungal cultures. Sixty of the 62 children (96.7%) who presented with scaling and occipital lymphadenopathy had positive fungal cultures. Of 100 children, only one child without adenopathy or alopecia had a positive fungal culture. Those who did not present with either scaling or occipital lymphadenopathy did not have positive fungal cultures.[194] Similarly, Coley et al[195] noted that when alopecia and hyperkeratosis of the scalp are noted (especially in children of color), there is an 82.1% chance that tinea capitis is present and oral antifungals should be started empirically. Alopecia alone in the absence of hyperkeratosis or lymphadenopathy had a less than 25% chance of being tinea capitis even in children of color but merits screening culture just the same.[195]

A scalp fungal culture should be performed for suspected tinea capitis. Use of a cotton-tipped applicator rubbed over the scalp and then onto media is the best technique for obtaining culture specimen. Pulling hairs or cutting hairs would include healthy uninfected hairs and can reduce specimen yield and be painful.[196] If there is a suppurative inflammatory reaction present, as in the setting of kerion, it is appropriate to perform a bacterial culture to rule out a bacterial superinfection. Potassium hydroxide 20% preparation can be used in office to identify hyphae in keratinocytes and spores in hairs. For patients using antifungal shampoos or pomades, spores can still be identified in fungal shafts. Calcofluor white can also be used as a preparation to identify fungi in scalp scrapings.

Wood's lamps were frequently used to examine the scalp of a person with suspected tinea capitis because zoonotic fluorescing *Microsporum* species (*Microsporum canis* and *Microsporum audouinii*) were the leading cause of infection in the United States in the 1950s. However, *T. tonsurans*, the most common cause of tinea capitis in the United States, does not fluoresce.[197] Kerions and inflammatory tinea capitis may still be caused by *Microsporum* species, and fluorescing the scalp with a Wood's lamp may be helpful in that setting. *M. canis* fluoresces white and *M. audouinii* fluoresces blue-green.[198]

Dermoscopy of the scalp may reveal comma-shaped hairs or corkscrew hairs.[199] Tinea capitis can be mistaken for a variety of other inflammatory conditions including atopic dermatitis, seborrheic dermatitis, alopecia areata, discoid lupus erythematosus, white piedra, bacterial infections, and favus.

To ensure treatment of all the keratinized hair extending into the follicles, systemic treatment is necessary to eradicate tinea capitis. **Table 84-2** outlines general systemic treatment guidelines. Griseofulvin has proven to be more efficacious for *Microsporum* species than terbinafine, whereas terbinafine is more efficacious for *Trichophyton* species.[200] In a study of 84 pediatric patients in New York City, the response rate to an initial course of griseofulvin treatment was 76%.[201] Second-line therapy options include crushed ultramicronized griseofulvin tablets, terbinafine sprinkles, itraconazole, and fluconazole.[195-197,200] In children with severe kerions, an oral prednisolone course may be necessary to decrease profound inflammation and possibly decrease the chances of permanent alopecia. Although griseofulvin is the gold standard, the bioavailability of griseofulvin is poor and can be enhanced by concurrent ingestion of fatty foods.

Prevention begins with avoidance of sharing hats, combs, brushes, and pillowcases. All such items should be washed or replaced weekly during active infection. Conditioners may be of benefit at prevention of tinea capitis and should be used for household contacts. Antifungal shampoos can be used for patients with tinea capitis and their household contacts to decrease transmissible fungal spores.[202] Adults, especially African American women,[203] with papulosquamous scalp disease and or alopecia should have scalp fungal cultures performed. Although

children are the most commonly affected by tinea capitis, consider undiagnosed adults in the home who many have tinea capitis in families with multiple episodes of tinea capitis.

Children diagnosed with tinea capitis may return to school after instituting systemic treatment. However, those engaged in contact sports with a lot of skin to skin contact, like wrestling or judo, require special "return to play" instructions. According to the National Collegiate Athletic Association and the National Federation of State High School Associations, athletes should only return to play after 2 weeks of systemic treatment.[204] Alternatively, use of a stocking cap or bandana to cover the contagious area may be of benefit.

Tinea capitis is a benign condition. The alopecia associated with tinea capitis is usually temporary and typically nonscarring. However, permanent alopecia may occur following extensive cases of kerion. Recurrence and reinfection are not uncommon, and vigilance in monitoring for signs of disease (especially hyperkeratosis and alopecia) is required even after successful therapy.

■ TINEA VERSICOLOR

Tinea versicolor is an overgrowth of *Malassezia* species in the seborrheic distribution, usually over the chest, back, and shoulders; uncommon sites of involvement include face, neck, forearms, lower back, groin, and inner thighs. Tinea versicolor is rarely seen in dark-skinned infants, with most cases occurring seasonally in warm weather in adolescence through young adulthood. Significant hypopigmentation and/or hyperpigmentation can be seen in adolescents of color. Therapy involves topical agents such as selenium sulfide or topical azole antifungals and, in more extensive cases, brief courses of oral antifungals. Continued use of weekly lotion or shampoo applications can be helpful at preventing recurrence in warmer months. Tanning while infected is ill advised due to aggravation of color disparity.

■ WHITE PIEDRA

White piedra (trichosporosis) is a superficial fungal/saprophytic yeast infection caused by *Trichosporon* species.[205,206] *Trichosporon* are found in soil, water, air, animal feces, and sewage.[207] Most cases of white piedra occur in tropical regions, but it can occur in any country, regardless of climate. Transmission to humans occurs, but the exact mechanism is unknown.[205-207]

Increased incidence of white piedra has been noted in patients who frequently use head coverings. Shivaprakash et al[207] suggest that the absence of hair's exposure to 'germicidal properties' of sunlight and humid temperature under head coverings may be contributory factors.

TABLE 84-2	Treatment of tinea capitis[232]			
Treatment	Dose	Course	Caveats	
First Line				
Griseofulvin microsize suspension	20–25 mg/kg/d (maximum of 500 mg twice daily)	6–8 weeks or more until fungal cultures are negative	Absorbs better with fatty foods (whole milk, eggs, cheese, ice cream)	
			Ultramicronized tablets can be used to increase bioavailability, especially in children over 50 lb	
Terbinafine	4–5 mg/kg/d 10–20 kg: 62.5 mg/d 20–40 kg: 125 mg/d >40 kg: 250 mg/d	2–4 weeks for *Trichophyton* 8–12 weeks for *Microsporum*	Sprinkles are the preferred formulation, to be poured over food once daily	
Second Line				
Fluconazole	5–6 mg/kg/d 8 mg/kg once per week	3–6 weeks 8–12 weeks		
Third Line				
Itraconazole Capsules Oral solution	5 mg/kg/d 3 mg/kg/d	3–6 weeks 8–12 weeks	Taking the medication with orange juice or iced tea may enhance absorption	

Kiken et al[205] reported eight children with white piedra, two of whom were siblings and seven of whom had long hair. Most of the children were from Latin America or the Middle East. Close contact and long hair may also be factors in developing white piedra.[205]

Upon examination of the hair shaft, white to tan/brown nodules are present. The white-tan nodules are irregularly shaped and feel gritty. Unlike pediculosis capitis and black piedra, white piedra can easily be removed from the hair shaft. White piedra may affect any hair-bearing area including the scalp, face (beard, mustache, eyebrows, eyelashes), axillae, and pubic area.[205]

Direct microscopy of the hair shaft with 10% potassium hydroxide mount helps to distinguish white piedra from pediculosis.[205,208] Hyphae and arthroconidia are visualized in white piedra.[206] White piedra does not fluoresce under Wood's lamp examination, in contrast to trichomycosis axillaris, which fluoresces coral pink. Fungal and bacterial cultures will distinguish white piedra from trichomycosis axillaris.[206]

The differential diagnosis includes pediculosis capitis, trichomycosis axillaris, monilethrix, and peripilar keratin cast.

Cutting off all of the hair is one treatment option. However, Kiken et al[205] report achieving clearance of white piedra with a combination of oral antifungals and antifungal shampoo, without cutting the hair. Therapeutic regimens that can be used include oral ketoconazole or oral fluconazole for a 1-month period accompanied by frequent use of topical ketoconazole 2% shampoo to eliminate the reservoir of fungus on the scalp. Shampoos should be continued until a month after fungal concretions have been eliminated.[205]

Trichosporon is ubiquitous in South America and the Middle East and is therefore difficult to avoid. Avoidance of sharing hats, combs, brushes, and pillowcases is the best prevention; however, the actual mode of transmission of the disease is unknown, so prevention is difficult. The prognosis is excellent. Most cases can be cleared with therapy similar to that of tinea capitis.

KELOIDS [FIGURE 84-6]

Keloids are reviewed elsewhere in this textbook; however, some specific clinical points in childhood bear review. Keloids are more common in individuals of color.[209] For children of color with a family history of keloids, careful evaluation regarding elective procedures is needed. Although younger children are less likely to form keloids, keloids can occur at any age.[209]

In the pediatric population, a complete history should be obtained. Keloids most commonly follow skin trauma; however, spontaneous keloid development may occur as a feature of a genetic syndrome like Rubstein-Taybi syndrome,[210] Dubowitz syndrome,[211] or nodular or keloidal scleroderma.[212]

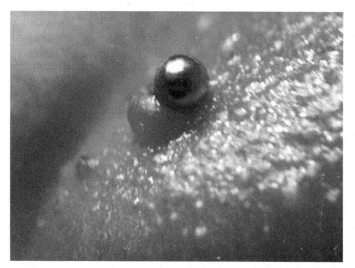

FIGURE 84-6. This 15-year-old African American girl developed a keloid adjacent to her nose piercing.

Often parents with keloids or a family history of keloids inquire about the risks of piercing their child's ears. One study found that children who pierced their ears early in life (before age 11 years) were less likely to develop keloids.[213] However, Tirgan et al[214] reported bilateral earlobe keloids in a 9-month-old child following ear piercing at age 3 months. The child had a family history of keloid development. Although early ear piercing is recommended if desired by parents, there is still no guarantee that keloids will not develop.

If keloids occur, treatments such as intralesional triamcinolone are appropriate, but special comfort measures should be taken in the pediatric population.[215] Topical numbing medication and/or distractors such as cellphone games or videos may reduce the child's anxiety about the procedure. In children who undergo surgical keloid repair, care must be taken to evaluate whether the child will be able tolerate postoperative measures (intralesional triamcinolone, pressure earrings, silicone dressings, or pressure dressings). If general anesthesia is used, the risks and benefits should be weighed.[216]

MUCOSAL PIGMENTATION

Mucosal pigmentation (also known as black gums),[217] particularly of the gingiva, is a prominent feature found in patients with skin of color (see Chapter 56).[218] The gingival and oral mucosal pigmentation often correlates with the cutaneous pigmentation.[11] In a study of 600 people of African descent, those with darkly pigmented skin were more likely to have darkly pigmented gingiva. However, many of the patients with darkly pigmented skin did not have darkly pigmented gingiva.[219,220]

Patients with this disease have confluent brown gingiva or brown patches present on gingiva. The pigmentation may even have a gray-blue hue.

The differential diagnosis includes benign pigmentation, Addison disease, Albright syndrome, blue nevi, melanocytic macule, oral melanoacanthoma, oral nevi, Peutz-Jeghers syndrome, smoker's melanosis, melanoma, and amalgam tattoo.[221]

Once underlying systemic conditions causing oral mucosal pigmentation have been excluded (eg, Addison disease), treatment options or reassurance can be discussed. Gingival hyperpigmentation in itself is not dangerous; therefore, medically, it requires no treatment.

However, adolescents or parents of children may be concerned about the cosmetic appearance. Various cosmetic techniques have been used to lighten the pigmentation of the gingiva including electrosurgery, scalpel surgical excision, surgical abrasion,[222] liquid nitrogen application,[10] and acellular dermal matrix with partial-thickness flap.[223]

Prevention is not possible if a child's mucosal pigment is due solely to the level of genetically predetermined cutaneous pigmentation. However, acquired gingival pigmentation has been seen in the children who have at least one parent who smokes.[224] In this case, limiting a child's exposure to secondhand smoke and discouraging teens from smoking may prevent not only acquired gingival pigmentation, but also exacerbation of other diseases, like asthma.

REFERENCES

1. Silverberg NB. *Atlas of Pediatric Cutaneous Biodiversity*. New York, NY: Springer, 2012.
2. Schachner LA, Hansen RG. Preface. In: Schachner LA, Hansen RC, eds. *Pediatric Dermatology*. 2nd ed. New York, NY: Churchill-Livingstone; 1995.
3. U.S. Census estimates. http://www.census.gov/compendia/statab/cats/population/estimates_and_projections_by_age_sex_raceethnicity.html. Accessed August 26, 2013.
4. Trowers A. Chapter 78: pediatric dermatology. In: Taylor S, Kelley P, eds. *Dermatology for Skin of Color*. 1st ed. New York, NY: McGraw Hill; 2009.
5. Cordova A. The Mongolian spot: a study of ethnic differences and a literature review. *Clin Pediatr (Phila)*. 1981;20:714-719.
6. Shih IH, Lin JY, Chen CH, Hong HS. A birthmark survey in 500 newborns: clinical observation in two northern Taiwan medical center nurseries. *Chang Gung Med J*. 2007;30:220-225.
7. Moosavi Z, Hosseini T. One-year survey of cutaneous lesions in 1000 consecutive Iranian newborns. *Pediatr Dermatol*. 2006;23:61-63.

8. Egemen A, Ikizoğlu T, Ergör S, Mete Asar G, Yilmaz O. Frequency and characteristics of Mongolian spots among Turkish children in Aegean region. *Turk J Pediatr.* 2006;48:232-236.

9. Rybojad M, Moraillon I, Ogier de Baulny H, Prigent F, Morel P. Extensive Mongolian spot related to Hurler disease. *Ann Dermatol Venereol.* 1999;126:35-37.

10. Sapadin AN, Friedman IS. Extensive Mongolian spots associated with Hunter syndrome. *J Am Acad Dermatol.* 1998;39:1013-1015.

11. Smalek JE. Significance of mongolian spots. *J Pediatr.* 1980;97:504.

12. Ho SG, Chan HH. The Asian dermatologic patient: review of common pigmentary disorders and cutaneous diseases. *Am J Clin Dermatol.* 2009;10:153-168.

13. Kagami S, Asahina A, Watanabe R, et al. Laser treatment of 26 Japanese patients with Mongolian spots. *Dermatol Surg.* 2008;34:1689-1694.

14. Van Praag MC, Van Rooij RW, Folkers E, Spritzer R, Menke HE, Oranje AP. Diagnosis and treatment of pustular disorders in the neonate. *Pediatr Dermatol.* 1997;14:131-143.

15. Wyre HW Jr, Murphy MO. Transient neonatal pustular melanosis. *Arch Dermatol.* 1979;115:458.

16. Ekiz O, Gül U, Mollamahmutoğlu L, Gönül M. Skin findings in newborns and their relationship with maternal factors: observational research. *Ann Dermatol.* 2013;25:1-4.

17. Kuo TT, Chan HL, Hsueh S. Clear cell papulosis of the skin. A new entity with histogenetic implications for cutaneous Paget's disease. *Am J Surg Pathol.* 1987;11:827-834.

18. Benouni S, Kos L, Ruggeri SY, North PE, Drolet BA. Clear cell papulosis in Hispanic siblings. *Arch Dermatol.* 2007;143:358-360.

19. Wysong A, Sundram U, Benjamin L. Clear-cell papulosis: a rare entity that may be misconstrued pathologically as normal skin. *Pediatr Dermatol.* 2012;29:195-198.

20. Sim JH, Do JE, Kim YC. Clear cell papulosis of the skin: acquired hypomelanosis. *Arch Dermatol.* 2011;147:128-129.

21. Tseng FW, Kuo TT, Lu PH et al. Long-term follow-up study of clear cell papulosis. *J Am Acad Dermatol.* 2009;63:266-273.

22. Foley P, Zuo Y, Plunkett A, Merlin K, Marks R. The frequency of common skin conditions in preschool-aged children in Australia: seborrheic dermatitis and pityriasis capitis (cradle cap). *Arch Dermatol.* 2003;139:318-322.

23. Williams JV, Eichenfield LF, Burke BL, Barnes-Eley M, Friedlander SF. Prevalence of scalp scaling in prepubertal children. *Pediatrics.* 2005;115:e1-e6.

24. Brodell RT, Patel S, Venglarcik JS, Moses D, Gemmel D. The safety of ketoconazole shampoo for infantile seborrheic dermatitis. *Pediatr Dermatol.* 1998;15:406-407.

25. Elish D, Silverberg NB. Infantile seborrheic dermatitis. *Cutis.* 2006;77: 297-300.

26. High WA, Pandya AG. Pilot trial of 1% pimecrolimus cream in the treatment of seborrheic dermatitis in African American adults with associated hypopigmentation. *J Am Acad Dermatol.* 2006;54:1083-1088.

27. Elewski B. An investigator-blind, randomized, 4-week, parallel-group, multicenter pilot study to compare the safety and efficacy of a nonsteroidal cream (Promiseb topical cream) and desonide cream 0.05% in the twice-daily treatment of mild to moderate seborrheic dermatitis of the face. *Clin Dermatol.* 2009;27:S48-S53.

28. Kiken DA, Silverberg NB. Atopic dermatitis in children, part 1: epidemiology, clinical features, and complications. *Cutis.* 2006;78:241-247.

29. Allen HB, Jones NP, Bowen SE. Lichenoid and other clinical presentations of atopic dermatitis in an inner city practice. *J Am Acad Dermatol.* 2008;58:503-504.

30. Julián-Gónzalez RE, Orozco-Covarrubias L, Durán-McKinster C, Palacios-Lopez C, Ruiz-Maldonado R, Sáez-de-Ocariz M. Less common clinical manifestations of atopic dermatitis: prevalence by age. *Pediatr Dermatol.* 2012;29:580-583.

31. Williams HC, Pembroke AC. Infraorbital crease, ethnic group, and atopic dermatitis. *Arch Dermatol.* 1996;132:51-54.

32. Hanifin JM, Reed ML A population-based survey of eczema prevalence in the United States. *Dermatitis.* 2007;18:82-91.

33. Janumpally SR, Feldman SR, Gupta AK, Fleischer AB Jr. In the United States, blacks and Asian/Pacific Islanders are more likely than whites to seek medical care for atopic dermatitis. *Arch Dermatol.* 2002;138:634-637.

34. Silverberg JI, Simpson EL, Durkin HG, Joks R. Prevalence of allergic disease in foreign-born American children. *JAMA Pediatr.* 2013;167:554-560.

35. Wegienka G, Havstad S, Joseph CL, et al. Racial disparities in allergic outcomes in African Americans emerge as early as age 2 years. *Clin Exp Allergy.* 2012;42:909-917.

36. Vachiramon V, Tey HL, Thompson AE, Yosipovitch G. Atopic dermatitis in African American children: addressing unmet needs of a common disease. *Pediatr Dermatol.* 2012;29:395-402.

37. Wesley NO, Maibach HI. Racial (ethnic) differences in skin properties: the objective data. *Am J Clin Dermatol.* 2003;4:843-860.

38. Hirano SA, Murray SB, Harvey VM. Reporting, representation, and subgroup analysis of race and ethnicity in published clinical trials of atopic dermatitis in the United States between 2000 and 2009. *Pediatr Dermatol.* 2012;29:749-755.

39. Fotoh C, Elkhyat A, Mac S, Sainthillier JM, Humbert P. Cutaneous differences between black, African or Caribbean mixed-race and Caucasian women: biometrological approach of the hydrolipidic film. *Skin Res Technol.* 2008;14:327-335.

40. Eichenfield LF, Lucky AW, Langley RG, et al. Use of pimecrolimus cream 1% (Elidel) in the treatment of atopic dermatitis in infants and children: the effects of ethnic origin and baseline disease severity on treatment outcome. *Int J Dermatol.* 2005;44:70-75.

41. Kim KH, Kono T. Overview of efficacy and safety of tacrolimus ointment in patients with atopic dermatitis in Asia and other areas. *Int J Dermatol.* 2011;50:1153-1161.

42. Silverberg NB. *Atlas of Pediatric Cutaneous Biodiversity.* New York, NY: Springer; 2013:83-85.

43. Silverberg NB, Licht J, Friedler S, Sethi S, Laude TA. Nickel contact hypersensitivity in children. *Pediatr Dermatol.* 2002;19:110-113.

44. Wu JJ, Black MH, Smith N, Porter AH, Jacobsen SJ, Koebnick C. Low prevalence of psoriasis among children and adolescents in a large multiethnic cohort in southern California. *J Am Acad Dermatol.* 2011;65:957-964.

45. Silverberg NB. Pediatric psoriasis: an update. *Ther Clin Risk Manag.* 2009;5:849-856.

46. McMichael AJ, Vachiramon V, Guzmán-Sánchez DA, Camacho F. Psoriasis in African-Americans: a caregivers' survey. *J Drugs Dermatol.* 2012;11:478-482.

47. Silverberg NB. *Atlas of Pediatric Cutaneous Biodiversity.* New York, NY: Springer; 2013:53-58.

48. Chiam LY, de Jager ME, Giam YC, de Jong EM, van de Kerkhof PC, Seyger MM.

49. Juvenile psoriasis in European and Asian children: similarities and differences. *Br J Dermatol.* 2011;164:1101-1103.

50. Tyring S, Mendoza N, Appell M, et al. A calcipotriene/betamethasone dipropionate two-compound scalp formulation in the treatment of scalp psoriasis in Hispanic/Latino and Black/African American patients: results of the randomized, 8-week, double-blind phase of a clinical trial. *Int J Dermatol.* 2010;49:1328-1333.

51. Shah SK, Arthur A, Yang YC, Stevens S, Alexis AF. A retrospective study to investigate racial and ethnic variations in the treatment of psoriasis with etanercept. *J Drugs Dermatol.* 2011;10:866-872.

52. Watanabe T, Kawamura T, Jacob SE, et al. Pityriasis rosea is associated with systemic active infection with both human herpesvirus-7 and human herpesvirus-6. *J Invest Dermatol.* 2002;119:793-797.

53. Amer A, Fischer H, Li X. The natural history of pityriasis rosea in black American children. How correct is the "classic" description? *Arch Pediatr Adolesc Med.* 2007;161:503-506.

54. Vano-Galvan S, Ma DL, Lopez-Neyra A, Perez B, Muñoz-Zato E, Jaén P. Atypical pityriasis rosea in a black child: a case report. *Cases J.* 2009;2:6796.

55. Centers for Disease Control and Prevention. http://www.cdc.gov/std/stats/STI-Estimates-Fact-Sheet-Feb-2013.pdf. Accessed March 8, 2015.

56. Kabbash C, Laude TA, Weinberg JM, Silverberg NB. Lichen planus in the lines of Blaschko. *Pediatr Dermatol.* 2002;19:541-545.

57. Walton KE, Bowers EV, Drolet BA, Holland KE. Childhood lichen planus: demographics of a U.S. population. *Pediatr Dermatol.* 2010;27:34-38.

58. Silverberg NB. *Atlas of Pediatric Cutaneous Biodiversity.* New York, NY: Springer; 2013:59-60.

59. Wain EM, Orchard GE, Whittaker SJ, Spittle M, Russell-Jones R. Outcome in 34 patients with juvenile-onset mycosis fungoides. A clinical, immunophenotypic, and molecular study. *Cancer.* 2003;98:2282-2290.

60. Pope E, Weitzman S, Ngan B, et al. mycosis fungoides in the pediatric population: report from an International Childhood Registry of Cutaneous Lymphoma. *J Cutaneous Med Surg.* 2010;14:1-6.

61. Veith W, Deleo V, Silverberg N. Medical phototherapy in childhood skin diseases. *Minerva Pediatr.* 2011;63:327-333.

62. McLaurin CI. Pediatric dermatology in black patients. *Dermatol Clin.* 1988;6:457-473.

63. Lane TN, Parker SS. Pityriasis lichenoides chronica in black patients. *Cutis.* 2010;85:125-129.

64. Boccara O, Blanche S, de Prost Y, Brousse N, Bodemer C, Fraitag S. Cutaneous hematologic disorders in children. *Pediatr Blood Cancer.* 2012;58: 226-232.

65. Mancini AJ, Frieden IJ, Paller AS. Infantile acropustulosis revisited: history of scabies and response to topical corticosteroids. *Pediatr Dermatol.* 1998;15:337-341.

66. Silverberg NB. *Atlas of Pediatric Cutaneous Biodiversity.* New York, NY: Springer; 2013:19-20.

67. Eichenfield LF, Krakowski AC, Piggott C, et al. Evidence-based recommendations for the diagnosis and treatment of pediatric acne. *Pediatrics.* 2013;131:S163-S186.

68. Laude TA, Kenney JA Jr, Prose NS, et al. Skin manifestations in individuals of African or Asian descent. *Pediatr Dermatol.* 1996;13:158-168.

69. Laude TA. Approach to dermatologic disorders in black children. *Semin Dermatol.* 1995;14:15-20.

70. Taylor SC, Cook-Bolden F, Rahman Z, Strachan D. Acne vulgaris in skin of color. *J Am Acad Dermatol.* 2002;46:S98-S106.

71. Silverberg NB. A brief primer on acne therapy for adolescents with skin of color. *Cutis.* 2013;92:20-26.

72. Green B, Morrell DS. Persistent facial dermatitis: pediatric perioral dermatitis. *Pediatr Ann.* 2007;36:796-798.

73. Urbatsch AJ, Frieden I, Williams ML, Elewski BE, Mancini AJ, Paller AS. Extrafacial and generalized granulomatous periorificial dermatitis. *Arch Dermatol.* 2002;138:1354-1358.

74. Shetty AK, Gedalia A. Sarcoidosis in children. *Curr Probl Pediatr.* 2000;30:149-176.

75. Shetty AK, Gedalia A. Childhood sarcoidosis: a rare but fascinating disorder. *Pediatr Rheumatol.* 2008;6:16.

76. Pattishall EN, Strope GL, Spinola SM, Denny FW. Childhood sarcoidosis. *J Pediatr.* 1986;108:169-177.

77. Kendig EL Jr. The clinical picture of sarcoidosis in children. *Pediatrics.* 1974;54:289-292.

78. Hetherington S. Sarcoidosis in young children. *Am J Dis Child.* 1982;136:13-15.

79. Kendig EL Jr. The clinical picture of sarcoidosis in children. *Pediatrics.* 1974;54:289-292.

80. Paller AS, Mancini A. *Hurwitz Clinical Pediatric Dermatology.* 3rd ed. New York, NY: Elsevier Saunders; 2006.

81. Kamphuis S, Silverman ED. Prevalence and burden of pediatric-onset systemic lupus erythematosus. *Nat Rev Rheumatol.* 2010;6:538-546.

82. Hiraki LT, Benseler SM, Tyrrell PN, Harvey E, Hebert D, Silverman ED. Ethnic differences in pediatric systemic lupus erythematosus. *J Rheumatol.* 2009;36:2539-2546.

83. Weston WL, Morelli JG, Lee LA. The clinical spectrum of anti-Ro-positive cutaneous neonatal lupus erythematosus. *J Am Acad Dermatol.* 1999;40(5 Pt 1):675-681.

84. Neiman AR, Lee LA, Weston WL, Buyon JP. Cutaneous manifestations of neonatal lupus without heart block: characteristics of mothers and children enrolled in a national registry. *J Pediatr.* 2000;137:674-680.

85. Buyon JP, Hiebert R, Copel J, et al. Autoimmune-associated congenital heart block: demographics, mortality, morbidity and recurrence rates obtained from a national neonatal lupus registry. *J Am Coll Cardiol.* 1998;31:1658-1666.

86. Lee LA. Cutaneous lupus in infancy and childhood. *Lupus.* 2010;19:1112-1117.

87. Salomonsson S, Strandberg L. Autoantibodies associated with congenital heart block. *Scand J Immunol.* 2010;72:185-188.

88. Brucato A. Prevention of congenital heart block in children of SSA-positive mothers. *Rheumatology (Oxford).* 2008;47:35-37.

89. Martin V, Lee LA, Askanase AD, Katholi M, Buyon JP. Long-term followup of children with neonatal lupus and their unaffected siblings. *Arthritis Rheum.* 2002;46:2377-2383.

90. Haggstrom AN, Drolet BA, Baselga E, et al. Prospective study of infantile hemangiomas: demographic, prenatal, and perinatal characteristics. *J Pediatr.* 2007;150:291-294.

91. Amrock SM, Weitzman M. Diverging racial trends in neonatal infantile hemangioma diagnoses, 1979-2006. *Pediatr Dermatol.* 2013;30:493-494.

92. Chiller KG, Passaro D, Frieden IJ. Hemangiomas of infancy: clinical characteristics, morphologic subtypes, and their relationship to race, ethnicity, and sex. *Arch Dermatol.* 2002;138:1567-1576.

93. Mehta NR, Shah KC, Theodore C, et al. Epidemiological study of vitiligo in Surat area, South Gujarat. *Indian J Med Res.* 1973;61:145-154.

94. Howitz J, Brodthagen H, Schwartz M, et al. Prevalence of vitiligo. Epidemiological survey on the Isle of Bornholm, Denmark. *Arch Dermatol.* 1977;113:47-52.

95. Boisseau-Garsaud AM, Garsaud P, Cales-Quist D, et al.. Epidemiology of vitiligo in the French West Indies (Isle of Martinique). *Int J Dermatol.* 2000;39:18-20.

96. Krüger C, Schallreuter KU. A review of the worldwide prevalence of vitiligo in children/adolescents and adults. *Int J Dermatol.* 2012;51:1206-1212.

97. Lerner AB. Vitiligo. *J Invest Dermatol.* 1959;32:285-310.

98. Halder RM, Grimes PE, Cowan CA et al. Childhood vitiligo. *J Am Acad Dermatol.* 1987;16:948-954.

99. Wang X, Du J, Wang T, et al. Prevalence and clinical profile of vitiligo in China: a community-based study in six cities. *Acta Derm Venereol.* 2013;93:62-65.

100. Lerner AB. Vitiligo. *J Invest Dermatol.* 1959;32:285-310.

101. Yamamah GA, Emam HM, Abdelhamid MF, et al. Epidemiologic study of dermatologic disorders among children in South Sinai, Egypt. *Int J Dermatol.* 2012;51:1180-1185.

102. Kovacs SO. Vitiligo. *J Am Acad Dermatol.* 1998;38:647-666.

103. Lee AY, Youm YH, Kim NH, et al. Keratinocytes in the depigmented epidermis of vitiligo are more vulnerable to trauma (suction) than keratinocytes in the normally pigmented epidermis, resulting in their apoptosis. *Br J Dermatol.* 2004;151:995-1003.

104. Wang X, Erf GF. Apoptosis in feathers of Smyth line chickens with autoimmune vitiligo. *J Autoimmun.* 2004;22:21-30.

105. Sun X, Xu A, Wei X, et al. Genetic epidemiology of vitiligo: a study of 815 probands and their families from south China. *Int J Dermatol.* 2006;45:1176-1181.

106. Alkhateeb A, Fain PR, Thody A, et al. Mapping of an autoimmunity susceptibility locus (AIS1) to chromosome 1p31.3-p32.2. *Hum Mol Genet.* 2002;11:661-667.

107. Jin Y, Birlea SA, Fain PR, et al. Genome-wide association analyses identify 13 new susceptibility loci for generalized vitiligo. *Nat Genet.* 2012;44:676-680.

108. Quan C, Ren YQ, Xiang LH, et al. Genome-wide association study for vitiligo identifies susceptibility loci at 6q27 and the MHC. *Nat Genet.* 2010;42:614-618.

109. Jin Y, Ferrara T, Gowan K, et al. Next-generation DNA re-sequencing identifies common variants of TYR and HLA-A that modulate the risk of generalized vitiligo via antigen presentation. *J Invest Dermatol.* 2012;132:1730-1733.

110. Ben Ahmed M, Zaraa I, Rekik R, et al. Functional defects of peripheral regulatory T lymphocytes in patients with progressive vitiligo. *Pigment Cell Melanoma Res.* 2012;25:99-109.

111. Lin X, Tian H, Xianmin M. Possible roles of B lymphocyte activating factor of the tumour necrosis factor family in vitiligo autoimmunity. *Med Hypotheses.* 2011;76:339-342.

112. Jalel A, Yassine M, Hamdaoui MH. Oxidative stress in experimental vitiligo C57BL/6 mice. *Indian J Dermatol.* 2009;54:221-224.

113. Liu L, Li C, Gao J, et al. Genetic polymorphisms of glutathione S-transferase and risk of vitiligo in the Chinese population. *J Invest Dermatol.* 2009;129:2646-2652.

114. D'Osualdo A, Reed JC. NLRP1, a regulator of innate immunity associated with vitiligo. *Pigment Cell Melanoma Res.* 2012;25:5-8.

115. Ruiz-Argüelles A, Brito GJ, Reyes-Izquierdo P, et al. Apoptosis of melanocytes in vitiligo results from antibody penetration. *J Autoimmun.* 2007;29:281-286.

116. Kumar R, Parsad D. Melanocytorrhagy and apoptosis in vitiligo: connecting jigsaw pieces. *Indian J Dermatolog Vener Lepr.* 2012;78:19-23.

117. Wu J, Zhou M, Wan Y, Xu A. CD8+ T cells from vitiligo perilesional margins induce autologous melanocyte apoptosis. *Mol Med Rep.* 2013;7:237-241.

118. Ghosh S. Chemical leukoderma: what's new on etiopathological and clinical aspects? *Indian J Dermatol.* 2010;55:255-258.

119. Hann SK, Kim YS, Yoo JH, Chun YS. Clinical and histopathologic characteristics of trichrome vitiligo. *J Am Acad Dermatol.* 2000;42:589-596.

120. Herane MI. Vitiligo and leukoderma in children. *Clin Dermatol.* 2003;21:283-295.

121. Halder RM, Grimes PE, Cowan CA, et al. Childhood vitiligo. *J Am Acad Dermatol.* 2003;20:207-210.

122. Pagovich OE, Silverberg JI, Freilich E, Silverberg NB. Thyroid abnormalities in pediatric patients with vitiligo in New York City. *Cutis.* 2008;81:463-466.

123. Iacovelli P, Sinagra JL, Vidolin AP, et al. Relevance of thyroiditis and of other autoimmune diseases in children with vitiligo. *Dermatology.* 2005;210:26-30.

124. Prćić S, Djuran V, Katanić D, et al. Vitiligo and thyroid dysfunction in children and adolescents. *Acta Dermatovenerol Croat.* 2011;19:248-254.

125. Kakourou T, Kanaka-Gantenbein C, Papadopoulou A, Kaloumenou E, Chrousos GP. Increased prevalence of chronic autoimmune (Hashimoto's) thyroiditis in children and adolescents with vitiligo. *J Am Acad Dermatol.* 2005;53:220-223.

126. Ezzedine K, Gauthier Y, Léauté-Labrèze C, et al. Segmental vitiligo associated with generalized vitiligo (mixed vitiligo): a retrospective case series of 19 patients. *J Am Acad Dermatol.* 2011;65:965-971.

127. Silverberg N. Segmental vitiligo may not be associated with risk of autoimmune thyroiditis. *Skinmed.* 2011;9:329-330.

128. Silverberg JI, Silverberg NB. Clinical features of vitiligo associated with comorbid autoimmune disease: a prospective survey. *J Am Acad Dermatol.* 2013;69:824-826.

129. Bilgiç O, Bilgiç A, Akiş HK, Eskioğlu F, Kiliç EZ. Depression, anxiety and health-related quality of life in children and adolescents with vitiligo. *Clin Exp Dermatol.* 2011;36:360-365.

130. Silverberg JI, Silverberg NB. Association between vitiligo extent and distribution and quality-of-life impairment. *JAMA Dermatol.* 2013;149:159-164.

131. Silverberg NB, Lin P, Travis L, et al. Tacrolimus ointment promotes repigmentation of vitiligo in children: a review of 57 cases. *J Am Acad Dermatol.* 2004;51:760-766.

132. Choi S, Kim DY, Whang SH, et al. Quality of life and psychological adaptation of Korean adolescents with vitiligo. *J Eur Acad Dermatol Venereol.* 2010;24:524-529.

133. Ongenae K, Dierckxsens L, Brochez L, et al. Quality of life and stigmatization profile in a cohort of vitiligo patients and effect of the use of camouflage. *Dermatology.* 2005;210:279-285.

134. Silvan M. The psychological aspects of vitiligo. *Cutis.* 2004;73:163-167.

135. Silverberg JI, Silverberg NB. Clinical features of vitiligo associated with comorbid autoimmune disease: a prospective survey. *J Am Acad Dermatol.* 2013;69-824-826.

136. Palit A, Inamadar A. Childhood vitiligo. *Indian J Dermatol Vener Lepr.* 2012;78:30-41.

137. Silverberg NB. *Atlas of Pediatric Cutaneous Biodiversity.* New York, NY: Springer; 2012:38.

138. Ezzedine K, Lim HW, Suzuki T, et al. Vitiligo Global Issue Consensus Conference Panelists. Revised classification/nomenclature of vitiligo and related issues: the Vitiligo Global Issues Consensus Conference. *Pigment Cell Melanoma Res.* 2012;25:E1-E13.

139. Taieb A. Vitiligo as an inflammatory skin disorder: a therapeutic perspective. *Pigment Cell Melanoma Res.* 2011;25:9-13.

140. Grimes PE, Soriano T, Dytoc MT. Topical tacrolimus for repigmentation of vitiligo. *J Am Acad Dermatol.* 2002;47:789-791.

141. Silverberg NB, Lin P, Travis L, et al. Tacrolimus ointment promotes repigmentation of vitiligo in children: a review of 57 cases. *J Am Acad Dermatol.* 2004;51:760-766.

142. Silverberg JI, Silverberg NB. Topical tacrolimus is more effective for treatment of vitiligo in patients of skin of color. *J Drugs Dermatol.* 2011;10:507-510.

143. Udompataikul M, Boonsupthip P, Siriwattanagate R. Effectiveness of 0.1% topical tacrolimus in adult and children patients with vitiligo. *J Dermatol.* 2011;38:536-540.

144. Ho N, Pope E, Weinstein M, et al. A double-blind, randomized, placebo-controlled trial of topical tacrolimus 0.1% vs. clobetasol propionate 0.05% in childhood vitiligo. *Br J Dermatol.* 2011;165:626-632.

145. Travis LB, Silverberg NB. Calcipotriene and corticosteroid combination therapy for vitiligo. *Pediatr Dermatol.* 2004;21:495-498.

146. Newman MD, Silverberg NB. Once-daily application of calcipotriene 0.005%-betamethasone dipropionate 0.064% ointment for repigmentation of facial vitiligo. *Cutis.* 2011;88:256-259.

147. Köse O, Arca E, Kurumlu Z. Mometasone cream versus pimecrolimus cream for the treatment of childhood localized vitiligo. *J Dermatolog Treat.* 2010;21:133-139.

148. Farajzadeh S, Daraei Z, Esfandiarpour I, et al. The efficacy of pimecrolimus 1% cream combined with microdermabrasion in the treatment of nonsegmental childhood vitiligo: a randomized placebo-controlled study. *Pediatr Dermatol.* 2009;26:286-291.

149. Hui-Lan Y, Xiao-Yan H, Jian-Yong F, et al. Combination of 308-nm excimer laser with topical pimecrolimus for the treatment of childhood vitiligo. *Pediatr Dermatol.* 2009;26:354-356.

150. Njoo MD, Bos JD, Westerhof W. Treatment of generalized vitiligo in children with narrow-band (TL-01) UVB radiation therapy. *J Am Acad Dermatol.* 2000;42:245-253.

151. Kanwar AJ, Dogra S. Narrow-band UVB for the treatment of generalized vitiligo in children. *Clin Exp Dermatol.* 2005;30:332-336.

152. Cho S, Kang HC, Hahm JH. Characteristics of vitiligo in Korean children. *Pediatr Dermatol.* 2000;17:189-193.

153. Lu-yan T, Wen-wen F. Topical tacalcitol and 308-nm monochromatic excimer light: a synergistic combination for the treatment of vitiligo. *Photodermatol Photoimmunol Photomed* 2006;22:310-314.

154. Hui-Lan Y, Xiao-Yan H, Jian-Yong F, et al. Combination of 308-nm excimer laser with topical pimecrolimus for the treatment of childhood vitiligo. *Pediatr Dermatol.* 2009;26:354-356.

155. Mohana D, Verma U, Amar AJ, Choudhary RKP. Reticulate acropigmentation of Dohi: a case report with insight into genodermatoses with mottled pigmentation. *Indian J Dermatol.* 2012;57:42-44.

156. Dhar S, Kanwar AJ, Jebraili R, Dawn G, Das A. Spectrum of reticular flexural and acral pigmentary disorder in Northern India. *J Dermatol.* 1994;21:598-603.

157. Hayashi M, Suzuki T. Dyschromatosis symmetrica hereditaria. *J Dermatol.* 2013;40:336-340.

158. Xing QH, Wang MT, Chen XD, et al. A gene locus responsible for dyschromatosis symmetrica hereditaria (DSH) maps to chromosome 6q24.2-q25.2. *Am J Hum Genet.* 2003;73:377-382.

159. Taki T, Kozuka S, Izawa Y, et al. Surgical treatment of speckled skin caused by dyschromatosis symmetrica hereditaria: case report. *J Dermatol.* 1986;13:471-473.

160. Gupta V, Kumar A. Dyskeratosis congenita. *Adv Exp Med Biol.* 2010;685:215-219.

161. Dokal I. Dyskeratosis congenita. *Hematology Am Soc Hematol Educ Program.* 2011;2011:480-486.

162. Rackley S, Pao M, Seratti GF, et al. Neuropsychiatric conditions among patients with dyskeratosis congenita: a link with telomere biology? *Psychosomatics.* 2012;5:230-235.

163. Keisham C, Sarkar R, Garg VK, Chugh S. Ashy dermatosis in an 8-year-old Indian child. *Indian Dermatol Online J.* 2013;4:30-32.

164. Silverberg NB, Herz J, Wagner A, Paller AS. Erythema dyschromicum perstans in prepubertal children. *Pediatr Dermatol.* 2003;20:398-403.

165. Torrelo A, Zaballos P, Colmenero I, Mediero IG, de Prada I, Zambrano A. Erythema dyschromicum perstans in children: a report of 14 cases. *J Eur Acad Dermatol Venereol.* 2005;19:422-426.

166. Schwartz RA, Centurian SA. Erythema dyschromicum perstans. *Medscape,* May 22, 2012. http://emedicine.medscape.com/article/1122807-overview. Accessed March 22, 2013.

167. Leung AK, Robson WL, Liu EK, et al. Melanonychia striata in Chinese children and adults. *Int J Dermatol.* 2007;46:920-922.

168. Leung AK, McLeod DR. Familial melanonychia striata. *J Natl Med Assoc.* 2008;100:743-745.

169. Hirata SH, Yamada S, Almeida FA, et al. Dermoscopy of the nail bed and matrix to assess melanonychia striata. *J Am Acad Dermatol.* 2005;53:884-886.

170. Lazaridou E, Giannopoulou C, Fotiadou C, Demiri E, Ioannides D. Congenital nevus of the nail apparatus: diagnostic approach of a case through dermoscopy. *Pediatr Dermatol.* 2013;30:e293-e294

171. Lilly E, Kundu RV. Dermatoses secondary to Asian cultural practices. *Int J Dermatol.* 2012;51:372-382.

172. Yoo SS, Tausk F. Cupping: East meets West. *Int J Dermatol.* 2004;43:664-665.

173. Children's Alliance. http://www.childally.org/courses/CAN101/CAN_S3physabuseother.html. Accessed March 9, 2015.

174. Fu JM, Price VH. Approach to hair loss in women of color. *Semin Cutan Med Surg.* 2009;28:109-114.

175. Silverberg NB, Silverberg JI, Wong ML. Trichoscopy using a handheld dermoscope: an in-office technique to diagnose genetic disease of the hair. *Arch Dermatol.* 2009;145:600-601.

176. Detwiler SP, Carson JL, Woosley JT, Gambling TM, Briggaman RA. Bubble hair. Case caused by an overheating hair dryer and reproducibility in normal hair with heat. *J Am Acad Dermatol.* 1994;30:54-60.

177. Savitha AS, Sacchidanand S, Revathy TN. Bubble hair and other acquired hair shaft anomalies due to hot ironing on wet hair. *Int J Trichol.* 2011;3:118-120.

178. Elston DM, Bergfeld WF, Whiting DA, et al. Bubble hair. *J Cutan Pathol.* 1992;19:439-444.

179. Lucky AW, Biro FM, Daniels SR, Cedars MI, Khoury PR, Morrison JA. The prevalence of upper lip hair in black and white girls during puberty: a new standard. *J Pediatr.* 2001;138:134-136.

180. Paller AS, Mancini A. *Hurwitz Clinical Pediatric Dermatology.* 3rd ed. New York, NY: Elsevier-Saunders; 2006.

181. Cordisco MR. An update on lasers in children. *Curr Opin Pediatr.* 2009;21:499-504.

182. Cantatore JL, Kriegel DA. Laser surgery: an approach to the pediatric patient. *J Am Acad Dermatol.* 2004;50:165-184.

183. Wendelin DS, Mallory GB, Mallory SB. Depilation in a 6-month-old with hypertrichosis: a case report. *Pediatric Dermatol.* 1999;16:311-313.

184. Heath CR, Taylor SC. Alopecia in an ophiasis pattern: traction alopecia versus alopecia areata. *Cutis.* 2012;89:213-216.

185. Silverberg NB. *Atlas of Pediatric Cutaneous Biodiversity.* New York, NY: Springer; 2012.

186. Haliasos EC, Kerner M, Jaimes-Lopez N, et al. Dermoscopy for the pediatric dermatologist part I: dermoscopy of pediatric infectious and inflammatory skin lesions and hair disorders. *Pediatr Dermatol.* 2013;30:163-171.

187. Laude TA. Approach to dermatologic disorders in black children. *Semin Dermatol.* 1995;14:15-20.

188. Wilmington M, Aly R, Frieden IJ. *Trichophyton tonsurans* tinea capitis in the San Francisco Bay area: increased infection demonstrated in a 20-year survey of fungal infections from 1974 to 1994. *J Med Vet Mycol.* 1996;34:285-287.

189. Elewski BE. Tinea capitis: a current perspective. *J Am Acad Dermatol.* 2000;42:1-20.

190. Sharma V, Silverberg NB, Howard R, Tran CT, Laude TA, Frieden IJ. Do hair care practices affect the acquisition of tinea capitis? A case-control study. *Arch Pediatr Adolesc Med.* 2001;155:818-821.

191. Garg AP, Muller J. Inhibition of growth of dermatophytes by Indian hair oils. *Mycoses.* 1992;35:363-369.

192. Kelly AP, Taylor SC, eds. *Dermatology for Skin of Color.* 1st ed. New York, NY: The McGraw-Hill Companies; 2009.

193. Paller AS, Mancini A. *Hurwitz Clinical Pediatric Dermatology.* 3rd ed. New York, NY: Elsevier Saunders; 2006.

194. Hubbard TW. The predictive value of symptoms in diagnosing childhood tinea capitis. *Arch Pediatr Adolesc Med.* 1999;153:1150-1153.

195. Coley MK, Bhanusali DG, Silverberg JI, Alexis AF, Silverberg NB. Scalp hyperkeratosis and alopecia in children of color. *J Drugs Dermatol.* 2011;10:511-516.

196. Friedlander SF, Pickering B, Cunningham BB, Gibbs NF, Eichenfield LF. Use of the cotton swab method in diagnosing tinea capitis. *Pediatrics.* 1999;104:276-279.

197. Laude TA, Shah BR, Lynfield Y. Tinea capitis in Brooklyn. *Am J Dis Child.* 1982;136:1047-1050.

198. Andrews MD, Burns M. Common tinea infections in children. *Am Fam Physician.* 2008;77:1415-1420.

199. Pinheiro AM, Lobato LA, Varella TC. Dermoscopy findings in tinea capitis: case report and literature review. *An Bras Dermatol.* 2012;87:313-314.

200. Gupta AK, Drummond-Main C. Meta-analysis of randomized, controlled trials comparing particular doses of griseofulvin and terbinafine for the treatment of tinea capitis. *Pediatr Dermatol.* 2013;30:1-6.

201. Bhanusali D, Coley M, Silverberg J, Alexis A, Silverberg N. Treatment outcomes for tinea capitis in a skin of color population. *J Drugs Dermatol.* 2012;11:852-856.

202. Greer DL. Successful treatment of tinea capitis with 2% ketoconazole shampoo. *Int J Dermatol.* 2000;39:302-304.

203. Silverberg NB, Weinberg JM, DeLeo VA. Tinea capitis: focus on African American women. *J Am Acad Dermatol.* 2002;46:S120-S124.

204. Grosset-Janin A, Nicolas X, Saraux A. Sport and infectious risk: a systematic review of the literature over 20 years. *Médecine et Maladies Infectieuses.* 2012;42:533-544.

205. Kiken DA, Sekaran A, Antaya RJ, Davis A, Imaeda S, Silverberg NB. White piedra in children. *J Am Acad Dermatol.* 2006;55:956-961.

206. de Almeida Júnior HL, Rivitti EA, Jaeger RG. White piedra: ultrastructure and a new microecological aspect. *Mycoses.* 1990;33:491-497.

207. Shivaprakash MR, Singh G, Gupta P, Dhaliwal M, Kanwar AJ, Chakrabarti A. Extensive white piedra of the scalp caused by *Trichosporon* inkin: a case report and review of literature. *Mycopathologia.* 2011;172:481-486.

208. Figueras MJ, Guarro J. Ultrastructural aspect of the keratinolytic activity of piedra. *Rev Iberoam Micol.* 2000;17:136-141.

209. Kelly AP. Update on the management of keloids. *Semin Cutan Med Surg.* 2009;28:71-76.

210. Goodfellow A, Emmerson RW, Calvert HT. Rubstein-Taybi syndrome and spontaneous keloids. *Clin Exp Dermatol.* 1980;5:369-371.

211. Halder R, Grimes P, McLaurin C, Kress M, Kenney J. Incidence of common dermatoses in a predominantly black dermatologic practice. *Cutis.* 1983;32:388-390.

212. Wriston CC, Rubin AI, Elenitsas R, Crawford GH. Nodular scleroderma: a report of 2 cases. *Am J Dermatopathol.* 2008;30:385-388.

213. Lane JE, Waller JL, Davis LS. Relationship between age of ear piercing and keloid formation. *Pediatrics.* 2005;115:1312-1314.

214. Tirgan MH, Shutty CM, Park TH. Nine-month-old patient with bilateral earlobe keloids. *Pediatrics.* 2013;131:e313-e317.

215. Hamrick M, Boswell W, Carney D. Successful treatment of earlobe keloids in the pediatric population. *J Pediatr Surg.* 2009;44:286-288.

216. Mellon RD, Simone AF, Rappaport BA. Use of anesthetic agents in neonates and young children. *Anesth Analg.* 2007;104:509-520.

217. Talebi M, Farmanbar N, Abolfazli S, Shirazi, AS. Management of physiological hyperpigmentation of oral mucosa by cryosurgical treatment: a case report. *J Dent Res Dent Clin Dent Prospects.* 2012;6:148-151.

218. Laude TA. Approach to dermatologic disorders in black children. *Semin Dermatol.* 1995;14:15-20.

219. Dummett CO. Colour changes in the oral mucosa. *J Can Dent Assoc.* 1967;33:206-212.

220. Dummett CO. Overview of normal oral pigmentations. *J Indiana Dent Assoc.* 1980;59:13-18.

221. Najjar T. Disorders of oral pigmentation. *Medscape.* http://emedicine.medscape.com/article/1078143-overview. Accessed March 16, 2013.

222. Kasagani SK, Nutalapati R, Muttthineni RB. Esthetic depigmentation of anterior gingiva. A case series. *N Y State Dent J.* 2012;78:26-31.

223. Pontes AEF, Pontes CC, Souza SLS, Novales AB, Grisi MFM, Taba M. Evaluation of the efficacy of the acellular dermal matrix allograft with partial thickness flap in the elimination of gingival melanin pigmentation. A comparative clinical study with 12 months of follow-up. *J Esthet Restor Dent.* 2006;18:135-143.

224. Hanioka T, Tanaka K, Ojima M, Yuuki K. Association of melanin pigmentation in the gingiva of children with parents who smoke. *Pediatrics.* 2005;116:e186.

225. Castelo-Soccio LA. Hair manifestations of systemic disease. *Curr Probl Pediatr Adolesc Health Care.* 2012;42:198-202.

226. Malinowska M, Jabobkiewicz-Banecka J, Kloska A, et al. Abnormalities in the hair morphology of patients with some but not all types of mucopolysaccharidoses. *Eur J Pediatr.* 2008;167:203-209.

227. Akcakus M, Koklu E, Kurtoglu S, Koklu S, Keskin M, Buyukkayhan D. Neonatal hypertrichosis in an infant of a diabetic mother with congenital hypothyroidism. *J Perinatol.* 2006;26:256-258.

228. Zaki SA, Lad V. Hypertrichosis due to congenital hypothyroidism. *Int J Trichol.* 2011;3:38-39.

229. Liu J, Baynam G. Cornelia de Lange syndrome. *Adv Exp Med Biol.* 2010;685:111-123.

230. Flannery DB, Fink SM, Francis G, Gilman PA. Hypertrichosis cubiti. *Am J Med Genet.* 1989;32:482-483.

231. Giannetti L, Consolo U, Bambini F. Tooth and oral mucosa hereditary anomalies in complex syndromes characterized by hyper- or hypotrichosis. *Minerva Stomatol.* 2003;52:25-30.

232. Kakourou T, Uksal U. Guidelines for the management of tinea capitis in children. *Pediatr Dermatol.* 2010;27:226-228.

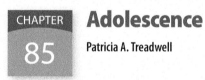

CHAPTER 85

Adolescence

Patricia A. Treadwell

KEY POINTS

- Dyspigmentation is often a major concern in adolescents with skin of color.

- Phytophotodermatitis can be misdiagnosed as ecchymoses from abuse.

- Epidermal nevus is the primary differential diagnosis for lichen striatus.

- The erythema in atopic dermatitis may be underestimated in skin of color.

- Adolescents with filaggrin mutations associated with atopic dermatitis have skin barrier dysfunction.

INTRODUCTION

This chapter will address selected dermatologic topics in skin of color pertaining to the age group from 13 to 19 years.[1]

ACNE

Acne is one of the most common dermatologic disorders in adolescence. The incidence in adolescents with skin of color is similar to that of adolescents with European ancestry; however, special attention is necessary for treatment choices and anticipating pigment changes.

Acne is an inflammatory dermatosis that is concentrated in areas of increased sebaceous glands. The four issues that are the major driving factors for acne development are: (1) abnormal keratinization leading to follicular plugging; (2) androgenic stimulation of sebaceous gland activity; (3) the effect of *Propionibacterium acnes* on sebum; and (4) inflammation.[2]

Characteristic acne lesions are open comedones (blackheads), closed comedones (whiteheads), inflammatory papules, pustules, nodules, and cysts.

Differential diagnoses include adenoma sebaceum, perioral dermatitis, rosacea, folliculitis, and drug-induced acneiform eruption.[3]

Treatment regimens are addressed in multiple articles[2,4,5] and Chapters 42 and 84 of this textbook. Of mention, topical retinoids (which are considered a first-line medical treatment for acne) should be prescribed cautiously in patients with skin of color.[5] Care should be taken to avoid irritation and subsequent dyspigmentation. Noncomedogenic facial moisturizers containing sunscreen are recommended for daily use along with acne therapies in any patient with a tendency to have dyspigmentation to specifically avoid further darkening of hyperpigmented areas.[6] Newer therapies with visible light, photodynamic therapy, and lasers have shown some efficacy.[7]

KAWASAKI DISEASE

Kawasaki disease is a disorder characterized by a systemic vasculitis that was first described by Dr. Tomisaku Kawasaki in 1967.[8] It is the leading cause of acquired cardiac disorders in children in the United States and other developed nations. Although Kawasaki disease typically occurs in young children, on occasion, adolescents can develop the disease. Because it is uncommon in adolescents and adolescents may have atypical clinical findings, proper diagnosis can be delayed.[9] It is crucial that the proper diagnosis be confirmed promptly because instituting treatment early with intravenous immunoglobulin has been shown to decrease the incidence of coronary artery aneurysms.[8]

Kawasaki disease affects children of color disproportionately. The incidence is highest in Japanese individuals and lowest in Caucasians with an intermediate incidence in African Americans and Hispanics. Recognizing the cutaneous signs of the disorder can assure that appropriate treatment regimens are initiated.

The criteria that compose the case definition for Kawasaki disease are fever persisting for 5 or more days; erythema and swelling of the palms and soles, with later desquamation; polymorphous exanthema; conjunctival injection; erythema of the lips and oral pharynx and strawberry tongue; and lymphadenopathy. Atypical or incomplete cases may not satisfy all of the criteria; thus, it is essential that practitioners consider Kawasaki disease in their differential diagnoses. Familiarity with the cutaneous findings is important for dermatologists so proper workup can be recommended[8] [**Figure 85-1**]. The cutaneous findings associated with Kawasaki disease are listed in **Table 85-1**.

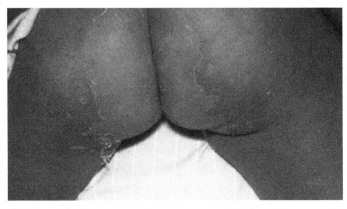

FIGURE 85-1. Desquamation on buttocks in a patient with Kawasaki disease.

TABLE 85-1	Cutaneous findings associated with Kawasaki disease

Conjunctival injection
Erythema of the lips and oral pharynx
Strawberry tongue
Fissures of the lips
Swelling of the hands and feet
Perineal desquamation
Desquamation of the hands and feet

Source: Adapted with permission from Fradin KN, Rhim HJ. An adolescent with fever, jaundice, and abdominal pain: An unusual presentation of Kawasaki disease. *J Adolesc Health* 2013;Jan;52(1):131-133.

All patients diagnosed with Kawasaki disease should receive a cardiology consultation, which typically includes an echocardiogram. Differential diagnoses include viral exanthem, staphylococcal scalded skin syndrome, scarlet fever, and toxic shock syndrome. Recommended treatment includes intravenous immunoglobulin and aspirin. Additional studies are needed on the use of corticosteroid therapy and other immunosuppressive agents.[10,11]

ACNE KELOIDALIS

Individuals who develop acne keloidalis may first experience this disorder in adolescence around puberty. It is much more common in males, but can also occur in female patients. This subject is covered more extensively in Chapter 34. Initially, a folliculitis with follicular-based pustules and papules develops, which can progress to form firm papules usually located in the occipital scalp and at the nape of the neck. In some cases, the papules coalesce to become keloidal plaques. Scarring alopecia may be a consequence. Some patients develop crusting, drainage, and secondary bacterial infection. Acne keloidalis lesions occur following a weakening of the follicular wall and subsequent exposure of the hair into the dermis, which then acts as a foreign body. Close shaving and tight collars contribute to the incidence of this disorder. A granulomatous foreign body reaction can be seen on histopathology.

Preventive measures include avoidance of close shaving of the occipital area and avoidance of tight-fitting clothing (especially collars) in the area. Medical treatments include benzoyl peroxide, retinoids, topical and intralesional strreoids. Antibiotics (topical or systemic) are prescribed if secondary infection is present. Imiquimod has been reported to be effective.[12] A comprehensive review of surgical treatments is presented in Chapter 34.

SEBORRHEIC DERMATITIS

Seborrheic dermatitis (SD) occurs in 3% to 10% of the population.[13] SD has been noted to be more common in males. The incidence has been described in the literature as both occurring more frequently[1] and less frequently[14] in skin of color. Further studies may be necessary to clarify this point. It is characterized by two different subtypes: infantile type and the adolescent and adult type. In adolescents and adults, the disorder is noted to have diffuse scale in the scalp and eyebrows along with erythematous patches with greasy scale located in the glabellar and paranasal areas. In individuals of color, the facial lesions may be annular or circular with some associated dyspigmentation[1] [**Figure 85-2**].

The inflammatory process in SD is mediated by free fatty acids in susceptible individuals.[13] Localized lipase activity has also been implicated

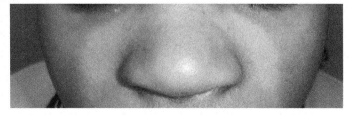

FIGURE 85-2. Hypopigmentation associated with seborrheic dermatitis.

in the pathogenesis of SD, which was demonstrated when *Malassezia* strains from healthy and SD skin were compared.[15] The incidence of SD is increased in acquired immunodeficiency syndrome, diabetes, malabsorption, and neurologic disorders. No association has been found between grooming practices and the incidence of SD in African American girls.[16]

Differential diagnoses for scalp involvement include psoriasis, tinea capitis, and eczema. Differential diagnoses for facial involvement include perioral dermatitis, secondary syphilis (when annular lesions are noted), psoriasis, tinea faciei, and tinea versicolor.

Ketoconazole shampoo has been found to be the most beneficial treatment for scalp involvement.[13] Ketoconazole cream likewise has been noted to be beneficial for lesions of the face and body. Topical anti-inflammatory agents (corticosteroids) and azoles are "likely to be beneficial."[13] There are also reports supporting the efficacy of topical calcineurin inhibitors.[17]

PITYRIASIS ROSEA

Pityriasis rosea is a self-limited papulosquamous condition. In light of seasonal variations and clustering, a viral etiology is probable.[18] Some literature has implicated human herpesvirus (HHV)-6 and HHV-7 as etiologic agents.[19] Seventy-five percent of patients are between the ages of 10 and 35 years. The condition can be preceded by symptoms of a viral illness.

Typically, the first lesion noted is the herald patch. This lesion is generally 2 to 5 cm and can be located anywhere on the body, especially on the proximal legs or arms, trunk, or neck.[20] The herald patch is often circular, erythematous, and has fine white scale. Within a few days, multiple smaller oval lesions with a similar morphology are noted. These lesions tend to be oriented parallel to the lines of skin cleavage. On the back, this is called a "fir tree" pattern, and on the flank, it is called a "school of minnows" pattern. In skin of color, the lesions may have an inverse pattern and be more papular and/or follicular centered.[21,22]

The eruption can persist for 6 to 8 weeks following the onset of the herald patch. Generally, the lesions are asymptomatic, but may be pruritic.

The differential diagnoses include tinea corporis (for the herald patch), guttate psoriasis, secondary syphilis, and pityriasis lichenoides chronica.

Treatment can be considered if the lesions are symptomatic. Topical corticosteroids and antipruritics have some efficacy. Treatment regimens using acyclovir have been published.[19,23] Erythromycin and ultraviolet light therapy have also been reported as efficacious.[24,25]

ATOPIC DERMATITIS

Atopic dermatitis in this age group has a similar clinical appearance to that in younger children. It tends to be more difficult to treat and often has widespread lichenification based on the chronic nature of the dermatitis.

In skin of color, the erythema may not be as evident when darker pigment is present. The severity of atopic dermatitis has been noted to be underestimated based on the underappreciation of erythema using all of the standard scoring instruments: Eczema Area and Severity Index (EASI), Scoring Atopic Dermatitis (SCORAD), Investigator Global Assessment (IGA), and Three-Item Severity Score (TIS). The erythema is less evident in more richly pigmented skin, thus leading to lower scores despite significant severity of the disorder.[26]

The distribution of lesions tends to vary with age. Adolescents and adults will tend to have lesions on the eyelids and genital areas in addition to fold areas.[28] Itching is a frequent accompanying feature of atopic dermatitis. Of note, the papular variant (consisting of discrete eczematous papules) of atopic dermatitis (also known as papular eczema) is more common in patients with skin of color [**Figure 85-3**]. In addition,

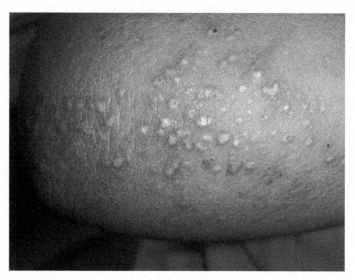

FIGURE 85-3. Papular eruption in a patient with atopic dermatitis.

pityriasis alba (irregular hypopigmented macules with fine scale) is more common in African Americans and Hispanics.[28] When the skin is pigmented, hypopigmentation and/or hyperpigmentation can also be a significant issue either following inflammation or associated with scarring[29] [**Figure 85-4**].

Filaggrin mutations have been identified in a subset of patients with atopic dermatitis and are associated with epidermal barrier dysfunction.[30] Patients in both African and European ancestry populations with filaggrin mutations have an increased propensity for developing eczema herpeticum.[31]

An extra rinse of the laundry and no dryer fabric softeners can minimize the effect of irritants in clothing. Trimming the fingernails can result in fewer linear erosions. Increases in the stratum corneum pH can be avoided by the use of mild cleansers.[32] Treatment of atopic dermatitis in adolescents includes repairing the epidermal barrier with daily short soaks and liberal use of moisturizers (especially while the skin is still damp). Topical corticosteroids are prescribed for the most affected patches. Topical calcineurin inhibitors are used for facial and intertriginous involvement. Oral antihistamines are useful for treating the pruritus, and in some cases, they can address the sleep disturbances present in up to 60% of individuals with atopic dermatitis.[33] Patients with atopic dermatitis are often colonized with bacteria, especially *Staphylococcus aureus*.[34] Dilute bleach baths and applying mupirocin intranasally and

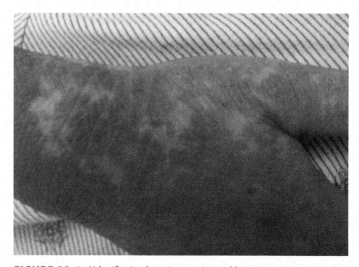

FIGURE 85-4. Lichenification, hypopigmentation, and hyperpigmentation in a patient with atopic dermatitis.

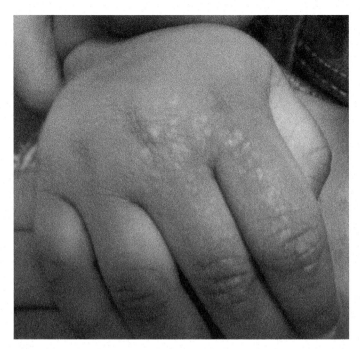

FIGURE 85-5. Hypopigmented papules of lichen striatus.

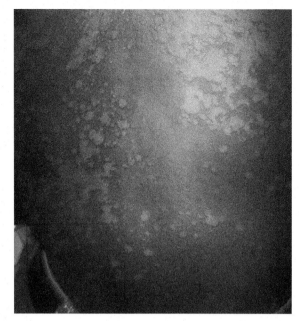

FIGURE 85-6. Tinea versicolor on the back.

under the fingernails can improve the atopic dermatitis.[35] Patients with eczema and secondary bacterial skin infections should also continue treatment with topical corticosteroids and/or other anti-inflammatories along with moisturizers to improve the epidermal barrier. Use of these agents alone (even without antibiotics) has been noted to decrease the level of skin colonization with *S. aureus*.[36]

More widespread cases of severe atopic dermatitis can be treated with narrowband ultraviolet B therapy and/or a variety of immunosuppressive agents.[37] A comprehensive discussion of treatment options can be found in Chapter 27.

Differential diagnoses include irritant dermatitis, psoriasis (especially guttate), and contact dermatitis.

LICHEN STRIATUS

Lichen striatus is a cutaneous disorder that is characterized by grouped papules in a linear pattern. The grouping follows embryonal migration patterns and Blaschko lines.[38] In adolescents of color, the papules often appear hypopigmented in contrast to the erythematous or hyperpigmented appearance in less pigmented individuals [**Figure 85-5**]. The disorder typically lasts for approximately 1 to 2 years and then spontaneously resolves.

If the fingers are involved, the nail bed may become involved and nail dystrophy can be seen.[39]

Differential diagnoses include epidermal nevus, lichen planus, papular eczema, and incontinentia pigmenti. Management include reassurance and expectant monitoring. If the patient is symptomatic, topical corticosteroids and antipruritics can be prescribed. The combination of topical retinoids and topical corticosteroids has been reported to be effective.[40]

TINEA VERSICOLOR

Tinea versicolor (TV) is a fungal infection of the skin caused by *Malassezia furfur* (aka *Pityrosporum ovale* and *Pityrosporum orbiculare*). *M. furfur* is part of the normal flora of the skin. The organism is nourished by the sebum and converts from the yeast form to the mycelial form and causes the disorder.[41] TV often occurs in adolescence. Additionally, the incidence is increased in settings of diabetes, pregnancy, immunosuppression, and hot, humid weather.

The patches with fine powdery scale are most frequently seen on the upper back, chest, and proximal arms in the same areas as the highest concentration of sebum. Adolescents of color are similarly affected as compared to Caucasian adolescents, but the clinical presentation may be different. The lesions are more often hypopigmented [**Figure 85-6**] and/or follicular centered in skin of color. Diagnosis can be made based on the clinical findings or through Wood's light examination. Short hyphae and spores ("spaghetti and meatballs") will be seen on a potassium hydroxide and India ink preparation [**Figure 85-7**]. Culture of the *M. furfur* is not feasible because the specific conditions necessary for growth are not easily achieved.

Differential diagnoses include vitiligo, pityriasis rosea, pityriasis rubra pilaris, and confluent and reticulated papillomatosis of Gougerot-Carteaud.[42]

A variety of treatment regimens have been described. Mechanical removal with a bath brush has some efficacy when other treatments may be contraindicated. If limited areas are noted, a topical antifungal such as ketoconazole cream or other azoles can be efficacious. Topical selenium

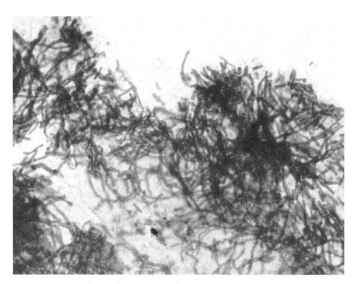

FIGURE 85-7. Potassium hydroxide and India ink preparation in tinea versicolor showing "spaghetti and meatballs."

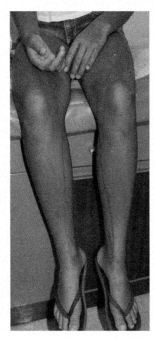

FIGURE 85-8. "Drip" pattern of hyperpigmentation in phytophotodermatitis.

sulfide lotion and ketoconazole shampoo can be applied to larger areas of involvement, left on for 5 to 10 minutes, and then washed off. They are applied nightly for a few weeks and subsequently used as needed. Oral medications including ketoconazole, itraconazole, and fluconazole have been used in a variety of treatment regimens.[43]

PHYTOPHOTODERMATITIS

Phytophotodermatitis often has a more prominent clinical appearance in adolescents with skin of color. Phytophotodermatitis is a phototoxic cutaneous reaction that results from exposure of the skin to furocoumarin derivatives (psoralens) and subsequent sun exposure. Furocoumarins can be found in lemons and limes, other citrus fruits, species of Umbelliferae (celery, cow parsley, giant hogweed, cowbane, carrot, parsnips, dill, fennel, and anise), rue, meadow grass, figs, and some perfumes.[44] Bullae can develop on exposed sites. The dermatitis may be painful, and ruptured bullae may be susceptible to secondary bacterial infection. A less intense reaction will result in pigment changes without bullae formation [**Figure 85-8**]. Phytophotodermatitis may on occasion be misdiagnosed as child abuse especially if there are handprints or streaks.[45] Protection from the sun following exposure to the derivatives can be preventative.[46]

BECKER NEVUS

Becker nevus, a benign cutaneous hamartoma, develops in the peripubertal period.[47] A higher prevalence is reported in individuals with skin of color.[48] Clinically, the hamartoma is typically unilateral and hyperpigmented, with an irregular outline and surface located on the shoulders, anterior chest, or scapula [**Figure 85-9**]. It is more frequent in males and in many cases has increased overlying hair and/or acne in the lesion.[49] In adolescents with more richly pigmented skin, the hyperpigmentation may be significant. The nevi tend to be asymptomatic; however, a Becker nevus syndrome has been described, which is characterized by associated abnormalities including breast hypoplasia, limb asymmetry, scoliosis, and supernumerary nipples.[49]

The histopathologic findings are acanthosis, papillomatosis, and increased pigmentation of the basal layer.

Differential diagnoses include congenital melanocytic nevus, café-au-lait macule, and hamartoma.[50]

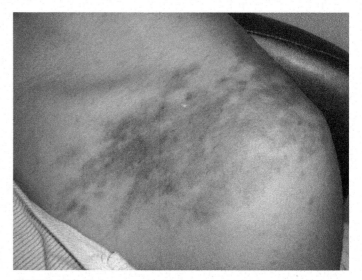

FIGURE 85-9. Becker nevus.

NEVUS SEBACEOUS

Nevus sebaceous of Jadassohn is a hamartomatous lesion that is present from birth but often becomes more raised and prominent in adolescence. The occurrence rate is 0.3% of newborns. The lesion is generally considered sporadic, but autosomal dominant cases have been noted.[51] The literature describes the lesions as yellow, yellow-brown, and orange. In skin of color, the lesions tend to be more pigmented. Clinically, nevus sebaceous is a hairless plaque with an irregular surface occurring most often on the scalp [**Figure 85-10**].

Basal cell carcinoma is the most common malignancy that may develop within these lesions, with an occurrence rate of approximately 1%. Other tumors, such as trichoblastoma, syringocystadenoma papilliferum, apocrine cystadenoma, squamous cell carcinoma, sebaceous epithelioma, and sebaceous carcinoma, have been reported.[52]

Histopathology shows increased sebaceous glands, papillomatosis, and hyperkeratosis.[53]

Differential diagnoses are aplasia cutis congenita (at birth) and epidermal nevus.

Sebaceous nevus syndrome is a subset of epidermal nevus syndrome. The syndromes are characterized by neurologic, ocular, and skeletal abnormalities associated with the nevus.[54]

Excision can be accomplished for tumors or cosmetic indications.[55]

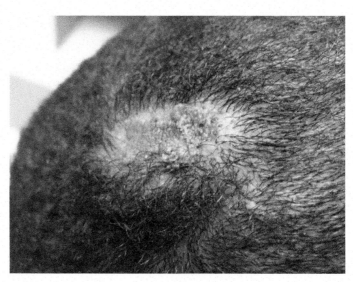

FIGURE 85-10. Nevus sebaceous of Jadassohn on the scalp.

REFERENCES

1. Woolfolk D, Treadwell PA. Dermatoses in adolescents of color. *Adolesc Med State Art Rev.* 2011;22:1-15.
2. Szczepaniak D, Treadwell P. Acne therapy in primary care: comprehensive review of current evidence-based interventions and treatments. *Adolesc Med State Art Rev.* 2011;22:77-96.
3. Poli F. Differential diagnosis of facial acne on black skin. *Int J Dermatol.* 2012;51(Suppl 1):24-26.
4. Strauss JS, Krowchuk DP, Leyden JJ, et al. Guidelines for care of acne vulgaris management. *J Am Acad Dermatol.* 2007;56:651-663.
5. Geria AN, Lawson CN, Halder RM. Topical retinoids for pigmented skin. *J Drugs Dermatol.* 2011;10:483-489.
6. Briley JJ, Lynfield YL, Chavda K. Sunscreen use and usefulness in African-Americans. *J Drugs Dermatol.* 2007;6:19-22.
7. Thiboutot D, Gollnick H, Bettoli V, et al. New insights into the management of acne: an update from the Global Alliance to Improve Outcomes in Acne group. *J Am Acad Dermatol.* 2009;60:S1-S50.
8. Rowley AH, Shulman ST. Recent advances in the understanding and management of Kawasaki disease. *Curr Infect Dis Rep.* 2010;12:96-102
9. Fradin KN, Rhim HJ. An adolescent with fever, jaundice, and abdominal pain: an unusual presentation of Kawasaki disease. *J Adolesc Health.* 2013;52:131-133.
10. Dominguez SR, Anderson MS. Advances in the treatment of Kawasaki disease. *Curr Opin Pediatr.* 2013;25:103-109.
11. Athappan G, Gale S, Ponniah T. Corticosteroid therapy for primary treatment of Kawasaki disease: weight of evidence: a meta-analysis and systemic review of the literature. *Cardiovasc J Afr.* 2009;20:233-236.
12. Shockman S, Paghdal KV, Cohen G. Medical and surgical management of keloids: a review. *J Drugs Dermatol.* 2010;9:1249-1257.
13. Naldi L. Seborrhoeic dermatitis. *Clin Evid (online).* 2010;2010:1713.
14. Breunig JA, de Almeida HL Jr, Duquia RP, et al: Scalp seborrheic dermatitis: prevalence and associated factors in male adolescents. *Int J Dermatol.* 2012;51:46-49.
15. Vlachos C, Gaitanis G, Alexopoulos EC, et al. Phospholipase activity after beta-endorphin exposure discriminates *Malassezia* strains isolated from healthy and seborrhoeic dermatitis skin. *J Eur Acad Dermatol Venereol.* 2013;27:1575-1578.
16. Rucker Wright D, Gathers R, Kapke A, et al. Hair care practices and their association with scalp and hair disorders in African American girls. *J Am Acad Dermatol.* 2011;64:253-262.
17. Poindexter GB, Burkhart CN, Morrell DS. Therapies for pediatric seborrheic dermatitis. *Pediatr Ann.* 2009;38:333-338.
18. Ayanlowo O, Akinkugbe A, Olumide Y. The pityriasis rosea calendar: a 7-year review of seasonal variation, age and sex distribution. *Nig Q J Hosp Med.* 2010;20:29-31.
19. Rassai S, Feily A, Sina N, et al. Low dose of acyclovir may be an effective treatment against pityriasis rosea: a random investigator-blind clinical trial on 64 patients. *J Eur Acad Dermatol Venereol.* 2011;1:24-26.
20. Polat M, Yildirim Y, Makara A. Palmar herald patch in pityriasis rosea. *Australas J Dermatol.* 2012;53:e64-e65.
21. Amer A, Fischer H, Li X. The natural history of pityriasis rosea in black American children: how correct is the "classic" description? *Arch Pediatr Adolesc Med.* 2007;161:503-506.
22. Zawar V, Chuh A. Follicular pityriasis rosea. A case report and a new classification of clinical variants of the disease. *J Dermatol Case Rep.* 2012;6:36-39.
23. Ehsani A, Esmaily N, Noormohammadpour P, et al. The comparison between the efficacy of high dose acyclovir and erythromycin on the period and signs of pityriasis rosea. *Indian J Dermatol.* 2010;55:246-248.
24. Drago F, Rebora A. Treatments for pityriasis rosea. *Skin Therapy Lett.* 2009;14:6-7.
25. Lim SH, Kim SM, Oh BH, et al. Low-dose ultraviolet A1 phototherapy for treating pityriasis rosea. *Ann Dermatol.* 2009;21:230-236.
26. Ben-Gashir MA, Hay RJ. Reliance on erythema scores may mask severe atopic dermatitis in black children compared to their white counterparts. *Br J Dermatol.* 2002;147:920-925.
27. Treadwell PA. Papulosquamous disorders: atopic dermatitis, psoriasis, seborrheic dermatitis, and nickel contact dermatitis. *Adolesc Med State Art Rev.* 2011;22:157-168.
28. Park JH, Hexsel D. Disorders of hypopigmentation. In: Kelly AB, Taylor S, eds. *Dermatology for Skin of Color.* New York, NY: McGraw Hill Medical; 2009:311.
29. Callender VD, St. Surin-Lord S, Davis EC, et al. Postinflammatory hyperpigmentation: etiologic and therapeutic considerations. *Am J Clin Dermatol.* 2011;12:87-99.
30. Cork MJ, Danby SG, Vasilopoulos Y, et al. Epidermal barrier dysfunction in atopic dermatitis. *J Invest Dermatol.* 2009;129:1892-1908.
31. Gao PS, Rafaels NM, Hand T, et al. Filaggrin mutations that confer risk of atopic dermatitis confer greater risk for eczema herpeticum. *J Allergy Clin Immunol.* 2009;124:507-513.
32. National Eczema Association. Bathing and moisturizing. http://www.nationaleczema.org/living-with-eczema/bathing-moisturizing. Accessed February 12, 2013.
33. Camfferman D, Kennedy JD, Gold M, et al. Eczema and sleep and its relationship to daytime functioning in children. *Sleep Med Rev.* 2010;14:359-369.
34. Friedman BC, Goldman RD. Anti-staphylococcal treatment in dermatitis. *Can Fam Physician.* 2011;57:669-671.
35. Huang JT, Abrams M, Tlougan B, et al. Treatment of *Staphylococcus aureus* colonization in atopic dermatitis decreases disease severity. *Pediatrics.* 2009;123:e808-e814.
36. Hung SH, Lin YT, Chu CY, et al. *Staphylococcus* colonization in atopic dermatitis treated with fluticasone or tacrolimus with or without antibiotics. *Ann Allergy Asthma Immunol.* 2007;98:51-56.
37. Ricci G, Dondi A, Patrizi A, et al. Systemic therapy of atopic dermatitis in children. *Drugs.* 2009;69:297-306.
38. Litvinov IV, Jafarian F. Lichen striatus and lines of Blaschko. *N Engl J Med.* 2012;367:2427.
39. Vozza A, Baroni A, Nacca L, et al. Lichen striatus with nail involvement in an 8-year-old child. *J Dermatol.* 2011;38:821-823.
40. Youssef SM, Teng JM. Effective topical combination therapy for treatment of lichen striatus in children: a case series and review. *J Drugs Dermatol.* 2012;11:872-875.
41. Haisley-Royster C. Cutaneous infestations and infections. *Adolesc Med State Art Rev.* 2011;22:129-145.
42. Berry M, Khachemoune A. Extensive tinea versicolor mimicking pityriasis rubra pilaris. *J Drugs Dermatol.* 2009;8:490-491.
43. Hu SW, Bigby M. Pityriasis versicolor: a systematic review of interventions. *Arch Dermatol.* 2010;146:1132-1140.
44. Sasseville D. Clinical patterns of phytodermatitis. *Dermatol Clin.* 2009;27:299-308.
45. Swerdlin A, Berkowitz C, Craft N. Cutaneous signs of child abuse. *J Am Acad Dermatol.* 2007;57:371-392.
46. Zhang R, Zhu W. Phytophotodermatitis due to wild carrot decoction. *Indian J Dermatol Venereol Leprol.* 2011;77:731.
47. Steiner D, Silva FA, Pessanha AC, et al. Do you know this syndrome? Becker nevus syndrome. *An Bras Dermatol.* 2011;86:165-166.
48. de Almeida HL Jr, Duquia RP, Souza PR, et al. Prevalence and characteristics of Becker nevus in Brazilian 18-year-old males. *Int J Dermatol.* 2010;49:718-720.
49. Criscione V, Telang GH. Becker nevus with ichthyotic features. *Arch Dermatol.* 2010;146:575-577.
50. Patrizi A, Medri M, Raone B, et al. Clinical characteristics of Becker's nevus in children: report of 118 cases from Italy. *Pediatr Dermatol.* 2012;29:571-574.
51. West C, Narahari S, Kwatra S, et al. Autosomal dominant transmission of nevus sebaceous of Jadassohn. *Dermatol Online J.* 2012;18:17.
52. Jo MS, Kwon KH, Shin HK, et al. Sebaceous carcinoma arising from the nevus sebaceous. *Arch Plast Surg.* 2012;39:431-433.
53. Ugras N, Ozgun G, Adim SB, et al. Nevus sebaceous at unusual location: a rare presentation. *Indian J Path Microbiol.* 2012;55:419-420.
54. Boger LS, Awasthi S, Eisen DB. Sebaceous nevus syndrome: a case report of a child with nevus sebaceous, mental retardation, seizures, and mucosal and ocular abnormalities. *Dermatol Online J.* 2012;18:5.
55. Chepla KJ, Gosain AK. Giant nevus sebaceous: definition, surgical techniques, and rationale for treatment. *Plast Reconstr Surg.* 2012;130:296e-304e.

Pregnancy

Daniel Butler
Kelly K. Park
Jenny Murase

KEY POINTS

- Striae gravidarum, keloids, melasma, and intrahepatic cholestasis of pregnancy have a predilection for pregnant women of color.

- Seventy percent of the world's patients with human immunodeficiency virus/acquired immunodeficiency virus live in sub-Saharan Africa, and African women of childbearing age have a heightened susceptibility for acquiring this infection.

- Mycosis fungoides, sarcoidosis, scleroderma, and lupus erythematosus are more aggressive and confer a poorer prognosis in pregnant women of color.

- It is important that patients understand that the risks associated with these diseases during pregnancy are largely due to poorly controlled disease.

- Planning a pregnancy 6 months after the disease has been controlled can help ensure the safety of the mother and child.

- It is important to stress contraception to patients whose disease is currently active or has been in remission for less than 6 months.

INTRODUCTION

Pregnant women of color constitute a unique population. It is important to note that there are dermatologic conditions that are seen exclusively in this group. Furthermore, there are special considerations when selecting and instituting therapies for pregnant women of color who have common dermatologic conditions.

DERMATOLOGIC CONDITIONS IN PREGNANT WOMEN OF COLOR

CONNECTIVE TISSUE CHANGES

Striae Gravidarum Striae gravidarum (SG) are striae distensae (SD), or stretch marks, that occur during pregnancy and are the most common connective tissue change observed during gestation. A risk factor for SG is race, specifically individuals of African American, Hispanic, East Asian, and South Asian descent.[1] Family history of striae, younger maternal age, maternal weight gain, premature birth, and newborn size are also factors.[2,3]

SG can appear in primigravidas or alternatively develop for the first time in subsequent pregnancies in any trimester, although they most commonly appear in the second and third trimesters. SG occurs most often on the abdomen and breasts. Initially, they appear as striae rubra and become longer, wider, and raised over time. They then become striae alba, or mature striae, which are wrinkled, white, and atrophic [**Figure 86-1**]. SG can be associated with pruritus, burning, and discomfort. SD in darker skin types are sometimes referred to as striae nigrae.[4] A mechanobiologic process is likely to activate or inhibit melanogenesis in this population, but there is no evidence of any topical preparation that would prevent SG.[5] However, topical vitamin A therapy with tretinoin (retinoic acid) 0.1% improves SG, but no study has been done exclusively in skin of color.[6] Combined therapies may improve striae alba in skin types I to V.[7]

Although not studied specifically for SG, various lasers have proved helpful for SD, including pregnancy-related striae. Fractional photothermolysis using the erbium-doped 1550-nm fractional laser is one such laser, but it comes with the risk of pigmentary changes.[8] Because melanin does not absorb the 1550-nm wavelength, the use of this laser

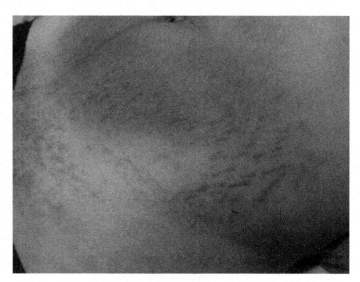

FIGURE 86-1. Stretch marks on an East Indian woman postpartum after her first pregnancy. In this patient, both striae rubra and evolving striae alba are present.

in skin of color has significantly less risk of postinflammatory pigmentation than other lasers.[8] The laser has been used in striae (both immature and mature) with graded improvement and better results in white rather than red striae.[9] For skin types IV to VI, the use of preoperative treatment may help in preventing or ameliorating pigmentary side effects.[8] The fractional nonablative 1540-nm erbium:glass laser has shown to be effective in skin types II to IV for striae rubra and alba, with transient side effects including postinflammatory hyperpigmentation.[10]

The 10,600-nm ablative carbon dioxide (CO_2) fractional (short-pulsed) laser has been studied in skin types IV to VI, with results ranging from lack of improvement in type IV skin to hyperpigmentation in type VI patients.[11] It is said that this treatment may be used only with great caution or should be avoided in these patients.[11,12]

The noncoherent, nonlaser, filtered intense pulsed light flashlamp, emitting broadband visible light, was studied in Hispanic women with skin types III to IV who had abdominal striae.[13] All patients showed clinical and microscopic improvement of their treated lesions. The 585-nm pulsed dye and nonablative 1450-nm diode lasers are also not recommended for use unless with great caution.[11]

The 1064-nm neodymium-doped yttrium-aluminum-garnet (Nd:YAG; Nd:Y3Al5O12) long-pulsed laser produces satisfactory results for SD in patients with skin types II to IV; however, although there was no report of its use in darker skin types, the authors suggested it may be safe in these patients.[14]

TriPollar radiofrequency has been shown to have promising results in women with SD in skin types IV and V with no lasting adverse effects.[15] Intradermal radiofrequency combined with autologous platelet-rich plasma has been found to produce improvement of striae (including due to pregnancy) in Asians with type IV skin, with no reports of postinflammatory pigmentation.[16]

The targeted narrowband ultraviolet B (UVB)/ultraviolet A1 (UVA1) device emitting noncoherent light with peaks at 313, 360, and 420 nm has been useful in skin types II to VI with striae alba for short-term repigmentation.[17]

The 308-nm excimer laser has been shown to help repigment striae alba but requires maintenance therapy and can lead to pigment splaying. Skin types III to VI were found to require less frequent maintenance treatments.[18]

A disk microneedle therapy system was found to improve SD in Koreans with type III and IV skin with both striae rubra and striae alba.[19]

Hypertrophic Scars and Keloids Hypertrophic scars and keloids (for a more in-depth discussion of keloids, see Chapter 33) are the result of abnormal wound healing and are common in African Americans, Hispanics, and Asians, along with those with a family history.[20] Formation

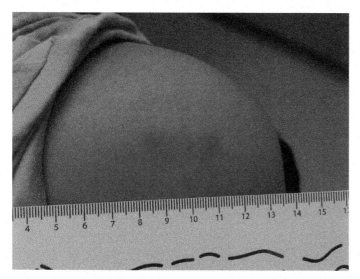

FIGURE 86-2. Keloid on the shoulder of an East Indian female that became inflamed during pregnancy, requiring intralesional triamcinolone injections.

occurs in areas of high melanocyte concentration, including the chest, shoulders [**Figure 86-2**], upper back, neck, and earlobes.[21] Keloid formation is a concern in surgical sites, particularly in cesarean sections. In a prospective study of 429 cesarean sections, keloids occurred in 1.6% of Hispanics, 5.2% of Asians, and 7.1% of African Americans, and those with keloid formation were found to have a higher risk of intraabdominal adhesions.[22]

There is no way to prevent hypertrophic scars and keloids; however, there are ways to reduce risk of occurrence. In pregnancy-related surgery, surgical technique should be atraumatic and precise with hemostasis and skin edge eversion closure. Proper wound care and debridement and infection prevention should be practiced. Cesarean sections using absorbable subcuticular stitch closure have better cosmetic results with reduced pain than surgical staples.[23] Bilayered closures of trunk and extremities with subcuticular running polyglactin 910 sutures left in place have better appearance and less erythema.

Intralesional corticosteroids are often first-line therapy. Simple excision and primary closure when caused by complicated wounds or delayed closure for hypertrophic scars is an option. However, complete surgical resection for keloids as monotherapy is associated with a high recurrence rate.

PIGMENTARY CHANGES

Hyperpigmentation, which is common in pregnancy, is seen in up to 90% of women and may be related to pregnancy hormones.[24] Commonly, it presents as a mild generalized hyperpigmentation with darkening of normally pigmented areas, such as in the areola, genital skin, nipples, axillae, and inner thighs, and at times, nevi, freckles, and scars. Linea alba can darken to become linea nigra [**Figure 86-3**].[25]

Melasma (chloasma), an acquired hyperpigmentation of the face, is commonly seen in women with skin of color, particularly those of African American, Hispanic, and Asian ancestry. A survey of Mexican women found that 66% developed melasma during pregnancy, of whom a third had persistent pigmentation. The gestational type may resolve in the postpartum period but is worsened by both visible and ultraviolet light. It may recur with another pregnancy or the use of oral contraceptives. Epidermal melasma, as opposed to dermal melasma, is treatable.

Treatment options include counseling regarding sun protection and the use of broad-spectrum sunscreens. For treatment of melasma, see Chapter 51.

Persistent melasma may be treated after delivery with topical agents such as hydroquinone, tretinoin, or azelaic acid. Glycolic acid peels are safe in patients with darker skin types because they are generally classified as superficial chemical peels. Intense pulsed light treatment combined with hydroquinone was studied in skin types III and IV with

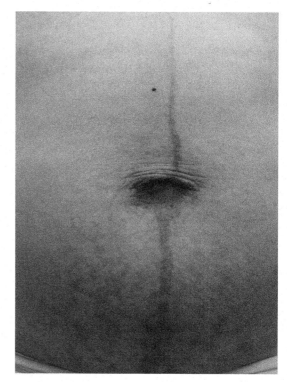

FIGURE 86-3. Linea nigra in a Chinese female that began to develop in the second trimester. Linea nigra appears in three quarters of pregnancies and is due to the increased melanocyte-stimulating hormone made by the placenta, which also results in melasma and darkening of the nipples.

noticeable improvement, although treatment should be given conservatively due to the risk of worsening melasma. Fractional thermolysis has been used in patients with skin types III to V with improvement and limited postinflammatory hyperpigmentation. However, those with type V skin did not respond to therapy. With any treatment, the risk in darker skin types of postinflammatory hyperpigmentation is high; therefore, patients should be adequately counseled.

DERMATOSES OF PREGNANCY

Certain skin diseases appear only in pregnant women and thus are known as the dermatoses of pregnancy. The specific dermatoses of pregnancy have been classified into four entities: pruritic urticarial papules and plaques of pregnancy (PUPPP), atopic eruption of pregnancy (AEP), pemphigoid gestationis formally known as herpes gestationis (PG), and intrahepatic cholestasis of pregnancy (ICP). Pustular psoriasis of pregnancy (PPP) is considered to be a fifth possible dermatosis of pregnancy. ICP is more common in women of color, and PUPPP is less common. PG [**Figure 86-4, A and B**] and AEP do not have a specific predilection for women with skin of color. It is important for the clinician to counsel patients on the safety of therapy when treating these conditions in pregnancy.

INTRAHEPATIC CHOLESTASIS OF PREGNANCY

This condition has been referred to by a variety of names including prurigo gravidarum, jaundice of pregnancy, and obstetric cholestasis. It is caused by genetic and hormonal effects on the gallbladder, which results in spillage of bile from the liver into the bloodstream. Patients present with significant pruritus and evidence of whole-body excoriation.

While this condition is seen across all population groups, an increased incidence has been appreciated in women with skin of color from several locales. Initially, South American Indians were identified to have an increased incidence of the condition during pregnancy, but subsequent studies have extended that demographic to both North and South American populations.[26,27] There appears to be a genetic predisposition for

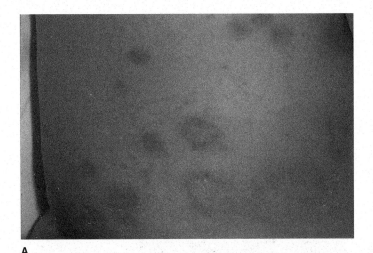

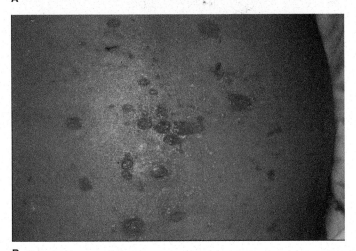

FIGURE 86-4. **(A)** Pemphigoid gestationis (PG) in pregnant African American female. **(B)** PG was originally called "herpes gestationis" because of the blistering appearance shown here, although it is not associated with the herpes virus.

these populations.[27] There is also increased prevalence in other populations including women of Indian and Pakistani descent.[28]

Assessment of jaundice can be difficult in skin of color patients. Ideal locations to assess color changes associated with jaundice are the buccal mucosa and the sclera of the eyes. Additionally, patients should be screened with questions regarding recent urine color changes or feelings of depression, both of which can indicate elevated bilirubin levels in the blood.

PRURITIC URTICARIAL PAPULES AND PLAQUES OF PREGNANCY

PUPPP is unique to pregnancy and typically appears in the third trimester of primigravid women [**Figure 86-5**]. When examining the prevalence of dermatoses of pregnancy in East Indian populations, PUPPP was the most common, representing close to 65% of cases.[29] While the condition is more frequently seen in Caucasian females, it is also seen in other populations including those of Asian descent as well as African and Afro-Caribbean descent.[30] Studies show that the condition is rarely associated with fetal or maternal complications and usually regresses 1 week postpartum.[31,32]

TREATMENT FOR SPECIFIC DERMATOSES OF PREGNANCY

Since the dermatoses of pregnancy rarely result in complications and often remit postpartum, the goal of treatment is the management of symptoms. The overriding complaint is pruritus, which is

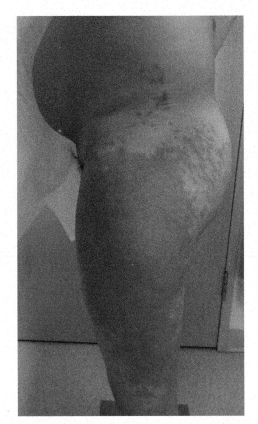

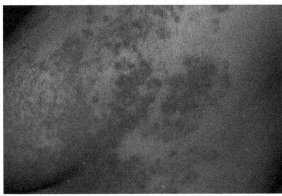

FIGURE 86-5. Pruritic urticarial papules and plaques of pregnancy, also known as polymorphic eruption of pregnancy, in a Taiwanese female. This often begins on the abdomen and subsequently can spread to the thighs, legs, feet, arms, chest, and neck.

effectively treated with first-line topical agents and oral medications when needed.

TOPICAL STEROIDS

Although the U.S. Food and Drug Administration (FDA) categorizes corticosteroids as a class C medication for use during pregnancy, there is enough evidence to warrant their safe use. Studies have shown no increase in congenital malformations or abnormalities including cleft palates for infants exposed in utero and no increase in preterm delivery. Conversely, there is evidence to support retarded fetal growth for those exposed to potent or superpotent topical corticosteroids. Studies have further classified the use of different strengths of topical corticosteroids. They found minimal growth retardation with high-strength steroids used in the first trimester, but there was a significant association of lower birth weight infants, smaller placental size, and lower plasma cortisol levels when the strongest topical steroids were used in the third trimester.[33,34] Additionally, an analysis of seven studies conducted over a 20-year span published in 2009 failed to show a statistically significant association between congenital malformations and topical corticosteroids in six of the seven studies.[35] From these data, recommendations were made regarding the use of topical corticosteroids during pregnancy. Potent and superpotent corticosteroids should be avoided, whereas mild to moderate-strength corticosteroids should be preferentially used. If potent or superpotent strengths are needed, they should be used for minimal time periods, and patients should be warned about potential fetal growth retardation.

ANTIHISTAMINES

First- and second-generation antihistamines can be used safely during pregnancy in low doses. Used in high doses in the third trimester, antihistamines have two potential toxicities: oxytocin-like effects, causing early uterine contractions and resulting in fetal hypoxia, and postpartum withdrawal in infants, which can result in seizure-like activity. Clinicians should make patients aware of the risk of retrolental fibroplasia, or retinopathy of prematurity, when using antihistamines within 2 weeks of delivery, specifically with preterm infants.[36]

When selecting an antihistamine, first-generation medications such as chlorpheniramine or diphenhydramine should be first line.[37] If the first-line agents cannot be tolerated, cetirizine and loratadine can be used after the first trimester.[38] It is important to absolutely avoid use of doxepin because of significant anticholinergic withdrawal effects including agitation, impaired cardiorespiratory function, and poor urinary and fecal continence.

URSODEOXYCHOLIC ACID

Used specifically for cholestatic disease of pregnancy, ursodeoxycholic acid proved to be both safe and effective in pregnancy. When pruritus is uncontrolled or liver enzymes are elevated, ursodeoxycholic acid, used in close to 500 patients, can improve liver function tests and diminish pruritus. In a study of over 500 pregnant women, maternal side effects were reported to be minimal, and fetal outcome was actually improved with respect to reducing fetal distress and premature births.[39]

NEOPLASTIC CONDITIONS

There are certain neoplastic conditions that appear more commonly in young females of color. Early-onset mycosis fungoides, defined as before age 40, is most common in African American and Hispanic women. Moreover, African American women diagnosed with early-onset disease have worse prognoses.[40]

Another rare but concerning cancer in skin of color patients is melanoma. While less prevalent in skin of color populations, melanoma is more likely to metastasize, resulting in worse survival rates. Among Asian, Pacific Island, and Latin American populations, the incidence of melanoma has steadily risen since 1996. Research continues to elucidate risks factors for skin of color populations, with the hope of establishing standard preventative and detection measures.[41]

SPECIAL CONSIDERATION WHEN TREATING PREGNANT WOMEN WITH SKIN OF COLOR

VITILIGO, PSORIASIS, AND ATOPIC DERMATITIS

Although no direct factors have been attributed to precipitating or exacerbating vitiligo (except the Koebner phenomenon), patients do report pregnancy as a cause [**Figure 86-6**]. Pregnancy in patients with vitiligo was not found to be associated with adverse pregnancy outcomes, including labor issues, and birth outcomes.[42] There are no guidelines for the treatment of vitiligo in pregnancy. The safest option may be simply camouflage using cosmetics and makeup. Low- to moderate-potency corticosteroids, narrowband UVB [Figure 86-6, A and B], and broadband UVB are also options. With UVB phototherapy, regardless of the condition being treated, folate supplementation should be provided to prevent folate deficiency, which would increase risk of neural tube defects in the first trimester.[43]

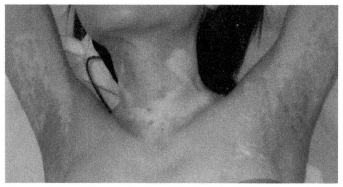

A

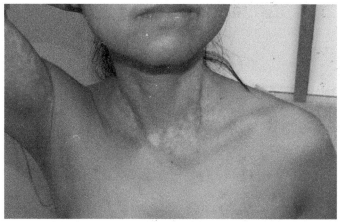

B

FIGURE 86-6. (A) Vitiligo initial presentation in a Japanese female. **(B)** The same patient following two to three times weekly narrowband ultraviolet B (UVB) therapy between 700 and 800 mJ after 72 weeks of therapy. Narrowband UVB therapy is a safe option for pregnant women who take adequate folic acid supplementation.

Psoriasis is a chronic inflammatory disorder that has characteristic erythematous plaques with scale. It is the sixth most common diagnosis of African American patient visits to the dermatologist, the fourth most common in Asian or Pacific Islander patient visits, and the third most common in Hispanic or Latino patient visits.[44] There are approximately 65,000 to 107,000 births to women with psoriasis annually.[45] Of pregnant women with psoriasis, 55% have reported improvement, 21% no change, and 23% worsening, whereas the majority have flaring in the postpartum period.[46,47] The Medical Board of the National Psoriasis Foundation released treatment options for pregnant and lactating women with psoriasis.[48] First-line treatments for pregnant women with mild psoriasis are emollients and low- to moderate-potency topical steroids. Second-line treatment is usually narrowband UVB phototherapy or broadband UVB phototherapy. UVB phototherapy can precipitate melasma, so patients should be counseled. Third-line therapies include tumor necrosis factor-α inhibitors (adalimumab, etanercept, infliximab) and cyclosporine. Systemic steroids for pustular psoriasis, which may occur in the later stages of pregnancy, can be used with caution in the second and third trimesters.

For lactating women, first-line treatment includes moisturizers and topical steroids. UVB phototherapy in lactating women is also safe. If unavoidable, systemic steroids should be ingested 4 hours prior to breastfeeding to minimize amounts found in breast milk.

Atopic dermatitis (AD) is the most common dermatosis during pregnancy, accounting for 36% to 49.7% of disorders.[49,50] It has been reported that up to 52% of pregnant patients with preexisting AD experienced worsening of disease [**Figure 86-7**].[51] It is reported that only 20% to 40% of patients have preexisting eczema.[49,50] Up to 2% of lactating mothers will develop areola and/or nipple eczema.[52] The basis of treatment should focus on emolliation and avoidance of irritants and allergens.[53] First-line therapy includes judicious use of topical corticosteroids and

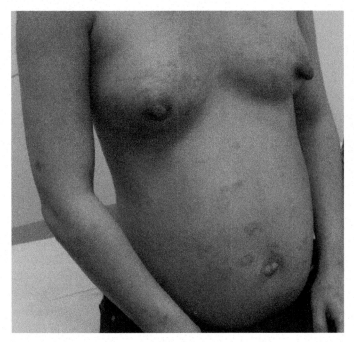

FIGURE 86-7. Atopic eruption of pregnancy in a Japanese female during the second trimester of pregnancy. This patient had longstanding atopic dermatitis and experienced a significant worsening of her condition during the latter half of her pregnancy.

oral antihistamines. UVB phototherapy is considered the safest second-line treatment in pregnancy. For very severe AD, oral corticosteroids may be used short term in the second and third trimester in low doses. Topical immunomodulators (pimecrolimus, tacrolimus) in small areas are also likely safe. Third-line therapy includes cyclosporine for severe AD. For bacterial superinfection, penicillin and cephalosporins are first line, and for herpetic superinfection, acyclovir is safe in pregnancy.

CONNECTIVE TISSUE DISEASE AND SARCOIDOSIS

◼ SYSTEMIC LUPUS ERYTHEMATOSUS

Systemic lupus erythematosus is a disease that typically presents in female patients during their fourth decade of life. Because disease onset occurs during the childbearing years, lupus appears regularly in pregnant females. Approximately 4500 women with lupus become pregnant each year in the United States alone.[54]

The literature supports a two- to three-fold increase in disease flares when patients are pregnant. The most common manifestation, which occurs in 25% to 90% of patients, is dermatologic, followed by lupus nephritis in up to 75% of patients.[55] While skin manifestations can be initial indicators of active disease, it is underlying kidney disease that carries significant comorbid consequences and requires prompt response. It is essential that nephritis be identified and properly evaluated. Differentiating preeclampsia from lupus nephritis can be difficult due to the overlap of hypertension, proteinuria, and hematuria in both disorders. This differentiation is paramount due to differences in treatment: eclampsia requires delivery, and lupus exacerbation can be managed pharmacologically.[54] Racial differences in pregnancy outcomes revealed that African American woman with lupus are more likely to have adverse outcomes, defined as hypertensive disorders, intrauterine growth retardation, or cesarean deliveries.[56] Because kidney disease is frequently responsible for fetal and maternal complications in lupus pregnancies, it is recommended that all clinicians carefully monitor for these serious complications.

◼ SARCOIDOSIS

Sarcoidosis is another disease that occurs commonly in skin of color populations [**Figure 86-8**]. African Americans have a three-fold higher

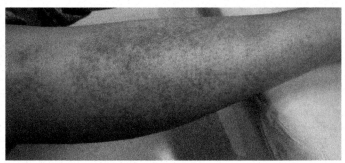

FIGURE 86-8. Cutaneous sarcoidosis in a Hispanic female. Note the numerous dermal papules with minimal epidermis surface change.

age-adjusted annual incidence than Caucasians. African American females between the ages of 30 and 39 are at highest risk of developing the disease.[57] Although lung disease is the most common presentation of sarcoidosis, there are a variety of dermatologic presentations as well, including erythema nodosum, lupus pernio, and macular, plaque, and subcutaneous nodular sarcoidosis.

Sarcoidosis rarely results in adverse pregnancy outcomes. However, the disease threatens pregnancy when there is significant uncontrolled disease including hypercalcemia, respiratory failure, or heart failure secondary to restrictive disease.[58,59] To avoid fetal compromise, pregnancy should be discouraged for patients with active disease. Pregnancy can be revisited once the disease is under appropriate medical control.

◼ SCLERODERMA

The scleroderma literature suggests a significant difference between African American and Caucasian patients in regard to increased incidence and severity of disease. A 20-year study revealed that African American females from the ages of 15 to 24 have the greatest incidence.[60] Additionally, it was found that women of color are more likely to develop multi-organ disease, be diagnosed at a younger age, have a higher incidence of inflammatory features, and have worse age-adjusted prognosis.[61]

Although active, multiorgan disease can be harmful during pregnancy due to placental vascular abnormalities, poor outcomes can be prevented with adequate disease control.[62] The first step is screening the patient during early pregnancy. It is proposed that clinicians, particularly dermatologists, ask general screening question regarding common rheumatologic disease manifestations including sun sensitivity, Raynaud phenomenon, and localized skin changes.[63] One study revealed that clinicians are 30% more likely to find undiagnosed rheumatic diseases if these simple screening questions are performed during the first trimester.[64]

◼ TREATMENT

The management of connective tissue disease and sarcoidosis can be challenging. It is important that patients understand that the risks associated with these diseases during pregnancy are largely due to poorly controlled disease. Planning a pregnancy 6 months after the disease has been controlled can help ensure the safety of the mother and child.[65] Toward this end, it is important to stress contraception to patients whose disease is currently active or has been in remission for less than 6 months. Patients may be reassured that they are likely to have more successful than unsuccessful pregnancies with these disorders, and with appropriate management and close follow-up, they can have a healthy pregnancy and good outcome.

ANTIMALARIALS

The antimalarial drugs, hydroxychloroquine and chloroquine, are used to treat cutaneous lesions of systemic and discoid lupus erythematosus because of their immune-modulating properties. Several studies support the safe use of hydroxychloroquine not only for malaria prophylaxis but also cutaneous disease in pregnancy. While animal models have shown some auditory and retinal effects of antimalarials, a 2009 meta-analysis found no increase in congenital defects, spontaneous abortions, fetal death, or even prematurity.[66] In addition to hydroxychloroquine's strong safety profile, it allows for decreased dosage of systemic steroids and diminishes the degree of lupus activity for patients during pregnancy. Other antimalarials, such as chloroquine, are also proven safe, but hydroxychloroquine has the lowest placental concentrations, which makes it the preferred choice. Its beneficial effects go beyond the skin by decreasing the risk of neonatal lupus and heart block in the mother.[67]

SYSTEMIC CORTICOSTEROIDS

Similar to topical corticosteroids, oral corticosteroids can be safe and effective to use during pregnancy, but due to greater bioavailability, there are increased risks to consider when using this medication. The literature shows evidence of intrauterine growth retardation, premature rupture of membranes, and preterm delivery in exposed infants and increases in cleft palates with exposure up to 12 weeks after conception. However, these results are challenged by much larger population studies that fail to show significant increases in cleft palates or other congenital malformations. There is also uncertainty as to whether the underlying disease, which is often associated with similar fetal outcomes, is the cause for these outcomes or if it is indeed a complication of the medication.[68]

Placental metabolism plays a role in which oral corticosteroid should be selected for treatment. Nonfluorinated corticosteroids, such as prednisone, are largely inactivated by placental enzymes and thus are minimally passed to the child. Fluorinated steroids such as betamethasone and dexamethasone pass freely through the placenta, which make them ideal for when fetal effects, such as promotion of lung maturity, are the desired outcome. In the case of a desired maternal effect, prednisone is the recommended medication. While there are challenges in using the oral corticosteroids, they remain an important option during pregnancy. However, they must be accompanied with a thorough assessment and discussion of the risk–benefit ratio with the patient.

HUMAN IMMUNODEFICIENCY VIRUS

Seventy percent of the world's human immunodeficiency virus (HIV)/acquired immunodeficiency (AIDS) patients live in sub-Saharan Africa, and this is the only region in the world where more females than males are infected. African women of childbearing age have a heightened susceptibility for acquiring this infection.[69] The infection is responsible for a unique group of skin manifestations that necessitate knowledge and skill for accurate diagnosis and management.

▣ INFECTIOUS

Coccidioidomycosis Pregnancy is known as a risk factor for a severe, diffuse form of coccidioidomycosis, a fungal infection that has a special predilection for immunosuppressed patients as well as African Americans. This puts HIV-positive females with skin of color at significantly heightened risk of this life-threatening disease for mother and child.[70,71] While the immunologic reason for the predilection is unknown, there is significant literature that shows that being of African descent is a risk factor for disseminated disease. Additionally, individuals of Filipino and Mexican descent are 175 and 3 times more likely, respectively, to have disseminated coccidioidomycosis.[72,73] While coccidioidomycosis has a variety of disease presentations, the most common presentations to a dermatologist include erythema nodosum or erythema multiforme.

Miscellaneous Infections Studies show that across HIV-positive populations, 90% of patients will have skin disease.[74,75] While not unique to pregnant patients, common infections include methicillin-resistant *Staphylococcus aureus*, human papilloma virus, herpes simplex virus, varicella zoster virus [**Figure 86-9**], scabies [**Figure 86-10, A and B**], molluscum contagiosum [**Figure 86-11**], and primary and secondary [**Figure 86-12**] syphilis.[76]

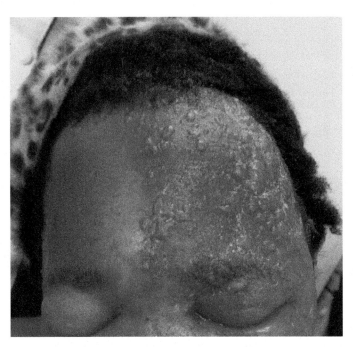

FIGURE 86-9. Human immunodeficiency virus (HIV)-positive African female with herpes zoster infection in a V_1 distribution. Unlike zoster in individuals without HIV infection, the dermatomal eruption may be particularly bullous, hemorrhagic, necrotic, and painful in HIV-infected persons. (Used with permission from Dr. Deepti Gupta.)

▣ PRURITUS AND INFLAMMATORY SKIN CONDITIONS

Pruritus Close to 30% of HIV-positive individuals will experience some degree of itching. Studies have shown a relationship between increased pruritus and HIV in pregnant females, but it is unclear if the pruritus is a product of the pregnancy itself or of HIV progression.[77,78] Chronic pruritus often leads to prurigo nodularis particularly when the itch-scratch cycle has continued for weeks to months. The goal of management is to identify the cause of the pruritus[79] with the ultimate goal of breaking the itch-scratch cycle.

Papular Pruritic Eruption Papular pruritic eruption is found more commonly in Africa and other tropical environments. This disease likely represents an exaggerated immune response to arthropod antigens in a subset of susceptible HIV-infected patients. Patients will often complain of pruritic lesions that last longer than a typical insect bite. The typical primary lesion is a firm, discrete, erythematous, urticarial papule.[80] In HIV patients, the condition can recur episodically and is often resistant to oral antihistamines and topical steroids. Most patients scratch the lesions because of the severe pruritus, leading to excoriated papules, marked postinflammatory hyperpigmentation, and, eventually, scarred nodules [**Figure 86-13, A and B**].[81]

Photodermatitis There can be several etiologic causes of photodermatologic reactions in pregnant patients with HIV. Not only can HIV itself have a photosensitizing effect, but several medications including azithromycin, tetracyclines, quinolones, and several antiparasitics taken for the infection can cause a similar reaction.[79]

Eczematous Dermatitis and Psoriasis These inflammatory skin disorders are common in African HIV-positive patients [**Figure 86-14**]. They can present with greater severity in HIV patients, such as new-onset erythroderma. Patients may or may not have a history of disease prior to HIV diagnosis.[79]

▣ CUTANEOUS DRUG REACTIONS IN HIV

Sulfonamides Sulfonamides are uniquely noted to cause drug eruptions, particularly trimethoprim-sulfamethoxazole, which is often used in HIV patients to treat pneumocystis pneumonia. Drug eruptions to sulfa-containing antibiotics can present in a variety of ways, with

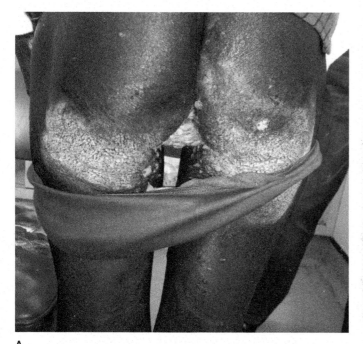

A

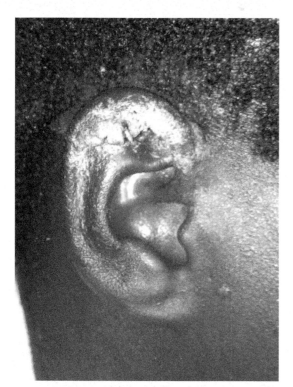

B

FIGURE 86-10. Scabies infection in human immunodeficiency virus (HIV)-positive African female. **(A)** HIV patients have higher likelihood of developing Norwegian crusted scabies. **(B)** Patients are also more likely to present with lesions on the head and neck, which is less common in immunocompetent individuals. Scabies can be treated safely with permethrin 5% cream, benzoyl benzoate in Europe, and topical sulfur 5% or 10% ointment in pregnancy. (Used with permission from Dr. Deepti Gupta.)

Stevens-Johnson syndrome and toxic epidermal necrolysis as the most severe presentations. The literature reveals that almost two-thirds of HIV-positive patients experience adverse reactions requiring discontinuation of the medication [**Figure 86-15**], and the rates of adverse reaction are particularly high in East Africa.[79,82] The medication can also contribute to hyperbilirubinemia and kernicterus in an unborn fetus; for that reason, sulfa antibiotics should be avoided 6 weeks prior to birth.

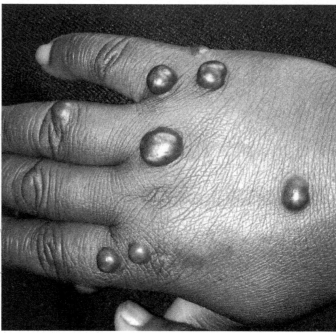

FIGURE 86-11. Molluscum contagiosum infection in a human immunodeficiency virus (HIV)-positive African female. Once CD4 count falls below 200/μL, the lesions tend to proliferate, and extensive molluscum contagiosum is a cutaneous marker of advanced HIV disease. (Used with permission from Dr. Deepti Gupta.)

Nevirapine While the side effect profile of this antiretroviral spans all HIV-infected individuals, it has a particular proclivity for causing reactions in pregnant HIV-positive females. It is associated with several adverse reactions, the most common being an erythematous drug rash that can precede liver toxicity. Two risk factors identified for a potentially life-threatening drug reaction include initiation of the drug late in pregnancy and those with a CD4 count greater than 250/μL upon initiation.[83] It is suggested to start the medication early in the pregnancy and only when HIV has progressed significantly.

Antiretroviral Therapy The World Health Organization recommends an initial antiretroviral regimen consisting of zidovudine, lamivudine, and nevirapine. If patients cannot tolerate zidovudine, stavudine, which has also proven safe in pregnancy, may be substituted. As previously mentioned, nevirapine has a significant adverse effect profile, but the

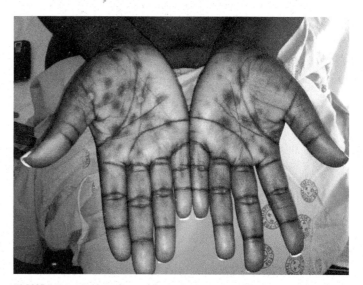

FIGURE 86-12. Secondary syphilis in a human immunodeficiency virus (HIV)-positive African female. The copper-colored maculopapular rash on the palms harbors bacteria and is contagious. (Used with permission from Dr. Deepti Gupta.)

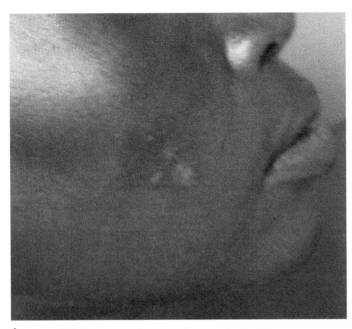

A

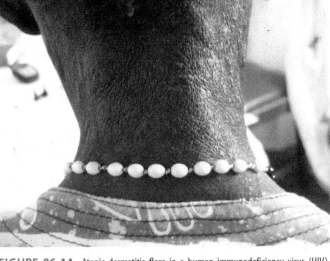

FIGURE 86-14. Atopic dermatitis flare in a human immunodeficiency virus (HIV)-positive female. HIV-infected adults with a previous history of atopic disease may note recurrence of atopy in advanced HIV disease as well as in pregnancy.

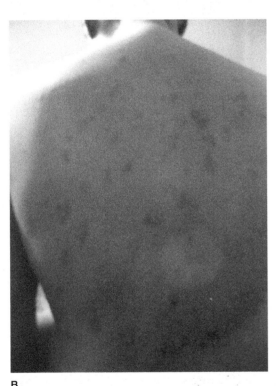

B

FIGURE 86-13. Pruritic papular eruption is thought to reflect an altered and exaggerated immune response to arthropod antigens in human immunodeficiency virus (HIV)-infected patients. The concentration of the lesions is highest on the extremities, but the face **(A)** and the trunk **(B)** are also involved in half of patients.

key is initiation of the medication early in pregnancy.[84] Efavirenz is commonly used in antiretroviral regimens, but it should be avoided given possible neural tube defects if administered in the first trimester. While the evidence is not overly compelling, it should be avoided in favor of the aforementioned therapies.[85,86]

SICKLE CELL DISEASE

Treatment of sickle cell disease (SCD) with hydroxyurea has been reported to result in in utero death or spontaneous abortion.[87] The National Toxicology Program expert program does not recommend

the use of hydroxyurea in pregnancy.[88] Chronic narcotic treatment for SCD patients is not uncommon, and it has been reported that pain control required for pregnant women with SCD has not been associated with congenital defects. Chronic narcotic treatment is associated with a risk of neonatal abstinence syndrome, but the risk was not found to be dependent on dose.[89]

In pregnancy, there is increased risk of the development of ulcers due to increased blood volume. Sickle cell ulceration is often recalcitrant to treatment and often recurs.[90] There have been two case reports of spontaneous healing of sickle cell ulcers during pregnancy, which was hypothesized to be due to fetal stem cell circulation. However, relapse occurred in both women 3 to 4 months after delivery.[91,92]

There is some research that suggests both micro- and macronutrient deficiencies are associated with SCD.[93] For SCD-related leg ulceration, zinc deficiency may play a role in pathogenesis.[93] In pregnant women with SCD, iron deficiency is common.[93] There are currently no specific

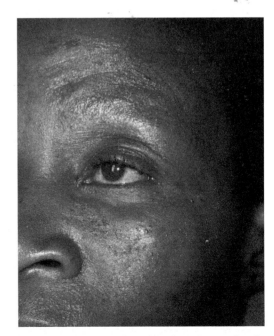

FIGURE 86-15. Photosensitivity secondary to sulfonamides in an African human immunodeficiency virus (HIV)-positive female. This patient was being treated for pneumocystis pneumonia.

recommended guidelines for zinc and iron supplementation for pregnant women with SCD, and clinicians must make decisions for patients on an individual basis.

CONCLUSION

SG, melasma, and ICP are disorders that occur not uncommonly in pregnant women of color. Additionally, serious systemic diseases including MF, sarcoidosis, scleroderma, and lupus appear to be more aggressive and confer a worse prognoses in pregnant women of color. The approach to these patients must include aggressive control of the underlying disease.

REFERENCES

1. Chang AL, Agredano YZ, Kimball AB. Risk factors associated with striae gravidarum. *J Am Acad Dermatol.* 2004;51:881-885.
2. Osman H, Rubeiz N, Tamim H, et al. Risk factors for the development of striae gravidarum. *Am J Obstet Gynecol.* 2007;196:62.e61-65.
3. Yamaguchi K, Suganuma N, Ohashi K. Quality of life evaluation in Japanese pregnant women with striae gravidarum: a cross-sectional study. *BMC Res Notes.* 2012;5:450.
4. Pierard-Franchimont C, Hermanns JF, Hermanns-Le T, et al. Striae distensae in darker skin types: the influence of melanocyte mechanobiology. *J Cosmet Dermatol.* 2005;4:174-178.
5. Brennan M, Young G, Devane D. Topical preparations for preventing stretch marks in pregnancy. *Cochrane Database Syst Rev.* 2012;11:CD000066.
6. Rangel O, Arias I, Garcia E, et al. Topical tretinoin 0.1% for pregnancy-related abdominal striae: an open-label, multicenter, prospective study. *Adv Ther.* 2001;18:181-186.
7. Ash K, Lord J, Zukowski M, et al. Comparison of topical therapy for striae alba (20% glycolic acid/0.05% tretinoin versus 20% glycolic acid/10% L-ascorbic acid). *Dermatol Surg.* 1998;24:849-856.
8. Sherling M, Friedman PM, Adrian R, et al. Consensus recommendations on the use of an erbium-doped 1,550-nm fractionated laser and its applications in dermatologic laser surgery. *Dermatol Surg.* 2010;36:461-469.
9. Bak H, Kim BJ, Lee WJ, et al. Treatment of striae distensae with fractional photothermolysis. *Dermatol Surg.* 2009;35:1215-1220.
10. de Angelis F, Kolesnikova L, Renato F, et al. Fractional nonablative 1540-nm laser treatment of striae distensae in Fitzpatrick skin types II to IV: clinical and histological results. *Aesthet Surg J.* 2011;31:411-419.
11. Nouri K, Romagosa R, Chartier T, et al. Comparison of the 585 nm pulse dye laser and the short pulsed CO2 laser in the treatment of striae distensae in skin types IV and VI. *Dermatol Surg.* 1999;25:368-370.
12. Lee SE, Kim JH, Lee SJ, et al. Treatment of striae distensae using an ablative 10,600-nm carbon dioxide fractional laser: a retrospective review of 27 participants. *Dermatol Surg.* 2010;36:1683-1690.
13. Hernandez-Perez E, Colombo-Charrier E, Valencia-Ibiett E. Intense pulsed light in the treatment of striae distensae. *Dermatol Surg.* 2002;28:1124-1130.
14. Goldman A, Rossato F, Prati C. Stretch marks: treatment using the 1,064-nm Nd:YAG laser. *Dermatol Surg.* 2008;34:686-691.
15. Manuskiatti W, Boonthaweeyuwat E, Varothai S. Treatment of striae distensae with a TriPollar radiofrequency device: a pilot study. *J Dermatolog Treat.* 2009;20:359-364.
16. Kim IS, Park KY, Kim BJ, Kim MN, Kim CW, Kim SE. Efficacy of intradermal radiofrequency combined with autologous platelet-rich plasma in striae distensae: a pilot study. *Int J Dermatol.* 2012;51:1253-1258.
17. Sadick NS, Magro C, Hoenig A. Prospective clinical and histological study to evaluate the efficacy and safety of a targeted high-intensity narrow band UVB/UVA1 therapy for striae alba. *J Cosmet Laser Ther.* 2007;9:79-83.
18. Alexiades-Armenakas MR, Bernstein LJ, Friedman PM, Geronemus RG. The safety and efficacy of the 308-nm excimer laser for pigment correction of hypopigmented scars and striae alba. *Arch Dermatol.* 2004;140:955-960.
19. Park KY, Kim HK, Kim SE, Kim BJ, Kim MN. Treatment of striae distensae using needling therapy: a pilot study. *Dermatol Surg.* 2012;38:1823-1828.
20. Shridharani SM, Magarakis M, Manson PN, Singh NK, Basdag B, Rosson GD. The emerging role of antineoplastic agents in the treatment of keloids and hypertrophic scars: a review. *Ann Plast Surg.* 2010;64:355-361.
21. Bayat A, Arscott G, Ollier WE, Ferguson MW, McGrouther DA. Description of site-specific morphology of keloid phenotypes in an Afrocaribbean population. *Br J Plast Surg.* 2004;57:122-133.
22. Tulandi T, Al-Sannan B, Akbar G, Ziegler C, Miner L. Prospective study of intraabdominal adhesions among women of different races with or without keloids. *Am J Obstet Gynecol.* 2011;204(2):132.e1-4.
23. Alderdice F, McKenna D, Dornan J. Techniques and materials for skin closure in caesarean section. *Cochrane Database Syst Rev.* 2003;2:CD003577.
24. Kroumpouzos G, Cohen LM. Dermatoses of pregnancy. *J Am Acad Dermatol.* 2001;45:1-19.
25. Cummings KDV. Dermatoses associated with pregnancy. *Cutis.* 1967;3:120-126.
26. Reyes H, Gonzalez MC, Ribalta J, et al. Prevalence of intrahepatic cholestasis of pregnancy in Chile. *Ann Intern Med.* 1978;88:487-493.
27. Reyes H, Wegmann ME, Segovia N, et al. HLA in Chileans with intrahepatic cholestasis of pregnancy. *Hepatology.* 1982;2:463-466.
28. Abedin P, Weaver JB, Egginton E. Intrahepatic cholestasis of pregnancy: prevalence and ethnic distribution. *Ethn Health.* 1999;4:35-37.
29. Kumari R, Jaisankar TJ, Thappa DM. A clinical study of skin changes in pregnancy. *Indian J Dermatol Venereol Leprol.* 2007;73:141.
30. Rudolph CM, Al-Fares S, Vaughan-Jones SA, Mullegger RR, Kerl H, Black MM. Polymorphic eruption of pregnancy: clinicopathology and potential trigger factors in 181 patients. *Br J Dermatol.* 2006;154:54-60.
31. Yancey KB, Hall RP, Lawley TJ. Pruritic urticarial papules and plaques of pregnancy. Clinical experience in twenty-five patients. *J Am Acad Dermatol.* 1984;10:473-480.
32. Alcalay J, Ingber A, Kafri B, et al. Hormonal evaluation and autoimmune background in pruritic urticarial papules and plaques of pregnancy. *Am J Obstet Gynecol.* 1988;158:417-420.
33. Mygind H, Thulstrup AM, Pedersen L, Larsen H. Risk of intrauterine growth retardation, malformations and other birth outcomes in children after topical use of corticosteroid in pregnancy. *Acta Obstet Gynecol Scand.* 2002;81:234-239.
34. Mahe A, Perret JL, Ly F, Fall F, Rault JP, Dumont A. The cosmetic use of skin-lightening products during pregnancy in Dakar, Senegal: a common and potentially hazardous practice. *Trans R Soc Trop Med Hyg.* 2007;101:183-187.
35. Chi CC, Lee CW, Wojnarowska F, Kirtschig G. Safety of topical corticosteroids in pregnancy. *Cochrane Database Syst Rev.* 2009;3:CD007346.
36. Zierler S, Purohit D. Prenatal antihistamine exposure and retrolental fibroplasia. *Am J Epidemiol.* 1986;123:192-196.
37. Kar S, Krishnan A, Preetha K, Mohankar A. A review of antihistamines used during pregnancy. *J Pharmacol Pharmacother.* 2012;3:105-108.
38. The use of newer asthma and allergy medications during pregnancy. The American College of Obstetricians and Gynecologists (ACOG) and The American College of Allergy, Asthma and Immunology (ACAAI). *Ann Allergy Asthma Immunol.* 2000;84:475-480.
39. Bacq Y, Sentilhes L, Reyes HB, et al. Efficacy of ursodeoxycholic acid in treating intrahepatic cholestasis of pregnancy: a meta-analysis. *Gastroenterology.* 2012;143:1492-1501.
40. Sun G, Berthelot C, Li Y, et al. Poor prognosis in non-Caucasian patients with early-onset mycosis fungoides. *J Am Acad Dermatol.* 2009;60:231-235.
41. Shoo BA, Kashani-Sabet M. Melanoma arising in African-, Asian-, Latino- and Native-American populations. *Semin Cutan Med Surg.* 2009;28:96-102.
42. Horev A, Weintraub AY, Sergienko R, Wiznitzer A, Halevy S, Sheiner E. Pregnancy outcome in women with vitiligo. *Int J Dermatol.* 2011;50:1083-1085.
43. Park KK, Murase JE. Narrowband UV-B phototherapy during pregnancy and folic acid depletion. *Arch Dermatol.* 2012;148:132-133.
44. Davis SA, Narahari S, Feldman SR, Huang W, Pichardo-Geisinger RO, McMichael AJ. Top dermatologic conditions in patients of color: an analysis of nationally representative data. *J Drugs Dermatol.* 2012;11:466-473.
45. Horn EJ, Chambers CD, Menter A, Kimball AB. Pregnancy outcomes in psoriasis: why do we know so little? *J Am Acad Dermatol.* 2009;61:e5-e8.
46. Murase JE, Chan KK, Garite TJ, Cooper DM, Weinstein GD. Hormonal effect on psoriasis in pregnancy and post partum. *Arch Dermatol.* 2005;141:601-606.
47. Boyd AS, Morris LF, Phillips CM, Menter MA. Psoriasis and pregnancy: hormone and immune system interaction. *Int J Dermatol.* 1996;35:169-172.
48. Bae YS, Van Voorhees AS, Hsu S, et al. Review of treatment options for psoriasis in pregnant or lactating women: from the Medical Board of the National Psoriasis Foundation. *J Am Acad Dermatol.* 2012;67:459-477.
49. Ambros-Rudolph CM, Mullegger RR, Vaughan-Jones SA, Kerl H, Black MM. The specific dermatoses of pregnancy revisited and reclassified: results of a retrospective two-center study on 505 pregnant patients. *J Am Acad Dermatol.* 2006;54:395-404.
50. Vaughan Jones SA, Hern S, Nelson-Piercy C, Seed PT, Black MM. A prospective study of 200 women with dermatoses of pregnancy correlating clinical findings with hormonal and immunopathological profiles. *Br J Dermatol.* 1999;141:71-81.

51. Kemmett D, Tidman MJ. The influence of the menstrual cycle and pregnancy on atopic dermatitis. *Br J Dermatol*. 1991;125(1):59-61.

52. Weatherhead S, Robson SC, Reynolds NJ. Eczema in pregnancy. *BMJ*. 2007;335:152-154.

53. Koutroulis I, Papoutsis J, Kroumpouzos G. Atopic dermatitis in pregnancy: current status and challenges. *Obstet Gynecol Surv*. 2011;66:654-663.

54. Clowse ME, Jamison M, Myers E, James AH. A national study of the complications of lupus in pregnancy. *Am J Obstet Gynecol*. 2008;199:127.e121-e126.

55. Clowse ME. Lupus activity in pregnancy. *Rheum Dis Clin North Am*. 2007;33:237-252.

56. Chakravarty EF, Nelson L, Krishnan E. Obstetric hospitalizations in the United States for women with systemic lupus erythematosus and rheumatoid arthritis. *Arthritis Rheum*. 2006;54:899-907.

57. Rybicki BA, Major M, Popovich J Jr, Maliarik MJ, Iannuzzi MC. Racial differences in sarcoidosis incidence: a 5-year study in a health maintenance organization. *Am J Epidemiol*. 1997;145:234-241.

58. Subramanian P, Chinthalapalli H, Krishnan M, et al. Pregnancy and sarcoidosis: an insight into the pathogenesis of hypercalciuria. *Chest*. 2004;126:995-998.

59. Ellafi M, Valeyre D. [Sarcoidosis and pregnancy]. *Rev Pneumol Clin*. 1999;55:335-337.

60. Steen VD, Oddis CV, Conte CG, Janoski J, Casterline GZ, Medsger TA Jr. Incidence of systemic sclerosis in Allegheny County, Pennsylvania. A twenty-year study of hospital-diagnosed cases, 1963-1982. *Arthritis Rheum*. 1997;40:441-445.

61. Laing TJ, Gillespie BW, Toth MB, et al. Racial differences in scleroderma among women in Michigan. *Arthritis Rheum*. 1997;40:734-742.

62. Rabhi M, Tiev KP, Genereau T, Cabane J. [Scleroderma and pregnancy]. *Ann Med Intern (Paris)*. 2002;153:193-200.

63. Spinillo A, Beneventi F, Ramoni V, et al. Prevalence and significance of previously undiagnosed rheumatic diseases in pregnancy. *Ann Rheum Dis*. 2012;71:918-923.

64. Spinillo A, Beneventi F, Epis OM, et al. Prevalence of undiagnosed autoimmune rheumatic diseases in the first trimester of pregnancy. Results of a two-steps strategy using a self-administered questionnaire and autoantibody testing. *BJOG*. 2008;115:51-57.

65. Lateef A, Petri M. Management of pregnancy in systemic lupus erythematosus. *Nat Rev Rheumatol*. 20128;710-718.

66. Sperber K, Hom C, Chao CP, Shapiro D, Ash J. Systematic review of hydroxychloroquine use in pregnant patients with autoimmune diseases. *Pediatr Rheumatol Online J*. 2009;7:9.

67. Izmirly PM, Costedoat-Chalumeau N, Pisoni CN, et al. Maternal use of hydroxychloroquine is associated with a reduced risk of recurrent anti-SSA/Ro-antibody-associated cardiac manifestations of neonatal lupus. *Circulation*. 2012;126:76-82.

68. Fitzsimons R, Greenberger PA, Patterson R. Outcome of pregnancy in women requiring corticosteroids for severe asthma. *J Allergy Clin Immunol*. 1986;78:349-353.

69. Glynn JR, Carael M, Auvert B, et al. Why do young women have a much higher prevalence of HIV than young men? A study in Kisumu, Kenya and Ndola, Zambia. *AIDS*. 2001;15(Suppl 4):S51-S60.

70. Woods CW, McRill C, Plikaytis BD, et al. Coccidioidomycosis in human immunodeficiency virus-infected persons in Arizona, 1994-1997: incidence, risk factors, and prevention. *J Infect Dis*. 2000;181:1428-1434.

71. Vaughan JE, Ramirez H. Coccidioidomycosis as a complication of pregnancy. *Calif Med*. 1951;74:121-125.

72. Smith CE, Beard RR. Varieties of coccidioidal infection in relation to the epidemiology and control of the diseases. *Am J Public Health Nations Health*. 1946;36:1394-1402.

73. Ruddy BE, Mayer AP, Ko MG, et al. Coccidioidomycosis in African Americans. *Mayo Clin Proc*. 2011;86:63-69.

74. Gibbs S. Skin disease and socioeconomic conditions in rural Africa: Tanzania. *Int J Dermatol*. 1996;35:633-639.

75. Mosam A, Irusen EM, Kagoro H, Aboobaker J, Dlova N. The impact of human immunodeficiency virus/acquired immunodeficiency syndrome (HIV/AIDS) on skin disease in KwaZulu-Natal, South Africa. *Int J Dermatol*. 2004;43:782-783.

76. Rodgers S, Leslie KS. Skin infections in HIV-infected individuals in the era of HAART. *Curr Opin Infect Dis*. 2011;24:124-129.

77. Alonso N, Lugo-Somolinos A, Torres-Paoli D, Sanchez JL. Prevalence of skin disease in HIV-positive pregnant women. *Int J Dermatol*. 2003;42:521-523.

78. Coopman SA, Johnson RA, Platt R, Stern RS. Cutaneous disease and drug reactions in HIV infection. *N Engl J Med*. 1993;328:1670-1674.

79. Amerson EH, Maurer TA. Dermatologic manifestations of HIV in Africa. *Top HIV Med*. 2010;18:16-22.

80. Resneck JS Jr, Van Beek M, Furmanski L, et al. Etiology of pruritic papular eruption with HIV infection in Uganda. *JAMA*. 2004;292:2614-2621.

81. Hevia O, Jimenez-Acosta F, Ceballos PI, Gould EW, Penneys NS. Pruritic papular eruption of the acquired immunodeficiency syndrome: a clinicopathologic study. *J Am Acad Dermatol*. 1991;24:231-235.

82. Gordin FM, Simon GL, Wofsy CB, Mills J. Adverse reactions to trimethoprim-sulfamethoxazole in patients with the acquired immunodeficiency syndrome. *Ann Intern Med*. 1984;100:495-499.

83. Kondo W, Carraro EA, Prandel E, et al. Nevirapine-induced side effects in pregnant women: experience of a Brazilian university hospital. *Braz J Infect Dis*. 2007;11:544-548.

84. Taylor GP, Clayden P, Dhar J, et al. British HIV Association guidelines for the management of HIV infection in pregnant women 2012. *HIV Med*. 2012;13(Suppl 2):87-157.

85. Ford N, Mofenson L, Kranzer K, et al. Safety of efavirenz in first-trimester of pregnancy: a systematic review and meta-analysis of outcomes from observational cohorts. *AIDS*. 2010;24:1461-1470.

86. Ford N, Calmy A, Mofenson L. Safety of efavirenz in the first trimester of pregnancy: an updated systematic review and meta-analysis. *AIDS*. 2011;25:2301-2304.

87. Thauvin-Robinet C, Maingueneau C, Robert E, et al. Exposure to hydroxyurea during pregnancy: a case series. *Leukemia*. 2001;15:1309-1311.

88. Lanzkron S, Strouse JJ, Wilson R, et al. Systematic review: hydroxyurea for the treatment of adults with sickle cell disease. *Ann Intern Med*. 2008;148:939-955.

89. Cleary BJ, Donnelly J, Strawbridge J, et al. Methadone dose and neonatal abstinence syndrome-systematic review and meta-analysis. *Addiction*. 2010;105:2071-2084.

90. Cackovic M, Chung C, Bolton LL, Kerstein MD. Leg ulceration in the sickle cell patient. *J Am Coll Surg*. 1998;187:307-309.

91. Droitcourt C, Khosrotehrani K, Girot R, Aractingi S. Healing of sickle cell ulcers during pregnancy: a favourable effect of foetal cell transfer? *J Eur Acad Dermatol Venereol*. 2008;22:1256-1257.

92. Cornbleet T. Spontaneous healing of sickle-cell anemia ulcer in pregnancy. *J Am Med Assoc*. 1952;148:1025-1026.

93. Reed JD, Redding-Lallinger R, Orringer EP. Nutrition and sickle cell disease. *Am J Hematol*. 1987;24:441-455.

CHAPTER

Geriatrics

87

Roopal V. Kundu
Neelam A. Vashi

KEY POINTS

- Aging changes in individuals with skin of color age typically occur 10 to 20 years later than those of age-matched white counterparts.

- Common clinical signs of photoaging in darker skinned individuals include lentigines, rhytides, telangiectasias, and loss of elasticity.

- Cleansers with lubricating products that contain emollients should also be employed, and appropriate photoprotection should be practiced.

- Maturational dyschromia (uneven skin tone) was a chief complaint in more than one-third of women with dark skin of color.

INTRODUCTION

In humans, aging refers to a multidimensional process of physical, psychological, and social change. Aging is an important part of all human societies reflecting not only biologic changes but also influences of cultural and societal standards. Although age is measured chronologically, the term *aging* is somewhat ambiguous, an organic process of growing older while showing the effects of increasing age. Understanding the fundamentals of mature skin is important to an aging population where individuals are expected to be productive into later years and hold a strong desire to maintain a youthful appearance.

RACIAL DIFFERENCES IN AGING

Across all skin types, the aging process involves photodamage, fat redistribution, bone shifting, and the loss of connective tissue. As life expectancy continues to increase, almost doubling over the past century, an aged appearance is often a presenting complaint for the Caucasian population. This particular group is often affected by the secondary effects of photoaging including fine lines, deep furrows, and age spots. Individuals with skin of color is less susceptible to sun-induced damage, so these clinical manifestations of aging are less severe and typically occur 10 to 20 years later than those of age-matched fairer-skinned counterparts.[1] Individuals with dark skin of color are overall thought to have firmer and smoother skin than individuals with lighter skin of the same age.[2]

STRUCTURAL AND FUNCTIONAL DIFFERENCES

Melanin is the major determinant of color in the skin, and the concentration of epidermal melanin in melanosomes is double in darker skin types compared to lightly pigmented skin types.[3] In addition, melanosome degradation within the keratinocyte is slower in darkly pigmented skin when compared to lightly pigmented skin. The melanin content and melanosomal dispersion pattern is thought to confer protection from accelerated aging induced by ultraviolet (UV) radiation.[1,4] Kaidbey et al[1] demonstrated that the epidermis of dark skin of color, on average, provided a sun protection factor (SPF) of 13.4, which provides a scientific basis for the observation of better aging in terms of reduced number of fine lines and wrinkles. Although the increased melanin provides protection from many harmful effects of UV radiation including photodamage and skin cancers, it also makes darkly pigmented skin more vulnerable to postinflammatory dyspigmentation. Therefore, more so than textural changes, inconsistent pigmentation with both hypopigmentation and hyperpigmentation is a sign of photoaging in people with skin of color.

Aging of the skin is also associated with progressive atrophy of the dermis and changes in the architectural organization leading to folds and wrinkles.[5] Asian and dark skin of color has a thicker and more compact dermis than fairer skin, with the thickness being proportional to the degree of pigmentation.[6] This likely contributes to the lower incidence of facial rhytides in Asians and African Americans.

The major cell type of the dermis is the fibroblast, which synthesizes the main structural elements of the dermis. Chronologic aging reduces the life of fibroblasts, with their potential for division being lower in the elderly.[5] Fibroblasts are more numerous, larger, and more multinucleated in dark skin of color than lighter-colored skin.[7] Fibroblast functionality and reactivity likely contribute to both the aging phenomena and also abnormal scarring, specifically keloid formation in those with skin of color.

KEY COMPONENTS OF AGING

There are many extrinsic and intrinsic factors that contribute to aging. Extrinsic aging relates to environmental exposures, health, and lifestyle. These factors are controllable and related to individual habits such as sun exposure, tobacco use, diet, and exercise.[8]

Cumulative exposure to sun is the most important extrinsic factor in aging skin, especially for lighter skin types. Patients with skin types III and IV may also suffer from dermatoheliosis. In skin types IV to VI, dyspigmentation is the most common feature of photoaging. Common clinical signs of photoaging include lentigines, rhytides, telangiectasias, and loss of elasticity.[8] Regardless of skin type, other extrinsic factors such as smoking, excessive alcohol use, and poor nutrition can contribute to premature skin aging.

Intrinsic aging reflects the genetic background of an individual and results from the passage of time. Intrinsically aged skin is typically smooth and unblemished, with exaggerated expression lines, fat atrophy with soft tissue redistribution, and bone remodeling.[8] People with skin of color exhibit less severe intrinsic facial aging, with signs of intrinsic aging appearing a decade later than in lighter skin types; however, there

is an overall paucity of literature discussing the relationship between darker pigmented skin and aging characteristics.

GENERAL SKIN CARE FOR AGING SKIN OF COLOR

Aging skin requires changes to overall regimens as mature and skin of color tend to be dryer than younger, lighter skin. Cleansing should occur less frequently, generally once daily or twice daily if heavy makeup is worn. Cleansers with lubricating products that contain emollients to moisturize as the skin is cleansed should also be employed. The face should be cleansed gently with a soft wash cloth or fingertips and pat dried. While cleansing should be decreased, moisturizing should be increased in the aging population. Richer creams should be applied two to three times a day, especially to damp skin immediately after cleansing. In addition, various forms of topical vitamin A can be used. Over-the-counter retinols can be used daily as long as they do not cause dryness or irritation. Prescription strength vitamin A derivatives can also be used, but care should be taken to ensure that these do not cause any irritation, which can worsen pigmentary alteration. Lastly, various forms of glycolic acid can be used to exfoliate dry, dull skin and improve overall skin tone.

PHOTOPROTECTION IN DARKER SKIN

To prevent or further discoloration, sun protection measures should be taken. Sunscreen, with a minimum of SPF 15, is still very important for aging skin because it can prevent further skin darkening and uneven skin tone. Furthermore, discussion of sun-protective clothing and hats and avoidance of direct sun should be discussed. Because photoprotection has not historically been targeted for communities with skin of color, it is important to give specific instructions on the type and use of photoprotection advised.

DYSPIGMENTATION

In skin types IV to VI, dyspigmentation in different forms is the most common feature of photoaging.

▌ IDIOPATHIC GUTTATE HYPOMELANOSIS

Idiopathic guttate hypomelanosis is an acquired, benign leukoderma of unknown etiology. It most commonly occurs in older dark-skinned people with a history of long-term sun exposure. The cause is not known, and treatment is difficult.

▌ POSTINFLAMMATORY HYPER- AND HYPOPIGMENTATION

Postinflammatory hyper- and hypopigmentation refers to the darkening or lightening of the skin that may occur after any inflammatory eruption or injury (see Chapter 52). The hyperpigmentation results from the melanocytes' response to the cutaneous insult, which causes an increased production and/or redistribution of melanin. Patients with darker skin are predisposed to this pigment alteration. As the skin in darker patients recovers from an acute inflammatory disease, it may become hyperpigmented (known as postinflammatory hyperpigmentation) or hypopigmented (known as postinflammatory hypopigmentation). Lightening or darkening of the skin is associated with many primary disorders including discoid lupus erythematosus, seborrheic dermatitis, tinea versicolor, atopic dermatitis, and sarcoidosis. History may include any type of prior inflammation or injury (eg, acne, arthropod assault, viral exanthems, eczema, psoriasis, trauma). Physical examination findings include small to large hyperpigmented macules and patches of varying sizes in any distribution. Although usually a clinical diagnosis, difficult cases can be aided with a biopsy for histopathologic evaluation. Disorders such as melasma, morphea, atrophoderma, and other rarer etiologies should be considered in patients without evidence of preceding inflammation by history or examination. The time required for the dyspigmentation to fade to normal is highly variable and relates to many factors including

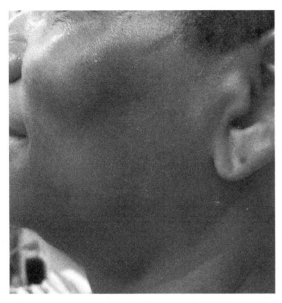

FIGURE 87-1. Maturational dyschromia: hyperpigmented ill-defined patches over the lateral zygoma in a middle-aged African American woman.

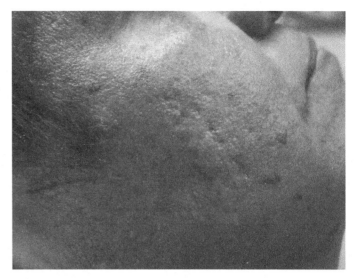

FIGURE 87-2. Seborrheic keratosis: hyperpigmented stuck-on, flat-topped papules over the cheeks in an older African American woman.

the patient's baseline skin tone, the type and intensity of the injury or inflammation, and the patient's sun exposure habits. Resolution of dyspigmentation can take years and can be psychologically distressing. Postinflammatory hypopigmentation generally recovers faster than postinflammatory hyperpigmentation; however, pigment alteration in scarred areas may be permanent. Treatments with topical bleaching agents, peeling agents, and lasers can be tried; however, they can also result in worsening of the original dyspigmentation and should always be used with caution.

MATURATIONAL DYSCHROMIA

Darkening of skin tone of the face, even outside of sunny months, can be an early sign of aging in mature dark skin. Maturational dyschromia, or a general uneven tone, can be described as diffuse hyperpigmentation that generally occurs on the lateral forehead and cheekbones [**Figure 87-1**]. One survey found that uneven skin tone was a chief complaint in more than one third of women with dark skin of color.[9] These changes in skin tone likely occur from chronic sun exposure over many years. Treatment options include topical bleaching agents, antioxidants, sunscreen, microdermabrasion, or chemical peels.

PERIORBITAL HYPERPIGMENTATION

Periorbital hyperpigmentation, also referred to as idiopathic cutaneous hyperchromia of the orbital region (ICHOR), periorbital melanosis, dark circles, or infraorbital pigmentation, is more frequently observed in the skin of color and aging population and can be of primary or secondary etiology.[10] The cause of secondary periorbital hyperpigmentation often has a multifactorial pathogenesis including genetic or constitutional pigmentation, dermal melanocytosis, postinflammatory hyperpigmentation secondary to atopic and/or allergic contact dermatitis, periorbital edema, excessive subcutaneous vascularity, and shadowing due to skin laxity and tear trough associated with aging.[10,11] Excessive sun exposure, drugs, hormonal causes, and extension of pigmentary demarcation lines have also been considered to be contributory.[10,12] ICHOR is characterized by bilateral darkening of the orbital skin and eyelid that is not secondary to systemic or local disease.[10] In a study by Ranu et al[13] on 200 patients with periorbital hyperpigmentation, possible causes were delineated according to history, physical examination, and assessment by dermatologists measuring with a Mexameter. They found the most common forms to be the vascular type (41.8%),

characterized by presence of erythema involving inner aspects of lower eyelids with prominent capillaries/telangiectasia or presence of bluish discoloration due to visible blue veins; the constitutional form (38.6%), characterized by the presence of brown-black hyperpigmentation of the lower eyelid skin along the shape of orbital rim; postinflammatory hyperpigmentation (12%); and shadow effects (11.4%) due to an overhanging tarsal muscle or deep tear trough.[13] Other causes included skin laxity, dry skin, hormonal disturbances, nutritional deficiencies, and other chronic illnesses.[13] Verschoore et al[14] confirmed that not only melanin deposits but also vascular stasis may play a role in the pathogenesis of ICHOR.

Regarding the localization of the pigmentation, earlier studies by Watanabe et al[15] and Malakar et al[12] have examined skin biopsies and found the presence of dermal melanocytosis and melanin pigment in upper dermal macrophages, respectively, thus partially explaining the recalcitrance of this condition to several treatments. Skin-lightening creams, chemical peels, intense pulsed light, Q-switched ruby laser, autologous fat transplantation, combinations of fat grafting and blepharoplasties, and fillers have all been tried, but none have provided long-term satisfactory treatment.[13]

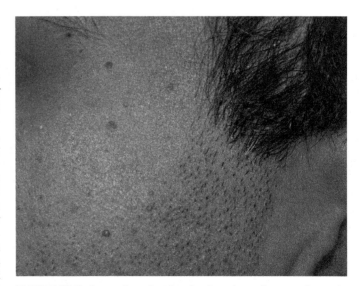

FIGURE 87-3. Dermatosis papulosa nigra: 1- to 2-mm brown discrete papules over the lateral cheek in an Asian man.

DERMATOSIS PAPULOSA NIGRA AND SEBORRHEIC KERATOSIS

Dermatosis papulosa nigra (DPN) is a common manifestation diagnosed primarily in African American, Afro-Caribbean, and sub-Saharan African individuals; however, it is also seen in other races. The cause and pathogenesis are unknown. DPN tends to have an earlier age of onset than that of seborrheic keratoses (SKs), but otherwise is similar and considered a variant of SK [**Figure 87-2**]. Among older East Asians, SKs on lateral aspect of face are common. DPN presents as 1- to 5-mm pigmented papules that are distributed bilaterally across the malar eminences, forehead, and, less often, the neck, chest, and back [**Figure 87-3**]. They appear during adolescence and increase in size and number over time, peaking in the sixth decade. Usually the lesions are asymptomatic but can occasionally be pruritic or irritated. The differential diagnosis includes skin tags, melanocytic nevi, lentigines, verrucae, and other adnexal tumors. Treatment is generally performed for cosmetic purposes and should be done with great care given the risks of dyspigmentation. Modalities include snip excision, curettage, electrodesiccation, light cryotherapy, and laser destruction.

MELASMA

Melasma is an acquired form of hyperpigmentation that is seen most commonly on the face (Chapter 51). The exact pathogenesis is unknown; however, it is hypothesized that following exposure to UV visible light, melanocytes produce increased amounts of melanin compared with uninvolved skin. Exacerbating factors include pregnancy, hormonal therapy such as oral contraceptives, and intense sun exposure. At least 90% of those affected are women. Clinically, there are light to dark brown patches with irregular borders most commonly distributed symmetrically on the centrofacial, malar, and mandibular regions; they can also be on the forearms. The differential diagnosis includes postinflammatory hyperpigmentation, solar lentigines, acanthosis nigricans, and other more rare pigmentary disorders including exogenous ochronosis, lichen planus pigmentosus, and erythema dyschromicum perstans. Treatment includes a combination approach with strict sun protection, topical depigmenting agents, chemical peels, and laser therapy.

EPHELIDES AND LENTIGINES

Ephelides and lentigines are a common manifestation of sun exposure in Caucasian patients and less so in those with skin of color.

Ephelides, or freckles, are the result of increased photo-induced melanogenesis and transport of an increased number of fully melanized melanosomes from melanocytes to keratinocytes. Ephelides occur only on sun-exposed areas of the body, particularly the face, dorsal hands, and upper trunk [**Figure 87-4**]. They are 1- to 3-mm well-demarcated macules that are round, oval, or irregular in shape. They may increase in number and distribution and show a tendency for confluence, but they can fade over time with aging. Ephelides are benign and show no propensity for malignant transformation.[16] Some ephelides may represent a subtype of solar lentigo.[17]

Solar lentigines are found in 90% of the Caucasian population older than 60 years of age, and their incidence increases with advancing age.[18] Lentigines are more common in Caucasians, but also occur in Asians. Inherited patterned lentiginosis favors more lightly pigmented African Americans, including those with mixed American Indian heritage. Solar lentigines are 3-mm to 2-cm well-circumscribed, round, oval, or irregularly shaped macules or patches that vary in color from tan to dark brown. They occur on sun-exposed areas, predominantly the dorsal aspects of hands and forearms, face, upper chest, and back.

Treatment options for ephelides and lentigines include sun protection measures, cryotherapy, and laser surgery.

HORI NEVI

Acquired bilateral nevus of Ota-like macules, or Hori nevi, are characterized by blue-gray to gray-brown macules primarily on the zygomatic area and less often on the forehead, temples, upper eyelids, and root and alae of the nose[19] [**Figure 87-5**]. It is a common dermal melanocytic hyperpigmentation in Asians, primarily Chinese and Japanese women from 20 to 70 years of age. The eye and oral mucosa are not involved. It may also be misdiagnosed as melasma. Treatment modalities, including cryotherapy, various Q-switched lasers including a combination of a 532-nm Q-switched Nd:YAG laser (QSNY) followed by a 1064-nm QSNY, or combined use of a scanned carbon dioxide laser or intense pulsed light with a Q-switched ruby laser, have been introduced with various clinical outcomes.[20,21]

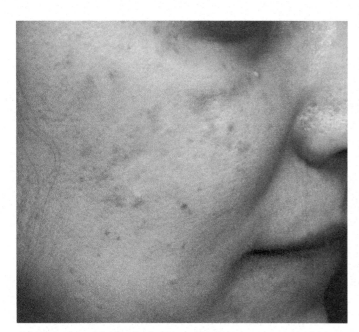

FIGURE 87-4. Ephelides: ill-defined matted light brown macules over the cheeks in a middle-aged Southeast Asian woman.

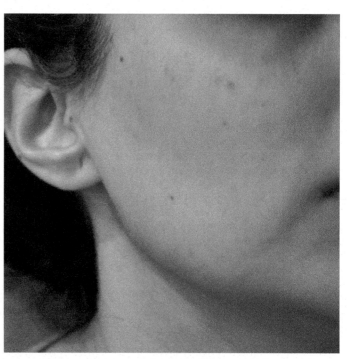

FIGURE 87-5. Hori nevi: small discrete grayish-brown macules over the malar eminences in an Asian woman.

RHYTIDES

The formation of crease lines, or rhytides, is a natural part of the aging process that can lead to deep furrows, frowns, and scowl lines. Dynamic rhytides occur over time and are caused by the repeated movement of hyperkinetic muscles, including the frontalis, corrugator supercilii, orbicularis oculi, procerus, and depressor supercilii. In darker skin types, differences in skin composition lead to less frequency of rhytides and wrinkling. In a study of adults living in Tucson, Arizona, most of the Caucasian women aged 45 to 50 years had wrinkles in the crow's feet and on the corners of the mouth, whereas none of the African American women of comparable age had obvious crow's feet wrinkles or perioral rhytides.[22] The skin of African Americans also felt firmer, and the histology of the dermal elastic fibers was similar to the appearance of these fibers in sun-protected Caucasian skin. Treatment with botulinum toxin is the gold standard in therapy, although topical retinoids can be used for finer rhytides for both treatment and prevention.

DEEP FURROWING AND SAGGING SKIN

As the face begins to age, fat atrophy and hypertrophy develop, ultimately producing demarcations between cosmetic units.[8] Features become concave, characterized by loss of volume in the lips (mainly the upper lip), sunken temple and cheek, scalloped mandible, and increased shadowing. Anatomic aging also occurs with differences based on facial location (ie, upper face, midface, and lower face). On the upper face, weakened brow muscles can be an early sign of aging. Ptosis can cause the brow arch to drop, creating a redundancy and hooding of the upper eyelid. This can lead to repetitive contractions of the frontalis muscle resulting in deep horizontal ridges on the forehead. Repeat movements of the corrugators can lead to a deep furrow of the glabella between the eyebrows.

Sagging under the eyes can be an early sign of aging in the midface region. As fat pads over the zygoma or cheekbone slowly descend, a deepening of the nasolabial folds occurs. For the lower face, repeat contractions of the orbicularis oris can lead to vertical wrinkles of the upper lip. The upper lip lengthens and both lips flatten with age.

With aging, the most significant change in appearance is the sagging of excess skin, which causes the conversion of primary arcs to straight lines.[8] Deep furrows and sagging skin are best treated with soft tissue fillers. Based on the particular skin type, some soft tissue fillers will achieve better results than others. Histologically, there is less thinning of collagen bundles and elastic tissue in darker skin types.[8] As a result, volumizers, fillers that stimulate collagen or elastin production or skin tightening, are more effective in skin of color. Volumizing is accomplished in the infraorbital, upper cheek, and lateral cheek regions using either cross-linked or larger particle hyaluronic acid, calcium hydroxylapatite, or poly-L-lactic acid.

Soft tissue fillers are excellent for minimizing cheek festooning, filling accentuated tear troughs, treating prejowl sulcus and temples, and lip augmentation. Over the years, the desire for full lips has gained widespread popularity, which has led to an increase in demand for lip augmentation. In African American women, changes in self-perception are motiving more women to emphasize the beauty of their lips and pursue procedures to rebuild the aging lip.[19] Whereas the typical goal of lip augmentation in Caucasian women is to increase the lip size beyond the original volume, people with skin types V or VI generally seek augmentation to only restore the size of the lip to the original volume and appearance. Subtle differences are important to note between the intrinsic aging process in African American and Caucasian patients. In Caucasian women, rhytides develop above and below the vermilion borders, because of thinning of the dermis, volume loss, loss of vermilion border, and overactivity of the perioral musculature. However, for African American women, rhytides occur predominantly below the vermilion border, in response to loss of volume of the upper lip. Also, the lower lip usually maintains the same appearance; however, it sometimes becomes flat and may appear to be more visible due to the loss of volume of the upper lip.[2]

Other treatment modalities for sagging skin include heat-producing technologies, including radiofrequency, long-wavelength laser, and broad-spectrum light sources. Heat-producing technology causes molecular and mechanical effects that tighten skin without injury to the overlying epidermis.

CONCLUSION

Persons of color will soon compose a majority of the international and domestic populations and, more so, will compose a majority of the aging population. A comprehensive knowledge and approach to assessment and treatment is necessary to properly care for our aging skin of color patients.

REFERENCES

1. Kaidbey KH, Agin PP, Sayre RM, Kligman AM. Photoprotection by melanin—a comparison of black and Caucasian skin. *J Am Acad Dermatol.* 1979;1:249-260.
2. Halder RM. The role of retinoids in the management of cutaneous conditions in blacks. *J Am Acad Dermatol.* 1998;39:S98-S103.
3. Iozumi K, Hoganson GE, Pennella R, Everett MA, Fuller BB. Role of tyrosinase as the determinant of pigmentation in cultured human melanocytes. *J Invest Dermatol.* 1993;100:806-811.
4. Taylor SC. Skin of color: biology, structure, function, and implications for dermatologic disease. *J Am Acad Dermatol.* 2002;46(2 Suppl):S41-S62.
5. Lapiere CM. The ageing dermis: the main cause for the appearance of 'old' skin. *Br J Dermatol.* 1990;122(Suppl 35):5-11.
6. Montagna WGP, Kenney JA. The structure of black skin. In: Montagna WGP, Kenney JA, eds. *Black Skin Structure and Function.* Houston, TX: Gulf Professional Publishing; 1993.
7. Montagna W, Carlisle K. The architecture of black and white facial skin. *J Am Acad Dermatol.* 1991;24:929-937.
8. Alam MBA, Kundu RV, Yoo S, Chan HH. *Cosmetic Dermatology for Skin of Color.* New York, NY: McGraw Hill; 2009.
9. Baumann L, Rodriguez D, Taylor SC, Wu J. Natural considerations for skin of color. *Cutis.* 2006;78(6 Suppl):2-19.
10. Sarkar R. Idiopathic cutaneous hyperchromia at the orbital region or periorbital hyperpigmentation. *J Cutan Aesthet Surg.* 2012;5:183-184.
11. Roh MR, Chung KY. Infraorbital dark circles: definition, causes, and treatment options. *Dermatol Surg.* 2009;35:1163-1171.
12. Malakar S, Lahiri K, Banerjee U, Mondal S, Sarangi S. Periorbital melanosis is an extension of pigmentary demarcation line-F on face. *Indian J Dermatol Venereol Leprol.* 2007;73:323-325.
13. Ranu H, Thng S, Goh BK, Burger A, Goh CL. Periorbital hyperpigmentation in Asians: an epidemiologic study and a proposed classification. *Dermatol Surg.* 2011;37:1297-1303.
14. Verschoore M, Gupta S, Sharma VK, Ortonne JP. Determination of melanin and haemoglobin in the skin of idiopathic cutaneous hyperchromia of the orbital region (ICHOR): a study of Indian patients. *J Cutan Aesthet Surg.* 2012;5:176-182.
15. Watanabe S, Nakai K, Ohnishi T. Condition known as "dark rings under the eyes" in the Japanese population is a kind of dermal melanocytosis which can be successfully treated by Q-switched ruby laser. *Dermatol Surg.* 2006;32:785-789.
16. Bliss JM, Ford D, Swerdlow AJ, et al. Risk of cutaneous melanoma associated with pigmentation characteristics and freckling: systematic overview of 10 case-control studies. The International Melanoma Analysis Group (IMAGE). *Int J Cancer.* 1995;62:367-376.
17. Rhodes AR, Albert LS, Barnhill RL, Weinstock MA. Sun-induced freckles in children and young adults. A correlation of clinical and histopathologic features. *Cancer.* 1991;67:1990-2001.
18. Rhodes AR, Harrist TJ, Momtaz TK. The PUVA-induced pigmented macule: a lentiginous proliferation of large, sometimes cytologically atypical, melanocytes. *J Am Acad Dermatol.* 1983;9:47-58.
19. Hori Y, Kawashima M, Oohara K, Kukita A. Acquired, bilateral nevus of Ota-like macules. *J Am Acad Dermatol.* 1984;10:961-964.
20. Ee HL, Goh CL, Khoo LS, Chan ES, Ang P. Treatment of acquired bilateral nevus of ota-like macules (Hori's nevus) with a combination of the 532 nm Q-Switched Nd:YAG laser followed by the 1,064 nm Q-switched Nd:YAG is more effective: prospective study. *Dermatol Surg.* 2006;32:34-40.
21. Cho SB, Park SJ, Kim MJ, Bu TS. Treatment of acquired bilateral nevus of Ota-like macules (Hori's nevus) using 1064-nm Q-switched Nd:YAG laser with low fluence. *Int J Dermatol.* 2009;48:1308-1312.
22. Stephens T. Ethnic sensitive skin: a review. *Cosmet Toiletries.* 1994;109:75-80.

CHAPTER 88

Africa

Ncosa C. Dlova
Anisa Mosam
Frances O. A. Ajose

INTRODUCTION

The African continent is the second largest continent in the world, at 11.7 million miles squared, which is 20.4% of the Earth's total land surface.[1] Fittingly, it is also the second most populous continent, with 853.6 million inhabitants, which is 14.72% of the world's human population.[1] The continent is divided into 54 recognized countries, and the average life expectancy at birth is 58 years.[2a] There are six African countries that lie directly on the equator, and this has implications on the inhabitants' exposure to ultraviolet (UV) rays. The Nile River is the longest river in the world and runs a course of 4.132 miles through Africa, providing a valuable source of nourishment, but at the same time acting as a breeding ground for transmittable skin diseases in certain regions.[2] This continent is considered by most paleoanthropologists to be the oldest inhabited place on Earth, with many considering Africa to be the area where the human species originated.[1]

The majority of common skin conditions in Africa are attributable to infections and infestations and hence are preventable. Transmissible skin conditions account for up to 85% of skin conditions in Tanzania, 78% in Malawi, 71.5% in Ethiopia, and 40% in Uganda.[2]

The aim of this chapter is to discuss conditions that either are unique to Africans or have an extremely high prevalence in Africa due to the high transmission rate of infections (eg, human immunodeficiency virus (HIV) and other infections that have always been endemic in Africa). In addition, the pigmentary conditions that have long plagued Africans will be highlighted. The conditions and diseases that will be focused on in this chapter are PPE, Kaposi sarcoma, acquired epidermodysplasia verruciformis syndrome, chromomycosis, leprosy, and albinism.

HUMAN IMMUNODEFICIENCY VIRUS

KEY POINTS

- With human immunodeficiency virus (HIV), the most common skin conditions are infections and infestations, which are preventable.

- Approximately 69% of the global total of HIV-infected individuals are in sub-Saharan Africa.

- HIV and acquired immunodeficiency syndrome have changed the landscape of skin diseases in Africa.

- The most common conditions stemming from HIV are Kaposi sarcoma, papular eruptions, herpes zoster, dermatophyte infections, and molluscum contagiosum.

- In children with HIV, the most common conditions are tinea capitis, molluscum contagiosum, verruca vulgaris, plane warts, and seborrheic eczema.

- Highly active antiretroviral therapies are associated with the increased prevalence of drug reactions and immune reconstitution inflammatory syndrome-related cutaneous events.

The HIV/acquired immunodeficiency syndrome (AIDS) endemic has wreaked havoc in Africa. Currently, there are 30.4 million infected people worldwide, with sub-Saharan Africa experiencing the greatest toll, with 69% of the global total and every 1 in 20 adults infected.[3] Of the 1.7 million people who died of AIDS-related causes in 2011, 70% were from Africa.[3] Sub-Saharan Africa is one of the regions that has shown the sharpest decline in the number of new infections (25% since 2001) and has one of the largest antiretroviral treatment programs worldwide. With these advances and the focus on antiretroviral programs, 9 million life years in sub-Saharan Africa have been saved since 1995, and the number of people included in treament progams increased by 59% (2.3 million people) in 2011 and 2012.[3]

HIV has changed the landscape of skin diseases on the continent. The most common skin conditions in Africa are Kaposi sarcoma, pruritic papular eruption of HIV (PPE), and drug reaction-related conditions, followed by herpes zoster, dermatophyte infections, and molluscum contagiosum, as documented in Nigeria.[4] In Ethiopian children, the most common dermatoses were those that were also common in the general population, for instance, tinea capitis, molluscum contagiosum, verruca vulgaris, plane warts, and seborrheic eczema.[5] In Tanzanian children with HIV, the prevalence of mucocutaneous disorders was high at 85%, despite the fact that 74% were on antiretroviral therapy.[6] The most common dermatosis was PPE, which was seen in 45% of children, followed by superficial fungal infections in 40%, viral infections in 23%, and bacterial infections in 12%. The most common fungal infections were tinea capitis and viral infectious plane warts.[6]

The prevalence and spectrum of skin diseases will change yet again in the future, as more HIV-infected patients are able to access antiretroviral therapy and the number of new HIV infections declines. However, highly active antiretroviral therapy (HAART) is a double-edged sword and is associated with the rising prevalence of drug reactions and immune reconstitution inflammatory syndrome-related events due to the high background prevalence of infections in Africa.

PRURITIC PAPULAR ERUPTION OF HIV

KEY POINTS

- PPE is one of the most common inflammatory skin conditions associated with HIV in Africa.

- It presents with pruritic urticarial papules, excoriated papules, and postinflammatory hyperpigmentation.

- The sites most often affected are the face, the 'V' of the neck, and the upper arms.

- Lesions are associated with cluster of differentiation 4 counts of <200 cells/μL.

- Resolution is a marker of good virologic control.

Pruritic papular eruption (PPE) of HIV has been documented as one of the most common inflammatory skin conditions associated with HIV in Africa.[7] It is a pruritic dermatosis initially presenting with erythematous papules on the extensors and trunk, progressing to excoriated papules (with repeated scratching, these can lead to prurigo), and eventually postinflammatory hyperpigmentation [**Figures 88-1 and 88-2**].

Urticarial lesions, when distributed on the face and in the 'V' of the neck area and when associated with an infiltration of eosinophils in

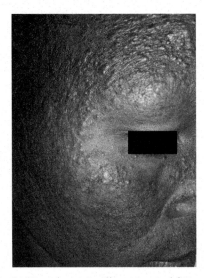

FIGURE 88-1. Pruritic papular eruption of human immunodeficiency virus with coalescing erythematous papules involving the face and background lichenification due to the pruritic nature of the disease.

the perifollicular region, are termed eosinophilic folliculitis. These two pruritic disorders are thought to be different manifestations of the same underlying disorder.[8] The pathogenesis is postulated to be related to insect bites, due to the pruritic nature of the disorders, the predilection for exposed sites, and the associated eosinophilia in both.[9]

Due to the pruritic nature of the disease, it is important to exclude scabies with an examination of a scraped skin lesion using a potassium hydroxide solution and/or a biopsy if necessary. In Africa, the other important confounder clinically is a papulonecrotic tuberculid, which presents with papules, pustules, and necrotic lesions on the extensors and the acral sites. A biopsy and Mantoux test will assist in differentiating scabies from PPE, which is primarily a pruritic disorder and leads to lichenification and hyperpigmentation.

PPE has been associated with advanced HIV infections, usually with cluster of differentiation (CD) 4 counts of <200 cells/μL, and can be used to monitor the virologic control of HIV.[3] Lesions have been known to disappear with HAART and subsequently reappear when there is resistance.[8] However, eosinophilic folliculitis can recur on HAART as a manifestation of immune reconstitution inflammatory syndrome and can be quite challenging to treat because it negatively affects adherence.

Therapy for PPE is primarily symptomatic with topical steroids and antihistamines. However, many patients will have persistent papules

and pruritus and will require the use of systemic tetracyclines or metronidazole. In recalcitrant cases, UVB radiation and tacrolimus may be effective.

KAPOSI SARCOMA

KEY POINTS

- The most common cancers in eastern and southern Africa are related to HIV.
- Kaposi sarcoma is the most common cancer in males and the second most common in females across Africa.
- Kaposi sarcoma presents as asymptomatic violaceous plaques, nodules, and lymphedema.
- Pulmonary involvement needs to be differentiated from tuberculosis.
- HAART is associated with a good 1-year survival rate.
- The best Kaposi sarcoma-specific response is seen with chemotherapy.

Cancers are becoming an increasingly important cause of morbidity and mortality globally, as well as in Africa specifically. The types of cancers in Africa differ from those in the West, with the most common cancers in eastern and southern Africa being those related to HIV/AIDS due to their high prevalence.[10] Kaposi sarcomas (KS), cervical cancers, and non-Hodgkin lymphomas are the most common forms, whereas in West Africa, cancers of the liver are more common.[10] KS is the most common tumor in many cancer registries across Africa, and the HIV epidemic has been responsible for the soaring incidence rates of KS, which are seen even in nonendemic areas. This has been documented in many countries in sub-Saharan Africa, such as Zimbabwe[11] and South Africa.[12]

KS can be classified into four types: classic, which is seen in the Mediterranean regions with a high prevalence in Jewish populations; African endemic, which is common in Central and West Africa; epidemic or HIV-associated; and iatrogenic, which is due to therapy-related immunosuppression. The prerequisite for the development of each type is the presence of the human herpesvirus type 8 infection.

The African endemic type can present as an indolent neoplasm, much like the classic type that presents in those living in the Mediterranean regions. These neoplasms present primarily on the feet and legs as hyperkeratotic plaques that respond well to radiotherapy [**Figures 88-3 and 88-4**]. These patients have an excellent 5-year survival rate. However, the African endemic type can present with aggressive clinical lesions that grow rapidly and exuberant nodules and plaques that progress deeper into the subcutaneous tissue, potentially affecting the underlying bone, and that

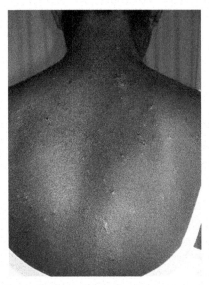

FIGURE 88-2. Pruritic papular eruption of human immunodeficiency virus. Note the scattered papules with excoriation on the trunk.

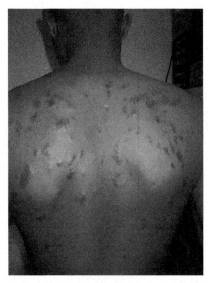

FIGURE 88-3. Violaceous plaques distributed symmetrically in Langer lines on the trunk of a patient with human immunodeficiency virus-associated Kaposi sarcoma.

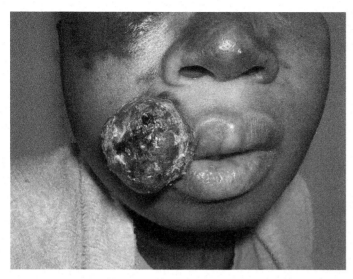

FIGURE 88-4. Periorbital edema and fungating tumor in human immunodeficiency virus-associated Kaposi sarcoma.

are not as susceptible to therapy. In children, this type presents primarily with lymphadenopathic disease and without cutaneous manifestations.

The importance of the epidemic or HIV-associated type lies in the fact that it is AIDS-defining and has been documented in several cancer registries as a public health concern in sub-Saharan Africa.[10,12] Even with the advances and upgrades in antiretroviral therapy, the incidence has remained unchanged; although in South Africa, this has been associated with improved diagnostic evaluations and greater access to chemotherapy, with more patients being retained in care and fewer lost to follow-up.[13] HAART is associated with improved survival for African patients with HIV-related KS, with a 1-year survival rate of 77%.[15] However, chemotherapy is also associated with the improved response of KS.[15]

The initial lesions of KS may go unnoticed by both patients and healthcare providers because they present initially as asymptomatic violaceous patches and plaques that then progress to nodules and lymphedema. It is usually the manifestation of pain due to dermal lymphatic infiltration, periorbital edema, or the involvement of exposed sites (eg, the face and hands) that is the cause for seeking treatment. Untreated lesions progress to massive lymphedema, extensive plaques and nodules, and visceral involvement. The gastrointestinal and pulmonary systems are the most common extracutaneous sites affected and are associated with a poor prognosis. In Africa, chest symptoms (including cough, hemoptysis, and dyspnea) require further investigation to differentiate KS from tuberculosis and other pneumonias associated with immunodeficiency.

The timely recognition and diagnosis of KS is important because the patient's prognosis is related to the extent of cutaneous and visceral involvement as well as the degree of immunosuppression. All patients with HIV-related KS should be treated with HAART. For lesions that are localized, radiation therapy is suitable; however, for visceral and extensive cutaneous lesions, chemotherapy is indicated instead. Patients initiating or changing HAART regimens are also at risk of the KS lesions worsening due to immune reconstitution inflammatory syndrome; furthermore, pulmonary lesions may be fatal and require immediate chemotherapy.

ACQUIRED EPIDERMODYSPLASIA VERRUCIFORMIS SYNDROME

KEY POINTS

- HIV-infected patients are predisposed to generalized verrucosis.
- These may include verruca vulgaris, verruca plana, and condylomata acuminata.
- Extensive plane warts, with pityriasis versicolor lesions seen in epidermodysplasia verruciformis, are common in children infected with HIV.

- This disorder is termed acquired epidermodysplasia verruciformis, and the warts contain group B human papillomavirus, similar to the genetic condition.
- Surveillance for the development of squamous cell carcinomas is important due to the high degree of sun exposure for patients in Africa and the immunosuppression from HIV.

Cutaneous viral infections are common in populations where overcrowding is rife, and unfortunately Africa is no exception. Human papillomavirus (HPV) infections present with common, flat, palmoplantar, and genital warts [**Figures 88-5 and 88-6**]. Due to immunosuppression, warts in HIV-positive patients are more numerous; furthermore, a number of HPV types can coexist, and these warts are more recalcitrant to therapy. In addition, surveillance is essential due to the known carcinogenic potential of HPV, especially in the face of the HIV-related immunosuppression.

Many African children are burdened with HIV from birth due to the vertical transmission of HIV. Although the rates of infection have been dramatically curbed in recent years, the sequelae of this mode of infection are still being seen. Children often present with a 'potpourri' of infections and inflammatory conditions due to their prolonged immunosuppression. Fortunately, many do reconstitute immunologically, and as their CD4 counts improve, they are able to better resist some of the common skin conditions associated with HIV.

However, children often present with a florid eruption of welldefined, hypopigmented, scaly plaques distributed over the sun-exposed areas (eg, the face, 'V' of the neck, extensors of the arms, and trunk), similar to the pityriasis versicolor lesions of epidermodysplasia verruciformis (EV). This has been documented in up to 25% of adolescents with HIV in Zimbabwe and is suggested as a marker of mother-to-child HIV transmission as opposed to horizontal transmission.[15] Although asymptomatic, these scaly plaques are particularly disfiguring and, in some cases, so extensive that only 'islands' of normal skin remain. This condition is particularly frustrating because these children often progress well on HAART; yet, unlike with other skin conditions, they do not see improvement of this rash.[16] However, glycolic acid has been used successfully to treat this extensive and persistent dermatosis.[17]

Histologically, many children present with epidermal dysplasia and large atypical nucleated cells in keeping with EV. In addition to this, all have been found to contain group B HPV consistent with EV. Because they are distinctly related to the immunosuppression of HIV/AIDS, the term acquired EV has been suggested.[18] Surveillance is imperative because there is a possibility of the development of malignancy in these lesions due to the underlying immunosuppression and exposure to the sun.

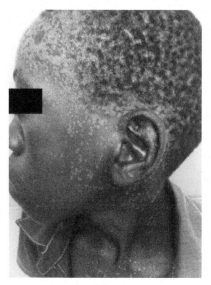

FIGURE 88-5. Acquired epidermodysplasia verruciformis in a child with extensive photo-distributed flat warts and koebnerization.

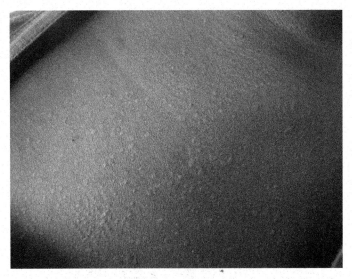

FIGURE 88-6. Hypopigmented scaly papules in acquired epidermodysplasia verruciformis seen in a patient with human immunodeficiency virus.

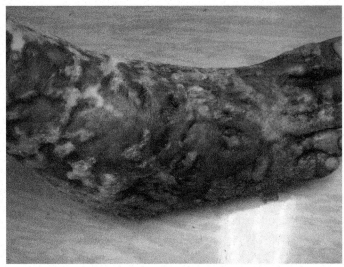

FIGURE 88-7. Chromomycosis with chronic plaques and nodules involving the foot.

CHROMOMYCOSIS

KEY POINTS

- Chromomycosis is a deep fungal infection affecting the skin and subcutaneous tissues.
- It has a worldwide distribution, with the majority of cases occurring in tropical and subtropical areas.
- Chromomycosis is common in rural agricultural workers.
- *Fonsecaea pedrosoi* is the most common causative organism.
- Treatment includes prolonged courses of chemotherapy with low cure rates.
- A few cases of squamous cell carcinoma complicating chromomycosis have been reported.

Chromomycosis is a chronic deep fungal infection that affects the skin and subcutaneous tissues with a tendency to involve the legs; however, it can occur in other areas.[19] Terra et al[20] coined the name chromoblastomycosis in 1922; the Greek prefix *chromo* means "color," referring to the dark color of the fungal cells in the tissues, and *blastos* means a "germ" or "bud," referring to yeast. However, this term is inaccurate because the fungus that causes the infection does not form buds but rather multiplies by splitting. The term chromomycosis was proposed by Moore and Almeida and subsequently replaced the term chromoblastomycosis.[19,21] The first cases were reported by Rudolph in Brazil in 1914.[22]

Chromomycosis has a worldwide distribution and has no racial predisposition; however, the majority of cases occur in tropical and subtropical areas, particularly in hot humid climates. The disease occurs particularly in patients who are regularly engaged in rural agricultural work. Thus far, only five species of dematiaceous (dark-colored) fungi have been attributed as causes of chromomycosis: *Fonsecaea pedrosoi*, *Fonsecaea compactum*, *Cladosporium carrionii*, *Phialophora verrucosa*, and *Rhinocladiella aquaspersa*.

F. pedrosoi remains the most common causative organism of chromomycosis in the world. It is found mainly in hot, humid tropical and subtropical regions, in contrast to *C. carrionii*, which is predominantly associated with dry, arid, and semi-arid regions.[21] Following traumatic inoculation, the fungus commonly penetrates the exposed areas of the skin on the lower limbs. The areas involved are frequently exposed areas of the skin (namely the feet, legs, and arms) even though other uncommon sites (such as the face, nose, neck, and genitalia) have also been described.[23] Most cases tend to evolve gradually over several years and with an average duration of 8 years, although they sometimes last for decades.[24] Various clinical types of lesions are seen, and these include nodular, plaques, atrophic, and verrucose, with the latter being the most common presentation.

The skin lesions present as slow-growing chronic papules and nodules that subsequently evolve into plaques that heal with scarring [**Figures 88-7 and 88-8**]. Complications include secondary infections, lymphatic obstruction with resultant lymphedema, and elephantiasis. A few cases of squamous cell carcinoma have also been reported.[25] Histopathologic features include pseudoepitheliomatous hyperplasia, background granulomatous inflammation, dematiaceous fungi, and microabscesses in the epidermis and dermis. Microscopy and cultures are used for the identification of the organisms. Patients require long-term antifungal therapy, which may be associated with poor response, numerous side effects, and exorbitant costs.

The treatment of chromomycosis includes prolonged courses of chemotherapy often combined with physical and surgical managements.[26] Cure rates for chromomycosis are low and range from 15% to 80%.[23]

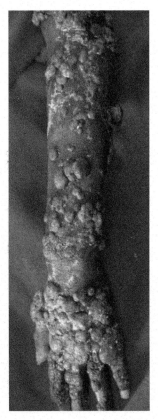

FIGURE 88-8. Chromomycosis with scattered nodules and plaques on the arm.

F. pedrosoi, the most common etiologic agent, is less sensitive to antifungal chemotherapy than *C. carrionii* or *P. verrucosa*.[27] For treatment, high doses of itraconazole and terbinafine for a minimum of 6 to 12 months have shown the best results.[28]

LEPROSY

KEY POINTS

- Leprosy remains endemic in all African countries.
- It is not a genetic disease.
- Infectiousness becomes negligible soon after the start of multidrug therapy.
- Leprosy reactions should be treated as an emergency.
- Close contact with multibacillary leprosy and paucibacillary leprosy sufferers indicates that an individual is 5 to 10 times and 2 to 3 times more likely, respectively, to contract leprosy than fellow community members.

Leprosy remains endemic in all countries in Africa.[29] However, significant progress has been made in controlling and reducing the physical, mental, and socioeconomic consequences of this infectious disease on patients and their families.

The causative organism is *Mycobacterium leprae*, which is an acid-fast, rod-shaped organism that closely resembles the tubercle bacillus.[30,31] The morphologic index (MI) and the bacteriologic index (BI) are useful in assessing the severity of the infection, the viability of the organisms, and the progress of patients under treatment. The BI is a count of the stained bacilli in a skin smear, while the MI is a count of the stained viable bacilli in this smear. A negative smear—or a BI of zero—indicates paucibacillary (PB) leprosy while all positive smear cases indicate multibacillary (MB) leprosy.[32]

DEFINITION OF A LEPROSY CASE

Leprosy is suspected in individuals with pale or reddish patches on the skin [**Figure 88-9**], associated with decreased or total loss of sensation in areas of the skin with patches; numbness or tingling of the digits; muscle weakness of the hands, feet, or eyelids; painful or tender nerves; swollen nodular face and earlobes [**Figure 88-10**]; or painless wounds or burns on the hands or feet. A diagnosis is made when, additionally, there is a thickened or enlarged peripheral nerve or the presence of acid-fast bacilli in a slit-skin smear.

The transmission of leprosy occurs by contact. Individuals in contact with MB and PB cases are 5 to 10 times and 2 to 3 times, respectively, more likely to contract clinical leprosy than individuals in endemic communities but with no known close contact with recognized cases. The familial

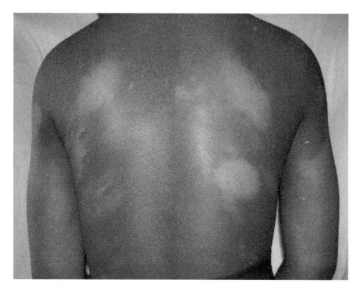

FIGURE 88-9. Hypopigmented anesthetic skin patches in borderline tuberculoid leprosy.

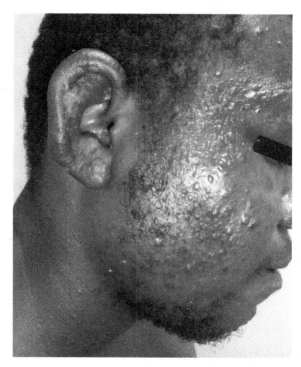

FIGURE 88-10. A 17-year-old male patient with multibacillary leprosy and severe erythema nodosum leprosum. He was febrile, with a temperature of 104°F (40°C), with pain in the joints and testicles.

clustering of leprosy cases is related to the contact and not the genetic factor; for this reason, leprosy should not be considered a genetic disease. The incubation period appears to be shorter for PB leprosy (approximately 2 to 5 years) than for MB leprosy (approximately 5 to 10 years, although it may sometimes take much longer).[33,34] A very high proportion of the bacilli are killed within days of starting multidrug therapy (MDT) for leprosy, and the infectiousness immediately becomes negligible.[35]

CHEMOTHERAPY AND MANAGEMENT WITH STANDARD MULTIDRUG THERAPY[29]

Rifampicin, clofazimine, and dapsone are three standard first-line drugs available for use in MDT regimens of fixed duration; however, none of these should be used as monotherapy.[29]

Second-line antileprosy drug classes include fluoroquinolones (pefloxacin and ofloxacin), a macrolide (clarithromycin), and a tetracycline (minocycline).[33,36-38] These may be substituted when patients, for whatever reason, are unable to use another drug (eg, rifampicin in liver disease, dapsone in glucose-6-phosphate dehydrogenase deficiency, or clofazimine when undesirable pigmentation is induced). A single dose of rifampicin 600 mg, ofloxacin 400 mg, and minocycline 100 mg is 99% leprostatic. Relapses after MDT can occur when new lesions appear with a significantly increased BI.[39]

MANAGEMENT OF LEPROSY REACTIONS

Leprosy reactions may affect 25% of African MB leprosy patients. The major clinical types of leprosy reactions are type 1, or a reversal reaction, and type 2, or an erythema nodosum leprosum (ENL) reaction.[40]

The inflammation associated with a leprosy reaction should be considered as a medical emergency because severe nerve injury may develop rapidly, with a subsequent loss of sensation, paralysis, and deformity.[41] Type 1 reactions occur across the whole leprosy spectrum and usually present as erythematous edema of skin patches. Type 2, or ENL, reactions are characterized by the appearance of tender, erythematous nodules in nonlesional areas in MB patients.

Guidelines for the Management of Severe Reactions A severe type 1 or reversal reaction should be treated with a course of prednisolone, usually lasting 3 to 6 months. Patients still on antileprosy treatment should continue the standard course of MDT. A severe type 2 or ENL reaction is treated with daily doses of prednisolone not exceeding 1 mg/kg (1 mg/2.2 lb) of the patient's body weight for 12 weeks, with adequate analgesics for pain and/or fever.[29] Patients should continue with MDT if the treatment is ongoing; however, if the MDT has been completed, they should not restart the treatment. If the patient is unresponsive to corticosteroids alone, clofazimine should be added, starting with 100 mg three times daily for a maximum of 12 weeks, with a gradual tapering of the dosage over the next 12 months.[29]

The prevention of disabilities begins with an early diagnosis of leprosy, as well as the recognition and treatment of complications such as neuritis and any reactions; the identification of patients at risk of developing secondary disabilities; and timely interventions.[29] Dermatologists should emphasize self-care and self-reliance, including the care of any dry, denervated skin on the palms and soles to prevent injury, care for burns and skin cracks, and care of the eyes to prevent keratitis and blindness.[29]

The stigmatization of those with leprosy, although on the decline, still has a strong social and psychological impact on all affected individuals, as well as their families and community. Socioeconomic rehabilitation of leprosy patients is important to improve their quality of life and increase their social integration.

ALBINISM

KEY POINTS

- Melanin is responsible for protection from the carcinogenic effects of UV radiation as well as the development of the visual apparatus.
- The consequences of albinism include accelerated aging, precancers, skin cancers, and poor vision.
- The African albino is 70 times more likely to develop skin cancer than other normally pigmented Africans.
- In Africa, an additional problem involves derogatory myths about the etiology of albinism; the sufferer and their family may be exposed to ridicule, stigmatization, and, in some cases, persecution or assault.
- Care of an albino patient should start from birth to give psychological support to the parents and education on sun avoidance or protection, with vision enhancement throughout school-age and adult life.

Albinism disorders are a heterogeneous group of inherited nonprogressive disorders of the melanin metabolism, manifesting a wide variety of phenotypes, limited number of genotypes, and rather complex genetics.[42] There is absence or defective production of melanin from its precursor, tyrosine. The main function of the melanin pigment is the filtering of UV radiation entering the skin to prevent sunburn, skin cancer, and the photolysis of folic acid in the skin.[43] This is done by forming a protective covering over the cellular DNA, which efficiently absorbs harmful UV radiation and transforms up to 99.9% of it into heat.[44] The fovea of the retina in the eye cannot reach full development in the absence of melanin.

Ocular albinism (OA) affects only the eyes, and oculocutaneous albinism (OCA) affects the eyes, skin, and hair. In OCA, there is little or no pigment in the eyes, skin, and hair, whereas in OA there is a lack of pigment in the eyes only, with the skin and hair color varying from very fair to dark. There are about nine different types of OCA; the most common type is OCA2, which is the most prevalent in Africans.

Albinism is found in all races with a worldwide frequency of about 1:17,000.[44] OCA2 occurs in 1:10,000 African Americans, but only in 1:36,000 Caucasian Americans.[45] Within Africa, the frequency ranges from as low as 1:15,000 in eastern Nigeria,[45] to as high as 1:1000 in the Tonga tribe of Zimbabwe.[46]

The tropical environment is unkind to the African albino. The reduction or complete lack of skin pigment in albinism leads to an intolerance of UV radiation, which predisposes the individual to early development of aggressive skin cancers [**Figure 88-11**], making them 70 times more likely to develop skin cancer than a nonalbino individual.[3] Albinos often start to develop basal cell carcinomas (BCC) and squamous cell

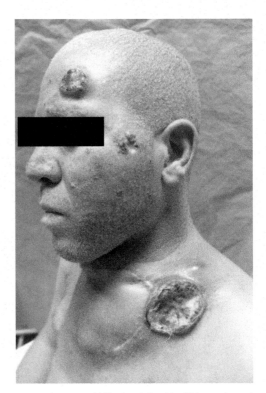

FIGURE 88-11. A 29-year-old Nigerian male with albinism and recurring squamous cell cancers.

carcinomas (SCC) by their teenage years, and the cancers may develop concurrently. However, albino individuals rarely develop melanomas. Many may have up to 50 actinic keratoses on areas of exposed skin by the age of 25 years old. Nonpigmenting albinos tend to develop cancers earlier, and these cancers are usually more aggressive. By the age of 40 years old, many albinos have had up to five skin cancers excised. One advantage is that albino patients demonstrate good healing, with scars that are neither hypertrophic nor result in the formation of keloids.

The visual abnormalities of albinism confer varying degrees of functional blindness that can significantly limit education. Other problems include limitations to both the patient's occupation and recreation.

An African with albinism [**Figure 88-12**] will generally have yellow to ivory-colored hair instead of the usual black hair, although the hair retains the 'kinky' hair texture. The skin color ranges from a very fair African complexion to very white Caucasian skin without any pigment at all. The pupils also lack pigment and may be gray or blue. In addition, the eyes are often crossed (strabismus) with constant rapid eye movements (nystagmus) and associated photophobia. In most types of OCA, the affected person must inherit the same type of mutated gene from both parents, making this condition an inherited autosomal recessive trait.[47,48] The parents of an albino child with OCA are therefore often two normally pigmented carriers of the same albinism gene. The OCA phenotype makes the African albino very conspicuous in any gathering.

In Africa, albinism is associated with social and cultural challenges that arise from the condition medically, as well as the many cultural and superstitious myths regarding the supposed etiology of the condition.[49,50] Both the affected child and mother may be at risk of mockery, stigmatization, discrimination, prejudice, and, in some cases, persecution and extermination.

In Nigeria and most parts of Africa, albinism is not recognized; it is often not indicated on birth records, and therefore the prevalence of the disorder is very difficult to assess. Genetic studies have only been done in South Africa, Tanzania, and a few other locations, and so the prevalent genotypes in many areas have yet to be evaluated.

The management of albinism consists mainly of preventive strategies to limit the damage to the skin and eyes from sun exposure, as well as maximizing visual competence to support educational and occupational

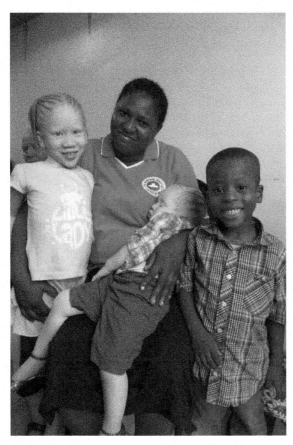

FIGURE 88-12. A Nigerian mother with her two albino daughters and normally pigmented son.

attainment. It is necessary that psychological support of the parents of an albino child should begin right from the child's birth because this period may be the most harmful to the child. Protection from sun exposure should start from birth, with hats and appropriate clothing, and the restriction of time spent outdoors while the sun is up. Regular skin surveillance is required for the early detection of skin cancers and precancers.

BCC and SCC are to be treated surgically and often require skin grafting.[51] Radiotherapy should be employed in cancers involving large areas. A few centers offer photodynamic therapy to treat multiple BCCs. Precancers should be treated with 5% fluorouracil ointments or imiquimod cream.

The use of chemical (ie, organic) sunscreens, although effective, is not yet very popular because of the requirement for frequent daily application, up to five times a day. Photosensitizing drugs are to be avoided in albinos, including sulfonamides, antihypertensive drugs, antifungals, and oral contraceptives. Career counseling is also necessary to avoid occupations that are skin and eye stressors. Patient support groups have been found useful and are encouraged in many parts of Africa. Marriage counseling should also be offered to albinos. Furthermore, carrier detection and prenatal diagnosis efforts should be intensified.

REFERENCES

1. Statistics Brain. Africa Continent statistics. http://www.statisticbrain.com/africa-continent-statistics/. Accessed April 9, 2013.
2a. World Health Organization. Global Health Observatory (GHO) data: Life expectancy. http://www.who.int/gho/mortality_burden_disease/life_tables/situation_trends_text/en/. Accessed October 10, 2015.
2. Gibbs S. Skin disease and socioeconomic conditions in rural Africa: Tanzania. *Int J Dermatol.* 1996;35:633-639.
3. UNAIDS, the Joint United Nations Programme on HIV/AIDS. 2012 UNAIDS Report on the Global AIDS Epidemic. http://www.unaids.org/en/resources/publications/2012/name,76121,en.asp. Accessed February 13, 2013.
4. Ukonu BA, Eze EU. Pattern of skin diseases at University of Benin Teaching Hospital, Benin City, Edo State, South-South Nigeria: a 12-month prospective study. *Glob J Health Sci.* 2012; 4:148-157.
5. Doni SN, Mitchell AL, Bogale Y, et al. Skin disorders affecting human immunodeficiency virus-infected children living in an orphanage in Ethiopia. *Clin Exp Dermatol.* 2012;37:15-19.
6. Umoru D, Oviawe O, Ibadin M, et al. Mucocutaneous manifestation of pediatric human immunodeficiency virus/acquired immunodeficiency syndrome (HIV/AIDS) in relation to degree of immunosuppression: a study of a West African population. *Int J Dermatol.* 2012;51:305-312.
7. Afonso JP, Tomimori J, Michalany NS, et al. Pruritic papular eruption and eosinophilic folliculitis associated with human immunodeficiency virus (HIV) infection: a histopathological and immunohistochemical comparative study. *J Am Acad Dermatol.* 2012;67:269-275.
8. Rosatelli JB, Roselino AM. Hyper-IgE, eosinophilia, and immediate cutaneous hypersensitivity to insect antigens in the pruritic papular eruption of human immunodeficiency virus. *Arch Dermatol.* 2001;137:672-673.
9. Castelnuovo B, Byakwaga H, Menten J, et al. Can response of a pruritic papular eruption to antiretroviral therapy be used as a clinical parameter to monitor virological outcome? *AIDS.* 2008;22:269-273.
10. Msyamboza KP, Dzamalala C, Mdokwe C, et al. Burden of cancer in Malawi; common types, incidence and trends: national population-based cancer registry. *BMC Res Notes.* 2012;5:149.
11. Chokunonga E, Borok MZ, Chirenje Z, et al. Trends in the incidence of cancer in the black population of Harare, Zimbabwe 1991-2010. *Int J Cancer.* 2013;1:721-729.
12. Mosam A, Carrara H, Uldrick TS, et al. Increasing incidence of Kaposi's sarcoma in black South Africans in KwaZulu-Natal, South Africa (1983–2006). *Int J STD AIDS.* 2009;20:553-556.
13. Mosam A, Uldrick TS, Shaik F, et al. An evaluation of the early effects of a combination antiretroviral therapy programme on the management of AIDS-associated Kaposi's sarcoma in KwaZulu-Natal, South Africa. *Int J STD AIDS.* 2011;22:671-673.
14. Mosam A, Shaik F, Uldrick TS, et al. A randomized controlled trial of highly active antiretroviral therapy versus highly active antiretroviral therapy and chemotherapy in therapy-naïve patients with HIV-associated Kaposi sarcoma in South Africa. *J Acquir Immune Defic Syndr.* 2012;60:150-157.
15. Lowe S, Ferrand RA, Morris-Jones R, et al. Skin disease among human immunodeficiency virus-infected adolescents in Zimbabwe: a strong indicator of underlying HIV infection. *Pediatr Infect Dis J.* 2010;29:346-351.
16. Lowe SM, Katsidzira L, Meys R, et al. Acquired epidermodysplasia verruciformis due to multiple and unusual HPV infection among vertically-infected, HIV-positive adolescents in Zimbabwe. *Clin Infect Dis.* 2012;54:e119-e123.
17. Moore RL, de Schaetzen V, Joseph M, et al. Acquired epidermodysplasia verruciformis syndrome in HIV-infected pediatric patients: prospective treatment trial with topical glycolic acid and human papillomavirus genotype characterization. *JAMA Dermatol.* 2012;148:128-130.
18. Daly ML, Hay RJ. Epidermodysplasia verruciformis and human immunodeficiency virus infection: a distinct entity? *Curr Opin Infect Dis.* 2012;25:123-125.
19. Lavalle P, Goncalves AP, Jardim ML, et al. Tropical deep fungal infections. In: Canizares O, Harman R, eds. *Clinical Tropical Dermatology.* 2nd ed. Oxford, United Kingdom: Blackwell Science Ltd; 1992:73-80.
20. Terra F, Torres M, da Fonseca O, et al. Novo typo de dermatite verrucosa mycose por Acrotheca com associacao de leishmaniosa. *Bras Med.* 1922;2:368-378.
21. McGinnis MR. Chromoblastomycosis and phaeohyphomycosis: new concepts, diagnosis, and mycology. *J Am Acad Dermatol.* 1983;8:1-16.
22. Richard-Yegres N, Yegres F. Chromomycosis: rural endemic in the northwestern region of Venezuela. *Rev Cubana Med Trop.* 2009;61:209-212.
23. Sharma NL, Sharma RC, Grover PS, et al. Chromoblastomycosis in India. *Int J Dermatol.* 1999;38:846-851.
24. Bansal AS, Prabhakar P. Chromomycosis: a twenty-year analysis of histologically confirmed cases in Jamaica. *Trop Geogr Med.* 1989;41:222-226.
25. Foster HM, Harris TJ. Malignant change (squamous carcinoma) in chronic chromoblastomycosis. *Aust N Z J Surg.* 1987;57:775-777.
26. Ameen M. Chromoblastomycosis: clinical presentation and management. *Clin Exp Dermatol.* 2009;34:849-854.
27. Ameen M. Managing chromoblastomycosis. *Trop Doct.* 2010;40:65-67.
28. Bonifaz A, Paredes-Solís V, Saúl A. Treating chromoblastomycosis with systemic antifungals. *Expert Opin Pharmacother.* 2004;5:247-254.
29. World Health Organization. WHO Expert Committee on Leprosy: Eighth report. http://www.searo.who.int/entity/global_leprosy_programme/publications/8th_expert_comm_2012.pdf. Accessed September 29, 2013.

30. World Health Organization. Leprosy elimination: microbiology of *M. leprae*. http://www.who.int/lep/microbiology/en/index.html. Accessed September 2, 2013.

31. World Health Organization. Leprosy elimination: WHO multidrug therapy (MDT). http://www.who.int/lep/mdt/en/. Accessed March 23, 2013.

32. Pannikar VK. Defining a case of leprosy. *Lepr Rev.* 1992;63:61s-65s.

33. Xiong JH, Ji B, Perani EG, et al. Further study of the effectiveness of single doses of clarithromycin and minocycline against *Mycobacterium leprae* in mice. *Int J Lepr Other Mycobact Dis.* 1994;62:37-42.

34. Boon NA, Colledge NR, Walker BR, et al, eds. *Davidson's Principles and Practice of Medicine.* Edinburgh, UK: Churchill Livingstone; 2006.

35. World Health Organization. *Report of the Tenth Meeting of the WHO Technical Advisory Group on Leprosy Control: New Delhi, India, 23 April 2009.* New Delhi, India: WHO Regional Office for South-East Asia; 2009.

36. Guelpa-Lauras CC, Perani EG, Giroir AM, et al. Activities of pefloxacin and ciprofloxacin against Mycobacterium leprae in the mouse. *Int J Lepr Other Mycobact Dis.* 1987;55:70-77.

37. Grosset JH, Guelpa-Lauras CC, Perani EG, et al. Activity of ofloxacin against Mycobacterium leprae in the mouse. *Int J Lepr Other Mycobact Dis.* 1988;56:259-264.

38. Ji B, Perani EG, Grosset JH. Effectiveness of clarithromycin and minocycline alone and in combination against experimental Mycobacterium leprae infection in mice. *Antimicrob Agents Chemother.* 1991;35:579-581.

39. Wu Q, Yin Y, Zhang L, et al. A study on a possibility of predicting early relapse in leprosy using a ND-O-BSA based ELISA. *Int J Lepr Other Mycobact Dis.* 2002;70:1-8.

40. Scollard DM, Adams LB, Gillis TP, et al. The continuing challenges of leprosy. *Clin Microbiol Rev.* 2006;19:338-381.

41. Walker SL, Lockwood DN. Leprosy type 1 (reversal) reactions and their management. *Lepr Rev.* 2008;79:372-386.

42. Zühlke C, Stell A, Käsmann-Kellner B. [Genetics of oculocutaneous albinism]. *Ophthalmologe.* 2007;104:674-680.

43. Brenner M, Hearing VJ. The protective role of melanin against UV damage in human skin. *Photochem Photobiol.* 2008;84:539-549.

44. Grønskov K, Ek J, Brondum-Nielsen K. Oculocutaneous albinism. *Orphanet J Rare Dis.* 2007;2:43.

45. Okoro AN. Albinism in Nigeria: a clinical and social study. *Br J Dermatol.* 1975;92:485-492.

46. Lund PM, Puri N, Durham-Pierre D, et al. Oculocutaneous albinism in an isolated Tonga community in Zimbabwe. *J Med Genet.* 1997;34:733-735.

47. Camand O, Boutboul S, Arbogast L, et al. Mutational analysis of the OA1 gene in ocular albinism. *Ophthalmic Genet.* 2003;24:167-173.

48. Winship IM, Babaya M, Ramesar RS. X-linked ocular albinism and sensorineural deafness: linkage to Xp22.3. *Genomics.* 1993;18:444-445.

49. Hong ES, Zeeb H, Repacholi MH. Albinism in Africa as a public health issue. *BMC Public Health.* 2006;6:212.

50. Arsene C. The Albino Paradox: faith, culture, and despair in contemporary Tanzania. http://www.african-politics.com/the-albino-paradox-%E2%80%93-faith-culture-and-despair-in-contemporary-tanzania/. Accessed January 28, 2013.

51. Mabula JB, Chalya PL, Mchembe MD, et al. Skin cancers among albinos at a University teaching hospital in northwestern Tanzania: a retrospective review of 64 cases. *BMC Dermatol.* 2012;12:5.

CHAPTER 89

Mainland Southeast Asia

Joyce Teng Ee Lim
Siew Eng Choon

KEY POINTS

- Multiple hospital-based surveys showed that the spectrum of skin disorders in Southeast Asia is similar to that seen in other regions except for an increase in pigmentary disorders such as nevus of Ota and Ito.

- Endemic subcutaneous mycoses such as chromoblastomycosis and sporotrichosis, which are prevalent in Southeast Asia, are not usually reported because of limited access to confirmatory laboratory tests.

- The diagnosis of chronic granulomatous skin infections such as chromoblastomycosis, sporotrichosis, lupus vulgaris, tuberculosis verrucosa cutis, and *Mycobacterium marinum* infection, which have similar clinical manifestations, is often only made retrospectively after successful therapeutic trial due to poor laboratory support.

- The incidence of systemic mycoses (mucormycosis, histoplasmosis, and penicilliosis) is increasing in tandem with the increasing number of immunocompromised patients, such as diabetic patients, organ transplant recipients, and patients with human immunodeficiency virus infection.

- Common dermatologic conditions seen in one part of this region may be different from those seen in another part because of the wide variation in ethnicity, skin types, hygienic practices, access to medical care, health-seeking behavior, and socioeconomic status.

- Preferences for alternative treatment and/or poor access to medical care often result in disease presentation in an advanced stage.

- Because most Southeast Asians have Fitzpatrick skin phototypes III to IV, skin cancers are not common but are increasingly seen in organ transplant recipients who are on long-term immunosuppressive therapy.

INTRODUCTION

Mainland Southeast Asia, comprising West Malaysia, Thailand, Vietnam, Cambodia, Laos, and Myanmar, has a population of about 0.6 billion.[1] Although there is no large-scale population-based study to determine the prevalence of skin diseases in this region, multiple hospital-based surveys showed that the spectrum of skin disorders is similar to that seen in other regions except for an increase in pigmentary disorders such as nevus of Ota and Ito.[2,3] However, endemic subcutaneous mycoses such as chromoblastomycosis and sporotrichosis, which are prevalent in Southeast Asia, are not usually reported because of limited access to confirmatory laboratory tests. Without good laboratory support, it is impossible to distinguish subcutaneous mycosis from cutaneous tuberculosis (especially lupus vulgaris and tuberculosis verrucosa cutis) and from *Mycobacterium marinum* infection, which have similar clinical manifestations. The incidence of systemic mycoses (mucormycosis, histoplasmosis, and penicilliosis) is increasing in tandem with the increasing number of immunocompromised patients, such as diabetic patients, organ transplant recipients, and patients with human immunodeficiency virus (HIV) infection.[4-6] Because most Southeast Asians have Fitzpatrick skin phototypes III to IV, skin cancers are not common but are increasingly seen in organ transplant recipients who are on long-term cyclosporine. Arsenic-induced nonmelanoma skin cancers are seen among patients with chronic exposure to arsenic found in well water and traditional Chinese medication.

Common dermatologic conditions seen in one part of this region may be different from those seen in another part because of the wide variation in ethnicity, skin types, hygienic practices, access to medical care, health-seeking behavior, and socioeconomic status. Preferences for alternative treatment and/or poor access to medical care often result in disease presentation in an advanced stage.

FUNGAL INFECTIONS

▦ SUPERFICIAL FUNGAL INFECTIONS

Superficial fungal infections are common worldwide and are mostly caused by dermatophytes, which are classified into three genera: *Trichophyton*, *Epidermophyton*, and *Microsporum*.[7-9] Dermatophytosis is characterized by annular plaques with active advancing edge [**Figure 89-1**]. The clinical types [**Figures 89-2 and 89-3**] and causative fungi of dermatophytosis in Southeast Asia are similar to those seen in other regions. However, a higher prevalence and more severe disease are commonly encountered, particularly in rural areas with poor access to care and in immunocompromised patients. White onychomycosis, a rare variant of

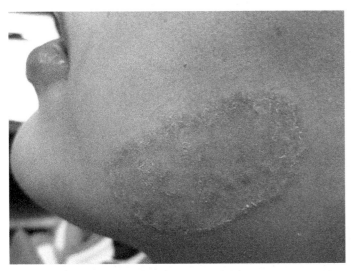

FIGURE 89-1. Classic annular plaque with active erythematous scaly edge and central clearing in a patient with tinea faciei. (Used with permission from Hospital Sultanah Aminah Johor Bahru, Malaysia.)

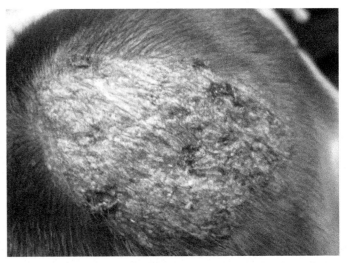

FIGURE 89-3. Kerion showing typical boggy crusted plaque in a child. (Used with permission from Hospital Sultanah Aminah Johor Bahru, Malaysia.)

onychomycosis caused mainly by *Trichophyton rubrum*, is seen mostly in immunocompromised patients[10,11] [**Figure 89-4**]. Diagnosis of dermatophytosis is established by microscopy or culture of infected skin, nail, or hair. Limited skin lesions may be treated by topical agents and more extensive involvement by systemic antifungal agents. Tinea unguium and tinea capitis need to be treated with systemic antifungal agents such as terbinafine or itraconazole.

Tinea versicolor, also known as pityriasis versicolor, is another common superficial infection caused by the yeast *Malassezia furfur*.[12] It is characterized by finely scaling thin plaques with variable pigmentation, occurring most commonly on the upper trunk and extremities. Hypo- and hyperpigmented plaques are usually seen in darker skin, whereas erythematous lesions are seen in fairer skin [**Figure 89-5**]. Definitive diagnosis is established by demonstrating the presence of the causative fungi in skin scrapings.

A recent systematic review on the treatment of tinea versicolor showed that both topical and systemic antifungal agents are effective.[13] Effective topical treatment includes using (1) ketoconazole, selenium sulfide, or zinc pyrithione shampoo, which is applied to affected areas for 5 to 10 minutes before showering off, once daily for 1 to 4 weeks, or (2) imidazole creams, which are applied once or twice daily for 1 to 4 weeks. Extensive tinea versicolor can be successfully and safely treated with the oral imidazole antifungal agents, including itraconazole, 200 mg/d for 7 days or 100 mg/d for 2 weeks or fluconazole, 300 mg/wk for 2 to 4 weeks.

SPOROTRICHOSIS

Sporotrichosis is the most prevalent subcutaneous mycosis caused by *Sporothrix schenckii*.[14,15] Infection occurs as a result of traumatic inoculation of the fungus through small cuts and scratches from thorns, barbs, wood splinters, wires, or animal bites/scratches.[14] Cats, in particular, have been shown to carry a large number of parasites in their nails and oral cavities. Cat bites/scratches are the main portal of entry for sporotrichosis in Malaysia, where cats are the most popular pets.[14-16] The three clinical presentations of cutaneous sporotrichosis are lymphocutaneous, fixed, and disseminated lesions. Extracutaneous disease, such as osteoarticular, pulmonary, mucosal, or systemic involvement, is rare. In Japan, fixed cases are the most commonly seen, whereas the lymphocutaneous variant predominates in Malaysia. In children, the fixed cutaneous form is more common than in adults.

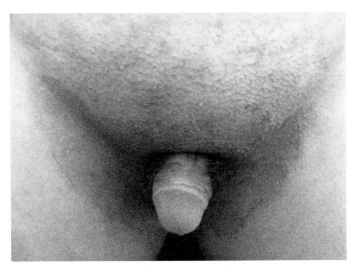

FIGURE 89-2. Tinea cruris with typical annular plaques on both groins. (Used with permission from Hospital Sultanah Aminah Johor Bahru, Malaysia.)

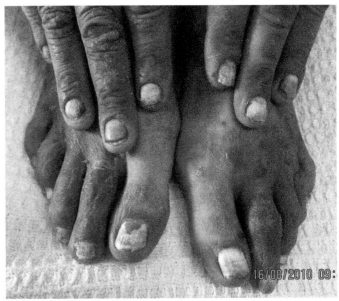

FIGURE 89-4. White superficial onychomycosis affecting toenails and fingernails in a patient with retroviral infection. (Used with permission from Hospital Sultanah Aminah Johor Bahru, Malaysia.)

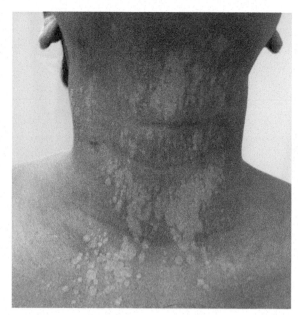

FIGURE 89-5. Tinea versicolor characterized by erythematous mildly scaly lesions. (Used with permission from Hospital Sultanah Aminah Johor Bahru, Malaysia.)

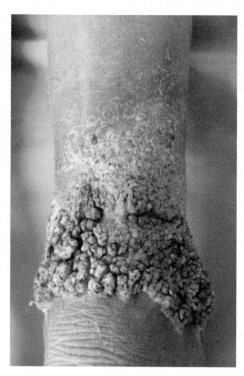

FIGURE 89-7. Verrucous variant of chromoblastomycosis with characteristic blackish spots. (Used with permission from Hospital Sultanah Aminah Johor Bahru, Malaysia.)

Fixed sporotrichosis is characterized by a painless, infiltrated, erythematous, or violaceous nodule or plaque that may become pustular or ulcerated. A linear row of violaceous nodules or plaques is typical of lymphocutaneous sporotrichosis [**Figure 89-6**]. Disseminated cutaneous sporotrichosis may occur in immunocompromised patients.

Positive culture of fungus is the gold standard for diagnosis. Direct microscopy of exudate or skin scraping is not useful, because fungal structures are not usually observed. Histology of a skin biopsy may show granulomatous microabscesses, but fungal structures are not commonly seen. Itraconazole (200 to 400 mg/d for 3 to 6 months) is the treatment of choice for fixed and lymphocutaneous sporotrichosis, although terbinafine (250 to 500 mg/d for 3 to 6 months) has been shown to be effective. Amphotericin B should be used in disseminated and extracutaneous sporotrichosis.

■ CHROMOBLASTOMYCOSIS

Chromoblastomycosis is a chronic progressive subcutaneous mycosis caused by several species of dematiaceous fungi mainly the *Fonsecaea*, *Phialophora*, or *Cladosporium* species.[17-21] The fungus is usually inoculated into the skin by a minor injury, for example, a cut by a splinter. Typically, a pink, grayish, or purplish scaly papule develops at the site of

inoculation, usually on the lower extremity. The lesion slowly enlarges and evolves into an erythematous (purplish in darker skin) psoriasiform or verrucous plaque or nodule that heals partially with scarring. The surface may resemble a cauliflower in the verrucous variant [**Figure 89-7**]. The commonly observed linear row of nodules/plaques may be due to lymphatic spread or autoinoculation through scratching. The affected limb may be swollen if left untreated, causing elephantiasis. Local complications include frequent recrudescence after therapy, a higher risk of squamous cell carcinoma, and disability from invasion of tendons, muscles, and joints.

The clinical diagnosis is readily clinched by looking for brownish sclerotic bodies in skin scrapings [**Figure 89-8**] or skin biopsy [**Figure 89-9**], although the fungus grows in culture within 4 weeks. Chromoblastomycosis is very difficult to treat. Small, localized lesions can be treated with

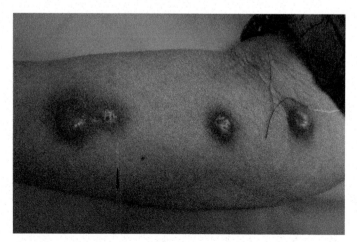

FIGURE 89-6. Linear row of purplish nodules seen in a patient with lymphocutaneous sporotrichosis. (Used with permission from Hospital Sultanah Aminah Johor Bahru, Malaysia.)

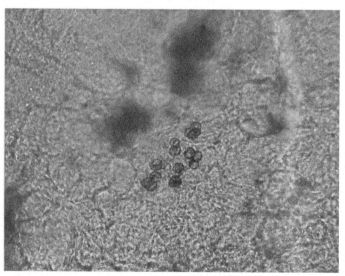

FIGURE 89-8. Chromoblastomycosis: characteristic brownish sclerotic spores on direct microscopy of skin scraping with potassium hydroxide. (Used with permission from Hospital Sultanah Aminah Johor Bahru, Malaysia.)

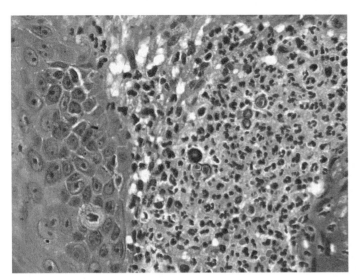

FIGURE 89-9. Chromoblastomycosis: characteristic dermal suppuration with double-walled brownish spores. (Used with permission from Hospital Sultanah Aminah Johor Bahru, Malaysia.)

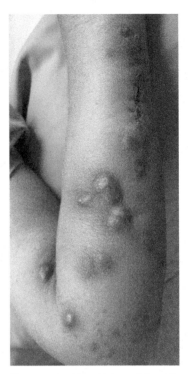

FIGURE 89-10. Mucormycosis with multiple purplish nodules on both upper limbs in a diabetic patient. (Used with permission from Hospital Sultanah Aminah Johor Bahru, Malaysia.)

wide surgical excision, cryotherapy, electrodessication, and curettage or through other destructive procedures.[17] More advanced lesions do respond to systemic antifungals given for at least 6 to 12 months, but lesions frequently relapse after stopping therapy. In general, itraconazole (300 to 400 mg/d) and terbinafine (250 to 500 mg/d) are effective, but the fungi are often resistant to fluconazole. A common approach is to combine cryosurgery with oral itraconazole (300 to 400 mg/d) for 6 to 8 months. There are also reports of successful treatment with flucytosine, amphotericin, and voriconazole.[17,22]

ZYGOMYCOSIS

Zygomycosis is a fungal infection caused by zygomycetes.[23-28] Zygomycetes are subdivided into two orders, the Mucorales and the Entomophthorales, which produce distinct patterns of disease. Mucorales, which encompass several genera (eg, *Rhizopus*, *Rhizomucor*, *Mucor*), cause rhinocerebral, pulmonary, gastrointestinal, and cutaneous infections in predominantly immunocompromised individuals and have a tendency to disseminate. The term *zygomycosis* is often used interchangeably with mucormycosis, whose incidence has increased to become the third most common invasive fungal infection after candidosis and aspergillosis.[25] Cutaneous mucormycosis is uncommon and may appear as pustules, blisters, nodules, necrotic ulcerations, ecthyma gangrenosum-like lesions, or necrotizing cellulitis [**Figure 89-10**]. Mortality is lowest in cutaneous mucormycosis, at 16%, compared to 67% in rhinocerebral, 83% in pulmonary, and 100% in disseminated and gastrointestinal mucormycosis. Tissue biopsy and culture are required for diagnosis. The mainstay of treatment is antifungal therapy with an amphotericin B preparation, debridement, and correction of the underlying medical condition if possible.

In contrast, the order Entomophthorales produces chronic cutaneous and subcutaneous infections in immunocompetent individuals that are almost exclusively limited to the tropics and rarely disseminate to internal organs.[25,27] The two clinically important species are *Basidiobolus ranarum* and *Conidiobolus coronatus*, which produce similar indolent infections of the skin and subcutaneous tissue, but at different anatomic sites. Basidiobolomycosis is characterized by a solitary, painless, indurated subcutaneous plaque predominantly on the trunk and limbs. Conidiobolomycosis, on the other hand, classically affects only the rhinofacial area. Infection generally starts as a unilateral swelling of the inferior turbinate and slowly extends into the surrounding subcutaneous tissues causing progressive enlargement of the nose and lips with subsequent formation of painless subcutaneous nodules on the cheeks, forehead, and glabella [**Figure 89-11**]. If left untreated, it can cause gross

facial disfiguration that is reminiscent of a tapir or hippopotamus. Diagnosis of conidiobolomycosis/basidiobolomycosis requires a close clinicopathologic correlation because culture of the fungi is often negative and it is impossible to differentiate the fungi of the Entomophthorales order histologically. Massive tissue eosinophilia with broad, nonseptate hyphae surrounded by intensely eosinophilic material, hence exhibiting Splendore-Hoeppli phenomenon, confirms the clinical diagnosis. Entomophthoramycosis does respond to most available antifungal agents, although response is better in early disease.[28]

PENICILLIOSIS

Penicilliosis, a systemic mycosis caused by *Penicillium marneffei*, is an endemic disease found only in East and Southeast Asia including

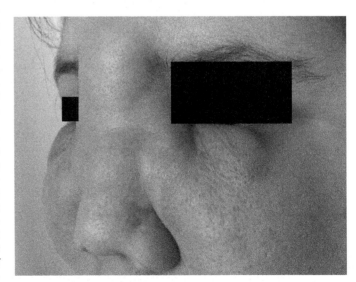

FIGURE 89-11. Conidiobolomycosis with characteristic subcutaneous rhinofacial nodules and swollen lip. (Used with permission from Hospital Sultanah Aminah Johor Bahru, Malaysia.)

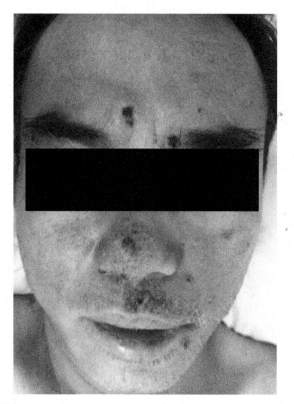

FIGURE 89-12. Penicilliosis: multiple umbilicated and crusted papules on forehead. (Used with permission from Hospital Sultanah Aminah Johor Bahru, Malaysia.)

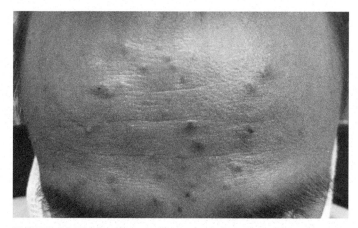

FIGURE 89-13. Histoplasmosis: extensive erythematous to purplish papules, some umbilicated, in a patient with retroviral infection. (Used with permission from Hospital Sultanah Aminah Johor Bahru, Malaysia.)

Thailand, China, Hong Kong, Laos, Cambodia, Malaysia, Myanmar, Vietnam, and Taiwan.[29-35] Sporadic cases have been reported from Manipur, Japan, and Korea.[36-38] International travel and migration have resulted in cases being diagnosed in individuals in Europe, Britain, the United States, and Australia.[35,36] Before the advent of human immunodeficiency virus (HIV) infection, penicilliosis was uncommon even in endemic areas, but it is now listed as the third most common opportunistic fungal infection after tuberculosis and cryptococcosis in patients with acquired immunodeficiency syndrome (AIDS) in northern Thailand.[39]

The natural hosts of *P. marneffei* are bamboo rats and human beings. Infection is believed to be via inhalation of the fungus.[36,40] Penicilliosis is a life-threatening systemic disease characterized by fever, weight loss, lymphadenopathy, hepatosplenomegaly, respiratory signs, and skin lesions. Cutaneous lesions usually start as umbilicated papules that may become necrotic papules or nodules [**Figure 89-12**]. Lesions are classically located on the face, upper chest, and arms. Diagnosis of penicilliosis is based on mycologic culture, which has the best yield for bone marrow samples (100%), followed by skin biopsies (90%) and blood (76%).[35] *P. marneffei* is a fast-growing fungus that often matures within 4 days when cultured at 25°C on Sabouraud dextrose agar (SDA). Characteristic fungal colonies are yellowish-green at the center with white rim that become folded, velvety, and membranous with distinctive diffusion of red pigment in SDA. Intravenous amphotericin B (0.6 mg/kg bodyweight/d) for 2 weeks followed by oral itraconazole (200 mg twice daily) for 10 weeks is the recommended treatment, but maintenance therapy with itraconazole (200 mg daily) is necessary to prevent relapse.

HISTOPLASMOSIS

Histoplasmosis is a common systemic mycosis caused by *Histoplasma capsulatum*, a dimorphic fungus of worldwide distribution.[4,41-43] The clinical spectrum ranges from asymptomatic, self-limited illness to a life-threatening progressive disseminated disease affecting the reticuloendothelial system. *Histoplasma* lives in soil and thrives in areas contaminated with bird or bat excrement. It has been isolated from bat and bird droppings. Infection is usually acquired after inhalation of microconidia from the environment following activities that disrupt soil such as cleaning chicken coups, cleaning attics and barns, caving, and construction. The majority of infected individuals are asymptomatic or have mild symptoms that are not diagnosed as histoplasmosis.

Acute pulmonary illness is the most common symptomatic disease followed by spleen and liver infection.[44] Disseminated histoplasmosis only occurs in approximately 10% of clinical cases, and risk factors include HIV infection, leukemia, lymphomas, alcoholism, organ transplants, impaired cellular immunity malignancies, dialysis, Cushing syndrome, and immunosuppressive therapies and use of biologics such as infliximab or etanercept.[41,42-48]

Cutaneous manifestations are seen in 10% to 25% of AIDS patients with disseminated histoplasmosis.[49] Skin lesions are common in endemic Latin America, being present in between 38% and 85% of these patients. The prevalence of histoplasmosis-induced skin lesions in HIV-infected East and Southeast Asians is not known, but it is seen in less than 10% of AIDS patients in the United States.[50,51] Umbilicated papules are commonly seen, but crusted papules, nodules, acneiform eruptions, and purplish plaques have been reported [**Figure 89-13**].

Definitive diagnosis is based on culture of *H. capsulatum* because the histologic features of granulomatous inflammation with fungal spores may be difficult to distinguish from penicilliosis. Measurements of *Histoplasma* polysaccharide antigen in urine and serum are useful tests for the diagnosis and monitoring of therapy in disseminated histoplasmosis, but these tests are not available in this region. The treatment of choice for severe disseminated histoplasmosis is amphotericin B at 0.7 to 1 mg/kg daily for 12 weeks. Itraconazole (200 mg twice daily) is a good alternative for moderate to mild disease. Fluconazole (800 mg daily) is less efficacious and should be reserved for treatment of histoplasmosis in patients who cannot tolerate itraconazole. Maintenance therapy is usually required lifelong with itraconazole (200 mg once or twice daily).

BACTERIAL INFECTIONS

LEPROSY

Leprosy is a chronic infectious disease caused by *Mycobacterium leprae* that affects primarily the skin and nerves. The prevalence of leprosy dropped dramatically with the implementation of multidrug therapy (MDT) recommended by the World Health Organization (WHO) in 1981, but it remains a major public health problem in economically disadvantaged countries in East and Southeast Asia. In 2011, 73% of total new leprosy cases (160,132 of 219,075 cases) reported to WHO by 105 countries were from Southeast Asia (India is classified under Southeast Asia by WHO).[52] China, Indonesia, Myanmar, and the Philippines were among the 18 countries that reported ≥ 1000 new cases per year. These 18 countries contributed 94% of the new cases detected globally in 2011.

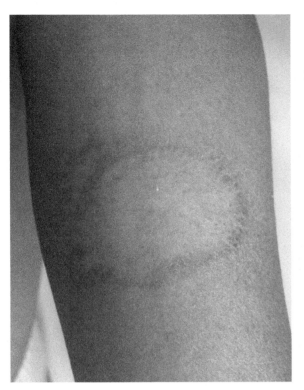

FIGURE 89-14. Tuberculoid leprosy with single anesthetic plaque. (Used with permission from Hospital Sultanah Aminah Johor Bahru, Malaysia.)

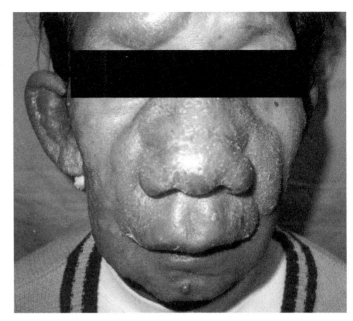

FIGURE 89-15. Severe reversal reaction in a leprosy patient with facial lesions. (Used with permission from Hospital Sultanah Aminah Johor Bahru, Malaysia.)

The mode of transmission of leprosy is not well understood, but it is believed to be acquired by person-to-person contact via nasal droplets. Leprosy may be a zoonosis in South America where nine-banded armadillos are natural reservoirs of infection.[53,54] *M. leprae* is acid-fast and is not very infectious, with a long regeneration time of 12 to 14 days. It has a long incubation period of 2 to 10 years. The clinical manifestations are dependent on the host immune reaction to the bacteria. At one end of the clinical spectrum, when a strong cell-mediated immunity (CMI) is mounted against *M. leprae*, patients developed tuberculoid leprosy, characterized by a few hypopigmented, anesthetic plaques [**Figure 89-14**]. At the other end, patients with lepromatous leprosy, who have poor or no CMI response, usually present with numerous skin lesions, infiltrated ears, loss of eyebrows, and high bacillary loads. Most patients have features between these two extreme groups and fall in the categories of borderline tuberculous, borderline borderline, or borderline lepromatous. The borderline cases are immunologically unstable and at greater risk of developing acute inflammatory episodes called leprosy reactions.[55,56]

Leprosy reactions are immunologic reactions to *M. leprae* antigen and can occur before therapy, during therapy, or after successful completion of MDT, but most occur within a year of starting therapy. Leprosy reactions are a major cause of nerve damage and morbidity. Hence, it is important to diagnose and treat leprosy reactions early to prevent nerve function impairment, deformity, and permanent disability. Leprosy reactions occur in 25% to 30% of patients with borderline or lepromatous leprosy. The two main leprosy reactions are type 1, or reversal reactions, and type 2, or erythema nodosum leprosum (ENL). These reactions occur separately but may arise at different times in the same patient. It is important to appreciate that both reactions can lead to permanent loss of nerve function.

Type 1 reaction occurs when existing lesions swell, redden, desquamate, or ulcerate [**Figure 89-15**]. Occasionally, new lesions may appear. Neuritis is common, but systemic upset is rare. ENL is a systemic disease characterized by fever and widespread crops of erythematous nodules and papules, which may ulcerate. Other features include neuritis, iritis/episcleritis, dactylitis, arthritis, orchitis, lymphadenopathy, and organomegaly.[55,56] There is a third type of reaction, called Lucio

phenomenon, that is rarely reported outside of Mexico and Costa Rica. However, cases have been reported from Singapore and Malaysia.[57,58]

Lucio phenomenon is an aggressive necrotizing variant of ENL that classically occurs in patients with undiagnosed and untreated nonnodular diffuse lepromatous leprosy known as Lucio leprosy. Patients with Lucio leprosy have diffusely infiltrated and shiny skin with madarosis (ie, loss of eyebrows and eyelashes). Lucio phenomenon is characterized by extensive, bizarrely shaped, painful purpuric skin lesions and ulcerations with a paucity of constitutional signs and symptoms. These lesions evolve into hemorrhagic bullae, infarcts, and subsequently ulcers that heal with atrophic stellate scars [**Figure 89-16**].

Diagnosis of leprosy is based on finding the bacteria on slit-skin smears or compatible histology, which usually shows granulomatous reaction with or without acid-fast bacilli. WHO recommends MDT with rifampicin and dapsone for paucibacillary disease (up to five skin lesions) or with rifampicin, dapsone, and clofazimine for multibacillary disease (more than five skin lesions). Recommended duration of treatment is 6 months for paucibacillary disease and 12 months for multibacillary disease. WHO recommends treatment of severe leprosy reactions with a course of steroids for 3 to 6 months. The WHO Global Strategy document does not give specific advice on the dosage of prednisolone in leprosy reactions. We commonly start prednisolone at a daily dose of 1 mg/kg body weight. The dose of prednisolone should be slowly reduced according to response. Patients with ENL require multiple or prolonged courses of prednisolone because the majority of them go on to develop several episodes over many years, as multiple acute episodes or chronic ENL. Thalidomide is very effective in the treatment of moderate to severe ENL but should be used with extreme caution due to its teratogenic potential.[59]

CUTANEOUS TUBERCULOSIS

Although Southeast Asian countries have at least a medium tuberculosis (TB) burden by WHO definition of having at least 50 new tuberculosis cases per 100,000 population per year, cutaneous TB is uncommon.[60] Cutaneous TB composes only a small proportion (<2%) of all cases of TB, with the highest incidence recorded in resource-poor countries.[61,62] In this region, TB verrucosa cutis, scrofuloderma, and lupus vulgaris, caused by *Mycobacterium tuberculosis*, are the more commonly seen types of cutaneous TB.[61,62]

TB verrucosa cutis, which is due to direct inoculation of mycobacteria into the skin, is characterized by a slowly progressive warty plaque located usually on the buttocks and lower limbs. Scrofuloderma, an

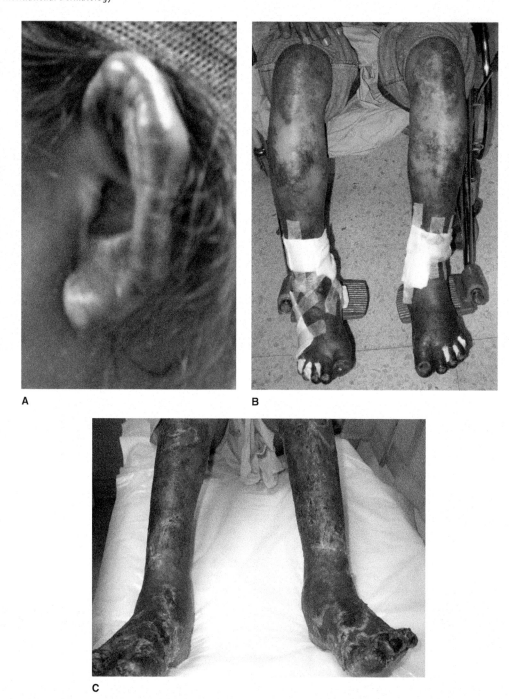

FIGURE 89-16. Lucio phenomenon. (**A**) Hemorrhagic blister affecting left ear helix. Diffuse painful cyanotic discoloration of both feet and multiple purpuric macules and patches on both lower limbs (**B**) that progressed to infarcts and ulcerations (**C**). (Used with permission from Hospital Sultanah Aminah Johor Bahru, Malaysia.)

extension into the skin of an underlying focus of TB, which may be a lymph node, an infected bone or joint, or a lacrimal gland or duct, usually presents as a bluish-red nodule or an undermined ulcer [**Figures 89-17 and 89-18**]. Lupus vulgaris, which usually occur in previously sensitized individuals, is characterized by a well-demarcated, skin-colored to reddish-brown plaque that shows areas of activity and also spontaneous healing with scarring [**Figure 89-19**]. Location on the knee, elbow, wrist, ear, and nose may result in disabling contractures and scarring. Diagnosis of skin TB is difficult in the resource-poor setting where common clinical differential diagnoses include cutaneous leishmaniasis, leprosy, fish-tank granuloma, chromoblastomycosis, sporotrichosis, and sarcoidosis. Many of these conditions also show granulomatous reactions on histology. The presence of underlying systemic TB, acid-fast bacilli in the skin lesion, and/or positive tuberculin reaction are supportive evidence of skin TB,

but definitive diagnosis is dependent on a positive culture of *M. tuberculosis* or identification of its DNA by polymerase chain reaction (PCR). Diagnosis is often only made retrospectively after a successful therapeutic trial because yield from tissue culture is low and PCR confirmation is not widely available.[63,64]

The standard recommended therapeutic regimen for pulmonary TB, which consists of an initial 2 months of four drugs (ie, isoniazid, rifampicin, pyrazinamide, and ethambutol) followed by a further 4 months of isoniazid plus rifampicin, is adequate for treating most cutaneous tuberculous.[60,61,64,65] Longer treatment courses are usually indicated only in cases where there is associated extrapulmonary disease involving the central nervous system, bone, or lymph nodes. A clinical response should be evident after 4 to 6 weeks of the therapeutic trial, with lupus vulgaris showing a faster response than scrofuloderma.[66]

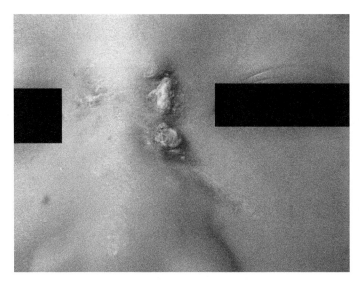

FIGURE 89-17. Scrofuloderma; likely extension from underlying lacrimal gland. (Used with permission from Hospital Sultanah Aminah Johor Bahru, Malaysia.)

FISH-TANK GRANULOMA

Fish-tank granuloma is caused by *Mycobacterium marinum*, which is usually introduced into the skin by minor trauma. *M. marinum* is ubiquitous in the aquatic environment and can be found in fresh, brackish, and salt water. It is also known as swimming pool granuloma, but swimming pools are a rare source of infection now due to effective chlorination/disinfection of public pools. Contact with contaminated aquarium water is the most common source of infection, although it may be acquired by handling infected fish or following fish bites. The majority of skin lesions are located on the upper limbs. An erythematous or bluish papule or nodule usually develops at the inoculation site after 2 to 3 weeks and slowly evolves into an erythematous or verrucous plaque [**Figure 89-20**].[67-69] Pustulations and ulceration may occur.

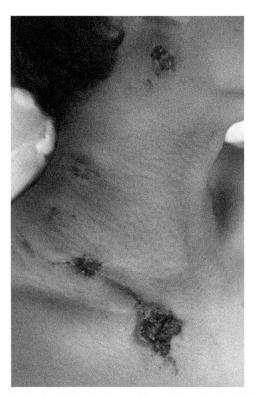

FIGURE 89-18. Scrofuloderma with cervical lymphadenopathy. (Used with permission from Hospital Sultanah Aminah Johor Bahru, Malaysia.)

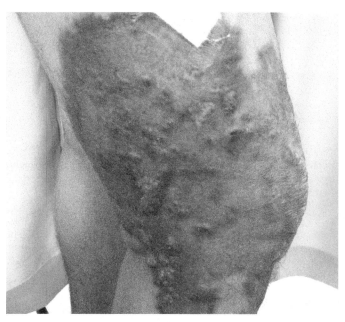

FIGURE 89-19. Lupus vulgaris. Reddish-brown plaque with active papules and areas of healing with scars. (Used with permission from Hospital Sultanah Aminah Johor Bahru, Malaysia.)

A sporotrichoid spread is seen in up to one-third of cases.[67] Lesions are usually localized to the skin, but tenosynovitis, arthritis, and osteoarthritis may rarely occur.[68] Localized pain and induration are common. Fever, lymphadenopathy, and systemic infection are rare but have been reported in immunosuppressed patients.

Diagnosis is often delayed because of unfamiliarity with this condition and difficulty in distinguishing it from other granulomatous infections such as cutaneous TB, sporotrichosis, chromomycosis, and mucormycosis. A definitive diagnosis is based on a positive tissue culture or by PCR technique. However, because PCR testing is not widely available and culture is only positive in 70% to 80% of *M. marinum* infections, a therapeutic trial should be offered if there is a history of aquatic exposure with consistent clinical findings. No optimal treatment has been established for this infection. Effective antibiotics include cotrimoxazole, doxycycline, minocycline, clarithromycin, rifampicin, ethambutol, and quinolones such as ciprofloxacin, levofloxacin, and moxifloxacin.[68]

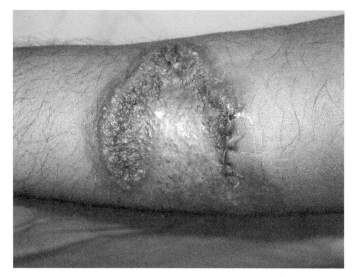

FIGURE 89-20. Fish-tank granuloma. This erythematous plaque with pustules on margin and central scarring on right forearm healed within 6 weeks with cotrimoxazole. (Used with permission from Hospital Sultanah Aminah Johor Bahru, Malaysia.)

Single-agent therapy with cotrimoxazole or doxycycline is usually adequate, but combination therapy with rifampicin and ethambutol is recommended for treating deep-seated infections. Treatment should be continued for at least 3 months or 2 months after lesions have subsided. Improvement should be evident after 6 weeks of therapeutic trial.

ECZEMATOUS DERMATOSES

ATOPIC DERMATITIS

Atopic dermatitis is one of the top 10 conditions seen in any dermatologic clinic in Southeast Asia (see Chapter 27). Most patients develop the condition before they reach 10 years of age. The prevalence rate among school children varies from 3.1% to over 20%.[70-77]

The clinical presentation of eczema in Southeast Asians resembles that seen in the rest of the world. Papular eczema is seen commonly. The itch can be intense, and the constant scratching often results in postinflammatory hypopigmentation. In children, patches of hypopigmentation with fine scales and indistinct borders are often seen on the face, a condition referred to as *pityriasis alba*. This is often seen after sun exposure when the surrounding normal skin becomes tanned, accentuating the contrast. Another common variant is prurigo nodularis. The most common infective complication is bacterial (eg, impetigo, folliculitis, furuncles), followed by viral (eg, herpes simplex infection, molluscum contagiosum).

Patient education is important because many myths abound in Asia. Trigger factors must be avoided and frequent baths discouraged. Moisturizers and topical steroids (titrated to disease activity) are the mainstay of therapy. Second-line therapeutic modalities such as topical calcineurin inhibitors, phototherapy, and oral immunosuppressants such as cyclosporine and azathioprine are available in the big cities but not the rural areas. A survey of dermatologists in Southeast Asia revealed that familiarity with diagnostic criteria, the early and judicious use of moisturizers and topical corticosteroids, and the treatment of *Staphylococcus aureus* superinfection with penicillinase-stable antibiotics should be emphasized in this region.[78]

CONTACT DERMATITIS

Traditional Folk Medications Traditional folk medications are still used widely in Southeast Asia. Investigation of contact dermatitis to these preparations can be difficult because ingredients may not be clearly labeled, and herbal preparations often do not come in standardized concoctions.[79]

Topical traditional Chinese medicaments are one example of such medications and include the following preparations:

1. *Wind oils.* These are used for the relief of headaches and abdominal pain. They contain menthol, camphor, and essential oils. The essential oils may cause allergic contact dermatitis.

2. *Rheumatism oils.* These are used for joint and muscle aches. They contain methyl salicylate, menthol, camphor, and essential oils.

3. *Oils and bonesetter's herbs.* These are used for musculoskeletal injuries such as sprains, contusions, and fractures. These contain mastic and myrrh, which are potential allergens.

4. *Medicated creams, balms, and plasters.*

Proflavine Proflavine, or flavine, is a common over-the-counter antiseptic. It is a yellow solution that can cause severe allergic contact dermatitis, including vesiculobullous, purpuric, and erythema-like reactions. It has a propensity for secondary spread.

Lime In Malaysia, lime has been used in traditional herbal baths and massage oils. Phototoxicity to the psoralen in lime juice may occur.

Contact Dermatitis to Plants Plants belonging to the Anacardiaceae and Compositae families are notorious for causing allergic contact dermatitis.[79]

- The sap of the mango (*Mangifera indica*) may cause allergic dermatitis, which may be erythema multiforme-like, in mango pickers.

- Rengas (*Gluta rengas*) is a hardwood indigenous to Malaysia and Indonesia. It is a potential allergen in wood workers.

- Black exudates from the fruit of the marking nut tree (*Semecarpus anacardium*) are used traditionally to mark laundry in Sri Lanka and India. Dermatitis to the laundry mark is known as *dhobie mark dermatitis* in these countries

- The Thai lacquer tree (*Melanrrhoea usitata*) and the Japanese lacquer tree (*Rhus verniciflua*) contain the resins thitsiol and urushiol, respectively. The resins may cause allergic contact dermatitis in lacquer workers.

- Cashew (*Anacardium occidentale*) nut oil derived from the shells may cause irritant and allergic contact dermatitis in cashew nut workers.

- Many species of the Anacardiaceae family are known to cross-react with poison ivy and poison oak.

- *Parthenium hysterophorus* is an important cause of allergic contact dermatitis in India. The allergen is a sesquiterpene lactone called *parthenin* that is present in all parts of the plant.

- The wild sunflower (*Tithonia diversifolia*) is a perennial shrub in Sri Lanka with bright yellow flowers that may cause an allergic contact dermatitis.

Contact Dermatitis to Cosmetics The bindi or kumkum is a colorful circular disc or spot applied to the central forehead of Hindu women. The adhesive or azo dye used may lead to allergic contact dermatitis, chemical leukoderma, or pigmented contact dermatitis.[79]

ACNE VULGARIS

Acne vulgaris, a multifactorial disorder of the pilosebaceous unit, is very common among adolescents in Southeast Asia. In some rural communities where acne is often viewed as a passage of adolescence that does not require medical treatment, it is not uncommon for patients to present late with nodulocystic acne and/or acne scars.

Asian patients have a higher risk of developing postinflammatory hyperpigmentation and acne keloid scars. In initiating therapy, physicians must choose between aggressive, effective treatments and the risk of skin irritation, which may lead to dyspigmentation. Topical treatments that are known to irritate the skin must be introduced slowly and titrated to response and skin irritation. A combination of medical and procedural treatments is often used.

MEDICAL TREATMENT

Patients often self-medicate with over-the-counter preparations containing benzoyl peroxide, salicylic acid, sulfur, or traditional herbs or oil.[80,81] For most physicians, topical retinoids and topical antibiotics are the mainstay of treatment. Generally, topical retinoids are well tolerated, although patients may complain of a burning sensation on sun exposure. Other topical agents are azelaic acid, glycolic acid, and retinaldehyde.[82-84] These topical agents can improve postinflammatory hyperpigmentation and therefore have an added advantage for use in Asian patients.

Oral antibiotics are given for moderate to severe inflammatory acne. The drug of choice is often doxycycline, because phototoxicity is not a major problem for most Asian patients due to their constitutive skin phototypes. Minocycline, on the other hand, is less popular because blue-black pigmentation sometimes is seen on acne scars, and some patients may have an overall darkening of their facial skin. Oral isotretinoin is the treatment of choice for nodulocystic acne, although it is often used for other less severe forms of acne. Because of cost constraints, there is a tendency to start the treatment late and for patients to stop treatment early, at the first sign of clinical improvement. The efficacy and relapse rates among Asian patients are comparable with those elsewhere.[85,86] Hormonal therapy in the form of oral contraceptive pills containing cyproterone acetate is available in Asia and effective for women with premenstrual acne flares or acne along the jawline.

PROCEDURAL TREATMENT

Procedural treatments are popular for treating acne and their sequelae. Chemical peels are effective in treating both inflammatory and comedonal acne. Glycolic acid, Jessner solution, and salicylic acid peels are equally effective and safe in Asian patients.[87-89] In addition to improving the acne lesions, chemical peels also improve the postacne hyperpigmentation that is commonly seen. Phototherapy using a combination of blue (415 nm) and red (630 to 660 nm) light-emitting diode (LED) lights is often added to the treatment regimen.[90] Aminolevulinic acid photodynamic therapy is another useful option.[91,92] It is not commonly used in rural Asia because of costs and potential side effects from the sun. The diode and pulsed dye lasers are useful in the treatment of inflammatory acne, but these are only available in the urban cities.[93-95]

TREATMENT OF ACNE SCARS

Acne scarring is common in rural Asia due to delay in seeking treatment, suboptimal control, or disease severity. Various treatment options are available to improve acne scars depending on the type of scar. Pitted or boxcar scars need surgical intervention like excision or subcision. Rolling scars can be improved with filler injections or resurfacing procedures like chemical peels, laser resurfacing, microdermabrasion, dermabrasion, and fractional resurfacing.[96-103] Chemical peels are popular because they are easily available and improve both acne and concomitant acne scars. Most physicians prefer to use superficial chemical peels because there is little risk of complications. However, such peels may not be as effective for deeper acne scars, which are commonly seen in Asians.

PIGMENTARY DISORDERS

MELASMA

Melasma is the most common acquired hyperpigmentary condition affecting Asian patients and is one of the top 10 conditions presenting to dermatologists in Southeast Asia. It is more common in women than in men (see Chapter 51).[104] Melasma usually develops in the third to fourth decade of life,[104] although it may start earlier in some darker racial groups. Several factors have been implicated in the pathogenesis of this disorder, including pregnancy, oral contraceptive use, sun exposure, genetic factors, cosmetics, and race.[104-107] A positive family history is common, with more than half of patients having a family history.[104,105] Individuals who work under the sun or in a hot environment tend to have worsening of their melasma. The same clinicopathologic factors are seen in both males and females.[106]

The main pathologic findings are in the epidermis. There is increased melanin and melanosomes in all layers of the epidermis. There is no change in keratinocytes proliferation. In the superficial and mid-dermis, melanin or melanophages are seen, but these findings are not present in all patients.[107,108] Flattening of the epidermis and solar elastosis are usually present, suggesting an association of melasma with sun exposure. It is still controversial whether the number of melanocytes is increased. Kang et al[107] reported an increase in melanocyte number as well as activity in facial melasma skin compared with adjacent normal skin. The melanocytes showed an increase in active protein synthesis and dopa-reactive tyrosinase formation, suggesting that they are responsible for the formation of melasma.

Melasma is seen on the face and, occasionally, on the arms, which are areas of sun exposure. The lesions are light to dark brown and occasionally may be gray. They are distributed symmetrically in three major patterns: centrofacial, malar, and mandibular patterns. Centrofacial melasma accounts for more than half of melasma seen, although in some communities, the malar pattern may be more common.[104,105,108]

In Asia, melasma is considered by most patients as a medical problem rather than a cosmetic nuisance. Some seek treatment for sociocultural reasons because the presence of melasma is often associated with "bad luck" for the patient, family, or family business. Treatment goals include removal or lightening of existing lesions and prevention of new pigment formation. Treatment is difficult because most modalities target epidermal pigment, and there is no effective treatment for dermal melasma. Effective treatment is complicated by the long-standing nature of the problem and the high rate of recurrence once treatment is discontinued. Usually, a combination of topical and procedural treatments is used for good results.

Medical Treatment   Patients should minimize sun exposure by using a broad-spectrum sunscreen during the day and physical protection in the form of broad-brimmed hats, sunglasses, umbrellas, or protective clothing when outdoors. For added protection, an oral agent containing *Polypodium leucotomos* (a fern extract marketed as Helioblock in Asia and Heliocare in the United States) can be taken before sun exposure. This agent is both an antioxidant and an immune modulator that downregulates actinic erythema and increases the skin's tolerance to the effects of ultraviolet (UV) radiation.[109]

Medical therapy of melasma includes topical agents that decrease synthesis of melanosomes (eg, tyrosinase inhibitors), agents that prevent the transfer of melanosomes to keratinocytes, and agents that accelerate cell turnover in the epidermis. A common formulation used in Asia is that proposed by Kligman and Willis in 1975, which combines hydroquinone 5%, tretinoin 0.1%, and dexamethasone 0.1%; variations of this original formulation are also used, with dermatologists substituting different corticosteroids and modifying the concentrations of tretinoin and hydroquinone.[110] These formulations are used until the melasma clears, and patients are often put on a maintenance regimen to prevent relapse of the melasma. A more stable formulation that contains hydroquinone 4%, tretinoin 0.05%, and fluocinolone acetonide 0.01% (Triluma cream) is also available in Asia.[111] In Southeast Asia, the rare side effect of acquired ochronosis from excessive use or misuse of hydroquinone has been reported.[112-114]

Azelaic acid is another commonly used agent, and when combined with glycolic acid, it is as effective as 4% hydroquinone.[115] Azelaic acid can be irritating, and this may lead to postinflammatory hyperpigmentation. Over-the-counter lightening agents like kojic acid or niacinamide are commonly used, but they are less effective than hydroqoquione.[116,117]

Procedural Therapy   Melasma is a therapeutic challenge for the dermatologist. Since most Asian patients with melasma have both epidermal and dermal pigmentation, topical therapy alone is often insufficient to clear their melasma. Chemical peels, microdermabrasion, lasers, and intense pulsed light are often used in combination with topical therapy.

Chemical peels can improve or clear melasma. In treating melasma in an Asian skin type, it is safer to use only superficial peeling agents like glycolic acids, Jessner solution, lactic acid, salicylic acid, pyruvic acids, and tretinoin and to start with lower concentrations to avoid the risk of causing postinflammatory hyperpigmentation. Glycolic acid peels (20% to 70%) performed every 3 weeks on one half of the face for a total of eight peels improved melasma in Chinese women from Singapore when compared with the side that did not receive any peeling.[118] However, these peels have a higher risk of postpeel hyperpigmentation in Asian skin. To reduce this risk and increase the effect of the chemical peel, the skin must be primed at least 2 weeks prior with either hydroquinone or tretinoin, with hydroquinone being superior as a priming agent.[119]

Intense pulsed light, Q-switched neodymium-doped yttrium-aluminum-garnet (Nd:YAG), and fractional erbium glass 1550-nm lasers have been used to treat melasma in Asian persons with some success.[120-131] Treatment is given at 4-week intervals until the melasma clears or improves. Patients will see an improvement in melasma as well as in skin texture. However, there is a risk of transient postinflammatory hyperpigmentation, hypopigmentation, and worsening of the melasma. Melasma tends to recur when laser treatments are stopped.

Tranexamic acid taken orally or as an intradermal injection has been shown to be safe and effective in lightening melasma.[125-131] It may not be effective when applied topically. Another popular treatment in Southeast Asia is the use of vitamin C iontophoresis or oral glutathione to treat melasma.[132] Further studies are warranted to determine the long-term efficacy and safety of these treatments.

◼ ACQUIRED BILATERAL NEVUS OF OTA–LIKE MACULES

Acquired bilateral nevus of Ota–like macule (ABNOM), or nevus fuscoceruleus zygomaticus, was first described by Hori and is often referred to as *Hori nevus*. It is often seen together with melasma and often mistaken for melasma. Sometimes ABNOMs may not be present clinically, but dermal melanocytes are visible on histology.[107]

Clinical Features The pigmentation initially starts as brown macules and later becomes darker and confluent. Onset is usually in the third to fourth decade and is more common among Chinese and Japanese women. There is usually a family history.[133] ABNOMs are distinguished from nevus of Ota by the late onset, the bilateral involvement of the zygoma, and the absence of mucosal involvement.

Pathology Histology shows the presence of melanocytes in the dermis. The intradermal melanocytes are clustered in groups and dispersed perivascularly in ABNOMs, unlike those in nevus of Ota, where they are scattered evenly throughout the dermis. This is one reason why the incidence of postinflammatory hyperpigmentation after laser treatment is higher in ABNOMs than in nevus of Ota.[134]

Treatment Unlike melasma, ABNOMs do not respond to topical agents or chemical peels. They can be cleared almost completely with dermabrasion,[135] which may leave scars. The Q-switched lasers are used to treat ABNOMs with relative success and few side effects, and the lesions remain clear at 3 to 4 years of follow-up.[135-138] A significant number of patients will develop postinflammatory hyperpigmentation (which needs to be addressed using topical lightening agents) or hypopigmentation, which will resolve spontaneously over time. There are no textural changes from the laser treatments. The number of treatment sessions varies from 2 to 11.

◼ POSTINFLAMMATORY HYPERPIGMENTATION

Postinflammatory hyperpigmentation (PIH) is common in Southeast Asians, especially in darker individuals such as Indians or Malays. It is often seen after an episode of acne, eczema, or insect-bite reaction and is made worse by constant picking or scratching at the lesion. PIH often follows interface dermatitis or lichenoid dermatitis. Exposure to UV rays tends to darken the areas of pigmentation.[139]

Diagnosis is usually made when there is a history of a preceding skin injury or skin inflammation, which may be iatrogenic, for example, after a laser procedure. Diagnosis may be difficult if the cutaneous inflammation is transient or mild, escaping the patient's notice.

Treatment Treatment of PIH is difficult. It often lasts for months and even up to a year. The currently available treatment modalities are often not effective. Minimizing sun exposure is important. Topical agents using tyrosinase inhibitors, tretinoin,[140] or glycolic acid can reduce PIH, especially the epidermal component. However, some patients may experience irritation from the treatment. In such instances, the addition of a low- to mid-potency topical steroid can reduce the risk of further PIH. Azelaic acid has been shown to be useful in treating patients with both acne and PIH from acne.[141]

Procedural therapy is often used in an attempt to reduce dermal PIH. Options include chemical peels, microdermabrasion, intense pulsed light, and lasers.[142-145] These must not be used too aggressively in order to prevent further PIH. The use of lasers is controversial; improvement is seen initially, but recurrence or worsening may occur as a result of trauma to the epidermis.

◼ NEVUS OF OTA

Nevus of Ota, or nevus fuscoceruleus ophthalmomaxillaris, is common among Chinese and Malays. It affects 0.014% to 0.034% of the Asian population.[146] Onset is in infancy for most patients; a third will present around puberty. Late onset in adults is rare. The hyperpigmentation is due to the presence of melanocytes in the upper or middle dermis. These melanocytes appear in the dermis during fetal life and fail to migrate to the epidermis.

Clinical Features Nevus of Ota presents as pigmented patches that vary in size from a few centimeters to larger ones that cover almost half

the face. Nevus of Ota appears as shades of brown to bluish-black. The lesion is usually unilateral (different from ABNOMs) and follows the distribution of the first two branches of the trigeminal nerve, that is, the periorbital region, temple, malar region, forehead, nose, and pre- and retroauricular regions. The infraorbital area is the most frequent site of involvement.[146] Extracutaneous involvement has been reported, especially ocular involvement. In two-thirds of patients, the ipsilateral sclera is involved. Other sites of involvement include the eye and the optic nerve, the tympanum and external auditory canal, the nasal mucosa, the lips, the palate, and the pharynx. Complications are rare. There are reports of associated glaucoma and optic melanomas, but these are rare in Asians.

Treatment The treatment of choice for nevus of Ota is the Q-switched laser. The Q-switched ruby laser, Q-switched alexandrite laser, and Q-switched Nd:YAG laser can effectively lighten nevus of Ota without significant side effects.[146-152] Treatment response depends on the age of the patient, the predominant color of the lesion, the thickness of the lesion, and the number of treatments. The mean number of treatments to achieve significant clearing is much fewer when treatment is started in a child as compared with starting treatment as an adult.[153] Fewer treatment sessions are needed to clear brown lesions (average of three sessions) than violet-blue or blue-green lesions (average of four to five sessions).[154] Lesions with a depth of 1 mm or less have a better treatment outcome.[155] Better results are obtained in patients with unilateral lesions and in patients who receive more treatment sessions. Complications are few, but transient hyperpigmentation or hypopigmentation is common. Scarring or textural change is rare.[155]

CHRONIC ARSENIC TOXICITY

Exposure to arsenic in Southeast Asia occurs due to ingestion of contaminated well water or contaminated traditional Chinese medications.[156,157] Symptoms of chronic arsenic toxicity usually develop after 6 months to 2 years of exposure. The time of onset depends on the arsenic concentration in the drinking water, cumulative intake, and the health status of the individual. Chronic arsenic toxicity is a multisystem disorder.

Areas of hyperpigmentation interspersed with hypomelanotic macules (the so-called "raindrops on a dusty road") are seen on the trunk, axillae, and groin. Other cutaneous manifestations include palmoplantar punctate keratoses (arsenical keratosis), guttate hypopigmentation, and skin neoplasms such as Bowen disease, squamous cell carcinoma, and basal cell carcinoma [**Figures 89-21 and 89-22**]. The mucosa is not

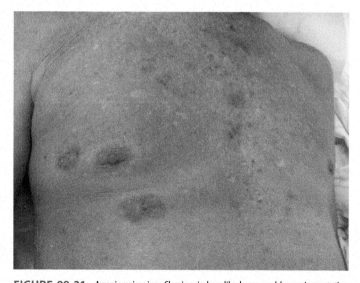

FIGURE 89-21. Arsenic poisoning. Classic raindrop-like hypo- and hyperpigmentation on chest with multiple ill-defined erythematous scaly plaques that were confirmed on biopsy to be Bowen disease. (Used with permission from Hospital Sultanah Aminah Johor Bahru, Malaysia.)

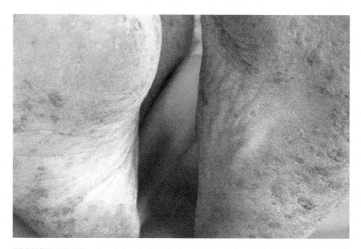

FIGURE 89-22. Arsenic keratosis on both soles in a patient with exposure to arsenic in traditional medication who succumbed to lung cancer. (Used with permission from Hospital Sultanah Aminah Johor Bahru, Malaysia.)

involved. Arsenical keratosis may progress to squamous cell carcinoma. Bowen disease occurs within 10 years of exposure and invasive carcinomas within 20 years.[158,159]

Patients may suffer from generalized weakness, loss of appetite and weight, anemia, sensory neuropathy, and other symptoms. Besides skin cancer, malignancies of the lung, liver, kidney, and bladder may develop. There is no effective treatment for chronic arsenic toxicity. Oral retinoids, curettage, and cryosurgery have been used to reduce arsenic keratoses, but these treatments are anecdotal or based on small series.[159] Treatment is mainly to detect and treat skin neoplasms as and when they arise.

REFERENCES

1. U.S. Census Bureau. World POPClock Projection. July 2012–July 2013 data. http://www.census.gov/population/popclockworld.html. Accessed November 10, 2012.
2. Taylor SC. Epidemiology of skin diseases in ethnic population. *Dermatol Clin.* 2002;21:601-607.
3. Taylor SC. Epidemiology of skin diseases in people of color. *Cutis.* 2003;71:271-275.
4. Chakrabarti A, Slavin MA. Endemic fungal infections in the Asia-Pacific region. *Med Mycol.* 2011;49:337-344.
5. Slavin MA, Chakrabarti A. Opportunistic fungal infections in the Asia-Pacific region. *Med Mycol.* 2012;50:18-25.
6. Drouhet E. Penicillosis due to *Penicillium marneffei:* a new emerging systemic mycosis in AIDS patients travelling or living in southeast-Asia. Review of 44 cases reported in HIV infected patients during the last 5 years compared to 44 cases of non AIDS patients reported over 20 years. *J Mycol Med.* 1993;4:195-224.
7. Havlickova B, Czaika VA, Friedrich M. Epidemiological trends in skin mycoses worldwide. *Mycoses.* 2008;51(Suppl 4):2-15.
8. Ameen M. Epidemiology of superficial fungal infections. *Clin Dermatol.* 2010;28:197-201.
9. Schwartz RA. Superficial fungal infections. *Lancet.* 2004;364:1173-1182.
10. Moreno-Coutino G, Toussaint-Caire S, Arenas R. Clinical, mycological and histological aspects of white onychomycosis. *Mycoses.* 2010;53:144-147.
11. Piraccini BM, Tosti A. White superficial onychomycosis. *Arch Dermatol.* 2004;140:696-701.
12. Gupta AK, Bluhm R, Summerbell R. Pityriasis versicolor. *J Eur Acad Dermatol Venereol.* 2002;16:19-33.
13. Hu SW. Bigby M. Pityriasis versicolor: a systematic review of interventions. *Arch Dermatol.* 2010;146:1132-1140.
14. Vásquez-del-Mercado E, Arenas R, Padilla-Desgarenes C. Sporotrichosis. *Clin Dermatol.* 2012;30:437-443.
15. Ramos-e-Silva M, Vasconcelos C, Carneiro S, Cestari T. Sporotrichosis. *Clin Dermatol.* 2007;25:181-187.
16. Tang MM, Tang JJ, Gill P, et al. Cutaneous sporotrichosis: a six-year review of 19 cases in a tertiary referral center in Malaysia. *Int J Dermatol.* 2012;51:702-708.

17. Torres-Guerrero E, Isa-Isa R, Isa M, Arenas R. Chromoblastomycosis. *Clin Dermatol.* 2012;30:403-408.
18. Bonifaz A, Carrasco-Gerard E, Saul A. Chromoblastomycosis: clinical and mycologic experience of 51 cases. *Mycoses.* 2001;44:1-7.
19. Kondo M, Hiruma M, Nishioka Y, et al. A case of chromomycosis caused by *Fonsecaea pedrosoi* and a review of reported cases of dematiaceous fungal infection in Japan. *Mycoses.* 2005;48:221-225.
20. Minotto R, Bernardi CD, Mallmann LF, et al. Chromoblastomycosis: a review of 100 cases in the state of Rio Grande do Sul. Brazil. *J Am Acad Dermatol.* 2001;44:585-592.
21. Silva JP, de Souza W, Rozental S. Chromoblastomycosis: a retrospective study of 325 cases on Amazonic Region (Brazil). *Mycopathologia.* 1998–1999;143:171-175.
22. Criado PR, Careta MF, Valente NY, et al. Extensive long-standing chromomycosis due to *Fonsecaea pedrosoi:* three cases with relevant improvement under voriconazole therapy. *J Dermatol Treat.* 2011;22:167-174.
23. Drouhet E, Ravisse P. Entomophthoromycosis. *Curr Top Med Mycol.* 1993;5:215-245.
24. Richardson M. The ecology of the zygomycetes and its impact on environmental exposure. *Clin Microbiol Infect.* 2009;15(Suppl 5):2-9.
25. Prabhu RM, Patel R. Mucormycosis and entomophthoramycosis: a review of the clinical manifestations, diagnosis and treatment. *Clin Microbiol Infect.* 2004;10(Suppl 1):31-47.
26. Mantadakis E, Samonis G. Clinical presentation of zygomycosis. *Clin Microbiol Infect.* 2009;15(Suppl 5):15-20.
27. Skiada A, Petrikkos G. Cutaneous zygomycosis. *Clin Microbiol Infect.* 2009;15(Suppl 5):41-45.
28. Choon SE, Kang J, RC Neafie, et al. Conidiobolomycosis in a young Malaysian woman showing chronic localized fibrosing leukocytoclastic vasculitis: a case report and meta-analysis focusing on clinicopathologic and therapeutic correlations with outcome. *Am J Dermatopathol.* 2012;34:511-522.
29. Supparatpinyo K, Khamwan C, Baosoung V, et al. Disseminated *Penicillium marneffei* infection in southeast Asia. *Lancet.* 1994;344:110-113.
30. Sirisanthana T, Supparatpinyo K, Chariyalertsak S, et al. Clinical presentation of 74 HIV-infected patients with disseminated *Penicillium marneffei* infection. *J Infect Dis.* 1998;15:65-68.
31. Duong TA. Infection due to *Penicillium marneffei,* an emerging pathogen: review of 155 reported cases. *Clin Infect Dis.* 1996;23:125-130.
32. Nittayananta W. Penicilliosis marneffei: another AIDS defining illness in Southeast Asia. *Oral Dis.* 1999;5:286-293.
33. Wu TC, Chan JW, Ng CK, et al. Clinical presentations and outcomes of *Penicillium marneffei* infections: a series from 1994 to 2004. *Hong Kong Med J.* 2008;14:103-109.
34. Nor-Hayati S, Sahlawati M, Suresh-Kumar C, Lee KCC. A retrospective review on successful management of Penicillium marneffei infections in patients with advanced HIV in Hospital Sungai Buloh. *Med J Malaysia.* 2012;67:66-70.
35. Vanittanakom N, Cooper CR Jr, Fisher MC, Sirisanthana T. *Penicillium marneffei* infection and recent advances in the epidemiology and molecular biology aspects. *Clin Microbiol Rev.* 2006;9:95-110.
36. Galimberti G, Torre AC, Baztán MC, Rodriguez-Chiappetta F. Emerging systemic fungal infections. *Clin Dermatol.* 2012;30:633-650.
37. Singh PN, Ranjana K, Singh YI, et al. Indigenous disseminated *Penicillium marneffei* infection in the State of Manipur, India: report of 4 autochthoctonous cases. *J Clin Microbiol.* 1999;37:2699-2702.
38. Jung JY, Jo GH, Kim HS, et al. Disseminated penicilliosis in a Korean human immunodeficiency virus infected patient from Laos. *J Korean Med Sci.* 2012;27:697-700.
39. Ustianowski AP, Sieu TPM, Day JN. *Penicillium marneffei* infection in HIV. *Infect Dis.* 2008;21:31-36.
40. Imwidthaya P. Update of penicillosis marneffei in Thailand. *Mycopathologia.* 1994;127:135-137.
41. Kauffman CA. Histoplasmosis: a clinical and laboratory update. *Clin Microbiol Rev.* 2007;20:115-132.
42. Knox KS. Hage CA. Histoplasmosis. *Proc Am Thorac Soc.* 2010;7:169-172.
43. Chang P, Rodas C. Skin lesions in histoplasmosis. *Clin Dermatol.* 2012;30:592-598.
44. Tobón AM, Agudelo CA, Rosero DS. Disseminated histoplasmosis a comparative study between patients with acquired immunodeficiency syndrome and non-human immunodeficiency virus-infected individuals. *Am J Trop Med Hyg.* 2005;73:576-582.
45. Wheat LJ, Kaufman CA. Histoplasmosis. *Infect Disease Clin North Am.* 2003;17:1-19.
46. Wheat LJ. Current diagnosis of histoplasmosis. *Trends Microbiol.* 2003;11:488-495.

47. Hajjeh RA, Pappas PG, Henderson HD. Multicenter case-control study of risk factor for histoplasmosis in human immunodeficiency virus infected people. *Clin Infect Dis.* 2001;32:1215-1220.

48. Lee JHR, Slifman NR, Gershon SK. Life-threatening histoplasmosis complicating immunotherapy with tumor necrosis factor antagonists infliximab and etanercept. *Arthritis Rheum.* 2002;46:2565-2570.

49. Eidbo J, Sanchez RL, Tschen JA. Cutaneous manifestations of histoplasmosis in acquired immunodeficiency syndrome. *Am J Surg Pathol.* 1993;17:110-116.

50. Porras B, Costner M, Friedman-Kien AE. Update on cutaneous manifestations of HIV infection. *Med Clin North Am.* 1998;82:1033-1037.

51. Karimi K, Wheat JL, Connoly P. Differences in histoplasmosis in patients with acquired immunodeficiency syndrome in United States and Brazil. *J Infect Dis.* 2002;186:1655-1660.

52. World Health Organization. Global leprosy situation, 2012. *Wkly Epidemiol Rec.* 2012;87:317-328.

53. Rodrigues LC, Lockwood DNJ. Leprosy now: epidemiology, progress, challenges, and research gaps. *Lancet Infect Dis.* 2011;11:464-470.

54. Suzuki K, Akama T, Kawashima A, et al. Current status of leprosy: epidemiology, basic science and clinical perspectives. *J Dermatol.* 2012;39:121-129.

55. Kahawita IP. Lockwood DN. Towards understanding the pathology of erythema nodosum leprosum. *Trans R Soc Trop Med Hyg.* 2008;102:329-337.

56. Van Veen NH, Lockwood DN, van Brakel WH, et al. Interventions for erythema nodosum leprosum. *Cochrane Database Syst Rev.* 2009;3:CD006949.

57. Ang P, Tay YK, Ng SK, Seow CS. Fatal Lucio's phenomenon in 2 patients with previously undiagnosed leprosy. *J Am Acad Dermatol.* 2003;48:958-961.

58. Choon SE, Tey KE. Lucio's phenomenon: a report of three cases seen in Johor, Malaysia. *Int J Dermatol.* 2009;48:984-988.

59. Walker SL, Waters MF, Lockwood DN. The role of thalidomide in the management of erythema nodosum leprosum. *Lepr Rev.* 2007;78:197-215.

60. World Health Organization. Global Tuberculosis Report 2012. http://www.who.int/tb/publications/global_report/gtbr12_main.pdf. Accessed on November 18, 2012.

61. Bravo F, Gotuzzo E. Cutaneous tuberculosis. *Clin Dermatol.* 2007;25:173-180.

62. Singal A, Sonthalia S. Cutaneous tuberculosis in children: the Indian perspective. *Indian J Dermatol Venereol Leprol.* 2010;76:494-503.

63. Sehgal VN, Sardana K, Bajaj P, Bhattacharya SN. Tuberculosis verrucosa cutis: antitubercular therapy, a well-conceived diagnostic criterion. *Int J Dermatol.* 2005;44:230-232.

64. Joint Tuberculosis Committee of the British Thoracic Society. Chemotherapy and management of tuberculosis in the United Kingdom: recommendations 1998. *Thorax.* 1998;53:536-548.

65. Blumberg HM, Burman WJ, Chaisson RE, et al. American Thoracic Society/Centers for Disease Control and Prevention/Infectious Diseases Society of America: treatment of tuberculosis. *Am J Respir Crit Care Med.* 2003;167:603-662.

66. Ramam M, Mittal R, Ramesh V. How soon does cutaneous tuberculosis respond to treatment? Implications for a therapeutic test of diagnosis. *Int J Dermatol.* 2005;44:121-124.

67. Tebruegge M, Curtis N. *Mycobacterium marinum. Adv Exp Med Biol.* 2011;719:201-210.

68. Cheung JP, Fung B, Wong SS, Ip WY. Review article: *Mycobacterium marinum* infection of the hand and wrist. *J Orthop Surg (Hong Kong).* 2010;18:98-103.

69. Ang P, Rattana-Apiromyakij N, Goh CL. Retrospective study of *Mycobacterium marinum* skin infections. Int *J Dermatol.* 2000;39:343-347.

70. Tay YK, Khoo BP, Goh CL. The profile of atopic dermatitis in a tertiary dermatology outpatient clinic in Singapore. *Int J Dermatol.* 1999;38:689-692.

71. Tay YK, Kong KH, Khoo L, et al. The prevalence and descriptive epidermiology of atopic dermatitis in Singapore school children. *Br J Dermatol.* 2002;146:101-106.

72. Al-Saeed WY, Al-Dawood KM, Bukhari IA, et al. Prevalence and pattern of skin disorders among female schoolchildren in eastern Saudi Arabia. *Saudi Med J.* 2006;27:227-234.

73. Yan DC, Ou LS, Tsai TL, et al. Prevalence and severity of asthma, rhinitis and eczema in 13-14 year-old children in Taipei, Taiwan. *Ann Allergy Asthma Immunol.* 2005;95:579-585.

74. Liao ME, Huang JL, Chiang LC. Prevalence of asthma, rhinitis and eczema from the ISAAC survey of schoolchildren in Central Taiwan, part I. *Asthma.* 2005;42:833-837.

75. Teeratakulpisarn J, Wiangnon S, Kosalaraksa P, Heng S. Surveying the prevalence of asthma, allergic rhinitis and eczema in school-children in Khon Kaen, northeastern Thailand using the ISSAC questionnaire, part III. *Asian Pacific J Allergy Immunol.* 2004;22:175-181.

76. Quah BS, Wan-Pauzi I, Ariffin N, Mazidah AR. Prevalence of asthma, eczema and allergic rhinitis: two surveys, 6 years apart, in Kota Bharu, Malaysia. *Respirology.* 2005;10:244-249.

77. Sugiura H, Umemoto N, deGuchi H, et al. Prevalence of childhood and adolescent atopic dermatitis in a Japanese population: comparison with the disease frequency examined 20 years ago. *Acta Dermatol Venereol.* 1998;78:293-294.

78. Chan YC, Tay YK, Sugito TL, et al. A study on the knowledge, attitudes and practices of Southeast Asian dermatologists in the management of atopic dermatitis. *Ann Acad Med Singapore.* 2006;35:794-803.

79. Ng SK, Goh CL, eds. *The Principles and Practice of Contact and Occupational Dermatology in the Asia-Pacific Region.* Singapore: World Scientific Publishing Company; 2001.

80. Sharquie KE, Al-Turfi IA, Al-Shimary WM. Treatment of acne vulgaris with 2% topical tea lotion. *Saudi Med J.* 2006;27:83-85.

81. Chomnawang MT, Surassmo S, Nukoolkarn VS, Gritsanapan W. Antimicrobial effects of Thai medicinal plants against acne-inducing bacteria. *J Ethnopharmacol.* 2005;101:330-333.

82. Spellman MC, Pinus SH. Efficacy and safety of azelaic acid and glycolic acid combination therapy compared with tretinoin therapy for acne. *Clin Ther.* 1998;20:711-721.

83. Dreno B, Nocera T, Verriere F, et al. Topical retinaldehyde with glycolic acid: study of tolerance and acceptability in association with anti-acne treatments in 1709 patients. *Dermatology.* 2005;210:22S-29S.

84. Poli F, Ribet V, Lauze C, et al. Efficacy and safety of 0.1% retinaldehyde/6% glycolic acid (diacneal) for mild to moderate acne vulgaris: a multicentre, double-blind, randomized vehicle-controlled trial. *Dermatology.* 2005;210:14-21.

85. Shahidullah M, Tham SN, Goh CL. Isotretinoin therapy in acne vulgaris: a 10 year retrospective study in Singapore. *Int J Dermatol.* 1994;33:60-63.

86. Ng PP, Goh CL. Treatment outcome of acne vulgaris with oral isotretinoin in 89 patients. *Int J Dermatol.* 1999;38:213-216.

87. Wang CM, Huang CL, Hu CT, et al. The effect of glycolic acid in the treatment of acne in Asian patients. *Dermatol Surg.* 1997;23:23-29.

88. Lee HS, Kim IH. Salicylic acid peels for the treatment of acne vulgaris in Asian patients. *Dermatol Surg.* 2003;29:1196-1199.

89. Kim SW, Moon SE, Kim JA, et al. Glycolic acid versus Jessner's solution: which is better for facial acne patients? A randomized, prospective clinical trial of split-face model therapy. *Dermatol Surg.* 1999;25:270-273.

90. Goldberg DJ, Russell BA. Combination blue (415 nm) and red (633 nm) LED phototherapy in the treatment of mild to severe acne vulgaris. *J Cosmet Laser Ther.* 2006;8:71-75.

91. Pollock B, Turner D, Stringer MR, et al. Topical aminolaevulinic acid photodynamic therapy for the treatment of acne vulgaris: a study of clinical efficacy and mechanism of action. *Br J Dermatol.* 2004;151:616-622.

92. Hongcharu W, Taylor CR, Chang Y, et al. Topical ALA-photodynamic therapy for the treatment of acne vulgaris. *J Invest Dermatol.* 2000;115:183-192.

93. Friedman PM, Jih MH, Kimyai-Asadi A, et al. Treatment of inflammatory facial acne vulgaris with the 1450 nm diode laser: Pilot study. *Dermatol Surg.* 2004;30:147-151.

94. Seaton ED, Charakida A, Mouser PE, et al. Pulsed-dye laser treatment for inflammatory acne vulgaris: randomised, controlled trial. *Lancet.* 2003;25:1347-1352.

95. Orringer JS, Kang S, Hamilton T, et al. Treatment of acne vulgaris with a pulsed dye laser: a randomized, controlled trial. *JAMA.* 2004;291:2834-2839.

96. Erbagci Z, Akcali C. Biweekly serial glycolic acid peels vs long-term daily use of topical low-strength glycolic acid in the treatment of atrophic acne scars. *Int J Dermatol.* 2000;39:789.

97. Al-Waiz MM, Al-Sharqi AI. Medium-depth chemical peels in the treatment of acne scars in dark-skinned individuals. *Dermatol Surg.* 2002;28:383-387.

98. Chan HH, Lam LK, Wong DS, et al. Use of 1320 nm Nd:YAG laser for wrinkle reduction and the treatment of atrophic acne scarring in Asians. *Laser Surg Med.* 2004;34:98-103.

99. Lipper GM, Perez M. Nonablative acne scar reduction after a series of treatments with a short-pulsed 1064 nm neodymium:YAG laser. *Dermatol Surg.* 2006;32:998-1006.

100. Nonablative 1450 nm diode laser in the treatment of facial atrophic acne scars in type IV to V Asian skin: a prospective clinical study. *Dermatol Surg.* 2004;30:1287-1291.

101. Woo SH, Park JH, Kye YC. Resurfacing of different types of facial acne scar with short-pulsed, variable-pulsed, and dual-mode Er:YAG laser. *Dermatol Surg.* 2004;30:488-493.

102. Jeong JT, Kye YC. Resurfacing of pitted facial acne scars with a long-pulsed Er:YAG laser. *Dermatol Surg.* 2001;27:107-110.

103. Tsai RY, Wang CN, Chang HL. Aluminum oxide crystal microderm-abrasion: a new technique for treating facial scarring. *Dermatol Surg.* 1995;21:539-542.

104. Goh CL, Diova CN. A retrospective study on the clinical presentation and treatment outcome of melasma in a tertiary dermatological referral centre in Singapore. *Singapore Med J.* 1999;40:455-458.

105. Moin A, Jabery Z, Fallah N. Prevalence and awareness of melasma during pregnancy. *Int J Dermatol.* 2006;45:285-288.

106. Vazquez M, Maldonado H, Benmaman C, et al. Melasma in men: a clinical and histologic study. *Int J Dermatol.* 1988;27:25-27.

107. Kang WH, Yoon KH, Lee ES, et al. Melasma: histopathological characteristics in 56 Korean patients. *Br J Dermatol.* 2002;146:228-237.

108. Sanchez NP, Pathak MA, Sato S, et al. Melasma: a clinical, light microscopic, ultrastructural, and immunofluorescence study. *J Am Acad Dermatol.* 1981;4:698-710.

109. Choudhry S, Bhatia N, Ceilley R, et al. Role of oral Polypodium leucotomos extract in dermatologic diseases: a review of the literature. *J Drugs Dermatol.* 2014;13:148-153.

110. Kligman AM, Willis I. A new formula for depigmenting human skin. *Arch Dermatol.* 1975;111:40-48.

111. Taylor SC, Torok H, Jones T, et al. Efficacy and safety of a new triple-combination agent for the treatment of facial melasma. *Cutis.* 2003;72:67-72.

112. Preya K, Suwirakorn O, Suwit S. Exogenous ochronosis and pigmented colloid milium induced by bleaching skin cream. *Environ Dermatol.* 1998;5:20-25.

113. Tan SK. Exogenous ochronosis in ethnic Chinese Asians: a clinicopathological study, diagnosis and treatment. *J Eur Acad Dermatol Venereol.* 2011;25:842-850.

114. Tan SK, Sim CS, Goh CL. Hydroquinone-induced exogenous ochronosis in Chinese: two case reports and a review. *Int J Dermatol.* 2008;47:639-640.

115. Fitton A, Goa KL. Azelaic acid: A review of its pharmacological properties and therapeutic efficacy in acne and hyperpigmentary skin disorders. *Drug.* 1991;41:780-798.

116. Lim JTE. Treatment of melasma using kojic acid in a gel containing hydroquinone and glycolic acid. *Dermatol Surg.* 1999;25:282-284.

117. Hakozaki T, Minwalla L, Ang JZ, et al. The effect of niacinamide on reducing cutaneous pigmentation and suppression of melanosome transfer. *Br J Dermatol.* 2002;147:20-31.

118. Lim JTE, Tham SN. Glycolic acid peels in the treatment of melasma. *Dermatol Surg.* 1997;23:177-179.

119. Nanda S, Grover C, Reddy BS. Efficacy of hydroquinone (2%) versus tretinoin (0.025%) as adjunct topical agents for chemical peeling in patients of melasma. *Dermatol Surg.* 2004;30:385-389.

120. Wang CC, Hui CY, Sue YM, et al. Intense pulsed light for the treatment of refractory melasma in Asian persons. *Dermatol Surg.* 2004;30:1196-1200.

121. Negishi K, Tezuka Y, Kushikata N, et al. Photorejuvenation for Asian skin by intense pulsed light. *Dermatol Surg.* 2001;27:627-632.

122. Na SY, Cho S, Lee SH. Intense pulse light and low fluence Q-Switched Nd-YAG laser treatment in Melasma patients. *Ann Dermatol.* 2012;24:267-273.

123. Kauvar AN. Successful treatment of melasma using a combination of microdermabrasion and Q-Switched Nd-Yag laser. *Laser Surg Med.* 2012;44:117-124.

124. Zhou X, Gold MH, Lu Z, Li Y. Efficacy and safety of Q-switched 1064nm laser treatment of melasma. *Dermatol Surg.* 2011;37:962-970.

125. Wattanakrai P, Mornchan R, Eimpurith S. Low fluence Q-switched Nd-YAG laser treatment of facial melasma in Asia. *Dermatol Surg.* 2010;36:76-87.

126. Tannous ZS, Astner S. Utilizing fractional resurfacing in the treatment of melasma. *J Cosmet Laser Ther.* 2005;7:39-43.

127. Rokhsar CK, Fitzpatrick RE. The treatment of melasma with fractional photothermolysis: a pilot study. *Dermatol Surg.* 2005;31:1645-1650.

128. Wu S, Shi H, Wu H, Yan S, Guo J, Sun Y, Pan L. Treatment of melasma with oral administration of tranexamic acid. *Aesthetic Plast Surg.* 2012;36:964-970.

129. Na JI, Choi SY, Yang SH, Choi HR, Kang HY, Park KC. Effect of tranexamic acid on melasma: a clinical trial with histological evaluation. *J Eur Acad Dermatol Venereol.* 2012;12:1468-1472.

130. Lee JH, Park JG, Lim SH, et al. Localized intradermal microinjection of tranexamic acid for the treatment of melasma in Asian patients: a preliminary clinical trial. *Dermatol Surg.* 2006;32:626-631.

131. Ayuthaya PK, Niumphradit N, Manosroi A, Nakakes A. Topical 5% tranexamine acid for the treatment of melasma in Asians: a double-blind randomised controlled clinical trial. *J Cosmetic Laser Ther.* 2012;14:150-154.

132. Huh CH, Seo KI, Park JY, et al. A randomized, double-blind, placebo-controlled trial of vitamin C iontophoresis in melasma. *Dermatology.* 2003;206:318-320.

133. Ee HL, Wong HC, Goh CL, et al. Characteristics of Hori's naevus: a prospective analysis. *Br J Dermatol.* 2005;154:50-53.

134. Lee B, Kim YC, Wang WH, et al. Comparison of characteristics of acquired bilateral nevus of Ota-like macules and nevus of Ota according to therapeutic outcome. *J Korean Med Sci.* 2004;19:554-559.

135. Kunachak S, Kunachakr S, Sirikulchayanonta V, et al. Dermabrasion is an effective treatment for acquired bilateral nevus of Ota-like macules. *Dermatol Surg.* 1996;22:559-562.

136. Kunachak S, Leelaudomlipi P. Q-switched Nd:YAG laser treatment for bilateral nevus of Ota-like macule: a long-term follow-up. *Lasers Surg Med.* 2000;26:376-379.

137. Suh DH, Han KH, Chung JH. Clinical use of the Q-switched Nd:YAG laser for the treatment of acquired bilateral nevus of Ota-like macules (ABNOM) in Koreans. *J Dermatol Ther.* 2001;12:163-166.

138. Polnikorn K, Tanrattanakorn S, Goldberg DJ. Treatment of Hori's nevus with the Q-switched Nd:YAG laser. *Dermatol Surg.* 200;26:477-480.

139. Lam AY, Wong DS, Lam LK, et al. A retrospective study on the complications of Q-switched alexandrite laser in the treatment of acquired bilateral nevus of Ota-like macules. *Dermatol Surg.* 2001;27:937-941.

140. Nordlund JJ. Postinflammatory hyperpigmentation. *Dermatol Clin.* 1988;6:185-192.

141. Bulengo-Ransby SM, Griffiths CEM, Kimbrough-Green CK, et al. Topical tretinoin (retinoic acid) therapy for hyperpigmented lesions caused by inflammation of the skin in black patients. *N Engl J Med.* 1993;328:1438-1443.

142. Lowe NJ, Rizk D, Grimes PE, et al. Azelaic acid 29% cream in the treatment of facial hyperpigmentation in darker-skinned patients. *Clin Ther.* 1998;20:945-959.

143. Burns RL, Prevost-Blank PL, Lawry MA, et al. Glycolic acid peels for post-inflammatory hyperpigmentation in black patients: a comparative study. *Dermatol Surg.* 1997;23:171-174.

144. Grimes PE. The safety and efficacy of salicylic acid chemical peels in darker racial-ethnic groups. *Dermatol Surg.* 1999;25:18-22.

145. Dierickx C, Goldman MP, Fitzpatrick RE. Laser treatment of erythematous, hypertrophic, and pigmented scars in 26 patients. *Plast Reconstr Surg.* 1995;95:84-90.

146. Chan HH, Kono T. Naevus of Ota: CLINICAL aspects and management. *Skinmed.* 2003;2:89-96.

147. Watanabe S, Takahashi H. Treatment of naevus of Ota with the Q-switched ruby laser. *N Engl J Med.* 1994;29: 1745-1750.

148. Chang CJ, Nelson JS, Achauer BM. Q-switched ruby laser treatment of oculodermal melanosis (nevus of Ota). *Plast Reconstr Surg.* 1996;98:1784-1790.

149. Yang HY, Lee CW, Ro YS, et al. Q-switched ruby laser in the treatment of nevus of Ota. *J Korean Med Sci.* 1996;11:165-170.

150. Alster TS, Williams CM. Treatment of naevus of Ota by the Q-switched alexandrite laser. *Dermatol Surg.* 1995;21:592-596.

151. Lu Z, Fang L, Jiao S, et al. Treatment of 522 patients with naevus of Ota with the Q-switched alexandrite laser. *Chin Med J.* 2003;116:226-230.

152. Kono T, Chan HH, Ercocen AR, et al. Use of Q-switched ruby laser in the treatment of nevus of Ota in different age groups. *Laser Surg Med.* 2003;32:391-395.

153. Ueda S, Isoda M, Imayama S. Response of naevus of Ota to Q-switched ruby laser treatment according to lesion colour. *Br J Dermatol.* 2000;142:77-83.

154. Kang W, Lee E, Choi GS. Treatment of Ota's nevus by Q-switched alexandrite laser: the therapeutic outcome in relation to clinical and histological findings. *Eur J Dermatol.* 1999;9:639-643.

155. Chan HH, Leung RS, Ying SY. A retrospective analysis of complications in the treatment of nevus of Ota with the Q-switched alexandrite and the Q-switched Nd:YAG lasers. *Dermatol Surg.* 2000;26:1000-1006.

156. Yeh S. Skin cancer in chronic arsenicism. *Hum Pathol.* 1973;4:469-485.

157. Agusa T, Kunito T, Fujihara J, et al. Contamination by arsenic and other trace elements in tube-well water and its risk assessment to humans in Hanoi, Vietnam. *Environ Pollut.* 2006;139: 95-106.

158. Miki Y, Kawatsu T, Matsuda K, et al. Cutaneous and pulmonary cancers associated with Bowen's disease. *J Am Acad Dermatol.* 1982;6:26-31.

159. Piamphongsant T. Chronic environmental arsenic poisoning. *Int J Dermatol.* 1999;38:401-410.

CHAPTER 90

Maritime Southeast Asia

Evangeline B. Handog
Maria Juliet E. Macarayo
Maria Suzanne L. Datuin

KEY POINTS

- Southeast Asia (SEA) is divided into mainland SEA and maritime SEA; maritime SEA, also known as island SEA or insular SEA, is composed of six regions: East Malaysia, Philippines, Brunei, East Timor, Singapore, and Indonesia.

- Maritime SEA has islands from very large to tiny pinpoints on the map, oceans that are generally shallow with few deep underwater trenches, active volcanoes making them vulnerable to earthquake activities, and a climate that is tropical.

- Situated in the typhoon belt, on average, around 20 typhoons enter the Philippines a year; the rest of the maritime SEA countries are generally free of hurricanes and typhoons.

- Cultural diversity is evident, as in mainland SEA; Muslims make up the majority of the Indonesian population, while the Philippines is a predominantly Catholic state.

- The majority of the population of both Indonesia and the Philippines belongs in the 15- to 64-year age group, and there are more males than females; skin phototype is usually between III and V.

- The common skin diseases are inflammatory dermatoses, the pigmentary disorder melasma, and diseases due to microbial agents and infestations.

Southeast Asia (SEA) is divided into mainland and maritime SEA. Six states (Myanmar, Thailand, Laos, Cambodia, West Malaysia, and Vietnam) compose mainland SEA. Maritime SEA, also known as island SEA or insular SEA, comprises of East Malaysia, Philippines, Brunei, East Timor, Singapore, and Indonesia. This chapter focuses on dermatoses commonly seen in maritime SEA.

SEA is a tropical region with similarities in climate as well as plant and animal life. Mainland SEA has long rivers, extensive lowland plains, and long coastlines.[1] Maritime SEA has islands that range from very large to tiny pinpoints on the map. Indonesia has 17,508 islands,[2] whereas the Philippines has 7107 islands.[3] Importantly, the seas of maritime SEA make it unique. The oceans are generally shallow with few deep underwater trenches. Except for the Philippines, the countries of maritime SEA are generally free of hurricanes and typhoons. Many active volcanoes are identified in this part of SEA, making them vulnerable to earthquakes.[1]

A distinctive feature of SEA is its cultural diversity. Migration into the region has a long history, playing a vital role in the existing cultural beliefs and practices.[1] Eighty-six percent of Indonesia's population are Muslims,[2] whereas in Singapore, Thailand, and the southern Philippines, Muslims are a minority.[1] The Philippines is a predominantly Catholic state.[3]

With a population of over a hundred million, 61.3% of Filipinos belong to the 15- to 64-year-old age group, and 34.3% are 0 to 14 years of age; there are more males than females. The Tagalogs are the largest (28.1%) of the 10 major ethnic groups in the country.[3] The Negritos were some of the earliest inhabitants, followed by successive waves of Austronesians and Chinese. With the arrival of the Japanese, Indians, Spaniards, Americans, and Europeans, intermarriages were inevitable, producing descendants known as the mestizos.[4] The Filipino culture is similar to that of other Asian countries with a Malay heritage, yet it also displays a significant amount of Spanish and American influences.

The Republic of Indonesia is inhabited by almost 250 million people, the majority of whom are the Javanese (40.6%). Like the Philippines, 66.5% of the population belongs to the 15- to 64-year-old age group, with 27.3% between 0 and 14 years old; similarly, males outnumber females. After decades of Dutch colonization and Japanese occupation,

TABLE 90-1 Common skin diseases in maritime Southeast Asia

Inflammatory skin disorders	Contact dermatitis
	Seborrheic dermatitis, psoriasis
	Acne vulgaris
Pigmentary disorder	Melasma
Diseases due to microbial agents and infestations	Tinea infections, verruca, impetigo, leprosy, scabies

Indonesia is now the world's third most populous democracy, the world's largest archipelagic state, and home to the world's largest Muslim population.[2]

With the maritime SEA region having a tropical climate and ethnic diversity, skin phototypes range from III to V, similar to other Asians. Cutaneous diseases common to the maritime SEA region are also seen in mainland SEA countries. Discussed in this chapter are inflammatory skin diseases, the pigmentary disorder melasma, and diseases due to microbial agents and infestations common to the region [**Table 90-1**].

CONTACT DERMATITIS

▧ EPIDEMIOLOGY

Contact dermatitis is one of the most common occupational inflammatory dermatoses in industrialized countries, affecting women more than men.[5-7] Gender differences may be attributed to social and environmental factors; females are more likely to have nickel sensitivity because of increased wearing of jewelry, whereas males are more likely to have chromate sensitivity from occupational exposure.[8,9] The study by Rui et al[9] showed interesting associations between some occupations and nickel, chromate, and cobalt allergy. The most common allergens in the Philippines (data from the Philippine Dermatological Society's training institutions) are nickel sulfate, p-phenylenediamine, colophony, formaldehyde, isopropyl-phenylenediamine, mercapto mix, fragrance mix, epoxy resin, potassium dichromate, thiuram, balsam of Peru, and cocamidopropylbetaine.[10] In a large population-based patch test study, nickel was the most common sensitizer in children.[11] The prevalence of allergic contact dermatitis (ACD) among children ranges from 14% to 77%.[12-15] Atopic dermatitis is a risk factor for allergic contact sensitization,[16] and ACD increases with age in atopics.[17] It is also common among the elderly due to impaired epidermal barrier function and delayed cutaneous recovery after injury. Medical comorbidities, including stasis dermatitis and venous ulcerations, further exacerbate this clinical picture.[18]

▧ PATHOPHYSIOLOGY

ACD is a type IV, delayed hypersensitivity reaction provoked by various exogenous substances.[19] The antigen complex formed from the linkage of epidermal proteins and haptens leads to sensitization.[20] Irritant contact dermatitis is a non–immune-modulated cutaneous inflammation; hence, previous sensitization is not required.[21] Direct contact with a chemical, physical, or biologic agent results in injury, direct cytotoxic effects, or cutaneous inflammation.[20,22]

▧ CLINICAL FEATURES

The clinical presentation of contact dermatitis varies. Acute ACD progresses from erythema to edema to papulovesiculation that occurs in the distribution of the contactant [**Figure 90-1**]. In situations where the allergen exposure is persistent, lichenification and scale predominate.[22] Resolution of ACD usually occurs 2 to 3 weeks after withdrawal of the offending agent.[23,24] Irritant contact dermatitis has a spectrum of clinical features, which can range from erythema to tissue necrosis.

▧ DIAGNOSIS

To establish the diagnosis of ACD, existence of contact allergy must be demonstrated by patch testing. The clinical relevance of a positive patch

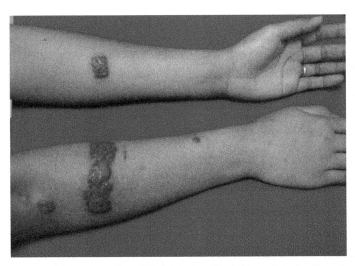

FIGURE 90-1. Contact dermatitis to henna tattoo. (Used with permission from Research Institute for Tropical Medicine, Department of Dermatology.)

test must be elicited by the dermatitis pattern and exposure history. The diagnosis of irritant contact dermatitis is one of exclusion, since there is no diagnostic test for this condition.

TREATMENT

Topical corticosteroids remain to be the gold standard in treatment and are generally well tolerated when used short term.[20] A topical corticosteroid/antibiotic combination may be used when there is superimposed bacterial infection.[22] Topical tacrolimus has been shown to be effective in ACD to nickel.[21] Psoralen plus ultraviolet (UV) A (PUVA) was shown to be superior to UVB in treating patients with recalcitrant dermatitis of the hands.[23] Oral antihistamines are used to relieve pruritus. Systemic corticosteroids are acceptable as treatment for moderate to severe acute cases and in refractory cases. Azathioprine can also be used as second-line treatment for contact dermatitis. Cyclosporine at 3 mg/kg/d was shown to be as effective as topical betamethasone 17,21-dipropionate in the treatment of chronic hand eczema.[24] Barrier creams, high-lipid-content moisturizing creams, fabric softeners, and cotton glove liners are effective for preventing irritant contact dermatitis. The application of a moisturizing cream containing 5% urea and 5% hydrogenated canola oil in preventing experimentally induced irritant contact dermatitis was found to be significantly better than the untreated control.[25]

SEBORRHEIC DERMATITIS

EPIDEMIOLOGY

Seborrheic dermatitis (SD) is a common, chronic relapsing inflammatory skin condition that presents with white to yellowish scales on oily areas of the face and body. The prevalence of adult SD is estimated at 1% to 5% in immunocompetent individuals but increases in immunocompromised patients such as those with acquired immunodeficiency syndrome (AIDS).[26-28] Although the exact etiopathogenesis of SD is not completely understood, the yeast *Malassezia*, androgens, degree of seborrhea, and the individual's immune response are key factors in its development.[26] There are two peaks in the incidence of SD, one during infancy and the other during the fourth to sixth decades of life.[27]

CLINICAL FEATURES

Infantile SD, called *cradle cap*, usually occurs at the age of 2 to 10 weeks and peaks at the third month of life.[28] It appears as thick, yellow or brown greasy scales over the vertex but may involve the entire scalp. Adult SD presents as white pityriasiform or yellowish greasy scales, with or without erythema, and primarily affects the scalp or oily areas of the

face and body. Pruritus is not a consistent feature but is common on the scalp and ear canal.[26] Sites of predilection include the anterior and posterior hairline, medial portion of the eyebrows, eyelids, glabellar region of the forehead, paranasal areas, nasolabial folds, ear canals, preauricular and retroauricular areas, central chest, and genitals.[26,29]

DIAGNOSIS

The diagnosis is made clinically based on the appearance and location of skin lesions.

TREATMENT

There is no cure for SD, but treatment reduces the redness, pruritus, and scaling and delays the relapse of the condition.

Infantile SD resolves spontaneously even without intervention. Thick scales can be softened with daily cleansing using a mild shampoo and application of mineral oil or other emollients. Low-potency topical corticosteroids may be applied to suppress the inflammation during the early part of therapy. For severe cases, topical antifungals may be used.

SD in adults, however, does not improve without treatment. Scalp SD is treated with medicated shampoos containing antifungals active against *Malassezia* species. Shampoos containing 2% ketoconazole or 1% ciclopirox are effective when used twice a week over a duration of 4 weeks.[26,29-32] Thereafter, intermittent usage of either, once or twice a week, was shown to prevent relapse.[26,29] Shampoos containing zinc pyrithione and selenium sulfide also have antifungal activity.

For inflamed or pruritic scalp lesions, a shampoo containing clobetasol propionate 0.05% may be used during the start of treatment.[29,33] Tar and salicylic acid in shampoos are useful in desquamating scaly areas.[32]

For SD on glabrous skin, topical imidazoles such as ketoconazole 2% or sertaconazole 2% cream significantly improve lesions when used twice a day; when used intermittently, they effectively maintain remission.[26,29,32,34] Topical calcineurin inhibitors (pimecrolimus 1% cream, tacrolimus 0.03%, and 0.1% ointment), topical metronidazole (0.75% gel, 1% gel), and azelaic acid 15% gel have been shown to be effective in patients with mild-to-moderate facial SD and may be used as corticosteroid-sparing agents.[26,29]

Coconut oil and guava extract have been used in the treatment of facial and scalp SD but only showed slight or minimal improvement.[35] Tea tree oil, honey, and cinnamic acid have antifungal activity against *Malassezia* species and may be used as alternative treatment options.[34]

In cases where SD is extensive, oral treatment with itraconazole and terbinafine may be a practical choice.[34]

PSORIASIS

EPIDEMIOLOGY

Psoriasis is a complex, chronic, recurrent inflammatory skin disorder that rarely is a threat to life but is associated with high morbidity rates and poor quality of life (see Chapter 24). The disease is more prevalent in countries farther from the equator.[36] Compared to Caucasians, it is less common among Asians,[37] with an overall prevalence rate in Asia noted to be <0.3%.[38] Male and females are equally affected,[39,41] but male predominance was noted among the Taiwanese and Chinese.[42,43] Local studies show greater occurrence in adults. Childhood cases among Chinese were noted to develop at a younger age among girls than boys.[44]

The strongest genetic link points to a locus within major histocompatibility complex (MHC) on chromosome 6p21 (*PSORS1*).[37,45,46] Early-onset psoriasis is associated with the presence of disease-associated human leukocyte antigens (HLAs) among Caucasians. However, presence of HLA-Cw1 and HLA-B46 noted among Southeast Asian and Taiwanese Chinese populations did not result in early onset of psoriasis.[47] Risk factors, such as streptococcal pharyngitis, stressful life events, low humidity, drugs, human immunodeficiency virus (HIV) infection, trauma, smoking, and obesity,[37] are also noted among Southeast Asians. Plaque-type psoriasis is seen in the majority of Asians,[40,41,43] with the scalp being a predominant site among Filipinos.[40,41] Familial occurrence varied from as low as 5.7% to 11% in our studies in the Philippines[40,41] to as high as 30% among the Chinese in China.[43]

CLINICAL FEATURES

The chronic plaque type is the most common form seen among Asians. Pruritus can be mild to moderate. Lesions may not always be symmetrical or multiple at the onset. In Asians, psoriatic nails manifest similarly as those seen in other races.[41] Scalp involvement was noted to occur in 75% to 90% of Asian patients. Among psoriatic children, 47% to 53% present with scalp lesions,[38] and this may be the first site of involvement, especially among Chinese children.[44] Ocular manifestations include eye discomfort and redness, flaking or crusting within the lashes, eyelid edema, psoriatic eyelid lesions, and visual changes. This may eventually lead to blepharitis, conjunctivitis, xerosis, corneal lesions, and uveitis.[48] Among the clinical patterns of joint involvement in psoriatic arthritis,[49] distal arthritis involving the distal interphalangeal joints was found to be more common among our patients. Psoriasis comorbidities noted in our studies in the Philippines were hypertension, diabetes mellitus, asthma/atopy, and arthritis.[40,41]

DIAGNOSIS

Diagnosis is mainly based on clinical presentation and history. A skin biopsy might be helpful when patients present with pustules or erythroderma.

TREATMENT

Treatment is individualized, depending on the severity of disease manifestation. Moisturization of the skin with virgin coconut oil, petroleum jelly, or other thick hydrating emollients is necessary to avoid the severe dryness that accompanies psoriasis. Topical treatments used in our setting are corticosteroids, the vitamin D analog calcipotriol with or without betamethasone ointment, tar preparations, tazarotene, and calcineurin inhibitors (tacrolimus and pimecrolimus). Phototherapy using broadband or narrowband UVB and PUVA are used for patients with extensive disease, alone or in combination with other treatments. Among the systemic therapies, methotrexate, cyclosporine, and etretinate are used to treat psoriasis when it involves more than 10% of the body surface area (BSA) and or involves <10% BSA but is debilitating or nonresponsive to topical medicaments. Biologicals are available, but due to the high cost of these drugs, they are reserved for very unresponsive or difficult-to-handle cases.

ACNE VULGARIS

EPIDEMIOLOGY

Acne vulgaris is a skin disorder that is common worldwide, including among Asian young adult populations.[50-52] It is the most common skin affliction seen in the Philippines[53,54] and Indonesia.

CLINICAL FEATURES

The multifactorial pathogenesis of acne exists in all races and ethnicities. Notable among Asians is the lesser incidence of the nodulocystic form of acne[55] and the greater tendency for acquiring postinflammatory hyperpigmentation (PIH).[55-58] Various classifications of acne vulgaris exist, but a simplified categorization based on disease severity is shown in **Table 90-2** (created by the Acne Board of the Philippines).[54]

TREATMENT

Asian skin encompasses skin phototypes II to V,[59,60] with skin tone varying from the lightest to the darkest shade of brown.[54] Treatment must therefore be individualized, not only in view of the patient's age, gender, and lifestyle but also considering how it affects the overall quality of life. Modalities being adapted in the Philippines [**Table 90-3**][54] are no

TABLE 90-2	Classification of acne severity created by the Acne Board of the Philippines[5]
Mild	Predominance of comedones (≤20) with few inflammatory papules (≤15)
Moderate	Predominance of inflammatory papules and pustules (≥15) with comedones and few nodules (≤3)
Severe	Primarily nodules and cysts (≥3) with presence of comedones, papules, and pustules

different from those of other Asian or Western countries. For mild cases of acne, topical retinoids remain the steady choice, varying only in the formulation and concentration. Benzoyl peroxide (BPO) reduces bacterial resistance and, as such, has been combined with other topical antibiotics with resultant increased efficacy of treatment.[61-63] Salicylic acid formulations, which are affordable and accessible in Asian countries, are popularly used because of their comedolytic properties. Azelaic acid is useful in treating acne and the accompanying PIH due to its low irritant potential and synergistic effect with other antiacne agents such as BPO, antibiotics, and retinoids.[64,65]

Combined topical agents in a fixed dose ratio are currently a popular option for acne treatment in Asia. Preparations available are combinations of adapalene/BPO gel, clindamycin/BPO gel, clindamycin/adapalene gel, and glycolic/retinaldehyde cream. Topical 5% dapsone gel has been shown to be safe and effective in acne treatment,[66,67] even in those with glucose-6-phosphate dehydrogenase deficiency.[68] Doxycycline (100 to 200 mg/d) or lymecycline (300 mg/d) is given for at least 12 weeks for moderate to severe acne vulgaris, usually in combination with topical agents. Oral isotretinoin is safe and effective in Asians.[69] However, relapse of acne with isotretinoin intake was noted among young patients, among those with severe and prolonged acne history, and with a cumulative dose of less than 100 mg/kg of body weight. Similarly, local patients who needed a second isotretinoin course were those taking mean cumulative doses of less than 120 mg/kg of body weight for 6.7 months.[70] Hormonal therapies commonly used are spironolactone and oral contraceptive pills containing cyproterone acetate.[58,64] Adjunctive therapies performed in our region are acne surgery, intralesional corticosteroid injection of cystic lesions, and superficial chemical peels. Because of the effectiveness and more reasonable cost of the aforementioned conventional approaches in our local practices, the use of radiofrequency, light, and lasers for acne treatment remains the least popular option for clinicians. Maintenance therapy with topical retinoids with or

TABLE 90-3	Acne Treatment Guidelines as recommended by the Acne Board of the Philippines[5]		
	Mild	Moderate	Severe
Comedonal	Papules/Pustules	Papulopustules/Nodules	Nodulocystic
Topical retinoids	Topical retinoids ± benzoyl peroxide ± antibiotic	Topical retinoids ± benzoyl peroxide or antibiotic	Oral isotretinoin
Salicylic acid	Azelaic acid	Oral antibiotics	Oral antibiotics + topical retinoids + benzoyl peroxide
		Hormonal therapy Isotretinoin	Hormonal therapy + topical retinoids ± benzoyl peroxide or topical antibiotic
Adjunctive Therapy			
Maintenance therapy: topical retinoids ± benzoyl peroxide			

without BPO is an important aspect in optimizing continued success in acne treatment. Patients are encouraged to practice photoprotection to minimize the development of PIH.

MELASMA

EPIDEMIOLOGY

The true incidence of melasma worldwide is still unknown, but incidence varies from as high as 33% to as low as 1.8%.[71] In the maritime Southeast Asian countries, it is one of patients' foremost concerns, especially among middle-aged females. Known causative factors (ie, UV radiation, hormonal changes, genetics, drugs, and cosmetics), alone or in combination, are the same among these regions (see Chapter 51).

CLINICAL FEATURES

Of the recognized three clinical patterns of melasma, malar presentation is seen most frequently, followed by the centrofacial and mandibular patterns. Brown or gray macules and patches are bilaterally and symmetrically distributed on sun-exposed areas (mainly on the cheeks, nose, cutaneous part of the upper lip, forehead, and mandibular areas) [**Figure 90-2**].

DIAGNOSIS

Diagnosis is mainly clinical. Epidermal melasma may be confirmed with a Wood lamp finding of enhanced pigmentation. Histopathology is mainly done to exclude other diagnoses when in doubt.

TREATMENT

Increased epidermal pigmentation is the hallmark of melasma and serves as the main target of treatment.[72] However, with the presence of hyperactive melanocytes[72,73] and evidence of degraded melanin molecules in the stratum corneum of lesional skin,[74] variability in treatment response exists. There is no fixed protocol for treatment of melasma, but adapting the following five-point strategy[75] maximizes success in treatment: (1) protection from the sun, including regular use of daily broad-spectrum topical sunscreen of sun protection factor (SPF) ≥30, with or without oral photoprotective agents (*Polypodium leucotomos*, see below), and physical protection (such as wide-brimmed hats and parasols); (2) reduction of melanocyte activity, including avoidance of exposure

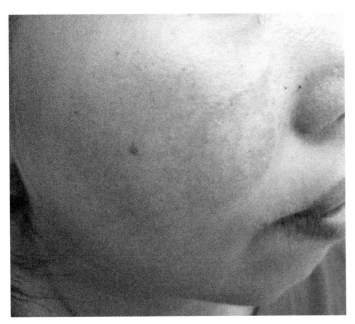

FIGURE 90-2. Melasma. (Used with permission from Research Institute for Tropical Medicine, Department of Dermatology.)

to sunlight and even indoor lights and precautionary measures regarding melasma-inducing factors such as oral contraceptive pills, scented cosmetics, and phototoxic drugs; (3) inhibition of melanin synthesis, including use of depigmenting compounds, alone or in combination; (4) removal of melanin, including procedural options like chemical peeling and microdermabrasion; and (5) disruption of melanin granules, including lasers, light therapy, and fractional resurfacing.

Maritime SEA countries are tropical, and the skin color of the population ranges from phototypes III to V; thus, sun protection against UVB, UVA, and visible light is a must. The application of broad-spectrum sunscreens, multiple times a day, both indoor and outdoor, is advocated. Among the available photoprotective systemic drugs,[75] *P. leucotomos* has gained popularity in the Philippines. Taken once daily at least 30 minutes before sun exposure, this drug acts as an antioxidant and an immune modulator, minimizing erythema and increasing cutaneous tolerance from sun exposure.[76,77] Several depigmenting agents, based on their action in the melanin pathway, are being used in the Philippines and Indonesia, either alone or in combination. The trend is not to rely on monotherapy but to optimize the effect on melasma by using several agents together in a fixed combination. Hydroquinone (HQ) 2% to 4% remains to an important part of our armamentarium against melasma. In current practice, it is usually combined with 0.025% to 0.1% tretinoin and a corticosteroid. A commercially available fixed triple-combination (TC) formula (HQ 4%, tretinoin 0.05%, and fluocinolone acetonide 0.01%) has undergone extensive multiracial, multicenter clinical trials and has been shown to be effective in the treatment of melasma.[75,78] Among Asians with moderate to severe melasma, TC was shown to have greater efficacy compared with HQ alone.[79] In an 8-week study on Thai women, TC was comparable to a similar homemade formula (4% HQ and 0.02% triamcinolone acetonide in a hydrophilic cream with a separate adjunct of 0.05% tretinoin cream).[80] A nightly application of TC is preferable in our setting with a maximum duration of 6 months of use.[81]

HQ and glycolic acid combined in different formulations are also often used. Other tyrosinase inhibitors used in these regions are azelaic acid 10% to 20%, kojic acid 2% to 4%, licorice extract, and arbutin 1%. Among the peroxidase inhibitors, topical indomethacin 8% was shown to be effective in Filipino women when applied twice daily for 12 weeks[75] and in Thai patients, especially on the cutaneous upper lip.[82] L-Ascorbic acid, which functions as an antioxidant,[75,83] is commonly used as an oral supplement alone or in combination with other vitamin supplements and also as a topical lightening agent. Its more stable derivative, Mg-L-ascorbly-2-phosphate (VC-PMG) is being used as an iontophoretic agent for melasma. Oral pycnogenol (with its active ingredient procyanidin) achieved significant skin lightening in melasma patients.[84,85] In a study of Filipino females, 24 mg of procyanidin combined with vitamins A, C, and E taken twice daily for 2 months resulted in a significant reduction in the melanin index and Melasma Area and Severity Index scores, with minimal adverse events.[86] Tetrahydrocurcumin, as a 0.25% cream, was comparable to 4% HQ in a local study among 50 Filipino women.[75] Tranexamic acid inhibits melanin synthesis by preventing the binding of plasminogen to the keratinocytes, thereby decreasing melanocyte tyrosinase activity.[87] Studies showed its applicability through intradermal microinjection,[88] topical formulations,[89,90] or intake of a 250-mg tablet twice daily for 6 months.[91] Another agent gaining popularity in this region is topical niacinamide, which has been shown to significantly decrease hyperpigmentation after 4 weeks of use compared to vehicle alone.[92] Retinoids (ie, tretinoin, retinaldehyde, isotretinoin, and adapalene), along with glycolic, mandelic, malic, lactic, and lactobionic acids, are skin-turnover accelerants popularly used alone or in combination with the other agents previously mentioned.

Chemical peeling every 2 to 4 weeks, using α-hydroxy acid, β-hydroxy acid, Jessner solution, tretinoin, or trichloracetic acid, is used, depending on the severity of melasma. Strong peels are generally avoided due to the possibility of PIH.[75] Microdermabrasion, when combined with topical application of depigmenting agents, was found to be effective in treating melasma.[93,94] Iontophoresis (with vitamin C solution, tretinoin

0.1% gel, and tranexamic acid solution), although painless and inexpensive, yields variable rates of effectiveness.[75,95]

Disruption of melanin granules is mainly done through the use of lasers, light therapy, or fractional resurfacing techniques. Variability of obtained results, the postprocedure PIH reported by dermatologists, and more importantly, the prohibitive cost of the machines make this option a last resort.

TINEA CORPORIS AND TINEA CRURIS

■ EPIDEMIOLOGY

Tinea corporis and tinea cruris are commonly encountered in most dermatologic clinics. These are caused by dermatophytes, with *Trichophyton rubrum, Trichophyton mentagrophytes*, and *Microsporum canis* being the most common etiologic agents.[96-98] Transmission mainly occurs from direct contact with an infected person or animal or from the soil, and infections occur more often in individuals with impaired cell-mediated immunity.[99,100] Tinea corporis and tinea cruris occur globally but are especially prevalent in areas with a warm, humid climate such as the Philippines and Indonesia.

■ CLINICAL FEATURES

Tinea corporis affects the skin of the trunk and extremities, while tinea cruris affects the groin and is commonly referred to as jock itch. In both cases, the infection usually begins as a small erythematous papule or plaque that becomes scaly and expands peripherally [**Figures 90-3**]. Central clearing results in the formation of the classic "ringworm" lesion. Vesicles and pustules may be present in very inflamed lesions.[100] Pruritus is the most common symptom and may be present even before the skin changes are visible.

■ DIAGNOSIS

Diagnosis is mainly clinical, but a Wood's lamp examination may be used to detect blue-green fluorescence emitted by some dermatophytes

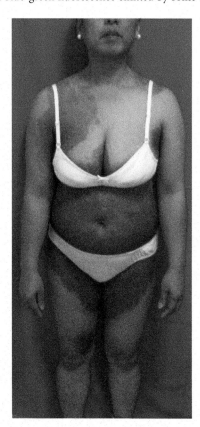

FIGURE 90-3. Extensive tinea corporis and cruris. (Used with permission from Research Institute for Tropical Medicine, Department of Dermatology.)

causing tinea corporis (*Microsporum audouinii* or *M. canis*).[97] Direct microscopy shows hyphae and conidia from skin scrapings in potassium hydroxide preparations. Fungal culture is definitive. Skin biopsies are mainly done when diagnosis is in doubt. Other diagnostic tests such as immunochemistry, polymerase chain reaction, restriction enzyme analysis, or flow cytometry are usually used for research purposes[97] and not routinely done in the clinics.

■ TREATMENT

For localized infections, topical antifungals applied once or twice a day are the first line of treatment. The allylamines, imidazoles, and triazoles are the most active against the dermatophytes.[98,101,102] Amorolfine and butenafine given for 2 to 4 weeks yielded high cure rates for tinea corporis, cruris, and pedis.[101,103,104] Application should be continued for 7 to 14 days beyond clinical clearance to prevent relapse.[97] Preparations containing a combination of an antifungal and a corticosteroid are sometimes given as initial treatment in cases with severe inflammation. However, these should be shifted to a plain antifungal once the inflammation has been adequately suppressed. For extensive disease where topical treatment is impractical or in cases of topical treatment failure, oral terbinafine, itraconazole, fluconazole, or griseofulvin may be given.[96,101,105,106] However, these are quite expensive and have more side effects.[96,97]

VERRUCA

■ EPIDEMIOLOGY

Cutaneous warts, specifically verruca vulgaris (common warts) and verruca plana (flat or plane warts), are consistently top causes for consult in most dermatologic clinics. These are caused by certain types of the human papillomavirus (HPV) and are common even in immunocompetent individuals. Plane warts are mainly caused by HPV-3 and HPV-10, while common warts are mainly caused by HPV-2 and HPV-4.[107] Common warts are more prevalent in young children, while plane warts are more prevalent in adults. Approximately 23% of warts regress spontaneously within 2 months, 30% within 3 months, and 65% to 78% within 2 years.[108]

■ CLINICAL FEATURES

Verruca vulgaris consists of well-circumscribed, grayish-white, rough papules, seen singly or in clusters, representing sites of autoinoculation. These are usually located on the fingers, hands, and feet, but may be seen on any part of the body. Lesions on the fingers sometimes involve the proximal and lateral nail folds, which are rather difficult to treat and have a higher rate of recurrence. Black dots may be seen on the warts, especially when there have been attempts by the patient to manually remove or debulk the lesion using nail clippers or scissors.

Verruca plana are flat-topped papules, pinpoint to a few millimeters in size, that may be flesh-colored, pink, or varying shades of brown. They are usually in clusters over an area or may be multiple and widespread in long-standing cases. Usually seen on the face, neck, and chest, they are also common on the hands and trunk.

■ TREATMENT

At present, there is no single treatment that has proven to be 100% effective in treating cutaneous warts.[107] While many warts spontaneously regress in 1 to 2 years, they can cause embarrassment and discomfort in some cases.[108] The most widely performed procedure in our setting is electrodessication with or without curettage for both common and plane warts. It is relatively inexpensive and widely available. However, treatment of young children continues to be a challenge because most are not able to tolerate this form of treatment. Cryotherapy, done mostly in tertiary hospitals or some private clinics, may only be suitable for older children or adults. It is also more expensive than electrodessication and requires multiple sessions (every 2-4 weeks). Side effects include hypopigmentation or hyperpigmentation, especially in individuals with darker skin types.[109] Ablation with carbon dioxide lasers is not commonly done in our region due to the high cost of treatment. Topical imiquimod, used on both common and flat warts, yielded varying degrees of success. In an open-label study in the Philippine General Hospital, use of imiquimod 5% cream revealed complete clearance of common warts in 31.8% of cases (n = 22), with improvement seen in 59%; only one of eight patients with plane warts demonstrated a response after nightly application for 16 weeks.[110] A local remedy used as an alternative treatment is a topical preparation using the extract of the cashew seed. The cream is applied directly on the lesion, causing necrosis, scabbing, and sloughing off of the wart. The exact component responsible for the therapeutic effect is unknown and the exact mechanism remains elusive, but it may be due to the necrotic destruction of the wart or through stimulating a cell-mediated response from the resulting inflammation. Side effects include burning sensation, erythema, and scarring.

For multiple and recalcitrant cases of facial plane warts, the use of low-dose oral isotretinoin has been shown to be of benefit.[107,111] Complete response was shown in 73% of patients (n = 26) after 2 months of treatment. Of this number, 78% had no recurrence within the 4-month follow-up period.[111] It should be noted that oral isotretinoin is not approved by the U.S. Food and Drug Administration for the treatment of verruca in the United States. The use of topical glycolic acid 15% and salicylic acid 2% was shown to be effective in clearing facial plane warts in 8 weeks with once-daily application.[112] More recently, immunotherapy with intralesional purified protein derivative and measles-mumps-rubella vaccine has been shown to be effective in treating multiple recalcitrant common warts in previously immunized patients.[113,114]

IMPETIGO

EPIDEMIOLOGY

Impetigo is a contagious bacterial skin infection caused predominantly by *Staphylococcus aureus*. *Streptococcus pyogenes* remains an important cause in developing countries, while community-acquired methicillin-resistant *S. aureus* (MRSA) is increasingly becoming a difficult pathogen to treat.[115] Impetigo is the most common bacterial infection in children[116] and is prevalent worldwide, with a peak age of incidence at 1 to 5 years old.[116,117] Spread of the infection is via direct contact with an infected person or through fomites.

CLINICAL FEATURES

Impetigo presents in two forms: nonbullous and bullous. Nonbullous impetigo is the more common form and starts as small erythematous macules that evolve into superficial vesicles or pustules that are eventually unroofed. It is common for patients to present already with erosions and the typical honey-colored crust. Spread to contiguous areas may be seen. Common locations are the central face and the extremities.

Bullous impetigo is less common and initially presents as a small superficial vesicle that enlarges into a thin-walled flaccid bulla before rupturing [**Figure 90-4**]. It is common to see the patient with a varnish-colored erosion with a collaret of scale when the bulla has ruptured. This form of impetigo is mediated by exfoliative toxins from *Staphylococcus aureus*. In immunocompromised individuals, this may disseminate hematogenously and result in the widespread form known as staphylococcal scaled skin syndrome.[118]

DIAGNOSIS

The diagnosis is usually made clinically. Gram stain and culture of blister fluid or exudates are done, especially if systemic therapy is to be given.[119] Susceptibility patterns should guide the clinician for definitive treatment.

TREATMENT

For limited disease, topical antibacterials are indicated. Mupirocin 2%, fusidic acid 2%, and retapamulin 1% ointment may be used.[120,121] While

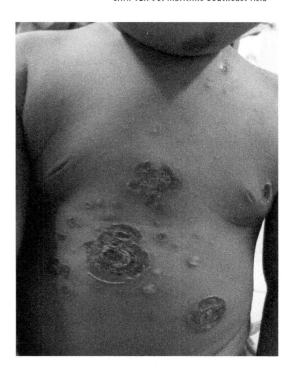

FIGURE 90-4. Bullous impetigo in a child. (Used with permission from Research Institute for Tropical Medicine, Department of Dermatology.)

effective for impetigo, there have been reports of resistance to mupirocin and fusidic acid.[122,123] In these cases, retapamulin may be used, as resistance has not yet been reported.[120,124] For otherwise healthy individuals with numerous or widespread lesions or treatment failure with topical therapy, a β-lactamase–resistant penicillin such as flucloxacillin or cloxacillin or a first-generation cephalosporin such as cephalexin may be used. Other options include erythromycin, clindamycin, and the macrolides.[125] If MRSA is suspected, β-lactam antibiotics should not be used, and local susceptibility patterns should guide empiric treatment.[115,125] In complicated cases, oral or intravenous antibiotics are indicated.

LEPROSY

EPIDEMIOLOGY

Leprosy, a chronic mycobacterial infection caused by *Mycobacterium leprae*, mainly damages the skin, nerves, and mucous membranes (see Chapter 66). Patients experience an array of cutaneous lesions, peripheral neuropathy with related disfigurement, deformity, and disability along with the social stigma associated with this disease.[126] Despite widespread implementation of multidrug therapy (MDT) in the mid-1980s, there were 228,474 new cases recorded in 2010 worldwide. Nine percent of these cases were in children, and 5.8% of cases presented with advanced grade 2 disability.[127] Of these new cases, 156,254 were from SEA; 2041 came from the Philippines, 93.92% of which were multibacillary cases.[127]

PATHOGENESIS

The Ridley-Jopling classification has identified five clinical spectrums of leprosy: polar tuberculoid (TT), borderline tuberculoid (BT), mid-borderline (BB), borderline lepromatous (BL), and polar lepromatous (LL). Multibacillary forms include BB, BL, and LL, while paucibacillary (PB) forms include TT and BT. The mildest form (TT) is characterized by a strong cell-mediated immune response against *M. leprae*, resulting in the reduction and eventual clearance of the infecting bacteria. At the other end of the spectrum is lepromatous leprosy, which presents with disseminated skin lesions and a weak immune response against *M. leprae* antigens.[128,129] The incubation period is between 3 and 10 years.[130] The exact mode of transmission is unknown but is believed to be via nasal secretions or sputum.

CLINICAL FEATURES[131-135]

The known cardinal signs of leprosy (hypoesthesia, skin lesions, and peripheral neuropathy) are evident among patients of all races. The first physical signs of leprosy are usually patches or plaques that are anesthetic or paresthetic. The neuropathy frequently presents as a stocking-glove pattern. Tuberculoid leprosy is usually nonprogressive with localized skin lesions, asymmetric nerve involvement, few bacilli, and a positive lepromin test. Lepromatous leprosy is progressive with nodular skin lesions [**Figure 90-5**], slow symmetric nerve involvement, numerous acid-fast bacilli, and a negative lepromin test. Five types of peripheral nerve abnormalities are common in leprosy: nerve enlargement, sensory impairment in skin lesions, nerve trunk palsies, stocking-glove pattern, and anhidrosis of palms or soles. Pure neuritic leprosy presents with asymmetrical involvement of peripheral nerve trunks and no visible skin lesions.

During treatment, the patient can develop reactions characterized by sudden acute inflammation. Type 1 reactions, where existing lesions become inflamed, are particularly seen in borderline leprosy forms. Type 2 erythema nodosum leprosum (ENL) reactions occur in patients with multibacillary disease, either spontaneously or while on treatment. Painful red nodules on the face and extensor surfaces of limbs appear in crops and subsequently desquamate. Peripheral neuritis and uveitis with its complications of synechiae, cataract, and glaucoma are the most serious complications of ENL. The Lucio phenomenon reaction, seen only in patients with Lucio leprosy, is due to necrotizing small-vessel vasculitis. Irregularly shaped erythematous patches or bullae may necrose, leaving slowly healing deep painful ulcers.

DIAGNOSIS[131-135]

Tactile and temperature sensations should be tested on every patient suspected of having leprosy. A lepromin test, although nondiagnostic, indicates host resistance to *M. leprae*. Tissue smear testing to determine bacterial index is done to assess treatment response in most of our institutions and health centers. Skin biopsy is performed to rule out other possible differential diagnoses and to determine the morphologic index. In pure neural leprosy, a nerve biopsy is necessary to establish the diagnosis. Polymerase chain reaction analysis to detect and identify *M. leprae* is not routinely done in our practice.

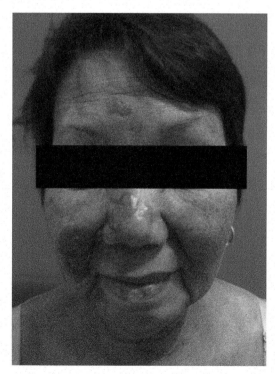

FIGURE 90-5. Lepromatous leprosy. (Used with permission from Research Institute for Tropical Medicine, Department of Dermatology.)

TREATMENT

Medical management of leprosy is directed at the infection itself and the reactional state if present.[132] MDT, composed of dapsone, rifampin, and clofazimine, has been the official recommended treatment of the World Health Organization (WHO) Study Group since 1981.[136] Alternatively, rifampin 600 mg, ofloxacin 400 mg, and minocycline 100 mg are given for a single paucibacillary (PB) lesion. In a study by Balagon et al,[137] an ofloxacin-containing regimen appeared generally efficacious compared with standard WHO-MDT in patients with PB and resulted in only a few relapses. Based on a local study, relapse rates among smear-positive leprosy patients who received 12 MDT blister packs were higher than those who received 24 blister packs, differing from previously published studies. Significant predictors were clinical spectrum, bacteriologic index of >3.5, and number of blister packs given.[138]

SCABIES

EPIDEMIOLOGY

Scabies is a common and highly contagious skin disease caused by the mite *Sarcoptes scabiei*. The prevalence worldwide is estimated at 300 million cases, affecting all ages and all socioeconomic groups.[139] It is prevalent in young children and in institutions where there is overcrowding (eg, prisons, homes for the elderly, orphanages). Transmission is generally from skin-to-skin contact with infested individuals; thus, it is common for family members or sexual partners to become concomitantly infected. Less commonly, fomites may be a route for transmission of the mite, especially for cases of crusted scabies.[140]

CLINICAL FEATURES

Scabies presents as intensely pruritic skin lesions characterized by a typical pattern of distribution known as the circle of Hebra. The pruritus is often worse at night and may be present even before the cutaneous lesions are apparent. The pathognomonic sign is the burrow, a thin threadlike tunnel in the epidermis. Other cutaneous lesions include erythematous and excoriated papules, vesicles, pustules, nodules, or a combination thereof.

Sites of predilection are the web spaces of the fingers and toes, flexor surface of the wrists, axillae, inguinal, waist, umbilicus, and buttocks. In children, the face and scalp may also be affected. In men, lesions are typically seen on the glans penis, shaft, or scrotum, while the breasts, nipples, and vulva are common sites in women.

DIAGNOSIS

Diagnosis is usually clinical and is reinforced by the presence of close personal contacts with the same condition. Confirmation of the diagnosis can be made by visualizing skin scrapings for mites or eggs using mineral oil preparations, dermoscopy, or a skin biopsy.

TREATMENT

Topical scabicides are the first line of treatment, with topical permethrin as the most effective based on randomized controlled trials.[141] Permethrin 5% is safe and effective in treating scabies in adults and in children 2 months and older. One treatment is usually curative, but a retreatment after 1 or 2 weeks is usually necessary.[142] Topical sulfur ointment (5% to 10%) is given to infants less than 2 months of age or to pregnant and nursing women. Treatment with 8% and 10% sulfur for 3 consecutive nights only was comparable to three consecutive whole-day treatments, with cure rates of 90.6% and 96.9%, respectively. Treatment for one 24-hour period resulted in a lower cure rate (42.4%). Side effects were mild burning sensation and irritant dermatitis.[143] Topical crotamiton is a second-line scabicide used mainly for its antipruritic effect. It produces clinical or parasitic cure after 28 days, but is less effective than permethrin.[139] Lindane has been withdrawn from the market due to resistance and central nervous system toxicity.[144] In a recent study, ivermectin 1% lotion was found to be as effective as permethrin 5% cream and may be used as an alternative treatment option.[144] Oral ivermectin, given as a single dose of 200 μg and repeated after 2 weeks, is useful as alternative treatment, especially in epidemics and where compliance to topical treatment may be difficult.[141,145] Compared to topical permethrin, oral ivermectin was found to be less effective.[141] Herbal medications for scabies include *Cassia alata* (akapulko) and *Gliridicia sepium* (kakawate). In a review of local Philippine studies, topical sulfur was shown to be more effective than topical *G. sepium*.[146] Antihistamines may be given to relieve the pruritus. Disinfection of clothing and bedding and concomitant treatment of household contacts are necessary to eradicate the mite.

REFERENCES

1. Introduction to Southeast Asia. http://asiasociety.org/countries/traditions/introduction-southeast-asia. Accessed March 3, 2013.
2. U.S. Central Intelligence Agency. Indonesia. https://www.cia.gov/library/publications/the-world-factbook/geos/id.html. Accessed March 3, 2013.
3. U.S. Central Intelligence Agency. Republic of the Philippines. https://www.cia.gov/library/publications/the-world-factbook/geos/rp.html. Accessed March 3, 2013.
4. Philippines. http://en.wikipedia.org/wiki/Philippines. Accessed March 3, 2013.
5. Coenraads PJ, Goncalo M. Skin diseases with high public health impact. Contact dermatitis. *Eur J Dermatol.* 2007;17:564-565.
6. Saint-Mezard P, Rosieres A, Krasteva M, et al. Allergic contact dermatitis. *Eur J Dermatol.* 2004;14:284-295.
7. García-Gavín J, Armario-Hita JC, Fernández-Redondo V, et al. Epidemiology of contact dermatitis in Spain. Results of the Spanish Surveillance System on Contact Allergies for the year 2008. *Actas Dermosifiliogr.* 2011;102:98-105.
8. Ruff CA, Belsito DV. The impact of various patient factors on contact allergy to nickel, cobalt, and chromate. *J Am Acad Dermatol.* 2006;55:32-39.
9. Rui F, Bovenzi M, Prodi A, et al. Nickel, cobalt and chromate sensitization and occupation. *Contact Dermatitis.* 2010;62:225-231.
10. Contact Dermatitis and Patch Testing: A Philippine Experience. 8th Asia Pacific Environmental and Occupational Dermatology Symposium, Philippines, 2005.
11. Mortz CG, Lauritsen JM, Bindslev-Jensen C, et al. Contact allergy and allergic contact dermatitis in adolescents: prevalence measures and associations. The Odense Adolescence Cohort Study on Atopic Diseases and Dermatitis (TOACS). *Acta Derm Venereol.* 2002;82:352-358.
12. Bruckner AL, Weston WL, Morelli JG. Does sensitization to contact allergens begin in infancy? *Pediatrics.* 2000;105:e3.
13. Fernández Vozmediano JM, Armario Hita JC. Allergic contact dermatitis in children. *J Eur Acad Dermatol Venereol.* 2005;19:42-46.
14. Seidenari S, Giusti F, Pepe P, et al. Contact sensitization in 1094 children undergoing patch testing over a 7-year period. *Pediatr Dermatol.* 2005;22:1-5.
15. Lewis VJ, Statham BN, Chowdhury MMU. Allergic contact dermatitis in 191 consecutively patch tested children. *Contact Dermatitis.* 2004;51:155-156.
16. Dotterud LK, Smith-Sivertsen T. Allergic contact sensitization in the general adult population: a population-based study from northern Norway. *Contact Dermatitis.* 2007;56:10-15.
17. Lammintausta K, Kalimo KM, Fagerlund VL. Patch test reactions in atopic patients. *Contact Dermatitis.* 1992;26:234-240.
18. Prakash AV, Davis MD. Contact dermatitis in older adults: a review of the literature. *Am J Clin Dermatol.* 2010;11:373-381.
19. Mark BJ, Slavin RG. Allergic contact dermatitis. *Med Clin North Am.* 2006;90:169-185.
20. Usatine RP, Riojas M. Diagnosis and management of contact dermatitis. *Am Fam Physician.* 2010;82:249-255.
21. Keil JE, Shmunes E. The epidemiology of work related skin disease in South Carolina. *Arch Dermatol.* 1983;119:650-654.
22. Cohen D, Jacob S. Allergic contact dermatitis. In: Wolff K, Goldsmith LA, Katz SI, eds. *Fitzpatrick's Dermatology in General Medicine.* 7th ed. New York, NY: McGraw Hill; 2008:135-146.
23. Belsito DV. Occupational contact dermatitis: etiology, prevalence and resultant impairment/disability. *J Am Acad Dermatol.* 2005;53:303-313.
24. Weedon D. *Weedon's Skin Pathology.* 3rd ed. Beijing, China: Churchill Livingstone Elsevier; 2010:102-105.
25. Astner S, Burnett N, Rius-Díaz F, et al. Irritant contact dermatitis induced by a common household irritant: a noninvasive evaluation of ethnic variability in skin response. *J Am Acad Dermatol.* 2006;54:458-465.
26. Bukvić Mokos Z, Kralj M, Basta-Juzbašić A, et al. Seborrheic dermatitis: an update. *Acta Dermatovenerol Croat.* 2012;20:98-104.
27. Kim GK. Seborrheic dermatitis and *Malassezia* species: how are they related? *J Clin Aesthet Dermatol.* 2009;2:14-17.
28. Gupta AK, Batra R, Bluhm R, et al. Skin diseases associated with *Malassezia* species. *J Am Acad Dermatol.* 2004;51:785-798.
29. Del Rosso JQ. Adult seborrheic dermatitis: a status report on practical topical management *J Clin Aesthet Dermatol.* 2011;4:32-38.
30. Peter RU, Richarz-Barthauer U. Successful treatment and prophylaxis of scalp seborrhoeic dermatitis and dandruff with 2% ketoconazole shampoo: results of a multicentre, double-blind, placebo-controlled trial. *Br J Dermatol.* 1995;132:441-445.
31. Abeck D. Rationale of frequency of use of ciclopirox 1% shampoo in the treatment of seborrheic dermatitis: results of a double-blind, placebo-controlled study comparing the efficacy of once, twice, and three times weekly usage. *Int J Dermatol.* 2004;43(Suppl 1):13-16.
32. Elewski BE. Safe and effective treatment of seborrheic dermatitis. *Cutis.* 2009;83:333-338.
33. Reygagne P, Poncet M, Sidou F, Soto P. Clobetasol propionate shampoo 0.05% in the treatment of seborrheic dermatitis of the scalp: results of a pilot study. *Cutis.* 2007;79:397-403.
34. Gupta AK, Nicol K, Batra R. Role of antifungal agents in the treatment of seborrheic dermatitis. *Am J Clin Dermatol.* 2004;5:417-422.
35. Villanueva CF, Henares-Esguerra EL, Dizon MEA, et al. Preparations for seborrheic dermatitis. Department of Dermatology, Makati Medical Center, Philippines, Unpublished manuscript.
36. Parisi R, Symmons DPM, Griffiths CEM, et al. Global epidemiology of psoriasis: a systematic review of incidence and prevalence. *J Inv Dermatol* 2013; 133: 377-385.
37. Chandran V, Raychaudhuri SP. Geoepidemiology and environmental factors of psoriasis and psoriatic arthritis. *J Autoimmunity.* 2010;34:314-321.
38. Frez MLF, Asawonda P, Gunasekara C, et al. Recommendations for a patient-centered approach to the assessment and treatment of scalp psoriasis: a consensus statement from the Asia Scalp Psoriasis Study Group. *J Dermatol Treat.* 2014;25:38-45.
39. Enamandram M, Kimball AB. Psoriasis epidemiology: the interplay of genes and the environment. *J Invest Dermatol.* 2013;133:287-289.
40. Tolentino JRG, Dizon JA. Sociodemographic and clinical profiles of psoriasis in Ospital ng Maynila Medical Center (1995-1999): a retrospective study. *J Phil Soc Cut Med.* 2003;71-77.
41. Kho JO, Pacheco CR, Serrano ACR. Epidemiological survey of psoriasis: clinical profile of 54 club members of the Psoriasis Foundation of the Philippines (Davao Medical Center's Department of Dermatology): a preliminary report. *J Phil Soc Cut Med.* 2001;40-46.
42. Tsai TF, Wang TS, Hung ST, et al. Epidemiology and comorbidities of psoriasis patients in a national database in Taiwan. *J Dermatol Sci.* 2011;63:40-46.
43. Ding X, Wang T, Shen Y, et al. Prevalence of psoriasis in China: a population-based study in six cities. *Eur J Dermatol.* 2012;22:663-667.
44. Wu Y, Lin Y, Liu HJ, et al. Childhood psoriasis: a study of 137 cases from central China. *World J Pediatr.* 2010;6:260-264.
45. Duffin KC, Chandran V, Gladman DD, et al. Genetics of psoriasis and psoriatic arthritis: update and future direction. *J Rheumatol.* 2008;35:1449-1453.
46. Oka A, Mabuchi T, Ozawa A, et al. Current understanding of human genetics and genetic analysis of psoriasis. *J Dermatol.* 2012;39:231-241.
47. Chiu HY, Huang PY, Jee SH, et al. HLA polymorphism among Chinese patients with chronic plaque psoriasis: subgroup analysis. *Br J Dermatol.* 2012;166:288-297.
48. Rehal B, Modjtahedi BS, Morse LS, et al. Ocular psoriasis. *J Am Acad Dermatol.* 2011;65:1202-1212.
49. Garg A, Gladman D. Recognizing psoriatic arthritis in the dermatology clinic. *J Am Acad Dermatol.* 2010;63:733-748.
50. Goh CL, Akarapanth R. Epidemiology of skin disease among children in a referral skin clinic in Singapore. *Pediatr Dermatol.* 1994;11:125-128.
51. Yeung CK, Teo LH, Xiang LH, et al. A community-based epidemiological study of acne vulgaris in Hong Kong adolescents. *Acta Derm Venereol.* 2002;82:104-107.
52. Shah SK, Bhanusali DG, Sachdev A, et al. A survey of skin conditions and concerns in South Asian Americans: a community-based study. *J Drugs Dermatol.* 2011;10:524-528.
53. Handog EB, Datuin MS, Singzon IA. Chemical peels for acne and acne scars in Asians: evidence based review. *J Cutan Aesthet Surg.* 2012;5:239-246.
54. Handog EB, Macarayo MJ, Gabriel MT. Acne scars in Asian patients. In: Tosti A, De Padova M, Beer K, eds. *Acne Scars: Classification and Treatment.* London, United Kingdom: Informa Healthcare; 2009:90-97.

55. Kim IH. Salicylic acid peel (acne peel). *Hong Kong J Dermatol Venereol.* 2005;13:83-85.

56. Dainichi T, Ueda S, Imayama S, et al. Excellent clinical results with a new preparation for chemical peeling in acne: 30% salicylic acid in polyethylene glycol vehicle. *Dermatol Surg.* 2008;34:891-899.

57. Taylor SC, Cook-Bolden F, Rahman Z, et al. Acne vulgaris in skin of color. *J Am Acad Dermatol.* 2002;46(2 Suppl):S98-S106.

58. Lim JT, Chan YC. Common skin diseases and treatments in Asia. In: Kelly AP, Taylor SC, eds. *Dermatology for Skin of Color.* New York, NY: McGraw Medical; 2009:613-615.

59. Leenutaphong V. Relationship between skin color and cutaneous response to ultraviolet radiation in Thai. *Photodermatol Photoimmunol.* 1995;11:198-203.

60. Youn JI, Oh JK, Kim BK, et al. Relation between skin phototype and MED in Korean brown skin. *Photodermatol Photoimmunol.* 1997;13:208-211.

61. Cunliffe WJ, Holland KT, Bojar R, et al. A randomized, double-blind comparison of a clindamycin phosphate/benzoyl peroxide gel formulation and a matching clindamycin gel with respect to microbiologic activity and clinical efficacy in the topical treatment of acne vulgaris. *Clin Ther.* 2002;24:1117-1133.

62. Dhawan SS. Comparison of 2 clindamycin 1%-benzoyl peroxide 5% topical gels used once daily in the management of acne vulgaris. *Cutis.* 2009;83:265-272.

63. Ko HC, Song M, Seo SH, et al. Prospective, open-label, comparative study of clindamycin 1%/benzoyl peroxide 5% gel with adapalene 0.1% gel in Asian acne patients: efficacy and tolerability. *J Eur Acad Dermatol Venereol.* 2009;23:245-250.

64. Davis EC, Callender VD. A review of acne in ethnic skin pathogenesis, clinical manifestations and management strategies. *J Clin Aesthet Dermatol.* 2010;3:24-38.

65. Webster G. Combination azelaic acid therapy for acne vulgaris. *J Am Acad Dermatol.* 2000;43(2 Pt 3):S47-S50.

66. Draelos ZD, Carter E, Maloney JM, et al. Two randomized studies demonstrate the efficacy and safety of dapsone gel 5% for the treatment of acne vulgaris. *J Am Acad Dermatol.* 2007;56:439.

67. Lucky AW, Maloney JM, Roberts J, et al. Dapsone gel 5% for the treatment of acne vulgaris: safety and efficacy of long-term (1 year) treatment. *J Drugs Dermatol.* 2007;6:981-987.

68. Piette WW, Taylor S, Pariser D, et al. Hematologic safety of dapsone gel 5% for topical treatment of acne vulgaris. *Arch Dermatol.* 2008;144:1564-1570.

69. Ng PP, Goh CL. Treatment outcome of acne vulgaris with oral isotretinoin in 89 patients. *Int J Dermatol.* 1999;38:213-216.

70. Haryati I, Jacinto SS. Profile of acne patients in the Philippines requiring a second course of oral isotretinoin. *Int J Dermatol.* 2005;44:999-1001.

71. Sheth VM, Pandya AG. Melasma: a comprehensive update part 1. *J Am Acad Dermatol.* 2011;65:689-697.

72. Kang HY, Ortonne JP. What should be considered in treatment of melasma. *Ann Dermatol.* 2010;22:373-378.

73. Kang HY, Bahadoran P, Suzuki I, et al. In vivo reflectance confocal microscopy detects pigmentary changes in melasma at a cellular level resolution. *Exp Dermatol.* 2010;19:e228-233.

74. Moncada B, Sahagún-Sánchez LK, Torres-Alvarez B, et al. Molecular structure and concentration of melanin in the stratum corneum of patients with melasma. *Photodermatol Photoimmunol Photomed.* 2009;25:159-160.

75. Handog EB, Macarayo MJE. Melasma. In: Tosti A, et al, eds. *Color Atlas of Chemical Peels.* Berlin, Germany: Springer-Verlag; 2011:123-139.

76. Alfonso-Lebrero JL, Dominguez-Jimenez C, Tejedor R, et al. Photoprotective properties of a hydrophilic extract of the fern *Polypodium leucotomos* on human skin cells. *J Photochem Photobiol B.* 2003;70:31-37.

77. Choudhry S, Bhatia N, Ceilley R, et al. Role of oral *Polypodium leucotomos* extract in dermatologic diseases: a review of the literature. *J Drugs Dermatol.* 2014;13:148-153.

78. Ball Arefiev KL, Hantash BM. Advances in the treatment of melasma: a review of recent literature. *Dermatol Surg.* 2012;38:971-984.

79. Chan R, Park KC, Lee MH, et al. A randomized controlled trial of the efficacy and safety of a fixed triple combination (fluocinolone acetonide 0.01%, hydroquinone 4%, tretinoin 0.05%) compared with hydroquinone 4% cream in Asian patients with moderate to severe melasma. *Br J Dermatol.* 2008;159:697-703.

80. Pratchyapruit W, Vashrangsi N, Sindhavananda J, et al. Instrumental analysis of the pattern of improvement and recurrence of melasma in Thai females treated with Kligman-Willis triple combination therapy. *Skin Res Technol.* 2011;17:226-233.

81. Grimes PE, Bhawan J, Guevara IL, et al. Continuous therapy followed by a maintenance therapy regimen with a triple combination cream for melasma. *J Am Acad Dermatol.* 2010;62:962-967.

82. Piamphongsant T. Treatment of melasma: a review with personal experience. *Int J Dermatol.* 1998;37:897-903.

83. Shweta K, Khozema S, Meenu R, et al. A systematic review on melasma: a review. *Int J Cur Bio Med Sci.* 2011;1:63-68.

84. Ni Z, Mu Y, Gulati O. Treatment of melasma with Pycnogenol. *Phytother Res.* 2002;16:567-571.

85. Shahrir M, Saadiah S, Sharifah I, et al. The efficacy and safety of French Maritime pine bark extract in the form of MSS Complex Actinosome on melasma. *Int Med J.* 2004;3:130-132.

86. Handog EB, Galang DA, De Leon-Godinez MA, et al. A randomized double-blind placebo controlled trial of oral procyanidin with vitamins A, C, E for melasma among Filipino women. *Int J Dermatol.* 2009;48:896-901.

87. Zhang X, Yang X, Yang H, et al. Study of inhibitory effect of acidum tranexamicum on melanin synthesis. *Chin J Dermatovenerol Integr Tradit West Med.* 2003;2:227-229.

88. Lee JH, Park JG, Lim SH, et al. Localized intradermal microinjection of tranexamic acid for treatment of melasma in Asian patients: a preliminary clinical trial. *Dermatol Surg.* 2006;32:626-631.

89. Na JI, Choi SY, Yang SH, et al. Effect of tranexamic acid on melasma: a clinical trial with histologic evaluation. *J Eur Acad Dermatol Venereol.* 2013;27:1035-1039.

90. Kanechorn N, Ayuthaya P, Niumphradit N. Topical 5% tranexamic acid for the treatment of melasma in Asians: a double-blind randomized controlled clinical trial. *J Cosmet Laser Ther.* 2012;14:150-154.

91. Wu S, Shi H, Wu S, et al. Treatment of melasma with oral administration of tranexamic acid. *Aesth Plast Surg.* 2012;36:964-970.

92. Hakozaki TL, Minwalla, Zhuang J, et al. The effect of niacinamide on reducing cutaneous pigmentation and suppression of melanosome transfer. *Br J Dermatol.* 2002;147:20-31.

93. Lim JTE, Chan YC. Melasma. In: Kelly AP, Taylor SC, eds. *Dermatology for Skin of Color.* New York, NY: McGraw Medical; 2009:615-617.

94. Roberts WE. Microdermabrasion dual therapy. *Skin Allergy News.* 2002;33:42.

95. Huh CH, Seo KI, Park JY, et al. A randomized, double-blind, placebo-controlled trial of vitamin C iontophoresis in melasma. *Dermatology.* 2003;206:318-320.

96. Dawson AL, Dellavalle RP, Elston DM. Infectious skin diseases: a review and needs assessment. *Dermatol Clin.* 2012;30:141-151.

97. Vander Straten MR, Hossain MA, Ghannoum MA. Cutaneous infections dermatophytosis, onychomycosis, and tinea versicolor. *Infect Dis Clin N Am.* 2003;17:87-112.

98. Gupta AK and Tu LQ. Dermatophytes: diagnosis and treatment. *J Am Acad Dermatol.* 2006;54:1050-1055.

99. Douri FE. Superficial fungal infection of the skin in patients with rheumatoid arthritis after methotrexate therapy. *Iraqi Postgrad Med J.* 2007;6:352-355.

100. Karakoca Y, Endoğru E, Erdemir AT, et al. Generalized inflammatory tinea corporis. *J Turk Acad Dermatol.* 2010;4:04402c.

101. Gupta AK, Cooper EA. Update in antifungal therapy of dermatophytosis. *Mycopathologia.* 2008;166:353-367.

102. Jerajani HR, Janaki C, Kumar S, et al. Comparative assessment of the efficacy and safety of sertaconazole (2%) cream versus terbinafine cream (1%) versus luliconazole (1%) cream in patients with dermatophytoses: a pilot study. *Indian J Dermatol.* 2013;58:34-38.

103. Das S, Barbhuniya JN, Biswas I, et al. Studies on comparison of the efficacy of terbinafine 1% cream and butenafine 1% cream for the treatment of tinea cruris. *Ind Dermatol Online J.* 2010;1:8-9.

104. Lesher JL, Babel DE, Stewart DM, et al. Butenafine 1% cream in the treatment of tinea cruris: a multicenter, vehicle-controlled, double-blind trial. *J Am Acad Dermatol.* 1997;36:S20-S24.

105. Rand S. Overview: the treatment of dermatophytosis. *J Am Acad Dermatol.* 2000;43:S104-S112.

106. De Doncker P, Gupta AK, Marynissen G, et al. Itraconazole pulse therapy for onychomycosis and dermatomycoses: an overview. *J Am Acad Dermatol.* 1997;37:969-974.

107. Miljkovic J. A novel therapeutic approach to plane warts: a report on two cases. *Acta Dermatovenerol Alp Panonica Adriat.* 2012;21:63-64.

108. Sterling JC, Handfield-Jones S, Hudson PM. British Association of Dermatologists. Guidelines for the management of cutaneous warts. *Br J Dermatol.* 2001;144:4-11.

109. Lipke MM. An armamentarium of wart treatments. *Clin Med Res.* 2006;4:273-293.

110. Chua MA, Pastorfide GC, Gonzales NM, et al. An open label efficacy study of topical imiquimod 5 percent cream in the treatment of verruca vulgaris and verruca plana in Filipinos. *J Phil Dermatolog Soc.* 2008;17:44-50.

111. Al-Hamamy HR, Salman HA, Abdulsattar NA. Treatment of plane warts with a low-dose oral isotretinoin. *ISRN Dermatol.* 2012;2012:163929.

112. Rodríguez-Cerdeira C, Sánchez-Blancob E. Glycolic acid 15% plus salicylic acid 2%: a new therapeutic pearl for facial flat warts. *J Clin Aesthet Dermatol.* 2011;4:62-64.

113. Abd-Elazeim F, Mohammed G, Fathy A, et al. Evaluation of IL-12 serum level in patients with recalcitrant multiple common warts, treated by intralesional tuberculin antigen. *J Dermatolog Treat.* 2014;25:264-267.

114. Nofal A, Nofal E. Intralesional immunotherapy of common warts: successful treatment with mumps, measles and rubella vaccine. *J Eur Acad Dermatol Venereol.* 2010;24:1166-1170.

115. Geria AN, Schwartz RA. Impetigo update: new challenges in the era of methicillin resistance. *Cutis.* 2010;85:65-70.

116. Cole C, Gazewood J. Diagnosis and treatment of impetigo. *Am Fam Physician.* 2007;75:859-864.

117. Parish LC, Parish JL. Retapamulin for the treatment of impetigo. *Expert Rev Dermatol.* 2008;3:141-149.

118. Hanakawa Y, Schechter NM, Lin C, et al. Molecular mechanisms of blister formation in bullous impetigo and staphylococcal scalded skin syndrome. *J Clin Invest.* 2002;110:53-60.

119. Sladden MJ, Johnston GA. Current options for the treatment of impetigo in children. *Expert Opin Pharmacother.* 2005;6:2245-2256.

120. Koning S, van der Sande R, Verhagen AP, et al. Interventions for impetigo. *Cochrane Database Syst Rev.* 2012;1:CD003261.

121. Shawar R, Scangarella-Oman N, Dalessandro M, et al. Topical retapamulin in the management of infected traumatic skin lesions. *Ther Clin Risk Manag.* 2009;5:41-49.

122. Howden BP, Grayson ML. Dumb and dumber: the potential waste of a useful antistaphylococcal agent: emerging fusidic acid resistance in *Staphylococcus aureus. Clin Infect Dis.* 2006;42:394-400.

123. Patel JB, Gorwitz RJ, Jernigan JA. Mupirocin resistance. *Clin Infect Dis.* 2009;49:935-941.

124. Weinberg JM, Tyring SK. Retapamulin: an antibacterial with a novel mode of action in an age of emerging resistance to *Staphylococcus aureus. J Drugs Dermatol.* 2010;9:1198-1204.

125. Jacobs MR, Jones RN, Giordano PA. Oral beta-lactams applied to uncomplicated infections of skin and skin structures. *Diagn Microbiol Infect Dis.* 2007;57(3 Suppl):55S-65S.

126. Scollard DM, Adams LB, Gillis TP, et al. The continuing challenges of leprosy. *Clin Microbiol Rev.* 2006;19:338-381.

127. World Health Organization. Leprosy update 2011. *Wkly Epidemiol Rec.* 2011;36:389-400.

128. Ridley DS, Jopling WH. Classification of leprosy according to immunity: a five group system. *Int J Lepr.* 1966;34:255-273.

129. Noto S, Schreuder P. Diagnosis of Leprosy. *Leprosy Mailing List.* 2010;1-25.

130. Pinheiro RO, De Souza Salles J, Sarno EN, et al. *Mycobacterium leprae*-host-cell interactions and genetic determinants in leprosy: an overview. *Future Microbiol.* 2011;6:217-230.

131. Krishnamurthy P, Kar HK, Bhattacharya SN, et al. Pathogenesis of leprosy. *Training Manual for Medial Officers: National Leprosy Eradication Program.* 2009;5:10-22.

132. Falanga V, Killoran C. Morphea. In: Wolff K, Goldsmith LA, Katz SI, eds. *Fitzpatrick's Dermatology in General Medicine.* 7th ed. New York, NY: McGraw-Hill; 2008:1786-1834.

133. James WD, Berger TG, Elston DM. *Andrew's Diseases of the Skin Clinical Dermatology.* 11th ed. Beijing, China: Elsevier; 2011:342-351.

134. Ramos-e-Silva M, de Castro MCR. Mycobacterial infections. In: Bolognia JL, Jorizzo JL, Schaffer JV, eds. *Dermatology.* 3rd ed. Beijing, China: Elsevier; 2012:1223-1227.

135. Lockwood DNJ. Leprosy. In: Burns T, Breathnach S, Cox N, et al, eds. *Rook's Textbook of Dermatology.* 8th ed. Singapore: Wiley-Blackwell; 2010:32.8-32.15.

136. WHO Study Group on Chemotherapy of Leprosy for Control Programmes. *Chemotherapy of Leprosy for Control Programmes: Report of a WHO Study Group.* Geneva, Switzerland: World Health Organization; 1982.

137. Balagon MF, Cellona RV, Abalos RM, et al. The efficacy of a four-week, ofloxacin-containing regimen compared with standard WHO-MDT in PB leprosy. *Lepr Rev.* 2010;81:27-33.

138. Chia CM, Gabriel MT, Hipolito R, et al. Relapse rate among smear-positive leprosy cases after 12 blister packs and 24 blister packs of multibacillary drug therapy in a tertiary hospital. Research Institute for Tropical Medicine, unpublished manuscript.

139. Johnstone PP, Strong M. Scabies. *Clin Evid (Online).* 2008:1707.

140. Monsel G, Chosidow O. Management of scabies. *Skin Therapy Lett.* 2012;17:1-4.

141. Strong M, Johnstone P. Interventions for treating scabies. *Cochrane Database Syst Rev.* 2007;3:CD000320.

142. Albakri L, Goldman RD. Permethrin for scabies in children. *Can Fam Physician.* 2010;56:1005-1006.

143. Sharquie KE, Al-Rawi JR, Noaimi AA, et al. Treatment of scabies using 8% and 10% topical sulfur ointment in different regimens of application. *J Drugs Dermatol.* 2012;11:357-364.

144. Chhaiya SB, Patel VJ, Dave JN, et al. Comparative efficacy and safety of topical permethrin, topical ivermectin, and oral ivermectin in patients of uncomplicated scabies. *Indian J Dermatol Venereol Leprol.* 2012;78:605-610.

145. Usha V, Gopalakrishnan Nair TV. A comparative study of oral ivermectin and topical permethrin cream in the treatment of scabies. *J Am Acad Dermatol.* 2000;42(2 Pt 1):236-240.

146. Lim CJ, Lui EC, Yaptinchay VC, et al. Systematic review on *Gliricidia sepium* in the treatment of scabies. Department of Dermatology, Jose R. Reyes Memorial Medical Center, Philippines, unpublished manuscript.

CHAPTER 91 South Asia

Rashmi Sarkar
Narendra Gokhale
Sudhanshu Sharma

KEY POINTS

- South Asia consists of Afghanistan, Bangladesh, Bhutan, India, Maldives, Nepal, Pakistan, and Sri Lanka.

- Dyspigmentation, infectious diseases and infections are commonly seen among patients in this region.

- Treatment modalities are similar to those used in other populations. However, treatment for dyspigmentation is still challenging.

INTRODUCTION

Dermatologic conditions commonly seen in South Asian patients include pigmentary disorders, eczemas, and infections. Other conditions seen, such as chemical leukoderma and bindi dermatitis, are specifically due to cultural practices in India.

ATOPIC DERMATITIS

EPIDEMIOLOGY

Atopic dermatitis is a chronic relapsing eczematous skin disease characterized by pruritus and inflammation and accompanied by cutaneous physiologic dysfunction, with a majority of the patients having a personal or family history of atopic diathesis (see Chapter 27).[1] Genetics has a great role to play and is one of the major diagnostic criteria.[2] The role of environmental factors, such as temperature, humidity, and clothing, and psychological factors is also gaining prominence.[3] The prevalence is greater in urban areas and among boys.[4] Prevalence and incidence are greater in north and central India, compared to the east and south, because these regions experience harsh winters with low humidity.[4]

CLINICAL FEATURES

The diagnosis of atopic dermatitis is based on well-defined clinical criteria.[5] Infantile atopic dermatitis patients generally present with facial involvements, whereas patients presenting in childhood have flexural involvement [**Figure 91-1**].

TREATMENT

Management is similar to that in patients seen in other parts of the world. The liberal use of emollients and moisturizers forms the backbone of therapy. Avoidance of aggravating environmental factors is beneficial.

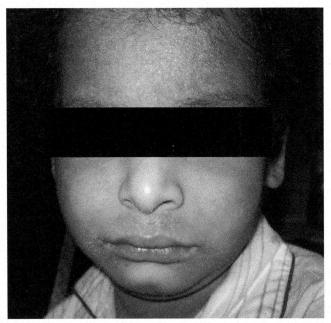

FIGURE 91-1. Atopic dermatitis showing generalized dryness of the face with Dennie-Morgan fold under lower eyelid.

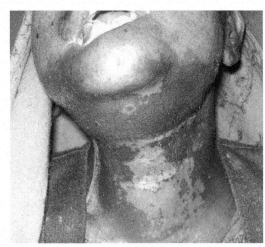

FIGURE 91-2. Contact irritant dermatitis secondary to alkali showing erythema, depigmentation, and vesiculation of affected area.

Topical corticosteroids form the first and, in most cases, the only pharmacologic therapy. In obviously secondarily infected limited area disease, in lesions close to anterior nares, and in flexures, corticosteroids may be combined with topical antibacterials.[6] The only concern is the high incidence of contact sensitivity, especially to neomycin, which is why it is avoided by dermatologists.[7] In extensive disease, a course of systemic antibiotics reduces the disease severity even if there is no obvious focus of infection in the skin or respiratory tract. Topical tacrolimus is a safer alternative to topical steroids for long-term use.[8]

Systemic therapy is reserved for severe and extensive cases. Systemic steroids can be used to control acute exacerbations. Oral cyclosporine is a good alternative for extensive cases for long-term use with proper monitoring.[9]

OCCUPATIONAL CONTACT DERMATITIS

EPIDEMIOLOGY

Occupational contact dermatitis (OCD) is the most significant and frequent dermatosis among all occupational skin diseases. OCD is a significant occupational hazard in some jobs, especially in the construction industry. Cement is one of the most important cause of occupational disease in construction workers.[10-12] Reported prevalence of allergic contact dermatitis to chromate among this population is usually more than 10%. The prevalence among symptomatic construction workers who were patch tested is more than 45%. Such high prevalence is in sharp contrast with the rate of around 1% among the general population.[13,14] Apart from chromate, epoxy resin, cobalt, nickel, and rubber, chemicals are also important allergens in the construction industry.[12]

CLINICAL FEATURES

Individuals with allergic contact dermatitis typically develop dermatitis, within a few days of exposure, in areas that were exposed directly to the allergen. Certain allergens (eg, neomycin) penetrate intact skin poorly, and the onset of dermatitis may be delayed up to a week following exposure.

The hallmark of the diagnosis of poison ivy is linear dermatitic lesions. The possibility of an external cause of dermatitis always must be considered if the dermatitis is linear or sharply defined. The immediate onset of dermatitis following initial exposure to material suggests either a cross-sensitization reaction, prior forgotten exposure to the substance, or nonspecific irritant contact dermatitis provoked by the agent in question [**Figure 91-2**].

TREATMENT

Topical corticosteroids are the mainstay of treatment, while a variety of symptomatic treatments can provide short-term relief of pruritus. However, the definitive treatment of allergic contact dermatitis is the identification and removal of any potential causal agents; otherwise, the patient is at increased risk for chronic or recurrent dermatitis. Topical soaks with cool tap water, Burow solution (1:40 dilution), or saline (1 tsp/pint) can be soothing. Cool compresses with saline or aluminum acetate solution are helpful for acute vesicular dermatitis. Some individuals with widespread vesicular dermatitis may obtain relief from lukewarm oatmeal baths.

Sedating oral antihistamines may help diminish pruritus via a central effect. Corticosteroid creams or ointments may reduce inflammation. Along with, or instead of, corticosteroids, tacrolimus ointment or pimecrolimus cream can be used. In severe cases, systemic corticosteroids may be needed. They should be started at a high dose, which is tapered gradually over about a few weeks.

AIRBORNE CONTACT DERMATITIS

EPIDEMIOLOGY

The prevalence of airborne contact dermatitis (ABCD) is difficult to estimate. This is primarily because of the fact that it can be very difficult and cumbersome to prove an ABCD, especially of irritant type, and secondly because the term *airborne* has been less often used in literature.[15,16]

In India, *Parthenium* dermatitis, caused by *Parthenium hysterophorus*, is an important cause of ABCD. It belongs to the family Compositae, subfamily Asteroide (tribe heliantheae), which itself is a large, diverse group of the plant kingdom. *P. hysterophorus* was accidentally introduced to India in a wheat shipment. It is a wind-pollinated plant and produces an enormous quantity of pollen (up to 624 million per plant) that can be carried away in clusters of 600 to 800 grains.[17] Lonkar and Jog were the first to report the epidemic of *Parthenium* dermatitis in agriculturists and field workers at Pune, Maharashtra, in 1968. Presently, it is the most common cause of plant dermatitis in India and is responsible for 40% of patients attending contact dermatitis clinics. Today, there is increased use of herbal ingredients in culinary, cosmetic, and medicinal products. Other members of the Compositae family that are in wide use are the ornamental annuals, like sunflowers, cosmos, marigold, and asters; herbaceous perennials, like dahlia, chrysanthemum, and marguerites; vegetables, like lettuce, chicory, and artichokes; herbal medicines, like feverfew (*Tanacetrim parthenium*) and pot marigold (*Calendula*); natural insecticides, like pyrethrum; and weeds like bindii (*Soliva ptero-sperma*), ragweed, fleabane, stinkwort, and capeweed.[18,19]

In a study by Agarwal and Souza,[20] from South India, 50 patients with a clinical picture and history consistent with *Parthenium* dermatitis due to exposure to *P. hysterophorus* were studied. Ninety percent of the patients were farmers, and 74.5% had exacerbations during summer. The most common type of dermatitis was the classic ABCD pattern (46%), followed by the mixed pattern (30%), erythroderma (14%), and chronic actinic dermatitis (10%). Of the 40 patients patch tested, 90% had patch test results positive for *Parthenium*.[20] In another study from Delhi, 75 patients with clinically suspected contact dermatitis were patch tested with the Indian Standard Series and indigenous antigens. *Parthenium* was the most common contact sensitizer (20%), followed by potassium dichromate (16%), xanthium (13.3%), nickel sulfate (12%), chrysanthemum (8%), and mercaptobenzothiazole and garlic (6.7% each).[18-20]

CLINICAL FEATURES

A person can be sensitised to airborne contactants by direct and indirect contact, or exposure to herbal cosmetics. Dooms-Goossens classified airborne dermatitis into five different types, namely, airborne irritant contact dermatitis, airborne allergic contact dermatitis, airborne phototoxic reactions, airborne photoallergic reactions, and airborne contact urticaria. Rare presentations include acneiform-like, lichenoid eruptions, fixed drug eruptions, exfoliative dermatitis, telangiectases, paresthesias, purpura, erythema multiforme-like eruption, pellagra-like dermatitis, and lymphomatoid contact dermatitis. In the classical allergic ABCD, there is involvement of exposed areas of the face, "V" of neck, hands and forearms, postauricular area ("Wilkinson triangle"), both eyelids, nasolabial folds, and under the chin. The involvement of both light-exposed and protected areas helps to differentiate ABCD from a photo-related dermatitis.

Cement dust usually presents as a dry, lichenified dermatitis due to its alkaline and hygroscopic properties. The eruption tends be dry rather than oozy even in cases of allergic contact dermatitis to the chromium or cobalt content in cement. Genital dermatitis due to indirect hand contact and accumulation of sawdust on the clothes is often seen in cabinet makers. Dermatitis from vapors is usually of occupational origin. In these cases, amines used as epoxy hardeners and resins are the most common culprits. Turpentine used to be the most frequent cause of airborne dermatitis, but is now rarely seen. Polyolefins, when heated, degrade and form aldehydes, ketones, and acids and very rarely induce airborne dermatitis. Additionally, plastic, rubber, glues, metals, insecticides, pesticides, solvents, and other industrial and pharmaceutical chemicals have been described as causing airborne dermatitis.

TREATMENT

Treatment of ABCD is difficult, with great emphasis on individualization. The severity of contact dermatitis depends on the degree of contact hypersensitivity and quantity of antigen to which the patient is exposed. For effective control of dermatitis, these two factors should be reduced. In cases of ABCD due to *Parthenium*, one should avoid going outdoors on days when pollen is present in high concentrations in air, especially in summer and in the months from September to November following the northeast monsoon showers. Air conditioning decreases indoor pollen counts. Simple routines like taking a bath after coming indoors, wearing fresh clothes, and eliminating weeds and grasses in the house garden can be of great help. Use of a barrier cream on the exposed areas after every wash is important to minimize penetration of antigen into skin. Other measures that can be used are photoprotection, sunscreens, change of job, change of residence, antihistamines, drying agents in cases of weeping eruptions, aluminum sulfate and calcium acetate, and emollients for lichenified areas.

Topical steroids are the mainstay of therapy as in other eczemas. Systemic steroids are indicated when there is more than 25% body surface area involvement and when dermatitis is suspected to be caused by allergens that persist in the skin for weeks after exposure (such as following exposure to *Toxicodendron* oleoresins). Immunosuppressives are indicated for severe, recalcitrant cases, and in those evolving into chronic actinic dermatitis. The most commonly used immunosuppressive agents are azathioprine, mycophenolate mofetil, and cyclosporine. Desensitization has been reported but is difficult to perform.[21]

ERYTHRODERMA

EPIDEMIOLOGY

The true incidence of erythroderma is unknown. Sehgal and Srivastava[22] performed a large prospective study in the Indian subcontinent, where they determined the incidence to be 35 per 100,000 dermatologic outpatients. In general, studies have shown a male predominance, with the male-to-female ratio ranging from 2:1 to 4:1 and the mean age between 40 and 60 years.[20-24] Rym et al[25] conducted a retrospective study of 80 erythrodermic adults, looking at patients examined between 1981 and 2000. The incidence of erythroderma from the study was 0.3%, the average age was 53.78 ± 18 years, and the male-to-female ratio was 2.2:1.[26,27] Psoriasis, eczemas, and drug-induced erythrodermas due to anticonvulsants and antitubercular drugs are the most common causes of erythroderma in South Asia.

CLINICAL FEATURES

The pattern observed is erythematous patches that increase in size and coalesce to form extensive areas of erythema and eventually spread to involve most of the skin surface. Some studies have shown sparing of the nose and paranasal areas, and this has been described as the "nose sign." The epidermis appears thin, giving a glossy appearance to the skin.[27] Once erythema has been established, white or yellow scales develop that progress to give the skin a dry appearance with a dull scarlet and gray hue. Induration and thickening of the skin from edema and lichenification may provoke a sensation of severe skin tightness in the patient. The skin is bright red, dry, scaly, and warm to touch.

Sometimes, the clinical presentation may be suggestive of the underlying cause. Typical psoriasiform plaques may be apparent in early erythrodermic psoriasis. Pityriasis rubra pilaris shows islands of sparing, orange-colored palmoplantar keratoderma, and hyperkeratotic follicular papules on juxta-articular extensor surfaces. The violaceous papules and reticulated buccal mucosal lesions of lichen planus may be evident.

The presence of lymphadenopathy and hepatosplenomegaly, particularly in association with liver dysfunction and fever, may suggest a drug hypersensitivity syndrome or malignancy such as cutaneous T-cell lymphoma. Gynecomastia has been reported in some patients, possibly reflecting a hyperestrogenic state, although the significance of this finding is unclear.

TREATMENT

The initial management of erythroderma is the same regardless of etiology. This should include replacement of nutritional, fluid, and electrolyte losses. Local skin care measures should be used, such as oatmeal baths and wet dressings applied to weeping or crusted sites followed by the application of bland emollients and topical corticosteroids. Known precipitants and irritants are to be avoided, and the underlying cause, with its complications, is to be treated. Secondary infections are treated with antibiotics. Edema in dependent areas, such as in periorbital and pedal areas, may require diuretics. Hemodynamic or metabolic instability should be addressed adequately. Serum protein, electrolyte, and blood urea levels should be monitored. This condition may resist therapy until the underlying cause is treated; hence, it is important to determine the underlying etiology early in its management.

INFECTIOUS DISEASES AND INFESTATIONS

LEPROSY

Epidemiology Leprosy currently affects approximately a quarter of a million people throughout the world, with 70% of these cases occurring in India (see Chapter 66). Cases of leprosy in India have decreased dramatically from 5,000,000 cases in 1985 to 213,000 cases in 2009. This significant decrease is largely due to the effectiveness of multidrug therapy (MDT), which was developed in 1981.[28,29] The prevalence of leprosy in India is now less than 1 case per 10,000 individuals, meeting the World Health Organization (WHO) criteria for leprosy elimination. Yet the WHO criterion for elimination is not met in all areas of the country; rural areas and urban slums continue to experience up to five times the number of leprosy cases as the national average.[30-32] The sex ratio of leprosy in children is nearly equal and skews toward males in adults.

A total of 135,000 new cases were detected during the year 2012 to 2013, which gives an annual new case detection rate (ANCDR) of 10.78 per 100,000 population. This is an increase in the ANCDR of 4.15% from 2011 to 2012 (10.35 per 100,000 in 2011). A total of 92,000 cases are on record as of April 1, 2013, giving a prevalence rate of 0.73 per 100,000 population. Detailed information on new leprosy cases detected during 2012 to 2013 indicates that there 49.92% of cases were multibacillary, 37.72% were female, 9.93% were children, and 3.45% had visible deformity. A total of 4650 cases with grade 2 disability (ie, visible deformity, severe visual impairment) were detected among the new leprosy cases during 2012 to 2013, indicating a grade 2 disability rate of 3.72 per million population. In addition, 5175 grade 1 cases were recorded, which indicates a rate of 4.14 per million population. A total of 13,387 child cases were recorded, which indicates a child case rate of 1.07 per 100,000 population. Thirty-three states/union territories had attained the level of leprosy elimination. A total of 542 of 640 districts (84.7%) also achieved elimination by March 2012.[33]

Clinical Features The signs and symptoms of leprosy can vary depending on the individual's immune response to *Mycobacterium leprae*. A painless skin patch accompanied by loss of sensation is seen in tuberculoid leprosy. Loss of sensation or paresthesia is observed where the affected peripheral nerves are distributed. Wasting and muscle weakness, foot drop, or clawed hands may result from neuritic pain and rapid peripheral nerve damage. Other features are ulcerations on hands or feet (such as ulcers at the metatarsal head), lagophthalmos, iridocyclitis, corneal ulceration, and/or secondary cataract due to nerve damage and direct bacillary skin or eye invasion.

Type 1 (reversal) reaction manifests as sudden onset of skin redness and new lesions with neuritis [**Figure 91-3**], and type 2 reaction (erythema nodosum leprosum) manifests as multiple skin nodules, fever, redness of eyes, muscle pain, and joint pain.

The WHO classification system uses clinical manifestations (the number of skin lesions and nerve involvement) as well as skin smear results to distinguish between forms of the disease. The two major WHO classifications are paucibacillary leprosy and multibacillary leprosy.

Treatment Prescription medications are the primary treatment for leprosy. Compliance with the full course of medications at home is crucial to successful treatment. Patients should also be educated to closely inspect their hands and feet for possible injuries that may go unnoticed because of the loss of sensation. Ulcers or tissue damage can result,

leading to skin infections and disability. Proper footwear and injury prevention should be encouraged.

The WHO currently recommends different treatment regimens for patients with paucibacillary leprosy and multibacillary leprosy. For paucibacillary leprosy, the WHO recommends 6 months of treatment using rifampicin (monthly) and dapsone. For multibacillary leprosy, WHO recommends 12 months of treatment using rifampicin (monthly), dapsone, and clofazimine.

■ CUTANEOUS TUBERCULOSIS

Epidemiology The overall prevalence of cutaneous tuberculosis (TB) in the study by Varshneya and Goyal[34] (0.7%) was a little higher than that found in other Indian studies, which have reported a prevalences of 0.59%, 0.50%, 0.28%, 0.24%, and 0.26%.[35,56]

The most common type of cutaneous TB seen in South Asia is lupus vulgaris (57.69%). The second most common type was scrofuloderma (21.2%), followed by TB verrucosa cutis (19.23%). Tuberculide (lichen scrofulosorum) was rarest (1.92%). Most of the patients were younger than age 25 years (61.52%), and males outnumbered females in a ratio of 2.25:1. The most common site of cutaneous TB varied from study to study, with the lower limbs being most common in one study, but the face being the most common in a study from western India and another study from north India.[37-39]

Clinical Features Cutaneous TB is classified into multibacillary and paucibacillary forms. The multibacillary forms include primary inoculation TB or tuberculous chancre (by direct inoculation), scrofuloderma, TB periorificialis (by continuity), and acute miliary TB and gumma (by hematogenous dissemination). These forms of the disease show abundant mycobacteria in the skin that can readily be seen by direct visualization of Ziehl-Neelsen–stained material and can be easily isolated by culture of biopsy material. The paucibacillary forms are those where there are sparse bacilli seen on histology and the microorganisms are difficult to isolate.

Lupus vulgaris may develop as a result of inoculation, or it may follow primary inoculation TB or bacillus Calmette-Guérin vaccination [**Figure 91-4**]. Some cases of lupus vulgaris are due to spread of tuberculosis from elsewhere in the body (often lung or cervical lymph nodes) via the lymphatic system or direct spread. It may also follow scrofuloderma or tuberculous infection of the mucous membranes. Rarely, it may follow hematogenous dissemination. Lupus vulgaris

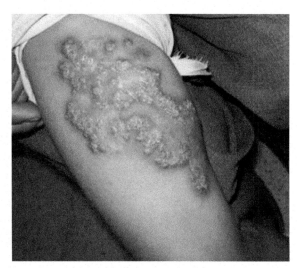

FIGURE 91-3. A patient with borderline tuberculoid leprosy with type 1 reaction showing well-defined erythematous annular plaque.

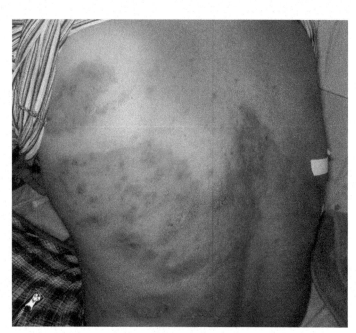

FIGURE 91-4. Lupus vulgaris showing well-defined plaque with bluish-violet borders and area of scarring as well as area of activity.

has been associated with tuberculous lymphadenitis in 40% of cases, scrofuloderma in 30% of cases, and TB of the lungs or bones in 10% to 20% of cases. Scrofuloderma is due to reactivation of dormant TB. There is contiguous involvement of overlying skin from an underlying tuberculous focus such as tuberculous lymphadenitis or tuberculous bone disease. Tuberculin test is usually positive. A cold abscess is formed, and the overlying skin is eroded. Scrofuloderma from tuberculous lymphadenitis often affects the parotid, submandibular, and supraclavicular and cervical lymph nodes.

Tuberculous gummata are due to hematogenous spread of tuberculosis from a primary source as a result of either breakdown of an old healed tubercle or reduced immunity. The lesions present as solitary or multiple subcutaneous abscesses that break down to form a discharging sinus. In immunocompetent patients, the lesions are solitary and may resolve spontaneously, but in immunocompromised cases, multiple lesions may occur and are associated with a poorer prognosis. The lesions begin as subcutaneous nodules, which become doughy in consistency. With progressive liquefaction, a cold abscess is formed and the skin erodes to form a discharging sinus. There may be healing with scarring and recurrence of disease over several years. In lichen scrofulosorum, there is a lichenoid eruption often in children with tuberculosis. The lesions are perifollicular and are yellow-brown or pink papules with a scaly or hyperkeratotic top. These are seen mainly on the trunk with a lichenoid distribution and persist for months before resolving spontaneously. Discoid plaques may be formed as the papules coalesce. The lesions resolve with antituberculous therapy within weeks to months.

Treatment Standard therapy regimens involving 2 months of antitubercular therapy (isoniazid, rifampicin, pyrazinamide, and ethambutol) followed by a further 4 months of isoniazid plus rifampicin have been adopted by most centers. Longer treatment courses are usually indicated only in cases where there is associated extrapulmonary disease involving the central nervous system or bone.

POST–KALA-AZAR DERMAL LEISHMANIASIS

Epidemiology Globally, 350 million people are estimated to be at risk of leishmaniasis, with an annual incidence of 1 to 1.5 million cases of cutaneous leishmaniasis and 200,000 to 400,000 cases of visceral leishmaniasis. More than 90% of the world's visceral leishmaniasis cases are located in India, Bangladesh, Brazil, Nepal, and Sudan. Kala-azar, which has led to a huge health burden in India, is endemic in eastern states, such as Bihar, eastern Uttar Pradesh, Jharkhand, and West Bengal. In India, 48 districts are endemic for visceral leishmaniasis.[40-42] An estimated 200 million people are at risk in four states. Cutaneous leishmaniasis cases are also reported from the states of Rajasthan and Kerala in India. Post–kala-azar dermal leishmaniasis (PKDL) occurs approximately in 5% to 10% of cases of visceral leishmaniasis in India.[41-43]

Clinical Features Leishmaniasis is a group of diseases caused by protozoan hemoflagellates of the genus *Leishmania*. The disease is transmitted by female sand flies (*Phlebotomus* or *Lutzomyia*) that feed on animal or human blood. In 1922, Brahmachari first described PKDL in Bengal. In India, PKDL develops in an otherwise asymptomatic individual, with a latent period of 1 to 2 years after treatment of visceral leishmaniasis. Patients may present with diverse skin manifestations including hypopigmented macules, erythematous papules, and nodules, sometimes in various combinations [**Figure 91-5**]. The number of parasites in the lesions depends on the cell-mediated immune status of the individual. In patients with predominantly macular lesions, cell-mediated immune status is high, with a positive leishmanin test and a scanty number of parasites, whereas in the nodular variety, cell-mediated immune status is low, with a negative leishmanin test and a significant number of parasites in the skin lesions.

In India, because there is no extrahuman reservoir of infection, PKDL is a recurrence of kala-azar that may appear on the skin of affected individuals up to 20 years after being partially treated, untreated, or even adequately treated. It manifests as hypopigmented macules, papules, nodules, or facial erythema. Although any organism causing kala-azar

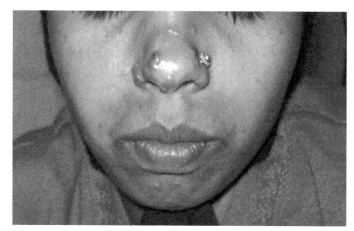

FIGURE 91-5. Post–kala-azar dermal leishmaniasis showing skin-colored papular and nodular lesions on the face.

can lead to PKDL, it is commonly associated with *Leishmania donovani*, which results in different disease patterns in India. In the Indian variant, nodules enlarge with time and form plaques but rarely ulcerate. Histology demonstrates a mixture of chronic inflammatory cells; there can be macrophage or epithelioid granuloma. Parasite concentration is not consistent among studies, perhaps reflecting low sensitivity of diagnostic methods used in earlier entries.

Treatment Injection of sodium stibogluconate (20 mg/kg body weight) for 90 to 120 days is the standard therapeutic regimen prescribed worldwide. Because it requires long duration of painful intramuscular or intravenous injections with resultant increased chance of toxicities like myalgia, arthralgia, cardiac conduction defects, and arrhythmias, other alternatives that have been used are miltefosine, and other, safer drugs.[40]

SCABIES

Epidemiology An epidemiologic survey was conducted in a population of 1727 persons living in 253 households in a semiurban area of Goa, India. The prevalence of scabies was 9.7% by persons, 22.5% by households, and 22.8% by families. Prevalence of scabies was highly associated with age. The highest prevalence (23.7%) was in school-age children.[44,45] Prevalence was higher for females than males aged 25 or older, but there was no significant difference in prevalence by sex for all ages. The first person to contact scabies in the family was generally a school child.[45-47]

Clinical Features The most common symptoms of scabies, itching and a skin rash, are caused by sensitization (a type of "allergic" reaction) to the proteins and feces of the parasite. Severe itching (pruritus), especially at night, is the earliest and most common symptom of scabies. Papular eruption, a pimple-like (papular) itchy (pruritic) "scabies rash," is also common. Itching and rash may affect much of the body or be limited to common sites such as between the fingers and the wrist, elbow, armpit, penis, nipple, waist, buttocks, and shoulder blades [**Figure 91-6**]. The head, face, neck, palms, and soles often are involved in infants and very young children, but usually not adults and older children.

Treatment In addition to the infested person, treatment also is recommended for household members and sexual contacts, particularly those who have had prolonged direct skin-to-skin contact with the infested person. Bedding, clothing, and towels used by infested persons or their household, sexual, and close contacts (as defined above) anytime during the 3 days before treatment should be decontaminated by washing in hot water and drying in a hot dryer, by dry cleaning, or by sealing in a plastic bag for at least 72 hours. Scabies mites generally do not survive more than 2 to 3 days away from human skin.

A commonly prescribed medication for scabies is permethrin 5% cream, which should be applied twice, with a week or so between each

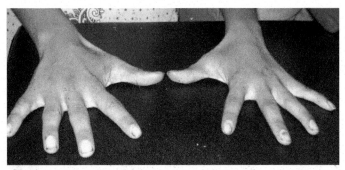

FIGURE 91-6. Scabies. Note excoriated hyperpigmented papules on finger web between right thumb and right index finger.

application. Permethrin is generally considered safe for children and adults of all ages, including women who are pregnant or nursing. Only permethrin, crotamiton, and sulfur ointment are considered safe for treating children younger than 2 years old. Oral ivermectin is use for treating crusted (Norwegian) scabies.

VITILIGO

EPIDEMIOLOGY

Vitiligo is an idiopathic, acquired, circumscribed hypomelanotic skin disorder, characterized by milky white patches of different sizes and shapes and affects 1% to 2% of the world population (see Chapter 49). Based on a few dermatologic outpatient records, the incidence of vitiligo is found to be 0.25% to 2.5% in India. The states of Gujarat and Rajasthan have the highest prevalence of approximately 8.8%.[48,49] The mean ages among males (24.8 years) and females (19.3 years) are significantly different.[49-51]

CLINICAL FEATURES

Vitiligo is a condition that causes depigmentation of sections of skin. It occurs when melanocytes, the cells responsible for skin pigmentation, die or are unable to function. The cause of vitiligo is unknown, but research suggests that it may arise from autoimmune, genetic, oxidative stress, neural, or viral causes. The most common form is nonsegmental vitiligo, which tends to appear in symmetric patches, sometimes over large areas of the body.

The most notable symptom of vitiligo is depigmentation of patches of skin that occurs on the extremities [**Figure 91-7**]. Although patches are initially small, they often enlarge and change shape. When skin lesions occur, they are most prominent on the face, hands, and wrists. Depigmentation is particularly noticeable around body orifices, such as the mouth, eyes, nostrils, genitalia, and umbilicus. Some lesions have hyperpigmentation around the edges. Patients who are stigmatized for their condition may experience depression and similar mood disorders.

TREATMENT

Although there is no cure for vitiligo, treatments are now available that can improve the disease. Some people may not be concerned about the white patches of skin if they are in areas not noticeable to others.

Management options generally fall into four groups. The first group is skin camouflage, which includes measures to cover or camouflage the affected skin. The second group involves treatments that aim to reverse the changes in the skin and includes medical and surgical treatments. Medical therapy includes topical corticosteroids, tacrolimus, pimecrolimus, narrowband ultraviolet (UV) B, psoralen with ultraviolet A (PUVA), oral corticosteroid. and other immunomodulators. Surgical therapy includes:

1. Tissue grafts:
   - Thin and ultra-thin split-thickness skin grafts
   - Suction blister epidermal grafts
   - Mini-punch grafts
   - Hair follicular grafts
   - Flip-top transplantation[52]
2. Cellular grafts:
   - Noncultured epidermal cell suspension
   - Cultured "pure" melanocytes
   - Cultured epithelial grafts

The third group involves treatments to depigment the skin completely. Finally, the fourth group consists of the use of sunscreens and other means of photoprotection to protect the pale skin.

PITYRIASIS ALBA

EPIDEMIOLOGY

Even though pityriasis alba is commonly encountered in dermatologic practice, there is a paucity of Indian studies on the subject. A clinico-epidemiologic study was carried out in 200 patients presenting to the skin department of Command Hospital, Air Force, Bangalore. Atopic background was detected in 85.5% of cases. Bacterial and fungal culture studies failed to reveal any infective etiology. Helminthiasis and iron deficiency anemia were detected in 15.5% and 16.5% of patients, respectively. However, no other nutritional deficiency was observed.[53]

CLINICAL FEATURES

The dry scaling appearance is most noticeable during the winter. During the summer, tanning of the surrounding normal skin makes the pale patches of pityriasis alba more prominent [**Figure 91-8**].

Individual lesions develop through the following three stages and are sometimes itchy:

1. Raised and red, although the redness is often mild and not noticed by parents or patients
2. Raised and pale
3. Smooth, flat, pale patches

Lesions are round or oval and 0.5 to 2 cm in size, although they may be larger if they occur on the body (up to 4 cm), and usually number from 4 or 5 to over 20. The patches are dry with very fine scales. They most commonly occur on the face (cheeks), but in 20% of patients, they also appear on the upper arms, neck, or shoulders.[54,55]

The diagnostic differential should consider tinea and vitiligo among other causative factors.

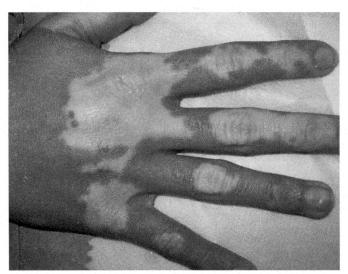

FIGURE 91-7. Well-defined depigmented patches in a patient with vitiligo.

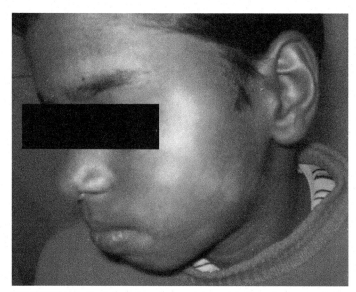

FIGURE 91-8. Pityriasis alba showing hypopigmented circular scaly plaque on the face of child.

TREATMENT

No treatment is required, and the patches in will settle time. The redness, scale, and itch, if present, may be managed with simple emollients and sometimes topical hydrocortisone. Because the patches of pityriasis alba do not darken normally in sunlight, effective sun protection helps minimize the discrepancy in coloration against the surrounding normal skin. Cosmetic camouflage may be required. Tacrolimus ointment has been reported as speeding resolution. In exceptionally severe cases, narrowband UVB or PUVA therapy may be considered.[55,56]

MELASMA

EPIDEMIOLOGY

Melasma is a common, acquired hypermelanosis that occurs in sun-exposed areas, mostly on the face, occasionally on the neck, and rarely on the forearms (see Chapter 51). The exact prevalence of melasma is unknown in most of the countries.[57-59] Melasma is a very common cutaneous disorder, accounting for 0.25% to 4% of the patients seen in dermatology clinics in Southeast Asia, and is the most common pigmentary disorder among Indians. The disease affects all races, but there is a particular prominence among Hispanics and Asians. Although women are predominantly affected, men are not excluded from melasma, representing approximately 10% of cases. It is rarely reported before puberty.[59,60]

CLINICAL FEATURES

The exact causes of melasma are unknown. However, multiple factors are implicated in its etiopathogenesis, mainly sunlight, genetic predisposition, and role of female hormonal activity. Exacerbation of melasma is almost inevitably seen after excessive sun exposure, and conversely, melasma gradually fades during a period of sun avoidance. Genetic factors are also involved, as suggested by familial occurrence and the higher prevalence of the disease among Hispanics and Asians. Other factors incriminated in the pathogenesis of melasma include pregnancy, oral contraceptives, estrogen–progesterone therapies, thyroid dysfunction, certain cosmetics, and phototoxic and antiseizure drugs.

The hyperpigmented patches may range from single to multiple and are usually symmetrical on the face and occasionally the "V" neck area [**Figure 91-9**]. According to the distribution of lesions, three clinical patterns of melasma are recognized. The centrofacial pattern is the most common pattern and involves the forehead, cheeks, upper lip, nose, and chin. The malar pattern involves the cheeks and nose. The mandibular pattern involves the ramus of the mandible.

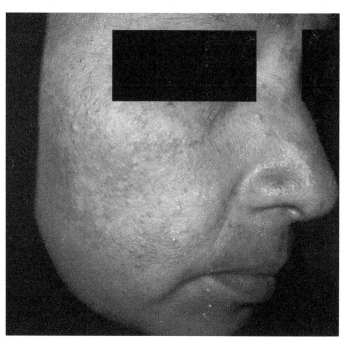

FIGURE 91-9. Melasma showing hyperpigmented macular lesion on the malar prominences.

TREATMENT

The discoloration usually disappears spontaneously over a period of several months after giving birth or stopping the oral contraceptives or hormone replacement therapy. Treatments are often ineffective because melasma recurs with continued exposure to the sun. Treatments to hasten the fading of the discolored patches include topical depigmenting agents, such as hydroquinone, triple-combination creams, 20% azelaic acid, kojic acid, and several newer botanicals and cosmeceuticals.[61] Procedural therapies such as chemical peels, dermabrasion, and laser treatment with intense pulsed light and fractional lasers have been tried.[61]

A Wood's lamp test should be used to determine whether the melasma is epidermal or dermal. Dermal melasma often proves difficult to treat. With all of these treatments, the effects are gradual, and a strict avoidance of sunlight is required. The use of broad-spectrum sunscreens containing inorganic (physical) UV filters (titanium dioxide and zinc dioxide), is preferred over those with only chemical filters. This is because UVA, UVB, and visible lights are all capable of stimulating pigment production. Cosmetic camouflage can also be used to hide melasma.

LICHEN PLANUS PIGMENTOSUS

EPIDEMIOLOGY

Lichen planus pigmentosus is a fairly common disorder of pigmentation in Indians, but reports comprising a sizeable number of patients are lacking in the literature. A study conducted by Kanwar et al[62] concluded that of the 124 patients (56 males, 68 females), the majority (48.4%) had the disease for 6 months to 3 years. The face and neck were the most common sites affected, with pigmentation varying from slate gray to brownish-black. The pattern of pigmentation was mostly diffuse (77.4%), followed by reticular (9.7%), blotchy (7.3%), and perifollicular (5.6%).[62]

CLINICAL FEATURES

Lichen planus pigmentosus was initially described in India and occurs in darker-skinned individuals, most commonly on the face, trunk, and upper extremities, with intertriginous involvement seen infrequently. The lesions generally present as hyperpigmented, sharply defined brown macules to patches, ranging in size from less than 1 cm to several centimeters. The condition is generally asymptomatic or only slightly pruritic. Mucosal, scalp, and nail involvement is absent.[63]

Reported biopsy findings have all been similar, showing an ortho-keratotic, atrophic epidermis with variably prominent lichenoid inflammation containing lymphocytes and histiocytes. There is prominent pigmentary incontinence and melanin-containing macrophages in the superficial dermis.

TREATMENT

The clinical course is variable, with some cases disappearing within weeks without therapy, whereas others can persist for years. Treatment with tacro-limus ointment, other calcineurin inhibitors, triple-combination therapy, and high potency steroids has had variable, but limited, success in isolated cases. Oral and topical retinoids have been used with variable outcomes. Photoprotection is essential.

PERIORBITAL HYPERPIGMENTATION

EPIDEMIOLOGY

A study was done by Ranu et al[64] to determine the primary cause of periorbital hyperpigmentation (POH) and classify it into five different types. The most common form of POH was the vascular type (41.8%), followed by constitutional (38.6%), postinflammatory hyperpigmentation (12%), shadow effects (11.4%), and other causes. The vascular type was seen predominantly in Chinese, whereas the constitutional type was most common in Indians and Malays.[64] Malakar et al,[65] in their study to identify the nature of pigmentation in periorbital melanosis, concluded that periorbital melanosis and pigmentary demarcation line of the face are not two different conditions; rather, they are two different manifestations of the same disease. POH has a multifactorial pathogenesis including genetic or constitutional pigmentation, excessive pigmentation akin to dermal melanocytosis, postinflammatory hyperpigmentation secondary to atopic and allergic contact dermatitis, periorbital edema, excessive subcutaneous vascularity, shadowing due to skin laxity, and tear trough associated with aging. Excessive sun exposure, drugs, hormonal causes, and extension of pigmentary demarcation lines, especially in Indian patients, have also been considered to be contributory.

CLINICAL FEATURES

POH is defined as bilateral, homogeneous, hyperchromic macules and patches primarily involving the lower eyelids but also sometimes extending toward the upper eyelids, eyebrows, malar regions, temporal regions, and lateral nasal root. The age of onset is usually after puberty or in early adulthood (16 to 25 years).

Whatever the cause, it is difficult to distinguish the cause clinically, and determination requires careful elimination by history and investigations. The complex nature of POH and lack of a clearly defined treatment regimen create a challenge for the treating physician.[66-68]

TREATMENT

POH is a generally benign, extremely common condition that is notoriously resistant to treatment. The key to successful treatment is determining the primary cause and complying with maintenance and preventive regimens.[66] A multimodal approach may be required, encompassing topical bleaching agents, chemical peels, laser therapy, and/or surgery. Chemical peels, intense pulsed light, Q-switched ruby laser, autologous fat transplantation, combinations of fat grafting and blepharoplasties, and fillers have all been tried for treatment, but none have provided satisfactory treatment.

POSTINFLAMMATORY HYPERPIGMENTATION

EPIDEMIOLOGY

Postinflammatory hyperpigmentation (PIH) tends to be more prevalent among Asians with darker skin, such as Malays and Indians, than those with lighter skin, such as the Chinese, suggesting that the degree

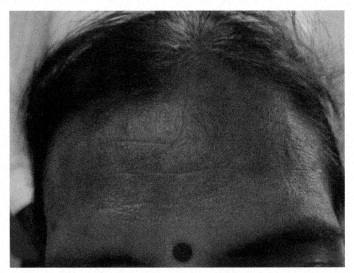

FIGURE 91-10. Postinflammatory hyperpigmentation manifesting as hyperpigmented patch on the forehead.

of pigmentation may be more contributory to the development of PIH. PIH occurs with equal incidence in males and females but is more common in darker skin types. The distribution of causative dermatoses determines the site of PIH. The lesions vary in color from light brown to bluish-gray and are irregularly shaped. PIH generally persists for months to years.[69,70]

CLINICAL FEATURES

PIH is the medical term given to discoloration of the skin that follows an inflammation or trauma to the skin [**Figure 91-10**]. It is the skin's natural response to inflammation. PIH presents as a flat area of macular discoloration on the skin (macule) ranging from pink to red, purple, brown, or black, depending on skin type and depth of discoloration. PIH is characterized by an acquired increase in cutaneous pigmentation secondary to an inflammatory process. Excess pigment deposition may occur in the epidermis or in both the epidermis and the dermis. PIH is very common among acne sufferers. PIH may be a sequela of conditions such as acne, allergic reactions, drug eruptions, papulosquamous disorders, eczematoid disorders, and vesiculobullous disorders.

TREATMENT

The treatment of PIH remains a challenge. The underlying disorder causing the hyperpigmentation should be treated. Patients should be advised on daily use of sunscreens and to practice photoprotection. Many topical medications have been used for PIH. These include hydroquinone, triple-combination creams, kojic acid, retinoids, corticosteroids, and vitamin C. Chemical peeling and dermabrasion have been tried with variable success. Combination therapies have shown good results.[71,72] Posttraumatic hyperpigmentation treated with 1550-nm erbium-doped Fraxel laser using a density of 880 to 1100 MTZ/cm showed more than 95% clearance with three treatment sessions.[72]

ACNE VULGARIS

EPIDEMIOLOGY

Acne vulgaris is a very common chronic inflammatory disease of the pilosebaceous units. The condition usually starts in adolescence, peaks at the ages of 14 to 19 years, and frequently resolves by the mid-twenties. It is more common in males but usually develops earlier in females than in males, which may reflect the earlier onset of puberty in females. The most severe forms of acne vulgaris occur more frequently in males, but the disease tends to be more persistent in females.[73] Most of the adults

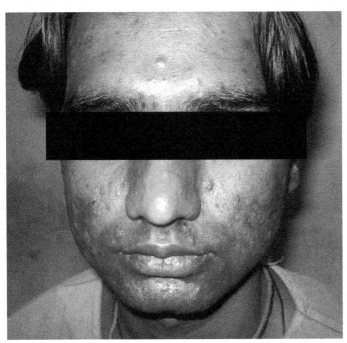

FIGURE 91-11. Acne vulgaris showing papulonodular lesions along with areas of scarring on the face.

seen with acne are adult males.[74] Acne can have a profound impact on the quality of life and lead to tremendous psychosocial complications.[75]

CLINICAL FEATURES

The lesions vary from comedones, papules, and pustules to nodulocystic lesions [**Figure 91-11**]. The sequelae can be devastating, with scarring and PIH. More so than active acne, in South Asia, it is the postacne hyperpigmentation that is most distressing. Associated conditions like obesity and signs of hyperandrogenism should be looked for, and such patients should be screened for hypothyroidism and polycystic ovarian disease.

TREATMENT

Mild forms are best treated with topical antibiotics, such as clindamycin and nadifloxacin,[76] topical benzoyl peroxide, and topical retinoids (like adapalene and tretinoin). Topical applications containing combinations of antibiotics and retinoids are very popular with dermatologists because of their relatively faster onset of effect.[76,77] According to the authors' personal experience, topical azelaic acid 20% is a good adjuvant to treatment.

Moderate forms are treated with oral antibiotics, such as macrolides (azithromycin) and tetracyclines (doxycycline and minocycline), in addition to the topical therapy.

Severe and resistant forms are best treated with oral isotretinoin, after careful patient selection and regular monitoring for side effects. Apart from the conventional doses, lower doses can be used with no loss of efficacy.[78] Chemical peels with glycolic acid, salicylic acid, and trichloroacetic acid are a useful adjuvant to the treatment regimen for faster resolution of lesions and to reduce scarring and PIH.[79] Micro-needling has become a useful tool to treat scars at a very low cost to the patient. It may be combined with subcision for deeper scars.[79,80] Fraction lasers, such as carbon dioxide, Eb:YAG, and erbium glass, reduce the scarring to a considerable extent.[81] Intense pulsed light can be used to reduce the lesions and reduce scarring.[82]

LICHEN PLANUS

Lichen planus has a worldwide distribution. The incidence in India appears to be around 0.6% to 0.8%.[83-85] The incidence among children in India is higher than in the rest of the world.[84]

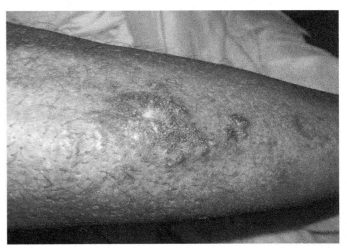

FIGURE 91-12. Lichen planus hypertrophicus showing violaceous irregular plaque on the shin.

CLINICAL FEATURES

The lesions are usually intensely itchy, bilaterally symmetrical, flat, polygonal, and violaceous or bluish black in color [**Figure 91-12**]. These are present more on the extremities than trunk.[83] They subside in weeks or months, leaving violaceous macules that last for months to years and cause lot of emotional distress. Actinic lichen planus is more common in India, similar to other tropical countries.[83] Children are more likely to develop hypertrophic lesions.[84] Oral lesions are quite common and should be differentiated from submucous fibrosis and smoker's melanosis following chewing of tobacco and smoking.[85] One study reported that oral lesions are more common than cutaneous lesions.[86]

TREATMENT

Oral corticosteroids form the mainstay of therapy in most of patients with extensive disease. These may be used daily or in "pulse doses" as biweekly therapy.[87] Pulse therapy has the advantage of a lower incidence of side effects. Cyclosporine is a good but expensive alternative to corticosteroids for resistant and widespread cases.

Topical therapy is suitable for limited area of involvement and for oral mucosal disease. Potent topical corticosteroids and tacrolimus ointment can be used.[88] Intralesional corticosteroids can be used for hypertrophic lesions.

Oral mucosal lesions can be treated with pastes of triamcinolone acetonide and with cyclosporine oral solution (swish and spit).

Other treatment modalities reported to be effective are dapsone, methotrexate, PUVA with sun exposure (PUVASOL), narrowband UVB, targeted phototherapy, mycophenolate mofetil, and oral retinoids.[89-92]

PITYRIASIS ROSEA

Pityriasis rosea is an acute exanthematous eruption of unknown etiology with a distinctive morphology. It affects all age groups, although it is most common in young adults. Incidence is maximum during winter and early summer, which leads to the belief that it may have an infective origin.[93]

CLINICAL FEATURES

The classical lesion is an erythematous annular plaque with a collarette of scales. The lesions are predominantly seen over the trunk along the lines of skin cleavage [**Figure 91-13**]. Exceptions are quite common (eg, only a herald patch, large lesions, papular rash, lesions in flexures, purpura).[93,94] Involvement of the face is more common in children. The rash is usually asymptomatic, and the biggest concern for the patient is the postinflammatory hypopigmentation that persists for weeks to months after the rash has subsided.

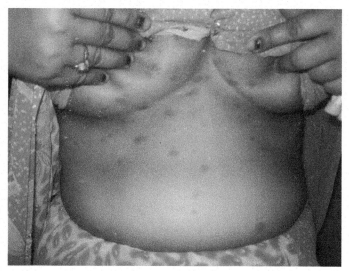

FIGURE 91-13. Pityriasis rosea showing multiple bilateral scaly annular lesions on the trunk.

TREATMENT

Many patients are empirically treated with oral macrolides, although convincing data about their effectiveness are lacking.[94,95] Acyclovir has also been reported to be effective.[96] Similar data have been published about the use of phototherapy.[96] Many dermatologists believe that treatment is unnecessary for a self-limiting disorder.

DISORDERS ATTRIBUTED TO FRICTION

SARI-INDUCED SKIN CHANGES

A sari is an elegantly worn piece of cloth traditionally worn by most Indian women. In recent times, a skirt-like petticoat is worn underneath it, which is tied by a string around the waist.[97] The very nature of tying the string tightly causes a plethora of problems.

Most of the women who wear a sari routinely have some hyperpigmentation and mild scaling at the site of tying the sari. Friction also causes hypo- and sometimes depigmentation. Occlusion leads to accumulation of sweat, leading to bacterial and superficial fungal infections. Disorders present elsewhere (eg, vitiligo, lichen planus) can become more pronounced at this site because of koebnerization.[98] Allergic contact dermatitis can develop at this site due to formaldehyde resins and dyes.[99] Asking the patient to wear gowns helps in rapid clearance of these conditions except the pigmentary changes, which take a long time to resolve.

FRICTION-INDUCED MELANOSIS AND AMYLOIDOSIS

It is a cultural practice in South Asia to rub the body well while bathing and afterward while drying the body. The perceived benefits are cleaner skin, removal of dead skin, and better blood circulation in the skin, which gives a good glow. But this practice results in increased melanization of the basal layer of the epidermis, melanin incontinence, and amyloid deposits.[100] Frictional melanosis resolves gradually with topical steroids and glycolic acid, but amyloidosis tends to persist.[101]

CHEMICAL LEUKODERMA

With hardly any quality control measures in place and rampant use of cheap imported products, chemical leukoderma due to consumer items is not uncommon. While this entity is reported in industrial settings in the Western countries, it is more common in the household setting in India. Patients suffer tremendous psychological stress on account of the perceived notions in society.

The various consumer items documented to cause contact depigmentation are sticker bindis, rain shoes, plastic chappals (sandals), hair dye/black henna (kali mehndi), alta (a red paste used by women in India to paint the borders of the feet), wallets, and even plastic cellphone covers.[102] The two possible mechanisms are either a direct cytotoxic effect on melanocytes causing cell death or inhibition of melanin synthesis by inhibition of tyrosinase.

The implicated chemicals are very commonly used in society, so this condition appears to develop in genetically predisposed individuals whose melanocytes are more susceptible.[103] With modernization, the substances used for ritualistic purposes have changed from the traditional vegetable dyes to factory-made products containing melano-toxic chemicals.[104] The chemicals include the following:

1. Hydroquinone, in bleaching creams[105]
2. Para-tertiary butylphenol (PTBP), in household adhesives, bindi, deodorants, spray perfumes, and household cleansers[104,106]
3. Paraphenylene diamine, in hair dyes and black hennas[107]
4. Azo dyes[108]
5. Mercurials and arsenicals[108]

BINDI/KUMKUM LEUKODERMA

Bindi is worn mostly by Hindu women as a cultural practice, and usually consists of a dot in the center of the forehead. Previously, it was made using vegetable dyes, but now it is worn as an adhesive patch. PTBP present in the adhesive is the culprit irritant. Initially an irritant dermatitis has been reported in a few patients. Depigmentation develops in weeks to years [**Figure 91-14**].[106]

LEATHER/RUBBER-INDUCED DEPIGMENTATION

Common items that can cause leather/rubber-induced depigmentation are rain shoes and slippers, synthetic leather wallets, watch straps, rubber gloves, and condoms. The usual culprit is monobenzyl ether of hydroquinone,[104,109] but in latex condoms, the culprit is mercaptobenzothiazole.[110]

MANAGEMENT

The diagnosis is usually easy. The most important step is to discontinue exposure to the offending substance as early as possible. This is often difficult because of deep-rooted religious beliefs.[111] Topical corticosteroids are effective, as is phototherapy. Resistant cases, particularly

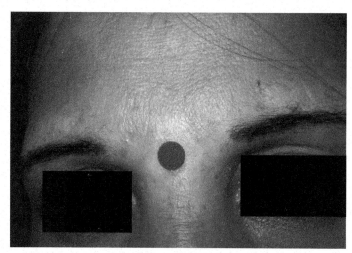

FIGURE 91-14. Bindi leukoderma showing depigmented circular macule on the forehead.

caused by cytotoxic chemicals, may need surgical treatment involving melanocyte transfer.

ABUSE OF TOPICAL CORTICOSTEROIDS

EPIDEMIOLOGY

Topical corticosteroids have made a significant contribution to the therapeutic armamentarium of the dermatologist. However, in recent years, they have been abused by doctors as well as patients. This is especially so in South Asia as drugs are freely available over the counter.[112-114] One multicenter study reported the use of topical steroids by 13% of the patients attending dermatologic outpatient departments. The most commonly abused agent is betamethasone valerate, available by the brand name Betnovate.[114] Recently, a combination of mometasone, tretinoin, and hydroquinone has also gained popularity as a skin-lightening cream and is likely to become commonly abused in the future.

Topical corticosteroids provide a prompt anti-inflammatory effect, ameliorating symptoms even without making a diagnosis and also inhibiting melanogenesis, contributing to lightening of the skin color.[114] Prolonged use of topical corticosteroids leads to a plethora of side effects (eg, atrophy, hypertrichosis).[115] Prolonged use on the face leads to a peculiar pattern variously known as steroid addiction[116] or as topical corticosteroid-dependent face,[114] which results in severe rebound erythema, burning, and scaling on the face when an attempt is made to stop the application.[114] This results in the patient continuing to use the corticosteroid and the development of increasingly severe atrophy, telangiectasia, and hypertrichosis.

TREATMENT

Treatment is gradually decreasing the potency of the corticosteroid applied over weeks to months, depending on the potency of the corticosteroid applied and the duration for which it has been applied. Also the burning associated with corticosteroid withdrawal is symptomatically treated with emollients, sunscreens, and topical calcineurin inhibitors. Systemic agents, including tetracyclines, isotretinoin, and antihistamines, have been shown to be beneficial.[117]

REFERENCES

1. Dhar S, Banerjee R. Atopic dermatitis in infants and children in India. *Indian J Dermatol Venereol Leprol.* 2010;76:504-513.
2. Dhar S, Kanwar AJ, Nagraja. Personal and family history of "atopy" in children with atopic dermatitis in north India. *Indian J Dermatol.* 1997;42:9-13.
3. Dhar S, Banerjee R, Dutta AK, Gupta AB. Comparison between the severity of atopic dermatitis in Indian Children born and brought up in UK and USA and that of Indian children born and brought up in India. *Indian J Dermatol.* 2003;48:200-202.
4. Sarkar R, Kanwar AJ. Clinico-epidemiological profile and factors affecting severity of atopic dermatitis in north Indian children. *Indian J Dermatol.* 2004;49:1171-1172.
5. Hanifin JM, Rajka G. Diagnostic features of atopic dermatitis. *Acta Derm Venereol (Stockh).* 1980;92:42-47.
6. Dhar S. Should topical antibacterials be routinely combined with topical steroids in the treatment of atopic dermatitis? *Indian J Dermatol Venereol Leprol.* 2005;71:71-72.
7. Sharma AD. Contact allergic dermatitis in patients with atopic dermatitis: a clinical study. *Indian J Dermatol Venereol Leprol.* 2005;71:97-99.
8. Saple DG, Torsekar RG, Pawanarkar V, et al. Evaluation of the efficacy, safety and tolerability of tacrolimus ointment in Indian patients of moderate to severe atopic dermatitis: a multicentric, open label, phase III study. *Indian J Dermatol Venereol Leprol.* 2003;69:396-400.
9. Harper JL, Ahmed I, Barclay G, et al. Cyclosporin for severe childhood AD: short course versus continuous therapy. *Br J Dermatol.* 2000;142:52.
10. Mahajan VK, Sharma NL. Occupational airborne contact dermatitis caused by *Pinus roxburghii* sawdust. *Contact Dermatitis.* 2011;64:110-111.
11. Sharma VK, Sethuraman G, Tejasvi T. Comparison of patch test contact sensitivity acetone and aqueous extracts of *Parthenium hysterophorus* in patients with airborne contact dermatitis. *Contact Dermatitis.* 2004;50:230-232.
12. Singhal V, Reddy BS. Common contact sensitizers in Delhi. *J Dermatol.* 2000;27:440-445.
13. Sharma VK, Asati DP. Pediatric contact dermatitis. *Indian J Dermatol Venereol Leprol.* 2010;76:514.
14. Sharma VK, Chakrabarti A. Common contact sensitizers in Chandigarh, India. A study of 200 patients with the European standard series. *Contact Dermatitis.* 1998;38:127-131.
15. Mahajan VK, Sharma NL, Sharma RC. *Parthenium* dermatitis: is it a systemic contact dermatitis or an airborne contact dermatitis? *Contact Dermatitis.* 2004;51:231-234.
16. Lakshmi C, Srinivas CR. *Parthenium* dermatitis caused by immediate and delayed hypersensitivity. *Contact Dermatitis.* 2007;57:64-65.
17. Verma KK, Manchanda Y, Pasricha JS. Azathioprine as a corticosteroid sparing agent for the treatment of dermatitis caused by the weed *Parthenium.* *Acta Derm Venereol.* 2000;80:31-32.
18. Sharma VK, Sethuraman G. *Parthenium* dermatitis. *Dermatitis.* 2007;18:183-190.
19. Sharma VK, Sethuraman G, Bhat R. Evaluation of clinical patterns of *Parthenium* dermatitis: a study of 74 cases. *Contact Dermatitis.* 2005;44:49-50.
20. Agarwal KK, Souza MD. Airborne contact dermatitis induced by *Parthenium*: a study of 50 cases in South India. *Clin Exp Dermatol.* 2009;34:e4-e6.
21. Handa S, Sahoo B, Sharma VK. Oral hyposensitisation in patients with contact dermatitis from *Parthenium hysterophorus.* *Contact Dermatitis.* 2001;44:279-282.
22. Sehgal VN, Srivastava G. Exfoliative dermatitis: a prospective study of 80 patients. *Dermatologica.* 1986;173:278-284.
23. Chakraborty. Lymphoma as a cause of exfoliative dermatitis. *Indian J Dermatol.* 1983;28:121-123.
24. Gupta R, Khera V. Erythroderma due to dermatophyte. *Acta Dermatol Venereol.* 2001;81:70.
25. Rym BM, Mourad M, Bechir Z, et al. Erythroderma in adults: a report of 80 cases. *Int J Dermatol.* 2005;44:731-735.
26. Sehgal VN, Srivastava G, Sardana K. Erythroderma/exfoliative dermatitis: a synopsis. *Int J Dermatol.* 2004;43:39-47.
27. Agarwal S, Khullar R, Kalla G, Malhotra YK. Nose sign of exfoliative dermatitis: a possible mechanism. *Arch Dermatol.* 1992;128:704.
28. Selvasekar A, Geetha AJ, Nisha K, et al. Childhood leprosy in an endemic area. *Lepr Rev.* 1999;70:21-27.
29. Rao S, Garole V, Walawalkar S, et al. Gender differentials in the social impact of leprosy. *Lepr Rev.* 1996;67:190-199.
30. Rao S, Announcement: India achieves national elimination of leprosy. *Ind J Lepr.* 2006;78:101.
31. Krishnamurthy P. Have we won the first battle against leprosy: guest editorial. *Ind J Lepr.* 2006;78:103-104.
32. Agarwal SP. Final push for elimination of leprosy in India. *Ind J Lepr.* 2005;77:213-215.
33. National Leprosy Eradication Programme. Progress Report for the year 2012-13 in India. Central Leprosy Division Directorate General of Health Services Nirman Bhawan, New Delhi, 110011.
34. Varshneya A, Goyal T. Incidence of various clinico-morphological variants of cutaneous tuberculosis and HIV concurrence: a study from the Indian subcontinent. *Ann Saudi Med.* 2011;31:134-139.
35. Pandhi D, Reddy BS, Chowdhary S, Khurana N. Cutaneous tuberculosis in Indian children: the importance of screening for involvement of internal organs. *J Eur Acad Dermatol Venereol.* 2004;18:546-551.
36. Singh G. Lupus vulgaris in India. *Indian J Dermatol Venereol Leprol.* 1974;40:257-260.
37. Kumar B, Rai R, Kaur I, Sahoo B, Muralidhar S, Radotra BD. Childhood cutaneous tuberculosis: a study over 25 years from northern India. *Int J Dermatol.* 2001;40:26-32.
38. Ramesh V, Misra RS, Beena KR, Mukherjee A. A study of cutaneous tuberculosis in children. *Pediatr Dermatol.* 1999;16:264-269.
39. Sehgal V, Sardana K, Sehgal R, Sharma S. The use of anti-tubercular therapy (ATT) as a diagnostic tool in pediatric cutaneous tuberculosis. *Int J Dermatol.* 2005;44:1-3.
40. Prasad R, Kumar R, Jaisawal BP, Singh UK. Miltefosine: an oral drug for visceral leishmaniasis. *Indian J Paediatr.* 2004;71:143-144.
41. Rathi SK, Pandhi RK, Chopra P, Khanna N. Post-kala-azar dermal leishmaniasis: a histopathological study. *Indian J Dermatol Venereol Leprol.* 2005;71:250-253.
42. Salotra P, Singh R. Challenges in the diagnosis of post kala-azar dermal leishmaniasis. *Indian J Med Res.* 2006;123:295-310.

43. Singh N, Ramesh V, Arora VK, Bhatia A, Kubba A, Ramam M. Nodular post-kala-azar dermal leishmaniasis: a distinct histopathological entity. *J Cutan Pathol.* 1998;25:95-99.

44. Thappa DM, Karthikeyan K. Exaggerated scabies in a child. *Indian Pediatr.* 2002;39:875-876.

45. Usha V, Gopalakrishnan TV. A comparative study of oral ivermectin and topical permethrin cream in the treatment of scabies. *J Am Acad Dermatol.* 2000;42:236-240.

46. Usha V. Review of ivermectin in scabies. *J Cutan Med Surg.* 2001;5:496-504.

47. Kaur P, Singh G. Community dermatology in India. *Int J Dermatol.* 1995;34:322-323.

48. Dutta AK, Mandal SB. A clinical study of 650 cases of vitiligo and their classification. *Indian J Dermatol.* 1969;14:103-105.

49. Koranne RV, Sehgal VN, Sachdeva KG. Clinical profile of vitiligo in North India. *Indian J Dermatol Venereol Leprol.* 1986;52:81-82.

50. Tawade YV, Parakh AP, Bharatia PR, et al. Vitiligo: A study of 998 cases attending KEM hospital in Pune. *Indian J Dermatol Venereol Lepr.* 1997;63:95-98.

51. Sarin RC, Kumar AS. A clinical study of vitiligo. *Indian J Dermatol Venereol Lepr.* 1977;83:190-194.

52. Sharma S, Garg VK, Sarkar R, Relhan V. Comparative study between flip-top transplantation and punch grafting in stable vitiligo patients. *Dermatol Surg.* 2013;39:1376-1384.

53. Vinod S, Singh G, Dash K, Grover S. Clinicoepidemiological study of pityriasis alba. *Indian J Dermatol Venereol Leprol.* 2002;68:338-340.

54. Vargas-Ocampo-F. Pityriasis alba: a histologic study. *Int J Dermatol.* 1993;32:870-873.

55. Du-Toit- MJ, Jordan HF. Pigmenting pityriasis alba. *Pediatric Dermatol.* 1993;10:1-5.

56. Wolf R, Wolf D, Tran H. Pityriasis alba in a psoriatic location. *Acta Derm Venereol (Stockh).* 1992;72:360.

57. Pasricha JS, Khaitan BK, Dash S. Pigmentary disorders in India. *Dermatol Clin.* 2007;25:343-522.

58. Thappa DM. Melasma (chloasma): a review with current treatment options. *Indian J Dermatol.* 2004;49:165-176.

59. Bandyopadhyay D. Topical treatment of melasma. *Indian J Dermatol.* 2009;54:303-309.

60. Achar A, Rathi SK. Melasma: a clinico-epidemiological study of 312 cases year. 2011;56:380-382.

61. Sarkar R, Chugh S, Garg VK. Newer and upcoming therapies for melasma. *Indian J Dermatol Venereol Leprol.* 2012;78:417-428.

62. Kanwar AJ, Dogra S, Handa S, Parsad D, Radotra BD. A study of 124 Indian patients with lichen planus pigmentosus. *Clin Exp Dermatol.* 2003;28:481-485.

63. Bhutani LK, Bedi TR, Pandi RK, Nayak NC. Lichen planus pigmentosus. *Dermatologica.* 1974;149:43-50.

64. Ranu H, Thng S, Goh BK, Burger A, Goh CL. Periorbital Hyperpigmentation in Asians: an epidemiologic study and a proposed classification. *Dermatol Surg.* 2011;37:1297-1303.

65. Malakar S, Lahiri K, Banerjee U, Mondal S, Sarangi S. Periorbital melanosis is an extension of pigmentary demarcation line-F on face. *Indian J Dermatol Venereol Leprol.* 2007;73:323-325.

66. Khanna N, Rasool S. Facial melanoses: Indian perspective. *Indian J Dermatol Venereol Leprol.* 2011;77:552-564.

67. Dhar S, Datta P, Malakar R. Pigmentary disorders. In: Valia RG, Valia AR, ed. *IADVL Text Book of Dermatology.* 3rd ed. Mumbai, India: Bhalani Publishing House;2008:773.

68. Gupta MA, Gupta AK. Dissatisfaction with skin appearance among patients with eating disorders and non-clinical controls. *Br J Dermatol.* 2001;145:110-113.

69. Yadalla HK, Aradhya S. Post acne hyperpigmentation: a brief review. *Dermatol Online J.* 2011;2:230-231.

70. Kubba R, Bajaj AK, Thappa DM, et al. Postinflammatory hyperpigmentation in acne. *Indian J Dermatol Venereol Leprol.* 2009;75:54.

71. Davis EC, Callender VD. A review of the epidemiology, clinical features, and treatment options in skin of color. *J Clin Aesthet Dermatol.* 2010;3:20-31.

72. Arora P, Sarkar R, Garg VK, Arya L. Laser for treatment of melasma and post inflammatory hyperpigmentation. *J Cutan Aesthet Surg.* 2012;5:93-103.

73. Adityan B, Thappa DM. Profile of acne vulgaris: a hospital-based study from South India. *Indian J Dermatol Venereol Leprol.* 2009;75:272-278.

74. Khunger N, Kumar C. A clinico-epidemiological study of adult acne: is it different from adolescent acne? *Indian J Dermatol Venereol Leprol.* 2012;78:335-341.

75. Pruthi GK, Babu N. Physical and psychosocial impact of acne in adult females. *Indian J Dermatol.* 2012;57:26-29.

76. Choudhury S, Chatterjee S, Sarkar DK, Dutta RN. Efficacy and safety of topical nadifloxacin and benzoyl peroxide versus clindamycin and benzoyl peroxide in acne vulgaris: a randomized controlled trial. *Indian J Pharmacol.* 2011;43:628-631.

77. Prasad S, Mukhopadhyay A, Kubavat A, et al. Efficacy and safety of a nano-emulsion gel formulation of adapalene 0.1% and clindamycin 1% combination in acne vulgaris: a randomized, open label, active-controlled, multicentric, phase IV clinical trial. *Indian J Dermatol Venereol Leprol.* 2012;78:459-467.

78. Agarwal US, Besarwal RK, Bhola K. Oral isotretinoin in different dose regimens for acne vulgaris: a randomized comparative trial. *Indian J Dermatol Venereol Leprol.* 2011;77:688-694.

79. Garg VK, Sinha S, Sarkar R. Glycolic acid peels versus salicylic-mandelic acid peels in active acne vulgaris and post-acne scarring and hyperpigmentation: a comparative study. *Dermatol Surg.* 2009;35:59-65.

80. Sharad J. Combination of microneedling and glycolic acid peels for the treatment of acne scars in dark skin. *J Cosmet Dermatol.* 2011;10:317-323.

81. Goel A, Krupashankar DS, Aurangabadkar S, et al. Fractional lasers in dermatology: current status and recommendations. *Indian J Dermatol Venereol Leprol.* 2011;77:369-379.

82. Mohanan S, Parveen B, Annie Malathy P, Gomathi N. Use of intense pulse light for acne vulgaris in Indian skin: a case series. *Int J Dermatol.* 2012;51:473-476.

83. Kachhawa D, Kachhawa V, Kalla G, et al. A clinico-aetiological profile of 375 cases of lichen planus. *Indian J Dermatol Venereol Leprol.* 1995;61:276-279.

84. Kanwar AJ, De D. Lichen planus in children. *Indian J Dermatol Venereol Leprol.* 2010;76:366-372.

85. Saraswathi TR, Ranganathan K, Shanmugam S, Sowmya R, Narasimhan PD, Gunaseelan R. Prevalence of oral lesions in relation to habits: cross-sectional study in South India. *Indian J Dent Res.* 2006;17:12.

86. Omal P, Jacob V, Prathap A, et al. Prevalence of oral, skin, and oral and skin lesions of lichen planus in patients visiting a dental school in southern India. *Indian J Dermatol.* 2012;57:107-109.

87. Ramesh M, Balachandran C, Shenoi SD, Rai VM. Efficacy of steroid oral mini-pulse therapy in lichen planus: an open trial in 35 patients. *Indian J Dermatol Venereol Leprol.* 2006;72:156-174.

88. Sonthalia S, Singal A. Comparative efficacy of tacrolimus 0.1% ointment and clobetasol propionate 0.05% *ointment* in oral lichen planus: a randomized double-blind trial. *Int J Dermatol.* 2012;51:1371-1378.

89. Kanwar AJ, De D. Methotrexate for treatment of lichen planus: old drug, new indication. *J Eur Acad Dermatol Venereol.* 2013;27:e410-e413.

90. Sharma L, Mishra MK. A comparative study of PUVASOL therapy in lichen planus. *Indian J Dermatol Venereol Leprol.* 2003;69:212-213.

91. Lavanya N, Jayanthi P, Rao UK, Ranganathan K. Oral lichen planus: an update on pathogenesis and treatment. *J Oral Maxillofac Pathol.* 2011;15:127-132.

92. Trehan M, Taylor CR. Low-dose excimer 308-nm laser for the treatment of oral lichen planus. *Arch Dermatol.* 2004;140:415-420.

93. Sharma L, Srivastava K. Clinicoepidemiological study of pityriasis rosea. *Indian J Dermatol Venereol Leprol.* 2008;74:647-649.

94. Chuh A, Lee A, Zawar V, Sciallis G, Kempf W. Pityriasis rosea: an update. *Indian J Dermatol Venereol Leprol.* 2005;71:311-315.

95. Sharma PK, Yadav TP, Gautam RK, Taneja N, Satyanarayana L. Erythromycin in pityriasis rosea: a double-blind, placebo-controlled clinical trial. *J Am Acad Dermatol.* 2000;42:241-244.

96. Chuh AA. Narrow band UVB phototherapy and oral acyclovir for pityriasis rosea. *Photodermatol Photoimmunol Photomed.* 2004;20:64-65.

97. Verma SB. Dermatological signs in South Asian women induced by sari and petticoat drawstrings. *Clin Exp Dermatol.* 2010;35:459-461.

98. Eapen BR, Shabana S, Anandan S. Waist dermatoses in Indian women wearing saree. *Indian J Dermatol Venereol Leprol.* 2003;69:88-89.

99. Rao S, Shenoy SD, Davis S, Nayak S. Detection of formaldehyde in textiles by chromotropic acid method. *Indian J Dermatol Venereol Leprol.* 2004;70:342-344.

100. Prabhakara VG, Chandra S, Krupa DS. Frictional pigmentary dermatoses: a clinical and histopathological study of 27 cases. *Indian J Dermatol Venereol Leprol.* 1997;63:99-100.

101. Yoshida A, Takahashi K, Tagami H, Akasaka T. Lichen amyloidosis induced on the upper back by long-term friction with a nylon towel. *J Dermatol.* 2009;36:56.

102. Bajaj AK, Saraswat A, Srivastav PK. Chemical leucoderma: Indian scenario, prognosis, and treatment. *Indian J Dermatol.* 2010;55:250-254.

103. Boissy RE, Manga P. On the etiology of contact/occupational vitiligo. *Pigment Cell Res.* 2004;17:208-214.

104. Ghosh S, Mukhopadhyay S. Chemical leucoderma: a clinico-aetiological study of 864 cases in the perspective of a developing country. *Br J Dermatol.* 2009;160:40-47.

105. Jimbow K, Obata H, Pathak MA, Fitzpatrick TB. Mechanism of depigmentation by hydroquinone. *J Invest Dermatol.* 1974;62:436-449.

106. Bajaj AK, Gupta SC, Chatterjee AK. Contact depigmentation from free para-tertiary-butylphenol in bindi adhesive. *Contact Dermatitis.* 1990;22:99-102.

107. Valsecchi R, Leghissa P, Di Landro A, Bartolozzi F, Riva M, Bancone C. Persistent leucoderma after henna tattoo. *Contact Dermatitis.* 2007;56:108-109.

108. Bajaj AK. Chemical leucoderma. In: Valia RG, Valia A, eds. *What's New in Dermatology, STDs and Leprosy?* Mumbai, India: Fulford; 2004:3-5.

109. Bajaj AK, Gupta SC, Chatterjee AK. Contact depigmentation of the breast. *Contact Dermatitis.* 1991;24:58.

110. Banerjee R, Banerjee K, Datta A. Condom leukoderma. *J Dermatol Venereol Leprol.* 2006;72:452-3.

111. Lilly E, Kundu RV. Dermatoses secondary to Asian cultural practices. *Int J Dermatol.* 2012;51:372-379.

112. Rathi SK, D'Souza P. Rational and ethical use of topical corticosteroids based on safety and efficacy. *Indian J Dermatol.* 2012;57:251-259.

113. Rathi S. Abuse of topical steroid as cosmetic cream: a social background of steroid dermatitis. *Indian J Dermatol.* 2006;51:154-155.

114. Saraswat A, Lahiri K, Chatterjee M, et al. Topical corticosteroid abuse on the face: a prospective, multicenter study of dermatology outpatients. *Indian J Dermatol Venereol Leprol.* 2011;77:160-166.

115. Hengge UR, Ruzicka T, Schwartz RA, Cork MJ. Adverse effects of topical glucocorticosteroids. *J Am Acad Dermatol.* 2006;54:1-15.

116. Kligman AM, Frosch PJ. Steroid addiction. *Int J Dermatol.* 1979;18:23-31.

117. Ljubojeviæ S, Basta-Juzbasiæ A, Lipozenèiæ J. Steroid dermatitis resembling rosacea: etiopathogenesis and treatment. *J Eur Acad Dermatol Venereol.* 2002;16:121-126.

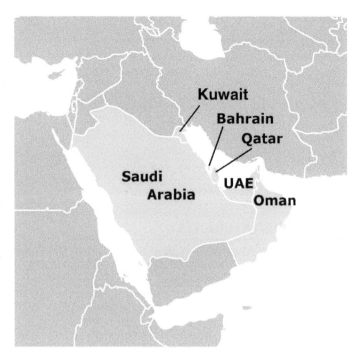

FIGURE 92-1. Arabic states that are members of the Gulf Cooperation Council. The region is also called the Arabian Gulf. UAE, United Arab Emirates.

CHAPTER

92

The Arabian Gulf

Nawal A. Habiballah Joma

KEY POINTS

- Atopic dermatitis is one of the most frequent cutaneous diagnoses in Arabian Gulf countries; rosacea is also a common concern.

- There has been a sharp rise in the incidence of eczema within this region, which is possibly due to environmental factors.

- A vitamin D deficiency is associated with many dermatologic conditions and is highly prevalent in individuals from the Arabian Gulf.

- There is a high rate of consanguineous marriages within the Gulf region. These marriages have resulted in an increase of rare genetic disorders throughout the Arab Gulf. However, more research needs to be done on the role of consanguinity on the dermatologic disorders described in this chapter.

- Melasma has a multifactorial pathogenesis and different modalities of presentation within the Arabian population.

- Skin-lightening products, some of which are potentially dermatologically damaging, are used extensively by those living in the Arabian Gulf.

- Psoriasis has a genetic basis, but is also influenced by the climate. It is less common in the tropics and in individuals with darker skin of color.

INTRODUCTION

The Arabian Gulf countries—Kuwait, Oman, the United Arab Emirates (UAE), Qatar, Yemen, Bahrain, and Saudi Arabia—make up a part of the Middle East. This southwestern section of Asia is situated just to the east of Africa [**Figure 92-1**]. In the past, the majority of these populations were nomadic. However, at present, more than 90% of the individuals in this region are settled, due to the rapid economic and urban growth that has occurred in the last 50 years.[1]

The total estimated population living in the Arabian Gulf is 74.8 million,[2] with a 75% Arab (Fitzpatrick skin types III and IV) and 25% Afro-Arab (Fitzpatrick skin types V and VI) distribution within the national populations. What is interesting, however, is that a large percentage of the Gulf's total population is made up of nonnational residents [**Table 92-1**] who have come to the Gulf for employment and, in some cases, have stayed on for generations.[2] Despite the lengthy stays that many of these nonnationals undertake and the fact that some were born in the Gulf and have lived there for their entire lives, very few of them will ever obtain citizenship in a Gulf nation state. These countries have instituted laws that prohibit the majority of nonnationals from ever obtaining citizenship, regardless of the duration of their residency.[3]

The unique demography that exists in the Arabian Gulf ranges widely between countries. For example, in Yemen, the nonnational population is very small. In contrast, in the UAE and Qatar, more than 80% of the population is made up of nonnationals, most of whom are from South Asian countries such as India and Bangladesh.[1] The nonnational population also consists of Middle Easterners from, for example, Egypt and Jordan; Southeast Asians, predominantly Filipinos and Indonesians; Africans, such as Sudanese and Somalis; and those of European descent [**Table 92-2**].

TABLE 92-1	Estimated national versus non-national populations in the Arabian Gulf in 2014

- Saudi Arabia: 29 million people with 31% nonnationals
- United Arab Emirates: 9.4 million people with 87% nonnationals
- Qatar: 2.2 million people with 85% nonnationals
- Oman: 4 million people with 44% nonnationals
- Bahrain: 1.3 million people with 55% nonnationals
- Kuwait: 3.4 million people with 37% nonnationals
- Yemen: 25.5 million people with a very small nonnational population

Source: Data from World Population Review. http://worldpopulationreview.com/countries/. Accessed May 18, 2014.

TABLE 92-2	Majority non-national populations living in Arabian Gulf countries, in descending order of population size

- Indians/Pakistanis/Bangladeshi/Sri Lankans
- Egyptians/ Jordanians/Palestinians/Syrians/Yemenis
- Filipinos
- Indonesians
- Sudanese/Somalis
- Turks
- Westerners

Source: Data from United Nations Statistics Division. Demographic Yearbook. http://unstats.un.org/unsd/demographic/products/dyb/dyb2008/Table04.pdf. Accessed September 20, 2013.

GENETIC DETERMINANTS

Consanguinity is a typical genetic feature of the Arabian Gulf countries. In a clinical genetics context, a consanguineous marriage commonly refers to a union between individuals related as second cousins or closer.[4] It has been estimated that 10.4% of the global population of 6.7 billion people are the progeny of consanguineous parents.[5]

Consanguinity rates vary around the world according to religion, culture, and geographic localization. The highest prevalence of consanguineous marriage has been recorded in northern Africa, the Middle East, and central and southern Asia [**Figure 92-2**].[4]

Among the Arab population, intrafamilial unions include double first cousins, first cousins, first cousins once removed, and second cousins. Unlike some other consanguineous societies, uncle-niece marriage is prohibited in Islam and, therefore, is largely absent among Arabs.

The impact of consanguinity on the predisposition to genetic disorders is sometimes misinterpreted or overstated. However, there has been a well-documented increase in rare genetic disorders among the offspring of consanguineous parents.[4] This can occur when both consanguineous parents are carriers of a particular genetic disorder, meaning their children have a 25% probability of being affected by this disorder.

These rare disorders are called autosomal recessive diseases, and they are caused by a mutation in a single gene. The dermatologic disorders described in this chapter are influenced by different genetic and environmental causes (and are, therefore, called complex genetic disorders). As such, the relevance of consanguinity to these disorders is not yet clear, although this factor is always worthy of consideration.

For the reasons just summarized, the prevalence of rare autosomal recessive diseases is higher in the Gulf than the rest of the world.[6] Among these are hemoglobin disorders and metabolic and neurogenetic disorders, all of which may have cutaneous manifestations of which dermatologists should be aware.

Additionally, the nationals of the Arabian Gulf face a number of unique dermatologic conditions that are attributable to causes unique to the Middle East. Rapid modernization, recent changes in dietary and social habits, extreme weather patterns, and cultural practices all contribute to the cutaneous manifestations seen commonly in the Gulf's population.

VITAMIN D DEFICIENCY

In recent years, vitamin D deficiency has become an issue for the Gulf's residents, which, given the climate, seems counterintuitive.[7] Due to the high temperatures and arid winds throughout most of the year, as well as cultural and religious reasons, the men and women of the Gulf cover their heads and leave little sun-exposed skin. In addition, in recent years, urbanization has lessened the need to go outside during the day. Offices, homes, and shopping centers are air-conditioned, discouraging residents from facing the sun, and outings generally happen in the late afternoon or evening when there is little sunlight left. Further contributing to a vitamin D deficiency, the Gulf's nationals have naturally dark skin but work hard to maintain a lighter skin tone. Therefore, they avoid sun exposure to prevent the darkening of their skin. The Gulf's most common skin types (primarily Fitzpatrick skin types III and IV) have higher levels of melanin, which acts as extremely efficient protection by absorbing solar ultraviolet rays. The angle of the sun, its distance from the equator, cloud cover,

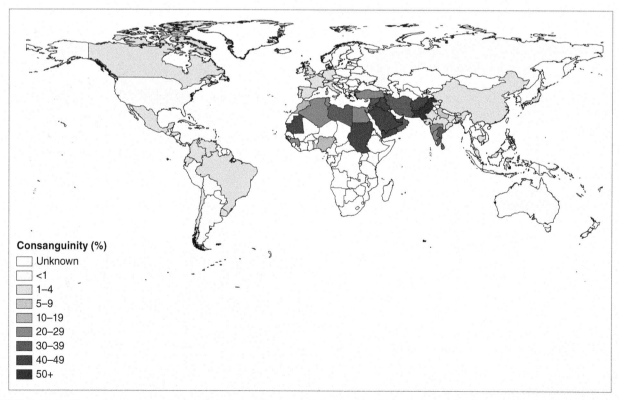

Consanguinity (%)
- Unknown
- <1
- 1–4
- 5–9
- 10–19
- 20–29
- 30–39
- 40–49
- 50+

FIGURE 92-2. The world map of consanguinity summarizes the frequency of consanguineous marriages throughout the world in 2014. (Used with permission from Professor Alan H. Bittles, Center for Human Genetics, Perth, Australia via Dr. Giovanni Romeo, Professor of Medical Genetics, Director, European School of Genetic Medicine, Bologna, Italy.)

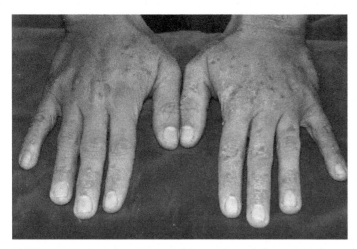

FIGURE 92-3. Atopic dermatitis is one of the most frequently diagnosed skin diseases in the Arabian Gulf. It is most likely caused by the hot, dry climate found in this geographic region.

use of sunscreens, diet, particulate matter, and latitude may also influence vitamin D levels.[8] It is therefore not just the cultural requirement to cover that is causing a vitamin D deficiency. Thus, all the aforementioned factors should be taken into account when investigating this phenomenon, especially considering that vitamin D deficiency has been associated with in a number of inflammatory and atopic skin diseases.[9]

ATOPIC DERMATITIS

Atopic dermatitis (AD) is one of the most frequently diagnosed skin diseases in the Arabian Gulf [**Figure 92-3**].[10] Its high prevalence is most likely a result of rapid urbanization and industrialization, and the corresponding exposure to harsh weather, high heat, pollutants, irritants, and other external allergens.[11] It is now generally accepted that the disease presents as the result of a combination of genetic and environmental factors.[12]

In the past decade, there has been a significant surge in the incidence of skin disease in Saudi Arabia, with almost 20% of children between the ages of 6 and 18 suffering from eczema [**Figure 92-4**].[8] This sharp rise is possibly due to environmental factors.

One study suggests the possible role and influence of a vitamin D deficiency in the prevalence, pathogenesis, and exacerbation of AD; however, those results have not been confirmed.[13] In addition, some data suggest that a premature abruption of breastfeeding may be one of the major factors contributing to the development of AD.[14]

Particularly for the Gulf's sun-avoiding population, vitamin D supplements should be considered in the treatment of AD. The use of oral vitamin D may correct a defect in the immune system, resulting in fewer infections and the prevention of dry skin.[13] Many kinds of medication for the treatment of AD, including homeopathic and herbal medications, are available over the counter in Saudi Arabia and in other Arabian Gulf countries. Similarly, all consultations and medications are free for Gulf citizens in government hospitals, including those from the UAE, Qatar, and Saudi Arabia. Prescription medications for eczema are also easily available.

MELASMA

Because the risk of developing melasma is much greater in harsh weather and in individuals who are subject to constant sun exposure,[15] this is a condition that is commonly seen among Arabian Gulf nationals [**Figure 92-5**]. Its precise etiopathogenesis is unknown; however, associations with genetic influences, sun exposure, pregnancy, oral contraceptives, estrogen–progesterone therapies, thyroid dysfunction, cosmetics, and drugs have been proposed.[15,16]

It has been theorized that people of Asian, African, and Arab descent are slow to respond to treatments for hyperpigmentation due to the nature of their Fitzpatrick skin of color variations (III through VI).[17]

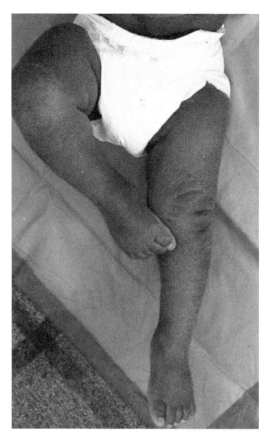

A

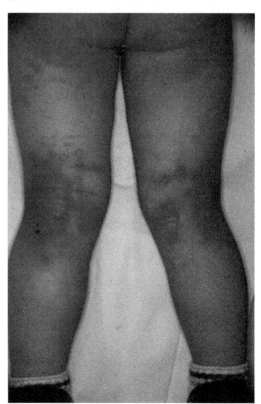

B

FIGURE 92-4. **(A)** A skin of color infant with poorly defined, mild erythematous scaling patches, bilaterally involving the lower limbs. **(B)** Well-defined erythematous scaling patches that symmetrically involve the gluteal and popliteal areas.

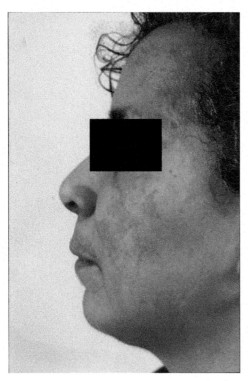

FIGURE 92-5. Centrofacial mixed melasma in a female patient with skin of color.

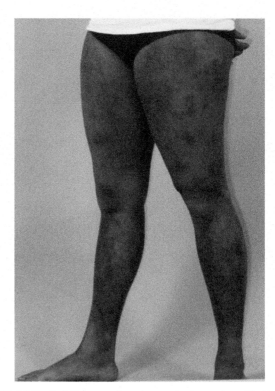

FIGURE 92-6. Postinflammatory hyperpigmentation in a patient with skin of color, demonstrating ashy pigmentation with areas of erythema and grayish-brown hyperpigmented patches.

The treatment of melasma should include education about sun avoidance, the use of sunscreen, and the use of hydroquinone and other bleaching medications. However, for some populations in the Gulf, sunscreen application may not be easily accepted due to the commonly held belief that their darker skin color, culturally mandated full-body attire, and indoor lifestyle will provide the necessary protection. Although this is unsubstantiated by research, the author has observed that many residents of the Gulf are concerned about the possible side effects of using sunscreen, including the development of an allergy or a skin irritation. Some patients believe that its ingredients can cause cancer. In contrast, a study in Kuwait showed that women wear sunscreen more commonly than men and have a greater awareness of sunscreen's protective effects, but not to the same extent as Westerners.[18]

POSTINFLAMMATORY HYPERPIGMENTATION

Postinflammatory hyperpigmentation (PIH) is a universal response of the skin that is most common in Fitzpatrick skin types III to VI [**Figure 92-6**].[19] A probable new variant of PIH, which is occasionally seen in Saudi Arabian women, is facial pigmentary demarcation lines. This is a chronic pigmentary problem.[20] When working with the Arab population, these pigmentary demarcation lines should be recognized and differentiated from other similar diseases, such as melasma.[21]

BEAUTY STANDARDS IN THE ARABIAN GULF

Beauty in the Arabian Gulf is more often than not associated with a preference for fairer skin. As such, skin-lightening creams and soaps have become popular in the Gulf, and they are promoted heavily within the media [**Figure 92-7**]. Some patients may attempt to treat their PIH with these skin-lightening products,[22] a number of which contain toxic ingredients, such as mercury, high-potency steroids, and high levels of hydroquinone. These products are easily available for over-the-counter purchase in Arabian Gulf countries. Glutathione, in particular, has captured a large portion of the market as a skin tone lightener. Healthcare professionals, dermatologists, and consumers should be aware of the use

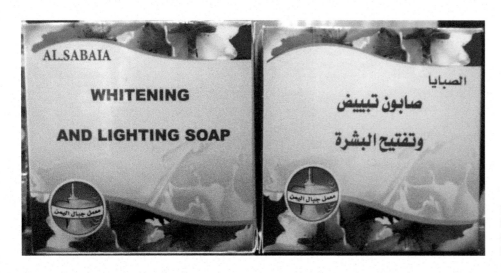

FIGURE 92-7. A skin-lightening soap product used by some women in the Arabian Gulf to lighten their skin. (Used with permission from Nassir Masoud and Zayna Saud Al Habsi.)

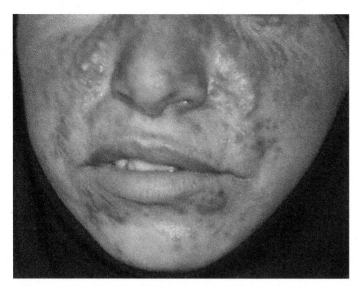

FIGURE 92-8. Rosacea with erythema, inflammatory papules, and pustules on the face of a young female from the Arabian Gulf, prior to treatment.

of these ingredients in skin-lightening products, as well as their possible effects on users.

ROSACEA

Rosacea is one of the most common skin diseases treated by dermatologists, even in the Arabian Gulf [**Figure 92-8**].[23] The etiology of rosacea is unknown; however, several factors that are prevalent in the Gulf region are likely to play a role in its development. These include climatic exposure to wind and sun, which can cause damage to blood vessels and dermal connective tissues.[24] Before the initiation of rosacea treatment, the triggering factors that exacerbate the patient's condition should be identified and avoided, if possible. This may prove difficult in the Arabian Gulf if the trigger is related to weather or diet. Common triggering factors include hot or cold temperatures, wind, hot drinks, caffeine, exercise, spicy food, alcohol, extreme emotions, topical products that irritate the skin and decrease its barrier function, and medications that cause flushing.[24]

The use of daily broad-spectrum sunscreen containing protective silicones, such as dimethicone or cyclomethicone, is recommended for all patients with rosacea. Physical blockers such as titanium dioxide and zinc oxide are generally well tolerated, and green-tinted sunscreens can provide coverage of the erythema.[25] However, as noted previously, an aversion to sunscreen for a variety of cultural or social reasons may be common among patients in the Gulf.

Oral contraceptive therapy has also been helpful for female patients whose rosacea worsens with their hormonal cycle.[26] However, in some cases, prescribing clinicians may encounter a reluctance for oral contraceptives due to religious or cultural prohibitions.

PSORIASIS

Psoriasis is a chronic inflammatory skin disorder that is one of the most common dermatoses worldwide [**Figure 92-9**].[27] It is characterized by dry, reddish, scaly patches, papules, and plaques that are usually pruritic. The incidence of psoriasis is dependent on the climate and the genetic heritage of a population.[28] There is a lack of data about the prevalence of psoriasis in the Gulf populations. However, it is known that the condition is less common in the tropics and in individuals with darker skin of color.[29,30] The lowest prevalence of psoriasis is found in populations from Africa, East Asia, India, and Samoa, and among indigenous Indian Americans.[31-38] Although it is less common in individuals with darker skin of color, psoriasis still appears to be a common dermatologic complaint within countries of the Gulf. The treatment for psoriasis is similar

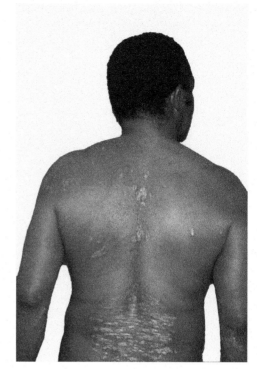

FIGURE 92-9. Plaque psoriasis on the back of a patient with darker skin of color.

across all racial groups and includes medication, light therapy, stress reduction, and climatotherapy, as well as various adjuncts such as solar radiation, sea bathing, moisturizers, and salicylic acid.[39]

CONCLUSION

While the dermatologic conditions observed in the Arabian Gulf countries are not unique, there are certain matters of interest that should be considered when treating patients from this area. Cultural practices within the region, including the high rate of consanguineous marriages and the population's predilection for avoiding sun exposure, as well as recent demographic shifts and dietary changes brought on by rapid economic development, affect the dermatology of Arab Gulf nationals. Physicians must keep these factors in mind when treating patients within the Arabian Gulf countries.

ACKNOWLEDGMENTS

A special thanks to Dr. Giovanni Romeo, Professor of Medical Genetics, Director, European School of Genetic Medicine, Bologna, Italy, who so graciously acted as a consultant on genetics for this chapter.

REFERENCES

1. United Nations Statistics Division. Demographic Yearbook. http://unstats .un.org/unsd/demographic/products/dyb/dyb2008/Table03.pdf. Accessed September 20, 2013.
2. World Population Review. Country Populations 2014. http://worldpopulation-review.com/countries/. Accessed May 18, 2014.
3. Naithani P. Challenges faced by expatriate workers in Gulf Cooperation Council countries. *IJBM*. 2010;1:98-103.
4. Bittles A. Consanguinity and its relevance to clinical genetics. *Clin Genet*. 2001;60:89-98.
5. Bittles AH, Black ML. The impact of consanguinity on neonatal and infant health. *Early Hum Dev*. 2010;86:737-741.
6. Tadmouri GO, Nair P, Obeid T, et al. Consanguinity and reproductive health among Arabs. *Reprod Health*. 2009;6:17.

7. Muhairi SJ, Mehairi AE, Khouri AA, et al. Vitamin D deficiency among healthy adolescents in Al Ain, United Arab Emirates. *BMC Public Health.* 2013;13:33.

8. Al-Zoman AY, Al-Asmari AK. Pattern of skin diseases at Riyadh Military Hospital. *Egyptian Dermatol Online J.* 2008;4:4.

9. Libon F, Cavalier E, Nikkels AF. Vitamin D and the skin. *Rev Med Liege.* 2013;68:458-464.

10. Bittles AH, Black ML. Evolution in health and medicine. Sackler colloquium: consanguinity, human evolution and complex diseases. *Proc Natl Acad Sci USA.* 2010;107:1779-1786.

11. Kim HO, Kim JH, Cho SI, et al. Improvement of atopic dermatitis severity after reducing indoor air pollutants. *Ann Dermatol.* 2013;25:292-297.

12. Lee JY, Seo JH, Kwon JW, et al. Exposure to gene-environment interactions before 1 year of age may favor the development of atopic dermatitis. *Int Arch Allergy Immunol.* 2012;157:363-371.

13. Peroni DG, Piacentini GL, Cametti E, et al. Correlation between serum 25-hydroxyvitamin D levels and severity of atopic dermatitis in children. *Br J Dermatol.* 2011;164:1078-1082.

14. Kuhnyar A, Egyud K, Szabo I, et al. Prevalence of atopic dermatitis among children under 19 in an East-Hungarian agricultural county. *Clin Dev Immunol.* 2006;13:395-399.

15. Passeron T. Melasma pathogenesis and influencing factors: an overview of the latest research. *J Eur Acad Dermatol Venereol.* 2013;1:5-6.

16. Handel AC, Lima PB, Tonolli VM, et al. Risk factors for facial melasma in women: a case-control study. *Br J Dermatol.* 2014;171:588-594.

17. British Association of Dermatologists. Melasma. www.bad.org.uk. Accessed September 20, 2013.

18. Al-Mutairi N, Issa BI, Nair V. Photoprotection and vitamin D status: a study on awareness, knowledge and attitude towards sun protection in general population from Kuwait, and its relation with vitamin D levels. *Indian J Dermatol Vernerol Leprol.* 2012;78:342-349.

19. Taylor S, Grimes P, Lim J, et al. Postinflammatory hyperpigmentation. *J Cutan Med Surg.* 2009;13:183-191.

20. Al-Samary A, Al Mohizea S, Bin-Saif G, et al. Pigmentary demarcation lines on the face in Saudi women. *Indian J Dermatol Venereol Leprol.* 2010;76:378-381.

21. Lynde CB, Kraft JN, Lynde CW. Topical treatments for melasma and postinflammatory hyperpigmentation. *Skin Therapy Lett.* 2006;11:1-6.

22. Ebanks JP, Wickett RR, Boissy RE. Mechanisms regulating skin pigmentation: the rise and fall of complexion coloration. *Int J Mol Sci.* 2009;10:4066-4087.

23. Al-Abdulla HA, Kamal AM, Mansour K. Pattern of skin disease in Qatar: a pilot study. *Gulf J Dermatol.* 1995;2:1-13.

24. Goldberg DJ, Berlin A. *Acne and Rosacea: Epidemiology, Diagnosis and Treatment.* London, United Kingdom: Manson Publishing; 2012:56-61.

25. Badreshia-Bansal S, Bansal V. Acne rosacea. In: Taylor SC, Gathers RC, Callender VD, et al, eds. *Treatments for Skin of Color: Expert Consult.* Philadelphia, PA: Saunders Elsevier; 2011:14-19.

26. Pelle MT, Crawford GH, James WD. Rosacea: II. Therapy. *J Am Acad Dermatol.* 2004;51:499-512.

27. Centre for Arab Genomic Studies. Psoriasis susceptibility. http://www.cags.org.ae/FMPro?-DB=ctga.fp5&-Format=ctga/ctga_detail.html&-RecID=34865&-Find. Accessed May 24, 2013.

28. Chandran V, Raychaudhuri SP. Geoepidemiology and environmental factors of psoriasis and psoriatic arthritis. *J Autoimmun.* 2010;34:J314-J321.

29. Alexis AF, Blackcloud P. Psoriasis in skin of color: epidemiology, genetics, clinical presentation, and treatment nuances. *J Clin Aesthet Dermatol.* 2014;7:16-24.

30. Farber EM, Nall L. Psoriasis in the tropics: epidemiologic, genetic, clinical, and therapeutic aspects. *Dermatol Clin.* 1994;12:805-816.

31. Cimmino M. Epidemiology of psoriasis and psoriatic arthritis. *Reumatismo.* 2007;59(Suppl 1):19-24.

32. Cheng L, Zhang SZ, Xiao CY, et al. The A5.1 allele of the major histocompatibility complex class I chain-related gene A is associated with psoriasis vulgaris in Chinese. *Br J Dermatol.* 2000;143:324-329.

33. Aoki T, Yoshikawa K. Psoriasis in Japan. *Arch Dermatol.* 1971;104:328-329.

34. Lin XR. Psoriasis in China. *J Dermatol.* 1993;20:746-755.

35. Ding X, Wang T, Shen Y. Prevalence of psoriasis in China: a population-based study in six cities. *Eur J Dermatol.* 2012;22:663-667.

36. Raychauduri SP, Farber EM. The prevalence of psoriasis in the world. *J Eur Acad Dermatol Venerol.* 2001;15:16-17.

37. Dogra S, Yadav S. Psoriasis in India: prevalence and pattern. *Indian J Dermatol Venereol Leprol.* 2010;76:595-601.

38. Campalani E, Barker JN. The clinical genetics of psoriasis. *Curr Genomics.* 2005;6:51-60.

39. National Psoriasis Foundation. Psoriasis treatments. http://www.psoriasis.org/about-psoriasis/treatments. Accessed May 24, 2014.

CHAPTER **93**

North America: Mexico

93A

Common Skin Diseases and Treatments in North America: Mexico

María-Ivonne Arellano-Mendoza
Amado Saúl-Cano

KEY POINTS

- The population with skin of color in Mexico is an amalgamation of modern-day ethnolinguistic groups with origins in Latin American countries. The Mexican population consists of indigenous Indians, Caucasians from a variety of European countries, individuals of European and indigenous Indian ancestry, and individuals of African descent. The Mexico population is used here as an example to represent Hispanics and those who come from other Latin American countries.

- The Hispanic population is the fastest-growing ethnolinguistic group in the United States, facilitated by immigration from Mexico, Central America, and other Latin American countries. This necessitates an understanding by dermatologists and healthcare providers of skin disorders that occur in patients from these countries.

- Pigmentary conditions are one of the most widely shared dermatologic occurrences seen in individuals with skin of color from Mexico.

- Cutaneous diseases commonly seen in Mexico include those of infectious, malignant, pigmentary, and photocutaneous etiology.

- Solar dermatitis, melasma, and facial postinflammatory hyperpigmentation are some of the most frequently occurring dermatoses in Mexico and throughout Latin America.

INTRODUCTION

Mexico is an ethnically and racially diverse country of approximately 120 million people.[1] The Mexican population consists of indigenous Indians, Caucasians from a variety of European countries, individuals of European and indigenous Indian ancestry, and individuals of African descent. Cutaneous diseases commonly seen in Mexico are quite varied and include those of infectious, malignant, pigmentary, and photocutaneous etiology [**Table 93A-1**]. Because the Hispanic population is rapidly growing in the United States and its growth is greatly facilitated

TABLE 93A-1 Common dermatoses in Mexico
Solar dermatitis
Ashy dermatitis
Melasma
Tinea imbricata
Mycetomas
Sporotrichosis
Cutaneous tuberculosis
Leprosy
Mexican leishmaniasis
Cutaneous larva migrans
Nonmelanoma skin cancers
Melanomas

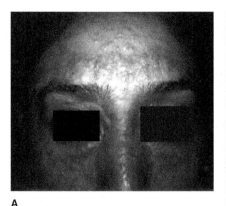 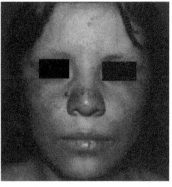 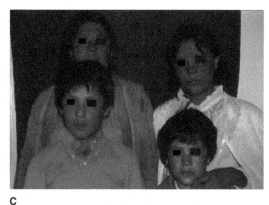

A   B   C

FIGURE 93A-1. **(A)** A case of solar dermatitis (actinic prurigo) in a female with intense conjunctivitis and chronic papular lesions. **(B)** Solar dermatitis in a female with conjunctivitis, cheilitis, and scarring. **(C)** Familial solar dermatitis in four family members.

by immigration from Mexico and other Latin American countries, it is important for dermatologists to have a working knowledge of common cutaneous diseases that occur in Mexico. This chapter reviews these common diseases.

SOLAR DERMATITIS

Solar dermatitis is one of the 10 most frequently occurring dermatoses in Mexico, representing approximately 3% to 5% of all cutaneous diseases [**Figure 93A-1**]. Also known as actinic prurigo, summer prurigo, and polymorphous light eruption, solar dermatitis tends to predominate in people who live in higher elevations. Onset may occur during childhood, with improvement occurring during the adolescent years. It is seen primarily in patients with skin of color and in women (2:1). Patients frequently seek dermatologic treatment during the third or fourth decade of life.

Solar dermatitis is induced by exposure to ultraviolet (UV) radiation, primarily UVB and, less often, UVA.[2] Hojyo-Tomoka et al[3] demonstrated that 92.8% of patients with actinic prurigo were human leukocyte antigen (HLA) D-related (DR) 4 positive. Furthermore, 80% of the HLA-DR4-positive patients were positive for the HLA-DRB1*0407 allele. HLA-A28 and HLA-B39 (B16) were also significantly increased, possibly explaining the higher frequency in the Mexican population.[3,4]

Treatment of solar dermatitis is often successful but requires both preventative measures and aggressive therapy. One of the most important aspects is a full explanation of the disease to the patient, stressing the fact that even low amounts of sun exposure exacerbate this dermatosis. Sun protection with hats, sunglasses, and umbrellas, as well as a broad-spectrum sunscreen, is mandatory, especially in the Mexican climate, which is characterized by high UV exposure. Emollients and mild cleansers should be applied as part of nightly adjuvant treatment. Sedating antihistamines are often necessary to control pruritus during exacerbations. Topical steroids are used occasionally to control acute eczematous lesions, but in severe or acute cases, oral treatment is preferred. Antimalarial agents (eg, chloroquine phosphate and hydroxychloroquine) are widely used in Mexico as a treatment for solar dermatitis. Ophthalmologic examinations are necessary at baseline and every 6 months until the drug is discontinued. Thalidomide has produced outstanding results and is prescribed in refractory or severe cases at 100 mg/d.[4]

ASHY DERMATOSIS

Ashy dermatosis, also known as dermatosis cenicienta, erythema chronicum figuratum melanodermicum, and pintoid, was first described by Oswaldo Ramírez in El Salvador in 1957.[5] The term erythema

dyschromicum perstans was subsequently suggested by Marion B. Sulzberger in the early 1960s. This disorder is seen most commonly in those of Latin American or Asian descent, but there have also been well-documented cases in patients of European or Turkish origin. There is a slightly higher predominance in women [**Figure 93A-2**].[6]

MELASMA

Although Mexico is located geographically in North America, many of its cultures, traditions, and diseases are similar to those described in Mesoamerica.[7] Melasma is one such disease; this very common facial dyschromia is the third most frequent reason for a dermatology consultation and the second most frequent facial hyperchromia. Arellano-Mendoza et al[8] reported that this condition was outnumbered only by facial postinflammatory hyperpigmentation (PIH) cases in a general hospital in Mexico. Although asymptomatic, disorders of facial pigmentation have profound social and psychological impacts in Mexican culture.

Melasma pigmentation may be distributed in one of three patterns: malar, mandibular, or centrofacial, which is the pattern seen most frequently in the Mexican population [**Figure 93A-3**].[9-11] Melasma represents a therapeutic challenge because treatment will not be successful without daily photoprotection strategies. Patients should use a broad-spectrum sunscreen and a hat while outdoors and avoid direct sun exposure; this is specifically applicable to Mexicans living in an environment with strong UV radiation.

POSTINFLAMMATORY HYPERPIGMENTATION

Some Mexican dermatologists consider PIH to be the most common type of hypermelanosis.[8] Its duration and severity correlate with skin color (Fitzpatrick skin types III to VI) and an individual's predisposition to the disease. The course of PIH is not predictable and can be stressful for patients who perceive it as an aesthetic imperfection. It is not yet well understood, and treatment is difficult because it consists of treating the original disease as well as avoiding procedures that might result in additional inflammatory insults to the skin. Patients usually respond after 4 to 8 weeks of using depigmenting agents and photoprotective measures [**Figure 93A-4**].

TINEA IMBRICATA

Tinea imbricata, also known as Tokelau or elegant/laced tinea, is a chronic dermatophyte infection that involves hairless skin.[2,12] First observed among the native inhabitants of Polynesia, it is caused by an

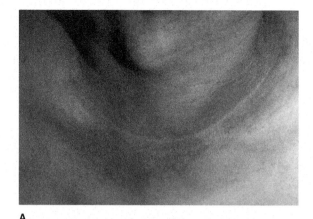

FIGURE 93A-2. Ashy dermatosis on the **(A)** neck and **(B)** trunk regions of a patient with skin of color. Note the grayish color of the pigmented lesions.

anthropophilic fungus, *Trichophyton concentricum,* that is transmitted from person to person through direct skin contact. Tinea imbricata is found in Africa, Asia, and Central and Latin America. There are several endemic areas in Mexico, including the states of Guerrero, Puebla, and Chiapas.[12,13] Genetic factors may determine its geographic distribution. Additionally, environmental factors, including heat and humidity, are strong determinants of distribution [**Figure 93A-5**].[14,15]

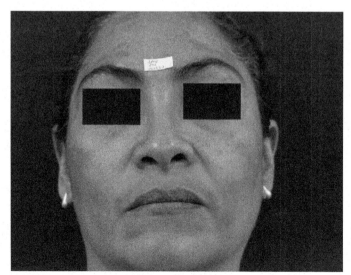

FIGURE 93A-3. Facial melasma in a Hispanic female.

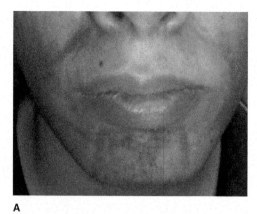

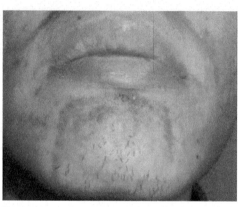

FIGURE 93A-4. (A and B) Postinflammatory hyperpigmentation occurring in a patient after a chemical peel.

MYCETOMAS

Mycetomas occur frequently in the tropical and subtropical countries of Asia and Africa and the Latin American countries of Mexico, Venezuela, Colombia, Brazil, and Argentina. In Mexico and Central America, mycetomas due to *Actinomycetes* predominate, whereas in Africa, Asia and Latin America, eumycetomas are more frequent.[16]

Mycetomas are more common in males than females (5:1) and during the third and fifth decades of life. This skin disease is uncommon in children before puberty because it is believed that androgens influence its development.[16-18] Mycetomas commonly occur on the lower extremities (ie, feet, legs, knees, thighs, and hips), which are more susceptible to

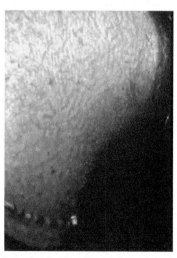

FIGURE 93A-5. Typical 'laced' pattern of tinea imbricata (sometimes known as Tokelau).

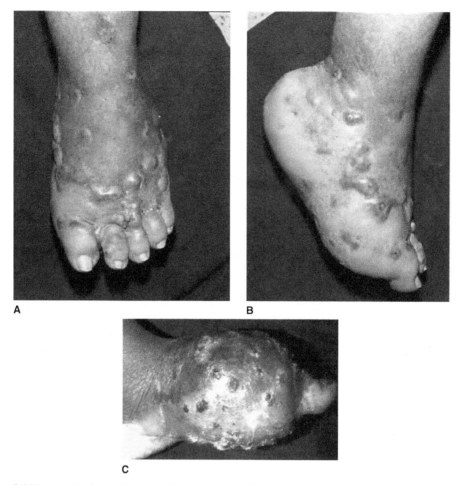

A

B

C

FIGURE 93A-6. **(A, B and C.)** Long-standing lesions of mycetomas. The feet are the most frequent location.

injury and inoculation [**Figure 93A-6**]. Person-to-person or site-to-site transmission does not occur.[19] In Mexico, this skin disease is seen primarily in workers who wear sandals or walk barefoot and in those who carry wood on their bare backs; this practice usually results in thoracic involvement [**Figure 93A-7**]. Other less common areas of involvement include the hands, elbows, arms, shoulders, neck, and head.

Diagnosis is often obvious from the clinical presentation, but confirmation with a mycologic examination is required. Direct examination of the exudate reveals the presence of grains that differ according to the species: *Nocardia* bacteria are 150 to 300 μm, round or bean shaped, colorless grains with clubs; *Actinomadura madurae* are up to 1 mm in diameter, with geographic boundaries; *Streptomyces pelletieri* are red; and *E*umycetes are either white or black. A biopsy allows for better agent identification through affinity of the granules and evaluation of their morphology. Culture identifies the species and, in the case of *Nocardia brasiliensis,* cultures grown in casein-enriched media are needed to differentiate it from other *Nocardia* species because only *N. brasiliensis* hydrolyzes casein.[20,21]

In addition to a complete examination of the patient, radiographic examination is required to determine the depth and aggressiveness of the disease. Prognosis depends on the location of the infection, the depth of involvement, and the etiologic agent.[2]

Treatment of actinomycetoma is achieved using several regimens. One regimen is diaminodiphenyl sulfone (100 g/d) plus sulfamethoxazole/trimethoprim (2 tablets per day). Severe long-standing cases require sulfamethoxazole/trimethoprim (2 tablets per day) plus pulse therapy with amikacin (15 mg/kg for 15 to 20 days). Close follow-up of this regimen is required with audiometric and renal function monitoring. Amoxicillin/clavulanate plus sulfamethoxazole/trimethoprim for

3 to 6 months is another regimen. Repeated treatments are sometimes necessary.[17,18,22]

Other drugs used for actinomycetoma therapy include fosfomycin, streptomycin, rifampin, and imipenem. Therapy for eumycetomas

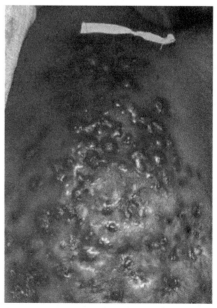

FIGURE 93A-7. Case of advanced thoracic mycetoma. The patient was inoculated after carrying wood on their shoulders.

includes itraconazole, fluconazole, and amphotericin B. In advanced cases, amputation may be required. Disease prevention includes education of agricultural workers about the disease and adequate protection with proper clothing and footware.[2]

SPOROTRICHOSIS

Sporotrichosis is caused by the ubiquitous fungus *Sporothrix schenckii,* which is found in vegetables, wood, straw, and flowers. Sporotrichosis occurs in tropical and subtropical regions of the world, although cases have been described in temperate and cold regions. In Mexico, it predominates in the central portion of the country. Men and women are equally affected, and it may be observed in any age group from childhood through old age. In Mexico, sporotrichosis has been considered an occupational disease.[23,24]

S. schenckii penetrates the host's skin through an abrasion and then produces cutaneous manifestations that vary due to the patient's immune response.[25] The clinical presentation may be divided into hyperergic and anergic forms. The two hyperergic forms, lymphangitic and fixed, are the most common [**Figure 93A-8**]. The lymphangitic presentation accounts for 70% of patients, with nodules and gummas distributed along the lymphatic vessels of the face and upper or lower limbs.[26] The fixed form, which consists of only one lesion, is generally located on the face and is found in 25% of Mexican patients. The lesion may be an erythematous, nodular, infiltrated, or limited plaque covered by thin scales. The course may be chronic and asymptomatic.[27]

Approximately 2% to 3% of patients present with an anergic form of sporotrichosis, but it is increasingly diagnosed in association with acquired immunodeficiency syndrome. Several clinical forms are recognized, including superficial erythematous-squamous, nodular hematogenous, osteoarticular, and systemic (affecting mainly the lung). The differential diagnosis of the fixed-plaque form of sporotrichosis includes cutaneous tuberculosis (TB) (lupus vulgaris) [**Figure 93A-9**] and leishmaniasis.

Cutaneous sporotrichin skin tests (read at 48 hours) can be a useful and fast determinative tool. However, the sporotrichin test is no longer routinely used for a diagnosis of sporotrichosis because it can yield false-positive and false-negative results.[28-30] Despite this, many international epidemiologic studies still use it to test groups of individuals living or working in a specific location. Attempts are then made to isolate the fungus from soils found locally. Nevertheless, despite the relative ease of use of this test, antigens adopted in sporotrichin tests currently lack standardization.[25] The intradermal reaction is therefore not diagnostic of sporotrichosis but identifies the immunologic response to this fungus and helps to classify the case as anergic or hyperergic.[25,31]

Diagnosis is made via culture, in which the white colony observed 8 days later turns black in color. Microscopic examination of the colony shows characteristic microconidial structures. Direct smears are not useful diagnostically because it is difficult to visualize the levaduriform structures, with the exception of some anergic patients.

Histopathologic features of sporotrichosis include nonsuppurative granulomas, in which yeast and structures resembling stars, known as asteroid bodies, can be found. Of note is the fact that asteroid bodies are not exclusive to sporotrichosis.

A very effective, well-tolerated, and inexpensive treatment for sporotrichosis is oral potassium iodide. In adults, this first-line treatment is administered at 3 to 6 g daily; in children, the dosage is 1 to 3 g daily for 3 months. Other effective but more expensive medications include griseofulvin, itraconazole, terbinafine, and sulfamethoxypyridazine. Local heat is another treatment modality. Amphotericin B is indicated for anergic forms of sporotrichosis.[32]

CUTANEOUS TUBERCULOSIS

In Mexico, TB remains a public health concern, with an incidence of 26 cases per 100,000 inhabitants; 4% of patients are under 15 years old and the male-to-female ratio is 1:6.[33] Pulmonary TB is the most

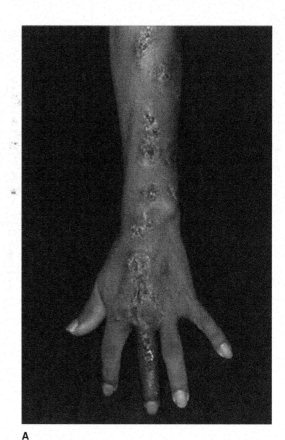

A

B

FIGURE 93A-8. (A) Lymphangitic sporotrichosis. (B) Fixed-plaque sporotrichosis.

frequently observed type, followed by osteoarticular, genital, and digestive TB. Cutaneous TB represents approximately 2% of all clinical forms of TB.[34]

Primary cutaneous infection is extremely rare, but when it occurs, it may appear as a cutaneous nodule with associated lymphangitis and adenopathy. Most cases are considered reinfected, with patients having previously had a pulmonary infection with *Mycobacterium tuberculosis bovis* or *hominis* and a positive purified protein derivative test. Patients can be reinfected endogenously from the original disease or from external sources. There are several classifications of the cutaneous forms of TB in Mexico. The one described by Latapí and colleagues (based on observations from Foch, an outstanding Austrian dermatologist and director of the Lupus Hospital in Vienna, who spent his last years in Mexico) is commonly followed [**Table 93A-2**].[2]

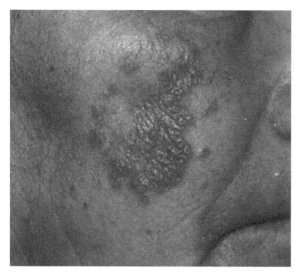

FIGURE 93A-9. Typical case of lupus vulgaris of the cheek.

The most common form of cutaneous TB in Mexico is colliquative TB [**Figure 93A-10**], also known as scrofuloderma or scrofulosis. Affecting primarily children and young adults, it is usually secondary to ganglion, bone, or articular infection. Lesions occur in the supraclavicular, axillary, groin, elbow, knee, and malleolar regions, where bones are in close proximity to the skin. Clinically, nodules and gummas form, beginning as small lesions that then enlarge over several weeks and become confluent and erythematous. The lesions subsequently become fluctuant and drain a yellow purulent material. Several lesions often evolve simultaneously until the entire region is affected with nodules, fistulas, and cold abscesses. Scarring invariably occurs, which leads to restriction of movement and deformity of the affected area. Systemic symptoms include fever, malaise, and anorexia. Pulmonary infection may occur simultaneously, with coughing, expectorations, thoracic pain, and dyspnea.

Differential diagnosis includes cervicofacial actinomycosis, sporotrichosis, and mycetomas.[2,35-37] Orificial, miliary, vegetant, and fungous varieties of TB are extremely rare in Mexico.[38] Nodular-necrotic TB, also termed papulonecrotic TB, occurs primarily on the elbows, knees, and gluteal area and rarely involves the face and earlobes. Morphologically, it presents as tiny nodules that ulcerate, crust, and heal with varioliform scars [**Figure 93A-11**].

LEPROSY

In 2013, the World Health Organization (WHO) estimated that there were 181,941 people with leprosy worldwide, distributed mostly among the poorest countries of Africa, Asia, and Latin America.[39] In Mexico, the prevalence is estimated to be 480 cases, with 215 new cases detected

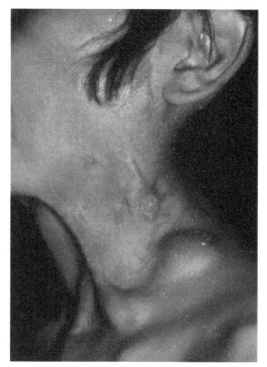

FIGURE 93A-10. Colliquative tuberculosis in a malnourished patient.

in 2011.[39,40] According to the WHO, this prevalence rate indicates that leprosy is no longer a public health issue.[41] However, there are areas of higher prevalence, such as the states of Sinaloa, Colima, Nayarit, Morelos, and Guanajuato.[2,40] Leprosy occurs more often among males and middle-aged persons, but it has been seen in children, including infants. Leprosy has been a curable disease since 1941, but, in patients in whom leprosy has been cured, physical, psychological, and social rehabilitation is mandatory.[42,43] There is no longer a need for the measures that were formerly used, such as the complete isolation of patients and their belongings.

MEXICAN LEISHMANIASIS

Leishmaniasis, also known as kala-azar, is a parasitic disease caused by protozoa from the *Leishmania* genus; several species exist depending on the region of the world. *Leishmania donovani* causes the disease frequently seen in Asia; *Leishmania tropica* causes the disease in

TABLE 93A-2	Cutaneous tuberculosis

Rare primary infection

Endogenous reinfection

Exogenous

I. Chronic forms (normergic)
   Colliquative tuberculosis, scrofuloderma: endogenous reinfection
   Verrucous tuberculosis (warty tuberculosis): endogenous reinfection
   Lupus tuberculosis, lupus vulgaris: endogenous and exogenous reinfection
   Orificial tuberculosis: endogenous reinfection
   Acute miliary tuberculosis: endogenous reinfection
II. Hematogenous forms (hyperergic)
   Deep nodular tuberculosis, erythema induratum of Bazin
   Nodular-necrotic tuberculosis, papulonecrotic
   Micronodular or liquenoid tuberculosis, lichen scrofulosus

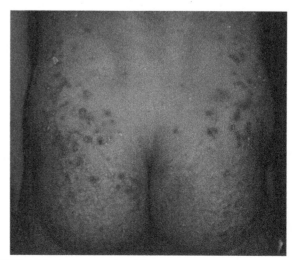

FIGURE 93A-11. Patient with nodular-necrotic tuberculosis. Note the varioliform scarring.

Mediterranean countries; the *Leishmania mexicana* complex includes the causal agents from Texas to Costa Rica; and *Leishmania braziliensis* and *Leishmania peruviana* produce leishmaniasis in Latin America.[2] The infectious agent is inoculated through a bite from *Phlebotomus* or *Lutzomyia* mosquitos that affects skin, mucosa, and viscera.

In Mexico, leishmaniasis is caused by *L. mexicana* transmitted by the mosquito *Lutzomyia olmeca*. These mosquitoes carry the amastigote, the nonflagellated form of the parasite, in their blood. The amastigote turns into the flagellated form, the promastigote. The insects then bite a healthy person or a reservoir (eg, dogs, wolves, or foxes) and introduce the infective form, the promastigotes, into the organism. The promastigote loses its flagellum and is phagocytosed by macrophages and subsequently invades other cells.[2] In Mexico, mucocutaneous cases are not seen.

In Mexico, the states most affected by leishmaniasis are Yucatán, Chiapas, Veracruz, and Oaxaca, but some cases have been reported in northern regions, such as Coahuila and Nayarit.[2,44] The disease is frequently found in agriculture workers, consisting mostly of men between the second and fourth decades of life who live in jungle or forest zones where gum and wood are exploited. Some cases have been described in the children and wives of agricultural workers who take their families to live with them in camps located in the zones where vectors exist.[45]

The most frequent clinical presentation of leishmaniasis is the so-called gumma ulcer, which is located asymmetrically mainly on the helix of ears, where mosquitoes bite most often. A nodule appears and rapidly turns into an ulcer with purulence and well-demarcated and infiltrated borders. The disease then runs an asymptomatic and chronic course, enlarging and destroying the ear. Lesions on the ears do not heal spontaneously, in contrast to those on the nose, cheeks, and upper limbs, which tend to heal spontaneously [**Figure 93A-12**].[46] In hyperergic cases, leishmaniasis is very difficult to demonstrate on biopsy, occasionally being found as puntiform structures inside giant cells or macrophages in tuberculoid infiltrates. In these patients, Montenegro reaction, or leishmanin skin test, is positive.

Cases of a diffuse, anergic, lepromatous form of leishmaniasis that resembles nodular lepromatous cases have been described in Venezuela and Mexico. These patients present with several disseminated ulcerated nodules affecting different parts of the body. Severe malaise is present. There is some controversy about these cases; some think that anergic diffuse cutaneous leishmaniasis is caused by *Leishmania pifanoi*, and others think that these cases are due to the immunologic status of the affected person.[47]

Intramuscular or intralesional pentavalent antimalarials are effective for treatment of leishmaniasis; chloroquine, ketoconazole, and itraconazole for 2 to 3 months have been used with good results. The Mexican forms of leishmaniasis can destroy the ear, which necessitates surgical reconstruction. Ulcers in other locations have been known to involute spontaneously after several months without treatment.[46,47]

CUTANEOUS LARVA MIGRANS

Cutaneous larva migrans is a disease caused by the larvae of nematodes that infect dogs and cats and occasionally can parasitize humans. It occurs frequently in tropical countries near the seashore or riversides. The superficial form of cutaneous larva migrans is the most common and is caused by *Ancylostoma* larvae from *Ancylostoma braziliense*, *Ancylostoma caninum*, *Ancylostoma duodenale* and *Necator americanus*. The adult worm is a parasite in the gut of dogs and cats; contaminated animal feces deposited on the ground can then infect patients via bare skin. The larva penetrates the skin, often through hair follicles, and immediately digs a tunnel, attempting to reach the surface of the skin.

Cutaneous larva migrans occurs on the limbs and back, areas that commonly come into contact with infected sand. Lesions consist of linear 'tracts' of different lengths that may assume a serpiginous form. Erythema, edema, and small vesicles may surround the lesions. Cutaneous larva migrans is an intensely pruritic disorder. Systemic symptoms do not occur because the larvae do not invade deeply. However, moderate eosinophilia may be observed [**Figure 93A-13**].[48] Lesions resolve

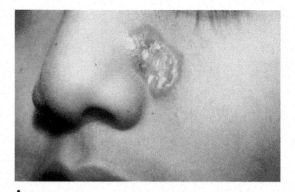

A

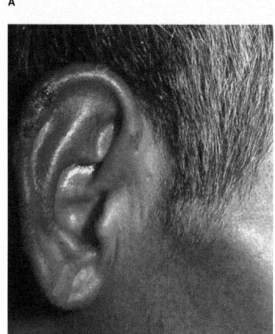

B

FIGURE 93A-12. **(A)** Leishmaniasis occurring on the face of a child. **(B)** Gumma ulcers, located on the ear in this patient, are the most frequent clinical presentation of leishmaniasis.

spontaneously once the larva dies, although the life span of the larva is several months.

The diagnosis of cutaneous larva migrans is made clinically. Histologic demonstration of larvae is very difficult because of the constant migration of the hookworms. Oral treatment is effective and includes ivermectin (150 to 250 mg/kg in a single dose), albendazole (400 mg in three doses), and thiabendazole (four weekly doses of 50 mg/kg). Preventative measures include wearing sandals and avoiding contact of bare skin with the sand in areas of disease prevalence.[48]

NONMELANOMA SKIN CANCERS

In Mexico, since 1998, nonmelanoma skin cancers (NMSC), notably basal cell carcinoma (BCC; representing 70% of cases) and squamous cell carcinomas (SCC; representing 17% of cases), are the second most common malignant tumors after cervical-uterine cancer.[49] According to data published by Peniche,[49] the ratio of BCC to SCC is 3 to 4:1. Analyzing a group of 2885 patients with BCC, most demonstrated signs of occupation-related chronic sun exposure (eg, employed as laborers, sailors, or salesmen), with 88% of BCCs located on the face (nose, 33.2%; eyelids, 18.3%; cheek, 14.7%; and frontal area, 8.5%).[49] The pigmented subtype of BCC occurs relatively frequently in Mexico. Lesions may be nodular, flat, or ulcerated, although dark pigmentation is

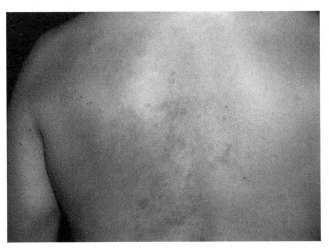

FIGURE 93A-13. A case of cutaneous larva migrans located on the back. This condition can occur after sleeping or lying down on contaminated sand.

almost always present [**Figure 93A-14**].[50] In Mexico, the most frequently observed histologic types are solid (33%), mixed solid-infiltrative (22%), infiltrative (8%), and pigmented (10%).[49,50]

In Mexico, SCC predominates in women in the 70- to 79-year-old age group, most of whom have a history of chronic and intense sun exposure.[51] In addition to SCCs, actinic keratoses [**Figure 93A-15**], solar lentigines, telangiectasias, and intense wrinkling may be present. Patients should be instructed on the use of sun protection, and an emphasis should be made on the importance of early detection of new lesions [**Figure 93A-16**].

MALIGNANT MELANOMAS

Although in some countries malignant melanomas (MMs) are an important public health issue due to a steady increase in incidence, epidemiologic data in Mexico reveal a different situation. According to data from the National Registry of Cancer and Histopathologic Registry of Malignant Neoplasms, the incidence of MM has remained at 1 per 100,000, with a mortality rate of 0.3 per 100,000.[50]

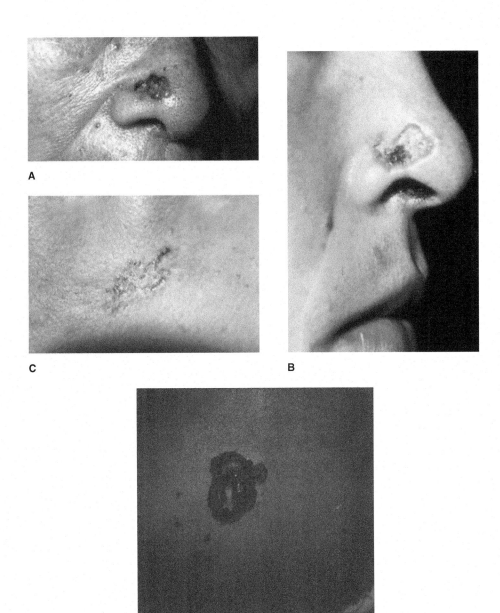

FIGURE 93A-14. (**A**) Typical pigmented basal cell carcinoma. (**B**) Scar-like basal cell carcinoma. (**C**) Superficial pearly basal cell carcinoma. (**D**) Superficial pigmented basal cell carcinoma.

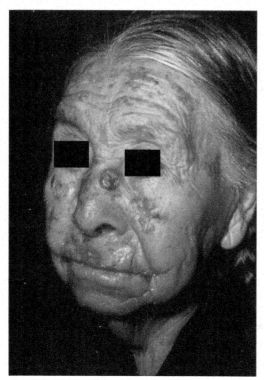

FIGURE 93A-15. Chronic actinic damage and skin cancers in a patient who has had extensive sun exposure.

In Mexico, 7.9% of skin tumors are cutaneous melanomas.[52] MMs occur slightly more often in women (57.1%), and the mean age at presentation is 54.3 years. The most common tumor site is the lower extremities.[53] In 252 Mexican patients, MMs were located as follows: 45% on the lower extremities, 27.4% on the head and neck, and 27.6% elsewhere (primarily the upper extremities and trunk).[52] These findings were consistent with series of patients in another hospital in Mexico.[54]

Nodular and acral lentiginous MMs are the most frequent types of melanoma in Mexico.[54,55] Acral lentiginous melanomas were the most common subtype among 165 Mexican patients; these are generally located on the palms and soles and affect subungual regions, primarily the first digit of the hands and feet [**Figures 93A-16(C) and 93A-17**].[54] Less frequently seen forms of melanoma include superficial spreading MMs, lentigo MMs, and oral MMs (which account for 1% to 8% of all MMs).[52,54-56] Patients are often misdiagnosed or initially undergo inappropriate treatments, thus necessitating referral to an oncology department. In Mexico, efforts are currently being made to assist patients in identifying and detecting suspicious pigmented lesions at an early, treatable stage.

CONCLUSION

Common skin disorders in Mexico are varied and include those of infectious, malignant, pigmentary, and photocutaneous etiology. Due to the climate, solar dermatitis is one of the 10 most frequent dermatoses among Mexicans. Patients are encouraged to use sun protection measures, including hats, sunglasses, umbrellas, and broad-spectrum sunscreens. Such photoprotective measures will also aid in the treatment of melasma, which, although asymptomatic, may have a social and psychological impact on individuals in the United States, Mexico, and other Latin American countries.

Because the Hispanic population is growing exponentially in the United States, it is important for dermatologists to understand common cutaneous diseases that occur in Mexico, a geographically contiguous country. Hispanic Americans are an ethnolinguistic group; the association with Mexico used here is an imperfect example that may be useful for dermatologists treating Hispanic patients, as well as for those treating patients living in other Latin American countries.

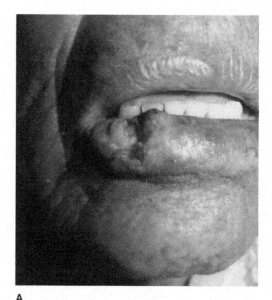

A

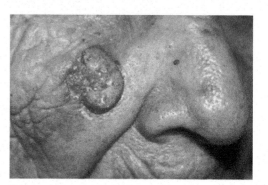

B

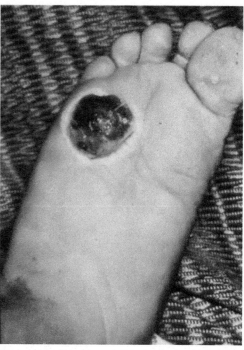

C

FIGURE 93A-16. **(A)** Squamous cell carcinoma of the lip. **(B)** Squamous cell carcinoma of the cheek. **(C)** Nodular distal melanoma of the sole.

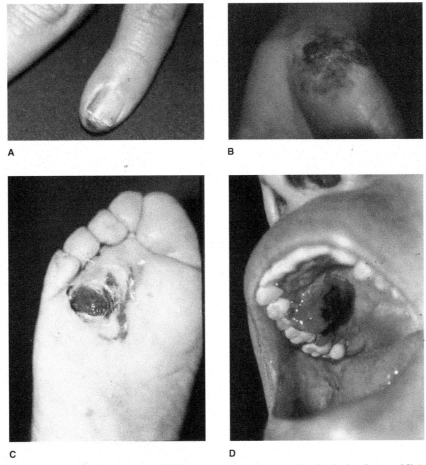

FIGURE 93A-17. (A) Acral lentiginous melanoma affecting the nail. **(B)** Acral lentiginous melanoma with a distal palmar location. **(C)** Acral advanced, ulcerated, lentiginous melanoma. **(D)** Mucosal oral melanoma.

REFERENCES

1. Central Intelligence Agency. The World Factbook: Mexico. www.cia.gov/library/publications/the-world-factbook/geos/mx.html. Accessed February 22, 2015.

2. Arellano I, Peniche A, eds. *Lecciones de Dermatología de Saúl.* 15th ed. Mexico City, Mexico: Mendez Editores; 2008.

3. Hojyo-Tomoka T, Granados J, Vargas-Alarcón G, et al. Further evidence of the role of HLA-DR4 in the genetic susceptibility to actinic prurigo. *J Am Acad Dermatol.* 1997;36:935-937.

4. Castañedo-Cazares JP. Actinic prurigo. www.emedicine.medscape.com/article/1120153-overview. Accessed January 22, 2013.

5. Ramírez CO, López L, Estado DG. Actual de la dermatosis cenicienta: sinonimia-erytema discromicum perstans. *Med Cutan Ibero Lat Am.* 1984;12:11.

6. Schwartz RA. Erythema dyschromicum perstans: the continuing enigma of Cinderella or ashy dermatosis. *Int J Dermatol.* 2004;43:230-232.

7. Saul A. La dermatología en los paises tropicales. *Dermatol Rev Mex.* 1989;2:3.

8. Arellano-Mendoza MI, Tirado Sánchez A, Mercadillo Pérez P, et al. Motivo de consulta: manchas hipercrómicas en la cara. *Dermatol Rev Mex.* 2011;54:180-184.

9. Grimes PE. Melasma: etiologic and therapeutic considerations. *Arch Dermatol.* 1995;131:1453-1457.

10. Navarrete-Solís J, Castanedo-Cázares JP, Torres-Álvarez B, et al. A double-blind, randomized clinical trial of niacinamide 4% versus hydroquinone 4% in the treatment of melasma. *Dermatol Res Pract.* 2011;2011:379173.

11. Katsambas A, Antoniou C. Melasma: classification and treatment. *J Eur Acad Dermatol Venereol.* 1995;4:217-223.

12. Bonifaz A, Archer-Dubon C, Saúl A. Tinea imbricata or Tokelau. *Int J Dermatol.* 2004;43:506-510.

13. Velasco-Castrejón O, González-Ochoa A. [Tinea imbricata in the mountains of Puebla, Mexico]. *Rev Invest Salud Publica.* 1976;35:109-116.

14. Cestari TF, Hexsel D, Viegas ML, et al. Validation of a melasma quality of life questionnaire for Brazilian Portuguese language: the MelasQoL-BP study and improvement of QoL of melasma patients after triple combination therapy. *Br J Dermatol.* 2006;156:13-20.

15. Hexsel D, Arellano I, Rendon M. Ethnic considerations in the treatment of Hispanic and Latin-American patients with hyperpigmentation. *Br J Dermatol.* 2006;156:7-12.

16. Bonifaz A, Tirado-Sánchez A, Calderón L, et al. Mycetoma: experience of 482 cases in a single center in Mexico. *PLoS Negl Trop Dis.* 2014;8:e3102.

17. López-Martínez R, Méndez-Tovar LJ, Bonifaz A, et al. [Update on the epidemiology of mycetoma in Mexico: a review of 3933 cases]. *Gac Med Mex.* 2013;149:586-592.

18. Bonifaz A, Ibarra G, Saúl A, et al. Mycetoma in children: experience with 15 cases. *Pediatr Infect Dis J.* 2007;26:50-52.

19. Cortez KJ, Roilides E, Quiroz-Telles F, et al. Infections caused by Scedosporium spp. *Clin Microbiol Rev.* 2008;21:157-197.

20. Novales J. [Dermatopathology's contribution to the knowledge of mycetomas]. *Med Cutan Ibero Lat Am.* 1995;23:248-252.

21. DermNet New Zealand Trust. Mycetoma. www.dermnetnz.org/fungal/mycetoma.html. Accessed February 22, 2015.

22. Welsh O. Mycetoma: current concepts in treatment. *Int J Dermatol.* 1991;30:387-398.

23. González Benavides J. La esporotricosis enfermedad ocupacional de los alfareros. *Rev Hosp Univ (Monterrey).* 1952;2:215-232.

24. Romero-Cabello R, Bonifaz A, Romero-Feregrino R, et al. Disseminated sporotricosis. *BMJ Case Rep.* 2011;2011.

25. Barros MB, de Almeida Paes R, Schubach AO. Sporothrix schenckii and sporotrichosis. *Clin Microbiol Rev.* 2011;24:633-654.

26. Vega ME, Waxtein L, Arenas R, et al. Ashy dermatosis and lichen planus pigmentosus: a clinicopathologic study of 31 cases. *Int J Dermatol.* 1992;31:90-94.

27. Baranda L, Torres-Alvarez B, Cortes-Franco R, et al. Involvement of cell adhesion and activation molecules in the pathogenesis of erythema dyschromicum perstans (ashy dermatitis): the effect of clofazimine therapy. *Arch Dermatol.* 1997;133:325-329.

28. Braun-Falco O, Plewig G, Wolff HH, et al. Fungal diseases. In: Braun-Falco O, Plewig G, Wolff HH, et al, eds. *Dermatology.* Berlin, Germany: Springer Science & Business Media; 2000:344-345.

29. Toriello C, Arjona-Rosado LC, Díaz-Gómez ML, et al. Efficiency of crude and purified fungal antigens in serodiagnosis to discriminate mycotic from other respiratory diseases. *Mycoses.* 1991;34:133-140.

30. Mahajan VK. Sporotrichosis: an overview and therapeutic options. *Dermatol Res Pract.* 2014;2014:272376.

31. Vásquez-del-Mercado E, Arenas R, Padilla-Desgarenes C. Sporotrichosis. *Clin Dermatol.* 2012;30:437-443.

32. Saúl A. Sporotrichosis. In: Jacobs P, Nail L, eds. *Antifungal Drug Therapy: A Complete Guide for the Practitioner.* New York, NY: Marcel Dekker Inc.; 1990:53-60.

33. World Health Organization. Tuberculosis profile: Mexico. https://extranet. who.int/sree/Reports?op=Replet&name=%2FWHO_HQ_Reports%2FG%2 2FPROD%2FEXT%2FTBCountryProfile&ISO2=MX&LAN=EN&outtype= pdf. Accessed February 24, 2015.

34. Hernández Solis A, Herrera González NE, Cazarez F, et al. Skin biopsy: a pillar in the identification of cutaneous *Mycobacterium tuberculosis* infection. *J Infect Dev Ctries.* 2012;6:626-631.

35. Saul A. La tuberculosis ayer y hoy. *Dermatol Rev Mex.* 1996;40:249-250.

36. Dias MF, Bernardes Filho F, Quaresma MV, et al. Update on cutaneous tuberculosis. *An Bras Dermatol.* 2014;89:925-938.

37. Almaguer-Chávez J, Ocampo-Candiani J, Rendón A. [Current panorama in the diagnosis of cutaneous tuberculosis]. *Actas Dermosifiliogr.* 2009;100:562-570.

38. Nachbar F, Cassen V, Nachbar T, et al. Orificial tuberculosis: detection by polymerase chain reaction. *Br J Dermatol.* 1996;135:106-109.

39. World Health Organization. Weekly epidemiological record: global leprosy: update on the 2012 situation. www.who.int/wer/2013/wer8835.pdf?ua=1. Accessed February 25, 2015.

40. Larrea MR, Carreño MC, Fine PE. Patterns and trends of leprosy in Mexico: 1989-2009. *Lepr Rev.* 2012;83:184-194.

41. World Health Organization. Leprosy elimination: leprosy today. www.who. int/lep/en. Accessed February 25, 2015.

42. National Institute of Allergy and Infectious Diseases. Leprosy (Hansen's disease): history of the disease. www.niaid.nih.gov/topics/leprosy/Understanding/Pages/history.aspx. Accessed February 25, 2015.

43. Rafferty J. Curing the stigma of leprosy. *Lepr Rev.* 2005;76:119-126.

44. World Health Organization. Leishmaniasis: Mexico. www.who.int/leishmaniasis/resources/MEXICO.pdf. Accessed February 25, 2015.

45. Hernández-Rivera MP, Hernández-Montes O, Chiñas-Pérez A, et al. Study of cutaneous leishmaniasis in the State of Campeche (Yucatan Peninsula), Mexico, over a period of two years. *Salud Publica Mex.* 2015;57:58-65.

46. World Health Organization. Control of the leishmaniases: report of a WHO Expert Committee. http://whqlibdoc.who.int/trs/WHO_TRS_793.pdf. Accessed February 25, 2015.

47. Silveira FT, Lainson R, Corbett CE. Clinical and immunopathological spectrum of American cutaneous leishmaniasis with special reference to the disease in Amazonian Brazil: a review. *Mem Inst Oswaldo Cruz.* 2004;99:239-251.

48. Caumes E. Treatment of cutaneous larva migrans. *Clin Infect Dis.* 2000;30: 811-814.

49. Peniche J. Tumores de la piel. In: Arellano I, Peniche A, eds. *Lecciones de Dermatología de Saúl.* 14th ed. México City, Mexico: Mendez Editores; 2001:650.

50. Miller S, Moresi JM. Actinic keratosis, basal cell carcinoma and squamous cell carcinoma. In: Bolognia JL, Jorisso JL, Rapini RP, eds. *Dermatology.* St Louis, MO: Mosby; 2003:1677.

51. Pinedo JL, Castañeda R, McBride LE, et al. Estimates of the skin cancer incidence in Zacatecas, México. *Open Dermatol J.* 2009;3:58-62.

52. Alfeiran Ruiz A, Escobar Alfaro G, de la Barreda BF, et al. Epidemiología del melanoma de piel en México. *Rev Inst Nac Cancerol (Mex).* 1998;44:168-174.

53. Schmerling RA, Loria D, Cinat G, et al. Cutaneous melanoma in Latin America: the need for more data. *Rev Panam Salud Publica.* 2011;30:431-438.

54. Káram-Orantes M, Toussaint-Caire S, Domínguez-Cherit J, et al. [Clinical and histopathological characteristics of malignant melanoma cases seen at "Dr. Manuel Gea González" General Hospital]. *Gac Med Mex.* 2008;144:219-223.

55. Gutiérrez Vidrio RM. Cáncer de piel. *Rev Fac Med UNAM.* 2003;46:166-171.

56. González Cervantes JG, Mora Tiscareño A, Beltrán Ortega A. [261 cases of cutaneous malignant melanoma: general characteristics and prognostic factor values]. *Rev Inst Nac Cancerol (Mex).* 1990;36:1103-1112.

Cosmetic Procedures and Treatments in North America: Mexico

Francisco Pérez-Atamoros
Claudio Cayetano Martinez

KEY POINTS

- The Mexican population is used here as an example of a Latin American population. This population is used as an example of the dermatologic cosmetic procedures that may be used among Hispanics in the United States and other populations of Latin American origin living elsewhere.

- Many Latin American individuals have darkly pigmented skin; this means that the clinical manifestations of photoaging are less apparent than among fairer-skinned individuals.

- In Mexican patients with Fitzpatrick skin types III, IV, and V, the most frequently obtained cosmetic procedures are chemical peels (for treating melasma and dyspigmentation), botulinum toxin, and laser therapy.

- The cosmetic use of botulinum toxin has become more accessible. Patients are interested in procedures that will not only improve their facial features but also ensure a more youthful appearance without permanent side effects.

- Superficial chemical peels are used to increase the results of cosmetic procedures because they are a low-cost adjuvant treatment. However, for treating depigmentation, these peels should not be used by themselves.

- The main challenge of treating patients with skin phototypes III, IV, or V with laser therapy is to deliver efficacious and reproducible results while minimizing unwanted adverse reactions.

INTRODUCTION

The term Latino denotes an ethnolinguistic group with origins in the countries of Latin America as well as individuals in the United States who self-identify as Hispanic. Although many people blend racial and ethnic categories in describing Latino/Hispanic individuals interchangeably, these terms actually indicate an ethnic category, rather than a particular race. It is therefore important to understand the differences between these two terms. According to Coon[1] in a 1962 publication called *The Origin of Races*, there are four major races of humans: Asian/ Mongoloid; Australoid; Black/Negroid; and White/Caucasian.

However, in 1950, in the first of four statements on issues of race commonly known as *The Race Question*, the United Nations Educational, Scientific, and Cultural Organization (UNESCO) stated that "National, religious, geographic, linguistic and cultural groups do not necessarily coincide with racial groups and the cultural traits of such groups have not demonstrated genetic connection with racial traits."[2] UNESCO then went on to suggest that the term race should be dropped altogether and that ethnic groups be used instead.[2] Subsequently, the 1951 revised version of the UNESCO statement went on to clarify the issue. While it was still agreed that "race, as a word, has become coloured by its misuse in connexion with national, linguistic and religious differences, and by its deliberate abuse by racialists,"[2] experts nevertheless were of the opinion that the term was still needed as an anthropologic classification of groups showing definite and characteristic combinations of biological, physical, and physiological traits.[2]

In 1964, the third UNESCO statement proposed that differences between individuals within a race were often greater than the average differences between races; they continued by stating that no national, religious, geographic, linguistic, or cultural group constituted a race and that the concept of race was purely biological.[2] In a final statement in 1967, experts were of the opinion that the division of human beings into races was based on conventional and arbitrary classifications, even stating that many scientists believed racial divisions to be of limited scientific interest and potentially inviting risky generalizations.[2]

With this information in mind, the terms Latino and Hispanic are used as indicators of ethnic groups for the purposes of this chapter. According to a study in 1998, there are more than 5000 ethnic groups globally.[3] In the United States, a "brown" category has been informally constructed for describing Hispanics; however, this is not an anthropologically based group.

The Mexican population is used here as an example of a Latin American population. This chapter focuses on this population in order to give an approximate idea of the dermatologic cosmetic procedures that may be used among Hispanics and people of Latin American origin who live in other countries.

Mexico is located in the southern part of North America, bordered to the north by the United States and in the southeast by Belize and Guatemala.

Its geography is associated with excessive solar radiation. Mexico receives high levels of ultraviolet (UV) radiation almost all year round according the Global Solar UV Index [**Figure 93B-1**].[4,5] Mexico's urban climate is also influenced by its elevation, which is about 2000 m above sea level. The high UV levels are also augmented by latitude, cloud cover, altitude, ozone, and ground reflection.

SUN DAMAGE IN THE MEXICAN POPULATION

In Mexico, sunscreen is prescribed by many medical specialists, including dermatologists, rheumatologists, pediatricians, and gynecologists. However, the therapeutic properties of different sunscreens are unknown because sun protection creams are not considered a prescription drug but, instead, a beauty product. The sun protection factor in some of these products has been found to be lower than that stated on the label, resulting in patients potentially using these products with a false sense of security.[6,7] High UV radiation and lack of effective sun protection

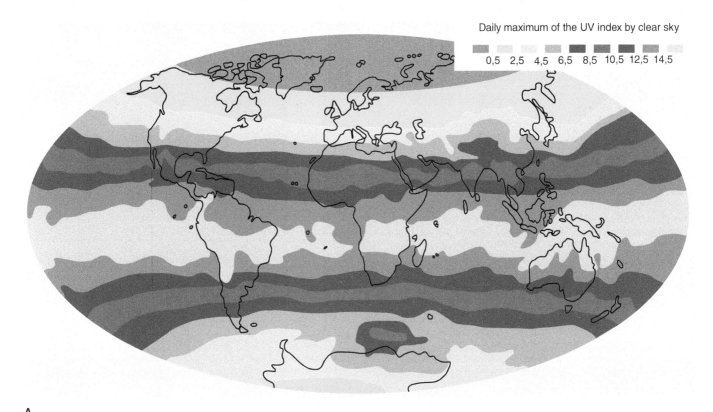

A

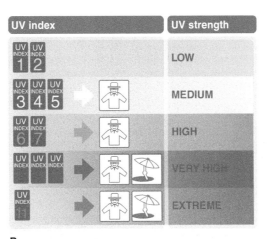

B

FIGURE 93B-1. **(A)** Global Solar Ultraviolet (UV) Index. (Reproduced with permission from Emmanuelle Bournay, GRID-Arendal. UV Index Worldmap. Found at http://www.grida.no/graphicslib/detail/uv-index-worldmap_1582.[4]) **(B)** General sun protection measures according to solar UV exposure. (Reproduced with permission from World Health Organization, World Meteorological Organization, United Nations Environment Programme and International Commission on Non-Ionizing Radiation Protection. Global Solar UV Index: A Practical Guide.[5])

accelerate the aging process; this may also be exacerbated by the higher rate of cigarette use, poor nutrition, and exposure to airborne particles in Mexico.[8]

The process of aging involves a progressive decrease in the maximal functioning and reserve capacity of all organs in the body, including the skin. Photoaging, which dermatologists can control, is the superposition of chronic UV-induced damage on intrinsic aging and accounts for most age-associated changes in skin appearance. With advancing years, an aged appearance is often the presenting complaint for people with lighter skin. This group is often affected by the secondary effects of photoaging: fine wrinkles, deep furrows, hyperpigmentation, and age spots. However, a high percentage of Latinos/Hispanics have darkly pigmented skin; hence, clinical manifestations of photoaging are less apparent clinically, and photoaging may become obvious 10 or 20 years later than in lighter-skinned individuals of the same age.[9]

All Fitzpatrick skin phototypes are represented within Latino/Hispanic populations, but phototypes III, IV, and V are the most prevalent. Despite the lack of precision in the Fitzpatrick classification system, it helps to express the great variability in Mexico's population as well as among the greater Latino/Hispanic population. At a more fundamental level, the descendants of Mexico's indigenous population have a certain advantage in that the photoprotective response stimulated by exposure to DNA-damaging UV irradiation creates skin pigmentation.

BOTULINUM TOXIN

The advent of botulinum toxin (BTX) in the 1990s effectively launched the modern era of nonsurgical aesthetic medicine. Many of the undesirable components of a senescent face, which previously required surgical intervention, are now readily addressed with neurotoxins. The wide acceptance of BTX has paved the way for the adoption of numerous other injectables, which are now common in dermatologists' offices.[10] Latin American patients increasingly demand the most common cosmetic procedures available. Cosmetic procedures have become more accessible, and more patients are looking to not only improve their facial features but also to get a more youthful appearance without permanent side effects.

BTX was brought by Francisco Pérez-Atamoros to Mexico and then broadcasted by his colleagues to the rest of the country and others in Latin America. Practically speaking, the application of BTX in this population results in few of the side effects suffered by other populations. Additionally, since this substance acts directly within the muscles, there is little risk of dyspigmentation. Of the small percentage of dermatologists and plastic surgeons in Mexico who have the ability to apply BTX, 90% focus the treatment in the upper third of the face, despite the more common technique of applying BTX in the middle and lower thirds of the face.

Latino/Hispanic males represent a very low percentage of the total number of patients receiving BTX applications; this may be in part due to the concept of machismo, which is very common among this social group. However, many patients among the rest of the population choose to return for a "free" reapplication of the neurotoxin following the initial successful BTX application, no matter the outcome. This means that the majority of patients lack experience with this procedure and often hold erroneous beliefs regarding the effectiveness of BTX if the reapplication is not performed.

This chapter focuses on some of the BTX application procedures that Pérez-Atamoros first implemented to improve lip wrinkles (upper and lower), nose tip lifting, and breast lifting in 1997, 2000, and 2002, respectively. Special considerations need to be given to Latino/Hispanic patients when injecting BTX, because some patients have individual characteristics or special requirements that must be taken into consideration when working with this neurotoxin.

FACE

BTX should be used in the middle and lower areas of the face. Additionally, it is important to remember that lower concentrations will encourage the spread of the toxin [**Figure 93B-2**].[11,12]

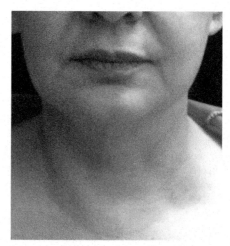

A

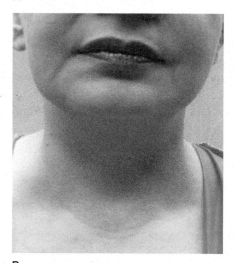

B

FIGURE 93B-2. The border depressor anguli oris area and neck in a female patient (**A**) before the application of botulinum toxin and (**B**) after.

FOREHEAD AND GLABELLA AREAS

In Latino/Hispanic patients, BTX must be injected in the medial area or upper part of the forehead and in the upper part of the corrugators. This is due to the anatomy of these muscles, as they have more volume in the lower part of the muscles and a lower insertion point. The application must be at least 2 or 3 cm over the brows to avoid bruising in the upper lid and lion's wrinkle [**Figure 93B-3**].[11]

CROW'S FEET

Application of BTX for these wrinkles can be undertaken using the standard technique; however, dermatologists should be very careful when dealing with the lower application point of the eyelid, because insertions in the zygomaticus major are very high and sometimes entwine with the orbicularis oculi. For that reason, it can be easy to accidentally paralyze the zygomaticus major by diffusion and create an asymmetric face [**Figure 93B-4**].[11]

MEDIAL AND LOWER FACE

Latino/Hispanic patients need fewer units of BTX in this region than in the rest of the face because the muscles of these areas are more sensitive to the neurotoxin. For example, to treat wrinkles in the lips, the general recommendation is to apply 4 to 8 IU. However, for the upper lip, a dose of 2 to 4 IU for the same area is enough to guarantee 100% effectiveness and duration. Aging can result in the loss of soft tissue. By using injectable fillers after botulinum toxin application, dermatologists can lift the cheeks and restore lost volume [**Figure 93B-5**].[11]

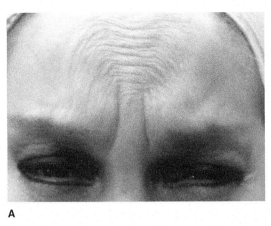

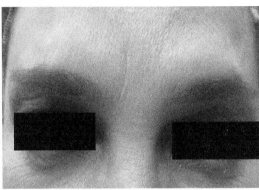

FIGURE 93B-3. The glabella/forehead area in a female patient **(A)** before the application of botulinum toxin and **(B)** after.

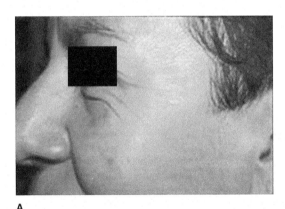

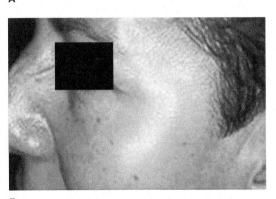

FIGURE 93B-4. Photographs demonstrating the reduced effect of crow's feet **(A)** before and **(B)** after the application of botulinum toxin.

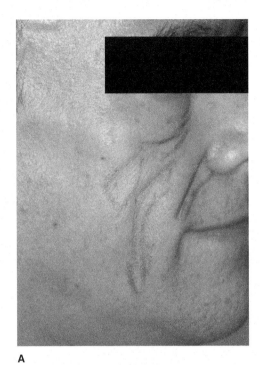

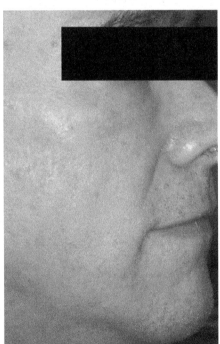

FIGURE 93B-5. Photographs showing a male patient **(A)** before and **(B)** after the application of a hyaluronic acid filler.

LIPS

There are two principal techniques to apply BTX to the lips. The first involves the application of the neurotoxin directly to the orbicularis oris muscle, with the dose depending on the number and depth of the wrinkles and, of course, the size of the lip. For the upper lip, the range is 2 to 4 IU of onabotulinum toxin A or 4 to 8 IU of abobotulinum toxin A; for the lower lip, the range is 2 to 6 IU of onabotulinum toxin A or 4 to 12 IU of abobotulinum toxin A. The second technique is to apply the BTX to the border of the lip to create a full aspect, similar to the filler application. The application of several injection points with 0.5 IU of onabotulinum toxin A or 1 IU of abobotulinum toxin A, similar to the upper and lower lips, is strongly recommended [**Figure 93B-6**].[11]

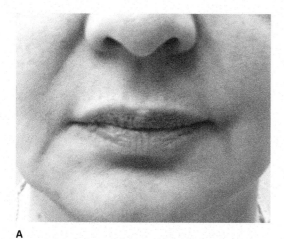

A

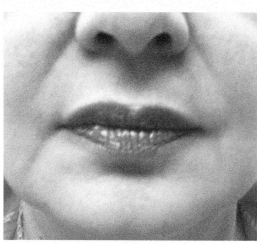

B

FIGURE 93B-6. The border lips and depressor anguli oris in a female patient (**A**) before the application of botulinum toxin and (**B**) after.

NOSE TIP LIFTING

The technique for lifting up the apex of the nose is to inject BTX in three points of the nose, including the alar portion of the nasalis bilaterally and the depressor septi nasi. If the BTX is just applied to the depressor septi muscle, the fixing action of the allar portion of the nasalis will stop this lifting. Depending of the anatomy of the patient's nose, the nose tip lifting can also be performed by using fillers alone **Figure 93B-7**, BTX alone, or in combination of both. Age-related loss of soft tissue is most noticable in the lips and the nasolabial and melolabial folds.[11]

BREAST LIFTING

The application of BTX to the pectoralis major is the most popular technique to lift the breasts. The pectoralis major is the largest muscle in the chest with a contraction vector from the diaphragm muscle to the shoulder; the application of BTX to the inferior and parasternum part of the pectoralis major will paralyze this area, promoting the contraction of the shoulder and moving the breast in an upward direction [**Figure 93B-8**].[11,13]

CHEMICAL PEELS

Increasingly, Latino/Hispanic individuals with melanocompetent skin are seeking out cosmetic measures to provide epidermal and color enhancement to their skin. Pigmentary conditions are some of the most frequent dermatologic concerns among Latino/Hispanic patients, with melasma being the most common [**Figure 93B-9**]. Although chemical peels may improve disorders like hyperpigmentation by removing

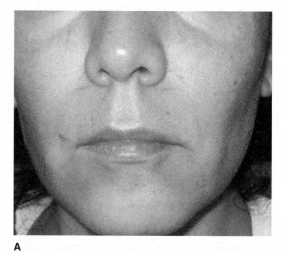

A

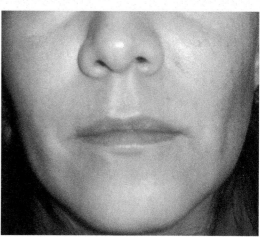

B

FIGURE 93B-7. Photographs showing a female patient (**A**) before and (**B**) after the application of a hyaluronic acid filler in the nasolabial and melolabial folds to restore volume in these areas.

unwanted melanin and signs of photoaging, they can also cause irritation that can lead to postinflammatory hyperpigmentation or hypopigmentation if not performed expertly. Therefore, superficial chemical peels may be used as a low-cost adjuvant treatment for treating dyspigmentation, although they should not be used as a single measure.

The depth of the peel depends on two main factors: the amount of solution used and the duration of time that the solution remains on the skin. Typically, chemical peels are performed monthly using gradually increasing concentrations. Titrating the concentration to the desired effect needs to be balanced with the patient's tolerance to the chemical peel—increasing the depth of the peel increases the risk of developing dyspigmentation and scarring. To avoid undesired consequences, the patient's complete medical history should be taken, including any history of keloid scarring, herpes simplex viral infections, and any recent isotretinoin therapy, in addition to asking about sensitivity to photosensitizing drugs.

RESORCINOL PEELS

Superficial chemical peels can be accomplished via the application of many agents. Resorcinol peels are one of the most commonly used substances for hyperpigmentation disorders in Latino/Hispanic patients and are considered the gold standard by many dermatologists. Resorcinol is related to phenol both structurally and chemically and is a highly effective tyrosinase inhibitor for the topical treatment of hyperpigmentation.

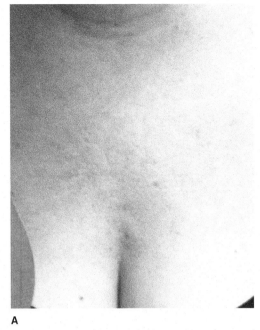

A

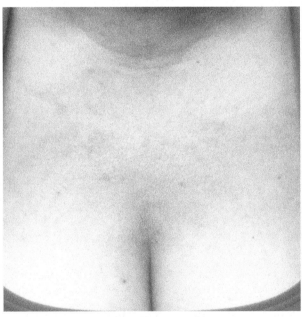

B

FIGURE 93B-8. The décolleté of a female patient **(A)** before the application of botulinum toxin and **(B)** after.

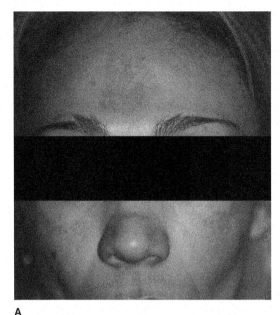

A

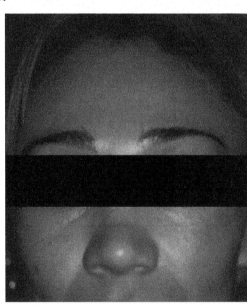

B

FIGURE 93B-9. Melasma is a common skin condition that results in facial discoloration. The photographs demonstrate the marked reduction in dyspigmentation in a young woman **(A)** before and **(B)** after a chemical peel.

The best results are achieved in patients with Fitzpatrick skin types I to IV.[14] Resorcinol combined with sulfur is considered a superficial peel that can be applied more than once over a short time period so as to achieve superior results. Consequently, this combination is considered a rewarding medium-depth peel to diminish oleaginous skin and ameliorate dyspigmentation.[15]

GLYCOLIC ACID PEELS

Glycolic acid peels (GAPs) are α-hydroxy acids with low to moderate short-term effects for melasma and pigmentary disorders. Using increasing concentrations, GAPs may be useful as an adjuvant for topical therapy, especially if patients are pretreated with hydroquinone for 2 weeks before the procedure, or when used in combination with a modified Kligman-Willis formula (hydroquinone 5%, tretinoin 0.05%, and hydrocortisone acetate 0.1%).[16-22]

SALICYLIC ACID PEELS

Salicylic acid peels are β-hydroxy acids; however, they have not been shown to add any significant benefit to topical therapy alone in patients with melasma and do not appear to be effective as a monotherapy.[23,24]

OTHER CHEMICAL PEELS

Other chemical peels include tretinoin 1%, Jessner solution (composed of salicylic acid, lactic acid, and ethanol), and 10% to 50% trichloroacetic acid. Tretinoin and Jessner solution peels have not been shown to be any more efficacious than GAPs in clinical studies, although this is controversial.[25-28]

LASER AND LIGHT THERAPIES

The challenge of treating patients with skin phototypes III to V with laser therapy is to deliver efficacious and reproducible results while minimizing unwanted adverse reactions. The use of longer wavelengths is

TABLE 93B-1   Common lasers used to treat patients with skin of color in Mexico

Laser	Wavelength (nm)	Target chromophore	Skin phototypes	Applications
Vascular				
Variable-pulsed KTP	532	Oxyhemoglobin (long-pulsed) Melanin/pigment (Q-switched)	All phototypes	Facial telangiectasias; venous malformations; cherry angiomas
Pulsed dye	585, 590, 595, 600	Oxyhemoglobin	All phototypes	Port wine stains; telangiectasias; scars; verrucae
Long-pulsed Nd:YAG	1064	Oxyhemoglobin	All phototypes	Venulectasias; telangiectasias; blue reticular veins
Diode	800	Oxyhemoglobin	All phototypes	Spider leg veins; venulectasias
Hair removal				
Diode	800, 810	Melanin	All phototypes	
Nd:YAG	1064	Melanin	All phototypes	
Fractional				
Fractional Er-doped fiber	1550	Water	Use with caution in phototypes IV and above	Resurfacing; scars; rhytides/wrinkles; dyspigmentation
Nonablative				
Nd:YAG	1064	Dermal collagen Water	All phototypes	Resurfacing; scars; keloids
Ablative				
CO_2	10,600	Water	Use with caution in phototypes IV and above	Total ablative resurfacing
Er:YAG	2940	Water	Use with caution in phototypes IV and above	Total ablative resurfacing

Abbreviations: CO_2, carbon dioxide; Er, erbium; Er:YAG, erbium-doped yttrium-aluminum-garnet; KTP, potassium titanyl phosphate; Nd:YAG, neodymium-doped yttrium-aluminum-garnet.

Source: Adapted with permission from Rossi AM, Perez MI. Laser therapy in Latino or Hispanic skin. *Facial Plast Surg Clin North Am*. 2011 May;19(2):389-403.[29]

essential when treating these skin phototypes. Laser treatments should be patiently tailored for each melanocompetent patient, and the use of test spots is encouraged before commencing treatment because there is no "one parameter fits all" approach. Learning curves are different for each laser, so dermatologists should become familiar with each system before starting treatment [**Table 93B-1**]. For that reason, ablative and fractional laser procedures should be used by experienced physicians only, and with caution in any patients with pigmented skin. Furthermore, these lasers should be used carefully on individuals with skin types V and VI [**Figure 93B-10**].[29]

Various limitations are noted in the availability of certain lasers and the cost of treatments, as well as restrictions and parameters related to each patient's phototype. In the experience of the authors, therapy for recalcitrant melasma combines high doses of hydroquinone (ranging from 8% to 20%) with intense pulsed light therapy every 2 weeks, along with neodymium-doped yttrium-aluminum-garnet (Nd:YAG) therapy at 1064 nm.[30] This controversial but effective treatment provides modest to excellent results and photoprotective measures. Several studies have shown that the 1064-nm Q-switched (QS) Nd:YAG is well absorbed by melanin and, being a longer wavelength, causes minimal damage to the

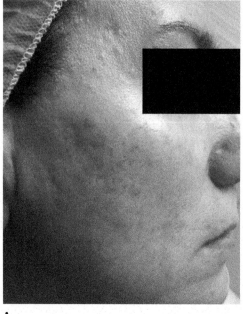
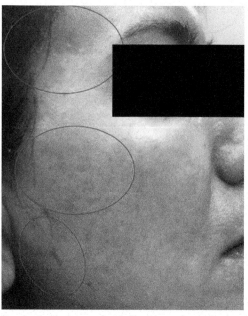

A   B

FIGURE 93B-10. Lasers are sometimes used to reduce the appearance of acne scars. The photographs demonstrate the efficacy of fractional carbon dioxide laser therapy in the reduction in scarring in a young woman **(A)** before and **(B)** after treatment.

epidermis and is not absorbed by hemoglobin. The deeper skin penetration is also helpful to target dermal melanin.

Low-dose QS-Nd:YAG laser also induces sublethal injury to melanosomes, causing fragmentation and rupture of the melanin granules into the cytoplasm. This effect is highly selective for melanosomes, because this wavelength is well absorbed by melanin relative to other structures.[31] The use of pulsed dye laser (PDL) therapy for the treatment of melasma is based on the theory that skin vascularization plays an important role in the pathogenesis of melasma. Melanocytes express vascular endothelial growth factor receptors 1 and 2, which are involved in the pigmentation process. The PDL, which is mainly used for vascular lesions, targets the vascular component in melasma lesions, decreasing the melanocyte stimulation and reducing subsequent melasma relapses.[32,33]

CONCLUSION

Although the term Hispanic is used in reference to individuals of Latin American origin currently residing in the United States, the term Latino denotes the overall ethnolinguistic group. There are many Latino individuals worldwide, residing in the United States as well as in the various countries of Latin America and elsewhere around the globe. In the United States, the Hispanic patient population is one of the fastest-growing demographics. As a result, physicians of all specialties, including dermatologists, should familiarize themselves with the specific patient concerns and commonly seen conditions of this population. This chapter has focused on the most common cosmetic dermatologic procedures and concerns in Mexico, as an example of Latin Americans who are multi-ethnic and multi-racial.

In Mexico, as well as in other Latin American countries, the most frequently obtained cosmetic procedures are chemical peels, BTX, and laser therapy. While many Latino/Hispanic individuals have darkly pigmented skin, ensuring that the clinical manifestations of photoaging are less apparent than among fairer-skinned individuals, there are still many dermatologic concerns among this population, including wrinkles, melasma, and dyspigmentation. Although UV protective measures such as sunscreen are routinely prescribed by medical specialists in Mexico, sun protection creams are not regulated and are sometimes ineffective. This factor, coupled with the high UV radiation characteristic of the country, can accelerate the aging process.

REFERENCES

1. Coon CS. *The Origin of Races*. New York, NY: Alfred A. Knopf Inc.; 1962.
2. United Nations Educational, Scientific and Cultural Organization. Four statements on the race question. http://unesdoc.unesco.org/images/0012/001229/122962eo.pdf. Accessed February 28, 2015.
3. Doyle R. Ethnic groups in the world. www.scientificamerican.com/article/ethnic-groups-in-the-world/. Accessed February 28, 2015.
4. Emmanuelle Bournay, UNEP/GRID-Arendal. UV Index Worldmap. www.grida.no/graphicslib/detail/uv-index-worldmap_1582. Accessed February 28, 2015.
5. World Health Organization, World Meteorological Organization, United Nations Environment Programme and International Commission on Non-Ionizing Radiation Protection. Global Solar UV Index: a practical guide. www.who.int/uv/publications/en/UVIGuide.pdf. Accessed February 28, 2015.
6. Norma Oficial Mexicana. NOM-141-SSAI-1995. Bienes y servicios. Etiquetado para productos de perfumería y belleza preenvasados. www.salud.gob.mx/unidades/cdi/nom/141ssa15.html. Accessed February 28, 2015.
7. Castanedo-Cázares JP, Torres-Alvarez B, Araujo-Andrade C, et al. [Ultraviolet absorption of prescription sunblocks in Mexico]. *Gac Med Mex.* 2008;144:35-38.
8. Carter-Pokras O, Zambrana RE, Poppell CF, et al. The environmental health of Latino children. *J Pediatr Health Care.* 2007;21:307-314.
9. Elsaie ML, Lloyd HW. Latest laser and light-based advances for ethnic skin rejuvenation. *Indian J Dermatol.* 2008;53:49-53.
10. Carruthers JD, Carruthers JA. Treatment of glabellar frown lines with C. botulinum: a exotoxin. *J Dermatol Surg Oncol.* 1992;18:17-21.
11. Pérez-Atamoros FM, Enriquez Merino J. *Dermatología Cosmética*. Federal District, Mexico: Elsevier; 2011:263-305.
12. Atamoros FP. Botulinum toxin in the lower one third of the face. *Clin Dermatol.* 2003;21:505-512.
13. Benedetto AV, ed. *Botulinum Toxin in Clinical Dermatology*. London, United Kingdom: CRC Press; 2006:219-236.
14. Karam PG. 50% resorcinol peel. *Int J Dermatol.* 1993;32:569-574.
15. Hernandez-Perez E. Different grades of chemical peel. *Am J Cosmetic Surg.* 1990;7:67-70.
16. Usuki A, Ohashi A, Sato H, et al. The inhibitory effect of glycolic acid and lactic acid on melanin synthesis in melanoma cells. *Exp Dermatol.* 2003;12:43-50.
17. Gupta RR, Mahajan BB, Garg G. Chemical peeling: evaluation of glycolic acid in varying concentrations and time intervals. *Indian J Dermatol Venereol Leprol.* 2001;67:28-29.
18. Javaheri SM, Handa S, Kaur I, et al. Safety and efficacy of glycolic acid facial peel in Indian women with melasma. *Int J Dermatol.* 2001;40:354-357.
19. Sarkar R, Kaur C, Bhalla M, et al. The combination of glycolic acid peels with a topical regimen in the treatment of melasma in dark-skinned patients: a comparative study. *Dermatol Surg.* 2002;28:828-832.
20. Erbil H, Sezer E, Taştan B, et al. Efficacy and safety of serial glycolic acid peels and a topical regimen in the treatment of recalcitrant melasma. *J Dermatol.* 2007;34:25-30.
21. Hurley ME, Guevara IL, Gonzales RM, et al. Efficacy of glycolic acid peels in the treatment of melasma. *Arch Dermatol.* 2002;138:1578-1582.
22. Garg VK, Sarkar R, Agarwal R. Comparative evaluation of beneficiary effects of priming agents (2% hydroquinone and 0.025% retinoic acid) in the treatment of melasma with glycolic acid peels. *Dermatol Surg.* 2008;34:1032-1039.
23. Grimes PE. The safety and efficacy of salicylic acid chemical peels in darker racial-ethnic groups. *Dermatol Surg.* 1999;25:18-22.
24. Ahn HH, Kim IH. Whitening effect of salicylic acid peels in Asian patients. *Dermatol Surg.* 2006;32:372-375.
25. Khunger N, Sarkar R, Jain RK. Tretinoin peels versus glycolic acid peels in the treatment of melasma in dark-skinned patients. *Dermatol Surg.* 2004;30:756-760.
26. Lawrence N, Cox SE, Brody HJ. Treatment of melasma with Jessner's solution versus glycolic acid: a comparison of clinical efficacy and evaluation of the predictive ability of Wood's light examination. *J Am Acad Dermatol.* 1997;36:589-593.
27. Sharquie KE, Al-Tikreety MM, Al-Mashhadani SA. Lactic acid chemical peels as a new therapeutic modality in melasma in comparison to Jessner's solution chemical peels. *Dermatol Surg.* 2006;32:1429-1436.
28. Chun EY, Lee JB, Lee KH. Focal trichloroacetic acid peel method for benign pigmented lesions in dark-skinned patients. *Dermatol Surg.* 2004;30:512-516.
29. Rossi AM, Perez MI. Laser therapy in Latino skin. *Facial Plast Surg Clin North Am.* 2011;19:389-403.
30. Nordlund J, Grimes P, Ortonne JP. The safety of hydroquinone. *J Cosmet Dermatol.* 2006;5:168-169.
31. Arora P, Sarkar R, Garg VK, et al. Lasers for treatment of melasma and post-inflammatory hyperpigmentation. *J Cutan Aesthet Surg.* 2012;5:93-103.
32. Plonka PM, Passeron T, Brenner M, et al. What are melanocytes really doing all day long? *Exp Dermatol.* 2009;18:799-819.
33. Passeron T, Fontas E, Kang HY, et al. Melasma treatment with pulsed-dye laser and triple combination cream: a prospective, randomized, single-blind, split-face study. *Arch Dermatol.* 2011;147:1106-1108.

CHAPTER

94

South America: Brazil

Marcia Ramos-e-Silva
Gabriela Munhoz-da-Fontoura
Dóris Hexsel

KEY POINTS

- Latin America has the largest skin of color population outside of the countries of Africa and Asia. Currently, Brazil and other Latin American countries have diverse populations composed of descendants from Europe, Africa, and Asia, along with Brazilian indigenous people.

- Brazilian and other Latin American skin of color populations experience cutaneous problems specific to or more common in people with skin of color. Problems that are due to skin color assume different characteristics from those found in Caucasians.

- Dry skin is a frequent complaint among Latin Americans with skin of color, and large amounts of emollients are often necessary.

- Tropical diseases such as scabies, syphilis, pityriasis versicolor, and tinea corporis may have a different clinical expression in Latin Americans than in other populations.

- Acral lentiginous melanoma is much more common in Latin American skin of color patients and older age groups compared with Caucasian patients and younger age groups.

INTRODUCTION

South America is as varied climatically as it is linguistically and racially [**Figure 94-1**]. Its history as a whole is one that has been affected by indigenous movements as well as colonial influences, and no country reflects this as colorfully as Brazil. Therefore, in this chapter, Brazil has been highlighted as a reflection and representation of South America as a whole.

It is estimated that approximately 2.5 million Amerindians were living in Brazil when the Portuguese first arrived in the country in 1500 and that Portuguese-Amerindian admixing began almost immediately.[1] Brazil originally had a population made up of countless indigenous tribes, and many of these tribes exist even today. The native population was small and dispersed compared to the indigenous population of the Spanish-dominated American regions, which included the Mayans, Incas, and Aztecs. Due to factors resulting from colonization, such as slavery, ethnic cleansing, newly introduced diseases, hunger, and marginalization, the native population has since been reduced to some 200,000 individuals.[2]

After 1550, many Africans were shipped to Brazil as slaves. It is uncertain how many arrived at Brazilian ports, with estimates ranging from 3 to 18 million. Due to the great number of slaves and their widespread miscegenation, Brazil is presently the country with the largest darker skin of color population outside of any country in Africa. As Father Antonio Vieira said in the seventeenth century, "Brazil's body is in America, but its soul is in Africa."[3] Additionally, Brazil experienced a great influx of immigrants from many diverse regions of the world during the nineteenth and twentieth centuries.

Brazilians today can trace their origins from four main sources—Amerindians, Europeans (mostly of Portuguese/Spanish origin), Africans, and Asians—but it is difficult to think of any racial or ethnic groups on Earth whose genetic heritage is not represented in the DNA of Brazilians. This has resulted in immense ethnic and racial variety within Brazilians with all shades of skin color.

In 2010, Brazil had a population of approximately 203,429,773; of these, 47.7% identified themselves as Caucasian, 43.1% as mulatto (a cultural term denoting individuals of mixed European and African ancestry), 7.6% as black or of African origin, 1.1% as Asian, and 0.4% as other ethnicities.[4] However, it is important to note that many individuals classified as Caucasian may also be identified as *mestizo* (individuals of mixed European and Native American ancestry).[5] Additionally, another common cultural term, *zambo*, is used to define people of mixed African and Native American ancestry.[5] It is, therefore, very difficult to characterize Brazilian people with a specific type of skin. Brazilians' *chiaroscuro* skin color population is one of the greatest challenges for those involved in studying the human genome.[6]

The skin of color populations in Brazil suffer from some of the cutaneous problems specific to those descended from Africa. As a matter of fact, Brazilians suffer more than other populations with skin of color in other geographic areas of the world. Additionally, in some cases, specific diseases or lesions in individuals with skin of color assume different characteristics from those found in the skin of individuals of European descent. Some of the problems that affect this large and important segment of the population are discussed below.[3,7]

HYPERTROPHIC SCARS AND KELOIDS

Keloids [**Figure 94-2**] and hypertrophic scars [**Figure 94-3**] represent cicatrization defects that are the result of excessive production by the extracellular matrix and high rate of mitoses of the dermal fibroblasts.[8]

Local tissue tension plays a very important role in the quality of the scars formed after trauma, and keloids are the result of an imbalance in fibroblast proliferation and production by the extracellular matrix in response to trauma.

This growth happens equally in men and women as a result of trauma, burns, surgical excisions, vaccinations, and acne, and keloids are a very frequent problem in Brazil due to the large skin of color and miscegenated population.[8-10] Young skin of color individuals are more prone to scar development,[11] presenting characteristic keloids mainly in the presternal region, but this phenomenon can also be observed among Brazilians of Asian descent. It is uncommon in Brazilians of European descent. In individuals with skin of color, keloids may become large. The patients seek treatment to relieve pain, itching, and restriction of movement; however, the aesthetic aspect is always the most important factor when considering treatment.[10,12]

Familial predisposition may be involved, especially in cases of multiple lesions, which have been reported as more common in individuals with blood type A, and the familial predisposition seems to be related to gene histocompatibility. Prevention is fundamental in patients with a known tendency to develop abnormal and excessive growth.

DRY SKIN

Dry skin, or xerosis [**Figures 94-4** and **94-5**], is a skin condition caused by a reduction of the lipidic mantle, which constitutes the barrier of the stratum corneum, determining increased water loss through the skin.[13-15] Dry skin usually presents scales at the surface and a clear loss of elasticity. If not treated, it may display signs such as cracks, fissures, itching, and the formation of lesions.[16] The probable cause for the reduction of sebum production in females during aging is reduced ovarian activity, which may lead to xerosis. Eccrine sweat glands also become less functional. The aging process makes the skin fragile, as functions of the cutaneous appendixes diminish and weaken.[17] Dry skin is more common in the elderly because, with aging, the stratum corneum tends to reduce the lipidic mantle, weakening the ability to retain water and reducing skin efficiency in maintaining corneous flexibility and elasticity.[18,19]

Xerosis occurs in individuals of both genders regardless of age and is a frequent complaint among skin of color patients, especially when occurring in the lower limbs and face, where the skin becomes grayish (ashy) due to extreme dryness. Often the use of inappropriate emollients and moisturizers, oils, and comedogenic products and inadequate bathing habits lead to worsening of the skin condition, with onset of allergies and acneiform eruptions, among other manifestations common in this group.

Dry skin can be intrinsic or acquired. If intrinsic, dry skin is genetically determined or related to pathologies such as atopic dermatitis,[19-21] hypothyroidism,[22,23] hypoparathyroidism,[24] nontreated diabetes, and kidney problems,[15] among others. When acquired, the skin becomes dry due to external factors such as climate, pollution, and exposure to chemical products that dissolve the lipidic mantle; very hot water and air conditioning, among others factors, can also contribute to dry skin. In Brazil, complaints about dry skin among skin of color patients are very frequent. In most patients, dry skin is related to pathologies, as mentioned above. External factors can worsen the condition, and, in Brazil, climatic factors are most commonly involved.

DYSCHROMIAS

Dyschromias in skin of color may be classified as melanic (with a melanocytic component) or nonmelanic (of other origin). Melanic dyschromia may be subdivided as hyperpigmentation or hypopigmentation that may be caused by natural factors (linked to race), primary factors (due to disorders such as acquired hyperpigmentation, which can be idiopathic familial), and secondary factors (usually entailing the postinflammatory processes).[25-28]

Examples of natural hyperpigmentation of skin of color include hyperpigmentation of the oral mucosa, which can often be confused with

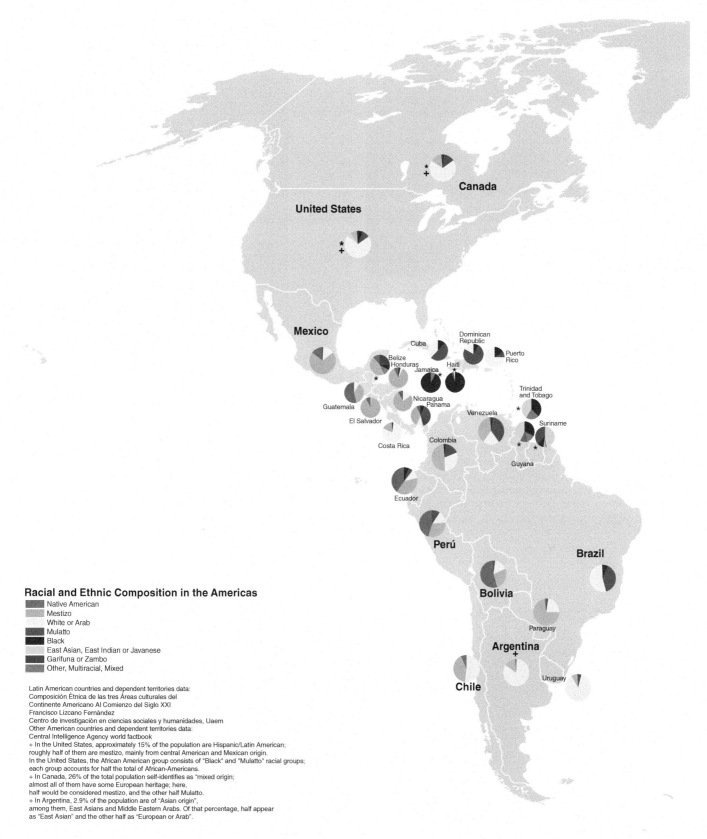

Racial and Ethnic Composition in the Americas

- Native American
- Mestizo
- White or Arab
- Mulatto
- Black
- East Asian, East Indian or Javanese
- Garifuna or Zambo
- Other, Multiracial, Mixed

Latin American countries and dependent territories data:
Composición Ètnica de las tres Áreas culturales del
Continente Americano Al Comienzo del Siglo XXI
Francisco Lizcano Fernàndez
Centro de investigaciòn en ciencias sociales y humanidades, Uaem
Other American countries and dependent territories data:
Central Intelligence Agency world factbook
+ In the United States, approximately 15% of the population are Hispanic/Latin American;
roughly half of them are mestizo, mainly from central American and Mexican origin.
In the United States, the African American group consists of "Black" and "Mulatto" racial groups;
each group accounts for half the total of African-Americans.
+ In Canada, 26% of the total population self-identifies as "mixed origin;
almost all of them have some European heritage; here,
half would be considered mestizo, and the other half Mulatto.
+ In Argentina, 2.9% of the population are of "Asian origin",
among them, East Asians and Middle Eastern Arabs. Of that percentage, half appear
as "East Asian" and the other half as "European or Arab".

FIGURE 94-1. Map of the racial and ethnic composition of the Americas.

diseases that cause areas of dark pigmentation,[29] palmoplantar hyperpigmentation, melanonychia striata, Mongolian macula (observed in 40% to 90% of newborns), and dermatosis papulosa nigra (which is extremely common in Brazil). Melasma is the main hyperpigmentation disorder. Secondary hyperpigmentation may be caused by trauma, allergy, acne vulgaris, psoriasis, pityriasis rosea, lichen planus, seborrheic dermatitis,

atopic dermatitis, keratosis pilaris, superficial fungal infections, topical and systemic medications, and ochronosis induced by hydroquinone, among others, leading to postinflammatory hyperpigmentation.

Skin of color can be affected by natural hypopigmentation, such as the hypochromic mask that can be seen in the middle of the face, the hypochromic triangle of the trapezius area, and linea alba. Primary

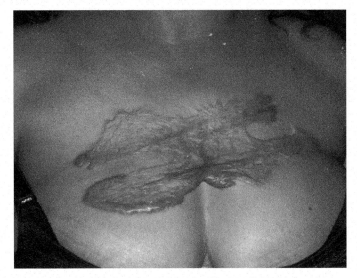

FIGURE 94-2. Keloid fanning beyond the original borders on a female's chest.

depigmented disorders include vitiligo, which is very common in Brazil, and albinism. Hypopigmented disorders include hypopigmented sarcoidosis, which occurs almost exclusively in those of African descent, achromatic pityriasis versicolor, pityriasis alba, pityriasis lichenoides chronica, and idiopathic guttate hypomelanosis, which is most common in those of African descent living in tropical countries.

Examples of secondary hypochromia include iatrogenic hypochromia and hypochromia caused by cosmetics containing depigmenting agents. Among the nonmelanic examples are angiomas, varicosities and telangiectasiaa, tattoos, and hemosiderotic deposits.[28]

All of the above disorders and conditions are extremely frequent in skin of color Brazilians; most people with skin of color with hyperpigmentation, when exposed to sunlight, find that their lesions become darker, whereas those with hypochromia and achromia can experience serious sunburns which are a risk throughout the whole year in most parts of Brazil.

MELASMA

In Brazil and other South American countries, there is a strong racial miscegenation with a high prevalence of melasma in higher phototypes [**Figure 94-6**]. In most Latin American countries, exposure to sunlight

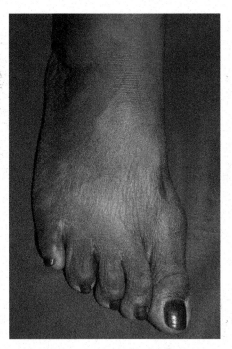

FIGURE 94-4. Senile xerotic skin, or dry skin, can be seen on the foot of this patient.

occurs year-round, usually for professional reasons, such as farming, or as a result of leisure, where, culturally, a tan is considered healthy and beautiful by most of the population. These facts explain the high incidence of melasma in tropical regions.[30]

TRACTION ALOPECIA

Traction alopecia is very common in Brazilian skin of color women who may prefer hairstyles that strain the hair stems, causing hair traction [**Figure 94-7**]. Alopecia is more common in the temporal region or in scalp margins, called marginal alopecia.

Also recognized are cosmetic alopecias, which are caused by vigorous brushing, heat straightening, excessive massage, and curling irons.[31] In

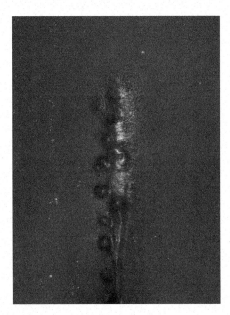

FIGURE 94-3. Postoperative linear hypertrophic scar.

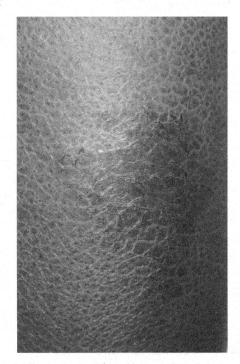

FIGURE 94-5. Xerotic eczematous dermatitis.

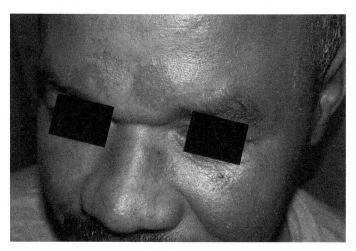

FIGURE 94-6. Melasma in a skin of color male.

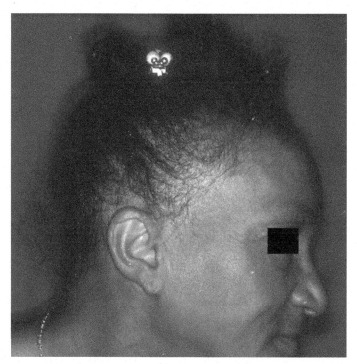

FIGURE 94-7. Traction alopecia in a Brazilian female, which can be the result of hairstyles that strain the hair stems.

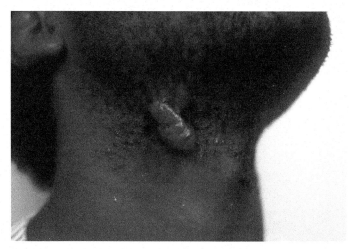

FIGURE 94-8. Pseudofolliculitis of the beard with keloid.

Brazil, it is also very common to make indiscriminate use of chemical products such as formol, which is widely applied in hair styling to straighten curly hair.

PSEUDOFOLLICULITIS OF THE BEARD AND GROIN

Pseudofolliculitis of the beard [**Figure 94-8**] occurs in people who shave frequently. It is a common occurrence in skin of color individuals due to the curly (ulotrichous) hair that penetrates the skin after shaving, leading to secondary folliculitis. Because the hair of those of European descent is not as curly, pseudofolliculitis is infrequent among that population.

In recent years, pseudofolliculitis has been observed in the groin of Brazilian women, occasionally also occurring in the thighs and legs. This is due to the use of ever-shorter bathing suits at Brazilian beaches,[32] leading to depilation of that area, a widespread habit among Brazilian women. To avoid this condition, there is currently an increased demand for definitive depilatory methods, such as laser application.

TROPICAL DISEASES

SCABIES

Scabies, a common disease in developing countries throughout the world, but mainly among poorer populations, is caused by the mite *Sarcoptes scabiei*. It is transmitted through personal contact, without preference for age, gender, or race.[33] In those with skin of color, scabies often becomes a diagnostic challenge because the erythematous papules are hardly visible; the diagnosis should be based on the intense itching, occurring mainly at night, as well as involvement of other family members. In Brazil, as in other countries, scabies occurs commonly in shelters, childcare centers, prisons, and other places with poor hygiene.

SYPHILIS

Syphilis is a contagious venereal treponematosis that leads to internal and cutaneous alterations. It is a universal disease, still frequent in Brazil, without preference for race or gender, caused by *Treponema pallidum*, which is transmitted through sexual contact, congenital transmission, transfusion, and other less frequent means. Its presence increases or decreases with changes of human sexual behavior. The disease can be congenital or acquired and develops in phases (recent and late, or primary, secondary, and tertiary).

In skin of color patients, a circinated or ring configuration may appear, with morphology of the lesions reminding one of geometric forms and associated with hyperchromia; these are called elegant syphilides [**Figures 94-9** and **94-10**]. Hyperchromia frequently persists after the efficient treatment of the disease, remaining an unaesthetic and stigmatizing aspect.

PITYRIASIS VERSICOLOR

Pityriasis versicolor is a superficial mycosis caused by *Malassezia furfur*. It is usually asymptomatic, of universal distribution, and found more frequently in countries with hot and humid tropical climates like Brazil's. It affects both genders of all ages with predominance in young adults. The condition is usually observed after solar exposure, and in Brazil, for this reason, it is known popularly as beach mycosis. It can acquire several shades, which is why it is called versicolor. In individuals with lighter skin, brownish, erythematous, or hypochromic macules are observed, while in darker skin, the lesions are generally hypochromic and often less visible, making their diagnosis more difficult and often leading to the fungus spreading over large areas of skin.

TINEAS

Dermatophytoses are caused by a group of keratinophylic fungi called dermatophytes and affect skin, hair, nails, and mucous membranes. In Brazil, dermatophytoses are common, and the term tinea is frequently used.

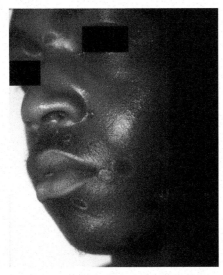

FIGURE 94-9. Elegant syphilides appear as ring configurations on the skin and frequently persist even after successful treatment of the disease.

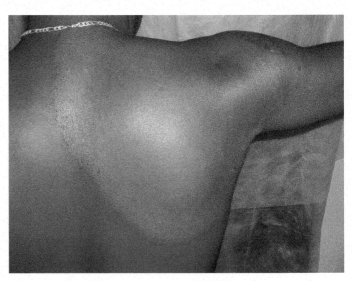

FIGURE 94-11.   Tinea corporis exhibiting a raised erythematosus active border.

They are more common in summer and autumn, with their distribution influenced by geographic factors such as vegetation type and density, the variety of animals present, the density of the human population, soil type, and pluvial region. According to the area of the body affected, tineas are classified as tinea cruris (groin), tinea corporis (body), or tinea pedis (foot), among others. Tineas can involve large areas if not treated and diagnosed promptly, and the lack of clinical signs in skin of color patients, in whose skins the erythema is less apparent, contributes to its spread [**Figure 94-11**].

MELANOMA AND OTHER SKIN CANCERS

Melanoma epidemiology is seldom studied in Brazil, and being a country of continental dimensions and varied racial and ethnic groups, it is difficult to characterize the epidemic profile of this type of cancer. According to Brazil's National Cancer Institute, skin cancer has a greater incidence than any other cancer in Brazil.[34] The main risk factor for melanoma is race.[35] In Brazil, the estimate of melanoma incidence is approximately 4 cases per 100,000 inhabitants, with an increase of 30% from 1978 to 1991.[36] Most patients who seek public health services for melanoma treatment are already in a phase of vertical growth or even of metastases. A 2002 study highlighted public hospital statistics, as most of the Brazilian population is treated in public institutions.[37] The study showed a significantly higher frequency of skin cancers in noncaucasian patients and older age groups. The study demonstrated a high percentage

of acral lentiginous melanomas in public hospitals [**Figure 94-12**], whereas in private clinics, a predominance of Caucasian patients was observed, with fewer patients in the older age groups and a smaller percentage of acral lentiginous melanomas.[37]

In November 2003, the Brazilian Dermatology Society showed that among 37,853 people, 69.9% revealed that they exposed themselves to sunlight without any sort of protection.[38] A total of 3108 new cases of melanoma were detected (8.2%), most of them in men and the 60-year-old age group. Those with skin of color were also polled (n = 2591), with 78.9% stating a failure to use sunscreen or any other sun protection.[38] Of those, 1.7% presented with skin cancer. Of the total skin cancers, 209 cases of melanoma (0.5%), 2448 cases of basal cell carcinoma (6.4%), and 446 cases of squamous cell carcinoma (1.2%) were found[38] [**Figures 94-13** and **94-14**].

According to data from that survey, the northern and northeast regions of Brazil presented the lowest rates of skin cancer, perhaps due to the preponderance of skin of color in those regions, since the higher amount of melanin in darker skin is a natural protection against the disease.[38]

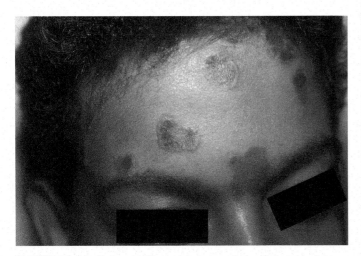

FIGURE 94-10. Elegant syphilides persisting as unaesthetic and stigmatizing lesions.

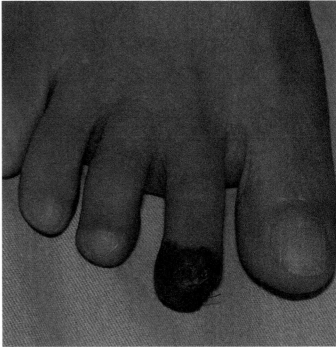

FIGURE 94-12. Melanoma appearing on the toe of a patient with skin of color.

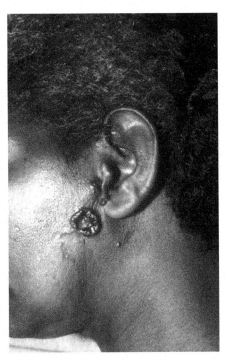

FIGURE 94-13. Basal cell carcinoma in a skin of color female.

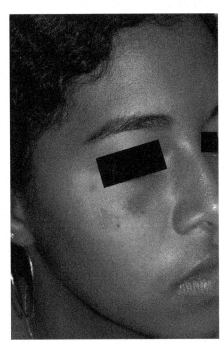

FIGURE 94-15. Postinflammatory hyperpigmentation on the face of a young girl with skin of color.

Because skin cancer is a malignant neoplasia occurring with high incidence in Brazil, it should be considered a public health problem, taking into account the need of resources for its diagnosis and treatment. Campaigns for prevention of skin cancer need to address and put more emphasis on guidance as to protection of skin of color. This information already has been given to lighter-skinned individuals, and individuals with skin of color need to be aware that solar exposure also causes damage to dark skin.

SPECIFIC COSMETIC PRODUCTS FOR SKIN AND HAIR

Skin of color in Brazil has the same characteristics as that in other parts of the world; therefore, data found in the literature may be applied here. The enormous number of individuals with skin of color is reflected in

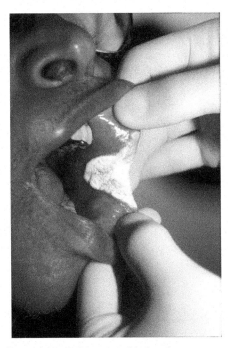

FIGURE 94-14. Squamous cell carcinoma of the buccal mucosa.

the market for cosmetics aimed at those with skin of color.[39] Products specific to those with skin of color have become a market necessity, and the cosmetic industry today is conscientious about development of suitable products for all types of skin during the formulation of cosmetics.[40]

In Brazil, medical and cosmetic products specific to skin of color increasingly arrive on the market and respond to the same problems experienced by skin of color individuals of other countries, while taking into consideration the climate of the country.

A very specific situation requires the need for photoprotection in those with skin of color because they also suffer the damaging effects of sun rays, which are responsible for photoaging and skin cancer,[40] although to a lesser degree than those with lighter skin. Because sun exposure is the main triggering and aggravating factor of melasma and other hyperpigmentation disorders, it is important that people of any skin color always use broad spectrum sunscreens with high sun protection factor.[33,41,42] The amount of melanin in the skin does not completely provide solar protection, and individuals with skin of color must be made aware of the need for photoprotection in the treatment of melasma and postinflammatory hyperpigmentation [**Figure 94-15**].[30,43] This photoprotection should be maintained after the lesions become lighter to avoid recurrence. Individuals should also consider other protective measures, such as the use of photoprotective clothings and hats.

CONCLUSION

Latin America has the largest skin of color population outside of the countries of Africa and Asia. The population is diverse and, like the rest of South America, is composed of descendants from Europe, Africa, and Asia, as well as the Brazilian indigenous people.

Problems that are due to skin of color assume different characteristics from those found in Caucasian individuals. Dry skin, or xerosis, is a frequent complaint in skin of color Brazilians. Typically, the use of inappropriate emollients and moisturizers, oils, and comedogenic products and inadequate bathing habits lead to worsening of the skin condition. In Latin American populations, tropical disease such as scabies, syphilis, pityriasis versicolor, and tinea corporis may exhibit different clinical expressions.

Acral lentiginous melanoma is much more common in Brazilian skin of color patients and older age groups compared with Caucasian patients and younger age groups.

REFERENCES

1. Pena SDJ, Bastos-Rodrigues L, Pimenta JR, et al. DNA tests probe the genomic ancestry of Brazilians. *Braz J Med Biol Res.* 2009;42:870-876.

2. Cáceres F. Os primeiros habitantes do Brazil. In: Cáceres F, ed. *História do Brazil.* São Paulo, Brazil: Editora Moderna; 1995:21-24.

3. Bueno E. *Brazil: Uma História—A Incrível Saga de um País.* São Paulo, Brazil: Ática; 2003:112-123.

4. Central Intelligence Agency. The World Factbook: Brazil. www.cia.gov/library/publications/the-world-factbook/geos/br.html. Accessed June 19, 2014.

5. Fernández FL. Composición Étnica de las Tres Áreas Culturales del Continente Americano al Comienzo del Siglo XXI. *Revista de Ciencias Sociales.* 2005;12:185-232.

6. Azevedo AL. Todas as cores do mundo. *Revista O Globo.* 2010;1:42-45.

7. Cáceres F. O mundo do açúcar. In: Cáceres F, ed. *História do Brazil.* São Paulo, Brazil: Editora Moderna; 1995:42-49.

8. Carneiro SCS, Ramos-e-Silva M. Cicatrização. In: Kede MP, Sabatovich O, eds. *Dermatologia Estética.* Rio de Janeiro, Brazil: Atheneu; 2003:11-20.

9. Sampaio S, Rivitti EA. Tumores mesenquimais e neurais. In: Sampaio S, Rivitti EA, eds. *Dermatologia.* 2nd ed. São Paulo, Brazil: Artes Médicas; 2001:847-868.

10. Martins S. Manejo dos quelóides. In: Gadelha AR, Costa IMC, eds. *Cirurgia Dermatológica em Consultório.* São Paulo, Brazil: Atheneu; 2003:219-222.

11. Barr RJ, Stegman SJ. Delayed skin test reaction to injectable collagen implant (Zyderm). The histopathologic comparative study. *J Am Acad Dermatol.* 1984;10:652-658.

12. Fitzpatrick RE. Treatment of inflamed hypertrophic scars using intralesional 5-FU. *Dermatol Surg.* 1999;25:224-232.

13. Mazereeuw J, Bonafe JL. Xerosis. *Ann Dermatol Venereol.* 2002;129:137-142.

14. Baumann L. Dry skin. In: Baumann L, ed. *Cosmetic Dermatology—Principles and Practice.* New York, NY: McGraw-Hill; 2002:29-32.

15. Magalhães L, Hofmeister H. Avaliação e classificação da pele sã. In: Kede MPV, Sabatovich O, eds. *Dermatologia Estética.* São Paulo, Brazil: Atheneu; 2003:23-42.

16. Norman RA. Xerosis and pruritus in the elderly recognition and management. *Dermatol Ther.* 2003;16:254-259.

17. Cestari TF, Trope BM. The mature adult. In: Parish LC, Brenner S, Ramos-e-Silva M, eds. *Women's Dermatology from Infancy to Maturity.* Lancaster, PA: Parthenon; 2001:72-80.

18. Maibach HI. Pele seca e envelhecimento: O que é verdade e o que não é. *Cosmetic Toiletries.* 1991;3:15-16.

19. Uehara M, Uehara M, Miyauchi H. The morphologic characteristics of dry skin in atopic dermatitis. *Arch Dermatol.* 1984;120:1186-1190.

20. Linde YW. Dry skin in atopic dermatitis. I. A clinical study. *Acta Dermatol Venereol.* 1989;69:311-314.

21. Tagami H. Causas da pele seca. *Cosmetic Toiletries.* 1992;4:26-28.

22. Westphal SA. Unusual presentations of hypothyroidism. *Am J Med Sci.* 1997;314:333-337.

23. Heymann WR, Gans EH, Manders SM, et al. Xerosis in hypothyroidism: a potential role for the use of topical thyroid hormone in euthyroid patients. *Med Hypotheses.* 2001;57:736-739.

24. Jabbour AS. Cutaneous manifestations of endocrine disorders: a guide for dermatologists. *Am J Clin Dermatol.* 2003;4:315-331.

25. McDonald CJ. Structure and function of the skin: are there differences between black and white skin? *Dermatol Clin.* 1988;6:343-347.

26. Grimes PE, Davis LT. Cosmetics in black. *Dermatol Clin.* 1991;9:53-68.

27. Westerhof W. A few more grains of melanin. *Int J Dermatol.* 1997;36:573-574.

28. Kede MPV, Britz M. Discromias em pele negra. In: Kede MPV, Sabatovich O, eds. *Dermatologia Estética.* São Paulo, Brazil: Atheneu; 2003:269-299.

29. Ramos-e-Silva M, Fernandes NC. Afecções das mucosas e semimucosas. *J Bras Med.* 2001;80:50-66.

30. Sacre RC. Melasma. In: Kede MPV, Sabatovich O, eds. *Dermatologia Estética.* São Paulo, Brazil: Atheneu; 2003:255-264.

31. Bakos L, Bakos RM, Azulay DR. Afecções dos pêlos. In: Azulay R, Azulay D, eds. *Dermatologia.* Rio de Janeiro, Brazil: Guanabara Koogan; 2003:484-493.

32. Sampaio SAP, Rivitti EA. Piodermites e outras dermatoses por bactérias. In: Sampaio SAP, Rivitti EA, eds. *Dermatologia.* 2nd ed. São Paulo, Brazil: Editora Artes Médicas; 2001:435-452.

33. Cardoso AC. Dermatoses zooparasitárias. In: Talhari S, Neves RG, eds. *Dermatologia Tropical.* Rio de Janeiro, Brazil: Medsi; 1995:1-21.

34. Cumberland S, Jurberg C. From Australia to Brazil: sun worshippers beware. *Bull World Health Organ.* 2009;87:574-575.

35. Gohara M, Perez M. Skin cancer and skin of color. http://www.skincancer.org/prevention/skin-cancer-and-skin-of-color. Accessed August 13, 2013.

36. Konrad P, Fabris MR, Melao S, et al. Histopathological and epidemiological profile of cases of primary cutaneous melanoma diagnosed in Criciuma-SC between 2005 and 2007. *An Bras Dermatol.* 2011;86:457-461.

37. Moreno M, Schmitt RL, Lang MG, et al. Epidemiological profile of patients with cutaneous melanoma in a region of Southern Brazil. http://www.hindawi.com/journals/jsc/2012/917346/. Accessed February 26, 2013.

38. Campanha Nacional de Prevenção ao Cêncer da Pele. SaúdeAgora. http://www.revistasaudeagora.com.br/htm/materia.asp?material=422. Accessed October 13, 2005.

39. Schlossman ML. Formulação de produtos étnicos para maquilagem. *Cosmetic Toiletries.* 1996;8:60.

40. Rocha Filho PA. Cosméticos étnicos: aspectos fisiológicos. *Cosmetic Toiletries.* 1996;8:34-38.

41. Pandya AG, Guevara IL. Disorders of hyperpigmentation. *Dermatol Clin.* 2000;18:91-98.

42. Baumann L. Disorders of pigmentation. In: Baumann L, ed. *Cosmetic Dermatology—Principles and Practice.* New York, NY: McGraw-Hill; 2002:63-71.

43. Verallo-Rowell VM. The tropics: Q&A. In: Verallo-Rowell VM, ed. *Skin in the Tropics—Sunscreens and Hyperpigmentation.* Pasig City, Philippines: Anvil Publishing; 2001:1-14.

| CHAPTER | **International Atlas: Africa, Asia, and Latin America** |

95

Ana Maria Anido Serrano
Allison Nicholas Metz
Ahmed Al Waily

INTRODUCTION

Studying the different aspects and manifestations of cutaneous diseases in people with skin of color is an important area of research for many reasons, not just because of the need to provide informed healthcare to all patients. Today, cultural diversity, global migration, and shifting demographic patterns have all contributed to the fact that populations with skin of color are an important and rapidly growing segment of the global community. This second edition of the textbook *Dermatology for Skin of Color* is an important work of reference that sets out to tackle this vital topic.

This chapter aims to provide clear and succinct information accompanied by high-quality images of a selected range of cutaneous diseases. Definitions, etiologic explanations, clinical perspectives, differential diagnoses, and treatment options are provided for 23 of the most common conditions affecting patients with skin of color. Using the information outlined in this atlas, dermatologists, medical students, and other medical professionals will be able to accurately recognize cutaneous diseases in patients with skin of color and learn appropriate and effective management techniques to treat them. Additionally, the chapter focuses on the distinctive clinical variations and manifestations encountered in patients with skin of color.

One of the most obvious skin changes seen in individuals with skin of color, as well as being one of the most distressing to experience for the patient, is pigmentary alteration. This clinical skin change often takes the form of either hyper- or hypopigmented skin disorders. Many postinflammatory conditions and photosensitive reactions can cause hyperpigmentation, such as melasma. Some of the diseases causing hypopigmentation include leukoderma, idiopathic guttate hypomelanosis, and pityriasis alba. Additionally, lesions that may seem yellowish-brown or red in fairer-skinned individuals, may instead appear in shades ranging from gray to purple in individuals with darker skin of color. This variation and color difference can be seen in several conditions, for instance in pityriasis rosea, psoriasis, and lichen planus.

Patients with skin of color often display distinctive reaction patterns that may manifest in their skin and hair. While there are no biochemical differences among African, Asian, and Caucasian hair types, hair phenotypes vary among the skin of color population, ranging from tightly coiled to very straight. Therefore, the inherent hair properties of certain patients with skin of color may result in their hair being more dry and brittle. As a result, these patients may need to use certain emollient or oil-based hair products to groom their hair without causing breakage of the hair shaft. The use of these products on the hair may sometimes lead to cutaneous disorders.

Various common diseases have different clinical manifestations among individuals in the patient population, for example acne vulgaris. Additionally, skin of color may react differently in relation to the treatment option chosen by the dermatologist. The treatment for skin disorders may need to be adjusted according to the patient and their individual skin type—for example, when using lasers, chemical peels, or microneedling therapy in patients with skin of color. Furthermore, dermatologists should be aware of different priorities with regard to advising their patients about skin care. While certain precautions should be advised to all patients regardless of skin variation, such as the importance of sunscreen protection and moisturizers, other factors may need to be emphasized according to the individual patient.

In conclusion, the study and understanding of skin of color are imperative for all physicians. Skin of color may demonstrate normal and natural variations that can cause concerned patients to seek medical attention for an otherwise benign condition. If these are unknown to the less experienced physician, these variants may cause patient distress and run the risk of unnecessary treatments or incorrect diagnoses. The same is true for the variations in clinical manifestations and the differences in treatment options and management that are applicable to this patient population. Therefore, education is required to ensure that clinicians can accurately and reliably diagnose cutaneous diseases among patients with skin of color. As the percentage of the population with skin of color increases all over the world, it is vital that the clinical needs of this group are not only met and addressed but become part of the routine education of physicians everywhere.

ACNE

DEFINITION

Acne vulgaris [**Figures 95-1, 95-2,** and **95-3**] occurs mainly during adolescence and presents with pleomorphic lesions that can leave severe scarring.

ETIOLOGY

Acne vulgaris is a multifactorial condition involving increased sebum production, the hypercornification of the pilosebaceous duct, abnormality of the microbial flora (especially colonization of the duct with *Propionibacterium acnes*), and the production of inflammation.

CLINICAL PERSPECTIVE

Acne vulgaris lesions are seen mainly on the face, midchest, back, shoulders, and upper arms, and can be inflammatory or noninflammatory. Comedones are pathognomic lesions that are conical and raised with a broad base and a plugged apex. Pustular and nodular lesions are commonly seen in Asian patients. The sequelae of acne, which include hyperpigmentation and scarring, are often more socially and psychologically distressing for the patient than the disease itself.

DIFFERENTIAL DIAGNOSIS

Rosacea may be considered in the differential diagnosis.

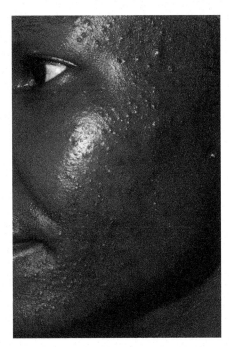

FIGURE 95-1. Africa. Acne. Greasy skin with open and closed comedones. (Used with permission from Barbara Leppard.)

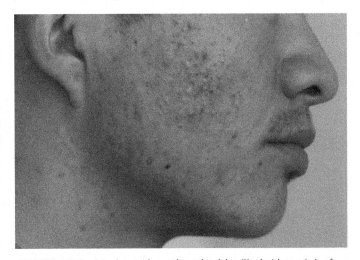

FIGURE 95-2. Asia. Acne with pustules and nodules. (Used with permission from Dr. Diqing Luo.)

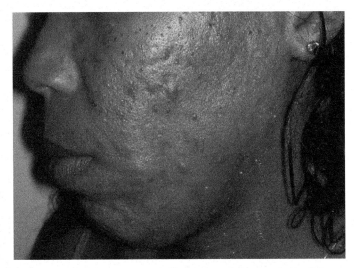

FIGURE 95-3. Latin America. Acne. (Used with permission from Dr. Marcia Ramos-e-Silva.)

TREATMENT

Patient education is an important element of acne treatment. Topical benzoyl peroxide or retinoic acid, topical antibiotics, topical therapy, systemic antibiotics, antiandrogens, and isotretinoin may be used. For cystic acne, aspiration, intralesional steroids, and dapsone should be prescribed. Scars may be treated surgically, and adapalene or azelaic acid cream can be used for postacne pigmentation.

ATOPIC DERMATITIS

DEFINITION

Atopic dermatitis (AD) [**Figures 95-4, 95-5,** and **95-6**] is a common chronic or relapsing dermatitis. Patients with AD may have a personal or family history of asthma, allergic rhinitis, or AD.

ETIOLOGY

This disease is caused by a complex interplay between various genetic and immunologic factors, and it is exacerbated by a genetic predisposition and environmental factors.

CLINICAL PERSPECTIVE

AD is usually seen in its mild and moderate forms, and rarely in its severe form. In individuals with darker skin of color, the lesions may have a follicular distribution, or the seemingly unaffected skin may have a dry, lackluster appearance. In the infantile phase, the face, scalp, extensor surfaces, and trunk are commonly affected. From 18 to 24 months onward, eczema may be observed on the flexural surfaces, including the neck, antecubital and popliteal fossae, wrists, and ankles.

DIFFERENTIAL DIAGNOSIS

Contact dermatitis and scabies should be considered in the differential diagnosis for AD. Infantile seborrheic dermatitis, which presents as more well-defined lesions and lesions in the diaper area, should be considered in infants.

TREATMENT OPTIONS

The first measure should be the identification and avoidance of provoking factors. Bathing, moisturizers, antibiotics for secondary infections, and antihistamines are important AD treatments. Topical corticosteroids

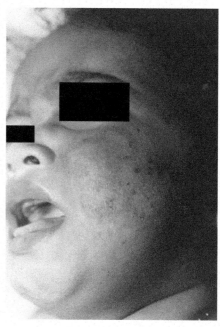

FIGURE 95-5. Asia. Atopic dermatitis on the cheeks. (Used with permission from Dr. Rashmi Sarkar.)

and topical calcineurin inhibitors such as tacrolimus and pimecrolimus are the mainstays of AD therapy. Severe cases may require treatment with phototherapy, photochemotherapy, cyclosporine, azathioprine, or interferons.

DRUG-INDUCED PHOTOSENSITIVITY REACTION

DEFINITION

Drug-induced photosensitivity reactions [**Figures 95-7, 95-8,** and **95-9**] are abnormal skin reactions to sunlight and artificial sources of ultraviolet and visible radiation. These reactions are induced by external or internally ingested photosensitizing drugs and other chemicals.

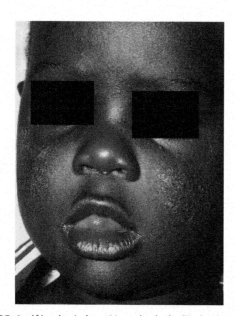

FIGURE 95-4. Africa. Atopic dermatitis on the cheeks. (Used with permission from Barbara Leppard.)

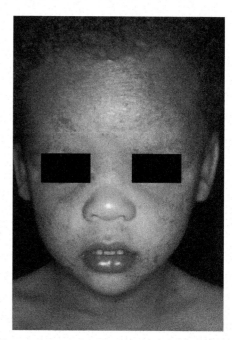

FIGURE 95-6. Latin America. Atopic dermatitis. (Used with permission from Dr. Tania Cestari.)

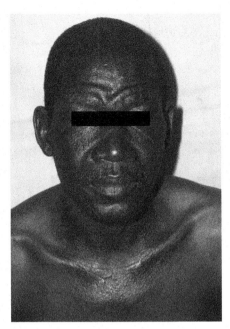

FIGURE 95-7. Africa. Photosensitivity reaction. (Used with permission from Barbara Leppard.)

ETIOLOGY

Most systemic photosensitizers are phototoxic in mechanism (exogenous: antibiotics, antidepressants, diuretics, psoralens, dyes, coal tars, anthracene, and chemical sunscreens; endogenous: porphyrins). The less common mechanisms include drug-induced lupus, pellagra, and photoallergy. Photoallergy is commonly caused by topical exposure to nonsteroidal anti-inflammatory drugs, fragrances, and sunscreens. Photoallergic reactions are cell-mediated, whereas phototoxic reactions are nonimmunologic.

CLINICAL PERSPECTIVE

Acute phototoxic reactions to drugs and chemicals can produce an immediate erythema and burning sensation in the light-exposed areas and are sometimes followed by blistering. Common sites of involvement are the forehead, nose, malar region, neck, 'V' of the chest, extensor forearms, and dorsal hands. The upper eyelids, nasolabial folds, upper lip,

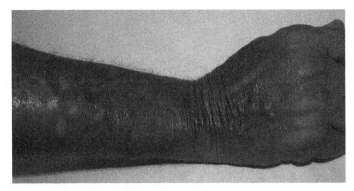

FIGURE 95-9. Latin America. Drug-induced photosensitivity reaction. (Used with permission from Dr. Marcia Ramos-e-Silva.)

and submental regions are characteristically spared. Photoallergic eruptions are itchy, eczematous, or vesicular. Among the Asian population, photoallergic reactions are more common than phototoxic reactions.

DIFFERENTIAL DIAGNOSIS

Photoallergic reactions may have to be differentiated from airborne contact dermatitis (involvement of the upper eyelid and submental region, typical history), atopic dermatitis (history of atopy), and polymorphous light reactions (absence of drug intake history). Phototoxic reactions have to be differentiated from severe sunburn, which is common in Asians.

TREATMENT OPTIONS

The best option is to replace the offending drug with a nonphototoxic alternative. Sun avoidance and broad-spectrum sunscreens are an important part of the treatment. Topical and oral corticosteroids, antihistamines, and ultraviolet B or psoralen plus ultraviolet A (PUVA) desensitization therapy may be required.

LEISHMANIASIS

DEFINITION

Leishmaniasis [**Figures 95-10, 95-11,** and **95-12**] is a protozoan disease with diverse clinical manifestations that are dependent on both the infective species of *Leishmania* and the immune response of the host. The disease is transmitted through the bite of a sandfly infected with *Leishmania* parasites.

ETIOLOGY

Post–kala-azar dermal leishmaniasis (PKDL) is a type of leishmaniasis that is caused primarily by *Leishmania donovani*. PKDL frequently follows an attack of kala-azar, or visceral leishmaniasis (VL), after 1 to 2 years. It is considered a dermal extension of the disease after the spontaneous or treatment-induced healing of VL.

CLINICAL PERSPECTIVES

In Indian patients, hypopigmented macules are usually the first manifestation. Widespread erythematous papules and nodular and noduloulcerative lesions involving the skin, nasal, oral, oropharyngeal, and laryngeal mucosa are also seen. Unusual forms include annular, hypertrophic, and xanthomatous leishmaniasis .

DIFFERENTIAL DIAGNOSIS

Diseases that can simulate PKDL are leprosy, diffuse cutaneous leishmaniasis, secondary syphilis, and sarcoidosis. In patients with macules, pityriasis/tinea versicolor and vitiligo should be ruled out.

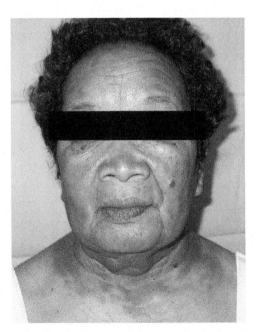

FIGURE 95-8. Asia. Griseofulvin-induced photosensitivity reaction. (Used with permission from Dr. Siew Eng Choon, Johor Bahru, Malaysia.)

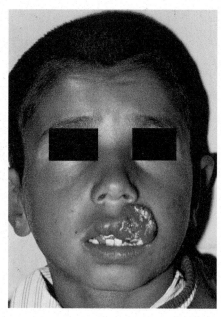

FIGURE 95-10. Africa. Cutaneous leishmaniasis on the lip. (Used with permission from Barbara Leppard.)

TREATMENT

PKDL is refractory to treatment. Sodium antimony gluconate, at a dose of 20 mg/kg and up to a maximum of 850 mg/d, is usually given intramuscularly for 4 months. Ketoconazole, allopurinol, and amphotericin B can be added to improve the response. If the hypopigmented macules persist, they may require PUVA therapy (also known as PUVAsol) to aid their resolution.

LEPROSY

DEFINITION

Leprosy [**Figures 95-13, 95-14,** and **95-15**] is a chronic granulomatous disease caused by *Mycobacterium leprae*. It primarily affects the

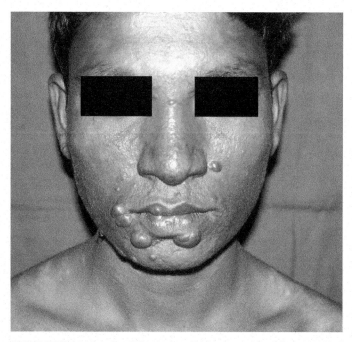

FIGURE 95-11. Asia. Post–kala-azar dermal leishmaniasis with nodular lesions. (Used with permission from Dr. V. Ramesh.)

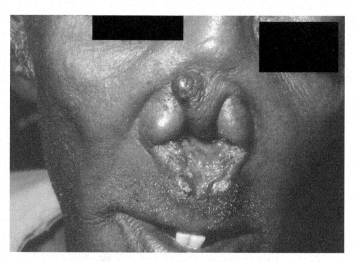

FIGURE 95-12. Latin America. Late-stage mucocutaneous leishmaniasis. (Used with permission from Dr. Marcia Ramos-e-Silva.)

peripheral nerves, skin, and other tissues such as the eye, the mucosa of the upper respiratory tract, the reticuloendothelial system, and the testes.

ETIOLOGY

Leprosy is caused by *M. leprae* bacteria.

CLINICAL PERSPECTIVE

The characteristic clinical manifestations of leprosy are numb hypopigmented or erythematous patches on the skin and thickened or enlarged peripheral nerves. Another indication is the demonstration of acid-fast bacilli on a slit-skin smear examination of the skin lesions. The reactions in leprosy may present as type 1, in which there is neuritis and a sudden edema of existing lesions, or they may present as type 2, erythema nodosum leprosum lesions, where there is a sudden appearance of erythematous, evanescent lesions, as well as fever, arthritis, orchitis, and

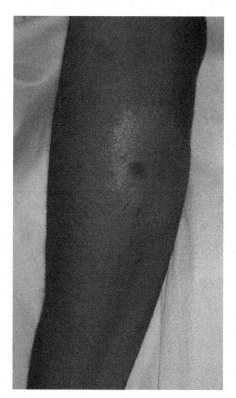

FIGURE 95-13. Africa. Tuberculoid leprosy presenting as a single anesthetic plaque. (Used with permission from Barbara Leppard.)

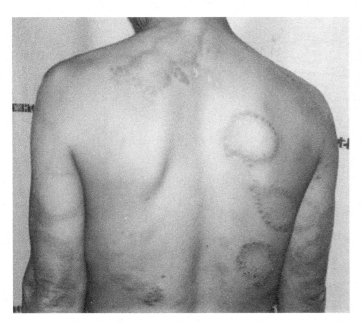

FIGURE 95-14. Asia. Borderline leprosy. (Used with permission from Dr. Rashmi Sarkar.)

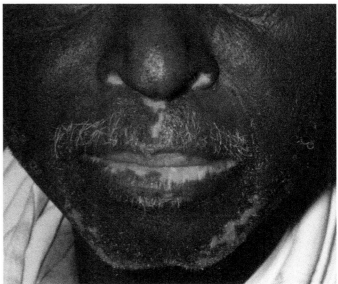

FIGURE 95-16. Africa. Vitiligo. (Used with permission from Barbara Leppard.)

visual disturbances. Pure neuritic leprosy is the form of leprosy that only involves the nerves with no skin lesions.

DIFFERENTIAL DIAGNOSIS

Vitiligo can be differentiated by depigmented macules with a normal sensation. Other granulomatous disorders, such as lupus vulgaris, sarcoidosis, syphilis, and leishmaniasis, should be ruled out.

TREATMENT OPTIONS

Multidrug therapy (MDT) is given for paucibacillary (PB) leprosy as once-a-month rifampicin, 600 mg orally, and dapsone, 100 mg daily, for 6 months. Alternatively, MDT for multibacillary leprosy consists of clofazimine given as 300 mg once monthly and 50 mg daily, in addition to the drugs of the PB MDT regimen, for 1 year. Steroids, antimalarial agents, and thalidomide are often given for reactions.

LEUKODERMA

DEFINITION

Any condition characterized by hypomelanotic or amelanotic lesions is known as leukoderma **Figures 95-16, 95-17,** and **95-18**]. Vitiligo, a form

of leukoderma, is a primary, usually progressive, symmetrical disorder of depigmentation with an unknown etiology.

ETIOLOGY

A genetic role is implicated in the pathogenesis of leukoderma. The mode of inheritance is autosomal dominant, although autosomal recessive or polygenic inheritance has also been suggested. There have been theories of an autoimmune etiology, as well as a neural autotoxic self-destructive mode.

CLINICAL PERSPECTIVE

A typical vitiligo lesion is a well-defined depigmented macule that is often associated with leukotrichia. Trichrome vitiligo describes a depigmented area surrounded by a comparatively hypopigmented zone that is separated from normal skin by a thin hyperpigmented rim. Vitiligo vulgaris is one of the most common types of vitiligo seen in Asia.

DIFFERENTIAL DIAGNOSIS

Bilateral lesions of vitiligo have to be differentiated from piebaldism. Chemical leukoderma can be differentiated because it will be confined

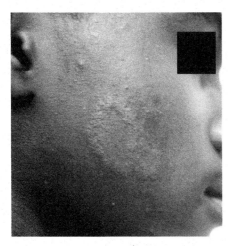

FIGURE 95-15. Latin America. Tuberculoid leprosy. (Reproduced with permission from Ramos-e-Silva M, Rebello P. Leprosy: Recognition and treatment. *Am J Clin Dermatol.* 2001;2:203-211.)

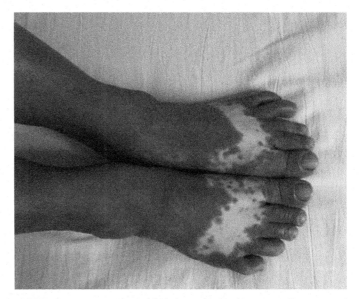

FIGURE 95-17. Asia. Chemical leukoderma. (Used with permission from Dr. Prasad Kumarasinghe.)

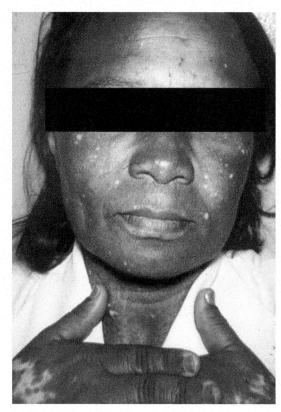

FIGURE 95-18. Latin America. Leukoderma punctate due to 10% hydroquinone. (Used with permission from Dr. Marcia Ramos-e-Silva.)

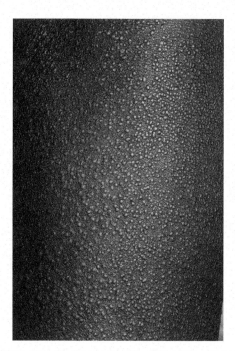

FIGURE 95-19. Africa. Tiny flat-topped papules of lichen nitidus. (Used with permission from Barbara Leppard.)

to the area of contact with certain chemicals. It is common to observe chemical leukoderma due to the bindi (a decorative mark worn on the forehead of Indian women) and footwear. Pityriasis alba is slightly scaly and primarily affects the face.

TREATMENT OPTIONS

For localized vitiligo, topical corticosteroids and topical calcineurin inhibitors (such as tacrolimus or pimecrolimus) are usually given. For generalized vitiligo, the common treatment options are oral pulse corticosteroids, narrowband ultraviolet B, PUVA therapy, khellin therapy, phenylalanine, placental extract, cyclophosphamide, and levamisole. In selected cases of stable vitiligo, surgery may be attempted. Psychological counseling is an important part of therapy, along with cosmetic camouflage.

LICHEN NITIDUS

DEFINITION

Lichen nitidus [**Figures 95-19, 95-20,** and **95-21**] consists of tiny, nonpruritic, shiny, flat-topped papules which present on the arms, abdomen, and penis.

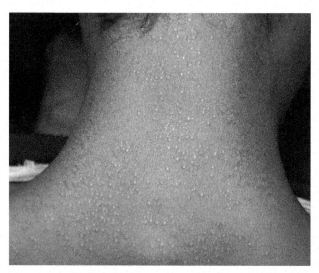

FIGURE 95-20. Asia. Lichen nitidus. (Used with permission from Dr. Sudhanshu Sharma.)

ETIOLOGY

Some believe lichen nitidus to be a variant of lichen planus, while others believe it to be a distinct entity. Most cases occur in children and young adults. There are also reports of familial lichen planus. It seems to occur more frequently in patients with darker skin of color. It has also been associated with Crohn disease and atopic dermatitis.

CLINICAL PERSPECTIVE

Lichen nitidus consists of pinhead-sized, round or polygonal, skin-colored papules that are present on the shaft and glans of the penis, lower abdomen, groin, breasts, and flexor surfaces of the arms and wrists. Oral and nail lesions are rare.

FIGURE 95-21. Latin America. Lichen nitidus. (Used with permission from Dr. Marcia Ramos-e-Silva.)

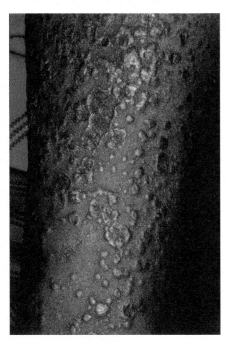

FIGURE 95-22. Africa. Lichen planus. Note the distinctive navy blue hyperpigmentation. (Used with permission from Barbara Leppard.)

DIFFERENTIAL DIAGNOSIS

Lichen planus can be differentiated by the presence of pruritic, violaceous papules. Those with keratosis pilaris have lesions on the extensor surfaces of their arms. Lichen scrofulosorum results in both follicular and interfollicular lesions and a positive tuberculin test.

TREATMENT OPTIONS

Patients with lichen nitidus can experience spontaneous resolution after many years, and no treatment is required in most cases. However, the primary treatment options include topical steroids, photochemotherapy, astemizole, cetirizine, and levamisole.

LICHEN PLANUS

DEFINITION

Lichen planus [**Figures 95-22, 95-23,** and **95-24**] is a distinctive papulosquamous disorder that is characterized by pruritic, violaceous papular lesions involving the skin, mucous membranes, hair, and nails.

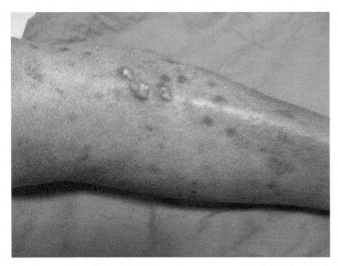

FIGURE 95-23. Asia. Classic lichen planus. (Used with permission from Dr. Rashmi Sarkar.)

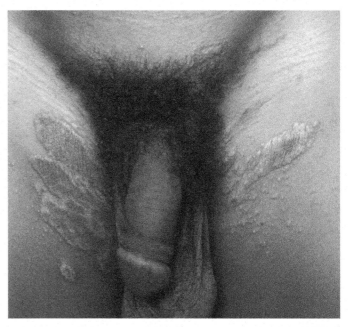

FIGURE 95-24. Latin America. Lichen planus. (Used with permission from Dr. Marcia Ramos-e-Silva.)

ETIOLOGY

The etiology of lichen planus is unknown. The precipitating causes may include viruses, drugs, and contact with certain chemicals such as color film developer.

CLINICAL PERSPECTIVE

Lichen planus lesions are intensely pruritic, violaceous, polygonal, shining, flat-topped papules involving the flexural areas, wrists, lumbar region, and ankles. The clinical variants are hypertrophic, actinic, oral, linear, annular, atrophic, guttate, follicular, ulcerative, bullous, forms, and Graham-Little syndrome. Two characteristic types that are seen among the Asian population are lichen planus pigmentosus and actinic lichen planus. The former has been mainly reported in Indian patients. It presents as multiple, discrete, hyperpigmented macules on the trunk, upper limbs, and face. The latter also displays a predilection for individuals from the Middle East, India, and East Africa. Sunlight appears to be a precipitating factor in lichen planus.

DIFFERENTIAL DIAGNOSIS

Other papulosquamous disorders, such as psoriasis, need to be ruled out.

TREATMENT OPTIONS

Since the disease is benign and self-limiting, treatment is symptomatic. Typical treatments include topical, intralesional, and systemic corticosteroids, while retinoids, cyclosporine, PUVA, dapsone, and griseofulvin are other options.

LUPUS VULGARIS

DEFINITION

Lupus vulgaris [**Figures 95-25, 95-26,** and **95-27**] is the most common form of cutaneous tuberculosis that is caused by *Mycobacterium tuberculosis* bacteria.

ETIOLOGY

This type of post–primary cutaneous tuberculosis is acquired from an exogenous source, although it may also arise from hematogenous

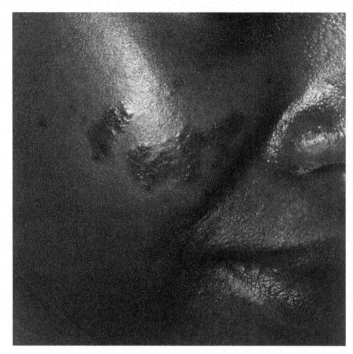

FIGURE 95-25. Africa. Lupus vulgaris. (Used with permission from Barbara Leppard.)

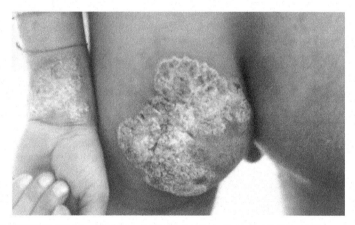

FIGURE 95-26. Asia. Lupus vulgaris. (Used with permission from Dr. V. Ramesh.)

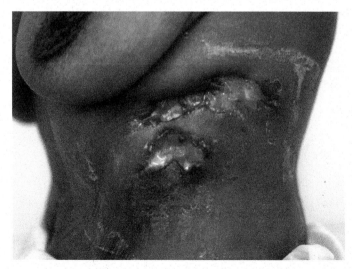

FIGURE 95-27. Latin America. Cutaneous tuberculosis. (Used with permission from Dr. Marcia Ramos-e-Silva.)

dissemination of *M. tuberculosis* in the body. Additionally, the disease can be caused by the progress of tuberculosis, by chance, or, rarely, as a result of the bacillus Calmette-Guérin (BCG) vaccination.

CLINICAL PERSPECTIVE

The face, buttocks, thighs, and legs are the most common sites of involvement. The lesions start as a few soft, 'apple jelly' nodules, which can coalesce to form a plaque, although the plaque may not be visible in those with darker skin of color. The disease progresses with irregular extension of the plaque, which sometimes heals with superficial scarring. Sometimes there can be ulceration, crusting, and scarring with destruction of the underlying tissues and cartilage.

DIFFERENTIAL DIAGNOSIS

Lupus vulgaris has to be differentiated from other granulomatous conditions. The differential diagnosis should include an analysis of the clinical features, tuberculin reaction, and histology, as well as the demonstration of acid-fast bacilli and the presence of active tuberculosis elsewhere in the body.

TREATMENT OPTIONS

Antitubercular therapy is the primary treatment for lupus vulgaris. This consists of a 2-month initial phase of rifampicin, isoniazid, pyrazinamide, and ethambutol, followed by a 4-month continuation phase with isoniazid and rifampicin as a short-course regimen. The period of treatment is usually 7 to 8 months.

MELASMA

DEFINITION

Melasma [**Figures 95-28, 95-29,** and **95-30**] is a common, acquired, hyperpigmentation condition that is characterized by symmetrically distributed medium to dark patches on sun-exposed areas, including the forehead, cheeks, temples, and upper lip.

ETIOLOGY

It is commonly seen in patients with darker skin of color such as Asians, Hispanics, and Africans, although individuals from any racial group

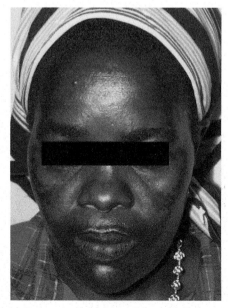

FIGURE 95-28. Africa. Melasma on the cheeks. Note the well-defined but irregular outline of the hyperpigmentation. (Used with permission from Barbara Leppard.)

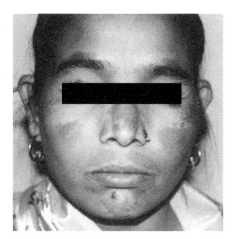

FIGURE 95-29. Asia. Melasma. (Used with permission from Dr. Rashmi Sarkar.)

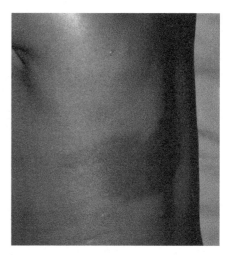

FIGURE 95-31. Africa. Mongolian spot. (Used with permission from Barbara Leppard.)

may be affected. It is most common in women of childbearing age (90%), but up to 10% of cases have been reported in males. Melasma occurs in genetically predisposed individuals. In addition, sunlight exposure, pregnancy, hormones, cosmetics, and drugs are important factors in the development of this condition.

CLINICAL PERSPECTIVE

The light to dark brown hyperpigmentation may be distributed in a centrofacial (63%), malar (21%), or mandibular (16%) pattern. A Wood lamp examination and histopathology will help to determine whether the lesions are epidermal, dermal, mixed, or indeterminate types.

DIFFERENTIAL DIAGNOSIS

This disease needs to be differentiated from other types of facial hyperpigmentation. This includes lichen planus pigmentosus, which presents as violaceous or slate-gray lesions, and toxic melanosis, which commonly occurs in Asians and in those who work with tar, coal tar products, and mineral oils.

TREATMENT OPTIONS

The epidermal variety of melasma is readily responsive to treatment. The discontinuation of provoking factors and the use of broad-spectrum sunscreens are the cornerstones of treatment. Topical depigmenting agents have been used, as well as chemical peels, either alone or in combination with topical therapy and fractional laser therapy.

MONGOLIAN SPOT

DEFINITION

The Mongolian spot [**Figures 95-31, 95-32,** and **95-33**] is a congenital blue-gray patch that is usually located in the lumbosacral region.

ETIOLOGY

The pigmentation is due to melanocytes in the dermis, as a result of their failure to complete the migration from the developing embryo's neural crest to their proper location in the basal layer of the epidermis. The affected areas have a slate-brown or blue color (ceruloderma) due to an optical effect from the pigment lying in the dermis. Mongolian spot is a congenital condition and is found in up to 90% of Asian babies.

CLINICAL PERSPECTIVE

The lesions are poorly circumscribed areas of slate-brown or blue-black pigmentation that are sometimes extensive. Multiple lesions may also be located in sites other than the lumbosacral region. They may fade in early childhood, although aberrant extrasacral spots can persist.

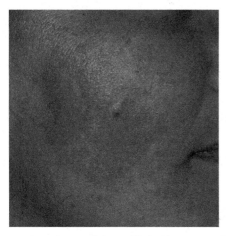

FIGURE 95-30. Latin America. Melasma. (Used with permission from Dr. Marcia Ramos-e-Silva.)

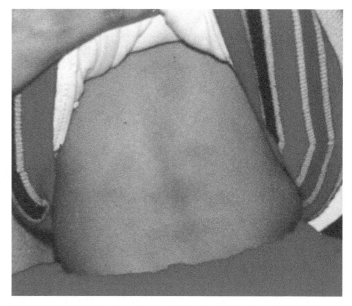

FIGURE 95-32. Asia. Mongolian spot. (Used with permission from Dr. Rashmi Sarkar.)

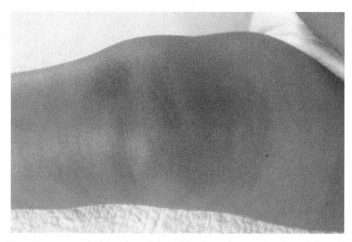

FIGURE 95-33. Latin America. Mongolian spot.

DIFFERENTIAL DIAGNOSIS

Mongolian spots may need to be differentiated from a bruise.

TREATMENT OPTIONS

No treatment is necessary. The parents of a baby with this condition should be reassured that the lesions will disappear with time.

NEVUS OF OTA

DEFINITION

Nevus of Ota [**Figures 95-34, 95-35,** and **95-36**] is a benign hyperpigmentation condition that affects one side of the face, in the region supplied by the ophthalmic and maxillary divisions of the trigeminal nerve.

ETIOLOGY

The lesion occurs because of an arrest in the migration of melanocytes from the neural crest to the epidermis. Most cases are congenital, although some patients may present in early adolescence. It is more prevalent in the Japanese but can also be observed in those from other population groups.

CLINICAL PERSPECTIVE

The lesion may be bilateral and is usually slate-brown or blue in color. The sclerae are often involved, and the cornea, iris, retina, ocular

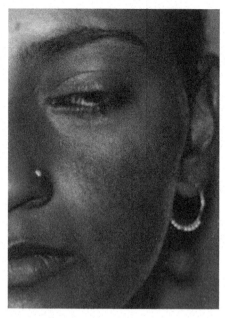

FIGURE 95-35. Asia. Nevus of Ota. (Used with permission from Dr. Rashmi Sarkar.)

muscles, and orbit may be pigmented. This condition does not resolve with time. Although malignant change in the cutaneous lesion is rare, melanomas are common in the choroid, iris, orbit, and brain.

DIFFERENTIAL DIAGNOSIS

A bilateral acquired dermal melanosis of the face may have to be considered in the differential diagnosis.

TREATMENT OPTIONS

The Q-switched ruby laser has shown good results in the treatment of this condition.

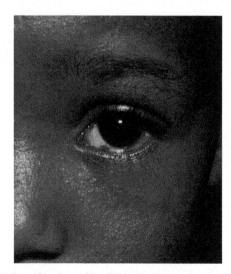

FIGURE 95-34. Africa. Nevus of Ota. (Used with permission from Barbara Leppard.)

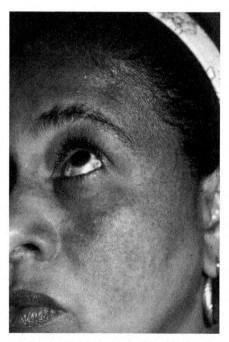

FIGURE 95-36. Latin America. Nevus of Ota. (Used with permission from Dr. Marcia Ramos-e-Silva.)

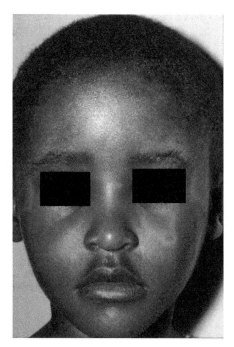

FIGURE 95-37. Africa. Pityriasis alba. (Used with permission from Barbara Leppard.)

PITYRIASIS ALBA

DEFINITION

Pityriasis alba (PA) [**Figures 95-37, 95-38,** and **95-39**] is a pattern of dermatitis in which erythema and scaling usually precede the development of conspicuous hypopigmentation.

ETIOLOGY

PA is sometimes a manifestation of atopic dermatitis, but it may not be confined to only atopic individuals. It is believed to result from either a

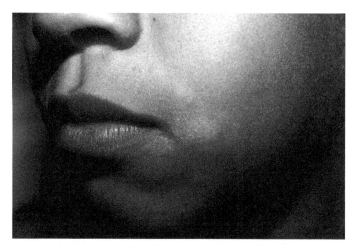

FIGURE 95-39. Latin America. Pityriasis alba. (Used with permission from Dr. Marcia Ramos-e-Silva.)

decrease in the number of active melanocytes or from a reduced capacity of the epidermal cells to acquire melanin during inflammation. This condition is extremely common in Asian and African children.

CLINICAL PERSPECTIVE

PA occurs commonly in children between 3 and 16 years of age. The lesions are round, oval, or irregular plaques that are red, pink, or skin-colored with fine, branny scaling. The lesions can occur singly or in multiples. In patients with darker skin of color, PA presents mainly as persistent fine scaling and hypopigmentation. The lesions are usually confined to the face; however, the neck, arms, and trunk may also be involved. The lesions can be persistent, and the hypopigmentation may last for a year or more.

DIFFERENTIAL DIAGNOSIS

Conspicuous hypopigmentation can mean that PA appears similar to vitiligo. However, the age at incidence, the scaling, and the distribution should point to the correct diagnosis.

TREATMENT OPTIONS

The scaling can be reduced by the use of a bland emollient. Topical tar or topical corticosteroids are beneficial in the inflammatory phase of PA. Topical tacrolimus and pimecrolimus are useful for facial lesions.

PITYRIASIS ROSEA

DEFINITION

Pityriasis rosea (PR) [**Figures 95-40, 95-41,** and **95-42**] is an acute, self-limiting disease that is characterized by a distinctive eruption of oval scaly papules and plaques and minimal constitutional symptoms.

ETIOLOGY

PR is common throughout the world, especially in tropical countries. Most cases occur in patients between the ages of 10 and 35 years. An infective agent may be implicated in the pathogenesis, although the etiology is largely unknown.

CLINICAL PERSPECTIVE

In Asians, PR presents as dull-red or reddish-brown scaly papular and oval-shaped medallions distributed on the trunk in a 'Christmas tree' pattern. In patients with darker skin of color, it presents as a hyper-pigmented scaly eruption. Occasionally, a slight fever, malaise, and lymphadenopathy may be present. Papulovesicular, vesicular, pustular,

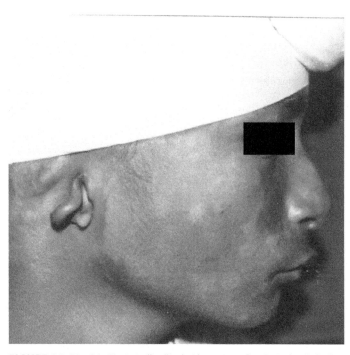

FIGURE 95-38. Asia. Pityriasis alba. (Used with permission from Dr. Rashmi Sarkar.)

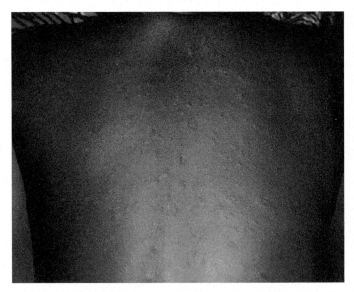

FIGURE 95-40. Africa. Pityriasis rosea. (Used with permission from Barbara Leppard.)

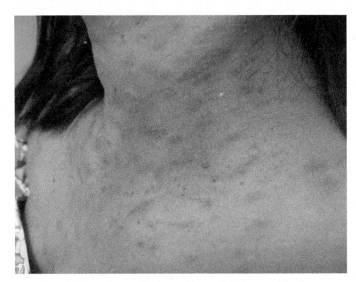

FIGURE 95-41. Asia. Pityriasis rosea. (Used with permission from Dr. Siew Eng Choon.)

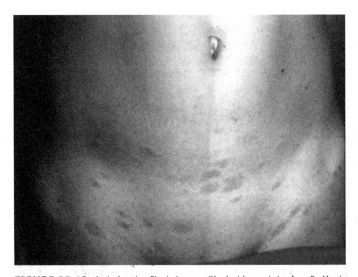

FIGURE 95-42. Latin America. Pityriasis rosea. (Used with permission from Dr. Marcia Ramos-e-Silva.)

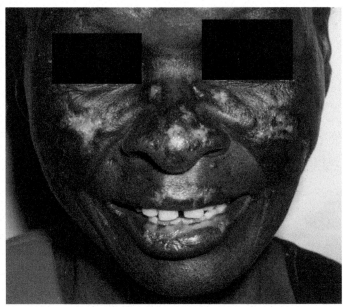

FIGURE 95-43. Africa. Postinflammatory hyper- and hypopigmentation of discoid lupus erythematosus. (Used with permission from Barbara Leppard.)

follicular, and erythema multiforme-like lesions are commonly seen in PR patients. The skin lesions usually fade in 3 to 6 weeks, leaving behind temporary hyperpigmentation or hypopigmentation.

DIFFERENTIAL DIAGNOSIS

Guttate psoriasis may have to be differentiated from PR, and secondary syphilis will also need to be excluded.

TREATMENT OPTIONS

Asymptomatic patients do not require treatment; however, it has been shown that a moderately potent topical steroid or ultraviolet B treatment can be useful. Oral erythromycin, given in a dose of 200 mg four times a day, may hasten the clearance of the lesions.

POSTINFLAMMATORY HYPER-/HYPOPIGMENTATION

DEFINITION

Postinflammatory hyper-/hypopigmentation [**Figures 95-43, 95-44, and 95-45**] is an acquired disorder of excess or decreased pigment deposition, respectively. It usually follows the resolution of various cutaneous disorders, as well as therapeutic interventions (such as laser therapy, chemical peels, and dermabrasion).

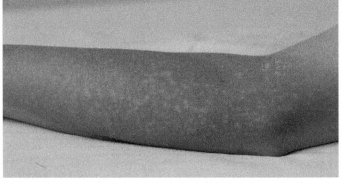

FIGURE 95-44. Asia. Postinflammatory hyperpigmentation. (Used with permission from Dr. Diqing Luo.)

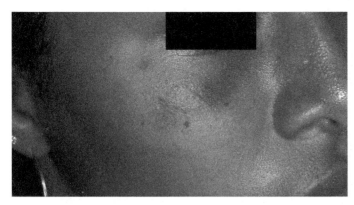

FIGURE 95-45. Latin America. Postinflammatory hyperpigmentation. (Used with permission from Dr. Marcia Ramos-e-Silva.)

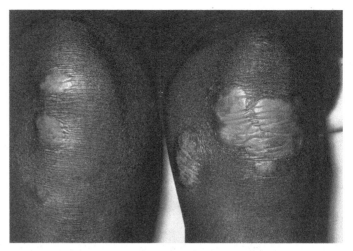

FIGURE 95-46. Africa. Psoriasis vulgaris on the knees. The red color plaques are obvious, even in darker skin of color. (Used with permission from Barbara Leppard.)

ETIOLOGY

Postinflammatory hyperpigmentation/hypopigmentation is more severe in patients with darker skin of color. Hyperpigmentation follows diseases such as contact dermatitis, lichen planus, phototoxic eruptions, acne vulgaris, atopic dermatitis, fixed drug eruptions, pityriasis rosea, secondary syphilis, and sarcoidosis. In darker skin of color patients, the hyperpigmentation worsens with ultraviolet exposure. Hypopigmentation is caused by atopic dermatitis, contact dermatitis, seborrheic dermatitis, secondary syphilis, discoid lupus erythematous, pityriasis alba, scleroderma, and lichen striatus. Physical therapies such as chemical peeling, laser therapy, cryosurgery, and dermabrasion may also lead to hypopigmentation or hyperpigmentation. Additionally, hypopigmentation can be a sequela of topical, intralesional, and intramuscular corticosteroid administration.

CLINICAL PERSPECTIVE

Postinflammatory hyper-/hypopigmentation may be more noticeable and distressing to patients with skin of color than the actual disease itself. Many of these pigmentary disturbances normalize with time.

DIFFERENTIAL DIAGNOSIS

Postinflammatory hypopigmentation may need to be differentiated from vitiligo. However, a history of the original skin lesions that led to the pigmentary alterations may establish the diagnosis.

TREATMENT OPTIONS

To achieve repigmentation, postinflammatory hypopigmentation may require treatment with topical steroids, topical calcineurin inhibitors, and topical PUVA therapy. A broad-spectrum sunscreen should also be included in the treatment. Epidermal postinflammatory hyperpigmentation can be treated with topical depigmenting agents alone or in combination with other therapies.

PSORIASIS VULGARIS

DEFINITION

Psoriasis [**Figures 95-46, 95-47,** and **95-48**] is a common inflammatory disease of the skin, hair, and nails recognized by characteristic red scaly plaques on the skin.

ETIOLOGY

Psoriasis may be caused by a genetic predisposition, but may also be triggered, *inter alia*, by injury to the skin, streptococcal throat infections, certain drugs, and physical and emotional stress.

CLINICAL PERSPECTIVE

The well-defined red scaly plaques can appear anywhere on the body. If the patient scratches the surface of the plaques, they become more obvious. Psoriasis is frequently located on the elbows and knees. Thick scaly plaques can occur on the scalp, which may extend down onto the forehead. Nail changes such as pitting, salmon patches, onycholysis, and subungual hyperkeratosis are prevalent.

DIFFERENTIAL DIAGNOSIS

The differential diagnosis could include other scaly rashes such as eczema and tinea. The diagnosis is usually obvious due to the well-defined border, the erythema, and the prolific scale of psoriasis.

ASSOCIATIONS

Associations include psoriatic arthritis, which is usually less severe than rheumatoid arthritis. It characteristically affects the distal interphalangeal joints. In rare cases, it can cause a mutilating arthritis that is clinically indistinguishable from severe rheumatoid arthritis, although patients will not have a positive rheumatoid factor. In extensive or hyperkeratotic psoriasis cases, associated human immunodeficiency virus (HIV)/acquired immunodeficiency syndrome (AIDS) should be considered.

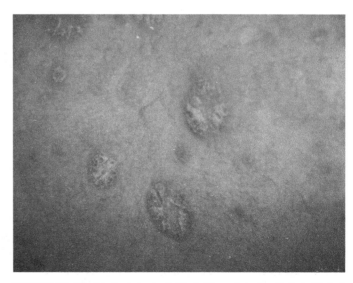

FIGURE 95-47. Asia. Psoriasis vulgaris. (Used with permission from Dr. Rashmi Sarkar.)

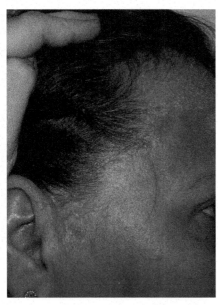

FIGURE 95-48. Latin America. Psoriasis vulgaris. (Used with permission from Barbara Leppard.)

TREATMENT OPTIONS

Topical therapy such as emollients, coal tar, corticosteroids, dithranol, calcipotriol, PUVA therapy, and tazarotene can be used to treat psoriasis vulgaris. Extensive cases will require phototherapy and photochemotherapy (eg, ultraviolet B, PUVA, and PUVAsol), methotrexate, acitretin, or cyclosporine.

SARCOIDOSIS

DEFINITION

Sarcoidosis [**Figures 95-49, 95-50,** and **95-51**] is a disease characterized by the formation of epithelioid cell tubercles in all or several affected organs. A cutaneous involvement affects 10% to 30% of sarcoidosis patients. This condition is less common in Asian individuals compared with the African population.

ETIOLOGY

The cause of sarcoidosis is unknown; however, the disease could possibly represent an unusual host reaction to infectious agents. It is likely that genetic factors are also involved. Depression of cell-mediated immunity is the hallmark of this disease.

CLINICAL PERSPECTIVE

Two types of cutaneous lesions are recognized: specific cutaneous sarcoid lesions and nonspecific reactive lesions. The common specific lesions in sarcoidosis are papules, plaques, and nodules. The plaques that are usually seen in Asian patients are irregular, infiltrated lesions that may be annular or serpiginous.

DIFFERENTIAL DIAGNOSIS

Lupus vulgaris, generalized granuloma annulare, secondary syphilis, and lymphomas may all mimic sarcoidosis. The histopathology will confirm the diagnosis.

TREATMENT OPTIONS

Sarcoidosis treatment depends on the extent of the involvement. Corticosteroids are the mainstay of therapy. Topical and intralesional steroids and cryotherapy are used for disfiguring cutaneous lesions. For cases of systemic sarcoidosis, the lesions involving the eyes and lungs will

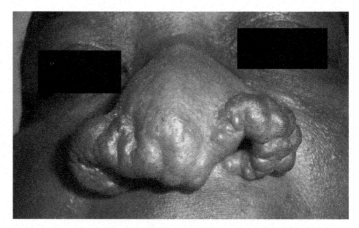

FIGURE 95-49. Africa. Sarcoidosis. (Used with permission from Dr. Anisa Mosam.)

require oral steroids or cytotoxic drugs. Allopurinol, antimalarials, and oxyphenbutazone have been used with limited success.

SCABIES

DEFINITION

Scabies [**Figures 95-52, 95-53,** and **95-54**] is characterized by intense itching and is caused by the mite, *Sarcoptes scabiei* var. *hominis.*

ETIOLOGY

Scabies affects individuals of all races and social classes throughout the world. It is usually transmitted by close physical contact, such as prolonged bed sharing or hand-holding. In developing countries, overcrowding, poverty, and poor hygiene encourage the spread of this condition. Scabies epidemics occur in 30-year cycles.

CLINICAL PERSPECTIVE

Intense itching, especially at night, is usually the main characteristic of scabies. The eruption consists of inflammatory papules, vesicles, excoriations, and crusting with the onset occurring 3 to 4 weeks after the infection is acquired. The pathognomonic lesions are burrows, which occur on the wrists, the finger web spaces, the sides of the fingers, the genitalia, and the feet. The pruritic papules occur predominantly around the axillae, periareolar and periumbilical areas, buttocks, and thighs. Postscabetic nodules may persist in the axillae, groin, scrotum, and penis. Eczematous changes and secondary infections are common.

DIFFERENTIAL DIAGNOSIS

Scabies with eczematization may be difficult to differentiate from atopic eczema.

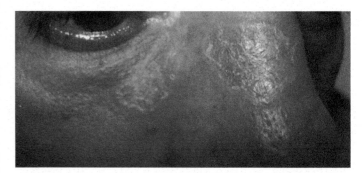

FIGURE 95-50. Asia. Sarcoidosis. (Used with permission from Dr. Rashmi Sarkar.)

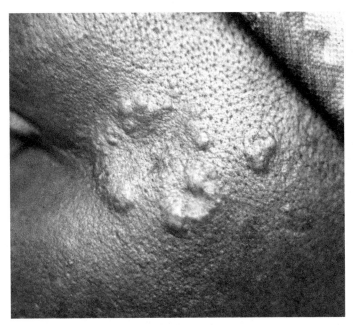

FIGURE 95-51. Latin America. Sarcoidosis. (Used with permission from Dr. Marcia Ramos-e-Silva.)

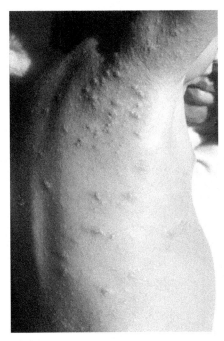

FIGURE 95-54. Latin America. Scabies in an 18-month-old child. (Used with permission from Dr. Marcia Ramos-e-Silva.)

▇ TREATMENT OPTIONS

Scabicides should be chosen based on efficacy, potential toxicity, cost, ease of application, secondary eczematization, and patient age. Permethrin 5% cream, 1% γ-benzene hexachloride lotion, 25% benzyl benzoate, monosulfiram, malathion, and crotamiton are all effective and safe topical treatment options. Sulfur and crotamiton or permethrin cream should be used for infants. At present, oral ivermectin is useful for ordinary scabies and institutional outbreaks of scabies.

SYPHILIS

▇ DEFINITION

Syphilis [**Figures 95-55, 95-56,** and **95-57**] is caused by the bacteria *Treponema pallidum.*

▇ ETIOLOGY

Syphilis is transmitted through direct sexual contact with an infected individual.

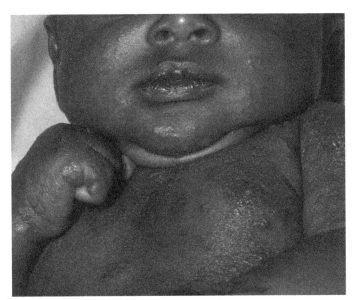

FIGURE 95-52. Africa. Scabies manifesting as an itchy rash in a 9-month-old boy. At this age, there can be involvement of the face. (Used with permission from Barbara Leppard.)

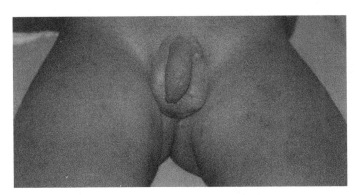

FIGURE 95-53. Asia. Scabies. Genital lesions. (Used with permission from Dr. Rashmi Sarkar.)

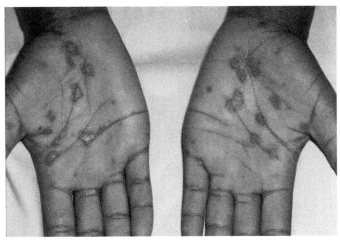

FIGURE 95-55. Africa. Secondary syphilis macules and papules on the palms. (Used with permission from Barbara Leppard.)

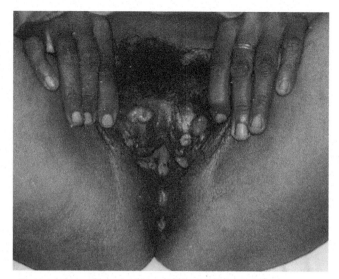

FIGURE 95-56. Asia. Condylomata lata of secondary syphilis. (Used with permission from Dr. Rashmi Sarkar.)

CLINICAL PERSPECTIVE

About 10 to 90 days after the infection, a firm, painless ulcer (primary chancre) occurs at the site of inoculation. At this primary stage, the diagnosis can be confirmed by finding the spirochetes on a smear taken from the ulcer and looked at under darkfield microscopy. This ulcer will usually heal spontaneously after 4 to 6 weeks if left untreated.

As the primary chancre is healing, or up to 6 months later, the patient may begin to feel unwell and develop secondary syphilis. This is marked by the presentation of a painless rash made up of macules, papules, or plaques, with an involvement of the palms and soles and erosions in the mouth and on the genitalia. Flat warty lesions (condylomata lata) are seen on the genitalia with patchy hair loss. The diagnosis can be confirmed by a positive serologic test, a Venereal Disease Research Laboratory (VDRL) test, or the more specific *T. pallidum* particle agglutination assay (TPHA) or fluorescent treponemal antibody absorption (FTA-ABS) test. Without treatment, this stage also will pass after approximately 6 months.

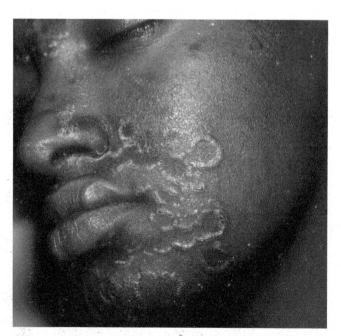

FIGURE 95-57. Latin America. Secondary syphilis. (Reproduced with permission from Parish LC, Brenner S, Ramos-e-Silva M, Parish JL. *Atlas of Women's Dermatology.* London, United Kingdom: Taylor & Francis; 2006.)

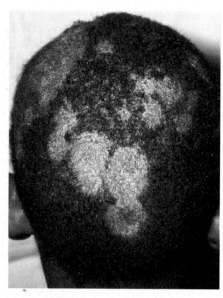

FIGURE 95-58. Africa. Tinea capitis with multiple bald patches on a child's scalp. (Used with permission from Barbara Leppard.)

DIFFERENTIAL DIAGNOSIS

Primary syphilis should be differentiated from herpes simplex and chancroid, whereas secondary syphilis should be differentiated from guttate psoriasis and PR. Syphilis can be associated with any other sexually transmitted disease and HIV/AIDS.

TREATMENT

Syphilis should be treated with a single dose of penicillin G benzathine, 2.4 MU intramuscularly. If the patient is HIV-positive, he or she should take three weekly doses of penicillin G benzathine, 2.4 MU intramuscularly.

TINEA CAPITIS

DEFINITION

Tinea capitis [**Figures 95-58, 95-59,** and **95-60**] is a fungal infection of the hair and scalp. The infection is most commonly caused by the *Trichophyton* and *Microsporum* species of dermatophytes.

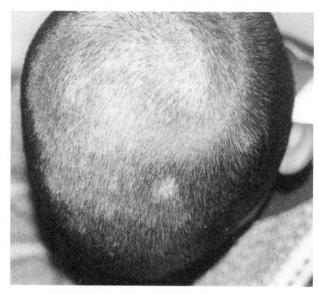

FIGURE 95-59. Asia. Gray patch of tinea capitis. (Used with permission from Dr. Rashmi Sarkar.)

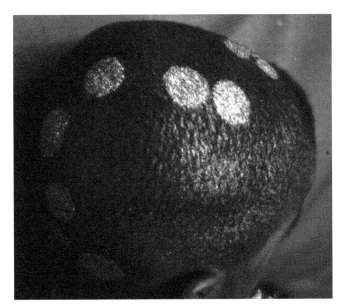

FIGURE 95-60. Latin America. Tinea capitis. (Used with permission from Dr. Marcia Ramos-e-Silva.)

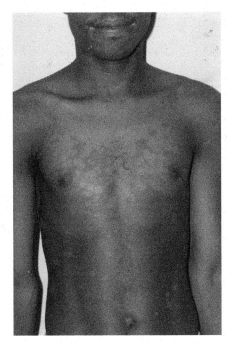

FIGURE 95-61. Africa. Tinea versicolor. (Used with permission from Barbara Leppard.)

 ETIOLOGY

The disease mainly affects children from 4 to 14 years of age and can be transmitted by infected combs, brushes, and caps. It has been shown that *Trichophyton violaceum* is the main cause of tinea capitis in Indian school children. Trauma to the scalp, due to head shaving for religious purposes, also seems to be an important contributory factor.

CLINICAL PERSPECTIVE

The clinical appearance of tinea capitis is extremely variable and is determined by the species of dermatophyte that is responsible for the infection. The immunity of the host is also a determining factor. Some tinea capitis cases will present as a few dull gray, broken-off hair strands with a little scaling. Other cases will be an inflammatory type with a boggy, indurated swelling that is studded with broken or unbroken hairs, vesicles, and pustules, known as kerions. The black dot type of tinea capitis consists of broken hairs along the scalp, whereas the favus type has yellow cup-shaped crusts that are pierced by hair strands.

DIFFERENTIAL DIAGNOSIS

Alopecia areata, psoriasis, and seborrheic dermatitis must be differentiated. When in doubt, a potassium hydroxide (KOH) preparation and/or a fungal culture will aid in the diagnosis.

TREATMENT OPTIONS

Oral griseofulvin, ketoconazole, itraconazole, and terbinafine are the mainstays of treatment. Selenium sulfide shampoo and other topical antifungal agents are also commonly prescribed.

TINEA VERSICOLOR

DEFINITION

Tinea versicolor [**Figures 95-61, 95-62,** and **95-63**] is a superficial fungal infection of the skin that is characterized by discrete or confluent, scaly, discolored or hypopigmented areas on the upper trunk.

ETIOLOGY

The causative organism is a lipophilic yeast, *Malassezia furfur*. It is commonly seen in tropical climates and in Asia.

CLINICAL PERSPECTIVE

The primary lesions are sharply demarcated macules, which may be pink, tan, or white (versicolor), and are covered by fine scaling. In patients with darker skin of color, large confluent areas of gray-brown pigmentation with scaling may be seen on the upper trunk, upper arms, neck, and abdomen, or extending to the groin and thighs. Facial and scalp involvement is common in Indian patients. The residual hypopigmentation, without any scaling, may persist for months.

DIFFERENTIAL DIAGNOSIS

Vitiligo and melasma are differentiated due to a lack of scaling. Seborrheic dermatitis would have yellow greasy scales, and pityriasis rosea consists of papules with a collarette of scales. Syphilis can be differentiated by the frequent involvement of the palms and soles and a positive Venereal Disease Research Laboratory (VDRL) test.

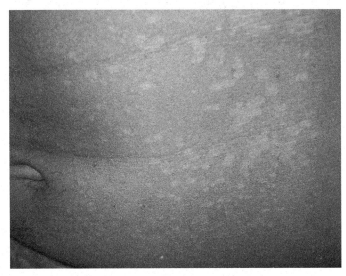

FIGURE 95-62. Asia. Tinea versicolor. (Used with permission from Dr. Sudhanshu Sharma.)

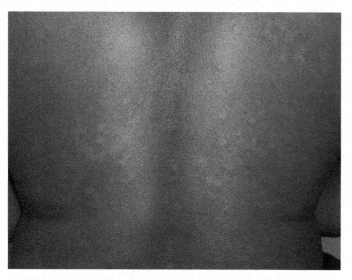

FIGURE 95-63. Latin America. Tinea versicolor. (Used with permission from Dr. Marcia Ramos-e-Silva.)

■ TREATMENT OPTIONS

Topical azole antifungals and 1% terbinafine cream work well in the treatment of tinea versicolor, and recovery usually takes 2 to 3 weeks. Ketoconazole lotions and shampoos and 2.5% selenium sulfide are other alternatives. It has been shown that oral ketoconazole and itraconazole are also effective in treating tinea vesicular. Itraconazole should be given in a total dose of 800 to 1000 mg over 5 days.

ACKNOWLEDGMENTS

Special thanks to Drs. Barbara J. Leppard, Rashmi Sarkar, and Marcia Ramos-e-Silva for providing the majority of the figures of the African, Asian, and Latin American skin diseases for this atlas.

We also appreciate the additional figures of African, Asian, and Latin American skin diseases from Drs. M. Bello, Tania Cestari, Siew Eng Choon, Diqing Luo, Anisa Mosam, V. Ramesh, and Sudhanshu Sharma.

CHAPTER 96

African American Pioneers in Dermatology

Angela D. Dillard
Frederick N. Quarles

INTRODUCTION

In his famous "I Have a Dream" speech in 1963, the Reverend Martin Luther King, Jr., spoke with hope of the day when people would be judged according to the content of their character rather than the color of their skin. In attacking the causes and consequences of discrimination, inequality, and injustice, it was certainly not King's intent to play down the importance of the objective study of skin of color itself. While many theorists locate the roots of racial prejudice in the color of skin, the darker skin of color has also inspired numerous men and women to dedicate their lives to the study, treatment, and care of dermatologic conditions and diseases. Race may be only skin deep—and not, that is to say, a matter of genetics and blood—but this skin holds many characteristics, oddities, benefits, and mysteries peculiar unto itself.

HISTORICAL CONTEXT

Today, African American dermatologists practice across the country, hold positions in major research universities and corporate institutions, and serve as advocates in public health organizations. Institutionally, most belong to the American Academy of Dermatology (AAD), and many of these dermatologists are among the 25,000 members of the National Medical Association (NMA), the oldest and largest national organization of African American physicians. The study and practice of skin of color dermatology is currently well established in a variety of medical schools and hospitals; however, this was not always the case. Indeed, writing a history of African American dermatology presents some interesting historical challenges, not the least of which is deciding what "counts" as dermatology and who can be regarded as a dermatologist. The practice and knowledge of African American dermatology undoubtedly existed in various forms long before the existence of officially trained and board-certified practitioners.

The first phase of modern dermatology in the United States (as well as in Continental Europe and Great Britain) dates from roughly 1850 to 1900, coinciding with periods of virulent racism and systemic racial exclusion in America. The first regional dermatologic associations began appearing in the United States at least as early as 1869, with the first national organization, the American Dermatological Association, holding its first annual meeting in 1877. Yet the specialty did not receive full official recognition until 1932, with the formation of the American Board of Dermatology as the first incorporated entity charged with setting and maintaining the standards for the practice of dermatology and syphilology. Shortly after this, the American Academy of Dermatology made its appearance in 1939; with over 19,000 members, it is the largest member-based organization for dermatologists in America and worldwide. As was the case in other medical specialties and within the professions at large, African Americans were pointedly excluded from these organizations for many years and were forced to establish their own separate associations and networks.

The men who met during the Cotton States and International Exposition in 1895 to call the NMA into existence knew the power of racial prejudice even as they sternly rejected its associations of inferiority. As was the case with other African American professional and fraternal organizations founded during the "nadir" of African American history, the NMA grew out of the patterns of racism and segregation that marginalized African American professionals—indeed all African Americans—from the mainstream of American society. However, these professionals were considered far from marginal within their own communities. Charles V. Roman captured the spirit of this duality in a statement that has become the historical manifesto of the organization:

> Conceived in no spirit of racial exclusiveness, fostering no ethnic antagonism, but born of the exigencies of the American environment, the National Medical Association has for its object the banding together for mutual cooperation and helpfulness, the men and women of African descent who are legally and honorably engaged in the practice of the cognate professions of medicine, surgery, pharmacy and dentistry.[1]

African American professionals were collectively denied admission to the ranks of the American Medical Association, which maintained a strict policy of racial exclusivity; in response to this, they turned inward to the mutual support and solidarity of their own associations. Such professional, fraternal, and religious organizations founded due to racism became the central components in the creation and maintenance of a vibrant African American public sphere. Thus this era of gross discrimination was also an age of institution and community-building that helped erect the infrastructure—one might say the bones and muscle—of African American communities.

And where there are bones and muscle, there is also skin—the largest organ of the human body. There were no dermatologists among the charter members of the NMA, but the Dermatology Section was founded in 1940 and has a distinctive history, and numerous dermatologists have served in various capacities within the NMA throughout the twentieth century. What follows is far from a definitive history of African American dermatologists in the United States, but is rather a brief overview of some of the men and women who can be regarded—and celebrated—as pioneers in the field; as institution-builders and educators; as trailblazers and mentors; and as those who are helping to shape the profession as we move further into the twenty-first century.

THE PIONEERS

THEODORE K. LAWLESS, MD

The first generation of African American dermatologists included a handful of mavericks and pioneers. Among the earliest and most emblematic of this group was Theodore K. Lawless, MD (1892–1971) [**Figure 96-1**]. Shortly after his birth in Thibodeaux, Louisiana, the family moved to New Orleans at a time when members of the African American community were struggling against the rising tide of racial segregation. Known to his friends as "T. K.," Lawless attended Straight College, a historically African American college that operated from 1868 to 1934, after which it merged with New Orleans University to form Dillard University. Years later, in 1955, he would remember his roots and honor his father, a former reverend, by establishing the Lawless Chapel at Dillard University with a $500,000 gift.[2]

After graduating from Straight College, he received his BA degree at Talladega College in Alabama in 1914. Lawless attended the University

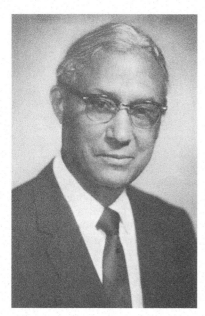

FIGURE 96-1. Theodore K. Lawless, MD (1892–1971), the grandchild of slaves, distinguished himself early on as an exemplary student and went on to amass an enormous clientele on the south side of Chicago, Illinois. People would wait hours to see this "doctor of humanity." (Used with permission from Marisol LLC, Muscat, Sultanate of Oman.)

of Kansas Medical School, and earned an MD from Northwestern University, Illinois, in 1919 and an MSc in 1920. After a 1-year fellowship in dermatology and syphilology at Massachusetts General Hospital in Boston, Lawless completed his postgraduate training at the University of Paris, France. Given the hostile racial climate within the United States, it was hardly unusual for aspiring African American professionals to seek further education in Europe.

By 1924, Lawless had returned to the United States and established a private practice in a predominantly African American neighborhood in Southside, Chicago, Illinois, during the years of the "Great Migration" that drew thousands of African American migrants from the South to northern cities. In the same year, he began teaching dermatology at Northwestern's medical school, where he served until 1941. As an instructor and researcher, Lawless made a number of contributions to the field of dermatology. His research was published in scholarly publications such as the *American Journal of Dermatology, Journal of Laboratory and Clinical Medicine*, and *Journal of the American Medical Association*. He worked to find a cure for leprosy and made several strides in the treatment of both leprosy and syphilis. As a dermatologist, Lawless was often consulted by other doctors, and he was noted for his egalitarian treatment of patients regardless of class or race. Lucius C. Earles, III, MD, who trained with Lawless in the late 1960s after completing his residency at Howard University, Washington, D.C., recalled that his patients included figures from "all walks of life, a heavy influx of folks from the lily-white suburbs as well as African Americans from Chicago."[3]

Although Lawless was a tireless professional and a major philanthropist—his several donations included the establishment of a dermatology department at Belinson Hospital in Tel-Aviv, Israel—he was also an educator, serving on the faculty of the University of Illinois. Another associate recalls that Lawless was "a doctor in the old sense of the word," and that he "dealt in humanity." The more people he could see, the more he felt he accomplished, and at $3 a visit (a substantial discount at a time when others were charging between $10 and $15), he amassed a fortune due to the sheer volume of patients he was able to accommodate.[4,5]

PAUL PRINCE BOSWELL, MD

At this time, Chicago was emerging as one of the early hubs of African American dermatology; another prominent Southside dermatologist,

Paul Prince Boswell, MD (1906–1982), was in private practice. A native of Pittsburgh and a graduate of Lincoln University in Pennsylvania, he received his MD at the University of Minnesota. While it is not clear where he did his residency in dermatology, he became a staff physician at Chicago's Provident Hospital and was also on the staff of both the Michael Reese and Michigan Avenue hospitals. In 1947, he was elected as a member of the AAD, becoming one of only three African American members at the time. As was the case with many of these early figures, Boswell's influence extended beyond the profession. For years, Boswell was a fixture in the African American society pages of the *Chicago Defender* and was deeply engaged in civic work. In the mid-1960s, he even served a term in the Illinois legislature.[6]

HAROLD THATCHER, MD

Lawless and Boswell were joined by Harold Thatcher, MD (1908–1995). A native of Kansas City, Kansas, and a 1929 graduate of the University of Minnesota Medical School, Thatcher's dermatologic training included an internship at Provident Hospital in Chicago and 4 years of study at Billings Hospital, Montana, with grants from both the Rockefeller and Rosenwald Foundations. Additionally, he spent a year at the New York University and Bellevue hospitals in New York, where he worked in dermatology and syphilology.

In 1942, Thatcher volunteered for military service and entered the U.S. Army with the rank of Major in the medical corps, serving his entire tenure as Chief of Medical Services and of regional and station hospitals, while based at Fort Huachuca in Arizona. In 1944, he was promoted to Lieutenant Colonel, and in 1945, he was awarded the Legion of Merit. As a civilian, he returned to Chicago and entered private practice, with an affiliation with Provident Hospital's Department of Dermatology. He was also a member of the Board of Trustees of Cook County Hospital's nursing school and a member of numerous civic and civil rights organizations.

Thatcher, who continued to play a role in the NMA, lived until 1995; his papers have been collected and are available in the archives of the Chicago Public Library.

HOMER E. HARRIS, JR., MD

One of Lawless's former students, Homer E. Harris, Jr., MD (1916–2007), became a pioneer in his own right. Born in Seattle, Washington, Harris was the first African American to venture into practice in the Pacific Northwest region. Harris, Jr., attended Meharry Medical College in Nashville, Tennessee, and interned in Kansas City, Missouri. He completed his dermatology residency at Illinois under Lawless's guidance.

Returning home to Seattle, he set up private practice in 1955 and remained there for over 40 years with a practice reputed to be the largest west of the Rockies. Harris, Jr., became a fixture within Seattle's African American community and found that the practice of dermatology provided him with "a sense of independence in not having to rely on hospitals or physicians for referrals." He was well-liked by his patients and highly regarded by the Seattle community, so much so that an anonymous donor contributed $1.3 million to be used for the creation of a half-acre park named in his honor.[7,8]

MADAM C. J. WALKER, PIONEER IN THE HAIR AND BEAUTY INDUSTRY

Within the category of pioneers and mavericks, one could also arguably include Sarah Breedlove, known as Madam C. J. Walker (1867–1919) [**Figure 96-2**], who was an entrepreneur in the burgeoning hair and beauty industry. A self-made millionaire, Walker invented several hair care products, including Madam Walker's Wonderful Hair Grower and a hair softener that could be used with a hot comb. Bald patches and scalp diseases functioned as the scarlet letter of poverty for many women of this era, and the famous Walker System offered them both social and physical relief. Although she was not a trained professional in the conventional sense, Walker nonetheless revolutionized the ways in which African American women styled and cared for their hair; she went on

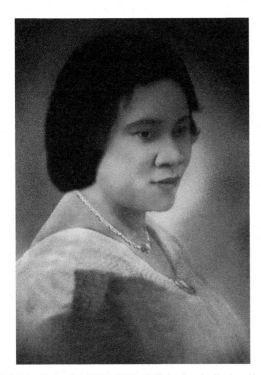

FIGURE 96-2. Madam C. J. Walker (1867–1919) developed sulfur-based hair products that responded to the ubiquitous scalp diseases of her time. She, in part, helped to establish Chicago, Illinois, as the "home of African American dermatology." (Used with permission from Marisol LLC, Muscat, Sultanate of Oman.)

to open a school—Lelia College, in Pittsburgh—where hundreds of "beauty culturists" were trained. This would have been one of the only major institutions where large numbers of women received any sort of training in the care of hair and skin. While Madam Walker eventually would relocate to New York, her empire was firmly rooted in the African American communities of Chicago, giving this city a fair bid for the title of "home of African American dermatology."[9]

THOMAS OBADIAH SENIOR, MD

The challenges of training African American professionals in a climate of racial hostility and segregation were substantial. Many of these pioneers looked to Europe or to the ranks of the military for training, and most spent some amount of time at historically African American institutions, either for their undergraduate or medical school education. Some came from other countries across the African American diaspora to attend these institutions. Thomas Obadiah Senior, MD (1883–1937), for example, was born in Broughton, Jamaica, and came to New York from Havana, Cuba, in 1919. Senior graduated from Meharry Medical College in 1923 and spent the bulk of his career there, first as an instructor and later as a professor in the fields of dermatology, genitourinary diseases, and syphilodermatology.[10]

THE PIONEERING ROLE OF THE DEPARTMENT OF DERMATOLOGY, HOWARD UNIVERSITY COLLEGE OF MEDICINE AND HOWARD UNIVERSITY HOSPITAL

There is one institution in particular that deserves special mention for its pioneering role. The history of the Department of Dermatology of the Howard University College of Medicine and Howard University Hospital (formerly Freedmen's Hospital) stretches back to 1906, when Henry H. Hazen, MD (1879–1951), conducted weekly dermatology clinics at Freedmen's Hospital and gave a regular course in dermatology to medical students. Hazen continued these efforts almost single-handedly until 1927, when Charles Wendell Freeman, MD (1900–1980), graduated

from the Howard University College of Medicine and began work in the dermatology clinic.

Freeman, a native of Washington, DC, traveled to Europe for advanced training in the specialty. From 1934 to 1935, he studied dermatology in Germany, Vienna, and other European medical centers as a fellow of the Oberlander Trust of Philadelphia. In subsequent years, Hazen's visits became less frequent, and Freeman's duties at the hospital expanded. By the early 1940s, he had become a clinical Assistant Professor at Howard University, and in 1941 was made a diplomate of the American Board of Dermatology and Syphilology after passing the board's examination. He was also widely known for his efforts to educate the general populace and specialists about the perils of syphilis. In 1942, for example, he embarked on a four-state lecture tour designed to bring the latest advancements to the general practitioner.[11,12] At various times over the next two decades or so, the Division of Dermatology at Freedmen's Hospital would be augmented by Drs. John C. Payne, Peter D. Johnson, Jocelyn Mitchell, and eventually, Jesse A. Kenne and Joseph G. Gathings.

Gathings (1898–1965), who also was among the earliest African American diplomates of the American Board of Dermatology and Syphilology, had 2 years of special training, from 1941 to 1943, as a Rosenwald Fellow at the New York Skin and Cancer Hospital. He would serve for some 15 years in the Division of Dermatology at Freedmen's Hospital and the Howard University College of Medicine, first as a clinical instructor and later advancing to a clinical Assistant Professor. He also had been a president of the NMA. At the time of his death in 1965, he was conducting a research project, supported by the Shriners, in the skin condition known as vitiligo. In 1961, he had been instrumental in obtaining the services of John A. Kenney, Jr. (1914–2003), who, in continuing the work of these pioneers, would go on to leave a distinctive mark on the African American study and practice of dermatology as one of the field's most noted institution builders.

INSTITUTION BUILDING: AFRICAN AMERICAN DERMATOLOGY COMES OF AGE

New fields of study, professional practice, and human endeavor need pioneers and trailblazers to search out new opportunities and to enlarge our sense of possibilities. However, as these avenues develop and grow, becoming more established, there must be a second generation willing to take on the vast responsibilities of building and sustaining these institutions and networks. It is this generation, straddling the divide between pioneers and builders, that is awarded more official recognition than their predecessors and that contains members who were able to make use of a wider arena in which to develop their talents and practice their craft.

VERNAL GORDON CAVE, MD

Vernal Gordon Cave, MD (1918–1997) [**Figure 96-3**], was born in Colón, Panama, and was raised primarily in Brooklyn, New York. This journey is a reminder of the "Great Migration" that brought thousands of African Americans from the South to the North and is dovetailed with the sizable wave of immigration to urban centers such as New York. Cave earned a BSc at City College (City University of New York) and an MD at Howard University College of Medicine in 1944. He served as a medical officer in the U.S. Army and Air Force and was a member of the renowned Tuskegee Airmen from 1947 to 1952; he was honorably discharged after obtaining the rank of Captain. His postgraduate studies were pursued at a number of hospitals, including the Harlem Hospital Center in New York City, Freedmen's Hospital in Washington, DC, the North Carolina Sanatorium for the Treatment of Tuberculosis in Wilson, North Carolina, and the Bellevue Hospital Center in New York, as well as the New York University Post-Graduate Medical School. In 1956 he became a diplomate of the American Board of Dermatology and Syphilology, thus becoming the first board-certified African American dermatologist in Brooklyn. The earliest dermatologist with skin of color across the river in New York City seems to have been Thomas L. Day, MD, who had a practice in Harlem, followed by Gerald Spencer, MD.

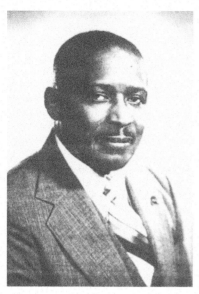

FIGURE 96-3. Vernal Cave, MD (1918–1997), who, during his term of leadership within the New York City Department of Health, implemented equal rights policies and policies that led to a decline in the incidence of infectious syphilis in the city.

For 16 years, ending in 1975, Cave served as Deputy Director, Acting Director, and Director of the Bureau of Venereal Disease Control of the New York City Department of Health. During his tenure of leadership within the Department of Health, not only did the incidence of infectious syphilis in New York City decline, but he also successfully implemented a policy of equal rights and opportunities for the positions and promotion of women.

Cave authored or coauthored some 35 scientific articles and chapters in scientific journals and medical textbooks. He was one of the original members of the Board of Directors at the inception of the New York City Health and Hospitals Corporation, exerting his efforts toward improved healthcare for all Americans regardless of race or economic status. Cave was a career member of the NMA, of which he was a past president, and was a member of the Board of Trustees of the Brooklyn Branch of the National Association for the Advancement of Colored People (NAACP). He was also a member of the Tuskegee Syphilis Study Ad Hoc Advisory Panel appointed by the federal government and held the position of Chairman of the NMA Tuskegee Syphilis Study Ad Hoc Committee. It was through the investigative work of these committees that the atrocities of the Tuskegee Syphilis Study were documented and exposed.

JOHN A. KENNEY, JR., MD

Born in Tuskegee, Alabama, John A. Kenney, Jr., MD (1914–2003) [**Figure 96-4**], was the son of John A. Kenney, Sr., the Medical Director and Chief Surgeon of the general hospital at the Tuskegee Institute, and personal physician to the institute's founder, Booker T. Washington. Kenney, Sr., was also a co-founder of the NMA. When his activities on behalf of African American doctors and nurses led to a Ku Klux Klan-initiated cross-burning on the Kenney family's lawn, Kenney, Sr., moved the family to Montclair, New Jersey, where Kenney, Jr., and his three siblings grew up and pursued their educations. Kenney, Jr., graduated from Bates College, Maine, and was a member of the class of 1945 at the Howard University College of Medicine.

While interning at Cleveland City Hospital in Ohio (then one of the first city hospitals to admit African American residents), Kenney, Jr., had a transformative experience: an influential doctor at the hospital persuaded him to choose dermatology as his specialty. At the time, none of the other 80 African American physicians in Cleveland were dermatologists, and many Caucasian dermatologists refused to treat African American patients—a situation that was painfully ubiquitous in most regions of the country. Inspired by the older doctor, Kenney, Jr., pursued dermatologic training at the University of Pennsylvania and

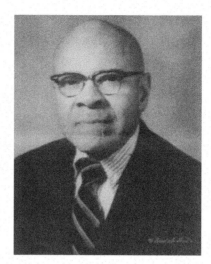

FIGURE 96-4. John A. Kenney, Jr., MD (1914–2003). During his over 30 years at Howard University, Washington, D.C., he is estimated to have trained and mentored one-third of all dermatologists with skin of color practicing at the time of his death.

the University of Michigan, returning in 1954 to Cleveland to join the staff at University Hospital and the faculty at Case Western Reserve. As the city's only African American dermatologist, he built a sizable practice that was not solely confined to patients with skin of color. Despite this success, he felt the lure of academia and the rigors of research and training new dermatologists. In accepting a teaching and administrative position at Howard University, Kenney, Jr., moved from the category of pioneer in the field to institution builder.

Kenney, Jr., came to Freedmen's Hospital and the Howard University College of Medicine in 1961 as Associate Professor of Dermatology and was selected as Chief of the Division when Charles Wendell Freeman retired in 1963. It was a position Kenney, Jr., would hold until 1981. In these crucial decades in which the study and practice of African American dermatology fully came of age, Kenney, Jr., not only trained residents but also gave dermatology lectures to medical students. Indeed, many of the "next generation" of dermatology specialists would cite these lectures as one of the reasons they were attracted to the specialty. During his nearly four decades at Howard University, Kenney, Jr., established a full Dermatology Department, a 3-year residency program, and a research laboratory in dermatology. Above all, he was instrumental in training numerous students pursuing careers in dermatology; by one reckoning, he trained and mentored one third of all African American dermatologists practicing at the time of his death.

OTHER AFRICAN AMERICAN DERMATOLOGISTS WHO CARRIED ON THE LEGACY

Kenney, Jr., was not the only major figure at Howard University during this period and not the only person responsible for the institutional growth and expansion of its dermatology program. There was also, among others, Harold E. Pierce, Jr., MD (1922–2006) [**Figure 96-5**], who served as an Assistant Professor of Dermatological Surgery at Howard University for 17 years. Pierce, Jr., had been a graduate of Howard University College of Medicine in 1946 and had gone on to intern at Harlem Hospital in New York and to complete a residency in dermatology at the Philadelphia General Hospital. In 1951, he accepted a commission as a Captain in what would become the U.S. Air Force Medical Service and served with distinction until officially retiring from the Air Force National Guard in 1976. As a dermatologist, Pierce, Jr., built his practice and reputation on his diagnoses and treatment of people with skin of color who suffered from complex skin disorders that his fellow clinicians were unable to solve.

During his long and varied career, Pierce, Jr., performed the first dermabrasion procedure on an African American patient, as well as hair

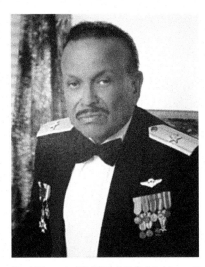

FIGURE 96-5. Harold Pierce, Jr., MD (1922–2006), built his practice upon his ability to diagnose and treat individuals with complex skin disorders that others could not diagnose or manage.

transplants and scar revision surgery. Years later he participated in the first liposuction. He was among the first and most prominent African American cosmetic surgeons in the country and is widely regarded as the "father of African American cosmetic surgery." The author of more than 50 medical articles and editor of *Cosmetic Surgery in Non-White Patients* (New York: Grune & Stratton, 1982), Pierce, Jr., trained numerous students, including Mershiler Allen, his medical-surgical assistant, at the Philadelphia College of Osteopathic Medicine and at Howard University. His daughter, Sandra E. Vause, MD, is a practicing dermatologist in New Jersey and has established the Harold E. Pierce, Jr., M.D. Scholarship Trust Fund to support resident doctors in the training and advancement of dermasurgery.[13] She is also the first African American woman dermatologist with dual board certification in dermatology and cosmetic surgery. She completed the American Board of Dermatology certification in November 1989 and subsequently completed a 1-year fellowship in cosmetic surgery with Drs. Farber and Bridenstein and then sat for and successfully completed the written and oral boards in cosmetic surgery through the American Board of Cosmetic Surgery in November 1991.

Freedmen's Hospital, which changed its name to Howard University Hospital in 1975, and the College of Medicine also had the good fortune to secure the presence of Harold R. Minus, MD (b. 1940) [**Figure 96-6**], who took over as Chairman of the Department of Dermatology from Kenney in 1980. He served in this capacity until 1992, when the department's current Chair, Rebat M. Halder, MD (b. 1953) [**Figure 96-7**], succeeded him. Halder, of Indian ancestry, is a 1978 graduate of Howard University College of Medicine. He completed a residency at Howard University Hospital, joining the faculty at Howard University in 1982, and has been Chairman of the Dermatology Department since 1992. Halder established and is the Director of the Ethnic Skin Research Institute within the department and is an authority on pigmentary disorders of the skin and in dermatology for skin of color. In 1999, he directed the first session on dermatology for skin of color at the annual meeting of the AAD and is the author of the first textbook on this subject entitled *Dermatology and Dermatological Therapy of Pigmented Skins* (2006). While the next generation of dermatologists was trained at several different institutions, including predominantly Caucasian universities such as the University of Michigan and within the ranks of the U.S. Armed Forces, Howard University nonetheless stands out as a virtual powerhouse in the field.

William Coffey, MD, and Lucius C. Earles, MD, were graduates of the Howard Medical School class of 1963, and both credit Kenney, Jr., for influencing them in choosing careers in dermatology. William Coffey went on to help develop the dermatology program at King-Drew Medical Center in Los Angeles, California, which includes the Charles Drew University of Medicine and Science, incorporated in 1966 after decades of militant community-based advocacy for improved medical services.

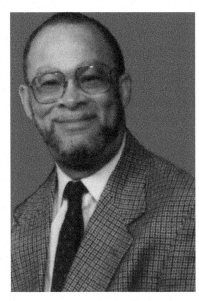

FIGURE 96-6. Harold Minus, MD (b. 1940), took over as Chairman of the Department of Dermatology at Howard University, Washington, D.C., in 1980 from John A. Kenney, Jr., MD, and served there until 1992.

Earles has been in private practice in Chicago for over 40 years and is a past president of the NMA.

Earles reflects on his residency training:

When I began the program ... the total number of those choosing dermatology in our class of about 88 at Howard University, 1963, was four. During those most interesting and informative two years, Charles Thurston, the second African American at [the] University of Michigan, generally came to our Friday morning sessions. It was at that time that I discovered that Dr. Kenney was the first African American dermatologist trained at the University of Michigan, and I didn't have the slightest idea that I would in time be the third.... During my residency at HU, I had the pleasure also of first meeting Greta Clarke, then a student rotating through dermatology as one of her electives. It was during this time in the program at Howard, when we attended the American Academy of Dermatology convention, that I came to realize actually how miniscule the number of African Americans was in dermatology. Present at the meeting were Dr. Kenney and his flock, John Carney from Los Angeles, John Butler of Detroit, Tommy Williams of D.C., a dermatologist who worked at D.C. General Hospital, and of course our own Carnot Evans.... To sum things up, it was apparent that there was minimal representation at that meeting of those who looked like us.

This situation, however, was dramatically altered by the increase in dermatology residents in the late 1960s and early 1970s, which forever changed the field.

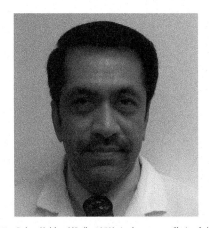

FIGURE 96-7. Rebat Halder, MD (b. 1953), is the current Chair of the Department of Dermatology at Howard University, Washington, D.C.

THE NEXT GENERATION OF AFRICAN AMERICAN DERMATOLOGISTS IN THE 1960's AND 1970's: THE "MAGNIFICENT SEVEN" AND OTHERS

By 1965, the post–World War II Civil Rights Movement had accomplished at least two of its major legislative goals: the Civil Rights Act of 1964 and the Voting Rights Act of 1965. Secured at a painfully high price in terms of human life and after nearly a decade of sustained organization and activism, the social and political environment of the nation was forever changed. Legalized racial segregation was now a thing of the past, and despite the lingering effects of institutional racism, African Americans were granted an unprecedented level of access and opportunity in education and professional life. At this moment, when change was in the air and a new militancy was gripping young African Americans across the nation, Howard University College of Medicine was privileged to receive the dermatology class of 1965. Kenney, Jr., was still relatively new to his post at Howard University, and it was his first full year teaching. In 1966, dermatology became an elective, and during these years, the program was home to a group of students dubbed by A. Paul Kelly, MD (1938–2014) [**Figure 96-8**], as the "Magnificent Seven": Robert Heidelberg, Boyd Savoy, Ike Willis, O. G. Rodman, Fletcher Robinson, James Hobbs, and Kelly himself, who notes that when this group completed their residencies, they "almost doubled the number of practicing African American dermatologists."[14,15]

Kelly, the son and grandson of physicians, was born in Ashville, North Carolina, and arrived at Howard University Medical School after earning an undergraduate degree at Brown University, Rhode Island. He was in his third-year clinical rotations when he heard a lecture on dermatology by Kenney, Jr., and was inspired to choose dermatology as his area of specialization. "Close your eyes and stick a pin in a map of the USA," he recalls Kenney, Jr., intoning. "Wherever the pin lands, you can go there and probably be the only African American dermatologist." For Kelly and his classmates, the pins landed in several different locations, making them in many instances "African American firsts."

Kelly was the first African American resident trained in dermatology at Henry Ford Hospital in Detroit, Michigan. His first faculty position was at the Brown University Department of Dermatology from 1971 to 1973, chaired by Charles McDonald, MD (b. 1932) [**Figure 96-9**], the first African American chairman of a dermatology program at an institution where the majority of people were Caucasians.

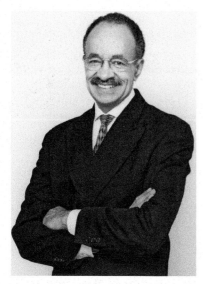

FIGURE 96-8. A. Paul Kelly, MD (1938–2014), the son and grandson of physicians, was heavily influenced by John A. Kenney, Jr., to become one of the "Magnificent Seven." After training in Detroit, Michigan, and achieving many other African American firsts, he went on to train dozens of other dermatologists. (Used with permission from Jim Dennis, Photographer, Oakland, California.)

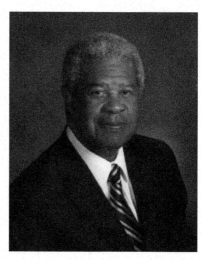

FIGURE 96-9. Charles McDonald, MD (b. 1932), who was the first Chairman of Dermatology Emeritus at Brown University, Rhode Island was the first African American chairman of a dermatology program at a Caucasian-dominant institution.

After leaving Brown University, Kelly went to Los Angeles and eventually became Chief of the Division of Dermatology at King-Drew Medical Center/Charles Drew University School of Medicine and Science from 1975 to 2006. The dermatology program at King-Drew Medical Center was the only program, other than the one at Howard University, that was specifically developed for the training of minority dermatologists. In many ways, and under very different circumstances, Kelly sought to do at King-Drew Medical Center what Kenney, Jr., and other pioneers had done at Howard University. Kelly has over 60 former residents who are grateful for their training in dermatology under his guidance. Kelly is well-known nationally and internationally for his research on keloids and has enjoyed a career marked by several "African American firsts." He was the first African American President of the American Dermatological Association, the Pacific Dermatologic Association, and the Association of Professors of Dermatology. He was also active in the NMA, having served as Editor-in-Chief of the *Journal of the National Medical Association* between 1997 and 2005. Lastly, he co-edited the textbook, Taylor and Kelly's Dermatology for Skin of Color, for both the 1st and 2nd editions.

Although Robert Heidelberg, MD (1939–2013), was not the first African American dermatologist in Detroit—that distinction goes either to John Butler, MD, or Edward W. Kelly, Jr., MD—he had one of the largest private practices in Detroit for over 40 years. In the tradition of Lawless, and other major contributors to the practice of dermatology, Heidelberg, known as "Dr. Bob" to his community, was strongly devoted to his patients. His focus was not on earning money from his patients but on giving them high-quality dermatologic care. At one point, when it was suggested that he move his practice to a more lucrative location outside of Detroit, Heidelberg responded by saying, "Then who will take care of our people?"[16] His daughter, Karen Heidelberg, MD (b. 1967) [**Figure 96-10**], is also a dermatologist and practiced with her father. She continues to serve Detroit's patients with her father's classmate, L. Boyd Savoy, MD, and other associates.

James Hobbs, MD (b. 1940), has been in private practice in Los Angeles for over 40 years. He, too, has a daughter, Lori Hobbs, MD (b. 1963), who is a dermatologist also practicing in Los Angeles [**Figure 96-11**]. Orlando G. Rodman, MD (b. 1940), was a member of Howard University's famous dermatology class of 1965 but left school to join the Army in 1966, serving as a paratrooper until 1969. Following the footsteps of Drs. Cave, Pierce, Thatcher, and others, he trained in dermatology while in the armed services. Board-certified in dermatology and dermatopathology, in 1974 he was named Chief of Dermatology at the Walter Reed Army Medical Center. After retiring from the Army as a Colonel in 1987, he joined the AAD's scientific program as Director of its Gross and Microscopic Symposium and was Vice Chairman of the Department of

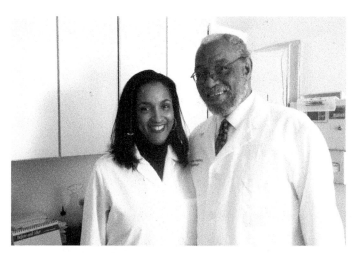

FIGURE 96-10. Robert P. Heidelberg, MD (1939–2013), and Karen Heidelberg, MD (b. 1967), set up a private practice that has been one of the largest in Detroit, Michigan, for over 40 years.

Dermatology at the Henry Ford Hospital in Detroit from 1987 to 1993. In 1993, he relocated to Macon, Georgia, where, until his retirement in 2005, he was part of the Georgia Dermatology Group.

Isaac "Ike" Willis, MD (1940–2007), was trained in dermatology at the University of Pennsylvania, where he worked closely with Albert Kligman, MD. Through their joint efforts, they developed the first combination "fading" cream that consisted of hydroquinone, retinoic acid, and a corticosteroid. Today, this combination fade cream is patented as Tri-Luma Cream® by the Galderma Pharmaceutical Company, Lausanne, Switzerland. After completing his training at the University of Pennsylvania, Willis relocated to his hometown of Atlanta, Georgia, joining the practice of Wesley Wilborn, MD, who is credited as the first African American dermatologist in the state of Georgia. Willis has written numerous scientific papers, mainly pertaining to melanin metabolism and the treatment of dyschromia. He remained in private practice in Atlanta for over 30 years until his death.

Leonard Boyd Savoy, MD (b. 1934), is a faculty member within the Department of Dermatology at Wayne State University in Detroit and was Chairman of the Dermatology Department at the Veteran Affairs

(VA) Medical Center in Allen Park, Michigan, for several years. He has written numerous scientific papers mostly relating to urticaria and the inflammatory and chemotactic responses in atopic dermatitis. Savoy practiced part-time with Robert Heidelberg and continues practicing with Karen Heidelberg. James Fletcher Robinson, MD (b. 1947), the last of the "Magnificent Seven," is the first and only African American dermatologist to have had a private practice for over 25 years in both St. Thomas, U.S. Virgin Islands, and Washington, DC.

Adding to the geographic diversity of the "Magnificent Seven" were a number of individuals who made their mark as the first to set up private practices in various locations, including Drs. Norman Walton (Alabama), Errol Quintal (Louisiana), Richard Gibbs (Tennessee), William Anderson (East Orange, New Jersey), and Raymond Blackburn (Texas), as well as Drs. Claude Vernon Caver (Hawaii) and, a little later, John H. Bocachica (Alaska).

As this generation came of age within the profession, they were both the cause and the beneficiaries of racial integration and the increased liberalization of American society in the late 1960s and 1970s. Educated and trained during the era of sit-ins, Freedom Rides, and Civil Rights marches, they entered the profession of dermatology as the calls for "Freedom Now" were replaced with the demands for "Black Power." "Black" was beautiful, and militant activists began to organize processes of community control and empowerment. By the late 1970s and early 1980s, the study and practice of skin of color dermatology had truly come into its own. The dermatology program at Howard University continued to turn out dozens of new dermatologists and was joined, in 1975, by the newly founded residency program at King-Drew Medical Center in Los Angeles.

At the same time, students with skin of color were being increasingly admitted to programs at institutions such as the University of Michigan and Brown University where McDonald has been such an important presence since 1968. While McDonald and Algin Garrett, MD (b. 1952) [**Figure 96-12**], a specialist in Mohs micrographic surgery and Chair of the dermatology program at Virginia Commonwealth University, are the rare African American heads of programs at majority institutions, this generation has had the benefit of education and mentoring from inspiring specialists beyond the cultural boundaries of race and ethnicity. Many of those who would later go on to play leading roles in staking out new geographic territories, in researching and engaging in new techniques, and in providing leadership for professional organizations, such as the NMA's Dermatology Section, were educated during this period.

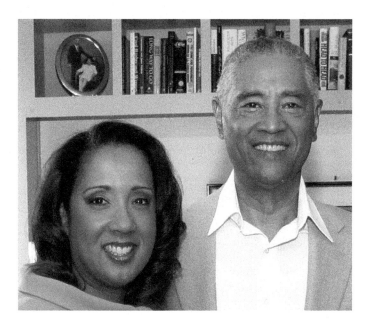

FIGURE 96-11. James Hobbs, MD (b. 1940), and Lori Hobbs, MD (b. 1963), have owned private dermatologic practices in Los Angeles, California, throughout the past 40 years.

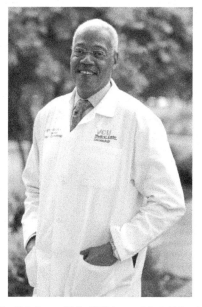

FIGURE 96-12. Algin Garrett, MD (b. 1952), is a specialist in Mohs micrographic surgery and Chair of the Dermatology Program of Virginia Commonwealth University.

The experiences of Frederick Quarles, MD (b. 1955), are to some extent emblematic of this generation. Born in Detroit in 1955, he has known many inspirational pioneers and institution builders personally, such as Drs. Cave, Pierce, and Kenney, Jr., and yet is still young enough to have witnessed and helped to encourage the transformation of the field in terms of gender, setting up a private practice in Norfolk, Virginia, with Katherine Treherne in 1985. Quarles received his MD degree from Howard University in 1981 and then completed his residency in dermatology at the same university under the guidance of Drs. Kenney, Minus, Pierce, Carnot Evans, and Halder, as well as Pearl Grimes and Cassandra McLaurin. His career has been shaped by both the liberalization of race relations in the United States since the mid-1960s and the continuing existence of our nation's racial polarization. His concern over the latter has propelled his involvement over the years with the Old Dominion Medical Society in Virginia (as a past president) and with the NMA, especially the Dermatology Section, of which he served as Chairman from 2005 to 2007. As a student of history, and distressed by the lack of attention to African American men and women in the histories of national organizations such as the American Dermatological Association, the AAD, and the American Board of Dermatology, this present history chapter was initiated as part of his service to the NMA.

Andrew F. Alexis, MD, MPH (b. 1974) [**Figure 96-13**] succeeded Susan Taylor, MD, as Director of the Skin of Color Center at St. Luke's Roosevelt Hospital Center, New York. Alexis credits his mother, Mercy Alexis, who has practiced dermatology for over 35 years in Toronto, Canada, as being his first mentor. After his dermatology residency at Weill Cornell Medical Center and his research fellowship in dermatopharmacology at New York University, he joined the Skin of Color Center in 2004 as Associate Director and went on to become Director in 2005. In his current position, he has expanded educational initiatives at national and international meetings and has mentored clinical research fellows and residents who have contributed to numerous research projects and publications on dermatologic disorders that are more prevalent in skin of color. His own work has focused on the treatment of hair and scalp disorders, performing cosmetic procedures in darker skin types, and the racial/ethnic differences in the treatment of common dermatologic disorders.

As the barriers of race became less daunting to dermatologists and other professionals with skin of color, so too did the traditional gender-based limitations of the field. With Minus as Chairman and Grimes and McLaurin as Assistant Professors within the Dermatology Department at Howard University during the 1980s, the door for women with skin of color to enter into the field of dermatology was opened, both at the historic Howard University and at a host of other institutions.

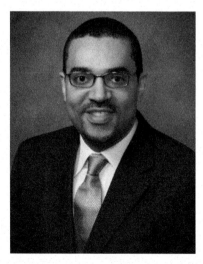

FIGURE 96-13. Andrew F. Alexis, MD, MPH (b. 1974), is the Director of the Skin of Color Center and Chairman, Department of Dermatology, Mount Sinai St. Luke's Hospital in New York, where he has mentored fellows and residents and expanded educational initiatives.

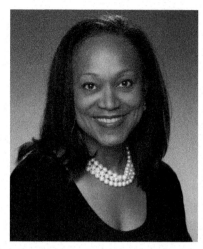

FIGURE 96-14. Pearl Grimes, MD (b. 1950), maintains a practice in Los Angeles, California, is a researcher and lecturer, and is known by many as "Mother Pearl" for her encouragement toward women and as an icon in dermatology.

AFRICAN AMERICAN WOMEN PIONEERS IN DERMATOLOGY

PEARL GRIMES, MD

Pearl Grimes, MD (b. 1950) [**Figure 96-14**], is fondly referred to by some as "Mother Pearl" for her leadership, mentoring, and encouragement of women in dermatology within the NMA and AAD. Since 1990, she has been the Medical Director of the Vitiligo and Pigmentation Institute of Southern California and maintains a full-time private practice in Los Angeles. Grimes is also a Clinical Professor of Dermatology at the David Geffen School of Medicine, Los Angeles, and lectures extensively on issues pertaining to her research on vitiligo—a topic she first developed an interest in from the direct mentoring she received from Kenney, Jr., while at Howard University. Grimes completed her medical education at Washington University in St. Louis, Missouri, (1970–1974) and her residency training in dermatology at Howard University Hospital (1975–1978), where she was Chief Resident (1978–1979). Grimes credits much of her success to a number of pioneers and institution builders, including Kenney, Jr., "who recognized strengths that I did not recognize myself." Kenney, Jr., she continues, "built the walls for an academic foundation that was laid at Washington University," and her experiences with Drs. Minus and Kelly "were the mortar and wood that completed the process."[17]

Grimes has been an important mentor in her own right to dermatologists of both genders, although she is particularly an inspiration for women in dermatology. She was first an instructor and later an Assistant Professor at Howard University's College of Medicine, as well as Director of the Vitiligo Research Center. In 1984, she left Howard University for a position at Charles R. Drew University of Medicine and Science, where she was an Assistant Professor until 1992 and an Associate Professor until 2005. As a teacher within and beyond the walls of academia, she has also played a leading role in broadly disseminating the histories of the profession, including such video productions as *The Women's Dermatologic Society: A Historical Perspective* (2005), *The Measure of a Great Man: The Life and Legacy of Dr. John A. Kenney, Jr.* (2004), and *History of the American Society of Dermatologic Surgery* (2006).

GRETA CLARK, MD

Greta Clark, MD (b. 1941), was one of the first African American women in private practice in Oakland, California, where she has been located for over 30 years and has served as a regional trustee for the NMA. Born in Detroit, Michigan, she received her MD degree in 1967 from Howard University; she completed a residency in internal medicine at Harlem Hospital, followed by a residency in dermatology at New York University in 1972. She was greatly influenced by Kenney, Jr., at Howard University and by Thomas Day in New York, as well as by Hilda Germaine Straker, MD, who maintained a private practice in Manhattan, New York, while heading the Division of Dermatology at Harlem Hospital.

HILDA GERMAINE STRAKER, MD

Hilda Germaine Straker, MD, is more than likely the first African American woman to be board-certified in dermatology. A native of New York and a 1940 graduate of Howard University, she completed an internship at Harlem Hospital and further dermatologic training at the Bellevue Medical Center. She was a member not only of the NMA but also of the American Medical Association, the AAD, and the American Women's Medical Association. After she retired from private practice, she became a consultant for the Revlon Cosmetics Company.[18-20]

CASSANDRA McLAURIN, MD

Cassandra McLaurin, MD (1948–2010), was at Howard University for over 30 years as an instructor (1978–1979), an Assistant Professor (1979–1984), and an Associate Professor (1984–2010) in the Department of Dermatology. She chose an academic career initially due to Kenney, Jr., having recruited her to Howard University, and remained there afterward because of her dedication to the training and empowerment of the next generation of dermatologists. Specializing in pediatric dermatology, she had a long publications record on topics ranging from keloids to pediatric dermatoses. She claimed Drs. Kenney and Minus as important mentors and published studies with colleagues such as Grimes. As a student, she especially admired Bernett Johnson, MD, "for his expertise in the arts and balanced approach to medicine and life"; this was a balance that she sought to help her own students and residents achieve.

YVONNE KNIGHT, MD, AND MARGERY SCOTT, MD

Yvonne Knight, MD (b. 1950) [**Figure 96-15**], heads the Aesthetic Clinique and the West End Dermatology Associates and Medi Spa West Clinic, in Richmond, Virginia. Knight graduated from the University of Michigan in premedical studies and trained at Howard University, and she is a board-certified dermatologist and an Assistant Clinical Professor in the Department of Dermatology of the Virginia Commonwealth University Medical Center. Margery Scott, MD (b. 1945), completed her dermatology residency at the Thomas Jefferson University Hospital

and her dermatopathology fellowship at Temple University's Skin and Cancer Hospital in Philadelphia. She then returned home to Norfolk, Virginia, and became one of the first African American female dermatologists to practice in Virginia—an honor she shares with Knight. Scott was Chief of the Division of Dermatology at the VA Medical Center in Hampton, Virginia, for over 30 years before retiring and accepting a full-time faculty position within the newly formed Department of Dermatology at Eastern Virginia Medical School (EVMS) in Norfolk, Virginia, from which she is also now retired. Scott has a daughter, Kimberly "Scott" Salkey, who completed a dermatology residency at EVMS and is a faculty member within its Department of Dermatology, making them the first mother–daughter dermatologists to work in tandem.

SUSAN C. TAYLOR, MD

Outside strictly academic circles, Susan C. Taylor, MD (b. 1958) [**Figure 96-16**], has become a highly visible leader in the field of dermatology. She serves on the Board of Directors for the AAD, and she is also a founding board member for the Skin of Color Society established in 2004. Under the auspices of the Skin of Color Society, Taylor helped to originate and institute an annual competition in skin of color dermatology for students, residents, and fellows, as well as a research competition and award for young investigators in the field of skin of color. Born in Philadelphia and educated at the University of Pennsylvania (gaining her BA in 1979) and Harvard University Medical School (gaining her MD in 1983), Taylor completed an internship and residency at Pennsylvania Hospital and a residency in dermatology at Columbia Presbyterian Medical Center in New York. She holds certifications in both internal medicine and dermatology. She has been in private practice in Philadelphia since 1989, and in 1999, she was appointed as Director and founder of the Skin of Color Center at St. Luke's Hospital Center. The Skin of Color Center, which is the first of its kind in the nation, is dedicated to the investigation, diagnosis, and treatment of diseases in individuals with skin of color, inclusive of those of African American, Hispanic, and Asian ancestry. As the third African American member of the Board of the AAD and the first African American woman in its 73-year history, Taylor served as a catalyst for change within the profession at large. She led physician colleagues to consensus over important issues including those related to diversity, as well as guiding the AAD Board to affirm its commitment to, and definition of, diversity. As part of her seminal work in defining the parameters of diversity, Taylor also convened a Skin of Color Classification Summit, incorporating dermatologists from Asia, Africa, and North and South America who gathered to discuss and revise the skin classification system.

Researchers, mentors, and teachers such as Drs. Taylor and Alexis sit at the heart of one of the major new trends in the field, one that involves the broadening of the former category of "black dermatology" in the direction of the science, study, and treatment of skin of color. Howard

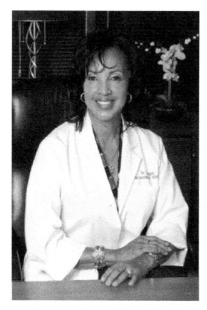

FIGURE 96-15. Yvonne Knight, MD (b. 1950), heads the Aesthetic Clinique and the West End Dermatology Associates and Medi Spa West Clinic and is an Assistant Professor at Virginia Commonwealth University Medical Center.

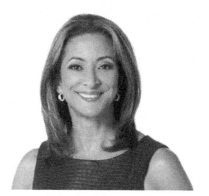

FIGURE 96-16. Susan C. Taylor, MD (b. 1958), well-known in both academic and non-academic circles, is the Founding Director of the one-of-a-kind Skin of Color Center at St. Luke's Roosevelt Hospital Center in New York. She endeavors to reconfigure the idea of skin of color and raise awareness of skin diseases in these populations.

University's Medical School and Hospital have a history of noncaucasian and non-African American students, particularly Indian students, and its present Chair, Halder, is of Indian ancestry. Kelly, moreover, has trained Hispanic, Asian, and Euro-American residents within the King-Drew Medical Center program. Consciously working under the rubric of "skin of color," promoting its study and care in societies, publications, websites, and lecture tours, Dr. Taylor and colleagues are helping to reconfigure the very idea of skin of color. Drs. Kelly and Taylor, editors of this textbook, *Taylor and Kelly's Dermatology for Skin of Color*, 2nd edition, seek to further develop awareness of the cutaneous manifestations of skin diseases in people with skin of color, while giving both younger and more mature dermatologists a platform for writing about these subjects.

LYNN McKINLEY-GRANT, MD, VALERIE CALLENDER, MD, AND CHERYL BURGESS, MD

Women with skin of color have come to occupy the very center of the study of dermatology of skin of color and are simply too numerous to mention and document in these pages. A representative sample drawn from academic and private practice, national organizations such as the NMA and the Women's Dermatologic Society (WDS), and the continuing tradition of highlighting "African American firsts" would include the women in the following paragraph.

Lynn McKinley-Grant, MD (b. 1948) [**Figure 96-17**], is a board-certified dermatologist and has over 20 years of experience in private practice and academic medicine. McKinley-Grant is an Associate Clinical Professor of Dermatology and an attending physician at the Melanoma Center at the Washington Hospital Center, Washington, DC. She attended Harvard University Medical School, has a Master's degree from Columbia University Teacher's College, and did her residency at New York University. She is a diplomate of both internal medicine and dermatology. Valerie Callender, MD (b. 1961), trained under Minus, lectures frequently at the national and international levels and has served as a past Chairman of the Dermatology Section of the NMA. Positioning herself at the nexus of the NMA, the WDS, and the Skin of Color Society, of which she served as president in 2013–2014, she also heads the Callender Skin and Laser Center in Mitchellville, Maryland. Similarly, Cheryl Burgess, MD (b. 1958), practices in the Washington, DC, area and was also trained at Howard University under Minus. She received an MD degree from Howard University in 1984 and completed her residency in 1988, during which time she was greatly influenced by Drs. Beverly Johnson, Treherne, and Quarles, all of whom allowed her to rotate with them and learn the various aspects and skills needed to run a dermatology practice. Burgess is the founder, Medical Director, and President of the Center for Dermatology and Dermatologic Surgery, the Professional Aesthetic Image Center, P.C., in Washington, DC. Additionally, she is an Assistant Clinical Professor at Georgetown University Medical Center and George Washington Hospital and is also the Director of an Allegan-sponsored Botox® Cosmetic Training Center, as well as author and senior editor of the book *Cosmetic Dermatology* (2005).

WENDY ROBERTS, MD, AND DENISE BUNTIN, MD

Wendy Roberts, MD (b. 1959), who was trained at the King-Drew Medical Center under Kelly, is currently in private practice in Desert Palms, California, and serves as a regional trustee for the AAD. Born in East Orange, New Jersey, she received an MD degree at Stanford University, California, in 1984 and completed her residency in 1991 and a dermatopathology fellowship at the New York University Medical Center in 1993. She is the founding Director of the Section of Dermatopathology, Division of Dermatology, Loma Linda University Medical Center, California, and is currently a Clinical Assistant Professor of Medicine at Loma Linda; she is the first African American dermatologist on the faculty. In addition to her practice in cosmetic dermatology, geriatric dermatology, and dermatopathology, she is active in numerous regional associations and in the WDS, serving as that organization's first African American president in 2009.

Another female dermatologist who was the first to venture into private practice in the state Tennessee is Denise Buntin, MD (b. 1954). She was also the first African American resident in dermatology at the University of Tennessee, where she served as Chief Resident (1982–1983). In addition to this, Buntin was one of the first woman to chair the Dermatology Section of the NMA.

PATRICIA TREADWELL, MD, AND GLORIA CAMPBELL-D'HUE, MD

Patricia Treadwell, MD (b. 1953) [**Figure 96-18**], a pediatric dermatologist in Indiana, became interested in dermatology during a residency in pediatrics at Riley Hospital, Indiana. Spending time in the office of Arthur Sumrall, MD, solidified her devotion to the field, and she completed her residency at the Indiana School of Medicine in 1983. She continues to hold faculty positions at Indiana in the Departments of Pediatrics and Dermatology. While attending a meeting of the AAD as a resident, Treadwell met and befriended Gloria Campbell-D'Hue, MD (b. 1948). A graduate of Emory University School of Medicine, Georgia, who did her dermatology residency at Cincinnati Hospital, Ohio, Campbell-D'Hue has been in private practice in Atlanta since 1983.

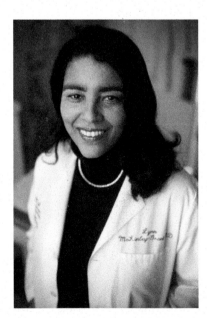

FIGURE 96-17. Lynn McKinley-Grant, MD (b. 1948), has come to occupy the very center of dermatology of skin of color, with over 20 years of experience in academic medicine and private practice.

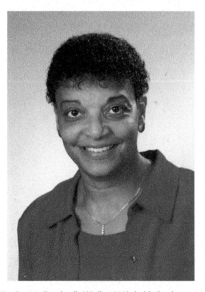

FIGURE 96-18. Patricia Treadwell, MD (b. 1953), holds faculty positions at the Indiana School of Medicine, where she also did her residency.

LORNA LACEN THOMAS, MD, KATHERINE TREHERNE, MD, AND JACQUELYN B. GARRETT, MD

Lorna Lacen Thomas, MD (b. 1942), received her medical degree from the University of Michigan and completed her internship and residency training at the Henry Ford Hospital. The first African American President of the Michigan Dermatological Society and a member of numerous boards and associations, Thomas maintains a thriving practice in Detroit. Katherine Treherne, MD (1955–2010), was a graduate of Meharry Medical College in 1980. She completed her dermatologic training at Howard University Hospital before moving to the Tidewater area of Virginia in 1985, where she remained in private practice until her death. Over the years, Treherne served as President of the Tidewater Dermatological Society, just one of many regional associations, and as Chairman of the Dermatology Section of the NMA (1993–1995). Jacquelyn B. Garrett, MD (b. 1961), graduated at the top of her class of 1985 at Howard University. The first lecture in dermatology she attended was delivered by Grimes, and she benefited from the tutelage and support of Drs. Halder and Minus. She moved to St. Louis to intern at Barnes Hospital, where she also completed her residency in dermatology in 1989, serving as Chief Resident during her last year. Garrett maintains a busy practice in the northern suburbs of St. Louis, and has served as president of a regional medical society (Mound City Medical Forum) and as head of the Dermatology Section of the NMA (1999–2001).

AMY McMICHAEL, MD

To round out the field and this segment of the history of African American dermatologists, four additional representative women have been selected: an academic, leaders in the arenas of cosmetics and pharmaceuticals, and a woman committed to what might be called "dermatologic community service." Very few "new-era" women have chosen to pursue full-time careers in academic dermatology, unlike Amy McMichael, MD (b. 1965) [**Figure 96-19**], who is Professor and Chair of dermatology at Wake Forest University in Winston Salem, North Carolina. Born and raised in Philadelphia, she is a graduate of the University of Pennsylvania School of Medicine and did her residency training at the University of Michigan. The professional experiences that McMichael finds most memorable include becoming a faculty member, her advanced training in epidemiology, and finishing her first book. She selected a career in university academia over private practice in order to teach others and encourage more people with skin of color to enter academia.

VICTORIA HOLLOWAY BARBOSA, MD

Victoria Holloway Barbosa, MD (b. 1969) [**Figure 96-20**], is a graduate of the Yale University School of Medicine. She completed an internship

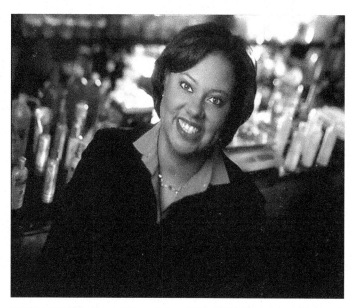

FIGURE 96-20. Victoria Holloway Barbosa, MD (b. 1969), left a long-time industry position with L'Oréal, USA to return to academia in a position with the Dermatology Department at Rush University Medical Center, Illinois and to a private dermatology practice.

in internal medicine at the Massachusetts General Hospital in Boston and her dermatology residency at Yale University, Connecticut, serving as Chief Resident. While she has been an instructor at Johns Hopkins University, Maryland, and a Clinical Assistant Professor at Howard University, Barbosa has spent the majority of her career as Vice President in Research and Development at the cosmetics and beauty company L'Oréal, USA, where she built and ran the L'Oréal Institute for Ethnic Hair and Skin Research in Chicago—the birthplace of the hair and beauty industry originally generated by Madam C. J. Walker in the early decades of the twentieth century. Board-certified since 1998, Barbosa specializes in general dermatologic conditions such as acne and eczema, as well as dermatology for skin of color and hair disorders. In 2006, she decided to leave the industry and return to academia, accepting a position as an Assistant Professor and Assistant Attending Physician for the Dermatology Department at Chicago's Rush University Medical Center. She also has a private dermatology practice in Chicago.

ALLISON NICHOLAS METZ, MD

Allison Nicholas Metz, MD (b. 1944) [**Figure 96-21**], was the first African American female dermatologist in the Northern California Permanente Medical Group, where she practiced for over 30 years until

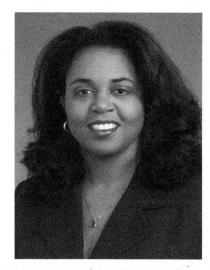

FIGURE 96-19. Amy McMichael, MD (b. 1965), selected a university career over private practice in order to teach others and encourage more people with skin of color to enter into academia. She is professor and chair of dermatology at Wake Forest University.

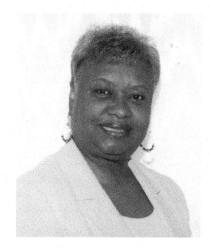

FIGURE 96-21. Allison Nicholas Metz, MD (b. 1944), was the first African American female dermatologist in the Northern California Permanente Medical Group from which she retired in 2007.

her retirement in 2007. A native of Jamaica, West Indies, she moved to Nashville and subsequently received an MD degree from Meharry Medical College in 1969, where she ranked first in her medical school class.. After an internship at Letterman Army Medical Center, San Francisco, California, she completed a residency in dermatology at the University of California San Francisco Medical Center in 1976. Drs. Willis and Arthur Mayo certainly influenced her choice of dermatology as a specialty, but as a resident, she became greatly inspired by Drs. Kenney and Kelly in their training of so many African American dermatologists.

■ STELLA BULENGO, MD

Stella Bulengo, MD (b. 1960), received BA and MD degrees and residency training from the University of Michigan after finishing high school in Nairobi, Kenya. Board-certified in dermatopathology as well as dermatology, she has worked to educate others—both at home and abroad—about the prevention of skin diseases. Since 1996, she has worked with her father (also a physician) in Tanzania on human immunodeficiency virus/acquired immunodeficiency syndrome (HIV/AIDS) prevention and has worked with that nation's Regional Dermatology Training Center, which trains doctors from Tanzania and other African countries. Over the years, she also has taught skin hygiene in Arusha, Tanzania, and has participated in similar programs in the United States. Bridging cultures and continents, Bulengo's experiences and commitments are representative of the range of community and outreach efforts that dermatologists with skin of color have been associated with for nearly a century. At present she is an adjunct clinical professor in the Department of Pathology, Medical College of Georgia in Agusta.

FACING THE FUTURE: AFRICAN AMERICAN DERMATOLOGY IN THE TWENTY-FIRST CENTURY

Many of the women and men—as well as the fathers, sons, mothers, and daughters—highlighted in the preceding sections are helping to define the future of skin of color dermatology at the close of the first decade of the twenty-first century. A quick survey of several practitioners identified a number of major trends. First and foremost is the shift from primarily "African American dermatology" to the study and care of skin of color, as discussed earlier. From Halder's Ethnic Skin Research Institute at Howard University; to Rush University's Ethnic Skin and Hair Clinic under the direction of Drs. Ella Tooms and Barbosa; to the Skin of Color Society, whose executive officers include Drs. Taylor, Halder, Callender, Barbosa, Kelly, Grimes, and others, this shift is beginning to make itself felt in the training and practice of dermatologists across the nation and throughout the world.

The choice of where dermatologists of skin of color train has also undergone a shift in more recent decades. The program at King-Drew Medical Center trained roughly 60 to 64 residents of various racial and ethnic backgrounds before its recent closing, whereas Howard University's program exists alongside other programs at majority institutions, with which it must compete. The question of what the future holds for one of the other major sites for training dermatologists of skin of color— the U.S. Armed Forces—also remains open. As this historical chapter makes clear, many of the earliest dermatologists with skin of color, such as Drs. Thatcher and Cave, served and practiced in the military, as did several second-generation specialists such as Rodman. So too did Charles S. Thurston, MD (b. 1934), a 1958 graduate of the Meharry Medical College, who did his internship at the William Beaumont Army Hospital, Texas, his residency at the University of Michigan (1963–1966), and advanced training at the School of Aviation Medical School, Alabama, before going on to pursue an academic career in and out of the U.S. Air Force. He is a retired Colonel and remains a member of the Association of Military Dermatologists.

Bernett L. Johnson, Jr., MD (1933–2009) [**Figure 96-22**], was also a graduate of Meharry Medical College. He did his dermatology residency at the University of Pennsylvania and the Naval Hospital in Philadelphia. He spent 23 years in the U.S. Navy's Medical Corps in a mixture of clinical,

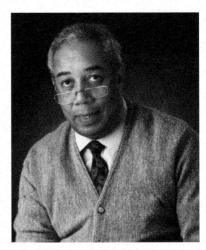

FIGURE 96-22. Bernett L. Johnson, Jr., MD (1933–2009), was a Professor at the University of Pennsylvania after serving 23 years in the U.S. Navy's Medical Corps.

academic, and administrative positions before returning to civilian life. He was a Professor of Pathology and Laboratory Medicine at the University of Pennsylvania. Brian Johnson, MD (b. 1960), the son of Johnson, Jr., has followed in his father's footsteps, continuing something of a pattern of intergenerational pairings. Brian Johnson received his dermatologic training in the Navy and is now in practice as a Mohs surgeon in Norfolk, Virginia.

One also could point to the career of Norvell V. Coots, MD (b. 1958) [**Figure 96-23**]. Coots is a Colonel and Commander of the Keller Army Community Hospital at West Point, New York, and the 52nd Command Surgeon for the U.S. Military Academy. He did part of his medical training at Howard University but finished his MD degree at the Oklahoma College of Medicine. After performing a transitional internship at the William Beaumont Army Medical Center in El Paso, Texas, and a 2-year tour as a General Medical Officer in Korea, he completed his dermatology residency at the Brooke Army Medical Center in San Antonio, Texas. As mentors, he claims, among others, Drs. Rodman and Thurston, as well as Clarence Wiley, MD (b. 1951), a civilian in private practice in Oklahoma. Coots's military assignments have included both clinical and operational positions and have taken him around the world in the service of the nation.

Coots is a highly decorated military man with numerous publications to his name. He was a Chairman of the Dermatology Section of the NMA and was selected to become the Assistant Deputy for Health Policy for the Assistant Secretary of the Army for Manpower and Reserve

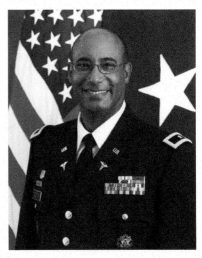

FIGURE 96-23. Norvell V. Coots, MD (b. 1958), is a Colonel, highly decorated for his military service, and is a published researcher as well.

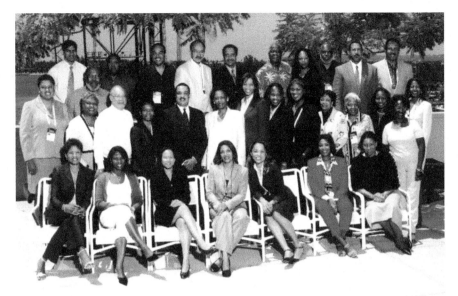

FIGURE 96-24. The National Medical Association Section of Dermatology in San Diego, California, in 2004. *First row seated from left to right:* Katherine Treherne, Cheryl Burgess, Dawna Shabazz, Shari Hicks-Graham, Kim Nichols, Tina Baisden-Pickett, Jacquelyn Garrett. *Second row from left to right:* Victoria Barbosa, Allison Nichols Metz, Harold Minus, Yolanda Holmes, Eliot Battle, Terry Dunn, Nicole DeYampert, Yolanda Lenzy, Denise Buntin, Brenda Vaughn, Cassandra McLaurin, Kimberly Scott, Denise Cook. *Third row from left to right:* Pavan Nootheti, William Coffey, Roland Hart, Moses Elam, A. Paul Kelly, Rebat Halder, George Cohen, Valerie Callender, Sidey Thompson, Fred Quarles, A. Melvin Alexander.

Affairs in July 2008. Upon being asked whether he had advice for persons considering a career in dermatology, he said:

> It is the best career decision that one can make. It offers immense rewards in terms of scope of practice, personal time and family time management; in essence it is a lifestyle specialty, and it is financially rewarding as well. Being an Army dermatologist is an issue in-and-of itself; and it is particularly rewarding to be able to treat service members and their family members for both common dermatoses and the unusual diseases contracted from world-wide deployments and travel.[21]

As the U.S. Armed Forces are called on many fronts and in numerous, often exotic locations, the arena for dermatologists to serve the needs of men and women in the Armed Forces seems destined to continue to attract new practitioners.

Another notable trend is the move from medical dermatology toward cosmetic dermatology. Facial contouring via the use of dermal fillers is being demonstrated and taught nationally and internationally by Grimes, Callender and Burgess. In terms of invasive procedures such as body contouring via liposuction, Ella Toombs, MD (b. 1951), has been performing and lecturing on this procedure since first being introduced to liposuction by Pierce in the mid-1980s. She has also played a leading role at the Ethnic Skin and Hair Clinic at Rush University Medical Center in Chicago and has been associated with an additional trend within the field: the development and testing of drug applications. Before joining the faculty at Rush University, she followed in the of Carnot Evans, MD, and served for years as a Dermatology Medical Officer at the U.S. Food and Drug Administration (FDA). At the FDA, Toombs oversaw the approval of drug applications that have transformed the practice of dermatology, including Dovonex® (calcipotriol for psoriasis), Ortho Tri-Cyclen® (ethinyl estradiol and norgestimate, the first birth control pill approved for acne), Sinequan® (doxepin, the first tricyclic antidepressant approved for pruritus), and Renova® (tretinoin emollient cream 0.05%, the first and only FDA-approved antiwrinkle cream).

In the growing field of laser surgery in skin of color, trendsetters include Arthur Sumrall, MD, from Indiana, who was one of the first eight American physicians to travel to France to learn the liposuction process from the French creator. These eight physicians also included Clarence Wiley, MD (b. 1951), from Oklahoma, who specializes in dermatologic, cosmetic, and laser surgery, photomedicine, and cosmetic products research; Seymour Weaver, MD (b. 1952), from Texas, who studied dermatologic surgery with Pierce in Philadelphia during his residency at Martin Luther King, Jr., General Hospital in Los Angeles; and Eliot Battle, MD (b. 1956), from Washington, DC. Battle did his dermatology fellowship at Howard University and his pioneering laser research at Harvard University's Wellman Laboratories of Photomedicine under the tutelage of Rox Anderson, MD (b. 1951), who helped to invent the new generation of noninvasive cosmetic lasers that are safe and effective on skin of color. A past Chairman of the Dermatology Section of the NMA, he is also co-founder and Director of Laser Surgery for Washington, DC's Cultura Cosmetic Medical Spa, a medical practice that merges dermatology, laser surgery, plastic surgery, and spa therapy.

The rise of "medi-spas" such as Cultura Dermatology and Laser Center and Odyssey Medispa in Marina del Rey, California, owned by Marcia Glenn, MD (b. 1961), represents yet another important developing trend in the field—one that will no doubt continue to offer new challenges and opportunities, new advancements in patient care (and comfort), and new avenues of research and innovation.

CONCLUSION

Researchers, mentors, and teachers sit at the heart of one of the major new trends in the field, one that involves the broadening of the category "black dermatology" in the direction of the science, study, and treatment of skin of color. Whether a pioneer, institution builder, academic, or the head of a department, center, institute, organization, board, or section, dermatologists of skin of color in all fields and subspecialties continue to contend with misconceptions about skin of color in terms of both diagnosis and treatment. While the dark days of exclusion and marginalization are happily over, the profession—and the nation—still struggle with the legacy of racial and gender discrimination. The men and women of the NMA still have an important role to play in moving us toward a future in which all forms of discrimination and prejudice are consigned to the distant past.

Many of the women and men who have served as Chairs of the NMA Dermatology Section have met this challenge head on. Some of their accomplishments have been noted in this historical overview, including those of Drs. McDonald, Willis, Grimes, Wilborn, Wiley, Kelly, Taylor, Treadwell, Buntin, Treherne, Garrett, Callender, Battle, Quarles, and Coots. To this list should also be added Thomas Johnson, MD, former Chief of Dermatology at Meharry College of Medicine, and Lindley Mordecai, MD, of San Francisco, as well as Drs. Earl Walker and Oscar Saffold.

No history is ever completely written, and the process of "making history" (in the dual sense of the phrase) is an ongoing one. Above all, as Dr. Garrett expressed so succinctly, "Given the increasing percentage of people worldwide with skin of color, there will be an increasing need for dermatologists who are sensitive and knowledgeable about the special needs of those patients" [**Figure 96-24**]. We hope that the past and the future of these dedicated dermatologists will continue to be chronicled and shared. The authors would like to thank the many members of the Dermatology Section of the NMA for their assistance in the collection of materials needed to complete this chapter, and we welcome their continued participation as this historical project grows and develops.[22]

REFERENCES

1. National Medical Association. Introduction. http://www.nmanet.org./index.php?option=com_content&view=article&id=2&Itemid=3. Accessed August 24, 2013.
2. Chicago Defender Writing Staff. Dillard Names Chapel for Lawless, Dad. *Chicago Defender*, 1965.
3. Correspondence with Earles LC III. November 20, 2005.
4. Mabley J. Profile on Lawless. *Chicago Tribune*, 1967.
5. Answers.com. Gale Contemporary Black Biography: Theodore K. Lawless. http://www.answers.com/topic/theodore-k-lawless. Accessed August 24, 2013.
6. Chicago Defender Writing Staff. Dr. Paul Boswell honored. *Chicago Defender*, 1947.
7. Clarridge C. Donor honors Seattle legend with $1.3 million park. *Seattle Post-Intelligencer*, 2002.
8. Smith C. Homer Harris, 1916-2007: dermatologist a sports pioneer. *Seattle Times*, 2007.
9. Baldwin DL. *Chicago's New Negroes: Modernity, The Great Migration, and Black Urban Life*. Chapel Hill, NC: University of North Carolina Press; 2007.
10. Correspondence with Nelson F and the Public Service Librarian at Meharry Medical College, January 13, 2008.
11. Chicago Defender Writing Staff. Howard instructor passes skin specialist exams. *Chicago Defender*, 1941, p. 3.
12. Pittsburgh Courier Writing Staff. Dermatologist. *Pittsburgh Courier*, 1942, p. 14.
13. Unknown author. Obituary of Dr. Harold E. Pierce, Jr., MD, Brigadier General (USAF, PANG, ret.), unknown publisher, 2006.
14. Dawson G. A quiet pioneer: an interview with A. Paul Kelly, MD, Editor in Chief Emeritus. *J Nat Med Assoc*. 2004;96:1404.
15. E-mail correspondence with Frederick Quarles with A. Paul Kelly, editor, April 28, 2008.
16. Spratling C. Dr. Robert P. Heidelberg dies at 74; dermatologist's focus wasn't on money. *Detroit Free Press*. http://www.freep.com/article/20130321/NEWS08/303210234/Dr-Robert-P-Heidelberg-dies-at-74-Dermatologist-s-focus-wasn-t-on-money. Accessed March 21, 2013.
17. Correspondence with Grimes P, January 8, 2008.
18. Chicago Defender Writing Staff. Dr. Hilda Straker fashions enviable career as New York skin specialist. *Chicago Defender*, 1960.
19. Callender VD. Dermatology section of the National Medical Association. *Women's Dermatologic Association Newsletter* 2002;6:8.
20. Correspondence with Clarke G, August 1, 2007.
21. Correspondence with Coots NV, January 13, 2008.
22. Correspondence with Kelly AP, April 28, 2008. He sent a partial list of noteworthy African American Dermatologists: A. Melvin Alexander, MD; William Anderson, MD; Saundrette G. Arrindell, MD; Tina Baisden-Pickett, MD; Victoria Holloway Barbosa, MD; Eliot Battle, MD; Michael Bigby, MD; Mavis V. Billups, MD; Raymond Blackburn, MD; John H. Bocachica, MD; Paul Prince Boswell, MD; Khari Bridges, MD; Stella Bulengo, MD; Cheryl Burgess, MD; Denise Buntin, MD; John Butler, MD; Valerie Callender, MD; Gloria Campbell-D'Hue, MD; John Carney, MD (deceased); Claude Vernon Cave, MD (deceased); Greta Clark, MD; Earl Claiborne, MD (deceased); William Coffey, MD; Fran Cook-Bolden, MD; Denise Cook, MD; George Cohen, MD; Norvell Vandervall Coots, MD; Linda Davis, MD; Thomas L. Day, Jr., MD; Thomas L. Day, Sr., MD; Kwame Deniake, MD; Nicole DeYampert; Angela Dillard, PhD; Terri Dunn, MD; Lucius C. Earles, III, MD; Rene Earles, MD; Moses Elam, MD; Roselyn E. Epps, MD; Carnot Evans, MD; C. Wendell Freeman, MD; Madeleine E. Gainers, MD; Algin Garrett, MD; Jacquelyn B. Garrett, MD; Raechele Gathers, MD; Joseph G. Gathings, MD; Yvette George, MD; Richard Gibbs, MD; Marcia Glenn, MD; William Grier, MD; Pearl Grimes, MD; Rebat M. Halder, MD; Jennifer Haley, MD; Roland Hart, MD; Carla Herriford, MD; Homer E. Harris, Jr., MD; Candrice Heath, MD; Karen Heidelberg, MD; Robert P. Heidelberg, MD; Shari Hicks-Graham, MD; Stacey Hunt, MD; James Hobbs, MD; Lori Hobbs, MD; Yolanda Holmes, MD; Robert Jackson, MD; Bernett L. Johnson, Jr., MD; Beverly Johnson, MD; Brian Johnson, MD; Bernett Johnson, MD; Peter D. Johnson, MD; Thomas Johnson, MD; William D. Keith, MD; Jesse

A. Kenne, MD; A. Paul Kelly, MD; Edward W. Kelly, Jr., MD; John A. Kenney, Jr., MD; Yvonne Knight, MD; Theodore K. Lawless, MD (1892–1971) (deceased); Yolanda Lenzy, MD; Charles McDonald, MD; Lynn McKinley-Grant, MD; Cassandra McLaurin, MD; Amy McMichael, MD; Arthur Mayo, MD; Allison Nicholas Metz, MD; Harold R. Minus, MD; Jocelyn Mitchell, MD; Lenley Mordecai, MD; Fern Nelson, MD; Lamar Nelson, MD; Kim Nichols, MD; Pavan Nootheti MD; John C. Payne, MD; Sherri Peace, MD; Harold E. Pierce, Jr., MD (deceased); Frederick N. Quarles, MD; Chemene R. Quinn, MD; Errol Quintal, MD; Wendy Roberts, MD; Fletcher Robinson, MD; Orlando G. Rodman, MD (deceased); Charles V. Roman, MD; Oscar Saffold, MD; Darlene Sampson, MD; Leonard Boyd Savoy, MD; Kimberly Scott, MD; Margery Scott, MD; Thomas Obadiah Senior, MD; Dwana Shabazz, MD; Ralph Skull, MD (deceased); Silvan Soden, MD; Gerald Spencer, MD; Hilda Germaine Straker, MD; Antoinette Stockton, MD; Pamela Summers, MD; Arthur Sumrall, MD; Susan Taylor, MD; Harold Thatcher, MD; Lorna Thomas, MD; Sidney Thompson, MD; Charles S. Thurston, MD; Ella Toombs, MD; Patricia Treadwell, MD; Katherine Treherne, MD; Andrea Trowers, MD; Phillip Valentine, MD; Sandra E. Vause, MD; Earl Walker, MD; Norman Walton, MD; Carl V. Washington, MD; Seymour M. Weaver, III, MD; Wesley Wilborn, MD; Clarence Wiley, MD; Isaac Willis, Sr., MD; Vernon Wilson, MD; Johnnie Woodson, Jr., MD; Linda Woodson, MD; and Dakara Wright, MD.

CHAPTER 97

Asian American Pioneers in Dermatology

Jasmine Yun

Justine Park

INTRODUCTION

Due to the increasing numbers of Asian Americans of both Asian and mixed Asian race, the responsibility of Asian American dermatologists to serve and educate this population is considerable. According to the 2010 U.S. Census, the Asian American population grew faster from 2000 to 2010 than any other racial group in the United States.[1] As of 2012, Asian Americans had the highest educational achievement level and median household income of any racial demographic in the country.[2,3] In 2008, Asian Americans held the highest median personal income of any other demographic group in the United States.[4,5] Adjusting for the proportion of the population, Asians and Caucasians had greater numbers of dermatologic encounters than African Americans and Native Americans in 1990. This correlates with the disparity in the median family income that exists between those racial groups.[6] From 1993 to 2009, the top five dermatologic conditions seen by dermatologists in Asian or Pacific Islander patients were acne, unspecified dermatitis or eczema, benign neoplasms of the skin, psoriasis, and seborrheic keratoses.[7] A retrospective cohort study of health-plan pediatric patients from 1997 to 2007 showed that the three most common diagnoses for Asian pediatric patients were dermatitis (29.1%), acne (22.2%), and warts (12.6%).[8] In 2009, a survey of 'westernized' Asian Americans in California indicated that they were more likely to view behaviors promoting sun exposure (tanned skin, increased weekend sun exposure, or actively lying out in the sun to get a tan) in a positive way.[9] This suggests that the Asian American population needs to be targeted by dermatologists for education regarding sun protection and the risks of skin cancer.

According to a census analysis from the American Medical Association in 2010, the percentage of dermatologists in the United States who reported that they were Asian (9.9%) was disproportionately low compared to the overall percentage of Asian physicians (17.4%).[10] The data also showed that this disproportionately low representation of Asian physicians within the field of dermatology was most noticeable among Asian Americans, relative to their African American colleagues or Hispanic American colleagues.[10] It should be noted that according to the 2012 Association of American Medical Colleges survey, 17% of dermatology residents were Asians, compared to 5% African Americans, and 5% Hispanics.

HISTORICAL CONTEXT

In 11,000 B.C., the first Asians came to inhabit the Americas by crossing the Bering Sea land bridge from Asia to Alaska. Evidence of Asian influence is apparent in Native American pottery dating from 800 B.C. From 300 to 750 A.D., Polynesian sailors settled the islands known as Hawaii. From 1565 to 1815, Filipinos were coerced by Spanish rule to serve in the Manila Galleon trade between the Philippines and North America. They are thought to be the first Asians to have traveled the Pacific Ocean to North America. In 1802, a Chinese sugar trader landed in Hawaii bringing boiling pans and other paraphernalia for making sugar.[11]

In 1830, the U.S. Census noted for the first time the number of Asians (at that time only Chinese) in America. In the nineteenth century, Chinese, Japanese, and Korean immigrants arrived in Hawaii to work on the sugar plantations. At the same time, numerous Chinese and Japanese were immigrating to the mainland United States to work as laborers on the transcontinental railroad.[11] However, from the 1880s to 1965, there was much legislation restricting Asians from immigrating to the United States. The Hart-Celler Act of 1965 permanently eliminated highly restrictive quotas preventing Asians from immigrating to the United States. Since this legislation was passed in 1965, the population of Asian Americans has been steadily increasing.

In the 1960s and 1970s, the United States invited physicians from Asia to address the needs of the growing general population and the shortage of physicians. Most immigrated from India and the Philippines. The influx of Asian physicians proved to be a solution to the chronic, long-term predicament the United States faced from the shortage of physicians. Asian physicians were recruited to serve the needs in rural areas and in primary care specialties. It is believed that the United States healthcare delivery crisis has been averted due to the influx of Asian physicians during the last 30 years. Also, the recognition of Asian physicians is thought to have increased acceptance of nonphysician Asians into mainstream society.[12-14]

THE PIONEERS

Most of the pioneering Asian American dermatologists are first- or second-generation immigrants and are ethnically diverse; countries of origin include Japan, China, Korea, India, Sri Lanka, and the Philippines. Their contributions have been important in the fields of the basic sciences, clinical research, education, leadership, politics, and the media.

KENZO SATO, MD, PHD

Kenzo Sato, MD, PhD (1939–2010) [**Figure 97-1**], received his master's and PhD degrees from the University of Hokkaido School of Medicine in Sapporo, Japan, and the University of Tohoku School of Medicine in Sendai, Japan. Sato graduated in 1964 and trained at the dermatology programs of the University of Oregon and the State University of New York in Buffalo. He was on faculty at the Department of Dermatology at the University of Iowa from 1978 to 1997. He worked at the Human Gene Therapy Research Institute (HGTRI) in Iowa until 2000. The HGTRI strives to revolutionize medical treatment by developing new methods and applications of human gene therapy for prevention, treatment, and cure. Sato's research was centered on eccrine gland pathology, and he was the first to describe the mechanism of action of the eccrine, apoeccrine (the modified apocrine gland), and apocrine glands. His work uncovered the abnormal function of sweat glands in cystic fibrosis. Sato's key findings led to the development of cystic fibrosis gene modification therapy. He had 49 years of experience in the field and was a dedicated dermatologist.

ALLAN KENJI IZUMI, MD

Allan Kenji Izumi, MD (1939–2012) [**Figure 97-2**], was born in Kula, Maui, Hawaii. He attended medical school at the University of California in San Francisco and completed his residency in dermatology at the University of Pennsylvania Health System. He did further study in dermatology at Moffitt Hospital, University of California and in internal medicine at San Francisco General Hospital Medical Complex. Izumi was board-certified in both dermatology and dermatopathology. His areas of expertise included contact dermatitis, granulomas, skin cancer, and skin diseases. He had 40 publications in these various subspecialties. Notably, he was instrumental in the founding of the Division of Dermatology at the University of Hawaii and served as its chief from 1973 to 2010. Izumi was also President of the Hawaii Dermatological Society in 1975 and was also very active in the Pacific Dermatological Society (now the Pacific Dermatologic Association), serving as President from 1995 to 1996. He was an active member of the American Dermatological Association and had 44 years of experience in the medical field. He was a key figure in the dermatologic community in Hawaii.

BRIAN V. JEGASOTHY, MD

Brian V. Jegasothy, MD (1943–2001) [**Figure 97-3**], attended medical school in Sri Lanka and completed his dermatology residency at Yale University, Connecticut, in 1974 and remained there to complete a 2-year postdoctorate fellowship in immunology. It was at Yale that he developed a lifelong dedication to 'bench' research. His work as an intern and resident in the Department of Medicine at Yale earned him a Best Intern Award. Known as "Dr. Brian", Jegasothy is revered by the Sri Lankan-American medical community as their pioneer. Jegasothy was on the faculty of the Department of Dermatology at Duke University, North Carolina, was Vice Chair of the Department of Dermatology at

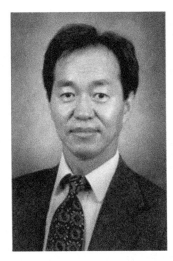

FIGURE 97-1. Kenzo Sato, MD, PhD (1939–2010), worked for a number of notable institutions throughout his career, including the Human Gene Therapy Institute, Iowa. His findings led to the development of cystic fibrosis gene modification therapy.

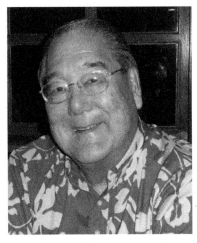

FIGURE 97-2. Allan Kenji Izumi, MD (1939–2012), was instrumental in establishing the Division of Dermatology at the University of Hawaii, serving as chief from 1973 until 2010.

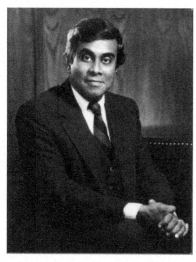

FIGURE 97-3. Brian V. Jegasothy, MD (1943–2001), held many academic posts throughout his career and was among the first to study the efficacy of extracorporeal photochemotherapy (photopheresis) for the treatment of systemically disseminated cutaneous T-cell lymphoma.

the University of Pennsylvania, and was Chairman of the Department of Dermatology at the University of Pittsburgh, Pennsylvania, from 1987 to 1999. Widely recognized for his work in basic science research he, along with Richard Edelson's group, was the first to study the efficacy of extracorporeal photochemotherapy (photopheresis) for the treatment of systemically disseminated cutaneous T-cell lymphoma, published in the *New England Journal of Medicine* in 1987. He also did some of the first studies on tacrolimus (FK506) for the treatment of recalcitrant psoriasis. His daughter, Manjula Jegasothy, MD, also a dermatologist, established the Brian V. Jegasothy, M.D., Endowed Basic Science Research Award at the University of Miami Miller School of Medicine, Florida, in celebration of her father's achievements.

LENORE KAKITA, MD

Lenore Kakita, MD (b. 1940) [**Figure 97-4**], was born in Oakland, California, and attended medical school at the University of California, San Francisco. She trained in dermatology at the University of California from 1968 to 1971. Kakita was active in the Los Angeles Dermatological Society and was President in 1982. At the state level, she actively worked

for the California Society of Dermatology and Dermatologic Surgery (CSDDS; previously the Congress of California Dermatologic Societies) and served as President. As a leader of the CSDDS, she helped to shape a number of bylaw amendments to change the structure of the American Academy of Dermatology (AAD) so as to include more practitioners. Due to her work, the slate of candidates for the AAD elections today is a diverse pick of academicians and private practitioners, thus representing the views of more dermatologists. Kakita was active on the Advisory Board of the AAD, a member of the Board of Directors, and became Chair in 1998. Kakita was also active in the Women's Dermatologic Society (WDS) and became its President in 2002. She was instrumental in the formation of the Legacy Foundation (now called the WDS Legacy Council) and also served as its Chair.

W. P. DANIEL SU, MD

W. P. Daniel Su, MD (b. 1943) [**Figure 97-5**], attended medical school at the National Taiwan University and completed his dermatology training at the Mayo Clinic, Minnesota. He was on the faculty at the Mayo Clinic from 1975 until 2008 and is currently Professor Emeritus there. Together with his colleagues at the Mayo Clinic, Su set the diagnostic criteria for Sweet syndrome and pyoderma gangrenosum. Enthusiastic in teaching and cultivating young people, he was elected as Teacher of the Year by dermatology residents and fellows of the Mayo Clinic three times and was also put in the Hall of Fame in the Mayo Graduate School of Medicine.

Su recognized the need to promote dermatopathology teaching in developing countries. He initiated and coordinated the Regional Clinicopathologic Colloquium in Egypt in 1990, followed by India, Columbia, Mexico, and other Asian countries. He was the President of the International Society of Dermatopathology from 1994 to 1997. Su was also the organizer or moderator of more than 65 national or international clinicopathologic sessions and has been visiting professor or invited speaker to more than 30 countries around the world. He also served as the Chairman of the Membership Committee, International Society of Dermatology, from 1990 to 2000 and was its Honorary Chairman from 2001 to 2009.

BEATRIZ COQUILLA-CANETE, MD

Beatriz Coquilla-Canete, MD (b. 1948) [**Figure 97-6**], was born in the Philippines but grew up in San Francisco. She and her family moved back to the Philippines in 1966, where she later attended medical school at the Faculty of Medicine and Surgery of the University of Santo Tomas in Manila. She joined the U.S. Army in 1979 and completed her dermatology residency at the Brooke Army Medical Center, Texas. She later completed her Master's degree in Healthcare Administration at

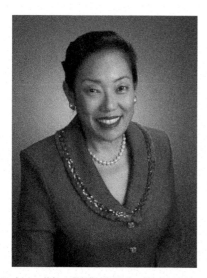

FIGURE 97-4. Lenore Kakita, MD (b. 1940), has been instrumental in making the American Academy of Dermatology more inclusive and has helped influence national policy in Washington, DC.

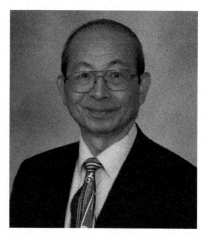

FIGURE 97-5. W. P. Daniel Su, MD (b. 1943), is currently Professor Emeritus at the Mayo Clinic, Minnesota. He was one of the first to recognize the need to promote dermatopathology teaching in developing countries and has coordinated colloquia to achieve this end.

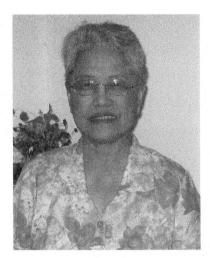

FIGURE 97-6. Beatriz Coquilla-Canete, MD (b. 1948), served in the U.S. Army for 20 years. She has been recognized and decorated for her dermatologic service around the world.

the prestigious U.S. Army-Baylor University at Fort Sam Houston in San Antonio, Texas. During her military career, she served as Chief of Dermatology Service at the Womack Army Community Hospital in Fort Bragg, North Carolina; Deputy Commander for Clinical Services at the Bayne Jones Army Community Hospital in Fort Polk, Louisiana; and Chief of Dermatology at the 67th Combat Support Hospital in Germany. One of only five physicians in the European Command to get promoted to colonel, Coquilla-Canete was then assigned to be Commander of the Vicenza Army Community Hospital in Italy. Coquilla-Canete's last assignment, prior to her retirement, was as Chief of Dermatology and Chief of Medicine, in Seoul, South Korea. Coquilla-Canete has received numerous decorations and medals from her years as a medical officer. In 1992, she received the Order of Military Medical Merit, a coveted award given to U.S. Army medical personnel for significant and exemplary contributions to the U.S. Army Medical Department.

HENRY LIM, MD

Henry Lim, MD (b. 1949) [**Figure 97-7**], received his medical degree from the State University of New York Downstate Medical Center in Brooklyn and completed his dermatology residency at the New York

University (NYU) School of Medicine. Lim is currently Chairman and C.S. Livingood Chair of the Department of Dermatology at Henry Ford Hospital, and Senior Vice President for Academic Affairs at the Henry Ford Health System in Detroit, Michigan. Prior to coming to Henry Ford Hospital, he was Professor of Dermatology at NYU School of Medicine, as well as Chief of Staff of the New York Veterans Affairs Medical Center. He has published more than 350 articles and is a recognized authority in photodermatology. Lim has served as co-founder and President of the Photomedicine Society, President of the American Society for Photobiology, President of the Michigan Dermatological Society, President of the American Board of Dermatology, and President of the American Dermatological Association. He is the president-elect of the American Academy of Dermatology (2016). He was an Associate Editor of the *Journal of Investigative Dermatology*, and was Editor-in-Chief of *Photodermatology, Photoimmunology & Photomedicine*. He is a Senior Editor of *Journal of Drugs in Dermatology*, and a member of the Editorial Board of *Photodermatology, Photoimmunology & Photomedicine*. He is an elected honorary member of dermatology organizations in Austria, the Philippines, and China. Lim is the Editor/Co-Editor of five textbooks: *Clinical Photomedicine*; *Photoaging*; *Photodermatology*; *Clinical Guide to Sunscreens and Photoprotection*; and *Cancer of the Skin*. He is also a Co-Editor of *Dermatology for Skin of Color* (second edition) with Drs. Kelly, Taylor, and Serrano.

CONTEMPORARY PIONEERS

JOHN KOO, MD

John Koo, MD (b. 1955) [**Figure 97-8**], received his medical degree from Harvard Medical School, Massachusetts, and completed a residency in psychiatry at the University of California in the Los Angeles Neuropsychiatric Institute before training in dermatology at the University of California, San Francisco (UCSF). He is Vice Chairman of the Department of Dermatology at UCSF and Director of the UCSF Psoriasis Day Care Center and Phototherapy Unit. He is also Director of the UCSF Psychodermatology Clinic and Director of the UCSF Dermatology Drug Research Unit. Koo is a nationally recognized expert on psoriasis and psychodermatology. He is Chairman of the Psoriasis Expert Resource Group, a psoriasis task force that is a joint function of the American Academy of Dermatology and the National Psoriasis Foundation. He is also a Medical Advisory Board Member of the National Psoriasis Foundation and a founding member of the Association for

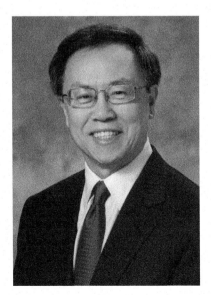

FIGURE 97-7. Henry Lim, MD (b. 1949), has researched, written, and edited an immense body of work on photodermatology throughout his career. He currently chairs the large Department of Dermatology at Henry Ford Hospital in Detroit, Michigan.

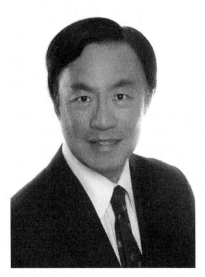

FIGURE 97-8. John Koo, MD (b. 1955), is a recognized expert on psoriasis and psychodermatology and a co-developer of the Koo-Menter Psoriasis Instrument to aid in identifying psoriasis patients warranting systemic therapy.

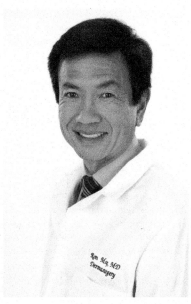

FIGURE 97-9. Ronald Moy, MD (b. 1957), was President of the American Academy of Dermatology. During his tenure, he worked as an advocate for dermatologists and their patients. He is the author of more than 200 scientific publications and 6 textbooks.

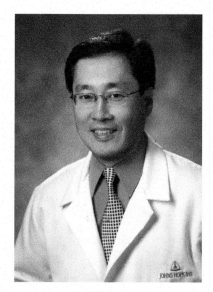

FIGURE 97-10. Sewon Kang, MD, MPH (b. 1958), is currently at the Department of Dermatology at Johns Hopkins University, Maryland, and is a highly regarded expert on skin aging.

Psychoneurocutaneous Medicine of North America. He is Co-Editor of *Contemporary Diagnosis and Management of Psoriasis* and *Psychocutaneous Medicine*. Koo, along with Alan Menter, Steven Feldman, and Jerry Bagel, developed the Koo-Menter Psoriasis Instrument as a diagnostic algorithm and a formal measure to aid in the identification of patients warranting systemic therapy due to the impact of psoriasis on their quality of life.

RONALD MOY, MD

Ronald Moy, MD (b. 1957) [**Figure 97-9**], earned his Bachelor's degree and medical degree from a combined program at the Rensselaer Polytechnic Institute and Albany Medical College in New York. He trained in dermatology at the Medical Center of the University of California, Los Angeles (UCLA). Moy completed his Mohs micrographic surgery fellowship at the University Center for the Health Sciences Montefiore Hospital in Pittsburgh under John Zitelli. Moy served as President of the AAD from 2011 to 2012. During his tenure, the healthcare reform law created a challenging healthcare delivery landscape for dermatologists. As president of the AAD, Moy was actively engaged with the U.S. Congress, Department of Health and Human Services, the Centers for Medicare and Medicaid Services, the Agency for Healthcare Research and Quality, and the Food and Drug Administration (FDA) as an advocate for dermatologists and their patients. Moy is a past member of the AAD's Board of Directors, past Chair of the Core Curriculum Committee, and a past Chair of the Coding and Reimbursement Task Force. He is former President of the American Society for Dermatologic Surgery, the Pacific Dermatologic Association, and the Los Angeles Metropolitan Dermatologic Society. In addition, he is past President of the Division of Medical Quality for the Medical Board of California. He is a past Editor-in-Chief of *Dermatologic Surgery* and has authored more than 200 scientific publications and 6 textbooks, including *Principles and Techniques of Cutaneous Surgery*. He has served as the Director of the Mohs Micrographic Surgery and Cutaneous Oncology Fellowship at UCLA and has served as Co-Chief of the Division of Dermatology at UCLA. Moy is also a recipient of the NIH/R0-1 and VA Merit Grants.

SEWON KANG, MD, MPH

Sewon Kang, MD, MPH (b. 1958) [**Figure 97-10**], was born in Seoul, Korea. He is a Haystack Scholar and graduate of the Williams College in Massachusetts, with a BA *cum laude* in chemistry, and the University of

Michigan, with an MD and an MPH in epidemiology. He trained at the University of Rochester, New York, in Internal Medicine and then did his dermatology residency along with a research fellowship at Harvard Medical School, where he was Chief Resident. He is currently Noxell Professor of Dermatology, Chair of the Department of Dermatology, and Dermatologist-in-Chief at the Johns Hopkins School of Medicine in Baltimore, Maryland. Prior to Johns Hopkins, he was an Arthur C. Curtis Professor of Dermatologic Translational Research scholar at the University of Michigan Medical School and a tenured Professor in the Department of Dermatology. He has served on the Board of Directors of the Society for Investigative Dermatology and the Association of Professors of Dermatology and the Board of Trustees of the Dermatology Foundation. Kang is also a member of the American Dermatological Association and the Korean Dermatologic Association of America. He is currently President of the Photomedicine Society and is a highly regarded expert on skin aging, having conducted extensive research involving retinoids and other treatments to inhibit photoaging and the natural aging of skin. He has authored numerous articles on skin aging, photomedicine, and psoriasis. Kang's many awards include the Presidential Citation from the American Academy of Dermatology and the Diversity Recognition Award from Johns Hopkins University.

YOUNGER CONTEMPORARY PIONEERS

JESSICA WU, MD

Jessica Wu, MD (b. 1968) [**Figure 97-11**], received her medical degree from Harvard Medical School and trained in dermatology at the University of Southern California (USC). She is currently an Assistant Clinical Professor of Dermatology at the USC School of Medicine. She was the principal investigator in several studies of cosmetic products that have resulted in FDA approval, including Juvéderm® and Latisse®. Wu is a member of the Medical Nutrition Council of the American Society for Nutrition and is the author of *Feed Your Face: Younger, Smoother Skin & A Beautiful Body in 28 Delicious Days*. A seasoned media expert, Wu has been interviewed on many television and radio programs including *Good Morning America*, *Fox News*, *Entertainment Tonight*, and *National Public Radio*, and has written for *CNN.com*. She has co-hosted episodes of the syndicated talk show, *The Doctors*, and regularly appears on the KTLA morning news in Los Angeles. She has been featured in publications such as the *New York Times*, *Los Angeles Times*, *Wall Street Journal*, and *People* magazine. Wu is also Co-Founder of BeautyShares Inc., a nonprofit organization dedicated to building confidence and self-esteem

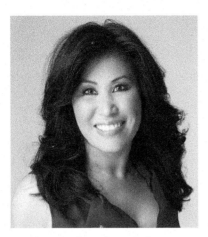

FIGURE 97-11. Jessica Wu, MD (b. 1968), is currently an Assistant Professor of Dermatology at the University of Southern California School of Medicine, and is well-known for her media appearances related to dermatologic concerns.

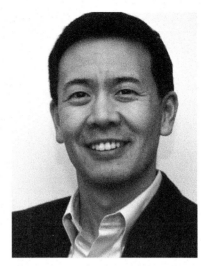

FIGURE 97-13. David Peng, MD (b. 1973), is among the youngest Asian American dermatologists to serve as a chair of a dermatology department and currently works at the University of Southern California Keck School of Medicine.

in disadvantaged teens and young women through after-school workshops that teach grooming and healthy lifestyle choices. In the field of cosmetic dermatology, she has raised awareness about the unique skin characteristics of Asian patients. Additionally, Wu has given multiple lectures and written numerous articles about the treatment of Asian skin.

HOWARD Y. CHANG, MD, PHD

Howard Y. Chang, MD, PhD (b. 1972) [**Figure 97-12**], is Professor of Dermatology at the Stanford University School of Medicine and an Early Career Scientist of the Howard Hughes Medical Institute. Dr. Chang received his PhD degree in Biology from the Massachusetts Institute of Technology, and his medical degree from Harvard Medical School. He completed his dermatology residency at Stanford University, California, and his postdoctoral fellowship with Professor Patrick Brown, and joined the faculty in 2004. His research addresses the ways in which individual cells know where they are located in the human body, which is important in normal development and in cancer metastasis. Chang discovered that a new class of genes, termed long noncoding ribonucleic acids, can control gene activity throughout the genome, illuminating a new layer of

biological regulation that has been hailed as an "Insight of the Decade" by *Science* magazine. Chang's honors include the Damon Runyon Scholar Award, American Cancer Society Research Scholar Award, California Institute for Regenerative Medicine New Faculty Award, elected membership to the American Society for Clinical Investigation, the Vilcek Prize for Creative Promise, the CERIES Award, and the Alfred Marchionini Prize.

DAVID PENG, MD

David Peng, MD (b. 1973) [**Figure 97-13**], received his medical degree at the University of California, San Diego (UCSD). He completed an internship in internal medicine at the UCLA, followed by a Master's in Public Health. Peng then went on to complete his residency in dermatology at UCSD. He was an Associate Professor and the Director of the Department of Dermatology's Residency Training Program at Stanford University School of Medicine, where he served from 2009 to 2013. Peng is among the youngest Asian American dermatologists to serve as a chair of a dermatology department; his most recent appointment in 2013 as Chair of the Dermatology Department at the University of Southern California Keck School of Medicine is a culmination of a career that has been dedicated to the teaching of dermatology residents and an academic focus on melanoma and contact dermatitis research. In 2008, Peng and his colleague Myles Cockburn conducted a study with the Kaiser Permanente consortium, Southern California, to promote accurate skin self-examinations among its more than two million members. He is also involved with the community-based SunSmart program, which educates hundreds of thousands of Los Angeles school-aged children on healthy sun exposure behaviors. In addition, he is currently a co-investigator for a major study funded by the National Institute of Environmental Health Sciences that seeks to define the effects of environmental ultraviolet exposure in melanogenesis.

CONCLUSION

The field of dermatology has greatly benefited from the diverse and inspirational contributions of Asian American dermatologists, in areas ranging from psoriasis to cosmetic dermatology, photodermatology to eccrine glands, and politics to education. Looking to the future, there should be an increase in the recruitment of Asian American physicians to the field of dermatology as the population of Asian Americans increases in the United States. We know that the leaders recognized here as pioneers in their field will serve as excellent role models for all dermatologists, including future Asian American dermatologists.

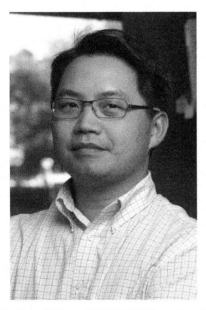

FIGURE 97-12. Howard Y. Chang, MD, PhD (b. 1972), has performed important cellular research, which led to his discovery of a new class of genes—long noncoding ribonucleic acids. He is currently on the faculty at Stanford University, California.

REFERENCES

1. U.S. Census Bureau. The Asian population: 2010-2010 census briefs. http://www.census.gov/prod/cen2010/briefs/c2010br-11.pdf. Accessed July 28, 2013.
2. White M. Asian-American population on the rise, Pew Research Center survey says. http://www.deseretnews.com/article/865571191/Asian-American-population-on-the-rise-Pew-Research-Center-survey-says.html. Accessed January 23, 2013.
3. Taylor P, Cohn D, Wang W, et al. The rise of Asian-Americans: Pew Research social & demographic trends. http://www.pewsocialtrends.org/files/2013/01/SDT_Rise_of_Asian_Americans.pdf. Accessed July 12, 2012.
4. U.S. Census Bureau. Educational attainment in the United States: 2007 – population characteristics. http://www.census.gov/prod/2009pubs/p20-560.pdf. Accessed August 15, 2012.
5. U.S. Census Bureau. Income, poverty, and health insurance coverage in the United States: 2008 – Current population reports – Consumer income. http://www.census.gov/prod/2009pubs/p60-236.pdf. Accessed July 18, 2012.
6. Fleischer AB Jr, Feldman SR, Bradham DD. Office-based physician services provided by dermatologists in the United States in 1990. *J Invest Dermatol.* 1994;102:93-97.
7. Davis SA, Narahari S, Feldman SR, et al. Top dermatologic conditions in patients of color: an analysis of nationally representative data. *J Drugs Dermatol.* 2012;11:466-473.
8. Henderson MD, Abboud J, Cogan CM, et al. Skin-of-color epidemiology: a report of the most common skin conditions by race. *Pediatr Dermatol.* 2012;29:584-589.
9. Gorell E, Lee C, Muñoz C, et al. Adoption of western culture by Californian Asian Americans: attitudes and practices promoting sun exposure. *Arch Dermatol.* 2009;145:552-556.
10. Association of American Medical Colleges. Diversity in the physician workforce: facts and figures 2010. https://members.aamc.org/eweb/upload/Diversity%20in%20the%20Physician%20Workforce%20Facts%20and%20Figures%202010.pdf. Accessed July 12, 2012.
11. Baron DG, Gall SB, eds. *Asian American Chronology.* New York, NY: U.X.L.; 1996.
12. Koehn NN, Fryer GE Jr, Phillips RL, et al. The increase in international medical graduates in family practice residency programs. *Fam Med.* 2002;34:468-469.
13. Mick SS, Lee SY. Are there need-based geographical differences between international medical graduates and U.S. medical graduates in rural U.S. counties? *J Rural Health.* 1999;15:26-43.
14. Saha S, Guiton G, Wimmers PF, et al. Student body racial and ethnic composition and diversity-related outcomes in US medical schools. *JAMA.* 2008;300:1135-1145.

HISTORICAL CONTEXT

Many of the premier Hispanic American dermatologists in the United States today were born in Central or South America and trained there before immigrating to the United States. To understand their influence, it is important to understand the origins of dermatology in the Southern Hemisphere.

Modern dermatology in Latin America began in the early twentieth century, when a few committed individuals opened dermatologic schools. The field attracted bright students and scholars, many of whom spent extensive time studying in Europe under Drs. Kaposi, Riehl, Sezary, Hallopeau, and Sabouraud, to name a few. They made major advances and published extensively in the fields of mycology, leprosy, cutaneous tuberculosis, and psoriasis. These physicians were from Argentina (for instance, Drs. Sommer, Aberastury, Baliña, Fidanza, and Puente), Brazil (Drs. Rabello, Lindenberg, Araujo, and Machado), Colombia (Dr. Uribe), Cuba (Dr. Menocal), Ecuador (Dr. Gault), Mexico (Drs. Lucio y Nájera, Cicero, and Ureña), Peru (Drs. Carrión and Escomel), Uruguay (Dr. Foresti), and Venezuela (Dr. Diaz). Their quest to advance dermatology helped establish Latin Americans as premier leaders in dermatology, and helped elevate dermatology in Central and South America into a position of importance.[3] Today, the Colegio Ibero Latino Americano de Dermatologia (CILAD) is the largest Spanish-speaking dermatology society in the world, with more than 4000 members in 22 countries.

THE PIONEERS

Despite the large number of Hispanic dermatologists in CILAD and the rapid growth of the Hispanic population in the United States, the number of Hispanic dermatologists practicing in the United States is disproportionately small; however, they constitute an important group. The following pioneering Hispanic American dermatologists, all master clinicians, have made and continue to make important contributions in basic science, clinical research, field research, education, and medical leadership.

◼ PEDRO BARQUIN, MD

Pedro Barquin, MD (1916–2002) [**Figure 98-1**], graduated from the School of Medicine of the University of La Habana, Cuba, in 1943. After finishing his dermatology residency, he went into private practice and was also Professor and Chairman of Dermatology and Leprosy at the Finlay Hospital of the Armed Forces in La Habana. He was President of

---

CHAPTER 98

Hispanic American Pioneers in Dermatology

Marta I. Rendon
Chere Lucas Anthony

INTRODUCTION

As the population of the United States diversifies at an increasingly rapid rate, the need for healthcare providers skilled in treating skin conditions for patients of all ethnic and racial groups continues to grow. As a result, Hispanic American dermatologists have become key players in the dermatology community. Hispanic dermatologists account for only 4.8% of all dermatologists in the United States.[1] Given the rise in the Hispanic population, this figure is disproportionately low. From 2012 to 2060, the Hispanic population in the United States is expected to grow from 53.3 million to 128.8 million.[2] By the end of that period, nearly one in every three U.S. residents will be of Hispanic descent, up from about one in six today.[2]

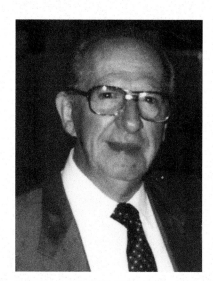

FIGURE 98-1. Pedro Barquin, MD (1916–2002), served as a Professor and Chairman of Dermatology and Leprosy in Havana, Cuba. After settling in the United States, he was a founding member of the Cuban Society of Dermatology in Exile.

the Cuban Society of Dermatology and Leprosy. In 1965, Barquin left Cuba and settled in Miami, Florida, where he became Clinical Professor in the Department of Dermatology of the University of Miami School of Medicine, with his last appointment as Professor Emeritus. Barquin was a member of both the American Academy of Dermatology and CILAD. He was a founding member of the Cuban Society of Dermatology in Exile. As a member of the Florida Society of Dermatology and the Miami Dermatological Society, Barquin promoted and made popular a lecture series for the dermatology community. In 1995, he was chosen as Dermatologist of the Year by the Florida Society of Dermatology and was awarded the University of Miami Practitioner of the Year Award in the same year. He is one of the most senior and revered Hispanic American dermatologists for his dedication to his profession and to his community at large.

NARDO ZAIAS, MD

Nardo Zaias, MD (b. 1931) [**Figure 98-2**], a Cuban native, received his dermatology training at the University of Miami, Florida; he subsequently served there as Professor of Dermatology. He has been at Mount Sinai Medical Center in Miami Beach since 1972, Chief of the Dermatology Department since 1992, and is still going strong today. Zaias set out to be a biologist and finished his Master's degree in fish parasitology when friends urged him to attend the newly opened medical school at the University of Miami. He chose to enter dermatology because the field allowed him to deal with parasites, fungi, and bacteria. It was his good fortune that Dr. Harvey Blank was Chairman of the Department of Dermatology, at the time, as Blank was also a biologist and was performing research using griseofulvin, the first systemic antimycotic. It was at the urging of Dr. Guido Matoltsky that Zaias embarked on a systematic study of the nail. After spending 1960 in Venezuela studying tropical mycoses, he returned to Miami and joined with the preeminent nail expert—a Cuban professor named Dr. Pardo Castello—who was then in the Department of Dermatology. Zaias was the first to describe the nail bed matrix as a separate entity from the nail plate matrix. He discovered that nail bed matrix stem cells move along the nail bed and that the entire structure is homologous to the hair root sheath. He also discovered that the most common toenail abnormality is caused by closed-toe shoes pressing on the toes in ways that reflect the asymmetry of an individual's gait.

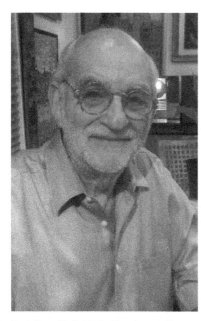

FIGURE 98-2. Nardo Zaias, MD (b. 1931), although originally interested in fish parasitology, was the first to discover that the most common toenail abnormality is caused by closed-toe shoes.

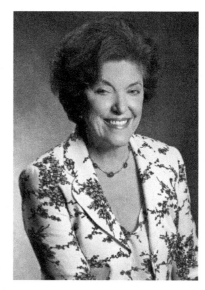

FIGURE 98-3. Irma Gigli, MD (b. 1932), was the first woman in the United States to lead the dermatology department at a major university (the University of California, San Diego School of Medicine). She also co-founded the Brown Foundation Institute of Molecular Medicine Center for the Prevention of Human Diseases in Texas.

IRMA GIGLI, MD

Irma Gigli, MD (b. 1932) [**Figure 98-3**], was born in Cordoba, Argentina, in 1931. She did her training in dermatology at Cook County Hospital, Chicago, Illinois, and in immunology at the Howard Hughes Medical Institute in Miami, Florida. Her appointment at the Peter and Robert Brigham Hospital marked the first time that dermatology was recognized as a separate division. She was also on the faculty at Harvard Medical School and then at New York University School of Medicine before becoming Chief of the Division of Dermatology at the University of California, San Diego School of Medicine in 1982. This was the first time a woman in the United States led a dermatology department at a major university. In 1995, Gigli moved to the University of Texas in Houston where she founded the Brown Foundation Institute of Molecular Medicine Center for the Prevention of Human Diseases with her late husband, Hans J. Muller-Eberhard, MD. She has been honored by election to a number of prestigious organizations, among them the American Academy of Arts and Sciences and the Institute of Medicine of the National Academy of Sciences. She was president of the Society of Investigative Dermatology. She is a fellow of the American Association for the Advancement of Science, and of the Association of American Physicians. Gigli has been honored as a teacher with a number of awards, and she takes special pride in the number of today's leaders in dermatology she trained and guided in their careers.

ERNESTO GONZALEZ-MARTINEZ, MD

Ernesto Gonzalez-Martinez, MD (b. 1939) [**Figure 98-4**], a native of Puerto Rico, attended the University of Puerto Rico for both college and medical school. He then trained in dermatology at Harvard Medical School, as a mentee of Dr. Thomas Fitzpatrick, before joining the staff of Massachusetts General Hospital (MGH) at Boston where he is still employed. His widowed mother did domestic work to provide for the family and was his guiding light and the inspiration to persevere in his medical career after his father died when he was only 5 years old. Gonzalez organizes goodwill clinics for the homeless population in the Boston Health Care for the Homeless Program, where he has developed a comprehensive dermatologic academic service, incorporating dermatology residents as part of their curriculum. He has also developed free telemedicine services in Puerto Rico and Honduras for underserved populations, where faculty members at MGH serve as teleconsultants. Gonzalez started the first mentorship program in the country for

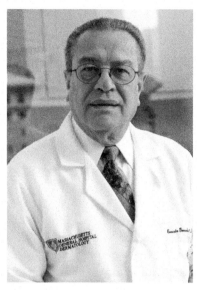

FIGURE 98-4. Ernesto Gonzalez-Martinez, MD (b. 1939), was trained in dermatology at Harvard Medical School, Connecticut. He is well-known for his contributions in the fields of contact dermatitis and phototherapy and for his philanthropic/educational services in dermatology.

Hispanic students at all four medical schools in Massachusetts. His contributions to the fields of contact dermatitis and phototherapy have been outstanding. He was one of the founders of photochemotherapy in the United States and started the first contact dermatitis clinic in New England. In 2005, MGH recognized his achievements by establishing the Ernesto Gonzalez Award for Outstanding Services to the Hispanic Community.

JORGE L. SANCHEZ, MD

Jorge L. Sanchez, MD (b. 1942) [**Figure 98-5**], was born in Puerto Rico, received his medical degree from the University of Puerto Rico, and trained in dermatology at the University Hospital in Rio Piedras, Puerto Rico. He then completed a dermatopathology fellowship at New York University. Sanchez is a leader in the field of dermatopathology and has authored three books and countless publications on the topic. His extensive research in the histopathology of the skin in the Hispanic population includes histopathologic diagnosis of the patch stage of

mycosis fungoides and clinicopathologic correlations in pigmentary disorders, especially melasma. Together with A. B. Ackerman, Sanchez co-authored the second edition of the book *Histopathological Diagnosis of Inflammatory Diseases of the Skin*. In addition to clinical contributions, his leadership ability has been recognized through numerous positions on editorial boards, committees, and appointments. He served as Chairman of the Department of Dermatology at the University of Puerto Rico for 20 years, Chancellor of the Medical Sciences campus at the same university, and President of the Puerto Rico Medical Board, and he has been president of more than one international dermatopathology societies. Although Sanchez's career has been based primarily in Puerto Rico, he has been a visiting professor at many U.S. medical schools and dermatology residency programs. His original pigmentation studies are considered landmark works for Hispanic American physicians in the United States.

LUIS A. DIAZ, MD

Luis A. Diaz, MD (b. 1942) [**Figure 98-6**], was born in Peru and received his medical degree from the Universidad Nacional de Trujillo, Peru. He completed his dermatology and immunology training at the State University of New York, Buffalo, and the Mayo Clinic, Minnesota. He is board-certified in dermatology and dermatologic immunology. Since 1976, Diaz has dedicated his professional career to education, patient care, and research. He has held faculty positions at the University of Michigan and Johns Hopkins University, Maryland. He was the Chairman of Dermatology at the Medical College of Wisconsin, Milwaukee, for 10 years, and since 2000, he has been serving as Chairman of Dermatology at the University of North Carolina, Chapel Hill. As an educator, Diaz has left his imprint on several generations of dermatology residents; as a clinician, he has been often listed on the Best Doctors of America. A leader in basic research, Diaz has authored more than 200 publications, primarily focusing on pemphigus, pemphigoid, and other autoimmune diseases of the skin. His contributions were recognized by his election as President of the Society for Investigative Dermatology (2001) and President of the Association of Professors of Dermatology (2014–2016) and the Institute of Medicine (2002). He was also elected to the Alpha Omega Alpha Honors Medical Society (2010).

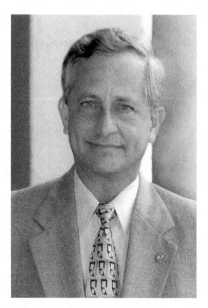

FIGURE 98-5. Jorge L. Sanchez, MD (b. 1942), is a leader in the field of dermatopathology, and his pigmentation studies are considered landmark works.

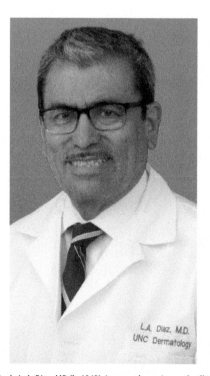

FIGURE 98-6. Luis A. Diaz, MD (b. 1942), is currently serving as the Chairman of Dermatology at the University of North Carolina Chapel Hill and has made bounteous contributions to the field of dermatology, focusing on the autoimmune diseases of the skin.

CONTEMPORARY PIONEERS

In the late twentieth and early twenty-first centuries, Hispanic American physicians were on the cutting edge of the explosive growth of the Latin American population in the United States. With the fundamental knowledge that Hispanics are a diverse group encompassing all six of the Fitzpatrick skin types, these physicians contributed to creating awareness of this diversity and the importance of understanding cultural differences in healthcare, and promoting as well as conducting research in diseases relating to Hispanic skin types. These pioneers have worked as university professors, chaired dermatology training programs, organized and founded regional and national societies, and brought outstanding medical care to their communities. All have made significant strides in their fields.

MIGUEL SANCHEZ, MD

Miguel Sanchez, MD (b. 1953) [**Figure 98-7**], a Cuban American, received his medical degree from the Albert Einstein College of Medicine in New York, and served residencies in pediatrics and family medicine at Montefiore Medical Center. He then completed his dermatology residency at New York University, where he currently holds the title of Professor of Dermatology. He is the Director of Dermatology and Syphilology at Bellevue Hospital Medical Center. Bellevue Hospital is one of the oldest public hospitals in the United States and one of the largest public hospitals in the world; importantly, the hospital has played a historic role in the emergence of dermatology as a specialty. From the time its doors first opened, Bellevue Hospital was the first institution in the city to respond to the challenges of epidemics like syphilis, measles, and other infectious diseases. The hospital squarely met the emerging acquired immunodeficiency syndrome epidemic by creating the first Dermatology Clinic for the care of human immunodeficiency virus patients in the country. More recently, Bellevue Hospital was selected as the main referral site by the New York City Department of Health for evaluating patients with possible bioterrorism-induced infectious diseases. Sanchez's research has led to many publications on skin disorders in skin of color; these include an extensive review on sarcoidosis in skin of color and cultural influences on healthcare practices.

FRANCISCO KERDEL, MD

Francisco Kerdel, MD (b. 1954) [**Figure 98-8**], was born in New York but spent his formative years either in Venezuela with his parents or in a leading independent school in London, UK. After completing medical school training at St. Thomas Hospital Medical School at London University, he took a fellowship in immunodermatology before doing his dermatology residency at Harvard Medical School, where he was Chief Resident, followed by a fellowship in immunodermatology at New

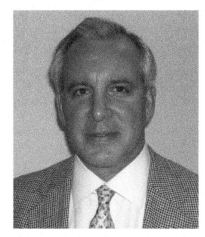

FIGURE 98-8. Francisco Kerdel, MD (b. 1954), is one of the key opinion leaders in immunodermatology and is a prolific writer and researcher as well as a highly sought after clinician.

York University. Since 1986, he has been at the University of Miami, where he is now a Professor of Dermatology and is currently Director of Dermatology Inpatient Services. Kerdel is one of the key opinion leaders in immunodermatology and psoriasis. He has authored almost 160 scientific articles and 37 books or book chapters. He has held leadership positions in the International Society of Dermatology, culminating as its President. Currently, he is the treasurer of the Foundation for International Dermatological Education and is a corresponding member of the Venezuela Academy of Medicine, as well as being an honorary member of the Argentinian and Chilean Societies of Dermatology. Considered an exceptional clinician, he has been an invited speaker at meetings worldwide and has been a visiting professor in Japan, Portugal, Italy, Australia, Brazil, Chile, Spain, England, Venezuela, Colombia, Uruguay, and Mexico. In 2001, Kerdel was awarded the Florida Society of Dermatology Practitioner of the Year. At present, he is also Vice Chair of the Department of Dermatology at the Florida International University in Miami, Florida's first public medical school.

DAVID A. RODRIGUEZ, MD

David A. Rodriguez, MD (b. 1955) [**Figure 98-9**], earned his medical degree from the University of Illinois College of Medicine in Chicago

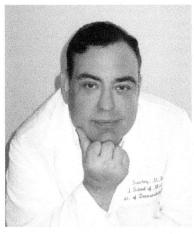

FIGURE 98-7. Miguel Sanchez, MD (b. 1953), is currently Professor of Dermatology at New York University and has published on the influence of culture on healthcare practices.

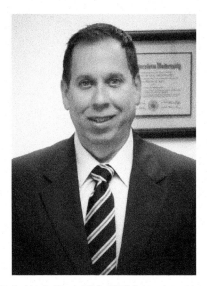

FIGURE 98-9. David A. Rodriguez, MD (b. 1955), frequently participates in clinical studies; the experience he has gained in the field of dermatology for skin of color has made him a much sought after speaker.

and completed his internship and residency in internal medicine at the Illinois Masonic Medical Center and at a University of Illinois-affiliated hospital, both in Chicago. The Cuban-born physician then served his residency in dermatology at the University of Illinois College of Medicine. Since his formative years, Rodriguez has been interested in dermatologic research. He was awarded the Adolph J. Rosenberg Award for research in dermatology while at the University of Illinois. Since that time, he has participated in more than 100 clinical studies on tinea pedis, tinea versicolor, psoriasis, rosacea, atopic dermatitis, onychomycosis, actinic keratosis, and acne vulgaris. His expertise has made him a popular speaker, and he has presented more than 100 lectures on topics such as actinic keratosis, atopic dermatitis, rosacea, psoriasis, and basal cell carcinoma at conferences and seminars. He is a board member of the Skin of Color Society, where his expertise in hyperpigmentation and aging in racial and ethnic populations is highly valued. Recently, he served as contributing editor for the textbook *Treatments for Skin of Color*, and authored a chapter in the book *Skin of Color*. Rodriguez is currently the Medical Director at Dermatology Associates and Research in Coral Gables, Florida. He serves as a voluntary Associate Professor in the Department of Dermatology and Cutaneous Surgery at the University of Miami and is on the staff at Metropolitan Hospital and Hialeah Hospital in Florida.

MARITZA I. PEREZ, MD

Maritza I. Perez, MD (b. 1957) [**Figure 98-10**], was born in Puerto Rico and graduated from the University of Puerto Rico School of Medicine with high honors, where she also did her residency in dermatology. Perez completed her postdoctoral training in immunodermatology at the Columbia College of Physicians and Surgeons in New York, and in dermatologic surgery, including Mohs micrographic surgery, laser surgery, and cosmetic dermatologic surgery, at New York University. She is certified by the American Board of Dermatology and the College of Mohs Micrographic Surgery. Currently, Perez is an attending physician, Department of Dermatology, Mount Sinai Beth Israel and Mount Sinai St. Luke's in New York City.

Perez's research experience is extensive and includes skin transplantation technology, cell culture and cell cloning techniques, and other clinical trials. A noted expert in the surgical treatment of melanomas, Perez has authored more than 100 publications, including academic articles, chapters, case reports, abstracts, and a book entitled *Understanding Melanoma*. She received the Teacher of the Year Award by the dermatology residents at St. Luke's Roosevelt Medical Center and was featured in

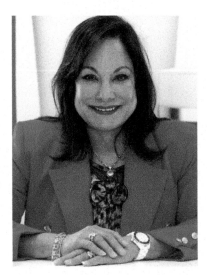

FIGURE 98-10. Maritza I. Perez, MD (b. 1957), has twice been voted one of America's top physicians for her work in dermatology.

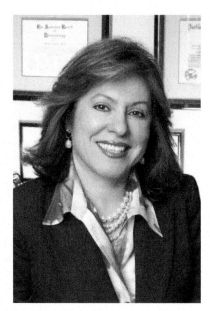

FIGURE 98-11. Marta I. Rendon, MD (b. 1957), is currently in private practice in Boca Raton, Florida. She is a highly skilled and accomplished clinician who is devoted to the care of skin of color patients suffering from skin disorders.

How to Find the Best Doctor—The New York Metro Area edition, twice being voted one of America's top physicians. She was elected to the Alpha Omega Alpha Honor Medical Society and has her own dermatology and cosmetic dermatology practice in Danbury, Connecticut.

MARTA I. RENDON, MD

Marta I. Rendon, MD (b. 1957) [**Figure 98-11**], is a native of Colombia, South America. She attended medical school in Puerto Rico and did her residency in internal medicine at the Albert Einstein Medical Center and in dermatology at the Parkland Memorial Hospital in Dallas, Texas. Rendon is the former Chair of the Department of Dermatology at the Cleveland Clinic, Florida. She has also served as a voluntary Clinical Associate Professor in the Department of Dermatology at the University of Miami School of Medicine for more than 20 years. Rendon has earned a national and international reputation as a researcher and lecturer specializing in acne, psoriasis, hyperpigmentation disorders, cosmetic dermatology, and hair loss. She has published more than 150 peer-reviewed abstracts and scientific articles and 10 book chapters and has also conducted 80 clinical studies in dermatology as principal investigator. She is a founding member of the Skin of Color Society and of the American Society of Cosmetic Dermatology and Aesthetic Medicine. She was also appointed to the 15-member International Board of the Pigmentary Disorders Academy. In the mid-1990s she began focusing on aesthetic dermatology and is currently in private practice at the Rendon Center for Dermatology and Aesthetic Medicine in Boca Raton, Florida, while serving as a Clinical Associate Professor in the Department of Biomedical Sciences at the Florida Atlantic University. She is devoted to the care of skin of color patients and has made important contributions to the development of skin of color as a distinct area in dermatology.

CONCLUSION

This chapter has focused on a few of the academic dermatologists whose leadership is widely recognized. There are countless other dermatologists who provide outstanding care for their patients, including Hispanics, and have made quiet contributions of their own. Yet the number of Hispanic dermatologists remains small, despite rapid growth in the Hispanic American population. This begs two questions: How prepared are dermatologists to deal with the disparities existing in dermatology? and, how can the number of Hispanics entering this field be increased?

There are two possibilities. First, it is incumbent upon dermatologists to encourage Hispanic youth to take an interest in medicine and, ultimately, in dermatology. To achieve this goal, mentorship programs are key. Second, leaders who can continue the efforts of the pioneers described in this chapter are also needed. Better ways to identify and treat skin conditions in the diverse Hispanic patient population is essential. Therefore, ongoing research and the education of future generations of dermatologists is necessary. Once every dermatologist understands Hispanic skin, the accomplishment will transcend all racial and ethnic groups and benefit patients everywhere.

REFERENCES

1. American Medical Association. Hispanic Physician Outreach Initiative. https://www.ama-assn.org/ama/pub/about-ama/our-people/member-groups-sections/minority-affairs-section/about-us/hispanic-physician-outreach-initiative.page. Accessed January 9, 2013.
2. U.S. Census Bureau. U.S. Census Bureau projections show a slower growing, older, more diverse nation a half century from now. https://www.census.gov/newsroom/releases/archives/population/cb12-243.html. Accessed January 9, 2013.
3. Canizares O. Dermatology in Latin America. *JAMA Dermatol*. 1956;74:648-658.

Index

Note: Page numbers followed by *f* and *t* indicate figures and tables, respectively.